W9-APO-206

HANDBOOK OF PHYSIOLOGY

Section 12: Exercise: Regulation and Integration of Multiple Systems

HANDBOOK OF PHYSIOLOGY

A critical, comprehensive presentation of physiological knowledge and concepts

Section 12: Exercise: Regulation and Integration of Multiple Systems

Edited by

LORING B. ROWELL
Department of Physiology and Biophysics
University of Washington

JOHN T. SHEPHERD
Department of Physiology and Biophysics
Mayo Clinic and Foundation

Associate Editors
Jerome A. Dempsey
John M. Johnson
Judith L. Smith
Ronald Terjung
Peter D. Wagner

New York Oxford
Published for the American Physiological Society
by Oxford University Press
1996

Oxford University Press

Oxford New York
Athens Auckland Bangkok Bombay
Calcutta Cape Town Dar es Salaam Delhi
Florence Hong Kong Istanbul Karachi
Kuala Lumpur Madras Madrid Melbourne
Mexico City Nairobi Paris Singapore
Taipei Tokyo Toronto

and associated companies in

Berlin Ibadan

Published for the American Physiological Society by Oxford University Press, Inc.,
198 Madison Avenue, New York, New York 10016

Library of Congress Cataloging-in-Publication Data
Exercise: Regulation and integration of multiple systems /
edited by Loring B. Rowell and John T. Shepherd ;
associated editors, Jerome A. Dempsey . . . [et al.].
p. cm.—(Handbook of physiology ; section 12)
Includes bibliographical references and index.
ISBN 0-19-509174-4
1. Exercise—Physiological aspects. I. Rowell, Loring B.
II. Shepherd, John T. (John Thompson), 1919– . III. American
Physiological Society (1887–) IV. Series: Handbook of Physiology
(Bethesda, Md.) ; section 12.
[DNLM: 1. Exercise—physiology. 2. Movement—physiology.
3. Blood Circulation—physiology. 4. Respiration—physiology.
5. Energy Metabolism—physiology.
QT 104 H236 1977 sect 12] QP6.H25 1977 sect. 12
[QP301] 599′.01 s–dc20 [612′.044]
DNLM/DLC for Library of Congress 95-13973

9 8 7 6 5 4 3 2 1

Printed in the United States of America
on acid-free paper

Preface

TRADITIONALLY the Handbook of Physiology series sponsored by the American Physiological Society has provided scholarly, comprehensive, and critical analyses of specific organ systems including the nervous, cardiovascular, and respiratory systems. Complex physiological processes such as aging or adaptation to the environment have also been analyzed. Some previous Handbooks dealt with responses of different organ systems to muscular exercise, but different systems were covered in different volumes so that the continuity and integration of multiple systems provided by the present volume could not be attained.

In the past decade or so, our understanding of physiological regulation during exercise has increased greatly and in parallel with progress in the medical sciences in general. The systematic investigation of this regulation draws from almost every area of physiology as well as from biochemistry, pharmacology, cellular and molecular biology, and medicine. Exercise continues to be a uniquely powerful means for exploring the integrative aspects of whole body function. It is this advantage that made muscular exercise the raison d'être of this Handbook with its emphasis on integration, which is perhaps the feature of physiology that best distinguishes it from the other basic medical sciences.

Background

In 1990 the American Physiological Society and Oxford University Press decided to produce a Handbook on the physiology of exercise. The goal was to provide in-depth analysis of regulatory mechanisms, including the signals responsible for the close matching of motor, cardiovascular, respiratory, and metabolic control during exercise. Unsolved problems concerning the origin of these signals have captured the imagination of investigators for over a century. A particular challenge was to examine both the functional and structural limits to the performance of organs and organ systems under severe stress.

By combining studies of control at cellular and molecular levels with studies on whole animals, this Handbook provides the natural and logical integration that is a hallmark of physiology. This dispels any notion that scientific progress is unidirectional, proceeding only to increasingly detailed investigation of smaller and smaller parts of the system down to its molecules. Despite the current enthusiasm for scientific reductionism, we hold to the view that physiology must also proceed in the reverse direction from a molecular level to analysis of responses in whole animals. As Blaise Pascal stated: "I hold it equally impossible to know the parts without knowing the whole and to know the whole without knowing the parts in detail."

After some debate, the consensus was to produce a single volume of specified length that covered the neural control of movement, control of the cardiovascular and respiratory systems, and of energy metabolism. Although page limitations sometimes restricted the expansive treatments that typified previous Handbooks, it forced the chapters to be focused and current. The scientific history underlying our present understanding is not covered here but is well documented in earlier Handbooks. Instead the focus is on where we are now and how we might proceed in the future. The requirements for brevity coupled with clarity, up-to-date analyses, in-depth interpretation and synthesis plus discussion of unsolved problems and future directions demanded insight, knowledge and perspicacity. In our view the authors and associate editors, all acknowledged experts in their fields, have succeeded splendidly in meeting these requirements and coping with the limitations.

With these limitations in mind, some things had to be excluded. There are no chapters devoted to age or gender-related differences in regulation, but these have been discussed wherever feasible. Nor are any chapters devoted to adaptations that accompany physical conditioning and their mechanisms; but some of the most important and recent information is included where it is relevant to the theme.

In summary, the reader is offered an organized synthesis of current ideas and a critical analysis of the mechanisms that govern control of movement, of breathing and pulmonary gas exchange, of blood flow and blood pressure and of skeletal muscle metabolism. The objective is to show how these mechanisms operate together during exercise and to look beyond current knowledge to new ideas currently under investigation.

Scope

This handbook is organized into three sections: neural control of movement, control of the respiratory and cardiovascular systems, and control of energy metabolism.

Neural Control of Movement

The eight chapters in this section consider the role of the nervous system at several different levels of the neuraxis in the control and regulation of voluntary limb movements, whole body posture, and equilibrium. Stereotypical limb motions such as walking and reflex actions, as well as the perception of afferent signals from proprioceptors in skeletal-articular structures, are discussed.

The lower motoneuron, called the "final common pathway" by Sir Charles Sherrington, provides the output signal to skeletal muscles. The properties of these neurons and the muscle fibers they innervate, motor units, must be understood in order to grasp how motion of different types and intensity is regulated. Commands to lower motoneurons are provided by such sources as 1) segmental afferents that establish spinal reflexes, 2) networks of interneurons within spinal circuits that provide stereotypical motor patterns, and 3) descending fibers from supraspinal centers, including projections from the brain stem and the cerebrum.

Spinal reflexes rely on fixed circuits that set up protective responses, such as flexion withdrawal, and do not require learning. The notion that reflexes are predictable (i.e., a specific stimulus always yields a specific response) is challenged. Actions of some spinal reflexes depend on the state of the animal and on the ongoing motor response.

The control of stereotypical movements, such as walking and breathing, may depend on circuits in the spinal cord and brain stem that provide a series of motor commands. Current research seeks to determine the design of these networks and the role of motion-dependent and supraspinal input in modifying the output of the intrinsic circuits.

Descending input from supraspinal centers is complex. Not only are there several distinct areas within the cerebrum, from which input is critical for providing the motor programs necessary for planning and executing voluntary motor responses, but there are also extensive interactions between these areas. Research today asks what areas of the cerebrum contribute motor commands and why there is need for such complex reciprocal connections among the many sensorimotor areas of the cerebrum.

Control of Respiratory and Cardiovascular Systems

The nine chapters in this section examine the regulation of the respiratory and cardiovascular systems. The most recent concepts regarding the central and peripheral neural and humoral control of these two systems as well as the mechanics of breathing and of pulmonary gas exchange are described. The continuing debate on the local and neural factors regulating the blood flow to the active muscles is discussed. The physical and functional limitations of these two systems and the questions as to which of these limits may be expanded by adaptation or reduced by age are assessed. Despite recent advances in physiology, we still lack full explanations of how the respiratory and circulatory systems are controlled during exercise. The authors offer new ideas to aid the search for fuller explanations.

The central neural control of respiratory and cardiovascular systems during exercise and the functional importance of centrally generated motor command signals as feed-forward controllers are described along with the peripheral feedback controllers originating from chemo- and mechanosensitive afferent nerve fibers in active skeletal muscle. The activation of muscle chemoreflexes appears to require that muscle perfusion declines sufficiently to compromise its oxygen supply, whereas mechanoreflexes can be activated by normal dynamic contractions. Although the relative importance of these reflexes in evoking responses to exercise is still unknown, new findings that offer important clues are presented.

Reflexes from active muscle as well as from the heart, lungs, and carotid bodies also can affect the respiratory system, but none of these peripheral afferent mechanisms appears to be the primary mediator for exercise hyperpnea. Nevertheless, these afferent systems may "fine-tune" ventilation by modulating either the pattern of breathing or the mechanical status of breathing so as to minimize its oxygen cost.

The breathing pattern during exercise is regulated by mechanical interactions between the lung and chest wall and by neural control of respiratory muscles. Locomotion and ventilation are coupled by complex combinations of mechanical and neural influences. Force development by the diaphragm is reduced during exhaustive exercise and respiratory muscles demand an increasing percentage of cardiac output as the cost of breathing increases. Possibly the sympathetic nervous system curtails the perfusion of respiratory muscles just as it curtails that of locomotor muscles when their total demands for oxygen begin to exceed their supply.

The factors that govern pulmonary gas exchange and acid-base regulation are examined; these range from chemical alteration of hemoglobin molecules to gas mixing in the lung, and to factors that determine the exchange of O_2 and CO_2 between the alveoli and pulmonary capillaries. Interactions between alveolar ventilation and pulmonary capillary blood flow are analyzed to distinguish among potential causes of alveolar-end capillary oxygen disequilibrium during severe exercise (e.g., postpulmonary arteriovenous shunts, alveolar-capillary diffusion limitation, and inequalities in alveolar ventilation:perfusion ratios). Among the potential limitations to maximal exercise performance, hypoxemia may be important in some athletes. A comprehensive analysis of acid-base balance benefits from a recent innovative approach in which $[H^+]$ is the dependent variable and the "strong ion difference" (SID) is an independent variable. This treatment provides a better understanding of what is regulated, and how, in order to restore this vital balance when it is disrupted by exercise.

The hemodynamics of the pulmonary circulation during exercise are presented so that the complex interactions among the heart, the lung and its vasculature are clarified. Factors both inside and outside of the lung microcirculation that determine the volume of fluid exchanged across the pulmonary capillaries are discussed, including those that protect against pulmonary edema and those that cause it.

The transport and metabolism of lactate during exercise are explored with emphasis on the shuttle of lactate via a carrier-mediated transport system between the tissue compartments that produce it and consume it. This includes the transport of lactate between active and passive muscles via blood and the regulation of lactate consumption by these muscles.

The physical and mechanical properties of the heart and vascular system including the complex mechanical coupling between the heart, the pericardium, the lung and the chest wall are analyzed to determine their hemodynamic interactions. Traditional determinants of cardiac output are reconsidered in the light of new insights about (1) how the structures that surround the heart can influence its performance and (2) how the skeletal muscle pump and the autonomic nervous system determine the relationships between cardiac output and venous return during exercise. This Handbook provides the first integrated look at these important physical, mechanical and neural determinants of cardiac performance during dynamic exercise. Control of the skeletal muscle circulation and the hyperemia of exercise can no longer be explained simply by metabolic feedback; the muscle pump by itself also increases muscle blood flow. Roles of endothelial-derived vasoactive factors are also important and like potential metabolic vasodilators can vary among muscle types and phases of exercise. Furthermore increased sympathetic activity in both muscle and coronary circulations adds important limits to their vasodilation. Possible mechanisms of vasodilation in both the skeletal muscle and coronary circulations during exercise are still disputed, partly because both redundancy and competition among mechanisms controlling blood flow to these organs make it difficult to evaluate the importance of any single mechanism. Nevertheless the authors present new information that improves our perspective.

Neural control of the peripheral circulation is treated in a new fashion that seeks to explain how the effects of cardiac and muscle pumps in series are balanced and also how the negative influences of heart-vascular coupling on cardiac filling and performance are counteracted. Factors that initiate reflex responses to exercise are examined and include the roles of central command, resetting of the arterial baroreflex, and afferent feedback from active muscles. A vital reflex adjustment is the active limitation of vasodilation in both active muscle and in skin; without this adjustment the heart could not maintain adequate arterial pressure.

Control of Energy Metabolism

This set of nine chapters deals with those biochemical and physiological events that are regulated in skeletal muscle to permit the great range of metabolism from rest to maximal exercise. Factors determining provision and oxidation of substrate and interactions among carbohydrates, fatty acids, and amino acids are emphasized. The adaptations of muscle to many influences involve the modification of molecules and subcellular elements within the myocyte, conversions among different muscle fiber types, and a redesign of the entire muscle to a different phenotype. The molecular and cellular events underlying muscle plasticity are considered and they are related by the authors to muscle performance and to its decline during fatigue. Among the most important are the processes that control energy metabolism within the myocyte, the determinants of adenosine triphosphate utilization during contractions, and metabolic regulation during steady state energy flux as well as cellular responses to transient and extreme metabolic demands. How glycolysis, glycogen metabolism and enzymes of the glycolytic pathway may be controlled in various muscle fiber types is explored as is the molecular basis for glucose transport and its control by insulin and other hormones.

The uptake and processing of fatty acids by active muscle and their transendothelial and transsarcolemmal movement and transport within the myocyte are described. Free fatty acid sources from circulating and intracellular triglyceride pools provide a major energy source that interacts with carbohydrate metabolism to enhance muscle endurance. Amino acid and protein transport and metabolism have an impact on critical metabolic pools and/or pathways within active muscles. Protein synthesis and degradation during exercise and the regulation of extramuscular substrate supply are examined. These processes require the integration of diverse metabolic support functions among multiple organ systems. Extramuscular fuel sources that are discussed include lipid and glucose and their endocrine regulation plus the regulation of lipid metabolism and glucose production by the liver.

A broad view of the plasticity of skeletal muscle as it 'remodels' with exercise is offered. This encompasses muscle mitochondrial content, oxidative enzyme capacity, optimal supply of metabolic substrate and also the interrelationships between these cellular adjustments and muscle perfusion, aerobic metabolism and the overall "design" of muscle function. Related to 'remodeling' are factors that control gene expression, such as contractile activity, contractile proteins, enzymes, mitochondria, transcription factors, growth factors, and receptors. Muscle fatigue is examined as a loss of peak force and as a function of muscle fiber composition, intensity, type and duration of exercise, physical conditioning and the events associated with excitation-contraction coupling and metabolic factors.

This Handbook was conceived with three primary objectives in mind. The first objective was to assemble the best available data and present our current understanding of motor, cardiovascular, respiratory and metabolic control during exercise. The second was to provide a clear picture of the current outstanding problems that limit our understanding of how these multiple systems function during dynamic exercise. The third objective was to present exciting new ideas that could provide the best basis for solving these problems in the future. The authors have fulfilled these objectives and in doing so, offer to medical and sports scientists and practitioners, and others concerned with exercise in health and disease, a current, in-depth view of modern integrative physiology. This view encompasses the ways in which molecular and cellular mechanisms are coordinated with central neural control, autonomic reflexes and chemical and humoral mechanisms. By presenting ideas on unsolved problems the authors invite all with the interest and skills to advance our understanding of this important challenge to body function.

It has been a pleasure and a privilege for us to work with internationally recognized individuals who organized the sections, chose distinguished authors, and fashioned the chapters that suit the overall concept of this volume. This Handbook would not have succeeded without the constructive interaction among the five Associate Editors and the authors, who wrote superb chapters under constraints that limited both their time and the size of their chapters. We feel honored by their willingness to make the enormous effort required, and we are grateful to them. We also acknowledge the foresight and efforts of Dr. Douglas Stuart who, as Chair of the Handbook Committee, initiated and explored the feasibility of this project.

Also, our thanks are due to Mr. Jeffrey House of Oxford University Press, who was a consistent source of advice, help and encouragement throughout the preparation of this volume.

April, 1995

L. B. R.
J. T. S.

Contents

Contributors

Lewis Adams
Department of Medicine
Charing Cross and Westminster Medical School
London, United Kingdom

Dorothy M. Ainsworth
Department of Clinical Science
College of Veterinary Medicine
Cornell University
Ithaca, New York

Robert J. Bache
Department of Medicine
Cardiovascular Division
University of Minnesota Medical School
Minneapolis, Minnesota

Kenneth M. Baldwin
Department of Physiology and Biophysics
University of California, Irvine
Irvine, California

Marc D. Binder
Department of Physiology and Biophysics
University of Washington
Seattle, Washington

S. Bodine-Fowler
Division of Orthopedics
VA Medical Center
San Diego, California

Frank W. Booth
Department of Integrative Biology
University of Texas Medical School
Houston, Texas

Alan D. Cherrington
Department of Molecular Physiology and Biophysics
Vanderbilt University School of Medicine
Nashville, Tennessee

Richard J. Connett
Department of Physiology
University of Rochester School of Medicine and Dentistry, and
Department of Biological Sciences
Monroe Community College
Rochester, New York

Jerome A. Dempsey
Department of Preventive Medicine
University of Wisconsin-Madison
Madison, Wisconsin

Richard P. Dum
Departments of Neurosurgery and Physiology
SUNY Health Science Center at Syracuse
Syracuse, New York

Dirk J. Duncker
Experimental Cardiology, Thoraxcenter
Erasmus University
Rotterdam, The Netherlands

V. R. Edgerton
Department of Physiological Science
University of California, Los Angeles
Los Angeles, California

Frederic L. Eldridge
Departments of Medicine and Physiology
University of North Carolina
Chapel Hill, North Carolina

Robert H. Fitts
Department of Biology
Marquette University
Milwaukee, Wisconsin

Jeanne M. Foley
Departments of Physiology, and Physical Education and Exercise Science
Michigan State University
East Lansing, Michigan

Hubert V. Forster
Department of Physiology
Medical College of Wisconsin
Milwaukee, Wisconsin

Ralph F. Fregosi
Department of Physiology
University of Arizona Health Sciences Center
Tucson, Arizona

Charles G. Gallagher
Division of Respiratory Medicine
Royal University Hospital
University of Saskatchewan
Saskatoon, Saskatchewan, Canada

Simon C. Gandevia
Prince of Wales Medical Research Institute
University of New South Wales
Sydney, Australia

L. Bruce Gladden
Department of Health and Human Performance
Auburn University
Auburn, Alabama

Abe Guz
Department of Medicine
Charing Cross and Westminster Medical School
London, United Kingdom

C. J. Heckman
Department of Physiology
Northwestern University
Chicago, Illinois

George J. F. Heigenhauser
Department of Medicine
McMaster University Health Sciences Center
Hamilton, Ontario, Canada

J. A. Hodgson
Brain Research Institute
University of California, Los Angeles
Los Angeles, California

Fay B. Horak
R. S. Dow Neurological Sciences Institute
Legacy Good Samaritan Hospital & Medical Center
Portland, Oregon

Connie C. W. Hsia
Department of Internal Medicine
University of Texas Southwestern Medical Center
Dallas, Texas

A. Ishihara
Laboratory of Neurochemistry
Faculty of Integrated Human Studies
Kyoto University
Kyoto, Japan

Gary A. Iwamoto
Department of Veterinary Biosciences
University of Illinois
Urbana, Illinois

Joseph S. Janicki
Department of Physiology and Pharmacology
Auburn University
Auburn, Alabama

Bruce D. Johnson
Division of Cardiovascular Diseases
Mayo Clinic and Foundation
Rochester, Minnesota

John M. Johnson
Department of Physiology
University of Texas Health Science Center
San Antonio, Texas

Robert L. Johnson, Jr.
Departments of Internal Medicine and Pulmonary Research
University of Texas Southwestern Medical Center
Dallas, Texas

Norman L. Jones
Department of Medicine
McMaster University Health Sciences Center
Hamilton, Ontario, Canada

Marc P. Kaufman
Division of Cardiovascular Medicine
Departments of Internal Medicine and Human Physiology
University of California, Davis
Davis, California

Dean L. Kellogg, Jr.
Departments of Physiology and of Medicine
University of Texas Health Science Center at San Antonio
San Antonio, Texas

Ronald J. Korthuis
Department of Physiology and Biophysics
Louisiana State University Medical Center
Shreveport, Louisiana

M. Harold Laughlin
Department of Veterinary Biomedical Sciences
University of Missouri
Columbia, Missouri

Jane M. Macpherson
R. S. Dow Neurological Sciences Institute
Legacy Good Samaritan Hospital & Medical Center
Portland, Oregon

Ronald A. Meyer
Departments of Physiology and Radiology
Michigan State University
East Lansing, Michigan

Jere H. Mitchell
Department of Internal Medicine
University of Texas Southwestern Medical School
Dallas, Texas

P. Darrell Neufer
Departments of Internal Medicine and Biochemistry
University of Texas Southwestern Medical Center
Dallas, Texas

Donal S. O'Leary
Department of Physiology
Wayne State University School of Medicine
Detroit, Michigan

Randall K. Powers
Department of Physiology & Biophysics
University of Washington
Seattle, Washington

Scott K. Powers
Departments of Exercise Science and Physiology
University of Florida
Gainesville, Florida

Arthur Prochazka
Division of Neuroscience
University of Alberta
Edmonton, Alberta, Canada

John T. Reeves
Departments of Medicine and Pediatrics
Developmental Lung Biology Laboratory
University of Colorado Health Sciences Center
Denver, Colorado

Robert S. Reneman
Departments of Physiology and Motion Sciences
Cardiovascular Research Institute Maastricht
University of Limburg
Maastricht, The Netherlands

Michael J. Rennie
Department of Anatomy and Physiology
University of Dundee
Dundee, Scotland

Erik A. Richter
Copenhagen Muscle Research Centre
August Krogh Institute
University of Copenhagen
Copenhagen, Denmark

James L. Robotham
Department of Anesthesiology and Critical Care Medicine
Johns Hopkins University
Baltimore, Maryland

Serge Rossignol
Center for Research in Neurological Sciences
Department of Physiology
Université de Montréal
Montréal, Québec, Canada

Loring B. Rowell
Departments of Physiology and Biophysics and of Medicine (Cardiology)
University of Washington School of Medicine
Seattle, Washington

R. R. Roy
Brain Research Institute
University of California, Los Angeles
Los Angeles, California

Kent Sahlin
Department of Physiology and Pharmacology
Karolinska Institute and
Department of Sports and Health Sciences
University College of Physical Education
Stockholm, Sweden

John T. Shepherd
Department of Physiology and Biophysics
Mayo Clinic and Foundation
Rochester, Minnesota

Don D. Sheriff
Division of Cardiovascular Research
St. Elizabeth's Medical Center
Boston, Massachusetts

Judith L. Smith
Department of Physiological Science
University of California, Los Angeles
Los Angeles, California

Peter L. Strick
Research Service
VA Medical Center
Departments of Neurosurgery and Physiology
SUNY Health Science Center at Syracuse
Syracuse, New York

Aubrey E. Taylor
Department of Physiology
University of South Alabama School of Medicine
Mobile, Alabama

Ronald Terjung
Department of Physiology
SUNY Health Science Center Syracuse
Syracuse, New York

Ger J. van der Vusse
Departments of Physiology and Motion Sciences
Cardiovascular Research Institute Maastricht
University of Limburg
Maastricht, The Netherlands

Peter D. Wagner
Department of Medicine
University of California-San Diego
La Jolla, California

Tony G. Waldrop
Department of Molecular and Integrative Physiology
University of Illinois
Urbana, Illinois

David H. Wasserman
Department of Molecular Physiology and Biophysics
Vanderbilt University School of Medicine
Nashville, Tennessee

R. Sanders Williams
Departments of Internal Medicine and Biochemistry
University of Texas Southwestern Medical Center
Dallas, Texas

Robert A. Wise
Department of Medicine
Johns Hopkins University
Baltimore, Maryland

Ronald F. Zernicke
Department of Surgery
University of Calgary
Calgary, Alberta, Canada

I

Neural Control of Movement

Associate Editor Judith L. Smith

1. The physiological control of motoneuron activity

MARC D. BINDER | *Department of Physiology & Biophysics, University of Washington, Seattle, Washington*
C. J. HECKMAN | *Department of Physiology, Northwestern University, Chicago, Illinois*
RANDALL K. POWERS | *Department of Physiology & Biophysics, University of Washington, Seattle, Washington*

CHAPTER CONTENTS

SHERRINGTON REFERRED TO THE MOTONEURON as the "final common pathway" to emphasize the axiom that every part of the nervous system involved in the control of movement must do so by acting either directly or indirectly on motoneurons (219). Thus, this first chapter in the section devoted to the neural control of movement will focus on the physiology of motoneurons. It is not our intention to provide a comprehensive review of motoneuron anatomy and physiology, nor to review the vast literature on motor unit properties and their patterns of utilization. Rather, we have been deliberately parochial in both our choice of topics and our point of view. Our goals are to describe the most salient, common features of motoneuron recruitment and rate modulation; to review the physiological properties of motoneurons and their synaptic inputs that underlie these features; and finally to consider the aggregate behavior of a pool of motoneurons as a neural system.

We have concentrated our efforts on the literature of the past decade and have avoided whenever possible discussing material so ably reviewed in the last *Handbook of Physiology* on motor control (43). The reader is therefore remanded to the following chapters in that volume: *Motor Units* by R.E. Burke (49); *Functional Organization of the Motoneuron Pool and Its Inputs* by E. Henneman and L.M. Mendell (156); and *Integration in Spinal Neuronal Systems* by F. Baldissera, H. Hultborn, and M. Ilert (14).

The motoneuron's response to synaptic inputs can be recorded at three locations: at the motoneuron soma with an intracellular electrode, at the motoneuron axon with either an intra- or extracellular electrode placed in the ventral roots or the muscle nerve, and at the muscle with an intramuscular electrode. The resultant force or motion is measured via force and position transducers placed either on the muscle tendon or in contact with the bone on which the tendon inserts.

Recordings made at these various locations have provided the values for a number of electrophysiological and mechanical parameters that have been used to describe the transformation of synaptic inputs into muscle force. Intracellular recordings from motoneurons have provided measures of the effective synaptic current reaching the somatic recording site (I_N; see later under Effective Synaptic Currents) as well as descriptions of the relation between injected (or synaptic) current and firing rate (*f-I* relation). Under isometric conditions, the force produced by the muscle unit (*F*) at a given motoneuron firing rate is specified by the muscle unit's force-frequency (*F-f*) relation and by its force-length (*F-L*) relation. When the muscle is free to move, the motor unit's force will also be governed by its force-velocity (*F-V*) relation. The force produced by the entire muscle will depend on the summed effects of its constituent motor units. The entire transformation of synaptic input (I_N) to muscle force (*F*) under steady-state isometric conditions can be described on the basis of the distribution of effective synaptic current (I_N) to the constituents of the motoneuron pool, the *f-I* relations of these motoneurons, and the *F-f* relations of their muscle units.

The population of motor units within an individual muscle exhibits a wide range of both mechanical and electrophysiological properties (25, 48, 192, 362). In terms of mechanical outputs, motor unit tetanic forces (F_{max}) have as much as a 100-fold range, contraction times have a five-fold range, and fatigue resistances at least a ten-fold range (reviewed in 49, 156). These mechanical properties are interrelated, and together with the profile of an unfused tetanus [i.e., "sag"; (50)] are frequently used to separate the population into motor unit types [i.e., type S: slow-twitch, low force, nonfatigable; type FR: fast-twitch, intermediate force, fatigue resistant; type FI: fast-twitch, intermediate force, intermediate fatigue resistance; and type FF: fast-twitch, high force, low fatigue resistance; (reviewed in (49)]. The electrophysiological properties of motoneurons also exhibit a wide range of variation that is correlated with the mechanical properties of their muscle units (see later under MOTONEURON PROPERTIES). The covariances between electrophysiological and mechanical properties of motor units and the relationship of synaptic input to these properties profoundly influence the input–output function of the motoneuron pool (see later under THE MOTONEURON POOL AND ITS MUSCLE AS A NEURAL SYSTEM).

The behavioral data describing the relation of motor unit activation patterns to whole-muscle force or electromyography (EMG) will be covered first, since our overall model of the motoneuron pool attempts to explain these data. The relationship of motoneuron behavior to intrinsic motoneuron properties will be described next. Subsequently, we will review the definition and measurement of effective synaptic current (I_N), along with what is presently known about the distribution of I_N from various presynaptic sources. Finally, we will describe steady-state models of the motoneuron pool that attempt to incorporate known features of synaptic input distributions, intrinsic motoneuron properties, and muscle unit mechanical properties into a neural system that can account for the observed steady-state motor unit behavior.

PATTERNS OF MOTOR OUTPUT

Orderly Recruitment of Motor Units

Our current understanding of motor unit recruitment is based on the seminal work of Henneman and colleagues in the 1960's (158), who proposed that motor units are always recruited in order of increasing size (reviewed in 49, 60, 156). After three decades of research, this "size principle" remains a valid description of recruitment order in many movement conditions, as long as the size of the motor unit is defined in rather broad terms. Motor unit size-related properties that directly correlate with recruitment threshold include twitch tension (TT), tetanic force (F_{max}), axonal conduction velocity (CV), and the amplitude of an extracellularly recorded axonal action potential [see reviews in Binder and Mendell (29)]. Because of the great wealth of data supporting this size-based recruitment order in a variety of conditions, it is often referred to as the "normal sequence of recruitment" or just as "orderly recruitment" (e.g., 110, 147, 151).

Two functional advantages of the normal recruitment sequence were originally postulated (157): *(1)* motor units are recruited in order of increasing fatigability, so that fatigable units are reserved for brief, forceful contractions; and *(2)* the relative precision of force control is the same at all force levels, since each newly recruited unit contributes approximately the same percentage increment in force to the total level of force. In addition, Henneman and colleagues (154, 155) have emphasized the simplicity inherent in an invariant recruitment sequence, as it allows the input–output properties of the motor units in a pool to be combined into a single, whole-system function. Despite this solid foundation, many important questions about recruitment order remain unresolved.

Measurement Techniques. The main problem in determining the consistency of recruitment order is measurement error, which itself induces randomness into the data (151). New techniques for recording from and stimulating single motor axons in animals have provided the most reliable data on recruitment order (364). These techniques yield accurate measurements of both the recruitment order of units and their mechanical properties, whereas previous studies were limited to measurements of axon action potential amplitude and conduction velocity. Subsequent refinements now allow routine and successful sampling of five to ten pairs of motor units per experiment (35, 75, 84, 85).

In humans, single motor unit recruitment and repetitive discharge have most often been studied by recording muscle fiber action potentials. Whereas the recent work in the decerebrate cat has focused on pairwise comparisons of recruitment order (e.g., 75, 84, 85), the standard analysis of recruitment in human subjects is based on the level of whole-muscle force at which a single motor unit is first activated (hereafter referred to as the unit's recruitment threshold). The mechanical properties of the recorded motor unit can be estimated by averaging the force fluctuations associated with the motor unit spike (224, 225). However, a number of factors may distort the amplitude and time course of the spike-triggered averaged twitch (59, 60, 227, 334). Microneurographic techniques have recently been adapted to allow direct stimulation of motor axons in humans (334, 335, 359), but the human recruitment data collected thus far lack the measurement accuracy of motor unit mechanical properties achieved in the animal preparations.

Precision and Stereotypy of the Normal Sequence. Recent studies in the decerebrate cat have provided further support for the normal, size-based recruitment sequence: Motor units with low forces are usually recruited before units with high forces (75, 84, 85, 364). During the stretch reflex, both F_{max} and CV, as well as several other motor unit properties, are equally good predictors of recruitment order. With each parameter, recruitment reversals occur in ~10% of trials (75, 84, 85), although the degree of randomness in recruitment can vary with the source of the synaptic input activating the pool (cf. 73). It has also been proposed that recruitment is ordered by motor unit type (49, 326). While there is no doubt the normal overall sequence is type S → type FR → type FF, recruitment has also been found to be orderly within type categories (19, 27, 364).

Studies of motor unit recruitment in human subjects during slow, voluntary changes in isometric force have generally also reported a size-based recruitment sequence [i.e., a positive correlation between the amplitude of the spike-triggered averaged twitch and recruitment threshold (reviewed in 60)]. Recent data also indicate that transcortical stimulation generates normal orderly recruitment (20, 61). Similarly, studies of recruitment driven by reflex inputs have generally supported the normal orderly pattern (58, 281), but the correspondence between volitional and phasic reflex recruitment orders may not be precise (91). Overall, the degree of precision in the recruitment sequence varies widely between studies (e.g., 225, 278, 337) and indeed among the subjects within a single study [Fig. 1.1*A*; (278)]. Random variations in recruitment threshold also occur from trial to trial within subjects using volitional control, possibly because the net joint forces are generated by multiple muscles (279, 280).

The qualitative impression formed from these findings is that recruitment order in humans is less precise than in the decerebrate cat preparation. However, the correlation statistics used in the human work are not directly comparable to the pairwise analysis used in the animal studies cited above. Computer simulation techniques have recently been used to compare the human and animal recruitment data quantitatively (151) and are considered later in this chapter (see later under Control of Orderly Recruitment).

The technical difficulties associated with single-unit recordings at high forces in humans and the difficulty in generating controlled high forces in reduced animal preparations limit the accuracy with which the upper limit of the range of recruitment can be established. In the intrinsic muscles of the hand, recruitment appears to be essentially complete

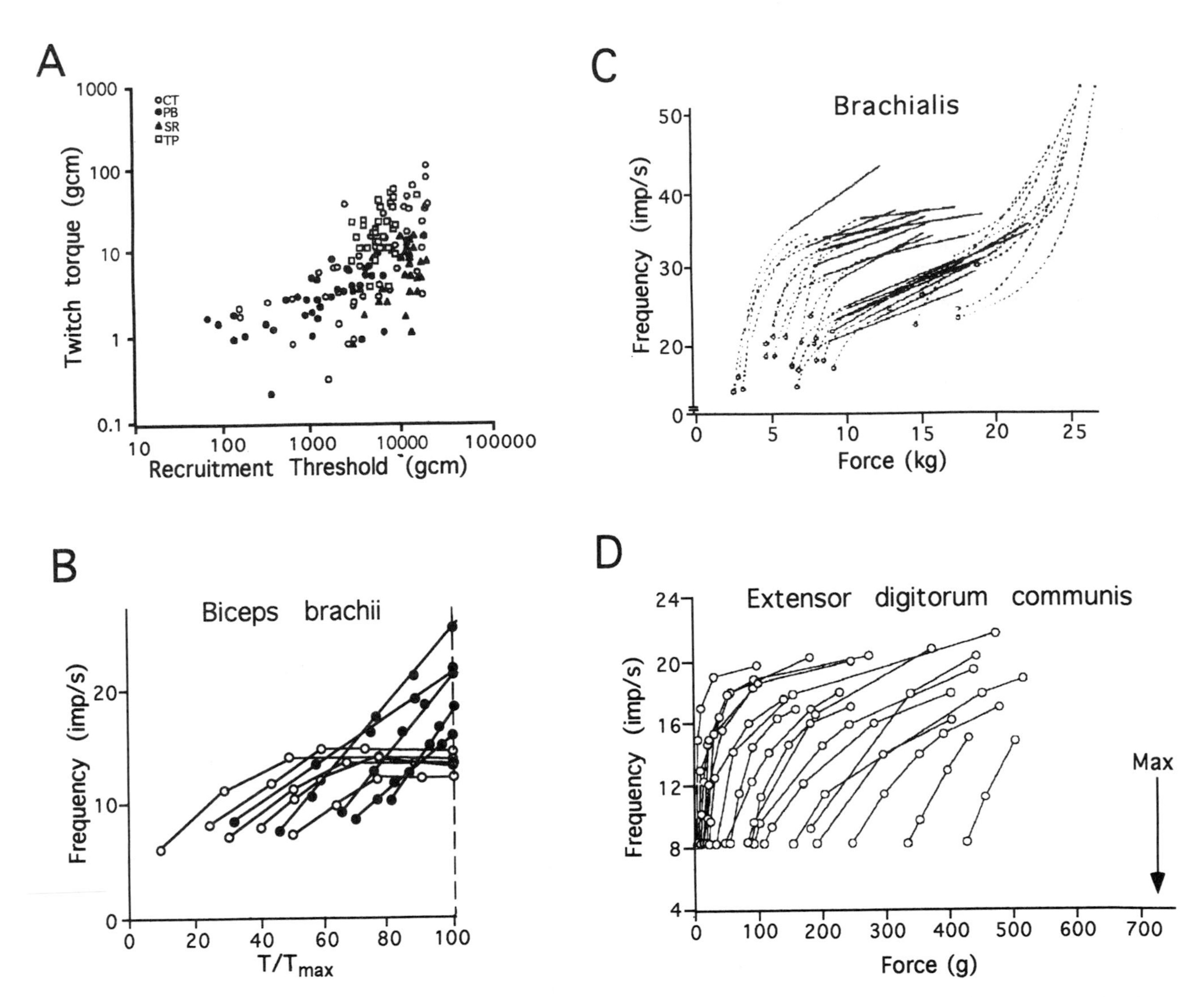

FIG. 1.1. Recruitment and rate-modulation patterns in human subjects. *A*, Recruitment order in four different human subjects for wrist extension of the extensor digitorum communis muscle (278). Relation between peak torque of the spike triggered average twitch and recruitment threshold. Symbols indicate different data for four different subjects. Correlation coefficients: subject CT (*open circles*): 0.63; PB (*filled circles*): 0.61; SR (*filled triangles*): 0.37; TP (*open squares*): 0.50. *B–D*, Rate-limiting patterns in human subjects in three different arm muscles: biceps brachii (141), brachialis (183), and extensor digitorum communis (227). In each case, the y-axis is single-unit discharge rate and the x-axis is muscle force, with maximum indicated. The data in *D* were originally displayed on semilog coordinates and have been digitized and replotted on a linear scale like that of the other two studies.

at about 50% of maximal force, but recruitment in the biceps, brachialis, and deltoid muscles may continue until more than 80% of maximal force is attained (92, 141, 183, 214, 225). Thus, there may be differences in recruitment ranges in intrinsic muscles of the hand vs. muscles of the elbow and shoulder.

Evidence for Systematic Recruitment Reversals. The demonstration of systematic recruitment reversals requires a statistically significant trend for high-force units to be recruited before low-force ones. The recruitment reversals must exceed 50% and the correlation coefficients between twitch force and recruitment threshold must be negative. In human subjects, electrical stimulation of the skin degrades the orderliness of recruitment but does not generate an overall reversed pattern (127). In the cat medial gastrocnemius (MG) muscle, cutaneous stimulation has been shown to sometimes reduce or even silence the discharge rate of type S motor units while increasing the discharge rate of type F units (75, 182), but this does not seem to be associated with consistent and repeatable recruitment reversals (75, 84).

Selective recruitment of type F units has been most clearly demonstrated by comparing different types of contractions of the human gastrocnemius and soleus muscles (239). Units with low recruitment thresholds measured during concentric (shortening) contractions were apparently suppressed during eccentric (lengthening) contractions. Given the reasonable assumption that the high-threshold units are mainly within the type F category, these data provide good evidence that a reversed recruitment sequence is utilized in a specific task.

Static vs. Dynamic Conditions. As movement speed increases, the force supplied by type S units decreases much more rapidly than that supplied by type F units because of differences in their force-velocity relations (see later under Dynamic Properties of Motor Units). This means that during rapid movements, type S units become superfluous as their forces fall to zero. As a consequence, it has been proposed that rapid motions may be accomplished by selective recruitment of type F units (316).

Studies in humans have generally not supported this idea. The normal sequence of recruitment occurs in "ballistic" increases in isometric force (e.g., 94) and in slow shortening movements (336). The activation patterns of the close synergists MG (75% type F units) and soleus (100% type S units) in freely moving animals are also consistent with normal recruitment, except during rapid paw shakes, in which MG is active while soleus is clearly suppressed (316). It has yet to be determined whether or not the type S units in MG are also suppressed in the paw shake.

Ideally, selective recruitment of type F units might be used in a movement in which recruitment of type S units is not just superfluous, but is an actual impediment. During isovelocity stretches, the slow-twitch soleus muscle tends to yield, giving a sharp reduction in stiffness (e.g., 180). In a predominantly fast-twitch muscle like MG, yielding is much less drastic (355). In a task in which a load needs to be smoothly lowered, the yielding behavior of slow-twitch units could be an impediment. This might explain the apparent selective use of type F units in lengthening contractions (239).

Orderly Recruitment in Multifunctional Muscles. The definition of the motoneuron pool has been debated vigorously over the last 20 years. To a large extent this debate was initiated by the "sensory partitioning hypothesis" of Stuart, Windhorst, and their colleagues, and by the anatomical description of muscle compartments by English and colleagues (reviewed in 361). Shortly thereafter, the "task group" hypothesis of Loeb and colleagues (71) focused on the motor output side, pointing out that the functional groupings of motoneurons during movements do not necessarily coincide with traditional anatomical boundaries between muscles. These findings prompted the question of how orderly recruitment is in complex or multifunctional muscles. Subpopulations of motor units within anatomically complex muscles can be activated independently in some behaviors. In humans, these include subpopulations for flexion vs. supination torques in elbow muscles (332, 348) and for movement of different fingers by the extensor digitorum communis (EDC) muscle (278). In animal studies, subpopulations have been demonstrated for hip muscles such as sartorius and biceps femoris during locomotion (261, 262), cutaneous flexion reflexes (261, 262), and responses to postural disturbances (70). Furthermore, a muscle can exhibit subpopulations for one behavior but not another (261, 262). It is not clear whether all of these diverse behaviors are consistent with the original "task group" notion (71).

An important component of the task group hypothesis is that the motor units within a subpopulation are recruited in an orderly fashion (71). Only one study has tested this directly. In EDC, the motor units within a subpopulation that was utilized solely for generation of isometric force at a single finger were recruited in the normal sequence (278). Moreover, when the subpopulations were combined for simultaneous activation of two fingers, the combined population of motor units still followed the normal pattern. In both cases, the ratios of stereotypy to randomness were similar to those in muscles without separate subpopulations. Because recruitment is orderly within each population, differences in unit recruitment across subpopulations do not provide evidence for recruitment reversals any more than would differences for units in separate muscles.

Rate Modulation of Motor Units

Slowly Varying Isometric Contractions. In contrast to the work on recruitment order, our understanding of motor unit rate modulation is based largely on recordings from human subjects. It is clear that motor units fire at rather low rates at their recruitment thresholds and then undergo rapid increases in firing rate as force is increased (reviewed in 49, 156). Two important questions regarding the behavior of type S vs. type F motor units have received considerable attention: *(1)* Which motor units exhibit a greater range of rate modulation?; and *(2)* Which motor units undergo the more rapid increase in discharge rate with increasing force?

In steady-state conditions, type S units reach tetanic force at much lower firing rates than do type F units (34, 198). Firing rates in excess of 20–30 imp/s are energetically wasteful for type S units, but are necessary for type F units to reach their maximal forces. Thus, one would expect type S units to have the most restricted range of rate modulation (197). Figure 1.1*B–D* shows single-unit discharge patterns across a wide range of forces from three different studies (141, 183, 227). In each case, the rates of low-threshold units tended to saturate as higher threshold units were recruited and increased their discharge rates. This phenomenon has been referred to as "rate limiting" (149, 150).

There are wide differences in the steepness of the initial firing rate-force slopes and in the maximal rates of the low-threshold units (Fig. 1.1*B–D*). In some cases, the maximum rates of high-threshold units exceeded those of low-threshold units [Fig. 1.1*B* and *C*; (see also 26, 135)] and in others they did not [Fig. 1.1*D*; (see also 118)]. There are also differences in the reported range of unit discharge rates at recruitment threshold (i.e., minimal rates), with some studies reporting that the minimal rates of motor units increase systematically with recruitment threshold [e.g., Fig. 1.1*C*; (see also 92)] but others not [Fig. 1.1*D*; (see also 330)]. The reasons for these interstudy differences in rate limiting, minimal firing rates, and maximal firing rates are unclear, but two technical issues must be kept in mind: *(1)* problems in maintaining secure unit isolation as muscle force increases means that the maximal discharge rates of low threshold units are difficult to measure; and *(2)* the force measured in many studies (including all of those illustrated in Fig. 1.1) reflects the combined actions of several muscles.

The question of whether type S or F units undergo the more rapid increases in firing rate cannot be directly answered from data on the relation between single-unit discharge rate and whole-muscle force, because this relation is strongly affected by the input–output function of the whole pool [(149, 150); see later under Input–Output Function of the Motoneuron Pool]. However, if the firing rates of single units are plotted against one another (226), the relative slope is the product of only two factors: the slopes of the frequency-current (*f-I*) relations of each motoneuron and the relative proportions of the synaptic drive (I_N; cf. 149) received by each motoneuron. These rate–rate plots indicate that higher threshold units tend to increase their rates of discharge more rapidly than do low-threshold units (226, 227).

Rate modulation in hindlimb motor units studied in the decerebrate cat appears to be qualitatively similar to that reported in humans. The increase in motor unit firing rates during the stretch reflex is clear (86), as it is for most units during various isometric forces generated by the crossed-extension reflex (260). The minimal rates of discharge tend to increase with recruitment threshold (35, 260), but maximum rates have not been studied due to the inability to generate controlled maximum forces. Severe rate limiting occurs during contractions evoked by simulation of the mesencephalic locomotor region (35, 45), but the generality of these findings is not clear.

Static vs. Dynamic Conditions. Rate modulation during rapid changes in motor command and muscle length has not been well documented. During locomotion in the intact cat, low-threshold units exhibit no rate limiting and attain higher discharge rates than do high-threshold units (162). In fact, the pattern of rate modulation of all units matched the smoothed envelope of the electromyogram (EMG), suggesting that the synaptic input to all motor units was similar. It is not yet known whether the discharge rates of the low-threshold units remain greater than those of the high-threshold units as the speed of locomotion increases. A very different pattern emerges from studies of locomotion induced by brainstem stimulation in the decerebrate cat, where rate modulation often begins with a very short interspike interval (a "doublet"), is maintained at a moderately high rate, and then rather abruptly ceases (365).

Motor unit rate modulation has been studied in human subjects during dynamic variations in isometric force. With moderate rates of change in isometric force, low-threshold units in the first dorsal interosseous displayed no rate limiting (92). In contrast, the low-threshold units in the deltoid muscle exhibited clear rate limiting, but the rates of low-threshold units still remained above those of high-threshold units (92). Rate limiting during ramp-like increases in forces has also been found in motor units in the wrist muscle, extensor carpi radialis (279). In this muscle, the time required for low-threshold units to reach a constant discharge rate was independent of the rate of rise of the force ramp, whereas high-threshold units required less time to do so as rate of rise of force increased (279). These data suggest that, as is the case for recruitment order (see above), rate modulation may be different in distal vs. proximal muscles.

MOTONEURON PROPERTIES

This section will describe the physiological features of motoneurons that may affect their control by synaptic inputs. The emphasis will be on information that has become available since motoneuron properties were last reviewed in the *Handbook* (49, 156), including: *(1)* reevaluations of the passive electrical properties of motoneurons based on the presence of real or artifactual nonuniformities in membrane properties, *(2)* descriptions of active conductances based on somatic voltage-clamp studies, *(3)* descriptions of the physiological modulation of active conductances by monoaminergic and peptidergic systems, and *(4)* computer simulations that relate the intrinsic properties of motoneurons to their physiological functions.

A motoneuron is recruited when its somatic membrane potential is displaced from its resting value (V_r) to the threshold value for initiating an action potential (V_{thr}). For a given injected or synaptic current (I), the change in somatic voltage (ΔV) will depend upon the effective input resistance of the cell (R_N) according to Ohm's law:

$$\Delta V = R_N * I \tag{1}$$

An action potential will be produced if ΔV exceeds the difference between the threshold voltage and the resting potential:

$$\Delta V > V_{thr} - V_r \tag{2}$$

Subsequent firing rate modulation will depend upon the relation between injected or synaptic current and the discharge rate (f), which is linear over a large range of currents:

$$f = f_0 + [f\text{-}I] * (I - I_0) \tag{3}$$

where I_0 is the minimum current needed to elicit steady repetitive discharge [generally about 1.5 times the current needed to produce a single action potential I_{rh}; (189)], f_0 is the minimum firing rate, and f-I is the slope of the frequency-current relation. As described below, the instantaneous firing rate is also a function of the rate of change of current and of the time since the onset of a current step.

Equations 1–3 provide a sufficient set of parameters to relate motoneuron output (firing rate, f) to input (synaptic or injected current, I). The intrinsic biophysical and morphological features of motoneurons that determine the values of V_r and R_N will be considered next. This will be followed by a discussion of the determinants of I_0, f_0, and f-I, as well as the effects of neuromodulators on each of these parameters. The last subsection on motoneuron properties will address the application of computer models to the study of the relation between motoneuron properties and function.

Both the subthreshold and suprathreshold behavior of motoneurons are affected by the properties and distribution of voltage-sensitive and calcium-sensitive ionic conductances. The active conductances known or likely to exist in mammalian motoneurons are summarized in Table 1.1. Each conductance is broadly characterized in terms of its primary charge carrier (i.e., potassium, sodium, or calcium ions), the voltage range over which it is activated, and its kinetics. Both the voltage activation range and speed of activation are presented in relative rather than absolute terms (see Table 1.1 for details). The characteristics and functional roles of individual conductances are discussed in more detail below.

The Ionic Basis of the Resting Potential

The resting potential (V_r') that is measured with an intrasomatic electrode depends on the activity of several ionic conductances. Its value may differ from the true (i.e., preimpalement) resting potential (V_r) because of an artifactual conductance resulting from the leak of ions around the microelectrode. As in other neurons, the resting potential of motoneurons is determined primarily by a resting potassium conductance in combination with a relatively high internal concentration of potassium (82, 116). Part of the potassium conductance active at rest is apparently distinct from other potassium conductances in that it is reduced by external barium ions and is insensitive to a number of blocking agents that affect other potassium channels (23, 244). The magnitude of this barium-sensitive leak conductance (G_{Krest}) is independent of voltage over a large range (244). Its spatial distribution in motoneurons is not known, but recent work suggests that an analogous conductance in rat sympathetic ganglion cells is not uniformly distributed across the somatodendritic membrane (274). Part of the resting potassium conductance may also result from current flow through a hyperpolarization-activated mixed cation conductance (G_h) and a calcium-activated potassium conductance (G_{KCa}, see Table 1.1 and below).

Although the potassium equilibrium potential has been estimated to be −80 to −100 mV in motoneurons (15, 82, 116, 367), average resting potentials obtained from large samples of cat spinal motoneurons recorded in vivo with sharp microelectrodes range from around −65 mV (249, 366) to around −75 mV (137, 138), depending upon the selection criteria used. The difference between the resting and potassium equilibrium potentials in motoneurons depends in part upon some resting permeability to sodium ions (116), resulting both from resting activation of G_h channels and from the artifactual leak conductance produced by an imperfect seal around

TABLE 1.1. *Conductances in Mammalian Motoneurons*

Conductance	Ion(s)	Activation Threshold	Activation Maximum	Inactivation Threshold	Inactivation Maximum	Activation Kinetics[a] (Inactivation Kinetics)	References
Krest	K	$<V_r$	$>V_{thr}$	—	—	Fast	23, 243, 244
KCa	K	$>V_r$ & $<V_{thr}$	$>>V_{thr}$[b]	—	—	Slow	15, 72, 167, 211, 235, 243, 306, 328, 349, 367
KCa_f	K	$\cong V_r$ & $<V_{thr}$	$>V_{thr}$[b]			Medium	346
KA_f	K	$\cong V_r$	$>V_{thr}$	$<V_r$	$>V_{thr}$	Fast (medium)	72, 303, 328
KA_s	K	$>V_r$ & $<V_{thr}$	$>V_{thr}$	$<V_r$	$>V_{thr}$	Slow (slow)	72
Kdr	K	$>V_{thr}$	$>>V_{thr}$	—	—	Medium	15, 305, 328
h	K, Na	$>V_r$ & $<V_{thr}$	$<V_r$[c]	—	—	Slow	15, 22, 72, 217, 327
Na_T (Soma)	Na	$>V_{thr}$	$>>V_{thr}$	$\cong V_{thr}$	$>V_{thr}$	Fast (medium)	1, 18, 307
Na_T (Init. Seg.)	Na	$\cong V_{thr}$	$>V_{thr}$	$>V_r$ & $<V_{thr}$	$>V_{thr}$	Fast (medium)	1, 18, 277, 307
Na_p	Na	$>V_r$ & $<V_{thr}$	$>V_{thr}$	—	—	Medium[d]	72, 235, 243, 276
i	Ca	$>V_r$ & $<V_{thr}$	$>V_{thr}$	—	—	Slow	298, 302, 303
Ca_T[e]	Ca	$>V_r$ & $<V_{thr}$	$>>V_{thr}$	$<V_r$	$>V_{thr}$	Medium (slow)	238, 346, 349
Ca_L	Ca	$>V_{thr}$	$>>V_{thr}$			Medium	237, 238, 346, 349
Ca_N	Ca	$>V_{thr}$	$>>V_{thr}$	$>V_r$ & $<V_{thr}$	$>V_{thr}$	Medium (slow)	238, 346, 349
Ca_p	Ca	$>V_{thr}$	$>>V_{thr}$	—	—	Medium	346

Conductances present in mammalian motoneurons. Conductances are characterized in terms of the abbreviated label used in the text, the ion species carrying the current, the relative voltage ranges over which activation and inactivation occurs, and the relative time constants of activation and inactivation. The last column lists the references pertaining to each conductance. Whenever possible the characteristics presented in the table are appropriate for adult cat motoneurons. Characteristics often differ across species and developmental stages. [a]Kinetics are characterized in terms of the range of time constants reported: fast, <1 ms; medium, 1–10 ms; slow, >10 ms. [b]Since KCa and KCa_f are sensitive to internal calcium, their activation ranges and kinetics reflect those of the triggering calcium currents. [c]The h conductance is increased by membrane hyperpolarization and decreased by depolarization. [d]Na_p kinetics are not well characterized in motoneurons, but time constants of <5 ms have been reported in cat neocortical neurons (cf. 319). [e]The T-type calcium conductance is more prominant in neonatal than in adult motoneurons (349).

the recording microelectrode. Measured values of resting potential do not differ significantly in different motor unit types (366) and are not correlated with measured R_N values (137, 138).

Determinants of Input Resistance

Contribution of Morphology and Membrane Resistivity. Our current understanding of how the biophysical and geometrical properties of motoneurons relate to input resistance (R_N) is based on the application of cable theory to passive (i.e., linear, voltage-independent) motoneuron behavior. This approach was originally introduced by Rall (268) and has subsequently been the subject of numerous theoretical and experimental studies (for reviews, see 175, 269, 270). Only a few aspects of the theory and its application will be presented here. For a more complete description, the reader should consult the cited reviews.

For a spherical neuron with no dendritic processes, input resistance (R_N) will be determined by the ratio of specific resistivity (R_m in $\Omega \cdot cm^2$) to the neuronal surface area (A_N). α-Motoneurons, however, have extensive dendritic trees, so that their geometrical and electrical properties are not well approximated by an isopotential sphere. Rall (268) demonstrated that the motoneuron could be represented as a lumped soma consisting of a resistance and capacitance in parallel attached to a uniform diameter cylinder of finite length, provided that intrinsic membrane properties are uniform over the entire somatodendritic surface and that the geometrical features of dendritic trees meet certain constraints. The electrical behavior of this model is determined by the values of four parameters: R_N, the membrane time constant ($\tau_m = R_m * C_m$, where C_m is the specific membrane capacitance), the ratio of dendritic to somatic input conductance (ρ), and the electrotonic length of the dendritic cylinder (L). The electrotonic length of the cylinder is its actual length divided by the space constant (λ), which is the length over which a steady-state voltage applied to a point on an infinitely long cylinder with the same properties would decay to $1/e$ of its initial value.

The validity of the approach described above depends on the degree to which the idealized equivalent cylinder model provides a reasonable approximation to the electrical properties of real motoneurons. The model's limitations were acknowledged at the outset (268), and a number of studies have been devoted to developing and applying more complicated models. The actual geometry of motoneuron dendrites does not strictly satisfy the constraints necessary to collapse all of the dendrites into a single cylinder of constant diameter. Figure 1.2*A* shows a reconstruction of an HRP-filled cat ankle extensor motoneuron. A single axon and anywhere from 6–19 dendritic trees project outward from the motoneuron soma (77, 88, 204, 229, 283, 343). The size and branching complexity of individual dendritic trees are correlated with the diameter of the stem dendrite arising from the soma (63, 77, 88, 204, 283, 343, 345); that is, larger stem dendrites give rise to larger and more complex dendritic trees than do smaller stem dendrites. The dendrites arising from the soma can exhibit a three- to four-fold range in their stem diameters and the various associated size-related measures (38, 39, 63, 88, 229) leading to marked differences in the electrical behavior of different dendrites of the same motoneuron (38, 39, 229).

Figure 1.2*B* and *C* show two different schematic representations of a single dendritic tree. At increasing distance from the soma, the number of branch points first increases then decreases sharply. The opposite pattern is observed for the number of branch terminations. The dendritic surface area changes as a function of radial distance from the soma, first increasing and then decreasing with increasing somatofugal distance (38, 77, 88, 205, 229, 283). As shown in Figure 1.2*C*, it is still possible to represent the average behavior of the dendrites with a single cable, but in order to more closely approximate the true structure of motoneuron dendrites, this cable should have a variable diameter, first increasing slightly and then tapering sharply as a function of distance from the soma (77, 115, 270).

A more serious problem with the idealized equivalent cylinder model is the assumption that R_m is uniform across the somatodendritic membrane. Recent work indicates that this is not the case and that some of the nonuniformity is likely to arise from a leak conductance introduced by inserting a microelectrode into the motoneuron soma [somatic shunt; (98)]. For a given magnitude of electrode-induced shunt conductance, the relative effect on the measured input conductance of a neuron will depend upon the magnitude of its "true" (i.e., uninjured) input conductance. Since motoneurons are relatively large, their "true" input conductance is also likely to be large and the shunt effect might be expected to be minor. Nonetheless, a number of recent studies suggest that the effects of electrode leak on measured motoneuron properties can be significant.

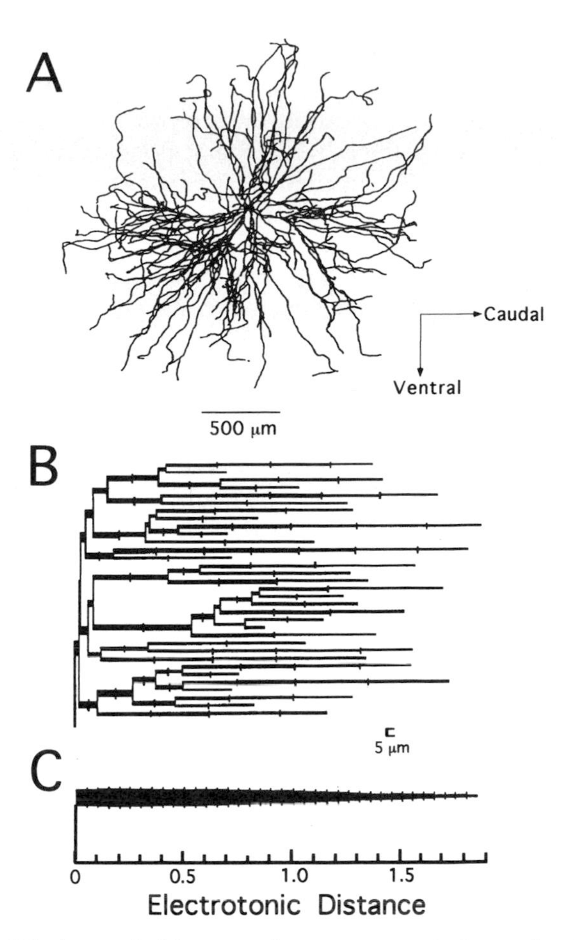

FIG. 1.2. Anatomical features of motoneurons. *A*, Camera lucida drawing of an HRP-filled cat medial gastrocnemius motoneuron (type FF), projected without perspective in the sagittal plane. [From Cullheim et al. (89).] *B* and *C*, Two different schematic plots of a single reconstructed dendritic tree. [From Rall et al. (270).] Distance scale is in units of electronic distance from the soma, calculated using a uniform specific membrane resistivity (R_m) of 11 kΩ·cm^2 and cytoplasmic resistivity (R_i) of 70 Ω·cm. Individual dendritic segments are represented in *B*, while in *C* the entire dendritic tree has been collapsed into a single unbranched "equivalent" cable.

Effects of Impalement-Induced Leak. Several methods have been used to estimate the magnitude of the leak conductance around the recording micropipette. However, all of these methods are based on untested assumptions and they can give rise to quite different estimates of the magnitude of the leak conductance. The first method is based on the premise that after impalement the measured resting potential is determined by an equilibrium between current flowing across the neuron's true resting conductance (G_N) and that flowing across the leak conductance around the electrode (G_{Lelec}). The measured resting potential (V'_r) will approach the "true" resting potential (V_r) when the relative magnitude of the electrode leak (G_{Lelec}/G_N) is small and will approach the equilibrium potential for the impalement-induced leak current (V_{Lelec}) when G_{Lelec} is large. If this leak conductance is relatively nonspecific for different ion species, V_{Lelec} should be around 0 mV. Gustafsson and Pinter (138) estimated that if the true motoneuron resting potential is −80 mV (and $V_{Lelec} = 0$), then the range of resting potentials measured in their sample were consistent with a maximum leak conductance that was 30% of the true input conductance. Their analysis suggests leak conductances on the order of 0.05–0.5 μS (resistances of 2–20 MΩ), which are similar to previous estimates derived from experiments on frog muscle fibers (161, 322).

A strong inverse relation between the measured values of R_N and resting potential would be expected if variations in leak conductance were the sole cause of variations in measured R_N (and if V_{Lelec} is significantly more depolarized than V_r). However, no significant correlations between either R_N or estimated shunt conductance and resting potential have been reported (e.g., 138, 285), and the differences in mean R_N among different motor unit types are not associated with differences in their average resting potentials (366). It is possible that the lack of correlation between measures of V_r and R_N is due to the fact that V_{Lelec} is close to the measured resting potential. This could occur if the electrode-induced leak led to an influx of calcium ions of sufficient magnitude to overwhelm the cells' intrinsic buffering and pumping capacity and to turn on a calcium-activated potassium conductance. However, neither the intracellular injection of calcium nor calcium chelators markedly alters the resting potential of motoneurons (212, 213, 282, 369).

The second method of estimating the leak conductance induced by electrode impalement requires anatomical reconstruction of the motoneuron in combination with measurements of R_N and the time course of the voltage response to a current step, together with assumed values of specific membrane capacitance (C_m) and internal cytoplasmic resistivity (R_i). If R_m is assumed to be uniform across the dendritic surface, matching the electrophysiological data with the measured geometry requires the R_m value for the somatic membrane to be severalfold smaller than that for the dendritic membrane (77, 115, 285; see also 204, 229). If the lower somatic R_m value is attributed entirely to an electrode-induced leak conductance, values of leak conductance of over 1 μS are often obtained.

The final method of estimating electrode-induced leak is based on comparisons of R_N measurements obtained with sharp and patch electrodes in the same cells under the same experimental conditions. If patch electrodes are assumed to form a perfect seal with the cell membrane, so that there is no electrode-induced leak, the mean leak conductance induced by sharp microelectrodes is simply the difference between the mean values of input conductance obtained with sharp and patch electrodes. Recent comparisons of this type are available for a number of neuron types (309, 318, 320), including neonatal rat lumbar motoneurons (compare 122 and 328). Differences in the two types of input conductance measurements range from 0.015–0.05 μS (i.e., electrode shunt resistances of 20–67 MΩ). However, the sharp electrodes employed in these studies had much higher resistances (and presumably smaller tip diameters) than the intracellular electrodes typically used to record from adult cat motoneurons, and the larger electrodes may well introduce a larger leak conductance.

In summary, estimates of the electrode-induced leak conductance based on measurements of V_r and R_N and from comparisons of R_N values obtained with sharp and patch electrodes are quite small. Considerably larger estimates are obtained from analyses of neuron models with R_m uniform everywhere except at the impalement site. The various approaches to estimating electrode leak might be reconciled if it is assumed that even in the absence of electrode impalement R_m is nonuniform across the somatodendritic membrane, perhaps increasing as a function of somatofugal distance (cf. 115). Electrode impalement might exaggerate this nonuniform R_m by adding a nonspecific leak conductance to the soma on the order of 0.05–0.01 μS. Thus, the extent to which the leak depolarizes the neuron from resting potential and reduces the measured input resistance and membrane time constant below their true values will depend on: *(1)* the relative magnitudes of the "true" neuron conductance and resting potential; and *(2)*, the electrode leak conductance and its reversal potential.

How does our present understanding of the passive, linear behavior of motoneurons differ from the idealized equivalent cylinder model (268)? The motoneuron can still be represented as a soma attached to an equivalent dendritic cable, but the diameter of the cable varies with somatofugal distance due to the observed patterns of dendritic branching, tapering, and termination. R_m varies across the surface of the neuron, and although the actual values are unknown, the dendritic R_m is likely to be significantly higher than the somatic R_m. Although the tips of the longest dendritic branches in this model may be more electrically distant from the soma than originally thought, the bulk of the dendritic membrane is relatively close electrically (cf. 270).

Variation in Input Resistance among Different Motoneurons. Equations 1 and 2 imply that, other factors being equal, motoneurons will be recruited in order of decreasing input resistance. Input resistances measured in cat lumbar motoneurons in vivo exhibit about a tenfold range from about 0.4–4.0 MΩ (e.g., 138, 366). Average R_N values are largest in type S, smaller in type FR, and smallest in type FF motoneurons (114, 366). The original formulation of the "size principle" implied that size is the most important factor in determining input resistance (158), and there is anatomical evidence for the existence of systematic differences in the sizes of motoneurons comprising a pool (e.g., 51, 87, 203). The myelinated motor axon diameters of type-identified cat gastrocnemius motoneurons are smallest in type S motoneurons and of approximately equal size in type FR and FF motoneurons (90). Soma size is positively correlated with axonal conduction velocity (87, 203), which is in turn proportional to axon diameter (87). Total dendritic surface area is also weakly correlated with conduction velocity (17, 51, 203). However, it is now generally accepted that systematic differences in specific membrane resistivity are at least equally important in producing variations in input resistance.

Within a motoneuron pool, cell surface area only varies over at most a fourfold range, regardless of whether A_N is estimated from electrophysiological measurements alone (138, 285), from estimates of dendritic surface area based on dendritic stem diameter (51, 345), or from complete anatomical reconstructions (17, 88). While these dimensional arguments suggest that variations in R_m contribute to variations in R_N, this contribution can be demonstrated more directly by plotting measures of R_N against estimates of A_N made in the same cells, and attempting to fit these plots using idealized equivalent cylinder models with a range of values for R_m and electronic length (51, 138). This approach indicates that the observed variation in R_N is likely to be associated with a three- to fivefold variation in R_m and that R_m is systematically higher in type S than in type F motoneurons. Analysis of motoneuron properties based on more complicated models support this conclusion. If dendritic R_m is assumed to be uniform, both somatic and dendritic R_m have been found to be correlated with R_N (204), and even if R_m is assumed to vary continuously across the somatodendritic membrane, a spatially weighted average of R_m is also correlated with the measured R_N (115).

Effects of Active Conductances. The effective input resistance of a motoneuron is likely to depend not only on R_m and geometry but also on the conductances active at rest, together with conductances activated or deactivated by changes in membrane potential. In the voltage range from close to the resting potential to more hyperpolarized potentials, the most prominent voltage-sensitive current is a hyperpolarization-activated mixed cation current with a reversal potential positive to the resting potential (I_h). The conductance underlying this current (G_h) is slowly activated by hyperpolarization with a half-activation voltage that is 20–30 mV negative to the resting potential [(15, 22, 72, 217, 327); cf. Table 1.1]. The contribution of G_h to the resting potential will depend upon the degree to which its activation range overlaps the measured resting potential: A significant steady-state activation would be expected at −70 mV, whereas little or no activation should take place at −60 mV (22, 217).

Additional slow, persistent inward and outward currents are activated over the voltage range from about 5–10 mV positive to rest through suprathreshold voltages. The slow outward current is probably due to the same calcium-activated potassium conductance (G_{KCa}) underlying the postspike afterhyperpolarization (see further on). Motoneurons may also exhibit a transient outward current [A-type current; (78)], but its properties in motoneurons have not been extensively studied [(72, 303); cf. Table 1.1].

The persistent inward current was first identified in cat lumbar motoneurons based on the clamp current recorded during slow-ramp, depolarizing voltage-clamp commands. The steady-state $I-V$ curve exhibits an "N-shape" (298) including a region of negative slope conductance at about 10–20 mV above the resting potential, which subsequently reverses to a positive slope due to the increasing activation of conductances mediating outward currents. Voltage-clamp commands encompassing the region of negative-slope conductance reveal a slowly activating inward current that is enhanced by external Ba^{2+} (303), and is not blocked by intracellular injection of lidocaine derivatives that block the fast sodium currents (303, 304). Based on this evidence, the persistent inward current in cat motoneurons is probably calcium mediated, although in other motoneurons, a negative-slope region in the $I-V$ curve may be produced by a persistent sodium current [Na_P; (72, 235, 243, 276].

The presence of these subthreshold conductances causes the measured input resistance of motoneurons to be both time- and voltage-dependent. Over the voltage range where G_h is active, depolarization of the membrane by an injected current step reduces G_h, and the slow deactivation of this conductance leads to a hyperpolarizing sag in the membrane trajectory. The opposite sequence of events (i.e., G_h activation and depolarizing sag) occurs in response to hyperpolarizing injected current steps. The presence of G_h reduces the effective input resistance, and because of its slow kinetics, the reduction of input resistance is most apparent in response to relatively long (>50 ms) current steps. At slightly more depolarized voltages, activation of G_{KCa} may contribute to the hyperpolarizing sag produced by depolarizing injected currents. Near spike threshold, a persistent inward current begins to predominate, leading to an increase in membrane depolarization and effective input resistance. This corresponds to the decrease in the slope of the steady-state $I-V$ relation measured under voltage-clamp conditions.

Although a number of techniques have been used to minimize or account for the effects of these subthreshold active conductances in order to obtain a measure of the "passive" properties of motoneurons (115, 138, 366), it is the effective value of R_N (rather than some ideal, linear R_N value) that determines the response of the motoneuron under physiological conditions. In spite of the inherently nonlinear nature of active conductances, a quantitative analysis of the time and voltage dependence of R_N can be obtained without sacrificing the analytical power of linear cable theory. This is accomplished by applying a piecewise linear, frequency-domain analysis of the neuron's response to small perturbations applied at different mean levels of membrane potential (210). The dependent variable of interest is then the frequency-dependent input impedance [$Z_N(\omega)$, $\omega = 2\pi f$] or admittance [$Y_N(\omega)$] rather than R_N or G_N, respectively.

Linearized frequency-domain descriptions have now been obtained for a number of different types of neurons including trigeminal ganglion cells and thalamic neurons from the guinea pig (263, 264), interneurons and motoneurons in the lamprey spinal cord (46, 232, 233), and cultured neuroblastoma cells (234, 363). A completely passive neuron behaves as a low-pass filter whose impedance decreases and phase lag approaches 90 degrees with increasing input current frequency due to the increasing fraction of the current that is shunted through the membrane capacitance (175). Moreover, the magnitude and phase of the impedance function are independent of the mean membrane potential. Voltage-dependent active conductances can alter the input impedance functions in a manner that is dependent upon the mean membrane potential. In lamprey motoneurons, activation of an inward current by membrane depolarization increases the magnitude of the steady-state impedance and produces a steeper fall-off in impedance and increase in phase lag with increasing frequencies (46). Blocking this inward current with tetrodotoxin (TTX) causes the behavior of the motoneuron to resemble that expected for a completely passive membrane. The increased steady-state impedance at more depolarized membrane potentials is analogous to the increased R_N measured near spike threshold from steady-state voltage-clamp analyses of cat lumbar motoneurons (see earlier). The frequency-dependent effects of the inward current act to exaggerate the neuron's low-pass filter characteristics (210). In a variety of other types of neurons, voltage-dependent activation of outward currents (e.g., 263) or inactivation of inward currents (264) reduces the steady-state impedance and produces a resonant peak in the frequency response function.

In summary, the subthreshold response of a motoneuron to voltage or current perturbations applied to the soma depends upon passive membrane properties and their spatial variation; the geometrical structure and size of the motoneuron; and the time, voltage-dependence and spatial distribution of any conductances showing significant activation in the subthreshold voltage range.

Threshold Behavior

Mechanisms of the Action Potential and Afterpotentials. Depolarizing synaptic or injected current of sufficient magnitude elicits a fast, sodium-dependent (Na_T; see Table 1.1) action potential that is followed by a prolonged afterhyperpolarization (AHP). The rising phase of the action potential consists of two components, which are thought to reflect a two-stage invasion of the motoneuron, starting at the axon segment next to the soma (initial segment) and continuing into the soma and probably the proximal dendrites (41, 81, 123). The transition between the axon and soma is called the axon hillock. In cat lumbar motoneurons, the base of the axon hillock is 6–15 μm in diameter and tapers over a length of 6–25 μm to join the initial segment of the axon (79, 80, 186, 187). The initial axon segment is unmyelinated and relatively long and narrow [3–5 μm in diameter × 23–35 μm in length (79, 80, 186, 187)]. A two-stage invasion of the motoneuron during the conduction of an antidromic action potential occurs as a consequence of the depolarizing current supplied by the initial segment action potential encountering the resistive load of the much larger soma. The initial segment also has a lower threshold for excitation in response to orthodromic (synaptic) activation, further suggesting that it is intrinsically more excitable than the soma. The increased excitability of the initial segment might be due to a higher density of sodium channels (68, 96, 230), or to the presence of a distinct subtype of sodium channels (69).

Although the extent of sodium channel distribution across the somatodendritic membrane is uncertain, several lines of evidence suggest that sodium channels are confined to the soma and portions of the dendritic membrane that are electronically close to the soma (1, 18, 241). Nonetheless, it is possible that there is some active propagation of a somatic action potential into the proximal dendrites (333).

The kinetics and voltage dependence of activation and inactivation of the somatic sodium current are qualitatively similar to those described by Hodgkin and Huxley (160) for the squid axon, although the time course of inactivation is slower than that predicted from a simple scaling of the Hodkgin-Huxley rate constants according to their temperature dependence (18; see also 230). In addition, the steady-state relations between voltage and both activation and inactivation are shifted to more depolarized values than those generally reported for axons (18, 307). There is relatively little steady-state inactivation of the somatic sodium current from the resting potential to its activation threshold (307).

The properties of the initial segment sodium current have not been studied directly, but they can be inferred from variations in firing level (the somatic voltage at which the rapid upstroke of the action potential begins) during repetitive discharge in motoneurons, and from voltage-clamp studies on axons. The somatic voltage at which the initial segment spike is elicited exhibits a delayed dependence on somatic membrane potential (55, 62), which can take the form of rapid fluctuations in threshold (62), as well as slower rises in firing level during prolonged suprathreshold current steps (307). This behavior is known as accommodation, and is thought to be produced in part by sodium channel inactivation (117, 296, 347). Experiments on cat motor axons suggest inactivation time constants in the range of 2–4 ms (277), and similar sodium inactivation kinetics have been described in other excitable membranes (reviewed in 159). However, a much slower component has also been described (e.g., 40, 169), which may underlie the slow increase in firing level observed during repetitive discharge (307). Over the entire range of repetitive discharge frequencies, spikes arise at somatic voltages below those needed to directly activate somatic sodium channels, demonstrating that the initial segment is always the trigger zone for the action potential (307).

Repolarization of the membrane following the peak of the action potential is produced by a combination of sodium inactivation, leak current, and delayed activation of potassium currents. Voltage-clamp recordings in cat lumbar motoneurons indicate the presence of two, kinetically distinguishable potassium currents [fast and slow (15, 305)]. The fast component is probably analogous to the delayed rectifier current described in a variety of neuron types (K_{dr}) [Table 1.1; (288)] and can be blocked by external tetraethylammonium (TEA) (305). Slowing of spike repolarization by TEA can be quite profound in many types of motoneurons (e.g., 72, 166, 235, 243, 350) but is relatively slight in cat lumbar motoneurons, perhaps because the leak conductance makes a large contribution to action potential repolarization (305). Spike repolarization is also prolonged by 4-aminopyridine (4-AP) (72, 243, 350), suggesting that one or more transient A-type potassium conductances (K_A) [Table 1.1; (288)] may also contribute. The limited voltage-clamp data on A-currents in motoneurons suggests that although they may contribute to the repolarization of action potentials evoked from the resting potential, their contribution may be minimal during repetitive discharge when the more depolarized membrane potential leads to their inactivation (72, 243, 302, 328). In neonatal rat motoneurons, a fast, high conductance subtype of calcium-activated potassium channel (K_{Caf}) [Table 1.1; (288)] has also been shown to contribute to action potential repolarization (346).

A brief, depolarizing afterpotential often follows the fast repolarization phase of the spike. There is still some controversy regarding the mechanisms of this delayed depolarization (DD). It was originally attributed to the active or passive spread of depolarization from the soma into the proximal dendrites following a somatic action potential (188, 240), but the DD has also been attributed to the spread of current from the initial segment (6). Finally, in neonatal motoneurons the DD is at least partially due to calcium entry triggered by the somatic spike (142, 349, 356).

The prolonged AHP that follows the delayed depolarization has been attributed to the activation of the slow potassium current component (15). This slow component first appears with depolarizing voltage steps that are subthreshold for an initial-segment spike, and increases in amplitude with increasing depolarization up to about 100 mV from rest, where it begins to decrease (15, 306). Its kinetics and voltage-dependence are likely to reflect those of the calcium currents that trigger it, since there is now a large body of evidence that this slow potassium current is due to an apamin-sensitive, calcium-activated potassium conductance [G_{KCa} in Table 1.1 (cf. 288)]. AHPs are completely or partially blocked by external application of divalent cations that block calcium conductances (72, 166, 211, 235, 243, 350, 368), and the AHP is also depressed by intracellular injection of calcium chelators (213, 350, 368).

In neonatal rat hypoglossal motoneurons, it has been demonstrated (346, 350) that the calcium influx responsible for triggering the AHP enters through two types of high-threshold calcium channels that are blocked by ω-conotoxin and ω-agatoxin, respectively (i.e., N-type and P-type calcium channels) [see Table 1.1; 308)]. Calcium entry through a low-threshold channel (T-type) [see Table 1.1; (308)] may contribute to action potential repolarization by activating a separate type of Ca-activated potassium conductance (346) (see K_{Caf} in Table 1.1). The fact that the AHP is unaffected by blocking other calcium conductances suggests that these N- and P-type calcium channels must be in close proximity to the calcium-activated potassium channels responsible for the AHP, but separated from other calcium channels. The activation of G_{KCa} by calcium is therefore likely to depend upon the local concentration of calcium, which will in turn depend upon the calcium entering through calcium channels and the location of these channels. The deactivation of G_{KCa} will not only depend upon the rate constants for calcium binding to the channel, but also on the rate at which calcium leaves the vicinity of the channel due to diffusion, binding to intracellular proteins, and pumping across the membrane.

Variation in Threshold Behavior among Motoneurons. The current thresholds for eliciting action potentials with long intracellular current steps [rheobase (I_{rh})] exhibit a tenfold range across individual motoneurons within a single motoneuron pool (66, 114, 137, 252) and vary systematically according to motoneuron type in the order type S < FR < FF (114, 366). The somatic voltage threshold for spike initiation (V_{thr}) exhibits a much smaller range of variation (66, 137, 249), suggesting that variations in rheobase are largely the result of variations in input resistance. The range of variation of rheobase also exceeds that of input conductance, suggesting that other factors may contribute (136). There is some tendency for V_{thr} to be lowest in low-rheobase, high-resistance (presumably type S and type FR) motoneurons (66, 137). In addition, the value of V_{thr} is greater than that predicted by the product of input resistance (R_N) and rheobase, reflecting the fact that the additional depolarization to threshold may be provided by a persistent inward current (see earlier). The difference between V_{thr} and the product of I_{rh} and R_N is also correlated with R_N, suggesting that the magnitude of the persistent inward current is similar in different motoneurons, and therefore that its relative effect is most prominent in small, high-R_N motoneurons (137). This conclusion is also supported by voltage-clamp data (304). Although changes in membrane properties subsequent to electrode impalement make differences in V_{thr} difficult to interpret (137), the lower value of V_{thr} in small motoneurons may reflect a higher relative density of initial segment sodium channels or perhaps a difference in their accommodative properties (55).

The magnitude and duration of the AHP following a single spike vary according to motoneuron size (371) and motor unit type: larger and longer AHPs are recorded in type S than in type F motoneurons (197, 366). It is not known whether these differences in AHP characteristics reflect differences in the properties or density of G_{KCa} channels or differences in the various factors controlling the time course of the calcium concentration in the vicinity of the channels. Gustafsson and Pinter (139) proposed that the kinetics of the AHP conductance may be similar across different motoneurons, but that a more developed sag conductance (G_h) in type F motoneurons provides an inward current that decreases the measured AHP duration. However, AHP characteristics measured at the resting potential are correlated with repetitive discharge behavior (see further on), even though G_h should be largely deactivated over the range of membrane potentials encountered during steady-state repetitive discharge.

Repetitive Discharge Behavior

Basic Characteristics and Mechanisms. Motoneurons respond to a suprathreshold injected current step with a series of action potentials whose instantaneous frequency is a function of both time and current intensity. Firing rate decreases as a function of time after the onset of the current step, a process called spike-frequency adaptation. The largest decrease in rate takes place in the first few interspike intervals [*initial adaptation*; (189, 190, 294, 295)] and a near steady-state frequency is reached by 0.5–1 s after current onset. If current injection is prolonged beyond 1 s, a more gradual decline in frequency takes place that continues over tens of seconds or even several minutes [*late adaptation*; (131, 166, 189, 201, 294, 295)]. A more quantitative analysis of the time course of adaptation in rat hypoglosssal motoneurons revealed three distinct phases of adaptation (294, 295). The *initial*, rapid phase of adaptation is characterized by a linear relation between instantaneous frequency and time, and is complete within the first few interspike intervals. The subsequent decline in frequency often exhibits two components: an *early* phase of adaptation that is typically complete within the first 2 s of discharge; and a *late* phase of adaptation that continues for the duration of firing.

In cat lumbar motoneurons, the relation between the steady-state discharge rate (i.e., that measured at 0.5–1 s) and the magnitude of injected current (*f-I* relation) can be described by one or two linear segments, with the second segment (secondary range) having a slope two to six times steeper than that of the first segment [primary range; (10, 12, 190, 297, 299, 307)]. Further increments in current may reveal a third segment (tertiary range) that generally has a lower slope than that of the secondary range (297). The *f-I* relations for the initial interspike intervals can also be described by two or three line segments, but the slopes of these segments are much steeper than those describing the steady-state *f-I* relation. The *initial* adaptation over the first few interspike intervals generates a progressive fall in the steepness of the *f-I* relations until they approach the steady-state relation. In some cells the true steady-state *f-I* relation may not be reached until 2 s or longer (294, 295). Qualitatively similar behavior has been described in a number of other types of motoneurons (166, 179, 228, 243, 350), although the steady-state *f-I* relation typically shows just one linear segment over the range of currents studied.

The conductance underlying the AHP is one of the primary determinants of the steady-state repetitive discharge properties of motoneurons. The minimum steady firing rate (f_0) is approximately equal to the reciprocal of AHP duration (191), although the two measures are not always tightly correlated (67, 179). The steady-state frequencies attained at the end of the primary and secondary ranges of firing are also correlated with the reciprocal of AHP duration (191). Finally, comparisons of steady-state *f-I* relations before and after pharmacological manipulations of the AHP conductance (72, 166, 243, 350), indicate that the steady-state *f-I* slope is inversely proportional to the magnitude of the AHP conductance.

A variety of evidence suggests that two other biophysical features described earlier make important contributions to motoneuron discharge behavior: *(1)* the low threshold, persistent inward current (I_i) (see Table 1.1) and *(2)* variations in spike threshold resulting from the accommodative properties of the initial segment. The presence of a persistent inward current is likely to have important effects on steady-state discharge behavior, provided that the somatic membrane potential can traverse voltage ranges over which this current is significantly activated. The increase in spike threshold at increasing rates of discharge allows this condition to occur (250, 307). Figure 1.3, which shows current-clamp and voltage-clamp recordings obtained in the same motoneuron, indicates that some inward current activation takes place at the membrane voltage reached at the end of the interspike interval at the lowest firing rate (denoted with *P* in Fig. 1.3) and that it is likely to be continuously activated throughout the interspike interval at the maximum primary range firing rate (denoted with *T* in Fig. 1.3). The upward bend in the steady-state *f-I* curve (secondary range firing) may result from the predominance of the inward current.

Initial adaptation, which is complete within the first few interspike intervals, has been previously correlated with increases in AHP amplitude (13) and duration (15, 175, 202). Summation of AHP currents could occur if the calcium concentration in the vicinity of the G_{KCa} channels does not return to resting levels at the end of the interspike intervals. *Initial* adaptation is also associated with an increase in firing level resulting from changes in the inactivation of initial segment sodium channels (307). Finally, depending upon its activation range and kinetics, I_h could contribute to *initial* adaptation: if it is partly activated at rest, it will provide an inward current that will increase discharge rate at the onset of a current step and then deactivate at the more depolarized voltages encountered during maintained repetitive discharge (cf. 317).

The slow decline in firing rate seen during *early* and *late* adaptation could reflect a progressive increase in outward currents, a progressive decrease in inward currents, or some combination of these two mechanisms (294, 295). Slow increases in the calcium concentration near the G_{KCa} channels would prolong the increase in G_{KCa} beyond the period of *initial* adaptation. Alternatively, progressive increases in other potassium currents might also contribute to *early* and *late* adaptation, although the activation of the Na^+-K^+ pump does not appear to contribute (292). A progressive decrease in inward sodium currents could result from slow inactivation processes (see earlier). Finally, more complex interactions between inward and outward currents might underlie *late* adaptation. For example, reducing or eliminating G_{KCa} by replacing external Ca^{2+} with

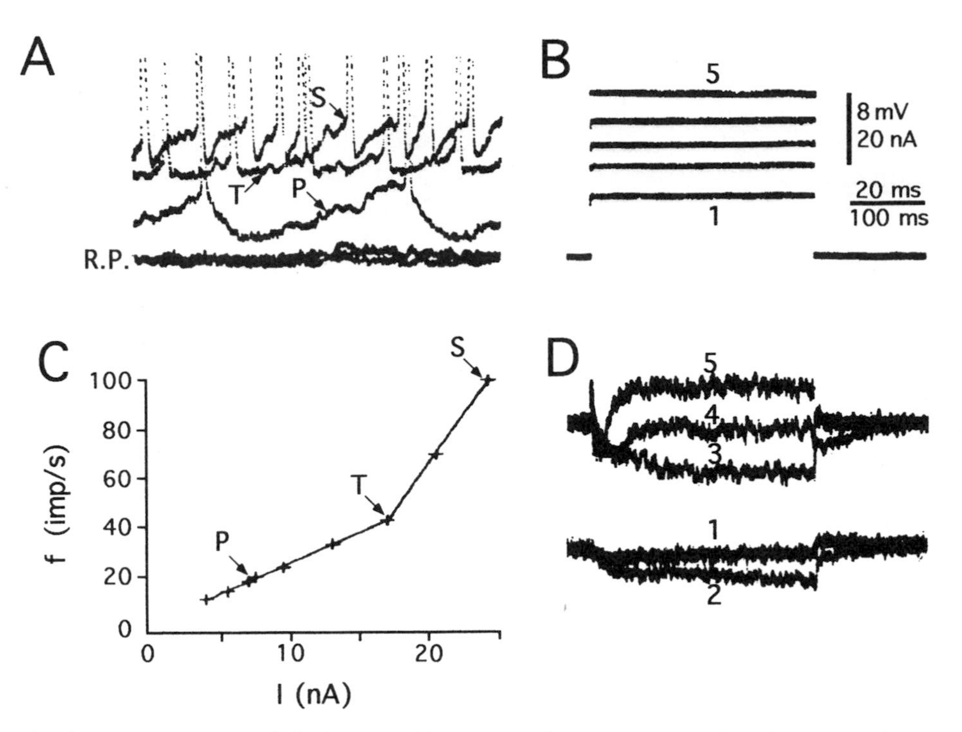

FIG. 1.3. Relation of voltage range traversed during repetitive discharge to the voltage dependence of the persistent inward current recorded under voltage-clamp conditions in the same cell. *A*, Voltage trajectories during repetitive discharge in the primary range (*P*) at the transition to thedary range (*T*) and at the upper end of the secondary range (*S*). Top of spikes (65 mV) are clipped. *B* and *D*, Voltage step commands (*B*) and the recorded membrane currents (after electronic subtraction of the leak current and the longest capacitative charging transient). (The baseline of traces 1 and 2 in the lower right panel are identical to those of traces 3–5 but have been shifted downward for clarity.). C, Average steady firing rate (f) vs. injected current (I) for the cell. [From Schwindt and Crill (307).]

Mn^{2+} leads to an initial increase in discharge rate for a given current level, and yet the magnitude of *late* adaptation is increased (291, 293). It is possible that under these conditions, an increase in the mean level of membrane depolarization during the interspike interval accelerates the development of sodium channel inactivation.

Variation in Discharge Behavior among Different Motoneurons. A number of aspects of the current-to-frequency transformation vary systematically across the motoneuron pool. The tenfold variation in rheobase (I_{rh}) is associated with a similar range in the minimum current needed to elicit steady repetitive discharge [I_0; (200)], which is about 1.5 times the rheobase value on average (191). Variations in the *f-I* relations among different motoneuron types also arise from type-related differences in AHP characteristics (see earlier). Due to their longer AHP durations, type S motoneurons begin to discharge at significantly lower rates than type F motoneurons (196), and the steady-state frequencies attained at the end of the primary and secondary ranges of firing are also lower in motoneurons with long AHP durations [presumably type S motoneurons; (191)]. In contrast, the primary and secondary range *f-I* slopes do not vary systematically with either motoneuron type (196) or input resistance (297; but see 192). Nonetheless, the systematic differences between minimum and maximum primary range discharge rates are matched to differences in motor unit force-frequency (*F-f*) relations, so that the rate modulation within the primary range regulates force output along the steepest portion of the muscle unit's force-frequency curve (191, 196).

Motoneuron discharge rate depends on both the amplitude and the rate of change of injected current (7, 8). The dynamic sensitivity of motoneurons to current injection also varies with motor unit type: it is highest in cells with low rheobase and long AHP durations [i.e., presumably type S motoneurons; (8, 9)]. This increased dynamic sensitivity in putative type S motoneurons may help compensate for the slower contraction speed of their muscle units. Direct measurement of motor unit force output in response to ramp current injection into their motoneurons suggests that the weakest motor units not only need less current to be recruited, but also reach their maximum rate of force development with less additional current than is required for stronger motor units (9).

Effects of Neuromodulators on Motoneuron Behavior

The preceding description of the mechanisms underlying motoneuron behavior was based on intracellular recordings obtained from intact, anesthetized animals or from in vitro preparations in which neuromodulators were not present in the bathing solution. In unanesthetized animals, activity in brainstem neurons with descending monoaminergic projections to the spinal cord leads to the release of noradrenaline and serotonin and the co-localized peptides TRH and substance P (176). Neuromodulators can act by altering both the sub- and suprathreshold behavior of motoneurons (28).

Effects of Neuromodulators on Subthreshold Behavior. The most extensively documented action of neuromodulators on the subthreshold behavior of vertebrate motoneurons is a reduction of the resting, barium-sensitive potassium leak conductance (G_{Krest}), producing increases in input resistance of around 50% and membrane depolarizations of up to 30 mV (23, 105, 112, 217, 221, 244). Two other effects have been ascribed to serotonin: *(1)* an enhancement of the hyperpolarization-activated conductance (G_h) in both adult and neonatal mammalian motoneurons (217, 329) and *(2)* a decrease in G_{KCa} activation in motoneurons from a number of different species (24, 165, 208, 351). The enhancement of G_h may be associated with a depolarizing shift in its half-activation voltage, leading to an increase in the resting level of G_h with a consequent membrane depolarization (208, 217). In crustacean motor neurons, G_{KCa} is significantly activated at the resting potential, so that the reduction of G_{KCa} by serotonin also contributes to membrane depolarization (208, 209).

The combination of the serotonin-induced increase in G_h and decrease in G_{Krest} and G_{KCa} will affect the time and voltage dependence of the motoneuron's input resistance. The somatic voltage change produced by a brief current pulse will be enhanced due to the decrease in G_{Krest}, while the steady-state input resistance will be reduced due to the enhanced G_h (217). At voltages negative to resting potential, the effects on G_h will predominate, while at voltages positive to rest, the reductions in both G_{Krest} and G_{KCa} will contribute to an increase in input resistance. The net effect on motoneuron excitability will also depend upon the amount of depolarization produced by the neuromodulator. Both serotonin and TRH have been found to decrease the minimum current for repetitive discharge (23, 221).

Even though the actions of neuromodulators have been assessed through intrasomatic recordings, the spatial distribution of monoaminergic synaptic terminals (see later under Transfer of Synaptic Current to the Soma) suggests that neuromodulators may control the properties of active conductances on dendrites. However, the spatial distribution of the various active ionic conductances are not known with any certainty in motoneurons, so that it is difficult to predict the effects of neuromodulators on dendritic processing. Reductions in dendritic G_{Krest} would make the dendrites more electrotonically compact, thereby increasing the relative efficacy of distally located synapses. Neuromodulator-induced alterations in the balance of dendritic conductances mediating inward and outward currents will affect the filtering properties of the dendrites, and may provide a means of "tuning" the dendrites to selectively enhance the efficacy of synaptic inputs occurring at particular frequencies (cf. 46, 233).

Effects of Neuromodulators on Repetitive Discharge. The suprathreshold behavior of motoneurons can also be altered by neuromodulators, primarily through their reduction of potassium conductances. Serotonin has been found to reduce the AHP following a single spike (24, 165, 351, 360). In lamprey motoneurons, the reduction of the AHP by serotonin does not appear to result from a reduction in calcium entry. It must either act directly on the channels responsible for G_{KCa} or exert its effects by altering the intracellular handling of calcium (351). In contrast, in neonatal rat hypoglossal motoneurons the reduction of the AHP by serotonin is associated with inhibition of the calcium currents responsible for evoking the AHP (21). AHP amplitude and duration could also be reduced through an enhancement of I_h (139, 217), but as discussed above, the negative voltage activation range of I_h should prevent it from exerting a prominent effect on repetitive discharge. In fact, the reduction of the AHP by neuromodulators is often associated with a significant increase in the slope of the *f-I* relation (e.g., 24, 165, 351), as occurs following pharmacological reduction of the AHP (see earlier).

The reduction of potassium currents by neuromodulators also allows the expression of plateau potentials and bistable discharge behavior, in which maintained depolarizations (plateaus) or repetitive discharge outlast the duration of depolarizing injected or synaptic current. Schwindt and Crill (304) reported that such behavior was invariably associated with an N-shaped steady-state *I–V* curve, in which the negative slope region crossed the zero current axis to yield a region of net inward current, reflecting the predominance of a persistent inward current (I_i) (cf. Table 1.1). Such an *I–V* curve and the associated discharge behavior can be induced in motoneurons of anesthetized animals by displacing intracellular potassium to reduce its equilibrium potential (304). Figure 1.4*A* illustrates *I–V* curves obtained before and after intracellular injection of tetramethylammonium (TMA), an impermeant cation that displaces intracellular potassium. Prior to TMA injection, a suprathreshold depolarizing current pulse elicits discharge only for the duration of current injection (Fig. 1.4*B*). After TMA injection has produced a net inward current region in the steady-state *I–V* curve, depolarizing current pulses elicit discharge that outlasts the period of current injection and can only be terminated by a hyperpolarizing current pulse (Fig. 1.4*C*).

Serotonin-induced bistable firing patterns have been reported in both turtle and cat motoneurons (reviewed in 171, 206). Bistable discharge behavior is often spontaneously present in motoneurons in unanesthetized decerebrate cats, presumably due to tonic activity in brainstem neurons with descending serotonergic fibers. It disappears following a spinal transection, but reappears following intravenous administration of serotonergic precursors (5-HTP). Figure 1.4*D* shows an example of bistable discharge behavior obtained after 5-HTP administration in an acutely spinalized cat. The plot of instantaneous discharge rate (*upper trace*) illustrates that instead of the typical adaptation of firing rate following the onset of the current step (see earlier), the discharge accelerates, reflecting the increasing predominance of inward over outward currents. The predominance of inward currents and the resultant discharge continues after the termination of the injected current pulse. The appearance of this type of behavior is critically dependent upon the stimulus parameters and is typically seen only if subthreshold depolarizing bias current is applied prior to the suprathreshold current pulse. A more typical reflection of increasing activation of an inward current is a counterclock-

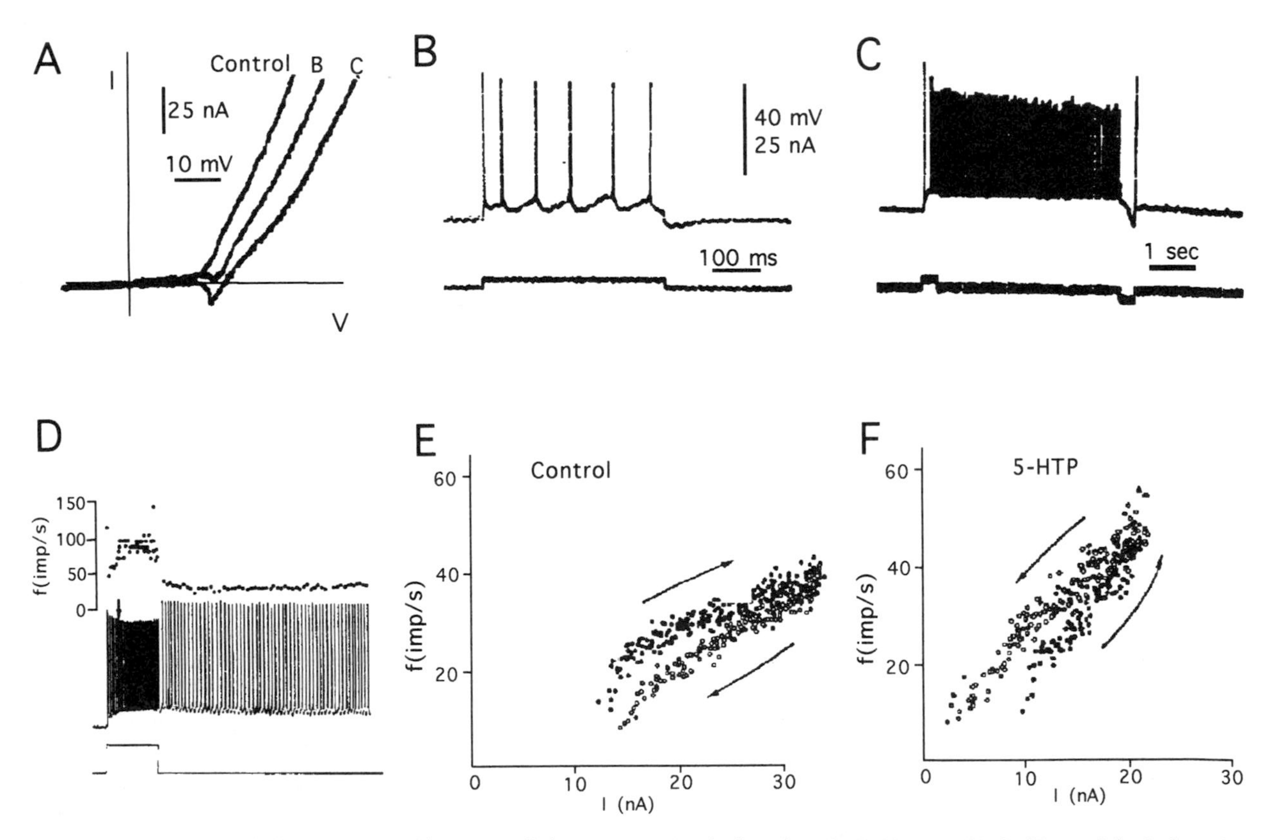

FIG. 1.4. Bistable discharge behavior induced by intracellular injection of TMA (*C*) or by the intravenous injection of the serotonergic precursor 5-HTP (*D* and *F*). *A*, *I–V* curves generated by a slow voltage-clamp ramp before (control), during (*B*), and after (*C*) TMA injection. *B*, Response to a suprathreshold depolarizing current pulse obtained just after the (*B*) *I–V* curve in *A*. *C*, Response of the same motoneuron to injected current obtained after the (*C*) *I–V* curve in *A*. [From Schwindt and Crill (304).] *D*. Bistable discharge behavior of a lumbar motoneuron in an acutely spinalized decerebrate cat following intravenous administration of 5-HTP. [From Hounsgaard et al. (164).] *E* and *F*, Response of a motoneuron to triangular current injection before (*E*) and after (*F*) 5-HTP administration. [From Hounsgaard et al. (164).]

wise hysteresis in the frequency response to triangular current pulses. Under control conditions, the discharge rate is higher on the ascending limb of the *f-I* curve than on the subsequent descending limb, reflecting the process of spike-frequency adaptation (Fig. 1.4*E*). Following 5-HTP administration, the discharge rate is higher on the descending limb of the current ramp, reflecting a slow increase in the predominance of inward currents (Fig. 1.4*F*).

The expression of bistable behavior rests on the voltage dependence, amplitude, and kinetics of the underlying persistent inward current. The deactivation time constant of the inward current must be long to prevent it from being turned off by voltage- or calcium-dependent potassium currents (303). Alternatively, a low sensitivity to hyperpolarizing current could reflect a distal location (140). In turtle motoneurons, bistable behavior has been attributed to the presence of a nifedipine-sensitive, low-threshold calcium conductance (165). A similar conductance is thought to underlie analogous behavior in cat motoneurons (164), although a persistent sodium current may contribute in other motoneurons (see earlier). However, very little is known about either the kinetics or the spatial location of persistent inward currents in motoneurons.

The functional significance of bistable discharge behavior in motoneurons is not well understood. The discharge activity of brainstem neurons with descending serotonergic projections suggests that these neurons function to facilitate motor output in both postural and rhythmic tasks (176). Abrupt jumps in motoneuron discharge rate have been observed during tonic stretch reflexes in decerebrate cats (164) and during quiet standing in rats (104), and have been attributed to the underlying bistable behavior of motoneurons. The recent demonstration that selective depletion of spinal monoamines (207) results in a dramatic decrease in the tonic activity of soleus motoneurons suggests that monoamine-induced, bistable discharge patterns may normally support tonic activity in certain postural muscles.

Neuromodulators may also act to support rhythmic patterns of motoneuron activation. During fictive locomotion in the decerebrate cat, AHPs are reduced and alterations in discharge behavior occur that suggest the predominance of an active inward current (45). It is possible that the combined activation of serotonin and *N*-methyl-D-aspartate (NDMA) receptors facilitate rhythmic oscillations in motoneuron discharge rate. Modeling work (see further on) suggests that rhythmic oscillations in lamprey neurons during fictive locomotion depend upon calcium entry through NMDA channels and the consequent activation of G_{KCa}, and that serotonin affects the frequency of oscillation through its effects on G_{KCa}. It is not known whether similar mechanisms contribute to locomotion in higher vertebrates. Locomotor drive potentials recorded in motoneurons during fictive locomotion in the cat increase in amplitude when the membrane is depolarized by current injection, but it is not known whether this property reflects NMDA receptor activation or the effect of an intrinsic inward current (44).

Motoneuron Models

Compartment Models. The development of motoneuron models has been critical to our understanding of how the behavior of motoneurons relates to their morphological and biophysical features. As discussed earlier, interpretations of measurements of input resistance and synaptic potentials have been facilitated by analytical approaches based on the idealized equivalent cylinder representation of the motoneuron. Because of the restrictive assumptions of the equivalent cylinder representation, compartmental models (i.e., representations in which the neuron is represented as a series of interconnected compartments) have been widely used to model a variety of processes involved in the input–output properties of motoneurons, including subthreshold responses to somatically injected current, transfer of charge from synaptic sites to the soma, initiation and somatodendritic spread of action potentials, and repetitive discharge properties.

Figure 1.5 represents the effects of several active conductances on the subthreshold behavior of a 17-compartment motoneuron model consisting of a spherical soma and a tapering dendritic cable. Figure 1.5*A* illustrates the response of the model without voltage-dependent conductances to a series of 250-ms depolarizing and hyperpolarizing current steps. The relation between the magnitude of injected current and the steady-state voltage is linear (Fig. 1.5*C*) and the slope of the relation yields a value for effective input resistance of 1.24 MΩ. Figure 1.5*B* illustrates the effects of inserting hyperpolarization-activated cation channels (G_h), slowly-activated potassium channels (G_{KCa}), and channels carrying a persistent inward current (G_i) on the soma compartment. The voltage response now exhibits depolarizing sag in response to hyperpolarizing current pulses, a less prominent hyperpolarizing sag in response to depolarizing current pulses, and an increase in effective input resistance near spike threshold. The change in the time course of the voltage response near the threshold reflects the dominant influence of the persistent inward current. Figure 1.5*D* shows the relation between the voltage measured at two differ-

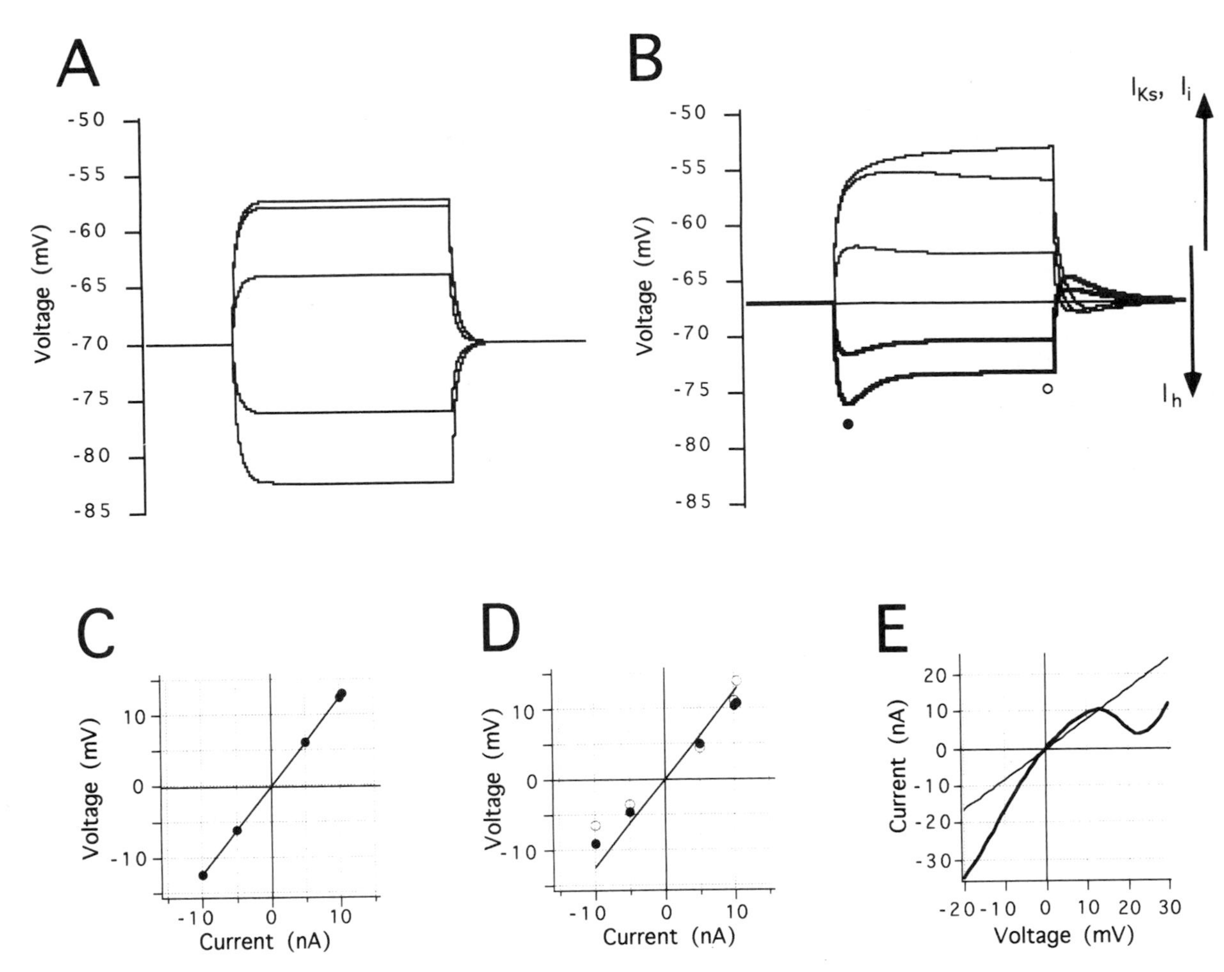

FIG. 1.5. Effects of active conductances on subthreshold behavior of motoneurons. *A*, Response of a passive neuron model to 250 ms injected current steps of different magnitude. The model consisted of a spherical soma (60 μm diameter) attached to a tapering, 16-compartment dendritic cylinder with a total membrane surface area of 622,000 μm^2. Specific membrane capacitance was 1 $\mu F \cdot cm^{-2}$ and specific membrane resistance varied from 2 $k\Omega \cdot cm^2$ in the soma up to 25 $k\Omega \cdot cm^2$ in the distal dendritic compartments. A nonspecific electrode leak conductance of 100 nS was placed in the soma to represent impalement-induced leak. All simulations were performed with Nodus software [DeShutter (93)] on a Macintosh computer. *B*, Effects of inserting active conductances on the somatic compartment. Three conductances were inserted: *(1)* a hyperpolarization-activated mixed cation conductance, *(2)* a slow potassium conductance, and *(3)* a conductance mediating a persistent inward current. Their steady-state voltage dependencies were specified by equations of the form: $G(V) = G_{max}/\{1 + \exp[(V - V_h)/S]\}$ for the first, $G(V) = G_{max}/(\{1 + \exp[(V_h - V)/S]\})^2$ for the second, and $G(V) = G_{max}/\{1 + \exp[(V_h - V)/S]\}$ for the third conductance. G_{max} is the maximum conductance and was equal to 500, 2,200, and 220 nS for the three conductances. V_h is the half-activation voltage and had values of −75, −25, and −48 mV, whereas S affects the steepness of the activation curve and had values of 5.3, 15, and 3 mV^{-1}. The conductance time constants were voltage independent and were set equal to 50, 40, and 20 ms. *C*, Voltage-current plots for simulated voltage traces shown in *A*. *D*, Voltage-current plots for simulated voltage traces shown in *B*. *Filled* and *open circles* represent voltages measured at two different times as indicated in *B*. *E*, Current-voltage relation (*curved line*) calculated by summing the leak current in the passive model (*straight line*) with the current-voltage relations of the three active conductances.

ent times during the course of current injection, and illustrates that when active conductances are present, the effective value of R_N differs from that obtained in the passive model (indicated by the line) and varies both with the duration of current injection and with membrane voltage. As shown in Figure 1.5*E*, the calculated steady-state relation between total membrane current and voltage exhibits the expected N-shape (see earlier).

A number of studies have used compartmental models incorporating Hodgkin-Huxley–type descriptions of active conductances to understand the relative contributions of sodium channel properties and motoneuron geometry to the features of intracellularly recorded action potentials. The inflection in the antidromic action potential can be produced by both experimental and computer simulations of a sudden increase in axon diameter (96, 230, 231). Computer simulations also suggest that the difference in excitability between the soma and the initial segment may depend upon differences in the properties of their sodium channels (96, 230, 339, 340). Finally, these studies suggest that the low initial segment threshold in response to synaptic input is not consistent with a high level of excitability of the dendritic tree (96, 230).

Although these multicompartment models with active conductances have been useful for studying single action potentials, relatively little work of this type has been devoted to understanding the repetitive discharge properties of motoneurons. All of the published models incorporating a range of active conductances were developed before the presence of a persistent inward current was established (202, 339, 340). However, even the presently available current- and voltage-clamp data are insufficient to specify model parameters. For example, modeling the behavior of calcium-activated conductances requires the specification of a number of parameters representing the processes of calcium entry, binding, diffusion, and active extrusion (e.g., 289). Although the time course of the AHP can be reproduced by simulating these processes (289, 340), many of the important parameters, such as the concentration and mobility of calcium-binding proteins and the spatial proximity of calcium and G_{KCa} channels, are not well specified for motoneurons. In fact, relatively little is presently known about the exact spatial distribution of any of the active ionic conductances of motoneurons. Finally, replication of the changes in firing threshold and spike shape during repetitive discharge is likely to require a more complicated model of sodium channel inactivation than that originally proposed by Hodgkin and Huxley (*cf.* 169).

The complexity of compartment models can be reduced by using a few relatively large dendritic compartments and by simplifying the representation of intracellular calcium dynamics. Models of this type have recently been used to describe the contribution of cellular properties to oscillations in discharge in lamprey neurons (42, 103, 352). A network of model neurons in which calcium entry through NMDA channels elicits a depolarization that is terminated by the activation of G_{KCa} can replicate the effects of 5-hydroxytryptamine (5-HT) and NMDA on the locomotor rhythm in the lamprey (42, 352).

Threshold-Crossing Models. Analysis of the mechanisms underlying repetitive discharge has often been based upon even simpler "threshold-crossing" models, in which many of the morphological and biophysical features of motoneurons are not explicitly represented. Motoneuron models that do not represent spike conductances explicitly, but simply produce a stereotyped action potential whenever a certain voltage threshold is crossed, have provided useful insights into repetitive discharge behavior. A number of the correlations between AHP and discharge properties can be explained on the basis of a threshold-crossing model in which the conductance underlying the AHP is a time-dependent process that reaches a peak value during the spike and then decays exponentially (194). Under conditions of steady-state current injection, a spike occurs whenever the depolarizing injected current overcomes the AHP current so that the membrane potential crosses a fixed voltage threshold (V_{thr}). This model not only provides an explanation for the correlation between the minimum steady discharge rate and the reciprocal of AHP duration, but also generates steady-state *f-I* curves that roughly approximate the experimental data (194). In addition, based on an inverse relation between the AHP decay time constant and the estimated peak value of AHP current, the model can also account for the increased dynamic sensitivity of motoneurons with long AHP durations (7, 8). Finally, the model predicts that the slope of the steady-state *f-I* relation will be inversely proportional to the magnitude of the AHP conductance, as has been observed experimentally (see earlier).

A number of variations of the basic threshold-crossing model have been developed in order to incorporate additional biophysical features of motoneurons and to explain a wider range of motoneuron discharge behaviors. It has been reported that the time course of the AHP conductance following a spike cannot be described by a single exponential function (10). A threshold-crossing model incorporating this estimated AHP time course was able to replicate the first-interval *f-I* relations measured in the same motoneurons (12). Spike-frequency adaptation and steady-state discharge behavior in this model depend upon the way in which the AHP conductance summates across successive interspike intervals (11, 13). Estimates of AHP conductance following successive spikes suggests that the summation is often not linear (13), and saturation of the AHP conductance was proposed as a mechanism for steady-state repetitive discharge in the secondary range.

Although models with a strictly time-dependent AHP conductance and fixed spike threshold can account for a wide range of discharge behaviors in both motoneurons and other central neurons (136), these models do not incorporate the persistent inward current or the variations in spike threshold known to exist in motoneurons. A one-compartment threshold-crossing model that incorporates an inward current and variable spike threshold in addition to the AHP conductance can effectively reproduce the relation between inward current activation and steady-state *f-I* behavior as well as bistable discharge behavior under conditions of reduced potassium conductance (250). Furthermore, the use of relatively simple motoneuron models together with a representation of the mechanical and/or electrical properties of motor units can be used to simulate the dynamic input–output properties of a pool of motoneurons (e.g., 315).

ORGANIZATION OF SYNAPTIC INPUTS TO THE MOTONEURON POOL

Understanding how synaptic inputs from segmental and descending systems shape motor output from the spinal cord requires detailed descriptions of the relative magnitudes of the synaptic currents produced by the different systems and their patterns of distribution within a motoneuron pool (49, 147). Equally important are knowledge of how distinct synaptic inputs interact when they are activated concurrently (28), and quantitative expressions for how synaptic currents are transduced into spike trains by motoneurons (255, 256, 258).

In this section, we will first discuss the processes by which currents generated at synapses are transferred to the soma where they affect the spike-generating conductances of the motoneuron. Next, we will review the available data on the distributions of synaptic inputs from identified systems within motoneuron pools. At the end of this section, we will briefly discuss the effects of synaptic inputs on motoneuron discharge.

Transfer of Synaptic Current to the Soma

Influence of Synaptic Location and Dendritic Membrane Resistivity. Under physiological conditions, displacement of the somatic membrane potential toward threshold is achieved by synaptic current rather than by current injected through an intrasomatic electrode. Motoneuron recruitment and rate modulation will therefore depend on the distribution of synaptic boutons as well as upon the intrinsic properties of motoneurons. Approximately half of the total surface area of the motoneuron is covered by synaptic boutons (36, 37, 79, 80, 186, 187, 284). Although the initial segment is not contacted by synaptic boutons, boutons are found with approximately equal density on the axon hillock and the motoneuron soma (79). The vast majority of synaptic contacts are made upon the dendrites, since they collectively account for 93%–99% of the total surface area of the motoneuron (38, 88, 283). Given a synaptic packing density of roughly 10 boutons/100 μm^2 of motoneuron surface area (36, 37, 79, 80, 186, 187, 284) and total surface areas in the range of 500,000 μm^2 (e.g., 88), individual motoneurons are likely to be contacted by approximately 50,000 synaptic boutons (342). Since different types of presynaptic fibers may each provide an average of from three (124) to nine (53) synaptic contacts on a motoneuron, the output of each motoneuron can be influenced by the activity of about 10,000 presynaptic neurons.

The limited data available comparing synaptic covering in motoneurons of different motor unit type suggest that the total synaptic covering of the soma and proximal dendrites is similar across motor unit types (36, 80, 186, 187), although slow motoneurons have a higher proportion of presumed inhibitory boutons than do fast motoneurons (36). Synaptic covering of the distal dendrites is higher in slow than in fast motoneurons, and while the ratio of presumed inhibitory to excitatory boutons decreases somatofugally in fast motoneurons, it remains relatively constant in slow motoneurons (36).

Conductance changes resulting from synaptic transmitter release will cause localized synaptic currents (I_{syn}) whose time course and amplitude depend on the conductance time course and the synaptic driving potential:

$$I_{syn}(t) = G_{syn}(t) * (V_m(t) - V_{eq}) \tag{4}$$

where $G_{syn}(t)$ is the conductance time course, $V_m(t)$ is the time course of the local membrane potential change, and V_{eq} is the synaptic reversal potential, which has been estimated to be +5 mV for excitatory synapses (111) and −81 mV for inhibitory synapses (325). The current transferred to the soma from a given synaptic site will be influenced by the geometrical features of the dendritic tree and by the effective value of R_m for the dendritic membrane interposed between the synapse and the soma. Variations in the geometry of different branches of the same dendritic tree will lead to variations in the relative current transfer from synapses at the same anatomical distance from the soma. Calculations based on an assumed uniform value of dendritic R_m and the actual geometry of different dendritic trees of the same motoneuron indicate that there could be up to a tenfold range in the amount of current transfer for synapses located at the same anatomical distance from the soma (38).

The amount of current transferred to the soma from a given synaptic site declines with decreases in the effective specific resistivity of the dendritic membrane. The recent finding that dendritic R_m is higher than previously thought (see earlier) suggests that many of the synapses are electrotonically close to the soma (cf. 77). However, as illustrated below, during high tonic levels of background synaptic activity the effective resistivity of the dendritic membrane shows relatively little dependence on the resting value of R_m, since it is dominated by the synaptic conductance. This implies that unless current transfer from distal synapses is "boosted" by an active process, much of the distally-generated charge will be shunted by tonic activity in more proximally located synapses.

The effective R_m of a dendritic compartment will be decreased during synaptic activity by an amount that depends upon the resting value of R_m, the conductance change produced by activating a single synapse and the net synaptic activation rate:

$$R'_m = 1/(G_m + G_{syn}) \quad (5)$$

where R'_m is the effective specific membrane resistivity during synaptic activation, G_m is the resting specific membrane conductance, and G_{syn} is the net conductance change during repetitive activation of a set of synapses. For large values of G_{syn} (i.e., $G_{syn} >> G_m$), the value of the effective membrane resistance (R'_m) is approximately equal to the reciprocal of G_{syn}. Figure 1.6 shows the estimated effect of synaptic activity on R'_m (cf. 16). The calculations are based on estimates of unitary excitatory and inhibitory conductance changes derived from voltage-clamp measurements of unitary synaptic currents (111, 325) and an average synaptic density of ten synaptic boutons/100 μm^2 (see earlier). For simplicity, it is further assumed that half of the synaptic boutons are excitatory and half inhibitory, and that the resting specific resistivity of the dendrites (R_m) is uniform and equal to 10 $k\Omega \cdot cm^2$. It can be seen that a fivefold decrease in R'_m occurs when all of the excitatory boutons release transmitter at a rate of 30 quanta/s (*open circles*). Inhibitory synaptic activity causes a more marked drop in R'_m due to a larger unitary conductance for inhibitory synaptic boutons (*filled circles*). Since the effective space constant of a cylindrical dendritic compartment (λ) is proportional to the square root of R_m (269), decreases in R_m increase the effective electrotonic distance between dendritic synapses and the soma.

Synaptic activity can also diminish synaptic charge transfer by reducing the driving force for synaptic current flow $[V_m(t) - V_{eq}]$. The combined effects of changing driving potential and R_m suggest that the summed effects of activating two synaptic inputs should be markedly less than the linear sum of their

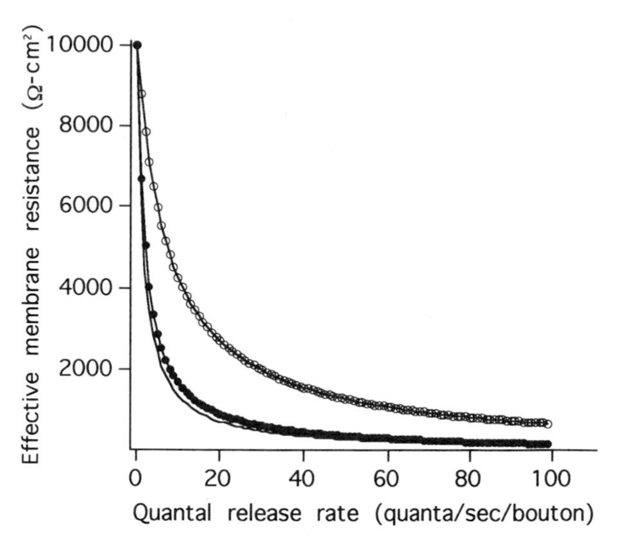

FIG. 1.6. Effects of activating all of the synaptic boutons on the effective membrane resistance of a dendritic compartment. The resting specific membrane resistance was 10 $k\Omega \cdot cm^2$. The quantal conductance change was calculated by fitting an equation of the form: $G(t) = A^*t^*\exp(-t/t)$ to published voltage-clamp data (111, 325; cf. 310) and then integrating conductance over time. The total synaptic conductance was calculated by multiplying this quantal conductance change (in Siemans-seconds per quantum) times the quantal release rate (in quanta per second per bouton) times the bouton density (in boutons/cm^2, assumed to be 5 million/cm^2 for both excitatory and inhibitory boutons) to yield the conductance change per unit area (Siemans/cm^2). The reciprocal of the sum of this value and the resting conductance yields the effective membrane resistance. *Open circles*, Effects of activating excitatory boutons alone. *Filled circles*, Effects of activating inhibitory boutons alone. *Solid line*, Effects of activating both excitatory and inhibitory boutons. [For a similar analysis, see Barrett (16)].

individual effects. Comparisons of the sizes of somatically recorded postsynaptic potentials (PSPs) in response to combined stimulation of different groups of afferent fibers have indeed shown some less-than-linear summation, although PSP amplitudes recorded on combined stimulation are generally 80% or more of the amplitude predicted from the linear sum of the individual PSPs (47, 52, 76, 271). These relatively small departures from linearity could be due to the fact that the synaptic boutons activated in the cited experiments were rather widely distributed, so that there was relatively little interaction between adjacent synapses. Alternatively, less-than-linear summation could be masked by the presence of voltage-dependent inward currents in the dendrites that add to the charge transferred to the soma (76).

The compartmental models of motoneurons discussed earlier (see under Compartmental Models) have provided insight into the transfer of synaptic current from subsynaptic sites to the soma. Simulation studies based on such models suggest that the amplitude and time course of a composite Ia EPSP are consistent with the measured morphological features of the distribution of Ia boutons on the motoneuron dendrites and the absence of active dendritic conductances (218, 310). These studies also suggest that near-linear summation of unitary Ia EPSPs occurs. However, the small departure from linearity is not surprising in this case because of the wide distribution of Ia boutons and the fact that all of the Ia afferents from a single muscle provide only about 1% of the total number of synaptic boutons on a motoneuron (53, 310). Saturation of synaptic effects is more likely to occur during high-frequency activation of a large number of synapses.

Figure 1.7 illustrates the magnitude of excitatory synaptic current reaching the soma of the motoneuron model used in Figure 1.5 as a function of the average quantal release rate. (For simplicity all active conductances have been removed.) The values for the density of excitatory synaptic boutons and the quantal excitatory conductance change are the same as those used in Figure 1.6. The relation between quantal release rate and the synaptic current delivered to the soma is clearly nonlinear. Moreover, the current delivered to the soma is reduced as the soma is clamped at more depolarized membrane potentials. However, this analysis suggests that even moderate quantal release rates can provide sufficient depolarizing current to drive motoneuron discharge

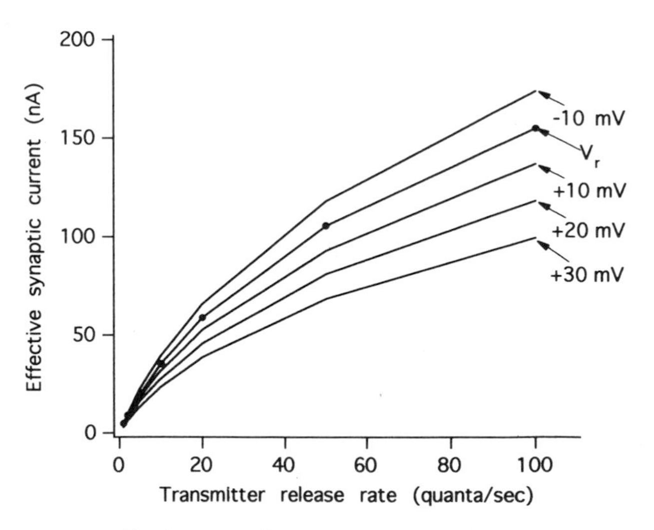

FIG. 1.7. Effective synaptic current vs. quantal release rate in a passive motoneuron model (same as that used in Fig. 1.5*A*). Excitatory synaptic boutons were assigned to each compartment with a density of 5/100 μm^2. The quantal conductance change was the same as that used in Figure 1.6. The effective synaptic current is measured in the soma compartment with the soma clamped at different voltages relative to the resting potential.

rates over the observed physiological range (190, 297, 307).

Effects of Active Dendritic Conductances. The presence of active dendritic conductances mediating inward currents would significantly enhance the delivery of synaptic current to the soma. Although there is abundant evidence for the presence of such conductances in the dendrites of a variety of other central neurons (for references, see 167), there is much less evidence for their presence in motoneuron dendrites. However, synaptic boutons containing neuromodulatory transmitters that are known to influence active conductances (see earlier) are found on both the dendritic and somatic membrane of motoneurons (2, 125, 266, 290, 341).

The presence of active dendritic conductances is also suggested by significant deviations of the observed shapes and amplitudes of PSPs from those predicted from a passive model of the dendrites. Because of the low-pass filter characteristic of the dendrite, distally generated PSPs should have longer rise-times, longer half-widths, and smaller peak amplitudes than proximally generated PSPs (175, 271, 273). Deviations from this pattern have been observed in neurons in which active dendritic conductances have been established on other grounds (242, 363).

In motoneurons, the predicted relations between rise-time and half-width are observed (275), but the peak amplitudes of distal Ia EPSPs are just as large as those of proximal ones (173, 174). This finding suggests either that the conductance change is greater at distal synapses or that current transmission from distal synapses is enhanced by some active membrane process. Redman and colleagues (76) reported that intracellular injection of tetraethylammonium (TEA) ions, which blocks voltage-sensitive K^+ channels (288), produced an increase in the amplitude and duration of single-fiber Ia EPSPs with a presumed distal location. Although the increased amplitude could have resulted from a direct effect of TEA on the relative permeability of K^+ in the subsynaptic channels (since it was associated with a shift in the synaptic reversal potential), its effect on the time course of distal EPSPs could be due to the presence of an active, dendritic inward current that was unmasked by the TEA-induced reduction of dendritic outward currents. This conclusion was supported by the observation of greater-than-linear summation of composite Ia EPSPs in TEA-injected motoneurons, which could not occur if the dendrites were passive.

Hounsgaard and Kiehn (168) have recently provided a more direct demonstration of the presence of active dendritic conductances in turtle motoneurons. In the presence of external tetrodotoxin (TTX) and TEA to block voltage-gated Na^+ and K^+ channels, respectively, externally applied polarizing fields that depolarized the dendrites (and hyperpolarized the soma) produced calcium-dependent spikes. The amplitude of the calcium spikes increased with increasing magnitudes of dendritic polarization, suggesting the recruitment of regenerative activity in an increasing proportion of the dendritic tree. More prolonged calcium plateaus were generated by dendritic depolarization in the presence of apamin, a specific blocker of calcium-activated potassium channels.

Although these results show that regenerative activity can be initiated in motoneuron dendrites in the presence of K^+ channel blockers, dendritic spikes are probably not a normal feature of adult mammalian motoneurons. There is evidence for dendritic spikes in neonatal (356) and axotomized motoneurons (215, 311), and they could theoretically occur in adult motoneurons when K^+ conductances are reduced by neuromodulators (see further on). Even if active dendritic conductances are not normally potent enough to support dendritic spikes, their presence will affect synaptic charge transfer to the soma. It is difficult to assess the magnitude of this effect based on the presently available data.

Enhanced transfer of excitatory synaptic current to the soma could arise from voltage dependence of the synaptic conductance itself, as is the case for the N-methyl-D-asparate (NMDA) glutamate receptor (223). The monosynaptic excitatory connection from Ia afferents to motoneurons is partially mediated by NMDA receptors in neonatal animals (248, 370; see, however, 177), but the density of NMDA receptors on motoneurons decreases during development (181) and the NMDA contribution to the Ia EPSP is minimal in adult motoneurons (109, 113). However, several investigators have reported direct excitatory effects of NMDA on adult vertebrate motoneurons (99–101, 353), and focal application of NMDA antagonists can suppress the excitatory effects produced in motoneurons by activating certain segmental and descending pathways (32, 184, 185). The voltage dependence of the excitatory current through NMDA-activated channels behaves like the intrinsic voltage-dependent conductances that induce a region of negative-slope conductance into the motoneuron's I–V relation (353). In addition, NMDA-activated channels are permeable to calcium as well as sodium (223), and calcium entry can activate a calcium-dependent potassium conductance. The resultant mixture of inward and outward currents is reflected in resonant behavior in the impedance function measured under voltage-clamp conditions (233) and membrane oscillations and bursting behavior under current-clamp conditions (99, 100, 353). Further discussion of the possible contribution of NMDA receptors to the rhythmic activation of motoneurons was presented earlier (see under Effects of Neuromodulators on Motoneuron Behavior).

Effective Synaptic Currents

We have recently proposed that measuring the synaptic current that reaches the soma of a motoneuron provides a more useful means of quantifying a synaptic input than does measuring the synaptic potentials alone (146, 147). We have called this measure the effective synaptic current [I_N (146); previously referred to as "effective somatic current" (273)]. Direct measurements of effective synaptic current obviate the effects of motoneuron input resistance and membrane potential that confound the analysis of synaptic potentials (147, 149) and may lead to a simple, quantitative expression for the relationship between synaptic input magnitude and synaptically evoked changes in motoneuron discharge rate (147, 256, 258). In addition, measurements of I_N have revealed features of the distribution of synaptic input from identified afferent systems that were unresolved in the earlier analyses of synaptic potential amplitudes (reviewed in 30).

The amount of synaptic charge that reaches the soma (Q_N) of a motoneuron can be calculated from the time integral of the postsynaptic potential (PSP) and the input resistance measured at the soma:

$$Q_N = [\int V_{PSP}(t)]/R_N \qquad (6)$$

In steady-state conditions, the integral in this equation is unnecessary and Ohm's law applies: the synaptic current reaching the soma equals the PSP divided by R_N. This quotient has been referred to as the effective somatic current (273) or the effective synaptic current (I_N; 146). From the foregoing, it is clear that the I_N and the PSP generated by an input system are both determined by the amount of current injected at each synapse and the factors influencing current transfer to the soma. But I_N has two important advantages. First, I_N provides a measure of synaptic efficacy that is not confounded by the tenfold range of R_N values across the motoneuron pool. Second, as both Redman (273) and Schwindt and Calvin (300) pointed out, because injected and synaptic currents usually have equivalent effects on motoneuron firing frequencies, I_N provides a direct measure of the effect of synaptic inputs on motor output.

Effective synaptic currents (I_N) can be readily measured in motoneurons by combining injected current with concurrent, repetitive activation of an identified source of synaptic input as shown in Figure 1.8. I_N is defined as the current required to clamp the membrane at the resting potential during the activation of the synaptic input [Fig. 1.8*B* and *E*; (146, 220, 258, 259)]. These recordings also yield measurements of the input resistance during synaptic activation (R_{Nsyn}), as well as the steady-state input resistance (R_{Nss}) in the absence of synaptic activation (Fig. 1.8*B*). A significant difference between these values indicates that the synaptic input altered the conductance of the motoneuron measured at the soma [Fig. 1.8*E*; (148, 220, 259)]. The relation between the amplitude of the steady-state synaptic potential (ΔV_s) and the membrane potential relative to rest just prior to the onset of synaptic activation (V_i) is used to determine the reversal potential and the dependence of I_N on somatic voltage [Fig. 1.8*C* and *F*; (220, 259)].

Distribution of Effective Synaptic Current from Identified Input Systems

Thus far, effective synaptic currents for five different input systems have been systematically analyzed. Results from these studies are reviewed below and summarized in Figure 1.9.

Monosynaptic Ia Input. The synaptic contacts between Ia afferent fibers and motoneurons have been more extensively studied than those of any other input system (reviewed in 236). The observed covariance between Ia EPSPs and motoneuron input resistance has generally been assumed to result from an approximately constant synaptic current applied to cells of varying R_N values (reviewed in 147), in keeping with the original *size principle* of recruitment (see earlier under Orderly Recruitment of Motor Units). Although the amplitudes of steady-state Ia EPSPs are highly correlated with R_N, measurements of the underlying effective synaptic currents indicate that this covariance results from systematic variance in both I_N and R_N. Within the cat MG motoneuron pool, the effective synaptic currents (I_N) generated by homonymous Ia afferents display a wide range of values that covary with R_N and other motoneuron properties: I_N is about twice as large on average in motoneurons with high R_N values as in those with low R_N values (146). Combining Ia afferent fibers from the synergist lateral gastrocnemius and soleus muscles approximately doubles the magnitude of I_N [mean value of MG Ia afferents, 2 nA; mean value of triceps surae Ia afferents, 4.2 nA; (357)].

Reciprocal Ia Inhibition. Comparisons of reciprocal Ia IPSPs with homonymous Ia EPSPs generated in cat hindlimb motoneurons have revealed the existence of a strong correlation between these two synaptic input systems (57). As is the case for Ia EPSPs, the amplitudes of composite reciprocal Ia IPSPs vary systematically in type-identified motoneurons: Ia IPSPs in type S are larger than those in type FR, which in turn are larger than those in type FF (57, 97). However, there is a steeper gradient of synaptic strength across the motoneuron pool for the Ia excitation than for the Ia inhibition (323); thus one would expect that differences in the effective synaptic currents underlying Ia inhibition within a motoneuron pool would be considerably less than those found for the excitatory Ia input. This appears to be the case, as the amplitudes of the inhibitory effective synaptic currents generated in antagonist motoneurons by the activation of MG Ia afferent fibers were not correlated with intrinsic motoneuron properties or with putative motor unit type (148). The average value of the steady-state Ia inhibitory synaptic current in the putative type F motoneurons was 1.60 ± 0.64 nA, while that for putative type S motoneurons was 1.65 ± 0.71 nA.

Since the synaptic boutons of Ia inhibitory interneurons lie predominantly on the soma of motoneurons (52; Fyffe, personal communication), as expected, they generate substantial changes in motoneuron input resistance. As was the case for the effective synaptic currents, there was no systematic relationship between the steady-state change in conductance and the electrical properties of the motoneuron (148).

Recurrent Inhibition. The role of recurrent inhibition in motor control remains uncertain. One long-held hypothesis is that recurrent inhibition acts to suppress the activity of low-threshold motoneurons when higher threshold motoneurons are recruited (102, 119, 132). Recent support for this hypothesis came from the demonstration that recurrent IPSP amplitude varies systematically with motor unit type in the order FF<FR<S (119) and the anatomical finding that the number of end branches and "swellings" (presumed synaptic boutons) of recurrent axon collaterals of type F motoneurons are greater than those of type S motoneurons (90). An alternative hypothesis has been offered by Hultborn and colleagues (172), who proposed that recurrent inhibition (and its modulation by descending systems) provides a variable-gain regulator of the overall output of a motoneuron pool. This hypothesis is predicated on a uniform distribution of recurrent inhibition within a motoneuron pool.

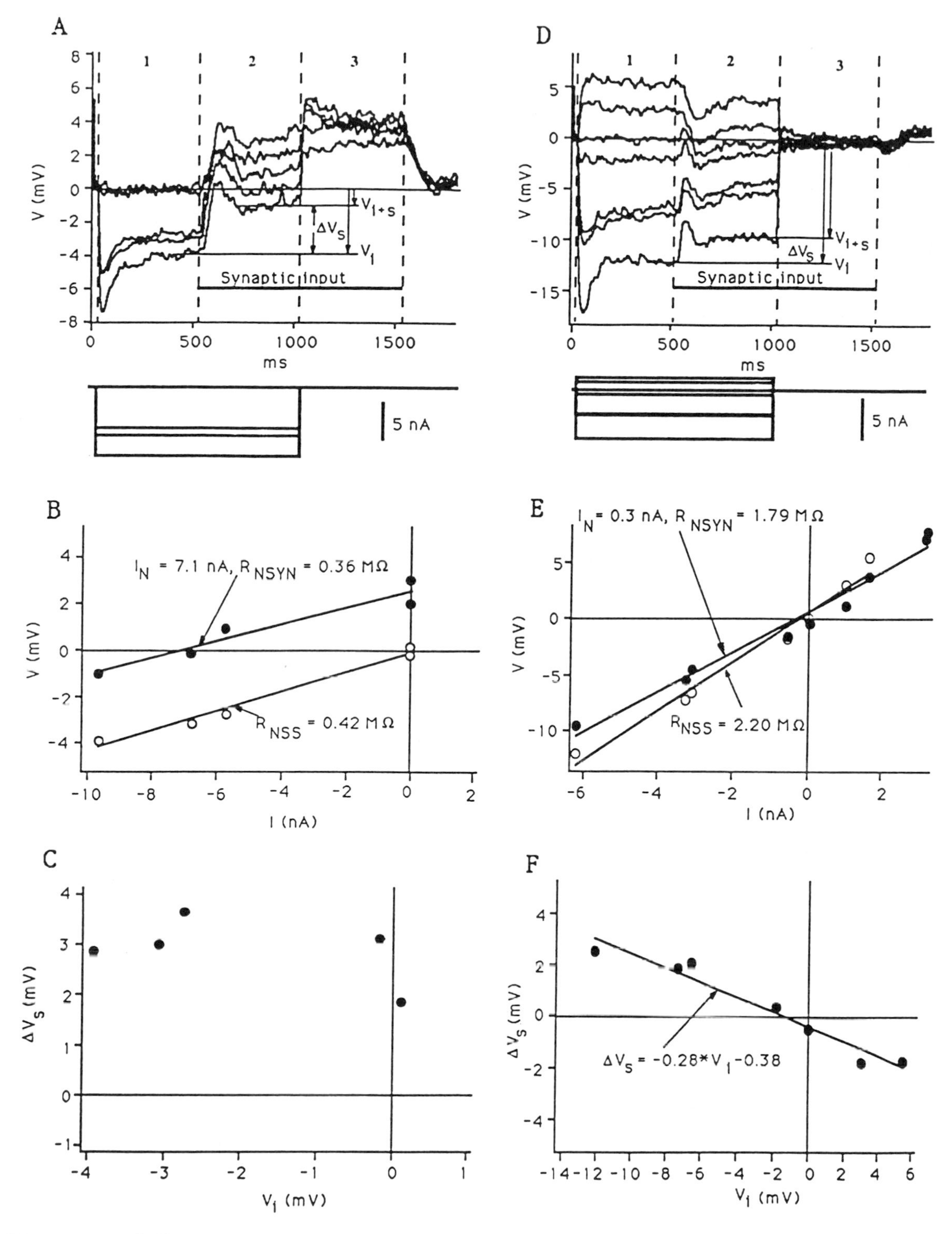

FIG. 1.8 Measurement of effective synaptic current (I_N). *A* and *D*, Membrane voltage responses of two triceps surae motoneurons to injected currents (*lower traces*) and synaptic current (*solid bar*). The experimental protocol consists of three 500 ms epochs (injected current alone, injected + synaptic current, and synaptic current alone), which are numbered and separated by *vertical dotted lines*. The mean resting potential (measured prior to current injection) has been subtracted from each trace and the traces have been digitally low-pass-filtered (100 Hz cutoff) for clarity. Voltage measurements are indicated for the bottom voltage trace in each set. V_i, steady-state voltage response to injected current alone; V_{i+s}, steady-state voltage response to synaptic and injected current; ΔV_s, change in voltage due to synaptic current = $V_{i+s} - V_i$. *B* and *E*, Steady-state voltage responses vs. injected current (*I*). *Solid lines* indicate best linear fit to the data points. The effective synaptic current (I_N) is taken to be equal in magnitude and opposite in sign to the current at which $V_{i+s} = 0$ (estimated from the zero intercept of the fit to V_{i+s} vs. *I*). The slope of the linear fit to V_i vs. *I* gives the steady-state input resistance (R_{NSS}), while the slope of the linear fit to V_{i+s} vs. *I* gives the steady-state input resistance during synaptic activation (R_{NSYN}). *C* and *F*, Dependence of steady-state synaptic potential (ΔV_s) on somatic membrane potential (V_i). [Adapted from Powers et al. (258).]

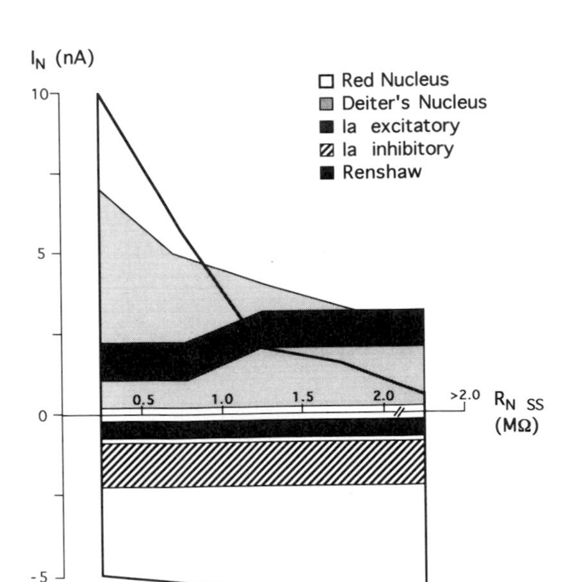

FIG. 1.9. Graphical representation of the magnitude and distribution of the effective synaptic currents at resting potential (I_N) from five different input systems. The *dark stippled band* represents I_N from homonymous Ia afferent fibers [Heckman and Binder (146)]; the *stripped band* represents I_N from Ia-inhibitory interneurons [Heckman and Binder (148)]; the *black band* represents the I_N from Renshaw interneurons [Lindsay and Binder (220)]; the *thick lines* outline the I_N from contralateral rubrospinal neurons [Powers et al. (259)]; and the *light stippled band* represents I_N from ipsilateral Deiter's nucleus [Westcott et al. (358)].

The distribution of effective synaptic currents underlying recurrent inhibition (RC I_N) in triceps surae motoneurons does appear to be uniform (220). RC I_N was entirely independent of all intrinsic motoneuron properties measured, although the amplitudes of the steady-state recurrent IPSPs (ΔV_s) were correlated with motoneuron input resistance (R_N), rheobase (I_{rh}), and afterhyperpolarization half-decay time ($AHP_{t1/2}$), as has been previously reported for transient recurrent IPSPs (119, 170). The mean RC I_N measured at rest was only 0.4 nA, considerably smaller than comparable values derived for other input systems (cf. Fig. 1.9). Since the Renshaw input was activated in this study by stimulating the synergist motor axons at 100 Hz, which produces steady-state IPSPs that are about 50% maximum value (Lindsay, Heckman, and Binder, unpublished data), the maximal RC I_N at rest is still likely to be less than 1 nA on average.

Motoneurons are more likely to receive recurrent inhibition while they are firing repetitively than when they are quiescent, and several hypotheses of the role of recurrent inhibition in motor control emphasize the possible effects of recurrent inhibition on firing frequency (e.g., 172). The mean RC I_N calculated at threshold was still only 1.25 nA, and the distribution within the pool was no different from that measured at resting potential (220). These results suggest that the effect of recurrent inhibition on the firing frequencies of motoneurons are uniform and quite modest. Using an average value for the slope of the motoneuron firing rate-injected current relationship (*f-I* curve) of 1.5 imp/s per nA (196), the average change in firing frequency produced by maximal recurrent inhibition (2.5 nA) should be less than 4 spikes/s. Since the slope of the *f-I* curve does not appear to covary with other motor unit properties (196), the change in firing frequency should not vary systematically within a motoneuron pool. The maximum effective synaptic current calculated at threshold (4.6 nA) would only decrease firing frequency by about 7 imp/s, a value similar to that observed in the experiments of Granit and Renkin (133) in which whole ventral roots were stimulated to activate the Renshaw cells (see later under Effects of Synaptic Inputs on Motoneuron Discharge).

Rubrospinal Input. The rubrospinal system is one of several oligosynaptic pathways in the cat that generate qualitatively different synaptic potentials within hindlimb motoneuron pools (54; see also 108, 163). Both excitatory and inhibitory last-order interneurons are activated by the contralateral red nucleus, leading to short-latency EPSPs and IPSPs, respectively. Low-threshold motoneurons receive predominantly inhibitory input, whereas the high-threshold motoneurons receive predominantly excitatory input.

The effective synaptic currents produced by stimulating the hindlimb projection area of the contralateral magnocellular red nucleus have been recently studied in cat triceps surae motoneurons (259). At resting potential, the distribution of effective synaptic currents from the red nucleus was qualitatively similar to the distribution of synaptic potentials: 86% of the putative type F motoneurons received a net depolarizing effective synaptic current from the red nucleus stimulation, whereas only 38% of the putative type S units did so. However, at threshold the distribution was markedly altered. Inhibition continued to predominate in the type S cells, but among the type F cells, half received net excitatory effective synaptic currents and half received net inhibitory effective synaptic currents. Other surprising features of these data are the enormous range of effective synaptic currents observed in different cells and the fact that they are often three times larger than comparable inputs from segmental pathways (Fig. 1.9). Activation of red nucleus synaptic input reduced motoneuron input resistance by 40%, on average (259). The effect on input resistance was most pronounced in those motoneurons that received hyperpolarizing effective synaptic currents.

The data on effective synaptic currents indicate that the red nucleus input may provide a powerful source of synaptic drive to some high-threshold motoneurons while concurrently inhibiting low-threshold cells. Thus, this input system can potentially alter the gain of the input–output function of the motoneuron pool, change the hierarchy of recruitment thresholds within the pool, and mediate rate limiting of discharge in low-threshold motoneurons (49, 54, 147, 149, 151, 259) (see also later under, Control of Orderly Recruitment and Control of Rate Modulation).

Lateral Vestibulospinal (Deiter's Nucleus) Input. In cats, the lateral vestibulospinal or Deiter's nucleus (DN) neurons project primarily to neck and forelimb motoneurons, but a small percentage descend to the lumbosacral area (121, 313, 314). Mono- and disynaptic DN EPSPs have been recorded in cat triceps motoneurons (134). Although all of monosynaptic EPSPs were quite small (< 2.2 mV), they did display a wide range of amplitudes that were not correlated with the duration of the AHP. Similarly, the amplitudes of monosynaptic EPSPs produced by stimulation of DN axons within the ipsilateral ventral funiculus were not related to motor unit type (57).

Based on the dependence of PSP amplitude on R_N, the data on DN synaptic potentials suggest that the underlying effective synaptic currents are inversely related to R_N. Recent direct measurements of the effective synaptic currents produced by DN stimulation in triceps surae motoneurons of the cat demonstrated that this is indeed the case (357, 358). The DN effective synaptic currents were primarily small and depolarizing in both MG and lateral gastrocnemius-soleus (LGS) motoneurons (mean, 2.5 nA). The DN input tended to be larger in putative type F motoneurons. The amplitudes of the steady-state DN synaptic potentials were similar to those previously reported for transient PSPs (57, 134). The DN PSP showed no correlation to rheobase, resting membrane potential, or either steady state or maximal input resistance of the cell. The DN synaptic input caused a small (average 15%) decrease in motoneuron input resistance.

Comparison of the DN input to that of the red nucleus (259) shows that the ranges of effective synaptic currents are similar (Fig. 1.9). Also both descending systems produce the largest depolarizing currents in the putative type F motoneurons. However, the mean depolarizing red nucleus I_N was twice as large as that from DN, and the difference in distribution of red nucleus I_N between putative type F and S motoneurons was more significant.

Other Synaptic Inputs. Synaptic inputs to spinal motoneuron pools from several other systems have been studied by recording synaptic potentials produced by transient electrical stimulation (reviewed in 49, 156, 236). Although it is difficult to draw strong inferences from these data as to the efficacy and distribution of the inputs, three distinct patterns of the synaptic potentials have appeared that are consistent with the different patterns of I_N described above. Measured at the motoneuron's resting potential, the synaptic potentials are either: *(1)* scaled to the input resistance of the motoneurons (e.g., Ia EPSPs, Ia IPSPs, Renshaw IPSPs), *(2)* independent of input resistance and of roughly equal magnitude in all cells (e.g., Deiter's nucleus EPSPs), or *(3)* predominantly inhibitory to low-threshold motoneurons and predominantly excitatory to high-threshold motoneurons (rubrospinal PSPs). The first pattern could arise from either a uniform distribution of I_N (Ia inhibition, recurrent inhibition) or a distribution skewed toward larger I_N amplitudes in low-threshold motoneurons (Ia excitation). The second pattern suggests a distribution skewed toward larger I_N amplitudes in high-threshold motoneurons, while the third pattern implies qualitative differences in I_N in different motoneurons.

Group II afferent fibers that innervate muscle spindles make monosynaptic connections with homonymous and synergist hindlimb motoneurons (237, 321). The afferent fibers appear to make relatively few contacts with the motoneurons in that the average projection frequency and average single-fiber EPSP amplitude are much lower than the comparable values for Ia afferent fibers. From their data, Munson and colleagues (237) estimated that activating all the spindle group II afferents at 100 imp/s would generate a steady-state EPSP of about 0.3 mV in a homonymous MG motoneuron. Activating the group Ia afferent fibers in a similar fashion generates an average steady-state EPSP that is more than eightfold larger [2.6 mV; (146)]. Moreover, Munson and colleagues (237) found that the amplitude of the single group II fiber EPSPs did not vary systematically with motoneuron input resistance, suggesting that the high-threshold motoneurons with low input resistances may receive more effective synaptic current from the group II afferent fibers than do the low-threshold cells. This pattern is similar to that from the ipsilateral Deiter's nucleus, and the converse of that from the homonymous Ia afferent fibers (see earlier). Group II muscle afferent fibers also generate disynaptic excitatory and inhibitory inputs to cat lumbar motoneurons mediated by interneurons in the intermediate zone/ventral horn [laminae VI–VIII: (reviewed in 178)]. However, neither the magnitude nor the pattern of distribution of these effects within individual motoneuron pools have been evaluated yet.

Several input systems have been examined that generate predominantly inhibitory synaptic potentials in low-threshold motoneurons and predominantly excitatory synaptic potentials to high-threshold motoneurons when measured at rest. These inputs include corticospinal neurons (108), low-threshold cutaneous afferents (54, 97, 216, 252; see however, 152), and group Ib afferents (251, 252), in addition to the rubrospinal system that was discussed earlier (54, 259). However, because the actions of these "mixed" inputs can be highly dependent on membrane potential (259), and responses of the excitatory and inhibitory pathways to repetitive activation can vary considerably (152), it is difficult to predict how these input systems will effect recruitment and rate modulation within a motoneuron pool.

Effects of Synaptic Inputs on Motoneuron Discharge

The functional significance of a synaptic input system should ideally be assessed in terms of its effects on both motoneuron recruitment and firing rate modulation. In general, previous analyses of the input–output properties of motoneuron pools have concentrated on motoneuron recruitment alone. However, since nearly 75% of motor unit force modulation is generally achieved through changes in discharge rate (197), understanding how synaptic inputs alter the discharge rates of activated motoneurons is of critical importance.

There is a considerable body of experimental work supporting the utility of synaptic current measurements in predicting synaptic effects on discharge rate. Experiments in which injected current was combined with steady-state synaptic currents demonstrated that synaptic and injected currents are usually entirely equivalent with respect to their effects on repetitive firing within the primary range. Moreover, during motoneuron discharge, input currents normally sum algebraically (130, 300, 301). Even synaptic inputs leading to large changes in motoneuron input resistance simply shift the *f-I* relation along the current axis, without producing a change in slope (195, 300, 301), indicating that synaptic inputs add a constant amount of depolarizing or hyperpolarizing current regardless of the background firing rate (see, however, 193 and 312 in which some synaptic inputs alter the slope of the *f-I* relation, indicating nonequivalence of synaptic and injected current).

Based on these results, Schwindt and Calvin (300) postulated that one could infer the effective, steady-state current delivered by any synaptic input from the slope of the motoneuron's *f-I* relation and the change in discharge produced by activating the synaptic input. This inference leads to a simple, quantitative expression for steady-state motoneuron behavior: the change in motoneuron discharge is equal to the product of the net effective synaptic current and the slope of the frequency-current curve in the primary range [$\Delta F = I_N * f\text{-}I$; (258)].

The validity of this expression has been tested by measuring each of these three quantities (ΔF, I_N, and *f-I*) in the same motoneuron (256, 258). As illustrated in Figure 1.10*A* and *B*, the actual firing rate increase produced in an MG motoneuron by activating the contralateral red nucleus is in excellent agreement with the predicted change in firing rate based on the product of effective synaptic current and the slope of the *f-I* relation. Similar results for a motoneuron that received an inhibitory input from the red nucleus are shown in Figure 1.10*C* and *D*.

Completely analogous results have been obtained for synaptic input from Ia afferents, Ia-inhibitory interneurons, Renshaw interneurons, interneurons activated by low-threshold cutaneous afferents from the sural nerve, flexor reflex afferent (FRA) input from the common peroneal nerve, and vestibulospinal input from the ipsilateral Deiter's nucleus. The results from all of these inputs are generally consistent with those reported earlier (258), although motoneuron output is generally greater than predicted under conditions in which the input contains a strong transient component (255, 256).

The correspondence between the observed changes in motoneuron discharge rate and those predicted based on the product of net effective synaptic current and *f-I* slope validates the measurement of effective synaptic current as a quantitative index of synaptic efficacy. This expression also simplifies quantitative analysis of neural circuitry, since the effective synaptic current already subsumes all of the factors governing current delivery from the dendrites to the soma, and therefore does not require any detailed information about the electronic architecture of the postsynaptic cell (115, 310) or information about the precise location of the presynaptic boutons (111, 271, 325).

Summation of Synaptic Inputs

Since the physiological activation and control of motoneurons clearly involves the concurrent activity of

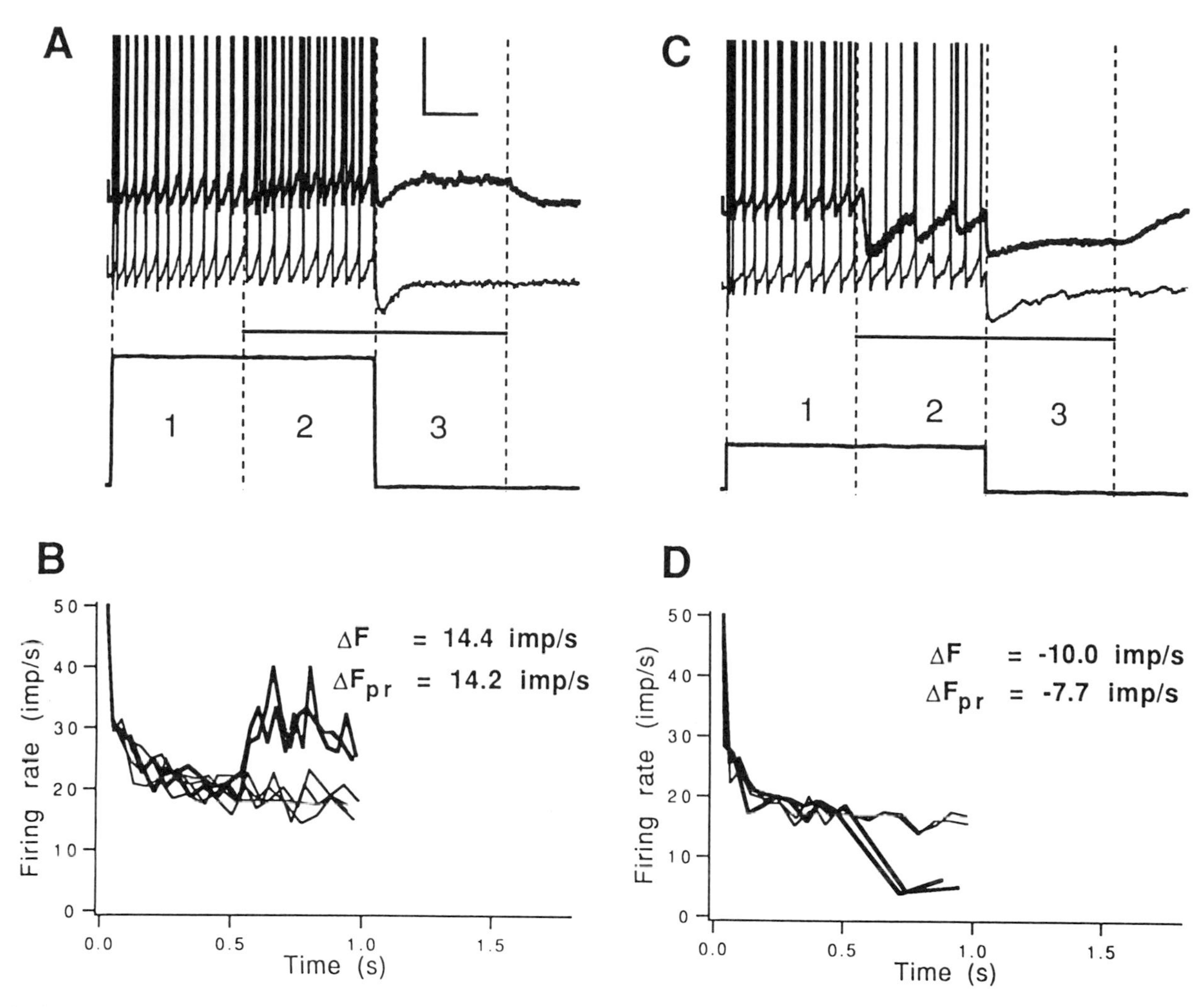

FIG. 1.10. Firing rate modulation produced by steady-state synaptic current. *A* and *C*, Responses of two different triceps surae motoneurons to injected current alone (*thin voltage traces*) and injected + synaptic current (*thick voltage traces*). *Bottom traces* are injected current; synaptic activation indicated by *solid bar*. The three experimental epochs are indicated by *dotted lines*. *B* and *D*, Instantaneous firing rate vs. time, calculated from the spike trains in *A* and *C*, and additional current alone and current + synaptic activation trials. The *thin traces* are the firing rate responses to injected current alone, while the current + synaptic activation responses are shown by the *thick traces*. The firing rate modulation produced by synaptic activation (ΔF) is equal to the difference in mean discharge rate (over the last 300 ms of current injection) between current + synaptic activation and current alone trials. [Modified from Powers et al. (258).]

many different synaptic input systems, knowledge of how synaptic inputs interact is critical for our understanding of input–output function. However, there are very few data available on the summation of effective synaptic currents during concurrent activation of two or more inputs or on the summation of the firing rate changes they induce (257). The theoretical framework for considering the summation of synaptic currents was presented earlier along with a review of the limited available data on the summation of transient synaptic potentials (see earlier under Transfer of Synaptic Current to the Soma).

The summation of excitatory synaptic inputs generated by muscle vibration [Ia excitation; (146)] and by red nucleus stimulation is demonstrated in Figure 1.11*A*. When the red nucleus was stimulated while the triceps surae muscles were vibrated concurrently, the net effective synaptic current measured in the MG motoneuron was quite close to the algebraic sum of the two individual currents. Moreover, the observed change in the firing rate produced by the concurrent stimulation was quite close to that predicted based on both the measured effective synaptic current and the algebraic sum of the changes in firing rate produced by the two inputs individually.

Not all combinations of synaptic inputs behave as simply and predictably as in this example. In those cases in which a synaptic input has both excitatory

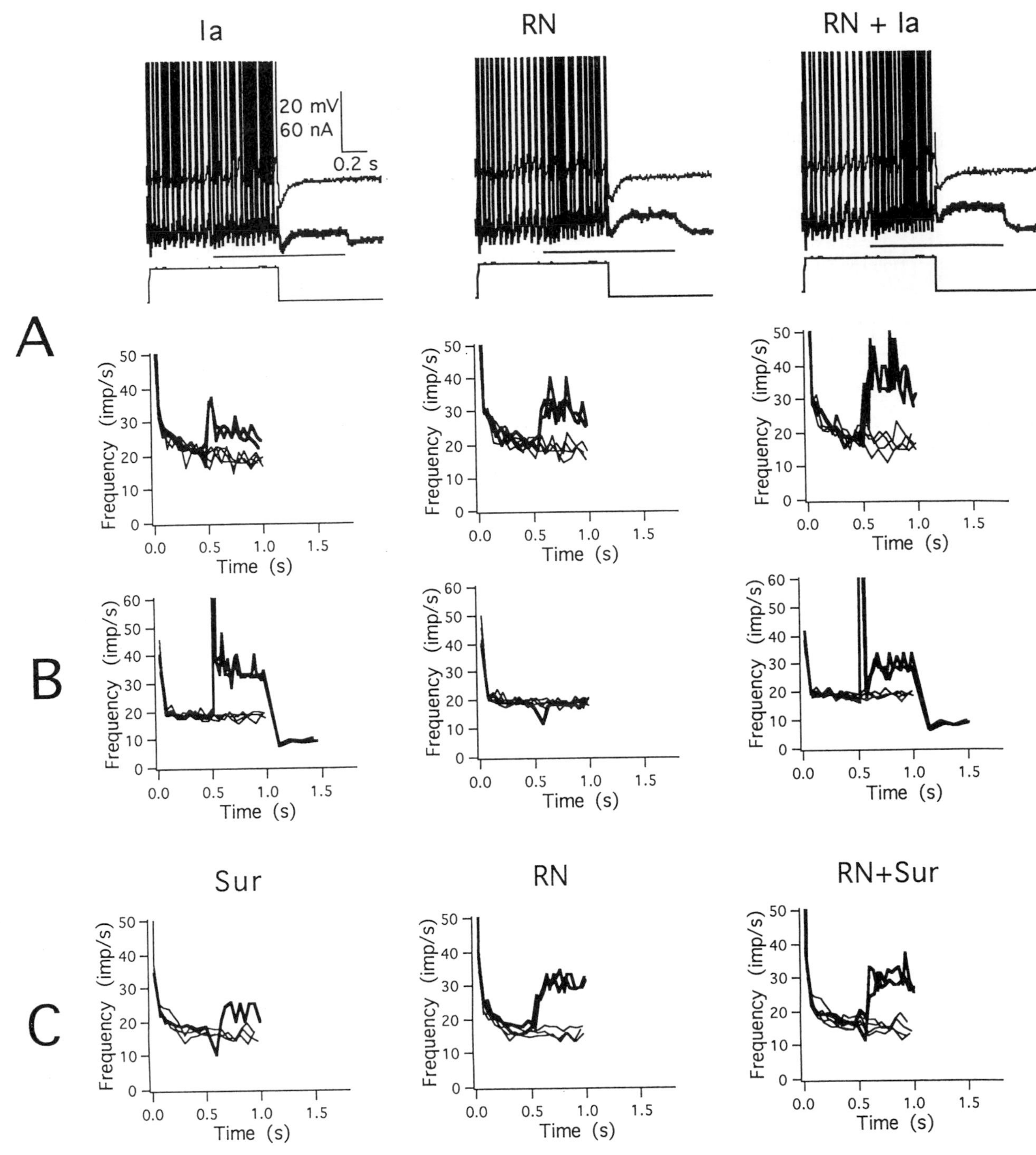

FIG. 1.11. The summation of synaptic inputs. *A*, Linear summation of synaptic inputs generated by Ia afferents and by red nucleus stimulation. In each panel the *upper voltage traces* show the responses of an MG motoneuron to injected current alone; the *lower traces* show the responses to the same amount of injected current plus the steady-state synaptic current. This MG cell had an *f-I* slope of 1.2 imp·s^{-1}·nA^{-1}. The Ia effective synaptic current was estimated to be 5.8 nA at threshold, and as shown in the *left panels*, it produced an average increase of 7.8 imp/s in the motoneuron's steady-state discharge. The predicted change was 7 imp/s. Stimulation within the contralateral red nucleus produced an estimated effective synaptic current at threshold of about 11.6 nA, which was predicted to produce an increase in the cell's firing rate of 14 imp/s. The actual measured change was 13.5 imp/s as shown in the *middle panels*. When the red nucleus was stimulated and the triceps surae muscles vibrated concurrently (*right panels*), the net effective synaptic current measured in the cell was 18.3 nA at rest, which was quite close to the algebraic sum of the two individual, effective synaptic currents (7.2 nA + 14.5 nA). Moreover, the observed change in the average firing rate produced by the concurrent stimulation (19.6 imp/s) was quite close to that predicted based on both the measured effective synaptic current (17.5 imp/s) and the algebraic sum of the changes in firing rate produced by the two inputs individually (21.3 imp/s). *B*, Nonlinear summation of the effects of synaptic inputs on motoneuron discharge. The *left-hand* panel shows that activating homonymous Ia afferent fibers produced about a 14 imp/s increase in discharge rate in this MG motoneuron. As indicated in the *middle panel*, stimulating within the red nucleus had virtually no effect on the steady-state firing rate of the same cell, although there is an indication of a transient inhibition at the onset. *Figure continues*

and inhibitory components, the net effective synaptic current is critically dependent on membrane potential (259); thus, it is difficult to predict how it will sum with other inputs because of the difficulty in determining the underlying membrane potential during repetitive firing. Figure 1.11*B* shows such an example. As indicated in the *middle panel*, stimulating within the red nucleus had virtually no effect on the steady-state firing rate of this MG motoneuron, although there is an indication of a transient inhibition at its onset. The *left panel* shows that activating homonymous Ia afferent fibers in the same cell produced a pronounced increase in firing rate. However, as shown on the right, when the Ia afferents and red nucleus were stimulated together, there was a marked reduction in the increase in firing rate produced by the Ia afferents alone. Although the result suggests nonlinear summation of the underlying effective synaptic currents from the two inputs, this may not have been the case. The additional depolarization generated by the Ia input presumably increased the inhibitory effective synaptic current provided by the red nucleus input, such that it decreased the net depolarizing current acting on the motoneuron.

A different type of nonlinear interaction, occlusion, is demonstrated in Figure 1.11*C*, which depicts the effects of stimulating the sural nerve and the red nucleus on the discharge rate of an MG motoneuron. Stimulation of both of these inputs produced clear depolarizing effective synaptic currents and increases in motoneuron discharge. However, when the two inputs were stimulated concurrently, the effective synaptic current and discharge rate modulation were no greater than those produced by red nucleus stimulation alone (*right panel*). These results suggest the absence of a subliminal fringe within the interneuronal pools upon which these two inputs converge, and thus a saturation of the currents they are able to deliver to the motoneuron.

It is quite likely that there are additional types of interactions between synaptic inputs other than those described above. Moreover, the summation of synaptic inputs is likely to depend on a number of other factors including the action of presynaptic inhibitory inputs, the spatial distribution of the synaptic inputs within the dendritic tree, and the action of neuromodulatory inputs.

THE MOTONEURON POOL AND ITS MUSCLE AS A NEURAL SYSTEM

The goal of this section is to consider to what degree the extensive data on individual motoneuron properties and synaptic inputs can account for the recruitment and rate modulation of motor units observed both in the cat and in man. We begin with a brief overview of the mechanical properties of motor units. This is followed by a consideration of how synaptic inputs and neuromechanical properties can be interlinked in a simple model of the motor unit input–output function under steady-state conditions. Finally, the single-unit input–output functions are used to generate an operational model of the entire motoneuron pool, allowing investigation of how whole-system behaviors arise from single-unit properties and inputs.

Mechanical Properties of Motor Units

The wide variation in the morphological and electrophysiological properties of the individual motoneurons comprising a motoneuron pool is matched by an equally wide range in the mechanical properties of the muscle units they innervate. The mechanical properties of motor units were extensively reviewed by Burke (49). This section is not a general review of recent data, but instead focuses on those motor unit properties and interactions that are especially relevant to the function of the motoneuron pool as a whole.

Neuromechanical Correlations. The correlations between the electrical and mechanical properties of motor units within a pool are essential for understanding the mechanisms for orderly recruitment and rate modulation. For recruitment order, the important correlations are those between the conduction velocities (CV), input resistances (R_N), and rheobases (I_{rh}) of the motoneurons, and the forces, contraction speeds, and fatigue resistances of their

FIG. 1.11. *Continued* However, as shown on the right, when the Ia afferents and red nucleus were stimulated together, the total increase in firing rate was much less than that produced by the Ia afferents alone. *C*, Occlusion of excitatory synaptic inputs mediated by common interneurons. Stimulation of the sural nerve at $5 \times T$ generated an effective synaptic current of 5.6 nA at threshold and a change in discharge of 7.3 imp/s in this MG motoneuron (*right panel*). In the same cell, stimulation within the red nucleus generated an effective synaptic current of 11.6 nA at threshold and a change in its discharge rate of 13.5 imp/s (*left-hand panel*). However, when the two inputs were stimulated concurrently (*right-hand panel*), the effective synaptic current and discharge rate modulation were no greater than those produced by red nucleus stimulation alone.

muscle units (5, 97, 106, 114, 126, 366). For rate modulation, the important correlations are those between the time courses of the motoneuron AHPs and the muscle-unit twitch contractions (5, 83, 97, 126, 366). However, the strength of the correlation between individual electrical and mechanical properties is highly variable, with *r* values ranging from 0.3–0.9. Much of this may be due to measurement error and interanimal variation. Conduction velocity measurements are sensitive to pooling data from different experiments (106). Motoneuron–muscle unit correlations can only be carried out in nonparalyzed preparations, where the overall quality of the intracellular penetrations is probably not as good as in paralyzed preparations. Correlations between different motoneuron properties improve when the sample is restricted to cells with the largest resting and action potentials (66, 138). Under optimal measurement conditions, motoneuron–muscle unit correlations across the whole pool can be as high as 0.9 (106), and combinations of motoneuron properties can be used to type-identify greater than 95% of motor units correctly (366).

There are two exceptions to the general pattern of covariance. First, Bakels and Kernell (4) found no systematic correlation between AHP and twitch characteristics for rat tibialis anterior motor units. They attributed this to the restricted range of unit mechanical properties, because this muscle contains primarily fast-twitch units. Second, correlations among motor unit mechanical properties in human muscles are weaker than those reported in animal studies (335), but this may be due to difficulties in resolving single-unit forces in large human muscles.

Effects of Stimulation Rate during Isometric Conditions. As with the whole muscle, the relation between the isometric force produced by a motor unit and the frequency at which it is activated (i.e., the *F-f* relation) is approximately sigmoid shaped (34, 56, 198). The *F-f* functions of type S and F units vary systematically because of differences in contraction time, with type F units requiring considerably higher discharge rates to achieve maximal force (34, 56, 198). During prolonged or repeated stimulation, the frequency required to generate a given isometric force first decreases due to potentiation (31, 33) and then dramatically increases as fatigue ensues (33). Furthermore, fatigue can occur even at low frequencies of stimulation (253).

Isometric behavior is normally studied at one muscle length, namely the optimal length for whole-muscle twitch or tetanic tension. There have only been a few studies of the force-length (F-L) relations of individual motor units (e.g., 324). A recent study of motor unit *F-L* relations showed that the effect of stimulation frequency on the *F-L* relations of type S and type F units was similar (153). For all units, optimal lengths for unit force generation shifted to longer lengths as stimulation rate was reduced, as previously observed in the whole soleus muscle (265). The effect of this phenomenon on steady-state isometric behavior is presented in a subsequent section (see later under Input–Output Function of the Motoneuron Pool).

Summation of Motor Unit Forces. Models of motoneuron pool behavior generally assume that motor unit forces sum linearly to generate whole-muscle force (e.g., 149). However, several recent studies have shown that summation of the forces of pairs or small groups of motor units is nonlinear: The actual multiunit force is in fact greater than the algebraic sum of the individual unit forces (74, 107, 254). This positive nonlinearity is reduced by small stretching or shortening movements (254). A related finding is that the forces of the smallest motor units in the MG muscle are actually potentiated with respect to the isometric state by prior or concurrent slow movements (153). Both positive nonlinear summation and movement potentiation appear to reflect nonlinear viscous interactions between the fibers of the active motor units and the surrounding matrix of connective tissue and passive muscle fibers (153, 254).

Because these interactions are likely to be confined to very low forces, neither of these nonlinearities is probably an important factor in normal motor control. For example, movement potentiation was restricted to units with forces of less than 200 mN (i.e., 20 g-wt) and thus was absent in many FR and all FF units and, of course, in whole-muscle forces (153). However, linearity of summation of motor unit forces across a wide range of total muscle force has yet to be investigated, and the effect of tendon compliance and muscle architecture on force summation is as yet unknown.

Dynamic Properties of Motor Units. Although the dynamic behavior of whole muscle has been well studied (reviewed in 245), much less is known about the behavior of individual motor units under nonisometric, dynamic conditions. The first studies of dynamic unit behaviors focused on small-amplitude stretches, showing that type S units generated relatively larger stretch-evoked forces than type F units and that stretching and shortening movements could modify subsequent isometric force levels by as much as 40% (247, 254). For larger scale movements, the force-velocity (*F-V*) function is the fundamental measure of dynamic behavior (245). Recent studies have successfully measured the *F-V* functions of single motor units and have found that the isometric measure of contraction "speed," twitch contraction time, is a good predictor of *F-V* behavior (153, 246). Thus, there is an inverse relation between contraction time and the maximum velocity of shortening in motor units in the cat lumbrical muscle (246), with type F units exhibiting considerably higher maximal velocities than type S units. The inverse correlation between contraction time and tetanic force gives a direct relation between tetanic force and maximal velocity. The absence of a contraction time-maximum velocity relation in motor units of the rat soleus muscle may have resulted from the rather restricted range of contraction times in this muscle (95). These data predict that the maximal velocity of shortening of the whole muscle will increase as recruitment proceeds in the normal sequence of S → FR → FF units. Computer simulations of this process are presented in a later section (see under Input–Output Function of the Motoneuron Pool).

Single Motor Unit Input–Output Function

In steady-state conditions, the coupling of effective synaptic current (I_N) and the motoneuron *f-I* function provides a simple depiction of the steady-state input–output processing of the motoneuron (149) that is consistent with experimental results [(256, 258); see earlier under Effects of Synaptic Inputs on Motoneuron Discharge]. By applying the motoneuron *f-I* function to the sigmoidal shaped *F-f* function of its muscle unit, one obtains an expression for the complete transduction of effective synaptic current to isometric force, the I_N-*F* function, under steady-state conditions (149). The simplicity of this expression is a consequence of the biology, rather than a compromise for computational efficiency (see earlier under MOTONEURON PROPERTIES).

Three examples of simulated motor unit I_N-*F* functions based closely on the *f-I* and *F-f* functions of cat MG motor units (149) are illustrated in Figure 1.12*A*. The type S and type FF units on the left and right, respectively, set the extremes of the population and the FR unit in the center illustrates the population midrange. The systematic differences in I_0 values are clear (i.e., the distances between the functions along the x-axis), but the force scale on the y-axis has been normalized to allow shape comparisons. The smooth approach to maximum is provided by the saturation of each unit's *F-f* function. Each unit produces a similar fraction of maximal force at threshold and at the transition to the secondary range (see later under Control of Rate Modulation).

Input–Output Function of the Motoneuron Pool

Models of the motoneuron pool based on the properties of single motor units can provide considerable insight into how the ensemble behavior of the system arises from its constituent elements. The earliest pool models were designed to examine the relationship between electrical stimulation of group I afferents and monosynaptic reflex outputs (267, 272, 286), but these did not consider motor unit force nor take orderly recruitment into account. Following Henneman's initial work (e.g., 157), orderly recruitment of motor units at their tetanic forces was incorporated into several models designed to provide estimates of the input–output function of the motoneuron pool and how various synaptic inputs affected this function (3, 57, 97, 114, 143, 144, 199). More recently, several modeling studies have also taken motor unit rate modulation into account (65, 120, 128, 145, 149, 150, 315, 339).

In steady-state conditions, plausible models of the input–output function of the motoneuron pool that include recruitment and rate modulation can be achieved using sets of realistically simulated single motor unit I_N-*F* transforms (120, 145, 149). Figure 1-12*B* illustrates the I_N-*F* transform that results from linear summation of the single-unit I_N-*F* functions for the cat MG muscle shown in Figure 1.12*A*. The shape of this system function is sigmoidal, with a low-gain region at low forces, a high-gain region over the midrange, and a smooth saturation at the highest forces (149; see also 120). Henneman and colleagues' proposal (157) that the skew in distributions of thresholds and forces of motor unit results in a constant force increment for each newly recruited unit does not seem to hold at low forces, even with all units generating the same percentage of their maximum force at threshold. However, above 5%–20% of maximum force, constancy does appear to be a good approximation. A similar conclusion applies to noise sensitivity. At very low forces, noisy inputs produced extremely noisy outputs, but once a substantial fraction of the pool is recruited, the noise is obscured by the summed activity of many units and the sensitivity of the input–output function to noise is greatly reduced (145, 149).

Results from recent studies of motor unit force-length (*F-L*) and force-velocity (*F-V*) functions in the cat MG muscle can be used to extend these simulations to nonisometric conditions. In single motor

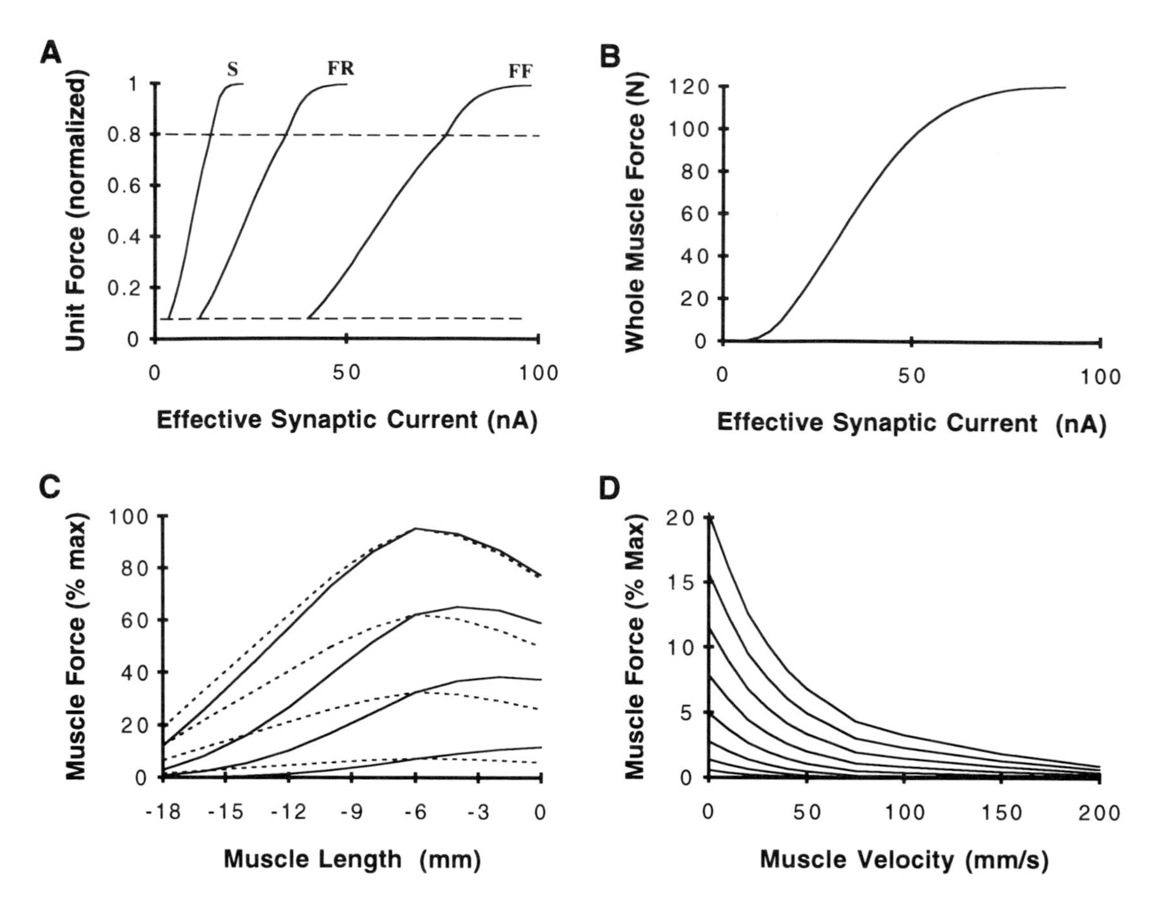

FIG. 1.12. Computer simulations of the input–output function of the mammalian motoneuron pool. *A*, Representative single-unit force-current (*F-I*) functions. *Dashed lines* indicate forces at the limits of the primary range of the motoneuron frequency-current (*f-I*) functions (i.e., threshold and at the transition to the secondary range). *B*, The whole pool input–output function that results when a uniform input is applied to the single-unit *F-I* functions and their forces are linearly summed. *C*, The pool force-length relation at various levels of synaptic input, with realistic recruitment and rate patterns. *Dashed lines* indicate force-length relations that occur in the absence of the interaction between stimulus rate and optimal length. *D*, The pool force-velocity functions at various levels of input, with realistic recruitment and rate patterns. (Data from in *A* and *B* from Heckman and Binder (149), in *C* and *D* from Heckman et al. (153).]

units (153) and whole muscles (265), increasing the stimulation rate decreases the optimal length for force production. Figure 1.12*C* shows that this phenomenon persists during normal recruitment and rate modulation of a motor unit population. Figure 1.12*D* shows that for *F-V* functions, the reduced V_{max} due to the initial recruitment of type S units (~50 mm/s) is evident only at the very lowest forces (153) because the tetanic forces of type S units are so small compared to those of type FR and FF units. By the time 10% of maximum force is attained, recruitment of type FR units provides a substantial portion of the total force and V_{max} for the system exceeds 200 mm/s. Further studies are needed in muscles with a larger proportion of S units than the cat MG (25% S).

The relation of whole-muscle EMG to motoneuron activity has also been simulated (120, 128, 315). Generally, the EMG-*F* relation is fairly linear (120, 128), because *I*-EMG and EMG-*F* functions tend to have opposite curvatures (120). However, this linearity is sensitive to the range of recruitment, with limited ranges (<50% of maximal force) being associated with nonlinear, unrealistic functions (120).

The slope of the input–output function of the motoneuron pool largely determines the gain for spinal reflexes (145). The initial curvature of the input–output function yields a roughly linear increase in reflex gain (145), consistent with the notion of automatic gain compensation (e.g., 222). However, this only occurs for the initial 10%–15% of the total force range, after which the gain becomes constant (15%–50%) and then declines to zero as maximum force is approached. These simulations were confined to steady-state force outputs, but simulations of the EMG output produced by H-reflex input showed a similar saturation (65, 315), as do the experimental data on the EMG responses to H-reflex inputs and muscle stretches (e.g., 129, 338).

Mechanisms Controlling Motor Outflow

When the effective synaptic current (I_N) is distributed uniformly to a motoneuron pool, the discharge patterns of the motoneurons are determined solely by their intrinsic properties. However, nonuniform distributions of I_N can alter these discharge patterns. With respect to recruitment order, a synaptic input system can overcome the normal sequence generated by the intrinsic differences in motoneuron current thresholds (I_0) by supplying high-threshold cells with a much greater amplitude of I_N than low-threshold cells (147, 151). The same general effect applies to rate modulation: the differences in rate modulation between units are dependent on the slopes of their intrinsic *f-I* functions and the relative proportion of the synaptic input they receive (145, 147). Neuromodulators and presynaptic inhibition may also affect discharge patterns. The neuromodulators studied thus far increase the excitability of motoneurons and the slopes of their *f-I* functions (see earlier under Effects of Neuromodulators on Motoneuron Behavior). It has been argued that these neuromodulatory actions are similar to those exerted by the concurrent actions of two or more synaptic input systems (28). For example, an increase in the hyperpolarization-activated inward current (I_h) produces a shift in the *f-I* function that is quite similar to that produced by constant activation of a synaptic system (28). Similarly, changes in *f-I* slope produced by actions on G_{KCa} are functionally equivalent to the effect of proportional activation of a synaptic input system, and presynaptic inhibition will simply reduce the I_N generated by its target input system by a constant percentage (145). Thus, in steady-state conditions, the effects of all three types of inputs (postsynaptic, neuromodulatory, and presynaptic inhibition) on the motor unit input–output function can be modeled in terms of their effects on the I_N–*f-I* combination.

The following sections have two related goals: *(1)* to use simulation results to show how motor unit intrinsic properties and various synaptic inputs shape motor outflow, and *(2)* to compare simulation results with normal behavior patterns in order to estimate the underlying organization of synaptic input. Thus, although synaptic input cannot be directly measured during normal motor behavior, it is possible to use realistic computer simulation techniques to make reasonable estimations. Steady-state conditions and linear summation of synaptic inputs and motor unit forces are assumed unless otherwise stated.

Control of the Pool Input–Output Function. The initial curved region of the sigmoid pool input–output function is produced primarily by the orderly recruitment of motor units of increasing force, while the linear region is dominated by force increases due to rate modulation with some continued role for recruitment [Fig. 1.12*B*; (149)]. The final smooth approach to maximum force reflects the saturation in *F-f* functions of the larger units. For the most part, this overall sigmoidal shape is unaffected by alterations in motor unit properties. However, the initial upward curvature is affected by variations in the skew in the distributions of current thresholds and muscle unit forces (149; cf. 120, 331, 339). Although linear summation of both input and output was assumed in these simulation studies, it turned out that the overall shape of the input–output function was actually insensitive to rather large amounts of nonlinear summation (149).

Burke (49) suggested that synaptic input systems that generate greater input in type F than type S units could be used to increase the input–output gain of the motoneuron pool. This idea was supported by the simulations performed by Kernell and Hultborn (199), using a recruitment-only model of the pool. However, computer simulations that include rate modulation suggest that synaptic inputs skewed toward excitation of type F units produce only modest changes in steady-state input–output slope and in reflex gain (145). Even the rubrospinal system, which generates approximately five times as much I_N in type FF vs. type S units (259), produced at most a 30% increase in gain. Furthermore, this change in gain was accompanied by deficits in the precision of force control and fatigue resistance expected from heavy reliance on type FF units. Thus, nonuniform distributions of synaptic inputs do not appear to provide a flexible means of gain control.

It seems reasonable to suppose instead that gain control is usually accomplished by neuromodulators (cf. 176) and presynaptic inhibition. For example, Capaday and Stein (64, 65) have hypothesized that the reduction in gain of the monosynaptic reflex in going from a stable posture to locomotion is due to presynaptic inhibition. This hypothesis illustrates a well-known advantage of gain control by presynaptic inhibition, namely its specificity to particular afferent inputs (287). In contrast, postsynaptic neuromodulatory actions will increase the output for all synaptic inputs (145). At present, the main limitation to understanding gain control via neuromodulators is the lack of information on their relative effects on type S vs. type F motor units. However, simulations based on the actions of monoamines suggest that gain control would be most effective when neuromodulatory actions are equipotential in all motoneurons. This allows significant gain increases while maintaining orderly recruitment, as well as actually improving both precision and fatigue resistance at low force levels (145).

Control of Orderly Recruitment. A model motoneuron pool based on the available experimental data on the cat medial gastrocnemius muscle has also been used to simulate recruitment order experiments (151). Monte Carlo techniques were employed to add random variance to the motor unit parameter values and to systematically sample the resulting recruitment sequences. The correlations between motoneuron excitability and various muscle unit properties such as force strongly support the normal, size-ordered recruitment sequence. The tenfold range of motoneuron I_{rh} (e.g., 137, 366) and I_0 (200) values is sufficient to maintain a robust, size-ordered sequence even when rather large amounts of random variance (i.e., noise) are added to degrade the motoneuron–muscle unit correlations [see Fig. 1.13; (151)]. These studies strongly support a fundamental role for the intrinsic properties of motoneurons in establishing the normal sequence of recruitment, much as originally envisioned by Henneman and colleagues (reviewed in 147, 156).

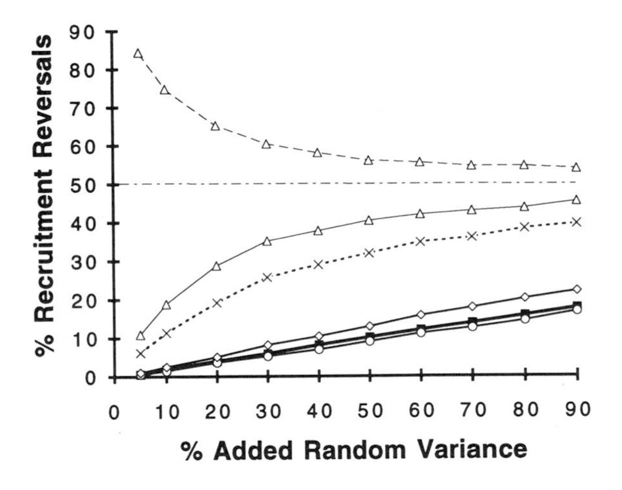

FIG. 1.13. Computer simulations of the effect of synaptic input on recruitment order. As random variance (i.e., noise) increased, the percentage of reversals generally increases. The uniform input allows recruitment to be specified by the intrinsic properties of the motor units. Only the rubrospinal combined excitation and inhibition gives a reversed sequence. Uniform distribution: *thick line, filled squares*; Ia input: *thin line, open circles*; vestibular input: *open diamonds*; rubrospinal excitation: *open triangles*; combined rubrospinal excitation and a constant 2 nA of rubrospinal inhibition: *dashed line, open triangles*; combined rubrospinal excitation, 2 nA of rubrospinal inhibition, and 2 nA of Ia excitation: *dashed line with x*'s. [From Heckman and Binder (151).]

Synaptic inputs that generate larger values of I_N in type S than in type F motor units expand the range of motoneuron recruitment thresholds, whereas those with the opposite pattern of I_N distribution tend to compress the range. Figure 1.13 shows that the Ia system, which produces more I_N in type S than in type F motor units (146), generates only a small improvement in simulated recruitment order. The vestibulospinal input, which has a distribution almost exactly opposite that of the Ia system (358), generates only a slightly degraded recruitment sequence.

In contrast, the rubrospinal system, which generates about five times as much excitatory I_N in type FF as in type S motor units (259), greatly destabilizes recruitment order. The distribution of larger effective synaptic currents to type F units by the rubrospinal system was not sufficient to reverse the normal recruitment sequence, rather it produced a near random recruitment pattern (151). Reversals could only be produced in these simulations when a source of inhibition was combined with the rubrospinal input. The amplitude of this inhibition could be quite small. Figure 1.13 shows that the −2 nA inhibitory component of the rubrospinal system was sufficient to create an entirely reversed sequence. The larger the inhibition, the greater the tendency for the sequence to reverse. However, superimposing a small Ia bias of only +2 nA could maintain normal recruitment when as much as −6 nA of inhibition was present. This finding is particularly interesting because activation of γ-motoneurons produces a background of Ia afferent activity in many movements (see Chapter 3). One role of such a Ia drive may be to maintain normal, size-ordered recruitment when other synaptic input systems with potentially disruptive distribution patterns are impinging on the motoneuron pool concurrently.

These simulation results suggest that suppression of type S units during eccentric contractions (239) should only occur when three conditions are met: (*1*) an input system organized like the rubrospinal excitation generates a substantial portion of the synaptic drive; (*2*) a source of inhibition is present; and (*3*) the amplitude of the inhibition is much greater than the amplitude of any background Ia excitation. These requirements may explain why activation of low-threshold, sural nerve afferents failed to cause systematic reversals in recruitment order of cat MG motoneurons (75, 84). Even though this input is probably organized like the rubrospinal input, the high level of Ia activity in the decerebrate cat and the tendency for the sural inhibition to diminish with repetitive activation (152) result in a normal recruitment sequence.

The large number of trials required for Monte Carlo simulations of recruitment order experiments (151) also provided a means of relating correlation coefficients between recruitment thresholds and mechanical properties (typically used in humans studies) to the percentage recruitment reversals observed in simultaneously recorded units (used in decerebrate cat studies). In terms of recruitment reversals, the results of this analysis showed a range of 0%–15% reversals for the decerebrate cat studies vs. 10%–35% reversals for the human studies. Whether the tendency for human data to show greater recruitment disorder reflects the greater measurement errors in human studies or a species difference in the organization of synaptic inputs is not yet known.

Control of Rate Modulation. The motoneuron *f-I* relation plays a major role in the rate modulation of motor units as muscle force increases above their recruitment thresholds. Kernell (196) has shown that the minimal firing rates of motoneurons in response to injected current vary systematically with the contraction times of their muscle units (see earlier under Repetitive Discharge Behavior). As a result, all motor units generate roughly the same proportion of their maximal force at threshold (5%–10%; see Fig. 1.12*A*). Similarly, at the transition between the primary and secondary ranges of firing, both fast- and slow-twitch motor units generate about 70%–90% of their maximal forces (Fig. 1.12*A*). Thus, most of the force generation of the motor unit occurs within the primary range of firing. The basis of the striking match between the motoneuron *f-I* function and the muscle unit *F-f* function is the strong covariation between the time courses of the motoneuron AHP and the muscle unit twitch contraction speed (e.g., 5, 126).

One would predict that human motor units should also display a systematic increase in minimal firing rates with recruitment threshold, but, as noted above, the available data are contradictory (see earlier under Rate Modulation of Motor Units). Furthermore, the rate limiting observed in steady-state conditions in human subjects (Fig. 1.1*B* and *C*) cannot be explained by the intrinsic properties of motor units (150, 197). This remains true even if it is assumed that type F units have higher *f-I* slopes than type S units (Heckman, unpublished results). This suggests that the synaptic input organization plays a crucial role in normal steady-state rate modulation (150).

Computer simulations of rate modulation have been performed using a variety of I_N distributions (150; Heckman, unpublished results). No single input system nor any linear combination of these systems could reproduce rate limiting. The only input organization that achieved a reasonable approximation of rate limiting was based on a two-tier structure, in which low levels of synaptic drive were generated by an input system that produced greater I_N in type S than in type F units, and then, above a certain activation level, all further increases in pool output were generated by synaptic inputs with the opposite distribution [I_N to type F > to type S; (150)]. Recent simulations have also shown that adding systematic differences in primary range *f-I* slopes to this "crossover" organization helps to maintain a wide range of recruitment thresholds (Heckman, unpublished results). At present, the experimental data are contradictory on this point (cf. 192 with 196) and further studies of this issue are clearly needed.

Figure 1.14 shows the rate modulation pattern that results from a crossover organization using distributions of I_N patterned after the homonymous Ia afferent and vestibulospinal systems (cf. Fig. 1.9) to drive the motoneuron pool. Rate limiting is clearly present and recruitment continues until about 60% of maximal force is attained. In addition, this simulation replicates the steeper rate modulation observed in high-threshold motor units seen by Monster and Chan (226, 227). It should be emphasized that Ia and vestibulospinal inputs used to generate the crossover scheme presented in Figure 1.14 are meant to represent general types of input distributions. Both low and high levels undoubtedly require multiple input systems (see 150). These results show that reasonable rate limiting can be achieved with a

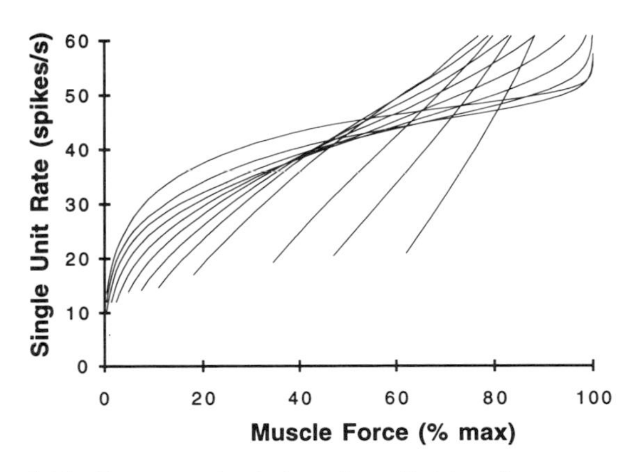

FIG. 1.14. Computer simulation of rate limiting, for comparison with the experimental data in Figure 1.2. See text for details of the "crossover" synaptic input organization used to produce this pattern. [cf. Heckman and Binder (150).]

relatively simple organization of synaptic input, but this certainly does not exclude other mechanisms.

Stimulation of the cat mesencephalic locomotor region (MLR) produces a very severe rate limiting (35, 45). This may involve neuromodulator effects (45), but the relation of these findings to human isometric contractions is unclear. Nonlinear input summation has also been hypothesized to play a role in rate limiting (149, 150). If sharp nonlinear summation began at the upper limit of the primary range of motoneurons, each unit would just reach its maximal force before undergoing limiting, thus giving near ideal energy optimization. However, simulations based on this hypothesis generate firing rates in each high-threshold unit that greatly exceed those of lower threshold units (150), a pattern not seen in most human subjects (Fig. 1.1*B–D*). Further studies of nonlinear input summation are needed to clarify its potential role in regulating motoneuron discharge.

Control of Motor Unit Utilization. Henneman and colleagues first proposed that the pattern of motor outflow from the spinal cord ensured optimal fatigue resistance by exploiting the diversity of motor unit mechanical properties (154, 156, 157). This view was supported by a comparison of the predicted input–output behavior of the cat MG motoneuron pool based on a size-ordered recruitment model and data obtained from the MG muscles of freely moving cats (354). The modeling results suggested that all postural and locomotor forces in this muscle could be produced solely by fatigue-resistant type S and type FR units (354). However, the contribution made by rate modulation to muscle force was not taken into account. Figure 1.15 allows the same comparisons to be made with a model of the motoneuron pool that included realistic rate modulation. The simulated pool output was based on the *f-I, F-f*, and *F-V* functions of the motor units of the cat MG muscle (145, 149, 153). Plotting synaptic input (y-axis) vs. muscle velocity of shortening (x-axis) and normalized whole-muscle force (z-axis) generated a curved, three-dimensional surface. The surface shading indicates the percentage of total muscle force generated by type FF units (lighter in-

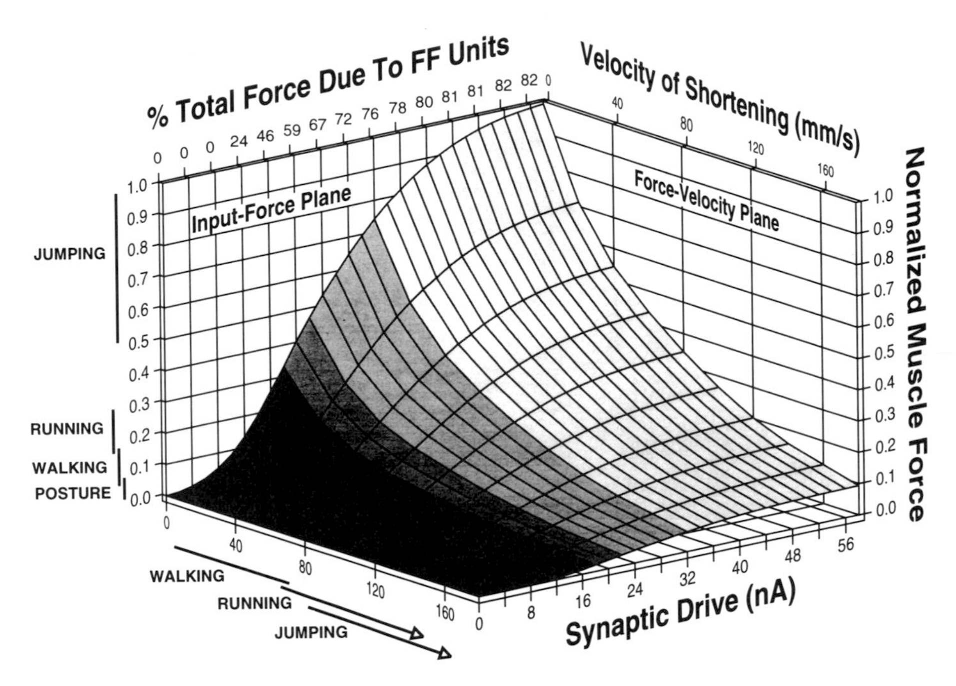

FIG. 1.15. Computer simulations of input–output relations between synaptic input (y-axis) to the motoneuron pool and muscle force (z-axis) and velocity of shortening (x-axis). Surface shading and y-axis labels at upper left indicate the percentage of muscle force generated by type FF units. Single motor unit *f-I, F-f*, and *F-V* functions based on the cat MG muscle (145, 149, 153). Lines labeled with various motor tasks indicate approximate ranges of forces (z-axis) and velocities (x-axis) measured in MG with chronically implanted devices. Force ranges were estimated from the peak during stance, which occurs in near isometric conditions as muscle velocity undergoes the transition between the extension and flexion phases of the stance [data from Walmsley et al. (354)]. Velocity ranges were taken from the peak velocities of shortening during the later portion of the stance phase, when rapid flexion is developing but the muscle is still active. Velocities for slow walking were taken from Weytjens (unpublished data). For faster speeds and jumping, velocities were estimated from the length records of Walmsley and colleagues (354). Jump heights ranged from about 0.5–1.2 m (354). Arrows for running and jumping indicate that the fastest velocities probably exceed the range of the figure, which falls well short of the maximum velocity for MG.

dicates greater type FF utilization), which provides an approximate index of fatigability. The lines along the z- and x-axes indicate the approximate ranges of forces and shortening velocities involved in posture, locomotion, and jumping in the cat (see legend for the limitations on the accuracy of these estimations; see also Chapters 5 and 8 for descriptions of cat locomotor behavior).

As illustrated in Figure 1.15, when rate modulation is taken into account along with orderly recruitment, the type FF units contribute to whole-muscle force at surprisingly low levels of output (145). The activation of type FF units begins just below 10% of maximal force and then rises steeply with increasing output. These modeling results suggest that only postural tasks can be achieved without the activation of type FF units (indicated by *dark band* across lower left of the figure). The type FF units generate as much as 25% of the force in walking and as much as 50% during running. It should be emphasized that a modest level of activity in descending monoaminergic fibers was assumed in Figure 1.15, sufficient to double motoneuron *f-I* gains. In the absence of such monoaminergic input, the participation of type FF units at low forces is even more dramatic (145). The key factor is the steepness of rate modulation: as the slope of motoneuron *f-I* functions increases, the activation pattern of type FF units approaches that predicted by a recruitment-only model (e.g., 354).

These simulation results suggest that a fundamental aspect of motor behavior, minimization of fatigue, may require modification of motoneuron intrinsic properties by monoamines. Results of other simulations using this model indicate that monoamines also enhance input–output gain and precision (see earlier under Control of the Pool Input–Output Function), supporting the hypothesis that descending brainstem monoaminergic systems play an important role in controlling posture (206, 207) and other basic movement patterns (176).

SUMMARY

The effects of activity in descending and peripheral afferent fibers on muscle force and length depend on the distribution of their synaptic terminals among the constituent motoneurons innervating the muscle, and on the intrinsic properties of the motoneurons and their innervated muscle fibers. Although the organization of synaptic inputs to motoneurons and the intrinsic motoneuron properties are among the most thoroughly studied aspects of the neural control of movement, it is not yet possible to account for all of the observations on motoneuron and muscle behavior in terms of the underlying physiology. We believe that the problem can be simplified by describing the transformation of synaptic inputs into motor output in three stages: *(1)* the delivery of synaptic current from the synaptic boutons to the motoneuron soma, where it can be measured as I_N; *(2)* the transduction of that synaptic current into motoneuron firing rate (*f-I* relation); and *(3)* the transformation of motoneuron firing rate to muscle unit force (*F-f* relation). Even though many of the biophysical mechanisms underlying these three processes are not completely understood, the relevant quantities and relations can be empirically determined. Given measurements of I_N, *f-I*, and *F-f* relations, it is possible to predict the relation between synaptic input and motor output under certain restricted conditions.

It is not yet possible to measure directly synaptic input to motoneurons during normal motor behavior. However, the computer simulation results discussed above provide a basis for reasonable speculations about the roles of various synaptic inputs in the generation of normal, steady-state motor outflow. A similar estimation for dynamic conditions awaits more sophisticated simulations and new experimental techniques.

We thank Drs. A. J. Berger, R. E. Burke, J. S. Carp, P. C. Scwindt, T. C. Cope, O. Kiehn, J. L. Smith, and L. B. Rowell for reviewing this chapter. Our experimental work and modeling studies have been supported by grants NS 26840, NS 31592, and NS 31925 from the National Institutes of Health and by the Medical Research Service of the Department of Veteran Affairs.

REFERENCES

1. Araki, T., and C. A. Terzuolo. Membrane currents in spinal motoneurons associated with the action potential and synaptic activity. *J. Neurophysiol.* 25: 772–789, 1962.
2. Arvidsson, U., S. Cullheim, B. Ulfhake, G. W. Bennett, K. C. Fone, A. C. Cuello, A. A. Verhofstad, T. J. Visser, and T. Hokfelt. 5-Hydroxytryptamine, substance P, and thyrotropin-releasing hormone in the adult cat spinal cord segment L7: immunohistochemical and chemical studies. *Synapse* 6: 237–270, 1990.
3. Bagust, J., S. Knott, D. M. Lewis, J. C. Luck, and R. A. Westerman. Isometric contractions of motor units in a fast twitch muscle of the cat. *J. Physiol. (Lond.)* 231: 87–104, 1973.
4. Bakels, R., and D. Kernell. Average but not continuous speed match between motoneurons and muscle units of rat tibialis anterior. *J. Neurophysiol.* 70: 1300–1306, 1993.
5. Bakels, R., and D. Kernell. Matching between motoneurone and muscle unit properties in rat medial gastrocnemius. *J. Physiol. (Lond.)* 463: 307–324, 1993.
6. Baldissera, F. Relationships between the spike components and the delayed depolarization in cat spinal neurones. *J. Physiol. (Lond.)* 259: 325–338, 1976.

7. Baldissera, F. Impulse frequency encoding of the dynamic aspects of excitation. *Arch. Ital. Biol.* 122: 43–58, 1984.
8. Baldissera, F., P. Campadelli, and L. Piccinelli. Neural encoding of input transients investigated by intracellular injection of ramp currents in cat α-motoneurones. *J. Physiol. (Lond.)* 328: 73–86, 1982.
9. Baldissera, F., P. Campadelli, and L. Piccinelli. The dynamic response of cat gastrocnemius motor units investigated by ramp-current injection into their motoneurones. *J. Physiol. (Lond.)* 387: 317–30, 1987.
10. Baldissera, F., and B. Gustafsson. Afterhyperpolarization time course in lumbar motoneurones of the cat. *Acta Physiol. Scand.* 91: 512–527, 1974.
11. Baldissera, F., and B. Gustafsson. Firing behaviour of a neuron model based on the afterhyperpolarization conductance time-course and algebraical summation. Adaptation and steady state firing. *Acta Physiol. Scand.* 92: 27–47, 1974.
12. Baldissera, F., and B. Gustafsson. Firing behaviour of a neuron model based on the afterhyperpolarization conductance time-course. First interval firing. *Acta Physiol. Scand.* 91: 528–544, 1974.
13. Baldissera, F., B. Gustafsson, and F. Parmiggiani. Saturating summation of the afterhyperpolarization conductance in spinal motoneurones: a mechanism for 'secondary range' repetitive firing. *Brain Res.* 146: 69–82, 1978.
14. Baldissera, F., H. Hultborn, and M. Illert. Integration in spinal neuronal systems. In: *Handbook of Physiology, The Nervous System, Motor Control*, edited by V. B. Brooks. Bethesda, MD: Am. Physiol. Soc., 1981, p. 509–595.
15. Barrett, E. F., J. N. Barrett, and W. E. Crill. Voltage-sensitive outward currents in cat motoneurones. *J. Physiol. (Lond.)* 304: 251–276, 1980.
16. Barrett, J. N. Motoneuron dendrites: role in synaptic integration. *Federation Proc.* 34: 1398–1407, 1975.
17. Barrett, J. N., and W. E. Crill. Specific membrane properties of cat motoneurones. *J. Physiol. (Lond.)* 239: 301–324, 1974.
18. Barrett, J. N., and W. E. Crill. Voltage clamp of cat motoneurone somata: properties of the fast inward current. *J. Physiol. (Lond.)* 304: 231–249, 1980.
19. Bawa, P., M. D. Binder, P. Ruenzel, and E. Henneman. Recruitment order of motoneurons in stretch reflexes is highly correlated with their axonal conduction velocity. *J. Neurophysiol.* 52: 410–420, 1984.
20. Bawa, P., and R. N. Lemon. Recruitment of motor units in response to transcranial magnetic stimulation in man. *J. Physiol. (Lond.)* 471: 445–464, 1993.
21. Bayliss, D. A., M. Umemiya, and A. J. Berger. Serotonin inhibits N- and P-type calcium channels and the after hyperpolarization in rat motoneurones. *J. Physiol. (Lond.)* 485: 635–647, 1995.
22. Bayliss, D. A., F. Viana, M. C. Bellingham, and A. J. Berger. Characteristics and postnatal development of a hyperpolarization-activated inward current in rat hypoglossal motoneurons in vitro. *J. Neurophysiol.* 71: 119–128, 1994.
23. Bayliss, D. A., F. Viana, and A. J. Berger. Mechanisms underlying excitatory effects of thyrotropin-releasing hormone on rat hypoglossal motoneurons in vitro. *J. Neurophysiol.* 68: 1733–1745, 1992.
24. Berger, A. J., D. A. Bayliss, and F. Viana. Modulation of neonatal rat hypoglossal motoneuron excitability by serotonin. *Neurosci. Lett.* 143: 164–168, 1992.
25. Bessou, P., F. Emonet-Dênand, and Y. Laporte. Relation entre la vitesse de conduction des fibres nerveuses mortices et le tempe de contraction de leurs unites motrices. *C. R. Acad. Sci. Ser. D.* 256: 5625–5627, 1963.
26. Bigland, B., and O. C. J. Lippold. Motor unit activity in the voluntary contraction of human muscle. *J. Physiol. (Lond.)* 125: 322–335, 1954.
27. Binder, M. D., P. Bawa, P. Ruenzel, and E. Henneman. Does orderly recruitment of motoneurons depend on the existence of different types of motor units? *Neurosci. Lett.* 36: 55–58, 1983.
28. Binder, M. D., C. J. Heckman, and R. K. Powers. How different afferent inputs control motoneuron discharge and the output of the motoneuron pool. *Curr. Opin. Neurobiol.* 3: 1028–1034, 1993.
29. Binder, M. D., and L. M. Mendell. *The Segmental Motor System*. New York: Oxford University Press, 1990.
30. Binder, M. D., and R. K. Powers. Effective synaptic currents generated in cat spinal motoneurones by activating descending and peripheral afferent fibres. In: *Alpha and Gamma Motor Systems*, edited by A. Taylor and M. Gladden. New York: Plenum Press, 1995.
31. Binder-Macleod, S. A., and H. P. Clamann. Force output of cat motor units stimulated with trains of linearly varying frequency. *J. Neurophysiol.* 61: 208–217, 1989.
32. Bohmer, G., K. Schmid, and W. Schauer. Evidence for an involvement of NMDA and non-NMDA receptors in synaptic excitation of phrenic motoneurons in the rabbit. *Neurosci. Lett.* 130: 271–274, 1991.
33. Botterman, B. R., and T. C. Cope. Motor-unit stimulation patterns during fatiguing contractions of constant tension. *J. Neurophysiol.* 60: 1198–1214, 1988.
34. Botterman, B. R., G. A. Iwamoto, and W. J. Gonyea. Gradation of isometric tension by different activation rates in motor units of cat flexor carpi radialis muscle. *J. Neurophysiol.* 56: 494–506, 1986.
35. Botterman, B. R., and K. E. Tansey. Recruitment order and discharge patterns among pairs of motor units evoked by brainstem stimulation. *Soc. Neurosci. Abstr.* 15: 919, 1989.
36. Brannstrom, T. Quantitative synaptology of functionally different types of cat medial gastrocnemius alpha-motoneurons. *J. Comp. Neurol.* 330: 439–454, 1993.
37. Bras, H., J. Destombes, P. Gogan, and S. Tyc-Dumont. The dendrites of single brain-stem motoneurons intracellularly labelled with horseradish peroxidase in the cat. An ultrastructural analysis of the synaptic covering and the microenvironment. *Neuroscience* 22: 971–981, 1987.
38. Bras, H., P. Gogan, and S. Tyc-Dumont. The dendrites of single brain-stem motoneurons intracellularly labelled with horseradish peroxidase in the cat. Morphological and electrical differences. *Neuroscience* 22: 947–970, 1987.
39. Bras, H., S. Korogod, Y. Driencourt, P. Gogan, and S. Tyc-dumont. Stochastic geometry and electronic architecture of dendritic arborization of brain stem motoneuron. *Eur. J. Neurosci.* 5: 1485–1493, 1993.
40. Brismar, T. Slow mechanism for sodium permeability inactivation in myelinated nerve fibre of *Xenopus laevis*. *J. Physiol. (Lond.)* 270: 283–297, 1977.
41. Brock, L. G., J. S. Coombs, and J. C. Eccles. Intracellular recording from antidromically activated motoneurons. *J. Physiol. (Lond.)* 122: 429–461, 1953.
42. Brodin, L., H. G. Trav'en, A. Lansner, P. Wallén, O. Ekeberg, and S. Grillner. Computer simulations of *N*-methyl-D-aspartate receptor–induced membrane properties in a neuron model. *J. Neurophysiol.* 66: 473–484, 1991.
43. Brooks, V. B. (Ed). *Handbook of Physiology, The Nervous System, Motor Control*. Bethesda, MD: Am. Physiol. Soc., 1981.
44. Brownstone, R., and H. Hultborn. Regulated and intrinsic properties of the motoneurone: effect on input-output re-

lations. In: *Muscle Afferents and Spinal Control of Movement*, edited by L. Jami, E. Pierrot-Deselligny, and D. Zytnicki. New York: Pergamon Press, 1992, p. 175–181.

45. Brownstone, R. M., L. M. Jordan, D. J. Kriellaars, B. R. Noga, and S. J. Shefchyk. On the regulation of repetitive firing in lumbar motoneurones during fictive locomotion in the cat. *Exp. Brain Res.*, 90: 441–455, 1992.
46. Buchanan, J. T., L. E. Moore, R. Hill, P. Wallén, and S. Grillner. Synaptic potentials and transfer functions of lamprey spinal neurons. *Biol. Cybern.* 67: 123–131, 1992.
47. Burke, R. E. Composite nature of the monosynaptic excitatory postsynaptic potential. *J. Neurophysiol.* 30: 1114–1137, 1967.
48. Burke, R. E. Motor unit types of cat triceps surae muscle. *J. Physiol. (Lond.)* 193: 141–160, 1967.
49. Burke, R. E. Motor units: anatomy, physiology, and functional organization. In: *Handbook of Physiology, The Nervous System, Motor Control*, edited by V. B. Brooks. Bethesda, MD: Am. Physiol. Soc., 1981, p. 345–422.
50. Burke, R. E. Motor unit types: some history and unsettled issues. In: *The Segmental Motor System*, edited by M. D. Binder and L. M. Mendell. New York: Oxford University Press, 1990, p. 207–221.
51. Burke, R. E., R. P. Dum, J. W. Fleshman, L. L. Glenn, T. A. Lev, M. J. O'Donovan, and M. J. Pinter. A HRP study of the relation between cell size and motor unit type in cat ankle extensor motoneurons. *J. Comp. Neurol.* 209: 17–28, 1982.
52. Burke, R. E., L. Fedina, and A. Lundberg. Spatial synaptic distribution of recurrent and group Ia inhibitory systems in cat spinal motoneurones. *J. Physiol. (Lond.)* 214: 305–326, 1971.
53. Burke, R. E., J. W. Fleshman, and I. Segev. Factors that control the efficacy of group Ia synapses in alpha-motoneurons. *J. Physiol. (Paris)* 83: 133–140, 1988.
54. Burke, R. E., E. Jankowska, and G. ten Bruggencate. A comparison of peripheral and rubrospinal input to slow and fast twitch motor units of triceps surae. *J. Physiol. (Lond.)* 207: 709–732, 1970.
55. Burke, R. E., and P. G. Nelson. Accommodation to current ramps in motoneurons of fast and slow twitch motor units. *Int. J. Neurosci.* 1: 347–356, 1971.
56. Burke, R. E., P. Rudomin, and F. E. Zajac. The effect of activation history on tension production by individual muscle units. *Brain Res.* 109: 515–529, 1976.
57. Burke, R. E., W. Z. Rymer, and J. V. Walsh. Relative strength of synaptic input from short-latency pathways to motor units of defined type in cat medial gastrocnemius. *J. Neurophysiol.* 39: 447–458, 1976.
58. Calancie, B., and P. Bawa. Firing patterns of human flexor carpi radialis motor units during the stretch reflex. *J. Neurophysiol.* 53: 1179–1193, 1985.
59. Calancie, B., and P. Bawa. Limitations of the spike triggered averaging technique. *Muscle Nerve* 9: 78–93, 1986.
60. Calancie, B., and P. Bawa. Motor unit recruitment in humans. In: *The Segmental Motor System*, edited by M. D. Binder and L. M. Mendell. New York: Oxford University Press, 1990, p. 75–95.
61. Calancie, B., M. Nordin, U. Wallin, and K. E. Hagbarth. Motor-unit responses in human wrist flexor and extensor muscles to transcranial cortical stimuli. *J. Neurophysiol.* 58: 1168–1185, 1987.
62. Calvin, W. H. Three modes of repetitive firing and the role of threshold time course between spikes. *Brain Res.* 59: 341–346, 1974.
63. Cameron, W. E., D. B. Averill, and A. J. Berger. Quantitative analysis of the dendrites of cat phrenic motoneurons stained intracellularly with horseradish peroxidase. *J. Comp. Neurol.* 231: 91–101, 1985.
64. Capaday, C., and R. B. Stein. Difference in the amplitude of the human soleus H reflex during walking and running. *J. Physiol. (Lond.)* 392: 513–522, 1987.
65. Capaday, C., and R. B. Stein. A method for simulating the reflex output of a motoneuron pool. *J. Neurosci. Methods* 21: 91–104, 1987.
66. Carp, J. S. Physiological properties of primate lumbar motoneurons. *J. Neurophysiol.* 68: 1121–1132, 1992.
67. Carp, J. S., R. K. Powers, and W. Z. Rymer. Alterations in motoneuron properties induced by acute dorsal spinal hemisection in the decerebrate cat. *Exp. Brain Res.* 83: 539–548, 1991.
68. Catterall, W. A. Localization of sodium channels in cultured neural cells. *J. Neurosci.* 1: 777–783, 1981.
69. Catterall, W. A. Cellular and molecular biology of voltage-gated sodium channels. *Physiol. Rev.* 72: S15–S47, 1992.
70. Chanaud, C. M., and J. M. Macpherson. Functionally complex muscles of the cat hindlimb. 3. Differential activation within biceps-femoris during postural perturbations. *Exp. Brain Res.* 85: 271–280, 1991.
71. Chanaud, C. M., C. A. Pratt, and G. E. Loeb. Functionally complex muscles of the cat hindlimb. 5. The roles of histochemical fiber-type regionalization and mechanical heterogeneity in differential muscle activation. *Exp. Brain Res.* 85: 300–313, 1991.
72. Chandler, S. H., C. Hsaio, T. Inoue, and L. J. Goldberg. Electrophysiological properties of guinea pig trigeminal motoneurons recorded in vitro. *J. Neurophysiol.* 71: 129–145, 1994.
73. Clamann, H. P., A. C. Ngai, C. G. Kukulka, and S. J. Goldberg. Motor pool organization in monosynaptic reflexes: responses in three different muscles. *J. Neurophysiol.* 50: 725–742, 1983.
74. Clamann, H. P., and T. B. Schelhorn. Nonlinear force addition of newly recruited motor units in the cat hindlimb. *Muscle Nerve* 11: 1079–1089, 1988.
75. Clark, B. D., S. M. Dacko, and T. C. Cope. Cutaneous stimulation fails to alter motor unit recruitment in the decerebrate cat. *J. Neurophysiol.* 70: 1433–1439, 1993.
76. Clements, J. D., P. G. Nelson, and S. J. Redman. Intracellular tetraethylammonium ions enhance group Ia excitatory post-synaptic potentials evoked in cat motoneurones. *J. Physiol. (Lond.)* 377: 267–282, 1986.
77. Clements, J. D., and S. J. Redman. Cable properties of cat spinal motoneurones measured by combining voltage clamp, current clamp and intracellular staining. *J. Physiol. (Lond.)* 409: 63–87, 1989.
78. Connor, J. A., and C. F. Stevens. Voltage clamp studies of a transient outward membrane current in gastropod neural somata. *J. Physiol. (Lond.)* 213: 21–30, 1971.
79. Conradi, S. Ultrastructure and distribution of neuronal and glial elements on the motoneuron surface in the lumbosacral spinal cord of the adult cat. *Acta Physiol. Scand. Suppl.* 332: 5–48, 1969.
80. Conradi, S., J. Kellerth, C. Berthold, and C. Hammarberg. Electron microscopic studies of serially sectioned cat spinal α-motoneurons: IV. Motoneurons innervating slow-twitch (type S) units of the soleus muscle. *J. Comp. Neurol.* 184: 769–782, 1979.
81. Coombs, J. S., D. R. Curtis, and J. C. Eccles. The generation of impulses in motoneurones. *J. Physiol. (Lond.)* 139: 232–249, 1957.

82. Coombs, J. S., J. C. Eccles, and P. Fatt. The specific ionic conductances and the ionic movements across the motoneuronal membrane that produce the inhibitory postsynaptic potential. *J. Physiol. (Lond.)* 130: 326–373, 1955.
83. Cope, T. C., S. C. Bobine, M. Fournier, and V. R. Edgerton. Soleus motor units in chronic spinal transected cats: physiological and morphological alterations. *J. Neurophysiol.* 55: 1202–1220, 1986.
84. Cope, T. C., and B. D. Clark. Motor-unit recruitment in the decerebrate cat—several unit properties are equally good predictors of order. *J. Neurophysiol.* 66: 1127–1138, 1991.
85. Cope, T. C., and B. D. Clark. Motor-unit recruitment in self-reinnervated muscle. *J. Neurophysiol.* 70: 1787–1796, 1993.
86. Cordo, P. J., and W. Z. Rymer. Motor-unit activation patterns in lengthening and isometric contractions of hindlimb extensor muscles in the decerebrate cat. *J. Neurophysiol.* 47: 782–796, 1982.
87. Cullheim, S. Relations between cell body size, axon diameter and axon conduction velocity of cat sciatic α-motoneurons stained with horseradish peroxidase. *Neurosci. Lett.* 8: 17–20, 1978.
88. Cullheim, S., J. W. Fleshman, L. L. Glenn, and R. E. Burke. Membrane area and dendritic structure in type-identified triceps surae alpha motoneurons. *J. Comp. Neurol.* 255: 68–81, 1987.
89. Cullheim, S., J. W. Fleshman, L. L. Glenn, and R. E. Burke. Three-dimensional architecture of dendritic trees in type-identified alpha-motoneurons. *J. Comp. Neurol.* 255: 82–96, 1987.
90. Cullheim, S., and J. Kellerth. A morphological study of the axons and recurrent axon collaterals of cat α-motoneurones supplying different functional types of muscle unit. *J. Physiol. (Lond.)* 281: 301–313, 1978.
91. Davies, L., A. W. Wiegner, and R. R. Young. Variation in firing order of human soleus motoneurons during voluntary and reflex activation. *Brain Res.* 602: 104–110, 1993.
92. De Luca, C. J., R. S. LeFever, M. P. McCue, and A. P. Xenakis. Behavior of human motor units in different muscles during linearly varying contractions. *J. Physiol. (Lond.)* 329: 113–128, 1982.
93. DeShutter, E. Computer software for development and simulation of compartmental models of neurons. *Comput. Biol. Med.* 19: 71–81, 1989.
94. Desmedt, J. E., and E. Godaux. Ballistic contractions in man: characteristic recruitment pattern of single motor units of the tibialis anterior muscle. *J. Physiol. (Lond.)* 264: 373–393, 1977.
95. Devasahayam, S. R., and T. G. Sandercock. Velocity of shortening of single motor units from rat soleus. *J. Neurophysiol.* 67: 1133–1145, 1992.
96. Dodge, F. A., and J. W. Cooley. Action potential of the motoneuron. *IBM J. Res. Dev.* 17: 219–229, 1973.
97. Dum, R. P., and T. T. Kennedy. Synaptic organization of defined motor unit types in cat tibialis anterior. *J. Neurophysiol.* 43: 1631–1644, 1980.
98. Durand, D. The somatic shunt cable model for neurons. *Biophys. J.* 46: 645–653, 1984.
99. Durand, J. NMDA actions on rat abducens motoneurones. *Eur. J. Neurosci.* 3: 621–633, 1991.
100. Durand, J. Synaptic excitation triggers oscillations during NMDA receptor activation in rat abducens motoneurons. *Eur. J. Neurosci.* 5: 1389–1397, 1993.
101. Durand, J., I. Engberg, and S. Tyc-Dumont. L-Glutamate and *N*-methyl-D-asparatate actions on membrane potential and conductance of cat abducens motoneurones. *Neurosci. Lett.* 79: 295–300, 1987.
102. Eccles, J. C., R. M. Eccles, A. Iggo, and M. Ito. Distribution of recurrent inhibition among motoneurons. *J. Physiol. (Lond.)* 159: 479–499, 1961.
103. Ekeberg, O., P. Wallén, A. Lansner, H. Trav'en, L. Brodin, and S. Grillner. A computer based model for realistic simulations of neural networks. I. The single neuron and synaptic interaction. *Biol. Cybern.* 65: 81–90, 1991.
104. Eken, T., and O. Kiehn. Bistable firing properties of soleus motor units in unrestrained rats. *Acta Physiol. Scand.* 136: 383–394, 1989.
105. Elliott, P., and D. I. Wallis. Serotonin and L-norepinephrine as mediators of altered excitability in neonatal rat motoneurons studied in vitro. *Neuroscience* 47: 533–544, 1992.
106. Emonet-Denand, F., C. C. Hunt, J. Petit, and B. Pollin. Proportion of fatigue-resistant motor units in hindlimb muscles of cat and their relation to axonal conduction velocity. *J. Physiol. (Lond.)* 400: 135–158, 1988.
107. Emonet-Denand, F., Y. Laporte, and U. Proske. Summation of tension in motor units of the soleus muscle of the cat. *Neurosci. Lett.* 116: 112–117, 1990.
108. Endo, K., T. Araki, and Y. Kawai. Contra- and ipsilateral cortical and rubral effects on fast and slow spinal motoneurons of the cat. *Brain Res.* 88: 91–98, 1975.
109. Engberg, I., I. Tarnawa, J. Durand, and M. Ouardouz. An analysis of synaptic transmission to motoneurons in the cat spinal cord using a new selective receptor blocker. *Acta Physiol. Scand.* 148: 97–100, 1993.
110. Enoka, R., and D. G. Stuart. Henneman's "size principle": current issues. *Trends Neurosci.* 7: 266–228, 1984.
111. Finkel, A. S., and S. J. Redman. The synaptic current evoked in cat spinal motoneurones by impulses in single group 1a axons. *J. Physiol. (Lond.)* 342: 615–632, 1983.
112. Fisher, N. D., and A. Nistri. Substance P and TRH share a common effector pathway in rat spinal motoneurones: an in vitro electrophysiological investigation. *Neurosci. Lett.* 153: 115–119, 1993.
113. Flatman, J. A., J. Durand, I. Engberg, and J. D. C. Lambert. Blocking the monosynaptic EPSP in spinal cord motoneurones with inhibitors of amino-acid excitation. *Neurol. Neurobiol.* 24: 285–292, 1987.
114. Fleshman, J. W., J. B. Munson, G. W. Sypert, and W. A. Friedman. Rheobase, input resistance, and motor-unit type in medial gastrocnemius motoneurons in the cat. *J. Neurophysiol.* 46: 1326–1338, 1981.
115. Fleshman, J. W., I. Segev, and R. B. Burke. Electrotonic architecture of type-identified alpha-motoneurons in the cat spinal cord. *J. Neurophysiol.* 60: 60–85, 1988.
116. Forsythe, I. D., and S. J. Redman. The dependence of motoneurone membrane potential on extracellular ion concentrations studied in isolated rat spinal cord. *J. Physiol. (Lond.)* 404: 83–99, 1988.
117. Frankenhaeuser, B., and A. B. Vallbo. Accommodation in myelinated nerve fibres of *Xenopus laevis* as computed on the basis of voltage clamp data. *Acta Physiol. Scand.* 63: 1–20, 1964.
118. Freund, H.-J., H. J. Budingen, and V. Dietz. Activity of single motor units from human forearm muscles during voluntary isometric contractions. *J. Neurophysiol.* 38: 933–946, 1975.
119. Friedman, W. A., G. W. Sypert, J. B. Munson, and J. W. Fleshman. Recurrent inhibition in type-identified motoneurons. *J. Neurophysiol.* 46: 1349–1359, 1981.

120. Fuglevand, A. J., D. A. Winter, and A. E. Patla. Models of recruitment and rate coding organization in motor-unit pools. *J. Neurophysiol.* 70: 2470–2488, 1993.
121. Fukushima, K., B. W. Peterson, and V. J. Wilson. Vestibulospinal, reticulospinal and interstitiospinal pathways in the cat. *Prog. Brain Res.* 50: 121–136, 1979.
122. Fulton, B. P., and K. Walton. Electrophysiological properties of neonatal rat motoneurones studied in vitro. *J. Physiol. (Lond.)* 370: 651–678, 1986.
123. Fuortes, M. G. F., K. Frank, and M. C. Becker. Steps in the production of motoneuron spikes. *J. Gen. Physiol.* 40: 735–752, 1957.
124. Fyffe, R. E. Spatial distribution of recurrent inhibitory synapses on spinal motoneurons in the cat. *J. Neurophysiol.* 65: 1134–1149, 1991.
125. Fyffe, R. E. W., F. J. Alvarez, J. C. Pearson, D. Harrington, and D. E. Dewey. Modulation of motoneuron activity: distribution of glycine receptors and serotonergic inputs on motoneuron dendrites. *Psychologist* 36: A11, 1993.
126. Gardiner, P. F. Physiological properties of motoneurons innervating different muscle unit types in rat gastrocnemius. *J. Neurophysiol.* 69: 1160–1170, 1993.
127. Garnett, R., and J. A. Stephens. Changes in the recruitment threshold of motor units produced by cutaneous stimulation in man. *J. Physiol. (Lond.)* 311: 463–473, 1981.
128. Gemperline, J. J. Disturbances of muscle activation in hemiparetic spasticity in man: an experimental and theoretical investigation into the contribution of abnormal motor unit discharge patterns to muscular weakness. Ph.D, Northwestern University, 1993.
129. Gottlieb, G. L., and G. C. Agarwal. Effects of initial conditions on the Hoffman reflex. *J. Neurol. Neurosurg. Psychiatry* 34: 226–230, 1971.
130. Granit, R., D. Kernell, and Y. Lamarre. Algebraical summation in synaptic activation of motoneurones firing within the 'primary range' to injected currents. *J. Physiol. (Lond.)* 187: 379–399, 1966.
131. Granit, R., D. Kernell, and G. K. Shortess. Quantitative aspects of repetitive firing of mammalian motoneurones, caused by injected currents. *J. Physiol. (Lond.)* 168: 911–931, 1963.
132. Granit, R., J. E. Pascoe, and G. Steg. The behavior of tonic α and γ motoneurones during stimulation of recurrent collaterals. *J. Physiol. (Lond.)* 138: 381–400, 1957.
133. Granit, R., and B. Renkin. Net depolarization and discharge rate of motoneurones, as measured by recurrent inhibition. *J. Physiol. (Lond.)* 158: 461–475, 1961.
134. Grillner, S., T. Hongo, and S. Lund. The vestibulospinal tract. Effects on alpha-motoneurones in the lumbosacral spinal cord in the cat. *Exp. Brain Res.* 10: 94–120, 1970.
135. Grimby, L., and J. Hannerz. Disturbances of voluntary recruitment order of low and frequency motor units on blockades of proprioceptive afferent activity. *Acta Physiol. Scand.* 96: 207–216, 1976.
136. Gustafsson, B. Afterpotentials and transduction properties in different types of central neurones. *Arch. Ital. Biol.* 122: 17–30, 1984.
137. Gustafsson, B., and M. J. Pinter. An investigation of threshold properties among cat spinal alpha-motoneurones. *J. Physiol. (Lond.)* 357: 453–483, 1984.
138. Gustafsson, B., and M. J. Pinter. Relations among passive electrical properties of lumbar alpha-motoneurones of the cat. *J. Physiol. (Lond.)* 356: 401–431, 1984.
139. Gustafsson, B., and M. J. Pinter. Factors determining the variation of the afterhyperpolarization duration in cat lumbar alpha-motoneurones. *Brain Res.* 326: 392–395, 1985.
140. Gutman, A. M. Bistability of dendrites. *Int. J. Neural Syst.* 1: 291–304, 1991.
141. Gydikov, A., and D. Kosarov. Physiological characteristics of the tonic and phasic motor units in human muscles. In: *Motor Control*, edited by A. Gydikov, N. Tankov, and D. Kosarov. New York: Plenum Press, 1973, p. 75–94.
142. Harada, Y., and T. Takahashi. The calcium component of the action potential in spinal motoneurones of the rat. *J. Physiol. (Lond.)* 335: 89–100, 1983.
143. Harrison, P. J. The relationship between the distribution of motor unit mechanical properties and the forces due to recruitment and to rate coding for the generation of muscle force. *Brain Res.* 264: 311–315, 1983.
144. Harrison, P. J., and A. Taylor. Individual excitatory post-synaptic potentials due to muscle spindle Ia afferents in cat triceps surae motoneurones. *J. Physiol. (Lond.)* 312: 455–470, 1981.
145. Heckman, C. J. Computer simulations of the effects of different synaptic input systems on the steady-state input-output structure of the motoneuron pool. *J. Neurophysiol.* 71: 1717–1739, 1994.
146. Heckman, C. J., and M. D. Binder. Analysis of effective synaptic currents generated by homonymous Ia afferent fibers in motoneurons of the cat. *J. Neurophysiol.* 60: 1946–1966, 1988.
147. Heckman, C. J., and M. D. Binder. Neural mechanisms underlying the orderly recruitment of motoneurons. In: *The Segmental Motor System*, edited by M. D. Binder and L. M. Mendell. New York: Oxford University Press, 1990, p. 182–204.
148. Heckman C. J., and M. D. Binder. Analysis of Ia-inhibitory synaptic input to cat spinal motoneurons evoked by vibration of antagonist muscles. *J. Neurophysiol.* 66: 1888–1893, 1991.
149. Heckman, C. J., and M. D. Binder. Computer simulation of the steady-state input-output function of the cat medial gastrocnemius motoneuron pool. *J. Neurophysiol.* 65: 952–967, 1991.
150. Heckman, C. J., and M. D. Binder. Computer simulations of motoneuron firing rate modulation. *J. Neurophysiol.* 69: 1005–1008, 1993.
151. Heckman, C. J., and M. D. Binder. Computer simulations of the effects of different synaptic input systems on motor unit recruitment. *J. Neurophysiol.* 70: 1827–1840, 1993.
152. Heckman, C. J., J. F. Miler, M. Munson, and W. Z. Rymer. Differences between steady-state and transient post-synaptic potentials elicited by stimulation of the sural nerve. *Exp. Brain Res.* 91: 167–170, 1992.
153. Heckman, C. J., J. L. Weytjens, and G. E. Loeb. Effect of velocity and mechanical history on the forces of motor units in the cat medial gastrocnemius muscle. *J. Neurophysiol.* 68: 1503–1515, 1992.
154. Henneman, E. Comments on the logical basis of muscle control. In: *The Segmental Motor System,* edited by M. D. Binder and L. M. Mendell. New York: Oxford University Press, 1990, p. vi–x.
155. Henneman, E., H. P. Clamann, J. D. Gillies, and R. D. Skinner. Rank order of motoneurons within a pool: law of combination. *J. Neurophysiol.* 37: 1338–1349, 1974.
156. Henneman, E., and L. M. Mendell. Functional organization of motoneuron pool and its inputs. In: *Handbook of Physiology, The Nervous System, Motor Control,* edited by V. B. Brooks. Bethesda, MD: Am. Physiol. Soc., 1981, p. 423–507.

157. Henneman, E., and C. B. Olson. Relations between structure and function in the design of skeletal muscle. *J. Neurophysiol.* 28: 581–598, 1965.
158. Henneman, E., G. Somjen, and D. O. Carpenter. Excitability and inhibitability of motoneurons of different sizes. *J. Neurophysiol.* 28: 599–620, 1965.
159. Hille, B. *Ionic Channels of Excitable Membranes*, 2nd ed. Sunderland, MA: Sinauer Associates, Inc., 1992.
160. Hodgkin, A. L., and A. F. Huxley. A quantitative description of membrane current and its application to conduction and excitation in nerve. *J. Physiol. (Lond.)* 116: 500–544, 1952.
161. Hodgkin, A. L., and S. Nakajima. The effect of diameter on the electrical constants of frog skeletal muscle fibres. *J. Physiol. (Lond.)* 221: 105–120, 1972.
162. Hoffer, J. A., N. Sugano, G. E. Loeb, W. B. Marks, M. J. O'Donovan, and C. A. Pratt. Cat hindlimb motoneurons during locomotion. II. Normal activity patterns. *J. Neurophysiol.* 57: 530–553, 1987.
163. Hongo, T., E. Jankowska, and A. Lundberg. The rubrospinal tract. I. Effects on alpha-motoneurones innervating hindlimb muscles in cats. *Exp. Brain Res.* 7: 344–364, 1969.
164. Hounsgaard, J., H. Hultborn, B. Jespersen, and O. Kiehn. Bistability of alpha-motoneurones in the decerebrate cat and in the acute spinal cat after intravenous 5-hydroxytryptophan. *J. Physiol. (Lond.)* 405: 345–367, 1988.
165. Hounsgaard, J., and O. Kiehn. Serotonin-induced bistability of turtle motoneurones caused by a nifedipine-sensitive calcium plateau otential. *J. Physiol. (Lond.)* 414: 265–282, 1989.
166. Hounsgaard, J., O. Kiehn, and I. Mintz. Response properties of motoneurones in a slice preparation of the turtle spinal cord. *J. Physiol. (Lond.)* 398: 575–589, 1988.
167. Hounsgaard, J., and J. Midtgaard. Dendrite processing in more ways than one. *Trends Neurosci.* 12: 313–315, 1989
168. Hounsgaard, J., and O. Kichn. Calcium spikes and calcium plateaux evoked by differential polarization in dendrites of turtle mononeurones in vitro. *J. Physiol. (Lond.)* 468: 245–259, 1993.
169. Howe, J. R., and J. M. Ritchie. Multiple kinetic components of sodium channel inactivation in rabbit Schwann cells. *J. Physiol. (Lond.)* 455: 529–566, 1992.
170. Hultborn, H., R. Katz, and R. Mackel. Distribution of recurrent inhibition within a motor nucleus. II. Amount of recurrent inhibition in motoneurons to fast and slow units. *Acta Physiol. Scand.* 134: 363–374, 1988.
171. Hultborn, H., and O. Kiehn. Neuromodulation of vertebrate motor neuron membrane properties. *Curr. Opin. Neurobiol.* 2: 770–775, 1992.
172. Hultborn, H., S. Lindstrom, and H. Wigstrom. On the function of recurrent inhibition in the spinal cord. *Exp. Brain Res.* 37: 399–403, 1979.
173. Iansek, R., and S. J. Redman. The amplitude, time course and charge of unitary excitatory post-synaptic potentials evoked in spinal motoneurone dendrites. *J. Physiol. (Lond.)* 234: 665–688, 1973.
174. Jack, J. J., S. J. Redman, and K. Wong. The components of synaptic potentials evoked in cat spinal motoneurones by impulses in single group Ia afferents. *J. Physiol. (Lond.)* 321: 65–96, 1981.
175. Jack, J. J. B., D. Noble, and R. W. Tsien. *Electric Current Flow in Excitable Cells.* Oxford: Clarendon Press, 1975.
176. Jacobs, B. L., and C. A. Fornal. 5-HT and motor control: a hypothesis. *Trends Neurosci.* 6: 346–352, 1993.
177. Jahr, C. E., and K. Yoshioka. Ia afferent excitation of motoneurones in the in vitro new-born rat spinal cord is selectively antagonized by kynurenate. *J. Physiol. (Lond.)* 370: 515–530, 1986.
178. Jankowska, E. Interneuronal relay in spinal pathways from proprioceptors. *Prog. Neurobiol.* 38: 335–378, 1992.
179. Jodkowski, J. S., F. Viana, T. E. Dick, and A. J. Berger. Repetitive firing properties of phrenic motoneurons in the cat. *J. Neurophysiol.* 60: 687–702, 1988.
180. Joyce, G. C., P. M. H. Rack, and D. R. Westbury. The mechanical properties of cat soleus muscle during controlled lengthening and shortening movements. *J. Physiol. (Lond.)* 204: 461–474, 1969.
181. Kalb, R. G., M. S. Lidow, M. J. Halsted, and S. Hockfield. *N*-Methyl-D-aspartate receptors are transiently expressed in the developing spinal cord ventral horn. *Proc. Natl. Acad. Sci. U. S. A.* 89: 8502–8506, 1992.
182. Kanda, K., R. E. Burke, and B. Walmsley. Differential control of fast and slow twitch motor units in the decerebrate cat. *Exp. Brain. Res.* 29: 57–74, 1977.
183. Kanosue, K., M. Yoshida, K. Akazawa, and K. Fuji. The number of active motor units and their firing rates in voluntary contraction of human brachialis muscle. *Jpn. J. Physiol.* 29: 427–444, 1979.
184. Katakura, N., and S. H. Chandler. An iontophoretic analysis of the pharmacologic mechanisms responsible for trigeminal motoneuronal discharge during masticatory-like activity in the guinea pig. *J. Neurophysiol.* 63: 356–369, 1990.
185. Katakura, N., and S. H. Chandler. Iontophoretic analysis of the pharmacologic mechanisms responsible for initiation and modulation of trigeminal motoneuronal discharge evoked by intra-oral afferent stimulation. *Brain Res.* 549: 66–77, 1991.
186. Kellerth, J., C. Berthold, and S. Conradi. Electron microscopic studies of serially sectioned cat spinal a-motoneurons: III. Motoneurons innervating fast-twitch (type FR) units of the gastrocnemius muscle. *J. Comp. Neurol.* 184: 755–768, 1979.
187. Kellerth, J., S. Conradi, and C. Berthold. Electron microscopic studies of serially sectioned cat spinal α-motoneurons: V. Motoneurons innervating fast-twitch (type FF) units of the gastrocnemius muscle. *J. Comp. Neurol.* 214: 451–458, 1983.
188. Kernell, D. The delayed depolarization in cat and rat motoneurons. *Prog. Brain Res.* 12: 42–55, 1964.
189. Kernell, D. The adaptation and the relation between discharge frequency and current strength of cat lumbosacral motoneurones stimulated by long-lasting injected currents. *Acta Physiol. Scand.* 65: 65–73, 1965.
190. Kernell, D. High frequency repetitive firing of cat lumbosacral motoneurones stimulated by long-lasting injected currents. *Acta Physiol. Scand.* 65: 74–86, 1965.
191. Kernell, D. The limits of firing frequency in cat lumbosacral motoneurones possessing different time course of afterhyperpolarization. *Acta Physiol. Scand.* 65: 87–100, 1965.
192. Kernell, D. Input resistance, electrical excitability and size of ventral horn cells in cat spinal cord. *Science* 152: 1637–1640, 1966.
193. Kernell, D. The repetitive discharge of motoneurones. In: *Muscular Afferents and Motor Control. Nobel Symp. I,* edited by R. Granit. Stockholm: Almqvist and Wiksell, 1966, p. 351–362.
194. Kernell, D. The repetitive impulse discharge of a simple neurone model compared to that of spinal motoneurones. *Brain Res.* 11: 685–687, 1968.

195. Kernell, D. Synaptic conductance changes and the repetitive impulse discharge of spinal motoneurones. *Brain Res.* 15: 291–294, 1970.
196. Kernell, D. Rhythmic properties of motoneurones innervating muscle fibres of different speed in m. gastrocnemius medialis of the cat. *Brain Res.* 160: 159–162, 1979.
197. Kernell, D. Functional properties of spinal motoneurons and gradation of muscle force. *Adv. Neurol.* 39: 213–226, 1983.
198. Kernell, D., O. Eerbeek, and B. A. Verhey. Relation between isometric force and stimulus rate in cat's hindlimb motor units of different twitch contraction time. *Exp. Brain Res.* 50: 220–227, 1983.
199. Kernell, D., and H. Hultborn. Synaptic effects on recruitment gain: a mechanism of importance for the input-output relations of motoneurone pools? *Brain Res.* 507: 176–179, 1990.
200. Kernell, D., and A. W. Monster. Threshold current for repetitive impulse firing in motoneurones innervating muscle fibres of different fatigue sensitivity in the cat. *Brain Res.* 229: 193–196, 1981.
201. Kernell, D., and A. W. Monster. Time course and properties of late adaptation in spinal motoneurones of the cat. *Exp. Brain Res.* 46: 191–196, 1982.
202. Kernell, D., and H. Sjoholm. Repetitive impulse firing: comparisons between neurone models based on 'voltage clamp equations' and spinal motoneurones. *Acta Physiol. Scand.* 87: 40–56, 1973.
203. Kernell, D., and B. Zwaagstra. Input conductance, axonal conduction velocity and cell size among hindlimb motoneurones of the cat. *Brain Res.* 204: 311– 26, 1980.
204. Kernell, D., and B. Zwaagstra. Dendrites of cat's spinal motoneurones: relationship between stem diameter and predicted input conductance. *J. Physiol. (Lond.)* 413: 255–269, 1989.
205. Kernell, D., and B. Zwaagstra. Size and remoteness: two relatively independent parameters of dendrites, as studied for spinal motoneurones of the cat. *J. Physiol. (Lond.)* 413: 233–254, 1989.
206. Kiehn, O. Plateau potentials and active integration in the 'final common pathway' for motor behaviour. *Trends Neurosci.* 14: 68–73, 1991.
207. Kiehn, O., E. Erdal, T. Eken, and T. Bruhn. Selective depletion of spinal monoamines changes for the soleus EMG from a tonic to a more phasic pattern *J. Physiol. (Lond.)* in press, 1995.
208. Kiehn, O., and R. M. Harris-Warrick. 5-HT modulation of hyperpolarization-activated inward current and calcium-dependent outward current in a crustacean motor neuron. *J. Neurophysiol.* 68: 496–508, 1992.
209. Kiehn, O., and R. M. Harris-Warrick. Serotonergic stretch receptors induce plateau properties in a crustacean motor neuron by a dual-conductance mechanism. *J. Neurophysiol.* 68: 485–495, 1992.
210. Koch, C. Cable theory in neurons with active, linearized membranes. *Biol. Cybern.* 50: 15–33, 1984.
211. Krnjević, K., Y. Lamour, J. F. MacDonald, and A. Nistri. Effects of some divalent cations on motoneurones in cats. *Can. J. Physiol. Pharmacol.* 57: 944–956, 1979.
212. Krnjević, K., and A. Lisiewicz. Injections of calcium ions into spinal motoneurones. *J. Physiol. (Lond.)* 225: 363–390, 1972.
213. Krnjević, K., E. Puil, and R. Werman. EGTA and motoneuronal after-potentials. *J. Physiol. (Lond.)* 275: 199–223, 1978.
214. Kukulka, C. G., and H. P. Clamann. Comparison of the recruitment and discharge properties of motor units in human brachial biceps and adductor pollicis during isometric contractions. *Brain Res.* 219: 45–55, 1981.
215. Kuno, M., and R. Llinas. Enhancement of synaptic action in chromatolyzed motoneurones of the cat. *J. Physiol. (Lond.)* 210: 807–821, 1970.
216. LaBella, L. A., J. P. Kehler, and D. A. McCrea. A differential synaptic input to the motor nuclei in triceps surae from the caudal and lateral cutaneous sural nerves. *J. Neurophysiol.* 61: 291–301, 1989.
217. Larkman, P. M., and J. S. Kelly. Ionic mechanisms mediating 5-hydroxytryptamine- and noradrenaline-evoked depolarization of adult rat facial motoneurones. *J. Physiol. (Lond.)* 456: 473–490, 1992.
218. Lev-Tov, A., J. P. Miller, R. E. Burke, and W. Rall. Factors that control amplitude of EPSPs in dendritic neurons. *J. Neurophysiol.* 50: 399–412, 1983.
219. Liddell, E. G. T., and C. S. Sherrington. Recruitment and some other factors of reflex inhibition. *Proc. R. Soc. Lond. B* 97: 488–518, 1925.
220. Lindsay, A. D., and M. D. Binder. Distribution of effective synaptic currents underlying recurrent inhibition in cat triceps surae motoneurons. *J. Neurophysiol.* 65: 168–177, 1991.
221. Lindsay, A. D., and J. L. Feldman. Modulation of respiratory activity of neonatal rat phrenic motoneurones by serotonin. *J. Physiol. (Lond.)* 461: 213–233, 1993.
222. Matthews, P. B. C. Observations on the automatic compensation of reflex gain on varying the pre-existing level of motor discharge in man. *J. Physiol. (Lond.)* 374: 73–90, 1986.
223. Mayer, M. L., and G. L. Westbrook. The physiology of excitatory amino acids in the vertebrate central nervous system. *Prog. Neurobiol.* 28: 197–276, 1987.
224. Milner-Brown, H. S., R. B. Stein, and R. Yemm. The contractile properties of human motor units during voluntary isometric contractions. *J. Physiol. (Lond.)* 228: 285–306, 1973.
225. Milner-Brown, H. S., R. B. Stein, and R. Yemm. The orderly recruitment of human motor units during voluntary isometric contractions. *J. Physiol. (Lond.)* 230: 359–370, 1973.
226. Monster, A. W. Firing rate behavior of human motor units during isometric voluntary contraction: relation to unit size. *Brain Res.* 171: 349–354, 1979.
227. Monster, A. W., and H. Chan. Isometric force production by motor units of extensor digitorum communis muscle in man. *J. Neurophysiol.* 40: 1432–1443, 1977.
228. Moore, J. A., and K. Appenteng. The membrane properties and firing characteristics of rat jaw-elevator motoneurones. *J. Physiol. (Lond.)* 423: 137–153, 1990.
229. Moore, J. A., and K. Appenteng. The morphology and electrical geometry of the rat jaw-elevator motoneurones. *J. Physiol. (Lond.)* 440: 325–343, 1991.
230. Moore, J. W., N. Stockbridge, and M. Westerfield. On the site of impulse initiation in a neurone. *J. Physiol. (Lond.)* 336: 301–311, 1983.
231. Moore, J. W., and M. Westerfield. Action potential propagation and threshold parameters in inhomogeneous regions of squid axons. *J. Physiol. (Lond.)* 336: 301–311, 1983.
232. Moore, L. E., and J. T. Buchanan. The effects of neurotransmitters on the integrative properties of spinal neurons in the lamprey. *J. Exp. Biol.* 175: 89–114, 1993.

233. Moore, L. E., R. H. Hill, and S. Grillner. Voltage-clamp frequency domain analysis of NMDA-activated neurons. *J. Exp. Biol.* 175: 59–87, 1993.
234. Moore, L. E., K. Yoshii, and B. N. Christensen. Transfer impedances between different regions of branched excitable cells. *J. Neurophysiol.* 59: 689–705, 1988.
235. Mosfeldt-Laursen, A., and J. C. Rekling. Electrophysiological properties of hypoglossal motoneurons of guinea-pigs studied in vitro. *Neuroscience* 30: 619–637, 1989.
236. Munson, J. B. Synaptic inputs to type-identified motor units. In: *The Segmental Motor System*, edited by M. D. Binder and L. M. Mendell. New York: Oxford University Press, 1990, p. 291–307.
237. Munson, J. B., J. W. Fleshman, and G. W. Sypert. Properties of single-fiber spindle group II EPSPs in triceps surae motoneurons. *J. Neurophysiol.* 44: 713–725, 1980.
238. Mynlieff, M., and K. G. Beam. Characterization of voltage-dependent calcium currents in mouse motoneurons. *J. Neurophysiol.* 68: 85–92, 1992.
239. Nardone, A., C. Romano, and M. Schieppati. Selective recruitment of high-threshold human motor units during voluntary isotonic lengthening of active muscle. *J. Physiol. (Lond.)* 409: 451–471, 1989.
240. Nelson, P. G., and R. E. Burke. Delayed depolarization in cat spinal motoneurons. *Exp. Neurol.* 17: 16–26, 1967.
241. Nelson, P. G., and K. Frank. Orthodromically produced changes in motoneuronal extracellular fields. *J. Neurophysiol.* 27: 928–941, 1964.
242. Nicoll, A., A. Larkman, and C. Blakemore. Modulation of EPSP shape and efficacy by intrinsic membrane conductances in rat neocortical pyramidal neurons *in vitro*. *J. Physiol. (Lond.)* 468: 693–710, 1993.
243. Nishimura, Y., P. C. Schwindt, and W. E. Crill. Electrical properties of facial motoneurons in brainstem slices from guinea pig. *Brain Res.* 502: 127–142, 1989.
244. Nistri, A., N. D. Fisher, and M. Gurnell. Block by the neuropeptide TRH of an apparently novel K^+ conductance of rat motoneurones. *Neurosci. Lett.* 120: 25–30, 1990.
245. Partridge, L. D., and L. A. Benton. Muscle, the motor. In: *Handbook of Physiology, The Nervous System, Motor Control,* edited by V. B. Brooks. Bethesda, MD: Am. Physiol. Soc., 1981, p. 43–106.
246. Petit, J., M. Chua, and C. C. Hunt. Maximum shortening speed of motor units of various types in cat lumbrical muscles. *J. Neurophysiol.* 69: 442–448, 1993.
247. Petit, J., G. M. Filippi, F. Emonet-Denand, C. C. Hunt, and Y. Laporte. Changes in muscle stiffness produced by motor units of different types in peroneus longus muscle of cat. *J. Neurophysiol.* 63: 190–197, 1990.
248. Pinco, M., and Lev-Tov, A. Synaptic excitation of alpha-motoneurons by dorsal root afferents in the neonatal rat spinal cord. *J. Neurophysiol.* 70: 406–417, 1993.
249. Pinter, M. J., R. L. Curtis, and M. J. Hosko. Voltage threshold and excitability among variously sized cat hindlimb motoneurons. *J. Neurophysiol.* 50: 644–657, 1983.
250. Powers, R. K. A variable-threshold motoneuron model that incorporates time-dependent and voltage-dependent potassium and calcium conductances. *J. Neurophysiol.* 70: 246–262, 1993.
251. Powers, R. K., and M. D. Binder. Determination of afferent fibers mediating oligosynaptic group I input to cat medial gastrocnemius motoneurons. *J. Neurophysiol.* 53: 518–529, 1985.
252. Powers, R. K., and M. D. Binder. Distribution of oligosynaptic group I input to the cat medial gastrocnemius motoneuron pool. *J. Neurophysiol.* 53: 497–517, 1985.
253. Powers, R. K., and M. D. Binder. Effects of low-frequency stimulation on the tension-frequency relations of fast-twitch motor units in the cat. *J. Neurophysiol.* 66: 905–918, 1991.
254. Powers, R. K., and M. D. Binder. Summation of motor unit tensions in the tibialis posterior muscle of the cat under isometric and nonisometric conditions. *J. Neurophysiol.* 66: 1838–1846, 1991.
255. Powers, R. K., and M. D. Binder. Quantitative analysis of motoneurone firing rate modulation in response to simulated synaptic inputs. In: *Alpha and Gamma Motor Systems*, edited by A. Taylor and M. Gladden. New York: Plenum Press, in press, 1995.
256. Powers, R. K., and M. D. Binder. Effective synaptic current and motoneuron firing rate modulation. *J. Neurophysiol.* 74: 793–801, 1995.
257. Powers, R. K., F. R. Robinson, M. A. Konodi, and M. D. Binder. Summation of effective synaptic currents and firing rate modulation in cat triceps surae motoneurons produced by concurrent stimulation of different synaptic input systems. *Soc. Neurosci. Abstr.* 17: 645, 1991.
258. Powers, R. K., F. R. Robinson, M. A. Konodi, and M. D. Binder. Effective synaptic current can be estimated from measurements of neuronal discharge. *J. Neurophysiol.* 68: 964–968, 1992.
259. Powers, R. K., F. R. Robinson, M. A. Konodi, and M. D. Binder. Distribution of rubrospinal synaptic input to cat triceps surae motoneurons. *J. Neurophysiol.* 70: 1460–1468, 1993.
260. Powers, R. K., and W. Z. Rymer. Effects of acute dorsal spinal hemisection on motoneuron discharge in the medial gastrocnemius of the decerebrate cat. *J. Neurophysiol.* 59: 1540–1556, 1988.
261. Pratt, C. A., C. M. Chanaud, and G. E. Loeb. Functionally complex muscles of the cat hindlimb. 4. Intramuscular distribution of movement command signals and cutaneous reflexes in broad, bifunctional thigh muscles. *Exp. Brain Res.* 85: 281–299, 1991.
262. Pratt, C. A., and G. E. Loeb. Functionally complex muscles of the cat hindlimb. 1. Patterns of activation across sartorius. *Exp. Brain Res.* 85: 243–256, 1991.
263. Puil, E., B. Gimbarzevsky, and I. Spigelman. Primary involvement of K+ conductance in membrane resonance of trigeminal root ganglion neurons. *J. Neurophysiol.* 59: 77–89, 1988.
264. Puil, E., H. Meiri, and Y. Yarom. Resonant behavior and frequency preferences of thalamic neurons. *J. Neurophysiol.* 71: 575–582, 1994.
265. Rack, P. M. H., and D. R. Westbury. The effects of length and stimulus rate on tension in the isometric cat soleus muscle. *J. Physiol. (Lond.)* 204: 443–460, 1969.
266. Rajaofetra, N., J. L. Ridet, P. Poulat, L. Marlier, F. Sandillon, M. Geffard, and A. Privat. Immunocytochemical mapping of noradrenergic projections to the rat spinal cord with an antiserum against noradrenaline. *J. Neurocytol.* 21: 481–494, 1992.
267. Rall, W. A statistical theory of monosynaptic input-output relations. *J. Cell. Comp. Physiol.* 46: 373–412, 1955.
268. Rall, W. Branching dendritic trees and motoneuron membrane resistivity. *Exp. Neurol.* 1: 491–527, 1959.
269. Rall, W. Core conductor theory and cable properties of neurons. In: *Handbook of Physiology, The Nervous System, Cellular Biology of Neurons*, edited by E. R. Kandel. Bethesda, MD: Am. Physiol. Soc., 1977, p. 39–97.
270. Rall, W., R. E. Burke, W. R. Holmes, J. J. Jack, S. J. Redman, and I. Segev. Matching dendritic neuron models to

experimental data. *Physiol. Rev.* 72, No. 4 (Suppl.): S159–S186, 1992.
271. Rall, W., R. E. Burke, T. G. Smith, P. G Nelson, and K. Frank. Dendritic location of synapses and possible mechanisms for the monosynaptic EPSP in motoneurons. *J. Neurophysiol.* 30: 1169–1193, 1967.
272. Rall, W., and C. C. Hunt. Analysis of reflex variability in terms of partially correlated excitability fluctuations in a population of motoneurons. *J. Gen. Physiol.* 39: 397–422, 1956.
273. Redman, S. A. quantitative approach to the integrative function of dendrites. In: *International Review of Physiology: Neurophysiology,* edited by R. Porter. Baltimore: University Park Press, 1976, p. 1–35.
274. Redman, S. J., E. M. McLachlan, and G. D. Hirst. Nonuniform passive membrane properties of rat lumbar sympathetic ganglion cells. *J. Neurophysiol.* 57: 633–644, 1987.
275. Redman, S. J., and B. Walmsley. The time course of synaptic potentials evoked in cat spinal motoneurones at identified group Ia synapses. *J. Physiol. (Lond.)* 343: 117–133, 1983.
276. Rekling, J. C. Interaction between thyrotropin-releasing hormone (TRH) and NMDA-receptor-mediated responses in hypoglossal motoneurones. *Brain Res.* 578: 289–296, 1992.
277. Richter, D. W., W. R. Schlue, K. H. Mauritz, and A. C. Nacimiento. Comparison of membrane properties of the cell body and the initial part of the axon of phasic motoneurones in the spinal cord of the cat. *Exp. Brain Res.* 21: 193–206, 1974.
278. Riek, S., and P. Bawa. Recruitment of motor units in human forearm extensors. *J. Neurophysiol.* 68: 100–108, 1992.
279. Romaiguere, P., J.- P. Vedel, S. Pagni, and A. Zenatti. Physiological properties of the motor units of the wrist extensor muscles in man. *Exp. Brain Res.* 78: 51–61, 1989.
280. Romaiguere, P., J. P. Vedel, and S. Pagni. Fluctuations in motor unit recruitment threshold during slow isometric contractions of wrist extensor muscles in man. *Neurosci. Lett.* 103: 50–55, 1989.
281. Romaiguere, P., J. P. Vedel, and S. Pagni. Effects of tonic vibration reflex on motor unit recruitment in human wrist extensor muscles. *Brain Res.* 602: 32–40, 1993.
282. Rose, P. K., and P. Brennan. Somatic shunts in neck motoneurons of the cat. *Soc. Neurosci. Abstr.* 15: 922, 1989.
283. Rose, P. K., S. A. Keirstead, and S. J. Vanner. A quantitative analysis of the geometry of cat motoneurons innervating neck and shoulder muscles. *J. Comp. Neurol.* 238: 89–107, 1985.
284. Rose, P. K., and H. M. Neuber. Morphology and frequency of axon terminals on the somata, proximal dendrites, and distal dendrites of dorsal neck motoneurons in the cat. *J. Comp. Neurol.* 307: 259–280, 1991.
285. Rose, P. K., and S. J. Vanner. Differences in somatic and dendritic specific membrane resistivity of spinal motoneurons: an electrophysiological study of neck and shoulder motoneurons in the cat. *J. Neurophysiol.* 60: 149–166, 1988.
286. Rosenblueth, A., N. Wiener, W. Pitts, and J. Garcia-Ramos. A statistical analysis of synaptic excitation. *J. Cell. Comp. Physiol.* 34: 173–205, 1949.
287. Rudomin, P. Presynaptic control of synaptic effectiveness of muscle spindle and tendon organ afferents in the mammalian spinal cord. In: *The Segmental Motor System*, edited by M. D. Binder and L. M. Mendell. New York: Oxford University Press, 1990, p. 349–380.
288. Rudy, B. Diversity and ubiquity of K channels. *Neuroscience* 25: 729–749, 1988.
289. Sah, P. Role of calcium influx and buffering in the kinetics of $Ca(2^+)$ activated K^+ current in rat vagal motoneurons. *J. Neurophysiol.* 68: 2237–2247, 1992.
290. Saha, S., K. Appenteng, and T. F. Batten. Light and electron microscopical localisation of 5-HT-immunoreactive boutons in the rat trigeminal motor nucleus. *Brain Res.* 559: 145–148, 1991.
291. Sawczuk, A. Adaptation in sustained motoneuron discharge. PhD., University of Washington, 1993.
292. Sawczuk, A., and M. D. Binder. Reduction of Na^+–K^+ activity does not reduce the late adaptation of motoneuron discharge. *Soc. Neurosci. Abstr.* 18: 512, 1992.
293. Sawczuk, A., and M. D. Binder. Reduction of the AHP with Mn^{++} decreases the initial adaptation, but increases the late adaptation in rat hypoglossal motoneuron discharge. *Physiologist* 36: A23, 1993.
294. Sawczuk, A., R. K. Powers, and M. D. Binder. Intrinsic properties of motoneurons: implications for muscle fatigue. In: *Fatigue: Neural and Muscular Mechanisms*, edited by S. Gandevia, R. Enoka, A. McComas, D. Stuart, and C. Thomas. New York: Plenum, 1995, p. 123–134.
295. Sawczuk, A., R. K. Powers, and M. D. Binder. Spike-frequency adaptation studied in hypoglossal motoneurons of the rat *J. Neurophysiol.* 73: 1799–1810, 1995.
296. Schlue, W. R., D. W. Richter, K. H. Mauritz, and A. C. Nacimiento. Mechanisms of accommodation to linearly rising currents in cat spinal motoneurones. *J. Neurophysiol.* 37: 310–315, 1974.
297. Schwindt, P. C. Membrane-potential trajectories underlying motoneuron rhythmic firing at high rates. *J. Neurophysiol.* 36: 434–439, 1973.
298. Schwindt, P. C., and W. E. Crill. A persistent negative resistance in cat lumbar motoneurons. *Brain Res.* 120: 173–178, 1977.
299. Schwindt, P. C., and W. H. Calvin. Membrane potential trajectories between spikes underlying motoneuron rhythmic firing. *J. Neurophysiol.* 35: 311–325, 1972.
300. Schwindt, P. C., and W. H. Calvin. Equivalence of synaptic and injected current in determining the membrane potential trajectory during motoneuron rhythmic firing. *Brain Res.* 59: 389–394, 1973.
301. Schwindt, P. C., and W. H. Calvin. Nature of conductances underlying rhythmic firing in cat spinal motoneurons. *J. Neurophysiol.* 36: 955–973, 1973.
302. Schwindt, P. C., and W. E. Crill. Effects of barium on cat spinal motoneurons studied by voltage clamp. *J. Neurophysiol.* 44: 827–846, 1980.
303. Schwindt, P. C., and W. E. Crill. Properties of a persistent inward current in normal and TEA-injected motoneurons. *J. Neurophysiol.* 43: 1700–1724, 1980.
304. Schwindt, P. C., and W. E. Crill. Role of a persistent inward current in motoneuron bursting during spinal seizures. *J. Neurophysiol.* 43: 1296–1318, 1980.
305. Schwindt, P. C., and W. E. Crill. Differential effects of TEA and cations on outward ionic currents of cat motoneurons. *J. Neurophysiol.* 46: 1–16, 1981.
306. Schwindt, P. C., and W. E. Crill. Negative slope conductance at large depolarizations in cat spinal motoneurons. *Brain Res.* 207: 471–475, 1981.
307. Schwindt, P. C., and W. E. Crill. Factors influencing motoneuron rhythmic firing: results from a voltage-clamp study. *J. Neurophysiol.* 48: 875–890, 1982.

308. Scott, R. H., H. A. Pearson, and A. C. Dolphin. Aspects of vertebrate neuronal voltage-activated calcium currents and their regulation. *Prog. Neurobiol.* 36: 485–520, 1991.
309. Scroggs, R. S., S. M. Todorovic, E. G. Anderson, and A. P. Fox. Variation in I_H, I_{IR}, and I_{LEAK} between acutely isolated adult rat dorsal root ganglion neurons of different size. *J. Neurophysiol.* 71: 271–279, 1994.
310. Segev, I., J. W. J. Fleshman, and R. E. Burke. Computer simulation of group Ia EPSPs using morphologically realistic models of cat alpha-motoneurons. *J. Neurophysiol.* 64: 648–660, 1990.
311. Sernagor, E., Y. Yarom, and R. Werman. Sodium-dependent regenerative responses in dendrites of axotomized motoneurons in the cat. *Proc. Natl. Acad. Sci. U. S. A.* 83: 7966–7970, 1986.
312. Shapovalov, A. I. Extrapyramidal monosynaptic and disynaptic control of mammalian alpha-motoneurons. *Brain Res.* 40: 105–115, 1972.
313. Shinoda, Y., T. Ohgaki, T. Futami, and Y. Sugiuchi. Structural basis for three-dimensional coding in the vestibulospinal reflex. *Ann. N. Y. Acad. Sci.* 545: 216–227, 1988.
314. Shinoda, Y., T. Ohgaki, T. Futami, and Y. Sugiuchi. Vestibular projections to the spinal cord: the morphology of single vestibulospinal axons. *Prog. Brain Res.* 76: 17–27, 1988.
315. Slot. P. J., and T. Sinkjær. Simulations of the alpha motoneuron pool electromyogram reflex at different preactivation levels in man. *Biol. Cybern.* 70: 351–358, 1994.
316. Smith, J. L., B. Betts, V. R. Edgerton, and R. Zernicke. Rapid ankle extension during paw shakes: selective recruitment of fast ankle extensors. *J. Neurophysiol.* 43: 612–620, 1980.
317. Spain, W. J., P. C. Schwindt, and W. E. Crill. Post-inhibitory excitation and inhibition in layer V pyramidal neurones from cat sensorimotor cortex. *J. Physiol. (Lond.)* 434: 609–626, 1991.
318. Spruston, N., and D. Johnston. Perforated patch-clamp analysis of the passive membrane properties of three classes of hippocampal neurons. *J. Neurophysiol.* 67: 508–529, 1992.
319. Stafstrom, C. E., P. C. Schwindt, M. C. Chubb, and W. E. Crill. Properties of persistent sodium conductance and calcium conductance of layer V neurons from cat sensorimotor cortex in vitro. *J. Neurophysiol.* 53: 153–170, 1985
320. Staley, K. J., T. S. Otis, and I. Mody. Membrane properties of dentate gyrus granule cells: comparison of sharp microelectrode and whole-cell recordings. *J. Neurophysiol.* 67: 1346–1358, 1992.
321. Stauffer, E. K., D. G. Watt, A. Taylor, R. M. Reinking, and D. G. Stuart. Analysis of muscle receptor connections by spike-triggered averaging. 2. Spindle group II afferents. *J. Neurophysiol.* 39: 1393–1402, 1976.
322. Stefani, E., and A. B. Steinbach. Resting potential and electrical properties of frog slow muscle fibers. Effect of different external solutions. *J. Physiol. (Lond.)* 203: 383–401, 1969.
323. Stein, R. B., and R. Bertoldi. The size principle: A synthesis of neurophysiological data. In: *Progress in Clinical Neurophysiology. Motor Unit Types, Recruitment and Plasticity in Health and Disease*, edited by J. E. Desmedt. Basel: Karger, 1981, p. 85–96.
324. Stephens, J. A., R. M. Reinking, and D. G. Stuart. The motor units of cat medial gastrocnemius: electrical and mechanical properties as a function of muscle length. *J. Morphol.* 146: 495–512, 1975.
325. Stuart, G. J., and S. J. Redman. Voltage dependence of Ia reciprocal inhibitory currents in cat spinal motoneurones. *J. Physiol. (Lond.)* 420: 111–125, 1990.
326. Sypert, G. W., and J. B. Munson. Basis of segmental motor control: motoneuron size or motor unit type? *Neurosurgery* 8: 608–621, 1981.
327. Takahashi, T. Inward rectification in neonatal rat spinal motoneurones. *J. Physiol. (Lond.)* 423: 47–62, 1990.
328. Takahashi, T. Membrane currents in visually identified motoneurones of neonatal rat spinal cord. *J. Physiol. (Lond.)* 423: 27–46, 1990.
329. Takahashi, T., and A. J. Berger. Direct excitation of rat spinal motoneurones by serotonin. *J. Physiol. (Lond.)* 423: 63–76, 1990.
330. Tanji, J., and M. Kato. Firing rate of individual motor units in voluntary contraction of abductor digiti minimi muscle in man. *Exp. Neurol.* 40: 771–783, 1973.
331. Tax, A. A. M., and J. J. Denier van der Gon. A model for neural control of gradation of muscle force. *Biol. Cybern.* 65: 227–234, 1991.
332. ter Haar Romeny, B. M., J. J. van der Gon, and C. C. Gielen. Relation between location of a motor unit in the human biceps brachii and its critical firing levels for different tasks. *Exp. Neurol.* 85: 631–650, 1984.
333. Terzuolo, C. A., and T. Araki. An analysis of intra- versus extracellular potential changes associated with activity of single spinal motoneurons. *Ann. N.Y. Acad. Sci.* 94: 547–558, 1961.
334. Thomas, C. K., B. Bigland-Ritchie, G. Westling, and R. S. Johansson. A comparison of human thenar motor-unit properties studied by intraneural motor-axon stimulation and spike-triggered averaging. *J. Neurophysiol.* 64: 1347–1351, 1990.
335. Thomas, C. K., R. S. Johansson, G. Westling, and B. Bigland-Ritchie. Twitch properties of human thenar motor units measured in response to intraneural motor-axon stimulation. *J. Neurophysiol.* 64: 1339–1346, 1990.
336. Thomas, C. K., B. H. Ross, and B. Calancie. Human motor-unit recruitment during isometric contractions and repeated dynamic movements. *J. Neurophysiol.* 57: 311–324, 1987.
337. Thomas, C. K., B. H. Ross, and R. B. Stein. Motor-unit recruitment in human first dorsal interosseous muscle for static contractions in three different directions. *J. Neurophysiol.* 55: 1017–1029, 1986.
338. Toft, E., T. Sinkjær, S. Andreassen, and K. Larsen. Mechanical and electromyographic responses to stretch of the human ankle extensors. *J. Neurophysiol.* 65: 1402–1410, 1991.
339. Traub, R. D. Motoneurons of different geometry and the size principle. *Biol. Cybern.* 25: 163–176, 1977.
340. Traub, R. D., and R. Llinas. The spatial distribution of ionic conductances in normal and axotomized motoneurons. *Neuroscience* 2: 829–849, 1977.
341. Ulfhake, B., U. Arvidsson, S. Cullheim, T. Hokfelt, E. Brodin, A. Verhofstad, and T. Visser. An ultrastructural study of 5-hydroxytryptamine-, thyrotropin-releasing hormone- and substance P-immunoreactive axonal boutons in the motor nucleus of spinal cord segments L7-S1 in the adult cat. *Neuroscience* 23: 917–929, 1987.
342. Ulfhake, B., and S. Cullheim. Postnatal development of cat hind limb motoneurons. III: changes in size of motoneurons supplying the triceps surae muscle. *J. Comp. Neurol.* 278: 103–20, 1988.
343. Ulfhake, B., and J. O. Kellerth. A quantitative light microscopic study of the dendrites of cat spinal alpha-motoneu-

rons after intracellular staining with horseradish peroxidase. *J. Comp. Neurol.* 202: 571–583, 1981.

344. Ulfhake, B., and J. O. Kellerth. A quantitative morphological study of HRP-labelled cat alpha-motoneurones supplying different hind limb muscles. *Brain Res.* 264: 1–19, 1983.
345. Ulfhake, B., and J. O. Kellerth. Electrophysiological and morphological measurements in cat gastrocnemius and soleus alpha-motoneurones. *Brain Res.* 307: 167–179, 1984.
346. Umemiya, M., and A. Berger. Properties and function of low- and high-voltage activated Ca^{2+} channels in hypoglossal motoneurons. *J. Neurosci.* 14: 5652–5660, 1994.
347. Vallbo, A. B. Accommodation related to the inactivation of the sodium permeability in single myelinated nerve fibres from *Xenopus laevis. Acta Physiol. Scand.* 61: 429–444, 1964.
348. van Zuylen, E. J., J. J. Denier van der Gon, and C. C. A. M. Gielen. Coordination and inhomogeneous activation of human arm muscles during isometric torques. *J. Neurophysiol.* 60: 1523–1548, 1988.
349. Viana, F., D. A. Bayliss, and A. J. Berger. Calcium conductances and their role in the firing behavior of neonatal rat hypoglossal motoneurons. *J. Neurophysiol.* 69: 2137–2149, 1993.
350. Viana, F., D. A. Bayliss, and A. J. Berger Multiple potassium conductances and their role in action potential repolarization and repetitive firing behavior of neonatal rat hypoglossal motoneurons. *J. Neurophysiol.* 69: 2150–2163, 1993.
351. Wallén, P., J. T. Buchanan, S. Grillner, R. H. Hill, J. Christenson, and T. Hokfelt. Effects of 5-hydroxytryptamine on the after hyperpolarization, spike frequency regulation, and oscillatory membrane properties in lamprey spinal cord neurons. *J. Neurophysiol.* 61: 759–768, 1989.
352. Wallén, P., O. Ekeberg, A. Lansner, K. Brodin, H. Traven, and S. Grillner. A computer-based model for realistic simulations of neural networks. II. The segmental network generating locomotor rhythmicity in the lamprey *J. Neurophysiol.* 68: 1939–1350, 1992.
353. Wallén, P., and S. Grillner. *N*-Methyl-D-aspartate receptor–induced, inherent oscillatory activity in neurons active during fictive locomotion in the lamprey. *J. Neurosci.* 7: 2745–2755, 1987.
354. Walmsley, B., J. A. Hodgson, and R. E. Burke. Forces produced by medial gastrocnemius and soleus muscles during locomotion in freely moving cats. *J. Neurophysiol.* 41: 1203–1216, 1978.
355. Walmsley, B., and U. Proske. Comparison of stiffness of soleus and medial gastrocnemius muscle in cats. *J. Neurophysiol.* 46: 250–259, 1981.
356. Walton, K., and B. P. Fulton. Ionic mechanisms underlying the firing properties of rat neonatal motoneurons studied *in vitro. Neuroscience* 19: 669–683, 1986.
357. Westcott, S. L. Comparison of vestibulospinal synaptic input and Ia afferent synaptic input in cat triceps surae motoneurons. Ph.D, University of Washington, 1993.
358. Westcott, S. L., R. K. Powers, F. R. Robinson, and M. D. Binder. Distribution of vestibulospinal synaptic input to cat triceps surae motoneurons. *Exp. Brain Res.* 107: in press, 1995.
359. Westling, G., R. S. Johansson, C. K. Thomas, and B. Bigland-Ritchie. Measurement of contractile and electrical properties of single human thenar motor units in response to intraneural motor-axon stimulation. *J. Neurophysiol.* 64: 1331–1338, 1990.
360. White, S. R., and S. J. Fung. Serotonin depolarizes cat spinal motoneurons *in situ* and decreases motoneuron afterhyperolarizing potentials. *Brain Res.* 502: 205–213, 1989.
361. Windhorst, U., T. M. Hamm, and D. G. Stuart. On the function of muscle and reflex partitioning. *Brain Behav. Sci.* 12: 629–681, 1989.
362. Wuerker, R. B., A. M. McPhedran, and E. Henneman. Properties of motor units in a heterogeneous pale muscle (m. gastrocnemius) in the cat. *J. Neurophysiol.* 28: 85–99, 1965.
363. Yoshii, K., L. E. Moore, and B. N. Christensen. Transfer impedances between different regions of branched excitable cells. *J. Neurophysiol.* 59: 706–716, 1988.
364. Zajac, F. E., and J. S. Faden. Relationship among recruitment order, axonal conduction velocity, and muscle-unit properties of type-identified motor units in cat plantaris muscle. *J. Neurophysiol.* 53: 1303–1322, 1985.
365. Zajac, F. E., and J. S. Young. Discharge properties of hindlimb motoneurons in decerebrate cats during locomotion induced by mesencephalic stimulation. *J. Neurophysiol.* 43: 1221–1235, 1980.
366. Zengel, J. E., S. A. Reid, G. W. Sypert, and J. B. Munson. Membrane electrical properties and prediction of motor-unit type of medial gastrocnemius motoneurons in the cat. *J. Neurophysiol.* 53: 1323–1344, 1985.
367. Zhang, L., and K. Krnjevi'c. Effects of 4-aminopyridine on the action potential and the after-hyperpolarization of cat spinal motoneurons. *Can. J. Physiol. Pharmacol.* 64: 1402–1406, 1986.
368. Zhang, L., and K. Krnjevi'c. Effects of intracellular injections of phorbol ester and protein kinase C on cat spinal motoneurons in vivo. *Neurosci. Lett.* 77: 287–292, 1987.
369. Zhang, L., and K. Krnjevi'c. Intracellular injection of Ca^{2+} chelator does not affect spike repolarization of cat spinal motoneurons. *Brain Res.* 462: 174–180, 1988.
370. Ziskind-Conhaim, L. NMDA receptors mediate poly- and monosynaptic potentials in motoneurons of rat embryos. *J. Neurosci.* 10: 125–135, 1990.
371. Zwaagstra, B., and D. Kernell. The duration of after-hyperpolarization in hindlimb alpha motoneurones of different sizes in the cat. *Neurosci. Lett.* 19: 303–307, 1980.

2. Neuromuscular adaptation

V. R. EDGERTON | *Department of Physiological Science, University of California, Los Angeles, Los Angeles, California*

S. BODINE-FOWLER | *Division of Orthopaedics, VA Medical Center, San Diego, California*

R. R. ROY | *Brain Research Institute, University of California, Los Angeles, Los Angeles, California*

A. ISHIHARA | *Laboratory of Neurochemistry, Faculty of Integrated Human Studies, Kyoto University, Kyoto, Japan*

J. A. HODGSON | *Brain Research Institute, University of California, Los Angeles, Los Angeles, California*

CHAPTER CONTENTS

THE EXTENT TO WHICH THE DIVERSITY of the biochemical, physiological, and morphological properties of skeletal muscle fibers can be attributed to motoneurons has been a point of active debate. The classic experiments (24) demonstrating that speed-related properties of slow and fast muscles reversed when the muscles were denervated and reinnervated by a foreign nerve (i.e., when a slow muscle was reinnervated by a nerve that normally innervated a fast muscle or vice versa) brought this issue into focus. These experiments raised several critical issues. For example, is the neural influence complete (i.e., does the motoneuron completely control the level of every protein associated with muscle fiber diversity)? Is the neural influence, regardless of its level of regulation of skeletal muscle properties, manifested via differential amounts or patterns of activity imposed on muscle fibers? Is the neural influence exerted via some neurotrophic phenomenon (i.e., some non–activity related means of neuronal control of muscle fibers)?

Many experimental approaches have been used to address these questions. One approach has been to determine how muscle fiber diversity evolves during development. Does the muscle fiber diversity become evident before or after muscle cells are innervated? Are there differential activity levels imposed by motoneurons during development that generate the muscle fiber diversity observed in the adult? In the first section of this chapter, evidence is presented that demonstrates that skeletal muscle fiber diversity precedes functional innervation. However, it appears that the level of diversity observed in the adult does not occur without functional innervation.

A second approach to understanding the neural control of skeletal muscle fibers has been to alter the activity imposed on the muscle fibers either during development or in the adult. One of the more common means of accomplishing this has been to chronically stimulate muscles via the muscle nerve or by direct stimulation via electrodes either placed on the surface of the muscle or implanted intramuscularly. The advantage of this approach is that it hypothetically eliminates the diversity of activation patterns (i.e., all muscle fibers are assumed to receive the same amount and pattern of stimulation). This may be true if the muscle nerve is cut, thereby eliminating the differential activity that normally occurs among muscle fibers and motor units. But the muscle nerve often is not transected and it is assumed (not necessarily correctly) that the amount of normally occurring stimuli is insignificant relative to the prolonged chronic artificial stimulation. Nevertheless, these chronic stimulation experiments have provided significant insight into the problems addressed in this chapter. These experiments have been the focus of several previous reviews (134, 191, 192, 212) and are not covered in this chapter. The essence of these reviews, however, is considered in our conclusions regarding the role of differential activity levels as a modulator of muscle fiber diversity. In addition, chronic exercise has been used to study the extent to which skeletal muscle fibers can adapt to an increase in natural physiological stimuli (see Chapter 25). However, exercise studies do not provide insight into the role of differential neuromuscular activity levels in producing muscle fiber diversity because differential patterns of activation occur normally in the intact neuromuscular system.

In this chapter we also discuss studies in which the strategy has been the antithesis of the chronic stimulation studies (i.e., the imposition of a common level of activation of all muscle fibers by eliminating all neural activation). These experiments allow us to address the following question: If the diversity in activation is eliminated, will the diversity among skeletal muscle fibers also be eliminated? These kinds of studies have been reported only recently and have not been the focus of previous reviews. Thus, these experiments will be discussed in this chapter. In general, they show a persistence of adult-like skeletal muscle fiber diversity in the absence of any significant level of activation for prolonged periods.

A common approach of presumably altering muscle activity patterns has been to reinnervate a slow muscle with a fast nerve and/or a fast muscle with a slow nerve. Although there is evidence suggesting that the activation patterns of the muscles change following cross-reinnervation (180), these experiments cannot control mechanisms that are not directly related to neuromuscular activity (e.g., neurotrophic factors). We have reviewed these studies in this chapter for several reasons. First, the questions of which properties of the skeletal muscle fibers are neurally regulated or modulated and to what degree neural control has been demonstrated for any given property are addressed. Because the degree of control can be a function of the duration of the experimental perturbation, we have also considered this issue carefully and have taken this into account in our interpretation of the results from the literature. These studies support the general conclusions that *(1)* there is a strong, although not complete, neural control of most of the muscle fiber properties that characterize muscle fiber diversity; *(2)* the duration of the cross-reinnervation experiments, at least between 6 months to 3 years, does not seem to be a critical factor in the completeness of conversion of the properties that determine fiber types; and *(3)* muscle fiber types can be converted from slow to fast less readily than fast to slow, at least in response to the presumed modulation in activation level associated with cross-reinnervation.

The third general topic related to muscle fiber diversity included in this chapter is the adaptability of motoneurons. This topic was selected because the differential activity patterns of the motoneurons may play a key role in the muscle fiber diversity. The question being addressed is: Do those properties of the motoneurons associated with differential activation (e.g., soma size and oxidative capacity) adapt when the muscle fibers they innervate change their function? It is concluded that there is a striking resistance to change of the motoneurons in either of these properties or in the relationship that exists between them. For example, motoneuron soma size and oxidative capacity do not change in response to prolonged absence of the generation of action potentials or to prolonged hyperactivity associated with functional overload of a muscle (35, 36).

Other topics related to muscle fiber diversity that are clearly relevant to the topic of this chapter are not addressed. Most notable is the regulatory potential of growth factors on skeletal muscle fibers.

These types of mechanisms are only beginning to be recognized as an important source of regulation of skeletal muscle properties (17, 53, 109, 140, 219, 264). The potential for nerve growth factors to regulate skeletal muscle properties directly or via glia or neurons in the spinal cord is largely unexplored.

The overall conclusion from this review is that the level and kind of proteins expressed and maintained in skeletal muscle fibers are regulated by multiple sources, many of which are probably interactive. Muscle fiber diversity is a characteristic of skeletal muscles that begins to develop prenatally in the absence of functional innervation. In general, the results of cross-reinnervation studies have not been interpreted rigorously. The significance of the absence of a total conversion from slow to fast properties or from fast to slow properties after prolonged cross-reinnervation has generally been overlooked. Likewise, muscle chronic stimulation studies generally have focused on what changed without adequately considering the significance of what did not change in the muscle. These studies, however, have clearly demonstrated that the level of activation, and/or closely associated events, of a muscle fiber is a key factor in the regulation of gene expression. Some regulatory mechanisms are not activity dependent. Hormonal and localized growth factors interacting with the forces and strains generated within and among muscle fibers with a given genetic predisposition must be integrated into a complex conceptual framework that encompasses the activity and neural-dependent mechanisms already known to play a role in skeletal muscle diversity. The significance of the morphological and physiological diversity of neurons and the adaptation of motoneurons and sensory neurons in inducing and sustaining muscle diversity remains largely undefined.

MATCHING OF MOTONEURONS AND MUSCLE FIBER PROPERTIES DURING NORMAL DEVELOPMENT

Muscle Development

Adult muscles contain multiple types of fibers as demonstrated by myosin ATPase histochemistry, immunohistochemical distinction of myosin heavy chain (MHC) isoforms, and histochemical and biochemical evaluation of the activities of enzymes related to energy metabolism (27, 190, 191). Muscle fibers of a motor unit in adult vertebrate muscles have similar (although not identical) metabolic and physiological properties (25, 193). Monoclonal antibodies for MHC isoforms have been used to show that, within a cross section, all the fibers innervated by a single motoneuron express the same MHC protein (148, 193). Until recently, fiber type generally has been thought to be imposed on a developing myofiber by the activity pattern of the innervating motoneuron, thus yielding homogeneous motor units. Recent studies, however, reveal that multiple types of intrinsically different myoblasts appear at different stages of development, giving rise to multiple fiber types even in the absence of innervation (169). This finding has raised the possibility that motoneurons innervate fibers of a specific type during development. Conversely, the initial innervation may be random and, through the process of synapse elimination and conversion of all fibers within each unit to the same fiber type may enable the muscle fibers of a motor unit to become more homogeneous.

Emergence of Fiber Type Diversity. The development of skeletal muscle involves a sequence of cellular changes including commitment of mesenchymal stem cells to a muscle lineage (i.e., myoblasts), withdrawal of myoblasts from the cell cycle and initiation of differentiation, fusion of myoblasts to form multinucleated myotubes, expression of muscle-specific genes, and innervation and formation of the neuromuscular junction. These steps are under the complex control of oncogenes, growth factors, myogenic regulatory factors, hormones, and neural activity (for recent reviews, see 182, 214).

Myoblasts have been classified into three major types: embryonic or primary myoblasts, fetal or secondary myoblasts, and adult myoblasts or satellite cells based primarily on the developmental stage at which they migrate to the limb bud [Fig. 2.1; (233)]. The first myoblasts to migrate from the somites are the embryonic or primary myoblasts, which appear in the limb bud of the mouse, for example, at embryonic days 13–14. Fetal or secondary myoblasts migrate several days later and are found in the limb bud at embryonic days 16–17. The last generation of myoblasts to populate the limb bud are the adult myoblasts, more commonly referred to as satellite cells, which are distinct from the embryonic and fetal myoblasts. Existing evidence suggests that the embryonic, fetal, and adult myoblasts are not lineal descendants of one another (169). Myoblasts differ not only in the timing of their appearance in the limb but also in their growth requirements in culture (44) and the morphological characteristics and myosin expression of the myotubes they form (168, 258).

The first muscle fibers to form in the limb are the primary muscle fibers, which form as a result of the fusion of embryonic myoblasts. In avians, two major and one minor subtype of myotubes can be cloned

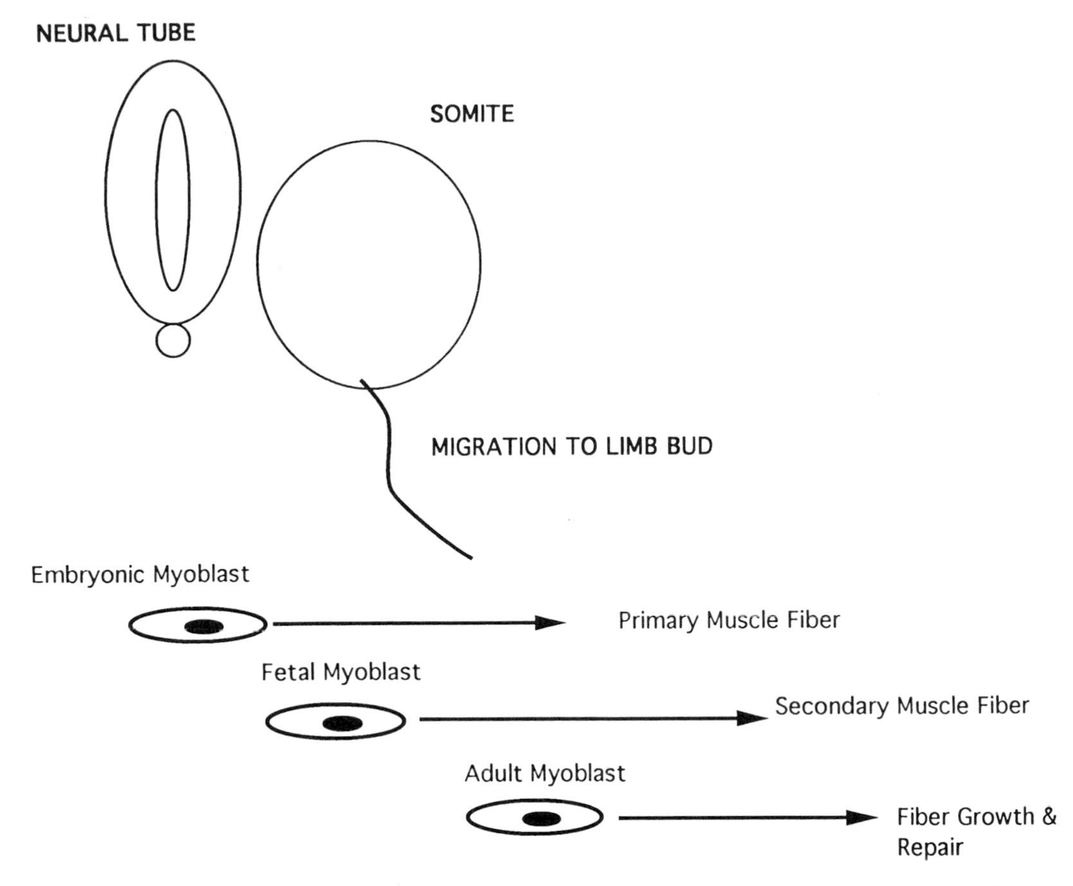

FIG. 2.1. The three major types of myoblasts—embryonic or primary myoblasts, fetal or secondary myoblasts, and adult myoblasts or satellite cells—are separated primarily by the developmental stage at which they migrate from the somite to the limb bud.

from embryonic myoblasts (46). The major primary fibers formed in vivo are *(1)* those that express a fast MHC isoform and slow MHC1 (originally designated fast) (168, 169); and *(2)* those that express a fast MHC isoform, slow MHC1, and slow MHC3 (originally designated fast/slow) (168, 169, 187). In mammals, subtypes of embryonic myoblasts have not been found (258), although they form fibers that eventually express either fast or slow adult MHC isoforms [Fig. 2.2; (41, 55, 175)]. Initially, all primary fibers express embryonic MHC and slow MHC. The majority of primary fibers will remain slow; however, in predominantly fast muscles, some of the primary fibers will begin to express the neonatal MHC and eventually one of the adult fast MHC isoforms (i.e., 2A, 2B, or 2X) (42). The location of the primary fiber within the muscle cross section appears to have a role in determining whether it will switch from slow to fast or remain slow. For example, all the primary fibers in the superficial region (i.e., that region farthest away from the bone) of the extensor digitorum longus (EDL) and tibialis anterior (TA) muscles of the rat switch from slow to fast, whereas only a few primary fibers in the deep region (i.e., that region closest to the bone) become fast (41).

The development of fiber type diversity among primary fibers appears to be independent of neural innervation. When spinal motoneurons are removed or prevented from innervating the limb bud prior to primary fiber formation, fibers expressing different MHC isoforms develop and the gradient of slow and fast fibers from superficial to deep within the cross section still occurs (29, 42, 46). This suggests that factors intrinsic to the myoblast or to the architecture of the muscle and independent of innervation determine the type in primary fibers.

The fetal period of muscle development is marked by a change in the predominant type of myoblast that can be isolated from muscles of the limb. Fetal myoblasts can be isolated from muscle at the time that secondary fibers are being formed (82). Consequently, it is accepted that fetal myoblasts form secondary fibers in vivo. Fetal myoblasts predominate only in early fetal development, whereas midfetal development is characterized by the appearance of

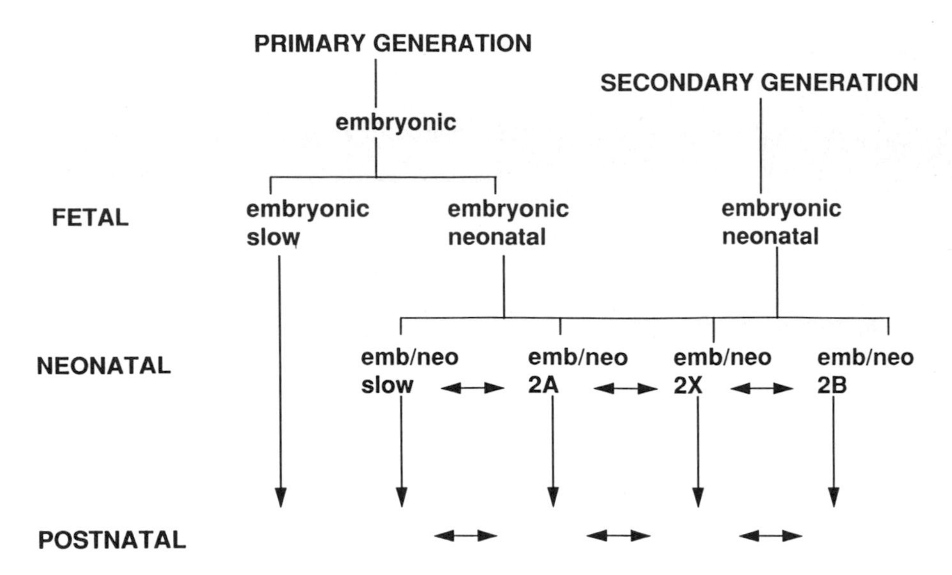

FIG. 2.2. A schematic of the emergence of myosin heavy chain types from primary and secondary myotubes at the fetal, neonatal, and postnatal stages of development.

adult myoblasts. Adult myoblasts are the only type found in late fetal development and postnatally, when they are commonly referred to as satellite cells. Like embryonic myoblasts, fetal and adult myoblasts both form long, highly nucleated myofibers but, unlike embryonic myoblasts, do not require conditioned media for clonal growth. Furthermore, secondary fibers express a different sequence of MHCs than primary fibers.

During normal fetal development, secondary fibers initially express both embryonic and neonatal MHC isoforms in mammals (41), and in most muscles will develop into adult fast fibers. One exception is the soleus, where a majority of the secondary fibers become slow (41, 175). This is likely to be the case in other predominantly slow muscles like the adductor longus and vastus intermedius, although this issue has not been investigated. Although myoblasts are determined cells in that they will form muscle and not other tissue, the types of adult MHCs (i.e., 2A, 2B, or 2X) they express are dependent on many factors, including their location within the muscle and thyroid hormone levels.

DeNardi et al. (55) showed that the expression of 2A, 2B, and 2X MHC transcripts occurs shortly after birth in rat hindlimb muscles and displays a specific regional distribution from the onset. For example, the mRNAs for types 2X and 2B MHCs are not expressed in the soleus, but are highly expressed in the TA and EDL. Moreover, fibers that co-expressed mRNAs for all of the fast MHCs were not found, suggesting that all fast fibers do not go through a common initial phase. When a small percentage of fibers in each muscle were found to co-express mRNAs of two MHCs, however, the co-expression was usually limited to the following pairs: slow/2A, 2A/2X, or 2X/2B. The adult distribution of fiber types was apparent in hindlimb muscles of the rat by postnatal days 14–21.

Proliferation and differentiation of embryonic and fetal myoblasts contributes to the formation and growth of muscle fibers during early development. Continued growth and repair of muscle fibers requires a third population of myoblasts, since differentiated myoblasts or myonuclei that express contractile proteins are postmitotic. Satellite cells or adult myoblasts are undifferentiated mononuclear cells with myogenic potential that reside between the basal lamina and plasma membrane of a muscle fiber. All skeletal muscles of adult vertebrates contain satellite cells, which become activated and proliferate in response to injury or disease. An activated satellite cell can continue to divide or it can differentiate and fuse into existing fibers or form new myofibers. The signals that activate satellite cells are unknown; however, growth factors such as fibroblast growth factor and tumor growth factor-β can stimulate proliferation of satellite cells in vitro [see Florini (87) for review].

Predetermination of Protein Expression. The existence of fibers that express different isoforms of the contractile proteins raises the question of whether satellite cells within specific fibers are *(1)* predetermined to express proteins of the corresponding type or *(2)* multipotential cells that express proteins of a specific isoform under the influence of exogenous factors. In avians and rodents there is evidence for at least two distinct types of satellite cells. Feldman and Stockdale (81) isolated satellite cells from a fast muscle (the pectoralis) and a slow tonic muscle (the anterior latissimus dorsi) of the chick and found two distinct populations of satellite cells. Myofibers formed in high-density cultures of satellite cells isolated from the pectoralis always expressed fast MHCs, whereas fibers formed from satellite cells from the anterior latissimus dorsi were either fast or fast/slow. Dusterhoft and Pette (67) found heterogeneous populations of satellite cells when they extracted satellite cells from the slow soleus and fast TA muscles of the rat. Additional evidence that satellite cells may be predetermined came from Hoh et al. (117), who found that myoblasts transplanted from the cat superfast jaw muscle into a fast-twitch leg muscle expressed superfast myosin but not the fast myosin isoforms of the host muscle. More recently, however, Hughes and Blau (120) demonstrated that extrinsic signals may override the intrinsic commitment of myoblast nuclei to express a particular set of contractile proteins. They injected clones of genetically labeled primary myoblasts into adult mouse and rat muscles. They observed that those myoblasts which fused to form new fibers expressed MHCs typical of their differentiation in vitro. However, when myoblasts fused with preexisting fibers, they expressed myosins characteristic of the host fiber. This suggests that undifferentiated myoblasts, (i.e., satellite cells) are committed to a specific program, but that this program can be overridden by extrinsic factors in the host environment.

Importance of Innervation. Primary myotubes form in the limb bud and differentially express MHC isoforms before the arrival of motor axons into the ventral and dorsal muscle masses. As noted previously, the initial fiber type differentiation and spatial distribution of types within the muscle can occur despite total denervation, blockade of neural activity, or innervation by foreign motoneurons (29, 41, 42, 46). Secondary myotubes, however, form after all of the motoneurons have arrived in the limb and after the period of cell death (145). Several studies have suggested that secondary fibers fail to form when innervation or neural activity is abolished (106, 205). Consequently, primary myogenesis is often described as a neurally independent process and secondary myogenesis as a neurally dependent process. Recent investigations (41, 42, 90), however, suggest that nerve-independent and nerve-dependent processes are involved in both primary and secondary fiber formation. Fredette and Landmesser (90) demonstrated that blockade of neural activity with *d*-tubocurare and denervation did not prevent secondary fibers from forming, although there was a 75% reduction in the number of secondary muscle fibers that formed. Moreover, there was a 50% reduction in the number of primary fibers found in the muscle that may have contributed to the loss of secondary fibers. In addition, the diversity of fiber types and pattern formation still occurred, although there was a loss in the number of slow fibers due to degeneration of some primary fibers and a loss of slow MHC expression in some primary and secondary fibers (42, 90). Clearly, innervation is required for normal muscle growth and fiber type diversity during the fetal period of development. However, the role of innervation in the initiation of primary and secondary lineages and fiber type distributions within the muscle is complex.

In summary, myogenesis and the differentiation of fibers into specific types are controlled by a combination of intrinsic myoblast properties and epigenetic factors including innervation. Nerve-dependent processes are less apparent during the early stages of development and become more prominent at later stages, especially postnatally. The relative importance of and the exact interrelationships between the many variables associated with these processes remain to be determined.

Specificity of Neuronal Connections to Muscle. A muscle is innervated by a pool of motoneurons located in a specific and spatially discrete region in the ventral horn of the spinal cord. The motor pool (i.e., those motoneurons innervating a specific muscle) forms a longitudinal column extending over two to four spinal segments. Although the axons that innervate a specific muscle may exit the spinal cord through different spinal nerves, they eventually converge to form a single muscle nerve. The outgrowth of motor axons has been studied in detail in the chick hindlimb [see reviews by Lance-Jones and Landmesser (141, 147)], revealing that motoneurons are able to find their appropriate targets with remarkable accuracy. The pathway taken by a nerve to a muscle is discrete, with few projection errors occurring during the developmental process. This precise patterning of neuronal connections emerges, in part, from the interactions between the growing tips of the axons, the growth cone, and the cellular environment through which they grow [see Dodd and Jessell (61)].

Projection Patterns. The location of the motoneurons innervating individual muscles has been determined using retrogradely transported tracers (28, 145). Generally speaking, there is a somatotopic relationship between the position of the individual motor pools within the spinal cord and the position of their target in the limb. More proximal muscles in the limb are innervated by more rostral motoneurons, and muscles formed from the ventral muscle mass are innervated by more medially located motoneurons in the spinal cord. Analysis of the projection pattern of axons going to a particular muscle shows that, at the spinal nerve level, axons from many motor pools are intermingled. Axons to individual muscles begin to sort into spatially discrete groups within and beyond the plexus (143).

To determine whether axons follow specific cues or are passively channeled down certain paths, Lance-Jones and Landmesser (142, 143) rotated the spinal cord along the anteroposterior axis in chick embryos so that motoneurons projecting to a specific muscle would exit the cord at a different level than normal. Although motoneurons exited the cord via the wrong spinal nerve, they were able to change their path in the plexus region so that they projected into the proper nerve trunk and innervated the correct muscle. These findings suggest that motoneurons are capable of following specific cues in order to project to the correct target. These specific guidance cues, however, appear not to operate over long distances, since motoneurons forced into the wrong plexus after cord reversals involving five or more segments are unable to find their correct muscle and instead project to a foreign muscle in general accord with their new position within the plexus (143). In some instances, however, motoneurons forced into the wrong plexus are capable of finding their correct target by taking totally aberrant paths within the limb, suggesting that motoneurons may be interacting with some diffusible factor released from the muscle.

Positional Guidance Cues. In the vertebrate hindlimb, each muscle is derived from myoblasts that originate from somites located directly adjacent to the region of the cord where motoneurons destined to innervate them originate (39). A topographical relationship between the location of the motor pool in the spinal cord and the location of the muscle it innervates suggests that motoneurons within a segment have an affinity for myogenic cells from the adjacent somites. However, muscles can be innervated with normal specificity when they are derived from somites from foreign levels. This observation suggests that somites are not prelabeled with specific proteins that attract motor axons from a specific level (139, 141).

When axons are forced into a foreign region of the limb, the innervation pattern that forms is appropriate for the limb region in question. For example, if axons from the anterior lumbar plexus are forced into the posterior sacral plexus, a normal sciatic nerve pattern will emerge even though these axons originally belonged to the femoral nerve. In addition, limbs that are made muscleless by irradiating the corresponding somites form the appropriate plexuses and nerve branches (248). Thus, it appears that the gross anatomical pattern of plexuses and nerve branches in the limb are determined by the surrounding extracellular tissue matrix (38, 138).

Contact-Mediated Cues. Segmental patterning of motor nerves may be determined by contact-mediated inhibition as well as selective adhesion between developing neurons (51). For example, the segmentation of spinal nerves appears to be influenced by inhibitory/adhesive molecules in the adjacent somites. Before axons reach the plexus region they must travel through the somites. Tosney (247) has shown that axons selectively project through the anterior half of the somite and actively grow away from the posterior half of the somite. Recently, lectin peanut agglutin staining has been localized to the posterior half of the somite (52). Davies et al. (52) used lectin-affinity chromatography and identified two molecules of molecular weight 48 kDa and 55 kDa from posterior somite tissue. When dorsal root ganglion cells growing on laminin were confronted with a substrate containing these peanut agglutin–binding proteins, growth cone extension stopped (52). Chick embryos stained with antibodies against the 48 kDa and 55 kDa proteins showed selective staining of the posterior half of the somites. Proteins that cross-react with these antibodies are also found in the gray, but not the white, matter of adult chick brains (217). Consequently, these studies suggest that a negative signal for growth cone extension exists in the posterior half of the somite.

Chemotrophic Cues. In addition to contact-mediated cues, growth cones may be oriented by diffusible chemotrophic molecules that are secreted by restricted populations of intermediate or final cellular targets. For example, avian motoneurons can find their appropriate muscle target even after displacement of motoneurons in the cord or after muscles in the limb are repositioned by embryonic surgery (144). Nerve growth factor is a diffusible factor that is required for the survival of embryonic sympathetic and sensory neurons. Furthermore, it is the only defined molecule that has been shown to act as a diffusible axonal chemoattractant (152). Evidence for this was provided by Levi-Montalcini and co-workers (166) when they injected large doses of nerve growth factor into the brainstem, causing sympathetic axons from all segmental levels to change their course and project into the central nervous system. Target-derived chemoattractants have been implicated in directing the growth of *(1)* trigeminal sensory axons to their epithelial targets (158), *(2)* spinal commissural axons to midline spinal floor plate cells (238), and *(3)* cortical projection neurons to subcortical targets (108).

Formation of Neuromuscular Junctions. The formation of the neuromuscular junction has been studied during normal development, in culture systems, and during reinnervation of mature muscles. This is a complex process involving reciprocal interactions between the muscle and nerve (see reviews in 37, 103, 216). Development of the mature mammalian neuromuscular junction in which each muscle fiber is innervated by a single motoneuron involves multiple stages that take weeks to occur.

The acetylcholine receptor (AChR) is a pentamer composed of four homologous transmembrane subunits with the stoichiometry α_2, β, γ, δ. In some species, such as the rat and calf, the γ-subunit is replaced by the ϵ-subunit in the adult (19). The AChR contains the acetylcholine (ACh) binding sites, the ion channels, and all of the structural elements required for the regulation of its opening by ACh (for review, see 37). AChRs are found in the membrane of mononucleated myoblasts and their expression is linked to the expression of myogenic regulatory factors and the differentiation of myoblasts. Upon fusion of myoblasts, the transcription of AChRs increases dramatically, reaching a density of 100–500 molecules/μm^2 throughout the myotube membrane (103). Small clusters of AChRs soon form along the membrane independent of innervation. Axonal growth cones within the muscle grow along and across the surface of the myotubes and spontaneously release ACh. The site of contact of the growth cone on the myotube appears to be influenced primarily by the point of entry of the nerve trunk into the muscle mass. The growth of the myotube at both ends results in the neuromuscular junction being located approximately in the middle of the fiber. After the initial contact is made, the growth cones of other motor axons make synapses at the initial site only.

Upon contact of the growth cone with the myotube, the rate of transmitter release increases dramatically and a series of nerve-dependent changes are initiated in the synaptic and extrasynaptic sites along the muscle fiber. Soon after innervation occurs, AChRs become clustered at the synaptic site and the nuclei near the synapse are stimulated to increase both the transcription and translation of the AChR subunits (reviewed in 103). Other proteins also become co-localized at the synaptic site including the 43 kDa protein and spectrin in the cytoskeleton and S-laminin, ACh esterase, and a heparin sulphate proteoglycan in the basal lamina. Soon after AChR clustering occurs at the synaptic site, AChRs disappear from the extrasynaptic membrane.

The clustering of AChRs at the synaptic site and the induction of nuclei near the synapse to selectively produce AChR mRNA subunits are nerve-dependent processes (Fig. 2.3). Although the initial clustering of the AChRs on the myotube is nerve-independent, following innervation the only AChRs to remain are those associated with the area in contact with the nerve. Those receptors present on the muscle surface at the site of nerve contact and newly synthesized receptors are anchored into the membrane. Agrin is one molecule that is involved in the clustering of AChRs in cultured myotubes (164). Agrin is synthesized by both motoneurons and muscles; however, it is the neurally derived form that appears to be required for AChR cluster formation (199).

Innervation of the muscle fiber causes not only a redistribution of AChRs throughout the membrane but also an increase in their number (83). The accumulation of the AChR subunit mRNAs occurs specifically under the motor nerve ending (167). Several mechanisms were proposed to explain this phenomenon including *(1)* a directed transport of the mRNA from the extrajunctional regions of the muscle fiber to the synaptic site; *(2)* an increased stability of AChR mRNA near the end-plate, or *(3)* an increased transcription of AChR genes in nuclei underlying the end-plate. To distinguish between these alternatives, transgenic mice were generated in which regions of AChR ϵ- and δ-subunit genes were used to direct the expression of a reporter gene (213, 225). Both subunits were used to show that the reporter product accumulated in or near the nuclei that lie directly beneath the motor end-plate. When the same reporter genes were controlled by other muscle-specific promoters, the reporter product was widely distributed within the muscle fiber. These results demonstrate that AChR genes are selectively transcribed by the synaptic nuclei (Fig. 2.3).

The induction of nuclei near the synaptic site to increase their expression of AChR subunits may be influenced by factors released by the nerve terminal. For example, AChR clusters appear on myotubes that are near to but not yet contacted by motor axons (50). Two candidates for this role are calcitonin gene–related peptide (CGRP) and a peptide of 42 kDa molecular weight referred to as acetylcholine receptor–inducting activity (ARIA). CGRP is present in spinal cord motoneurons (95) and motor nerve endings, where it is stored in dense-coated ves-

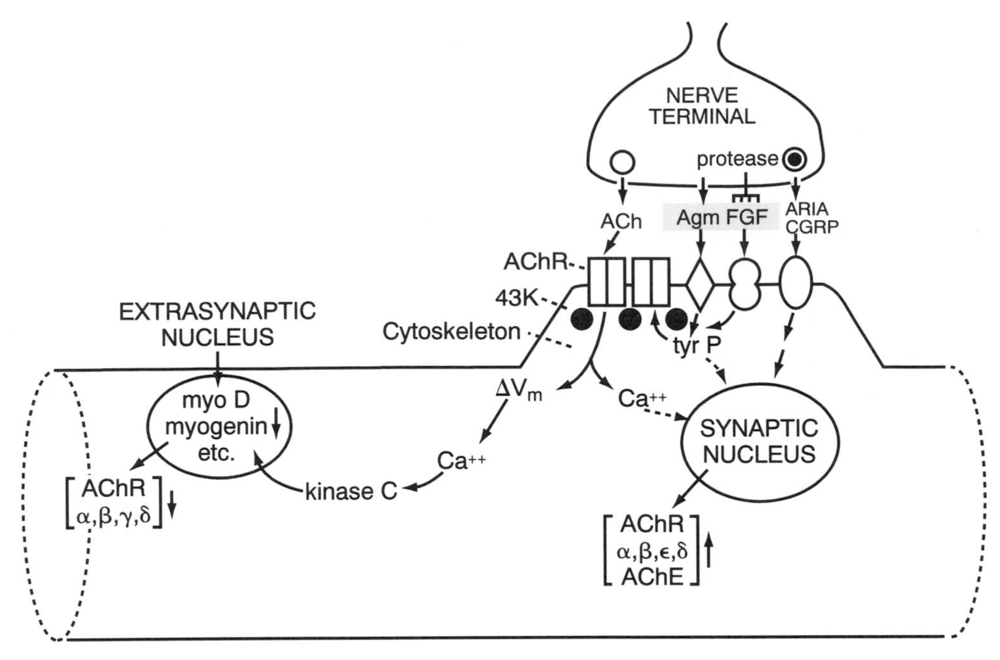

FIG. 2.3. A schematic of some of the factors potentially involved in the neural control of expression of AChR via the neuromuscular junction. Note that AChR transcription is repressed in extrajunctional nuclei by activity, perhaps via protein kinase C and Myo-D–like transcription factors. Activity may also affect the junctional nuclei via receptors involving agrin and FGF, which may cause AChR clustering by stimulating tyrosine phosphorylation and AChR-43KDa interactions; ARIA and CGRP could also affect junctional nuclei via separate receptors.

icles and can be released upon electrical stimulation of the motor nerve (254). Addition of CGRP to primary cultures of chick myotubes causes a 1.3- to 1.5-fold increase in total surface AChR levels and an approximate threefold increase in α-subunit mRNA levels (186). The effect of CGRP on AChR biosynthesis appears to be mediated by cyclic adenosine monophosphate (cAMP), since CGRP elevates intracellular levels of cAMP and activates muscle adenylate cyclase (151). CGRP-immunoreactive neurons are detected in the chick ventral spinal cord at embryonic day 6, and their numbers reach a peak between embryonic days 12 and 18. Furthermore, CGRP binding sites are present on embryonic muscle fibers, reaching a peak specific activity between embryonic days 11 and 14, when the neuromuscular junctions are formed (257). These data suggest that CGRP contributes to the motor end-plate morphogenesis. Another peptide that may have an important role in the development of the motor end-plate is ARIA. ARIA is present in brain and spinal cord anterior horn cells; however, it is not known whether it is present in or released from motoneurons (256). When added to myotube cultures, ARIA stimulates the accumulation of α-subunit mRNAs (79, 162). ARIA also has been shown to increase selectively the expression of ϵ-subunit mRNA in cultured cells (162).

The metabolic and channel properties of the AChR change during maturation of the motor endplate. Newly formed synaptic and extrasynaptic AChRs have a half-life in the membrane of 10–20 h (80). After nerve contact and AChR clustering occurs at the synaptic site, the turnover time of the AChR subunits at the synaptic site increases to about 10 days (198). This stabilization appears to be influenced by muscle activity, since the turnover time of the receptors decreases after denervation. There are two populations of AChRs following denervation: one whose turnover time is stabilized to the adult values after reinnervation, and a second population that does not change its turnover time but which disappears upon reinnervation (220).

The early subsynaptic receptors and extrasynaptic receptors have average open times of about 4 ms. Over the first few weeks after synaptic clustering of the receptors, the kinetics of the receptor current charge and the average open time of the junctional receptors is reduced to about 1 ms (216). This change has been shown to be due to the specific replacement of γ-subunit with the ϵ-subunit in the rat (19, 262). The switch occurs at the level of transcription, with a decrease in the production of γ-subunit mRNA and an increase in the production of ϵ-subunit mRNA among the synaptic nuclei (163, 262).

At the same time that these changes are occurring, acetylcholine esterase (AChE) is deposited in the subsynaptic membrane. Like the AChR, AChE is concentrated at the neuromuscular junctions of developing and adult muscle fibers. AChE in skeletal muscle can be present in two forms, globular and asymmetric (102, 249). Low levels of enzymatic activity can be detected throughout the length of the fiber; however, the end-plate contains a specialized form (the A form) that is composed of catalytic subunits linked to a collagen-like tail that attaches to the basal lamina (249). Although the nerve can produce AChE, the majority of the AChE found at the end-plate is produced by myonuclei (54) and, once assembled, inserted into the membrane overlying the nuclei (206). Recently, it was also demonstrated that AChE mRNA and protein are selectively expressed in innervated regions of muscle fibers much like the AChR (129). Unlike the AChR, the increased accumulation of AChE at the end-plate results primarily from stabilization of the mRNA, rather than from enhanced transcription of the gene (91).

Following the subsynaptic location of AChRs and AChE, extrajunctional receptors are lost. This loss is neurally mediated and is the result of repression of the transcription of AChR subunits. For example, denervation of adult muscles causes a reappearance of AChRs extrasynaptically (251), whereas there is a loss of these receptors upon reinnervation of the muscle. Upon transection of the sciatic nerve in the rat there is a 30- to 50-fold increase in the levels of α- and δ-subunit–specific mRNA and a fivefold increase in the levels of β-subunit–specific mRNA within the soleus muscle (97, 263). Increases in the γ- and ϵ-subunit–specific mRNAs are also found after denervation. In situ hybridization with cDNA probes specific to the different AChR subunits was used to determine that the increase in ϵ-subunit mRNA was localized to the synaptic nuclei. Conversely, the increase in γ-subunit mRNA was due to an increase in transcription by the extrasynaptic nuclei (263).

Electrical activity of the nerve appears to influence the distribution of extrasynaptic receptors. Direct electrical stimulation of the muscle prevents the upregulation of extrajunctional receptors (96) and ACh hypersensitivity (156) following denervation. Blockage of synaptic transmission in innervated muscle by tetrodotoxin (TTX) also increases the number of extrajunctional receptors by approximately twofold within 48 h of the block (14). Neural activity exerts its effect by regulating the level of transcription of the receptor subunits. The transactivation factors that mediate the effect of activity may include members of the MyoD family of transcription activators, which are also involved in the initial induction of AChR genes during myogenesis. Levels of MyoD and myogenin increase in parallel with levels of AChR after denervation in the adult (72, 178). The regulation of these transcription factors may involve changes in nuclear protein kinase C activity by intracellular Ca^{2+} (see 37 for review).

In summary, the amount and distribution of AChR subunits in muscle fibers appears to be regulated by mechanisms that control the level of transcription of the AChR subunit genes. Evidence supports the existence of three overlapping mechanisms: *(1)* activation of the AChR genes by the MyoD family of myogenic factors, *(2)* repression of the genes by electrical activity, and *(3)* local induction of the nuclei at the synapse by neural factors.

Motoneuron Development

Regulation of Neuronal Population Size. Naturally occurring neuronal cell death is a developmental process that is characterized by a substantial loss of embryonic neurons (as much as 40%–70% of a population) that occurs during a relatively well-defined period during embryogenesis (see 183 for review). Two well-characterized systems that undergo developmental cell death are the dorsal root ganglia (105) and the lateral motor column of the chick (103). The actual role that neuronal cell death plays during the development of the neuromuscular system is unknown. It is unlikely that cell death is used as a mechanism to correct errors in the projection of axons to their target. For example, in ciliary and limb innervating motoneurons, those cells that were removed by cell death *(1)* successfully innervated the correct target, *(2)* underwent normal biochemical and ultrastructural differentiation prior to death, and *(3)* became functionally innervated (146, 181). Furthermore, motoneurons experimentally forced to innervate a foreign muscle do not exhibit additional cell death.

The exact mechanisms that determine motoneuron survival or death are still undefined. Two general types of cellular degeneration have been described based on morphological changes. Necrotic cell death is characterized by cellular edema and culminates in the rupture of plasma and internal membranes and leakage of cellular contents (60). A second type of degeneration, called apoptosis, involves the loss of cell volume and a chromatin condensation with initial preservation of the integrity of cytoplasmic organelles. Electron microscopic examination of naturally occurring cell death has shown that the initial morphological alterations include chromatin condensation and has suggested that the morphological degeneration is more similar to apoptosis than necrosis (40, 48).

The common assumption has been that the loss of some required trophic support causes the cell to shut down its metabolism and undergo a passive process of necrotic degradation. Based on this assumption, one would predict that inhibition of protein and RNA synthesis should mimic the effect of the loss of trophic factor and increase cell death. If, however, cell death is an active process whereby the loss of trophic factor induces new gene expression, which triggers a series of events that actively induces cellular degradation and death, then the inhibition of protein and RNA synthesis should reduce cell death. The death of sympathetic neurons in culture after nerve growth factor removal was prevented by the addition of compounds that inhibit RNA or protein synthesis (161). In vivo, the death of neurons induced by the removal of limbs prior to the cell death period and the death of motoneurons following peripheral nerve axotomy in the embryo following the cell death period was prevented by treatment with cyclohexamide and actinomycin D, agents that inhibit RNA and protein synthesis (185). These findings support the hypothesis that, during development, naturally occurring cell death is an active process that involves the activation of "cell death genes" following the removal of some essential signal (possibly trophic factors).

Target Size and Trophic Factors. Based on evidence collected from experiments that alter the amount of target tissue, it has been proposed that neuronal survival is dependent on the ability of the neuron to compete for a limited amount of trophic factor released by the target tissue. A proportional or linear relationship between the number of surviving neurons and the size of the target would be expected based on this size-matching hypothesis (183). As an example in the chick, removal of a muscle or target organ has resulted in the death of 40%–90% of all associated neurons (104, 184), whereas increasing the size of the target (e.g., by grafting of a supernumerary limb) increased the number of neurons that survived by 25%–40% (117). The number of surviving motoneurons is proposed to match the number of muscle fibers present in the target at the time of cell death. At the time of cell death, only clusters of primary myotubes are present within the muscles and they can account for only a small percentage of the final number of muscle fibers. Secondary fibers, generated after the cell death period, account for the majority of fibers within a muscle. Tanaka and Landmesser (236) used chick-quail chimeras to show a close correlation ($R = 0.996$) between the number of primary myotubes present and the number of motoneurons that survived the cell death period. This result may seem surprising given that primary fibers make up such a small percentage of the final target; however, Fredette and Landmesser (90) recently found a close correlation between the number of primary fibers and the number of secondary fibers that form. These results suggest that other target-associated factors also affect neuronal survival [e.g., the number of muscle fibers (primary myotubes or final number of fibers), myofiber size, the number of synaptic sites, the amount of trophic factor, and the amount of nonmuscle mesenchymal tissue].

If trophic factors are produced by the target, how do neurons interact with the target to get access to the trophic factors? The general view has been that the amount of trophic factor produced by the target is limited. Blocking neuromuscular activity with *d*-tubocurare or α-bungarotoxin during the normal cell death period can rescue all limb-innervating motoneurons (195), suggesting an up-regulation of a target-derived trophic factor in inactive muscle. Recent experiments on embryonic muscles, however, have revealed that some putative trophic factors are not increased after denervation or paralysis (119, 235), and therefore the limitation may not be in the amount produced but in the neuron's access to the trophic factor. If motoneurons gain access to trophic factors through their synapses with the AChR on the muscle fibers, then a motoneuron with a large number of branches would make more synapses, receive more trophic factor, and have a greater chance for survival than a motoneuron with fewer branches. Alternatively, if the number of AChRs increased, then the number of potential sites for synaptogenesis and trophic factor uptake would increase. This can be achieved with curare treatment or denervation. For example, Dahm and Landmesser (49) showed that blockage of neuromuscular activity in embryos with curare resulted in an increase in intramuscular branching and synapse formation, as well as a decrease in neuronal cell death. Furthermore, they demonstrated that a decrease in motoneuron branching due to treatment with an endosialidase, which did not affect neuromuscular activity, decreased motoneuron survival (237). These results support the hypothesis that neurons gain access to target-derived trophic factors through synapse formation.

Nerve growth factor is the best characterized molecule that meets all the criteria for a neurotrophic factor (9). Several other putative neurotrophic factors have been described and proposed to promote the survival of other neuron populations (9, 226).

Nevertheless, nerve growth factor remains the only characterized molecule that meets all of the criteria for a neurotrophic factor involved in regulating the survival of discrete populations of developing neurons in vivo. The addition of nerve growth factor to rat sympathetic and sensory neurons in vitro prevents cell death and stimulates axonal outgrowth. Furthermore, administration of anti–nerve growth factor antisera to newborn rats causes the death of almost all sympathetic neurons, suggesting that nerve growth factor is required for neuronal survival (see 152 for review). Brain-derived neurotrophic factor (BDNF) is another molecule that has been shown to promote the survival of embryonic chick sensory neurons in vitro (9) and quail sensory neurons in vivo (114). A factor purified from rat skeletal muscle, ChAT development factor (CDF), also has been shown to promote the survival of motoneurons in vivo and in vitro (165).

Motoneuron Physiology. When motoneurons innervate the limb bud, the dorsal and ventral muscle masses are composed only of primary muscle fibers that usually develop into slow fibers. The extent to which the motoneurons that innervate the limb at this time are differentiated into slow and fast types characteristic of the adult is unknown.

Heterogeneity of Motoneuron Properties. In the adult, motoneurons innervating each of the muscle unit types differ in their electrophysiological and morphological properties (25, 234). The diameter of a motor axon has been directly correlated with the conduction velocity and the size of the parent cell body and total cell membrane area (11). Since the motor axons innervating the slow (S) units are smaller and conduct more slowly than the motor axons innervating the fast motor unit types [i.e., fast fatigue resistant (FR) and fast-fatigable (FF)], it was assumed that the motoneurons innervating the slow motor units were smaller in size than the motoneurons innervating the fast motor units. Burke et al. (28) used retrograde tracers to label the motor pools of the soleus and medial gastrocnemius (MG) muscles of the cat and found considerable overlap between the size of slow and fast motoneurons. The average soma diameter of slow motoneurons in the soleus, composed of only type S units, was only slightly smaller than the average soma diameter of motoneurons in the MG, composed of both slow and fast motor units (mean, 50.1 and 53.1 μm for the soleus and MG, respectively). Subsequently, Burke et al. (26) used intracellular techniques to record the electrophysiological properties of single motoneurons and to label them with horseradish peroxidase (HRP) and found that type S motoneurons had smaller soma diameters (43 μm) and fewer primary dendritic branches (seven dendrites) on average than the type FF motoneurons (diameter of 54 μm and 11 dendrites). In general there is a weak correlation between the total cell membrane area of motoneurons and the type of muscle unit innervated (i.e., FF > FR > S), suggesting that factors in addition to size determine the firing patterns of motoneurons.

There is also an inverse correlation between the size of motoneurons and their input resistance (11). Input resistance is a complex function of membrane area, membrane resistance, and the time and length constants of the neuron (25). In general, slow motoneurons have a higher input resistance than fast motoneurons. Consequently, the same amount of current injected into a slow and a fast motoneuron will cause a greater change in the membrane potential of the slow motoneuron than the fast motoneuron because of Ohm's law ($E=IR$). This results in systematic differences in their susceptibility to generate action potentials during intracellular current injection (see 110 for review). In general, less current is required by slow motoneurons to reach threshold for action potential generation. Lastly, slow and fast motoneurons differ in the duration of after hyperpolarization (AHP). The AHP is important in determining the maximum frequency that a motoneuron can fire. Slow motoneurons have a longer AHP than fast motoneurons and also fire at a lower maximum frequency. The AHP duration of the motoneuron is inversely related to the contraction time of the muscle unit. In general, the intrinsic properties of the motoneurons vary such that there is a gradient of decreasing excitability that has the following sequence: S > FR > FF.

There is relatively little known about the electrical properties of embryonic motoneurons. Ziskind-Conhaim (265) reported that rat lumbar motoneurons become electrically excitable at 14 days of gestation. At 16–18 days of gestation, excitatory synaptic potentials can be evoked in response to dorsal root stimulation. Prior to birth there are increases in the resting membrane potential, the input resistance, and the maximum rate of rise of the action potential. It is unknown, however, whether differences exist between motoneurons within the same motor pool at the time of birth. At what stage motoneurons differentiate into types is still relatively unknown, although it appears that differences in the morphological and electrical properties of motoneurons arise primarily during the first 2 weeks of postnatal development.

Electrophysiologically, AHP duration is the best discriminator between slow and fast motoneurons

(234). In the kitten, Huizar et al. (121) reported no significant difference in the AHP duration between soleus and MG motoneurons at postnatal days 16–21. By postnatal day 60, however, there was a significant difference between the two populations. Interestingly, the AHP duration in both soleus and MG motoneurons of the kitten is significantly shorter (~60 ms) than in the adult (150 ms in the soleus and 75 ms in the MG). In contrast, the AHP duration of rat lumbar motoneurons at postnatal days 3–12 is longer (range, 65–178 ms) compared with adult (range, 35–76 ms) (92). Navarrette et al. (177) have suggested that there is a difference in the AHP duration of motoneurons in the slow soleus and the fast TA in rats at postnatal days 0–12. At birth, Navarette and Vrbova (176) have reported that the aggregate electromyographic (EMG) activity of the soleus, an extensor, is not significantly different from that of flexors such as the TA or EDL. During the first 2 weeks postnatally, the flexors and extensors are often co-activated. Distinct differences in the EMG activity patterns between the soleus and flexors become evident at about 14 days postnatally, which coincides with the elimination of polyinnervation within the muscle and the acquisition of adult fiber types.

As noted previously, a significant level of heterogeneity of muscle fibers is evident during development prior to innervation. Significant changes in motoneuron morphology and physiology that affect the excitation patterns of the motor units continue to occur after innervation. Similarly, the diversity of muscle fiber properties continues toward that observed in the adult. In mammals, at no stage during development or during several weeks after birth are the activation patterns similar to those in the adult. Because both neural and muscular properties are changing rapidly during development, it has become difficult to determine the extent to which the activity patterns imposed on muscle fibers influence the expression of proteins.

Synapse Elimination

Mammalian muscle fibers are initially innervated by multiple motoneurons (polyinnervation) at the same end-plate. For example, at birth, each of the ~25 soleus motoneurons innervates about 25% of the ~2,800 fibers in the soleus of rats. Consequently, each soleus muscle fiber receives an input from about five motoneurons (244). The number of inputs per fiber varies for different muscles. Of the muscles that have been examined, the soleus has the largest number of inputs per fiber (five inputs per fiber) at birth, whereas predominantly fast muscles such as the EDL, diaphragm, lumbricals, and intercostals have about three inputs per fiber (128).

Over the course of weeks, all but one input is lost, a process referred to as synapse elimination (see 128 for review). The timing of the loss of polyinnervation and the rate of loss of terminals differs among muscles, suggesting that some systemic factor is not the signal for synapse elimination. In the rat diaphragm and intercostal muscles the number of inputs per fiber is at a peak 1 day prior to birth and is dramatically reduced by birth (56). In contrast, in the rat soleus a net loss of terminals cannot be demonstrated until postnatal day 6, and the first singly innervated terminals are not detected until the second postnatal week (23). The timing of synapse elimination appears to be influenced by many factors including the timing of the myogenesis, the pattern of neuromuscular activity, and the fiber type composition of the muscle. The end result of synapse elimination is that each motoneuron innervates fewer muscle fibers than initially contacted and that each muscle fiber is innervated by only one motor axon.

Available evidence suggests that the loss of terminals is not a random process, but one that is dependent in part on a competitive process. It was initially postulated that the mechanism of loss of terminals at the synapse was due to competition between the presynaptic terminals and the eventual degeneration of all but one of the presynaptic terminal nerve branches. Numerous investigations, however, failed to find degenerating terminals, and the observations were more in line with retraction and resorption of the terminal branches by the parent axon (16, 203). More recently, it has been demonstrated that synapse elimination involves the loss of the postsynaptic receptors prior to the withdrawal of the nerve terminals overlying the depleted postsynaptic sites (4). These observations were made with a technique that allows visualization of the presynaptic terminals of multiple axons with vital fluorescent dyes and postsynaptic receptors with rhodamine-labeled α-bungarotoxin (5). These data suggest that the postsynaptic terminal mediates elimination of presynaptic inputs. Little is known, however, about what factors the postsynaptic terminals might be competing for and what mechanism results in their ultimate withdrawal from the postsynaptic membrane.

Competition vs. Intrinsic Withdrawal. The primary evidence for the role of competition during synapse elimination has come from partial denervation experiments performed just after birth in the soleus of the rat and mouse (23, 84, 245) and in the lumbricals of the rat (13). The initial experiments were performed in the rat soleus (23, 245). At birth, the soleus that normally is innervated by 20–30 motoneurons was partially denervated, sparing 2–16 motor axons. The average size of the remaining motor units, measured several weeks later, was smaller than at birth, but 40% larger than units in control mature animals. The results suggested that two mechanisms were acting during synapse elimination: *(1)* competition between axons innervating the same synapse, and *(2)* an intrinsic program within the motoneuron to withdraw synapses. Similar experiments were performed in the rat lumbricals in which it was possible to cut all but one of the motor axons to the muscle, thus eliminating all competition between axons (13). After 2 weeks the average size of the single remaining motor unit was about the same as prior to the partial denervation (~50% larger than normal), suggesting that without competition synapse elimination did not occur. Consequently, Betz and colleagues (13) proposed that in the lumbricals withdrawal of synapses can be fully explained by competition.

These results motivated Fladby and Jansen (85) to repeat the experiments in the mouse soleus, which contains fewer motor units than the rat soleus. By cutting the fifth lumbar ventral root they produced soleus muscles with varying numbers of motor units. When more than seven motor units remained, all the muscle fibers were innervated and the average size of the motor units was larger than normal. With less than seven units the number of innervated fibers was reduced and was directly related to the number of remaining motor units. Interestingly, with fewer than seven units, the average motor unit size remained the same, ~80 fibers per unit. These results reconfirmed the early suggestion that motoneurons have some intrinsic limit to the number of terminals that can be maintained. Consequently, during synapse elimination it appears that both a noncompetitive and a competitive mechanism are involved in determining the distribution of motor unit sizes observed in the adult.

Activity and Synapse Elimination. The activity level of muscle fibers influence the formation and elimination of synapses. Blockage of nerve activity by TTX on postnatal day 9 or 10, when soleus muscle fibers are still polyneuronally innervated, slows down the rate of synapse elimination during the first few days of the block (241). However, 6–7 days after the block, 70%–90% of the muscle fibers are polyneuronally innervated compared to only 5% or less on the contralateral side (241). The polyinnervation is eliminated within a few days of removing the TTX block (243). The same effects of inactivity also have been demonstrated by Brown et al. (22) using α-bungarotoxin to inactivate the muscle fibers and by Caldwell et al. (30) using neonatal spinal cord isolation (i.e., transection of the spinal cord at two levels and dorsal rhizotomy between the transection sites).

Increasing the activity of muscle fibers has the opposite effect on synapse elimination. Imposed electrical stimulation of the neonatal rat sciatic nerve (179) or the soleus muscle (240) via intramuscular electrodes accelerates synapse elimination in the soleus. Interestingly, the effect appears to be dependent on the pattern of activity. The same number of stimuli given as a 100 Hz train of 1 s duration delivered every 100 s over the course of a day was more effective in eliminating synapses than a continuous 1 Hz train (240). Although these experiments indicate that activity has a dramatic effect on the development of neuromuscular connectivity, they do not address the role of activity in the competition between axons innervating the same fiber. To address this issue, several models of differential activation of axons to the same muscle have been tested.

Role of Competition between Axons. Ribchester and Taxt (200, 201) explored the effects of a differential block of nerve activity on synapse formation and elimination in the adult rat lumbrical muscle during reinnervation. The lumbrical receives its innervation from two separate nerves: the sural (SN) and lateral plantar (LPN) nerve. The majority of the innervation (5–10 of the 11 motor axons) comes from the LPN. In the initial experiments, both the LPN and SN were crushed and the activity in the LPN was blocked with TTX. After 2 weeks of LPN block, the SN motor units were twice as large as control SN units and the LPN units were smaller than normal. These results supported the hypothesis that more active presynaptic terminals have a competitive advantage over less active presynaptic terminals. However, additional experiments revealed that the process is very complex and that activity may not be the only important variable to consider. For example, when the SN was left intact and the LPN was crushed and its activity blocked, the SN nerve sprouted to reinnervate the entire muscle while the LPN was regenerating. However, even though the LPN was blocked it was able to displace some SN innervation and establish exclusive innervation of some fibers. Consequently, presynaptic activity does not invariably decide the outcome of competitive interactions.

Ridge and Betz (202) attempted to examine in neonatal rats the effects of increased activity of either the SN or LPN motor axons on synapse elimination in the lumbrical. They found no significant difference in the sizes of SN motor units in response to stimulation. In contrast to these results, Callaway et al. (31, 32) reported that inactive terminals were at a selective advantage over active terminals. In the neonatal rat, they selectively blocked one of the three ventral roots (L7, S1, or S2) supplying motor axons to the soleus. The effect of selective nerve root block was that motor units innervated by the inactive root were about 50% larger than normal and units innervated by the remaining active roots were significantly smaller than normal. These results are interesting in light of the fact that in adults the largest motor units are the least activated while the smallest motor units are the most activated (see 110 for review).

It is clear that neuromuscular activity has a profound effect on synapse elimination; however, the mechanisms by which activity exerts its control are still poorly understood. Recently, much has been learned about the molecular processes underlying synapse formation and the role of activity (see 103 for review). A better understanding of the roles of pre- and postsynaptic cells in the decision-making process will help identify the signals that control synapse elimination.

Innervation of Muscle Fiber Types and the Role of Synapse Elimination. As mentioned previously, muscle fibers can differentiate into slow and fast fibers independent of innervation. Moreover, the number and location of slow and fast fiber types within a muscle in the neonate is similar, if not identical, to that in the adult, suggesting that fibers do not undergo nerve-induced transformations in type during the period of synapse elimination. This observation has led to the hypothesis that the role of synapse elimination is to match motoneurons with the appropriate type of fiber. Experiments to address this hypothesis have been performed in the mouse, rat, and rabbit.

Thompson et al. (246) used the glycogen depletion technique to identify the fibers belonging to a single motor unit in the soleus of the neonatal rat when each fiber was innervated by approximately two to three axons. They found that the fiber type composition of each unit was highly biased toward one type. In a muscle composed of 55% slow and 45% fast fibers, motor units were composed of at least 70% of one fiber type, and in some cases greater than 90% of one type. These data suggested that motoneurons selectively innervate fibers of a particular type (i.e., slow or fast) initially. Gordon and Van Essen (99) came to a similar conclusion based on the contractile properties of motor units in the soleus of the neonatal rabbit. They found a bimodal distribution of contraction times during the period of polyinnervation and concluded that slow and fast fibers were preferentially innervated prior to the conclusion of synapse elimination. More recently, Fladby and Jansen (86) examined the fiber type composition of motor units in the soleus of the 5-day-old mouse. They used micropipettes filled with Lucifer yellow to impale and record the end-plate potentials from fibers belonging to a single unit and then filled them with the dye. The dye-filled motor unit fibers were identified and typed by immunohistochemical methods. They found that each unit was composed of predominantly one type of fiber at a time when each fiber was innervated by approximately six inputs. Moreover, the twitch contraction times matched the fiber type composition of each motor unit.

The results found in the lumbrical by Jones et al. (135, 136) are in contrast to the findings previously mentioned. They used glycogen depletion to examine single motor unit fibers in the lumbrical of 3-day-old rats and found that 11 of 12 motor units identified were nonselectively innervated based on the fiber type composition of each of the units. The lumbricals of 3-day-old rats contain about 12% slow fibers, and 11 of the 12 gycogen-depleted units contained an average of 13% slow fibers. Consequently, they concluded that the initial innervation was random and that synapse elimination served to sharpen the selectivity of innervation of fiber types. The reasons for the differences between the results obtained in the soleus and the lumbrical are unclear; the differences may be related to the relative immaturity of the lumbrical muscle at birth. Secondary myogenesis continues into the second week of postnatal life in the lumbrical, whereas it is complete in the soleus within days after birth. From these data it is obvious that there are still many questions with regard to the development of motor units from different muscles composed of fibers expressing the same MHC isoform. Withdrawal of synapses based on fiber type mismatches cannot account for all of the synapse elimination, since a fiber innervated by two axons of the same type should theoretically maintain both inputs unless other factors account for the competition.

Positional Cues and Synapse Elimination. In some muscles there is a topographical projection of motoneurons onto the muscle (i.e., motoneurons specifically innervate select regions of the muscle, thereby establishing functional compartments) (78). Segmental innervation has been shown most convincingly in broad, sheet-like muscles such as the diaphragm, serratus anterior, and intercostals (149). Laskowski and Sanes (150) demonstrated that the segmentotopic innervation found in the adult diaphragm was reestabished after transection of the phrenic nerve. These observations lead to the proposal that synapse elimination may serve to sharpen the boundaries of these compartments by matching motoneurons to a specific topographical location within the muscle. Similar types of matching occur during development between the sensory compartments of muscles and the motor pools (261).

In the neonatal rat soleus, Miyata and Yoshioka (171) reported a greater loss of terminals from axons originating from lumbar root 4 than axons from lumbar root 5. However, these results could not be confirmed in the soleus of the rat (242), the rabbit (98), or the mouse (85). Each of these investigations showed no preferential loss of terminals in the soleus based on segmental innervation. These results are not surprising because the soleus is a uniarticulate muscle that has a relatively even distribution of fast and slow fibers throughout the muscle cross section. Similarly, somatotopic innervation and sharpening of compartments during synapse elimination has not been demonstrated in the rat EDL (6) or lumbrical (15).

The hypothesis of synapse elimination based on positional information has been supported by studies in the mouse gluteus maximus (21) and the rat lateral gastrocnemius (LG) (12). In the gluteus maximus, Brown and Booth (21) observed that at birth motor units innervated fibers scattered over ~40% of the muscle cross section. After synapse elimination, the motor unit territory was markedly smaller, decreasing from about 40% to 15% of the cross section of the muscle. In addition, a stronger topographical relationship emerged as synapse elimination proceeded (i.e., rostral motoneurons innervated the posterior region of the muscle and caudal motoneurons innervated the anterior region of the muscle). These results were confirmed and extended by Bennett and Lavidis (12), who used glycogen-depletion techniques. In the rat LG at birth, the muscle is evenly innervated by motor axons from the L4 and L5 ventral roots. After a week or more, the innervation pattern has changed such that the medial edge is innervated equally by both roots, but the lateral edge is exclusively innervated by L4. Consequently, it appears that a segmental preference was established during the synapse elimination period. However, Donahue and English (62) found that the compartmentalization of the rat LG was well established at the time of birth. During the first postnatal week, 8% of the muscle fibers received inputs from more than one compartment, whereas after postnatal day 7 no cross-compartmental inputs could be detected. Furthermore, delaying synapse elimination in the LG by tenotomy did not change the rate at which the small percentage of cross-compartmentalization was eliminated (62, 63). These results suggest that the innervation territories of compartmentalized nerve branches are largely established at birth and that postnatal synapse elimination does not serve to sharpen the boundaries of the compartments.

Summary

The fact that synapse elimination occurs postnatally in the neuromuscular system is well established. The exact role that synapse elimination plays, however, remains undefined. Synapse elimination could serve to eliminate mismatches with regard to fiber type, to sharpen compartmental boundaries within a muscle, or to sharpen motor unit territories. Synapse elimination could also serve to establish the distribution of motor unit sizes that is apparent in adult muscles and allows for the orderly recruitment of motor units during movement. Recent work by Lichtman and co-workers (155) has provided new information on how synapses may be lost; however, at the molecular level little is known about what determines which motor inputs will be eliminated. For example, are motoneurons differentiated into fast and slow types at the time of innervation? If so, do they selectively innervate fibers of a specific type or is the initial innervation random with regard to fiber type? To what extent can a motoneuron distinguish between fibers of different types, since at the time of innervation the adult fast MHC isoforms are not expressed? If loss of postsynaptic receptors precedes the loss of the presynaptic terminals, how does a muscle fiber distinguish between different inputs? What are the underlying molecular events that lead to the elimination of all but one input? How does a motoneuron make the decision to sustain innervation ratios that will be highly ordered with respect to maximum force and order of recruitment?

Given the extensive amount of motoneuron death, multiple innervation of single fibers and the complete withdrawal of multiple inputs to motoneurons during development, the precision that exists in adult motor pools with respect to the recruitment order defined within an accuracy of 2%–3% of the tetanic tension between motor units represents an exquisite regulation of development of the neuromuscular system.

NEURAL AND NONNEURAL SOURCES OF CONTROL OF ADULT SKELETAL MUSCLE PROPERTIES

Cross-Reinnervation

By 1960 there was a range of studies pointing to the possibility of the matching of neural and muscular properties and that the matching could result from a neural regulation of muscle properties (45, 57, 68). It was not, however, until Buller et al. (24) reported that a slow muscle became faster (shorter isometric twitch contraction and relaxation times) after reinnervation by a nerve that normally innervated a fast muscle (and vice versa) that it became evident that the nervous system could modulate skeletal muscle properties. In this same study (24), it was concluded that the matching of the characteristics of the motoneuron and muscle fibers "occurs very largely, if not exclusively, in the reverse direction from motoneurons to muscle fibers." This conclusion was based principally on the observations that the duration of AHP and the conduction velocity of the slow soleus motoneurons that reinnervated the fast flexor digitorum longus (FDL) did not change toward that more typical of a fast muscle. Within the next 5 years, other experiments suggested that much of the diversity in the physiological properties of muscle occurred at the motor unit level (58, 111). For example, the slower contracting motor units generally had slower conduction velocities and lower recruitment thresholds compared to the faster contracting units (111). Furthermore, the biochemical properties of muscle fibers of the slow soleus and fast MG (e.g., low staining for myosin ATPase) matched the motor unit contractile properties.

Some of the key issues raised by the results of these studies were: *(1)* Does the nervous system modulate all physiological properties associated with skeletal muscle fiber diversity? *(2)* Does the nervous system have complete control of some or all of these properties of diversity? *(3)* If the neural control is manifested via the motoneuron, is it derived from the activation characteristics of the neuron or is it via non-activity associated events (i.e., a neurotrophic mechanism)? *(4)* Is the motoneuron itself the conduit for the neural control of skeletal muscle properties or is it via some other cell types (e.g., Schwann cells)? Most of the studies of reinnervated or cross-reinnervated muscles since the pioneer studies of Buller and colleagues (24) have attempted to answer questions 1, 2, and 3. Little attention has been given to the last question and consequently the following section focuses on the first three issues.

There have been many studies of muscle properties following cross-reinnervation in adults. The reports cited are ones that permit an assessment of *(1)* the completeness of the conversion of multiple physiological and biochemical fiber type characteristics, and *(2)* the adequacy of the length of the postoperative periods. Based on the results of these studies, we conclude that the nervous system has partial control (i.e., some influence on most properties of skeletal muscle fibers that contribute to their diversity). At least some of this influence seems to be manifested via the pattern and/or amount of activity from a given motoneuron. It has become equally apparent that the neural influence is manifested in conjunction with other sources of control, some of which are only beginning to be recognized.

Physiological Properties. The observations of Buller and colleagues (24) that slow muscles can become faster and fast muscles can become slower when the nerves to a slow and a fast muscle are crossed have been confirmed many times. The majority of these studies have used the soleus muscle for two reasons. First the soleus muscle of the rabbit, cat, and guinea pig is usually comprised exclusively of slow muscle fibers. Therefore, an adaptation from slow to fast in any fiber or muscle property can be detected easily. Second, the soleus anatomically is in a convenient position to be reinnervated with any of a number of predominantly fast nerves (e.g., the EDL, FDL, MG, or peroneal nerve). These fast nerves, however, differ in their "pureness" with respect to the percentage of fast fibers in the muscle that they originally innervated and in matching numbers of axons relative to the number of fibers in the soleus muscle. This factor complicates the interpretation of the results of reinnervation of the "pure" soleus muscle with a mixed nerve. One of the limiting factors in innervating fast muscles with the slow soleus nerve may be that the ratio of available muscle fibers to motoneurons is extremely high. Furthermore, motoneurons may innervate more muscle fibers than normal and/or there may be some selective processes related to type that may be operating. In general, fast muscles have heterogeneous type-related properties, and this may contribute to the differential responsiveness observed in fast muscles cross-reinnervated by a "purely" slow population of axons, at least with respect to the completeness of the conversion.

The results from these studies indicate that all of the muscle properties studied following cross-reinnervation are modulated by the nervous system. The whole-muscle physiological properties studied include isometric twitch contraction and relaxation times and the maximum velocity of shortening per sarcomere.

The magnitude of the physiological changes have varied widely. One of the earliest and most thorough examinations of the physiological properties of cross-reinnervated muscles was the work of Sreter and colleagues in rabbits (228, 229). They found that the contraction times in both the soleus and the EDL were 100% converted; that is, the values for the slow and fast cross-reinnervated muscles were similar to those for fast and slow self-reinnervated muscles, respectively, 12 months after surgery. The conversion in the maximum velocity of shortening, on the other hand, was 75% and 90% complete for the soleus and EDL, respectively. Luff (157) reported that the maximum velocity of shortening of the EDL was almost 100% converted to slow in the cat, whereas the soleus was only 63% converted to fast in the rat after 12 months of cross-reinnervation. Only a 33% and 41% conversion was observed in the contraction and half-relaxation times, respectively, of the crossed EDL in rats (157), while both properties were about 90% converted in the crossed soleus after 12 months. In a similar study, Barany and Close (8) found about 50% conversion in the contraction and half-relaxation times in the crossed EDL and about 85% conversion of both parameters in the soleus after 13–14 months of cross-reinnervation. Muntener et al. (174) reported that the contraction time of the crossed EDL was converted by about 60% toward slow values, whereas the soleus contraction time was actually faster than that of the normal EDL in the rat. Mommaerts et al. (173) reported conversions of the cat soleus contraction times that were 75%–96% complete 14–23 months after crossing with the flexor hallucis longus (FHL) nerve and only 4%–55% complete in the FHL. Lesser levels of conversion were observed in the maximum velocity of shortening and in the myosin ATPase activity measured biochemically (see below).

In summary, some conversion of several physiological properties related to speed of muscle contraction has been observed following cross-reinnervation. The level of conversion has varied widely for both slow and fast muscles. However, in no experiment has there been complete conversion of all speed-related contractile properties following cross-reinnervation. It can always be hypothesized that the duration of the cross-reinnervation was insufficient, but little difference has been observed in the level of conversion in studies lasting from 3–4 months to about 3 years. We conclude that there is little evidence that complete conversion of the speed-related muscle contractile properties following cross-reinnervation occurs in the rat, cat, or rabbit. Some remaining questions are: *(1)* Which muscle proteins are under neural control? *(2)* How complete is the neural control of these proteins? and *(3)* What are the sources and mechanisms of the neural control?

Biochemical Properties. Evidence for the complete control of the nervous system of the expression of those proteins associated with muscle fiber diversity is even less convincing than that for the physiological properties. The incompleteness of the conversion of the biochemical properties from fast to slow or from slow to fast following cross-reinnervation has been demonstrated in a variety of species and for a range of contractile and metabolic enzymes. The type of biochemical properties examined and the methods used have varied widely.

Contractile proteins. Those biochemical properties associated with the dynamics of excitation-contraction coupling and the properties of the contractile event are of particular interest because they relate to the physiological properties discussed above. Calcium-activated ATPase activity, an enzyme highly correlated with speed of shortening in control muscles (7), was 80% converted in the rabbit soleus cross-reinnervated with the EDL nerve, but the conversion was only 46% complete in the EDL cross-reinnervated with the soleus nerve (229). Furthermore, Mommaerts et al. (173) found a poor relationship between the amount of conversion based on the velocity of shortening compared to the myosin ATPase activity. For example, in one animal 19 months after cross-reinnervation of the soleus, the conversion of the maximum rate of shortening was 93% complete, while the myosin ATPase activity was only 38% complete. In another animal the conversion was 75% and 15% complete for these same measures. Guth and Samaha (101) reported that the cat soleus, normally 100% slow, contained only 30% fast myosin after cross-reinnervation. On the other hand, no slow myosin remained in the rat soleus after 12–16 months of cross-reinnervation with the EDL nerve (116). This latter observation, however, was based on visual observations of electrophoretic gels separating isoforms of slow and fast myosin (i.e., not separated into light and heavy chains associated with slow and fast muscle). This is the only report that has suggested that a complete conversion of myosin can occur in a cross-reinnervated muscle.

Different types of light and heavy chains of myosin also have been examined after cross-reinnervation. Both slow and fast light chains of myosin were found in the soleus and EDL muscles after nerve crossing, reflecting an incomplete conversion of the myosin types expressed (229). Secrist and Kerrick (218) found that about one-third of the light chains in the rabbit soleus were of the fast type after cross-reinnervation with the EDL nerve.

Regulatory proteins. Proteins related to calcium regulation also have been studied. Both troponin and tropomyosin isoforms are affected by cross-reinnervation. For example, about 90% of the fibers in the rabbit soleus contained the fast troponin complex (based on antibody reactions) 4 to 7 months after cross-reinnervation with the EDL or TA nerve (59).

The amount of conversion was "much less complete" in the fast muscles cross-reinnervated with the soleus nerve: 98% and 93% of the fibers in the TA and EDL reacted with the fast troponin I antibody in control, whereas 69% and 21% reacted after cross-reinnervation. In the rabbit soleus, 8–27 months after cross-reinnervation with the lateral popliteal nerve, 65% of the troponin I was of the fast type in the crossed compared to 31% in the control muscles (1). There is some evidence based on two-dimensional gel electrophoresis that the δ- and γ-, but not the α- and β-, subunits of tropomyosin changed after cross-reinnervation (107). It was concluded that the type of innervation markedly affected the polymorphic form of troponin I but did not affect tropomyosin or troponin C. These authors (107) speculated that multiple factors were involved in regulating the genes of these proteins (i.e., that there were other sources of regulation in addition to the nervous system).

Proteins related to oxidative phosphorylation. Malate and isocitrate dehydrogenase activities of muscle homogenates remained high in the cross-reinnervated soleus, while in the cross-reinnervated FDL these enzyme activities increased. These data demonstrated that the high oxidative capacity of the soleus was maintained when innervated by motoneurons that normally innervated muscle fibers that have very low oxidative capacities. Some of the slow fibers became fast and high glycolytic after reinnervation, but the oxidative capacity was not down-regulated as might have been expected assuming the very low levels of stimulation characteristic of fast glycolytic (FG) fibers (113). In fact, based on histochemical analyses there were no fibers with low oxidative capacity in the cross-reinnervated soleus. The reverse was not true in the FDL cross-reinnervated by the soleus nerve; that is, the low oxidative capacity of most of the FDL muscle fibers was modulated upward when reinnervated by motoneurons that are normally highly active.

Margreth et al. (160) allowed reinnervation for 3–4 months in the rat after cutting the sciatic nerve. The soleus showed ~24% conversion with respect to calcium ATPase activity, but no change in the amount of myoglobin and succinate cytochrome *c* reductase. In the cross-reinnervated soleus muscle, there was a reduction in β-hydroxyacyl CoA dehydrogenase and citrate synthase activity. However, the decrease was similar to that observed following self-reinnervation. Some evidence for a down-regulation of the oxidative capacity of the crossed soleus, however, has been reported. For example, the activities of the mitochondrial enzymes malate and citrate dehydrogenase in the crossed rabbit soleus (6–17 months) decreased about 20% and that of β-hydroxyacyl CoA dehydrogenase activity decreased by 40%–60% compared to the soleus in the contralateral, unoperated leg. In general, these findings demonstrate a bias toward high oxidative capacity, manifested by the retention of oxidative capacity in cross-reinnervated slow muscle and the up-regulation of oxidative enzymes in cross-reinnervated fast muscle.

Glycolytic proteins. An examination of enzymes related to glycolysis is interesting, not because of their role in determining fatigability, but because they are so tightly linked to the types of myosin and speed-related properties of muscles (27). Margreth et al. (160) found about a 20%–30% conversion of the soleus based on glycerol phosphate, glucose-3-phosphate, and lactate dehydrogenase (LDH) activities in muscle homogenates 3–4 months after sciatic nerve transection and reinnervation in the rat. These results were similar to those observed by Prewitt and Salafsky (196) in the cat. Pyruvate kinase and aldolase were about 30% and 18% converted in the crossed soleus, respectively, whereas they were converted by 86% and 65% in the crossed FDL, respectively. Mommaerts et al. (173) showed a 48% and 31% conversion of pyruvate kinase and aldolase activities, respectively, in the soleus 11 months after cross-reinnervation with the EDL nerve. Lactate dehydrogenase activity was about 54% converted in the crossed rat soleus and 47% in the cat soleus. The crossed FDL muscle in the cat was 63% converted based on LDH activity. A significant increase in the muscle type isoform of LDH and decrease in the heart type LDH activity was observed in the cat after cross-reinnervation (i.e., there was a qualitative change in the relative expression of one isoform vs. another).

Jobsis (133) studied metabolic proteins in the soleus and FDL of the rat 6–9 months after cross-reinnervation. In addition, two rats were studied after 2 years of cross-reinnervation. During the 6- to 9-month period the percentage conversion of the soleus toward that observed in the self-reinnervated FDL was 96% and 90%, respectively, for phosphofructokinase and glycerol phosphate oxidase activities. Similar comparisons for the convertibility of these enzyme activities in the FDL toward the values observed in the soleus were 68% and 55%. The authors state, however, that after 2 years the conversion appeared to be complete. Unfortunately, this conclusion was based on biochemical data from only two animals. The histochemical data on these same rats, in contrast, suggested incomplete conversion after 2 years. For example, 37% of the fibers in the control soleus had high glycerol phosphate oxidase staining compared to 53% in the cross-reinnervated soleus. In comparison, the normal FDL muscle had 78% of the fibers staining darkly for the glycolytic enzyme.

Reichmann et al. (197) studied two soleus muscles after 6 months and two after 17 months of cross-reinnervation with the peroneal nerve in the rabbit. The activities of seven glycolytic enzymes were markedly increased in the crossed soleus, but the percentage conversion could not be estimated because no data were reported for any fast muscles nor for any self-reinnervated soleus muscles. The cross-reinnervated soleus expressed fast myosin light chains (none were observed in controls) and a higher proportion of the LDH isoform of the skeletal muscle type as opposed to the heart type than in controls. The glycolytic enzymes studied showed a two-fold increase in activity. No changes in enzyme activities were found in the cross-reinnervated fast muscles and the authors suggested that this was due to the relatively few slow motoneurons available to innervate the fast muscles.

In summary, these results demonstate that the glycolytic properties are up-regulated in the crossed soleus by the presence of motoneurons that normally innervate fast muscles, and are down-regulated in crossed fast muscles by the presence of motoneurons that normally innervate slow muscles. The conversions are not complete in either direction.

Histochemical and Immunohistochemical Properties. Further insight into the question of the completeness of the neural control of muscle properties has been gained using histochemical and immunohistochemical techniques. Advantages of these procedures are that enzyme activities or the presence of a given protein or peptide within individual fibers can be examined and that a series of enzymes can be studied easily in the same fibers. A disadvantage in most cases is that the measures are qualitative. Based on these approaches, the incompleteness of the conversion of the physiological and biochemical properties of the muscle can be related to the percentage of the fibers that undergo a conversion in type. This was first indicated by staining muscle cross sections for myofibrillar ATPase activity after alkaline preincubation (i.e., activating the fast and inhibiting the slow ATPase isoforms) and acid preincubation (i.e., activating the slow and inhibiting the fast ATPase isoforms) (20). Based on these staining procedures, it is clear that some fibers change myosin types while others do not following cross-reinnervation. For example, after cross-reinnervation of the soleus the percentage of fibers that remained slow (type I) was: 48% in the rat (239); 34% (218), 82% (204), and 15% (197) in the rabbit; and 70% (100), 61% (154), and 91%–100% (89) in the cat. In one study (197), the cross-reinnervated soleus contained only 15% type I fibers compared to 100% in control animals. It is clear, however, from the photomicrographs obtained from sandwiched tissue blocks in which cross-reinnervated and contralateral, unoperated muscles were processed simultaneously, that the intensities of the myofibrillar ATPase histochemical staining reactions were not strictly comparable (197). These observations emphasize one of the limitations in qualitative histochemistry, particularly the myofibrillar ATPase assay, which is highly pH sensitive as noted above (20). It does not appear that these staining properties accurately reflect differences in the myosin isoforms or combinations of myosins that are being expressed in a fiber. Thus, from the standpoint of identifying specific myosins expressed per fiber and associating this expression with fiber type based on myofibrillar ATPase activity, the conversion of many fibers was incomplete following cross-reinnervation.

An important feature of the diversity of skeletal muscles is the coordination of the expression of enzymes related to metabolic support and contractile activity. The enzymes of glycolysis and oxidative phosphorylation have been categorized and correlated with the speed and fatigue properties in normal muscle fibers. FG fibers contract rapidly, fatigue rapidly, and have a low oxidative and a high glycolytic capacity (27, 190). Fast oxidative glycolytic fibers (FOG) also contract rapidly and have a high glycolytic capacity, but also have a high capacity to sustain oxidative phosphorylation. FOG fibers have a high density of mitochondria and are more resistant to fatigue than are the FG fibers. Slow oxidative (SO) fibers contract slowly, have a low glycolytic capacity and a high oxidative capacity, and are very resistant to fatigue. Unlike the comparisons made between the closely linked speed-related and the biochemical properties, there are no data to compare at the whole-muscle level between the metabolically related proteins and fatigability. The relationship between fatigability and biochemical properties will be addressed in a later section when examining motor unit properties.

Are the metabolically related enzymes in skeletal muscle under complete neural control? Prewitt and Salafsky (196) reported that the cross-reinnervated soleus contained 44% slow fibers (probably equivalent to SO fibers) compared to 89% in control, with the remaining fibers in both the control and cross-reinnervated soleus being equivalent to FOG fibers. The normal FDL had 23%, 32%, and 39% SO, FG, and FOG fibers, respectively, as identified by qualitative histochemical techniques. (Note that 6% of the fibers had light phosphorylase and SDH activities and could not be classified.) The crossed FDL contained 83%, 4%, and 12% SO, FG, and FOG fibers, respectively. Dum and co-workers showed that although the mean contraction time of the cat soleus was reduced considerably after reinnervation by the gastrocnemius nerve, only 7% of the soleus muscle fibers were type II (fast) as defined by myofibrillar ATPase staining 30 to 50 weeks after cross-reinnervation (65, 66). A resistance to conversion of some slow fibers in the soleus also was evident 3 years after cross-reinnervation in one study (154). The conclusion from these studies is that the fast nerve is limited in its ability to transform the slow soleus muscle fibers and that the changes occur rather rapidly (within ~4 months).

Less information has been reported on fiber type adaptations in fast muscles. Almost complete transformation in the contractile and histochemical properties of the FDL cross-reinnervated with the soleus nerve was observed with 95% of the fibers having ATPase staining characteristics similar to that of self-reinnervated or normal soleus muscles (65, 66). When the LG and soleus muscles were reinnervated with the MG nerve, the resistance of soleus muscle fibers to transformation to fast fibers was quite evident (89). After 9–11 months of reinnervation, the LG contained the normal proportion of motor unit types found in the MG. This contrasting effect (i.e., almost complete transformation of a fast muscle to slow, but almost no conversion of a slow muscle toward fast following cross-reinnervation) is particularly striking considering that the experiments were performed by the same investigators.

Immunohistochemical analyses provide a clear demonstration of the difference in susceptibility of individual fibers to change the expression from one myosin isoform to another. For example, Gauthier et al. (94) reported that the majority of soleus fibers after cross-reinnervation reacted with a fast type of myosin light chain as well as with an antibody for slow myosin, indicating a considerable level of co-expression of fast and slow myosin isoforms within the same muscle fiber. Several other authors have reported that the myosin types did not change in most fibers after the soleus was reinnervated by a fast nerve (89, 153).

In summary, the histochemical and immunohistochemical analyses of cross-reinnervated muscle demonstrate that the soleus nerve can exert considerable influence on a fast muscle, but that the slow muscle is less influenced by a fast nerve. The results also suggest that there are significant differences among fibers within a muscle in their susceptibility to conversion following cross-reinnervation. This differential response is particularly evident in the soleus, where the muscle fibers normally appear to be quite homogeneous in their properties.

Motor Unit Properties. Studies of motor units following cross-reinnervation have been particularly useful in defining the level of influence that the motoneuron has on adult skeletal muscle fibers. Luff (157) studied 15 units in the control soleus of rats and 15 units in soleus muscles reinnervated by the FHL nerve. The mean contraction times for the control soleus motor units were 15 and 25 ms for fast and slow units, while the mean for all 15 units in the cross-reinnervated soleus was 25 ms (range, 16–46 ms). Lewis et al. (154) studied motor units in the cat soleus 3 years after cross-reinnervation with either the FHL or FDL nerve. The mean contraction time of the soleus motor units was reduced, but remained much longer than that of typical fast units in the FHL or FDL. Bagust et al. (2) also found that the contraction times of motor units in the crossed cat soleus were not completely converted to the fast profile of FDL motor units. All of these results suggest some resistance to a neurally induced modification of motor unit twitch contraction times.

Edgerton et al. (70) demonstrated that, when the cat soleus was reinnervated by the FHL nerve for 12–14 months, the soleus motor units that were reinnervated by the FHL motoneurons maintained their resistance to fatigue. Thus, these motor units retained the characteristics of the normal soleus rather than acquiring the more fatigable profile that typified the normal FHL units. The maintenance of a high resistance to fatigue of soleus motor units after cross-reinnervation with a fast nerve subsequently has been shown in several reports (88, 96). Furthermore, the histochemical profiles of the fibers in cross-reinnervated muscles match those of fibers having a high resistance to fatigue (i.e., showing high oxidative enzyme staining) (66, 70, 153). Dum et al. (66) classified all 23 cross-reinnervated motor units isolated in the soleus cross-reinnervated by the FDL as slow based on the sag test and fatigue resistance (although many of the motor units had fast contraction times).

In summary, these studies demonstrated that the source of innervation of the muscle fibers of a motor unit in a cross-reinnervated soleus muscle was derived from a motoneuron that normally innervated a predominantly fast muscle. In spite of the maintenance of functional connections between the foreign motoneuron and the slow muscle for up to 3 years, most properties of most fibers of these crossed motor units retained many properties of slow fibers.

These data also demonstrate that the degree of conversion can differ substantially among the cross-reinnervated units.

Limitations. What is the appropriate control for cross-reinnervated muscles? Several studies have shown that the contralateral, unoperated muscle does not serve as an adequate control (130, 173, 197). For example, the mean percentages of fibers in the rabbit soleus classified as type II were 0%, 30%, and 85% in control, contralateral unoperated, and cross-reinnervated muscles, respectively. The authors interpretation of the changes in the contralateral control muscles was that a unilateral denervation of the peroneal and soleus nerves imposed an altered use of the contralateral leg that in turn induced changes in muscle fiber phenotype (197).

In almost every experimental paradigm involving crossed nerves, it is difficult to draw firm conclusions regarding the extent to which muscle fibers can be converted when innervated by an axon that originally innervated another muscle fiber phenotype. One reason for this limitation is that the number of available axons following nerve crossing is often not proportional to the number of muscle fibers in the muscle being reinnervated. It is perhaps unreasonable to presume that the soleus nerve could successfully innervate all of the fibers in the TA or EDL, given that the number of fibers in these muscles is several times greater than the number of muscle fibers in the soleus. In addition to the large number of muscle fibers in the fast muscles relative to the few axons in the soleus nerve, slow motoneurons do not innervate as many muscle fibers as do fast motoneurons (43, 255), further limiting the amount of conversion that could be expected. Another complication in most of the cross-reinnervation studies has been the presence of severe atrophy of the cross-reinnervated muscles, suggesting among other things that there may be many denervated fibers in these muscles (173). Rarely is there verification that all or even most muscle fibers were reinnervated (i.e., some muscle fibers may remain denervated). The "pureness" of the cross-reinnervation is a factor that is only occasionally taken into account. A "pure" nerve cross means that stimulation of the crossed nerve proximal to the original transection site results in no contraction of the original muscle (i.e., there was no self-reinnervation).

It also should be recognized that all muscle fibers are denervated for some period of time before the axons can reach the new target. For this as well as other reasons, one necessary control for a cross-reinnervated study is a self-reinnervated muscle. Ideally, the self-reinnervation would be performed in animals in which the contralateral leg would be unoperated. This is usually not feasible, however, given the large number of animals that would be required. In any case, because muscle properties change in unoperated and self-reinnervated muscles contralateral to the cross-reinnervated muscles, there are some effects of the cross-reinnervation process that are not due only to the source of the innervating axon. Whether these effects are transmitted neurally or humorally or can be attributed to altered "use" is unknown.

Prolonged Electrical Silence

The question being asked in these experiments is: Can the motoneuron modulate protein expression in skeletal muscle fibers by mechanisms that are independent of neuromuscular activity? In these experiments, the innervation of the muscle fibers remains intact, but action potentials are not allowed to reach the muscle fibers. Two aproaches have been useful in determining whether the nervous system can modulate muscle properties in the absence of activity: *(1)* a surgical strategy and *(2)* a pharmacological strategy.

Surgically Induced Inactivity. The surgical model of inactivity eliminates *(1)* descending signals to the lumbar spinal cord, *(2)* ascending input, and *(3)* all afferent input that enters the lumbar cord via the dorsal roots. This model is commonly referred to as the "Tower preparation" (74–77, 193, 194, 209, 250). Tower's (250) original studies on three dogs led her to conclude that the dependence of skeletal muscle on its innervation to alter protein expression was not completely dependent on the activity in its motoneurons. This activity independence is commonly viewed as evidence for a neurotrophic mechanism. Many of the results on the spinal isolated preparation, performed mainly in adult cats, have been summarized recently (207). The results have been rather straightforward, but surprising.

The atrophic response to prolonged electrical silence appears to be specific to the muscle type: the degree of fiber atrophy is proportional to the percentage of slow fibers in a given muscle. Predominantly slow muscles, such as the soleus, atrophy most (~60%), whereas predominantly fast flexors, such as the TA, atrophy least (~10%) (211).

Many fibers co-expressed fast and slow isoforms of troponin I after 8 months of spinal isolation. For example, about 60% of the fibers in the cat soleus expressed fast troponin I compared to less than 1% for unoperated control cats (75). Nevertheless, after 2–3 years of spinal isolation, the slow forms of myosin light chains and tropomyosin appeared to be absent in the cat soleus (232). In the cat MG there were few fibers that still expressed slow myosin after 6 months of electrical silence (131), whereas in the soleus 45% of the fibers were type I based on alkaline ATPase staining (100). About 10% of the soleus fibers expressed both slow and fast types of MHCs. These experiments show that although there was a greater expression of the fast isoforms of myosin and/or troponin I after spinal isolation, some heterogeneity in myosin expression among fibers in most if not all muscles persisted (75, 207, 211).

The maximum velocity of shortening increased by about 75% in the soleus and 15% in the MG after 6 months of inactivity (3). The metabolic profiles in the soleus for the slow and fast myosin fiber types remained normal, with there being no loss of SDH activity after 6 months of spinal isolation (100). Similarly, citrate synthase activity in whole-muscle homogenates was unchanged in the soleus after 8 months of electrical silence (208). However, a significant decrease in the mean SDH activity of individual fibers was observed in the MG (131).

A normal complement of fatigue-resistant units, both FR and S, persist in the cat TA following 6 months of electrical silence (193). Although mean fiber sizes decreased in the fast units, but not in the slow units, the specific tension and spatial distribution patterns of all motor units were similar in the silent and the normal muscles. Variations in fiber cross-sectional area, and in SDH and α-glycerophosphate dehydrogenase (GPD) activities among fibers of the same motor unit in the cat TA were similar in control and in 6-month spinal isolated cats (194). All of these results indicate that differential levels or patterns of neuromuscular activity are not essential to maintain the range of histochemical and physiological motor unit types found in the TA of normal adult cats.

These results, particularly from the soleus muscle, indicate that many physiological, metabolic, and morphological properties of a muscle that contribute to muscle fiber diversity have considerable independence from neuromuscular activity. The degree of independence, however, appears to be closely associated with the initial fiber type composition of the muscle and may also be related to the primary function of the muscle. One must conclude from these results that all fibers do not respond identically to the same stimuli (i.e., the absence of action potentials). Thus, there seems to be inherent differences in the gene expression among fibers of a muscle, even in one of the muscles considered to have the most uniform population of fibers in mammals (i.e., the soleus). An alternative interpretation is, of course, that the period of silence imposed in these experiments has not been maintained for a sufficiently long period to have "forgotten" the pattern of gene expression imposed, perhaps neonatally, by differential activity patterns. Evidence against this, however, is that the normal heterogeneity in enzyme properties persisted in the MG of young adult cats that had been spinalized (T12) at 2 weeks of age. Thus, these muscles never had normal levels of activity, but the diversity in the biochemical and physiological properties of muscle fibers and motor units developed normally (73, 115).

Pharmacologically Induced Inactivity. Pharmacological blockade of nerve impulses to the muscles provides another approach to differentiate between the neural effects that are activity dependent and those that are not activity dependent. For example, TTX applied to a peripheral nerve will block conduction of action potentials distal to the site of application, theoretically without interfering with normal axonal transport mechanisms (18). Batrachotoxin (BTX), on the other hand, blocks action potentials and axonal transport (259). Denervation eliminates action potentials, axonal transport processes, and any other form of direct communication between the nerve and muscle. Thus, differences in the effects of TTX vs. BTX treatment may be attributable to those processes that are dependent on axonal transport.

Skeletal muscles atrophy in response to each of these treatments, but the severity of the atrophy differs markedly. The EDL atrophied by 26%, 16%, and 3% after 8 days of denervation, BTX, or TTX administration, respectively (259). In a subsequent study (260), soleus wet weights were 58%, 19%, and 8% less than control in 20-day denervated, BTX-treated or TTX-treated rats, respectively. After 40 days, comparable values were 66%, 46%, and 15%. Spector (227) reported about 50% and 60% atrophy in the rat soleus after 2 and 4 weeks of denervation compared to about 40% and 50% after TTX treatment, respectively. Mean fiber cross-sectional areas were smaller after denervation than after TTX treatment (227). These results demonstrate that *(1)* denervation and BTX treatment eliminate significant sources of regulation of skeletal muscle proteins that are not related to activity levels, *(2)* some of the neural regulation is linked to axoplasmic transport, *(3)* some component of the neural regulation can be attributed to the pattern or amount of activity of those axons, and (4) most of the atrophy occurs rapidly (within 2 weeks) and begins to plateau thereafter.

TTX treatment also changed the contractile properties of the skeletal muscles. Reductions in maximum tetanic tensions generally reflect the loss in muscle weight, although the tension losses may exceed the decrease in weight (93). Isometric twitch contraction and relaxation times were lengthened and the frequency-tension response reflected a "slowing" of fast muscles (93, 159, 231). Two and four weeks of denervation of the rat soleus resulted in longer contraction and half-relaxation times than TTX treatment (227). For example, the contraction time was 11% longer than control after TTX for 2 weeks, but 25% longer after denervation. The maximum velocity of shortening of the soleus, on the other hand, was faster than control after 2 and 4 weeks of TTX treatment. The combination of longer contraction and relaxation phases of an isometric twitch and a faster maximum shortening velocity during an isotonic contraction is an unusual response to any experimental perturbation of a skeletal muscle. It is not so rare, on the other hand, for either the isometric twitch contraction time or the maximum rate of shortening to change independently. These data are consistent with the view that the mechanisms involved in the isometric and isotonic contractile properties differ. They further emphasize that elimination of the nerve supply to a muscle is radically different from simply blocking or eliminating neuromuscular activation.

The changes in isometric twitch contractile properties are consistent with the reported depressed rate of calcium uptake and release of the fragmented sarcoplasmic reticulum after 40 days of TTX treatment in slow and fast muscles (259, 260). The prolonged twitch properties also could be related to rapid changes in the resting membrane potential (18). Within 10 days of TTX treatment, the resting membrane potential of the soleus fibers dropped from 80 mV to 71 mV. The resting membrane potential dropped even farther (i.e., to 63 mV) after 10 days of denervation. In the EDL, the membrane potential dropped from 76 mV to 72 mV after TTX treatment and to 64 mV after denervation. Thus, 53% of the drop in membrane potential of the soleus fibers 10 days after denervation might be attributed to TTX-induced inactivity, and in the EDL 33% could be attributed to inactivity. After 21 days of TTX treatment, the effects attributable to inactivity in the soleus and EDL were 49% and 61%, respectively. A five- and threefold larger increase in ACh receptors was observed after denervation than after TTX treatment in the soleus and EDL, respectively. These membrane effects related to activation of muscle could contribute to the changes in twitch contractile properties, but this has not been demonstrated.

Few data on the adaptation of contractile proteins in pharmacologically blocked muscles exist. Spector (227) showed about a 15% decrease in the proportion of SO fibers in the soleus after either 2 or 4 weeks of TTX treatment, and a 10% increase in the speed (i.e., maximum velocity of shortening) potential of the soleus. On the other hand, calcium-activated myosin ATPase in the gastrocnemius declined after 2 weeks of TTX treatment (253) and developmental MHCs preferentially appeared in type IIa fibers of the TA (215).

The fatigability of whole muscle after TTX treatment also has been examined. As has now been demonstrated in a variety of models that reduce or eliminate neuromuscular activity (207), slow muscles remain relatively fatigue-resistant following TTX treatment. This observation, however, has been less consistent in mixed, fast muscles. After 14 days of TTX treatment, the fatigability of the rat plantaris and gastrocnemius were unchanged, even though a 25%–35% decrease in SDH activity was observed in the gastrocnemius (93, 230).

In summary, the experimental approach of modulating potential sources of neural control of muscle properties pharmacologically has provided a better understanding of the role of neuromuscular activity in maintaining normal properties of muscles and muscle fiber diversity. The differences in the effects of TTX treatment vs. BTX treatment or denervation on the physiological, morphological and biochemical properties of the muscle may be attributable to non–activity dependent processes (e.g., axonal transport processes that are still present following TTX treatment but not BTX treatment or denervation). One limitation of the pharmacological approach has been the relatively short periods of treatment use. This does not appear to be due to technical limitations even though experiments involving more prolonged periods are more difficult to conduct. In addition, those studies applying drug agents via "cuffs" implanted around the nerves should include sham implants, since it is difficult to avoid some nerve damage using these "cuffs." Another limitation has been that major nerves usually have been blocked pharmacologically. The effects of essentially paralyzing the entire limb may be different from those after a more localized block (i.e., on the specific nerve to one muscle). Certainly the mechanical interactions imposed on the muscles could be markedly different under these two conditions. Thus, muscle properties should be examined after more prolonged and more target-specific treatments. Based on the available data, however, the diversity among muscles and among muscle fibers appears to be minimally affected by electrically silencing the muscle nerves: there is little evidence that silent muscles become homogeneous following inactivity.

MORPHOLOGICAL AND METABOLIC PROPERTIES OF MOTONEURONS

Relationship of Soma Size and Metabolic Properties

The significance of the relationship between the size of the soma of neurons in the ventral horn and their electrophysiological properties (e.g., input resistance, axonal conduction velocity, and duration of AHP following an action potential) (10, 11, 47, 137, 266) continues to interest neurobiologists. Campa and Engel (33) observed high phosphorylase activity in the larger neurons of the ventral horn in the cat and high SDH activity in the smaller neurons. More quantitative enzyme histochemical analyses have enabled the relationship between soma size and metabolic properties to be examined more closely. The smaller ventral horn neurons have the higher oxidative enzyme activities (64, 189, 222), whereas the larger neurons have the higher glycolytic enzyme activities (221).

Chalmers and Edgerton (34) pointed out, however, that smaller neurons in the lumbar spinal cords of the rat and cat had a wide range in SDH activities, whereas larger neurons were generally limited to the lower SDH activities. They concluded that soma size is not the only determining factor for the level of metabolic activity of a neuron in the spinal cord; there is now general agreement on this. A high oxidative capacity seems particularly appropriate for the more easily recruited smaller motoneurons; it corresponds well with Henneman's size principle (112) whereby, as a rule, the smaller motoneurons are recruited before and more often than the larger motoneurons and are metabolically more active.

Skeletal muscle fibers are innervated by three categories of spinal motoneurons (i.e., α, β, γ). α-Motoneurons innervate the extrafusal muscle fibers that constitute the main mass of a muscle, in which the single axon of each motoneuron branches to supply a number of muscle fibers. An α-motoneuron and the muscle fibers that it innervates constitutes a motor unit. The motoneurons innervating a single muscle are collectively called a motor pool. γ-Motoneurons innervate the intrafusal muscle fibers that regulate the length and the tension of the intrafusal fibers of muscle spindles. A soma diameter of 25 μm in the rat (223) and 32.5 μm in the cat (28) often is used as an anatomical measure to distinguish between the larger α- and the smaller γ-motoneurons. β-Motoneurons are those that innervate both extrafusal and intrafusal muscle fibers, are observed infrequently, and little is known about their metabolic properties.

Are the differences in the enzyme activity of the ventral horn neurons related to the type of neuron and/or the type of muscle fibers that they innervate? To examine the enzyme activity of the motoneurons within a specific motor pool, Sickles and Oblak (222) retrogradely labeled motoneurons by exposing the muscle nerve to HRP. The nicotinamide adenine dinucleotide-diaphorase (NADH-D) activity of the motoneurons and muscle fibers in the rat tensor fascia latae (predominantly FG fibers), TA (predominantly FG and FOG fibers), and soleus (predominantly SO fibers) were determined. The mean enzyme activity of motoneurons in each motor pool corresponded closely with that of the muscle fibers innervated by each pool. This study was the first to report metabolic differences in motoneurons innervating muscles having different fiber type compositions. Similar conclusions have now been reached based on analyses of several oxidative enzymes, muscles and their motor pools and in several species (123, 126, 172). No relationship between soma size and GPD activity of motoneurons was found in these same motor pools (122).

The relationship between motoneuron properties and muscle fiber types was examined further by comparing the SDH activity of motoneurons innervating the deep compared to the superficial portion of the rat TA muscle. The TA has an increasing gradient of muscle fibers having a high oxidative enzyme activity proceeding from the superficial (away from the tibia) to the deep (close to the tibia) portion of the muscle. A large variation in the enzyme activity of motoneurons, especially among medium-sized motoneurons, was found in the TA motor pool, although an inverse relationship between soma size and SDH activity was evident when the total motor pool was considered (126). Similarly, Ishihara et al. (124, 125) observed a large variation in GPD activity of motoneurons in the TA motor pool, but the activities were independent of soma size, even when the neurons innervating the deep and superficial fibers were identified. The deep portion of the rat TA had, on average, higher SDH activities than motoneurons innervating the superficial portion. Similarly, Miyata and Kawai (170) used neuronal tracer techniques and compared the soma size and NADH-D activity of motoneurons innervating the superficial (predominantly low oxidative fibers) and deep (predominantly high oxidative fibers) portions of the rat gluteus medius muscle. A higher mean enzyme activity was observed in the motoneurons innervating the deep than the superficial portion of the muscle. Again, no differences were seen in the mean soma size of motoneurons innervating the two portions of the muscle. Together these results suggest that there is a close relationship between the oxidative enzyme activities of the motoneurons in a motor pool and the muscle fibers that they innervate and that this relationship appears to be tightly linked. No significant relationship is evident, however, between a glycolytic marker enzyme (GPD) or a glycogenolytic enzyme (phosphorylase) and soma size.

Adaptability of Soma Size and Metabolic Properties

The issue addressed in this section is whether the motoneurons and muscle fibers within a neuromuscular unit adapt similarly when the neuromuscular unit is perturbed. The effects of thyroid hormone on the NADH-D reductase activity of motoneurons in the rat soleus and tensor fascia latae motor pools were compared with changes in the enzyme activity of the muscles that they innervate (224). NADH-D activity of soleus motoneurons and the muscle fibers that they innervate increased after 7 weeks of thyroid hormone treatment. No adaptations were observed in the tensor fascia latae muscle fibers or motoneurons, leading the authors to conclude that the changes in oxidative metabolism in motoneurons were matched with those in the muscle fibers. Furthermore, Pearson and Sickles (188) found a parallel decrease in NADH-D activity in the motoneurons and the muscle fibers of the soleus motor pool after 60 days of functional overload in the rat.

Ishihara et al. (127) reported that the SDH activity of medium-sized motoneurons in the rat soleus motor pool increased after 7 weeks of continuous exposure to a hypoxic environment. Although the overall SDH activity of the total motor pool was unaffected, the medium-sized motoneurons only (probably the small α-motoneurons) had higher SDH activities than control. A marked loss of mass and an alteration in some metabolic properties of skeletal muscles, in particular predominantly slow muscles such as the soleus (69), occur in response to spaceflight (207). The percentage of small motoneurons with high SDH activities increased in the lumbar spinal cord of the rat after 14 days of spaceflight (132). Although the type of neuron affected was not identified, these data are consistent with the decrease in the mean fiber size and the maintenance of SDH activity of the fibers in the soleus muscle of these same rats following spaceflight (207). In general, all of these results (127, 188, 224) suggest that changes in the metabolic capacity of motoneurons and the muscle fibers they innervate remain coordinated.

The results from other studies of the morphological and metabolic plasticity of motoneurons to increased or decreased activation, however, are not consistent with this conclusion. The soma size and SDH activity of the motoneurons in the peroneal nerve of the cat did not show any changes after 8 weeks of chronic stimulation of the muscle nerve (64), whereas the muscle fibers show an increase in SDH activity following chronic stimulation (212). Chalmers et al. (36) also found that the soma size and SDH activity of lumbar motoneurons in the adult cat were unchanged after 6 months of either virtual electrical silence induced by spinal isolation or decreased activity resulting from low thoracic spinal cord transection. In contrast, the mean fiber size in the slow and fast muscles and the mean SDH activity of the fibers in the fast muscles were decreased (100, 130, 131, 207).

Functional overload, on the other hand, results in an increase or no change in the oxidative capacity of the overloaded muscle (see Chapter 24). Chalmers et al. (35) found an increase in the mean fiber size and a decrease in the mean fiber SDH activity after 12 weeks of functional overload of the cat plantaris. No change occurred in the size or SDH activity of the innervating motoneurons (HRP labeled). Thus, independence of the plasticity in the enzyme activities of muscle fibers and their innervating motoneurons was observed. Similarly, Chalmers et al. (36) found no change in the mean soma size 4 months after axotomy, but the mean SDH activity of lumbar motoneurons was reduced.

The absence of changes in soma size and/or enzyme activity of motoneurons after prolonged periods of elevation or elimination of electrical activity suggest that (*1*) the metabolic demands associated with motoneuron activity represents a small proportion of the total energy demand of a motoneuron, and/or (*2*) the enzyme activity of a motoneuron was unable to adapt to a large chronic change in energy demand (36, 71).

In summary, soma size and the oxidative potential of the motoneurons seem to have insignificant roles in the regulation of motor unit plasticity associated with chronic modulation in neuromuscular activity levels. The persistence of normal motoneuron properties even after extreme perturbations in neuromuscular activity could reflect the unusual intrinsic stability and apparent importance of sustaining these properties to maintain normal motor function. Furthermore, these data suggest that in spite of the functional interdependence of a motoneuron and the muscle fibers it innervates, the adaptations within the different components of the motor unit are not tightly coordinated. Furthermore, it seems likely that the diversity found in skeletal muscle is not attributable to the oxidative potential and soma size of motoneurons nor to its adaptability.

GENE AMPLIFICATION WITHIN A MOTOR UNIT

Regardless of the physiological and molecular mechanisms that influence, modulate, and regulate skeletal muscle properties there are astronomical levels of inter- and intracellular signaling that must occur in order for a motor unit to develop as a type (i.e., S, FR, or FF). A significant level of coordination of protein expression must occur between and within each muscle fiber. It is estimated that there are at least 2,000–5,000 myonuclei per slow muscle fiber assuming fiber lengths of only 1–2 cm (252). In most motor units of the rat hindlimb musculature, 100–400 muscle fibers are innervated by a single motoneuron having one nucleus. Thus the nucleus of one motoneuron can have an amplification factor of about 200,000 (2,000 × 100) to 2,000,000 (5,000 × 400) in its potential to exert control over these myonuclei. The level of interdependence between the single motoneuron nucleus and the thousands of myonuclei that it can influence is undefined. As discussed in the previous section on cross-reinnervation it is virtually certain, however, that the level of control of the neuron over the skeletal muscles is not complete.

OVERALL SUMMARY

During development some cells differentiate into motoneurons while others become muscle fibers. These two types of cells eventually interconnect with remarkable accuracy and predictability with respect to their physiological, morphological, and biochemical properties. This matching of neural and muscular properties emerges in animals that differ substantially in the rate of development and level of maturity of the neuromuscular system at birth. These developmental processes represent an "experiment of nature" that has provided important insight into some of the factors and mechanisms that may play important roles in the emergence of skeletal muscle diversity (i.e., more commonly recognized as muscle fiber types). It is clear that at least some of the diversity observed in the adult can be attributed to differentiating events that occur prior to motoneurons reaching the target muscle.

Although less conclusive, it appears that differential patterns and/or amounts of activation of individual motoneurons, as occurs during normal movement, are rarely observed by the developmental stage when almost full fiber type diversity has emerged. However, it is also clear that some neural influence, via activity and other mechanisms, is essential for the muscle to develop fully to the adult level. It remains unclear whether the differential activity patterns of the nervous system are necessary to achieve adult-like diversity.

A second experimental paradigm that reflects some level of neural control of muscle fiber diversity in adult animals is the cross-reinnervation of slow and fast muscles. Among the many published studies testing neural control hypotheses of muscle proteins following cross-reinnervation, the absence of rigor and consistency in interpreting the results are noteworthy. A common view that has evolved from these studies is that the motoneuron determines all properties of the target muscle by imposing a specific patter and/or amount of activation. However, convincing evidence for complete neural control of the physiological, morphological, or biochemical properties of the muscles by completely converting a fast muscle to slow or a slow muscle to fast has not been published. Although some studies have reported complete conversion of one property, other related parameters have consistently failed to convert completely. The absence of complete conversion following cross-reinnervation is often attributed to technical and biological limitations such as impureness of the nerve crosses, altered use of the muscles, and/or mismatching in the number of axons available relative to the number of muscle fibers to innervate. All of these points may be valid, but the fact remains that there is no convincing evidence of complete neural control of muscle diversity. There is, on the other hand, convincing evidence that there is a neural influence on muscle diversity. It appears that there are multiple and probably interactive sources from which influences on gene expression of skeletal muscle fibers can be derived; the motoneuron is one of these sources.

What are the mechanisms of the neural influence on skeletal muscle properties? There is considerable support from chronic stimulation studies for the hypothesis that the motoneuronal influences can be exerted via their differential activity patterns. However, several other factors should be considered relative to the interpretation of the chronic stimulation studies, such as interactions between the electrical and force-generating events of neuromuscular function. There is also evidence to support the hypothesis that the motoneuron influences muscle fibers via neurotrophic or non–activity dependent neural mechanism(s). For example, almost a normal level of skeletal muscle fiber and motor unit diversity persists during the complete and prolonged (months) absence of the generation of action potentials in motoneurons or muscle fibers. Thus, normal muscle fiber diversity can be readily sustained if there is normal motoneuron–muscle fiber connectivity in the absence of neuromuscular activity. These results emphasize the importance of searching for the non-activity dependent neural mechanisms of control of gene expression in skeletal muscles.

If the motoneuron is a primary source of influence on skeletal muscle properties, what are the features that permit the single nucleus of a motoneuron to tightly control and synchronize gene expression in the hundreds to millions of myonuclei in the muscle fibers it innervates? Attempts to identify such motoneuronal properties and to determine the plasticity of these properties within a unit are at a very early stage. Thus far, it appears that at least the soma size and the metabolic support system associated with oxidative phosphorylation are quite stable when challenged by extreme levels of chronic inactivity or hyperactivity.

A major breakthrough in understanding the mechanisms of neural control of muscle proteins would be the identification of the distinguishing elements of a motoneuron that influence the expression of either a slow or a fast myosin isoform in the muscle fibers it innervates. Other relevant and fundamental questions are: What are the regulatory events that define how many muscle fibers can and prefer to be innervated by a motoneuron? How does the relatively constant order of motoneuronal recruitment become so well matched with the force-generating potential of a motor unit? Is the matching of a motoneuron to its target size a reflection of activity recruitment–related phenomena? To what extent can this contribute to the type of muscle unit? Although these and many other questions remain unanswered, an understanding of motoneuronal diversity and plasticity will be a key element in understanding muscle fiber diversity and plasticity.

The authors wish to thank C. Rigmaiden and M. K. Day for their assistance in preparing the manuscript. The work presented from our laboratories were funded, in part, by NIH Grant NS16333 and NASA Grants NCC 2-535 and 199-26-12-09.

REFERENCES

1. Amphlett, G. W., S. V. Perry, H. Syska, M. D. Brown, and G. Vrbova. Cross innervation and the regulatory protein system of rabbit soleus muscle. *Nature* 257:602–604, 1975.
2. Bagust, J., D. M. Lewis, and R. A. Westerman. Motor units in cross-reinnervated fast and slow twitch muscle of the cat. *J Physiol. (Lond.)* 313:223–235, 1981.
3. Baldwin, K. M., R. R. Roy, V. R. Edgerton, and R. E. Herrick. Interaction of nerve activity and skeletal muscle mechanical activity in regulating isomyosin expression. In: *Advances in Myochemistry*, edited by G. Benzi. London: John Libbey Eurotext, Ltd., 1989, p. 83–92.
4. Balice-Gordon, R. J., C. K. Chua, C. C. Nelson, and J. W. Lichtman. Gradual loss of synaptic cartels precedes axon withdrawal at developing neuromuscular junctions. *Neuron* 11:801–815, 1993.
5. Balice-Gordon, R. J., and J. W. Lichtman. In vivo visualization of the growth of pre- and postsynaptic elements of neuromuscular junctions in the mouse. *J. Neurosci.* 10: 894–908, 1990.
6. Balice-Gordon, R. J., and W. J. Thompson. The organization and development of compartmentalized innervation in rat extensor digitorum longus muscle. *J. Physiol. (Lond.)* 398: 211–231, 1988.
7. Barany, M. ATPase activity of myosin correlated with speed of muscle shortening. *J. Gen. Physiol.* 50 (Suppl): 197–218, 1967.
8. Barany, M., and R. I. Close. The transformation of myosin in cross-innervated rat muscles. *J. Physiol. (Lond.)* 213: 455–474, 1971.
9. Barde, Y. A. Trophic factors and neuronal survival. *Neuron* 2: 1525–1534, 1989.
10. Barrett, J. N., and W. E. Crill. Specific membrane resistivity of dye-injected cat motoneurons. *Brain Res.* 28: 556–561, 1971.
11. Barrett, J. N., and W. E. Crill. Specific membrane properties of cat motoneurones. *J. Physiol. (Lond.)* 239: 301–324, 1974.
12. Bennett, M. R., and N. A. Lavidis. Development of the topographical projection of motor neurons to a rat muscle accompanies loss of polyneuronal innervation. *J. Neurosci.* 4: 2204–2212, 1984.
13. Betz, W. J., J. H. Caldwell, and R. R. Ribchester. The effects of partial denervation at birth on the development of muscle fibres and motor units in rat lumbrical muscle. *J. Physiol. (Lond.)* 303: 265–279, 1980.
14. Betz, H., and J. P. Changeux. Regulation of muscle acetylcholine receptor synthesis in vitro by cyclic nucleotide derivatives. *Nature* 278: 749–752, 1979.
15. Betz, W. J., R. R. Ribchester, and R. M. Ridge. Competitive mechanisms underlying synapse elimination in the lumbrical muscle of the rat. *J. Neurobiol.* 21: 1–17, 1990.
16. Bixby, J. L. Ultrastructural observations on synapse elimination in neonatal rabbit skeletal muscle. *J. Neurocytol.* 10: 81–100, 1981.
17. Bradshaw, R. A., T. L. Blundell, R. Lapatto, N. Q. McDonald, and J. Murray-Rust. Nerve growth factor revisited. *Trends Biochem. Sci.* 18: 48–52, 1993.
18. Bray, J. J., J. I. Hubbard, and R. G. Mills. The trophic influence of tetrodotoxin-inactive nerves on normal and reinnervated rat skeletal muscles. *J. Physiol. (Lond.)* 297: 479–491, 1979.
19. Brenner, H. R., V. Witzemann, and B. Sakmann. Imprinting of acetylcholine receptor messenger RNA accumulation in mammalian neuromuscular synapses. *Nature* 344: 544–547, 1990.
20. Brooke, M. H., and K. K. Kaiser. Three "myosin adenosine triphosphatase" systems: the nature of their pH lability and sulfhydryl dependence. *J. Histochem. Cytochem.* 18: 670–672, 1970.
21. Brown, M. C., and C. M. Booth. Postnatal development of the adult pattern of motor axon distribution in rat muscle. *Nature* 304: 741–742, 1983.

22. Brown, M. C., W. G. Hopkins, and R. J. Keynes. Short- and long-term effects of paralysis on the motor innervation of two different neonatal mouse muscles. *J. Physiol. (Lond.)* 329: 439–450, 1982.
23. Brown, M. C., J. K. Jansen, and D. Van Essen. Polyneuronal innervation of skeletal muscle in new-born rats and its elimination during maturation. *J. Physiol. (Lond.)* 261: 387–422, 1976.
24. Buller, A. J., J. C. Eccles, and R. M. Eccles. Interactions between motoneurones and muscles in respect of the characteristic speeds of their responses. *J. Physiol. (Lond.)* 150: 417–430, 1960.
25. Burke, R. E. Motor units: anatomy, physiology and functional organization. In: *Handbook of Physiology, The Nervous System, Motor Control*, edited by V. B. Brooks. Bethesda, MD: Am. Physiol. Soc., 1981, p. 345–422.
26. Burke, R. E., R. P. Dum, J. W. Fleshman, L. L. Glenn, A. Lev-Tov, M. J. O'Donovan, and M. J. Pinter. A HRP study of the relation between cell size and motor unit type in cat ankle extensor motoneurons. *J. Comp. Neurol.* 209: 17–28, 1982.
27. Burke, R. E. and V. R. Edgerton. Motor unit properties and selective involvement in movement. *Exerc. Sport Sci. Rev.* 3: 31–81, 1975.
28. Burke, R. E., P. L. Strick, K. Kanda, C. C. Kim, and B. Walmsley. Anatomy of medial gastrocnemius and soleus motor nuclei in cat spinal cord. *J. Neurophysiol.* 40: 667–680, 1977.
29. Butler, J., E. Cosmos, and J. Brierley. Differentiation of muscle fiber types in aneurogenic brachial muscles of the chick embryo. *J. Exp. Zool.* 224: 65–80, 1982.
30. Caldwell, J. H., and R. M. Ridge. The effects of deafferentation and spinal cord transection on synapse elimination in developing rat muscles. *J. Physiol. (Lond.)* 339: 145–159, 1983.
31. Callaway, E. M., J. M. Soha, and D. C. Van Essen. Competition favouring inactive over active motor neurons during synapse elimination. *Nature* 328: 422–426, 1987.
32. Callaway, E. M., J. M. Soha, and D. C. Van Essen. Differential loss of neuromuscular connections according to activity level and spinal position of neonatal rabbit soleus motor neurons. *J. Neurosurg. Sci.* 9: 1806–1824, 1989.
33. Campa, J. F., and W. K. Engel. Histochemistry of motor neurons and interneurons in the cat lumbar spinal cord. *Neurology* 20: 559–568, 1970.
34. Chalmers, G. R., and V. R. Edgerton. Single motoneuron succinate dehydrogenase activity. *J. Histochem. Cytochem.* 37: 1107–1114, 1989.
35. Chalmers, G. R., R. R. Roy, and V. R. Edgerton. Motoneuron and muscle fiber succinate dehydrogenase activity in control and overloaded plantaris. *J. Appl. Physiol.* 71: 1589–1592, 1991.
36. Chalmers, G. R., R. R. Roy, and V. R. Edgerton. Adaptability of the oxidative capacity of motoneurons. *Brain Res.* 570: 1–10, 1992.
37. Changeux, J. P. Compartmentalized transcription of acetylcholine receptor genes during motor endplate epigenesis. *New Biol.* 3: 413–429, 1991.
38. Chevallier, A., and M. Kieny. On the role of the connective tissue in the patterning of the chick limb musculature. *Roux Arch. Dev. Biol.* 191: 227–280, 1982.
39. Chevallier, A., M. Kieny, and A. Mauger. Limb-somite relationship: origin of the limb musculature. *J. Embryol. Exp. Morphol.* 41: 245–258, 1977.
40. Clarke, P. G. Developmental cell death: morphological diversity and multiple mechanisms. *Anat. Embryol.* 181: 195–213, 1990.
41. Condon, K., L. Silberstein, H. M. Blau, and W. J. Thompson. Development of muscle fiber types in the prenatal rat hindlimb. *Dev. Biol.* 138: 256–274, 1990.
42. Condon, K., L. Silberstein, H. M. Blau, and W. J. Thompson. Differentiation of fiber types in aneural musculature of the prenatal rat hindlimb. *Dev. Biol.* 138: 275–295, 1990.
43. Cope, T. C., and B. D. Clark. Motor-unit recruitment in self-reinnervated muscle. *J. Neurophysiol.* 70: 1787–1796, 1993.
44. Cossu, G., M. Pacifici, S. Adamo, M. Bouche, and M. Molinaro. TPA-induced inhibition of the expression of differentiative traits in cultured myotubes: dependence on protein synthesis. *Differentiation* 21: 62–65, 1982.
45. Creed, R. S., D. Denny-Brown, J. C. Eccles, E. G. T. Liddell, and C. S. Sherrington. In: *Reflex Activity of the Spinal Cord.* London: Oxford University Press, 1932.
46. Crow, M. T., and F. E. Stockdale. Myosin expression and specialization among the earliest muscle fibers of the developing avian limb. *Dev. Biol.* 113: 238–254, 1986.
47. Cullheim, S. Relations between cell body size, axon diameter and axon conduction velocity of cat sciatic alpha-motoneurons stained with horseradish peroxidase. *Neurosci. Lett.* 8: 17–20, 1978.
48. Cunningham, T. J. Naturally occurring neuron death and its regulation by developing neural pathways. *Int. Rev. Cytol.* 74: 163–186, 1982.
49. Dahm, L. M., and L. T. Landmesser. The regulation of intramuscular nerve branching during normal development and following activity blockade. *Dev. Biol.* 130: 621–644, 1988.
50. Dahm, L. M., and L. T. Landmesser. The regulation of synaptogenesis during normal development and following activity blockade. *J. Neurosci.* 11: 238–255, 1991.
51. Davies, J. A., and G. M. Cook. Growth cone inhibition—an important mechanism in neural development? *Bioessays* 13: 11–15, 1991.
52. Davies, J. A., G. M. Cook, C. D. Stern, and R. J. Keynes. Isolation from chick somites of a glycoprotein fraction that causes collapse of dorsal root ganglion growth cones. *Neuron* 4: 11–20, 1990.
53. Davis, S., T. H. Aldrich, D. M. Valenzuela, V. V. Wong, M. E. Furth, S. P. Squinto, and G. D. Yancopoulos. The receptor for ciliary neurotrophic factor. *Science* 253: 59–63, 1991.
54. De La Porte, S., F. M. Vallette, J. Grassi, M. Vigny, and J. Koenig. Presynaptic or postsynaptic origin of acetylcholinesterase at neuromuscular junctions? An immunological study in heterologous nerve-muscle cultures. *Dev. Biol.* 116: 69–77, 1986.
55. DeNardi, C., S. Ausoni, P. Moretti, L. Gorza, M. Velleca, M. Buckingham, and S. Schiaffino. Type 2X-myosin heavy chain is coded by a muscle fiber type-specific and developmentally regulated gene. *J. Cell Biol.* 123: 823–835, 1993.
56. Dennis, M. J., L. Ziskind-Conhaim, and A. J. Harris. Development of neuromuscular junctions in rat embryos. *Dev. Biol.* 81: 266–279, 1981.
57. Denny-Brown, D. On the nature of postural reflexes. *Proc. R. Soc. Lond. Ser. B* 104: 252–300, 1929.
58. Devanandan, M. S., R. M. Eccles, and R. A. Westerman. Single motor units of mammalian muscles. *J. Physiol. (Lond.)* 178: 359–367, 1965.

59. Dhoot, G. K., S. V. Perry, and G. Vrbova. Changes in the distribution of the components of the troponin complex in muscle fibers after cross-innervation. *Exp. Neurol.* 72: 513–530, 1981.
60. Dive, C., C. D. Gregory, D. J. Phipps, D. L. Evans, A. E. Milner, and A. H. Wyllie. Analysis and discrimination of necrosis and apoptosis (programmed cell death) by multiparameter flow cytometry. *Biochim. Biophys. Acta* 1133: 275–285, 1992.
61. Dodd, J., and T. M. Jessell. Axon guidance and the patterning of neuronal projections in vertebrates. *Science* 242: 692–699, 1988.
62. Donahue, S. P., and A. W. English. Selective elimination of cross-compartmental innervation in rat lateral gastrocnemius muscle. *J. Neurosci.* 9:1621–1627, 1989.
63. Donahue, S. P., A. W. English, R. L. Roden, and G. A. Schwartz. Tenotomy delays both synapse elimination and myogenesis in rat lateral gastrocnemius. *Neuroscience* 42: 275–282, 1991.
64. Donselaar, Y., D. Kernell, and O. Eerbeek. Soma size and oxidative enzyme activity in normal and chronically stimulated motoneurones of the cat's spinal cord. *Brain Res.* 385: 22–29, 1986.
65. Dum, R. P., M. J. O'Donovan, J. Toop, and R. E. Burke. Cross-reinnervated motor units in cat muscle. I. Flexor digitorum longus muscle units reinnervated by soleus motoneurons. *J. Neurophysiol.* 54: 818–836, 1985.
66. Dum, R. P., M. J. O'Donovan, J. Toop, P. Tsairis, M. J. Pinter, and R. E. Burke. Cross-reinnervated motor units in cat muscle. II. Soleus muscle reinnervated by flexor digitorum longus motoneurons. *J. Neurophysiol.* 54: 837–851, 1985.
67. Dusterhoft, S., and D. Pette. Satellite cells from slow rat muscle express low myosin under appropriate culture conditions. *Differentiation* 53: 25–33, 1993.
68. Eccles, J. C., R. M. Eccles, and A. Lundberg. The action potentials of the alpha motoneurones supplying fast and slow muscles. *J. Physiol. (Lond.)* 142: 275–291, 1958.
69. Edgerton, V. R., and R. R. Roy. Neuromuscular adaptations to actual and simulated spaceflight. In: *Handbook of Physiology, Environmental Physiology*, edited by M. J. Fregly and C. M. Blatteis. New York: Oxford University Press, 1995, p. 721–764.
70. Edgerton, V. R., G. Goslow, Jr., S. A. Rasmussen, and S. A. Spector. Is resistance of a muscle to fatigue controlled by its motoneurones? *Nature* 285: 589–590, 1980.
71. Edgerton, V. R., R. R. Roy, and G. R. Chalmers. Does the size principle give insight into the energy requirements of motoneurons? In: *The Segmental Motor System*, edited by M. D. Binder and L. M. Mendell. New York: Oxford University Press, 1989, p. 150–164.
72. Eftimie, R., H. R. Brenner, and A. Buonanno. Myogenin and MyoD join a family of skeletal muscle genes regulated by electrical activity. *Proc. Natl. Acad. Sci. U. S. A.* 88: 1349–1353, 1991.
73. Eldred, E., L. Smith, and V. R. Edgerton. Comparison of contraction times of a muscle and its motor units. *Neurosci. Lett.* 146: 199–202, 1992.
74. Eldridge, L. Lumbrosacral spinal isolation in cat surgical preparation and health maintenance. *Exp. Neurol.* 83: 318–327, 1984.
75. Eldridge, L., G. K. Dhoot, and W. F. Mommaerts. Neural influences on the distribution of troponin I isotypes in the cat. *Exp. Neurol.* 83: 328–346, 1984.
76. Eldridge, L., M. Liebhold, and J. H. Steinbach. Alterations in cat skeletal neuromuscular junctions following prolonged inactivity. *J. Physiol. (Lond.)* 313: 529–545, 1981.
77. Eldridge, L., and W. Mommaerts. Ability to electrically silent nerves to specify fast and slow muscle characteristics. In: *Plasticity of Muscle*, edited by D. Pette. Berlin: Walter de Gruyter, 1980, p. 325–337.
78. English, A. W., and W. D. Letbetter. Anatomy and innervation patterns of cat lateral gastrocnemius and plantaris muscles. *Am. J. Anat.* 164: 67–77, 1982.
79. Falls, D. L., D. A. Harris, F. A. Johnson, M. M. Morgan, G. Corfas, and G. D. Fischbach. Mr 42,000 ARIA: a protein that may regulate the accumulation of acetylcholine receptors at developing chick neuromuscular junctions. *Cold Spring Harb. Symp. Quant. Biol.* 55: 397–406, 1990.
80. Fambrough, D. M. Control of acetylcholine receptors in skeletal muscle. *Physiol. Rev.* 59: 165–227, 1979.
81. Feldman, J. L., and F. E. Stockdale. Skeletal muscle satellite cell diversity: satellite cells from fibres of different types in cell culture. *Dev. Biol.* 143: 320–334, 1990.
82. Feldman, J. L., and F. E. Stockdale. Temporal appearance of satellite cells during myogenesis. *Dev. Biol.* 153: 217–226, 1992.
83. Fischbach, G. D., and S. A. Cohen. The distribution of acetylcholine sensitivity over uninnervated and innervated muscle fibers grown in cell culture. *Dev. Biol.* 31: 147–162, 1973.
84. Fladby, T. Postnatal loss of synaptic terminals in the normal mouse soleus muscle. *Acta Physiol. Scand.* 129: 229–238, 1987.
85. Fladby, T., and J. K. Jansen. Postnatal loss of synaptic terminals in the partially denervated mouse soleus muscle. *Acta Physiol. Scand.* 129: 239–246, 1987.
86. Fladby, T., and J. K. Jansen. Selective innervation of neonatal fast and slow muscle fibres before net loss of synaptic terminals in the mouse soleus muscle. *Acta Physiol. Scand.* 134: 561–562, 1988.
87. Florini, J. R., D. Z. Ewton, and K. A. Magri. Hormones, growth factors, and myogenic differentiation. *Annu. Rev. Physiol.* 53: 201–216, 1991.
88. Foehring, R. C., and J. B. Munson. Motoneuron and muscle-unit properties after long-term direct innervation of soleus muscle by medial gastrocnemius nerve in cat. *J. Neurophysiol.* 64: 847–861, 1990.
89. Foehring, R. C., G. W. Sypert, and J. B. Munson. Motor-unit properties following cross-reinnervation of cat lateral gastrocnemius and soleus muscles with medial gastrocnemius nerve. I. Influence of motoneurons on muscle. *J. Neurophysiol.* 57: 1210–1226, 1987.
90. Fredette, B. J., and L. T. Landmesser. A reevaluation of the role of innervation in primary and secondary myogenesis in developing chick muscle. *Dev. Biol.* 143: 19–35, 1991.
91. Fuentes, M. E., and P. Taylor. Control of acetylcholinesterase gene expression during myogenesis. *Neuron* 10: 679–687, 1993.
92. Fulton, B. P., and K. Walton. Electrophysiological properties of neonatal rat motoneurones studied in vitro. *J. Physiol. (Lond.)* 370: 651–678, 1986.
93. Gardiner, P. F., M. Favron, and P. Corriveau. Histochemical and contractile responses of rat medial gastrocnemius to 2 weeks of complete disuse. *Can. J. Physiol. Pharmacol.* 70: 1075–1081, 1992.
94. Gauthier, G. F., R. E. Burke, S. Lowey, and A. W. Hobbs. Myosin isozymes in normal and cross-reinnervated cat skeletal muscle fibers. *J. Cell Biol.* 97: 756–771, 1983.

95. Gibson, S. J., J. M. Polak, S. R. Bloom, I. M. Sabate, P. M. Mulderry, M. A. Ghatei, G. P. McGregor, J. F. Morrison, J. S. Kelly, R. M. Evans, et al. Calcitonin gene-related peptide immunoreactivity in the spinal cord of man and of eight other species. *J. Neurosci.* 4: 3101–3111, 1984.
96. Gillespie, M. J., T. Gordon, and P. R. Murphy. Motor units and histochemistry in rat lateral gastrocnemius and soleus muscles: evidence for dissociation of physiological and histochemical properties after reinnervation. *J. Neurophysiol.* 57: 921–937, 1987.
97. Goldman, D., H. R. Brenner, and S. Heinemann. Acetylcholine receptor alpha-, beta-, gamma-, and delta-subunit mRNA levels are regulated by muscle activity. *Neuron* 1: 329–333, 1988.
98. Gordon, H., and D. C. Van Essen. The relation of neuromuscular synapse elimination to spinal position of rabbit and rat soleus motoneurones. *J. Physiol. (Lond.)* 339: 591–597, 1983.
99. Gordon, H., and D. C. Van Essen. Specific innervation of muscle fiber types in a developmentally polyinnervated muscle. *Dev. Biol.* 111: 42–50, 1985.
100. Graham, S. C., R. R. Roy, C. Navarro, B. Jiang, D. Pierotti, S. Bodine-Fowler, and V. R. Edgerton. Enzyme and size profiles in chronically inactive cat soleus muscle fibers. *Muscle Nerve* 15: 27–36, 1992.
101. Guth, L., and F. J. Samaha. Procedure for the histochemical demonstration of actomyosin ATPase. *Exp. Neurol.* 28: 365–367, 1970.
102. Hall, Z. W. Multiple forms of acetylcholinesterase and their distribution in endplate and non-endplate regions of rat diaphragm muscle. *J. Neurobiol.* 4: 343–361, 1973.
103. Hall, Z. W., and J. R. Sanes. Synaptic structure and development: the neuromuscular junction. *Cell* 10: 99–121, 1993.
104. Hamburger, V. Cell death in the development of the lateral motor column of the chick embryo. *J. Comp. Neurol.* 160: 535–546, 1975.
105. Hamburger, V., and R. Levi-Montalcini. Proliferation, differentiation and degeneration in the spinal ganglia of the chick embryo under normal and experimental conditions. *J. Exp. Zool.* 111: 457–502, 1949.
106. Harris, A. J. Embryonic growth and innervation of rat skeletal muscles. I. Neural regulation of muscle fibre numbers. *Philos. Trans. R. Soc. Lond. [Biol.]* 293: 257–277, 1981.
107. Heeley, D. H., G. K. Dhoot, N. Frearson, S. V. Perry, and G. Vrbova. The effect of cross-innervation on the tropomyosin composition of rabbit skeletal muscle. *FEBS Lett.* 152: 282–286, 1983.
108. Heffner, C. D., A. G. Lumsden, and D. D. O'Leary. Target control of collateral extension and directional axon growth in the mammalian brain. *Science* 247: 217–220, 1990.
109. Helgren, M. E., S. P. Squinto, H. L. Davis, D. J. Parry, T. G. Boulton, C. S. Heck, Y. Zhu, G. D. Yancopoulos, R. M. Lindsay, and P. S. DiStefano. Trophic effect of ciliary neurotrophic factor on denervated skeletal muscle. *Cell* 76: 493–504, 1994.
110. Henneman, E., and L. M. Mendell. Functional organization of motoneuron pool and its input. In: *Handbook of Physiology, The Nervous System, Motor Control*, edited by V. B. Brooks. Bethesda, MD: Am. Physiol. Soc., 1981, p. 423–507.
111. Henneman, E., and C. B. Olson. Relations between structure and function in the design of skeletal muscles. *J. Neurophysiol.* 28: 581–598, 1965.
112. Henneman, E., G. Somjen, and D. O. Carpenter. Functional significance of cell size in spinal motoneurons. *J. Neurophysiol.* 28: 560–580, 1965.
113. Hennig, R. and T. Lomo. Firing patterns of motor units in normal rats. *Nature* 314: 164–166, 1985.
114. Hofer, M. M., and Y. A. Barde. Brain-derived neurotrophic factor prevents neuronal death in vivo. *Nature* 331: 261–262, 1988.
115. Hoffman, S. J., R. R. Roy, C. E. Blanco, and V. R. Edgerton. Enzyme profiles of single muscle fibers never exposed to normal neuromuscular activity. *J. Appl. Physiol.* 69: 1150–1158, 1990.
116. Hoh, J. F. Neural regulation of mammalian fast and slow muscle myosins: an electrophoretic analysis. *Biochemistry* 14: 742–747, 1975.
117. Hoh, J. F., S. Hughes, and J. Hoy. Myogenic and neurogenic regulation of myosin gene expression in cat jaw-closing muscles regenerating in fast and slow limb muscle beds. *J. Muscle Res. Cell Motil.* 9: 59–72, 1988.
118. Hollyday, M., and V. Hamburger. Reduction of the naturally occurring motor neuron loss by enlargement of the periphery. *J. Comp. Neurol.* 170: 311–320, 1976.
119. Houenou, L. J., J. L. McManaman, D. Prevette, and R. W. Oppenheim. Regulation of putative muscle-derived neurotrophic factors by muscle activity and innervation: in vivo and in vitro studies. *J. Neurosci.* 11: 2829–2837, 1991.
120. Hughes, S. M., and H. M. Blau. Muscle fiber pattern is independent of cell lineage in postnatal rodent development. *Cell* 68: 659–671, 1992.
121. Huizar, P., M. Kuno, and Y. Miyata. Differentiation of motoneurones and skeletal muscles in kittens. *J. Physiol. (Lond.)* 252: 465–479, 1975.
122. Ishihara, A., H. Araki, and Y. Nishihira. Menadione-linked alpha-glycerophosphate dehydrogenase activity of motoneurons in rat soleus and extensor digitorum longus neuron pools. *Neurochem. Res.* 14: 455–458, 1989.
123. Ishihara, A., H. Naitoh, H. Araki, and Y. Nishihira. Soma size and oxidative enzyme activity of motoneurones supplying the fast twitch and slow twitch muscles in the rat. *Brain Res.* 446: 195–198, 1988.
124. Ishihara, A., R. R. Roy, and V. R. Edgerton. Succinate dehydrogenase activity and soma size of motoneurons innervating different portions of the rat tibialis anterior. *Neuroscience* 68: 813–822, 1995.
125. Ishihara, A., S. Taguchi, H. Araki, and Y. Nishihira. Oxidative and glycolytic metabolism of the tibialis anterior motoneurons in the rat. *Acta Physiol. Scand.* 141: 129–130, 1991.
126. Ishihara, A., S. Taguchi, H. Araki, and Y. Nishihira. Retrograde neuronal labeling of motoneurons in the rat by fluorescent tracers, and quantitative analysis of oxidative enzyme activity in labeled neurons. *Neurosci. Lett.* 124: 141–143, 1991.
127. Ishihara, A., S. Taguchi, M. Itoh, and K. Itoh. Oxidative metabolism of the rat soleus neuron pool following hypobaric hypoxia. *Brain Res. Bull.* 24: 143–146, 1990.
128. Jansen, J. K., and T. Fladby. The perinatal reorganization of the innervation of skeletal muscle in mammals. *Prog. Neurobiol. 34:* 39–90, 1990.
129. Jasmin, B. J., R. K. Lee, and R. L. Rotundo. Compartmentalization of acetylcholinesterase mRNA and enzyme at the vertebrate neuromuscular junction. *Neuron* 11: 467–477, 1993.
130. Jean, D. H., L. Guth, and R. W. Albers. Neural regulation of the structure of myosin. *Exp. Neurol.* 38: 458–471, 1973.

131. Jiang, B. A., R. R. Roy, C. Navarro, Q. Nguyen, D. Pierotti, and V. R. Edgerton. Enzymatic responses of cat medial gastrocnemius fibers to chronic inactivity. *J. Appl. Physiol.* 70: 231–239, 1991.
132. Jiang, B., R. R. Roy, I. V. Polyakov, I. B. Krasnov, and V. R. Edgerton. Ventral horn cell responses to spaceflight and hindlimb suspension. *J. Appl. Physiol.* 73 (Suppl.): 107S–111S, 1992.
133. Jobsis, A. C., A. E. Meijer, and A. H. Vloedman. Alteration of the maximal activity of the gluconeogenetic enzyme fructose-1,6-diphosphatase of skeletal muscle by cross-reinnervation. A histochemical and biochemical investigation of fatiguability-related aspects. *J. Neurol. Sci.* 30: 1–11, 1976.
134. Jolesz, F., and F. A. Sreter. Development, innervation, and activity-pattern induced changes in skeletal muscle. *Annu. Rev. Physiol.* 43: 531–552, 1981.
135. Jones, S. P., R. M. Ridge, and A. Rowlerson. The non-selective innervation of muscle fibres and mixed composition of motor units in a muscle of neonatal rat. *J. Physiol. (Lond.)* 386: 377–394, 1987.
136. Jones, S. P., R. M. Ridge, and A. Rowlerson. Rat muscle during post-natal development: evidence in favour of no interconversion between fast- and slow-twitch fibres. *J. Physiol. (Lond.)* 386: 395–406, 1987.
137. Kernell, D., and B. Zwaagstra. Input conductance axonal conduction velocity and cell size among hindlimb motoneurones of the cat. *Brain Res.* 204: 311–326, 1980.
138. Keynes, R. J., and C. D. Stern. Segmentation in the vertebrate nervous system. *Nature* 310: 786–789, 1984.
139. Keynes, R. J., R. V. Stirling, C. D. Stern, and D. Summerbell. The specificity of motor innervation of the chick wing does not depend upon the segmental origin of muscles. *Development* 99: 565–575, 1987.
140. Klein, R., I. Silos-Santiago, R. J. Smeyne, S. A. Lira, R. Brambilla, S. Bryant, L. Zhang, W. D. Snider, and M. Barbacid. Disruption of the neurotrophin-3 receptor gene trkC eliminates la muscle afferents and results in abnormal movements. *Nature* 368: 249–251, 1995.
141. Lance-Jones, C. Motoneuron axon guidance: development of specific projections to two muscles in the embryonic chick limb. *Brain Behav. Evol.* 31: 209–217, 1988.
142. Lance-Jones, C., and L. Landmesser. Motoneuron projection patterns to the chick hindlimb following early partial reversals of the spinal cord. *J. Physiol. (Lond.)* 301: 581–602, 1980.
143. Lance-Jones, C., and L. Landmesser. Motoneuron axon pathways in the developing hindlimb of the chick embryo. *Proc. R. Soc. Lond.* 214: 1–18, 1981.
144. Lance-Jones, C., and L. Landmesser. Motoneuron axon pathways in the embryonic chick hindlimb following early experimental manipulations of the spinal cord. *Proc. R. Soc. Lond.* 214: 19–52, 1981.
145. Landmesser, L. The distribution of motoneurones supplying chick hind limb muscles. *J. Physiol. (Lond.)* 284: 371–389, 1978.
146. Landmesser, L., and G. Pilar. Synaptic transmission and cell death during normal ganglionic development. *J. Physiol. (Lond.)* 241: 737–749, 1974.
147. Landmesser, L. T. The generation of neuromuscular specificity. *Annu. Rev. Neurosci.* 3: 279–302, 1980.
148. Larsson, L., L. Edstrom, B. Lindegren, L. Gorza, and S. Schiaffino. MHC composition and enzyme histochemical and physiological properties of a novel fast-twitch motor unit type. *Am. J. Physiol.* 261: C93–101, 1991.
149. Laskowski, M. B., and J. R. Sanes. Topographic mapping of motor pools onto skeletal muscles. *J. Neurosci.* 7: 252–260, 1987.
150. Laskowski, M. B., and J. R. Sanes. Topographically selective reinnervation of adult mammalian skeletal muscles. *J. Neurosci.* 8: 3094–3099, 1988.
151. Laufer, R., and J. P. Changeux. Calcitonin gene-related peptide elevates cyclic AMP levels in chick skeletal muscle: Possible neurotrophic role for a coexisting neuronal messenger. *EMBO J.* 6: 901–906, 1987.
152. Levi-Montalcini, R. Developmental neurobiology and the natural history of nerve growth factor. *Annu. Rev. Neurosci.* 5: 341–362, 1982.
153. Lewis, D. M., A. Rowlerson, and S. N. Webb. Motor units and immunohistochemistry of cat soleus muscle after long periods of cross-reinnervation. *J. Physiol. (Lond.)* 325: 403–418, 1982.
154. Lewis, S. E., P. Anderson, and D. F. Goldspink. The effects of calcium on protein turnover in skeletal muscles of the rat. *Biochem. J.* 204: 257–264, 1982.
155. Lichtman, J. W., and R. J. Balice-Gordon. Understanding synaptic competition in theory and in practice. *J. Neurobiol.* 21: 99–106, 1990.
156. Lomo, T., and J. Rosenthal. Control of ACh sensitivity by muscle activity in the rat. *J. Physiol. (Lond.)* 221: 493–513, 1972.
157. Luff, A. R. Dynamic properties of fast and slow skeletal muscles in the cat and rat following cross-reinnervation. *J. Physiol. (Lond.)* 248: 83–96, 1975.
158. Lumsden, A. G., and A. M. Davies. Chemotropic effect of specific target epithelium in the developing mammalian nervous system. *Nature* 323: 538–539, 1986.
159. MacIntosh, B. R., M. C. Roberge, and P. F. Gardiner. Absence of staircase following disuse in rat gastrocnemius muscle. *Can. J. Physiol. Pharmacol.* 66: 707–713, 1988.
160. Margreth, A., G. Salviati, and I. Mussini. Biochemical changes in slow muscle by reinnervation with fast nerve fibres. In: *Clinical Studies in Myology*, edited by B. A. Kakulas. Amsterdam: Excerpta Medica, 1973, p. 337–345.
161. Martin, D. P., R. E.. Schmidt, P. S. DiStefano, O. H Lowry, J. G. Carter, and E. Johnson, Jr. Inhibitors of protein synthesis and RNA synthesis prevent neuronal death caused by nerve growth factor deprivation. *J. Cell Biol.* 106: 829–844, 1988.
162. Martinou, J. C., D. L. Falls, G. D. Fischbach, and J. P. Merlie. Acetylcholine receptor-inducing activity stimulates expression of the epsilon-subunit gene of the muscle acetylcholine receptor. *Proc. Natl. Acad. Sci. U. S. A.* 88: 7669–7673, 1991.
163. Martinou, J. C., and J. P. Merlie. Nerve-dependent modulation of acetylcholine receptor epsilon-subunit gene expression. *J. Neurosci.* 11: 1291–1299, 1991.
164. McMahan, U. J. The agrin hypothesis. *Cold Spring Harb. Symp. Quant. Biol.* 55: 407–418, 1990.
165. McManaman, J. L., R. W. Oppenheim, D. Prevette, and D. Marchetti. Rescue of motoneurons from cell death by a purified skeletal muscle polypeptide: effects of the ChAT development factor, CDF. *Neuron* 4: 891–898, 1990.
166. Menesini Chen, M. G., J. S. Chen, and R. Levi-Montalcini. Sympathetic nerve fibers ingrowth in the central nervous system of neonatal rodent upon intracerebral NGF injections. *Arch. Ital. Biol.* 116: 53–84, 1978.
167. Merlie, J. P., and J. R. Sanes. Concentration of acetylcholine receptor mRNA in synaptic regions of adult muscle fibres. *Nature* 317: 66–68, 1985.

168. Miller, J. B., M. T. Crow, and F. E. Stockdale. Slow and fast myosin heavy chain content defines three types of myotubes in early muscle cell cultures. *J. Cell Biol.* 101: 1643–1650, 1985.
169. Miller, J. B., and F. E. Stockdale. Developmental origins of skeletal muscle fibers: clonal analysis of myogenic cell lineages based on expression of fast and slow myosin heavy chains. *Proc. Natl. Acad. Sci. U. S. A.* 83: 3860–3864, 1986.
170. Miyata, H., and Y. Kawai. Relationship between soma diameter and oxidative enzyme activity of alpha-motoneurons. *Brain Res.* 581: 101–107, 1992.
171. Miyata, Y., and K. Yoshioka. Selective elimination of motor nerve terminals in the rat soleus muscle during development. *J. Physiol. (Lond.)* 309: 631–646, 1980.
172. Mjaatvedt, A. E., and M. T. Wong-Riley. Double-labeling of rat alpha-motoneurons for cytochrome oxidase and retrogradely transported [3H]WGA. *Brain Res.* 368: 178–182, 1986.
173. Mommaerts, W. F., K. Seraydarian, M. Suh, C. J. Kean, and A. J. Buller. The conversion of some biochemical properties of mammalian skeletal muscles following cross-reinnervation. *Exp. Neurol.* 55: 637–653, 1977.
174. Muntener, M., A. M. Rowlerson, M. W. Berchtold, and C. W. Heizmann. Changes in the concentration of the calcium-binding parvalbumin in cross-reinnervated rat muscles. Comparison of biochemical with physiological and histochemical parameters. *J. Biol. Chem.* 262: 465–469, 1987.
175. Narusawa, M., R. B. Fitzsimons, S. Izumo, B. Nadal-Ginard, N. A. Rubinstein, and A. M. Kelly. Slow myosin in developing rat skeletal muscle. *J. Cell Biol.* 104: 447–459, 1987.
176. Navarrette, R., and G. Vrbova. Activity-dependent interactions between motoneurones and muscles: their role in the development of the motor unit. *Prog. Neurobiol.* 41: 93–124, 1993.
177. Navarrette, R., K. D. Walton, and R. R. Llinas. Postnatal changes in the electrical properties of muscle-identified rat motoneurons: an in vitro study. *Soc. Neurosci. Abstr.* 13: 1060, 1988.
178. Neville, C. M., M. Schmidt, and J. Schmidt. Response of myogenic determination factors to cessation and resumption of electrical activity in skeletal muscle: a possible role for myogenin in denervation supersensitivity. *Cell. Mol. Neurobiol.* 12: 511–527, 1992.
179. O'Brien, R. A., A. J. Ostberg, and G. Vrbova. Observations on the elimination of polyneuronal innervation in developing mammalian skeletal muscle. *J. Physiol. (Lond.)* 282: 571–582, 1978.
180. O'Donovan, M. J. M. J. Pinter, R. P. Dum, and R. E. Burke. Kinesiological studies of self- and cross-reinnervated FDL and soleus muscles in freely moving cats. *J. Neurophysiol.* 54: 852–866, 1985.
181. Okada, A., S. Furber, N. Okado, S. Homma, and R. W. Oppenheim. Cell death of motoneurons in the chick embryo spinal cord. X. Synapse formation on motoneurons following the reduction of cell death by neuromuscular blockade. *J. Neurobiol.* 20: 219–233, 1989.
182. Olson, E. N. Interplay between proliferation and differentiation within the myogenic lineage. *Dev. Biol.* 154: 261–272, 1992.
183. Oppenheim, R. W. Cell death during development of the nervous system. *Annu. Rev. Neurosci.* 14: 453–501, 1991.
184. Oppenheim, R. W., I. W. Chu-Wang, and J. L. Maderdrut. Cell death of motoneurons in the chick embryo spinal cord. III. The differentiation of motoneurons prior to their induced degeneration following limb-bud removal. *J. Comp. Neurol.* 177: 87–111, 1978.
185. Oppenheim, R. W., D. Prevette, M. Tytell, and S. Homma. Naturally occurring and induced neuronal death in the chick embryo in vivo rquires protein and RNA synthesis: evidence for the role of cell death genes. *Dev. Biol.* 138: 104–113, 1990.
186. Osterlund, M., B. Fontaine, A. Devillers-Thiery, B. Geoffroy, and J. P. Changeux. Acetylcholine receptor expression in primary cultures of embryonic chick myotubes—I. Discoordinate regulation of alpha-, gamma- and delta-subunit gene expression by calcitonin gene-related peptide and by muscle electrical activity. *Neuroscience* 32: 279–287, 1989.
187. Page, S., J. B. Miller, J. X. DiMario, E. J. Hager, A. Moser, and F. E. Stockdale. Developmentally regulated expression of three slow isoforms of myosin heavy chain: diversity among the first fibers to form in avian muscle. *Dev. Biol.* 154: 118–128, 1992.
188. Pearson, J. K., and D. W. Sickles. Enzyme activity changes in rat soleus motoneurons and muscle after synergist ablation. *J. Appl. Physiol.* 63: 2301–2308, 1987.
189. Penny, J. E., J. R. Kukums, J. H. Tyrer, and M. J. Eadie. Quantitative oxidative enzyme histochemistry of the spinal cord. Part 2. Relation of cell size and enzyme activity to vulnerability to ischaemia. *J. Neurol. Sci.* 26: 187–192, 1975.
190. Peter, J. B., R. J. Barnard, V. R. Edgerton, C. A. Gillespie, and K. E. Stempel. Metabolic profiles of three fiber types of skeletal muscle in guinea pigs and rabbits. *Biochemistry* 11: 2627–2633, 1972.
191. Pette, D., and R. S. Staron. Cellular and molecular diversities of mammalian skeletal muscle fibers. *Rev. Physiol. Biochem. Pharmacol.* 116: 1–76, 1990.
192. Pette, D., and G. Vrbova. Neural control of phenotypic expression in mammalian muscle fibers. *Muscle Nerve* 8: 676–689, 1985.
193. Pierotti, D. J., R. R. Roy, S. C. Bodine-Fowler, J. A. Hodgson, and V. R. Edgerton. Mechanical and morphological properties of chronically inactive cat tibialis anterior motor units. *J. Physiol. (Lond.)* 444: 175–192, 1991.
194. Pierotti, D. J., R. R. Roy, J. A. Hodgson, and V. R. Edgerton. Level of independence of motor unit properties from neuromuscular activity. *Muscle Nerve* 17: 1324–1335, 1994.
195. Pittman, R., and R. W. Oppenheim. Cell death of motoneurons in the chick embryo spinal cord. IV. Evidence that a functional neuromuscular interaction is involved in the regulation of naturally occurring cell death and the stabilization of synapses. *J. Comp. Neurol.* 187: 425–446, 1979.
196. Prewitt, M. A., and B. Salafsky. Effect of cross innervation on biochemical characteristics of skeletal muscles. *Am. J. Physiol.* 213: 295–300, 1967.
197. Reichmann, H., T. Srihari, and D. Pette. Ipsi- and contralateral fibre transformations by cross-reinnervation. A principle of symmetry. *Pflugers Arch.* 397: 202–208, 1983.
198. Reiness, C. G., and C. B. Weinberg. Metabolic stabilization of acetylcholine receptors at newly formed neuromuscular junctions in rat. *Dev. Biol.* 84: 247–254, 1981.
199. Reist, N. E., M. J. Werle, and U. J. McMahan. Agrin released by motor neurons induces the aggregation of acetylcholine receptors at neuromuscular junctions. *Neuron* 8: 865–868, 1992.

200. Ribchester, R. R. Activity-dependent and -independent synaptic interactions during reinnervation of partially denervated rat muscle. *J. Physiol. (Lond.)* 401: 53–75, 1988.
201. Ribchester, R. R., and T. Taxt. Repression of inactive motor nerve terminals in partially denervated rat muscle after regeneration of active motor axons. *J. Physiol. (Lond.)* 347: 497–511, 1984.
202. Ridge, R. M., and W. J. Betz. The effect of selective, chronic stimulation on motor unit size in developing rat muscle. *J Neurosci.* 4: 2614–2620, 1984.
203. Riley, D. A. Spontaneous elimination of nerve terminals from the endplates of developing skeletal myofibers. *Brain Res.* 134: 279–285, 1977.
204. Robbins, N., G. Karpati, and W. K. Engel. Histochemical and contractile properties in the cross-innervated guinea pig soleus muscle. *Arch. Neurol.* 20: 318–329, 1969.
205. Ross, J. J., M. J. Duxson, and A. J. Harris. Neural determination of muscle fibre numbers in embryonic rat lumbrical muscles. *Development* 100: 395–409, 1987.
206. Rossi, S. G., and R. L. Rotundo. Cell surface acetylcholinesterase molecules on multinucleated myotubes are clustered over the nucleus of origin. *J. Cell Biol.* 119: 1657–1667, 1992.
207. Roy, R. R., K. M. Baldwin, and V. R. Edgerton. The plasticity of skeletal muscle: effects of neuromuscular activity. *Exerc. Sport Sci. Rev.* 19: 269–312, 1991.
208. Roy, R. R., K. M. Baldwin, R. D. Sacks, L. Eldridge, and V. R. Edgerton. Mechanical and metabolic properties after prolonged inactivation and/or cross-reinnervation of cat soleus. *Med. Sci. Sports Exerc.* 19: 550, 1987.
209. Roy, R. R., J. A. Hodgson, S. D. Lauretz, D. J. Pierotti, R. J. Grayek, and V. R. Edgerton. Chronic spinal cord-injured cats: surgical procedures and management. *Lab. Anim. Sci.* 42: 335–343, 1992.
210. Roy, R. R., D. L. Hutchison, D. J. Pierotti, J. A. Hodgson, and V. R. Edgerton. EMG patterns of rat ankle extensors and flexors during treadmill locomotion and swimming. *J. Appl. Physiol.* 70: 2522–2529, 1991.
211. Roy, R. R., D. J. Pierotti, V. Flores, W. Rudolph, and V. R. Edgerton. Fibre size and type adaptations to spinal isolation and cyclical passive stretch in cat hindlimb. *J. Anat.* 180: 491–499, 1992.
212. Salmons, S., and J. Henriksson. The adaptive response of skeletal muscle to increased use. *Muscle Nerve* 4: 94–105, 1981.
213. Sanes, J. R., Y. R. Johnson, P. T. Kotzbauer, J. Mudd, T. Hanley, J. C. Martinou, and J. P. Merlie. Selective expression of an acetylcholine receptor-lacZ transgene in synaptic nuclei of adult muscle fibers. *Development* 113: 1181–1191, 1991.
214. Sassoon, D. A. Myogenic regulatory factors: dissecting their role and regulation during vertebrate embryogenesis. *Dev. Biol.* 156: 11–23, 1993.
215. Schiaffino, S., L. Gorza, G. Pitton, L. Saggin, S. Ausoni, S. Sartore, and T. Lomo. Embryonic and neonatal myosin heavy chain in denervated and paralyzed rat skeletal muscle. *Dev. Biol.* 127: 1–11, 1988.
216. Schuetze, S. M., and L. W. Role. Developmental regulation of nicotinic acetylcholine receptors. *Annu. Rev. Neurosci.* 10: 403–457, 1987.
217. Schwab, M. E., J. P. Kapfhammer, and C. E. Bandtlow. Inhibitors of neurite growth. *Annu. Rev. Neurosci.* 16: 565–595, 1993.
218. Secrist, D. J., and W. G. Kerrick. Associated changes in Ca^{2+} and Sr^{2+} activation properties and fiber proteins in cross-reinnervated rabbit soleus. *Pflugers Arch.* 384: 219–229, 1980.
219. Sekiya, S., S. Homma, Y. Miyata, and M. Kuno. Effects of nerve growth factor on differentiation of muscle spindles following nerve lesion in neonatal rats. *J. Neurosci.* 6: 2019–2025, 1986.
220. Shyng, S. L., and M. M. Salpeter. Effect of reinnervation on the degradation rate of junctional acetylcholine receptors synthesized in denervated skeletal muscles. *J. Neurosci.* 10: 3905–3915, 1990.
221. Sickles, D. W., and R. E. McLendon. Metabolic variation among rat lumbrosacral alpha-motoneurons. *Histochemistry* 79: 205–217, 1983.
222. Sickles, D. W., and T. G. Oblak. A horseradish peroxidase labeling technique for correlation of motoneuron metabolic activity with muscle fiber types. *J. Neurosci. Methods* 7: 195–201, 1983.
223. Sickles, D. W., and T. G. Oblak. Metabolic variation among alpha-motoneurons innervating different muscle-fiber types. I. Oxidative enzyme activity. *J. Neurophysiol.* 51: 529–537, 1984.
224. Sickles, D. W., T. G. Oblak, and J. Scholer. Hyperthyroidism selectively increases oxidative metabolism of slow-oxidative motor units. *Exp. Neurol.* 97: 90–105, 1987.
225. Simon, A. M., P. Hoppe, and S. J. Burden. Spatial restriction of AChR gene expression to subsynaptic nuclei. *Development* 114: 545–553, 1992.
226. Snider, W. D., and E. Johnson, Jr. Neurotrophic molecules. *Ann. Neurol.* 26: 489–506, 1989.
227. Spector, S. A. Trophic effects on the contractile and histochemical properties of rat soleus muscle. *J Neurosci.* 5: 2189–2196, 1985.
228. Sreter, F. A., and J. Gergely. The effect of cross reinnervation on the synthesis of myosin light chains. *Biochem. Biophys. Res. Commun.* 56: 84–89, 1974.
229. Sreter, F. A., A. R. Luff, and J. Gergely. Effect of cross-reinnervation on physiological parameters and on properties of myosin and sarcoplasmic reticulum of fast and slow muscles of the rabbit. *J. Gen. Physiol.* 66: 811–821, 1975.
230. St-Pierre, D. M., D. Leonard, and P. F. Gardiner. Recovery of muscle from tetrodotoxin-induced disuse and the influence of daily exercise. 1. Contractile properties. *Exp. Neurol.* 98: 472–488, 1987.
231. St-Pierre, D. M., D. Leonard, R. Houle, and P. F. Gardiner. Recovery of muscle from tetrodotoxin-induced disuse and the influence of daily exercise. 2. Muscle enzymes and fatigue characteristics. *Exp. Neurol.* 101: 327–346, 1988.
232. Steinbach, J. H., D. Schubert, and L. Eldridge. Changes in cat muscle contractile proteins after prolonged muscle inactivity. *Exp. Neurol.* 67: 655–669, 1980.
233. Stockdale, F. E. Myogenic cell lineages. *Dev. Biol.* 154: 284–298, 1992.
234. Sypert, G W., and J. B. Munson. Basis of segmental motor control: motoneuron size or motor unit type? *Neurosurgery* 8: 608–621, 1981.
235. Tanaka, H. Chronic application of curare does not increase the level of motoneuron survival-promoting activity in limb muscle extracts during the naturally occurring motoneuron cell death period. *Dev. Biol.* 124: 347–357, 1987.
236. Tanaka, H., and L. T. Landmesser. Cell death of lumbosacral motoneurons in chick, quail, and chick-quail chimera embryos: a test of the quantitative matching hypothesis of neuronal cell death. *J. Neurosci.* 6: 2889–2899, 1986.

237. Tang, J., L. Landmesser, and U. Rutishauser. Polysialic acid influences specific pathfinding by avian motoneurons. *Neuron* 8: 1031–1044, 1992.
238. Tessier-Lavigne, M., M. Placzek, A. G. Lumsden, J. Dodd, and T. M. Jessell. Chemotropic guidance of developing axons in the mammalian central nervous system. *Nature* 336: 775–778, 1988.
239. Thomas, P. E., and K. W. Ranatunga. Factors affecting muscle fiber transformation in cross-reinnervated muscle. *Muscle Nerve* 16: 193–199, 1993.
240. Thompson, W. Synapse elimination in neonatal rat muscle is sensitive to pattern of muscle use. *Nature* 302: 614–616, 1983.
241. Thompson, W., D. P. Kuffler, and J. K. Jansen. The effect of prolonged, reversible block of nerve impulses on the elimination of polyneuronal innervation of new-born rat skeletal muscle fibers. *Neuroscience* 4: 271–281, 1979.
242. Thompson, W. J. Lack of segmental selectivity in elimination of synapses from soleus muscle of new-born rats. *J. Physiol. (Lond.)* 335: 343–352, 1983.
243. Thompson, W. J. Activity and synapse elimination at the neuromuscular junction. *Cell. Mol. Neurobiol.* 5: 167–182, 1985.
244. Thompson, W. J., K. Condon, and S. H. Astrow. The origin and selective innervation of early muscle fiber types in the rat. *J. Neurobiol.* 21: 212–222, 1990.
245. Thompson, W. J., and J. K. S. Jansen. The extent of sprouting of remaining motor units in partly denervated immature and adult rat soleus muscle. *Neuroscience* 2: 523–535, 1977.
246. Thompson, W. J., L. A. Sutton, and D. A. Riley. Fibre type composition of single motor units during synapse elimination in neonatal rat soleus muscle. *Nature* 309: 709–711, 1984.
247. Tosney, K. W. Somites and axon guidance. *Scanning Microsc.* 2: 427–442, 1988.
248. Tosney, K. W., and L. T. Landmesser. Pattern and specificity of axonal outgrowth following varying degrees of chick limb bud ablation. *J. Neurosci.* 4: 2518–2527, 1984.
249. Toutant, J. P., and J. Massoulie. Acetylcholinesterase. In: *Mammalian Ectoenzymes*, edited by A. J. Kenny and A. J. Turner. New York: Elsevier Science Publishers, 1987, p. 289–328.
250. Tower, S. S. Function and structure in the chronically isolated lumbo-sacral spinal cord of the dog. *J. Comp. Neurol.* 67: 109–131, 1937.
251. Tsay, H. J., and J. Schmidt. Skeletal muscle denervation activates acetylcholine receptor genes. *J. Cell Biol.* 108: 1523–1526, 1989.
252. Tseng, B. S., C. E. Kasper, and V. R. Edgerton. Cytoplasm-to-myonucleus ratios and succinate dehydrogenase activities in adult rat slow and fast muscle fibers. *Cell Tissue Res.* 275: 39–49, 1994.
253. Turcotte, R., R. Panenic, and P. F. Gardiner. TTX-induced muscle disuse alters CA2+ activation characteristics of myofibril ATPase. *Comp. Biochem. Physiol. A* 100: 183–186, 1991.
254. Uchida, S., H. Yamamoto, S. Iio, N. Matsumoto, X. B. Wang, N. Yonehara, Y. Imai, R. Inoki, and H. Yoshida. Release of calcitonin gene-related peptide-like immunoreactive substance from neuromuscular junction by nerve excitation and its action on striated muscle. *J. Neurochem.* 54: 1000–1003, 1990.
255. Unguez, G. A., S. Bodine-Fowler, R. R. Roy, D. J. Pierotti, and V. R. Edgerton. Evidence of incomplete neural control of motor unit properties in cat tibialis anterior after self-reinnervation. *J. Physiol. (Lond.)* 472: 103–125, 1993.
256. Usdin, T. B., and G. D. Fischbach. Purification and characterization of a polypeptide from chick brain that promotes the accumulation of acetylcholine receptors in chick myotubes. *J. Cell Biol.* 103: 493–507, 1986.
257. Villar, M. J., M. Roa, M. Huchet, T. Hokfelt, J. P. Changeux, J. Fahrenkrug, J. C. Brown, M. Epstein, and L. Hersh. Immunoreactive calcitonin gene-related peptide, vasoactive intestinal polypeptide and somatostatin: distribution in developing chicken spinal cord motoneurons and role in regulation of muscle acetylcholine receptor synthesis. *Eur. J. Neurosci.* 1: 269–287, 1989.
258. Vivarelli, E., W. E. Brown, R. G. Whalen, and G. Cossu. The expression of slow myosin during mammalian somitogenesis and limb bud differentiation. *J. Cell Biol.* 107: 2191–2197, 1988.
259. Wan, K. K., and R. J. Boegman. Calcium uptake by muscle sarcoplasmic reticulum following neural application of batrachotoxin or tetrodotoxin. *FEBS Lett.* 112: 163–167, 1980.
260. Wan, K. K., and R. J. Boegman. Response of rat skeletal muscle to neural application of batrachotoxin or tetrodotoxin: effect on soluble proteins. *Exp. Neurol.* 74: 447–457, 1981.
261. Windhorst, U., T. M. Hamm, and D. G. Stuart. On the function of muscle and reflex partitioning. *Behav. Brain Sci.* 12: 629–681, 1989.
262. Witzemann, V., B. Barg, M. Criado, E. Stein, and B. Sakmann. Developmental regulation of five subunit specific mRNAs encoding acetylcholine receptor subtypes in rat muscle. *FEBS Lett.* 242: 419–424, 1989.
263. Witzemann, V., and B. Sakmann. Differential regulation of MyoD and myogenin mRNA levels by nerve induced muscle activity. *FEBS Lett.* 282: 259–264, 1991.
264. Yamada, S., N. Buffinger, J. DiMario, and R. C. Strohman. Fibroblast growth factor is stored in fiber extracellular matrix and plays a role in regulating muscle hypertrophy. *Med. Sci. Sports Exerc.* 21: S173–S180, 1989.
265. Ziskind-Conhaim, L. Electrical properties of motoneurons in the spinal cord of rat embryos. *Dev. Biol.* 128: 21–29, 1988.
266. Zwaagstra, B., and D. Kernell. The duration of after-hyperpolarization in hindlimb alpha motoneurons of different sizes in the cat. *Neurosci. Lett.* 19: 303–307, 1980.

3. Proprioceptive feedback and movement regulation

ARTHUR PROCHAZKA | *Division of Neuroscience, University of Alberta, Edmonton, Alberta, Canada*

CHAPTER CONTENTS

"YOU CAN ONLY CONTROL WHAT YOU SENSE." This statement summarizes the current view of sensorimotor control (243) and underlies most of the material in this chapter. As we will see, the removal of sensory feedback to the central nervous system (CNS) has long been known to impair, though not abolish, motor function, particularly in tasks requiring dexterity and context-dependent control. However, it is only in the last decade or two that the flexibility in the use of sensory feedback by the CNS has become fully apparent. In this period, the field of sensorimotor control has truly flourished. Guesswork regarding the nature of the feedback signals to the CNS in voluntary movement has been replaced by hard data on the activity of single afferents and ensembles of afferents of different sensory modalities. In many species the responses of CNS neurons to incoming information depend heavily on behavioral context and attentional mechanisms. Perhaps of most importance, there has been a major conceptual shift in formulating hypotheses of sensorimotor control. Models based on reflex arcs and servo loops controlling single muscles are now being augmented by multivariate models that incorporate state- and context-dependent rules. Technology, which 40 years ago provided the framework of servo-control theory for analyzing limb stretch reflexes and oculomotor control, now offers a rich diversity of additional options, including control structures ostensibly modeled on the CNS itself (e.g., expert systems, neural networks, "fuzzy" logic control systems). With fewer conceptual constraints in the way, the hunt is now on to identify the sensorimotor rules and neuronal circuitry that govern the control of movements in various animal species. It is understood that few of these rules are likely to be rigidly fixed. The CNS can clearly modify, modulate, or override any of its control subsystems to cope with changes in task and context. Furthermore, it is apparent that vertebrates and invertebrates share some basic mechanisms of sensorimotor control. Thus, although the focus of this chapter is on mammalian systems, invertebrate systems are discussed where appropriate.

SENSORY FEEDBACK: HISTORICAL BACKGROUND

Reflected Action: The "Sentient Principle"

Ideas regarding the sensory control of movement date back to Descartes in the mid seventeenth century. Interesting accounts of the historical development of the subject may be found in Brazier (45, 46). Briefly, Descartes posited that there was a flow of sensory "spirits" along the "marrow" of nerves leading to the CNS. Motor spirits were directed back toward the muscles along hollow canals in the same nerves. The sensory input supposedly opened valves or pores in the pineal gland, thus controlling motor output. Over the next 200 years, the idea of a "sentient principle" underlying motor actions was further developed and studied empirically. The existence of separate sensory and motor nerve fibers was suggesed by Jiři Prochazka in 1780 and then verified experimentally in the famous studies of Bell and Magendie. By the end of the nineteenth century, Hall and others had shown that the spinal cord had a considerable autonomy in its reflex responses.

Perhaps the most influential theory of all regarding reflexes was that of Sechenov (1863), who proposed that all animal and human behavior could essentially be reduced to reflex action (307). Sechenov asserted that higher brain function comprised three elements: sensory inflow, a central reflexive process governed by physical laws, and motor output. "Willed" movements were held to arise as a consequence of residual or remembered sensory inputs, triggered internally. Sechenov suggested that reflexive motor output could be evoked by small fractions of past sensory input. This led him to formulate the idea of conditioned reflexes, which his student Pavlov developed into a major field of inquiry. Complex, goal-directed actions were seen as chains of simple reflexes, each of which elicited the next reflex in sequence. Interestingly, Sechenov's views brought him into conflict with the government and judiciary of the time, because it was felt that criminal acts could potentially be defended on the grounds that they were reflex chains over which the accused had no control.

The study of reflexes entered the modern era of scientific measurement with the work of Horsley, Sherrington, Hughlings Jackson, Adrian, Magnus, Graham Brown, and others. This period has been extensively reviewed elsewhere (46, 84, 148, 238). By 1930 the following concepts and mechanisms had been identified and studied: action potential frequency code, proprioception, exteroception, neuronal excitation and inhibition, reflex integration and plasticity, decerebrate rigidity, righting reflexes, positive supporting reaction, reflex stepping, and motor functions of cerebellum and motor cortex. The midbrain reticular formation had been linked to attention and arousal (229). In the 1950s and 1960s, the advent of intracellular recording enabled Eccles, Lloyd, Lundberg, and Laporte to analyze reflex connections at the cellular level (reviewed in 19, 187). By the mid 1960s the signaling properties of muscle spindles and tendon organs, and the modulating action of fusimotor efferent fibers on muscle spindles, had been elucidated in great detail by B.H.C. Matthews, P.B.C. Matthews, Hunt, Kuffler, Boyd, Houk, and others (178). The wealth of new knowledge about the individual components of the motor system set the stage for the development of comprehensive hypotheses of sensorimotor control, an enterprise that continues to this day.

Motor Effects of Sensory Loss

One way to determine the role of sensory input is selectively to abolish it, for example, by transecting the sensory nerves entering the CNS, and then to look for deficits in motor performance. This was first done by Magendie (46), and has since been carried out in numerous different ways in animals ranging from insects, lobsters, and crabs (23, 71, 167, 350) to amphibia, reptiles, birds, fish, and mammals, including humans (157, 256, 257, 297, 298). In nearly all cases, purposeful or rhythmic motor action persisted after deafferentation, but accuracy and adaptability were diminished (see Chapter 4).

Although deafferentation experiments seem simple enough in principle, the results have been varied and confusing, engendering much controversy and debate. For example, Mott and Sherrington maintained that deafferentated monkeys had profound and enduring deficits in limb movements (250), but Munk strongly disagreed, claiming that after recovery the animals' motor performance was remarkably good (251). With hindsight, most of the inconsistencies in the published accounts can be attributed to the following factors. First, the full capability of a deafferentated limb is only expressed if the contralateral limb is also deafferentated or bound (251, 321). Second, tiny remnants of sensory input may suffice for reasonable control, especially of simple movements (140, 298). Third, nervous systems are good at developing new motor strategies to circumvent deficits, making these less obvious (75). Fourth, ischemic deafferentation generally produces pain and unusual sensations, which themselves can alter motor output (183, 205). Finally, deficits are prominent when tasks are complex (133). They may be missed if testing is too simple.

With these complications in mind, the following conclusions regarding deafferentation are now fairly secure:

1. the basic ability to produce voluntary force and move limbs is preserved after deafferentation. However, movements are generally uncoordinated and inaccurate, especially when visual guidance is absent (133, 257, 294, 297).

2. coordination of the different segments of the primate hand in precision tasks is particularly impaired (Fig. 3.1). The accuracy of spatial orientation, fractionated movements and anticipatory preshaping of the hand is reduced, and writing may be severely affected (79, 138, 205, 328).

3. Gait is possible after deafferentation, but again it tends to be irregular and uncoordinated. This holds true in vertebrates and invertebrates alike (23, 24, 25, 72, 137, 140). In humans who have lost limb proprioception, gait is severely impaired and requires conscious attention (75). If neck proprioception is also lost, gait becomes virtually impossible (328).

4. Control of tasks involving simultaneous changes in several variables, coordination of several limb segments, or adaptation to changes in the external environment is impaired. Thus, fastening buttons or holding a cup are difficult and sometimes impossible without visual guidance (133, 294, 298).

Central Pattern Generators and Sensory Feedback

A very important concept that emerged from deafferentation studies was the idea that there are neuronal assemblies in the CNS that can generate basic patterns of motor output for rhythmic activities such as walking, breathing, chewing, swimming, and flying, without sensory input (50, 157, 263, 350). In 1911, Graham Brown posited an "intrinsic factor"

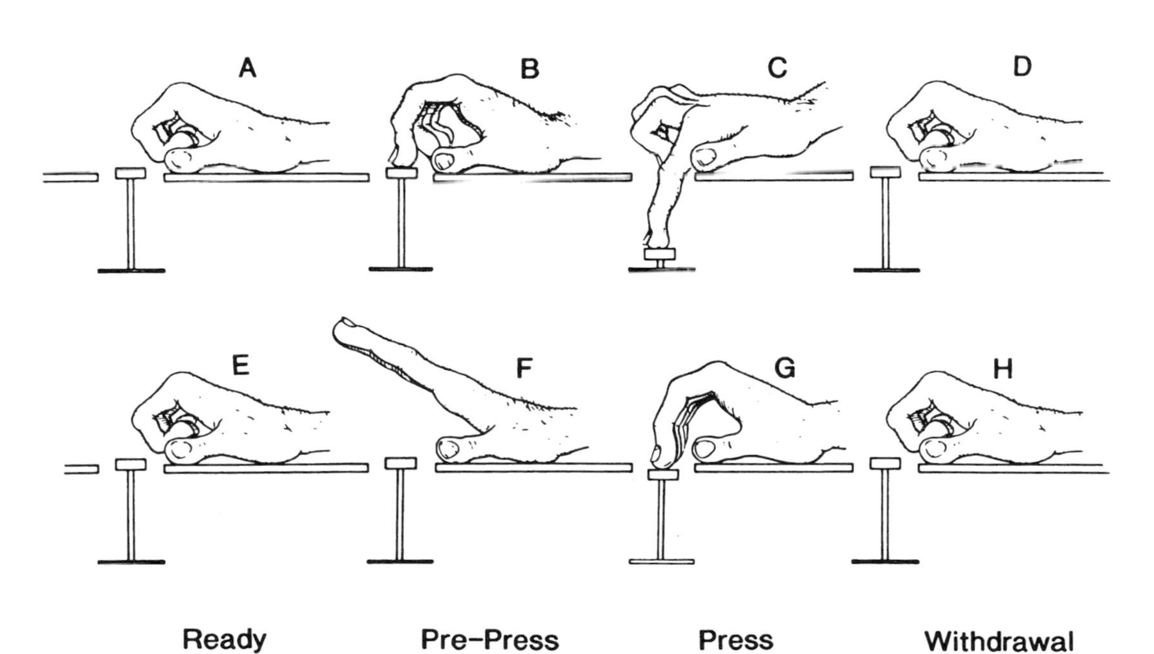

FIG. 3.1. Effect of selective deafferentation on hand control in a macaque monkey. Finger movements in a key-pressing task, before (*top*) and after (*bottom*) a cuneate fasciculus lesion. The premovement start position was similar in normal and lesioned animals (*A* and *E*), as was the final position (*D* and *H*). However, the individual control of fingers was dramatically lost after the lesion (compare *F* to *B*). The fingers extended, bore down on the key in unison (*G*) and finished in a tightly flexed power grip (*H*). From here a return to position *F*, with the fingers fully extended, was not uncommon, with multiple cycles of *F-G-H* in rapid succession. [Reproduced from Cooper et al. (79).]

for locomotion in the spinal cord, on the grounds that coordinated activation of flexors and extensors could be seen after the cord had been isolated from descending supraspinal input and from all afferent input (50). Grillner coined the term "central pattern generator" to describe the hypothetical intrinsic circuitry (157). Just how well the spinal central pattern generator functioned in isolation from sensory input became a matter of some debate. Most groups acknowledged that after deafferentation the locomotor rhythm was more labile [cats (160); crabs (167); stick insects (24)]. Yet many intricate details of normal muscle coordination could be found in selected recordings from muscle nerves in deafferentated walking cats (Fig. 3.2). Other authors stressed the variability of the data, particularly in relation to bifunctional muscles (23, 224, 263). It has even been

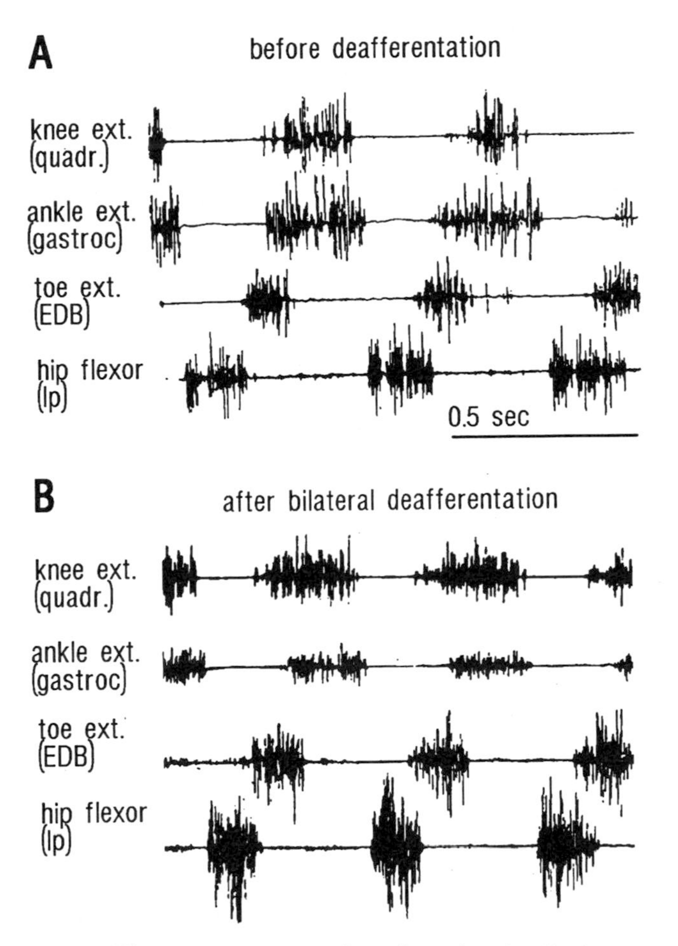

FIG. 3.2. Electromyogram recordings from four hindlimb muscles in a decerebrate cat induced to walk on a treadmill by electrical stimulation of the midbrain locomotor area. The relative timing of the bursts of activity is remarkably similar before (*A*) and after (*B*) bilateral hindlimb deafferentation. ext., extensor; quadr., quadriceps; gastroc, gastrocnemius; EDB, extensor digitorum brevis; Ip, iliopsoas. [Adapted from Grillner and Zangger (160).]

suggested that the activation patterns of the bifunctional muscles in 3:4-dihydroxyphenylalanine (DOPA)-induced fictive locomotion are those of backward rather than forward locomotion (51).

In certain specific cases, movements in a normal animal can be attributed fairly clearly to central programming. For example, in cockroaches, afferent feedback in fast walking is too delayed to have a reflex effect within a given cycle, the duration of which is 40 ms or less (88, 355). At most, the sensory input might affect the motor program in ensuing steps [one-step-ahead control; (195)]. In locusts, sensory input influences the wing-beat cycle *following* the one in which it was elicited (266). In rapid ballistic movements in humans, sensory feedback is also too slow to modify the motor output (90). Human subjects and monkeys must plan in advance the force of certain movements, based on visual judgment and prior memory (133). The neural activity involved in this planning has been recorded in several different ways. Indeed, even the simple co-contraction strategy that humans use to stiffen limbs when learning novel tasks may be viewed as a centrally generated motor program (32, 247).

Grillner (1975) suggested that in locomotion, reflexes are "prepared to operate but (are) without any effect so long as the movement proceeds according to the set central program" (157). This notion has its origins in the "Reafferenzprinzip" of von Holst (339) and remains influential to this day (6, 18, 22). Somewhat at odds with this view is the evidence that sensory input during gait can have a very strong effect indeed. For example, when a rhythmically air-stepping animal is lowered to the ground, the instant a limb gains firm ground support, the rhythm slows or ceases (23, 24, 102, 136). The hindlimbs of spinal cats walking on a split-belt treadmill adapt their cadence to each belt separately (125). Obstruction of hip movement (9, 159) or loading of extensor muscles (78, 102) can completely suppress rhythmicity in a leg, while the other legs continue to cycle. In the absence of sensory feedback, obstacles or inclines are not compensated for, and if the animal is not supported it falls (137, 140). Rossignol (see Chapter 5) deals in more detail with the relationship of sensory input to the locomotor pattern generator. For our present purposes, we may conclude that:

1. The CNS can autonomously generate detailed patterns of muscle activity that can form the substrate of complex movements.
2. To be useful, these motor patterns must be under direct feedback control. They are modulated and at times overruled by sensory-evoked control mechanisms in the CNS.

3. In some animals, generation of the locomotor rhythm depends entirely on sensorimotor interaction (i.e., sensory input is an integral and necessary part of the locomotor pattern generator) (23, 24).

STRUCTURE AND RESPONSE PROPERTIES OF PROPRIOCEPTORS

Many types of sensory receptor contribute to motor control in different animals, and several reviews detail the morphology and functional properties of these receptors in vertebrates (148, 178, 185, 189, 238, 280, 285) and invertebrates (22, 24, 56, 57, 71, 127). In the following summary, the emphasis will be on mammalian proprioceptors, although corresponding invertebrate analogs will be mentioned.

The word "proprioception" refers to the sensing of the body's own movements (see also Chapter 4). In 1821 Charles Bell assumed that muscles contained sensory elements that contributed both to conscious "muscle sense" and to the subconscious reflex control of movement (46). This view prevailed through the 1940s. However, by the 1950s, neurophysiologists had for various reasons rejected a conscious sensorial role for muscle proprioception. It was not until 1972, when it was shown that the selective activation of muscle receptors with vibration-evoked illusions of movement, that this role was reinstated (143). In the meantime, clinicians had continued to think of proprioception in kinesthetic terms, evaluating it according to their patients' perception of imposed movements of the extremities. In this chapter, we will take the broad view. Any receptor that can signal position or movement about joints qualifies as a proprioceptor, regardless of whether the information reaches consciousness, or for that matter whether it demonstrably contributes to movement control.

By and large, limb proprioceptors sense one of two variables: displacement and force. The transduction process generally introduces dynamic components of response and various nonlinearities. In mammals, limb displacement is sensed by muscle spindle, joint, ligamentous, and skin receptors (178, 189, 238, 349). The invertebrate displacement sensors are chordotonal organs, thoracicocoxal muscle receptor organs, and various hair sensilla (127). In receptors with efferent innervation (muscle spindles and thoracicocoxal muscle receptor organs), the CNS modulates the gain of the afferent response to muscle stretch and adds a tonic component of firing or a "bias" (57). Mammalian tendon organs signal the force produced by a few motor units (175). Small ensembles of tendon organs can provide information about whole-muscle force (283), but there is disagreement about the fidelity of this information (174, 185). The invertebrate analogs of tendon organs, campaniform sensilla, act like strain gauges, detecting strain in the external cuticle that gives indirect and nonlinear information about limb loading (127). Mammalian joint and ligamentous receptors respond best to extremes of joint angle, though some midrange signaling occurs (52, 118). It is debatable whether joint and ligamentous receptors make a significant contribution to the sensory input required for controlling normal movements (189).

Muscle Spindles

In the last 40 years, more effort has gone into understanding the structure, functioning, and reflex action of muscle spindles than of all the other mammalian mechanoreceptors combined. This is because it was long assumed that spindles were the most important proprioceptors for movement control. It is now apparent that the spindles' "poor relations," the tendon organs, may be just as important for controlling cyclical movements such as locomotion (78, 102). Spindle afferents make monosynaptic connections with α-motoneurons, so they offered an accessible portal for studying central synaptic action. Finally, the nature and function of the γ-fusimotor supply to spindles intrigued many researchers and continues to do so. Boyd, Gladden, and Hulliger have written excellent reviews on muscle spindles and fusimotor action (41, 42, 178). What follows is a brief and necessarily incomplete summary and update of certain aspects of this work, selected to facilitate the functional emphasis of this chapter.

Spindle Structure. Depending on its size, a mammalian muscle may contain up to 500 spindles (20, 42, 340). These are located amongst the extrafusal muscle fibers, sometimes in association with one or more tendon organs (1, 230, 290). Spindles range in length from 0.5–10 mm, corresponding to 10%–20% of extrafusal fiber length (287, 343). They consist of six to ten infrafusal muscle fibers attached at each end (pole) to the surrounding extrafusal fibers (Fig. 3.3). A central capsular enlargement that gives the spindle its fusiform shape and hence its name contains one or two primary and one to five secondary sensory endings spiralled around noncontractile portions of the intrafusal fibers (20, 41). The endings project into the muscle nerve via group Ia (primary) and group II (secondary) afferent axons (21, 42). The capsule protects the endings from the large swings in electrolyte concentrations that accompany extrafusal contractions. Each spindle is innervated

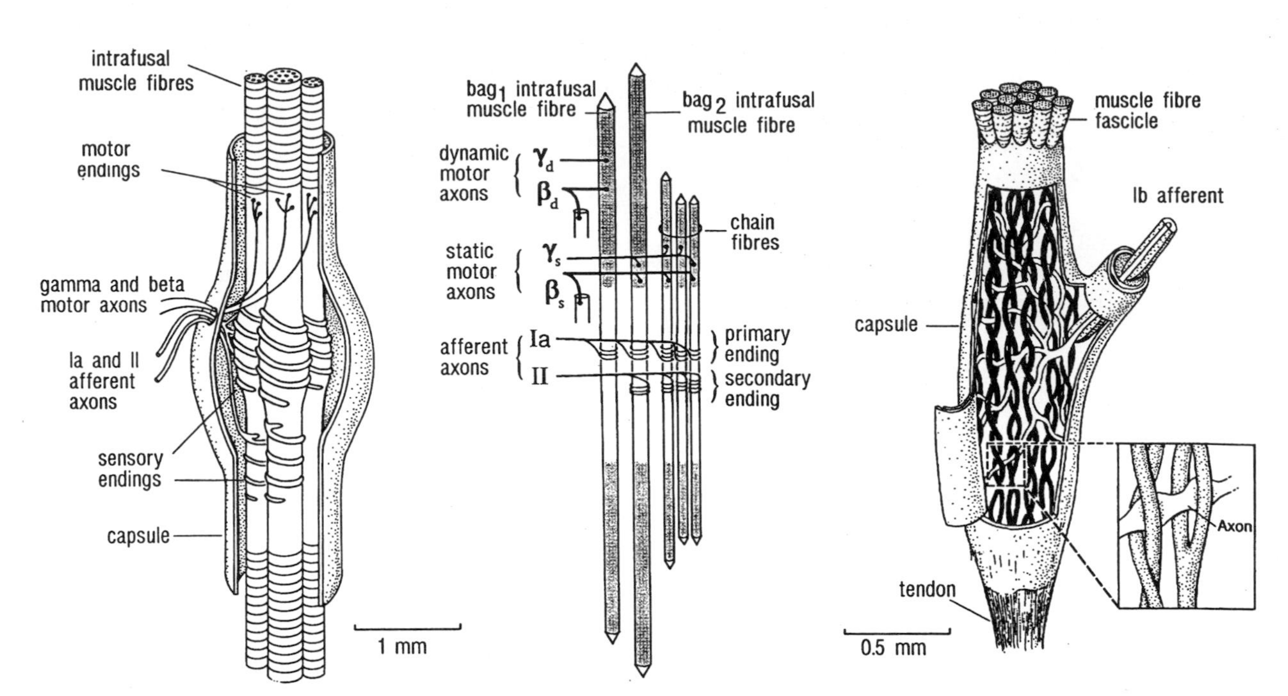

FIG. 3.3. Schematic of a mammalian muscle spindle (*A*) and Golgi tendon organ (*B*). The γ- and β-fusimotor axons innervate six to ten intrafusal muscle fibers (not all shown). The β-motoneurons also innervate extrafusal muscle fibers as indicated. The central regions of the intrafusal fibers, around which the group Ia and II sensory afferents spiral, are noncontractile. When the polar ends of the intrafusal fibers contract in response to γ and/or β activity, the sensory regions are stretched, causing increased Ia and II firing. Dynamic fusimotor action stiffens the bag_1 intrafusal muscle fiber, so that when the ends of the spindle are stretched, more of the stretch is imparted to the sensory region, thus sensitizing the Ia ending. The terminal branches of the tendon organ are entwined amongst the musculotendinous strands of 10–20 motor units, and "sample" the active force produced by them. [Adapted from Kandel et al. (193) and Zelena and Soukup (354).]

by 10–12 γ-fusimotor axons and often by a β-skeletofusimotor axon, which also innervates surrounding extrafusal muscle (114).

The morphological details of the sensory and motor innervation of muscle spindles were debated for many years, principally by Ian Boyd and David Barker (reviewed in 178). The consensus now is that the typical limb spindle in cats, monkeys, and humans contains three types of intrafusal muscle fiber: a dynamic bag_1 (DB1 or b_1), a static bag_2 (SB2 or b_2), and 2–11 chain (c) fibers. A functional separation of chain fibers into long and short has been suggested (201). Activation of each intrafusal fiber has specific effects on afferent responses to length changes. The b_1 fiber is selectively activated by dynamic fusimotor (γ_d) or skeletofusimotor (β_d) axons, although nonselective activation along with b_2 and chain fibers may sometimes occur (113). The b_2 and chain fibers are activated selectively or concomitantly by static fusimotor or skeletofusimotor (γ_s or β_s) axons. Some spindles, notably the minor members of tandem or compound spindles in neck muscles, lack b_1 fibers (1, 20, 201). Their primary afferents are consequently called b_2c afferents. Neck b_2c afferents have stretch-response properties and conduction velocities intermediate between those of limb primary and secondary spindle afferents (101, 290). In hindlimb muscles, up to 30% of primary endings may be of the b_2c type (326).

Spindle Response Properties. The length-response characteristics of spindle primary and secondary endings with and without fusimotor action have been characterized in great detail over the last 50 years (reviewed in 41, 113, 178, 238). Though there are some minor variations between species, basic spindle characteristics, elucidated in acute experiments and summarized in Figure 3.4, are remarkably similar in cats, monkeys, and humans (70, 256, 273). Both primary and secondary endings transduce length changes dynamically, the primary endings having somewhat larger velocity- and acceleration-sensitive components of response (i.e., slightly more phase advance for sinusoidal inputs and larger step-

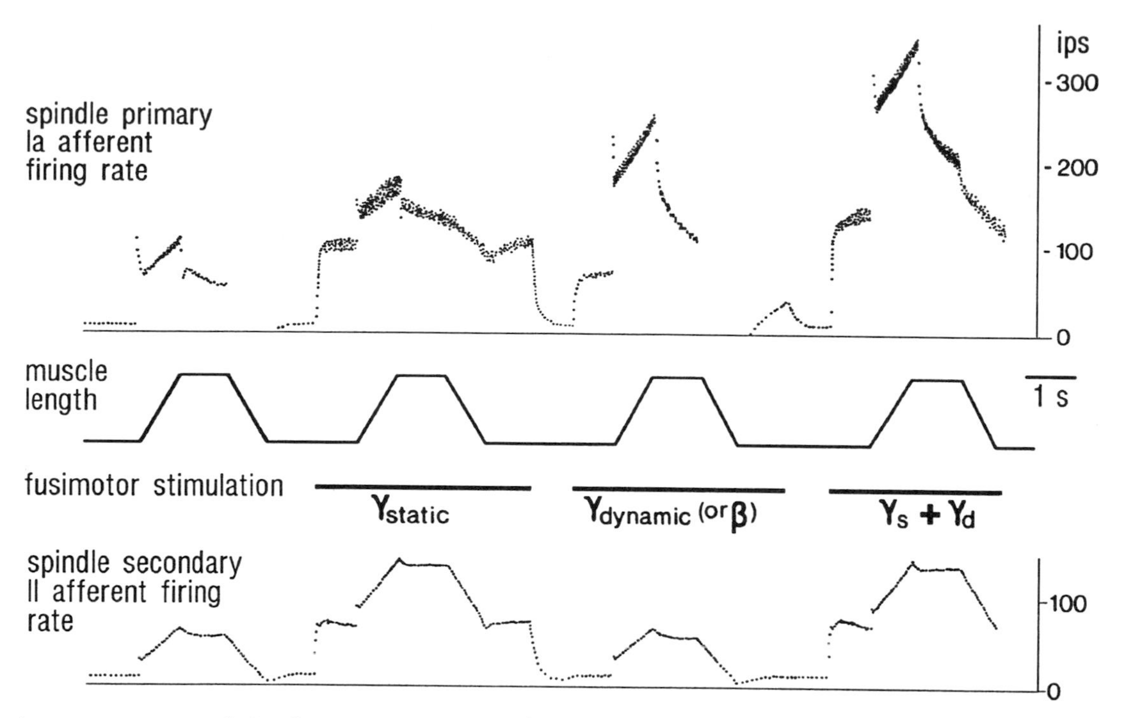

FIG. 3.4. Schematic summary of the firing rate responses of group Ia and II spindle afferents to trapezoidal length changes with and without concomitant fusimotor stimulation. The firing rates shown are typical of displacements of about 10% of rest-length and velocities of 0.05 rest-length/s. The *horizontal bars* indicate periods of fusimotor stimulation at 100/s. Note the big increase in Ia stretch sensitivity with γ_d stimulation and the strong biasing effect of γ_s stimulation. Combined γ_d and γ_s stimulation gives occlusion effects. ips, imp/s. [Adapted from Prochazka (278).]

changes in firing at the onset of ramp stretches). The responses of both types of ending show many nonlinearities, notably length-, velocity-, and amplitude-dependent sensitivity (27, 68, 180, 240); aftereffects of muscle contraction; history of length changes and fusimotor modulation (49, 249, 286, 346); nonlinear velocity scaling (176, 271, 299); irregularity of discharge intervals (154, 241); and local unloading effects of extrafusal muscle contraction (36, 170). There is a large range of stretch-sensitivities between individual group Ia and II afferents, notably in relation to the velocity-sensitive components of response. Effectively, there is a continuum of behavior from group II afferents with low displacement- and velocity-sensitivity, to group Ia afferents, which can be highly velocity-sensitive (17, 304, 347).

From a functional point of view, the most important aspects of fusimotor action can be summarized as follows. When muscle displacements are small (<0.5% of muscle rest length), pure γ_d action, mediated by b_1 fibers, slightly *decreases* the stretch-sensitivity or gain of Ia afferents and adds some bias (141). Phase advance, which in the absence of fusimotor action ranges from 45–90 degrees for sinusoidal length changes in the range 1–4 Hz, is slightly *reduced* by γ_d action. For larger amplitude length changes, γ_d action increases Ia stretch-sensitivity up to fivefold (43). Phase advance may increase slightly (180) or decrease slightly (68). Strong γ_s action adds a relatively large bias to both Ia and II firing and generally attenuates Ia stretch-sensitivity by 50% or more for all amplitudes of length change (68, 87, 180). Paradoxically, *weak* γ_s action can *increase* Ia sensitivity (179). In either case, phase appears to be little affected.

Although γ_d fibers occasionally have an intermediate (b_1b_2) action on primary endings, they rarely if ever activate secondary endings. Of the six to nine γ_s axons acting on a secondary ending, each adds some bias, most attenuate its sensitivity to very small dynamic stretches (<1% rest length), and two or three attenuate its response to large-amplitude stretches too (48, 68, 87). However, one or two of the γ_s axons may substantially *increase* the secondary ending's sensitivity to stretches greater than 4% rest length, presumably via b_2 intrafusal fibers (186). In some ways, the action of these γ_s fibers on secondary endings is quite similar to the action of γ_d fibers on primary endings. Indeed, one could even argue that the overall repertoire of fusimotor control of spindle primary and secondary endings differs in detail rather than in any fundamental way.

The internal disposition, strength, and sensory innervation of the three types of intrafusal muscle fiber presumably determine the particular type of fusimotor action on a given primary or secondary ending. This can range from "pure" chain-type action (biasing, driving of Ia's, reduced stretch-sensitivity) to b_2 action (strong biasing, stretch-sensitivity decreased in Ia afferents, increased in II afferents), to "pure" b_1 action (minimal effects on II's, moderate biasing, and large increases in stretch-sensitivity in Ia's) (41, 113, 326).

The terms *dynamic* and *static* fusimotor action are misleading, in that both types of action alter mainly the *gain* and *offset* rather than the *dynamics* of Ia and II responses to stretch. Matthews originally coined the terms to distinguish the strong γ_s biasing action on Ia afferents at constant (static) muscle length from the large increases in Ia response to (dynamic) length changes evoked by γ_d fibers (236). Subsequently, it was claimed that γ_d action selectively increases velocity-sensitivity of Ia afferents (208), but this was based on an association of velocity response with the *slopes* of firing rate in ramp stretches (a nonlinear property discussed below). In fact, if the *initial steps* in rate are taken as the velocity components, and the slopes are taken as the length responses, γ_d action does not significantly change the ratio, nor does it change the frequency of singularities in sinusoidal frequency–response plots (68).

Spindle Models. Various mathematical models of these properties have been developed. Though it has always been recognized that nonlinearities are a major problem, several very useful linear frequency–response analyses have been published (68, 87, 141, 166, 177, 241, 272). Representative transfer functions relating firing rate to input are as follows:

spindle Ia afferents, displacement inputs less than 0.5% rest-length (68):

$$\frac{K_1 s(s + 0.4)(s + 11)(s + 44)}{(s + 0.04)(s + 0.8)} \qquad (1)$$

spindle Ia afferents, displacement inputs greater than 0.5% rest-length (68):

$$\frac{K_2 s(s + 0.4)(s + 4)(s + 44)}{(s + 0.04)(s + 0.8)} \qquad (2)$$

spindle II afferents, all displacement inputs (68, 272):

$$\frac{K_3(s + 0.4)(s + 11)}{(s + 0.8)} \qquad (3)$$

where K_1, K_2, and K_3 are gain constants and s is the Laplace frequency-domain operator.

As we saw above, γ action, either static or dynamic, changes the gain of spindle afferent responses but has little effect on the dynamics. γ action can therefore be characterized by changes in the gain constants alone (γ_d: increased K_1 or K_2; γ_s: decreased K_1 or K_2, increased K_3). Ia afferents are more velocity-sensitive as temperature drops, and this may be represented by reducing the "44" parameter in the $(s + 44)$ terms (272). However, a limitation of the linear models is that velocity-sensitive components of Ia responses to ramps do not scale *linearly* with increasing velocity (237). Schäfer et al. (172, 299) and Houk et al. (176) proposed a power-law relationship between Ia responses and velocity of stretch:

$$\text{Ia firing rate} = \text{constant} \times \text{velocity}^n \qquad (4)$$

The mean value of the exponent n was 0.56 in Schäfer's hands or 0.3 according to Houk. Schäfer's analysis was restricted to the dynamic index (the decrement in firing at the end of a ramp stretch). Houk et al. (176) found that the addition of a length-dependent term:

$$\text{Ia firing rate} = \text{constant} \times \text{length} \times \text{velocity}^{0.3} \qquad (5)$$

characterized the response of Ia afferents during ramp stretches of different velocities. The initial step in Ia firing at the onset of a ramp stretch was represented by two more terms added to equation 5, specifying firing rate and muscle length offsets r_0 and l_0:

$$(\text{Ia firing rate} - r_0) = \text{constant} \times (\text{length} - l_0) \times \text{velocity}^{0.3} \qquad (6)$$

An interesting nonlinearity predicted by equation 6 is that the size of the initial step in firing rate depends on the muscle length at which the ramp stretch starts. This produces an increase in the ratio of the velocity response (step in firing rate at stretch onset) to the displacement response (slope of firing rate profile). Poppele (271) also reported changes in this ratio, but in relation to stretch velocity rather than initial length, a result that is *not* predicted by equation 6.

Details aside, the important point is that the Ia response is clearly a nonlinear function of length and velocity. Other nonlinear models have been published by Hasan (165) and Schaafsma et al. (300), the latter including muscle length-tension properties and spike-encoding mechanisms. So far, it is the linear transfer functions (68, 272) that have proved most accessible and practical to modelers, although the problem of nonlinearity, particularly in relation to velocity scaling, always lurks in the background. For all their lack of precision and generality, linear models are useful in revealing fusimotor modulation of muscle spindle firing in awake animals (see Fig. 3.9) and gain and stability in the stretch-reflex arc (28, 184, 291). Admittedly, the conclusions would be strengthened if they were validated with the more accurate but computationally demanding nonlinear models.

Tendon Organs

Structure and Response Properties. Tendon organs are encapsulated corpuscles 0.2–1 mm long. Over 90% are located at musculotendinous junctions or tendinous inscriptions (21). Their sensory endings, which project into the muscle nerve as group Ib axons, are entwined amongst the tendinous strands of 10–20 motor units, a given motor unit engaging one to six tendon organs (185, 285, 288). In the absence of muscle contraction, most tendon organs have a high threshold to imposed muscle stretch (235). Thus, tendon organs were initially considered to be "overload protectors," firing only when muscle force approached injurious levels. This idea was dispelled when it was shown that the adequate stimulus for tendon organs was active contraction of the motor units with which they were associated (175, 188). Even in the absence of active contraction, when the rates of applied muscle stretch were matched to those in the step cycle, 46 of 53 tendon organs were activated (319). Indeed, it is now quite clear that tendon organs as an ensemble respond over the full physiological range of muscle force (5, 83, 174).

Tendon Organ Models. Because it is impossible to monitor force from the small group of motor units that innervate a tendon organ, it is difficult to determine precise input–output characteristics for the receptor. Nonetheless, some frequency analyses have been performed by applying feedback-controlled force signals to whole muscle (8, 177). This indicated that tendon organs had a high-pass filtering property, or dynamic component of response, similar to that of spindle II endings (5). Tendon organ Ib afferents, all force inputs (177):

$$\frac{K(s + 0.15)(s + 1.5)(s + 16)}{(s + 0.20)(s + 2.0)(s + 37)} \tag{5}$$

where K is a gain constant. Another similarity with spindle II afferents is that Ib afferents tend to fire fairly regularly, except at low levels of active force, when unfused twitch contractions of newly recruited motor units summate and "beat," causing characteristic bursts of Ib firing (155, 174). The Anderson transfer function, used in conjunction with monitored force, gave a good fit to the firing profile of a Ib afferent recorded in a conscious cat (8, 15). There are various sources of nonlinearity in Ib transduction. First, a given ending may be unloaded by contractions of muscle fibers not inserting into the receptor capsule (175, 320, 354). Second, the relationship between whole-muscle force and the force produced by the tendon organ's cohort of motor units is unlikely to be perfectly linear. Third, at low active forces, the beating effects alluded to above are seen and, as each new motor unit is recruited, a characteristic step in firing rate occurs (15, 83, 334). Thus the attractive simplification that tendon organs provide a more-or-less linear representation of whole-muscle force is problematic and has been debated for some time (35, 83, 155, 174, 185).

Spindle and Tendon Organ Densities: A Clue as to Function?

There are 25,000–30,000 muscle spindles in the human body: 4,000 in each arm and 7,000 in each leg (42, 340). Muscles vary tremendously in the number of spindles and tendon organs they contain. This has often been seen as a clue to unraveling their function (1, 21, 59, 185, 238, 340). Some intrinsic hand muscles that contain large numbers of spindles have no tendon organs at all (185). Other muscles, notably the diaphragm, the digastric muscle, intrinsic muscles of the larynx, and extraocular muscles in some species, have no spindles (238).

One interpretation of these differences is that muscles engaged in fine control have the most proprioceptors. For example, in the cat forepaw, which can perform delicate manipulative tasks, the fifth interosseus has 119 spindles/g; whereas lateral gastrocnemius, a hindlimb extensor, has only five spindles/g (69). Some deep neck muscles have up to 500 spindles/g (1). Granit suggested that these muscles control precise movements and so they require elaborate spindle control (148). However, this was challenged by Banks and Stacey (20), who reviewed data on 75 muscles in different species and found that spindle density depended not so much on muscle function as on size. The average number of spindles n in a muscle of weight w grams was:

$$n = 38\, w^{0.32} \tag{8}$$

derived from:

$$\log_{10} n = 1.58 + 0.32 \log_{10} w \tag{9}$$

Roughly speaking, equation 8 says that the number of spindles = 38 × cube root of muscle weight in grams. Thus, a 64 g muscle should have about 152 spindles. On this basis, the cat fifth interosseus has only 5% more spindles than expected from its size, about the same as the hindlimb extensor soleus (20). Buxton and Peck (59) put an interesting slant on the issue. They claimed that the number of spindles acting about a joint correlated better with the summed range-of-motion or motor complexity of the joint than the net weight of the muscles. Contrary to previous ideas, it was argued that proximal muscles had more range-of-motion and were richer in spindles than distal ones (305). However, the numbers of spindles were calculated from summed muscle weights. This is probably invalid, as equation 9 applies only to individual muscles. Regardless of how the numbers are computed, however, it is true that the intervertebral neck muscles have a "bewildering number of spindles" (80). The spindles and tendon organs are arranged in complexes that in some cases stretch continuously from one end of a muscle to the other (1). Furthermore, the control of movements of the head is undoubtedly complex. Precise muscle contractions are required to hold the head upright and oriented; the head must provide a stable platform for the visual system, even during large movements of the trunk. In quadrupeds, the mouth is used for feeding, for grooming, and for manipulating objects, all of which require accurate head movement. The high spindle densities in neck muscles are therefore consistent with the idea that the greater the motor demands, the more spindles are required; however, in human psychophysical experiments, the resolution of head movements was found to be somewhat *lower* than that in the limbs, hands, and digits (327). In short, the hypothesis that spindle numbers are related to motor skill is simple and didactically appealing, but unfortunately it is not supported by all of the available evidence.

Proprioceptors in Joints, Ligaments, and Skin

Mechanoreceptors in joint capsules, joint ligaments, and skin are anatomically well placed to provide proprioceptive feedback, but it has been surprisingly difficult to establish their role precisely. Until the late 1960s, joint receptors were assumed to mediate position sense and to signal joint position over the full range of motion (44). However, in an important series of experiments, Burgess and Clark found that most joint receptors in the cat knee were actually quite unresponsive in the midrange (52, 73). This finding has been debated ever since. Ferrell (118), for example, disputed the emphasis of Burgess and Clark's results, claiming that a substantial proportion of units in the cat knee posterior articular nerve responded in the midrange. Tracey (332) recorded from 110 cat wrist joint receptors and obtained results in broad agreement with Burgess and Clark, in that the receptors started firing only when the wrist was pushed into a fairly flexed position, but Zalkind (353) found slowly adapting afferents in cat wrist joint that fired over the whole range of motion. Intercostal joint receptors (139), hip joint afferents (66), and temporomandibular joint receptors (219) were reported to signal across all joint angles. Some of the full-range afferents in the cat posterior knee joint nerve apparently originate in either muscle spindles or tendon organs in nearby muscles (73, 153, 245). Loading of the joint capsule by muscle contraction sensitizes joint receptors, in some cases enough to confer midrange responsiveness on them (156).

On balance, studies in reduced preparations indicated that joint capsular and ligamentous afferents are capable of signaling limb position and movement at the extremes of motion and in some joints over the full range of motion. Given that single-unit discharges are discernable in recordings from whole joint nerves (118), the total number of receptors signaling midrange movement is probably quite low compared to the number of surrounding muscle and skin receptors responding to the same movement. Joint afferents have conduction velocities mainly in the group II range (52), and their segmental reflex connections with α-motoneurons are less direct than those of muscle spindles (187, 189). Their contribution to kinesthesia and sensorimotor control probably complements that of the other proprioceptors (242, see Chapter 4) and they may have a special role in inhibiting muscles when joints are damaged (183).

Receptors in the glabrous or hairy skin overlying joints and muscle respond both phasically and tonically to movement (349) and so are good candidates for a role in proprioception. Furthermore, there is a huge number of skin receptors in the extremities. The human hand has an estimated 17,000 skin mechanoreceptors with myelinated afferent fibers (190), compared to a population in the whole arm of about 4,000 muscle spindles, 2,500 tendon organs, and perhaps a few hundred midrange joint receptors. The skin receptors best suited to signal position are slowly adapting type II receptors, which respond to stretching of the skin, in some cases several centimeters from the point of maximal strain (173). Slowly adapting type I skin receptors respond more locally, fire less regularly, and adapt more rapidly. Additionally, there are at least four kinds of hair follicle and rapidly adapting glabrous skin receptors that respond to the dynamic components of hair deflection or skin stretch (349).

Invertebrate Proprioceptors

The response properties of the invertebrate displacement sensors of the chordotonal organs and thoracicocoxal muscle receptor organs have been studied in several species. In general these receptors have high-pass characteristics comparable to those of mammalian muscle spindles. For example, in recordings from various single afferents innervating femoral chordotonal organs in stick insects, units were encountered that were predominantly length-sensitive, velocity-sensitive, acceleration-sensitive, or admixtures of the three (23, 24). Crustacean thoracicocoxal muscle receptor organs have two types of sensory afferents, T and S, which are analogous to mammalian spindle Ia and II afferents (57). They are nonspiking, transmitting signals to the CNS electrotonically, but in all other respects their responses to length changes and their efferent control by Rm1 and Rm2 motoneurons (equivalent to γ-and β-motoneurons) are astonishingly similar to those of muscle spindle endings. Campaniform sensilla, located in the external cuticle of many invertebrates, show high-pass characteristics comparable to those of their mammalian analogs, the tendon organs. High-pass frequency response characteristics have also been reported for other classes of invertebrate proprioceptors including locust forewing stretch receptors (266) and cockroach femoral tactile spines (274).

RESPONSE PROPERTIES OF PROPRIOCEPTORS DURING ACTIVE MOVEMENT

Methodology

Until the 1960s, no recordings had been obtained from sensory afferents during unrestrained voluntary movement in any species. Yet there was already a wealth of data on their passive properties in anesthetized animals and on their activity during reflexive hindlimb movements and respiration in lightly anesthetized, spinalized or decerebrate animals. In the 1960s, various theories were proposed on how the sensory endings might fire during normal movements and how the afferent input might be used by the CNS in controlling these movements. With hindsight, some of the assumptions were more or less right and some were more or less wrong. In the following, most of the emphasis will be on the data obtained since 1967 on the firing of proprioceptive afferents in normal voluntary movements.

Hagbarth and Vallbo (1967) pioneered the neurography technique of recording from single sensory nerve fibers using semimicroelectrodes inserted into peripheral nerves of awake human subjects (Fig. 3.5*A*). The importance of this work in elucidating natural sensory activity during movement cannot be overstated. It coincided with the studies of muscle receptors in decerebrate locomotor cats (309). Other methods have since been developed to record from first-order afferents in normal cats and monkeys [Fig. 3.5; (74, 124, 142, 216, 276, 301)]. A large body of information on sensory input during voluntary movement now exists. While much has been clarified, particularly with regard to tendon organ and skin receptor activity, the firing patterns of muscle spindles and the fusimotor activity that shapes them remain somewhat controversial. Nonetheless, for certain classes of movement such as slow, rhythmical muscle contractions in humans and locomotion in the cat, the firing profiles of spindles and tendor organs are now well characterized, allowing a fairly detailed analysis of sensorimotor interactions.

Although recordings from spindle afferents have been obtained during voluntary movement in humans, cats, and monkeys, it has been virtually impossible to obtain equivalent data on γ-motoneurons (but see 221, 289). In fact it is rather fortunate that spindle-afferents rather than γ-efferents are accessible, because spindles are innervated by up to a dozen γ-motoneurons and it would be difficult indeed to infer spindle afferent behavior from kinematics and the firing of single γ-motoneurons alone. This is not to say that γ recordings should not be pursued in the conscious animal; information about type-specific γ activity is of great interest in relation to arousal, sensory set, and central rhythm generation. But the resultant *sensory* signals are in fact more crucial for understanding the basics of the sensory control of movement.

Muscle Spindles

Involuntary Movements in Animals. The earliest clues regarding fusimotor control of muscle spindle sensitivity in active movements came from recordings in decerebrate cats (111). Spindles in reflexly activated muscles often increased their firing, even when the muscles shortened. This led to the notion of α-γ linkage (148), whereby γ action was posited to keep spindles taut and responsive in the face of extrafusal shortening (209, 238, 268). The early data also showed that γ-fusimotor neurons could fire spontaneously in the absence of detectable muscle activity

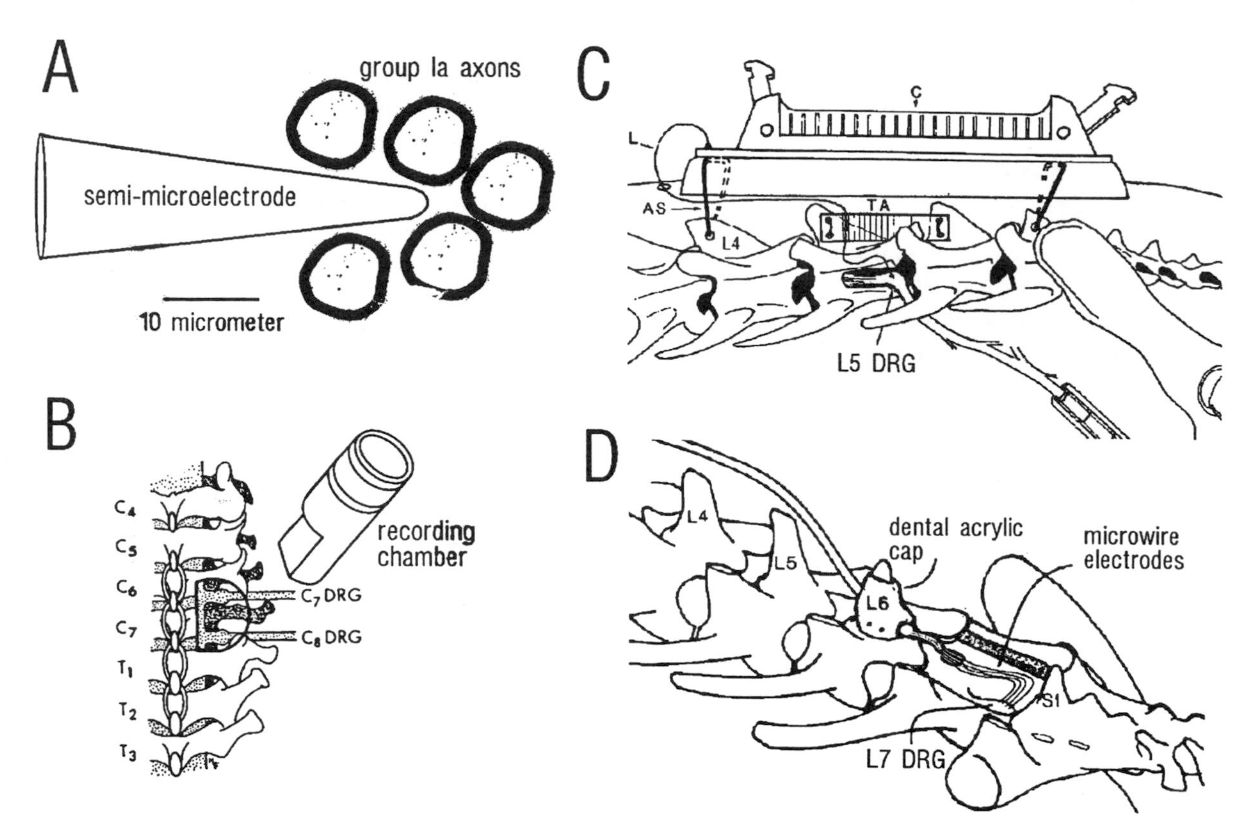

FIG. 3.5. Techniques to record from single nerve fibers in conscious humans (*A*), monkeys (*B*), and cats (*C* and *D*). *A*, Schematic profile of a neurography electrode pushed amongst Ia axons in a peripheral nerve (shown in cross section). The uninsulated portion of tip is about 30 μm long. Single-unit selectivity probably relies on proximity of tip to a node of Ranvier of an axon. [Adapted from Wall and McMahon (341).] *B*, Exploded view of recording chamber over monkey cervical (C7, C8) dorsal root ganglia (DRG). Holes drilled through the lateral vertebral processes allow access to DRG by microelectrodes lowered in chamber. [Adapted from Schieber et al. (302).] *C*, Loeb's "hatpin" microwire implants in cat lumbar (L5) dorsal root ganglion (DRG). Microwire lead from DRG is stabilized on a Silastic sheet sutured between L5 and L6 vertebral spinous processes, then tunneled up to connector back-pack. *D*, Floating microwire variant of *C*, showing stabilization of cable shield in dental acrylic cap on L7 spinous process. Microwires are also stuck and/or sutured to dura mater. [*C* and *D* adapted from Prochazka (276).]

and that they generally had lower thresholds than α-motoneurons to electrical stimulation within the CNS, particularly within the reticular formation (151), to mechanical stimuli such as twisting the ear (150), and to noxious stimulation (182, 189, 191).

Spindle afferent and γ-efferent firing was also recorded during involuntary *rhythmical* motor activity in many different reduced preparations. This material has been reviewed several times (148, 178, 222, 238, 275) and so only the salient points are summarized here. Recordings during *respiration* in anesthetized cats generally supported the idea of phasic, α-linked γ activity, but tonic γ firing was also observed (152). The first recordings from spindle afferents during *locomotor* movements were obtained in high decerebrate cats (309). Firing was closely linked to phasic bursts of muscle activity rather than stretch, again suggesting a dominance of α-linked γ action. But in subsequent recordings (308), length changes were the more powerful modulatory influence, so it was hard to draw firm conclusions from these studies. Several other research groups have recorded from spindles in decerebrate or decorticate cats generating locomotor rhythms. The experimental techniques, conditions, and constraints varied between laboratories (33, 60, 252, 267, 312). The picture that has emerged from the reduced locomotor preparations is that γ activity is partly linked to α activity and partly independent of it. This is neatly illustrated in Figure 3.6, which shows the neural traffic in a muscle nerve during locomotion in a thalamic cat. The afferent and efferent components of activity were separated analytically on the basis of delays between two recording sites (33). The spindle Ia and II firing profiles in this figure are somewhat distorted versions of the muscle length profile. γ Firing is modulated roughly in phase with α activity, about a "carrier" frequency (i.e., bias or offset). The phasic component of γ action presumably maintained the spindle afferent discharge dur-

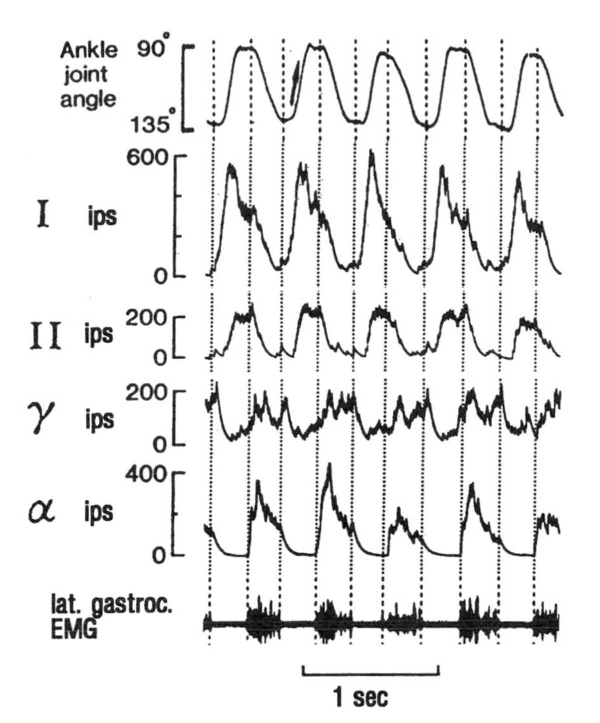

FIG. 3.6. Activity of group I and II afferent fibers and α and γ motor fibers during spontaneous air-stepping movements in high decerebrate cats. The mean firing rate profiles were estimated by electronically sorting afferent and efferent signals in a branch of the nerve to lateral gastrocnemius muscle. The technique does not differentiate between spindle Ia and tendon organ Ib afferent activity, but in this experiment Ia activity probably dominated the group I record, because there was no ground contact or weight bearing. Muscle lengthening is shown by the *arrow*. Both Ia and II afferents fired mainly during muscle stretch. The γ activity was modulated in time with the α bursts and whole-muscle electromyogram and there was an additional tonic offset or bias (i.e., there were both phasic and tonic components of γ discharge). [Adapted from Bessou et al. (33).]

ing extrafusal shortening and the tonic component set the underlying spindle afferent bias and sensitivity, depending on the admixture of γ_d and γ_s activity involved.

There has been much speculation on whether γ_d and γ_s fibers have distinct firing patterns during rhythmical movement. Some data indicate phasic α-γ_s linkage with tonic γ_d activity, some indicate α-γ_d linkage with γ_s tonic, and some indicate muscle-specific combinations (see Table 3.1, later). A case has also been made for coactivation of γ_d, β_d and fatigue-resistant type S motor units in "tonic" muscles and γ_s, β_s and fast-twitch type F motor units in "phasic" muscles (34). β-Motoneurons are α-motoneurons that innervate spindles, so they presumably fire at rates typical of motor units: 5–20 imp/s. Spindles are rarely innervated by more than one β-motoneuron, so β-fusimotor action, although guaranteed to be α-linked, is probably relatively weak compared to the action of a cohort of 10–12 γ-motoneurons firing at much higher rates. This weak β action may, however, be amplified or potentiated by concomitant γ action (112).

Voluntary Movements in Animals. The firing of spindle afferents recorded during chewing and other jaw movements in awake cats (74, 322) and monkeys (142, 204, 234) was generally related to muscle length, albeit with additional electromyogram (EMG)-linked components resulting from presumed α-linked γ and β action. Single-unit activity has also been recorded with microelectrodes from the cervical dorsal roots of awake cats and monkeys [Fig. 3.5*B,C,D*; (77, 124, 301, 302)]. Because the stability of the recording situation was precarious, the monkeys were not anesthetized during afferent identification. Several units with convincing spindle Ia-like responses to muscle twitches and vibration were characterized in slow tracking movements and self-paced rapid movements (330). In the rapid movements the afferents responded mainly to displacement, with phase advances consistent with the dynamic transfer characteristics of Ia afferents. However, during slow tracking (Fig. 3.7), some units fired as much during muscle shortening as lengthening. Although some of this could be ascribed to α-γ linkage, there were various features that indicated significant independence of α and γ activity (301, 302, 330). In contrast, the units recorded by Flament et al. (124) all increased their firing during isometric contractions, indicating α-γ linkage.

The firing of muscle afferents recorded in awake, walking cats (see Fig. 3.5*C* and *D*) has been combined in small ensembles according to muscle group and receptor type (Fig. 3.8). Some interesting facts and figures emerge from these data. First, the data showed that ensembles of as few as four or five afferents can provide the CNS with high-resolution information on muscle length and force. After the data of four or five afferents are averaged, the addition of more afferents does not substantially change the ensemble profile. Second, when the linear model of equation 2 is applied to the averaged length signals, the resulting profiles match the corresponding ensemble firing rates well (Fig. 3.9). This means that to a first approximation spindle afferents signal muscle length and velocity in the step cycle. Third, deviations from the modeled profiles suggest some α-linked γ action and mechanical transients related to tendon stretch, muscle "bounce," or muscle slackening (170, 287). Finally, if the firing of all the spindles in a typical cat hindlimb muscle is summed, the peak Ia input to the CNS in the step cycle is 20–40 kimp/s (283). The net monosynaptic reflex action of

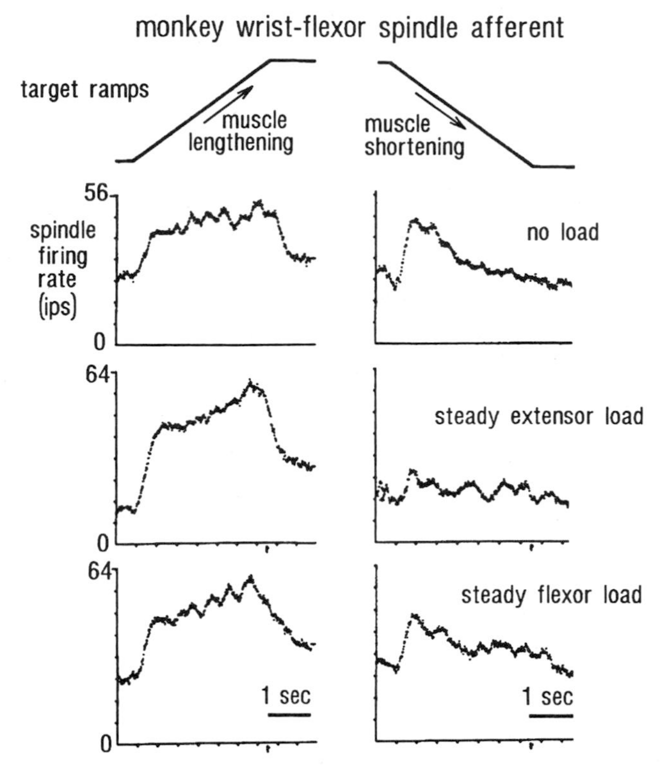

FIG. 3.7. Firing rate profiles of a monkey wrist-flexor spindle afferent recorded during voluntary wrist movements tracking a displayed ramp-and-hold target. Each profile is an average of several trials. Actual wrist movement was not shown, but it is assumed that tracking was good. Six combinations of movement and loading condition are shown. Left column, wrist extension trials (muscle lengthens); right column, wrist flexion (muscle shortens). Top row, no load; middle row, steady extensor load; bottom, flexor load. During muscle lengthening, afferent increases its firing rate. At onset of shortening, smaller increases in rate are seen, indicating some γ action. Relationship to loading conditions was interpreted as evidence for independence of γ and α activity. [Adapted from Schieber and Thach (302).]

this is nearly enough to depolarize low-threshold α-motoneurons from rest to firing threshold [(278); see also Chapter 1]. Note that if a 20 kimp/s signal were played through a loudspeaker, it would be so high pitched as to be inaudible.

Voluntary Movements in Humans. In the 1970s, Hagbarth and Vallbo did many neurography trials and trained students and visiting scientists in the technique. Neurography was independently developed in Munich (318) and Paris (292). As a result, hundreds of recordings from single muscle and skin afferents have now been documented by different groups around the world (131, 161, 178, 190, 349). Spindle afferents of various muscles of the hand, arm, and leg have been studied in different sensorimotor tasks and contexts. Certain basic firing properties have been observed repeatedly and are now established beyond reasonable doubt:

1. In relaxed muscles, spindle afferents behave like passive stretch receptors, increasing their firing in response to muscle stretch and decreasing it during shortening (Fig. 3.10*A*). The stretch-sensitivities of the afferents, expressed in terms of proportional changes in muscle length, are similar to those of deafferentated spindles in cats (107, 238, 334), baboons (70), and isolated human muscle (257, 273).
2. α-γ Coactivation: when muscles are voluntarily activated there are clear signs of accompanying fusimotor activation: increased spindle afferent firing in isometric contractions (Fig. 3.10*B*) or maintained firing if the muscle shortens (Fig. 3.11). This implies a "hard-wired" α-γ linkage, as posited by Granit (148) and reaffirmed by Hagbarth (161) and Rothwell et al. (293). In the early neurography work the EMG-linked component of γ action seemed to dominate spindle afferent responses, particularly in isometric data of the type in Fig. 3.10*B*. In the late 1970s, spindle afferent recordings in cats and monkeys performing normal movements indicated that changes in muscle length generally overrode the effect of α-linked γ action. Correspondingly, in the more recent human neurography experiments, when muscles contracting against loads were allowed to lengthen and shorten, the spindle firing also usually reflected the muscle length changes rather than the EMG (Fig. 3.11).
3. Firing rates of human spindles during active movements are quite low: usually in the range of 0–30 imp/s. Maximal rates of up to 85 imp/s have been seen in faster movements and tremor (336). By comparison, in cat gait, Ia firing rates of 50–200 imp/s were typical and rates greater than 600 imp/s occurred in imposed movements or unusual tasks (145, 217, 218, 283). Monkey jaw Ia afferents fired at 0 –250 imp/s during eating and up to 360 imp/s in rapid movements (142, 204).
4. Human spindles fire in segmented bursts during rapid muscle stretch (162). It was posited (109) that these bursts could cause the M1, M2, and M3 segments of EMG response to rapid stretch (207, 232). Data in awake cats lent support to this idea, showing Ia bursts during rapid stretch and corresponding EMG bursts at monosynaptic latencies (15, 284). However, this hypothesis has been overshadowed to some extent by new evidence that EMG responses at M2/M3 latency are mediated by long-loop transcortical pathways (62, 239).

Task-Related Fusimotor Set. Motor tasks with elements of novelty, difficulty, or arousal are often as-

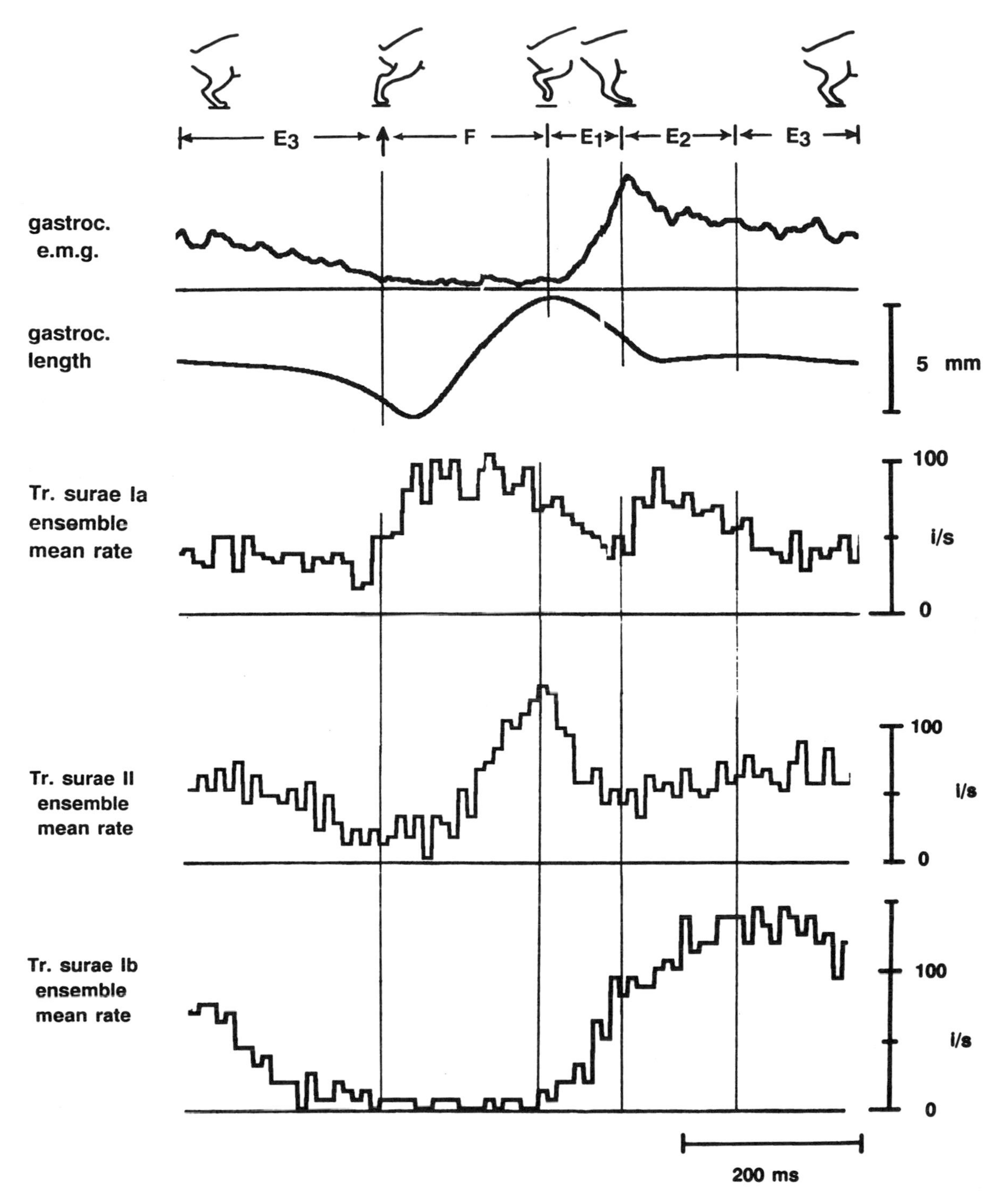

FIG. 3.8. Mean firing rate profiles of the three types of large-diameter afferents in cat triceps surae muscles in the step cycle. The ensemble data were averaged from chronic recordings of nine Ia afferents, two II afferents, and four Ib afferents. Each afferent contributed four step cycles. The firing rate profiles are event histograms of 10 ms bin width calibrated in terms of mean firing rate. The electromyogram and length averages were obtained from the Ia data only, but were similar for the II and Ib recordings. Note the high peak firing rate of tendon organ Ib afferents during the stance phase. [Adapted from Prochazka et al. (283).]

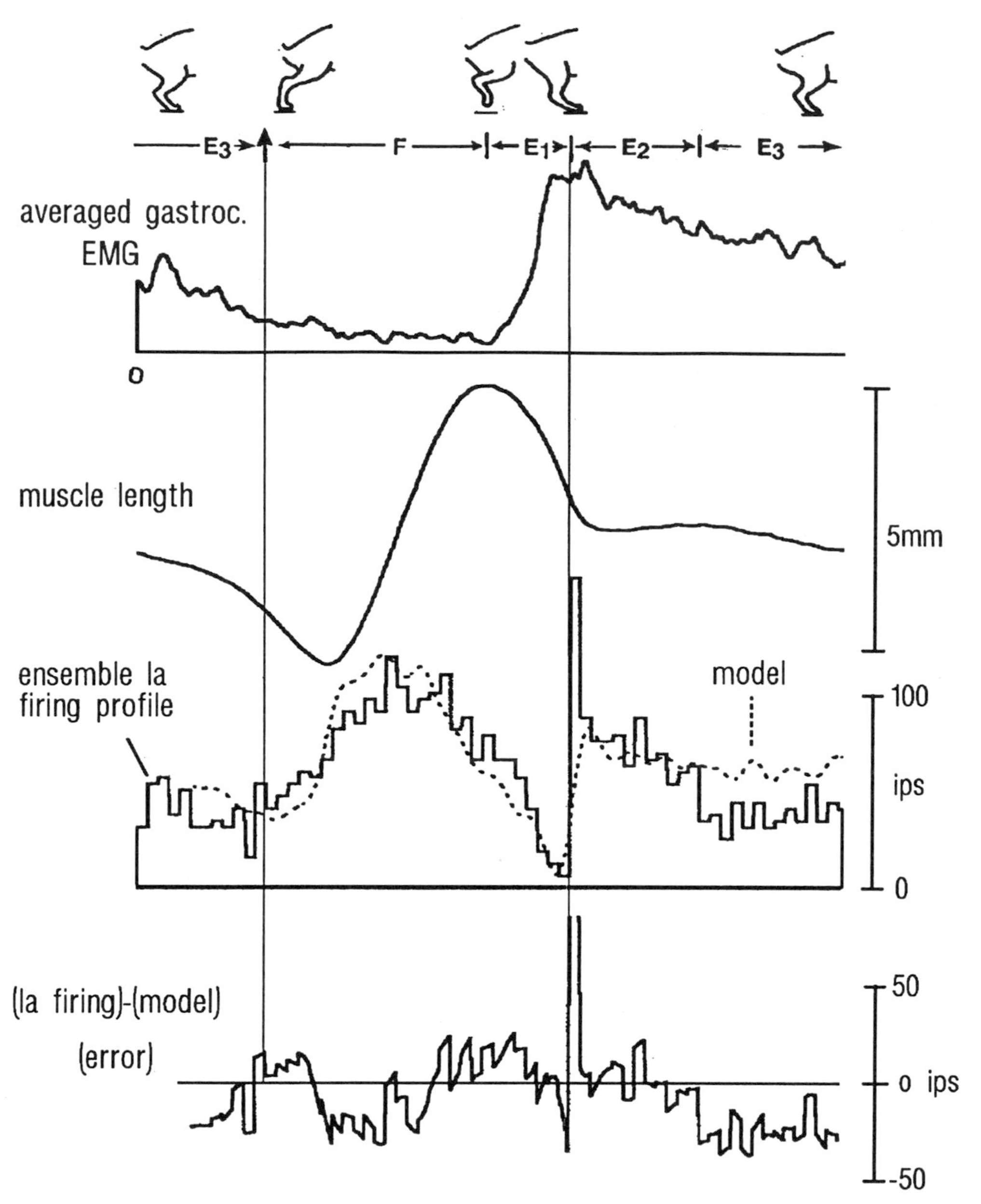

FIG. 3.9. Same Ia data as in Figure 3.8, but this time aligned to the moment of foot contact, thus exaggerating the contact-related Ia firing transient. *Dashed curve* was obtained by digitally filtering the length profile using equation 2. *Bottom trace* shows difference between ensemble profile and model (i.e., the firing rate not accounted for). The modulation depth of the ensemble profile is 108 imp/s; that of the error signal is 67 imp/s. The error reflects factors such as fusimotor modulation, tendon compliance effects, and muscle unloading. There is no clear relationship between the error and the electromyogram, indicating that α-linked components of γ action were not dominant.

sociated with high spindle Ia stretch-sensitivity and firing rates in cats [(282); Fig. 3.12]. The task- and context-dependence of γ_d activation that this implies has been associated with the general phenomenon of preparatory set (117). Elevated fusimotor set has been inferred in several tasks and contexts, but the most reliable way to evoke it in conscious cats is to impose movements on a limb. This presumably evokes a state of increased alertness or wariness in the animals. The Ia firing rates during imposed movements can be quite astonishing (>600 imp/s). With firing rates such as these, the net Ia input to the CNS from all of the spindles in the cat hindlimb may transiently exceed 0.2 Mimp/s (277).

The notion of fusimotor set presupposes α-γ independence, particularly in relation to γ_d-motoneurons. Consequently, in human neurography experiments, evidence for convincing and significant γ

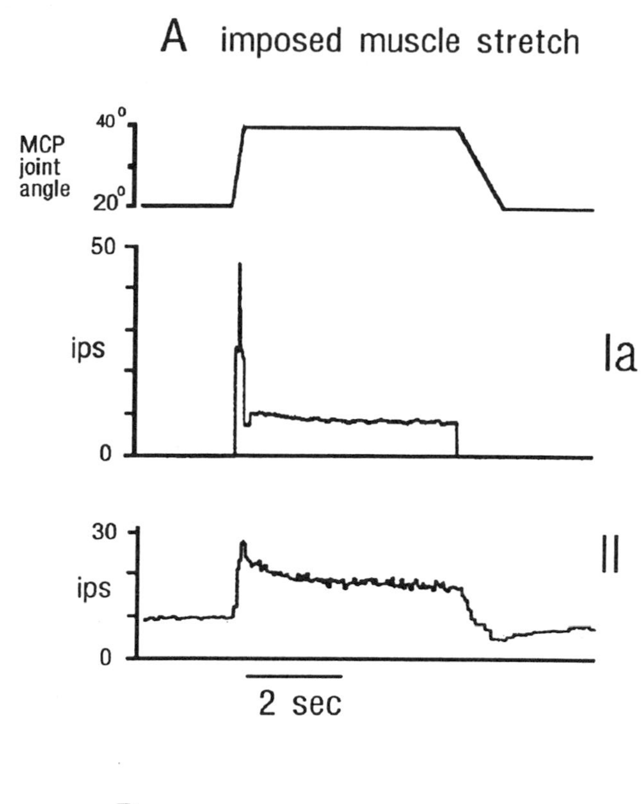

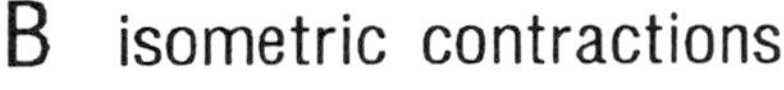

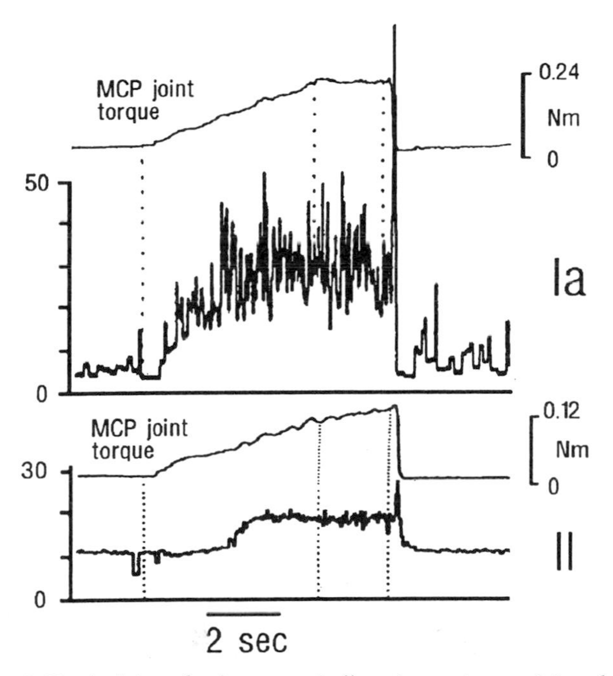

FIG. 3.10. Activity of a human spindle primary (group Ia) and secondary (group II) afferent of a finger extensor in imposed movements and voluntary isometric contractions. *A*, Both afferents responded to muscle stretch. As the muscle shortened, the group Ia afferent fell silent and the group II afferent reduced its firing rate. *B*, Both endings showed increased firing during isometric contractions of the receptor-bearing muscle, monitored as torque about the metacarpophalangeal (MCP) joint. [Adapted from Edin and Vallbo (108).]

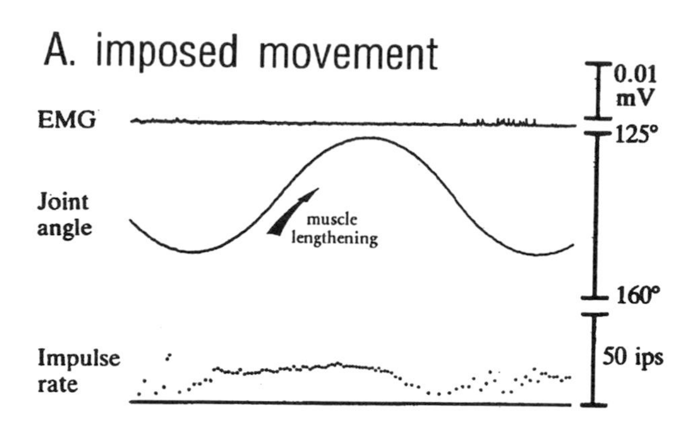

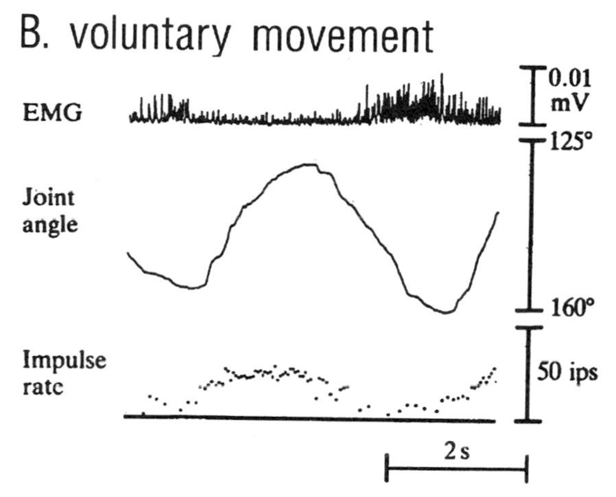

FIG. 3.11. Response of a human muscle spindle afferent of a finger extensor to imposed movements and voluntary movements against a small external load opposing finger extension. *A*, The afferent responded to the imposed sinusoidal displacement and maintained its firing during muscle shortening, indicating some fusimotor action. There was minimal electromyographic activity during the imposed movements. *B*, The spindle responded to the active movements in much the same way. There was no evidence in this case of additional firing linked to the voluntary electromyogram, as would be expected from α-γ co-activation. [Adapted from Al-Falahe et al. (4).]

action independent of α activity has been sought. So far little independence has been found (3, 10, 54, 55, 130, 289, 336). Table 3.1 summarizes the various hypotheses regarding the central control of γ_s- and γ_d-motoneurons. Clearly, both α-linked and tonic components of γ activity are implicated throughout. The tonic components of γ drive are task- or set-related in most cases.

As already mentioned, spindle firing rates are low in human neurography compared to those in the cat and monkey recordings. It is unclear at this stage whether this represents a genuine species difference, or whether it is merely a consequence of experimental design. In neurography, the risk of dislodging electrodes from their location in peripheral nerves places constraints on the speed and freedom of

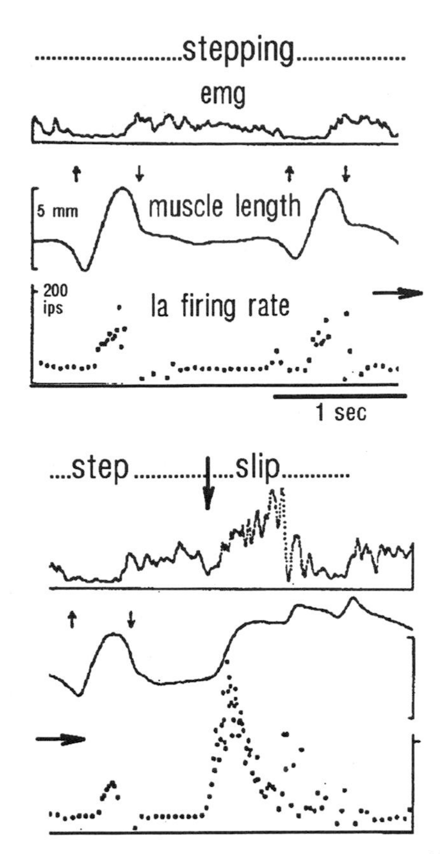

FIG. 3.12. Ankle extensor Ia firing illustrating a sudden change in stretch-sensitivity when the hindlimb of a cat walking along a table surface slipped on the edge of the table. The record is continuous from upper to lower panel. At the moment marked with the *arrow*, the cat slipped and crouched, the receptor-bearing muscle actively lengthened, and the spindle afferent responded with firing rates of nearly 400 imp/s. This was interpreted as a sudden task- or context-related increase in γ_d action, exemplifying "fusimotor set." [Adapted from Prochazka et al. (281).]

movement. When movement velocities are matched, the species differences are not so marked. Thus in slow hand movements, monkey spindles fired at 0–80 imp/s (124, 302). In alert cats performing slow hindlimb limb movements, firing rates were also often in the 0–80 imp/s range (personal observations). It should be remembered that animals brought into an unfamiliar laboratory for recording sessions are likely to be aroused, alert, and suspicious, whereas human subjects can rationalize the situation, and although discomfort is involved, they are unlikely to maintain a heightened state of motor readiness. The somewhat higher firing rates in animals performing comparable slow movements and the much higher rates associated with novel tasks and imposed forces may therefore be due to increased arousal and attention in the animal subjects. Equivalent states of arousal, alertness, and anxiety occur in normal daily life in humans, but it is difficult to reproduce them in the neurography setting. The question of whether humans exhibit fusimotor set is therefore still open.

Central Control of the Fusimotor System. Fusimotor set also presupposes that there are areas in the CNS that selectively activate γ-motoneurons. Granit and Kaada (1952) found that stimulation of the brainstem reticular formation produced fusimotor excitation along with generalized motor arousal (151). This association of γ activity with diffuse arousal was soon overshadowed by the theory of phasic, α-linked activation. However, Appelberg (11, 12) later found that stimulation of a region dorsal and caudal to the red nucleus selectively activated γ_d-motoneurons. Appelberg called this region the mesencephalic area for dynamic control (MesADC). Although the location of the MesADC and its specificity in controlling only *dynamic* fusimotor activity has been questioned, recent results have confirmed that γ_d action is readily elicited from regions both caudal and rostral to the red nucleus (324). This effect was seen in jaw muscle spindles as well as in hindlimb spindles (323), indicating that brainstem control of γ_d action is diffuse and widespread. In fact, the MesADC may be part of a larger subcortical system involved in attentional and orienting mechanisms (229), of which fusimotor set is but one example. Other areas implicated in γ_d control are the motor cortex (338) and habenular nucleus (95). γ_s Activity has been evoked from regions caudal and dorsal to the red nucleus (158, 324), the vestibular nuclei (65), and substantia nigra pars reticulata (345). Note that some of these putative fusimotor control centers may have neuromodulatory rather than direct motor functions.

Several lines of evidence have also implicated the cerebellum in fusimotor control (100, 110, 135, 149, 151, 302, 329, 330). Indeed, cerebellar hypotonia and ataxia are sometimes explained in terms of fusimotor dysfunction. However, these ideas have been undermined by a recent study in conscious cats, in which spindle afferents were monitored before and during ataxia resulting from lidocaine inactivation of the cerebellar nuclei (145). Task-dependent fusimotor modulation of spindle responses was not detectably changed during the ataxia. It was concluded that the cerebellum was not a major controller of the fusimotor system, and that the ataxia observed did not result from disordered fusimotion.

Spontaneous and reflex-evoked γ activity has been recorded in acute spinal cats (30). There was indirect evidence that γ_s and γ_d fibers were affected reciprocally by intravenous DOPA in this preparation. In acute DOPA-treated spinal locomotor cats, phasic γ

TABLE 3.1. *Summary of Hypotheses Regarding CNS Control of γ Activity*

Preparation	Muscles and Movement	γ-Fusimotor Profile		References
		γ_s	γ_d	
Decerebrate or anesthetized cat	Hindlimb, reflexive	α-Linked (γ_s?) + some tonic or reflex-evoked firing		149–151, 158
Decerebrate or anesthetized cat	Intercostal: respiration, coughing	α-Linked + tonic or reflex-evoked firing		81, 85, 115, 306
Decerebrate or spinal locomotor cat	Hindlimb extensors: locomotion	α-Linked		308, 309, 312
Anesthetized cat	Intercostal: respiration	Tonic	α-Linked	152
Anesthetized cat	Jaw closers: reflex chewing	α-Linked	Tonic	14, 95, 147
Decerebrate locomotor cat	Hindlimb *flexors*: locomotion	α-Linked	Tonic	33, 60, 252, 253, 267
Decerebrate locomotor cat	Hindlimb *extensors*: locomotion	Tonic	α-Linked	33, 60, 252, 253, 267
Normal monkey + cat	Jaw closers: chewing, lapping	Tonic & some α-linked		74, 142, 204, 234, 322
Normal cat	Hindlimb: locomotion	Tonic + some α-linked	Task-/set-related + some α-linked	145, 218, 277, 281, 282
Human	Hand, arm and leg: isometric and tracking	Mainly α-linked, some set-/task-related		3, 54, 108, 130, 161, 163, 289, 293
Normal monkey	Forearm: isometric and tracking	Task-related + some α-linked		110, 124, 301, 302

activity has been reported (312) and in chronic spinal locomotor cats, spindle firing patterns suggested intense, tonic γ_s activity (Pearson, personal communication). The fact that the spinal preparation shows generalized fusimotor activation that is in part independent of phasic α activity indicates that at least some of the interneuronal circuitry of fusimotor control resides in the spinal cord.

Tendon Organs

Animal Data. Hindlimb Ib afferents in the awake cat typically fire in the range 0–150 imp/s during active muscle contractions in stepping and greater than 400 imp/s in rapid imposed stretch (15, 215, 283). Extensor forces in slow cat gait usually reach about 15% of maximal isometric force (342). This is somewhat higher than the forces attained in the human Ib recordings mentioned above, where firing rates were in the range of 0–50 imp/s. Staircase firing increments (Fig. 3.13) and other nonlinearities are smoothed away in ensemble firing profiles of as few as four Ib endings (Fig. 3.8) but it has been argued that these discontinuities might actually convey useful information to the CNS about motor unit recruitment and local mechanical events in the muscle (1, 35).

Surprisingly, the ensemble data indicated that the net firing rates of all the tendon organ Ib afferents of ankle extensor muscles rivaled that of the corresponding spindle Ia and II populations during the stance phase of the step cycle (Fig. 3.8). There has recently been a complete reappraisal of the role of extensor Ib input in relation to reflexes and locomotor pattern generation and accordingly the details of Ib firing during the step cycle have assumed a greater importance (see below).

Human Neurography Data. Recordings from Ib afferents are scarce in the neurographic literature, as they are in the chronic animal data. Most human Ib afferents were silent in relaxed muscle and fired during active muscle contraction at rates in the range of 0–50 imp/s (4, 10, 107). Again, for stability reasons peak forces were low (~0.08 Newton meter at metacarpophalangeal joint: i.e., probably <15% maximal voluntary torque). Unlike spindle afferents, human Ib endings never showed signs of unloading in isometric contractions (108). An interesting property of Ib firing is the staircase nature of increases and decreases in firing rate during smooth increases and decreases in muscle force [Fig. 3.13; (108)]. This was first described by Vallbo (334) and was later corroborated in decerebrate cats (183) and then in awake cats (15). It presumably reflects progressive recruit-

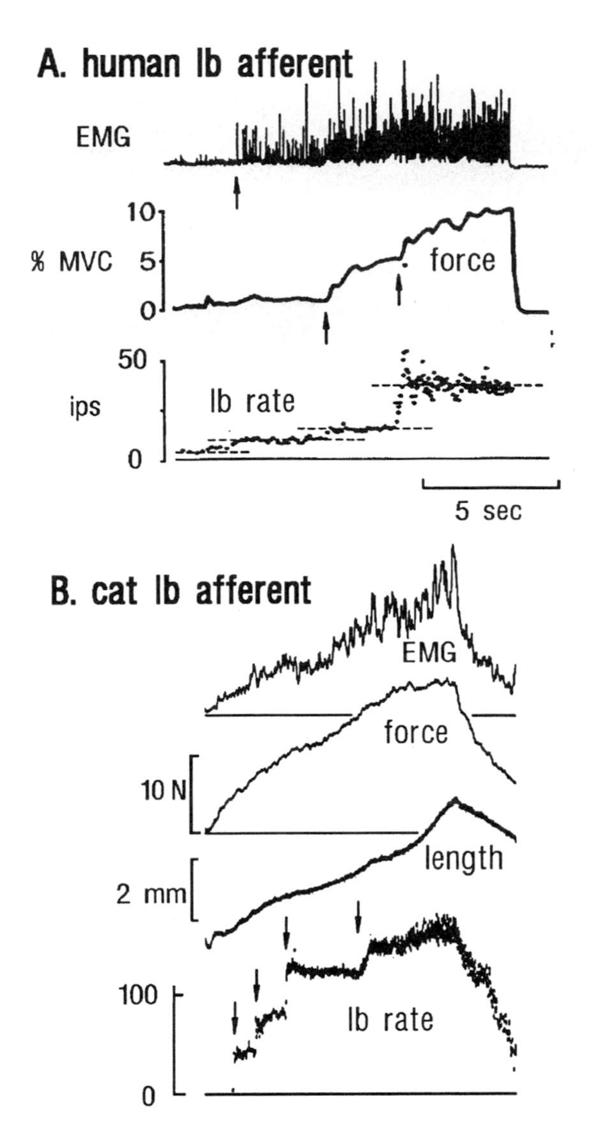

FIG. 3.13. Firing of single Golgi tendon organ afferents during slowly increasing muscle force in (*A*) a human finger extensor muscle and (*B*) an ankle extensor muscle in the awake cat. The *arrows* indicate increments in firing rate attributed to progressive recruitment of motor units. The rate increments and overall range of firing rate of the human tendon organ were smaller than in the cat: finger extensor force was expressed as a percentage of maximal voluntary contraction (% MVC). For comparison, in the cat 10 N measured at the footpads is roughly equivalent to 15% maximal force (343). [*A* Adapted from Edin and Vallbo (108), *B* from Appenteng and Prochazka (15).]

ment and derecruitment of motor units. As previously mentioned, this and other nonlinearities have raised the question of whether tendon organs can possibly signal whole-muscle force (185).

Skin and Joint Afferents

Animal Data. Although skin afferents have been encountered more often than muscle afferents in chronic animal studies, very few recordings have been documented in the literature. This may be because skin afferent firing during movement was perceived as being fairly predictable, though actually this is not always the case. Receptors in the skin in the vicinity of the jaw can signal jaw movement in a reproducible manner and could therefore provide proprioceptive information to the CNS (13). Not surprisingly, skin and hair follicle receptors in and around the footpad in the cat's paw signal foot touch-down and some fire throughout stance (171, 215, 216, 333).

Chronic data on the firing of joint receptors in animals is even more scanty (215, 216). This is not too surprising, as joint receptors are far outnumbered by skin and muscle receptors so the likelihood of encountering them in random samples of dorsal root fibers is low. Their afferents are smaller than many muscle and skin afferents, so they are less likely to produce discriminable action potentials. Finally, differentiating them from spindle afferents is problematic, especially if suxamethonium is not used. The few data that exist indicate that some joint afferents fire throughout the step cycle, while others scarcely fire at all in the midrange (216).

Human Data. Neurographic studies have shown that slowly adapting type II skin receptors signal the stretching of skin over nearby joints, which could provide proprioceptive signals to the CNS [(53, 105,106, 181, 196, 248); see also Chapter 4]. However, two objections must be dealt with before this can be accepted. First, slowly adapting type II afferents are rather nonspecific in their response to the direction of skin stretching. Edin (105) characterized this in vectorial terms, showing that although a given receptor has a preferred strain axis, it also responds, albeit at lower firing rates, to strain in all other directions (Fig. 3.14). Nonspecific directional sensitivity raises the problem of ambiguity in the information signaled, in that a given receptor, say over the metacarpals, may respond just as vigorously to being stretched by movement of one finger as it does to movement of another. Edin has an interesting answer to this objection. If convergence is allowed, the information from an ensemble of slowly adapting type II skin receptors on the back of the hand would in theory provide a sensory population vector that would reliably differentiate individual finger movements. Edin has shown this both by neurography and by measuring skin strain at a matrix of points on the back of the hand during finger movements (Edin, personal communication). In fact, by observing one's own hand during finger movements, and by focusing on the tactile sensation in the finger

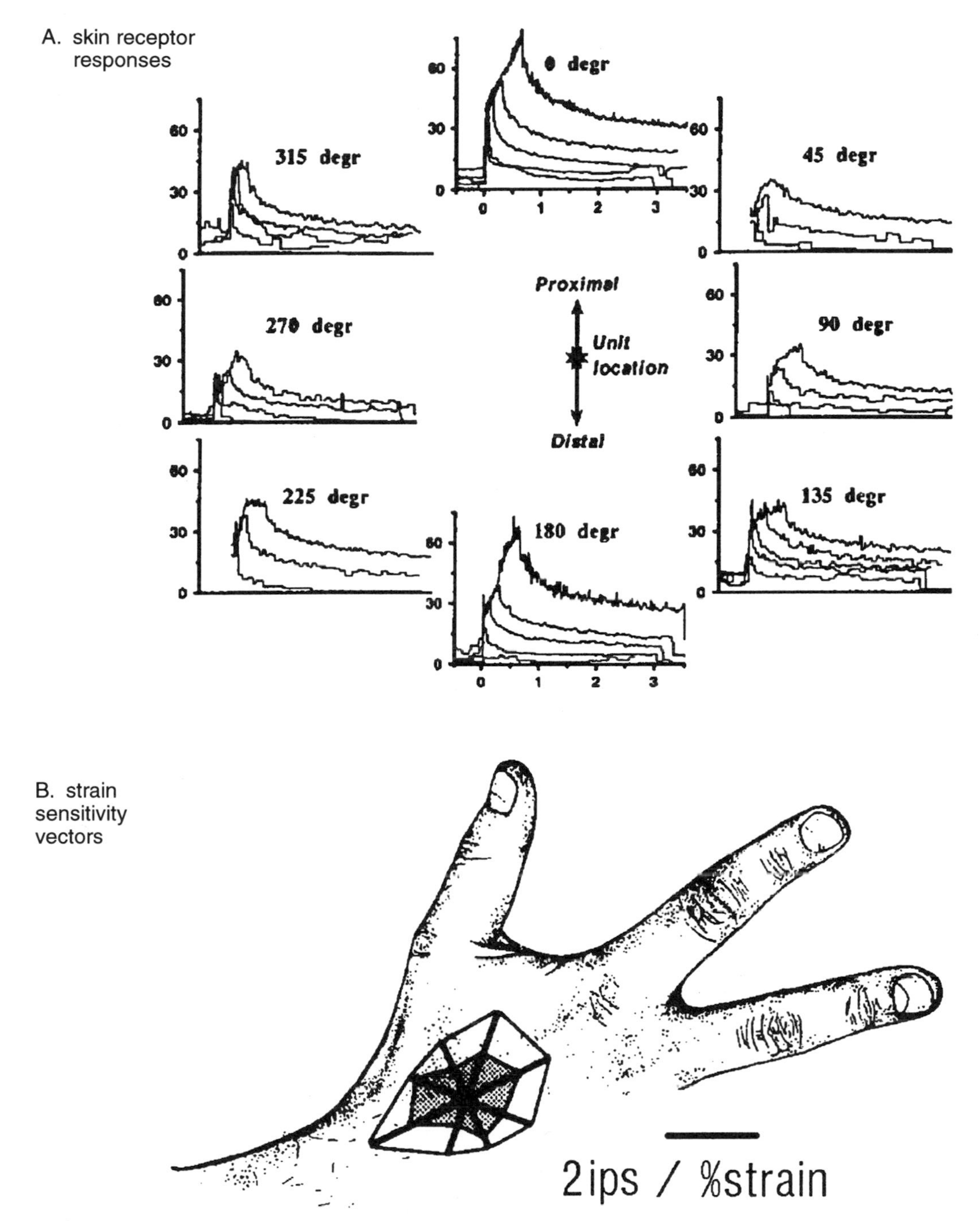

FIG. 3.14. SAII skin receptor responses to stretching the skin in the receptive field at the angles shown (0 degrees is along forearm axis). Each plot shows the firing rate responses to five skin stretches applied along the angular axis indicated and causing strains of 1.25%, 2.5%, 5%, 10%, and 20%, respectively. The sensitivity along a given axis was expressed as the adapted response per % strain (i.e., imp · s^{-1} · $\%strain^{-1}$), and superimposed on the diagram of the hand as a vector with appropriate length and orientation. This receptor would presumably respond best to flexion of the forefinger, but it might also respond to flexion of the other fingers and the thumb. [Adapted from Edin (105).]

webs, it is easy to convince oneself of Edin's argument.

The second objection is that some skin areas contain afferents that signal over the whole range of joint movement while others do not. For example, palmar glabrous skin afferents responded only at the extremes of finger joint displacement (53, 225), whereas nonglabrous receptors on the back of the hand responded over the full range of motion (10). Given that different joints are associated with different proportions of glabrous and hairy skin, skin-mediated proprioceptive acuity would be rather uneven.

If skin receptors contribute to *conscious* proprioception (248), one might expect that electrical stimulation of them would give rise to kinesthetic illusions. In human neurography it is claimed possible to stimulate through the recording needle and excite only the axon being recorded from (225, 335, but cf. 341). When this was done in 18 slowly adapting type II skin afferents, movement sensations resulted in two cases (225). In the same experiment stimulation of single spindle afferents did *not* give rise to kinesthetic sensations even though ensemble spindle input evoked by muscle vibration and whole-nerve electrical stimulation clearly does [(129); see also Chapter 4]. The positive result in single slowly adapting type II skin receptors is thus powerful evidence that skin afferents play an important role in proprioception. Recently, Edin's sensory vector matrix has been tested in reverse in the author's laboratory by D.F. Collins. Skin afferents at a set of points on the back of the hand and over the finger joints were stimulated electrically and mechanically. This produced weak illusions of finger movement, which were greatly augmented by tendon vibration.

Joint receptors have occasionally been recorded neurographically (53, 104, 181, 225), though it is worth noting that differentiating joint afferents from group II spindle afferents is problematic (280). The firing profiles indicated that the afferents signaled over a fair range of joint angle. Human psychophysical experiments designed to evaluate the contributions of muscle, skin, and joint receptors to kinesthesia have been somewhat inconsistent. Several groups found that local anesthesia of joint afferents did not interfere signficantly with position sense, whereas inactivation of muscle afferents did (73, 296). Position sense was fairly normal in patients who had undergone total replacement of knee joints (86), hip joints (194), finger joints, and toe joints (86). On the other hand, Ferrell and Smith (120) anesthetized the proximal interphalangeal joint in a human subject and found inaccuracies in position matching, particularly at the extremes of joint angle. Anesthetizing the knee joint capsule in cats led to marked motor and kinesthetic deficits (119). At this point the relative contributions of joint and skin receptors to kinesthesia and motor control are still unresolved.

Invertebrate Proprioceptors

There is very little information on the firing of proprioceptive afferents during free movement in invertebrates. Wilson and Gettrup (351) first recorded from wing stretch receptors during tethered flight in grasshoppers. Zill and his colleagues (211, 212, 355) found that tibial campaniform sensilla fired rhythmically in relation to force and cuticular strain in certain parts of the cockroach step cycle. As the cadence increased to 24 steps/s there was a progressive phase shift between bursts of afferent and efferent activity. This and other evidence suggested that proprioceptive feedback in rapid stepping was too delayed to contribute reflexly within the same step cycle. A switch to open-loop control in rapid gait was posited. Under these circumstances proprioceptive signals may be used to provide overall postural information and one-step-ahead control.

FEEDBACK CONTROL

Basic Concepts, Definitions, and Types of Control System

In the last few years there has been a move to integrate the mass of information on simple reflexes into an overall view of how multisegmented limbs are controlled. To gain some perspective, let us first summarize some basic concepts and design features of engineering control systems. In robotics, the essence of control is to guide actuators to move loads in a desired manner. The desired movement is termed the *input* and the actual movement is the *output*. In a closed-loop control system, the output produced by the actuator is monitored by a sensor, fed back and compared to the input, producing an *error* signal. The error signal is passed on through one or more elements back to the actuator, thus closing the loop. The signal transmitted around the loop is generally altered ("conditioned") by each element (e.g., dynamic filtering). This may be an unavoidable property of the element or it may be added to compensate for unwanted filtering elsewhere in the loop (269). In the simplest case, if the load-moving properties of the actuator are understood and there are no obstacles, it is enough to supply a predesigned input signal to the actuator, to move the load as required. Although there is no feedback as such and the system therefore operates "open-loop," the nature of the input signal derives from prior feedback comparisons of outputs and inputs. Most factory robots operate open-loop, their tasks being divided into stages, the sequential completion of which is sensed by switches or position sensors. In sophisticated robots, several variables may be sensed and used in complex ways to control actuators. As Levine and Loeb (210) entertainingly remarked, you need only look in a mirror "to see an example of a very satisfactory nonlinear MIMO control system." The similarity to neural sensorimotor control is compelling, so let us identify some basic control systems.

Proportional Control. Actuators are driven in proportion to the error between command signals and sensory signals. The error signal is usually filtered dynamically to improve performance [differentiation to speed up response, integration to attain zero final error, the combination being termed proportional-integral-differential (PID) control].

Finite State (Conditional) Control. Finite state systems were first formulated in relation to production-line processes. In these systems, actuators are driven according to rules such as: *IF* this sensory condition is satisfied *AND* that sensory condition is satisfied *THEN* do such-and-such (331). If one thinks of all the available sensory inputs as comprising a multidimensional vector, a rule or state is satisfied when the vector falls within a region of vector space "belonging" to that rule. In some systems, rules are derived using automatic induction algorithms in which the relative importance of different sensors emerges quantitatively [i.e., some sensors are more equal than others (195)].

Adaptive (Self-Organizing) Control. Internal transmission properties of the controller (e.g., compensation parameters) are modified or tuned on the basis of performance assessments or parameter identification in preceding time segments. In essence, a supervisory controller assesses performance and adjusts parameters in the basic controller (e.g., when the load changes). Because there are many ways to assess performance and to change parameters, adaptive controller design is virtually an art form (98, 269).

Predictive (Feedforward) Control. Parametric changes are generated in advance of expected loading conditions. For example, transmission delays (e.g., to and from extraterrestrial robots such as moon buggies) may be overcome by using an internal model of the actuator/load, which provides an immediate simulated output suitable for local closed-loop operation. A copy of the simulated output is passed through an analog delay line and compared with the "real" delayed output, allowing follow-up error correction (315, cf. 339).

Neural Networks: Sensorimotor Maps. An orderly array of artificial "neurons" with large numbers of "synaptic" interconnections is set up within a digital processor to transform sensory inputs into motor outputs. Appropriate transformations are "learnt" by strengthening or weakening the interconnections according to the success or failure of repeated trials of a sensorimotor task ("knowledge of results"). This process may be viewed as a form of feedback control. There are various types of network structure and numerous "teaching" algorithms (192). The map or engram thus learnt can subsequently be used open-loop (no feedback) to transform multivariate commands or sensory inputs into desired responses.

Fuzzy Logic. Inputs from sensors are assigned "membership" functions. A membership function translates a particular value from a sensor into a measure of the "truth" of a linguistic description of state such as "the leg is in early swing." For example, suppose leg extensor force is high. The likely truth of the statement "the leg is in early swing" is very low, whereas the likely truth of "the leg is in late stance" is quite high. Because the description of state is imprecise, it is termed "fuzzy." Each fuzzy sensory state is coupled with a corresponding fuzzy motor state such as "activate flexors strongly and extensors weakly." The corresponding *motor* membership function is scaled according to the "truth" accorded its related sensory state. Several motor membership functions are then condensed into a discrete value using a "defuzzification" algorithm. This discrete value drives the actuator(s) (98, 199). In "neuro-fuzzy" controllers, the membership functions themselves are adjusted to optimize performance criteria. In essence, fuzzy systems allow multiple sensory modalities to be weighted and combined according to linguistically recognizable rules. This feature makes them interesting in relation to neural control (see below).

From the 1950s to the mid-1980s, neurophysiologists were somewhat mesmerized by the first of the above schemes, proportional feedback control. This was partly due to successful modeling of the oculomotor system and partly to some basic structural similarities between the stretch reflex arc and servo loops (238). Proportional feedback models are useful in describing the control of one or two variables such as muscle length and force. But when multivariate, complex movements such as those in posture and locomotion are considered, they quickly become unmanageable (210). Some of the other systems may then be more applicable. It is interesting that all six control schemes listed above are now being applied to the practical problem of controlling human movements artificially (168, 270, 279).

Proprioceptive Control

This section deals with current and emerging views on proprioceptive control strategies and the way reflexes and higher level control are combined to produce normal movement. Several excellent and exhaustive reviews have appeared recently on reflex integration in the spinal cord [(19, 187, 244); see also Chapter 1]. The emphasis in what follows will therefore not be on spinal reflex mechanisms, but rather on current attempts to understand proprioceptive feedback in a general sense and in relation to the control schemes just summarized.

Proportional Control (Stretch Reflexes). It was recognized many years ago that the stretch reflex arc is analogous to a proportional feedback control loop. The length sensors, muscle spindles, feed back a signal related to muscle stretch. Motoneurons (the comparators) subtract this from the descending command for muscle shortening (the "input" signal). The difference (error) drives the muscle to shorten. Note that the descending command to *shorten* is opposite in sign to the *lengthening* signal from spindles; summing the two is equivalent to subtraction, which is consistent with negative feedback.

Given this compelling analogy and the many studies of the spindle-mediated stretch reflex over nearly a century, the role of the stretch reflex in controlling movement is still remarkably elusive. On the one hand, it is clear that a volley of action potentials evoked in the Ia afferents of a muscle by a tendon tap or nerve stimulus can produce a reflex twitch of homonymous and synergistic muscles that can move a limb. On the other hand, when displacements are applied to a limb, the components of EMG response attributable to spinal reflexes are relatively small (164, 207, 232). Perturbing forces are transmitted through skin and underlying tissue, simultaneously stretching, jarring, and unloading many receptors in skin, ligament, muscle, and tendon. Yet the afferents of the stretched muscles seem to dominate the responses, because inactivating or bypassing the other sensory modalities has little effect (28, 91, 231). The long-latency reflexes are larger and more forceful than the monosynaptic or short-latency oligosynaptic components. They are mediated partly via transcortical pathways (62, 238) and partly via segmental reflex action evoked by Ia activity that continues as the displacement unfolds (134, 162). They are also under volitional control, so their designation as reflexes is a loose one. The functional role of Ib input in load compensation in the human arm is unclear. In theory, concomitant force and length feedback of varying relative weight should result in spring-like behavior of varying compliance, but attempts to verify this in human subjects have been inconclusive (82). Ib feedback plays an important role in modulating postural and locomotor reflexes (93).

It is often said that reflex gains are low. What does this mean? In theory, gain around a feedback loop may be measured by detaching the sensor, applying a displacement to it, and measuring the actuator's response. The response-to-stimulus ratio is, by definition, the open-loop gain (i.e., the overall product of the gain of each element all the way around the loop). This experiment is possible in invertebrates whose proprioceptors are anatomically separate from muscles: thus stretch-reflex gain has been measured as a function of frequency in different behavioral states in stick insects (24). During load compensation the gains ranged from 1–11. Comparable indirect estimates have been derived in humans, gains being in the range of 0–2 (28). The gains in these very different species were similar in the sense that they were much lower than gains in electronic circuits or robotic devices. This is presumably because load-moving muscles develop phase lags greater than 180 degrees in a frequency range of 0–10 Hz, which restricts the gains attainable without reflexes becoming unstable.

Reflex gain should be seen in context. The function of the stretch reflex is to resist load perturbations and maintain stability. In general, the closed-loop operation of a feedback loop with an open loop gain x reduces the deflection otherwise caused by a force perturbation by $1/(1 + x)$. Thus an open loop gain of just 1 would reduce the deflection of a tonically activated muscle by 50% (i.e., muscle stiffness is effectively doubled). If the inherent muscle stiffness itself is high—for example, because of agonist-antagonist co-contraction (32)—the force resulting from the stretch reflex is also high because the reflex multiplies the effect of the inherent stiffness (28, 311). Thus although stretch reflex gains in animals are numerically low by technological standards, they are functionally significant in the biological context (61). In some cases they may be increased to cause a "useful" instability (26, 303). Animal movements are smooth rather than robotic (i.e., load compensation is compliant rather than stiff). It is therefore appropriate that stretch reflexes are not very strong.

Many experiments have shown that stretch reflex gain varies with intention, task, and sensory context (47, 117, 123, 164). The longer latency electromyographic responses in humans are under strong volitional control and in certain cases are inhibited or even reversed (63, 99, 202, 247, 254). Mono- or oligosynaptic H-reflexes during stepping are lower than in quiet stance, and in running they are lower still (63, 64). H-reflexes are also attenuated in difficult tasks (214) and when muscles are co-activated (258). Although it is generally assumed that gain is modulated by presynaptic inhibition as part of the central motor program, this may also be due to movement-evoked reafference (76).

Positive Force Feedback? In cats it has recently been shown that extensor Ib–mediated reflexes, which are inhibitory during quiet stance, completely reverse and become excitatory during the stance phase of gait (78, 264). In invertebrates reflexes also reverse when going from rest to active movement (25). In principle, positive force feedback should be destabilizing. However, provided that the open-loop gain of positive force feedback remains less than 1, the operation of a positive Ib reflex arc is stable and in fact mimics rather well the behavior of the cat limb during gait. This has been modeled in the author's laboratory with the help of Dr. David Bennett, using both physical actuators operating under positive force feedback and mathematical control-systems models (manuscript in preparation). As positive force feedback gain approaches 1, a force applied to the actuator is resisted, much as in a length servo. However, unlike a length servo, this occurs at whatever length the output happens to be when the system is turned on (cf. lead-pipe rigidity). In combination with weak negative length feedback (loop gain ~1), the system reproduces command displacements and responds to external perturbations like a spring whose stiffness rapidly increases as force feedback open-loop gain approaches 1.

At this stage it is unclear whether this excitatory Ib action during cat gait really does constitute positive force feedback or whether the Ib input acts at the level of the locomotor pattern generator, triggering the stance/swing transition in a finite-state manner (see below). The issue is currently being tackled in two or three laboratories: essentially, if *proportional* excitatory responses to Ib input can be demonstrated during gait, this would support the idea of proportional positive feedback. This is not to say that the two mechanisms are mutually exclusive; Ib input could still also "trigger" the pattern generator within a finite-state structure.

Inherent Feedback Due to Muscle Properties. In early feedback models of the stretch reflex, the actuator, muscle, was treated as a pure force generator. But it has long been known that in the absence of reflexes, contracting muscles respond to imposed stretch like stiff springs. Partridge (260) equated this to a sort of "intrinsic" length feedback. The great innovation of the equilibrium-point hypotheses of Feldman (31) and Bizzi (37) was to include this nonneural component of feedback explicitly. Feldman's concept is illustrated in simple form in Fig. 3.15. The load-bearing hand is at an equilibrium position, which results from a spring-like deflection from an internally set "virtual" position. The deflection depends on the load and the inherent muscle stiffness *augmented* by the stretch reflex. In theory, the "virtual" or unloaded position is revealed by removing the load (while distracting the subject and so avoiding adaptive responses). If the weight of the forearm is neglected, a notional position is reached which Feldman termed λ. Assuming that the nonreflexive com-

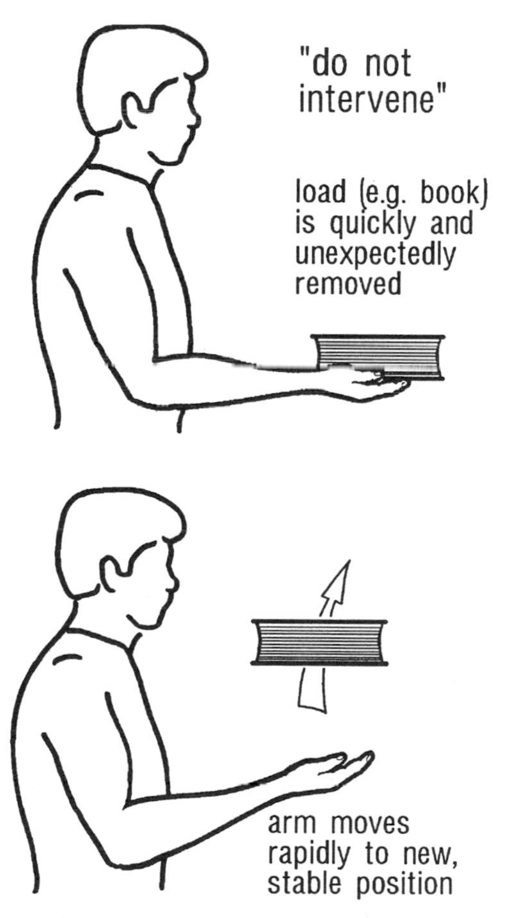

FIG. 3.15. Schematic illustrating the equilibrium point hypothesis. When the book is removed, the arm flexes to a new stable position, close to the threshold of the stretch reflex (the virtual position λ). [Adapted from McCloskey and Prochazka (243).]

mand is set constant throughout, λ corresponds to the muscle length at which the stretch reflex neither adds to nor subtracts from the set level of activation of motoneurons innervating the muscle. Feldman referred to this as the displacement threshold of the stretch reflex. Muscle length can clearly be changed either by changing the centrally generated set level, or by changing the reflex threshold. In fact it has been argued that these amount to the same thing (243).

There is no denying the basic appeal of the equilibrium-point concept: a notational command point moves along a centrally generated trajectory, dragging a load around via a spring (206, 316). In a sense, this is a general way of looking at any load-moving control system. However, some of the details are problematic and have caused a great deal of controversy. For example, in the λ theory, there has been an insistence on the invariance of reflex gain (31) in the face of overwhelming evidence that in fact reflex gain is modulated in relation to task and context, through the mechanisms of presynaptic inhibition, fusimotor activation, and muscle nonlinearities. Strongly activated muscles can only shorten so far, so when large loads are involved, one must assume that virtual trajectories are compressed into small regions close to the anatomical boundaries of the work space. Resolution then becomes a problem. Nonetheless, by placing intrinsic muscle properties in the center of the control scheme, equilibrium-point theories have had a major impact on the field.

Finite State Control: The Logic of Postural Constraints. In 1975, Forssberg and colleagues made the important discovery that during locomotion in the chronic spinal cat, responses elicited by mechanical stimuli impeding the forward swing of the leg actually reversed when the stimuli were applied during the stance phase (126). This was later confirmed in normal cats (97, 344) and humans (29). The topic is reviewed by Rossignol (Chapter 5) so we need only consider the broader ramifications here.

The phase-dependent reversal of reflexes may be viewed as a special case of finite-state control, the rules being of the type:

Rule 1. *IF* swing phase
AND skin stimulus
THEN lift and place leg;
IF stance phase
AND skin stimulus
THEN extend leg and prolong stance.

The rules developed in active prosthetic and orthotic devices show interesting parallels with those identified in animal species (270, 279). For example, the rule for switching from stance to swing in several designs of above-knee prostheses has the following form:

Rule 2. *IF* extensor force low
AND hip extended
THEN initiate swing.

The same rule was identified quite independently in cat, cockroach, lobster, and stick insect [(9, 24, 25, 71, 159, 265); Fig. 3.16]. The rule-base for flexion onset does not stop with the ipsilateral leg. If the contralateral leg has not ended *its* swing phase, ipsilateral flexion does not occur; *IF* stance *AND* contralateral swing *THEN* delay flexion and prolong stance. This is best illustrated in "foot-in-hole" experiments, where an unexpected absence of contralateral ground support causes a delay in swing-onset in the load-bearing leg (144.) Yet in a gallop, both legs can be in the air at the same time, indicating that the contralateral ground-support condition only applies in slow walking. A more complete version of rule 2 is therefore:

Rule 3: *IF* gait slow
AND contralateral limb loaded
AND extensor force low
AND hip extended
THEN initiate swing,
ELSE prolong stance.

Certain sensory combinations or motor tasks may trigger "override" rules. An obstacle impeding forward swing evokes skin input from the dorsum of the foot that causes the normal swing phase to be aborted and replaced with a stereotyped lifting and placing of the foot: rule 1, the stumble reaction. In above-knee prostheses this is specifically designated a "hazard" state (270). Nociceptive input and input from high-threshold joint afferents may terminate stance and so they may also be viewed as triggering override rules (183). Another type of override is presumably required in *backward* walking (see Chapter 8). Here, swing is initiated when the hip is maximally *flexed* and the gastrocnemii (but not soleus) are still loaded. It remains to be seen whether an entirely new rule is required or whether it is possible to modify rule 3 to fit this situation. Furthermore, the relative difficulty cats and dogs seem to have in walking backwards may indicate that the required variant of rule 3 is not "hard-wired."

The rules discussed so far relate largely to sensory input. Centrally generated programs must also be taken into account. As mentioned earlier, animals

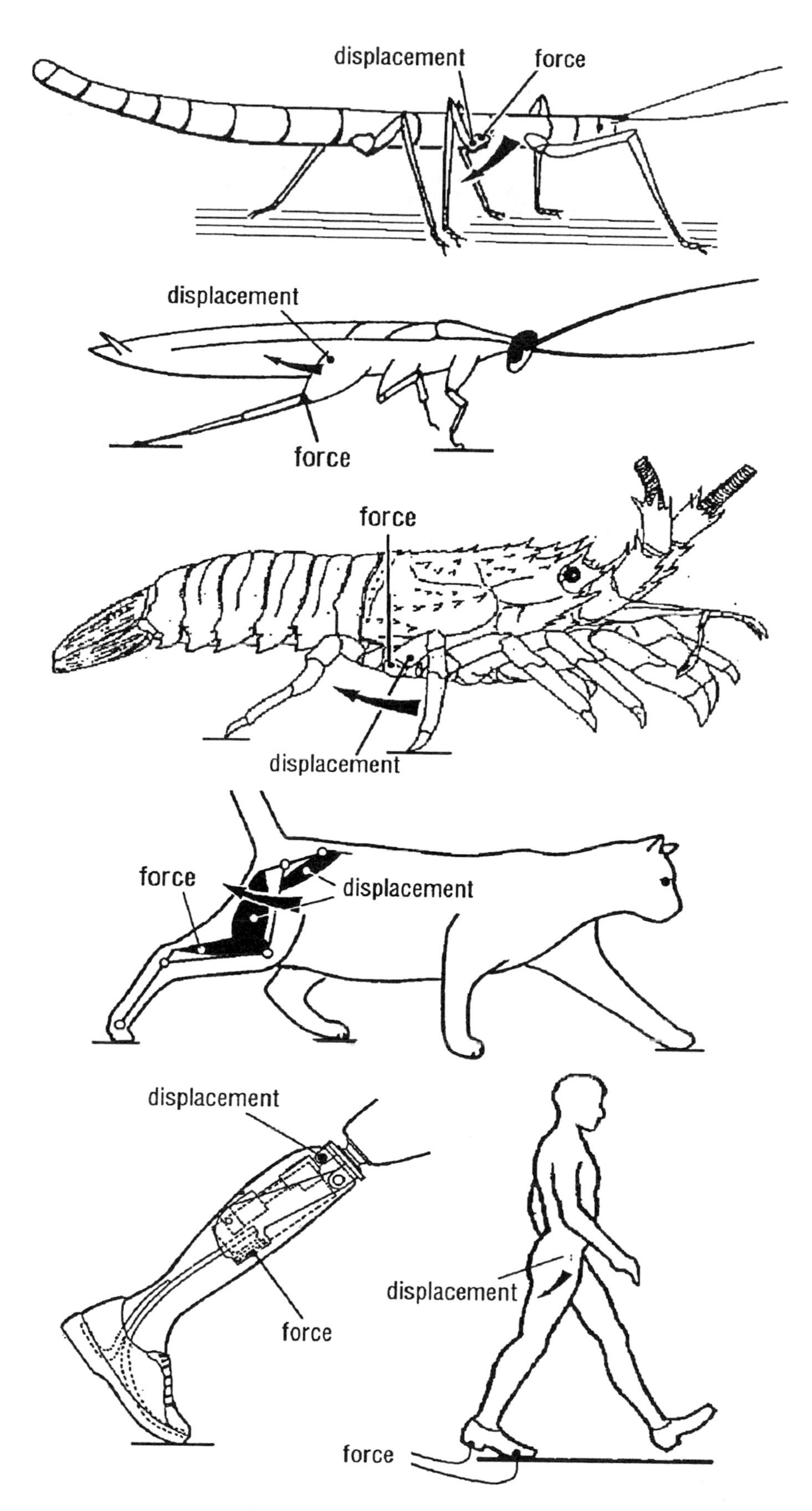

FIG. 3.16. Schematics of stick insect, locust, lobster, cat, active leg prosthesis, and man using functional electrical stimulation. In each case, pairs of sensory variables are indicated that have been shown to be used in a conditional way to initiate the swing phase of gait (i.e., *IF* displacement exceeds threshold *AND* force has declined below threshold, *THEN* initiate flexion). Approximate positions of identified sensors (natural and artificial) are shown. [Adapted from Prochazka (279).]

held above the ground may "air-step" (136). Swing phases are rhythmically and consistently triggered even though rule 3 is not satisfied. This may be explained in terms of the default operation of a central oscillator that cycles autonomously in the absence of sensory input. When the foot contacts the ground, sensory input is restored and the oscillator is dominated by it according to rule 3. A very similar relationship is seen in scratch responses in cats: if the hindlimb is held in an extended position, the scratching rhythm is suppressed (89). If the paw misses its target or only makes light contact, the extensor phase is relatively short. When firm contact is made, the extensor phase lengthens. In this case not only are limb sensors implicated, but so too are mechanoreceptors of the paw, head, and neck (67). Postural responses to translation of ground support may in fact also be viewed as default programs upon which sensory input is overlayed [(227, 228); Chapter 7]. Other pattern generators under sensory control include those for respiration, mastication (220), and paw-shaking (198). In all of these situations it is possible to identify proportional, finite state, adaptive, and/or predictive mechanisms interacting with basic pattern generators.

"*IF-THEN*" rules simply provide a description of the association of inputs and outputs in movements that have multiple phases and are subject to postural constraints. They are compatible with proportional control and the central generation of temporal patterns and synergies. Indeed, it is hard to see how "real" motor sequences such as those in gait could be described *without* combining some form of conditional logic with intrinsic central pattern generator and proportional control mechanisms. One can now also begin to speculate on how the logic might be implemented in the spinal cord. For example, rule 2 might be achieved by facilitation of the "swing generator" by hip flexor Ia feedback (200) and disinhibition of it by extensor Ib feedback (265). Alternatively, the extensor half-center might be held in the *ON* state by extensor Ib facilitation (in addition to direct positive Ib feedback to motoneurons). With the decline of Ib activity at the end of stance, the central oscillator is released, and swing is initiated with support from hip flexor Ia feedback (169). Hazard states such as the stumble corrective reaction and nociceptive gating would require powerful and direct reflex pathways that could override and reset the central pattern generator.

This approach is new in spinal cord research, which has hitherto focused largely on cellular mechanisms and isolated reflexes. Motor strategies and rules are inferred from studies of normal movement (e.g., 24, 144, 261). The neuronal circuitry that executes these rules is then sought in a goal-directed manner so that the functionally important circuits are targeted (6, 146, 244, 264, 325).

Proprioception and the Higher Centers: Adaptive and Predictive Control. A sign of *adaptive* control is that parameters are adjusted as movements proceed. A sign of *prediction* is that parameters are adjusted in advance of expected motor tasks or sensory input. It goes virtually without saying that nervous systems are adaptive/predictive controllers par excellence. Responses to external stimuli can change from one trial to the next according to performance. For example, Nashner (1976) showed that reflex responses to stance perturbations in humans were suppressed over three or four trials if they were arranged to destabilize posture (254). With simpler perturbations, responses actually reversed from one trial to the next, according to stimulus direction (255). The changes were too rapid to be explained in terms of preparatory set; instead, a fast selection of the appropriate synergy based on the evolving sensory input was posited. Selection may rely on feedback from particular groups of receptors, as suggested in a remarkable series of experiments by Dietz and colleagues in which underwater stance platforms or elastic straps were used to modify weight-bearing conditions (93, 94). Brooke and McIlroy (1990) found that when postural stimuli were unpredictable, whole portions of response could be deleted from one trial to the next (47). It was as though the responses of a given muscle were pieced together from prestored patterns, according to intent, uncertainty, and sensory information about the task and the postural conditions preceding it. Indeed, the common theme of much recent work is that the CNS has a repertoire of responses, synergies, and cyclical patterns, which it can modulate, select, and combine according to context and sensory state (161, 314). Some of this is done in a predictive manner, suggestive of preparatory set (117), and some is done as the movements evolve (76, 92, 314).

Where in the mammalian CNS does the prediction and selection occur? First, it should be understood that sensory input is generally gated or filtered before it reaches the higher centers. For example, routine or irrelevant *tactile* input to cortex is attenuated, while "relevant" signals are enhanced (2, 310). This modulation occurs at brainstem, thalamic, and cortical levels. Other than fusimotor effects, little is known about gating of *proprioceptive* input to higher centers (6, 122). Enhanced proprioceptive transmission has been posited, but not proved, in tasks that require attention and are associated with increased γ_d action (103, 277). The inferior olive may control proprioceptive transmission to the cerebellum: olivary neurons in conscious monkeys are most responsive to novel stimuli (132) and reafferent signals are attenuated in the spinoolivocerebellar pathway during locomotion, whereas novel stimuli are not (213). Cerebellar cortical neurons show activity in anticipation of skin and proprioceptive stimuli (313). Interestingly, the mesencephalic system implicated in γ_d control sends collaterals to parts of the olive (12). This is consistent with the idea that the rubrobulbospinal system is a general area for preparatory set, adaptation, and proprioceptive gain control.

Spinocerebellar tract neurons encode *combinations* of sensory input from a whole limb, global variables such as displacement of the foot with respect to the body (39, 337), or information on interneuronal state (223). After processing through the cortex, sensory responses in cerebellar nuclear cells are even more complex (38, 40, 226, 317, 337). At this stage, just how the cerebellum uses proprioceptive information is a matter of speculation, but much evidence points to predictive and adaptive functions (38, 246, 313).

Proprioceptive input reaches the motor cortex via the dorsal column nuclei, nucleus Z, the thalamus, area 3a, and somatosensory cortex (16, 203, 259, 262, 348). Stimulation of motor cortex produces illusions of movement (7). In monkeys, limb perturbations evoke responses in motor cortical cells (58, 116, 122, 128) and, in some cases, stimulation of the same cells excites motor units of the perturbed muscles, demonstrating a transcortical feedback loop (121). Like the cerebellum, the motor cortex has long been implicated in sensorimotor prediction and adaptation (96, 117, 197, 233). Mechanisms may include presynaptic inhibition (295), selection of motor programs, and fusimotor control (338).

Multivariate "Fuzzy" Logic. We have discussed proprioceptive control in terms of servo loops, conditional logic, and predictive mechanisms. In conclusion, we should consider analogies with connectionist systems, which perform adaptive feedback control and which have structures at least superficially analogous to neuronal circuitry. In neural nets, information is processed by virtue of learnt "synaptic" weights or connections of different strengths between large numbers of simple summing elements. In fuzzy logic the weighting takes the form of "membership functions." The way the weighting is determined varies from one system to another and need not concern us here. The important thing is to recognize some basic analogies with neural control:

1. Weighting functions are used to process and combine input from many sensors and to control many outputs simultaneously: "parliamentary principle" (24).
2. Performance is matched to task and context by altering the weighting of signals: "response selection" (47).
3. The relative importance of different types of sensor may vary: "task-dependent reflex reversal" (264, 325).
4. The activity of internal, "hidden layer" elements is poorly related either to sensory inputs or motor outputs: "unrelated" cortical neurons (121).
5. Executive circuits evaluate or predict performance on the basis of multimodal sensory input and make appropriate parametric modifications: cerebellum (329).
6. These circuits might be separate and discrete from the main control loops, but must have two-way links with them: "accessory gain control" (226, 255).

The neural net concept of "hidden layer" cells is useful because it offers an explanation for the fact that some cortical neurons fire in relation to motor tasks but neighboring neurons do not (121). However, a disadvantage of neural net models is that the way they function is hard to analyze and categorize in terms of a rule base. Fuzzy controllers are interesting because their sensorimotor mapping is more explicit. Furthermore, they are more "biological" than finite state systems in that they work with graded rather than all-or-nothing sensory states. Whereas the finite-state rule for switching from stance to swing might require extensor force to be less than 5 N *and* hip angle to exceed 120 degrees, a fuzzy system would assign weights to muscle force, joint angle, and other inputs, and would trigger swing if the mean of the corresponding output functions was close enough to the "swing" end of the scale. A strikingly similar mechanism was suggested by Bässler (24) for the control of locomotion in stick insects: "As in a parliament, the stimulus not only activates the coalition government responsible for the performance of the response but also activates the opposition." In other words, as extensor force declines and the hip extends, the votes for initiating swing increase while those for maintaining stance decline. Votes are weighted according to the population represented by each "seat." The switch occurs when the total number of votes and their relative weight crosses a threshold. Groups of interneurons could be viewed as belonging to a party with a particular policy: "If the leg is quite extended, we will turn the flexors on strongly and the extensors weakly." Votes for a party (membership in it) are maximal under certain political (sensory) circumstances.

Artificial systems in which available sensors are "awarded" weightings according to their importance in predicting or controlling motor tasks (168, 195) may be of great value in understanding proprioception. Among the interesting research topics in the future will be to establish the control logic and relative weighting accorded sensory input from skin, joint, ligament, muscle spindle, and tendon organ afferents in different sensorimotor contexts.

CONCLUSION

The last decade has seen a proliferation of new ideas on the nature and use of proprioceptive feedback in natural behavior. The notion of stereotyped, immutable reflexes somehow coordinated by a complex motor program has been overshadowed by the various control schemes described above, in which proprioception plays a variable but often crucial role. The empirical and theoretical possibilities have opened up tremendously. Because sensorimotor interactions provide one of the few accessible windows into the internal workings of nervous systems, progress in this area will continue to have an important impact on neuroscience as a whole.

This work was funded by the Alberta Heritage Foundation for Medical Research, the Canadian Medical Research Council, and the Networks of Centers of Excellence. I thank Patrick Trend, Josef Elek, Monica Gorassini, Janet Taylor, David Bennett, David Collins, Keir Pearson, and Richard Stein for help and support.

REFERENCES

1. Abrahams, V. C., and F. J. R. Richmond. Specialization of sensorimotor organization in the neck muscle system. *Prog. Brain Res.* 76: 125–135, 1988.
2. Ageranioti-Belanger, S. A., and C. E. Chapman. Discharge properties of neurones in the hand area of primary somatosensory cortex in monkeys in relation to the performance of an active tactile discrimination task. II. Area 2 as compared to areas 3b and 1. *Exp. Brain Res.* 91: 207–228, 1992.
3. Al-Falahe, N. A., M. Nagaoka, and A. B. Vallbo. Lack of fusimotor modulation in a motor adaptation task in man. *Acta Physiol. Scand.* 140: 23–30, 1990a.
4. Al-Falahe, N. A., M. Nagaoka, and A. B. Vallbo. Response profiles of human muscle afferents during active finger movements. *Brain* 113: 325–346, 1990b.
5. Alnaes, E. Static and dynamic properties of Golgi tendon organs in the anterior tibial and soleus muscles of the cat. *Acta Physiol. Scand.* 70: 176–187, 1967.
6. Alstermark, B., A. Lundberg, and L.-G. Pettersson. The pathway from Ia forelimb afferents to motor cortex: a new hypothesis. *Neurosci. Res.* 11: 221–225, 1991.
7. Amassian, V. E., R. Q. Cracco, and P. J. Maccabee. A sense of movement elicited in paralyzed distal arm by focal magnetic coil stimulation of human motor cortex. *Brain Res.* 479: 355–360, 1989.
8. Anderson, J. H. Dynamic characteristics of Golgi tendon organs. *Brain Res.* 67: 531–537, 1974.
9. Andersson, O., and S. Grillner. Peripheral control of the cat's step cycle. II. Entrainment of the central pattern generators for locomotion by sinusoidal hip movements during "fictive locomotion." *Acta Physiol. Scand.* 118: 229–239, 1983.
10. Aniss, A. M., H.-C. Diener, J. Hore, S. C. Gandevia, and D. Burke. Behavior of human muscle receptors when reliant on proprioceptive feedback during standing. *J. Neurophysiol.* 64: 661–670, 1990.
11. Appelberg, B. Central control of extensor muscle spindle dynamic sensitivity. *Life Sci.* 9: 706–708, 1963.
12. Appelberg, B. Selective central control of dynamic gamma motoneurones utilised for the functional classification of gamma cells. In: *Muscle Receptors and Movement*, edited by A. Taylor and A. Prochazka. London: Macmillan, 1981, p. 97–108.
13. Appenteng, K., J. P. Lund, and J. J. Seguin. Behavior of cutaneous mechanoreceptors recorded in mandibular division of gasserian ganglion of the rabbit during movements of lower jaw. *J. Neurophysiol.* 47: 151–166, 1982.
14. Appenteng, K., T. Morimoto, and A. Taylor. Fusimotor activity in masseter nerve of the cat during reflex jaw movements. *J. Physiol. (Lond.)* 305: 415–432, 1980.
15. Appenteng, K., and A. Prochazka. Tendon organ firing during active muscle lengthening in normal cats. *J. Physiol. (Lond.)* 353: 81–92, 1984.
16. Avendano, C., A. J. Isla, and E. Rausell. Area 3a in the cat. II. Projections to the motor cortex and their relations to other corticocortical connections. *J. Comp. Neurol.* 321: 373–386, 1992.
17. Awiszus, F., and S. S. Schäfer. Subdivision of primary afferents from passive cat muscle spindles based on a single slow-adaptation parameter. *Brain Res.* 612: 110–114, 1993.
18. Baev, K. V., and Y. P. Shimansky. Principles of organization of neural systems controlling automatic movements in animals. *Prog. Neurobiol.* 39: 45–112, 1992.
19. Baldissera, F., H. Hultborn, and M. Illert. Integration in spinal neuronal systems. In: *Handbook of Physiology, The Nervous System, Motor Control*, edited by V. B. Brooks. Bethesda, MD: Am. Physiol. Soc., 1982, p. 509–595.
20. Banks, R. W., and M. J. Stacey. Quantitative studies on mammalian muscle spindles and their sensory innervation. In: *Mechanoreceptors: Development, Structure and Function*, edited by P. Hnik, T. Soukup, R. Vejsada, and J. Zelena. London: Plenum, 1988, p. 263–269.
21. Barker, D. The morphology of muscle receptors. In: *Handbook of Sensory Physiol. Vol. 3, Part 2 (Muscle Receptors)*, edited by C. C. Hunt. Berlin: Springer, 1974, p. 1–190.
22. Barnes, W. J. P. Proprioceptive influences on motor output during walking in the crayfish. *J. Physiol. (Paris)* 73: 543–564, 1977.
23. Bässler, U. *Neural Basis of Elementary Behavior in Stick Insects. Studies of Brain Function.* Berlin: Springer, 1983, p. 169.

24. Bässler, U. The femur-tibia control system of stick insects—a model system for the study of the neural basis of joint control. *Brain Res. Rev.* 18: 207–226, 1993.
25. Bässler, U. The walking- (and searching-) pattern generator of stick insects, a modular system composed of reflex chains and endogenous oscillators. *Biol. Cybern.* 69: 305–317, 1993.
26. Bässler, U., and U. Nothof. Gain control in a proprioceptive feedback loop as a prerequisite for working close to instability. *J. Comp. Physiol. [A]* 175: 23–33, 1994.
27. Baumann, T. K., and M. Hulliger. The dependence of the response of cat spindle Ia afferents to sinusoidal stretch on the velocity of concomitant movement. *J. Physiol. (Lond.)* 439: 325–350, 1991.
28. Bennett, D. J., M. Gorassini, and A. Prochazka. Catching a ball: contributions of intrinsic muscle stiffness, reflexes and higher-order responses. *Can. J. Physiol. Pharmacol.* 72: 525–534, 1994.
29. Berger, W., V. Dietz, and J. Quintern. Corrective reactions to stumbling in man: neuronal coordination of bilateral leg muscle activity during gait. *J. Physiol. (Lond.)* 357: 109–125, 1984.
30. Bergmans, J., and S. Grillner. Reciprocal control of spontaneous activity and reflex effects in static and dynamic flexor alpha-motoneurones revealed by an injection of DOPA. *Acta Physiol. Scand.* 77: 106–124, 1969.
31. Berkinblit, M. B., A. G. Feldman, and O. I. Fukson. Adaptability of innate motor patterns and motor control mechanisms. *Behav. Brain Sci.* 9: 585–638, 1986.
32. Bernstein, N. A. Trends and problems in the study of investigation of physiology of activity. In: *The Coordination and Regulation of Movements.* Oxford: Pergamon, 1967 (Orig. *Questions of Philosophy, Vopr. Filos.* 6: 77–92, 1961).
33. Bessou, P., J.-M. Cabelguen, M. Joffroy, R. Montoya, and B. Pagès. Efferent and afferent activity in a gastrocnemius nerve branch during locomotion in the thalamic cat. *Exp. Brain Res.* 64: 553–568, 1986.
34. Bessou, P., M. Joffroy, R. Montoya, and B. Pagès. Evidence of the co-activation of Alpha-motoneurones and static gamma-motoneurones of the sartorius medialis muscle during locomotion in the thalamic cat. *Exp. Brain Res.* 82: 191–198, 1990.
35. Binder, M. D. Further evidence that the Golgi tendon organ monitors the activity of a discrete set of motor units within a muscle. *Exp. Brain Res.* 43: 186–192, 1981.
36. Binder, M. D., and D. G. Stuart. Responses of Ia and spindle group II afferents to single motor-unit contractions. *J. Neurophysiol.* 43: 621–629, 1980.
37. Bizzi, E., N. Hogan, F. A. Mussa-Ivaldi, and S. Giszter. Does the nervous system use equilibrium-point control to guide single and multiple joint movements? *Behav. Brain Sci.* 15: 603–613, 1992.
38. Bloedel, J. R., V. Bracha, and P. S. Larson. Real time operations of the cerebellar cortex. *Can. J. Neurol. Sci.* 20 (Suppl. 3): S7–S18, 1993.
39. Bosco, G., and R. E. Poppele. Broad directional tuning in spinal projections to the cerebellum. *J. Neurophysiol.* 70: 863–866, 1993.
40. Bourbonnais, D., C. Krieger, and A. M. Smith. Cerebellar cortical activity during stretch of antagonist muscles. *Can. J. Physiol. Pharmacol.* 64: 1202–1213, 1986.
41. Boyd, I. A. Intrafusal muscle fibres in the cat and their motor control. In: *Feedback and Motor Control in Invertebrates and Vertebrates*, edited by W. J. P. Barnes and M. H. Gladden. London: Croon Helm, 1985, p. 123–144.
42. Boyd, I. A., and M. Gladden. Morphology of mammalian muscle spindles. Review. In: *The Muscle Spindle*, edited by I. A. Boyd and M. Gladden. London: Macmillan, 1985, p. 3–22.
43. Boyd, I. A., P. R. Murphy, and V. A. Moss. Analysis of primary and secondary afferent responses to stretch during activation of the dynamic bag_1 fibre or the static bag_2 fibre in cat muscle spindles. In: *The Muscle Spindle*, edited by I. A. Boyd and M. Gladden. London: Macmillan, 1985, p. 153–158.
44. Boyd, I. A., and T. D. M. Roberts. Proprioceptive discharges from stretch receptors in the knee joint of the cat. *J. Physiol. (Lond.)* 122: 38–58, 1953.
45. Brazier, M. *A History of Neurophysiology in the 17th and 18th Centuries.* New York: Raven, 1984, p. 230.
46. Brazier, M. *A History of Neurophysiology in the 19th Century.* New York: Raven, 1988, p. 265.
47. Brooke, J. D., and W. E. McIlroy. Brain plans and servo loops in determining corrective movements. In: *Multiple Muscle Systems: Biomechanics and Movement Organization*, edited by J. M. Winters and S. L.-Y. Woo. Berlin: Springer, 1990, p. 706–716.
48. Brown, M. C., I. Engberg, and P. B. C. Matthews. Fusimotor stimulation and the dynamic sensitivity of the secondary ending of the muscle spindle. *J. Physiol. (Lond.)* 189: 545–550, 1967.
49. Brown, M. C., G. M. Goodwin, and P. B. C. Matthews. After-effects of fusimotor stimulation on the response of muscle spindle primary afferent endings. *J. Physiol. (Lond.)* 205: 677–694, 1969.
50. Brown, T. G. The intrinsic factor in the act of progression in the mammal. *Proc. R. Soc. Lond. B* 84: 308–319, 1911.
51. Buford, J. A., and J. L. Smith. Adaptive control for backward quadrupedal walking. II. Hindlimb muscle synergies. *J. Neurophysiol.* 64: 756–766, 1990.
52. Burgess, P. R., and F. J. Clark. Characteristics of knee joint receptors in the cat. *J. Physiol. (Lond.)* 203: 317–335, 1969.
53. Burke, D., S. C. Gandevia, and G. Macefield. Responses to passive movement of receptors in joint, skin and muscle of the human hand. *J. Physiol. (Lond.)* 402: 347–361, 1988.
54. Burke, D., B. McKeon, N. F. Skuse, and R. A. Westerman. Anticipation and fusimotor activity in preparation for a voluntary contraction. *J. Physiol. (Lond.)* 306: 337–348, 1980.
55. Burke, D., B. McKeon, and R. A. Westerman. Induced changes in the thresholds for voluntary activation of human spindle endings. *J. Physiol. (Lond.)* 302: 171–182, 1980.
56. Burrows, M. Local circuits for the control of leg movements in an insect. *Trends Neurosci.* 15: 226–232, 1992.
57. Bush, B. M. H. Non-impulsive stretch receptors in crustaceans. In: *Neurones Without Impulses*, edited by A. Roberts and B. M. H. Bush. Cambridge: Cambridge University Press, 1981, p. 147–176.
58. Butler, E. G., M. K. Horne, and J. Rawson. Sensory characteristics of monkey thalamic and motor cortex neurones. *J. Physiol. (Lond.)* 445: 1–24, 1992.
59. Buxton, D. F., and D. Peck. Neuromuscular spindles relative to joint movement complexities. *Clin. Anat.* 2: 211–224, 1989.
60. Cabelguen, J.-M. Static and dynamic fusimotor controls in various hindlimb muscles during locomotor activity in the decorticate cat. *Brain Res.* 213: 83–98, 1981.
61. Capaday, C., and J. D. Cooke. The effect of muscle vibration on the attainment of intended final position during

voluntary human arm movements. *Exp. Brain Res.* 42: 228–230, 1981.

62. Capaday, C., R. Forget, R. Fraser, and Y. Lamarre. Evidence for a contribution of the motor cortex to the long-latency stretch reflex of the human thumb. *J. Physiol. (Lond.)* 440: 243–255, 1991.
63. Capaday, C., and R. B. Stein. Amplitude modulation of the soleus H-reflex in the human during walking and standing. *J. Neurosci.* 6: 1308–1313, 1986.
64. Capaday, C., and R. B. Stein. Difference in the amplitude of the human soleus H reflex during walking and running. *J. Physiol. (Lond.)* 392: 513–522, 1987.
65. Carli, G., K. Diete-Spiff, and O. Pompeiano. Responses of the muscle spindles and the extrafusal fibres in an extensor muscle to stimulation of the lateral vestibular nucleus in the cat. *Arch. Ital. Biol.* 105: 209–242, 1967.
66. Carli, G., F. Farabollini, G. Fontani, and M. Meucci. Slowly adapting receptors in cat hip joint. *J. Neurophysiol.* 42: 767–778, 1979.
67. Carlson Kuhta, P., and J. L. Smith. Scratch responses in normal cats: hindlimb kinematics and muscle synergies. *J. Neurophysiol.* 64: 1653–1667, 1990.
68. Chen, W. J., and R. E. Poppele. Small-signal analysis of response of mammalian muscle spindles with fusimotor stimulation and a comparison with large-signal properties. *J. Neurophysiol.* 41: 15–27, 1978.
69. Chin, N. K., M. Cope, and M. Pang. Number and distribution of spindle capsules in seven hindlimb muscles of the cat. In: *Symposium on Muscle Receptors*, edited by D. Barker. Hong Kong: Hong Kong University Press, 1962, p. 241–248.
70. Cheney, P. D., and J. B. Preston. Classification and response characteristics of muscle spindle afferents in the primate. *J. Neurophysiol.* 39: 1–8, 1976.
71. Clarac, F. Decapod crustacean leg coordination during walking. In: *Locomotion and Energetics in Arthropods*, edited by C. F. Herreid and C. R. Fourtner. New York: Plenum, 1982, p. 31–71.
72. Clarac, F., and J. Ayers. Walking in crustacea: motor program and peripheral regulation. *J. Physiol. (Paris)* 73: 523–542, 1977.
73. Clark, F. J., R. C. Burgess, J. W. Chapin, and W. T. Lipscomb. Role of intramuscular receptors in the awareness of limb position. *J. Neurophysiol.* 54: 1529–1540, 1985.
74. Cody, F. W. J., L. M. Harrison, and A. Taylor. Analysis of activity of muscle spindles of the jaw-closing muscles during normal movements in the cat. *J. Physiol. (Lond.)* 253: 565–582, 1975.
75. Cole, J. D., and E. M. Sedgwick. The perceptions of force and of movement in a man without large myelinated sensory afferents below the neck. *J. Physiol. (Lond.)* 449: 503–515, 1992.
76. Collins, D. F., W. E. McIlroy, and J. D. Brooke. Contralateral inhibition of soleus H reflexes with different velocities of passive movement of the opposite leg. *Brain Res.* 603: 96–101, 1993.
77. Collins, D. F., M. Gorassini, and A. Prochazka. Forelimb proprioceptors recorded during voluntary movements in cats. In: *Alpha and Gamma Motor Systems*, edited by A. Taylor and M. H. Gladden. London: Macmillan, 1995 (in press).
78. Conway, B. A., H. Hultborn, and O. Kiehn. Proprioceptive input resets central locomotor rhythm in the spinal cat. *Exp. Brain Res.* 68: 643–656, 1987.
79. Cooper, B. Y., D. S. Glendinning, and C. J. Vierck. Finger movement deficits in the stumptail macaque following lesions of the fasciculus cuneatus. *Somatosens. Mot. Res.* 10: 17–29, 1993.
80. Cooper, S. The small motor nerves to muscle spindles and to extrinsic eye muscles. *J. Physiol. (Lond.)* 186: 28–29P, 1966.
81. Corda, M., C. V. Euler, and G. Lennerstrand. Reflex and cerebellar influences on alpha and "rhythmic" and "tonic" gamma activity in the intercostal muscle. *J. Physiol. (Lond.)* 184: 898–923, 1966.
82. Crago, P. E., J. C. Houk, and Z. Hasan. Regulatory actions of human stretch reflex. *J. Neurophysiol.* 39: 925–935, 1976.
83. Crago, P. E., J. C. Houk, and W. Z. Rymer. Sampling of total muscle force by tendon organs. *J. Neurophysiol.* 47: 1069–1083, 1982.
84. Creed, R. S., D. Denny-Brown, J. C. Eccles, E. G. T. Liddell, and C. S. Sherrington. In: *Reflex Activity of the Spinal Cord*. New York: Oxford University Press, 1972, p. 216.
85. Critchlow, V., and C. V. Euler. Intercostal muscle spindle activity and its gamma motor control. *J. Physiol. (Lond.)* 168: 820–847, 1963.
86. Cross, M. J., and D. I. McCloskey. Position sense following surgical removal of joints in man. *Brain Res.* 55: 443–445, 1973.
87. Cussons, P. D., M. Hulliger, and P. B. C. Matthews. Effects of fusimotor stimulation on the response of the secondary endings of the muscle spindle to sinusoidal stretching. *J. Physiol. (Lond.)* 270: 835–850, 1977.
88. Delcomyn, F. Perturbation of the motor system in freely walking cockroaches. I. Rear leg amputation and the timing of motor activity in leg muscles. *J. Exp. Biol.* 156: 483–502, 1991.
89. Deliagina, T. G., A. G. Feldman, I. M. Gelfand, and G. N. Orlovsky. On the role of central program and afferent inflow in the control of scratching movements in the cat. *Brain Res.* 100: 297–313, 1975.
90. Desmedt, J. E., and E. Godaux. Voluntary motor commands in human ballistic movements. *Ann. Neurol.* 5: 415–421, 1979.
91. Diener, H. C., J. Dichgans, B. Guschlbauer, and H. Mau. The significance of proprioception on postural stabilization as assessed by ischaemia. *Brain Res.* 296: 103–109, 1984.
92. Diener, H. C., F. B. Horak, and L. M. Nashner. Influence of stimulus parameters on human postural responses. *J. Neurophysiol.* 59: 1888–1905, 1988.
93. Dietz, V., A. Gollhofer, M. Kleiber, and M. Trippel. Regulation of bipedal stance: dependency on "load" receptors. *Exp. Brain Res.* 89: 229–231, 1992.
94. Dietz, V., M. Trippel, M. Discher, and G. A. Horstmann. Compensation of human stance perturbations: selection of the appropriate electromyographic pattern. *Neurosci. Lett.* 126: 71–74, 1991.
95. Donga, R., A. Taylor, and P. J. W. Jüch. The use of midbrain stimulation to identify the discharges of static and dynamic fusimotor neurones during reflex jaw movements in the anaesthetized cat. *Exp. Physiol.* 78: 15–23, 1993.
96. Drew, T. Motor cortical activity during voluntary gait modifications in the cat. I. Cells related to the forelimbs. *J. Neurophysiol.* 70: 179–199, 1993.
97. Drew, T., and S. Rossignol. Forelimb responses to cutaneous nerve stimulation during locomotion in intact cats. *Brain Res.* 329: 323–328, 1985.
98. Driankov, D., H. Hellendoorn, and M. Reinfrank. *An Introduction to Fuzzy Control*. New York: Springer, 1993, p. 316.

99. Dufresne, J. R., J. F. Soechting, and C. A. Terzuolo. Modulation of the myotatic reflex gain in man during intentional movements. *Brain Res.* 193: 62–84, 1980.
100. Durbaba, R., A. Taylor, J. F. Rodgers, and A. J. Fowle. Fusimotor effects of cerebellar outflow in the anaesthetized cat. *J. Physiol. (Lond.)* 479: 141–142P, 1994.
101. Dutia, M. B. The muscles and joints of the neck: their specialisation and role in head movement. *Prog. Neurobiol.* 37: 165–178, 1991.
102. Duysens, J., and K. G. Pearson. Inhibition of flexor burst generation by loading ankle extensor muscles in walking cats. *Brain Res.* 187: 321–333, 1980.
103. Dyhre-Poulsen, P. Perception of tactile stimuli before ballistic and during tracking movements. In: *Active Touch*, edited by G. Gordon. Oxford: Pergamon, 1978, p. 171–176.
104. Edin, B. B. Finger joint movement sensitivity of non-cutaneous mechanoreceptor afferents in the human radial nerve. *Exp. Brain Res.* 82: 417–422, 1990.
105. Edin, B. B. Quantitative analysis of static strain sensitivity in human mechanoreceptors from hairy skin. *J. Neurophysiol.* 67: 1105–1113, 1992.
106. Edin, B. B., and J. H. Abbs. Finger movement responses of cutaneous mechanoreceptors in the dorsal skin of the human hand. *J. Neurophysiol.* 65: 657–670, 1991.
107. Edin, B. B., and A. B. Vallbo. Dynamic response of human muscle spindle afferents to stretch. *J. Neurophysiol.* 63: 1297–1306, 1990.
108. Edin, B. B., and A. B. Vallbo. Muscle afferent responses to isometric contractions and relaxations in humans. *J. Neurophysiol.* 63: 1307–1313, 1990.
109. Eklund, G., K.-E. Hagbarth, J. V. Hagglund, and E. U. Wallin. The "late" reflex responses to muscle stretch: the "resonance hypothesis" versus the "long-loop hypothesis." *J. Physiol. (Lond.)* 326: 79–90, 1982.
110. Elble, R. J., M. H. Schieber, and W. T. Thach. Activity of muscle spindles, motor cortex and cerebellar nuclei during action tremor. *Brain Res.* 323: 330–334, 1984.
111. Eldred, E., R. Granit, and P. A. Merton. Supraspinal control of the muscle spindle and its significance. *J. Physiol. (Lond.)* 122: 498–523, 1953.
112. Emonet-Dénand, F., and Y. Laporte. Observations on the effects on spindle primary endings of the stimulation at low frequency of dynamic β-axons. *Brain Res.* 258: 101–104, 1983.
113. Emonet-Dénand, F., Y. Laporte, P. B. C. Matthews, and J. Petit. On the subdivision of static and dynamic fusimotor actions on the primary ending of the cat muscle spindle. *J. Physiol. (Lond.)* 268: 827–861, 1977.
114. Emonet-Dénand, F., J. Petit, and Y. Laporte. Comparison of skeleto-fusimotor innervation in cat peroneus brevis and peroneus tertius muscles. *J. Physiol. (Lond.)* 458: 519–525, 1992.
115. von Euler, C., and G. Peretti. Dynamic and static contributions to the rhythmic γ activation of primary and secondary spindle endings in external intercostal muscle. *J. Physiol. (Lond.)* 187: 501–516, 1966.
116. Evarts, E. V., and C. Fromm. Sensory responses in motor cortex neurons during precise motor control. *Neurosci. Lett.* 5: 267–272, 1977.
117. Evarts, E. V., Y. Shinoda, and S. P. Wise. *Neurophysiological Approaches to Higher Brain Functions*. New York: Wiley, 1984, p. 198.
118. Ferrell, W. R. The adequacy of stretch receptors in the cat knee joint for signalling joint angle throughout a full range of movement. *J. Physiol. (Lond.)* 299: 85–100, 1980.
119. Ferrell, W. R., R. H. Baxendale, C. Carnachan, and I. K. Hart. The influence of joint afferent discharge on locomotion, proprioception and activity in conscious cats. *Brain Res.* 347: 41–48, 1985.
120. Ferrell, W. R., and A. Smith. The effect of loading on position sense at the proximal interphalangeal joint of the human finger. *J. Physiol. (Lond.)* 418: 145–161, 1989.
121. Fetz, E. E. Are movement parameters recognizably coded in the activity of single neurons? *Behav. Brain Sci.* 15: 679–690, 1992.
122. Fetz, E. E., D. V. Finocchio, M. A. Baker, and M. J. Soso. Sensory and motor responses of precentral cortex cells during comparable passive and active joint movements. *J. Neurophysiol.* 43: 1070–1089, 1980.
123. Fitzpatrick, R. C., J. L. Taylor, and D. I. McCloskey. Ankle stiffness of standing humans in response to imperceptible perturbation: reflex and task-dependent components. *J. Physiol. (Lond.)* 454: 533–547, 1992.
124. Flament, D., P. A. Fortier, and E. Fetz. Response patterns and postspike effects of peripheral afferents in dorsal root ganglia of behaving monkeys. *J. Neurophysiol.* 67: 875–889, 1992.
125. Forssberg, H., S. Grillner, J. Halbertsma, and S. Rossignol. The locomotion of the low spinal cat. II. Interlimb coordination. *Acta Physiol. Scand.* 108: 283–295, 1980.
126. Forssberg, H., S. Grillner, and S. Rossignol. Phase dependent reflex reversal during walking in chronic spinal cats. *Brain Res.* 85: 103–107, 1975.
127. French, A. Transduction mechanisms of mechanosensilla. *Annu. Rev. Entomol.* 33: 39–58, 1988.
128. Fromm, C., S. P. Wise, and E. V. Evarts. Sensory response properties of pyramidal tract neurons in the precentral motor cortex and postcentral gyrus of the rhesus monkey. *Exp. Brain Res.* 54: 177–185, 1984.
129. Gandevia, S. C. Illusory movements produced by electrical stimulation of low-threshold muscle afferents from the hand. *Brain* 108: 965–981, 1985.
130. Gandevia, S. C., and D. Burke. Effect of training on voluntary activation of human fusimotor neurons. *J. Neurophysiol.* 54: 1422–1429, 1985.
131. Gandevia, S. C., and D. Burke. Does the nervous system depend on kinesthetic information to control natural limb movements? *Behav. Brain Sci.* 15: 614–632, 1992.
132. Gellman, R., A. R. Gibson, and J. C. Houk. Inferior olivary neurons in the awake cat: detection of contact and passive body displacement. *J. Neurophysiol.* 54: 40–60, 1985.
133. Ghez, C., J. Gordon, M. F. Ghilardi, C. N. Christakos, and S. E. Cooper. Roles of proprioceptive input in the programming of arm trajectories. *Cold Spring Harb. Symp. Quant. Biol.* 55: 837–847, 1990.
134. Ghez, C., and Y. Shinoda. Spinal mechanisms of the functional stretch reflex. *Exp. Brain Res.* 32: 55–68, 1978.
135. Gilman, S. The mechanism of cerebellar hypotonia. An experimental study in the monkey. *Brain* 92: 621–638, 1969.
136. Giuliani, C. A., and J. L. Smith. Development and characteristics of airstepping in chronic spinal cats. *J. Neurosci.* 5: 1276–1282, 1985.
137. Giuliani, C. A., and J. L. Smith. Stepping behaviors in chronic spinal cats with one hindlimb deafferented. *J. Neurosci.* 7: 2537–2546, 1987.
138. Glendinning, D. S., B. Y. Cooper, C. J. Vierck, and C. M. Leonard. Altered precision grasping in stumptail macaques after fasciculus cuneatus lesions. *Somatosens. Mot. Res.* 9: 61–73, 1992.
139. Godwin-Austen, R. B. The mechanoreceptors of the costovertebral joints. *J. Physiol. (Lond.)* 202: 737–753, 1969.

140. Goldberger, M. E. Locomotor recovery after unilateral hindlimb deafferentation in cats. *Brain Res.* 123: 59–74, 1977.
141. Goodwin, G. M., M. Hulliger, and P. B. C. Matthews. The effects of fusimotor stimulation during small-amplitude stretching on the frequency-response of the primary ending of the mammalian muscle spindle. *J. Physiol. (Lond.)* 253: 175–206, 1975.
142. Goodwin, G. M., and E. S. Luschei. Discharge of spindle afferents from jaw-closing muscles during chewing in alert monkeys. *J. Neurophysiol.* 38: 560–571, 1975.
143. Goodwin, G. M., D. I. McCloskey, and P. B. C. Matthews. The contribution of muscle afferents to kinaesthesia shown by vibration-induced illusions of movement and by the effects of paralysing joint afferents. *Brain* 95: 705–748, 1972.
144. Gorassini, M., A. Prochazka, G. W. Hiebert, and M. Gauthier. Adaptive responses to loss of ground support during walking. I. Intact cats. *J. Neurophysiol.* 71: 603–610, 1994.
145. Gorassini, M., A. Prochazka, and J. Taylor. Cerebellar ataxia and muscle spindle sensitivity. *J. Neurophysiol.* 70: 1853–1862, 1993.
146. Gossard, J.-P., R. M. Brownstone, I. Barajon, and H. Hultborn. Transmission in a locomotor-related group Ib pathway from hindlimb extensor muscles in the cat. *Exp. Brain Res.* 98: 213–228, 1994.
147. Gottlieb, S., and A. Taylor. Interpretation of fusimotor activity in cat masseter nerve during reflex jaw movements. *J. Physiol. (Lond.)* 345: 423–438, 1983.
148. Granit, R. *The Basis of Motor Control.* London: Academic, 1970, p. 346.
149. Granit, R., B. Holmgren, and P. A. Merton. The two routes for excitation of muscle and their subservience to the cerebellum. *J. Physiol. (Lond.)* 130: 213–224, 1955.
150. Granit, R., C. Job, and B. R. Kaada. Activation of muscle spindles in pinna reflex. *Acta Physiol. Scand.* 27: 161–168, 1952.
151. Granit, R., and B. R. Kaada. Influence of stimulation of central nervous structures on muscle spindles in cat. *Acta Physiol. Scand.* 27: 130–160, 1952.
152. Greer, J. J., and R. B. Stein. Fusimotor control of muscle spindle sensitivity during respiration in the cat. *J. Physiol. (Lond.)* 422: 245–264, 1990.
153. Gregory, J. E., A. K. McIntyre, and U. Proske. Tendon organ afferents in the knee joint nerve of the cat. *Neurosci. Lett.* 103: 287–292, 1989.
154. Gregory, J. E., D. L. Morgan, and U. Proske. Two kinds of resting discharge in cat muscle spindles. *J. Neurophysiol.* 66: 602–612, 1991.
155. Gregory, J. E., and U. Proske. The responses of Golgi tendon organs to stimulation of different combinations of motor units. *J. Physiol. (Lond.)* 295: 251–262, 1979.
156. Grigg, P., and B. J. Greenspan. Response of primate joint afferent neurons to mechanical stimulation of knee joint. *J. Neurophysiol.* 40: 1–8, 1977.
157. Grillner, S. Locomotion in vertebrates: central mechanisms and reflex interaction. *Physiol. Rev.* 55: 247–304, 1975.
158. Grillner, S., T. Hongo, and S. Lund. Descending monosynaptic and reflex control of γ-motoneurones. *Acta Physiol. Scand.* 75: 592–613, 1969.
159. Grillner, S., and S. Rossignol. On the initiation of the swing phase of locomotion in chronic spinal cats. *Brain Res.* 146: 269–277, 1978.
160. Grillner, S., and P. Zangger. The effect of dorsal root transection on the efferent motor pattern in the cat's hindlimb locomotion. *Acta Physiol. Scand.* 120: 393–405, 1984.
161. Hagbarth, K.-E. Microneurography and applications to issues of motor control: Fifth Annual Stuart Reiner Memorial Lecture. *Muscle Nerve* 16: 693–705, 1993.
162. Hagbarth, K.-E., J. V. Hägglund, E. U. Wallin, and R. R. Young. Grouped spindle and electromyographic responses to abrupt wrist extension movements in man. *J. Physiol. (Lond.)* 312: 81–96, 1981.
163. Hagbarth, K.-E., and A. B. Vallbo. Afferent response to mechanical stimulation of muscle receptors in man. *Acta Soc. Med. Upsalien* 72: 102–104, 1967.
164. Hammond, P. H., P. A. Merton, and G. G. Sutton. Nervous gradation of muscular contraction. *Br. Med. Bull.* 12: 214–218, 1956.
165. Hasan, Z. A model of spindle afferent response to muscle stretch. *J. Neurophysiol.* 49: 989–1006, 1983.
166. Hasan, Z., and J. C. Houk. Analysis of response properties of deefferented mammalian spindle receptors based on frequency response. *J. Neurophysiol.* 38: 663–672, 1975.
167. Head, S. I., and B. M. H. Bush. Proprioceptive reflex interactions with central motor rhythms in the isolated thoracic ganglion of the shore crab. *J. Comp. Physiol. [A]* 168: 445–459, 1991.
168. Heller, B. W., P. H. Veltink, N. J. M. Rijkhoff, W. L. C. Rutten, and B. J. Andrews. Reconstructing muscle activation during normal walking: a comparison of symbolic and connectionist machine learning techniques. *Biol. Cybern.* 69: 327–335, 1993.
169. Hiebert, G., M. Gorassini, W. Jiang, A Prochazka, and K. G. Pearson. Adaptive responses to loss of ground support during walking. II. Comparison of intact and chronic spinal cats. *J. Neurophysiol.* 71: 611–622, 1994.
170. Hoffer, J. A., A. A. Caputi, and I. E. Pose. Activity of muscle proprioceptors in cat posture and locomotion: relation to EMG, tendon force and the movement of fibres and aponeurotic segments. In: *Muscle Afferents And Spinal Control of Movement*, edited by L. Jami, E. Pierrot-Deseilligny, and D. Zytnicki. London: Pergamon, 1992, p. 113–122.
171. Hoffer, J. A., and M. K. Haugland. Signals from tactile receptors in glabrous skin for restoring motor function in paralyzed humans. In: *Neural Prostheses: Replacing Motor Function After Disease or Disability*, edited by R. B. Stein, P. H. Peckham, and D. B. Popovic. New York: Oxford University Press, 1992, p. 91–125.
172. Holm, W., D. Padeken, and S. S. Schäfer. Characteristic curves of the dynamic response of primary muscle spindle endings with and without gamma stimulation. *Pflugers Arch.* 391: 163–170, 1981.
173. Horch, K. W., R. P. Tuckett, and P. R. Burgess. A key to the classification of cutaneous mechanoreceptors. *J. Invest. Dermatol.* 69: 75–82, 1977.
174. Horcholle-Bossavit, G., L. Jami, J. Petit, R. Vejsada, and D. Zytnicki. Ensemble discharge from Golgi tendon organs of cat peroneus tertius muscle. *J. Neurophysiol.* 64: 813–821, 1990.
175. Houk, J., and E. Henneman. Responses of Golgi tendon organs to active contractions of the soleus muscle of the cat. *J. Neurophysiol.* 30: 466–481, 1967.
176. Houk, J. C., W. Z. Rymer, and P. E. Crago. Dependence of dynamic response of spindle receptors on muscle length and velocity. *J. Neurophysiol.* 46: 143–166, 1981.
177. Houk, J. C., and W. Simon. Responses of Golgi tendon organs to forces applied to muscle tendon. *J. Neurophysiol.* 30: 1466–1481, 1967.

178. Hulliger, M. The mammalian muscle spindle and its central control. *Rev. Physiol. Biochem. Pharmacol.* 101: 1–110, 1984.
179. Hulliger, M., F. Emonet-Dénand, and T. K. Baumann. Enhancement of stretch sensitivity of cat primary spindle afferents by low-rate static gamma action. In: *The Muscle Spindle*, edited by I. A. Boyd and M. H. Gladden. London: Macmillan, 1985, p. 189–193.
180. Hulliger, M., P. B. C. Matthews, and J. Noth. Static and dynamic fusimotor stimulation on the response of Ia fibres to low frequency sinusoidal stretching of widely ranging amplitudes. *J. Physiol. (Lond.)* 267: 811–838, 1977.
181. Hulliger, M., E. Nordh, A.-E. Thelin, and A. B. Vallbo. The responses of afferent fibres from the glabrous skin of the hand during voluntary finger movements in man. *J. Physiol. (Lond.)* 291: 233–249, 1979.
182. Hunt, C. C., and A. S. Paintal. Spinal reflex regulation of fusimotor neurones. *J. Physiol. (Lond.)* 143: 195–212, 1958.
183. Iles, J. F., M. Stokes, and A. Young. Reflex actions of knee joint afferents during contraction of the human quadriceps. *Clin. Physiol.* 10: 489–500, 1990.
184. Jacks, A., A. Prochazka, and P. St. J. Trend. Instability in human forearm movements studied with feedback-controlled electrical stimulation of muscles. *J. Physiol. (Lond.)* 402: 443–461, 1988.
185. Jami, L. Golgi tendon organs in mammalian skeletal muscle: functional properties and central actions. *Physiol. Rev.* 72: 623–666, 1992.
186. Jami, L., and J. Petit. Fusimotor actions on sensitivity of spindle secondary endings to slow muscle stretch in cat peroneus tertius. *J. Neurophysiol.* 41: 860–869, 1978.
187. Jankowska, E. Interneuronal relay in spinal pathways from proprioceptors. *Prog. Neurobiol.* 38: 335–378, 1992.
188. Jansen, J. K. S., and T. Rudjord. On the silent period and Golgi tendon organs of the soleus muscle of the cat. *Acta Physiol. Scand.* 62: 364–379, 1964.
189. Johansson, H., P. Sjölander, and P. Sojka. Receptors in the knee joint ligaments and their role in the biomechanics of the joint. *CRC Crit. Rev. Biomed. Eng.* 18: 341–368, 1991.
190. Johansson, R. S., and A. B. Vallbo. Tactile sensibility in the human hand: relative and absolute densities of four types of mechanoreceptive units in glabrous skin. *J. Physiol. (Lond.)* 286: 283–300, 1979.
191. Jovanovic, K., R. Anastasijevic, and J. Vuco. Reflex effects on gamma fusimotor neurones of chemically induced discharges in small-diameter muscle afferents in decerebrate cats. *Brain Res.* 521: 89–94, 1990.
192. Kalveram, K. T. A neural network model rapidly learning gains and gating of reflexes necessary to adapt to an arm's dynamics. *Biol. Cybern.* 68: 183–191, 1992.
193. Kandel, E. R., J. H. Schwartz, and T. M. Jessell. *Principles of Neural Science.* New York: Elsevier, 1991, p. 1135.
194. Karanjia, P. N., and J. H. Ferguson. Passive joint position sense after total hip replacement surgery. *Ann. Neurol.* 13: 654–657, 1983.
195. Kirkwood, C. A., B. J. Andrews, and P. Mowforth. Automatic detection of gait events: a case study using inductive learning techniques. *J. Biomed. Eng.* 11: 511–516, 1989.
196. Knibestöl, M., and A. B. Vallbo. Single unit analysis of mechanoreceptor activity from the human glabrous skin. *Acta Physiol. Scand.* 80: 178–195, 1970.
197. Kornhuber, H. H., and L. Deecke. Hirnpotentialänderungen bei Willkürbewegungen und passiven Bewegungen des Menschen: Bereitschaftspotential und reafferente Potentiale. *Pflugers Arch.* 284: 1–17, 1965.
198. Koshland, G. F., and J. L. Smith. Paw-shake responses with joint immobilization: EMG changes with atypical feedback. *Exp. Brain Res.* 77: 361–373, 1989.
199. Kosko, B., and S. Isaka. Fuzzy logic. *Sci. Am.* 269: 76–81, 1993.
200. Kriellaars, R. M., B. R. Brownstone, D. J. Noga, and L. M. Jordan. Mechanical entrainment of fictive locomotion in the decerebrate cat. *J. Neurophysiol.* 71: 2074–2086, 1994.
201. Kucera, J., and R. Hughes. Histological study of motor innervation to long nuclear chain intrafusal fibres in the muscle spindle of the cat. *Cell Tiss. Res.* 228: 535–547, 1983.
202. Lacquaniti, F., N. A. Borghese, and M. Carrozzo. Transient reversal of the stretch reflex in human arm muscles. *J. Neurophysiol.* 66: 939–954, 1991.
203. Landgren, S., and H. Silfvenius. Nucleus Z, the medullary relay in the projection path to the cerebral cortex of group I muscle afferents from the cat's hind limb. *J. Physiol. (Lond.)* 218: 551–571, 1971.
204. Larson, C. R., D. V. Finocchio, A. Smith, and E. S. Luschei. Jaw muscle afferent firing during an isotonic jaw positioning task in the monkey. *J. Neurophysiol.* 50: 61–73, 1983.
205. Laszlo, J. I., and P. J. Bairstow. Accuracy of movement, peripheral feedback and efference copy. *J. Mot. Behav.* 3: 241–252, 1971.
206. Latash, M. L. Virtual trajectories, joint stiffness, and changes in the limb natural frequency during single-joint oscillatory movements. *Neuroscience* 49: 209–220, 1992.
207. Lee, R. G., J. T. Murphy, and W. G. Tatton. Long-latency myotatic reflexes in man: mechanisms, functional significance, and changes in patients with Parkinson's disease or hemiplegia. In: *Motor Control Mechanisms in Health and Disease*, edited by J. E. Desmedt. New York: Raven, 1983, p. 489–508.
208. Lennerstrand, G., and U. Thoden. Position and velocity sensitivity of muscle spindles in the cat. II. Dynamic fusimotor single-fibre activation of primary endings. *Acta Physiol. Scand.* 74: 16–29, 1968.
209. Lennerstrand, G., and U. Thoden. Muscle spindle responses to concomitant variations in length and in fusimotor activation. *Acta Physiol. Scand.* 74: 153–165, 1968.
210. Levine, W. S., and G. E. Loeb. The neural control of limb movement. *IEEE Control Sys.* 12: 38–47, 1992.
211. Libersat, F., F. Clarac, and S. Zill. Force-sensitive mechanoreceptors of the dactyl of the crab: single-unit responses during walking and evaluation of function. *J. Neurophysiol.* 57: 1618–1637, 1987.
212. Libersat, F., S. Zill, and F. Clarac. Single-unit responses and reflex effects of force-sensitive mechanoreceptors of the dactyl of the crab. *J. Neurophysiol.* 57: 1601–1617, 1987.
213. Lidierth, M., and R. Apps. Gating in the spino-olivocerebellar pathways to the c1 zone of the cerebellar cortex during locomotion in the cat. *J. Physiol. (Lond.)* 430: 453–469, 1990.
214. Llewellyn, M., J. Yang, and A. Prochazka. Human H-reflexes are smaller in difficult beam walking than in normal treadmill walking. *Exp. Brain Res.* 83: 22–28, 1990.
215. Loeb, G. E. Somatosensory unit input to the spinal cord during normal walking. *Can. J. Physiol. Pharmacol.* 59: 627–635, 1981.
216. Loeb, G. E., M. J. Bak, and J. Duysens. Long-term unit recording from somatosensory neurons in the spinal gan-

glia of the freely walking cat. *Science* 197: 1192–1194, 1977.
217. Loeb, G. E., and J. Duysens. Activity patterns in individual hindlimb primary and secondary muscle spindle afferents during normal movements in unrestrained cats. *J. Neurophysiol.* 42: 420–440, 1979.
218. Loeb, G. E., J. A. Hoffer, and C. A. Pratt. Activity of spindle afferents from cat anterior thigh muscles. I. Identification and patterns during normal locomotion. *J. Neurophysiol.* 54: 549–564, 1985.
219. Lund, J. P., and B. Matthews. Responses of temporomandibular joint afferents recorded in the Gasserian ganglion of the rabbit to passive movements of the mandible. In: *Oral-Facial Sensory and Motor Functions*, edited by Y. Kawamura. Tokyo: Quintessence, 1981, p. 153–160.
220. Lund, J. P., K. Sasamoto, T. Murakami, and K. A. Olsson. Analysis of rhythmical jaw movements produced by electrical stimulation of motor-sensory cortex of rabbits. *J. Neurophysiol.* 52: 1014–1029, 1984.
221. Lund, J. P., A. M. Smith, B. J. Sessle, and T. Murakami. Activity of trigeminal alpha and gamma motoneurones and muscle afferents during performance of a biting task. *J. Neurophysiol.* 42: 710–725, 1979.
222. Lundberg, A. *Reflex Control of Stepping. Nansen Memorial Lecture V.* Oslo: University Forlaget, 1969, p. 42.
223. Lundberg, A. Function of the ventral spinocerebellar tract. A new hypothesis. *Exp. Brain Res.* 12: 317–330, 1971.
224. Lundberg, A. Half-centres revisited. In: *Regulatory Functions of the CNS, Motion and Organization Principles*, edited by J. Szentagothai, M. Palkovits, and J. Hamori. Budapest: Pergamon, 1980, p. 155–167.
225. Macefield, G., S. C. Gandevia, and D. Burke. Perceptual responses to microstimulation of single afferents innervating joints, muscles and skin of the human hand. *J. Physiol. (Lond.)* 429: 113–129, 1990.
226. Mackay, W. A., and J. T. Murphy. Cerebellar modulation of reflex gain. *Prog. Neurobiol.* 13: 361–417, 1979.
227. MacPherson, J. M. Strategies that simplify the control of quadrupedal stance. II. Electromyographic activity. *J. Neurophysiol.* 60: 218–231, 1988.
228. MacPherson, J. M., D. S. Rushmer, and D. C. Dunbar. Postural responses in the cat to unexpected rotations of the supporting surface: evidence for a centrally generated synergic organization. *Exp. Brain Res.* 62: 152–160, 1986.
229. Magoun, H. W., and R. Rhines. An inhibitory mechanism in the bulbar reticular formation. *J. Neurophysiol.* 9: 165–171, 1946.
230. Marchand, R., C. F. Bridgman, E. Schumpert, and E. Eldred. Association of tendon organs and muscle spindles in muscles of the cat's leg. *Anat. Rec.* 169: 23–32, 1971.
231. Marsden, C. D., P. A. Merton, and H. B. Morton. The sensory mechanism of servo action in human muscle. *J. Physiol. (Lond.)* 265: 521–535, 1977.
232. Marsden, C. D., J. C. Rothwell, and B. L. Day. Long-latency automatic responses to muscle stretch in man: origin and function. In: *Motor Control Mechanisms in Health and Disease*, edited by J. E. Desmedt. New York: Raven, 1983, p. 509–539.
233. Martin, J. H., and C. Ghez. Differential impairments in reaching and grasping produced by local inactivation within the forelimb representation of the motor cortex in the cat. *Exp. Brain Res.* 94: 429–443, 1993.
234. Matsunami, K., and K. Kubota. Muscle afferents of trigeminal mesencephalic tract nucleus and mastication in chronic monkeys. *Jpn. J. Physiol.* 22: 545–555, 1972.
235. Matthews, B. H. C. Nerve endings in mammalian muscle. *J. Physiol. (Lond.)* 78: 1–33, 1933.
236. Matthews, P. B. C. The differentiation of two types of fusimotor fibre by their effects on the dynamic response of muscle spindle primary endings. *Q. J. Exp. Physiol.* 47: 324–333, 1962.
237. Matthews, P. B. C. The response of de-efferented muscle spindle receptors to stretching at different velocities. *J. Physiol. (Lond.)* 168: 660–678, 1963.
238. Matthews, P. B. C. *Mammalian Muscle Receptors and their Central Actions.* London: Arnold, 1972, p. 630.
239. Matthews, P. B. C. The human stretch reflex and the motor cortex. *Trends Neurosci.* 14: 87–91, 1991.
240. Matthews, P. B. C., and R. B. Stein. The sensitivity of muscle spindle afferents to small sinusoidal changes of length. *J. Physiol. (Lond.)* 200: 723–743, 1969.
241. Matthews, P. B. C., and R. B. Stein. The regularity of primary and secondary muscle spindle afferent discharges. *J. Physiol. (Lond.)* 202: 59–82, 1969.
242. McCloskey, D. I., M. J. Cross, R. Honner, and E. K. Potter. Sensory effects of pulling or vibrating exposed tendons in man. *Brain* 106: 21–37, 1983.
243. McCloskey, D. I., and A. Prochazka. The role of sensory information in the guidance of voluntary movement. *Somatosens. Mot. Res.* 11: 69–76, 1994.
244. McCrea, D. A. Can sense be made of spinal interneuron circuits? *Behav. Brain Sci.* 15: 633–643, 1992.
245. McIntyre, A. K., U. Proske, and D. J. Tracey. Afferent fibres from muscle receptors in the posterior nerve of the cat's knee joint. *Exp. Brain Res.* 33: 415–424, 1978.
246. Miall, R. C., J. F. Stein, and D. J. Weir. The cerebellum as an adaptive Smith-predictor in visuomotor control. *Soc. Neurosci. Abstr.* 15: 180, 1989.
247. Milner, T. E., and C. Cloutier. Compensation for mechanically unstable loading in voluntary wrist movement. *Exp. Brain Res.* 94: 522–532, 1993.
248. Moberg, E. The role of cutaneous afferents in position sense, kinaesthesia, and motor function of the hand. *Brain* 106: 1–19, 1983.
249. Morgan, D. L., A. Prochazka, and U. Proske. The aftereffects of stretch and fusimotor stimulation on the responses of primary endings of cat muscle spindles. *J. Physiol. (Lond.)* 356: 465–478, 1984.
250. Mott, F. W., and C. S. Sherrington. Experiments upon the influence of sensory nerves upon movement and nutrition of the limbs. *Proc. R. Soc. Lond. B* 57: 481–488, 1895.
251. Munk, H. *Ueber die Funktionen von Hirn und Rückenmark.* Berlin: Hirschwald, 1909, p. 247–285.
252. Murphy, P. R., and H. A. Martin. Fusimotor discharge patterns during rhythmic movements. *Trends Neurosci.* 16: 273–278, 1993.
253. Murphy, P. R., R. B. Stein, and J. Taylor. Phasic and tonic modulation of impulse rates in motoneurons during locomotion in premammillary cats. *J. Neurophysiol.* 52: 228–243, 1984.
254. Nashner, L. M. Adapting reflexes controlling the human posture. *Exp. Brain Res.* 26: 59–72, 1976.
255. Nashner, L. M., M. Woollacott, and G. Tuma. Organization of rapid responses to postural and locomotor-like perturbations of standing man. *Exp. Brain Res.* 36: 463–476, 1979.
256. Nathan, P. W., M. C. Smith, and A. W. Cook. Sensory effects in man of lesions of the posterior columns and of some other afferent pathways. *Brain* 109: 1003–1041, 1986.

257. Newsom Davis, J. The response to stretch of human intercostal muscle spindles studied *in vitro*. *J. Physiol. (Lond.)* 249: 561–579, 1975.
258. Nielsen, J., and Y. Kagamihara. The regulation of disynaptic reciprocal Ia inhibition during co-contraction of antagonistic muscles in man. *J. Physiol. (Lond.)* 456: 373–391, 1992.
259. Padel, Y., and J. L. Relova. Somatosensory responses in the cat motor cortex. I. Identification and course of an afferent pathway. *J. Neurophysiol.* 66: 2041–2058, 1991.
260. Partridge, L. D. Signal-handling characteristics of load-moving skeletal muscle. *Am. J. Physiol.* 210: 1178–1191, 1966.
261. Patla, A. E. Visual control of human locomotion. In: *Adaptability of Human Gait*, edited by A. E. Patla. New York: Elsevier, 1991, p. 55–97.
262. Pavlides, C., E. Miyashita, and H. Asanuma. Projection from the sensory to the motor cortex is important in learning motor skills in the monkey. *J. Neurophysiol.* 70: 733–741, 1993.
263. Pearson, K. G. Common principles of motor control in vertebrates and invertebrates. *Annu. Rev. Neurosci.* 16: 265–297, 1993.
264. Pearson, K. G., and D. F. Collins. Reversal of the influence of group Ib afferents from plantaris on activity in medial gastrocnemius muscle during locomotor activity. *J. Neurophysiol.* 70: 1009–1017, 1993.
265. Pearson, K. G., and J. Duysens. Function of segmental reflexes in the control of stepping in cockroaches and cats. In: *Neural Control of Locomotion*, edited by R. M. Herman, S. Grillner, P. S. G. Stein, and D. G. Stuart. New York: Plenum, 1976, p. 519–537.
266. Pearson, K. G., and J. M. Ramirez. Influence of input from the forewing stretch receptors on motoneurones in flying locusts. *J. Exp. Biol.* 151: 317–340, 1990.
267. Perret, C., and P. Buser. Static and dynamic fusimotor activity during locomotor movements in the cat. *Brain Res.* 40: 165–169, 1972.
268. Phillips, C. G. Motor apparatus of the baboon's hand. The Ferrier Lecture, 1968. *Proc. R. Soc. Lond. B* 173: 141–174, 1969.
269. Phillips, C. L., and R. D. Harbor. *Feedback Control Systems*, 2nd ed. Englewood Cliffs, NJ: Prentice Hall, 1991, p. 664.
270. Popovic, D., R. Tomovic, D. Tepavac, and L. Schwirtlich. Control aspects of active above-knee prosthesis. *Int. J. Man. Mach. Stud.* 35: 751–767, 1991.
271. Poppele, R. E. An analysis of muscle spindle behavior using randomly applied stretches. *Neuroscience* 6: 1157–1165, 1981.
272. Poppele, R. E., and R. J. Bowman. Quantitative description of linear behavior of mammalian muscle spindles. *J. Neurophysiol.* 33: 59–72, 1970.
273. Poppele, R. E., and W. R. Kennedy. Comparison between behavior of human and cat muscle spindles recorded in vitro. *Brain Res.* 75: 316–319, 1974.
274. Pringle, J. W. S., and V. J. Wilson. The response of a sense organ to a harmonic stimulus. *J. Exp. Biol.* 29: 220–234, 1952.
275. Prochazka, A. Muscle spindle function during normal movement. In: *International Review of Physiology and Neurophysiology IV*, edited by R. Porter. Baltimore: MTP University Park, 1981, p. 47–90.
276. Prochazka, A. Chronic techniques for studying neurophysiology of movement in cats. In: *Methods for Neuronal Recording in Conscious Animals* (IBRO Handbook Ser.: Methods Neurosci. 4), edited by R. Lemon. New York: Wiley, 1983, p. 113–128.
277. Prochazka, A. Sensorimotor gain control: a basic strategy of motor systems? *Prog. Neurobiol.* 33: 281–307, 1989.
278. Prochazka, A. Ensemble inputs to α-motoneurons during movement. In: *The Motor Unit—Physiology, Diseases, Regeneration*, edited by R. Dengler. Munich: Urban Schwarzenberg, 1990, p. 32–42.
279. Prochazka, A. Comparison of natural and artificial control of movement. *IEEE Trans. Rehab. Eng.* 1: 7–17, 1993.
280. Prochazka, A., and M. Hulliger. Muscle afferent function and its significance for motor control mechanisms during voluntary movements in cat, monkey and man. In: *Motor Control Mechanisms in Health and Disease*, edited by J. E. Desmedt. New York: Raven, 1983, p. 93–132.
281. Prochazka, A., M. Hulliger, P. Trend, and N. Dürmüller. Dynamic and static fusimotor set in various behavioural contexts. In: *Mechanoreceptors: Development, Structure and Function*, edited by P. Hnik, T. Soukup, R. Vejsada, and J. Zelena. London: Plenum, 1988, p. 417–430.
282. Prochazka, A., M. Hulliger, P. Zangger, and K. Appenteng. "Fusimotor set": new evidence for α-independent control of γ-motoneurones during movement in the awake cat. *Brain Res.* 339: 136–140, 1985.
283. Prochazka, A., P. Trend, M. Hulliger, and S. Vincent. Ensemble proprioceptive activity in the cat step cycle: towards a representative look-up chart. In: *Afferent Control of Posture and Locomotion*, edited by J. H. J. Allum and M. Hulliger. Amsterdam: Elsevier, 1989b, *Prog. Brain Res.* 80: 61–74.
284. Prochazka, A., and P. Wand. Muscle spindle responses to rapid stretching in normal cats. In: *Muscle Receptors and Movement*, edited by A. Taylor and A. Prochazka. London: Macmillan, 1981, p. 257–261.
285. Proske, U. The Golgi tendon organ: properties of the receptor and reflex action of impulses arising from tendon organs. In: *Int. Rev. Physiol. 25, Neurophysiol. IV*, edited by R. Porter. Baltimore: MTP University Park, 1981, p. 127–171.
286. Proske, U., D. L. Morgan, and J. E. Gregory. Thixotropy in skeletal muscle and in muscle spindles: A review. *Prog. Neurobiol.* 41: 705–721, 1993.
287. Rack, P. M. H., and D. Westbury. Elastic properties of the cat soleus tendon and their functional importance. *J. Physiol. (Lond.)* 347: 479–495, 1984.
288. Reinking, R. M., J. A. Stephens, and D. J. Stuart. The tendon organs of cat medial gastrocnemius: significance of motor unit type and size for the activation of Ib afferents. *J. Physiol. (Lond.)* 250: 491–512, 1975.
289. Ribot, E., J.-P. Roll, and J.-P. Vedel. Efferent discharges recorded from single skeletomotor and fusimotor fibres in man. *J. Physiol. (Lond.)* 375: 251–268, 1986.
290. Richmond, F. J. R., and V. C. Abrahams. Physiological properties of muscle spindles in dorsal neck muscles of the cat. *J. Neurophysiol.* 42: 604–617, 1979.
291. Roberts, W. J., N. P. Rosenthal, and C. A. Terzuolo. A control model of stretch reflex. *J. Neurophysiol.* 34: 620–634, 1971.
292. Roll, J. P., and J. P. Vedel. Kinesthetic role of muscle afferents in man, studied by tendon vibration and microneurography. *Exp. Brain Res.* 47: 177–190, 1982.
293. Rothwell, J. C., S. C. Gandevia, and D. Burke. Activation of fusimotor neurones by motor cortical stimulation in human subjects. *J. Physiol. (Lond.)* 431: 743–756, 1990.

294. Rothwell, J. C., M. M. Traub, B. L. Day, J. A. Obeso, P. K. Thomas, and C. D. Marsden. Manual motor performance in deafferented man. *Brain* 105: 515–542, 1982.
295. Rudomin, P. Presynaptic inhibition of muscle spindle and tendon organ afferents in the mammalian spinal cord. *Trends Neurosci.* 13: 499–505, 1990.
296. Rymer, W. Z., and A. D'Almeida. Joint position sense: the effects of muscle contraction. *Brain* 103: 1–22, 1980.
297. Sanes, J. N., K.-H. Mauritz, M. C. Dalakas, and E. V. Evarts. Motor control in humans with large-fiber sensory neuropathy. *Hum. Neurobiol.* 4: 101–114, 1985.
298. Sainburg, R. L., H. Poizner, and C. Ghez. Loss of proprioception produces deficits in interjoint coordination. *J. Neurophysiol.* 70: 2136–2147, 1993.
299. Schäfer, S. S. The characteristic curves of the dynamic response of primary muscle spindle endings in the absence and presence of stimulation of fusimotor fibres. *Brain Res.* 59: 395–399, 1973.
300. Schaafsma, A., E. Otten, and J. D. Van Willigen. A muscle spindle model for primary afferent firing based on a simulation of intrafusal mechanical events. *J. Neurophysiol.* 65: 1297–1312, 1991.
301. Schieber, M. H., and W. T. Thach. Alpha-gamma dissociation during slow tracking movements of the monkey's wrist: preliminary evidence from spinal ganglion recording. *Brain Res.* 202: 213–216, 1980.
302. Schieber, M. H., and W. T. Thach. Trained slow tracking. II. Bidirectional discharge patterns of cerebellar nuclear, motor cortex, and spindle afferent neurons. *J. Neurophysiol.* 54: 1228–1270, 1985.
303. Schlapp, M. Observations on a voluntary tremor—violinist's vibrato. *Q. J. Exp. Physiol.* 58: 357–368, 1973.
304. Scott, J. J. A., J. E. Gregory, U. Proske, and D. L. Morgan. Correlating resting discharge with small signal sensitivity and discharge variability in primary endings of cat soleus muscle spindles. *J. Neurophysiol.* 71: 309–316, 1994.
305. Scott, S. H., and G. E. Loeb. The computation of position sense from spindles in mono- and multiarticular muscles. *J. Neurosci.* 14: 7529–7540, 1995.
306. Sears, T. A. Efferent discharges in alpha and fusimotor fibres of intercostal nerves of the cat. *J. Physiol. (Lond.)* 174: 295–315, 1964.
307. Sechenov, I. M. *Refleksy Golovnogo Mozga (1863)* English Translation: *Reflexes of the Brain.* In: *I. M. Sechenov, Selected Works*, by A. A. Subkov. Moscow: State Publ. House Biol. Med. Lit., 1935, p. 264–322.
308. Severin, F. V. The role of the gamma motor system in the activation of the extensor alpha motor neurones during controlled locomotion. *Biophysics* 15: 1138–1145, 1970.
309. Severin, F. V., G. N. Orlovsky, and M. L. Shik. Work of the muscle receptors during controlled locomotion. *Biophysics* 12: 575–586, 1967.
310. Sinclair, R. J., and H. Burton. Neuronal activity in the second somatosensory cortex of monkeys (*Macaca mulatta*) during active touch of gratings. *J. Neurophysiol.* 70: 331–350, 1993.
311. Sinkjaer, T., E. Toft, S. Andreassen, and B. C. Hornemann. Muscle stiffness in human ankle dorsiflexors: intrinsic and reflex components. *J. Neurophysiol.* 60: 1110–1121, 1988.
312. Sjöström, A., and P. Zangger. Alpha-gamma-linkage in the spinal generator for locomotion in the cat. *Acta Physiol. Scand.* 94: 130–132, 1975.
313. Smith, A. M., C. Dugas, P. Fortier, J. Kalaska, and N. Picard. Comparing cerebellar and motor cortical activity in reaching and grasping. *Can. J. Neurol. Sci.* 20 (Suppl. 3): S53–S61, 1993.
314. Smith, J. L., M. G. Hoy, G. F. Koshland, D. M. Phillips, and R. F. Zernicke. Intralimb coordination of the paw-shake response: a novel mixed synergy. *J. Neurophysiol.* 54: 1271–1281, 1985.
315. Smith, O. J. M. A controller to overcome dead time. *ISA J.* 6: 28–33, 1959.
316. St-Onge, N., H. Qi, and A. G. Feldman. The patterns of control signals underlying elbow joint movements in humans. *Neurosci. Lett.* 164: 171–174, 1993.
317. Strick, P. L. The influence of motor preparation on the response of cerebellar neurons to limb displacements. *J. Neurosci.* 3: 2007–2020, 1983.
318. Struppler, A., and F. Erbel. Analysis of proprioceptive excitability with special reference to the "unloading reflex." In: *Neurophysiology Studied in Man*, edited by G. Somjen. Amsterdam: Excerpta Medica, *Ex. Med. Congr. Ser. 253*, 1972, p. 298–304.
319. Stuart, D. G., G. E. Goslow, C. G. Mosher, and R. M. Reinking. Stretch responsiveness of Golgi tendon organs. *Exp. Brain Res.* 10: 463–476, 1970.
320. Stuart, D. G., C. G. Mosher, R. L. Gerlach, and R. M. Reinking. Mechanical arrangement and transducing properties of Golgi tendon organs. *Exp. Brain Res.* 14: 274–292, 1972.
321. Taub, E., I. A. Goldberg, and P. Taub. Deafferentation in monkeys: pointing at a target without visual feedback. *Exp. Neurol.* 46: 178–186, 1975.
322. Taylor, A., and F. W. J. Cody. Jaw muscle spindle activity in the cat during normal movements of eating and drinking. *Brain Res.* 71: 523–530, 1974.
323. Taylor, A., and R. Donga. Central mechanisms of selective fusimotor control. In: *Afferent Control of Posture and Movement*, edited by J. H. J. Allum and M. Hulliger. Amsterdam: Elsevier, 1989, p. 27–36.
324. Taylor, A., R. Donga, and P. J. W. Jüch. Fusimotor effects of midbrain stimulation on jaw muscle spindles of the anaesthetized cat. *Exp. Brain Res.* 93: 37–45, 1993.
325. Taylor, A., and S. Gottlieb. Convergence of several sensory modalities in motor control. In: *Feedback and Motor Control in Invertebrates and Vertebrates*, edited by W. J. P. Barnes and M. H. Gladden. London: Croon Helm, 1985, p. 77–92.
326. Taylor, A., J. F. Rodgers, A. J. Fowle, and R. Durbaba. The effect of succinylcholine on cat gastrocnemius muscle spindle afferents of different types. *J. Physiol. (Lond.)* 456: 629–644, 1992.
327. Taylor, J. L., and D. I. McCloskey. Proprioception in the neck. *Exp. Brain Res.* 70: 351–360, 1988.
328. Teasdale, N., R. Forget, C. Bard, J. Paillard, M. Fleury, and Y. Lamarre. The role of afferent information for the production of isometric forces and for handwriting tasks. *Acta Psychol.* 82: 179–191, 1993.
329. Thach, W. T., H. P. Goodkin, and J. G. Keating. The cerebellum and the adaptive coordination of movement. *Annu. Rev. Neurosci.* 15: 403–442, 1992.
330. Thach, W. T., J. G. Perry, and M. H. Schieber. Cerebellar output: body images and muscle spindles. *Exp. Brain Res.* 6 (Suppl.): 440–454, 1982.
331. Tomovic, R., and R. McGhee. A finite state approach to the synthesis of control systems. *IEEE Trans. Hum. Fac. Electron.* 7: 122–128, 1966.
332. Tracey, D. J. Characteristics of wrist joint receptors in the cat. *Exp. Brain Res.* 34: 165–176, 1979.
333. Trend, P. Gain control in proprioceptive reflex pathways. Ph.D. thesis, University of London, 1987.

334. Vallbo, A. B. Afferent discharge from human muscle spindles in non-contracting muscles. Steady state impulse frequency as a function of joint angle. *Acta Physiol. Scand.* 90: 303–318, 1974.
335. Vallbo, A. B. Sensations evoked from the glabrous skin of the human hand by electrical stimulation of unitary mechanosensitive afferents. *Brain Res.* 215: 359–363, 1981.
336. Vallbo, A. B., and N. A. Al-Falahe. Human muscle spindle response in a motor learning task. *J. Physiol. (Lond.)* 421: 553–568, 1990.
337. Van Kan, P. L. E., A. R. Gibson, and J. C. Houk. Movement-related inputs to intermediate cerebellum of the monkey. *J. Neurophysiol.* 69: 74–94, 1993.
338. Vedel, J. P. Cortical control of dynamic and static gamma motoneurone activity. In: *New Developments in Electromyography and Clinical Neurophysiology*, edited by J. E. Desmedt. Basel: Karger, 1973, p. 126–135.
339. Von Holst, E. Relations between the central nervous system and the peripheral organs. *Br. J. Anim. Behav.* 2: 89–94, 1954.
340. Voss, H. Tabelle der absoluten und relativen Muskelspindelzahlen der menschlichen Skelettmuskulatur. *Anat. Anz.* 129: 562–572, 1971.
341. Wall, P. D., and S. B. McMahon. Microneurography and its relation to perceived sensation. A critical review. *Pain* 21: 209–229, 1985.
342. Walmsley, B., J. A. Hodgson, and R. E. Burke. Forces produced by medial gastrocnemius and soleus muscles during locomotion in freely moving cats. *J. Neurophysiol.* 41: 1203–1216, 1978.
343. Walmsley, B., and U. Proske. Comparison of stiffness of soleus and medial gastrocnemius muscles in cats. *J. Neurophysiol.* 46: 250–259, 1981.
344. Wand, P., A. Prochazka, and K.-H. Sontag. Neuromuscular responses to gait perturbations in freely moving cats. *Exp. Brain Res.* 38: 109–114, 1980.
345. Wand, P., M. Schwarz, W. Kolasiewicz, and K.-H. Sontag. Nigral output neurons are engaged in regulation of static fusimotor action onto flexors in cats. *Pflugers Arch.* 391: 255–257, 1981.
346. Wei, J. Y., B. R. Kripke, and P. R. Burgess. Classification of muscle spindle receptors. *Brain Res.* 370: 119–126, 1986.
347. Wei, J. Y., J. Simon, M. Randic, and P. R. Burgess. Joint angle signalling by muscle spindle receptors. *Brain Res.* 370: 108–118, 1986.
348. Wiesendanger, M., and T. S. Miles. Ascending pathway of low-threshold muscle afferents to the cerebral cortex and its possible role in motor control. *Physiol. Rev.* 62: 1234–1270, 1982.
349. Willis, W. D., and R. E. Coggeshall. *Sensory Mechanisms of the Spinal Cord*, 2nd ed. New York: Plenum, 1991, p. 575.
350. Wilson, D. M. The central nervous control of flight in a locust. *J. Exp. Biol.* 38: 471–479, 1961.
351. Wilson, D. M., and E. Gettrup. A stretch reflex controlling wing-beat frequency in grasshoppers. *J. Exp. Biol.* 40: 171–185, 1963.
352. Young, R. R., and K.-E. Hagbarth. Physiological tremor enhanced by manoeuvres affecting the segmental stretch reflex. *J. Neurol. Neurosurg. Psychiatry* 43: 248–256, 1980.
353. Zalkind, V. I. Method for an adequate stimulation of receptors of the cat carpo-radialis joint. *Sechenov Physiol. J. USSR*, 57: 1123–1127, 1971.
354. Zelena, J., and T. Soukup. The in-series and in-parallel components in rat hindlimb tendon organs. *Neuroscience* 9: 899–910, 1983.
355. Zill, S. Proprioceptive feedback and the control of cockroach walking. In: *Feedback and Motor Control in Invertebrates and Vertebrates*, edited by W. J. P. Barnes and M. H. Gladden. London: Croon Helm, 1985, p. 187–208.

4. Kinesthesia: roles for afferent signals and motor commands

SIMON C. GANDEVIA | *Prince of Wales Medical Research Institute and University of New South Wales, Sydney, Australia*

CHAPTER CONTENTS

WHETHER A PERSON WALKS OR RUNS or adopts a static posture, the potential instability of the multiple joints, bones, and muscles must be inherently obvious to a physicist. Despite the body's physical instability, it is a surprisingly stable structure. The control of movement and posture is believed to involve particular neural signals, some of which have access to consciousness. Such signals, encompassed within the terms kinesthesia and proprioception proposed originally by Bastian and Sherrington, respectively, arise from activity in mechanoreceptors, from centrally generated motor commands, and from interactions between these afferent and efferent signals. The two terms have become virtually synonymous and have acquired a loose meaning that covers almost anything concerned with the control of movement. This expanded meaning is more than can be accommodated here, although it fits with Sherrington's "proprio-ceptive system," which encompassed reflex control of movement without the need to "predicate nor to preclude sensation" (293, 294).

This chapter considers neural mechanisms underlying components of kinesthesia; these include sensations of limb movement and position, sensations of force and heaviness, and sensations of the timing of muscular contractions. The final part of the chapter deals with functional issues, such as how global kinesthetic mechanisms operate and how they are disturbed by aging and disease.

HISTORICAL PERSPECTIVES

Debate about the roles of sensory inputs (i.e., afferent mechanisms) and the will (i.e., efferent mechanisms) has seen the demise of many terminologies which, in the nineteenth century, changed as much due to fashion as to experiment. Key points are summarized in Table 4.1 (for review, see 25, 173, 220, 221, 288, 289, 292). Due to widespread belief in "feelings of effort" or "sensations of innervation," it was generally assumed that at least some perceptual phenomena required the participation of efferent processes (289). Circumstances requiring them included: stabilization of vision despite eye movements, the effects of weak eye muscles on vi-

TABLE 4.1. *Summary of Milestones in the History of Kinesthesia*

1802:	J. T. Engel described a muscle sense, although uncertain if it was "afferent" or "efferent."
1807:	Maine de Biran founded a psychology based on "immediate apperception." The "will" represented a feeling of effort signaled by a "sens musculaire" (afferent or efferent).
1823:	Bell began interest in the "sixth" or "muscle" sense. His arguments centered on "consciousness of muscular exertion." He recognized both afferent and efferent components but did not always distinguish them. Visual location was determined by "consciousness of the degree of effort put upon the voluntary extraocular muscles."
1855:	Bain was a strong proponent of outflow and the "sense of effort."
1863:	Wundt introduced the term "innervation sensations" or "innervation feelings."
1865:	Donders described fractionation of reaction time into stages which were based on voluntary choice and cognitive processes.
1866:	Sechenov published *The Reflexes of the Brain*, in which he championed the role of reflexes in mental activities.
1866:	Helmholtz published *Handbuck der Physiologischen Optik*. He provided much evidence in favor of sensations of "effort" in visual localization.
1880:	Bastian introduced the term "kinaesthesis." It was thought to be afferent in origin (but carefully not specified) and to leave memory traces within the CNS.
1886:	Mach argued for a role of the will. He described effort sensations following his own transient complete motor "stroke."
1890:	William James argued forcefully against existence of all perceived efferent signals in *The Principles of Psychology*.
1900:	Sherrington reviewed "the muscular sense" and argued that muscle and joint receptors were critical, and, like James, that it was not necessary to consider "sensations of innervation." He proposed a role for extraocular muscle receptors.
1906:	Sherrington introduced the term "proprioception." It focused on internally generated movements of the body and included inputs from muscles and joints, usually in "reflex alliance" with vestibular inputs. Cutaneous inputs were excluded.
1950:	Von Holst specified a motor outflow or "efference copy" from which was subtracted the peripheral input or "reafferent" signal; this yielded an "exafferent" signal. If the reafferent signal matched the predicted value (efference copy), the animal behaved as if the environment were stationary.
1950:	Sperry introduced the term "corollary discharge" for a motor output signal that acted on visual centers to compensate for displacement of the retinal image.
1960:	Brindley and Merton confirmed there is poor sensation of eye position. Merton subsequently argued that muscle spindle signals would be too confusing to provide conscious signals (because of fusimotor drive). He erroneously reintroduced the notion that the "sense of effort" led to perception of limb movement.
1967:	Swett and Bourassa denied a cortical projection for group I muscle afferents based on their failure to condition behavior in response to electrical stimulation in cats.
1968:	Development of microneurography by Hagbarth and Vallbo. This led to measurement of the responses of human muscle, joint, and cutaneous afferents to vibration and natural stimulation, and in the early 1980s, to development of microstimulation for single axons. Beginning in the late 1980s, the kinesthetic potential of joint and cutaneous receptors was reinvestigated using both microneurographic recording and stimulation.
1972:	Goodwin, McCloskey, and Matthews described vibration-induced illusions of joint movement and position. Much additional evidence was provided to indicate that muscle spindle afferents contribute to perception of limb position and movement.
1974:	McCloskey, Goodwin, and Ebeling reassessed evidence that signals of motor command contribute to sensations of muscle force and heaviness. They distinguished between sensations of heaviness and absolute tension.
1970s:	Accumulation of evidence that muscle afferents project to the cerebral cortex in experimental animals including nonhuman primates, a finding confirmed for humans in the 1980s.
1983:	Experiments independently reveal that the perceived timing of muscle contraction can be generated from a motor command signal occurring before movement (Libet and colleagues: McCloskey and colleagues).
1984:	McIntyre, Proske, and Rawson described a specific cortical projection for Golgi tendon organ afferents.
1985:	Gandevia described illusions of movement and position following electrical stimulation of group I muscle afferents.
1987:	Gandevia and Rothwell showed that motor commands, below threshold for movement, could be learnt and consistently delivered in the absence of peripheral feedback.
1990:	Gauthier et al. confirmed the long-suspected role for extraocular muscle afferents in visual localization.

sual position, judgments of heaviness, observations in patients with paralysis, and the fractionation of reaction times.

Three developments brought on the temporary demise of the belief in sensations of innervation (289). First, the belief arose that reflexes subserved nearly all behavior, a position advocated by Sechenov that reduced the role of volition. Second, Darwinian evolution meant that use of the will was not only a human but an animal characteristic. Finally, the development of clinical neurology blurred the distinctions between motor and sensory disturbances. Volition, no longer spontaneous, was directed by reflex or imagined events.

Among psychologists, the views of G. E. Müller and William James held sway. While those for and against feelings of innervation usually agreed on the observations, the arguments arose in their explanation. Thus, if an observation could be explained by a difference in afferent input, a role for feelings of innervation was unnecessary. Hence, the greater accuracy in assessing weights lifted actively rather than passively was explained by the difference in sensory inputs and not in efferent signals.

Subsequently, roles for "outflow" diminished. Goldscheider used electrical stimulation around joints to show the role of joint receptors in position and movement sensation, and argued for an input from tendons in the sense of force (126). Before 1850, the skin had been considered important in the sense of weight. Reviewing the muscular sense in 1900, Sherrington included "all reactions or sense arising in motor organs," those related to "posture, active and passive movement, and resistance to movement" (292). Subsequently, he coined the term "proprio-ceptors" for inputs from muscles, joints, and the vestibular apparatus, though their central actions did not necessarily imply perception (294). These receptors responded to mechanical stimuli, particularly muscular contractions, initiated by the organism itself. The term "kinaesthesis" was adopted by Bastian and included "cutaneous impressions, impressions from muscles and other deep structures of the limbs (such as fasciae, tendons, and articular surfaces) all of which yield conscious impressions . . . in addition, there seems to be a highly important set of unfelt or but little felt impressions which guide the volitional activity" (17). The term "joint position sense" concurrently evolved in neurology.

In the twentieth century physiologists continued to emphasize the afferent side, spurred on by the study of reflexes and then the ability to record nerve impulses. The role of outflow resurfaced through two influential terminologies. To explain the circling of insects or fish when the eye or neck is rotated, Sperry (303) considered, but did not favor, the view that it resulted from the reversed "sign" of an oculomotor reflex. He regarded the circling as associated with an "illusory spinning of the visual field" due to the animal's movements and thus proposed "a corollary discharge into the visual centres to compensate for the retinal displacement." This was a "central adjustor" rather than direct cause of visual perception. Von Holst and Mittelstaedt (157, 158) devised the reafference principle whereby an exact signal of the motor output ("efference copy") was subtracted from the sensory input or "reafference" to yield a (error) signal or "exafference" that drove stabilization of the visual image. These signals did not necessarily evoke sensations, although they might be transmitted "upwards, sometimes to the highest centres" (158). Alternative views about corollary discharges and cancellation or reafference have been proposed (e.g., 229, 245). Nonetheless, the central nervous system (CNS) must determine whether a changed input derives from the external world (i.e., the visualized object moved) or directly from the motor system (i.e., the body, head, or eyes moved; see also KINESTHETIC MECHANISMS IN ISOLATION, later). Motor command signals provide a parsimonious solution. For example, the operation of a simple efference copy mechanism has been isolated in electric fish to detect the timing of environmental electric signals received by the knollenorgan class of electroreceptors (21). Signals generated by the fish's own electric organ are cancelled by a precisely timed inhibitory corollary of the motor command (Fig. 4.1). For other classes of electroreceptor, partial cancellation of the input caused by the fish's electric organ occurs using motor command corollaries that are modifiable by recent environmental inputs.

The term "efference copy" implied a replica of the motor command, whereas corollary discharge was not necessarily a replica but merely a signal derived from the command. Hence efference copies are a special case of corollary discharges, which in turn can be regarded as subsets of motor command signals. The latter term has been used here because it avoids the nuances of the original definitions.

In the latter part of this century researchers determined the perceptual roles for skin, joint, and muscle receptors. Following the discovery in 1972 that muscle spindle afferents contribute to sensations of limb position and movement (129; see also 81), the pendulum swung, perhaps too heavily, against joint and cutaneous afferents. Psychophysical studies have established the roles for motor command corollaries. Thus subjective timing of a muscle contraction can

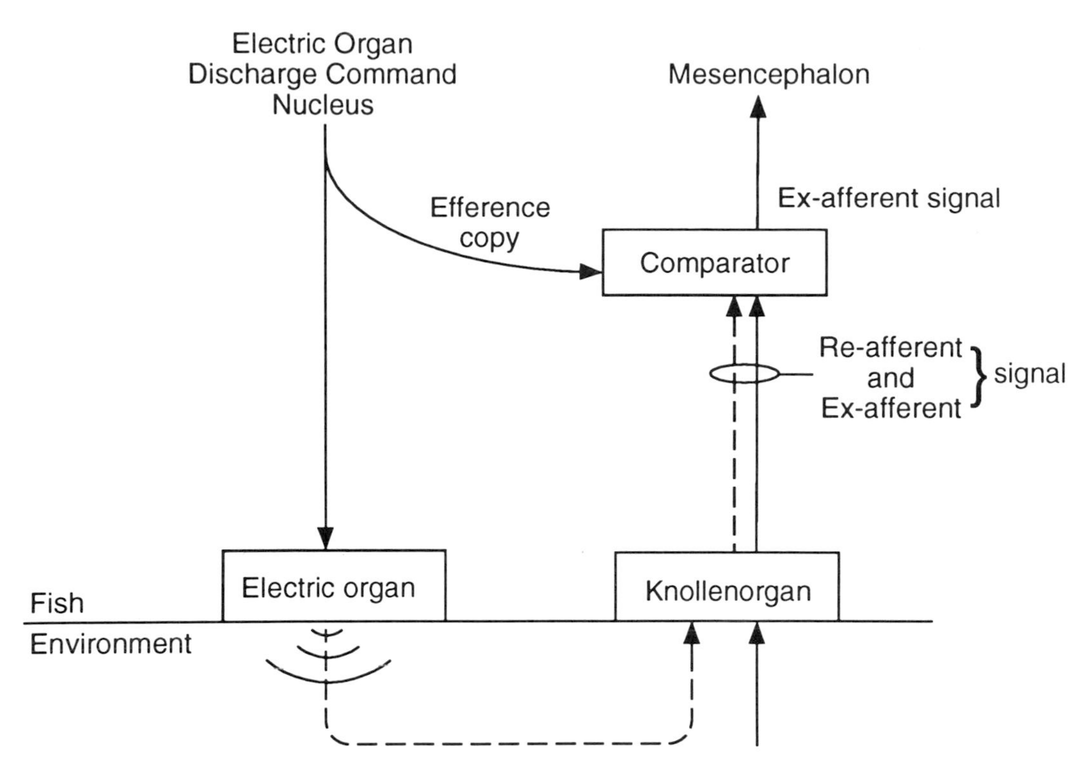

FIG. 4.1. Schematic representation of one efference copy mechanism used by mormyrid fish. The electric organ discharges in response to the command from the electric organ discharge nucleus and this evokes a reafferent signal in the knollenorgan receptor. Environmentally mediated events evoke exafferent signals in this receptor. The efference copy acts as an exact inhibitory template to block reafferent signals so that the fish can more easily detect the environmental signals. Here, the corollary discharge provides a precise template of the expected reafference (see text). [Adapted from Bell (21).]

occur by reference to a centrally generated signal (211, 222), and central commands, subthreshold for movement, can be directed to muscles (58, 119). Perception of the location of visual targets also relies in part on perceived motor commands (e.g., 121, 122).

CURRENT DEFINITIONS

Kinesthesia and proprioception encompass a group of sensations. First is the traditional sensation of position and movement of the limbs and trunk. Second, there are sensations related to muscle force, including effort, tension, heaviness, and stiffness. Third, sensations exist for timing muscle contractions. Fourth, there is a sensation of body posture and size as part of a "schema" encompassing more than one joint. The term "inputs" is used to refer to the discharge of afferents from muscle, joint, and muscle receptors. The term "kinesthetic signals" includes the contribution from motor command signals as well as the inputs from skin, joint, and muscle receptors. Motor commands encompass the general term corollary discharge as well as the specific form called an efference copy.

These sensations are all considered to evoke specific percepts that can be verbalized and studied with psychophysical and neurophysiological tools. This does not prevent kinesthetic signals from influencing motor control if a sensation is not evoked. Indeed, some patients with blindness due to a cortical lesion lose the ability to describe visualized objects but retain the ability to grasp them (127). This dissociation happens in normal subjects in that some movements within a sequence are performed so rapidly that perception cannot "keep up." Hence, motor commands will also operate at subconscious levels.

There has long been controversy about how to "reference" kinesthetic signals. Muscle afferents from the limbs (and the eye) were sometimes denied a kinesthetic role because unnatural pulling on a muscle failed to evoke a percept *referred to the muscle* (e.g., 32, 246). It is now clear that limb muscle receptors influence sensations of limb movement (and those from eye muscles influence sensations of visual movement) just as cutaneous inputs influence sensations of objects on the skin. Appropriate referencing of motor command signals must also occur.

PROPERTIES OF KINESTHETIC AFFERENTS

The full array of specialized muscle, joint, and cutaneous afferents are potential kinesthetic inputs. All can respond to passive or active joint movements, but response to a mechanical disturbance is not sufficient to prove that the afferent class has a kinesthetic role. An afferent class may have more than one kinesthetic role.

Muscle Spindles

Muscle spindles have a sensory and motor innervation. The sensory component consists of one primary and several secondary spindle receptors that are distinguished by numerous properties. Afferent and efferent control of spindles has been reviewed extensively (e.g., 28, 164, 213, 236, 237, 309; see also Chapter 3). Primary spindle endings give rise to group Ia afferents and secondary endings to slower conducting group II afferents. The motor innervation comprises purely fusimotor axons (or γ-motoneurons), which innervate several spindles; and the less frequent skeletofusimotor axons (or β-motoneurons), which innervate intrafusal *and* extrafusal muscle fibers. Fusimotor axons are distinguished by their innervation of particular types of intrafusal muscle fibers and their action on primary and secondary afferents. In the early 1960s, intrafusal fibers were separated into nuclear bag fibers and nuclear chain fibers based on their morphology. Usually there are two to three bag fibers and almost twice as many chain fibers. Later morphological, histochemical and functional studies subdivided the nuclear bag fibers into the bag_1 and bag_2 fibers (for references, see 72, 260).

The number, density, and location of spindles range widely between and within muscles. A few human muscles such as digastric and stapedius have no spindles (see 38). Spindle densities are higher in intrinsic hand muscles than proximal muscles, while the deep layers of neck muscles have the highest densities (e.g., 9, 71, 326). Densities are higher for small muscles that cross few joints than for larger muscles in parallel with them. Basic properties of cat and human spindles are similar, although there are some anatomical differences (see 38).

Spindle Afferent Properties. Primary spindle afferents discharge at higher rates to dynamic stimuli such as stretch or tendon taps than secondary afferents. The primary spindle ending can discharge in temporal relation to mechanical perturbations subthreshold for increasing the overall discharge rate, but a price for a highly sensitive length monitor is addition of biological noise to the signal that must be removed by central "averaging." The high sensitivity of primary spindle endings means that their exact intramuscular location modifies their response, as all regions of a muscle do not lengthen uniformly (242). The "partitioning" of input from part of a "muscle" has implications for kinesthesia (335). Subjects can use the inputs from portions of the long flexor and extensor muscles to deduce which finger is flexed when the whole hand is anesthetized (108, 129).

Distinction between primary and secondary spindle afferents can be aided by measurement of their conduction velocity in animal studies. However, in humans it is rarely feasible to assess this for single afferents. Nonetheless, recordings from afferents innervating finger extensors can be distinguished based on *a priori* combination of features, including responses to passive stretch and muscle contractions (80). The CNS should be able to extract a signal of movement by comparison of the behavior of primary and secondary afferents. Properties of vibration-induced illusions of movement are consistent with this view (218).

Spindle "Nonlinearities." Spindle primaries have long been known to behave in a nonlinear way to length changes. These nonlinearities include the "initial burst" at the onset of stretch. This "acceleration" response increases with the velocity of lengthening, but is abolished unless the muscle has been at a stable length for seconds. The so-called linear range of primary spindle behavior is defined by the small range of vibration amplitudes that produces steep and *proportional* modulation of spindle discharge. In cat muscles it extends to about 100 μm. Beyond this, the depth of spindle modulation increases less steeply with vibration amplitude. This provides high sensitivity to small intramuscular events with compression of the response range so that large perturbations are accommodated without saturation. The linear range is reestablished at a new muscle length. However, this depends on prevailing conditions [Fig. 4.2; (17, 18)]. Thus, the modulation of primary spindle endings by vibration (50 μm amplitude) was diminished to one-tenth or less during slow "triangular" stretches (<0.05 muscle lengths/s). If the vibration was large (1 mm), the modulation remained constant despite the background stretch. Because spindle sensitivity changes so much with the length history of the muscle, extraction by the CNS

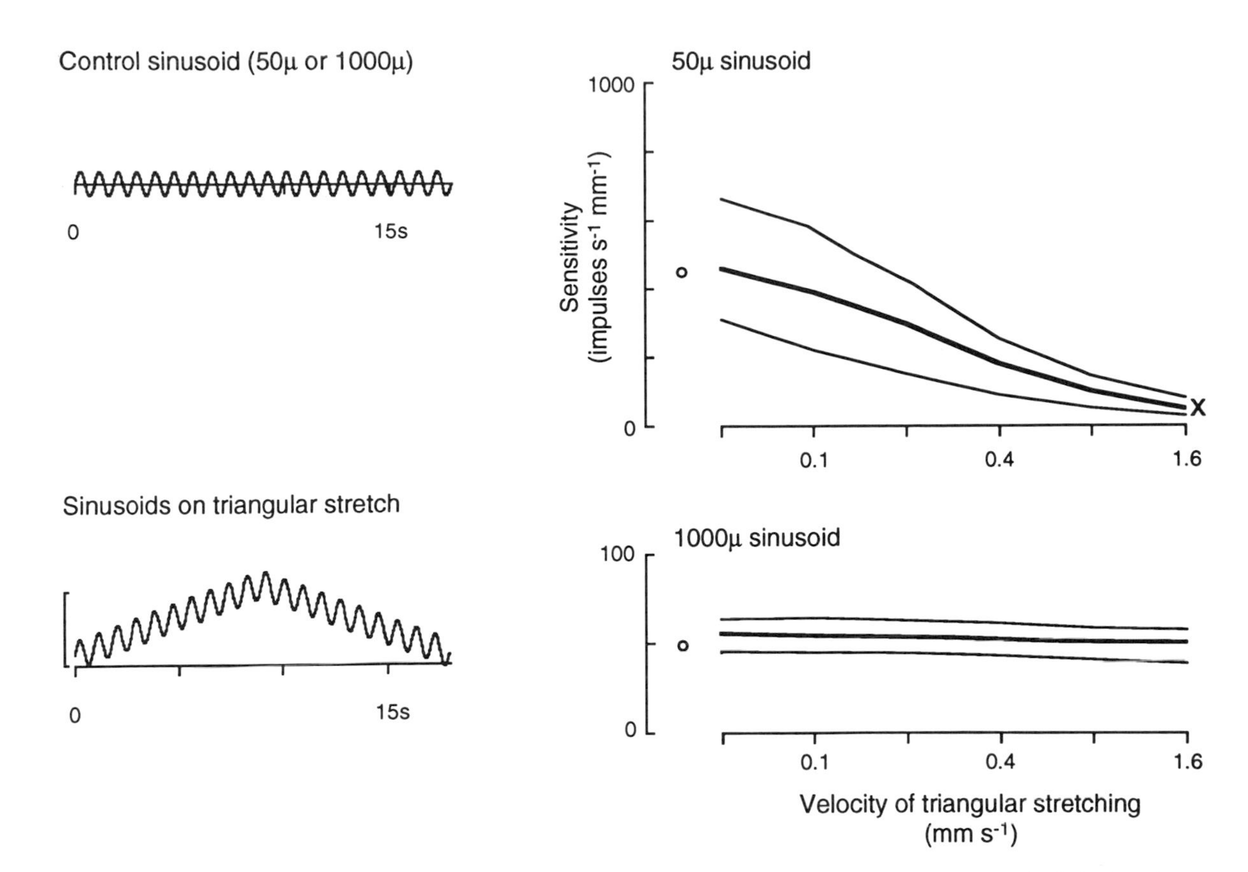

FIG. 4.2. Modulation of muscle spindle discharge by small length changes diminishes markedly when they are superimposed on slow movements. Data from a population of primary spindle afferents innervating the cat soleus muscle to illustrate the effects of an underlying slow movement on the sensitivity to sinusoidal stretch delivered at about 1 Hz. Panels at left show the control sinusoidal stretch (*upper trace*) and the sinusoidal stretch delivered during a slow "triangular" movement (*lower trace*). Panels at right show the responses for a 50 μm (*above*) and 1,000 μm sinusoid (*below*). Responses to combined sinusoidal and triangular stretch shown as the median (*thick line*) with interquartile ranges. *Open circle* indicates the control responses without slow movement. Sensitivity scale is enlarged in the *lower panel*, with the *cross* in the *upper panel* indicating the corresponding response to 1,000 μm sinusoid during the fastest movement. These results mean that primary spindle afferents will encode large changes in length faithfully but will only respond dynamically to very small perturbations when the movement is very slow or isometric. [Adapted from Baumann and Hulliger (18).]

of an *absolute* signal of muscle length or velocity will be impossible. Hence, alternative means must define the extremes of angular ranges.

The principal mechanism for the nonlinearities in spindle behavior is termed "thixotropy," a plastic, friction-like behavior of muscle (for review, see 268). It produces relatively greater resistance of muscle to small than large movements and a transition from high to low resistance after a large stretch. The resistance redevelops over several seconds, largely through the re-formation of some cross bridges between myosin and actin. As a result, about one-third of human muscle spindle endings discharge at higher rates after a weak voluntary isometric contraction (334).

Fusimotor Mechanisms. By the 1960s, static and dynamic fusimotor actions had been defined, based on the consistent effects produced by stimulation of single axons on the stretch responsiveness of primary spindle afferents. Dynamic axons produced little increase in primary afferent discharge but a marked increase in dynamic responsiveness, whereas static axons elevated background discharge rates (even "driving" the afferent at the stimulus frequency or a subharmonic) with reduced sensitivity to dynamic events. Static but not dynamic axons have an excitatory effect on secondaries. These findings were conveniently explained by innervation of bag fibers by dynamic axons and chain fibers by static ones, with chain fibers having a more rapid contraction time. Static axons innervate both nuclear chain and some nuclear bag fibers. When bag fibers were later subdivided into two types (bag_1 and bag_2), with dynamic axons innervating bag_1 fibers exclusively, it raised the question of whether the static system should be subdivided according to whether individual axons innervate bag_2 fibers, chain fibers, or both (26, 49, 72). The spindle is at least a two-compartment structure, with bag_1 and dynamic γ innervation separate from the remaining innervation of bag_2 and chain fibers. In passive spindles, the latter compartment is important, with the bag_2 fibers critical for setting the background discharge of primary spindle afferents, and with chain fibers setting it for the secondary spindle afferents (267). The perceptual consequences of this subdivision are unknown.

Skeletomotor or β innervation of muscles provides an obligatory mechanism for production of force and modulation of spindle sensitivity: dynamic β axons innervate bag_1 fibers (and extrafusal slow-twitch units) and static axons innervate chain fibers (and fast-twitch extrafusal units) almost exclusively (cf. 13). This system would provide a significant input under isometric conditions.

Central Actions on Fusimotor Neurons. If descending pathways preferentially recruit the dynamic system and subdivisions of the static system, it suggests that evolution of such systems is functionally important and provides an insight as to how complex the system of corollary discharges must be for accurate interpretation of muscle spindle signals. With electrical stimulation there is a mesencephalic site at which dynamic fusimotor activation occurs (see 6), and it may also be possible to activate output to bag_2 and chain fibers independently (73). Recordings from spindle afferents under natural conditions and fusimotor neurones in "reduced" animal preparations confirm that the static and dynamic systems can be differentially activated (for review, see 251; see also Chapter 3). Data are available for jaw, intercostal, and hindlimb muscles. For example, for a cat walking on a beam there is a high level of dynamic fusimotor drive on top of tonic static drive (e.g., 165). Recruitment of presumed static and dynamic fusimotor outflows occurs during stepping in the decerebrate cat and this pattern differs for plantar- and dorsiflexors of the ankle (251), but the extent to which this is reflexly driven is unknown. In humans, static fusimotor neurons seem to be recruited together with the command to α-motoneurons (for references, see 37, 105, 107, 320). During slow shortening contractions, fusimotor drive may be sufficient to keep pace with extrafusal unloading (e.g., 2).

Central interpretation of spindle discharge can be accomplished through a motor command that cancels or "allows for" the expected discharge, leaving only the additional exafference to be evaluated. The progressive attenuation of vibration-induced illusions of movement with voluntary contractions of increasing strength argues for such a mechanism (129, 218). Against this, the entrainment of spindle afferents by the vibration might be suboptimal during contraction [Fig. 4.3; (34, 41)]. "Cancellation" of all fusimotor drive is not trivial, particularly in human subjects, where natural spindle discharge rates are lower than those in the cat.

Tendon Organ Afferents

Golgi tendon organs are uniquely placed to record motor unit forces, and given that primary spindle endings evoke kinesthetic sensations, there is no reason to deny a similar privilege to tendon organs (for review, see 12, 174, 266). Over 90% of tendon organs are located at the musculotendinous junctions, with the remainder in the tendon (12). The latter group could signal whole-muscle force. Commonly fusiform, this encapsulated receptor (up to 1 mm in length and 0.2 mm in diameter) is "in series" with a few muscle fibers and "in parallel" with others inserting around it (338). More muscle fibers join the receptor than leave as collagen bundles at the tendon. The morphology of tendon organs is similar across species (see 174). The number of muscle fibers inserting into a tendon organ ranges from 5–50, with 10–20 being common in humans (30, 187). This innervation includes a mixture of muscle fibers of different motor unit types (137, for reference, see 174). The adequate stimulus for tendon organs seems to be contractile forces acting at the receptor rather than passive stretch. They have lower thresholds for active force than for that produced by passive stretch (e.g., 163). While up to a third may have a background discharge in the cat hindlimb, their discharge fails to increase with passive muscle stretch. Tendon organs in relaxed muscles (of humans and cats) respond poorly to muscle vibration compared with primary spindle endings [Fig. 4.3*B*; (34, 40)].

Each tendon organ is innervated by a single group I afferent, myelinated until close to the receptor, with 98% of receptors receiving one afferent and up to 15% of afferents innervating more than one receptor (12). These Ib afferents have conduction velocities that overlap those of primary muscle spindle afferents but with a fractionally lower mean value (see 236).

No significance has been placed on the ratio of tendon organs to muscle spindles being less than one, although a close anatomical relation between the two main intramuscular receptors has long been recognized. Tendon organ numbers should not be

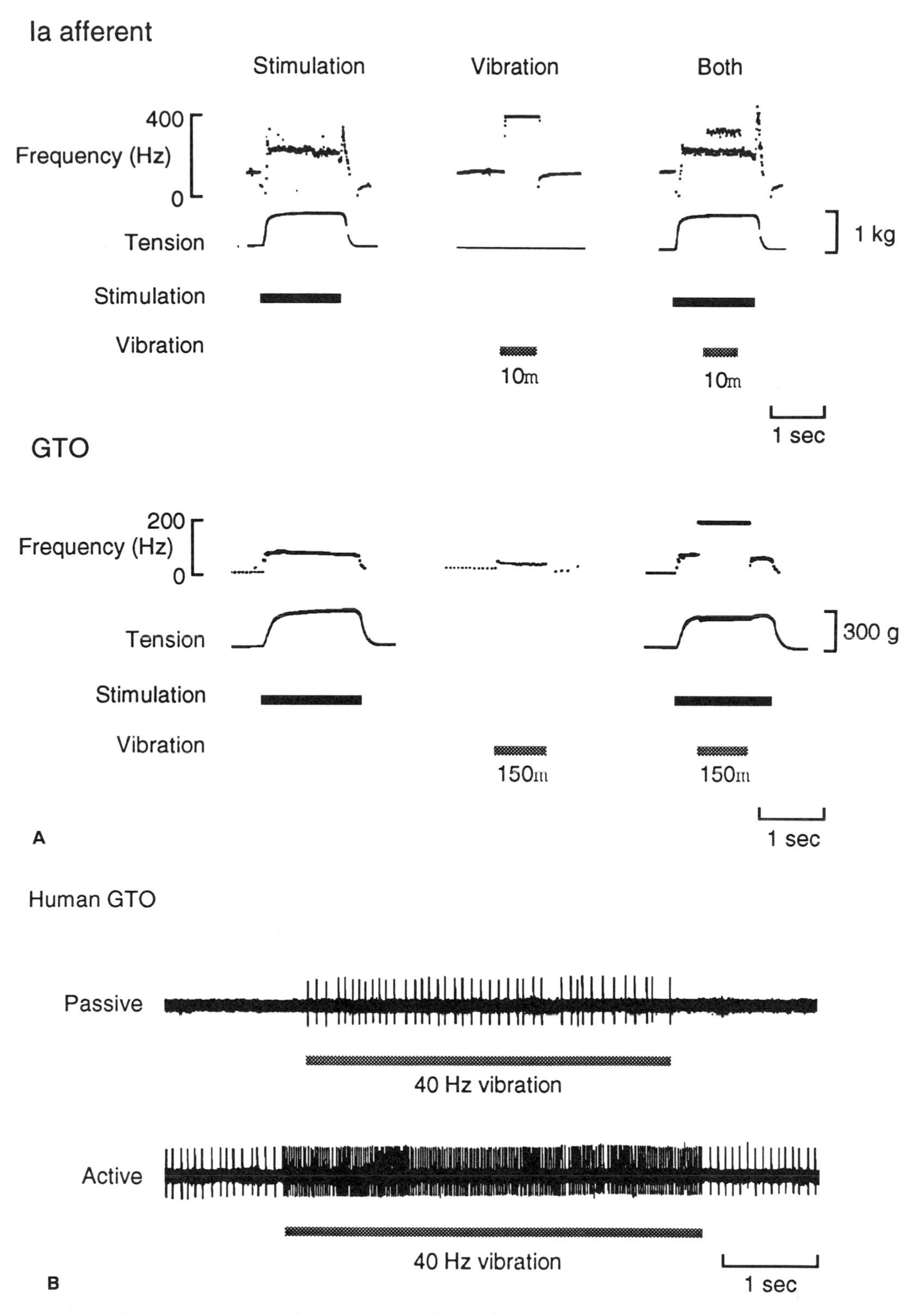

FIG. 4.3. *A*, Comparison between responses of a primary muscle spindle afferent and Golgi tendon organ in the cat soleus muscle to longitudinal vibration under control conditions and during a contraction produced by intense ventral root stimulation. The primary muscle spindle ending follows 1:1 the vibration at 400 Hz (10 m) under control conditions. Its discharge increases during contraction (due to fusimotor activation), but, during combined contraction and vibration, the response is less than under control conditions. The tendon organ requires larger amplitude vibration to respond at rest (200 Hz, 150 m), increases its discharge during muscle contraction, but, during combined contraction and vibration, the response is 1:1 and greater than under the control conditions. (Adapted from Brown, Engberg, and Matthews (34).] *B*, Behavior of a Golgi tendon organ afferent to vibration applied transversely to the tibialis anterior tendon at 40 Hz when the muscle is relaxed (*upper panels*) and during a weak voluntary contraction (*lower panels*). The unit responds at a subharmonic of the vibration frequency during relaxation but responds 1:1 with vibration during the contraction. [From Roll, Vedel, and Ribot (276).] While it is possible that the response of the Golgi tendon organ afferents shown in these two panels represents the extreme of their behavior, nonetheless, some will behave this way under natural conditions.

equated with fine motor control, for they are absent from lumbrical muscles in the monkey hand (71). Elsewhere, tendon organ numbers are crudely proportional to muscle spindle numbers, probably even in the diaphragm, a muscle previously believed to contain a paucity of spindles (11, see 107).

Encoding properties of single tendon organs will depend on several factors, some of which are "before" the receptor. These include the recruitment and discharge frequencies of motor units with fibers inserting into the receptor plus the interaction between focal in-series and in-parallel forces (e.g., 183). Studies on isolated tendon organs suggest that the in-series effect will be influenced by the stiffness of the receptor. Greater compliance confers a lower threshold and sensitivity to static force. Strain on the receptor rather than force is the critical variable (100). The receptor potential itself shows some dynamic sensitivity for small-amplitude stretches (333), with the probability that impulse initiation may occur at more than one site (134). Action potentials can be generated by the contraction of a single fiber in-series with the receptor. If an axon innervates more than one receptor, then discharge "resetting" may occur.

While there are many factors that might thwart a simple proportional relationship between force at the receptor and discharge frequency, this relationship may be relevant for the perception of muscle force. Loading produced by contraction of in-series motor units dominates the discharge of tendon organs and is only masked by unloading from other motor units at very short muscle lengths (135). While a tendon organ responds reproducibily to twitch forces, its discharge is not proportional to the tendon force produced by single motor unit contractions (for references, see 174). Motor units with small as well as large forces produce high discharge frequencies in tendon organs. Under natural conditions, when more than one motor unit contracts, the response of tendon organ and muscle spindle afferents is not the algebraic sum of the discharges produced by the individual motor units, nor do motor unit forces measured at the tendon always add linearly.

The tendon organ has a particular sensitivity to *changes* in contractile force: action potentials are generated as force rises, and unfused motor unit contractions affect their firing more than static forces (174, 175). Even during shortening contractions, tendon organs faithfully transduce force increments during unfused contractions (135, 160). Tendon organ frequency sometimes "steps" up, presumably reflecting recruitment of a new motor unit (e.g., 7, 64, 319). The conventional wisdom asserted that even if a single tendon organ did not respond proportionally to maintained force, the ensemble input from a muscle's complement of tendon organs would mirror active force in the tendon. Jami and colleagues checked this by simultaneously recording from all ten tendon organs innervating the cat peroneus tertius while motor units were stimulated singly or together [Fig. 4.4; 161]. Average discharge frequency fails to increase monotonically with tendon force: when both motor units were stimulated at 40 Hz, force almost doubled, but the average discharge rate was similar to that when motor unit B contracted alone. However, if the CNS monitored the total input from tendon organs, rather than the discharge of an "average" receptor, a near linear relationship between population input and force emerges (Fig. 4.4, *lower panel*). When force develops in contractions of many motor units, the total discharge of tendon organs usually rises smoothly and filters any step changes in frequency with motor unit recruitment (64). During human stance, most tendon organs in tibialis anterior are silent or have low discharge frequencies (<10 Hz) that increase during sway (4). Perhaps effectively high tendon compliance at low contraction forces contributes to the lower discharge rates of both tendon organ and muscle spindle afferents in humans compared with cats (154).

The discharge of tendon organs to muscle stretch during contraction is often overlooked. Once motor units inserting into a tendon organ are active, the receptor cannot distinguish between an increase in active force and that produced by stretch of the muscle. However, during shortening this relation might break down when receptor compliance and muscle length–tension properties contribute. During contractions produced by stimulation of ventral roots, longitudinal tendon vibration "appreciably" increases tendon organ responses, while the sensitivity of spindle primaries "regularly" diminishes despite fusimotor stimulation sufficient to offset any unloading [Fig. 4.3; (34)]. This implies, not just that vibration is an "unclean" stimulus for spindle afferents, but that extraction of pure signals of force and length by reference to inputs from an agonist muscle must require significant central processing. Indeed, psychophysical studies confirm that even with intact antagonist muscles, the two signals cannot be separated perfectly (e.g., 283, 329).

Overall, each tendon organ provides a picture of the static and dynamic force produced by motor units with which it is loaded. This gives an indirect corollary of the final motor command reaching the muscle.

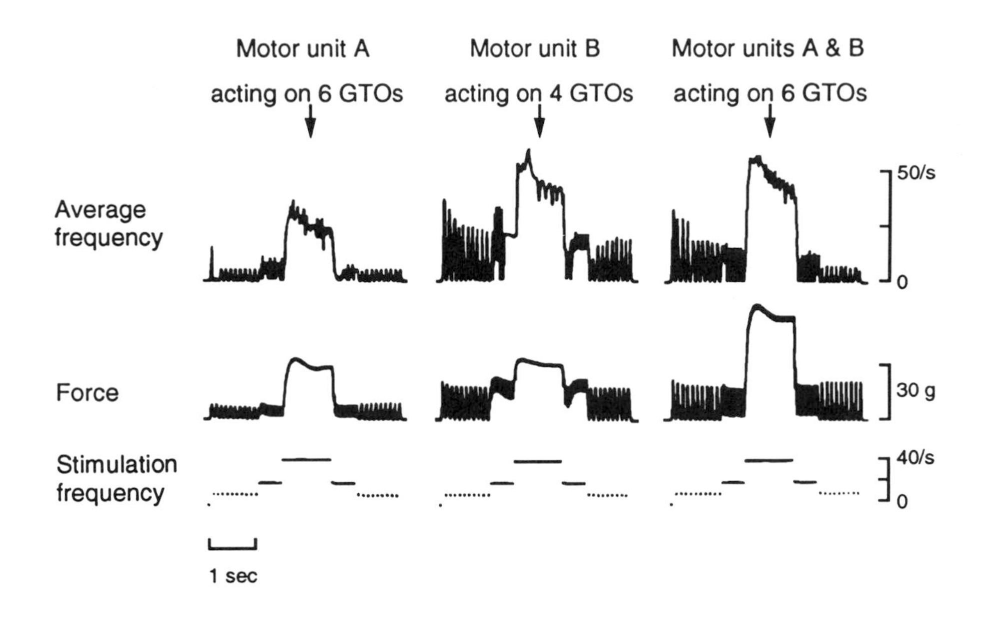

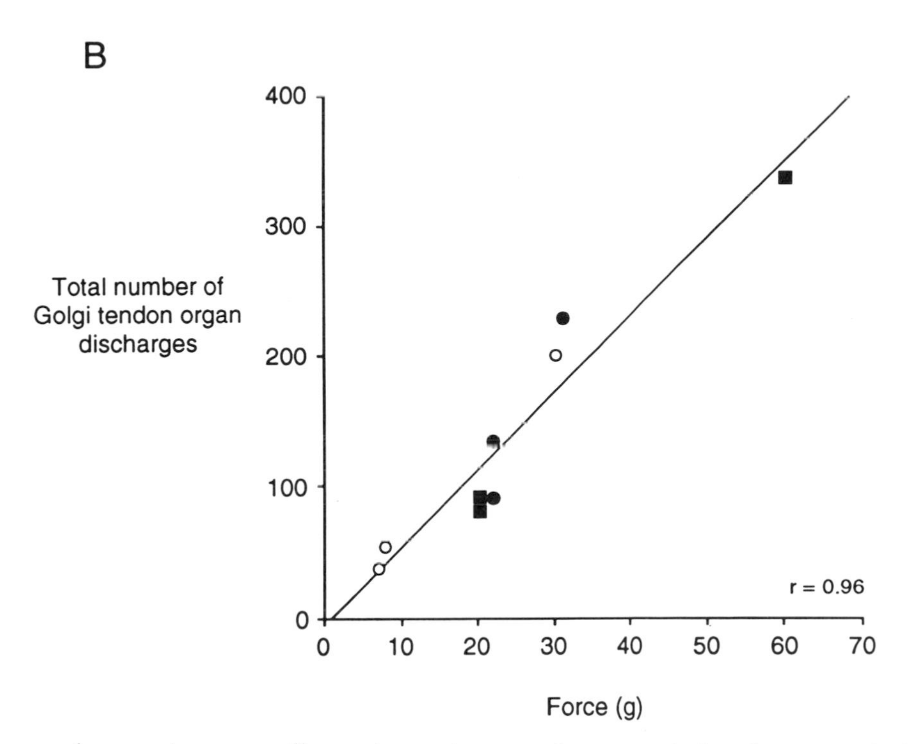

FIG. 4.4. Responses of ten tendon organ afferents innervating peroneus tertius muscle in the cat to motor unit forces produced by stimulation of one or two motor units. *A*, Average tendon organ responses to the forces from motor unit A (*left panel*), motor unit B (*middle panel*), and both motor units (*right panel*). Stimuli given at 10, 20, and 40 Hz. Motor unit A activated six tendon organs and motor unit B activated four tendon organs (shared with motor unit A). Average tendon organ response calculated from the responses of the activated tendon organs. When both motor units contract to 40 Hz stimulation, force at the tendon adds as expected from the algebraic sum of the force to each motor unit, but the average discharge frequency does not exceed that when unit 2 contracts alone. Note that in the *right panel* the average tendon organ response to stimulation of both motor units at 20 Hz is less after the tetanus at 40 Hz. [Adapted from Jami (174).] *B*, Predicted ensemble response for the data in part A of the figure when the *total number* of tendon organ discharges is calculated (from their average discharge and the number activated). This has been estimated for the tetani produced by 40 Hz stimuli and the two sets of 20 Hz stimuli. Total tendon organ input increases very well with tendon force.

Joint Afferents

All intra-articular structures such as ligaments, disks and menisci are innervated by small- and large-diameter afferents. The specialized receptors include varieties of Ruffini and Golgi endings, both slowly adapting, and Pacinian and smaller paciniform endings, which are rapidly adapting (for review, see 27, 269, 299, 339). Their distribution is nonuniform within a joint. This may reflect the location of stresses, and the type of receptor may match these stresses. For example, the articular parts of the larynx are innervated mostly by paciniform afferents. The major kinesthetic innervation will include some Golgi (tendon) organs in ligaments and subcapsular tissues, and predominantly Ruffini endings in the fibrous capsule. Golgi afferents respond to compressive forces normal to the capsular surface, while the Ruffini afferents respond to planar forces (141, 142).

Recordings while a joint is probed or moved have disclosed slowly and rapidly adapting discharges, even in unmyelinated afferents. In the cat, single-unit properties have been described for many joints including the knee, elbow, wrist, and temporomandibular joint (for references, see 220, 269). There has been much less study of single-joint afferents in primates.

Two limitations affect studies of the properties and projections of joint afferents. First, unless the joint capsule is exposed, it is hard to identify joint afferents definitively during neural recordings. This procedure is not feasible in human studies. Second, joint afferents run only short distances in their "own" nerve before joining conventional "muscle," "cutaneous," or "mixed" nerves. Hence, the purity of nerve trunks is questionable and "joint" nerves contain occasional large-diameter muscle afferents (226).

Responses Across the Angular Range. Joint afferents cannot contribute to sensations of joint position and movement if they do not discharge to these stimuli. Initial studies in the 1950s reported slowly adapting signals of absolute joint angle and velocity of passive movement in the middle of the range of knee movement in the cat. By contrast, Burgess and Clark (35, see also 52) found that less than 5% of joint afferents were active in this range and ascribed these to spindle afferents from the popliteus muscle. Ferrell (86) subsequently found that 18% of slowly adapting units discharged tonically in the midrange, even after removal of the fleshy part of the popliteus muscle [although this will not remove all its tendon organs; (133)]. Units that began to discharge within the midrange increased their firing towards one angular extreme and had receptive fields in the joint capsule or cruciate ligaments. Units that discharged predominantly at the extremes commonly had receptive fields in the capsule. While units with receptive fields in the anterior cruciate ligament discharged during movements within the working range of motion, they fired more with stresses against the resistance of joint structures (200). Fewer than 2% of knee joint afferents responded monotonically across the angular range in the monkey and they may have been popliteus muscle afferents (140). While discrepancies in the various studies remain, a consensus is that the "majority of slowly adapting receptors discharged near the extremes of movement and maintained a steady adapted discharge when the limb was held at an extreme position" (86).

Two microneurographic studies have examined the properties of human joint afferents. In the first, recordings were made from afferents in the median and ulnar nerve (39). Identification was based on a slowly adapting discharge to focal pressure (400 mN) over the known joint capsule but no response to cutaneous stimuli. Of 120 afferents, 15% fulfilled these criteria. One-third had a background discharge. Passive movement to the end of a range produced little change in firing unless hyperflexion or hyperextension was applied. Many could not signal joint angle unambiguously and responded at both ends of the physiological range (Fig. 4.5). A response to stress in more than one axis of rotation was common. A monotonic discharge across the usual angular range occurred in only two afferents. The population input from the digital joints projecting in the median and ulnar nerves would contain some information about position and movement in the normal range but much more on movement towards an abnormal extreme of joint motion. This study excluded units with receptive fields over joints that also responded to cutaneous stimuli, and this may have removed some afferents with a midrange discharge. Afferents in the superficial radial nerve behave differently (77). Of 148 afferents, 8 innervated joint receptors with tactile receptive fields "close" to joints. Seven were classified as subcutaneous afferents. All but one were related to the metacarpophalangeal joint of the thumb and responded to low focal forces (~10 mN) and increased their discharge monotonically with flexion beginning at 0–30 degrees of flexion, with little or no response to extension. The discrepancy between the two studies is not simply due to criteria for classification, because relatively few receptors in the glabrous skin respond across the movement range (39, 166). The simplest explanation is that the population of joint afferents

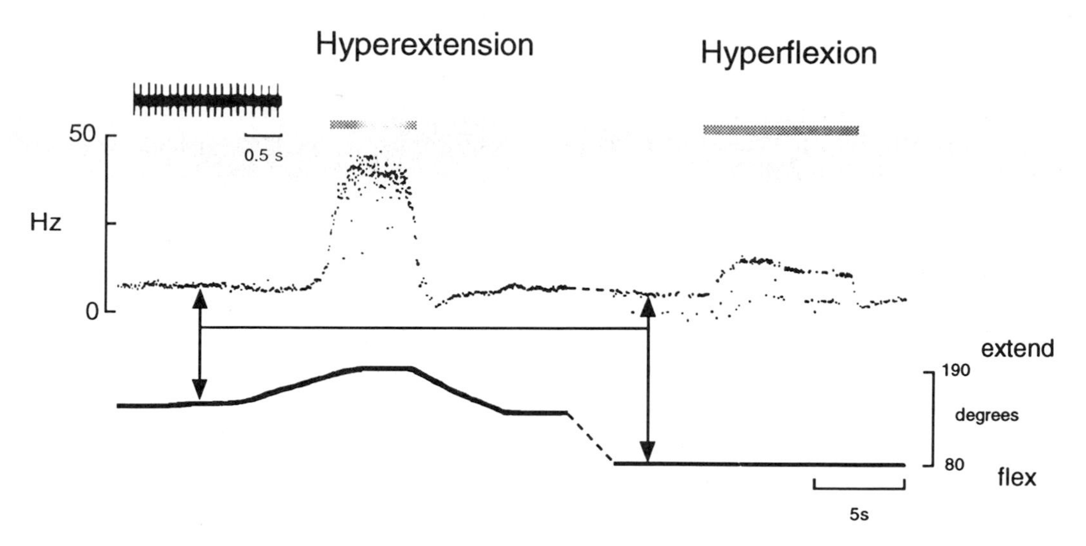

FIG. 4.5. Behavior of a joint afferent from the proximal interphalangeal joint of the index finger recorded from the median nerve. Responses during passive rotation in the flexion-extension axis. *Inset* shows a tonic discharge when the joint was in the rest position. *Upper trace*, Instantaneous frequency. *Lower trace*, Goniometer record. Note the sustained high-frequency discharge when the joint was moved into extreme extension, with no change in background discharge when it moved into flexion but a sustained discharge when forced into extreme flexion. Many receptors of this type also responded to movements in the abduction-adduction or extorsion-intorsion axis. [Adapted from Burke, Gandevia, and Macefield (39).]

in the radial nerve differs from that in the other nerves.

Effects of Muscle Contraction. An effect of muscle contraction on joint receptor discharge might be expected, given the anatomical proximity between muscles, tendons, and joints, although it would complicate the interpretation of their signals. Three changes have been reported. First, the background discharge increases monotonically with active or passive force with the joint fixed. For example, for the monkey knee, 68% of units active at the limit of extension responded to gastrocnemius contractions, and 29% responded to quadriceps contractions (140). Second, muscle contraction increases the angular range over which afferents respond to passive movement. Such receptors would signal not only joint angle but also muscle force. However, the magnitude of the effect is not accepted. Baxendale and Ferrell (19) found no effect of increased muscle tone on midrange discharge from elbow joint afferents in the cat. Joint afferents seem to need high muscle force for activation, although this varies depending on which muscles contract, receptor location, and joint angle. While the force thresholds at the knee exceed those usually associated with passive movement, they would not be outside the ranges during locomotion. The forces for the hand might be lower (77; Macefield and Johansson, unpublished results). Third, for joint afferents innervating the dorsum of the thumb, due to the location of the extensor tendon and the surface of the joint, half the units behaved oppositely to active and passive movements (77). Thus, they discharged during extension not flexion. This would severely degrade their ability to signal absolute joint position.

In conclusion, some specialized joint receptors signal angular position and movement within the usual range, but the population input will increase when stress on the joint is increased by reaching the extremes of movement. The majority of receptors respond to stresses in more than one axis of joint "movement," so that, in isolation, they do not provide unambiguous signals of joint position. Muscular contraction might further lessen their capacity to signal absolute position but cause more of them to discharge in the usual range and thus to encode muscle force.

Cutaneous Afferents

Cutaneous receptors embedded in a multilayered glove covering the skeleton are well placed to signal movement of the underlying skeleton. However, their capacity to generate perceived signals of joint position and movements is less well developed than for the other kinesthetic afferents. A brief description of the major cutaneous afferents follows, with emphasis on their kinesthetic potential (for review, see 70, 170, 250).

Human nonhairy (glabrous) skin contains four major specialized receptor classes: two rapidly adapting, one associated with Meissner's corpuscles (termed RA), and the other with Pacinian corpuscles (PC); together with two slowly adapting, one associated with Merkel disks (SA I) and the other with Ruffini endings (SA II). Innervation density increases along the extremity, being much higher for the finger pulp than the palm, a distribution that conforms with the gradient of tactile discrimination. The preponderance of specialized input from the pad of the digits occurs, especially for the SA I and RA units (e.g., 179, 210). In human digital nerves, these receptor classes have afferents with indistinguishable conduction velocities, all in the 20–60 m/s range (e.g., 234).

Human hairy skin contains (guard) hairs that are multiply innervated by nonencapsulated hair-follicle receptors (250). Hair units are rapidly adapting and have larger receptive fields than the two SA receptor types. An additional rapidly adapting "field" unit has been described but its endings have not been unequivocally identified. The SA receptors are Merkel cell receptors grouped under visible touch domes, and the Ruffini endings occur usually with hairs. Pacinian corpuscles occur rarely except around joints, tendon sheaths, and interosseous membranes. With the exception of afferents from hair follicles and Pacinian corpuscles, the specialized receptors have circumscribed receptive fields. The distribution and properties of receptors within the human hairy skin vary at different locations (321).

In primates, the Merkel cell afferent (SA I) is found within the epidermis of both glabrous and hairy skin, with the afferent branching to form the disk below the specialized epithelial Merkel cell. In glabrous skin, they attach to keratinocytes and are found near sweat ducts, the rete pegs at the bottom of the epidermal ridges, and in groups in the rete ridge. Each Merkel cell receives one afferent that innervates many cells. In human hairy skin, groups of Merkel cells with a single afferent occur below elevated touch pads. The afferent discharge is slowly adapting, and irregular. For the hand, the afferent fibers have multiple small, receptive fields (2–3 mm diameter) and respond poorly to remote skin stretch (see 170). Some show directional sensitivity. They have a low threshold to vertical indentation and are well suited to provide static and dynamic cues about surface texture and shape. While they can respond to local vibration of the skin over a similar bandwidth to the Pacinian corpuscle (325), central processing seems to exclude them from contributing to vibration sensibility.

The encapsulated receptors are found within the dermis and have variable numbers of lamellae, from three to four in Ruffini endings to 60–70 in Pacinian corpuscles. Ruffini endings (SA II) are innervated by a single afferent [6–12 mm diameter, (50)] that may supply other endings. The receptor, anchored via collagen fibers at its poles, allows dermal tension to reach the receptor. Their receptive fields are less well defined than the SA I units and are often oriented longitudinally in the limb. Their discharge to skin stretch is characteristically regular (for references, see 78). SA II units also respond faithfully to high frequencies of vibration, provided that the stimulus is precisely located (148). Under natural conditions they will respond to focal stimuli due to contact with the skin, plus local and remote stretch of the skin (Fig. 4.6).

The Pacinian corpuscle is the largest cutaneous receptor, up to 1–4 mm in length and 0.5–1 mm in diameter. The capsule and inner core act as high-pass filters, giving the receptor features suited to mediate the sensation of vibration (e.g., 249). It has a 1:1 fiber-to-receptor ratio, with about 600 in the human hand, 120/cm^2 of finger pulp (70). Their receptive fields are large and units will often discharge to a tap anywhere on the hand.

The recently evolved Meissner's corpuscles (RA) reside in dermal papillae and are innervated by two to nine fibers. In the finger pulp they occur every two to three ridges, less frequently in the palm, with rudimentary forms on the back of the digit. Their discharge is greater for stimuli along rather than across the dermal ridges and they adapt rapidly to focal pressure and are preferentially tuned to local vibration in the 30–40 Hz range (e.g., 307). Their sensitivity to the velocity of indentation makes them well suited to encode the sharpness of edges and to detect elevations such as Braille characters (see 207). The velocity of indentation required to generate an impulse is higher than that for SA units.

With the possible exception of SA II units, inputs from the other major cutaneous receptors provide perceptual information about the contact, shape, size, and texture of surfaces (e.g., 128). For many judgments of texture, no one class of cutaneous afferent responds to selectively that it alone explains the psychophysical capacities. This type of conclusion is likely to apply also to kinesthetic judgments.

Kinesthetic Properties of Cutaneous Afferents. Three studies have examined the possibility that cutaneous afferents signal joint position and movement. In the first, Hulliger and colleagues (166) examined the responses of afferents innervating the glabrous skin of the hand to voluntary movements of the fingers. Virtually all PC and SA II units, and two-thirds of RA and SA I units, responded to voluntary finger move-

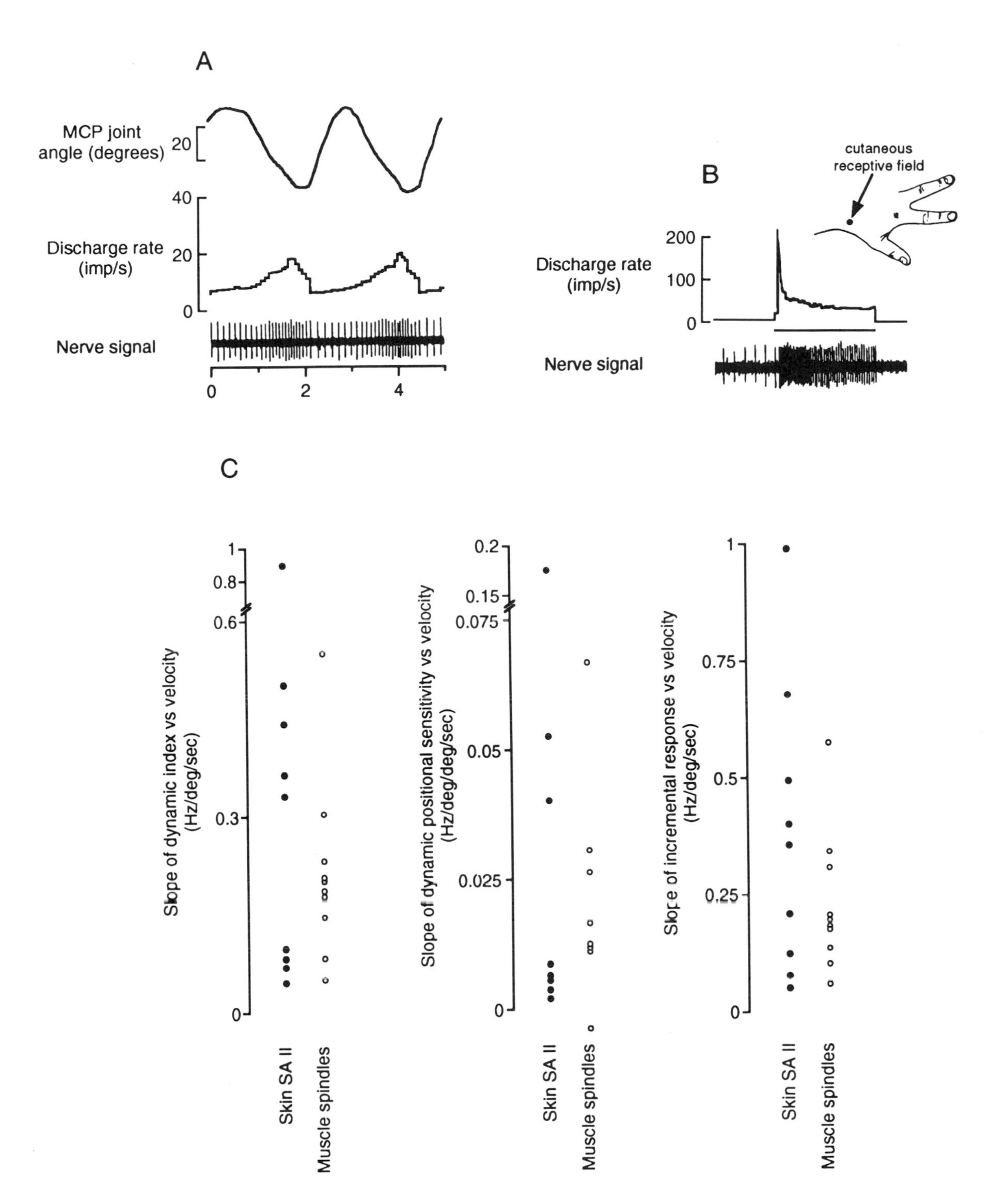

FIG. 4.6. *A*, Responses of a typical SA II afferent innervating the skin on the dorsum of the hand during voluntary flexion and extension of the metacarpophalangeal joint of the index finger. *B*, The receptive field and response to focal indentation of the skin. Despite its "remote" location, the afferent responds to the voluntary movements. [Adapted from Edin and Abbs (79).] *C*, Summary of the responsiveness of a sample of SA II cutaneous afferents innervating the dorsum of the hand and muscle spindle afferents from extensors of the index finger to movement of the metacarpophalangeal joint of the index finger with the muscles relaxed. The three vertical axes refer to different methods of measuring the static and dynamic sensitivity of the afferents to applied movements. [From Grill and Hallett (143).]

ments. Responses were similar for movements and for focal cutaneous stimuli in the receptive field. The total number of discharges decreased as the frequency of a cyclical voluntary movement increases from 1 Hz to 5 Hz, but many units still responded to slow movements (<0.75 Hz). Ramp movements of the whole finger from an intermediate position to full flexion or extension produced a mean discharge of only three to six impulses. Most RA and PC units (87%) responded to *both* flexion and extension, while half the SA population had directionally specific behavior. An estimate of movement responsiveness showed the ranking from greatest to least: PC, SA II, SA I, and RA. With the hand relaxed, the only cutaneous units with a background discharge were SA IIs, with one-third spontaneously active. A static response to ajoint position occurred for 81% of SA IIs and 17% of SA Is. Of 21 SA units, 12 increased their discharge towards full extension, 3 towards full flexion, and the remainder showed no change: increases in discharge occurred "only in extreme angular positions."

In a comparable study of passive movements, Burke and colleagues (39) confirmed that most SA units in the nonhairy skin of the hand were activated by movement and that their static responses to angular position occurred "towards the limits of joint rotation." Two-thirds of the SA units had directional specificity, but the remainder discharged in extreme flexion and extension. A quarter responded to movements in more than one movement axis. Thus, while many rapidly adapting units discharge to small movements and serve as peripheral timing markers, they lack directional and angular specificity. Slowly adapting responses, particularly from SA II units, occurred across the angular range, towards one or more extreme of movement. Central processing would be required to establish which extreme, given that some units respond multiaxially. During the static phase of holding an object with the fingers and thumb, the SA IIs show a tonic modulation with grasp force (see 331). Such behavior makes the glabrous skin afferents less attractive as monitors of joint angle and velocity.

As hairy skin moves freely with underlying bony movement, their receptors have a kinesthetic advantage. Receptors on the back of the hand discharge with finger movements. SA units discharged during flexion and reduced their discharge during extension (78, 79). Their cutaneous receptive fields were not necessarily directly over the joints whose movement excited them (Fig. 4.6). Of 42 SA units, 13 discharged only for movements of the metacarpophalangeal joint of the index, 9 for movement at only the adjacent joint of the middle finger, and 3 for the metacaropophalangeal joint of the thumb. The remaining 17 units discharged to movement at more than one joint in a digit (ten units) or to movement of more than one digit (seven units). Because of their location, some SA units discharged in a complex way, to flexion at the metacarpophalangeal joint but extension at the proximal interphalangeal joint. Hysteresis was marked. In terms of strict angular sensitivity, the SA IIs respond as well to movements at the index metacarpophalangeal joint as presumed primary spindle afferents [Fig. 4.6C; 143]. Both afferent sources may contribute to the ability to detect small changes in the thickness of objects held between the index finger and thumb, an ability initially ascribed to muscle afferents alone (180).

As passive muscle spindle afferents respond uniaxially across the angular range and as there are more than enough muscles to cover the degrees of freedom at a joint, they are probably better suited to provide kinesthetic signals of joint movement, although a contribution from remote SA IIs cannot be ruled out. However, their input is less able to provide specific information about one joint without central "solving" for possible ambiguities.

Possible Kinesthetic Role for Group III and IV Fibers

Small-diameter afferents conducting in the group III and IV range transduce mechanical, chemical, and thermal nociceptive stimuli, although many remain apparently unresponsive to natural stimuli. They represent a large fraction of skin, joint, and muscle afferents. Some small-diameter muscle inputs could provide information about the disposition of the limbs including the degree of muscle stretch, muscle force, and fatigue. This is hard to establish directly because it is difficult to stimulate them in a selective or natural way.

Group III muscle afferents, as characterized by Paintal (259) and others (57, 82), respond better to local pressure than muscle stretch, with their receptive fields preferentially near tendons or motor points in different muscles. Some afferents discharge during muscle contractions and respond to innocuous stimuli such as pressure (82). Stimuli for the group IV muscle afferents are multifarious, with some discharging seconds after muscle stretch, and others responding with different delays to muscle contractions (196). Even if sensitivity to innocuous pressure occurs rarely, it will recruit a large number of receptors. Most afferent units respond to more than one stimulus, so that any distinction between mechanoreceptive and chemosensitive units is problematic. Ischemic contractions are a potent stimulus for group IV afferents (240).

The skin contains C-fiber mechanoreceptive units with restricted receptive fields and lower mechanical thresholds than the more numerous C-nociceptor units. Some respond merely to brushing the skin and discharge on stimulus removal. For human hairy skin, about 40% of touch-sensitive units are low-threshold C fibers (323). Innocuous mechanical stimuli generated surprisingly high discharge rates (up to 100 Hz) despite conduction velocities of only 1 m/s. Subjects can accurately localize areas from which C-fiber activity is evoked (e.g., 186, 256). Thus these afferents are not excluded from providing some ancillary kinesthetic cues due to poor spatial coding. When the major kinesthetic inputs are lost, as in large-fiber sensory neuropathies, the small-fiber inputs will take on a larger role (see later under DEAFFERENTATION). Temperature changes in the armpit can signal that the arm is abducted.

Cortical Projections

Electrophysiological studies in the 1950s denied a cortical projection for muscle afferents and corroborated their exclusion from kinesthesia, while joint afferents had long been known to project to the cortex based on electrical stimulation of "joint" nerves. In 1958, Amassian and Berlin (3) demonstrated a cortical receiving area for group I inputs from the cat forelimb, and this was soon confirmed in primates (for review, see 220, 262, 332, 337). A specific projection for Ib afferents was also established in the cat (227). In brief, groups Ia, Ib, and II muscle afferents have short-latency projections to the contralateral somatosensory cortex, particularly area 3a (and thence to areas 1 and 2), but also to area 4 (motor cortex). The afferent route to the motor cortex is controversial but includes a projection from area 3a (see 264). The projection of muscle afferents from the lower limb involves the dorsolateral funiculus and thence to nucleus Z with collaterals to the cerebellum, while that from the upper limb includes the traditional dorsal column pathway.

Cells in the somatosensory and motor cortex of primates discharge to joint movement (for references, see 262, 264). Cells respond to static or dynamic components of muscle stretch (162). Whether this reflects differential projections of primary and secondary spindle endings is unknown. During voluntary contractions, the discharge of up to half the relevant motor cortical neurons encodes changes in force (see 177, 330), but this will not reflect only an afferent force signal. In humans, passive movement of joints as well as selective stimulation of muscle afferents evokes somatosensory cortical potentials (e.g., 42, 106). Attempts have followed to confirm a cortical projection from tendon organs with "selective" stimulation of Ib afferents (281), but the technique is insufficiently sensitive because the transverse vibration used to raise the electrical threshold of primary spindle afferents will not recruit them with certainty (see 63).

Features of the projections are becoming clear. First, it is impossible to deny any class of afferent a kinesthetic role on the basis of its projection to the cerebral cortex. Second, convergence along the afferent pathways and at cortical levels is the rule rather than the exception, particularly if intracellular recordings are used. Thus, the dorsal spinocerebellar tract, long believed to project modality-specific information from muscle receptors from the hindlimb, receives complex polysynaptic convergence from cutaneous and other inputs (e.g., 228, 257). Third, cortical cells and those at relay nuclei also receive corticofugal signals that alter their properties during movement. Cutaneous transmission diminishes in proportion to movement velocity (for references, see 178), but the degree to which this is due to subtle differences in attention or afferent input is hard to disentangle. Psychophysical studies confirm that cutaneous stimuli are harder to detect during and just before movement (for references, 243, 265, 290). Changes before movement must be due to corticofugal gating. Although the neural circuitry exists, enhancement of relevant kinesthetic and tactile signals during active movement has so far received only modest support from electrophysiological studies. Reductions in thresholds for movement detection during muscle contraction are explicable by an enhanced input from intramuscular receptors (see later under KINESTHETIC MECHANISMS IN ISOLATION).

KINESTHETIC MECHANISMS IN ISOLATION

Illusions Produced by Stimulation of Kinesthetic Afferents

Vibration of muscles and tendons activates muscle spindle afferents (see earlier under PROPERTIES OF KINESTHETIC AFFERENTS) and produces illusory changes in joint position. First reported in 1972, these illusions reestablished a kinesthetic role for muscle receptors [Table 4.1; (129)]. Major features of these illusions are set out below.

1. Vibration produces illusory movements consistent with perceived lengthening of the vibrated mus-

cle. They begin at short latency, continue as long as the input, and carry the limb into "impossible" positions (65). Thus, the CNS "extends" the body schema in response to the artificial barrage from muscle spindle afferents. The velocity of the illusion increases with vibration frequency (e.g., 129, 275, 276), but decreases at the highest frequency, presumably because fewer afferents stay "entrained" [Fig. 4.7*A*; (63)].

2. There is also an illusion of altered position with vibration. The distortion is about 10 degrees for elbow flexors vibrated at 100 Hz (129). This remains while the "velocity" component diminishes if vibration frequency decreases and amplitude increases (218). Such maneuvers enhance the contribution from secondary spindle endings.

3. Vibration-induced discharges in muscle afferents from agonist or antagonist muscles disturb motor tasks that depend upon knowledge of joint angle (e.g., 47). Errors are less obvious when the agonist is vibrated during shortening because the mechanical coupling to its spindles is insecure. The velocity of the final illusion reflects the difference in inputs from agonist and antagonist muscle spindles [Fig. 4.7*B*; (124)].

4. Voluntary contractions diminish or even abolish the vibration illusions (129, 218). It is as if the voluntarily induced fusimotor activation "occludes" the spindle response to vibration during strong contractions and the CNS considers only the discharge rate in excess of that from the voluntary contraction (i.e., a corollary motor command cancels a component of the spindle discharge) [Fig. 4.1; (see also 85)]. Reduced entrainment of spindle afferents and increased entrainment of Golgi tendon organs during vibration and contraction may also contribute (Fig. 4.3).

5. The abnormal spindle input is judged in its behavioral context (see later under FUNCTIONAL ASPECTS OF KINESTHESIA). Thus, if the elbow flexors are vibrated when the finger touches the nose, the nose appears to elongate (e.g., 202); if the neck extensors are vibrated, the head and visualized targets move down into flexion (e.g., 277); and if the arm is vibrated in the dark, a light projected from it appears to move (e.g., 74).

Electrical Stimulation of Muscle, Joint, and Cutaneous Afferents

Few studies have assessed kinesthetic illusions with electrical stimulation. However, in one study stimulation of the ulnar nerve produced complex illusory movements of the fingers, without cutaneous paresthesias or activation of motor axons (102). Illusions were consistent with lengthening of the intrinsic muscles. This extended results from muscle vibration. First, coding could be investigated without uncertainty as to the afferent discharge rate: the velocity of the illusion increased linearly with the stimulation frequency (Fig. 4.7C). Second, as even a single synchronized volley produced an illusory movement, spatial but not temporal summation was necessary. Third, as the illusions involved ulnar-innervated intrinsic muscles acting on the thumb, index finger, and middle finger, they must have been induced by muscle rather than cutaneous afferents. This counters the argument that the vibratory illusions reflect activation of remote cutaneous afferents (246). Finally, muscle afferents activated below motor threshold (presumably from primary endings) produce a simultaneous movement and position illusion. Thus, a muscle afferent input can be processed in terms of more than one physical variable.

Stimulation of digital nerves (innervating the skin and interphalangeal joints) produces an illusory twisting of joints or an oscillation: the joints do not move through a large angular range, a finding consistent with the paucity of cutaneous and joint afferents responding in this range (102). By contrast, stimulation of the superficial radial nerve (innervating skin on the dorsum of the hand and some underlying joints) produces illusions of smooth flexion, akin to a grasp, involving the metacarpophalangeal joints with or without flexion at the interphalangeal joints of the thumb and index finger (104). This may involve joint and/or cutaneous afferents given that, in this nerve, both discharge across the angular range (see earlier under PROPERTIES OF KINESTHETIC AFFERENTS).

Microstimulation of Single Afferents. Stimulation of a single identified afferent in a subject who reports the sensation is a way to check both the afferent's perceptual potency and specificity. Recordings from hair follicle afferents in the exposed superficial radial nerve of volunteers suggested that the stimulus for sensation was "of the same order" as for the afferent fibers and so "[a] few impulses, possibly even a single impulse, are sufficient to evoke a conscious sensation" (153). Microneurographic recordings from afferents innervating the fingertips supported this conclusion: thresholds for the detection of an indentation paralleled those for an action potential in PC and RA units. Proximal to the midpalm, units had similar mechanical thresholds but higher psychophysical thresholds; this implies that spatial summation was required (e.g., 179).

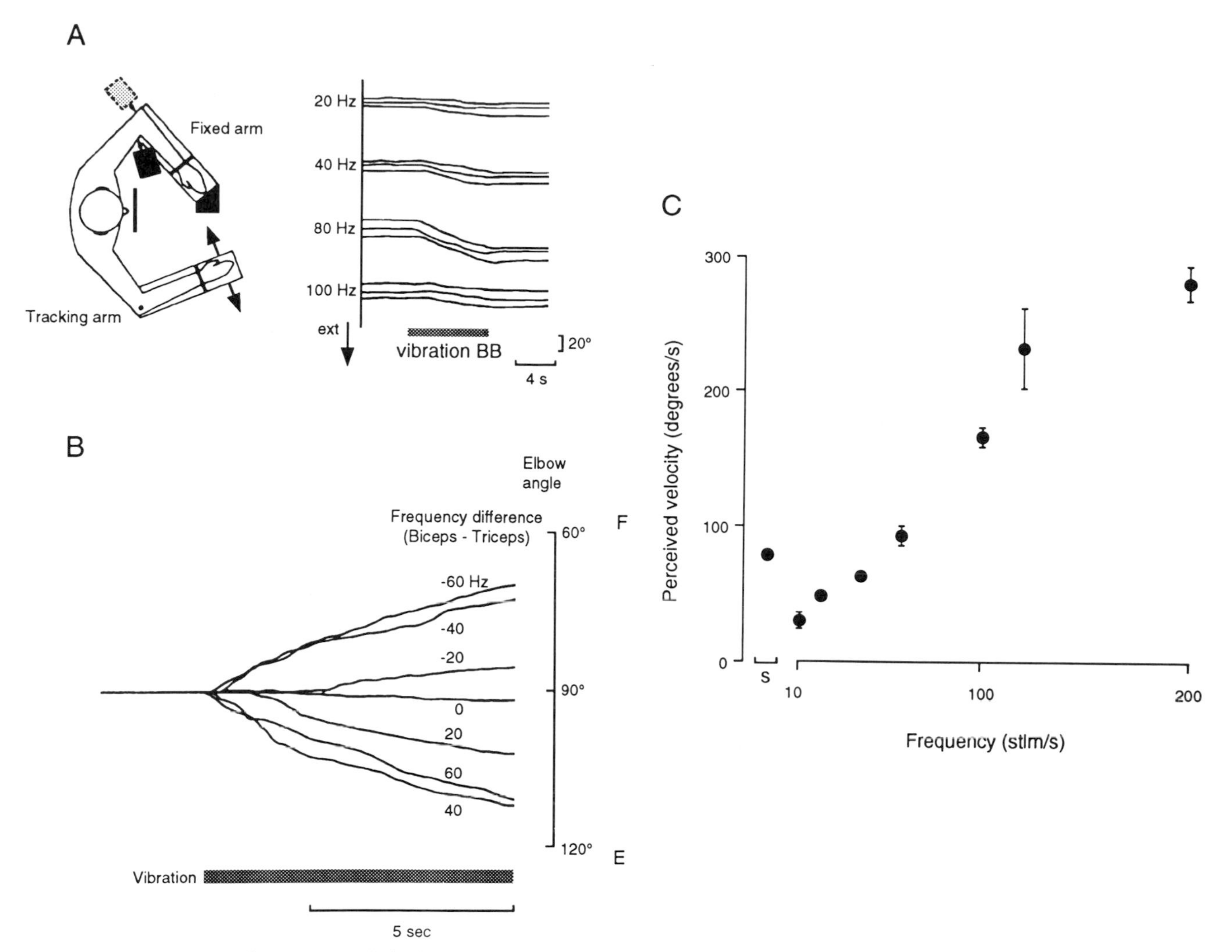

FIG. 4.7. *A*, Movement illusions recorded when vibrators are applied to the distal tendons of the left biceps brachii and triceps brachii. Left arm is fixed and the right (tracking arm) is mobile and connected to a goniometer. The subject matches the perceived movement during vibration of the biceps tendon at different frequencies. The speed of the illusory extension movement increases with vibration frequency but diminishes at the highest frequency, presumably because the primary spindle afferents no longer follow 1:1 the vibrator frequency. [Adapted from Roll and Vedel (275).] *B*, Superimposed data from one subject for combinations of vibration applied simultaneously to the biceps and triceps muscles. Perceived movement of the vibrated arm depends on the difference in frequencies of vibration, with an illusory movement of extension when the vibration frequency is greater for the flexors than extensors. [Adapted from Gilhodes, Roll, and Tardy-Gervet (124).] *C*, During trains of stimuli delivered to the ulnar nerve at the wrist (below motor threshold and without inducing cutaneous paresthesias), the subject experienced illusory flexion of the interphalangeal joints and extension of the metacarpophalangeal (MCP) joint. The complex illusory motion at three joints is consistent with perceived elongation of the interosseous and lumbrical muscles acting on the ring finger. The component at the MCP joint was measured with matching movements on the contralateral side. Relationship between stimulus frequency and perceived velocity for one subject. By comparison with *A*, the illusory movement (mean ± SEM) increases progressively even at stimulus frequencies above 100/s. This suggests that mechanical entrainment of spindle afferent discharge is impaired at higher vibration frequencies. [Reproduced from Gandevia (102) and Gandevia and Burke (107).]

Since proof that the mechanical stimuli activated only *one* afferent is lacking, electrical stimulation through the microelectrode was tried. Reports from two laboratories indicated that stimulus intensities of about 1 mA applied near large-diameter cutaneous afferents in the median nerve yielded consistent tactile sensations. Sensations were projected to the receptive fields of the afferents that were believed to be stimulated: a tap, flutter, or vibratory sensation depending on stimulus frequency for RA units; vibration or tickle for PC units; local pressure or indentation for SA I afferents; and no sensations for SA II afferents (see 255, 287, 322). RA but not SA I units evoked percepts with single stimuli. A third laboratory confirmed the results for cutaneous stimuli and reported that microstimulation of joint but not muscle spindle afferent sites evoked sensations (231). Single stimuli produced deep punctate sensations referred to the joint region and were consistent with the receptive field. At some sites trains of stimuli yielded movement sensations involving motion or joint twisting. The illusory movements were usually small and in the direction with the largest afferent response. They were in the midrange rather than at the limits of joint rotation where they discharged most vigorously (see earlier under PROPERTIES OF KINESTHETIC AFFERENTS).

Stimulation of spindle afferents from intrinsic hand muscles evoked no sensations at intensities subthreshold for movement. Despite stimulation within motor fascicles, the sensations sometimes had a tactile quality (e.g., the skin on the back of the hand stretched or fingertips touched) (231). Two SA II receptors near the fingernail responded to passive flexion of the terminal joint and produced illusory flexion on stimulation. Hence, some single-joint afferents and SA II cutaneous afferents definitely evoke kinesthetic sensations. As muscle spindle afferents produced no comparable sensations, spatial summation is necessary for their kinesthetic role.

Results obtained with microstimulation of cutaneous afferents ran contrary to pattern theories of cutaneous sensation, and the psychophysical and stimulus procedures were criticized (327). However, the stimulus intensity required for the sensations is identical to that for activation of a single axion in animals, the sensations occur whether microstimulation is performed before or after mapping the receptive fields (318), the stimulated axon develops post-tetanic hyperexcitability, and its discharge has been monitored proximally in simultaneous recordings (255). Finally, the probability that SA II afferents would be shown to elicit no cutaneous sensations by three independent investigators is remote. While microneurography electrodes undoubtedly produce conduction block in some afferents, stimulation of single axons remains a valid approach.

Sensations of Joint Position and Movement

Signals of both position and velocity are used to execute movement (22). Sensation of these signals has usually been measured by matching the position of homologous joints on both sides of the body or detecting applied movements and their direction. Because changes in movement and position cannot be dissociated, it is hard to separate the responsible neural mechanisms. Joint displacements can be detected with very slow rotations that cause no overt sensation of movement (155). If detection of a set angular displacement does not deteriorate at progressively lower velocities, then a "static-position" sense exists (53, 54) and must depend on kinesthetic signals with pure position sensitivity.

"Position" sense or detection of exceedingly slow movements (<2 degrees/min) has been measured at knee, ankle, and finger joints (53, 54, 88, 312). One group argued this depended on muscle spindle afferents because nerve blocks affecting some muscle afferents impaired it (54, 56). The sensation seemed absent for the proximal interphalangeal joint, but others disagreed. Both interphalangeal and metacarpophalangeal joints had similar detection thresholds (312). Co-contraction of finger muscles at the final position, or positioning the hand to disengage muscles acting on the distal joint, but did not change detection thresholds significantly (Fig. 4.8). Thus, cutaneous and joint afferents can signal static position.[1] If muscle receptors provide such a signal, it is duplicated by joint and cutaneous inputs. A true position sense will be heightened towards the angular extremes when more joint and cutaneous afferents discharge. Sometimes, perceptual conflict may arise: skin anesthesia around the knee improved accuracy in some judgments suggesting that cutaneous afferents activated by the device displacing the limb provided a false cue (56, 159). No specific role for cutaneous afferents in position sense has yet been shown although some contribution seems likely. An indirect argument against them is that sensations of cutaneous pressure adapt more rapidly than those of joint position (159).

Other Aspects of "position" Sense. Other aspects of the putative static position sense give clues about underlying neural mechanisms.

1. Disagreement still exists about the ability of muscle afferents to provide position and movement sensations based on the results of pulling exposed tendons (see 223, 246). This may reflect how much of the slack in the tendon was taken up before lengthening. Hence Moberg (246), who argued against a role for muscle receptors, found that pulling on a flexor tendon at the wrist gave illusory ex-

[1]Attempts to dissociate kinesthetic performance into a position-sense and movement-sense component are somewhat arbitrary because the latter is likely to depend upon the *extent* of position change. For a particular displacement, position- and movement-sense need not be equally sensitive to velocity. Measured with standard displacements, poor position sensation could be overcome by good movement sensation and vice versa: the properties of any velocity integrators would then be critical. As passive movements at velocities below 1 degree/s excite little sensation that the part is being moved, the term position sense is useful, even if the afferents signals do not encode only position.

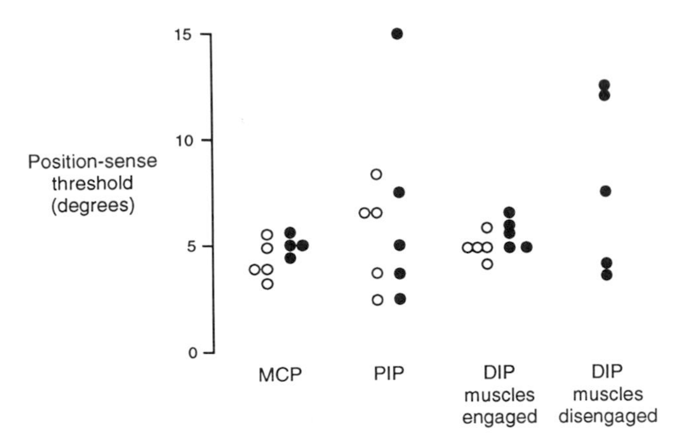

FIG. 4.8. Position-sense thresholds for detection of joint displacements at the metacarpophalangeal (MCP), proximal interphalangeal (PIP), and distal interphalangeal (DIP) joints of the middle finger in five subjects. Movements were delivered with the joint in the midrange at 2 degrees min (i.e., below the velocity at which movement sensations occur). Each point depicts data from one subject with *filled circles* for control performance under passive conditions and *open circles* for estimates when voluntary contraction of the flexors and extensors occurred *after* the final position had been reached. In one condition, the hand was postured so that the distal joint of the middle finger could not be moved by voluntary contractions and thus the joint was effectively disengaged from its attachments. [Adapted from Taylor and McCloskey (312).]

tension of the appropriate joints when the fingers were extended but not "semiflexed."

2. If subjects match the perceived joint position on one side with that on the other, systematic errors exist between trials and subjects (e.g., 92, 218, 247). Such deviations do not correlate with overt deficits in motor performance and are present even in congenitally blind subjects. The spine with its multiple joints shows great acuity, with errors of less than 1 degree in repositioning the trunk in the frontal plane (8, 172). Acuity for rotation may be higher for the trunk than for the neck (311, 313). Knowledge of absolute joint position, whether reached actively or passively, is less accurate for limb muscles. Detection threshold at the distal finger joint is about 5 to 10 degrees, a fair fraction of their angular range. This finding could have little impact on normal voluntary movements that generate *active* forces.

3. Perceived joint position changes if the background spindle discharge is varied via thixotropy (see earlier under PROPERTIES OF KINESTHETIC AFFERENTS). After an elbow flexor contraction at a short muscle length, an intermediate joint angle is perceived to be more extended than expected (136). Errors could be as large as 20 degrees. Spindles in relaxed muscles have been conditioned by preceding activity, and small voluntary contractions produce spindle aftereffects (334). Hence it is not surprising that contraction at a new joint position after passive movement does not enhance absolute position sense (312). Indeed, there are reports that active positioning produces little change in absolute position sense. When subjects are supine and any otolith input eliminated, subjects can position the thorax on the pelvis to within a degree under active or passive conditions (172). In contrast, greater accuracy with active movement has usually been reported for limb muscles[2] (e.g., 92, 93, 214, 258). The difficulty in keeping all spinal muscles relaxed would explain the lower thresholds for the spine and the failure of further contraction to improve them.

4. Apparent position of a joint may deviate even if its position is fixed. If the head is held to one side, it seems to return to the midline over 10 min (147, see also 328). As this occurred with active maintenance of head position, it may reflect a slow change in the body schema.

5. While angles at each joint could be computed to determine the full orientation of a limb, orientation, particularly in relation to gravity, is more acutely sensed than position at individual joints (301, 336). This would produce high acuity in estimates of spinal attitude, especially when standing (95, 146). It is as if the position of a body part is calculated relative to a frame of reference, such as the trunk, with single angles being imperfectly determined (see later under FUNCTIONAL ASPECTS OF KINESTHESIA).

Assessment of Movement Sensation

Since the studies of Goldscheider in the 1880s, thresholds for detection of passive movement have been measured for most limb joints. Proprioception has been analyzed in detail at the distal joint of the middle finger because this joint allows dissection of the joint, cutaneous, and muscle afferent contributions (55, 91, 108, 111, 149). Movements can be applied with the middle finger flexed and the adjacent ones extended so that the long flexor and the extensor mechanism are disengaged and unable to pull the joint. Detection of direction of applied movements to the joint is more difficult than when the adjacent fingers are flexed and only the long flexor can pull the joint (Fig. 4.9*A*). The input from

[2]Quantitative comparison between studies using different methods to assess sensations of position and movement is dangerous, not just because methods used to denote detection or measure a threshold often differ, but because the device that moves the joint and the restraints that limit movement to one joint inevitably generate extraneous cues about joint motion. Just because these signals are not reported by subjects does not signify their absence. This problem also applies to comparisons of performance at different joints.

muscle spindle afferents is responsible, given the poor stretch sensitivity of passive tendon organs. This improvement is more than can be explained by the addition of the input from long flexor afferents. Anesthesia of digital joint and cutaneous afferents isolates the muscle afferent input: performance is then between that when cutaneous and joint afferents contribute and when the full kinesthetic machinery acts. However, at lower angular velocities (~1 degree/s) the isolated muscle afferent contribution is not enough to explain the deterioration with muscle disengagement. When both extensors and flexors pull the joint, the muscle afferent contribution improves. Total proprioceptive performance is more than the sum of a muscle afferent component and a joint/skin component.

What subserves kinesthetic performance when the muscle afferent contribution is eliminated? Two groups silenced joint receptors with intracapsular anesthesia (55, 91). Performance deteriorated, although the effect was not large (Fig. 4.9*A*). Expansion of the joint space enhanced movement detection at intermediate velocities. Residual performance after intracapsular anesthesia signifies the best that can come from local (or remote) cutaneous afferents in isolation. Performance remained unchanged with anesthesia of the skin over the dorsum of the joint.

Given their sensitivity to movement at the metacarpophalangeal joint, the role of remote cutaneous afferents on the dorsum of the hand should be considered (79, 143). They may be unloaded by the posture used to disengage muscles and loaded when the digits adjacent to the middle one are flexed (at the metacarpophalangeal and proximal interphalangeal joints). If so, it is hard to explain the improved performance when the dorsal skin is unloaded with both proximal joints near full extension. This reengages the extensor muscle mechanism. Further evidence that remote cutaneous afferents do not mediate the full improvement is that acuity increases with a weak voluntary contraction when joint and local cutaneous afferents are blocked (Fig. 4.10*A*). This is easily explained by recruitment of specialized intramuscular receptors.

Local and remote cutaneous SA II afferents must have a small specific role that can be duplicated by other afferent sources. They may, like any receptor with a background discharge, facilitate the detection process. Detection of passive movements at the distal joint of the finger diminishes when the adjacent fin-

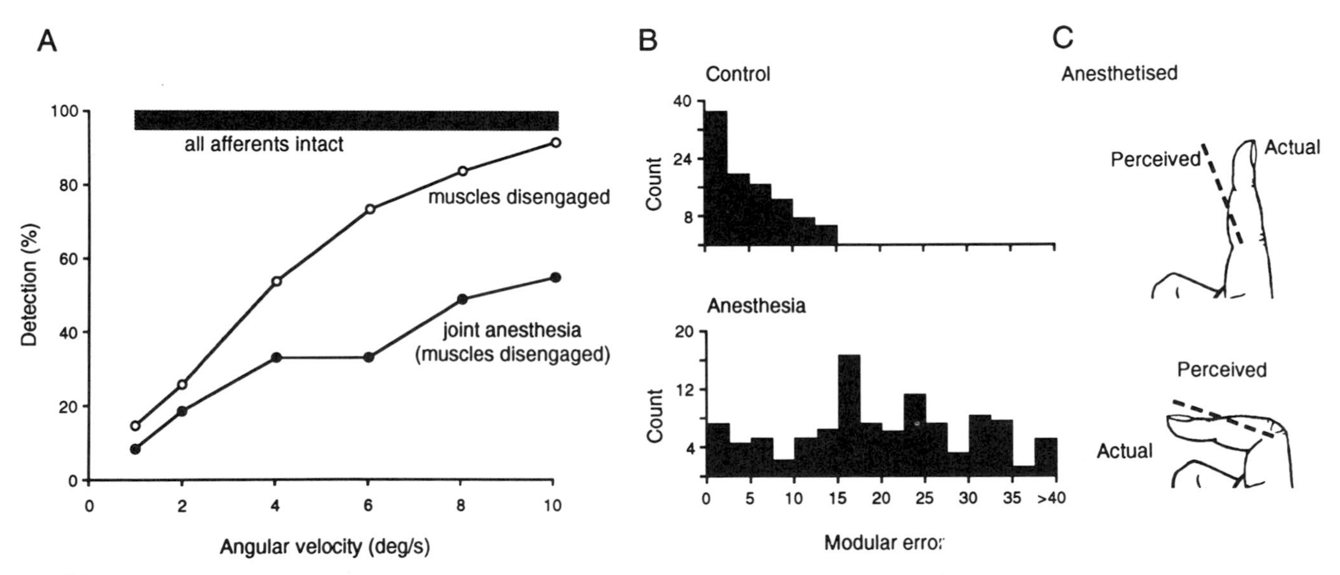

FIG. 4.9. *A*, Detection of 5-degree movements at different angular velocities from a midposition of the distal interphalangeal joint of the middle finger. Subjects had to nominate correctly the direction of the movement. Mean data from references 55 and 91 have been pooled. Data with the hand postured so as to disengage the flexor and extensor muscles are shown as *open circles* (111). *Filled circles* represent performance when the distal interphalangeal joint was injected with local anesthetic. Performance is best when the muscle, joint, and cutaneous afferents are all intact (*hatched horizontal bar*): it deteriorates when muscles cannot contribute to movement detection and deteriorates further when the joint space is injected with local anesthetic. (From Gandevia and Burke (107).] *B*, Distribution of modular errors for the perceived position of the proximal interphalangeal joint of the index finger under control conditions (*upper panel*) and when the digital nerves of the finger had been blocked with local anesthetic (*lower panel*). [Adapted from Ferrell and Smith (92).] A schematic view of the perceived position of the proximal joint of the finger during digital anesthesia shown by the *dashed lines*. The range of perceived positions of the joint was compressed when joint and cutaneous afferents were anesthetized. C, Schematic representation of the distortion of position sense induced by a digital nerve block.

gers are anesthetized (53, 111). However, the ability to match a passively produced *position* may not be impaired (92). This difference suggests that central facilitation is more apparent for detection of movements.

Comparisons between movement detection at different joints have often been used to support the view that distal joints have lesser acuity than proximal ones. However, angular movement need not be the critical variable (149). The large angular threshold for a finger joint can result in a smaller error in position of the fingertip than the small angular threshold for a proximal joint such as the shoulder. Indeed, for equal control of fingertip position, angular thresholds must be less for proximal joints. Thresholds for detection of passive movement at shoulder, elbow, and finger differed between joints when expressed in angles or final positions of the fingertip. For the elbow and distal joint of the finger the thresholds between joints seemed closer if expressed in terms of fractional changes in muscle length. Thus, the CNS behaves as if passive movement detection is related to muscle length changes. This argument requires major assumptions about tendon compliance and spindle behavior and cutaneous contributions. However, data for the lower limb provide some support (272). When only a few muscles cross joints, then passive movement detection will deteriorate (36, 149).

As truly passive movements are rare, one must ask if the threshold for detection of movement changes during muscular contractions (with the full kinesthetic machinery intact). The impairment in movement detection when the local cutaneous and joint inputs are blocked can be severe but is overcome if voluntary contraction is permitted [Fig. 4.10*A*; (111, 198)]. At the elbow joint, without any nerve blocks, movement detection during muscle contraction improves greatly for angular velocities below 1 degree/s [Fig. 4.10*B*; (315)]. Thresholds were lower for extension than flexion movements. The changes suggest a perceptual contribution from the population of elbow flexor spindle afferents, although the details are not simple, given tendon compliance (138, 270), co-contraction, and fusimotor effects. Joint and cutaneous receptors sensitive to contraction could theoretically contribute.

Senses of Force and Heaviness

Several mechanisms contribute to help judge the weight of an object. First, in the absence of any muscle contraction, the pressure of the object on skin will excite cutaneous receptors and possibly some local joint and muscle receptors. Second, during muscular contraction joint, muscle, and ligamentous receptors discharge. The tendon organ's sensitivity

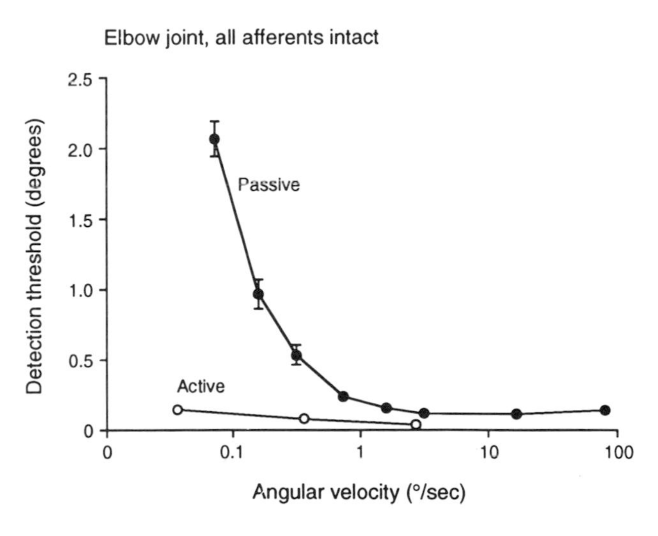

FIG. 4.10. *A*, Detection of the direction of movements applied to the distal interphalangeal joint of the middle finger when the digit was anesthetized at its base (*open circles*) and when the subject exerted a weak flexor contraction with the anesthetized finger (*filled circles*). The hand was postured so that only contraction of the long flexor moved the joint. Proprioceptive acuity was restored to within the normal range when muscle contraction occurred in the absence of local joint and cutaneous inputs (compare Fig. 4.9*A*). Remote cutaneous signals were available throughout. [Adapted from Gandevia and McCloskey (111).] *B*, Detection of the direction of movements applied to the elbow under passive conditions (*filled circles*) and during a voluntary contraction (*open circles*) in two groups of subjects. Data from the passive condition used a slightly different definition of threshold from that during contraction. [Adapted from Taylor and McCloskey (315).]

to active force is notable (see earlier under PROPERTIES OF KINESTHETIC AFFERENTS). Third, signals of motor command or effort generated within the CNS provide indirect information about the motor output. This century the latter two mechanisms have been disputed. However, the second follows from known receptor properties and their central projections. Evidence for the third mechanism is presented first.

How is it possible to define the role of a central command in the sensing of force and heaviness? The neurologist Gordon Holmes realized that "every paretic limb exaggerates the load it carries if its sensation be normal, and the asthenic cerebellar arm may similarly over-estimate the resistance that the test object opposes to its movement" (156). Eleven of 15 patients overestimated perceived heaviness due to "the greater effort which a patient suffering from a unilateral cerebellar lesion must put into all attempts to move the homolateral limb" (156). Reproducibility of judgments was relatively preserved. That perceived heaviness increases with effective weakness (despite normal sensation) has been documented in a variety of ways including studies of patients with other central lesions upstream of the motoneuron. An example that avoids some potential pitfalls is illustrated below. The location of the relevant motor command signal in force and heaviness judgments has been little studied, although some evidence points to a role for the sensorimotor cortex (101, 233; for review, see 103, 273; cf. 248).

Reflex inputs from the digital nerves containing only cutaneous and joint afferents alter the background "excitability" of low- and high-threshold motoneurons of an intrinsic muscle (5). When weights are matched from side to side but intense (almost painful) stimuli are delivered on the side lifting a reference weight, motoneurons are inhibited and perceived heaviness increases by 20%–30% (Fig. 4.11*A*). Muscle output is constant but the supraspinal drive required to overcome the spinal inhibition has increased. For weights requiring recruitment of higher threshold motoneurons, innocuous stimuli produced a small nett facilitation and a corresponding reduction in perceived heaviness. The functional relevance is that, irrespective of how central command signals are derived, the CNS has access to signals that covary directly with the excitation of the recruited motoneurons. As judged by changes in perceived heaviness, cutaneous inputs powerfully affect cooperative synergist movements. Stimulation of the thumb or index finger facilitates flexion and inhibits extension of the neighboring digit, while inputs from the hand facilitate elbow flexion (e.g., 113, 116; Kilbreath et al., unpublished observations). Thus, perceived effort is minimized for simple cooperative tasks.

An independent approach has established the perceptual access of motor commands and indicated how finely they can be graded (119). Intramuscular electrodes recorded the simultaneous discharge of the lowest threshold motor units in two nearby muscles. While the subject focused an effort on one muscle, subliminal for motoneuronal recruitment, the contralateral motor cortex received a weak transcranial stimulus. For pairs of intrinsic hand muscles, but not forearm muscles, subjects learned to transfer a subliminal effort from one motoneuron pool to the other (Fig. 4.12). Success was judged when the cortical stimulus recruited the low-threshold motor unit in the "focused" but not the "unfocused" muscle. This ability involves access to motor command signals because there is no motor unit recruitment at the time of testing or altered feedback from joint, cutaneous, or muscle afferents. Success in this task may parallel the divergence of corticospinal projections (see Chapter 6).

Muscle fatigue produced by sustained contractions increases perceived heaviness and force (115, 181, 183, 224). This does not conclusively favor a motor command component because the input from small-diameter muscle afferents will increase (see earlier under PROPERTIES OF KINESTHETIC AFFERENTS and later under FUNCTIONAL ASPECTS OF KINESTHESIA). While this can inhibit motoneurons, central interpretation of the input could also change. Experimentally induced weakness produced by local infusion of paralyzing agents adds more substance to Holmes' dictum (e.g., 112, 114). During such weakness, inputs from small-diameter muscle afferents should be unaltered, the nett tendon organ input unchanged, although the total spindle input is probably increased through increased fusimotor drive. The latter effect should decrease rather than increase perceived heaviness (224). Increases in perceived heaviness occur when the motor command should increase, such as changing the length–tension properties of the muscle (44, 68).

Experiments producing changes in perceived force when force is unchanged form the cornerstone of arguments that the CNS does not only use signals of muscle tension in judgment of force and heaviness (for reviews, see 43, 103, 182, 220, 221). However, they do not exclude a contribution from peripheral afferents to such judgments, and some results are consistent with perception of a tension signal. When isometric force during a voluntary contraction increases (via the tonic vibration reflex) or decreases (through reciprocal inhibition), subjects can attend to either the motor command required or the altered

A

Digital nerve stimuli 2T

Digital nerve stimuli ≥4T

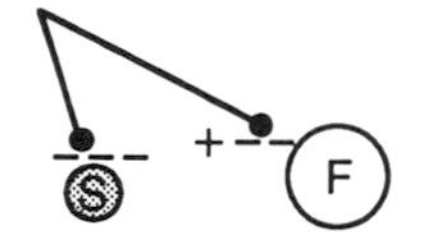

First dorsal interosseus

Lift 100g: Perceived heaviness unchanged | Perceived heaviness incresed **29%**

Lift 500g: Perceived heaviness decreased **4%** | Perceived heaviness increased **18%**

B

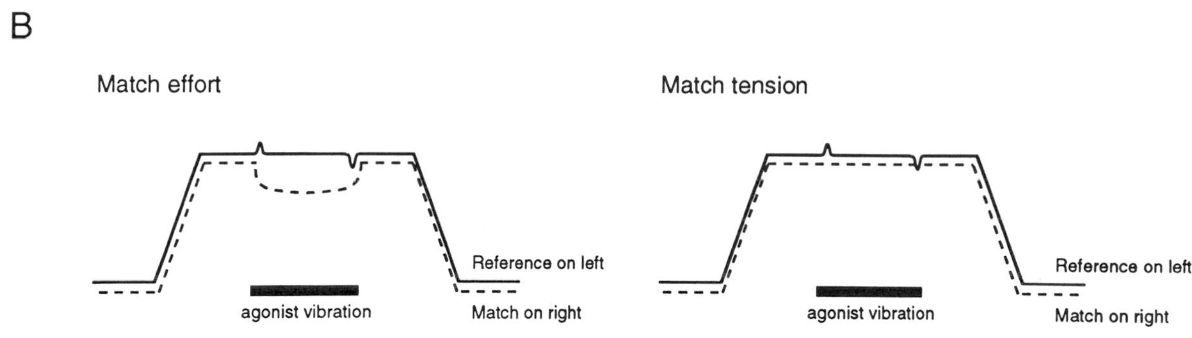

FIG. 4.11. *A*, Correlation between the reflex effects produced by digital nerve stimuli (*upper panels*) and the changes in perceived heaviness (*lower panels*). Stimuli at low intensity [twice sensory threshold (2T)] are innocuous and produce reflex inhibition of low-threshold motoneurons (type S) and excitation of high-threshold motoneurons (type F), whereas higher intensity stimuli (at 4T) are slightly painful and produce widespread inhibition of the motoneuron pool. Weights were lifted by abduction of the index finger (first dorsal interosseous muscle) with stimuli delivered to the digital nerves of the index finger. Nett reflex inhibition by cutaneous afferents increases perceived heaviness, although the absolute heaviness of the reference weight is unaltered. [Data from Aniss, Gandevia, and Milne (5).] *B*, Schematic representation of responses when subjects match the perceived effort (*left panel*) and perceived tension (*right panel*) produced by elbow flexion under isometric conditions. The reference force (*solid line*) was produced with the aid of visual feedback. A tonic vibration reflex was used to "assist" the contraction of the agonist elbow flexors as indicated by the *horizontal bars*. If the subject matched the perceived effort required to match the reference force, the matching force diminished, but if required, the subject could accurately match the perceived isometric force during the reflex assistance to movement when the effort required to maintain it had diminished. [Based on McCloskey, Ebeling, and Goodwin (224).]

muscle tension [Fig. 4.11*B*; (224, 274)]. During fatigue, as opposed to partial curarization (112, 113, 274), this is impossible (181, 183). During a weak voluntary contraction against a spring by elbow flexion, subjects can maintain either the tension constant or the angular position of the elbow: signals of very small changes in active force or position are detectable (61). A contributory role for motor commands is unlikely, given the difficulty in maintenance of constant force or position with complete deafferentation (see later under DEAFFERENTATION).

If signals of tension and position are usually accessible, then their interrelations provide insight into central mechanisms. Stiffness can be matched for springs compressed between index finger and thumb even after digital anesthesia (274). For the elbow flexors, the fractional change in the stimulus required for detection is highest for viscosity, intermediate for stiffness, and lowest for force (184, 185). This favors force (or a direct corollary) as the primary kinesthetic signal. Signals of position and force are not absolutely accurate, as position is overestimated in proportion to voluntary force during contraction against a spring, an effect explicable by an interaction among signals of force, position, and perhaps central commands (274, 283, 329), although the stretch of tendons could contribute to this misperception.

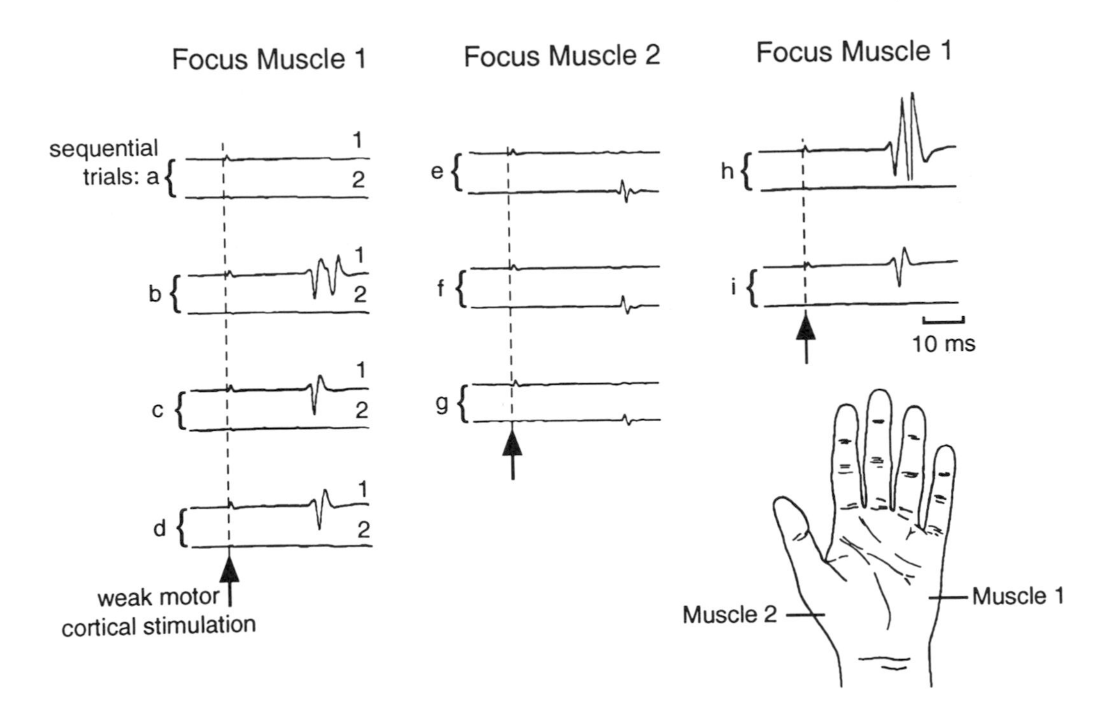

FIG. 4.12. Attempted "focusing" by one subject on either abductor digiti minimi (muscle 1) or abductor digiti minimi (muscle 2). Sketch at *lower right* shows the simultaneous recording from the two muscles. The subject attempted this without recruitment of the lowest threshold motor units (recorded with needle electrodes) and thus there was no movement-related feedback. At unpredictable times, a weak transcranial stimulus to the contralateral motor cortex tested the success of focusing. Nine trials from one continuous sequence are shown. *Upper trace* in each pair is from abductor digiti minimi (muscle 1) and *lower trace* from abductor pollicis brevis (muscle 2). *Upward arrow* and *dotted lines* indicate the timing of stimuli to the motor cortex (delivered only when both muscles were electromyographically silent). In the first column (*trials a–d*) the subject focused on muscle 1. On the first trial (*a*), the cortical stimulus failed to evoke activity in either muscle. On the next three trials, the subject successfully achieved activity in muscle 1 without discharging muscle 2. The instruction was then changed to focus on muscle 2. After three successful trials (*e–g*), the instruction was reversed. [Adapted from Gandevia and Rothwell (119).]

Movement-related inputs are presumed to mediate the greater accuracy in isometric than isotonic force matching. Absolute errors with isometric force matching are well recognized, although an afferent signal from intramuscular receptors alone allows recalibration of signals of motor command (115). To match an isometric force on one side, subjects generate a larger force (isotonically) against a spring on the other side (235). Reasons for this have not been addressed, but peripheral and central effects will be involved.

Decoding of Tension Signals. Signals of peripheral muscle tension require decoding. They originate in tendon organs, but contributions from contraction-sensitive joint afferents and cutaneous afferents excited via couplings to the limb are possible. However, reliance on cutaneous signals alone in the absence of voluntary muscle contraction provides poor weight acuity (e.g., 33, 94). The increase in perceived force during a sustained voluntary contraction is inconsistent with a cutaneous contribution.

1. If the CNS is to determine the size of an external weight based purely on signals of muscle tension, it needs information about how the load acts on the skeleton. For example, with the upper arm vertical and a mass added to the wrist, the intramuscular tension required to support it will be higher when the elbow is nearly fully extended than in the midrange. Intramuscular tension predicts external forces only when joint angles and the line of pull of the force are known. This reinforces the need for external calibration of central commands.

2. The senses of muscular force and heaviness have frequently been treated together without consideration of their physical differences. This oversight arose as both variables are biased by signals of motor command. It is only the sensation of heaviness of a *lifted* object that requires that the gravitational acceleration be overcome. Not surprisingly, a change in acceleration or mass changes perceived force (e.g., 279, 280). Weights feel lighter when lifted in space. Subjects signal neither the absolute weight nor the mass, although some adaptation to the altered force conditions occurs. A single kines-

thetic signal will be insufficient to explain these adaptations. Some role for corollary motor signals is inevitable to determine whether altered acceleration reflects a change in mass or motor drive. If corollaries of motor command bias tension perception, such signals cannot signal absolute force or weight. Without a kinesthetic, visual, or auditory input to indicate that a weight has been moved or force generated, command signals remain dimensionless. Nonetheless, such signals guide residual motor performance (see later under DEAFFERENTATION).

3. Tendon organ afferents have diminished stretch and force sensitivity after contractions (169, cf. 150) and a reference force is overestimated after a voluntary isometric contraction (168, 317). If subjects merely matched an intramuscular tension signal, the overestimation fits with tendon organ desensitization, although potentiation of muscle fibers and reflex changes favoring facilitation remain to be excluded.

4. The accuracy of force judgments changes little when a single weight in the hand is lifted by muscle groups at the shoulder, elbow, and wrist (109). This is a rare example of when more kinesthetic signals do not aid performance. For two muscles concurrently active to lift *separate* weights by simultaneous flexion at the distal interphalangeal joint of the finger, accuracy of weight judgment remains constant. The perceived heaviness of a reference weight increases despite digital anesthesia (Fig. 4.13). If, as is likely, this does not rely on reflexes biasing the motoneuron pools, then it denotes a limit on the ability of the CNS to specify the destination of commands sent simultaneously to nearby muscles.

5. When performance between muscles at constant fractions of maximal force was compared for hand muscles, the accuracy of repeated weight estimates was greatest for flexor pollicis longus, phylogenetically the newest muscle. It had greater accuracy than the intrinsic muscles or flexor digitorum profundus and it lacked the usual tendency for judgments to deteriorate at low forces [Fig. 4.14*B*; (195)]. Whether this specialization requires finer peripheral or central sensitivity is unknown, but it cautions against the assumption that kinesthesia is equivalent at all muscles.

6. Finally, the interpretation of motor commands and force signals must be fitted into central expectations. Thus, large objects are expected to feel heavy through visual and haptic cues (e.g., 83, 131, 219). Such expectation leads to altered kinesthetic inputs as larger forces are applied to the bigger object. Similarly, perceived body weight is calibrated to the usual gravitational acceleration, such that doubling the force on a foot by shifting all the body weight onto it produces little change in apparent weight (203).

Sense of Timing of Muscle Action

Determination of time differences with neurons acting as delay lines and coincidence detectors is phylogenetically old, but perception of the time of voluntary contractions has been little considered. Psychologists used the early reaction-time studies to measure cognitive processes rather than voluntary timing. The perceived timing of muscle action fits the definition of proprioception because it involves muscle actions generated by the organism itself. The cerebellum is a major neural structure contributing to motor and perhaps perceptual timing (e.g., 193), with the posterior parietal cortex implicated in temporal judgments of cutaneous stimuli (204). Coincidence of events is not only crucial to establish perceptual unity but also to execute sequences of rapid movement such as playing the piano or throwing a ball. In such sequences, peripheral signals of position and velocity must be used to help time later com-

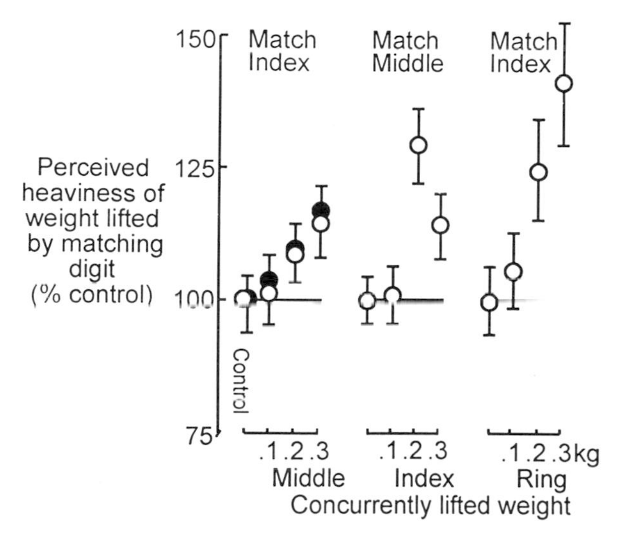

FIG. 4.13. Results from three lifting combinations in which flexor digitorum profundus lifted a reference weight of 200 g on the reference side. In experimental trials a weight was also lifted concurrently on the same side, and in control trials no concurrent weight was lifted. The perceived heaviness of the reference weight was always determined by matching it to a variable weight lifted by thumb flexion on the contralateral side. Data obtained when the fingers lifting the reference and concurrent weight were anesthetized (*open circles*), and for combination when sensation was intact (*filled circles*). Mean (± SEM) for a group of subjects. The finger that lifted the reference weight is indicated at the top of the panel, and the finger that lifted the concurrent weight at the bottom. Perceived heaviness of the reference weight increases when a neighboring finger lifts concurrently, even when the digits are anesthetized. [Adapted from Kilbrath and Gandevia (194).]

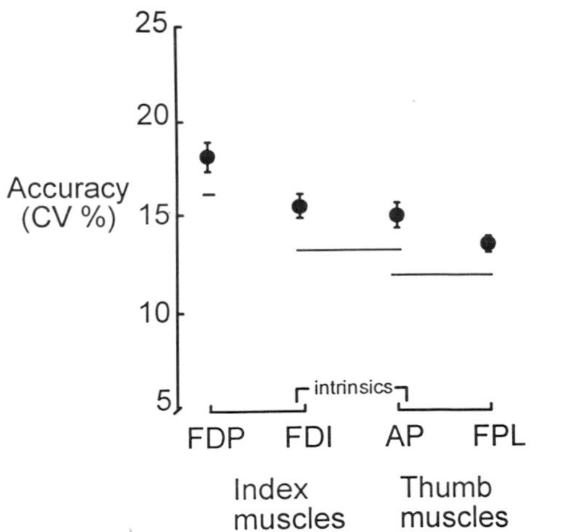

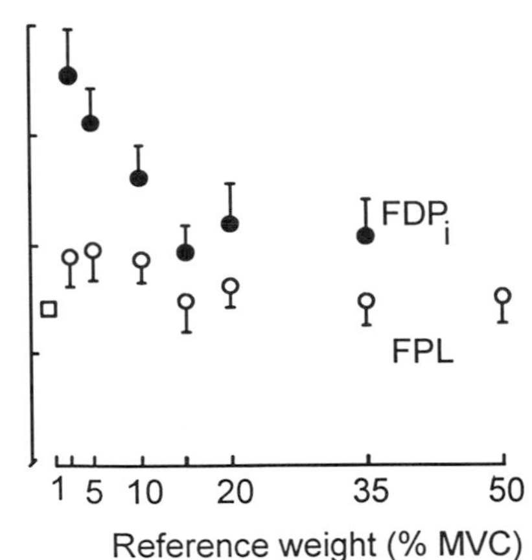

FIG. 4.14. Accuracy of matching weights in a group of subjects with four muscles [flexor pollicis longus (FPL), flexor digitorum longus acting on the index finger (FDP index), adductor pollicis (AP) and first dorsal interosseous (FDI)] at several fractions of maximal voluntary force (MVC). Reference weights lifted on one side were matched with variable weights lifted with the corresponding muscle on the contralateral side. Accuracy derived from the coefficient of variation of repeated lifts (mean ± SEM). *A*, Accuracy for the four different muscles. Flexor pollicis longus showed significantly higher accuracy than the other muscles. *B*, Matching over a wide range of weights for FPL (*open circles*) and FDP index (*filled circles*). Even at very low forces (< 1% MVC, *open square*) accuracy is maintained for FPL. [Adapted from Kilbreath and Gandevia (195).]

ponents of the movement (see 22). When moving more than one limb, the motor outputs commonly synchronize if there is no constraint for independent action. Just as with other kinesthetic sensations, it is not easy to tease out the components involved. Movements can be triggered by subliminal stimuli and corrections to voluntary movements initiated before the error requiring correction is perceived (48, 62, 314).

Although not yet measured formally, the ability of humans to determine the timing of voluntary commands when conscious but fully paralyzed is not in doubt. To some this indicates only that movement can be planned without reference to sensory inputs. However, it repudiates the view that only afferent inputs are relevant (see earlier under HISTORICAL PERSPECTIVES). The method adopted independently by McCloskey and Libet is to relate the perceived timing of an internally generated movement and another event such as a peripheral nerve stimulus or the movement on a clock (211, 222).

For an *actual movement* of the hand to seem simultaneous with a reference stimulus to the foot electromyographic (EMG) activity must begin about 100 ms *before* the stimulus [Fig. 4.15; (212)]. However, for the reference stimulus to seem simultaneous with the motor command to move the hand, the stimulus has to occur much earlier. Thus, if the stimulus and onset of EMG are simultaneous, the subject judges that the command to move is first, whereas the *movement* has to be underway for the subject to believe it is first. The differential attention to a command signal arising before movement or a kinesthetic input generated after it was surprisingly easy. For "simultaneous" movements of different parts of the body, some subjects align motor commands (i.e., EMG in a cranial muscle precedes that in the leg), whereas others align the actual movement. These kinesthetic judgments occur seamlessly through more than one neural mechanism despite temporal disparity. Libet reached similar conclusions (211) and also emphasized that cortical readiness potentials precede the earliest voluntary intent to move. As expected, a deafferented patient relied less on peripheral signals (10).

The "clock" experiments prove that some perceivable timing signals arise from motor commands before movement. Such signals are available to sequence movements, even at unconscious levels. Additional delays may be built into the absolute latency for evoking a sensation from kinesthetic inputs and also from motor commands (e.g., 212).

Other Roles for Motor Commands

Motor commands contribute to sensations of force, heaviness, and timing, but other roles have been proposed for them (see earlier under CURRENT DEFINITIONS), especially in the oculomotor system. They might signal that a movement has not only been commanded but that it has occurred. This view has long seemed attractive to explain visual displace-

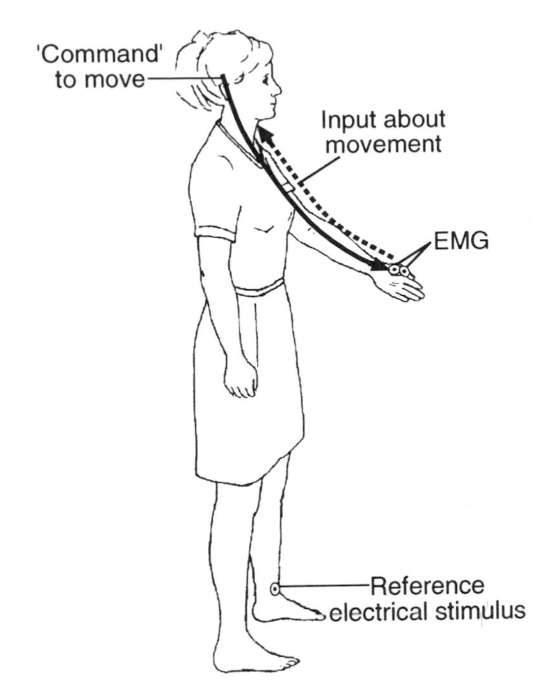

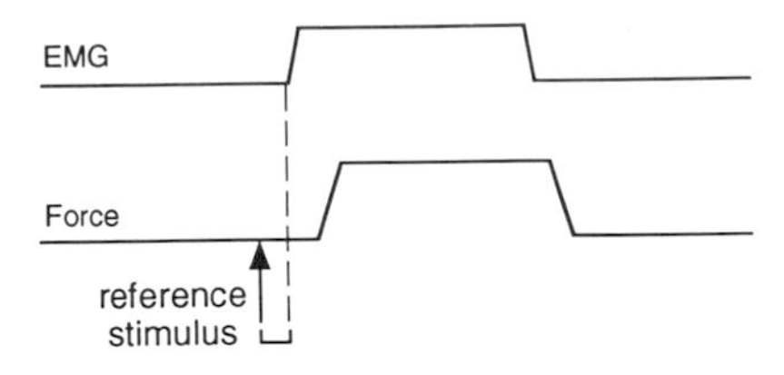

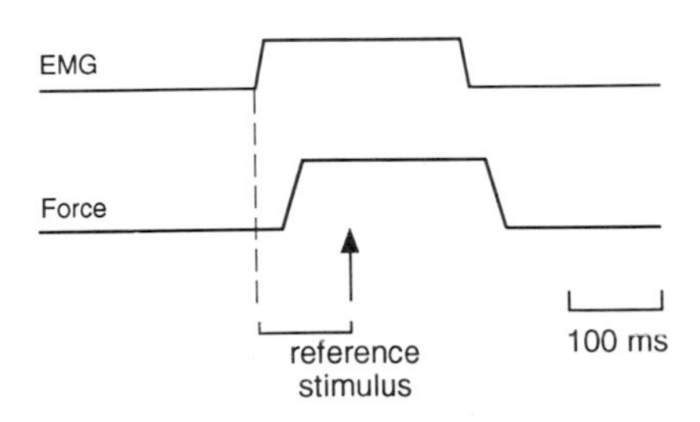

FIG. 4.15. Dissociation of the perceived command to move and the perceived time at which the muscle actually contracted. The subject makes intermittent contractions of a hand muscle, and around the time they occur a reference stimulus is delivered to the foot. Timing of the reference stimulus for perceived simultaneity can be deduced from repeated trials. *Upper panel* shows when the subject believes that the command to move and the stimulus occur simultaneously. *Lower panel* shows when the subject believes that the actual movement and the stimulus occur simultaneously. *Traces* in the two conditions aligned with the voluntary EMG to show that, for the command to move to occur at the same time as the reference stimulus, the stimulus precedes the EMG, but for the actual movement to seem first, the reference stimulus comes after the EMG. When the EMG coincided with the stimulus, the command to move was perceived to occur first, whereas the reference stimulus had to occur some 100 ms later (i.e., well into the contraction) for the actual movement to seem first. [Based on McCloskey et al. (222).]

ment on attempted movement with seemingly paralyzed eye muscles and even apparent limb movements. To one proponent, "There is no reason why we should not be able to judge the size of motor volleys as accurately as we can judge the size of sensory volleys arriving" (241).

Attempted movements with acutely paralyzed limb muscles do not generate a sensation that the joints moved, indeed the limb feels "heavy" and "stuck." Thus, isolated delivery of the command does not produce illusory motion. This observation has been confirmed in some circumstances in which feedback was abolished [e.g., spinal transection; (101, 155)], but in others some feedback remained and might have overidden any perceptual effect of the isolated motor command [e.g., paralysis with neuromuscular blocking drugs; pure motor strokes; (101, 110)].

The minimal peripheral signal that must coexist with a motor command to induce a voluntary movement sensation has not been formally established. When subjects try to contract muscles paralyzed with a local infusion of tubocurarine and a cutaneous signal consistent with movement, the paralyzed muscle is perceived to remain stationary (225). However, the possibility that a signal from muscle spindles could combine to provide the sense of a voluntary movement was raised in a recent study of total body paralysis (110). Subjects unexpectedly reported a vague sensation of ankle plantar flexion with attempted ankle dorsiflexion. If the intrafusal fibers had not been completely blocked, the unexpectedly large spindle input from the ankle dorsiflexors would be misinterpreted as a lengthening plantar flexion.

While isolated signals of motor command may not indicate that a movement has occurred, they can signal that the wrong movement has been initiated. When subjects must rapidly move in one of two directions or produce rapid accurate isometric forces, they correct occasional errors before a voluntary response could have been initiated (62, 132).

Ocular Kinesthesia and Motor Commands. Dispute about extraocular muscle signals and motor commands is not new. Helmholtz (152) showed that the

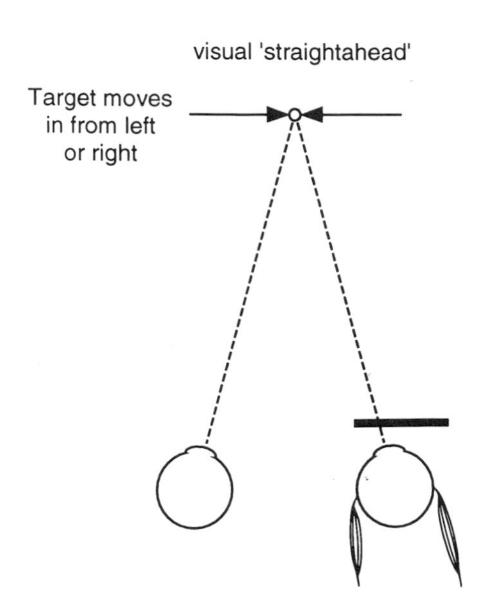

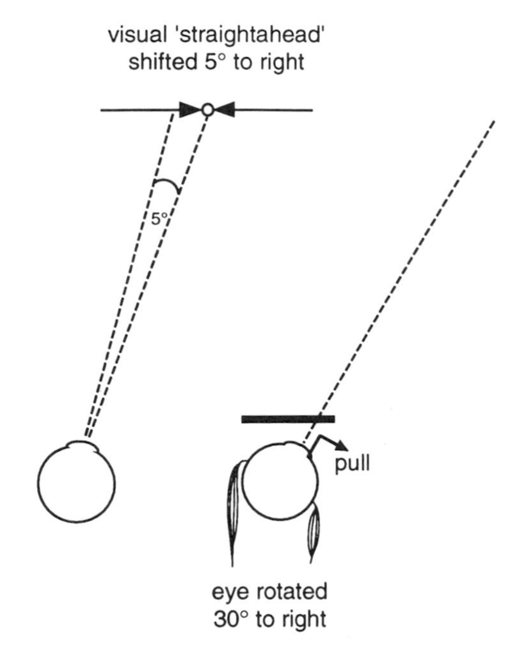

FIG. 4.16. *At left*, The two eyes are shown while the subject looks straight ahead but with vision prevented by a cover over the right eye. The subject viewed targets moving slowly from the left or right (*horizontal arrows*) and indicated when they appeared directly in front (i.e., straight ahead) (*open circle*). *At right*, The right eye has been rotated 30 degrees to the right via a corneal lens, but it remains covered. Visual "straight ahead" is now judged to be ~5 degrees to the right (i.e., in the direction of the deviated and covered eye). Note there was no reflex change in position of the uncovered left eye. Despite the deviation in visual localization, there was no sensation that eye position had changed. [Adapted from Gauthier, Nommay, and Vercher (122).]

position of objects viewed by the eye (perceived eye position) derived from a knowledge of outgoing commands, while Sherrington (295) argued that ocular muscle proprioception was adequate. Recent studies confirm that both signals influence sensation (29, 121, 122, 305). The simple mechanics of the eye and absence of joint receptors might suggest that oculomotor control is simple and well suited to rapid "feedforward" control. However, eye muscles are richly endowed with proprioceptors, and loss of their inputs impairs development of binocular vision.

Patients with sudden paralysis of extraocular muscles believe that apparent motion of the visual world occurs in the direction of the willed movement (e.g., 29, 152). Furthermore, willed movements of the eye were reported when eye movement was physically prevented. Passive eye movements were undetected when forceps pulled the muscle even for both eyes (32). Better psychophysical techniques have revealed that passive movements are detectable.

In darkness, trained subjects detected the direction of applied horizontal loads to the eye through a contact lens, presumably via a signal from extraocular muscles. Loading was initiated by the subject but its direction was unknown (296). Support came from vibration of eye muscles. This shifted perceived location of visual targets: vibration of the right lateral rectus induced a drift in position of a target to the left (277, 324). This illusion took into account input from both eyes and was abolished in a structured visual environment when purely retinal signals determine target location (324).

Not all evidence fitted Helmholtz's view that motor commands in isolation generated a sense of movement of the visual world. Complete paralysis with neuromuscular blocking agents prevents a perceptual shift in the visual world despite voluntary effort. However, visual shifts in the direction of gaze accompany attempts to contract *partially* paralyzed muscles (see 31, 306). Only if inputs from muscle spindles and other proprioceptors are ignored can these shifts be ascribed to a pure influence of motor commands.

Because patients with strabismus make errors pointing to visual targets in the direction of the nonfixing eye, Gauthier studied the localization of targets when a nonviewing eye had been displaced passively (121, 122). Sustained deviation of one eye of 30 degrees via a scleral lens caused errors of about 5 degrees in the perceived "straight ahead" position and in pointing at targets (Fig. 4.16). If a command signal determined the visual axis, no errors would have been expected. If proprioceptive inputs from the viewing eye are added, as much as one-third of

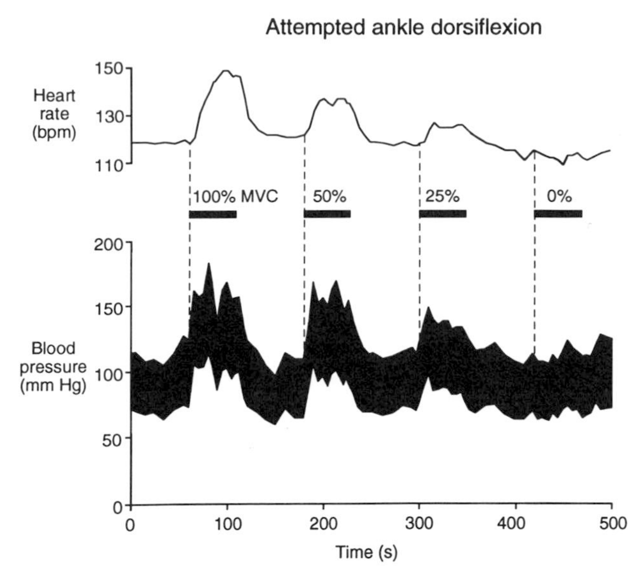

FIG. 4.17. Blood pressure and heart rate records in a subject with all muscles completely paralyzed with a high-dose infusion of atracurium during attempted contractions of the paralyzed dorsiflexors of the ankle. Supramaximal stimulation of the phrenic nerve confirmed that paralysis was complete. Attempted contractions at 100%, 50%, and 25% of maximum. The effect of a sham maneuver consisting of verbal encouragement but no attempted contraction is included ("0%"). *Solid bars* indicate the duration of each test period. Cardiovascular responses are graded with the level of motor command or effort. This effect must be due to motor commands and cannot be due to co-contraction of remote muscles. [From Gandevia et al. (110).]

the input required to elaborate the position of the eye derives from extraocular signals.

Another approach has yielded a similar conclusion, although the method is less sound. It relies on the change in localization of targets when subjects induced in themselves shifts in perceived target position by pushing on the edge of one eye (29). This was believed to increase the motor command for oculomotor stabilization while the input from intramuscular receptors remained constant, a view inconsistent with the responses of muscle spindles under fusimotor drive and of tendon organs. Other studies favoring a principal role for motor commands have relied on the dubious assumption that if eye position is maintained despite loading, kinesthetic input is constant (e.g., 297). Studies on limb muscles predict a perceptual "trade-off" between signals of force and length and so visual mislocalization is neither surprising nor definitive evidence for efferent commands as signals of ocular position.

In summary, motor commands to ocular muscles contribute to stabilize the visual world and to help the CNS predict how much of an object's movement in retinal coordinates reflects object movement and how much reflects eyeball movement. They may do this through cancellation of the expected visual shifts but they need not involve direct interpretation of the motor command as an index of movement. Mittelstaedt has documented many neural mechanisms through which this could be achieved (245).

Cardiovascular Control and Motor Commands. Motor command signals help control not only movement but also autonomic and automatic functions that change, for homeostatic reasons, with movement. Examples are the increases in blood pressure, heart rate, and pulmonary ventilation during exercise. Krogh and Lindhardt (201) originally envisaged that cortical outflow "irradiated" respiratory centers during effort to produce these changes, but the role of such signals has remained contentious despite studies supporting their role (e.g., 130, 171; for review, see 244). There is redundancy because group III and IV muscle afferents can evoke the required changes (e.g., 1), and even imagination of muscle contractions can contribute (69).

A crucial objection to a role for motor commands was raised over a century ago by Ferrier (94). He realized that any increased effort when attempting to contract a weak muscle may come not only from a central source: "In all instances the consciousness of effort is conditioned by the actual fact of muscular contraction." Because remote contractions occur in proportion to increased effort, it is necessary to establish the magnitude of their effects. This requires measurement of cardiorespiratory changes in the *presence* of motor commands but the *absence of any* movement. This has recently been achieved in completely paralyzed subjects who attempted to contract muscles (Fig. 4.17). Increases in blood pressure and heart rate were proportional to the level of motor command or effort (110). During fictive efforts, the increases were simlar to those with real contractions prior to paralysis. Hence the potential potency of these motor commands cannot now be denied, while the problem of remote contractions requires evaluation in each experimental situation.

DEAFFERENTATION

Removal of peripheral kinesthetic input forces the CNS to rely on motor commands together with any ancillary cues provided by the unaffected senses such as vision and audition. Founders of the "muscle" senses, Bell (20), Sherrington (294), and Bastian (17) soon realized that performance surviving true deafferentation was the least that isolated motor commands could produce, while deficits indicated the maximal contribution usually made by kinesthetic inputs. Indeed, Phillips recently argued that little voluntary movement of the hand may survive *acute* deafferentation (261).

Critical questions must be considered for all studies of "deafferentation." First, when is performance tested after deafferentation? The earlier the testing or more acute the pathology, the less relearning and use of trick stratagems. Second, how complete is the afferent loss and have other structures been affected? Coherent inputs from small numbers of afferent fibers provide useful perceptions (see earlier unrder KINESTHETIC MECHANISMS IN ISOLATION), while some discharge from afferent fibers can persist after complete nerve section. Attempts to section the dorsal roots may damage blood supply to the spinal cord. Third, what ancillary inputs are available to guide movement? A few afferents escape dorsal root section by traveling in ventral roots. Fourth, is movement performed under optimal conditions? No method of producing deafferentation is optimal. Methods include surgical division of the dorsal roots, peripheral neuropathies affecting large-diameter afferents, and central lesions, particularly the new rare tabes dorsalis (see 261, 286). Local anesthesia or ischemia produces reversible deafferentation (e.g., 209). Given the various methods and technical limitations, it is not surprising that results are discordant. Some deficits and positive aspects of performance are considered below. However, survival of a motor ability after deafferentation does not necessarily reveal how perceptual mechanisms are used.

Primates deprived of kinesthetic input by dorsal rhizotomies or lesions in sensory pathways have impaired ability to guide the arm without vision. Muscle tone is usually reduced and abnormal postures of the limbs occur. Recovery of purposeful reaching is hastened if the normal arm is restrained, or if both arms are affected (see 286, 308).

A study of elbow movements in monkeys following surgical deafferentation by Polit and Bizzi is commonly cited to highlight the ability to move to specified elbow positions despite loading (263). However, the movements were slow with large targets (10–15 degrees). Successful performance was limited as "Whenever we changed the usual spatial relationship between the animal and the arm apparatus or applied a constant bias load, the monkey's pointing response was inaccurate." After deafferentation, a pincer rather than precision grip characterizes movements of the fingers and thumb (e.g., 59, 97, 308). In a patient with partial deafferentation due to a parietal lesion that spared the motor cortex: "The reaching phase of the movement was correctly executed, although the grasping phase was misadapted due to the inability to shape the hand according to the spatial configuration of the object" (176).

Renewed interest in the role of muscle afferent feedback prompted a search for patients with large-fiber sensory neuropathies. Case studies (e.g., 60, 282) and small series have been investigated, with the study of seven patients by Sanes and colleagues being influential (284, 286; see also 98, 123). The patients developed a neuropathy over many years with "diminished" sensations of touch, temperature, pin prick, limb position, and cutaneous vibration, with relatively preserved motor power. In some, sensation was impaired to the shoulder and hip. Nerve biopsies showed loss of large myelinated fibers. Attempts to maintain a steady force with the wrist flexors and visual feedback of position generated a slow oscillation, presumably reflecting correction of visually determined errors. Drifts from the target position began once visual feedback was withdrawn, but usually remained within ±10 degrees over 20 s. Variations in the initial flexor load did not systematically alter positioning accuracy. Similar defects were present for movements against an elastic load, with the smallest movements showing the greatest relative errors. Thus fine movements rely critically on kinesthetic inputs (285). Movements missed the target if unpredictable loads were added (98).

There was a fair ability to match ascending but not descending forces (284; see also 316). Judgments of weight or force were relatively preserved if the patient saw the object move. With vision, a patient detected changes of 10% in the weight lifted by elbow flexors (60), which is about twice the usual threshold. Without vision, the weight had to be doubled. Any surviving input from small-diameter afferents provided only a minimally useful signal that force developed. Normal subjects lifting weights by thumb flexion when deprived of inputs from the skin and joint of the thumb show close to normal accuracy (115, 194); Kilbreath et al., unpublished observations). Hence an input from intramuscular receptors suffices to calibrate the motor command. Many kinesthetic inputs and ancillary signals can calibrate the motor command, so impaired weight-matching in a patient with neuropathy does not exclude the motor commands from such judgments.

The rhythm of alternating flexion and extension movements at the wrist was reasonably preserved, despite co-contraction (282, 286). Other motor programs persisted such as inhibition of tonic antagonist muscle activity prior to movement, triphasic EMG bursts in agonist and antagonist muscles, and anticipatory postural contractions of remote muscles (98, 99; see also 199). Full descriptions of attempts to stand and walk are rare in cases of (partial) deafferentation, but an ataxic, wide-based gait with straightened knees is likely.

If these abnormalities derive from a loss of muscle afferent input, they should occur with acute muscle deafferentation. To study this, motor output has been intercepted by recording proximal to a complete nerve block (117, 118, 230). Subjects can recruit and grade the discharge of motoneurons innervating acutely paralyzed muscles in the hand or leg (Fig. 4.18). Auditory or visual feedback helped performance but was not essential. Maintenance of a constant motor output, as in the patients, deteriorated with time, although subjects generated graded steps of motor command without ancillary feedback (Fig. 18*A* and *B*). Two differences between efferent control have emerged for the upper and lower limb. Cutaneous feedback often powerfully aided performance for the intrinsic muscles, but had less effect in the lower limb. Selective recruitment of single muscles was easier for the hand than for the leg muscles. As in patients with sensory neuropathy, there was asymmetry in slowly rising then falling motor commands (Fig. 4.18*C*). At the start of a rising "contraction," motor output increases too fast, as if "searching" for some afferent signal of "success," then falls away quickly (117). All subjects performed similarly with this acute deafferentation. Thus vari-

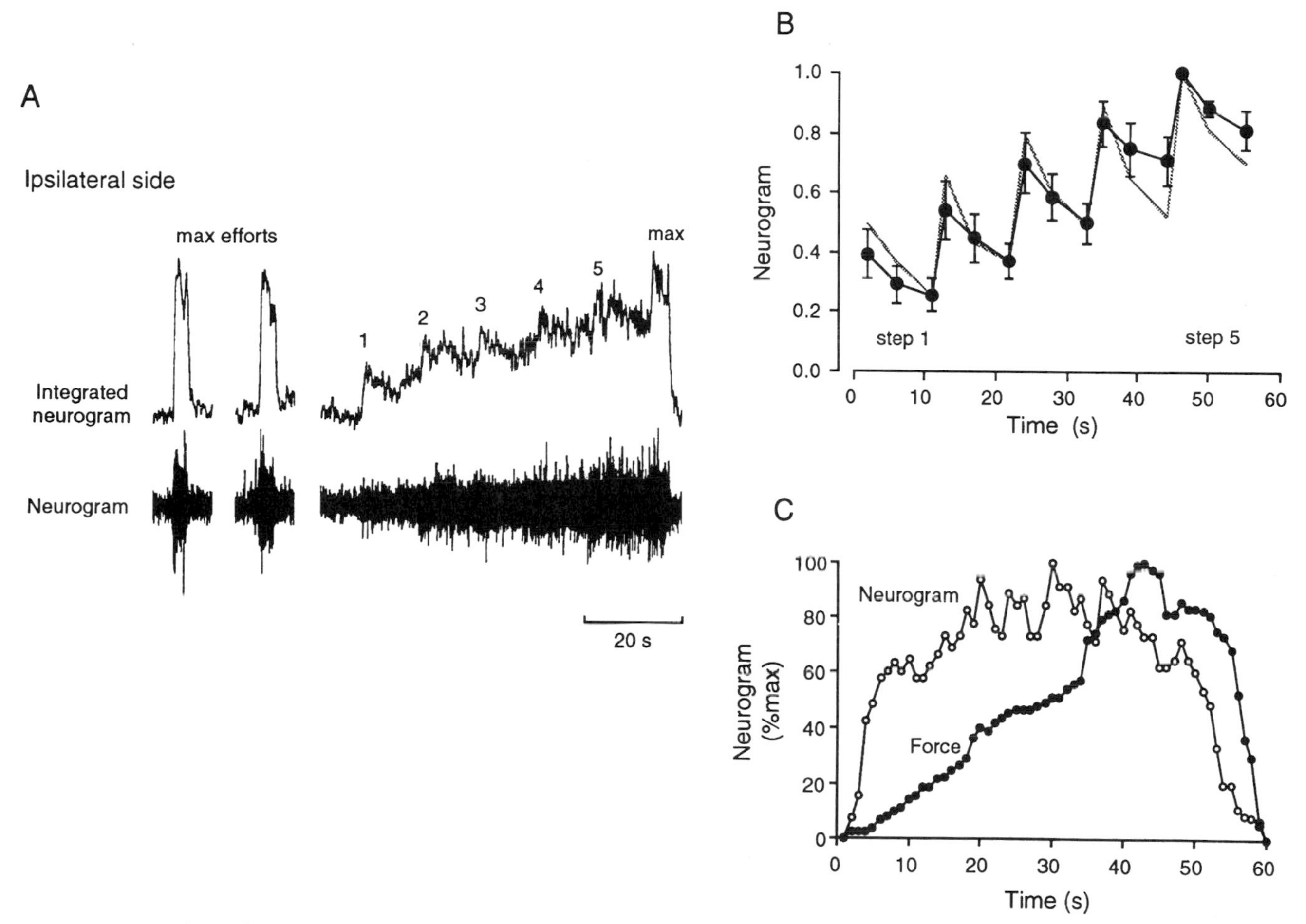

FIG. 4.18. Recording of the motor output to a completely paralyzed muscle. Microneurographic recordings were made from tibialis anterior motor axons when the whole common peroneal nerve was blocked distal to the recording site with local anesthetic. Muscle afferent feedback was thus acutely removed and attempted dorsiflexion of the ankle produced no movement. *A*, Raw and integrated neurogram directed to tibialis anterior during 2 rapid maximal efforts (*left*) and subsequently during a sequence of five steps of increasing effort (*right*). This sequence ended with a maximal effort. *B*, Pooled data for step sequences of effort with auditory feedback of the neurogram from five subjects (*open symbols, solid line*) and without (*hatched line*). Note that the initial step is larger in the absence of auditory feedback as is the decline in neurogram within each step. *C*, Performance when attempting a matching effort on the paralyzed and the normal side is not the same for rising and falling forces. Neurogram from the paralyzed side and force recorded simultaneously from the dorsiflexors on the contralateral side. For rising forces the neurogram is excessive, and for falling forces it is too low. Under control conditions subjects can produce closely correlated ramps of increasing then decreasing effort. (From Gandevia et al. (117), with permission).]

able performance among patients with neuropathies suggests variation in the afferent loss rather than in the ability to use motor commands.

Observations in primates with deafferentation support the view that motor commands can be accessed to time and grade contractions and reveal their limitations. These commands provide a dimensionless signal of the start and level of motor drive which, on its own, cannot signal joint angle, velocity, or force unless the particular starting conditions have been learned. Given a signal that a weight has been lifted, knowledge of motor commands can clearly aid simple tasks. Lacking calibration by vision or some other cue, it is difficult to sustain motor commands indefinitely, with or without cocontraction. Even if only provided before a movement, vision helps performance (123). Not surprisingly, multijoint movements are more severely affected following deafferentation, with standing, walking, and writing achieved with difficulty especially when neck muscles are also involved (e.g., 123, 316). Walking is a task patients with complete neuropathic deafferentation do not regain.

FUNCTIONAL ASPECTS OF KINESTHESIA

Body Schema

A sensation like kinesthesia that provides spatial information cannot be considered in isolation. Signals about the disposition of the body in space and of objects around it include visual, auditory, and vestibular cues. Since vision of the finger helps guide reaching to a target, Sherrington's division of spatial receptors into exteroceptive (visual, auditory, and cutaneous inputs) and proprioceptive (muscle, tendon, and joint) inputs is somewhat arbitrary. Strictly, vestibular receptors are proprioceptors. They provide a perceivable signal about the upright position when standing, but their threshold is well above that required to regulate normal stance (95, 96). Detection of rotation of the neck is no better when the head is moved on the body compared with when the trunk is moved and the head is still (311).

Knowledge of limb lengths, joint angles and forces, as well as vision is needed to position the fingers accurately. Hence kinesthesia should include the perceptual map of the segments of the body. Recordings from multiple cortical cells have allowed the neural substrates for these maps to be studied (see 189).

Head and Holmes (151) defined the body schema in 1911 to explain perceptual deficits after amputation and cortical lesions. First, they recognized a "standard" "against which all subsequent changes for posture [or movement] are measured before they enter consciousness." Second, this schema was "plastic" so that "Every recognizable change enters into consciousness already charged with its relation to something that has gone before, just as on a taximeter the distance is presented to us already transformed into shillings and pence." They also deduced there must be schemas for each major sense (including vision, kinesthesia, and tactile sensation) that can be interrogated independently but which are usually fused. These concepts remain disarmingly modern. Current evidence favors a genetically determined body map, modifiable by experience, which can be accessed following amputation and deafferentation even if body parts have never developed (see 192, 238). Reorganization of sensorimotor cortical maps follows amputation of parts of the hand within minutes and continues over weeks (e.g., 45, 188). Stimuli to the face evoke sensation referred to the amputated hand (e.g., 271).

Electrophysiological studies have defined the posterior parietal cortex as a site for body schemas that coalesce across sensory modalities (see 304). This fits with the clinical observations of hemineglect in patients with lesions in this area. Furthermore, this cortical area receives corollary inputs from the motor cortex.

Psychophysical studies have exposed the impermanence of the body schema. Changes in muscle and cutaneous inputs distort the whole body schema rather than simply the perceived position of joints. If, the elbow flexors are vibrated and the forearm is fixed horizontally against a wall, the body seems to rotate away from the forearm (202). This illusion takes longer to develop than the expected illusion of elbow extension because the CNS needs time to compute the "best" solution. Similarly, artificial activation of muscle afferents from the hand evokes impossible postures of the fingers (65, 102) and abolition of the usual sensory input with anesthesia of the thumb or arm increases the perceived size of the digits (104, 239).

A second approach has been to determine how the body schema is used. When asked to point at an object, the angle of the upper arm at the shoulder depends on whether the "frame of reference" is centered on the head (i.e., visual map) or on the shoulder (kinesthetic map) (see 300). If vision is allowed, the pointing finger lies on a line between the eyes and the object (i.e., head frame of reference), but without vision, the finger lies on a line between the shoulder and the object (i.e., shoulder frame of reference) (310). Subjects can apply the kinesthetic signals from the pointing movement to visual or kinesthetic maps. However, the visual frame of reference becomes dominant in patients with a sensory neuropathy. Unlike normal subjects, they trace mirror-reversed shapes without difficulty (24, 206).

Muscle Fatigue

Muscle fatigue is a series of processes, both peripheral and central, that reduce maximal voluntary force in exercise. It modifies kinesthesia through several mechanisms. Proprioceptive afferents change their discharge. In addition, the contraction and relaxation rates of muscle usually slow depending on the type of exercise (see 84), and group III muscle afferents are sensitized (150). The responsiveness to passive stretch increases in primary muscle spindle afferents and decreases in tendon organs (51, 169, 252, 317). The discharge of nonspindle group II and group III afferents increases with fatigue (150). Spindle discharge declines during fatiguing voluntary contractions (232). These kinesthetic inputs degrade as the quality of motor performance deteriorates and tremor begins. Position matching shows much variability and possibly a deterioration during fatigue (291, 298). Altered kinesthetic inputs and corticofugal commands modify transmission at spinal and supraspinal sites. Motivation and attentional factors also need consideration.

A familiar change with fatigue is that forces become more difficult to sustain and weights become characteristically heavy. This is easily documented in matching tasks (e.g., 115, 181, 224). Several factors will contribute. First, as fatigue develops at sites beyond the neuromuscular junction, force maintenance will require an increased command to recruit motor units. Second, the increased effort "irradiates" to synergist and remote muscle groups so that the illusory increase with concurrent contraction of related muscles will occur [Fig. 4.13; (194)]. Third, motoneurons are "inhibited" by small-diameter muscle afferents (23, 176, 120) (see earlier under KINESTHETIC MECHANISMS IN ISOLATION) and due to reduced muscle spindle facilitation (232). Finally, the afferents that evoke sensations of muscle pain may presumably signal the perceived level of muscle fatigue.

Altered Kinesthesia with Aging

The CNS drives a musculoskeletal system that alters with growth and senescence. Age-related changes in motor function vary widely among individuals. Beyond the fifth decade, cross-sectional studies reveal changes in receptor properties; nerve conduction velocities; and cutaneous, visual, and vestibular function. These changes, together with likely cognitive deficits, impair performance in proprioceptive testing. Errors in position matching and movement detection develop at distal, proximal, and spinal joints (e.g., 89, 147, 190, 197, 205, 215, 216). In a study of 550 women, proprioceptive and cutaneous sensation along with visual and vestibular performance deteriorated with age (217). The correlation was stronger for cutaneous vibration sense than for position-matching ability or judgments of vestibular "upright." With aging, relatively greater reliance might be placed on proprioceptive cues for motor performance.

On the output side, maximal isometric and dynamic strength declines, probably in all muscle groups but particularly in the ankle plantar flexors (67). These strength reductions derive from denervation and atrophy of type II muscle fibers, particularly above the age of 70 (e.g., 208), and perhaps also from a reduction in the number of motor units (46). The metabolic profile and response to electrical stimulation of aged muscle is consistent with impaired endurance, although tests of voluntary performance are less conclusive. Remodeling of the motor control system occurs as the relaxation rate of motor units slows with age and this is accompanied by an appropriate reduction in the firing rate of motor units (see 254).

Overall, position and movement sense is impaired, together with muscular strength and the capacity for coordination. Standing and other tasks become more difficult and less stable. Diminished proprioception for the toes, impaired cutaneous sensation, and reduced strength at the ankle predict the likelihood of falling in elderly subjects (196, 215, 216, 302). A corollary is that restoring strength and mobility would reduce this risk.

Changes in Kinesthesia with Joint Pathology

If joint afferents add their weight to key kinesthetic sensations (see earlier under KINESTHETIC MECHANISMS IN ISOLATION), then joint pathology may affect them. A critical point in patient studies is not only the control group, but also whether remote pathological changes exist, involving other afferents. In animals, an acute effusion enhances the movement responsiveness of some group II joint afferents due to the increase in intracapsular pressure (87). With an artificial effusion, movement detection improves at a finger joint when muscle afferents could not contribute [Fig. 4.10*A*; (55, 91)]. Injection of kaolin and carrageenan into the cat knee inflames the joint for up to 24 hours, during which the number of group II joint afferents with a background discharge increases, but their mechanical thresholds are unaltered (75). The number of group III and IV afferents with a background discharge doubles (from about 40% to 80%), and their mechanical thresholds decrease so that more than 90% respond to innocuous movements (Fig. 4.19*A*). Similar changes occur in chronic arthritis (e.g., 145). The altered movement-induced feedback from joint afferents produces not only arthritic pain but reflex limitations to movement and sensitization of central sites to which the afferents project (see 144, 167).

Artificial replacement of the knee, hip, metacarpophalangeal, and metatarsophalangeal joints offers an attractive way to assess the role of joint receptors. Most studies report a mild deficiency in kinesthetic performance relative to a control group (14–16), or when compared to the unoperated side (139, 191; cf. 66). For position rematching and detection of passive movements at the knee (<1 degree/s), no side-to-side difference in acuity was apparent (14), although acuity was lower than in a matched population (Fig. 4.19*B*). The slight deficiency had been unappreciated because joint function declines not only on the operated side in osteoarthritis, and because the changes are too small to detect with manual evaluation. If the remaining kinesthetic signals, such as those from local and remote cutaneous afferents, are enhanced by bandaging the knee, then acuity improves (16).

With knee replacement, thresholds for detection and reproduction of applied movements increased from about 5–6 degrees (in matched controls) to 8–10 degrees (Fig. 4.19*B*). Grigg and colleagues (139) concluded that hip joint receptors were largely redundant. However, detection of movements (0.15 degree/s) was impaired significantly in three of eight patients on the operated side. All patients judged small (<5 degree abduction) but not large passive movements (5–15 degrees) with greater precision on the nonoperated side, and patients consistently overestimated the size of applied movements on the operated side. One test showed no impairment on the operated side, but signals of motor commands could explain this.

Patients with rheumatoid arthritis have distorted position sense (89). The proximal joint of the fingers

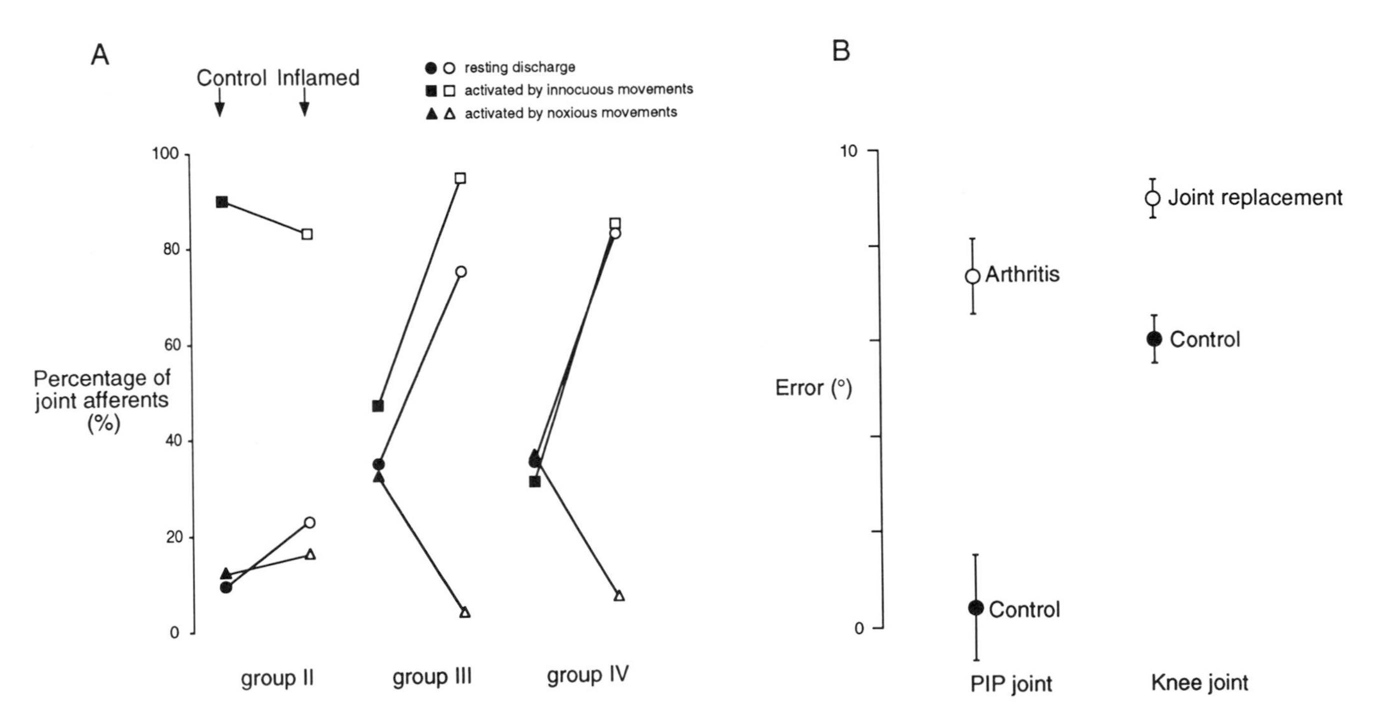

FIG. 4.19. *A*, Data from a model of acute arthritis in the cat knee. Joint afferents in the medial articular nerve, classified according to conduction velocity, studied under control conditions (*filled symbols*) and during acute inflammation (*open symbols*). The percentages of units with a background discharge in the midrange (*circles*), responsiveness to non-noxious (*squares*) and noxious movements (*triangles*) are shown. [Data from Dorn, Schaible, and Schmidt (75).] *B*, *At left*, Mean values (± SEM) for estimates of position sense at the proximal interphalangeal joint of the index finger (PIP) in subjects with rheumatoid arthritis and a matched control group. Subjects aligned a silhouette to the perceived position of the passively displaced joint (0.3 degree/s). Errors were usually in the direction of the flexion deformity. [Data from Ferrell, Crighton, and Sturrock (90).] *At right*, Mean values (± SEM) for estimates of position sense at the knee in subjects with knee replacement and an age-matched control group. The test relied on active reproduction of a passively imposed position. [Data from Barrack et al. (14).]

seems more flexed (Fig. 4.17*B*), with the matching error being 7 degrees in the patients and less than 1 degree in control subjects. This change may reflect not only joint afferent input but a perceptual remapping due to the flexion deformity. Patients with hypermobile joints, previous dislocations, and ligament rupture might also have a mild proprioceptive impairment.

CONCLUSIONS

Figure 4.20 depicts a simple scheme for kinesthetic signals. Afferent and efferent kinesthetic signals have no single role: they contribute to kinesthesia and motor learning; they also reflexly change movements. Their contribution to motor control proceeds with or without conscious awareness. In the short and long term, kinesthetic signals mold an adaptive model of the musculoskeletal system (253).

How much have we advanced since the debates in the nineteenth century? The neurophysiological background is clearer, even if the arguments are similar. Improved methods in psychophysics and the single-neuron recording in awake animals and humans have permitted a detailed examination of the role of each kinesthetic signal, although, as emphasized throughout, kinesthesia includes several sets of sensations and multiple mechanisms contribute to most of them. Inclusion of sensations of muscle timing and the body schema in the definition of kinesthesia recognizes their essential role in the control of movement.

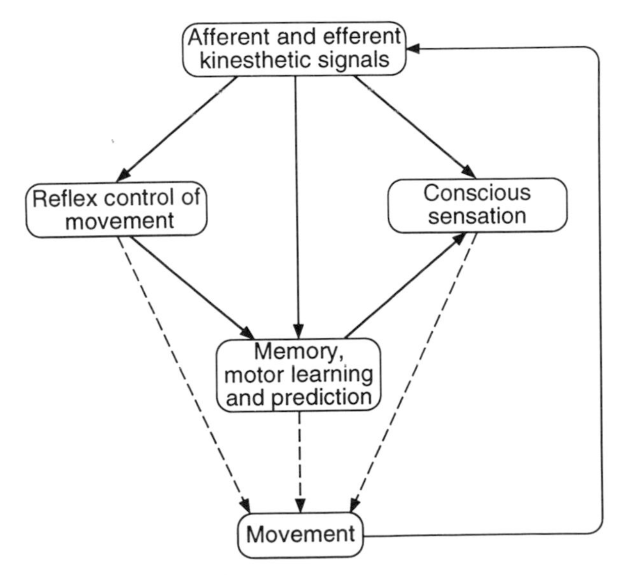

FIG. 4.20. Schematic representation of the destinations for both afferent and efferent kinesthetic signals.

Redundancy is rife among the kinesthetic inputs and they are used opportunistically in movement execution and perception. The production of an accurate kinesthetic map may require a multiplicity of inputs to cope with the different properties of each receptor class. Because most natural perturbations move contracting muscles, and as muscle spindles and tendon organs respond preferentially to such perturbations, their inputs must have a prime role. However, their capacities to deliver absolute information about position and loads are limited. The presence of multiple inputs tuned to different aspects of natural movements ensures that potential kinesthetic ambiguities can be resolved, with signals from passive antagonist and synergist muscles, and rapidly adapting "event detectors" in the skin likely to be important. Prediction of kinesthetic roles for particular afferents requires knowledge of their properties, although the discharge of an afferent to one variable is not sufficient to establish that the discharge causes a percept. Hence the potential of cutaneous afferents to contribute to movement sense is undeniable, but the magnitude of the contribution is small at some joints, although the full answer is awaited. Caution is also warranted in the interpretation of kinesthetic signals under extreme conditions: because a particular kinesthetic signal then contributes does not establish that it will do so under less extreme conditions.

Kinesthesia encompasses sensations from skin and joint inputs, sensations from intramuscular receptors, and sensations biased by motor command corollaries. However, as Wundt argued over a century ago, each of these three mechanisms involved in the so-called muscle sense "is insufficient, because none is capable of explaining the totality of the phenomenon we encounter in the domain of movement sensations" (278). Future studies will probe not simply the presence of the various signals but how they are combined, where they are formed within the CNS, and how they are used.

The author's work is supported by the National Health and Medical Research Council (of Australia) and the Asthma Foundation of New South Wales. I am most indebted to Ms. M. Sweet and Ms. J. Butler, who have helped in preparation of the text and illustrations. As the number of references that could be cited was restricted and the text required in early 1995, I apologize for the unavoidable omissions. I am grateful to colleagues who provided suggestions on drafts of the text, including Professors D. Burke, I. McCloskey, U. Proske, and Dr. T. Inglis, and to many others for interesting discussions and for allowing unpublished material to be cited.

REFERENCES

1. Adams, L., A. Guz, J. A. Innes, and K. Murphy. The early circulatory and ventilatory response to voluntary and electrically induced exercise in man. *J. Physiol. (Lond.)* 383: 19–30, 1987.
2. Al-Falahe, N. A., M. Nagaoka, and Å. B. Vallbo. Response profiles of human muscle afferents during active finger movements. *Brain* 113: 325–346, 1990.
3. Amassian, V. E., and L. Berlin. Early cortical projection of group I afferents in the forelimb muscle nerves of cat. *J. Physiol. (Lond.)* 143: 61P, 1958.
4. Aniss, A. M., H.-C. Diener, J. Hore, S. C. Gandevia, and D. Burke. Behavior of human muscle receptors when reliant on proprioceptive feedback during standing. *J. Neurophysiol.* 64: 661–670, 1990.
5. Aniss, A. M., S. C. Gandevia, and R. J. Milne. Changes in perceived heaviness and motor commands produced by cutaneous reflexes in man. *J. Physiol. (Lond.)* 397: 113–126, 1988.
6. Appelberg, B. Selective central control of dynamic gamma motoneurons utilised for the functional classification of gamma cells. In: *Muscle Receptors and Movement*, edited by A. Taylor and A. Prochzaka. London: Macmillan, 1981, p. 97–108.
7. Appenteng, K., and A. Prochazka. Tendon organ firing during active muscle lengthening in awake, normally behaving cats. *J. Physiol. (Lond.)* 353: 81–92, 1984.
8. Ashton-Miller, J. A., K. M. McGlashen, and A. B. Schultz. Trunk positioning accuracy in children 7–18 years old. *J. Orthopaed. Res.* 10: 217–225, 1992.
9. Bakker, D. A., and F. J. R. Richmond. Muscle spindle complexes in muscles around upper cervical vertebrae in the cat. *J. Neurophysiol.* 48: 62–74, 1982.
10. Bard, C., J. Paillard, Y. Lajoie, M. Fleury, N. Teasdale, R. Forget, and Y. Lamarre. Role of afferent information in the timing of motor commands: a comparative study with a deafferented patient. *Neuropsychologia* 30: 201–206, 1992.
11. Balkowiec, A., K. Kukula, and P. Szulczyk. Functional classification of afferent phrenic nerve fibres and diaphagmatic receptors in cats. *J. Physiol. (Lond.)* 483: 759–768, 1995.
12. Barker, D. The morphology of muscle receptors. In: *Handbook of Sensory Physiology, Muscle Receptors*, edited by C. C. Hunt. Berlin: Springer-Verlag, 1974, vol. III, part 2, p. 1–190.
13. Barker, D., J. J. Scott, and M. J. Stacey. A study of glycogen depletion and the fibre-type composition of cat skeletofusimotor units. *J. Physiol. (Lond.)* 450: 565–579, 1992.
14. Barrack, R. L., H. B. Skinner, S. D. Cook, and R. J. Haddad. Effect of articular disease and total knee arthroplasty on knee joint-position sense. *J. Neurophysiol.* 50: 684–687, 1983.
15. Barrett, D. S. Proprioception and function after anterior cruciate reconstruction. *J. Bone Joint Surg.* 73-B: 833–837, 1991.
16. Barrett, D. S., A. G. Cobb, and G. Bentley. Joint proprioception in normal, osteoarthritic and replaced knees. *J. Bone Joint Surg.* 73-B: 53–56, 1991.
17. Bastian, H. C. The "muscular sense"; its nature and localization. *Brain* 10: 1–136, 1888.
18. Baumann, T. K., and M. Hulliger. The dependence of the response of cat spindle Ia afferents to sinusoidal stretch on the velocity of concomitant movement. *J. Physiol. (Lond.)* 439: 325–350, 1991.
19. Baxendale, R. H., and W. R. Ferrell. Discharge characteristics of the elbow joint nerve of the cat. *Brain Res.* 261: 195–203, 1983.
20. Bell, C. *The Hand: Its Mechanism and Vital Endowments as Evincing Design*. London: Pickering, 1833.
21. Bell, C. C. Electroreception in mormyrid fish, central physiology. In: *Electroreception*, edited by T. H. Bullock and W. Heiligenberg. New York: John Wiley & Sons, Inc., 1986, p. 423–452.
22. Bevan, L., P. Cordo, L. Carlton, and M. Carlton. Proprioceptive coordination of movement sequences: discrimination of joint angle versus angular distance. *J. Neurophysiol.* 71: 1862–1872, 1994.
23. Bigland-Ritchie, B., N. J. Dawson, R. S. Johansson, and O. C. J. Lippold. Reflex origin for the slowing of motoneurone firing rates in fatigue of human voluntary contractions. *J. Physiol. (Lond.)* 379: 451–459, 1986.
24. Blouin, J., C. Bard, N. Teasdale, J. Paillard, M. Fleury, R. Forget, and Y. Lamarre. Reference systems for coding spatial information in normal subjects and a deafferented patient. *Exp. Brain Res.* 93: 324–331, 1993.
25. Boring, E. G. *Sensation and Perception in the History of Experimental Psychology*. New York: Appleton-Century-Crofts, 1942.
26. Boyd, I. A. Two types of static gamma-axon in cat muscle spindles. *Q. J. Exp. Physiol.* 71: 307–327, 1986.
27. Boyd, I. A., and Davey, M. R. *Composition of Peripheral Nerves*. Edinburgh: Livingstone, 1968.
28. Boyd, I. A., and M. H. Gladden. *The Muscle Spindle*, 1985. London: Macmillan, 1985.
29. Bridgeman, B., and L. Stark. Ocular proprioception and efference copy in registering visual direction. *Vision Res.* 31: 1903–1913, 1991.
30. Bridgeman, C. F. Comparisons of structure of tendon organs in the rat, cat, and man. *J. Comp. Neurol.* 138: 369–372, 1970.
31. Brindley, G. S., G. M. Goodwin, J. J. Kulikowski, and D. Leighton. Stability of vision with a paralysed eye. *J. Physiol. (Lond.)* 258: 65P–66P, 1976.
32. Brindley, G. S., and Merton, P. A. The absence of position sense in the human eye. *J. Physiol. (Lond.)* 153: 127–130, 1960.
33. Brodie, E. E., and H. E. Ross. Sensorimotor mechanisms in weight discrimination. *Percept. Psychophys.* 36: 477–481, 1984.
34. Brown, M. C. I. Engberg, and P. B. C. Matthews. The relative sensitivity to vibration of muscle receptors of the cat. *J. Physiol. (Lond.)* 192: 773–800, 1967.
35. Burgess, P. R., and F. J. Clark. Characteristics of knee joint receptors in the cat. *J. Physiol. (Lond.)* 203: 317–335, 1969.
36. Burgess, P. R., J. Y. Wei, F. J. Clark, and J. Simon. Signaling of kinesthetic information by peripheral sensory receptors. *Annu. Rev. Neurosci.* 5: 171–187, 1982.
37. Burke, D. The activity of human muscle spindle endings in normal motor behavior. *Int. Rev. Physiol.* 25: 91–126, 1981.
38. Burke, D., and S. C. Gandevia. Peripheral motor system. In: *The Human Nervous System*, edited by G. Paxinos. New York: Academic Press, 1990, p. 125–145.
39. Burke, D., S. C. Gandevia, and G. Macefield. Responses to passive movement of receptors in joint, skin and muscle of the human hand. *J. Physiol. (Lond.)* 402: 347–361, 1988.
40. Burke, D., K.-E. Hagbarth, L. Lofstedt, and B. G. Wallin. The responses of human muscle spindle endings to vibra-

tion of non-contracting muscles. *J. Physiol. (Lond.)* 261: 673–693, 1976.
41. Burke, D., K.-E. Hagbarth, L. Lofstedt, and B. G. Wallin. The responses of human muscle spindle endings to vibration during isometric contraction. *J. Physiol. (Lond.)* 261: 695–711, 1976.
42. Burke, D., N. F. Skuse, and A. K. Lethlean. Cutaneous and muscle afferent components of the cerebral potential evoked by electrical stimulation of human peripheral nerves. *Electroencephalogr. Clin. Neurophysiol.* 51: 579–588, 1981.
43. Cafarelli, E. Force sensation in fresh and fatigued human skeletal muscle. *Exer. Sport Sci. Rev.* 16: 139–168, 1988.
44. Cafarelli, E., and B. Bigland-Ritchie. Sensation of static force in muscles of different length. *Exp. Neurol.* 65: 511–525, 1979.
45. Calford, M. B., and R. Tweedale. Immediate and chronic changes in responses of somatosensory cortex in adult flying-fox after digit amputation. *Nature* 332: 446–448, 1988.
46. Campbell, M. J., A. J. McComas, and F. Petito. Physiological changes in ageing muscles. *J. Neurol. Neurosurg. Psychiatry* 36: 174–182, 1973.
47. Capaday, C., and J. D. Cooke. The effects of muscle vibration of the attainment of intended final position during voluntary human arm movements. *Exp. Brain Res.* 42: 228–230, 1981.
48. Castiello, U., Y. Paulignan, and M. Jeannerod. Temporal dissociation of motor responses and subjective awareness. A study in normal subjects. *Brain* 114: 2639–2655, 1991.
49. Celichowski, J., F. Emonet-Denand, Y. Laporte, and J. Petit. Distribution of static gamma axons in cat peroneus tertius spindles determined by exclusively physiological criteria. *J. Neurophysiol.* 71: 722–732, 1994.
50. Chambers, M. R., K. H. Andres, M. von Duering, and A. Iggo. The structure and function of the slowly adapting type II mechanoreceptor in hairy skin. *Q. J. Exp. Physiol.* 57: 417–445, 1972.
51. Christakos, C. N., and U. Windshorst. Spindle gain increase during muscle unit fatigue. *Brain Res.* 365: 388–392, 1986.
52. Clark, F. J., and P. R. Burgess. Slowly adapting receptors in cat knee joint: can they signal joint angle? *J. Neurophysiol.* 38: 1448–1463, 1975.
53. Clark, F. J., R. C. Burgess, and J. W. Chapin. Proprioception with the proximal interphalangeal joint of the index finger. Evidence for a movement sense without a static-position sense. *Brain* 109: 1195–1208, 1986.
54. Clark, F. J., R. C. Burgess, J. W. Chapin, and W. T. Lipscomb. Role of intramuscular receptors in the awareness of limb position. *J. Neurophysiol.* 54: 1529–1540, 1985.
55. Clark, F. J., P. Grigg, and J. W. Chapin. The contribution of articular receptors to proprioception with the fingers in humans. *J. Neurophysiol.* 61: 186–193, 1989.
56. Clark, F. J., K. W. Horch, S. M. Bach, and G. F. Larson. Contributions of cutaneous and joint receptors to static knee-position sense in man. *J. Neurophysiol.* 42: 877–888, 1979.
57. Cleland, C. L., L. Hayward, and W. Z. Rymer. Neural mechanisms underlying the clasp-knife reflex in the cat. II. Stretch-sensitive muscular-free nerve endings. *J. Neurophysiol.* 64: 1319–1330, 1990.
58. Cole, J. D., and W. L. Merton. Focusing of motor command in a subject with a large fibre sensory neuropathy below the neck. *J. Physiol. (Lond.)* 476: 85P, 1994.
59. Cole, J., and J. Paillard. Living without touch and peripheral information about body position and movement: studies upon deafferented subjects. *Can. J. Physiol. Pharmacol.* 1994 (in press).
60. Cole, J. D., and E. M. Sedgwick. The perceptions of force and of movement in a man without large myelinated sensory afferents below the neck. *J. Physiol. (Lond.)* 449: 503–515, 1992.
61. Colebatch, J. G., and D. I. McCloskey. Maintenance of constant arm position or force: reflex and volitional components in man. *J. Physiol. (Lond.)* 386: 247–261, 1987.
62. Cooke, J. D., and V. A. Diggles. Rapid error correction during human arm movements: evidence for central monitoring. *J. Motor Behav.* 16: 348–363, 1984.
63. Cordo, P., S. C. Gandevia, J. P. Hales, D. Burke, and G. Laird. Force and displacement-controlled tendon vibration in humans. *Electroencephalogr. Clin. Neurophysiol.* 89: 45–53, 1993.
64. Crago, P. E., J. C. Houk, and W. Z. Rymer. Sampling of total muscle force by tendon organs. *J. Neurophysiol.* 47: 1069–1083, 1982.
65. Craske, B. Perception of impossible limb positions induced by tendon vibration. *Science* 196: 71–73, 1977.
66. Cross, M. J., and D. I. McCloskey. Position sense following surgical removal of joints in man. *Brain Res.* 55: 443–445, 1973.
67. Davies, C. T. M., and M. J. White. The contractile properties of elderly human triceps surae. *Gerontology* 29: 19–25, 1983.
68. Davis, C. M. The role of effective lever length in the perception of lifted weights. *Percept. Psychophys.* 13: 238–240, 1974.
69. Decety, J., M. Jeannerod, D. Durozard, and G. Baverel. Central activation of autonomic effectors during mental simulation of motor actions in man. *J. Physiol. (Lond.)* 461: 549–563, 1993.
70. Dellon, A. L. *Evaluation of Sensibility and Re-education of Sensation in the Hand*. Baltimore: Williams & Wilkins, 1981.
71. Devanandan, M. S., S. Ghosh, and K. T. John. A quantitative study of muscle spindles and tendon organs in some intrinsic muscles of the hand in the bonnet monkey *(Macaca radiata)*. *Anat. Rec.* 207: 263–266, 1983.
72. Dickson, M., F. Emonet-Dénand, M. H. Gladden, J. Petit, and J. Ward. Incidence of non-driving excitation of Ia afferents during ramp frequency stimulation of static gamma-axons in cat hindlimbs. *J. Physiol. (Lond.)* 460: 657–673, 1993.
73. Dickson, M., and M. H. Gladden. Central and reflex recruitment of γ motoneurones of individual muscle spindles of the tenuissimus muscle in anaesthetised cats. In: *Muscle Afferents and Spinal Control of Movement*, edited by L. Jami, E. Pierrot-Deseilligny, and D. Zytnicki. Oxford: Pergamon, 1992, p. 37–42.
74. DiZio, P., C. E. Lathan, and J. R. Lackner. The role of brachial muscle spindle signals in assignment of visual direction. *J. Neurophysiol.* 70: 1578–1584, 1993.
75. Dorn, T., H.-G. Schaible, and R. F. Schmidt. Response properties of thick myelinated group II afferents in the medial articular nerve of normal and inflamed knee joints of the cat. *Somatosens. Mot. Res.* 8: 127–136, 1991.
76. Duchateau, J., and K. Hainaut. Behaviour of short and long latency reflexes in fatigued human muscles. *J. Physiol. (Lond.)* 471: 787–799, 1993.

77. Edin, B. B. Finger joint movement sensitivity of non-cutaneous mechanoreceptor afferents in the human radial nerve. *Exp. Brain Res.* 82: 417–422, 1990.
78. Edin, B. B. Quantitative analysis of static strain sensitivity in human mechanoreceptors from hairy skin. *J. Neurophysiol.* 67: 1105–1113, 1992.
79. Edin, B. B., and J. H. Abbs. Finger movement responses of cutaneous mechanoreceptors in the dorsal skin of the human hand. *J. Neurophysiol.* 65: 657–670, 1991.
80. Edin, B. B., and Å. B. Vallbo. Classification of human muscle stretch receptor afferents: a Bayesian approach. *J. Neurophysiol.* 63: 1314–1322, 1990.
81. Eklund, G. Position sense and state of contraction: the effects of vibration. *J. Neurol. Neurosurg. Psychiatry* 35: 606–611, 1972.
82. Ellaway, P. H., P. R. Murphy, and A. Tripathi. Closely coupled excitation of gamma-motoneurones by group III muscle afferents with low mechanical threshold in the cat. *J. Physiol. (Lond.)* 331: 481–498, 1982.
83. Ellis, R. R., and S. J. Lederman. The role of haptic versus visual volume cues in the size-weight illusion. *Percept. Psychophys.* 53: 315–324, 1993.
84. Enoka, R. M., and D. G. Stuart. Neurobiology of muscle fatigue. *J. Appl. Physiol.* 72: 1631–1648, 1992.
85. Feldman, A. G., and M. L. Latash. Interaction of afferent and efferent signals underlying joint position sense: empirical and theoretical approaches. *J. Mot. Behav.* 14: 174–193, 1982.
86. Ferrell, W. R. The adequacy of stretch receptors in the cat knee joint for signalling joint angle throughout a full range of movement. *J. Physiol. (Lond.)* 299: 85–99, 1980.
87. Ferrell, W. R. The effect of acute joint distension on mechanoreceptor discharge in the knee of the cat. *Q. J. Exp. Physiol.* 72: 493–499, 1987.
88. Ferrell, W. R., and B. Craske. Contribution of joint and muscle afferents to position sense at the human proximal interphalangeal joint. *Exp. Physiol.* 77: 331–342, 1992.
89. Ferrell, W. R., A. Crighton, and R. D. Sturrock. Age-dependent changes in position sense in human proximal interphalangeal joints. *Neuroreport* 3: 259–261, 1992.
90. Ferrell, W. R., A. Crighton, and R. D. Sturrock. Position sense at the proximal interphalangeal joint is distorted in patients with rheumatoid arthritis of finger joints. *Exp. Physiol.* 77: 675–680, 1992.
91. Ferrell, W. R., S. C. Gandevia, and D. I. McCloskey. The role of joint receptors in human kinaesthesia when intramuscular receptors cannot contribute. *J. Physiol. (Lond.)* 386: 63–71, 1987.
92. Ferrell, W. R., and A. Smith. Position sense at the proximal interphalangeal joint of the human index finger. *J. Physiol. (Lond.)* 399: 49–61, 1988.
93. Ferrell, W. R., and A. Smith. The effect of loading on position sense at the proximal interphalangeal joint of the human index finger. *J. Physiol. (Lond.)* 418: 145–161, 1989.
94. Ferrier, D. *The Functions of the Brain.* London: Smith, Elder & Co., 1876.
95. Fitzpatrick, R., and D. I. McCloskey. Proprioceptive, visual and vestibular thresholds for the perception of sway during standing in humans. *J. Physiol. (Lond.)* 478: 173–186, 1994.
96. Fitzpatrick, R., D. Burke, and S. C. Gandevia. Task-dependent reflex responses and movement illusions evoked by galvanic vestibular stimulation in standing humans. *J. Physiol. (Lond.)* 478: 363–372, 1994.
97. Foerster, O. Schlaffe und spastische Lähmung. In: *Handbuch der normalen und pathologischen Physiologie, Vol. 10*, edited by A. Berthe, G. V. Bergman, G. Embden, and A. Ellinger. Berlin, Heidelberg, New York: Springer, 1927, p. 900–901.
98. Forget, R., and Y. Lamarre. Rapid elbow flexion in the absence of proprioceptive and cutaneous feedback. *Hum. Neurobiol.* 6: 27–37, 1987.
99. Forget, R., and Y. Lamarre. Anticipatory postural adjustment in the absence of normal peripheral feedback. *Brain Res.* 508: 176–179, 1990.
100. Fukami, Y., and R. S. Wilkinson. Responses of isolated Golgi tendon organs of the cat. *J. Physiol. (Lond.)* 265: 673–689, 1977.
101. Gandevia, S. C. The perception of motor commands or effort during muscular paralysis. *Brain* 105: 151–159, 1982.
102. Gandevia, S. C. Illusory movements produced by electrical stimulation of low-threshold muscle afferents from the hand. *Brain* 108: 965–981, 1985.
103. Gandevia, S. C. Roles for perceived voluntary motor commands in motor control. *Trends Neurosci.* 10: 81–85, 1987.
104. Gandevia, S. C. Kinaesthetic illusions involving the hand which are not dependent on muscle afferents. *Proc. Aust. Physiol. Pharmacol. Soc.* 25: 31P, 1994.
105. Gandevia, S. C., and D. Burke. Effect of training on voluntary activation of human fusimotor neurons. *J. Neurophysiol.* 54: 1422–1429, 1985.
106. Gandevia, S. C., and D. Burke. Projection to the cerebral cortex from proximal and distal muscles in the human upper limb. *Brain* 111: 389–403, 1988.
107. Gandevia, S. C., and D. Burke. Does the nervous system depend on kinesthetic information to control natural limb movements. *Behav. Brain Sci.* 15: 614–632, 815–819, 1992.
108. Gandevia, S. C., L. A. Hali, D. I. McCloskey, and E. K. Potter. Proprioceptive sensation at the terminal joint of the middle finger. *J. Physiol. (Lond.)* 335: 507–517, 1983.
109. Gandevia, S. C., and S. Kilbreath. Accuracy of weight estimation for weights lifted by proximal and distal muscles of the human upper limb. *J. Physiol. (Lond.)* 423: 299–310, 1990.
110. Gandevia, S. C., K. Killian, D. K. McKenzie, M. Crawford, G. M. Allen, R. B. Gorman, and J. P. Hales. Respiratory sensations, cardiovascular control, kinaesthesia and transcranial stimulation during paralysis in humans. *J. Physiol. (Lond.)* 470: 85–107, 1993.
111. Gandevia, S. C., and D. I. McCloskey. Joint sense, muscle sense, and their combination as position sense measured at the distal interphalangeal joint of the middle finger. *J. Physiol. (Lond.)* 260: 387–407, 1976.
112. Gandevia, S. C., and D. I. McCloskey. Sensations of heaviness. *Brain* 100: 345–354, 1977.
113. Gandevia, S. C., and D. I. McCloskey. Effects of related sensory inputs on motor performances in man studied through changes in perceived heaviness. *J. Physiol. (Lond.)* 272: 653–672, 1977.
114. Gandevia, S. C., and D. I. McCloskey. Changes in motor commands, as shown by changes in perceived heaviness, during partial curarization and peripheral anaesthesia in man. *J. Physiol. (Lond.)* 272: 673–689, 1977.
115. Gandevia, S. C., and D. I. McCloskey. Interpretation of perceived motor commands by reference to afferent signals. *J. Physiol. (Lond.)* 283: 193–199, 1978.

116. Gandevia, S. C., D. I. McCloskey, and E. K. Potter. Alterations in perceived heaviness during digital anaesthesia. *J. Physiol. (Lond.)* 306: 365–375, 1980.
117. Gandevia, S. C., V. G. Macefield, B. Bigland-Ritchie, R. B. Gorman, and D. Burke. Motoneuronal output and gradation of effort in attempts to contract acutely paralysed leg muscles in man. *J. Physiol. (Lond.)* 471: 411–427, 1993.
118. Gandevia, S. C., G. Macefield, D. Burke, and D. K. McKenzie. Voluntary activation of human motor axons in the absence of muscle afferent feedback: the control of the deafferented hand. *Brain* 113: 1563–1581, 1990.
119. Gandevia, S. C., and J. C. Rothwell. Knowledge of motor commands and the recruitment of human motoneurons. *Brain* 110: 1117–1130, 1987.
120. Garland, S. J. Role of small diameter afferents in reflex inhibition during human muscle fatigue. *J. Physiol. (Lond.)* 435: 547–558, 1991.
121. Gauthier, G. M., D. Nommay, and J.-L. Vercher. Ocular muscle proprioception and visual localization of targets in man. *Brain* 113: 1857–1871, 1990.
122. Gauthier, G. M., D. Nommay, and J.-L. Vercher. The role of ocular muscle proprioception in visual localization of targets. *Science* 249: 58–61, 1990.
123. Ghez, C., J. Gordon, M. F. Ghilardi, C. N. Christakos, and S. E. Cooper. Roles of proprioceptive input in the programming of arm trajectories. *Cold Spring Harb. Symp. Quant. Biol.* 55: 837–847, 1990.
124. Gilhodes, J. C., J. P. Roll, and M. F. Tardy-Gervet. Perceptual and motor effects of agonist-antagonist muscle vibration in man. *Exp. Brain Res.* 61: 395–402, 1986.
125. Gilsing, M. G., C. G. Van den Bosch, S.-G. Lee, J. A. Ashton-Miller, N. B. Alexander, A. G. Schiltz, and W. A. Ericson. Association of age with the threshold for detecting ankle inversion and eversion in upright stance. *Age Ageing* 24: 58–66, 1995.
126. Goldscheider, A. (1889) Untersuchungen uber den Muskelsinn. *Arch. Anat. Physiol. (Liepzig)* 3: 369–502, 1889.
127. Goodale, M. A., and A. D. Milner. Separate visual pathways for perception and action. *TINS* 15: 20–25, 1992.
128. Goodwin, A. W., K. T. John, K. Sathian, and I. Darian-Smith. Spatial and temporal factors determining afferent fiber responses to a grating moving sinusoidally over the monkey's fingerpad. *J. Neurosci.* 9: 1280–1293, 1989.
129. Goodwin, G. M., D. I. McCloskey, and P. B. C. Matthews. The contribution of muscle afferents to kinaesthesia shown by vibration induced illusions of movement and by the effects of paralysing joint afferents. *Brain* 95: 705–748, 1972.
130. Goodwin, G. M., D. I. McCloskey, and J. H. Mitchell. Cardiovascular and respiratory responses to changes in central command during isometric exercise at constant muscle tension. *J. Physiol. (Lond.)* 226: 173–190, 1972.
131. Gordon, A. M., H. Forssberg, R. S. Johansson, and G. Westling. The integration of haptically acquired size information in the programming of precision grip. *Exp. Brain Res.* 83: 483–488, 1991.
132. Gordon, J., and C. Ghez. Trajectory control in targeted force impulses. III. Compensatory adjustments for initial errors. *Exp. Brain Res.* 67: 253–269, 1987.
133. Gregory, J. E., A. K. McIntyre, and U. Proske. Tendon organ afferents in the knee joint nerve of the cat. *Neurosci. Lett.* 103: 287–292, 1989.
134. Gregory, J. E., D. L. Morgan, and U. Proske. Site of impulse initiation in tendon organs of cat soleus muscle. *J. Neurophysiol.* 54: 1383–1395, 1985.
135. Gregory, J. E., D. L. Morgan, and U. Proske. The discharge of cat tendon organs during unloading contractions. *Exp. Brain Res.* 61: 222–226, 1986.
136. Gregory, J. E., D. L. Morgan, and U. Proske, Aftereffects in the responses of cat muscle spindles and errors of limb position sense in man. *J. Neurophysiol.* 59: 1220–1230, 1988.
137. Gregory, J. E., and U. Proske. The responses of Golgi tendon organs to stimulation of different combinations of motor units. *J. Physiol. (Lond.)* 295: 251–262, 1979.
138. Griffiths, R. I. Shortening of muscle fibres during stretch of the active cat medial gastrocnemius muscle: the role of tendon compliance. *J. Physiol. (Lond.)* 436: 219–236, 1991.
139. Grigg, P., G. A. Finerman, and L. H. Riley. Joint-position sense after total hip replacement. *J. Bone Joint Surg.* 55-A: 1016–1025, 1973.
140. Grigg, P., and B. J. Greenspan. Response of primate joint afferent neurons to mechanical stimulation of knee joint. *J. Neurophysiol.* 40: 1–8, 1977.
141. Grigg, P., and A. H. Hoffman. Properties of Ruffini afferents revealed by stress analysis of isolated sections of cat knee capsule. *J. Neurophysiol.* 47: 41–54, 1982.
142. Grigg, P., A. H. Hoffman, and K. E. Fogarty. Properties of Golgi-Mazzoni afferents in the cat knee joint capsule, as revealed by mechanical studies of isolated joint capsule. *J. Neurophysiol.* 47: 31–40, 1982.
143. Grill, S. E., and M. Hallett. Velocity sensitivity of human muscle spindle afferents and type II slowly adapting cutaneous mechanoreceptors. *J. Physiol. (Lond.)* (in press).
144. Grubb, B. D., R. U. Stiller, and H.-G. Schaible. Dynamic changes in the receptive field properties of spinal cord neurons with ankle input in rats with chronic unilateral inflammation in the ankle region. *Exp. Brain Res.* 92: 441–452, 1993.
145. Guilbaud, G., A. Iggo, and R. Tegner. Sensory receptors in ankle joint capsules of normal and anthritic rats. *Exp. Brain Res.* 58: 29–40, 1985.
146. Gurfinkel, V. S., M. I. Lipshits, and K. E. Popov. Thresholds for kinesthetic sensation in the vertical position. *Hum. Physiol.* 8: 439–445, 1982.
147. Gurfinkel, V. S., K. E. Popov, B. N. Smetanin, and V. Yu. Shlykov. Changes in the direction of vestibulomotor response in the course of adaptation to protracted static head turning in man. Translated from *Neurofiziologiya* 21: 210–217, 1989.
148. Gynther, B. D., R. M. Vickery, and M. J. Rowe. Responses of slowly adapting type II afferent fibres in cat hairy skin to vibrotactile stimuli. *J. Physiol. (Lond.)* 458: 151–169, 1992.
149. Hall, L. A., and D. I. McCloskey. Detections of movements imposed on finger, elbow and shoulder joints. *J. Physiol. (Lond.)* 335: 519–533, 1983.
150. Hayward, L., U. Wesselmann, and W. Z. Rymer. Effects of muscle fatigue on mechanically sensitive afferents of slow conduction velocity in the cat triceps surae. *J. Neurophysiol.* 65: 360–370, 1991.
151. Head, H., and G. Holmes. Sensory disturbances from cerebral lesions. *Brain* 34: 102–254, 1911.
152. Helmholtz, H. von. *Handbuch der Physiologischen Optik B. III.* Leipzig: Voss, English translation 3rd edition, 1925, edited by J. P. C. Southall. *A Treatise on Physiological Optics* (Vol. 3). New York: Dover, 1963.
153. Hensel, H., and K. K. A. Boman. Afferent impulses in cutaneous sensory nerves in human subjects. *J. Neurophysiol.* 23: 564–578, 1960.

154. Herbert, R. D., and S. C. Gandevia. Changes in pennation with joint angle and muscle torque: *in vivo* measurements in human brachialis muscle. *J. Physiol. (Lond.)* 484: 523–532, 1995.
155. Hobbs, S. F., and S. C. Gandevia. Cardiovascular responses and the sense of effort during attempts to contract paralysed muscles: role of the spinal cord. *Neurosci. Lett.* 57: 85–90, 1985.
156. Holmes, G. *Selected Papers of Sir Gordon Holmes*, edited by F. M. R. Walshe. London: Macmillan, 1956.
157. Holst, H. von. Relations between the central nervous system and the peripheral organs. *Br. J. Anim. Behav.* 2: 89–94, 1954.
158. Holst, H. von, and H. Mittelstaedt. The reafference principle. Interaction between the central nervous system and the periphery. (English translation) In: *Selected Papers of Erich von Holst: The Behavioural Physiology of Animals and Man* (1950). London: Methuen, 1973, p. 134–173.
159. Horch, K. W., F. J. Clark, and P. R. Burgess. Awareness of knee joint angle under static conditions. *J. Neurophysiol.* 38: 1436–1447, 1975.
160. Horcholle-Bossavit, G., L. Jami, J. Petit, R. Vejsada, and D. Zytnicki. Effects of muscle shortening on the responses of cat tendon organs to unfused contractions. *J. Neurophysiol.* 59: 1510–1523, 1988.
161. Horcholle-Bossavit, G., L. Jami, J. Petit, R. Vejsada, and D. Zytnicki. Ensemble discharge from Golgi tendon organs of the cat peroneus tertius muscle. *J. Neurophysiol.* 64: 813–821, 1990.
162. Hore, J., J. P. Preston, R. G. Durkovic, and P. D. Cheney. Responses of cortical neurons (areas 3a and 4) to ramp stretch of hindlimb muscles in the baboon. *J. Neurophysiol.* 39: 484–500, 1976.
163. Houk, J. C., J. J. Singer, and E. Henneman. Adequate stimulus for tendon organs with observations on mechanics of ankle joint. *J. Neurophysiol.* 34: 1051–1065, 1971.
164. Hulliger, M. The mammalian muscle spindle and its central control. *Rev. Physiol. Biochem. Pharmacol.* 101: 1–111, 1984.
165. Hulliger, M., N. Dürmüller, A. Prochazka, and P. Trend. Flexible fusimotor control of muscle spindle feedback during a variety of natural movements. *Prog. Brain Res.* 80: 87–101, 1989.
166. Hulliger, M., E. Nordh, A.-E. Thelin, and Å. B. Vallbo. The responses of afferent fibres from the glabrous skin of the hand during voluntary finger movements in man. *J. Physiol. (Lond.)* 291: 233–249, 1979.
167. Hurley, M. V., and D. J. Newham. The influence of arthrogenous muscle inhibition on quadriceps rehabilitation of patients with early, unilateral osteoarthritic knees. *Br. J. Rheumatol.* 32: 127–131, 1993.
168. Hutton, R. S., K. Kaiya, S. Suzuki, and S. Watanabe. Post-contraction errors in human force production are reduced by muscle stretch. *J. Physiol. (Lond.)* 393: 247–259, 1987.
169. Hutton, R. S., and D. L. Nelson. Stretch sensitivity of Golgi tendon organs in fatigued gastrocnemius muscle. *Med. Sci. Sports Exerc.* 18: 69–74, 1986.
170. Iggo, A., and K. H. Andres. Morphology of cutaneous receptors. *Annu. Rev. Neurosci.* 5: 1–31, 1982.
171. Innes, J. A., S. C. De Cort, P. J. Evans, and A. Guz. Central command influences cardiorespiratory response to dynamic exercise in humans with unilateral weakness. *J. Physiol. (Lond.)* 448: 551–563, 1992.
172. Jakobs, T., J. A. A. Miller, and A. B. Schultz. Trunk position sense in the frontal plane. *Exp. Neurol.* 90: 129–138, 1985.
173. James, W. *The Principles of Psychology*. New York: Holt & Co., 1890.
174. Jami, L. Golgi tendon organs in mammalian skeletal muscle: functional properties and central actions. *Physiol. Rev.* 72: 623–666, 1992.
175. Jami, L., J. Petit, U. Proske, and D. Zytnicki. Responses of tendon organs to unfused contractions of single motor units. *J. Neurophysiol.* 53: 32–42, 1985.
176. Jeannerod, M., F. Michel, and C. Prablanc. The control of hand movements in a case of hemianaesthesia following a parietal lesion. *Brain* 107: 899–920, 1984.
177. Jennings, V. A., Y. Lamour, H. Solis, and C. Fromm. Somatosensory cortex activity related to position and force. *J. Neurophysiol.* 49: 1216–1229, 1983.
178. Jiang, W., C. E. Chapman, and Y. Lamarre. Modulation of the cutaneous responsiveness of neurones in the primary somatosensory cortex during conditioned arm movements in the monkey. *Exp. Brain Res.* 84: 342–354, 1991.
179. Johansson, R. S., and Å. B. Vallbo. Tactile sensibility in the human hand: relative and absolute densities of four types of mechanoreceptive units in glabrous skin. *J. Physiol. (Lond.)* 286: 282–300, 1979.
180. John, K. T., A. W. Goodwin, and I. Darian-Smith. Tactile discrimination of thickness. *Exp. Brain Res.* 78: 62–68, 1989.
181. Jones, L. A. Role of central and peripheral signals in force sensation during fatigue. *Exp. Neurol.* 81: 497–503, 1983.
182. Jones, L. A. Motor illusions: what do they reveal about proprioception? *Psychol. Bull.* 103: 72–86, 1988.
183. Jones, L. A., and I. W. Hunter. Effect of fatigue on force sensation. *Exp. Neurol.* 81: 640–650, 1983.
184. Jones, L. A., and I. W. Hunter. A perceptual analysis of stiffness. *Exp. Brain Res.* 79: 150–156, 1990.
185. Jones, L. A., and I. W. Hunter. A perceptual analysis of viscosity. *Exp. Brain Res.* 94: 343–351, 1993.
186. Jorum, E., L. E. Lundberg, and H. E. Torebjörk. Peripheral projections of nociceptive unmyelinated axons in the human peroneal nerve. *J. Physiol. (Lond.)* 416: 291–301, 1989.
187. Jozsa, L., J. Balint, P. Kannus, M. Jarvinen, and M. Lehto. Mechanoreceptors in human myotendinous junction. *Muscle Nerve* 16: 453–457, 1993.
188. Kaas, J. H., M. M. Merzenich, and H. P. Killackey. The reorganization of somatosensory cortex following peripheral nerve damage in adult and developing mammals. *Annu. Rev. Neurosci.* 6: 325–356, 1983.
189. Kalaska, J. F., and D. J. Crammond. Cerebral cortical mechanisms of reaching movements. *Science* 255: 1517–1523, 1992.
190. Kaplan, F. S., J. E. Nixon, M. Reitz, L. Rindfleish, and J. Tucker. Age-related changes in proprioception and sensation of joint position. *Acta Orthop. Scand.* 56: 72–74, 1985.
191. Karanjia, P. N., and J. H. Ferguson. Passive joint position sense after total hip replacement surgery. *Ann. Neurol.* 13: 654–657, 1983.
192. Katz, J. Psychophysical correlates of phantom limb experience. *J. Neurol. Neurosurg. Psychiatry* 55: 811–821, 1992.
193. Keele, S. W., and R. Ivry. Does the cerebellum provide a common computation for diverse tasks? A timing hypothesis. *Ann. N.Y. Acad. Sci.* 608: 179–211, 1990.
194. Kilbreath, S. L., and S. C. Gandevia. Independent digit control: failure to partition perceived heaviness of weights lifted by digits of the human hand. *J. Physiol. (Lond.)* 442: 585–599, 1991.

195. Kilbreath, S. L., and S. C. Gandevia. Neural and biomechanical specialization of human thumb muscles revealed by matching weights and grasping objects. *J. Physiol. (Lond.)* 472: 537–556, 1993.
196. Kniffki, K.-D., S. Mense, and R. F. Schmidt. Responses of group IV afferent units from skeletal muscle to stretch, contraction and chemical stimulation. *Exp. Brain Res.* 31: 511–522, 1978.
197. Kokmen, E., R. W. Bossmeyer, and W. J. Williams. Quantitative evaluation of joint motion sensation in an aging population. *J. Gerontol.* 33: 62–67, 1978.
198. Konradsen, L., J. B. Ravn, and A. I. Sørensen. Proprioception at the ankle: the effect of anaesthetic blockade of ligament receptors. *J. Bone Joint Surg.* 75-B: 433–436, 1993.
199. Koshland, G. F., and J. L. Smith. Mutable and immutable features of paw-shake responses after hindlimb deafferentation in the cat. *J. Neurophysiol.* 62: 162–173, 1989.
200. Krauspe, R., M. Schmidt, and H.-G. Chaible. Sensory innervation of the anterior cruciate ligament. *J. Bone Joint Surg.* 74-A: 390–397, 1992.
201. Krogh, A., and J. Lindhadt. The regulation of respiration and circulation during the initial stages of muscular work. *J. Physiol. (Lond.)* 47: 112–136, 1913.
202. Lackner, J. R. Some proprioceptive influences on the perceptual representation of body shape and orientation. *Brain* 111: 281–297, 1988.
203. Lackner, J. R., and A. Graybiel. Perception of body weight and body mass at twice earth-gravity acceleration levels. *Brain* 107: 133–144, 1984.
204. Lacruz, F., J. Artieda, M. A. Pastor, and J. A. Obeso. The anatomical basis of somaesthetic temporal discrimination in humans. *J. Neurol. Neurosurg. Psychiatry* 54: 1077–1081, 1991.
205. Laidlaw, R. W., and N. A. Hamilton. A study of thresholds in apperception of passive movement among normal control subjects. *Bull. Neurol. Inst.* 6: 268–273, 1937.
206. Lajoie, Y., J. Paillard, N. Teasdale, C. Bard, M. Fleury, R. Forget, and Y. Lamarre. Mirror drawing in a deafferented patient and normal subjects: visuoproprioceptive conflict. *Neurology* 42: 1104–1106, 1992.
207. LaMotte, R. H., and J. Whitehouse. Tactile detection of a dot on a smooth surface: peripheral neural events. *J. Neurophysiol.* 56: 1109–1128, 1986.
208. Larsson, L. Morphological and functional characteristics of the ageing skeletal muscle in man. A cross-sectional study. *Acta Physiol. Scand.* 457 (Suppl.): 1–36, 1978.
209. Lazlo, J. I., and P. J. Bairstow. Accuracy of movement, peripheral feedback and efference copy. *J. Mot. Behav.* 3: 241–252, 1971.
210. Leem, J. W., W. D. Willis, and J. M. Chung. Cutaneous sensory receptors in the rat foot. *J. Neurophysiol.* 69: 1684–1699, 1993.
211. Libet, B., C. A. Gleason, E. W. Wright, and D. K. Pearl. Time of conscious intention to act in relation to onset of cerebral activity (readiness-potential). The unconscious initiation of a freely voluntary act. *Brain* 106: 623–642, 1983.
212. Libet, B., D. K. Pearl, D. E. Morledge, C. A. Gleason, Y. Hosobuchi, and N. M. Barbaro. Control of the transition from sensory detection to sensory awareness in man by the duration of a thalamic stimulus. The cerebral 'time-on' factor. *Brain* 114: 1731–1757, 1991.
213. Loeb, G. E. The control and responses of mammalian muscle spindles during normally executed motor tasks. *Exerc. Sport Sci. Rev.* 12: 157–204, 1984.
214. Loo, C. K., L. A. Hall, D. I. McCloskey, and M. J. Rowe. Proprioceptive contributions to tactile identification of figures: dependence on figure size. *Behav. Brain Res.* 7: 383–386, 1983.
215. Lord, S. R., R. D. Clark, and I. W. Webster. Physiological factors associated with falls in an elderly population. *J. Am. Geriatr. Soc.* 39: 1194–1200, 1991.
216. Lord, S. R., R. D. Clark, and I. W. Webster. Postural stability and associated physiological factors in a population of aged persons. *J. Gerontol. Med. Sci.* 46: M69–M76, 1991.
217. Lord, S. R., and J. A. Ward. Age-associated differences in sensori-motor function and balance in community dwelling women. *Age Aging* 23: 452–460, 1994.
218. McCloskey, D. I. Differences between the senses of movement and position shown by the effects of loading and vibration of muscles in man. *Brain Res.* 61: 119–131, 1973.
219. McCloskey, D. I. Muscular and cutaneous mechanisms in the estimation of the weights of grasped objects. *Neuropsychologia* 12: 513–520, 1974.
220. McCloskey, D. I. Kinesthetic sensibility. *Physiol. Rev.* 58: 763–820, 1978.
221. McCloskey, D. I. Corollary discharges: motor commands and perception. In: *Handbook of Physiology, The Nervous System, Motor Control*, edited by V. B. Brooks. Bethesda, MD: Am. Physiol. Soc., 1981, p. 1415–1447.
222. McCloskey, D. I., J. G. Colebatch, E. K. Potter, and D. Burke. Judgments about onset of rapid voluntary movements in man. *J. Neurophysiol.* 49: 851–863, 1983.
223. McCloskey, D. I., M. J. Cross, R. Honner, and E. K. Potter. Sensory effects of pulling or vibrating exposed tendons in man. *Brain* 106: 21–37, 1983.
224. McCloskey, D. I., P. Ebeling, and G. M. Goodwin. Estimation of weights and tensions and apparent involvement of a "sense of effort." *Exp. Neurol.* 42: 220–232, 1974.
225. McCloskey, D. I., and T. A. G. Torda. Corollary motor discharges and kinaesthesia. *Brain Res.* 100: 467–470, 1975.
226. McIntyre, A. K., U. Proske, and D. J. Tracey. Afferent fibres from muscle receptors in the posterior nerve of the cat's knee joint. *Exp. Brain Res.* 33: 415–424, 1978.
227. McIntyre, A. K., U. Proske, and J. A. Rawson. Cortical projection of afferent information from tendon organs in the cat. *J. Physiol. (Lond.)* 354: 395–406, 1984.
228. McIntyre, A. K., U. Proske, and J. A. Rawson. Pathway to the cerebral cortex for impulses from tendon organs in the cat's hindlimb. *J. Physiol. (Lond.)* 369: 115–126, 1985.
229. McKay, D. M. Perception and brain function. In: *The Neurosciences Second Study Program*, edited by F. O. Schmitt. New York: Rockefeller University Press, 1970, p. 303–316.
230. Macefield, V. G., S. C. Gandevia, B. Bigland-Ritchie, R. B. Gorman, and D. Burke. The firing rates of human motoneurones voluntarily activated in the absence of muscle afferent feedback. *J. Physiol. (Lond.)* 471: 429–443, 1993.
231. Macefield, G., S. C. Gandevia, and D. Burke. Perceptual responses to microstimulation of single afferents innervating joints, muscles and skin of the human hand. *J. Physiol. (Lond.)* 429: 113–129, 1990.
232. Macefield, G., K.-E. Hagbarth, R. Gorman, S. C. Gandevia, and D. Burke. Decline in spindle support to alpha motoneurones during sustained voluntary contractions. *J. Physiol. (Lond.)* 440: 497–512, 1991.
233. Mach, E. *The Analysis of Sensations* (1886). New York: Dover, 1959.

234. Mackel, R. Conduction of neural impulses in human mechanoreceptive cutaneous afferents. *J. Physiol. (Lond.)* 401: 597–615, 1988.
235. Mai, N., P. Schreiber, and J. Hermsdorfer. Changes in perceived finger force produced by muscular contractions under isometric and anisometric conditions. *Exp. Brain Res.* 84: 453–460, 1991.
236. Matthews, P. B. C. *Mammalian Muscle Receptors and Their Central Actions*. London: Arnold, 1972.
237. Matthews, P. B. C. Muscle spindles: their messages and their fusimotor supply. In: *Handbook of Physiology, The Nervous System, Motor Control*, edited by V. B. Brooks. Bethesda, MD: Am. Physiol. Soc., 1981, p. 189–227.
238. Melzack, R. Phantom limbs and the concept of a neuromatrix. *Trends Neurosci.* 13: 88–92, 1990.
239. Melzack, R., and P. R. Bromage. Experimental phantom limbs. *Exp. Neurol.* 39: 261–269, 1973.
240. Mense, S., and M. Stahnke. Responses in muscle afferent fibres of slow conduction velocity to contractions and ischaemia in the cat. *J. Physiol. (Lond.)* 342: 383–397, 1983.
241. Merton, P. A. The accuracy of directing the eyes and the hand in the dark. *J. Physiol. (Lond.)* 156: 555–577, 1961.
242. Meyer-Lohmann, J., W. Riebold, and D. Robrecht. Mechanical influence of the extrafusal muscle on the static behaviour of deefferented primary muscle spindle endings in the cat. *Pflugers Arch.* 352: 267–278, 1974.
243. Milne, R. J., A. M. Aniss, N. E. Kay, and S. G. Gandevia. Reduction in perceived intensity of cutaneous stimuli during movement: a quantitative study. *Exp. Brain Res.* 70: 569–576, 1988.
244. Mitchell, J. H. Neural control of the circulation during exercise. *Med. Sci. Sports Exerc.* 22: 141–154, 1990.
245. Mittelstaedt, H. Basic solutions to the problem of headcentric visual localization. In: *The Perception and Control of Self-Motion*, edited by R. Warren and A. Wertheim. Hillsdale, NJ: Lawrence Erlbaum Associates, 1990, p. 267–286.
246. Moberg, E. The role of cutaneous afferents in position sense, kinaesthesia, and motor function of the hand. *Brain* 106: 1–19, 1983.
247. Moberg, E. Two-point discrimination test. A valuable part of hand surgical rehabilitation, e.g. in tetraplegia. *Scand. J. Rehab. Med.* 22: 127–134, 1990.
248. Moore, A. P. Impaired sensorimotor integration in parkinsonism and dyskinesia: a role for corollary discharges? *J. Neurol. Neurosurg. Psychiatry* 50: 544–552, 1987.
249. Mountcastle, V. B., R. H. LaMotte, and G. Carli. Detection thresholds for stimuli in humans and monkeys: comparison with threshold events in mechanoreceptive afferent nerve fibres innervating the monkey hand. *J. Neurophysiol.* 35: 122–136, 1972.
250. Munger, B. L., and C. Ide. The structure and function of cutaneous sensory receptors. *Arch. Histol. Cytol.* 51: 1–34, 1988.
251. Murphy, P. R., and H. A. Martin. Fusimotor discharge patterns during rhythmic movements. *Trends Neurosci.* 16: 273–278, 1993.
252. Nelson, D. L., and R. S. Hutton. Dynamic and static stretch responses in muscle spindle receptors in fatigued muscle. *Med. Sci. Sports Exerc.* 17: 445–450, 1985.
253. Neilson, P. D. The problem of redundancy in movement control: the adaptive model theory approach. *Psychol. Res.* 55: 99–106, 1993.
254. Newton, J. P., R. Yemm, and M. J. N. McDonagh. Study of age changes in the motor units of the first dorsal interosseous muscle in man. *Gerontology* 34: 115–119, 1988.
255. Ochoa, J. L., and Torebjörk, H. E. Sensations evoked by intraneural microstimulation of single mechanoreceptor units innervating the human hand. *J. Physiol. (Lond.)* 342: 633–654, 1983.
256. Ochoa, J. L. and Torebjörk, H. E. Sensations evoked by intraneural microstimulation of C nociceptor fibres in human skin nerves. *J. Physiol. (Lond.)* 415: 583–599, 1989.
257. Osborn, C. E., and R. E. Poppele. Parallel distributed network characteristics of the DSCT. *J. Neurophysiol.* 68: 1100–1112, 1992.
258. Paillard, J., and M. Brouchon. Active and passive movements in the calibration of position sense. In: *The Neuropsychology of Spatially Oriented Behaviour*, edited by S. J. Freedman. Homewood, IL: Dorsey Press, 1968, p. 37–55.
259. Paintal, A. S. Functional analysis of group III afferent fibers of mammalian muscles. *J. Physiol. (Lond.)* 152: 250–270, 1960.
260. Patten, R. M., and W. K. Ovalle. Morphometry and histoenzymology of the hamster tenuissimus and its muscle spindles. *Anat. Rec.* 232: 499–511, 1992.
261. Phillips, C. G. *Movements of the Hand*. Liverpool: Liverpool University Press, 1987.
262. Phillips, C. G., and R. Porter. *Corticospinal Neurones. Their Role in Movement*. London: Academic Press, 1977.
263. Polit, A., and E. Bizzi. Characteristics of motor programs underlying arm movements in monkeys. *J. Neurophysiol.* 42: 183–194, 1979.
264. Porter, R., and R. Lemon. *Corticospinal Function and Voluntary Movement*. Oxford: Clarendon Press, 1993.
265. Prochazka, A. Sensorimotor gain control: a basic strategy of motor systems? *Prog. Neurobiol.* 333: 281–307, 1989.
266. Proske, U. The tendon organ. In: *Peripheral Neuropathy*, edited by P. J. Dyck, P. K. Thomas, J. W. Griffin, P. A. Low, and J. F. Poduslo, 3rd edition, Philadelphia: W. B. Saunders Co., 1993, p. 141–148.
267. Proske, U., J. E. Gregory, and D. L. Morgan. Where in the muscle spindle is the resting discharge generated? *Exp. Physiol.* 76: 777–785, 1991.
268. Proske, U., D. L. Morgan, and J. E. Gregory. Thixotrophy in skeletal muscle and in muscle spindles: a review. *Prog. Neurobiol.* 41: 705–721, 1993.
269. Proske, U., H.-G. Schaible, and R. F. Schmidt. Joint receptors and kinaesthesia. *Exp. Brain Res.* 72: 219–224, 1988.
270. Rack, P. M., and H. F. Ross. The tendon of flexor pollicis longus: its effects on the muscular control of force and position at the human thumb. *J. Physiol. (Lond.)* 351: 99–110, 1984.
271. Ramachandran, V. S., M. Stewart, and D. C. Rogers-Ramachandran. Perceptual correlates of massive cortical reorganization. *Neuroreport* 3: 583–586, 1992.
272. Refshauge, K. M., R. Chan, J. L. Taylor, and D. I. McCloskey. Detection of movements imposed on hip, knee, ankle and toe joints. *J. Physiol. (Lond.)* (in press).
273. Roland, P. E. Sensory feedback to the cerebral cortex during voluntary movement in man. *Behav. Brain Sci.* 1: 129–171, 1978.
274. Roland, P. E., and H. Ladegaard-Pedersen. A quantitative analysis of sensations of tension and kinaesthesia in man. Evidence for a peripherally originating muscular sense and for a sense of effort. *Brain* 100: 671–692, 1977.

275. Roll, J. P., and J. P. Vedel. Kinesthetic role of muscle afferents in man, studies by tendon vibration and microneurography. *Exp. Brain Res.* 47: 177–190, 1982.
276. Roll, J. P., J. P. Vedel, and E. Ribot. Alteration of proprioceptive messages induced by tendon vibration in man. *Exp. Brain Res.* 76: 213–222, 1989.
277. Roll, R., J. L. Velay, and J. P. Roll. Eye and neck proprioceptive messages contribute to the spatial coding of retinal input in visually oriented activities. *Exp. Brain Res.* 85: 423–431, 1991.
278. Ross, H. E., and K. Bischof. Wundt's views on sensations of innervation: a reevaluation. *Perception* 10: 319–329, 1981.
279. Ross, H. E., E. Brodie, and A. Benson. Mass-discrimination in weightlessness and readaptation to earth's gravity. *Exp. Brain Res.* 64: 358–366, 1986.
280. Ross, H. E., and M. F. Reschke. Mass estimation and discrimination during brief periods of zero gravity. *Percept. Psychophys.* 31: 429–436, 1982.
281. Rossi, A., R. Mazzocchio, and S. Parlanti. Cortical projection of putative group Ib afferent fibres from the human forearm. *Brain Res.* 547: 62–68, 1991.
282. Rothwell, J. C., M. M. Traub, B. L. Day, J. A. Obeso, P. K. Thomas, and C. D. Marsden. Manual motor performance in a deafferented man. *Brain* 105: 515–542, 1982.
283. Rymer, W. Z., and A. D'Almeida. Joint position sense: the effects of muscle contraction. *Brain* 103: 1–22, 1980.
284. Sanes, J. N. Motor representations in deafferented humans: a mechanism for disordered movement performance. In: *Attention and Performance Volume XIII: Motor Representation and Control*, edited by M. Jeannerod. Hillsdale, NJ: Lawrence Erlbaum Associates, 1990, p. 714–735.
285. Sanes, J. N., and E. V. Evarts. Effects of perturbations on accuracy of arm movements. *J. Neurosci.* 3: 977–986, 1983.
286. Sanes, J. N., K.-H. Mauritz, M. C. Dalakas, and E. V. Evarts. Motor control in humans with large-fiber sensory neuropathy. *Hum. Neurobiol.* 4: 101–114, 1985.
287. Schady, W. J. L., and H. E. Torebjörk. Projected and receptive fields: a comparison of projected areas of sensation evoked by intraneural stimulation of mechanoreceptive units, and their innervation territories. *Acta Physiol. Scand.* 119: 267–275, 1983.
288. Scheerer, E. Muscle sense and innervation feelings: a chapter in the history of perception and action. In: *Perspectives on Perception and Action*, edited by H. Heuer and A. F. Sanders. London: Lawrence Erlbaum Associates, 1987, p. 171–194.
289. Scheerer, E. On the will: an historical perspective. In: *Volitional Action*, edited by W. A. Hershberger. North-Holland: Elsevier Science Publishers B.V., 1989, p. 39–60.
290. Schmidt, R. F., W. J. Schady, and H. E. Torebjörk. Gating of tactile input from the hand. I. Effects of finger movement. *Exp. Brain Res.* 79: 97–102, 1990.
291. Sharpe, M. H., and T. S. Miles. Position sense at the elbow after fatiguing contractions. *Exp. Brain Res.* 94: 179–182, 1993.
292. Sherrington, C. S. The muscular sense. In: *Text-Book of Physiology*, edited by E. A. Schäfer. Edinburgh: Pentland, 1900, vol. 2, p. 1002–1025.
293. Sherrington, C. S. *The Integrative Action of the Nervous System.* New Haven: Yale University Press, 1906, 1947.
294. Sherrington, C. S. On the proprio-ceptive system, especially in its reflex aspects. *Brain* 29: 467–482, 1906.
295. Sherrington, C. S. Observations on the sensual role of the proprioceptive nerve supply of the extrinsic ocular muscles. *Brain* 41: 332–343, 1918.
296. Skavenski, A. A. Inflow as a source of extraretinal eye position information. *Vision Res.* 12: 221–229, 1972.
297. Skavenski, A. A., G. Haddad, and R. M. Steinman. The extraretinal signal for the visual perception of direction. *Percept. Psychophys.* 11: 287–290, 1972.
298. Skinner, H. B., M. P. Wyatt, J. A. Hodgdon, D. W. Conard, and R. L. Barrack. Effect of fatigue on joint position sense of the knee. *J. Orthopaed. Res.* 4: 112–118, 1986.
299. Skoglund, S. Joint receptors and kinaesthesis. In: *Somatosensory System*, edited by A. Iggo. New York: Springer-Verlag, 1973, p. 111–136.
300. Soechting, J. F., and M. Flanders. Moving in three-dimensional space: frames of reference, vectors, and coordinate systems. *Annu. Rev. Neurosci.* 15: 167–191, 1992.
301. Soechting, J. F., and B. Ross. Psychophysical determination of coordinate representation of human arm orientation. *Neuroscience* 13: 595–604, 1984.
302. Sorock, G. S., and D. M. Labiner. Peripheral neuromuscular dysfunction and falls in an elderly cohort. *Am. J. Epidemiol.* 136: 584–591, 1992.
303. Sperry, R. W. Neural basis of the spontaneous optokinetic response produced by visual neural inversion. *J. Comp. Physiol. Psychol.* 43: 482–489, 1950.
304. Stein, J. F. The representation of egocentric space in the posterior parietal cortex. *Behav. Brain Sci.* 15: 691–700, 1992.
305. Steinbach, M. J., and D. R. Smith. Spatial localization after strabismus surgery: evidence for inflow. *Science* 213: 1407–1409, 1981.
306. Stevens, J. K., R. C. Emerson, G. L. Gerstein, T., Kallos, G. R. Neufeld, C. W. Nichols, and A. C. Rosenquist. Paralysis of the awake human: visual perceptions. *Vision Res.* 16: 93–98, 1976.
307. Talbot, W. H., I. Darian-Smith, H. H. Kornhuber, and V. B. Mountcastle. The sense of flutter-vibration: comparison of the human capacity with response patterns of mechanoreceptive afferents from the monkey hand. *J. Neurophysiol.* 31: 301–334, 1968.
308. Taub, E., and A. J. Berman. Movement and learning in the absence of sensory feedback. In: *The Neuropsychology of Spatially Oriented Behavior*, edited by S. J. Freedman. Homewood, IL: Dorsey, 1968, p. 173–192.
309. Taylor, A., and A. Prochazka. *Muscle Receptors and Movement.* London: Macmillan, 1981.
310. Taylor, J. L., and D. I. McCloskey. Pointing. *Behav. Brain Res.* 29: 1–5, 1988.
311. Taylor, J. L., and D. I. McCloskey. Proprioception in the neck. *Exp. Brain Res.* 70: 351–360, 1988.
312. Taylor, J. L., and D. I. McCloskey. Ability to detect angular displacements of the fingers made at an imperceptibly slow speed. *Brain* 113: 157–166, 1990.
313. Taylor, J. L., and D. I. McCloskey. Proprioceptive sensation in rotation of the trunk. *Exp. Brain Res.* 81: 413–416, 1990.
314. Taylor, J. L., and D. I. McCloskey. Triggering of preprogrammed movements as reactions to masked stimuli. *J. Neurophysiol.* 63: 439–446, 1990.
315. Taylor, J. L., and D. I. McCloskey. Detection of slow movements imposed at the elbow during active flexion in man. *J. Physiol. (Lond.)* 457: 503–513, 1992.
316. Teasdale, N., R. Forget, C. Bard, J. Paillard, M. Fleury, and Y. Lamarre. The role of proprioceptive information for the

production of isometric forces and for handwriting tasks. *Acta Psychol.* 82: 179–191, 1993.
317. Thompson, S., J. E. Gregory, and U. Proske. Errors in force estimation can be explained by tendon organ desensitization. *Exp. Brain Res.* 79: 365–372, 1990.
318. Torebjörk, H. E., Å. B. Vallbo, and J. L. Ochoa. Intraneural microstimulation in man: its relation to specificity of tactile sensations. *Brain* 110: 1509–1529, 1987.
319. Vallbo, Å. B. Human muscle spindle discharge during isometric voluntary contractions. Amplitude relations between spindle frequency and torque. *Acta Physiol. Scand.* 90: 319–336, 1974.
320. Vallbo, Å. B., K.-E. Hagbarth, H. E. Torebjörk, and B. G. Wallin. Somatosensory, proprioceptive, and sympathetic activity in human peripheral nerves. *Physiol. Rev.* 59: 919–957, 1979.
321. Vallbo, Å. B., H. Olausson, J. Wessberg, and N. Kakuda. Receptive field characteristics of tactile units with myelinated afferents in hairy skin of human subjects. *J. Physiol. (Lond.)* 483: 783–795, 1995.
322. Vallbo, Å. B., K. Å. Olsson, K.-G. Westberg, and F. J. Clark. Microstimulation of single tactile afferents from the human hand. Sensory attributes related to unit type and properties of receptive fields. *Brain* 107: 727–749, 1984.
323. Vallbo, Å. B., K. Å. Olsson, J. Westberg, and U. Norrsell. A system of unmyelinated afferents for innocuous mechanoreception in the human skin. *Brain Res.* 628: 301–304, 1993.
324. Velay, J. L., R. Roll, G. Lenerstrand, and J. P. Roll. Eye proprioception and visual localization in humans: influence of ocular dominance and visual context. *Vision Res.* 34: 2169–2176, 1994.
325. Vickery, R. M., B. D. Gynther, and M. J. Rowe. Vibrotactile sensitivity of slowly adapting type I sensory fibres associated with touch domes in cat hairy skin. *J. Physiol. (Lond.)* 453: 609–626, 1992.
326. Voss, H. Tabelle der absoluten and relativen muskelspindelzhalen der menschlichen skelettmuskulatur. *Anat. Anz.* 129: 562–572, 1971.
327. Wall, P. D., and S. B. McMahon. Microneurography and its relation to perceived sensation. A critical review. *Pain* 21: 209–229, 1985.
328. Wann, J. P., and S. F. Ibrahim. Does limb proprioception drift? *Exp. Brain Res.* 91: 162–166, 1992.
329. Watson, J. D. G., J. G. Colebatch, and D. I. McCloskey. Effects of externally imposed elastic loads on the ability to estimate position and force. *Behav. Brain Res.* 13: 267–271, 1984.
330. Werner, W., E. Bauswein, and C. Fromm. Static firing rates of premotor and primary motor cortical neurons associated with torque and joint position. *Exp. Brain Res.* 86: 293–302, 1991.
331. Westling, G., and R. S. Johansson. Responses in glabrous skin mechanoreceptors during precision grip in humans. *Exp. Brain Res.* 66: 128–140, 1987.
332. Wiesendanger, M., and T. S. Miles. Ascending pathway of low-threshold muscle afferents to the cerebral cortex and its possible role in motor control. *Physiol. Rev.* 62: 1234–1270, 1982.
333. Wilkinson, R. S., and Y. Fukami. Responses of isolated Golgi tendon organs of cat to sinusoidal stretch. *J. Neurophysiol.* 49: 976–988, 1983.
334. Wilson, L., S. C. Gandevia, and D. Burke. Discharge rates of muscle spindle afferents in human tibialis anterior. *Proc. Aust. Neurosci. Soc.* 5: 104, 1994.
335. Windhorst, U., T. M. Hamm, and D. G. Stuart. On the function of muscle and reflex partitioning. *Behav. Brain Sci.* 12: 629–681, 1989.
336. Worringham, C. J., G. E. Stelmach, and Z. E. Martin. Limb segment inclination sense in proprioception. *Exp. Brain Res.* 66: 653–658, 1987.
337. York, D. H. Somatosensory evoked potentials in man: differentiation of spinal pathways responsible for conduction from the forelimb vs. hindlimb. *Prog. Neurobiol.* 25: 1–25, 1985.
338. Zelena, J., and T. Soukup. The in-series and in-parallel components in rat hindlimb tendon organs. *Neuroscience* 9: 899–910, 1983.
339. Zimny, M. L. Mechanoreceptors in articular tissues. *Am. J. Anat.* 182: 16–32, 1988.

5. Neural control of stereotypic limb movements

SERGE ROSSIGNOL | Center for Research in Neurological Sciences, Department of Physiology, Faculty of Medicine, Université de Montréal, Montréal, Québec, Canada

CHAPTER CONTENTS

The overall picture is an interaction between subtle volitional corrections and basic central and peripheral elements, all of which in a joint effort may produce movements ranging from ballet dance to a tight rope walk.

Sten Grillner, 1981.

THE OPENING QUOTE, taken from the concluding remarks of Grillner's landmark review (175), already expressed a view that has been enriched in the last 15 years by new findings and new perspectives. Reviewing the field of neural control of stereotypic movements raises many challenges, not the least of which is that this area has been competently reviewed many times over the last 15 years (14, 83, 175–177, 243, 265, 338) and has been the subject, in total or in part, of an equally large number of symposia and books (4, 6, 40, 180, 203, 290, 322, 341).

This intense activity has been largely driven by questions aimed at relating those properties of muscles, nerve cells, and pathways known from anatomical or physiological observations in static conditions to the dynamic conditions of cyclic behaviors. New preparations (chronic, fictive, in vitro preparations) have permitted investigators to study these questions in the real behavioral context or else in very reduced states. Chronically implanted preparations have allowed us to study how various muscles are utilized in such behaviors, how the various unit types in a given muscle can be selected in the different phases of the movement, and how the nervous system specifically selects various anatomical synergists in appropriate phases. Reflex studies have also revealed properties that appear only in rhythmic behaviors and cannot be predicted by physiological observations in static conditions. Some responses from afferent or descending inputs may be evoked in one phase and not in the other phase of the rhythmic movement. Moreover, inputs from some particular muscle receptors in ankle extensors (i.e., Golgi tendon organs), that normally exert an inhibitory action on their parent muscle, produce an excitatory effect during locomotion. Reduced preparations have permitted the identification of the membrane properties, the location, and the types of some of the cells that may participate in the generation of spinal rhythmic behaviors.

Neurotransmitters capable of triggering or modulating such rhythmic behaviors have also been studied. Elemental spinal circuits can be combined and triggered by specific sensory inputs, descending inputs, or neurotransmitters to generate various patterns. The spinal cord is capable of coupling the same muscles in different synergies, thereby generating many different behaviors (locomotion, scratching, paw shaking) and producing many forms of the same behavior (walking forward or backward, turning). Thus, one aim of this review is to integrate a number of studies on stereotypic patterns that have added considerably to our more general understanding of the nervous system by revealing that some of its functions appear only when the nervous system is engaged in particular tasks such as generating cyclic behaviors and adapting them to the environment in which they are produced.

Although a great deal of our knowledge on basic mechanisms of rhythm generation comes from work in invertebrates, insects, and low vertebrates, the present review will largely be focused on mammalian limb movements. The vast literature on human locomotion has not been reviewed either, although some findings in humans have been incorporated when they complement particular concepts. This chapter will first describe the kinematics and electromyographic (EMG) activity recorded during stereotypic movements in intact animals with an emphasis on locomotion. The potential of various reduced preparations (spinal, deafferentated, paralyzed) to express these patterns will be discussed in order to establish that the basic stereotypic patterns can be generated at the spinal level (i.e., without descending inputs) and centrally (i.e., without motion-related afferent feedback). Having established this, the last two sections will then be devoted to the interactions between these centrally generated patterns with afferent and descending inputs. This tripartite organization involving spinal circuits, afferent feedback, and descending inputs is central to our current understanding of how these cyclic patterns are continuously adapted to internal and external demands.

KINEMATICS AND MUSCLE ACTIVITY

The understanding of movements requires some knowledge of kinetics (forces), kinematics (movements), and EMG activity. Only the two last topics will be discussed in some detail, since a full chapter is devoted to kinetics (see Chapter 8). This review is largely based on cat data, although some data in dogs are also reported. The main purpose of this detailed section is that although the cyclic movements can be viewed, in a first approximation, as a simple alternation between flexion and extension, the actual expression of these motor patterns results from elaborate, detailed, and specific patterns of activity of various muscles.

Hindlimb Locomotor Movements

Kinematics. Each limb performs sequentially a complete step cycle during which the paw is in contact with the ground for some time (*stance* or support) and then brought forward again (*swing* or transfer) (Fig. 5.1*C*). It is traditional, since Philippson (278), to further subdivide these two main phases on events occurring at the ankle and knee (Fig. 5.1*B*). Swing starts by a flexion (F) of all joints; while the hip continues its flexion, the ankle and knee start extending (E1) until the paw touches the ground. At paw contact, the knee and ankle are passively flexed during weight acceptance (E2 or yield phase), the MTP joint continues the extension initiated in E1 whereas the proximal interphalangeal joint (PIP) flexes briskly (224). During the third extension phase (E3 or push-off), all joints extend to propel the body forward. This general description is still valid, although its limitations have been clearly pointed out (175), especially when the angular excursion of any particular joint is described in relation to paw contact or in relation to other joints. For instance, at the stance-swing transition, the knee starts flexing some 16–20 ms before toe-off (184); at the same time or even slightly earlier, the MTP joint starts to plantar-flex (135, 168, 224, 254) and the PIP joint to extend (224); the knee reaches its full flexion before the ankle; and the hip starts to extend some 20 ms before paw contact (184), which brings the leg backward slightly so that the paw does not stamp the ground.

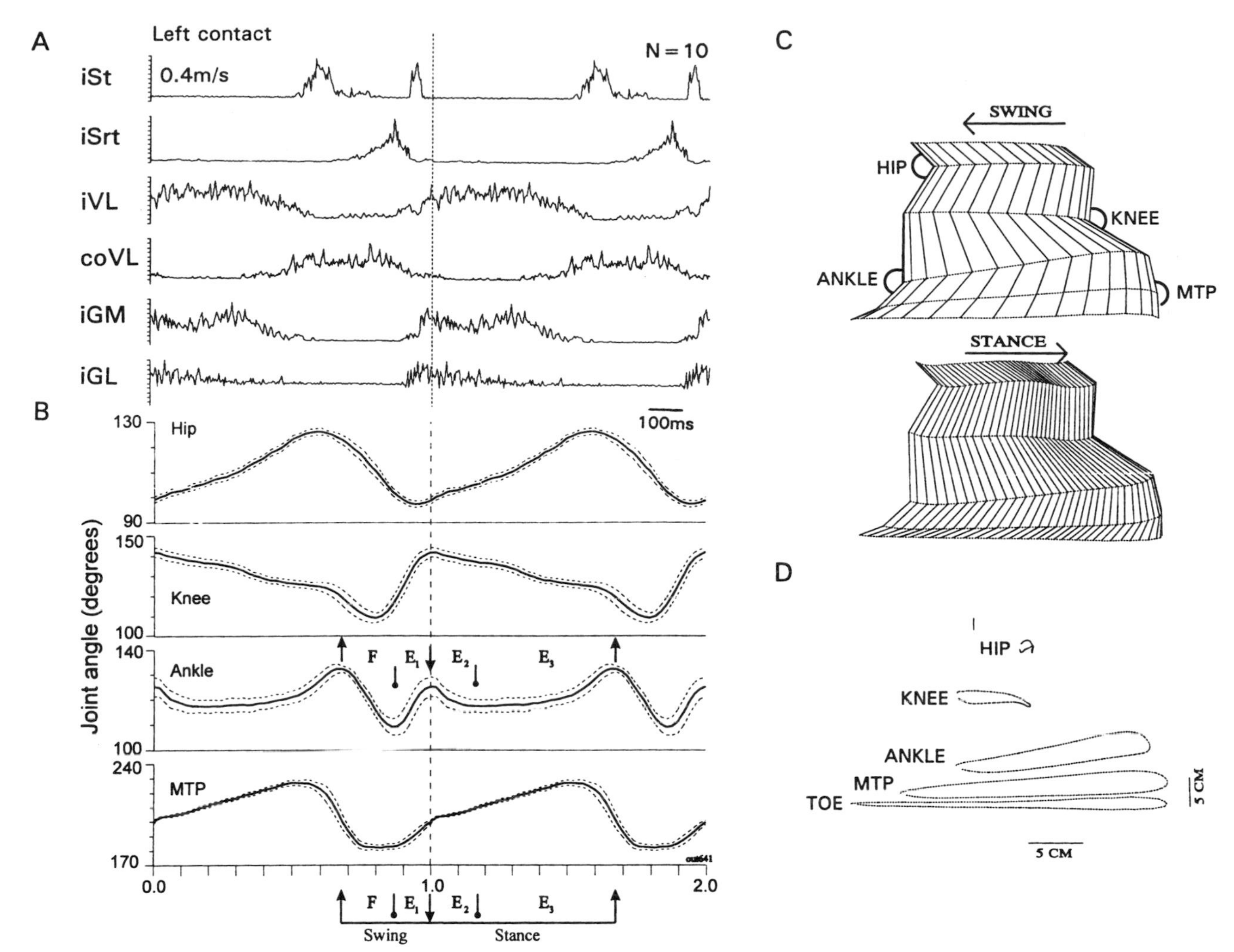

FIG. 5.1. Kinematic and synchronized EMG activity of locomotion in a chronically implanted cat walking on a treadmill at 0.4 m/s. *A*, The flexor and extensor EMGs rectified and filtered and aligned on paw contact (*dotted line*). The average cycle is repeated twice. St, semitendinosus; Srt, sartorius anterior; VL, vastus lateralis; GM, medial gastrocnemius; GL, lateral gastrocnemius. *B*, The angle plots are taken from ten successive cycles with the *dotted envelope* indicating 1 standard error. In the duty cycle, the *downward arrow* is aligned with the *vertical dotted line* to mark paw contact; the two *upgoing arrows* are two successive foot lifts; F1, F2, and E3 refer to the subdivisions of the swing and stance according to Philippson (278). *C*, One complete cycle is reconstructed as stick diagrams for swing and stance; *arrows* indicate the direction of movement. *D*, The trajectory of each marker is displayed during one step cycle. The calibration applies to both C and D.

EMGs. Describing in detail the "normal" pattern of EMG from published records is like describing all the little twigs of trees in a forest, but still it reveals the complexity of the mechanisms generating the locomotor pattern. Differences in EMG descriptions may depend on how the animal walked, in which conditions, on what part of the muscle was recorded, and on what kind of electrodes were used. However, some muscles have a more or less consistent pattern under various experimental conditions; others (small muscles acting around the ankle and foot) appear more whimsical and may be related to learned strategies by the animal (232). A schematic description of EMG activity during trot is given in Figure 5.2, which is intended to serve as a look-up table constructed from several sources by normalizing the periods of EMG discharges and aligning them on paw contact. The abbreviations used in the description can be found in Figure 5.2.

Stance phase. These "extensor" muscles have very similar patterns of activity (141, 282, 289). They are activated some 20–80 ms [depending on the speed (184)] before the actual paw contact so that their discharge cannot be triggered by sensory events associated with contact as emphasized by Engberg and Lundberg (135). Recent experiments confirmed this by demonstrating that the initial discharges in ankle extensors is similar whether the cat

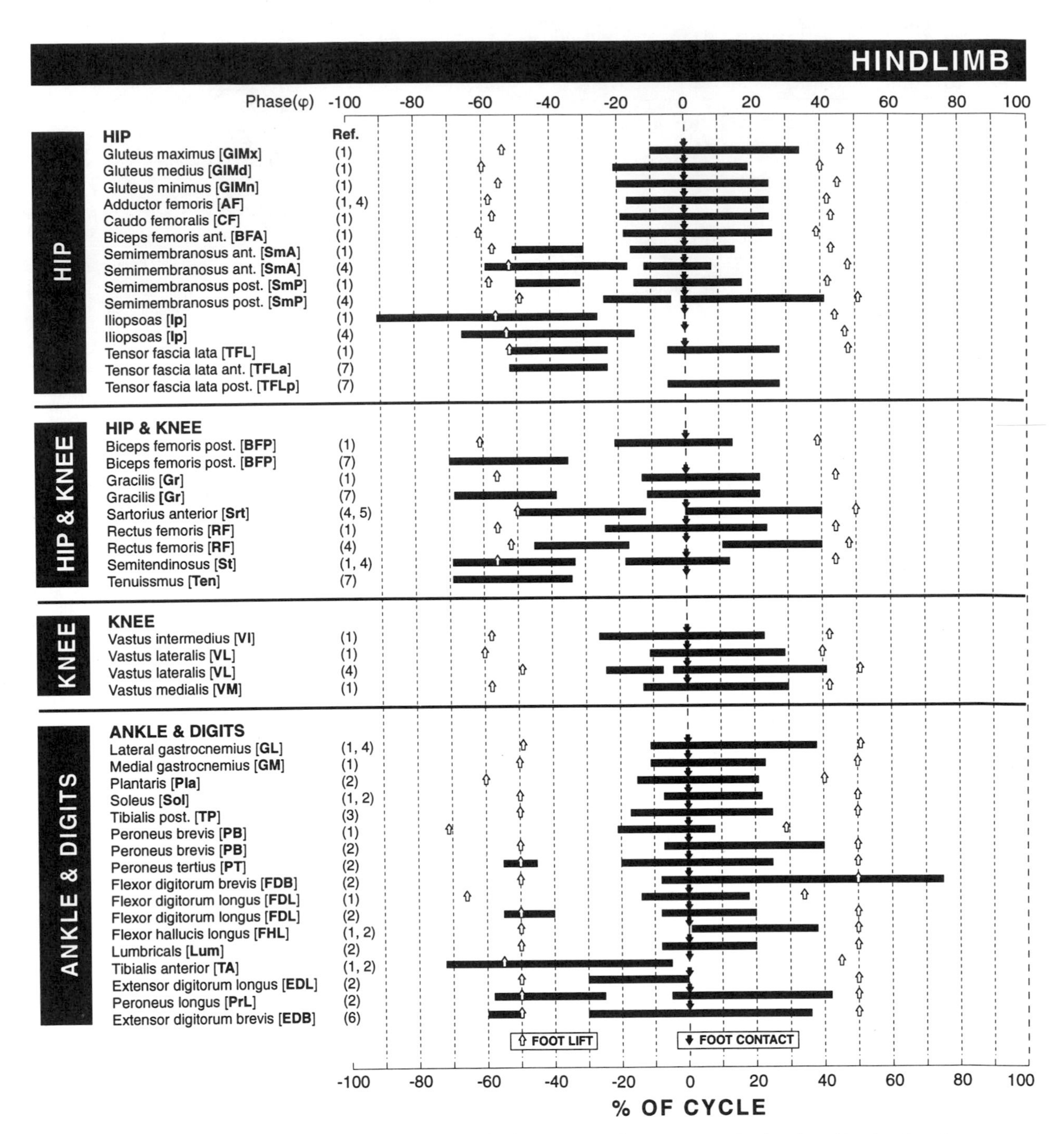

FIG. 5.2. Bar diagram of the activity of the principal hindlimb muscles during trot aligned on paw contact (*downward arrows*) with corresponding toe-off in the preceding and following cycles. The patterns of EMGs were obtained from various sources (by scanning typical records) or rearranged from published values and aligned on paw contact. The inaccuracy resulting from these manipulations was judged to be offset by the advantages of displaying the several recorded muscles in a single format. Names and abbreviations of muscles are given together with the source. The sources are: [1] = (289); [2] = (232); [3] = (1); [4] = (135); [5] = (284); [6] = (147) (spinal cat during walk); [7] = (282).

touches the ground or steps in a hole (164). Figure 5.1*A* shows that extensor muscles may have a different overall discharge profile: vastus lateralis (VL) is usually gradually recruited from E1 and peaks in E3, while the gastrocnemii medialis and lateralis (GM and GL) generally have a more abrupt onset and peak during E2 during their lengthening phase (164, 357, 360). In VL, another more variable (135) burst may be present even earlier in E1 (very small in Fig. 5.1*A*).

The uniarticular heads of quadriceps (vastus lateralis, vastus intermedius, vastus medialis) follow this general extensor pattern. The bifunctional rectus femoris (knee extensor and hip flexor) has a single long extensor burst (289) or a burst in E1 followed by a period of silence and then another distinct burst in E3 (344), particularly during trotting (135).

Although the gastrocnemii and soleus are synergist ankle extensors, the soleus, with its slow fiber composition, is recruited almost maximally at low speeds and generates a similar force at all speeds, whereas the dynamic range of force output for the gastrocnemii can be up to eight to ten times with increasing speeds (357). Using buckle force transducers on tendons of the triceps surae and estimates of muscle length changes (360), the amount of negative and positive work performed by various muscles during stepping was calculated. During E2, the gastrocnemii and soleus muscles perform negative work (they are lengthened while contracting); during E3, shortening of muscles during force development results in positive work. It was further proposed that individual compartments of GL could be recruited differentially during locomotion at different speeds. The most distal compartment of GL, containing mainly small slow-twitch motor units, is recruited at low speeds (low force) while more proximal compartments, containing larger, faster, and more fatigable motor units, are mainly activated at higher speeds of locomotion (139).

Extensor muscles acting around the ankle and digits are interesting in many respects since they have an important role in positioning and stabilizing the foot, as well as "flexing" (plantar-flexion) the digits. Flexor digitorum longus (FDL) and flexor hallucis longus (FHL), which are close anatomical synergists, are nonetheless differentially recruited during walking. FDL has a distinct short burst of activity very early on around toe-off (232, 254) and seems to produce the very early plantar-flexion of the digits needed to clear the paw from ground, whereas FHL is active only during stance. FDL is also sometimes recruited during stance (289), especially when the step cycle is perturbed (254) and may be related to a flexion of the PIP joint during stance (224). Although these two muscles have a similar action in the toe-in and toe-out direction (229), FHL produces a much greater plantar-flexion ankle torque than FDL, which may explain its predominant discharge during stance. This points to the importance of knowing the precise moment arm of action of the various muscles in the range of angular excursion during locomotion to understand their discharge pattern (372).

It should also be emphasized that the action of some muscles may vary among animals because of inherent variability, strategies, or anatomical variability (232) that can result in different moment arms for a given muscle. Peroneus longus (PrL) can be recruited mainly during swing (190), stance and swing in others, or throughout stance in some cats (1, 232). Similarly, peroneus tertius (PT) may have a particularly strong component in one phase in one cat and not in another cat. It is also of interest to mention that despite such variation in locomotor discharge, the reflex behavior of these muscles during locomotion may be more consistent (232).

Swing phase. Muscles related to the swing phase, especially biarticular muscles, may have a more complex and versatile discharge pattern (135, 175, 184, 289). Sartorius has two anatomically distinct portions: an anterior part that flexes the hip and extends the knee, and a medial part that flexes both the hip and knee. Although its activity is sometimes described as a single EMG burst starting before foot lift-off and peaking about at the same time as the hip flexor iliopsoas (IP) (184, 289), others have reported a consistent second burst in the anterior part during stance (135, 195). A more detailed study of single muscle units (195, 284) showed that some sartorius units fired in early swing to flex the hip and knee, others fired in late swing to extend the knee and flex the hip, and finally other units discharged to extend the knee during stance. The activation of the various subdivisions of the muscle differs according to different stereotypic motions such as locomotion, scratching, and the paw shake (284).

Semitendinosus (St), a knee flexor and hip extensor, has received much attention because of its particular discharge pattern (141, 202, 275, 276, 329). St discharges in late E3 and is involved in the earliest part of swing when the paw is lifted off the ground. St and its synergist semimembranosus posterior (SmP) both have a variable second burst of activity in E1 just before paw contact (135, 141, 275, 282, 289, 329). This E1 burst is more consistent at higher speeds and may be related to the need for a greater torque in flexion to decelerate both the hip and knee at the end of swing in preparation for foot contact (329, 363). The greater dependence of the second burst of activity in St on peripheral feedback (141, 284, 329, 363) is in keeping with the suggestion made by Perret (275, 276) that the pattern of discharge of bifunctional muscles, such as St, can be influenced by sensory stimulation (see later under CENTRAL GENERATION OF STEREOTYPIC PATTERNS).

Semitendinosus and tibialis anterior (TA) discharge differently according to the histochemically different regions recorded (80). The deep regions of these muscles contain mainly slow oxidative fibers and are recruited during slow walk, whereas the more superficial regions containing fast glycolytic muscle fibers are activated during most activities including fast locomotion, paw shake, and scratch.

Forelimb Locomotor Movements

Kinematics. The forelimb step cycle is also classically subdivided according to Philippson's scheme (see Fig. 5.3). Its description is somewhat more complex because of the added movement of the scapula relative to the rib cage (136, 137, 241). Functionally, the scapula is homologous to the femur, the humerus to the shank, the radius-ulna to the foot, and the wrist to the metatarsophalangeal (MTP) joint. Because the cat is aclavicular, the scapula is attached to the thorax and vertebral column only by muscles. During the swing phase of locomotion, the scapula is rotated which brings the glenoid cavity a few centimeters forward.

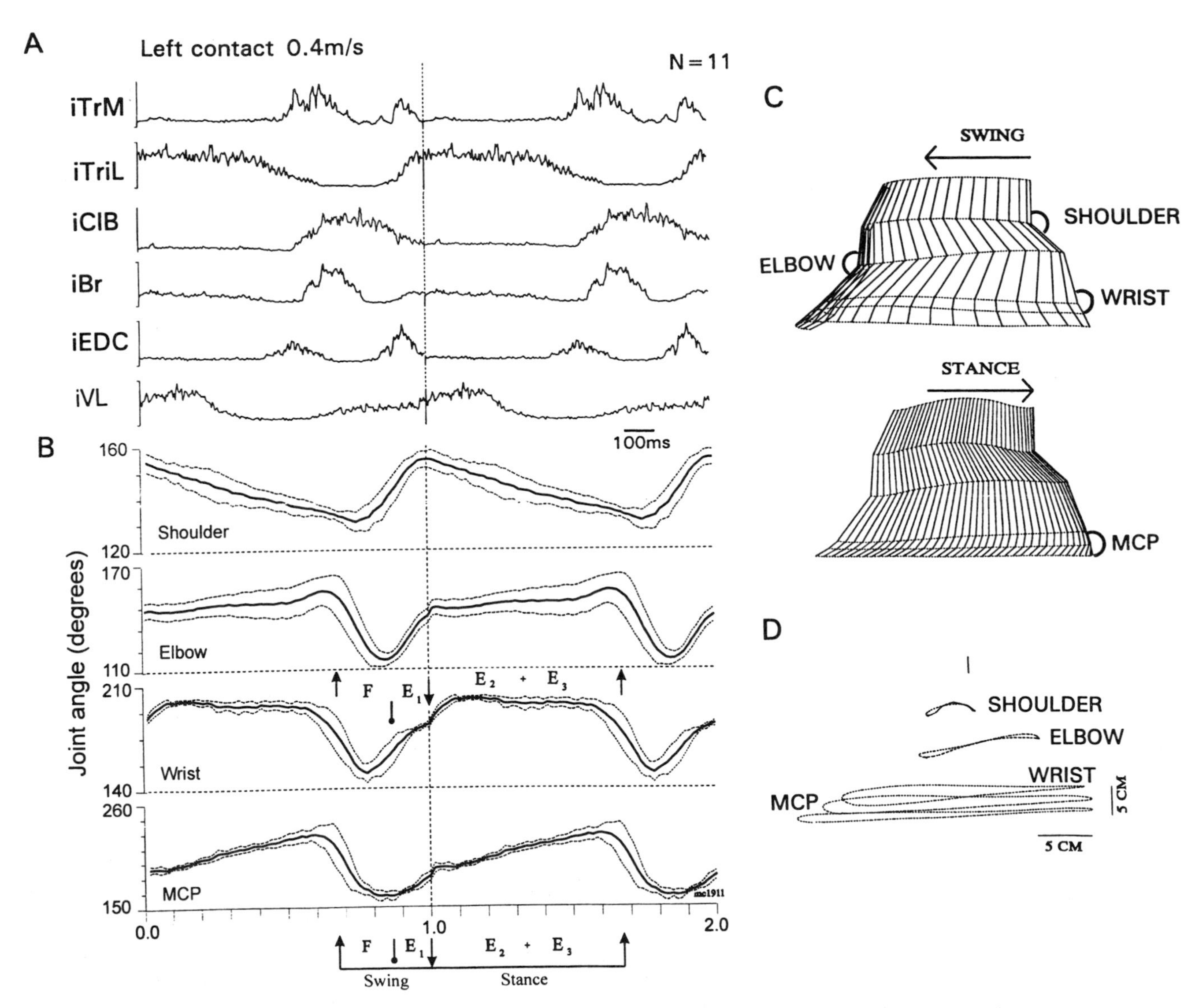

FIG. 5.3. Same as Figure 5.1 but for the forelimbs. In *A*, 20 cycles are averaged; in *B*, 6 cycles. These cycles are normal step cycles in between cycles where the cat steps over obstacles. (From T. Drew and B. Kably, unpublished observations.)

During the F phase of swing, the elbow and shoulder flex and the wrist plantar-flexes. In E1, while the shoulder and elbow extend, the wrist dorsiflexes. At paw contact (E2), a very small and short yield occurs in the elbow and shoulder. The wrist angle is about 180 degrees at paw contact and can reach 210 degrees toward the end of the yield phase. In the remainder of stance, the wrist is actively plantar-flexed and maintains an angle of about 200 degrees (see Fig. 5-3*B*). The finer movements of the distal joints were studied using a pulsed X-ray technique (70) that also permitted movements of the forefoot in other planes, such as supination-pronation, to be analyzed.

EMGs. A limited number of studies on forelimb muscles have been performed (107, 108, 136, 137, 197, 344, 368) and are summarized in Figure 5.4. Scapular muscles play a key role during stance, since the animal's weight is supported through these muscles. Extrinsic appendicular muscles attaching the humerus to the sternum (pectoralis muscles) or to the vertebrae (latissimus dorsi) move the shoulder girdle while pulling on the humerus during stance. The supraspinatus, infraspinatus, and subscapularis are active mainly during stance, although some activity of the subscapularis and infraspinatus may control the amount of mediolateral limb displacement in swing by imposing various degrees of adduction and abduction of the humerus. All parts of the deltoideus have been shown to have various amounts of activity related to stance and swing. Acromiodeltoideus and cleidodeltoideus discharge almost equally in both phases (107), whereas the spinodeltoideus has its main burst during swing (107). Teres major, which attaches the caudal border of the scapula to the humerus, discharge two short bursts at the onset and offset of swing [Fig. 5.3*A*; (104, 107)]. Some low-level activity is also seen throughout the initial part of stance (107, 137, 344).

The three heads of triceps (long head, lateral, and medial) start their discharge prior to paw contact as seen in Figure 5.3*A*. This precedence increases with speed, from practially null [see Fig. 5.4; (107)] during walk to several milliseconds during trot and gallop in dogs (344). The long head of triceps that attaches to the scapula often has a short distinct burst just prior to swing (107, 344). The EMG of the brachialis, biceps brachii, and cleidobrachialis start before paw-off and terminate before or at paw contact.

Muscles dorsiflexing the wrist and digits (extensor carpi radialis, extensor digitorum communis) have two bursts associated with toe-off and toe contact (Fig. 5.3*A*, EDC). Extensor carpi ulnaris, on the other hand, discharges throughout stance (104, 107), much as the plantar flexors of the wrist and digits (palmaris longus, flexor digitorum profundus, flexor carpi ulnaris).

The above descriptions suggest that there are sophisticated control mechanisms determining not only the timing of discharge but also the selection of heads of muscles, regions of muscles or units within a muscle that are activated in the various phases of step cycle.

Walking at Different Speeds, Slopes, and Directions

Figure 5.5, modified from Halbertsma (184), illustrates for one hindlimb the major changes occurring in the step cycle and its subcomponents as the cat moves from 0.1 m/s to 0.9 m/s on a motor-driven treadmill. Although collected on a limited speed range, these data generally agree with the data obtained by Goslow et al. (168) on a walkway, where cats moved at speeds ranging from 0.44 m/s (1 mph) to 7.1 m/s (16 mph). Cycle time (T_c) and support time (T_{su}) vary with speed as a hyperbolic function, whereas the swing time (T_{sw}) is almost invariant. The support time is linearly related to the cycle time. Most of the variation of the support time comes from variations of E3.

Speed can be increased by changing the cadence (steps per minute) or the step length. Thus increase in velocity is achieved by applying a greater force for a shorter time at a faster rate. In cats, the step length (or support length) increases slightly in the low-speed range. Whereas the paw is placed constantly at about 8 cm in front of the hip at the onset of stance, the paw is brought backward at an increasing distance as a function of velocity (Fig. 5.5*D*). This is mainly achieved through a greater hip excursion (184). At higher speeds, the hip excursion remains stable, even during gallop (168).

According to Goslow et al. (168), cats use a walking gait below 0.7 m/s, a trotting gait between 0.7 and 2.7 m/s, and gallop above 2.7 m/s. Goslow et al. (168) have shown that during high-speed galloping (7.3 m/s) there are large movements of the lower spine.

Several parameters of EMG (timing, burst duration and amplitude, pattern) change when an animal walks faster or walks on an incline or backward. The onset of extensor muscle activity before paw contact may be on the order of 10% during walk and may even reach 40% of the cycle during gallop (184). During gallop some extensor muscles are active for a longer time prior to paw contact than after (135, 289). The burst durations in extensors vary

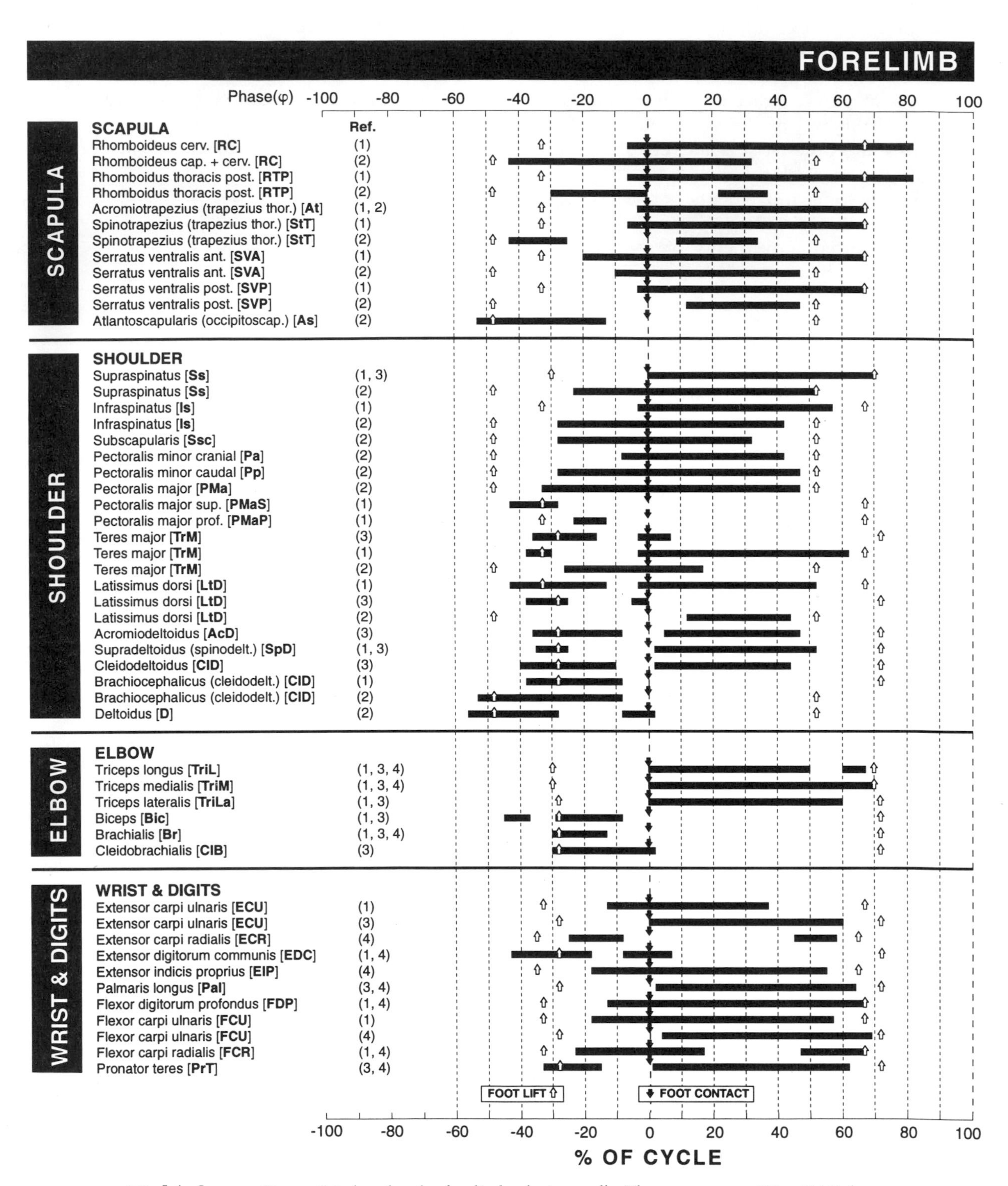

FIG. 5.4. Same as Figure 5.2, but for the forelimbs during walk. The sources are: [1] = (344) for the dog; [2] = (137); [3] = (107); [4] = (197).

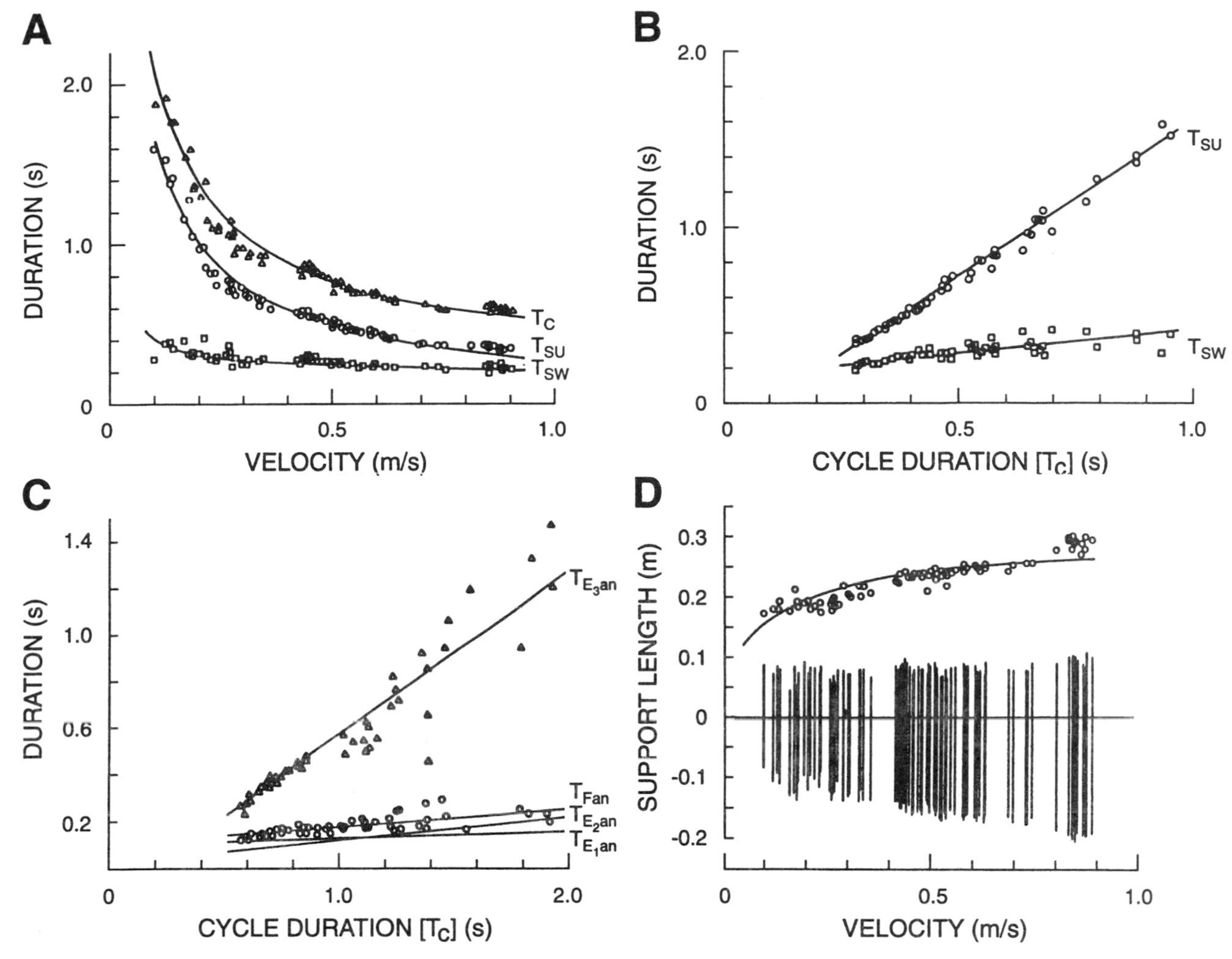

FIG. 5.5. Changes of the kinematics with walking speed of a normal intact cat walking on a treadmill [from (184)]. *A*, Adjustments in the step cycle with speed. The stride cycle duration (T_C; *triangles*), the support phase duration (T_{SU}; *circles*), and the swing phases duration (T_{SW}, *squares*) are plotted vs. the velocity of locomotion. *B*, Adjustments of the support (T_{SU}, *circles*) and swing (T_{SW}, *squares*) phase duration with the stride cycle duration (T_C). Each symbol represents one interval. The *straight lines* were fitted to the data. *C*, Adjustments of the phases of the ankle joint with the stride cycle duration. The duration of the flexion phase (T_{Fan}) and of the third extension phase (T_{E3an}; *triangles*) are plotted. Each symbol represents one interval. The *straight line* was fitted to these data and to the data of the duration of the first (T_{E1an}) and second (T_{E2an}) extension phase (data points not drawn for sake of clarity). Data from one cat. *D*, Adjustment of the amplitude of the limb movements—the support length—with speed. The support lengths are plotted as *circles*. The horizontal positions of the toe with respect to the hip during the support phase are plotted as *bars*. The *top* and *bottom* of the bars indicate the toe position at touch-down and lift-off, respectively. The support lengths are calculated from these positions. Each symbol represents data from a single stride. Approximately coinciding symbols are omitted for the sake of clarity.

linearly with cycle period, whereas flexors show little variation with speed. With increasing speed or when walking up an incline some ankle extensors (i.e., gastrocnemius) but not others (i.e., soleus) increase their mean discharge amplitude (279), whereas the ankle flexor tibialis anterior varies little. Back muscles do not discharge at slow speeds but are recruited in trot and gallop (374).

Change in direction from forward to backward walking is also accompanied by changes in the kinematics and kinetics and in the timing characteristics of EMGs. Work in cats has shown that backward walking is complex and involves not only a change in posture (the lower back is ventroflexed) (63) but also a change in weight transfer between forelimbs and hindlimbs (270) so that the hindlimbs carry more weight than the forelimbs. The knee plays the main propulsive role during backward walking rather than the hip as during forward walking (see Chapter 8). Other work in quadrupeds (such as in the mole rats, for which this is a more usual behavior) shows that backward and forward walking can be achieved without significant postural changes (133).

Interlimb Coordination

The coordination between the limbs of tetrapods has been well summarized in Grillner's review (175). One stride is defined as the time interval between two successive contacts of the same foot. One step is defined by the time of successive contacts between the left and the right foot or right and left foot. During walking, the right hindfoot contacts the ground at 50% of the left stride. The period of stance is longer than that of a single step, which results in two short periods of double support between periods of single support. These double-support phases gradually disappear with increasing speed. When considering distances, it is usual to refer to the stride length as the distance traveled during one complete stride. In the overground situation this distance is the sum of two steps (left-right and right-left). During treadmill locomotion, it is current to measure the support or stance length as the distance traveled by the foot of one limb, from its contact to its following lift-off; this is of course equal to stance duration × belt velocity. Similarly, the total step length (175) or stride length is the sum of the stance or support length and the distance traveled by the belt during the swing period of that limb; this is equal to the belt velocity × stride duration. In symmetrical gaits, both hindlimbs and both forelimbs are coupled out of phase. However, the coupling between the forelimbs and hindlimbs is speed related. In walk, the forelimb contacts the ground at about 25% of the hindlimb stride, whereas during trot, the forelimb touches ground at 50% of the hindlimb stride and is then coupled to the contralateral hindlimb (diagonal coupling). There seems to be a tendency to use more frequently an ipsilateral or parallel coupling between the forelimb and the hindlimb (pace) on the treadmill (51). During gallop, both hindlimbs are in phase (half-bound) or more or less in phase (transverse and rotatory gallop), while the forelimbs are more or less out of phase.

Although the limbs are generally either in phase or out of phase, intermediate-phase values are also observed to adapt to differential speeds of the limbs such as during turning. This situation was studied experimentally on a treadmill in which each belt could be controlled independently (split-belt). In decerebrate cats and chronic spinal cats (148) as well as in intact cats (184), when the speed differential is 2:1 up to 3:1, the hindlimbs maintain a symmetrical 1:1 coupling and the cycle duration of both limbs is intermediate between the fast and slow limb (i.e., the cycle of the fast limb is somewhat longer and the cycle of the slow limb somewhat shorter than at similar speeds in the tied belt situation). All subcomponents of the cycle structure can be altered to accommodate the cycle changes needed to maintain a 1:1 coupling. Although each limb can be regarded as an autonomous walking unit, when coupled to the fellow limb, the cycle of the limb is influenced by the cycle of the contralateral limb. Similar observations were also made in 7-month-old human infants walking on a split-belt treadmill (343) and in adults (99).

Many neural mechanisms may participate in the control of interlimb coupling through a variety of crossed pathways (204, 205, 306) and other interlimb reflexes (306), as well as through descending inputs to adapt to various contexts (51).

Other Stereotypic Movements

Scratching and Wiping. Scratching is another cyclic behavior of interest because it has specific features that can be evoked and identified in reduced preparations as will be illustrated later. In the cat, scratching (93, 223) is an episodic motor behavior that can be elicited, for example, by an irritant on the skin of the external meatus or pinna. Scratching includes a fairly complex sequence of movements. The head is turned and tilted so that the ipsilateral hindlimb can reach the irritated area. The hindlimb is first positioned by flexing the hip, knee, and ankle, and then the knee is extended to reach the pinna (postural, aiming, or approach phase). Then follows the scratching itself that consists of cyclical flexion and extension at all joints at a frequency of 4–8 Hz for about 10–15 cycles and then a return of the limb to its original position. During scratching, the knee motion is uncoupled from ankle and hip motions for a period while the knee rapidly extends and the ankle and hip are still flexing. The foot trajectory is largely circular and its speed of motion not uniform, being slower in the upper region of the trajectory when the actual contact occurs. Although there is a general alternation between flexors and extensors (Fig. 5.6), the extensors are often recruited sequentially: ankle, knee, and hip.

In intact cats (232, 254) the amplitude of ankle extensors soleus and GM are reversed, soleus being high during walk and low during scratch and vice versa for GM. FHL and FDL muscles also discharge prior to the ankle extensors. FHL, which produces claw protrusion, is most active during this behavior compared to walking and paw shake (1). Scratching develops at around 3 weeks after birth, at which

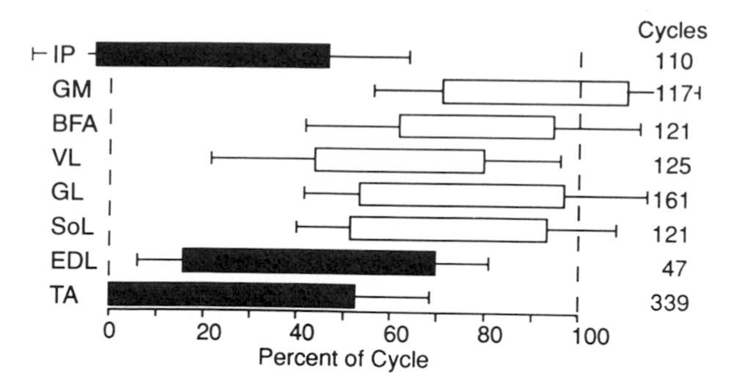

FIG. 5.6. Summary of muscles activities for cyclic scratching. For each muscle, the *bar* represents the average burst duration normalized to the TA cycle period. Standard deviation of onset and offset latencies for each burst duration are denoted by *horizontal lines* to the left and right of each bar, respectively. Flexor muscles are indicated by *shaded bars* and extensor muscles by *unshaded bars*. Number of cycles analyzed for each muscle is listed at the right. [Adapted from Kuhta and Smith (223) with permission.]

date kittens express already an adult EMG pattern (53).

Deliagina et al. (93) described the pattern of discharge of several hindlimb muscles in decerebrate cats. The flexor and extensor muscles at the knee are recruited somewhat prior to the muscles at the ankle, which is also consistent with the lead of the knee over the ankle and hip. The patterns fell largely in two groups: those discharging during the long phase, corresponding largely to the flexors in locomotion; and those during the short scratching phase (apparently shorter in decerebrate than intact cats), corresponding largely to the extensors in the stance phase. St whose main burst coincides with those of extensors [also in intact cat (223)] is an exception.

A number of detailed studies have been performed on turtle scratch and reviewed by Stein (337). This work stresses the ability of the turtle spinal cord to generate different forms of the scratch reflex depending on the location of an irritant. Thus, the turtle can generate a rostral scratch, a pocket scratch, and a caudal scratch using different parts of the scratching limb and different muscle synergies.

The wiping reflex is the equivalent of scratching in frogs, and even after spinalization, a frog can remove an irritant placed on the skin with precise movements of the leg and foot (151). Again, the forms of wiping and movement trajectories vary with the location of the irritant. Interestingly if the irritant is placed on the same spot of the forelimb (elbow) and the forelimb is retracted or protracted, the hindlimb of the spinal frog can accurately wipe the irritant regardless of the position of the forelimb, suggesting that the spinal cord can integrate complex proprioceptive inputs to plan the wiping accurately.

Fast Paw Shake. When a cat steps in water or when an irritant is stuck on its foot, it shakes its limb rapidly (8–12 Hz). Kinematic analysis of a paw shake sequence in the intact cat shows that the hip is first abducted and then the knee and ankle rapidly flex and extend, the knee and ankle becoming rapidly out of phase (327, 328, 330). Typically, the first few cycles have a higher frequency than the last. EMG recordings of such responses (1, 232, 254, 327) reveal that the small distal muscles (such as FDL) are powerfully activated during paw shake and that fast ankle extensors are not only preferentially recruited but slow muscles such as soleus appear derecruited (232, 327). New synergies, different from those observed in locomotion [see Fig. 5.7; (328, 330)], are organized during paw shake. Thus TA, the ankle flexor, is coactivated with VL, a knee extensor. During walking at slow speed (<0.7 m/s), a truncated form of paw shake can be observed during the swing phase when there is an irritant on the paw. Thus, during the swing phase of locomotion, three or four cycles are performed with the typical EMG synergies seen in paw shake (73). The locomotor structure is

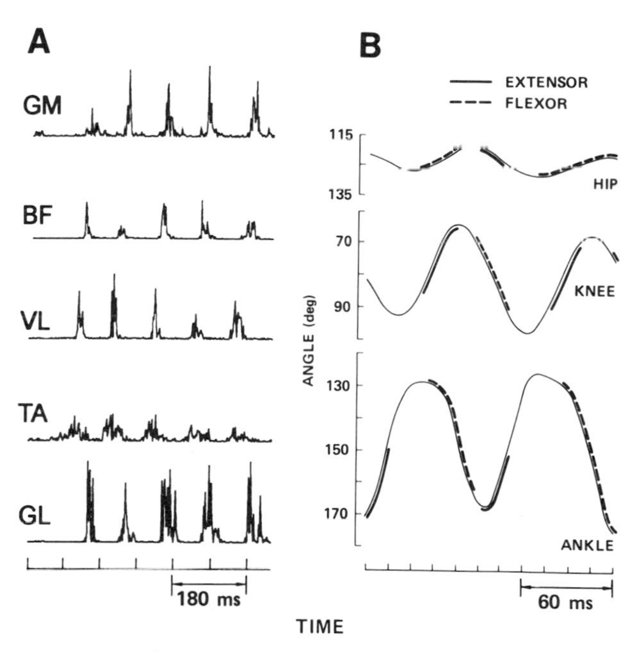

FIG. 5.7. Muscle synergies during paw shaking. In *A*, EMG of hip (GM, BF), knee (VL, BF), and ankle (GL, TA) muscles are shown for the beginning of a nine-cycle paw shake response with a mean cycle period of 86 ms. In *B*, activities of these muscles are related to hindlimb motions during steady-state cycles. [Adapted from Smith et al. (330).]

adjusted so that the swing phase during which paw shake occurs is longer than usual and the following recovery stance phase shorter.

STEREOTYPIC MOVEMENTS IN SPINAL ANIMALS

Stereotypic Movements after Complete Spinal Lesions

What is the ability of reduced preparations to express these complex stereotypic patterns? Since the celebrated accounts of Sherrington (317, 318) on reflexes, walking, standing, and scratching in spinal animals, there have been several reports on the reflex and motor capabilities of animals with a complete transection of the spinal cord. Work in the cat was rare before 1973, when an influential paper appeared (174) describing that kittens, spinalized within a few days after birth (before they had expressed any hindlimb locomotor pattern), could walk and gallop with their hindlimbs on a treadmill, provided their forelimbs stood on a platform. These "spinal kittens" not only could walk with the hindlimbs with correct paw placement and hindquarter support but could also place their paw on a surface when the dorsum of the foot touched an edge [placing reaction (150, 174)] and could hop sideways when the cat was leaned to one side.

A more complete account of the findings in chronic spinal kittens, published later (147, 148, 175), showed not only that the kinematics and the EMGs of spinal cats were very similar to normal cats but also that the spinal cats had the ability to adapt their locomotion to the various speeds of the treadmill and even to asymmetrical treadmill speeds. The age of spinalization and the amount of training on the treadmill (30 min five times a week) were shown to have important effects on the locomotor pattern (331). Chronic spinal cats can also perform paw shake during swing, showing that the spinal cord is capable of switching rapidly between such different synergies (74).

A report on cats spinalized as adults (129) stressed the fact that the interlimb coordination was lost when attempting to walk with all four limbs on a treadmill and that the step cycle was very disorganized. Work with adult cats spinalized at T13 (36, 296, 297) has shown that the quality of hindlimb locomotion is dramatically improved by training and that the spinal locomotor pattern evolves with time. Spinal cats made plantigrade paw contact and could maintain the weight of the hindquarters by the third week. Foot drag during the first part of swing was present in most cats. The timing of the EMGs observed was similar to those before spinalization in cats chronically implanted with EMG electrodes before the spinalization (44, 297).

The work of Lovely et al. (235) shows that the force level recorded, at least in soleus, is large enough to participate in propulsion as suggested for the spinal kittens (147) but that it declines rapidly during stance, which could facilitate the premature onset of swing [see later (119)] and could contribute to the foot drag.

The importance of regular daily training (even starting as late as 1 month after transection) has been supported by the work of many (123, 234, 235). This is, of course, of great interest in the clinical situation, where training may be started only late after the spinal injury (33, 39, 152, 359). Another remarkable effect appears to be in the specificity of training. Spinal cats received a specific training only for standing on a platform for several months. These cats had a very poor locomotor performance on the treadmill (123).

A locomotor-related behavior, airstepping, which is evoked by holding the cat by the thorax and letting the hindlimbs pendent, was studied in adult chronic spinal cats (161). A full sequence of airstepping (ten steps) could be elicited with strong pinching of the tail at day 19, while spontaneous airstepping could be observed at 33 days by just holding the cat in the air by the thorax. This is much longer than in spinal kittens, in which such behavior can be obtained a few days after spinalization.

The evolution of the spinal locomotor pattern has been studied as a function of age of spinalization in kittens (55, 292). Although normal kittens do not walk (or only exceptionally) within the first week after birth, kittens spinalized 1–2 days after birth can readily generate a locomotor pattern. Cats operated on at 2 weeks of age do not perform as well and apparently were able to walk only 3–5 days after the lesion, and their performance decreased after 3 months. The release of behavior and better performance of neonatal spinal cats was attributed to a decrease of spinal γ-aminobutyric acid (GABA) in the spinal neonate compared to the adult spinal (293).

What about spinal primates? Philippson (278) made some laconic comments on three spinal monkeys, although he clearly states that locomotor movements were observed. A major study was conducted by Eidelberg et al. (131) on macaque monkeys (spinalized at T8–T9). In acute spinal monkeys, dihydroxyphenylalanine (DOPA) did not induce locomotion; in the chronic state (up to 4 months), clonidine did not evoke locomotor movements. There is, however, recent evidence in marmosets (small New World monkeys) that fictive locomotor rhythm can be induced by DOPA (201).

Evidence for rhythm generation in the spinal human is also not very clear as reviewed by Vilensky et al. (354). The results of Bussel (65, 294), however, suggest that there might be some spinal circuits in humans capable of generating a basic rhythmicity. A recent report also claims that some rhythmicity can be obtained in complete paraplegics with assistance and the injection of noradrenaline in the intrathecal space (96).

Calancie et al. (69) relate the case of a patient with a 17-year history of a neurologically incomplete lesion of the cervical spinal cord who displayed involuntary well-organized rhythms in the legs when laying supine in bed, thus extending the hips (see later). These involuntary locomotor movements appeared in a period of particularly intense locomotor training and disappeared after the patient returned to a sedentary life. Although this does not prove without doubt that there is a central rhythm generator for locomotion in humans, it strongly suggests that, in humans as well as most other animals, well-organized locomotor movements may be generated at the spinal cord level and perhaps by other supraspinal structures and therefore offers great hope for the beneficial effects that training and pharmacotherapy could have in patients with partial spinal cord lesions (39, 295).

Stereotypic Movements after Partial Spinal Lesions

Bilateral pyramidotomy does not impair the production of locomotion in cats or monkeys; a bilateral pyramidotomy combined with medial brainstem lesions in monkeys induces a persistent inability to right, walk, and turn, whereas independent finger movements are preserved, suggesting a critical role of the medial reticular formation in the control of locomotion (15). Sparing of at least part of a ventrolateral quadrant in the cat [as shown by the associated labeling by horseradish peroxidase (HRP) of neurons in the pontine and medullary formation] was claimed to be essential for recovery of locomotion in chronically lesioned cats (84, 130) and monkeys (131) (see 128 for a review of early literature on different subtotal lesions in primates and nonprimates). However, evidence is mounting that cats (165–167; Brustein and Rossignol, unpublished observations) and monkeys (354) can walk with the hindlimbs after a chronic section of the ventrolateral pathways. These lesions often result in a perturbed coordination between forelimbs and hindlimbs (130, 166), the forelimbs and hindlimbs walking at times more or less independently or with various phase shifts. A reappraisal of the lesion data in monkeys (354) also suggests that locomotion is possible in primates after very extensive lesions involving the ventrolateral tracts. Studies in humans also indicate that the ventrolateral pathways surgically severed for pain control in cancer patients do not result in major motor impairments (247). Thus, the dorsolateral pathways are capable of triggering voluntary hindlimb movements in cats with a chronic lesion of the ventrolateral funiculi. However, complementary findings (Jiang and Drew, unpublished observations) indicate that section of the dorsolateral funiculi alone does not abolish locomotion but results in some permanent deficits such as foot drag during swing and the inability to clear an obstacle with the foot during walking, suggesting that locomotion can probably be triggered by various inputs coursing through different tracts (see later under Initiation of Locomotion).

Several months after a chronic hemisection of the spinal cord (12), monkeys recovered locomotor functions. In hemisected cats, the basic locomotor pattern recuperates within about 2 weeks, although there remain some permanent deficits in more demanding locomotor tasks such as walking on pegs (189). In another series on low thoracic hemisected cats, a second hemitransection was made at the contralateral midthoracic level. These cats could still regain voluntary locomotor functions overground, although the forelimb and hindlimb coupling could be lost (217), even when, in some cats, a good portion of propriospinal pathways remained. The rate of recovery depended on the time interval between the two hemisections: the shorter the interval, the longer it took to recover (216). This suggests that perhaps descending pathways known to collateralize at several levels such as the reticulospinal pathways (277) must be given sufficient time to compensate for the loss of other pathways.

After a longitudinal split of the lumbar cord from L2–3 to L7–S1, cats can, after about 1 month, stand and walk with bilateral hindlimb coordination, suggesting that the interlimb coordination can be ensured by descending pathways (214). After such a split and a further unilateral hemisection, the isolated spinal cord can eventually step even though it is isolated from supraspinal and contralateral inputs [the quality of such locomotion is difficult to assess (215)].

The neural pathways that could subserve forelimb–hindlimb coordination have been also studied with partial spinal lesions. Cats with a caudal thoracic lesion of the dorsal column (138) had normal modes of coupling between homolateral limbs, but these were labile and shifted from one to the other (but see 167). Other lesions—namely of the DSCT (140) tract, which does not produce these effects—suggested that long propriospinal pathways are probably involved. However, the experiments on serial hemisections of the cord suggested that propriospinal pathways are not crucial for interlimb coordination (217).

Pharmacology of Stereotypic Patterns

Whereas the previous section suggested that locomotor training is important for the recovery of locomotor function in the spinal state, it is also important to better understand how various neurotransmitters may control the expression of locomotor patterns (298) and could be used even in a clinical context as recently reviewed (39, 295).

Noradrenergic System. Early work indicated that ephedrine and D-amphetamine were capable of inducing some stepping in spinal animals (see 39). A series of papers published by the group of Lundberg in 1966–1967 on the effect of L-DOPA on the spinal cord (see 175) constitute the real starting point of a whole series of work on the pharmacological induction or the modulation of the spinal locomotor pattern, especially the noradrenergic system. The neuronal circuits activated in these conditions were thought to represent a physiological substratum for the half-centers model proposed by T. G. Brown (59). Soon afterward, Grillner and Zangger (see 175) showed that long sequences of alternating activities in flexor and extensor nerves could be observed by potentiating L-DOPA with nialamide, a monoamine oxidase inhibitor.

Similarly, clonidine, an α_2-noradrenergic receptor agonist, can induce hindlimb stepping on a treadmill in acutely spinalized cats (146). When clonidine was given intraperitoneally 24–48 h after spinalization, locomotor movements were performed with the hips often more extended than usual (38), and the flexor burst duration was almost equal to that of the extensors. When clonidine was given 6–7 days postlesion, the amplitude of hip excursion was nearly normal and the cat could support its weight; however, there could be a marked foot drag. In late spinal cats walking spontaneously, clonidine could exert a potent modulation of the locomotor pattern (35, 38, 296). The stance length, at the same speed as before drug injection, was much larger and so were the bursts of discharge in flexor muscles. There was no significant change in mean EMG amplitude. Under these conditions, cats could also be induced to walk backward on the treadmill.

After clonidine, there is a marked reduction in short-latency cutaneous reflex excitability, consistent with the findings of reduced excitability with L-DOPA. Thus, short-latency flexion reflexes, elicited by stimulating electrically the dorsum of the foot, are still present but have a much higher threshold. Fast paw shake, readily evoked by dipping the hindpaw in water before clonidine, is abolished after the drug. These effects of clonidine can be largely reversed by yohimbine, a noradrenergic blocker (163). Ongoing work is aimed at evaluating the various noradrenergic agonists, using an intrathecal approach. Figure 5.8 illustrates how a single intrathecal bolus of clonidine can induce a good locomotor pattern (Fig. 5.8*B*) in a cat spinalized 3 days earlier and which had no locomotor capacity just prior to the drug injection (Fig. 5.8*A*).

The possibility of initiating locomotion soon after the spinal transection with noradrenergic agonists allowed the evaluation, in a few cats, of the effect of early locomotor training on recovery (32) using a daily dose of clonidine and intensive training on the treadmill (about 60–90 min of actual walk in bouts of 15 min). The results suggest that within 8–12 days, the four spinal cats had reached their prespinalization locomotor performance (cycle duration vs. treadmill speed, weight support of the hindquarters) and could thereafter maintain this performance without drugs for several weeks.

Serotoninergic System. In neonatal rats, in either fictive conditions with ventral root recordings or in semi-isolated spinal cord with limbs attached, 5-hydroxytryptamine (5-HT) can induce slow (0.5–0.2 Hz) and fast (5–10 Hz) rhythmic activity (77, 333) that can be intermingled. A recent study in the same preparation (78) established that fictive locomotor pattern recorded in bilateral ventral roots can be evoked in a dose-dependent manner by 5-HT and can be blocked by 5-HT1 and 5-HT2 antagonists. In acutely spinalized rabbits, 5-hydroxytryptophan (5-HTP) was shown to evoke a fictive locomotor pattern and to facilitate the discharge of the extensors more than that of the flexor nerves (348, 349). In decerebrate cats (179), 5-HTP, the 5-HT precursor that crosses the blood-brain barrier, markedly increased the muscular activity tonically but did not induce locomotion. Similarly, in early-spinal cats, 5-HTP and two agonists, Quipazine and 5-methoxydimethyl-tryptamine (5-MeODMT), failed to induce locomotion when given intraperitoneally, although cats given the same preparation on the same day could walk very well with clonidine (38).

In late chronic spinal cats, 5-HTP, Quipazine, and 5-MeODMT had dramatic effects (37). At the same

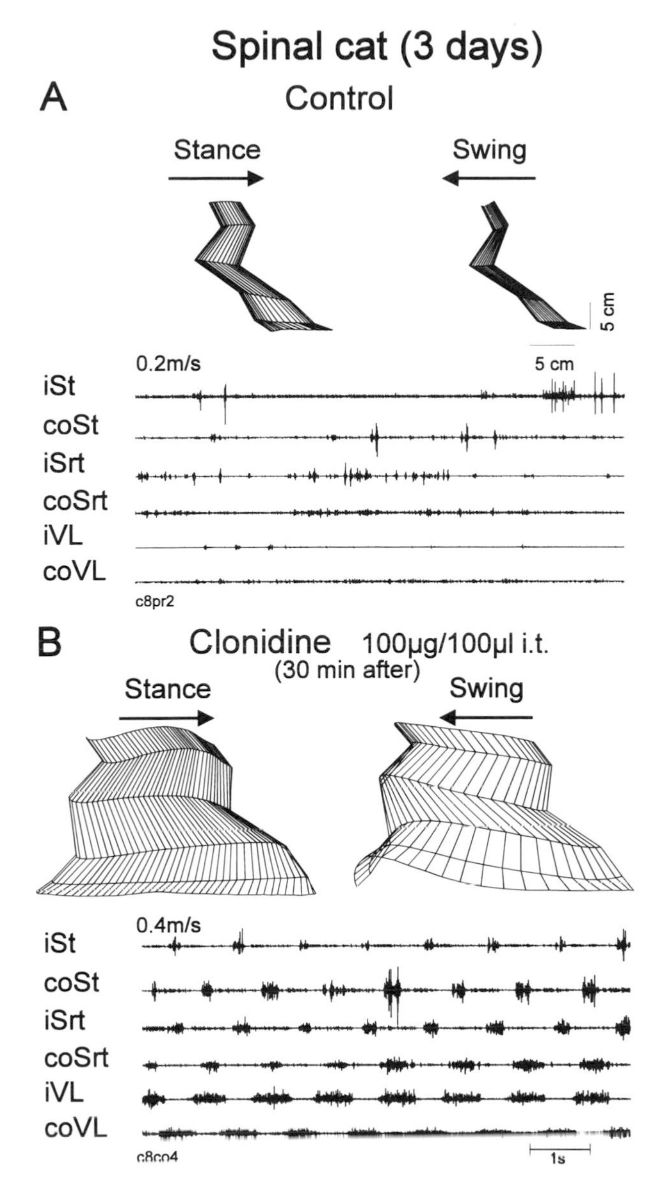

FIG. 5.8. Intrathecal injection of clonidine in an adult cat spinalized 3 days before. *A*, In the control period just before injecting clonidine, there is practically no rhythmic movement on the treadmill set at 0.2 m/s. *B*, About 30 min after the injection of clonidine (single bolus of 100 μg/100 μl) through the intrathecal cannula whose tip was around L5. Both the kinematics and EMG recordings show a nice pattern of walking. (From Chau, Barbeau, and Rossignol, unpublished observations.)

treadmill speed, stance lengths could be much larger as was the case with noradrenergic drugs. However, contrary to noradrenergic drugs that did not significantly increase the mean EMG amplitude, serotonergic drugs increased the amplitude of EMGs to more than three times the control level. Even the back muscles, which are generally silent or recruited at low levels in chronic spinal cats walking at slow speeds, were strongly activated after 5-HT drugs and discharged in the double-burst pattern seen in the normal cat walking at high speeds (374). Cats walked with long strides and, during stance, the legs pushed forcefully on the belt. Fast paw shakes were brisker after 5-HT drugs, in contrast to noradrenergic drugs. Cyproheptadine, a 5-HT2 blocker (34), largely reversed these effects on locomotion. In some experiments noradrenergic agonists and serotonergic agonists were combined; the cycle length was increased as well as duration and amplitude of the EMG bursts (38).

Other Neurochemical Systems. N-Methyl-D-aspartate (NMDA), quisqualate, and kainate receptors, activated by glutamate and related excitatory amino acids (EAA), have been studied for their capacity to trigger locomotion in in vitro preparations of lamprey (56, 57), Xenopus (90), and neonatal rats (77, 78, 222, 333). The combination of 5-HT and N-Methyl aspartate (NMA) was able to maintain a stable pattern for several minutes with a frequency intermediate between that of NMA or 5-HT alone (332). Sulphur-containing excitatory amino acids are potent activators of locomotion and GABA exerts a potent inhibitory control over the locomotor rhythm (79). Agonists of NMDA (aspartate, glutamate, NMA) and non-NMDA agonists (kainate) were very effective, whereas quisqualate/alpha-amino-3-hydroxy-5-methyl-4 isoxazole proprionic acid (AMPA) agonists were not (333). Other studies on the induction of rhythmic patterns by NMA, 5-HT, and acetylcholine (ACh) were performed in neonatal rats using recordings of peripheral nerves to monitor ankle flexor and extensor activity (87). Although ACh (with edrophonium), 5-HT, or NMA can generate rhythmic patterns, some of these are incompatible with locomotion (86). In the decerebrate cat, recent research (100) has shown that intrathecal application of 2-amino-5-phosphonovaleric acid (AP5) or 6-cyano-7-nitroquinoxaline-2,3 dione (CNQX), which are NMDA and non-NMDA receptor antagonists, respectively, can block the brainstem-evoked locomotion on the treadmill. NMDA coupled with the uptake inhibitor dihydrokainic acid (DHK) could elicit well-coordinated alternate activation of muscles in fictive conditions, whereas quisqualate and kainate were ineffective. Recent experiments with intrathecal injections of NMA in early-spinal cats (within 1 week of spinalization) did not induce locomotion but could trigger high-frequency discharges akin to fast paw shake; in the same animals clonidine could evoke locomotion as usual. In chronic spinal cats having recuperated locomotion, walking could be blocked by AP5 and could be reinstated by intrathecal NMA (Chau, Jordan, and Rossignol, unpublished observations).

Various other substances have been used to pharmacologically initiate locomotion. Strychnine, a glycine inhibitor, can trigger locomotion in chronic spinal dogs (186), whereas bicuculline, a GABA antagonist, can facilitate locomotion in chronic spinal cats (293). Finally, certain drugs have been used to potentiate fictive locomotion; 4-aminopyridine, a potassium channel blocker, was shown to facilitate DOPA-induced fictive locomotion in spinal cats (112, 269, 373) even if it is incapable of triggering the locomotor pattern by itself. Naloxone, an opioid antagonist, can facilitate locomotion induced in acute or chronic spinal cats by clonidine (267) or generate spinal rhythms by itself (307).

CENTRAL GENERATION OF STEREOTYPIC PATTERNS

Locomotion

The relative importance of afferent feedback in the generation of rhythmic movements has been widely debated (175, 236) (see later under AFFERENT CONTROLS; see also Chapter 3), and all arguments cannot be presented here in detail. However, that rhythmic activity can be generated in the absence of peripheral afferent inputs after deafferentation has been solidly established for locomotion (182), scratching in cats and rats (59, 93) and wiping in frogs (151). Similar conclusions have been reached with paralyzed preparations in which all phasic afferent feedback is removed and the pattern is recorded as discharges in identified cut muscle nerves ("fictive locomotion"). Such patterns were recorded in various preparations: acute and chronic spinal cats (30, 181, 269), spinal rabbits injected with nialamide and L-DOPA (349), lightly anesthetized paralyzed rabbits (348), thalamic (decorticate) cats (23, 276) and rabbits (353) that develop rhythmic activity spontaneously without drugs, and finally decerebrate cats with electrical stimulation of the mesencephalic locomotor region (MLR) (see later) (143, 212). Only in a few cases (181) was the pattern studied in a spinal, curarized, and deafferentated spinal cord. As mentioned before, in the spinal marmoset, a low-level primate, fictive locomotion can be induced with DOPA (201).

In the cat, a number of key features of locomotion are preserved in all conditions (intact, spinal, and fictive; Fig. 5.9): bilateral alternation, flexor bursts shorter than extensor bursts, knee flexor St of shorter duration than the hip flexor sartorius, double burst in St in spinal and fictive preparations. Thus, in agreement with a large body of evidence gathered in different species (92) and for different rhythmic

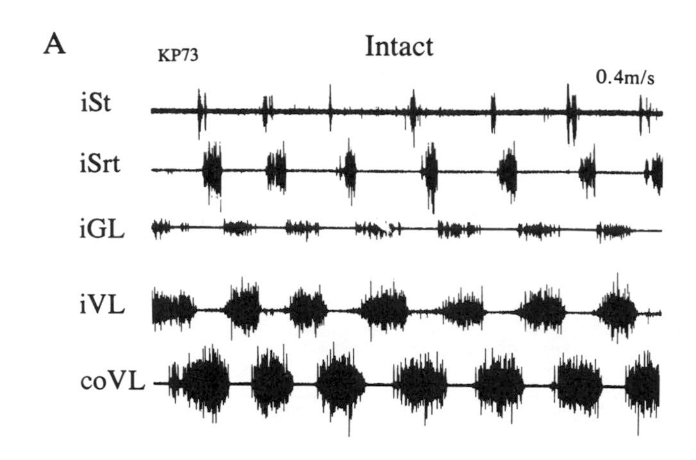

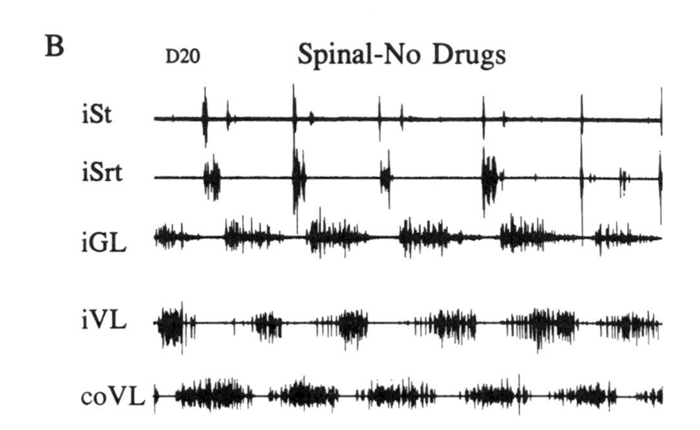

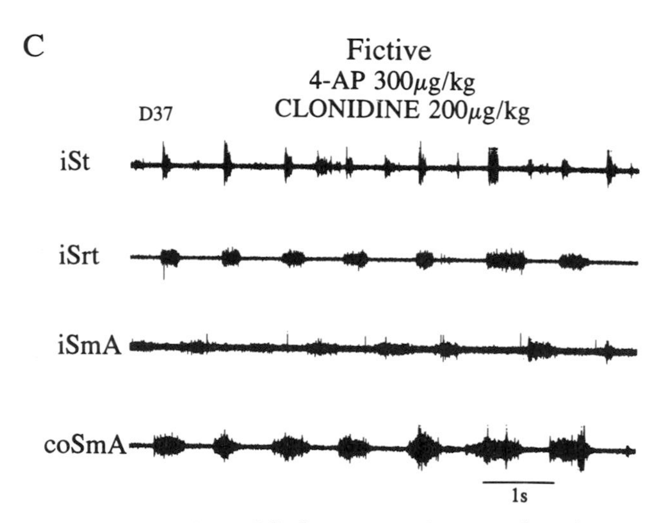

FIG. 5.9. Comparison of discharges in various muscle and muscle nerves in the same cat in three different conditions. In *A*, Normal cat, chronically implanted with EMG electrodes [see Drew and Rossignol (107) for details of implantation] walking on a motor-driven treadmill at 0.4 m/s. *B*, The same cat 20 days after spinalization and training [see Barbeau and Rossignol (36) for details of training]. *C*, Same cat, 37 days following spinalization; the cat was decerebrated anemically, paralyzed with gallamine triethiodide, and injected with 4-aminopyridine and clonidine. Nerve recordings are made with polymer cuff electrodes (269). [Reproduced with permission from Rossignol et al. (302).]

behaviors (237), locomotion and closely related patterns such as scratching and paw shake are generated centrally in the spinal cord in the absence of afferent feedback but are markedly influenced by such feedback. After reviewing these rhythmic patterns at the nerve and neuronal levels, some mechanisms of rhythmic generation will be discussed as well as how segmental and descending inputs interact with them.

Motor Nerves and Motoneurons (MNs). The fictive locomotor pattern in acute spinal cats injected with noradrenergic substances is often much slower than the slowest walk (0.1–0.2 m/s) used on a treadmill. In chronic spinal cats (225, 269) or decerebrate preparation with MLR stimulation or decorticate cats, the fictive cycle duration can often be on the order of 0.8–1 s, which is about the period of a normal cat walking at a speed of 0.4 m/s.

Hindlimbs. A number of muscles appear to discharge simply as flexors or extensors with one single burst of activity per cycle (23, 181, 276). Semitendinosus exhibited a double burst under various fictive conditions (23, 182, 269, 276, 353), including after spinalization, curarization, and deafferentation (181). The discharge can be quite labile and be influenced by the position of the leg during recording or on the presence of peripheral stimulation. Intracellular records of St MNs also show a double depolarization corresponding to the time where the motoneurons would be expected to discharge (261, 276).

Sartorius (Srt) MNs discharge in the flexion phase only (68, 182, 261, 276). Their period of activity is much longer than that of St MNs and may sometime occupy more than 60% of the cycle. Thus the phase of depolarization of certain Srt MNs can be significantly longer than the period of spike discharge (68, 261) corresponding to electroneurography (ENG) recordings. Recent work (269) has also indicated that activity in Srt nerve may occur not only during the flexion period but also during the extension period, and the amount of this activity may depend on the position of the limb at the time of recording.

TA nerve, as does Srt nerve, has a more prolonged burst of activity than St nerve (182), and both Srt and TA nerve activity peak at about the same time (269). This seems also the case for EDL (23). This corresponds very well to the intact situation in which the hip and ankle reach their maximal flexion later than the knee (see above). FDL and FHL, both physiological plantar flexors of the toes, are recruited differentially also in fictive conditions, FDL showing a characteristic well-developed early flexion burst with a variable amount of activity during the extension phase (23), whereas the FHL uniquely discharges during the extensor phase (143). Again, this is a very clear indication that two close synergists, with similar though not identical reflex organization, receive a detailed and specific central command during locomotion.

Rectus femoris (knee extensor–hip flexor) may also discharge two bursts of activity in the fictive state (276) depending on the presence of certain peripheral tonic stimuli. Intracellular recordings also clearly showed two phases of depolarization. Small ankle and toe muscles may be more variable, but generally their discharge is consistent with their EMG pattern (23, 276).

Forelimbs. Research by Viala and Vidal (350) demonstrated that paralyzed rabbits with spinal sections at C1 and T12 can display, after DOPA and nialamide, an in-phase and out-of-phase discharge in forelimb muscle nerves, clearly indicating that the cervical spinal cord is capable of generating a locomotor rhythm. Similar findings were reported in high spinal cats (242, 373). When the spinal cord is intact, the hindlimb circuitry appears to exert a powerful control on the forelimb rhythm and may even prevent it so that it is customary to section the cord at T13 to study forelimb fictive locomotion (21). Fictive locomotion in thalamic cats also produces a coordinated pattern of fore- and hindlimbs (68).

Elbow flexors (Br, Bic, CIB) always appear to have a simple flexor burst (68). The shoulder flexor teres major, which was shown to have a pure flexor activity in some cases and some extensor activity in others, may show two periods of activity in fictive conditions (68). Pinching of the skin of the distal forelimb can increase the flexor component and abolish completely the extensor component. Conversely, subscapularis, which discharges during stance in the intact conditions, may discharge one or two bursts in fictive conditions in flexion and extension. Pinching of the distal forelimb may abolish the flexor burst and enhance the extensor burst.

From the work of Cabelguen et al. (68) and others (367) the discharge of other muscle nerves can be summarized as follows. Flexor discharges were found in the various trapezius components, although these discharge mainly during stance in intact cats; extensor activity was observed in rhomboideus as in the intact. Appendicular muscle (P and LtD) discharge during the extensor phase, although LtD has a significant activity at the beginning of the flexor period. Flexors of the digits may have a main burst during the period of extensor activity, whereas extensor carpi ulnaris shows a significant burst in the flexor period.

Motoneurons from elbow flexors and extensors as well as from radial motor nuclei innervating the wrist and digits muscles were shown to have many characteristics of their intact patterns (162, 365, 366), the most distal muscles being the most variable.

Membrane properties of motoneurons. Different mechanisms could account for the rhythmicity of motoneurons. There could be an excitation during one phase and return to a normal resting potential in between or an inhibition between two successive excitatory periods. The cyclical depolarization could be due to a cyclical disinhibition or to a periodic increase of synaptic activity in excitatory pathways. These possibilities can be tested directly by measuring the input resistance of motoneurons with intracellular recordings of motoneurons during fictive locomotion. The work of Edgerton et al. (124) showed that motoneurons were cyclically depolarized and hyperpolarized during fictive locomotion and that, while some motoneurons discharged spikes during the depolarized phase, others did not, although they were also depolarized. Various studies in different preparations showed conclusively, with intracellular chloride injections in motoneurons, that the hyperpolarization reversed or that it was much reduced between two successive phases of depolarization (81, 124, 261, 274). This suggests that both the excitatory and inhibitory phases are actively generated by synaptic inputs and that one phase or the other is not the result of disinhibition or disfacilitation. This was further documented by measurements of input resistance of motoneurons during fictive locomotion induced by stimulation of the MLR (315). The somatic input resistance of most motoneurons did not change in the two opposite phases, in keeping with the notion that synaptic activity is responsible for both phases (see, however, 305 for contrary evidence).

It was suggested that the discharge of single motoneurons could be mimicked by injecting, in motoneurons of anesthetized and paralyzed cats, intracellular currents that followed an envelope of the activity of the parent muscle obained by filtering its EMG activity (196). However, the discharge of the motoneurons during the excitatory phase of the locomotor drive potential (LDP) does not appear to be completely explained on the basis of a simple somatic depolarization mimicking the current injected through an intracellular microelectrode (61). Rather, it is suggested that locomotor activation triggers special membrane properties such as plateau potentials (198) or other voltage-dependent excitation of motoneurons through a neurotransmitter-regulated regenerative process (60). In these conditions, there is a reduction in afterhyperpolarization (AHP) after spontaneous or electrically evoked spikes, consistent with the work in lampreys (355).

The above results suggest that motoneuronal membrane properties would participate in stabilizing their own rhythmicity. The question of whether motoneurons are part of the central pattern generator has been addressed more directly in different preparations (298). In neonatal rat motoneurons, NMDA induces oscillatory properties (332) that are tetrodotoxin (TTX) resistant (194), much as in the lamprey (356). In chick embryos, optical lesion of motoneurons filled with dextran-fluorescein, leaving interneurons intact, result in a much diminished albeit not abolished rhythmic motility, suggesting that motoneurons themselves may participate in the maintenance of the rhythmic pattern (252).

Interneurons

Identified interneurons (INs). The first study to investigate the discharge of single spinal interneurons was performed by Orlovsky and Feldman (259) in decerebrate cats induced to walk on a treadmill with MLR stimulation. After deafferentation, about two-thirds of the interneurons in the intermediate laminae were still phasically modulated and were considered to contribute to the actual generation of the pattern. Ia INs mediating reciprocal inhibition were recorded during real walking on the treadmill of decerebrate cats (142) and their discharges coincided with the activity of the muscle from which they receive their afferent input. Ia INs, which also receive recurrent Renshaw inhibition, were less inhibited during locomotion, consistent with the idea that recurrent inhibition is decreased during locomotion (see 175).

The role of Ia INs was further investigated in acute spinal cats injected with DOPA (124) and in decerebrate paralyzed cats with MLR stimulation (208, 240, 283). Injection of strychnine, a glycine antagonist that would abolish the efferent output of Ia INs, effectively decreased the hyperpolarization phase in motoneurons but failed to abolish the rhythmicity. Renshaw cells were found to be activated somewhat after the respective motoneurons (208, 240, 251) and well timed to decrease the activity of their parent motoneurons and associated Ia INs. Mecamylamine, a cholinergic blocker that reduces the activation of Renshaw cells and thus blocks recurrent inhibition on motoneurons and Ia INs, did not abolish the rhythmicity of either the motoneurons or of Ia INs (283). It is concluded that the rhythmicity of Ia INs is not essentially controlled by recurrent inhibitory inputs but rather is due to an excitatory central command from a pattern generator independent of motoneuron discharge and Renshaw cell activity.

L4 INs, receiving monosynaptic inputs from group II afferents of certain muscles (pretibial flexors, sartorius, quadriceps) as well as Ia inputs and articular and cutaneous inputs (125, 126) and inputs from corticospinal and rubrospinal tracts and projecting to L7 motor nuclei, were postulated to play a role during locomotion, perhaps in relation to hip position and the transition from stance to swing (127). MLR stimulation evoked EPSPs in these L4 INs and L-DOPA, injected in acute spinal cats, affected markedly the response of the interneurons as well as the field potentials in the intermediate regions and ventral horn by gr II stimulation. During MLR fictive locomotion (312), two-thirds of these L4 INs were active during the flexion phase, whereas the remaining INs were not rhythmically active but were subjected to a cyclical modulation of their responsiveness to peripheral inputs.

C3–C4 propriospinal interneurons sending their axon to forelimb motoneurons and a collateral to the lateral reticular nucleus were studied during fictive locomotion evoked by MLR stimulation (21). Most of these cells discharged rhythmically as did cells from the LRN even after cerebellar ablation. This modulation ceases after cooling of the cord at C7, suggesting that their modulation is related to the intraspinal process at this level. In another study in behaving cats (5), it was concluded that although these C3–C4 Ins can be labeled by the activity dependent WGA-HRP marker during reaching movements, they are not labeled during locomotion. Finally, another group of cervical interneurons located at the C6–C7 were also found to be rhythmically active during fictive locomotion (191, 342, 367, 369).

Localization of interneurons. A number of recent studies have used activity-dependent markers to try localizing neurons implicated in rhythm generation. 2-Deoxyglucose, an activity-dependent metabolic marker, has been used to label brainstem structures during active walking in mesencephalic cats with MLR stimulation (321) as well as spinal structures during DOPA-induced fictive locomotion in rabbits (347). The latter work reported marking in the intermediate gray of the cord. This is consistent with the findings of Dai et al. (89), who described (using *c-fos*, an activity-dependent genetic marker) cells around the central spinal canal that were labeled after a period of fictive locomotion. Similar findings were made with scratching in the paralyzed cats (31). Studies on the distribution of isopotential fields in the spinal cord after MLR stimulation (248) confirm the importance of this medial region. In the chick embryo, studies using a calcium-imaging technique as well as electrophysiological recordings during locomotion in the chick (253) have shown that the dorsal horn as well as the medial part of the cord are not essential for the generation of rhythmicity and that the ventral horn contains all the elements necessary for rhythmicity. However, the rostral segments have more potential for generating rhythmicity and interneurons activating motoneurons in lower segments are located dorsomedially in the ventral horn and their axon course through ventrolateral pathways (192). Similarly, in cats, upper lumbar segments (L3–L5) are more important for rhythmicity (94, 159), since fictive locomotion cannot be elicited after a section at caudal L5 (181). Finally, it has recently been shown, in in vitro neonatal rats induced to walk with NMDA and 5-HT, that cells located around the central canal are heavily labeled by the activity marker sulforhodamine after a period of locomotion and this even after dorsal rhizotomy (219). Using slice preparations of rat spinal cord, neurons that are ventrolateral to the central canal, in medial lamina VII, have been found to have pacemaker-like properties (membrane oscillations insensitive to TTX that are evoked by NMDA but not kainate, 5-HT, or noradrenaline); these conditional bursters are postulated to be implicated in the generation of locomotor rhythms (193).

Scratching and Paw Shake

Studies on reduced preparations have given very good insights on control mechanisms of scratching. An excellent account of the central regulation of locomotion and scratching and the possible sharing of neurons in locomotion and scratching has been published (159). By electrical stimulation at C1–C2 (with or without local application of D-tubocurarine chloride on the surface of C1), it was possible to elicit a scratching behavior (without the head movement, which was constrained) (93). This pattern could be evoked also after deafferentation. In fictive conditions, the hindlimb has to be manually positioned in flexion to elicit scratching (49, 93). Similar results have been obtained by Baev's group, who further showed modifications of the pattern with limb positions (25, 325) as was discussed for locomotion (269). The detailed studies of the muscle nerve discharge during fictive scratching again illustrates that while there are, broadly speaking, two phases, the details of the discharge pattern in terms of both timing and profile suggest that there is a central pattern generator for scratching, which may be a functional modification of the locomotion generator (49, 95, 159). Many interneurons are involved in generating this pattern, since their discharge is spread out throughout the entire scratch cycle (27, 50).

The various forms of scratch can also be evoked after paralysis in the turtle; in these preparations it was shown that motoneurons were depolarized and hyperpolarized in the opposite phase (291).

In semichronic spinal cats, we have studied fictive paw shake (269) by squirting water on the central pad. Well-developed paw shake sequence could be elicited, with the typical TA-VL synergies being preserved in such fictive conditions (see previous section).

Ontogeny of Stereotypic Movements

Locomotion and Paw Shake. One study has dealt with the development of motor behavior in cat embryos (362). The limb movements are initially passively coupled to squirming movements of the head and trunk (righting responses). Initially, the forelegs are synchronous and, at about 50 days, true alternate stepping appears in the forelimbs but not in the hindlimbs, so that at birth the hindlimbs are coupled in phase. More is known about the early development of locomotion in kittens (54, 292). Normal kittens generally do not make weight-bearing steps during the first postnatal week, although they can, even at 3 days, if for instance they rush to feed on their mother. Quadrupedal overground stepping on the digits is seen at the end of the second week. In weeks 3 and 4, the pattern dramatically improves and by the end of the fifth week a continuous pattern with a narrow base of support and appropriate swing is generated. Airstepping can be elicited as soon as day 3 but gradually disappears. EMG recordings (55) show a progressive out-of-phase coupling of the limbs, a correlation between the duration of extensors (not flexors) with the cycle duration, a strong synergy between knee and ankle extensors, and reciprocal pattern of activation between ankle extensor and flexor. This work suggests that the basic circuitry is present right at birth and its full manifestation is contingent upon the development of other intrinsic and extrinsic factors, a conclusion reached by work on chick embryo and tadpoles in which developmental issues can be studied on a wider developmental scale.

Hatching. For obvious reasons, the chick has been one of the favorite animals for the study of the development of cyclical behaviors (42). The spinal cord of the chick embryo offers also the possibility of an in-depth cellular analysis of rhythmic motor patterns using patch-clamp recording of neurons (311), as well as calcium imaging techniques to localize cells related to the generation of the rhythm (253). Electrical stimulation of the cord or the brainstem can elicit bouts of embryonic activity. Optical imaging using the membrane-permeant calcium indicator Fura-2 shows that during a rhythmic sequence ventrolateral neurons light up first, and this is followed by a calcium wave extending medially and dorsolaterally. The chick embryo also offers a very nice model for the study of functional regeneration of descending pathways after spinal lesions. Using open-field locomotion or brainstem-evoked locomotion as an indicator, it was shown that lesions made before E13 were anatomically and functionally repaired (187, 188). If the same lesion was made after the permissive period, which largely corresponds to the myelination, then there was no such repair. Using double-labeling methods, Steeves suggested that this functional recovery is indeed due to regeneration of brainstem cells whose axon was cut.

Central Pattern Generator(s)

It is legitimate to ask whether there is a multiplicity of pattern generators (i.e., distinct circuits) in the spinal cord for each observable motor pattern or whether the CNS assembles different subunits in practically unlimited combinations giving rise to the many motor patterns observed, as proposed by Grillner (unit burst generator) (175) and by Getting (building blocks) (160). There is obviously no definite answer to such a question, given the complexity of the circuitry involved. Furthermore, it also seems that rhythmic behaviors can be achieved in many different ways, so that a solution for one species may differ from another. The outputs may look the same but the generating network may be very different and can result from the different combinations of similar building blocks, these being defined as cellular, synaptic, and network properties. Activating some membrane properties with a neurotransmitter or including or excluding neurons through various external inputs may change the behavior of the networks [frequency as well as shifts between neurons giving rise to new or different patterns (185)]. These concepts must always be in the background when discussing the mechanisms of generation of stereotypic limb movements in higher vertebrates, in which the thousands of interneurons (the large majority being unidentified) and various membrane properties and connectivity are only starting to be unraveled. Grillner (124) proposed that not only each limb but each joint, and indeed each synergistic muscle group acting around a joint, could be controlled by a unit burst generator. The rhythmicity of the unit burst could be generated as suggested before by the combination of various building blocks of membrane, synaptic, and network interactions. The unit burst generators could be coupled in phase, out of phase, or with a variable phase and give rise to various behaviors (e.g., forward and backward walking). Work in humans shows that forward and backward walking have mirror trajectory images. This is achieved by major changes in the discharge of muscles so that, for instance, hamstring muscles, instead of discharging at the swing-stance transition now discharge at the stance-swing transition, the ankle flexor TA discharges during stance, and the knee extensor VL discharges throughout stance to produce propulsion. Similar findings were made in crustacea (82) and in mole rats for which the forward-backward behavior is very common as well as in the various forms of scratch in the turtle (338). Different conclusions were reached in studies on backward walking in cats that suggested that the basic EMG pattern is more or less the same in forward and backward walking but that the postural strategy of the animal is changed (see Chapter 8).

Attempts to identify how building blocks can be assembled to generate different stereotypic patterns have been made especially for locomotion and scratching (159). The two patterns have similarities: flexors and extensors alternate and the flexion phase is almost identical in both patterns. However, during scratching the extensor is very short (in fictive conditions), whereas during locomotion, the extensor phase is usually longer than the flexor phase during walk and trot (but not gallop). The rhythm of scratching is higher than locomotion and the postural bias of the hindlimbs is different, being in flexion for scratch and extension for locomotion. Also, all limbs are coupled during locomotion, whereas scratching involves mainly one limb. In fictive conditions there can be a smooth transition from one to the others, and interneurons discharging in one behavior keep the same relationship with the motor output in both behaviors.

The possibility of having two concomitant behaviors such as walking and fast paw shake also speaks in favor of common elements, some being similarly coupled and others differently coupled (328). Thus, whereas during locomotion the knee extensor VL is synergistically coupled to the ankle extensor GL, it is out of phase during fast paw shake. Fast paw shaking, however, when occurring during locomotion, alters the characteristics of locomotion so that the subcomponents of the cycle can be changed and the coupling between the hindlimbs may be altered, an adaptation also seen when the two hindlimbs are walking at different speeds on split belts.

Overall, the evidence suggests that stereotypic limb movements are generated by coupling various unit burst generators controlling the muscle synergists of each joint in different ways. These unit burst generators can themselves be made of various building blocks of membrane, synaptic, and network properties that can be brought into play by various transmitters released by segmental and suprasegmental inputs. These notions, developed over the years, offer a framework in which the limitless combinatorial properties of the nervous elements can be brought into action to produce "movements ranging from ballet dance to a tight rope walk" (175).

AFFERENT CONTROLS

The general role of afferents in relation to the central generation of rhythmic patterns has been alluded to in the previous section. Comparative aspects of afferent mechanisms in locomotion, mastication, and respiration have been reviewed elsewhere (301). The reflex control of stereotypic movements has been studied with various approaches such as recording the activity of afferents, inactivating the afferents through rhizotomies or neurectomy, and finally by stimulating the afferents either tonically throughout locomotion or in discrete phases of the cycle. This scheme will be used to discuss proprioceptive and cutaneous controls. The specific role of stretch receptors and other proprioceptors during locomotion and paw shake is described in more details in Chapter 3.

Proprioceptive Control

Lifting an otherwise quiescent spinal cat or dog by the thorax, thus extending passively the hindlimbs, triggers airstepping. This is largely due to stimulation of proprioceptors (especially at the hip), since removal of the skin does not abolish the response (318). In decerebrate cats, the effects of a weak stimulation of the MLR generating a rhythmic bursting in a ventral root filament can be abolished by positioning the limb forward or backward (260). Similarly, in chronic spinal cats walking on a treadmill, manually flexing one hip abolishes stepping in that limb (but not in the other), while stepping is resumed when the hip is extended to a degree of extension normally reached at the end of stance (178). During fictive locomotion (269), flexion of the hip abolishes rhythmicity, whereas extension markedly increases the vigor of the rhythm. Stimulation of proprioceptive afferents have also been performed in decerebrate cats walking on a treadmill and during fictive conditions (302). During real locomotion, protracting one forelimb shortens the flexor activity and increases markedly the duration of extensor activity and cycle time and can even lead to an arrest of locomotion. With retraction of one forelimb, there is a marked increase in the vigor of the locomotion, with high-amplitude activity in forelimb flexors. These changes are largely reproducible in fictive conditions, where the changes resulting from protraction or retraction of one limb only induces complementary changes bilaterally (increased flexion on one side is accompanied by an increase in contralateral extension). While stimulating C1–C2 segments electrically or chemically, a progressive manual flexion of the limb in flexion allows a scratching pattern to appear, whereas it disappears when the limb is pendent (93). Likewise, passive manipulation of the ankle joint can change the amplitude of the bursts in GL during scratching. These experimental situations reveal the complex interactions that must exist at all times between the central command and the afferent feedback. The final burst discharge is a composite of the central command and the instantaneous afferent feedback signaling the position of the limb.

Orlovsky (256) showed that retarding or accelerating the movement of the hip joint had widespread effects on more distal joints. These were not due to simple effects in a kinematic chain but suggested that the hip joint exerts a general control of the locomotor sequence in other joints. The importance of the hip joint has also been studied using sinusoidal movements (11) of the hip to entrain the rhythm as well as ramp stretches (10) at various points in the fictive locomotor cycle. A more recent study (221) on locomotor entrainment of the fictive MLR-induced locomotor pattern concluded that hip capsular afferents could not be responsible, since harmonic entrainment (1:1) persisted after specific hip joint deafferentation. The entrainment appears to be related to the periodic stretch of muscles, and even only a few muscles around the hip may be sufficient. Similar conclusions on distributed afferent feedback were reached when selective denervation of the hip and limb was performed to find the responsible afferents in positional reflex reversal (299).

Rhythmic stretch of ankle extensors can entrain the locomotor rhythm and the relation of the muscle nerve discharge with force parameter, suggesting a role for muscle load receptors in the entrainment phenomenon (85). This is consistent with the suggestion of Pearson and Duysens (119) that unloading of the ankle extensors is a crucial input that signals the effective termination of stance and triggers flexor muscles to initiate a new step. Furthermore, recent data (169, 266, 268) suggest that Golgi tendon organ inputs excite extensor motoneurons during the stance phase of locomotion through a pathway operating only during locomotor activity. These Ib inputs could then serve to reinforce the ongoing extensor activity during stance and prevent the initiation of a new flexor burst. The reduction of Ib input at the end of stance would then signal the time for a new step to occur.

The role of primary spindle afferents during locomotion was first postulated by Severin (see 175), who showed that selective block of γ axons in motor nerves significantly reduced the EMG amplitude, suggesting that the block would reduce a positive afferent feedback signal from stretch receptors. It was shown in various preparations that Ia afferents discharge during the phase when the muscles are passively stretched but also during the lengthening contraction of muscles (see Chapter 3). Although the α-γ activation may vary according to tasks (285), it was shown that dynamic and static γ-motoneuron discharges were linked to the central pattern generator, since α-γ coactivation was shown in decorticate or high decerebrate walking preparations (66, 246) as well as in paralyzed DOPA spinal cats (326). Recordings of spindle primary afferents from the forelimbs during locomotion in thalamic cats indicate a high degree of fusimotor control, since the spindle afferents discharged during the extrafusal discharge of the muscle and were even active in absence of such overt EMG activity (67).

The participation of stretch receptors in the regulation of motor output has been studied in walking decerebrate cats (3), fictive decerebrate cats (114), and thalamic and normal cats (113) as well as in humans (72). The response to stretch of soleus, as well as the H-reflex, is highest during stance and the monosynaptic Ia excitatory postsynaptic potentials (EPSPs) are largest in extensor motoneurons during their period of activity (316). It is likely, therefore, that the natural Ia afferent input normally contributes to maintain the activity or increase the activity in extensor muscles after the initial contact (164). Dietz (98) has shown that a brief ankle stretch in early stance in humans generates only a very small monosynaptic reflex compared to the response obtained with the same stimulus in the sitting position. However, Yang et al. (371), using a pneumatic device allowing stretch of the ankle in the early part of stance, have shown that the gain of the stretch reflex is high and may contribute substantially (30%–60%) to the activation of the soleus muscle. Whereas a muscle stretch in early stance may be useful to potentiate the ongoing activity of the muscle, a similar stretch of the muscle during flexion of the joint in the opposite phase could evoke an unwanted stretch reflex unless the afferent input is rendered less effective (see later under Presynaptic Mechanisms) or impinges on motoneurons, which are inhibited (114). The modulation of the monosynaptic pathway (Ia EPSPs in motoneurons) during fictive locomotion in relation to conductance changes is still controversial (316). Besides these monosynaptic effects, it appears that group I stimulation of ankle extensor (i.e., plantaris or MG) during fictive locomotion in the cat can have a widespread effect on many extensors of the limb, suggesting that such inputs, during real locomotion, could indeed serve to reinforce the stance phase as in a positive-feedback mechanism (183). Stimulation of group II afferent fibers from flexor muscles curtailed flexor bursts and initiated activity in extensors; stimulation during extension had little effect. It is suggested that this group of receptors may participate in determining the timing of the different subcomponents of the step cycle (271). Studies in the turtle monopodal swimming also show that the responses to proprioceptors is phase dependent and may serve either to strengthen the ongoing phase of the movement or else participate in the transition from one phase to the other (230).

The mechanisms discussed above would seem ideal to entrain the locomotor rhythm at different speeds or direction in, for instance, a spinal cat. During stance, stretch of extensor muscles (groups Ia and II inputs), load signals (Ib inputs), as well as inputs from muscles acting at around the hip joint would tend to maintain the ongoing extension activity (phase-promoting influences). Toward the end of stance, positional or directional signals from the hip muscles and joint, unloading of ankle muscles corresponding to a backward position of the limb would then facilitate the appearance of the next flexor burst. In normal cats, however, supraspinal commands must also participate in this regulation of the step cycle and could even override these reflex mechanisms as will be seen later.

Cutaneous Control

Tonic Stimulation. Neurectomy of cutaneous nerves innervating the foot and ankle does not alter the locomotor pattern (120, 318, 323), nor does infiltration of the central foot pad with a local anesthetic or other parts of the foot (149, 286).

Stimulation of the perineal region [scrotum, vulva and base of the tail, inguinal fold (318)], the face area (209), the pinnae (13) is most effective in triggering locomotion (see also later the relation between the fifth nerve nuclear complex and locomotor initiating areas). Stimuli of dorsal columns and dorsal roots (181) (undoubtedly also activating other afferents as well as cutaneous) are also very effective in inducing locomotion. In various preparations, tonic stimulation of the skin and cutaneous nerves of various regions can increase the locomotor rhythm (143, 352); stimulation of C fibers and, in DOPA spinal cats, stimulation of group III and IV afferents through intra-arterial injections of bradykinin or KCl in gastrocnemius as well as high-threshold stimulation of the superficial peroneal nerve (220) all lead to an enhancement of the ongoing rhythmic activity.

In turn, other types of tonic stimuli can completely inhibit these locomotor movements in both real and fictive conditions. Thus, pressure of the skin of the lumbar region (351) or controlled electrical stimulation (352) will, in the rabbit, abolish locomotion in a manner akin to the well-known hypnotic akinesia in which animals are rendered inactive by pressure over the back and the abdomen.

Phasic Stimulation. Although removal of the skin does not prevent entrainment when moving the hip (11), rhythmic stimulation of skin nerves can also entrain the fictive rhythm in spinal DOPA cats (300). There are several examples in the literature (299) of the adaptability of cutaneous reflexes to the static position of the limbs, such as hip flexion or extension, and several other examples of phase-dependent modulation in sign and amplitude of reflexes during locomotion where the limbs continually change position and direction. In some cases, the stimulus is effective in one phase of the step cycle and is ineffective in the opposite phase or else it excites (phase-dependent reversal) or inhibits the antagonist muscle groups in the opposite phase of the step cycle.

The initial studies on the modulation of cutaneous reflexes during locomotion were performed in chronic spinal cats (149) using a mechanical tapper to contact the dorsum of the foot in different phases of the step cycle. When the dorsum of the foot was tapped during swing as if the limb was meeting an obstacle, there was a well-organized response consisting first of a knee flexion rapidly withdrawing the foot and then a flexion of the ankle and hip to step in front of the obstacle. In intact cats, touching the dorsum of the foot with a stick or an air puff could evoke similar responses (145). Very short latency discharges in TA (10 ms) and GL (~25 ms) are thought to lock the ankle while the knee flexion withdraws the foot (145, 286, 358). After anesthesia of the dorsum of the foot, these responses are abolished (149, 286) and only responses induced by muscle stretch while the foot pushed against the obstacle remained. When the same mechanical stimulus is given during stance, in the chronic spinal cat, flexor muscles do not respond, but on the other hand there is a short-latency increase in the already active extensor muscles at the ankle and knee. Although the kinematic consequences are less dramatic than during swing, there is a distinct increase in the ankle and knee angular velocity in the extension direction (149).

Given the impossibility of applying exactly the same stimulation in all phases of the step cycle, electrical stimuli have been used to stimulate the skin (surface electrodes or indwelling subcutaneous electrodes) or the cutaneous nerves themselves. During swing, short-latency responses occur in the knee flexor St and ankle flexor TA (~10 ms, labeled *P1* in Fig. 5.10); very often a second response appears (~25 ms, labeled *P2* in Fig. 5.10) in the chronic spinal cat as well as in the intact cat. Several flexor muscles follow more or less this scheme (116, 145, 232). The short-latency P1 response and the long-latency P2 response can be modulated differentially (2), with the P2 response peaking in late stance (116, 145, 232). P2 responses can also occur without preceding P1 responses. A short-latency P1 response (10 ms) in GL was observed during swing in intact cats by Forssberg (145) and occasionally by others [see Fig. 5.10 for small GM response in F and (2, 232) but not by others (116, 286)]. The response latencies varied slightly within a given phase of the step cycle and were ordered according to the sequence mentioned before (knee, ankle, hip). A similar response pattern was also demonstrated in decerebrate cats (118, 145). In most of these studies, it was a consistent finding that the period of reflex responsiveness did not necessarily match the period of locomotor activity. Thus the long-latency P2 responses in St may be phase advanced and peak before the onset of the muscle activity; similarly, the short-latency P1 responses may very well exceed the initial St burst (149) and be absent during the second St burst. Perret and Cabelguen (276) have illustrated these discrepancies for several muscles, including St, FHL, and EDL, using stimulation of dorsal root filaments. These discrepancies undoubtedly reflect the underlying central changes in excitatory states that are detected only by reflex testing. Interestingly, a recent study shows that although the locomotor recruitment of distal hindlimb muscles may be significantly

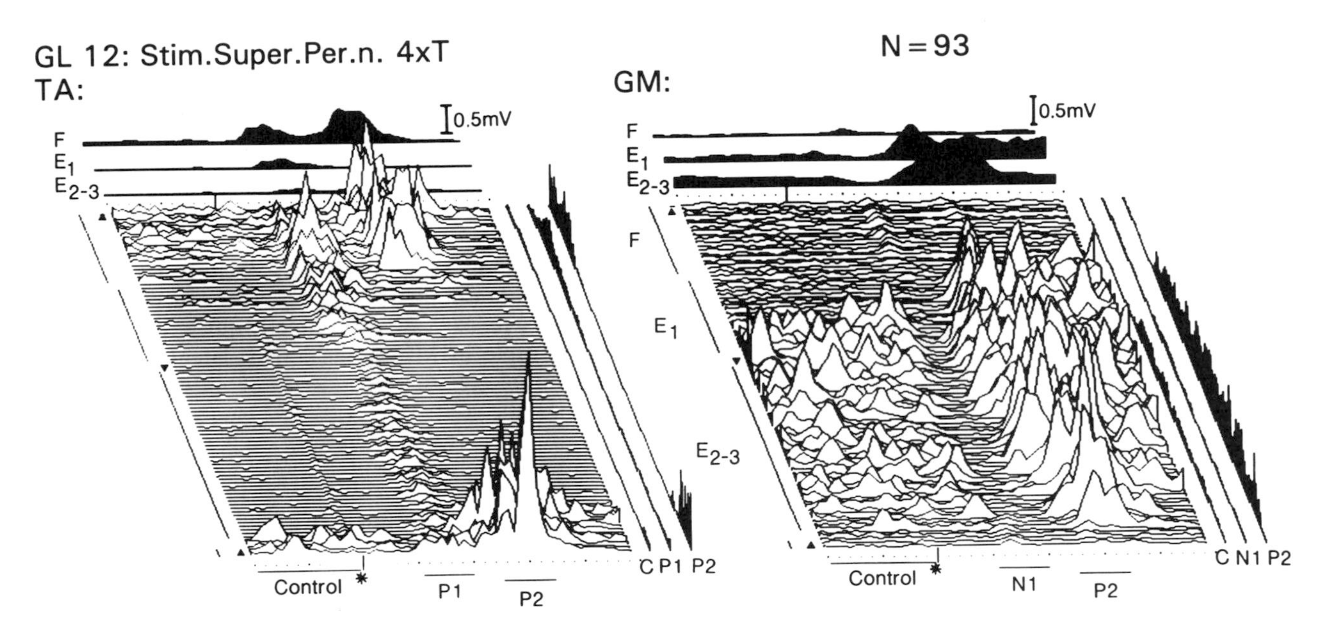

FIG. 5.10. Peristimulus rasters ordered by step cycle phase showing EMGs recorded simultaneously in tibialis anterior (TA) and gastrocnemius medialis (GM) muscles in response to 93 stimuli of superficial peroneal nerve at 4 × threshold for the fastest conducting afferents. *Time bar at bottom*, 20 ms before and 50 ms after stimulus presentation *(*)*; regions marked control (C), P1, P2, and N1 correspond to *diagonally oriented traces* at right edge of each raster in which data point represents the mean EMG value for the corresponding peristimulus period of adjacent EMG trace. *Bars along the left diagonal edge* indicate Philippson (278) step cycle phases during which stimulus was presented. F, flexion; E_1, swing phase extension; E_{2-3}, stance. *Small black triangles* indicate footlift (*upward*) and footfall (*downward*). The *traces bracketed by the bars* have been averaged to produce the correspondingly labeled, *filled plots at the top*; traces near the transitions have been excluded (note gaps between bars) because of uncertainty in their exact phasing. Bars have been phase-advanced slightly from Philippson phases because of EMG phase-lead (note *short bar* including the last few traces at the end of the stance period at the *bottom of the rasters*, with the *F bars* at the *top*. [Figure and legend modified from Loeb (232).]

different among animals, their reflex excitability in the step cycle is more reproducible (232).

There is a general agreement (2, 43, 116, 145, 149, 232, 233, 286) that, in the intact cat, stimulation of cutaneous nerves during stance gives a predominant short-latency inhibition (*N1* in Fig. 5.10) followed by a longer latency (~25–30 ms) excitatory response [*P2* in GM responses of Fig. 5.10, which is the equivalent of P3 in a former study (116)]. In chronic spinal cats, the short-latency inhibition is less pronounced (145) and even P2 (and P1?) excitatory responses can be seen in GM and FDL, especially with sural stimulation (2) and occasionally in VM motor units (233). This is consistent with previous observations on short-latency excitatory pathways to extensor motoneurons (143, 226, 227). Thus, although the short-latency responses in extensors may be dominated by inhibition, it is clear that, after this early inhibition, the dominant effect of cutaneous inputs from the pads and plantar surface as well as the sural territory during locomotion is excitatory during the stance phase. These long-latency responses could be due to a postinhibitory rebound (232) or to stretch reflexes occurring after a period of strong inhibition during which the muscles would lengthen. The latter possibility is unlikely, since the long-latency excitation in extensors is also seen in fictive preparations (9).

In the forelimbs, cutaneous reflexes are also highly phase dependent during walking in intact cats [see Fig. 5.11; (107, 108, 239)] and in thalamic cats (324). When the normal cat hits an obstacle with the forelimb, the elbow flexors and extensors are strongly coactivated (note the reflex coactivation of brachialis and triceps during the swing phase in Fig. 5.11C), thus locking the elbow, while the shoulder retracts the limb. This is followed by a long-latency protraction bringing the limb in front of the impeding obstacle. The very large out of phase excitatory response in triceps during swing (recall that the an-

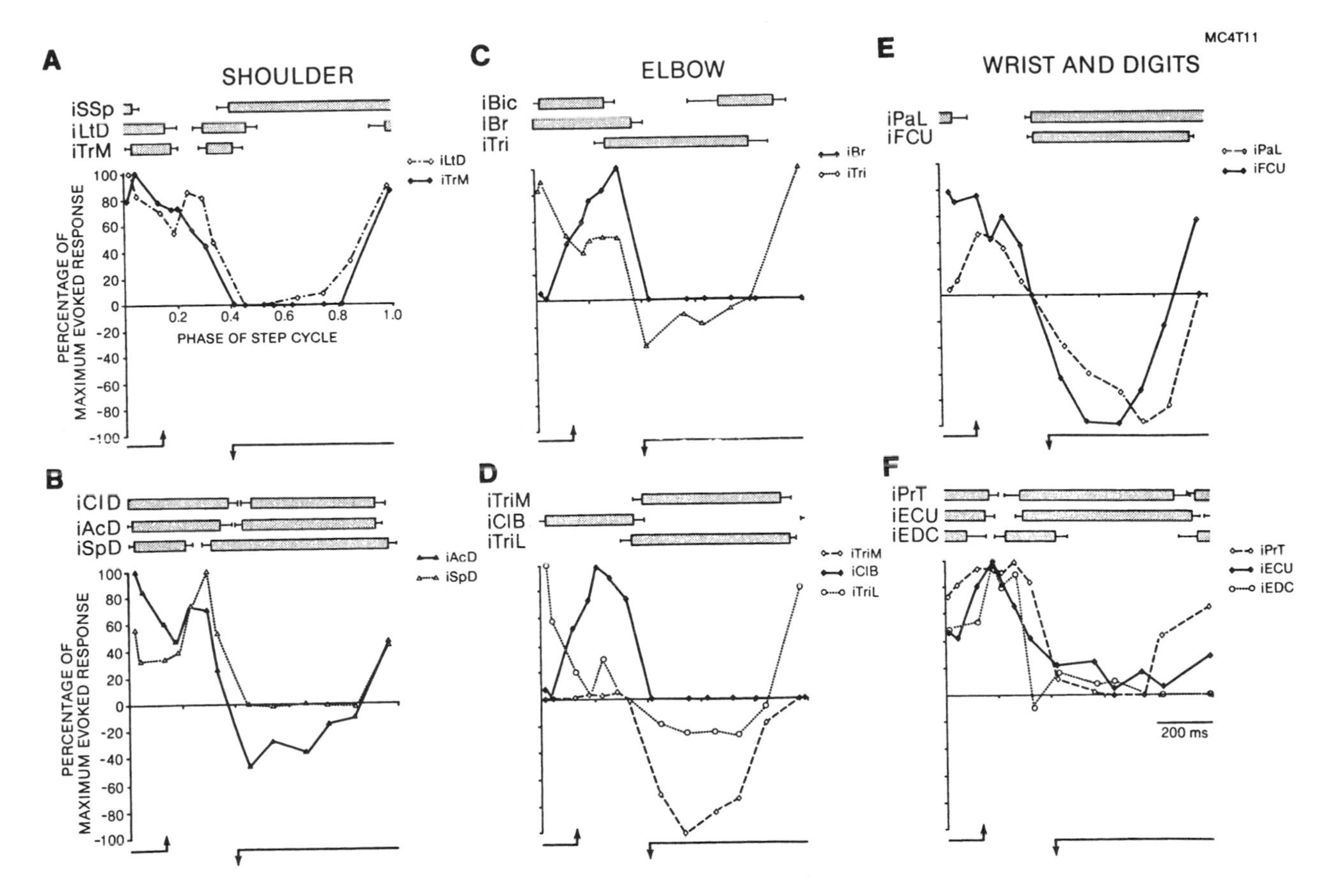

FIG. 5.11. Amplitude of the integrated responses as a function of the time of stimulus application in the normalized step cycle. The graphs are divided into the reflex effects on muscles of the shoulder (*A* and *B*), elbow (*C* and *D*), and wrist and digits (*E* and *F*). Note that the responses in each muscle are expressed as a percentage of the maximal response in that muscle, or for inhibitory responses, to the minimal value. The *stippled bars* above each graph show the normal activity of the muscles during more than 30 unstimulated step cycles aligned with respect to the onset of activity in Br. The *small horizontal lines* give the standard deviation of the average values of EMG activity. The average occurrence of foot contact and foot lift is also indicated under each graph. In this experiment, no short-latency effects were evoked in Biceps (Bic), cleidobrachialis (ClD), or supraspinatus (Ssp). [Reproduced from Drew and Rossignol (107).]

kle extensors are also activated during perturbations of the swing in the hindlimbs) is striking and illustrates how the CNS may control the reflex responsiveness separately from the locomotor activation of the same muscles. Thus, besides activating triceps during stance, the CNS must keep a high excitability level in interneuronal pathways, receiving cutaneous inputs and projecting to triceps so that such contingencies can be met efficiently. Figure 5.11, on the other hand, illustrates very well how the pattern of reflex modulation is not stereotyped for all flexor or extensor muscles. Rather, each muscle is specifically excited, inhibited, or unresponsive in the various phases of the step cycle. Even the exact time within a phase where, for instance, flexor muscles are responsive within a phase may vary. Note in Figure 5.11 that shoulder flexors (Fig. 5.11*A* and *B*) tend to be reflexly more responsive in late stance or very early swing, whereas elbow flexors are more responsive later in swing. Thus perturbations occurring in early swing can be compensated mainly by a shoulder flexion, whereas in later swing both shoulder and elbow flexions are needed.

Cutaneous inputs, during the swing phase, evoke complex organized responses that are well integrated and recruit flexors and extensors in a very precise sequence. Furthermore, during backward walking, cats generate very different responses during the backward swing to efficiently avoid the obstacle (62). Overall, this suggests that the control of "stumbling" corrective reactions (145) do not result from the simple activation of muscles that happen to discharge at that moment of the cycle.

Cutaneous inputs during the stance phase may play different roles depending on the location of the input and the strength of the input. Inputs from the pads have a dominant excitatory effect to extensor muscles after a brief inhibitory effect. This appears actually to be the most important effect by which cutaneous inputs from the foot could be used to partially regulate stance by providing positive feedback during stance (phase-promoting reflex) and delaying the onset of swing, perhaps in parallel with muscle proprioceptors of ankle and toe extensors (118). Excitatory responses in extensors following stimulation of the dorsum of the foot may serve to shorten the stance and thus minimize the period during which the foot would contact a moving object. These responses appear to be very localized so that, for instance, an object touching the laterally localized receptive field of the caudal cutaneous sural nerve may generate a response in medial gastrocnemius and would correspond to a specific excitatory pathway from sural nerve to GM (226). Stimulation of specific cutaneous nerves may also give a "local" sign during locomotion (116), with the sural and common peroneal nerve giving rise to a predominant extensor response, while the tibial nerve gives a predominant flexion response in premammillary and intact cats (115, 120). This is also consistent with recent work in the rat showing an elaborate set of reflexes that specifically moves the foot away from the stimulus given to different loci on the foot (309).

The intensity of stimulation and therefore the afferents recruited may be important in determining the response. Duysens and Loeb (116) showed that Aδ fibers produced the responses shown above; with recent improved methods it was also shown that fibers in the Aα and Aβ ranges were also involved (232, 282). Stronger stimulation of all cutaneous nerves or skin regions may evoke a more massive withdrawal response whatever the phase of the step cycle in which the stimulation is delivered in all studied preparations (115, 145, 149).

Contralateral responses at rather short latency (in the 20–25 ms range) were also observed in chronic spinal cats (116, 149). Although the distinction between P2 and P3 latencies is not very significant (25–30 ms), the crossed excitatory responses in extensors usually have a shorter latency than the ipsilateral excitatory responses. Crossed flexor as well as crossed extensor responses were observed in decerebrate (158) and intact cats (116, 117), strengthening the functional concept of phase-dependent reversal.

In humans, electrical stimulation of the skin or cutaneous nerves of the lower limbs has essentially shown a similar task dependency (64, 122, 339) and a similar phase dependency of reflex responses with the step cycle (45, 97, 213, 370). As was the case in the cat, the responses in several muscles are phase dependent, and the pattern of responses in ipsilateral and contralateral muscles cannot be explained on the basis of an automatic gain control, which would set the gain of the reflex simply on the locomotor EMG amplitude, but rather there is a premotoneuronal gain control (121, 122). Similar conclusions were reached with reflexes elicited during cycling (58, 264).

Mechanisms of Reflex Modulation

These reflex studies demonstrate a continuous modulation of the efficiency of afferent inputs on the locomotor pattern, an important fact to consider when thinking about the role of afferent feedback generated by the movements themselves. There are three levels at which the phasic modulation of spinal reflexes during locomotion can occur: motoneuronal, interneuronal, and presynaptic levels. In turn, the excitability of these three levels can change through the action of peripherally derived or centrally generated influences. For example, afferent inputs, signaling muscle stretch or muscle force, could determine the level of excitability of interneurons also receiving cutaneous inputs or change the presynaptic excitability of cutaneous afferents so that the movements themselves could participate in the selection of the appropriate reflex responses. However, there is a powerful gating of reflexes during fictive locomotion so that, without denying a potential role for afferent feedback in the control of reflexes, this feedback is generally not essential for the selection of reflexes (9, 149, 225, 300, 308). The central pattern generator (CPG) appears to set the appropriate excitability at each level to merge reflex responses with the muscle activity pattern in a given phase of locomotion so that the progression is maintained and there is an effective compensation. The following experiments indicate which of these mechanisms may, alone or in combination, participate in the organization and selection of the reflex responses.

Motoneuronal Mechanisms. Intracellular PSPs evoked from cutaneous inputs are phasically modulated in both flexor and extensor motoneurons (9). Early and late EPSPs in extensor motoneurons, corresponding to short- and long-latency responses (P1 and P2 responses in EMGs), are modulated independently within the cycle. Since no conductance changes could be observed in motoneurons during the fictive cycle, it was concluded that the increase in PSP amplitude, during the depolarizing phase of the motoneurons, is caused by a premotoneuronal mechanism. Since EPSP modulation can be as large as 40%, it is possible that the membrane depolarization of the motoneurons may also participate in the modulation of the reflex responses. In some cases, different patterns of modulation were observed with cutaneous stimulation. In flexor motoneurons, EPSPs were large during the depolarization and smaller in the opposite phase or else could be replaced by IPSPs; in extensor motoneurons, there could be either a pattern of modulation of EPSPs (larger during depolarization) or IPSPs (larger during hyperpolarization) or else a mixture of EPSPs during the active period and IPSPs in the opposite phase (308).

Other studies (304) using inputs from the superficial peroneal nerve during fictive locomotion showed that the EPSPs in FDL MNs were greatest during the depolarizing phase of the motoneurons. However, there is much specificity in the response organization to inputs of various cutaneous nerves (305). In a recent study (225), we have shown in fictive locomotion induced by noradrenergic drugs in semichronic spinal cats that a full repertoire of modulation of short-latency reflexes could be reproduced, including reflex reversal as in the walking spinal cat.

Interneuronal Mechanisms. As mentioned previously, FDL and FHL are partial anatomical synergists that have different activation patterns during locomotion [Fig. 5.2; (254)]. A study of afferent inputs (143) showed that Ia EPSPs in motoneurons of both muscles originated from both muscles and were similar (see also 52). During locomotion, superficial peroneal nerve produced maximal EPSPs in early flexion in FDL MNs, whereas EPSPs evoked by plantaris nerve are minimal during that phase. The latter are, however, maximal when FDL MNs occasionally discharge during the extension phase. Given the short latency of these reflexes, it was suggested that the CPG for locomotion exerts a differential control on interneuronal pathways carrying information from different afferents.

Whereas it is known that Ib inputs from Golgi tendon organs will classically generate disynaptic IPSPs in extensor motoneurons, the same input now becomes excitatory during locomotion (85, 169, 266, 268), presumably by the enhancement of Ib effects through excitatory INs.

From all these previous studies, it is possible to conclude that the excitability of a number of interneurons (see earlier under CENTRAL GENERATION OF STEREOTYPIC PATTERNS) is controlled directly by the CPG to ensure the balance between maintaining the progression and organizing appropriate corrective responses needed to adapt it to the real environment.

Presynaptic Mechanisms. Reflex modulation can also occur by changing the excitability of the afferent terminals at a presynaptic level. The presynaptic control appears to be a potentially effective mechanism to differentially modulate the efficacy of afferent inputs in different tasks and their different phases (88, 199, 200). For instance, in humans it was shown that the H-reflex is gradually decreased in amplitude as the subject goes from standing (where maximal ankle stability is required), to walking and to running, where the control may depend much less on feedback from spindle afferents. Since these changes in amplitude of the H-reflex occur when the EMG output is similar in the three tasks, it is postulated that the amplitude modulation depends on presynaptic controls (71, 340).

Animal experiments support the notion that there is a significant presynaptic inhibition during fictive scratching [see Fig. 5.12 (28)] and locomotion (24,

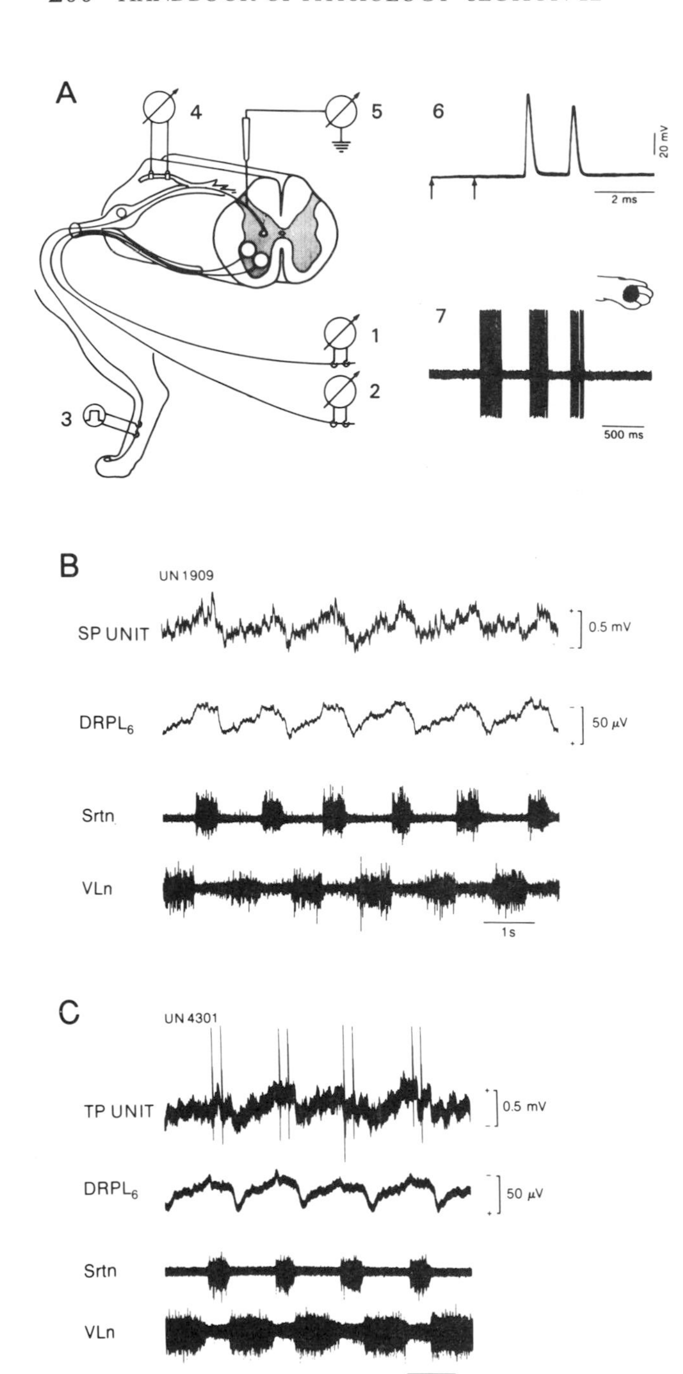

FIG. 5.12. Presynaptic events during fictive locomotion. *A*, Schematic representation of experimental procedures. *1* and *2*, Sartorius nerve and vastus lateralis nerve recorded with bipolar Ag/AgCl electrodes in paraffine oil. *3*, Electrical stimulation at a high frequency (>700 Hz) of peripheral superficial peroneal (SP) or tibial posterior (TA) nerves enclosed in polymer cuff electrodes. *4*, Proximal stump of a cut dorsal rootlet was recorded with a bipolar Ag/AgCl electrode for dorsal root potentials (DRPs) in paraffine oil. *5*, Micropipette filled with K^+ citrate inserted close to the dorsal rootlet's entrance in the cord, 0.5–1.0 mm deep. *6*, DC recording of the action potentials evoked by the high-frequency stimulation of 3. Note the short constant latency and the absence of prepotentials (two superimposed sweeps). *7*, AC recordings (100 Hz–10 KHz) of the responses to natural stimuli applied to the receptive field. The SP unit represented here is responding with bursts of action potentials (truncated) to three successive light air puffs on hair located on the dorsal aspect of the foot. Amplitude calibration of *6* does not apply to *7*. In *B* and *C*, intra-axonal recordings of cutaneous primary afferents during fictive locomotion. From top to bottom: intra-axonal recording of an SP primary afferent or TA primary afferent, DRP from an L7 dorsal rootlet, flexor (Srtn), and extensor (VLn). In *C*, the intra-axonal signal is thicker than in *B* because of the bandwidth (0.1 Hz–10 KHz) used to record action potentials. [From Gossard, Cabelguen, and Rossignol (170).]

29, 114) as measured directly with dorsal root potentials and Wall's technique for various types of afferents. During fictive locomotion in decorticate cats as well as in DOPA spinal cats (111), dorsal root potentials (DRPs) fluctuate rhythmically when the fictive rhythm starts, in both hindlimbs and forelimbs. The DRPs show two distinct peaks, the maximal peak largely corresponding to the period of flexor activity.

Intracellular recording of primary cutaneous (170) and muscle (172) afferents indicated that, although the general pattern of depolarization seen in DRPs was recognized, other patterns were observed in individual units suggesting that there might be a great variety of control that can influence the state of excitability of these afferents. Using Wall's technique (29, 114), it was shown that the depolarization of various groups of terminals (cutaneous, Ia, and 1b) are depolarized in the same phase as the maximum DRPs.

In many cases, rhythmic bursts of spikes were observed to coincide with one of the depolarizing peaks (111, 113). Since these are recorded in the proximal stump of cut dorsal rootlet, they represent antidromic discharges. These occur in various phases of the step cycle and the burst discharges were generally correlated with variations in the cycle duration (111). They were observed in intracellular recordings of cutaneous afferents (170) and muscle primary afferents (172). It has also been possible to record such antidromic discharges in cut dorsal rootlets (280, 364) in decerebrate cats during treadmill walking. Preliminary results (46) indicate that 80% of antidromic units discharge rhythmically and occur in equal proportion during swing and during stance. There is some evidence that such antidromic activity may also be present in intact cat (113).

It is still difficult to suggest how changes in presynaptic excitability may contribute to reflex gating, although some experiments have shown that presynaptic control between afferents may be important (113, 171, 173). It is interesting to note that similar presynaptic phenomena are found in lower preparations such as the crayfish (75, 76, 134) and even in humans (340). This control may be very useful in different tasks or in different phases of a task where the afferent inputs may acquire a very different "meaning," depending on the context.

SUPRASPINAL CONTROL

Supraspinal control of locomotion can be viewed from many aspects: initiation of locomotion, control of posture and propulsion, and corrections to adapt one or several steps to the environment. Several structures can be implicated in the initiation and can play a role in posture and correction. Some current views on various structures and mechanisms that may participate in the initiation of locomotion will first be reviewed. The role of other structures in posture and corrections based on lesion, recording, or stimulation studies will be reviewed separately. The role of the cerebellum during locomotion has been adequately reviewed (14, 15, 19, 258) and will not be covered here.

Initiation of Locomotion

The anatomical connectivity of mesodiencephalic structures involved in triggering locomotion, especially the subthalamic region (SLR) and the MLR has been reviewed in considerable detail by Armstrong (14), and the essentials are summarized in Figure 5.13. Early and more recent experiments involving stimulation of these structures have been reviewed (159, 320). In a decerebrate cat (precollicular-postmammillary section) placed on a moving treadmill belt, stimulation with a train of stimulus (usually < 100 μA, 20–60 Hz) of the MLR, a region just below the inferior colliculus and largely coincident with the cuneiformis nucleus and the pedunculopontine nucleus (PPN) (see later), will suddenly trigger a complete quadrupedal locomotor pattern; increasing the strength of the stimulus, as well as the treadmill speed, can evoke trot and gallop (320). Stimulation of the MLR also triggers a "fictive" locomotor pattern in the absence of afferent feedback (212). Without stimulation, "mesencephalic" preparations do not display spontaneous locomotion, contrary to cats with a premammillary section, the so-called thalamic preparations (175). Another more rostral region, the SLR, coincident with the field of Forel and which receives abundant cortical inputs and entopeduncular inputs (26), appears capable of inducing locomotion even after destroying most of the MLR. Cats with an SLR lesion will not locomote spontaneously; however, stimulation of the MLR can evoke locomotion (159) in these cats. Stimulation of the corticospinal tracts can evoke locomotion, presumably through activation of these structures and not directly, since the effect persists after a pyramidotomy (see 175).

How the MLR and structures that project to it induce locomotion is not clear yet. One view is that the action of the MLR is exerted through medial reticular formation (MRF) and ventrolateral spinal pathways (154, 155, 209–211, 243, 249, 250). The evidence in favor of that concept is the following. The MLR projects to the MRF (26, 335); cooling of the MRF blocks the MLR-induced locomotion (313); electrical stimulation (154, 243) of the MRF and chemical activation of the MRF with cholinergic agonists or substance P (154) or glutamic acid (249) can also evoke locomotion; destruction of ventrolateral pathways that contain the reticulospinal pathways in decerebrate cats prevent MLR-induced locomotion (334); and identified units in the MRF are activated during locomotion (see later).

The alternative view (218, 310, 319) is that locomotion is induced through an extensive polysynaptic propriospinal system, the pontomedullary locomotor strip (PLS) or region (PLR) that includes the lateral tegmentum from the MLR to propriospinal neurons (218) in the cervical cord (laminae V–VIII) through a dorsolateral pathway. These propriospinal interneurons located in the high cervical cord and low thoracic cord could activate locomotor circuits located more caudally through their axons traveling in ventrolateral pathways (159). Destruction of the cervical gray matter leaving intact the ventrolateral pathways abolished MLR-evoked locomotion. At the pontomedullary level, this strip is close to the spinal nucleus of the trigeminal complex (26, 249), and when activated chemically with glutamic acid or picrotoxin, locomotion is initiated. It was postulated that the locomotor activation is of sensory origin much as it is possible to induce locomotion by stimulation of dorsal roots or peripheral nerves (249). Stimulation of sensory sites whose projecting collaterals are closely associated with hypothalamic and MLR supports this idea of a sensory-associated triggering of locomotion (48).

The MLR can also be activated by iontophoretic applications of GABA antagonists such as bicuculline and picrotoxin (156) and can be inhibited by GABA and diazepam (156, 281). This and other findings suggested that the MLR is normally controlled by inhibitory regions such as the substantia nigra (157) and the entopeduncular nucleus, both output nuclei of the basal ganglia (see Fig. 5.13). The relations between the basal ganglia and the MLR were reviewed (153) and it was suggested that the

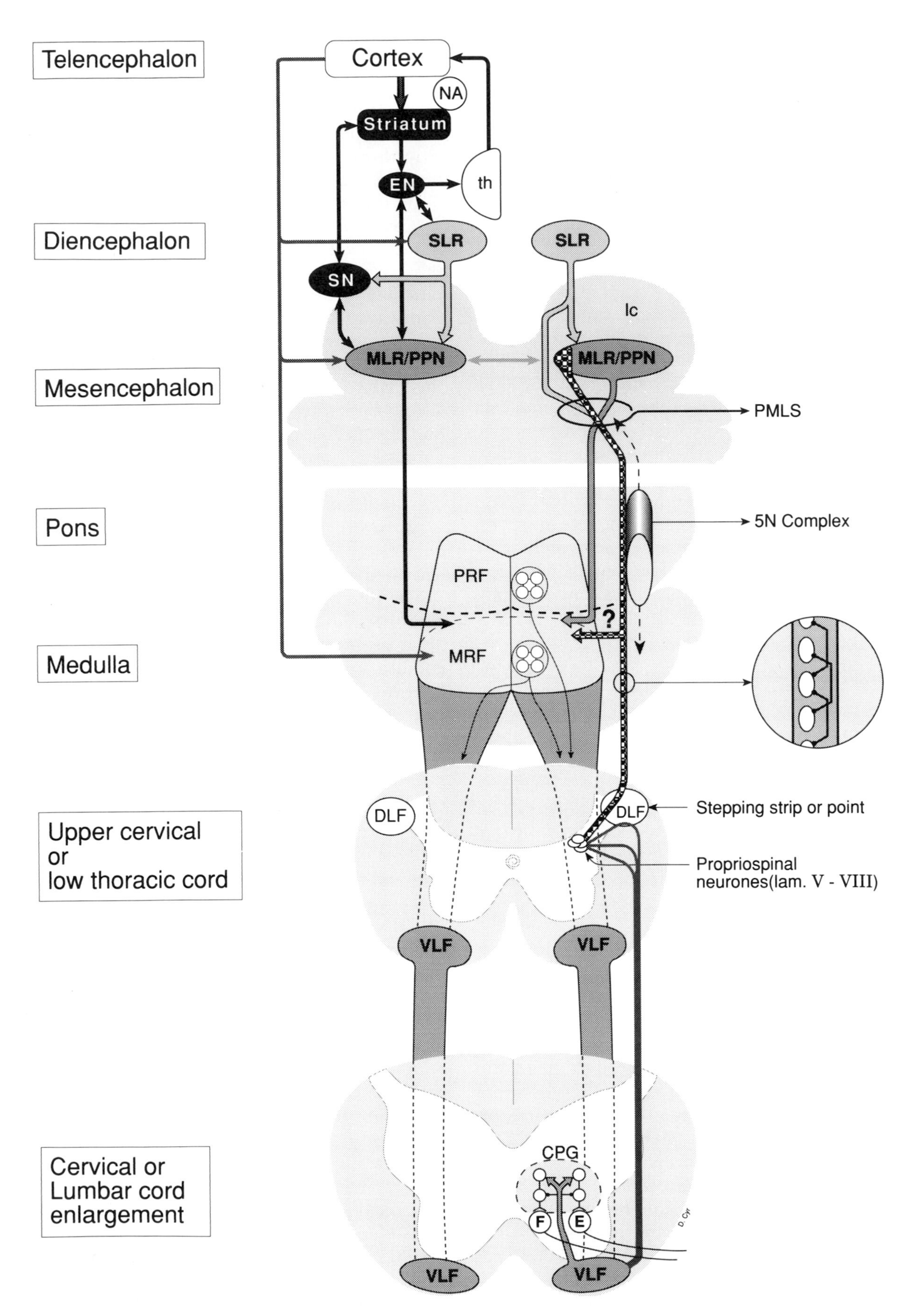

FIG. 5.13. An overview of the structures involved in the initiation of locomotion. This figure was largely inspired by Garcia-Rill (153), Gelfand et al. (159), and Jordan (210). 5N, trigeminal nuclear complex; CPG, central pattern generator; DLF, dorsolateral funiculus; EN, entopeduncular nucleus; IC, inferior colliculus; MLR, mesencephalic locomotor region; MRF, medullary reticular formation; NA, nucleus accumbens; PMLS, pontomedullary locomotor strip; PPN, pedonculopontine nucleus; PRF, pontine reticular formation; SLR, subthalamic locomotor region; SN, substantia nigra; Str, striatum; Th, thalamus; VLF, ventrolateral funiculus.

PPN, located ventrally to the MLR, could participate in the effects evoked from the stimulation of the MLR. In Figure 5.13, following Armstrong's suggestion (14), the expression MLR/PPN is used, although it should not be considered that the PPN is the only cell structure in this region that could participate in the MLR effect (e.g., cuneiformis nucleus).

Work by Shefchyk and Jordan (314) showed that stimulation of the MLR produced EPSPs and IPSPs in motoneurons in the two locomotor phases at latencies implicating an interneuronal relay in the cord. It is presumed that the MLR, through excitation of the MRF, excites spinal interneurons capable of generating these EPSPs and IPSPs in motoneurons and gives rise to the locomotor rhythm (see Fig. 5.13).

Given the proximity of the locus coeruleus (LC) to the MLR (209) and the well-known effects of noradrenergic mechanisms on locomotion (see earlier), the role of LC in triggering locomotion has been studied using 6-Hydroxy dopamine (6-OHDA) lesion of noradrenergic pathways in the cord (336). Locomotion could still be induced by MLR stimulation, suggesting that these pathways are not essential, although they may be one route by which locomotion is initiated. Recordings of LC cells during treadmill locomotion show a general increase of their firing frequency, although the mean firing rate remained comparatively low (2–3 Hz) (288). Serotonin-containing neurons in various raphe nuclei were also shown to discharge at a higher rate during walking and movements, although no indications are given as to the phasic relationship with components of the step cycle (287, 345).

Posture and Corrections

The Medial Reticular Formation. As discussed in a previous section, partial lesions of the cord in chronic animals suggest an important but not exclusive role of the reticulospinal pathways during locomotion. Following the pioneering work of Orlovsky, who recorded from reticulospinal (RS) neurons during locomotion in the mesencephalic and thalamic cat and stimulated the MRF during locomotion, the following picture emerged (see 175). With stimulation of the MLR, about 70% of RS neurons are activated after a certain latent period and about 50% of these become rhythmically modulated during actual walking. Stimulation of the MRF evoked phase-dependent responses: excitation of ipsilateral hindlimb flexors during or just before swing and inhibition of extensors during stance. Microstimulation of the MRF (30 ms trains at 35 μA) during locomotion in thalamic cats (106) could also evoke phase-dependent excitatory responses in flexor or extensor muscles of the forelimbs or the hindlimbs. Although many sites produced excitatory responses in extensors, some also evoked inhibitory responses. The excitatory responses were generally coordinated so that a short-latency (8–20 ms) ipsilateral flexor response was accompanied by a simultaneous extensor response in the contralateral limb of the same girdle. These short trains could have a significant effect on cycle duration, due to combined effects of ipsilateral flexor and contralateral extensor responses. Longer trains (200 ms) could actually reset the step cycle as also shown in fictive preparations with MLF stimulation (303) or stimuli within the MRF itself (273). The latter work also showed a marked effect on cycle time, with a clear prolongation of the ipsilateral flexor phase (in agreement with 91) and a decrease or increase of the extensor phase with stimuli given during that phase.

A detailed study of the stimulation of MRF in the intact cat was performed using a lightweight microdrive that allowed exploration of the whole MRF while monitoring the movement and EMG responses elicited at rest or during locomotion. At rest (109), movements elicited included head motions toward the side of the stimulation, with generally an ipsilateral forelimb flexion and contralateral extension. Hindlimb responses were less frequent and less predictable. Despite well-characterized movements in one direction or the other, EMG responses (110) also revealed a great deal of coactivation of muscles in the neck as well as in flexors and extensors of a given limb. With stimulation of the same sites during actual walking of cats on a treadmill (103), there were well-organized coactivation responses seen at rest replaced by well-organized phase-dependent responses. It is suggested that these responses are transmitted through interneurons whose excitability are closely regulated by the CPG. Recent work also suggests that the transmission through a short-latency disynaptic pathway from MLF to hindlimb motoneurons is phasically modulated during locomotion (144).

Recordings of identified RS cells in the MRF were also performed in chronic unrestrained cats walking on a treadmill (105). About one-third of the cells were found to discharge in rather strict relationship with one or two muscles such as a flexor in one limb and an extensor in the contralateral limb. Of those cells that were related to particular muscles, two-thirds were related to extensor muscles, in keeping with the microstimulation results reported above. Very similar results were obtained in fictive conditions (272).

Of related importance is the role of the MRF in the control of posture associated with locomotion and this has been reviewed elsewhere [(243–245); see also Chapter 7]. Electrical (243) or chemical (228) stimulation of the brainstem in various regions can facilitate [ventral tegmentum field (VTF)] or inhibit [dorsal tegmentum field (DTF)] the MLR-induced locomotion (243). Similar effects on posture are obtained during locomotion by stimulation of the same areas in chronically implanted cats.

Vestibulospinal and Rubrospinal Controls. Despite the fact that vestibular nuclei have some projections to the MLR as demonstrated by HRP studies (26), tonic stimulation of Deiter's nucleus does not apparently trigger locomotion. Ablation of Deiter's nucleus reduces or abolishes locomotion in MLR cats or has insignificant consequences (206, 257). Short trains of stimuli to Deiter's nucleus produce phase-dependent effects, increasing the amplitude of extensor activity during the period where they are normally recruited (257). Muscles such as sartorius, which discharges during both swing and stance, were generally excited only during stance.

In conditions in which the animals are fixed to a treadmill and walking at a constant speed, stimulation of Deiter's nucleus did not produce large changes in limb movements, although, had the cat been free to move, a change in speed could have occurred. The stabilizing role played by afferent feedback in such circumstances was suggested by the results obtained in fictive preparations (high decerebrate cats with DOPA) in which stimulation of vestibular nuclei had important effects on cycle timing and structure (303).

Vestibulospinal neurons discharge rhythmically during locomotion (255) and attain their maximal discharge on average during late swing and early stance of the ipsilateral hindlimb (note that the forelimbs are attached). Some cells were also found to have a double discharge pattern, and this pattern seems more frequent in decerebrate cats walking also with the forelimbs (346). The rhythmic discharge is greatly influenced by passive movements of the limb: *(1)* the cells stop firing if the ipsilateral limb is arrested even though the contralateral limb continues to walk, *(2)* passive flexion of all joints increase the rhythmic discharge, and *(3)* an upward tilt of the treadmill increases the discharge. The cells lose their rhythmicity after cerebellectomy, which suggests that modulation was linked to ascending signals through dorsal (DSCT) and ventral spinocerebellar pathway (VSCT) (20). Some studies on the discharge of VS cells in intact cats have been briefly reported (41).

Much less is known about the role of rubrospinal cells during stereotypic limb movements. Destruction of the red nucleus does not prevent locomotion in decerebrate cats (256). Stimulation of the red nucleus increases flexor activity in the contralateral hindlimb in a phase-dependent manner (257). Identified rubrospinal cells have their main discharge during contralateral hindlimb swing and their rhythmicity is abolished after cerebellectomy. Their activity is practically not affected by changing speed, which is commensurate with the fact that swing duration changes little with speed (256). To obviate this, Orlovsky (256) altered the swing phase using various mechanical devices and showed that the discharges of rubrospinal neurons were not altered when the changes were localized only at the knee or ankle but were modified when the perturbations involved the hip, with resulting reorganization of the overall pattern in the whole limb. It was postulated that the modulation of rubrospinal cells in such a circumstance could result from the inputs provided by VSCT cells, which may be more related to global events than to localized effects on joints. The sensory modulation of rubrospinal cells could also occur through other ascending afferents that travel through the lemniscal system and give off collaterals to the red nucleus (207, 262). Rubrospinal cells were also recorded during fictive locomotion (22) and showed a minimum of activity at the stance-swing transition and a peak in the second half of flexion.

Motor Cortex. After a pyramidal lesion, locomotor deficits in the contralateral limbs are transitory during ordinary or simple locomotion, but cats with such lesions have great difficulty in coping with more demanding locomotor skills such as walking on a ladder or on a narrow beam (132, 231). Recordings of the motor cortex with chronically implanted microwires showed that 80% of the cells were rhythmically modulated during walking in relation to stance or swing (16, 17, 263). Interestingly, the cell discharge characteristics varied little with increasing speed or increasing slope of the treadmill despite large changes in EMG characteristics, suggesting that these cells do not play a major role in the amplitude modulation of muscle discharge under these conditions. Intracortical microstimulation revealed phase-dependent responses in contralateral forelimb flexors and extensors, with flexors being excited during or just about at their period of activity, whereas extensors were generally inhibited (18).

Two further lines of study show that the motor cortex is involved in the control of locomotion, when cats step on a mobile rung (7, 8, 238) or when they step over an obstacle placed on the treadmill belt (101, 102, 104, 301). When the contralateral forelimb leads (i.e., is the first to step over the obstacle), there is first an increase in the limb flexors followed by an increase in elbow extensor activity and the digit dorsiflexors EDC. When the forelimb trails, the extensor activity has to be curtailed and flexors have to be recruited. Drew (361) showed that cortical cells recorded in the posterior bank of the cruciate sulcus (hindlimb region of area 4) modify their discharge in relation to the compensatory movements. Similar findings were made with recording of cortical cells in cats walking over a series of barriers with different spacing or on a horizontal ladder (47).

The combined results suggest that the motor cortex may be involved on the one hand in regulating the transition from stance to swing, and thus the timing of the step cycle and, on the other hand in controlling the precise positioning of the foot at the onset of stance.

CONCLUDING REMARKS

Over the last 15 years, studies of stereotypic movements have broadened our overall comprehension of motor control. We have learned that the nervous system utilizes muscles in a complex manner to take advantage of their biomechanical and histochemical properties and that movements can only be described by taking into account both the kinetics and the muscular activity. We have also extended much of the knowledge on the motor capabilities of the spinal animal, even in adulthood, and added new approaches to interact with motor programs through the use of neurotransmitters that can alter the characteristics of the stereotyped movements. This may lead to important pharmacological interventions in patients with spinal cord injuries. There is now a general consensus that the spinal cord can generate a rather detailed program in the absence of peripheral feedback and suprasegmental inputs. These pattern generators, however, are exquisitely sensitive to afferent feedback and descending inputs so that the picture is that of a tripartite system in constant interaction. The study of these interactions reveals at the same time the autonomy and the interdependence of the various parts. The CPG can be influenced by afferent and descending inputs but differently according to the phases of the cycle, so that appropriate corrections can be achieved without undue disruption of the ongoing cycle. We have also learned more about mechanisms of rhythmicity, how membrane properties are revealed in neurons during such cyclic activity, and how the nervous system may combine various elements at its disposal to generate the many forms of similar behaviors. We have learned about the ontogeny of these rhythmic activities. New preparations have been introduced that are bound to unravel some of the details of the neurons and their location so that a better understanding of the circuitry involved in generating stereotypic movements in mammals will be gained as it was so elegantly done in more primitive preparations.

I would like to dedicate this review to Céline and Elsa for their joyous companionship and to my precious colleagues, collaborators, students, technicians, and secretaries, without whom much of this would not have been possible. My particular thanks to J. Provencher and F. Lebel for their competent help and D. Cyr for his skillful graphics work. I would like to extend my gratitude to Drs. T. Drew, J.-P. Gossard, S. Grillner, L. Jordan, G. E. Loeb, A. Smith, and J. L. Smith for their comments and suggestions on earlier drafts. Some of the work reported here was supported unfailingly throughout the years by the Medical Research Council of Canada.

REFERENCES

1. Abraham, L. D., and G. E. Loeb. The distal hindlimb musculature of the cat. Patterns of normal use. *Exp. Brain Res.* 58: 580–593, 1985.
2. Abraham, L. D., W. B. Marks, and G. E. Loeb. The distal hindlimb musculature of the cat. Cutaneous reflexes during locomotion. *Exp. Brain Res.* 58: 594–603, 1985.
3. Akazawa, K., J. W. Aldridge, J. D. Steeves, and R. B. Stein. Modulation of stretch reflexes during locomotion in the mesencephalic cat. *J. Physiol. (Lond.)* 329: 553–567, 1982.
4. Allum, J. H. J., and M. Hulliger. *Afferent Control of Posture and Locomotion.* Amsterdam: Elsevier, 1989, p. 1–512.
5. Alstermark, B., and Kummel, H. Transneuronal labelling of neurones projecting to forelimb motoneurones in cats performing different movements. *Brain Res.* 376: 387–391, 1986.
6. Amblard, B., A. Berthoz, and F. Clarac. *Posture and Gait: Development, Adaptation and Modulation, Proc. of the IXth International Symposium on Postural and Gait Research.* North Holland: Elsevier, 1988, p. 1–456.
7. Amos, A., D. M. Armstrong, and D. E. Marple-Horvat. Responses of motor cortical neurones in the cat to unexpected perturbations of locomotion. *Neurosci. Lett.* 104: 147–151, 1989.
8. Amos, A., D. M. Armstrong, and D. E. Marple-Horvat. Changes in the discharge patterns of motor cortical neurones associated with volitional changes in stepping in the cat. *Neurosci. Lett.* 109: 107–112, 1990.
9. Andersson, O., H. Forssberg, S. Grillner, and M. Lindquist. Phasic gain control of the transmission in cutaneous reflex pathways in motoneurones during "fictive" locomotion. *Brain Res.* 149: 503–507, 1978.
10. Andersson, O., and S. Grillner. Peripheral control of the cat's step cycle. I. Phase dependent effects of ramp-movements of the hip during "fictive locomotion." *Acta Physiol. Scand.* 113: 89–101, 1981.

11. Andersson, O., and S. Grillner. Peripheral control of the cat's step cycle. II. Entrainment of the central pattern generators for locomotion by sinusoidal hip movements during "fictive locomotion." *Acta Physiol. Scand.* 118: 229–239, 1983.
12. Aoki, M., Y. Fujito, A. Mizuguchi, and H. Satomi. Recovery of hindlimb movement after spinal hemisection and collateral sprouting from corticospinal fibers in monkeys. In: *Neurobiological Basis of Human Locomotion*, edited by M. Shimamura, S. Grillner, and V. R. Edgerton. Tokyo: Japan Scientific Societies Press, 1991, p. 401–405.
13. Aoki, M., and S. Mori. Locomotor elicited by pinna stimulation in the acute precollicular-post-mammillary decerebrate cat. *Brain Res.* 214: 424–428, 1981.
14. Armstrong, D. M. Supraspinal contributions to the initiation and control of locomotion in the cat. *Prog. Neurobiol.* 26: 273–361, 1986.
15. Armstrong, D. M. The supraspinal control of mammalian locomotion. *J. Physiol. (Lond.)* 405: 1–37, 1988.
16. Armstrong, D. M., and T. Drew. Discharges of pyramidal tract and other motor cortical neurones during locomotion in the cat. *J. Physiol. (Lond.)* 346: 471–495, 1984.
17. Armstrong, D. M., and T. Drew. Locomotor-related neuronal discharges in cat motor cortex compared with peripheral receptive fields and evoked movements. *J. Physiol. (Lond.)* 346: 497–517, 1984.
18. Armstrong, D. M., and T. Drew. Forelimb electromyographic responses to motor cortex stimulation during locomotion in the cat. *J. Physiol. (Lond.)* 367: 327–351, 1985.
19. Arshavsky, Y. I., I. M. Gelfand, and G. N. Orlovsky. The cerebellum and control of rhythmical movements. *Trends Neurosci.* 6: 417–422, 1983.
20. Arshavsky, Y. I., I. M. Gelfand, G. N. Orlovsky, G. A. Pavlova, and L. B. Popova. Origin of signals conveyed by the ventral spino-cerebellar tract and spino-reticulo-cerebellar pathway. *Exp. Brain Res.* 54: 426–431, 1984.
21. Arshavsky, Y. I., G. N. Orlovsky, G. A. Pavlova, and L. B. Popova. Activity of C3–C4 propriospinal neurons during fictitious forelimb locomotion in the cat. *Brain Res.* 363: 354–357, 1986.
22. Arshavsky, Y. I., G. N. Orlovsky, and C. Perret. Activity of rubrospinal neurons during locomotion and scratching in the cat. *Behav. Brain Res.* 28: 193–199, 1988.
23. Baev, K. V. Central locomotor program for the cat's hindlimb. *Neuroscience* 3: 1081–1092, 1978.
24. Baev, K. V. Polarization of primary afferent terminals in the lumbar spinal cord during fictitious locomotion. *Neurophysiology* 12: 305–311, 1980.
25. Baev, K. V. The central program of activation of hind-limb muscles during scratching in cats. *Neurophysiology* 13: 38–44, 1981.
26. Baev, K. V., V. K. Beresovskii, T. G. Kebkalo, and L. A. Savoskina. Afferent and efferent connections of brainstem locomotor regions study by means of horseradish peroxidase transport technique. *Neuroscience* 26: 871–892, 1988.
27. Baev, K. V., A. M. Degtyarenko, T. V. Zavadskaya, and P. G. Kostyuk. Activity of lumbosacral interneurons during fictitious scratching. *Neurophysiology* 13: 45–52, 1981.
28. Baev, K. V., and P. G. Kostyuk. Primary afferent depolarization evoked by the activity of spinal scratching generator. *Neuroscience* 6: 205–215, 1981.
29. Baev, K. V., and P. G. Kostyuk. Polarization of primary afferent terminals of lumbosacral cord elicited by the activity of spinal locomotor generator. *Neuroscience* 7: 1401–1409, 1982.
30. Baker, L. L., S. H. Chandler, and L. J. Goldberg. L-Dopa induced locomotor-like activity in ankle flexor and extensor nerves of chronic and acute spinal cats. *Exp. Neurol.* 86: 515–526, 1984.
31. Barajon, I., J.-P. Gossard, and H. Hultborn. Induction of *fos* expression by activity in the spinal rhythm generator for scratching. *Brain Res.* 588: 168–172, 1992.
32. Barbeau, H., C. Chau, and S. Rossignol. Noradrenergic agonists and locomotor training affect locomotor recovery after cord transection in adult cats. *Brain Res. Bull.* 30: 387–393, 1993.
33. Barbeau, H., M. Dannakas, and B. Arsenault. The effects of locomotor training in spinal cord injured subjects: a preliminary study. *Restorative Neurol. Neurosci.* 12: 93–96, 1992.
34. Barbeau, H., M. Filion, and P. Bédard. Effects of agonists and antagonists of serotonin on spontaneous hindlimb EMG activity in chronic spinal rats. *Neuropharmacology* 20: 99–107, 1981.
35. Barbeau, H., C. Julien, and S. Rossignol. The effects of clonidine and yohimbine on locomotion and cutaneous reflexes in the adult chronic spinal cat. *Brain Res.* 437: 83–96, 1987.
36. Barbeau, H., and S. Rossignol. Recovery of locomotion after chronic spinalization in the adult cat. *Brain Res.* 412: 84–95, 1987.
37. Barbeau, H., and S. Rossignol. The effects of serotonergic drugs on the locomotor pattern and on cutaneous reflexes of the adult chronic spinal cat. *Brain Res.* 514: 55–67, 1990.
38. Barbeau, H., and S. Rossignol. Initiation and modulation of the locomotor pattern in the adult chronic spinal cat by noradrenergic, serotonergic and dopaminergic drugs. *Brain Res.* 546: 250–260, 1991.
39. Barbeau, H., and S. Rossignol. Spinal cord injury: enhancement of locomotor recovery. *Curr. Opin. Neurol.* 7: 517–524, 1994.
40. Barnes, W. J. P., and M. H. Gladden. Central control of sense organ excitability. In: *Feedback and Motor Control in Invertebrates and Vertebrates*, edited by W. J. P. Barnes and M. H. Gladden. London: Croom Helm, 1985, p. 1–496.
41. Batson, D. E., and D. M. Armstrong. Discharge of Deiters neurones during locomotion in the cat. *Proc. Int. Cong. Physiol. Sci.* 14: 315, 1980.
42. Bekoff, A. Neuroethological approaches to the study of motor development in chicks: achievements and challenges. *J. Neurobiol.* 23: 1486–1505, 1992.
43. Belanger, M., T. Drew, J. Provencher, and S. Rossignol. The study of locomotion and cutaneous reflexes in the same cat before and after spinalisation. *Soc. Neurosci. Abstr.* 12: 880, 1986.
44. Belanger, M., T. Drew, and S. Rossignol. Spinal locomotion: a comparison of the kinematics and the electromyographic activity in the same animal before and after spinalization. *Acta Biol. Hung.* 39: 151–154, 1988.
45. Belanger, M., and A. E. Patla. Phase-dependent compensatory responses to perturbation applied during walking in humans. *J. Mot. Behav.* 19: 434–453, 1987.
46. Beloozerova, I. N., and S. Rossignol. Antidromic activity of dorsal root filaments during treadmill locomotion in thalamic cats. *Soc. Neurosci. Abstr.* 20: 1755, 1994.
47. Beloozerova, I. N., and M. G. Sirota. The role of the motor cortex in the control of accuracy of locomotor movements in the cat. *J. Physiol. (Lond.)* 461: 1–25, 1993.

48. Beresovskii, V. K., and K. V. Baev. New locomotor regions of the brainstem revealed by means of electrical stimulation. *Neuroscience* 26: 863–870, 1988.
49. Berkinblit, M. B., T. G. Deliagina, A. G. Feldman, I. M. Gelfand, and G. N. Orlovsky. Generation of scratching. II. Nonregular regimes of generation. *J. Neurophysiol.* 41: 1058–1069, 1978.
50. Berkinblit, M. B., T. G. Deliagina, A. G. Feldman, and G. N. Orlovsky. Generation of scratching. 1. Activity of spinal interneurons during scratching. *J. Neurophysiol.* 41: 1040–1057, 1978.
51. Blaszczyk, J., and G. E. Loeb. Why cats pace on the treadmill. *Physiol. Behav.* 53 501–507, 1993.
52. Bonasera, S. J., and T. R. Nichols. Mechanical actions of heterogenic reflexes linking long toe flexors with ankle and knee extensors of the cat hindlimb. *J. Neurophysiol.* 71: 1096–1110, 1994.
53. Bradley, N. S., and J. L. Smith. Neuromuscular patterns of stereotypic hindlimb behaviors in the first postnatal months. I. Stepping in normal kittens. *Dev. Brain Res.* 38: 37–52, 1988.
54. Bradley, N. S., and J. L. Smith. Neuromuscular patterns of stereotypic hindlimb behaviors in the first postnatal months. III. Scratching and the paw-shake response in kittens. *Dev. Brain Res.* 38: 69–82, 1988.
55. Bradley, N. S., and J. L. Smith. Neuromuscular patterns of stereotypic hindlimb behaviors in the first postnatal months. II. Stepping in spinal kittens. *Dev. Brain Res.* 38: 53–67, 1988.
56. Brodin, L., and S. Grillner. The role of putative excitatory amino acid neurotransmitters in the initiation of locomotion in the lamprey spinal cord. I. The effects of excitatory amino acid antagonists. *Brain Res.* 360: 139–148, 1985.
57. Brodin, L., and S. Grillner. The role of putative excitatory amino acid neurotransmitters in the initiation of locomotion in the lamprey spinal cord. II. The effects of amino acid uptake inhibitors. *Brain Res.* 360: 149–158, 1985.
58. Brown, D. A., and C. G. Kukulka. Human flexor reflex modulation during cycling. *J. Neurophysiol.* 69: 1212–1224, 1993.
59. Brown, T. G. The intrinsic factors in the act of progression in the mammal. *Proc. R. Soc. Lond. B.* 84: 308–319, 1911.
60. Brownstone, R. M., J.-P. Gossard, and H. Hultborn. Voltage-dependent excitation of motoneurones from spinal locomotor centres in the cat. *Exp. Brain Res.* 102: 34–44, 1994.
61. Brownstone, R. M., L. M. Jordan, D. J. Kriellaars, B. R. Noga, and S. J. Shefchyk. On the regulation of repetitive firing in lumbar motoneurones during fictive locomotion in the cat. *Exp. Brain Res.* 90: 441–455, 1992.
62. Buford, J. A., and J. L. Smith. Adaptive control for backward quadrupedal walking. III. Stumbling corrective reactions and cutaneous reflex sensitivity. *J. Neurophysiol.* 70: 1102–1114, 1993.
63. Buford, J. A., R. F. Zernicke, and J. L. Smith. Adaptive control for backward quadrupedal walking. I. Posture and hindlimb kinematics. *J. Neurophysiol.* 64: 745–755, 1990.
64. Burke, D., H. G. Dickson, and N. F. Skuse. Task-dependent changes in the responses to low-threshold cutaneous afferent volleys in the human lower limb. *J. Physiol. (Lond.)* 432: 445–458, 1991.
65. Bussel, B. C., A. Roby-Brami, A. Yakovleff, and N. Bennis. Evidences for the presence of a spinal stepping generator in patients with a spinal cord section. In: *Posture and Gait: Development, Adaptation and Modulation*, edited by B. Amblard, A. Berthoz, and F. Clarac. North Holland: Elsevier, 1988, p. 273–278.
66. Cabelguen, J.-M. Static and dynamic fusimotor controls in various hindlimb muscles during locomotor activity in the decorticate cat. *Brain Res.* 213: 83–97, 1981.
67. Cabelguen, J.-M., D. Orsal, and C. Perret. Discharges of forelimb spindle primary afferents during locomotor activity in the decorticate cat. *Brain Res.* 306: 359–364, 1984.
68. Cabelguen, J.-M., D. Orsal, C. Perret, and M. Zattara. Central pattern generation of forelimb and hindlimb locomotor activities in the cat. In: *Regulatory Functions of the CNS, Principles of Motion and Organization. Adv. Physiol. Sci. 1*, edited by J. Szentagothai, M. Palkovits, and J. Hamori. Budapest: Akadamiai Kiado, 1981, p. 199–211.
69. Calancie, B., B. Needham-Shropshire, P. Jacobs, K. Willer, G. Zych, and B. A. Green. Involuntary stepping after chronic spinal cord injury. Evidence for a central rhythm generator for locomotion in man. *Brain* 117: 1143–1159, 1994.
70. Caliebe, F., J. Häußler, P. Hoffmann, M. Illert, J. Schirrmacher, and E. Wiedemann. Cat distal forelimb joints and locomotion: an x-ray study. *Eur. J. Neurosci.* 3: 18–31, 1991.
71. Capaday, C., and R. B. Stein. Amplitude modulation of the soleus H-reflex in the human during walking and standing. *J. Neurosci.* 6: 1308–1313, 1986.
72. Capaday, C., and R. B. Stein. Difference in the amplitude of the human soleus H reflex during walking and running. *J. Physiol. (Lond.)* 392: 513–522, 1987.
73. Carter, M. C., and J. L. Smith. Simultaneous control of two rhythmical behaviors. I. Locomotion with paw-shake response in normal cat. *J. Neurophysiol.* 56: 171–183, 1986.
74. Carter, M. C., and J. L. Smith. Simultaneous control of two rhythmical behaviors. II. Hindlimb walking with paw-shake response in spinal cat. *J. Neurophysiol.* 56: 184–195, 1986.
75. Cattaert, D., A. El Manira, and F. Clarac. Direct evidence for presynaptic inhibitory mechanisms in crayfish sensory afferents. *J. Neurophysiol.* 67: 610–624, 1992.
76. Cattaert, D., A. El Manira, A. Marchand, and F. Clarac. Central control of the sensory afferent terminals from a leg chordotonal organ in crayfish in vitro preparation. *Neurosci. Lett.* 108: 81–87, 1990.
77. Cazalets, J. R., P. Grillner, I. Menard, J. Cremieux, and F. Clarac. Two types of motor rhythm induced by NMDA and amines in an in vitro spinal cord preparation of neonatal rat. *Neurosci. Lett.* 111: 116–121, 1990.
78. Cazalets, J. R., Y. Sqalli-Houssaini, and F. Clarac. Activation of the central pattern generators for locomotion by serotonin and excitatory amino acids in neonatal rat. *J. Physiol. (Lond.)* 455: 187–204, 1992.
79. Cazalets, J. R., Y. Sqalli-Houssaini, and F. Clarac. GABAergic inactivation of the central pattern generators for locomotion in isolated neonatal rat spinal cord. *J. Physiol. (Lond.)* 474: 173–181, 1994.
80. Chanaud, C. M., C. A. Pratt, and G. E. Loeb. Functionally complex muscles of the cat hindlimb. V. The roles of histochemical fiber-type regionalization and mechanical heterogeneity in differential muscle activation. *Exp. Brain Res.* 85: 300–313, 1991.
81. Chandler, S. H., L. L. Baker, and L. J. Goldberg. Characterization of synaptic potentials in hindlimb extensor motoneurons during L-dopa-induced fictive locomotion in acute and chronic spinal cats. *Brain Res.* 303: 91–100, 1984.

82. Clarac, F. Spatial and temporal co-ordination during walking in crustacea. *Trends Neurosci.* 7: 293–298, 1984.
83. Cohen, A. H., S. Rossignol, and S. Grillner. *Neural Control of Rhythmic Movements in Vertebrates.* New York: John Wiley & Sons, 1988, p. 1–500.
84. Contamin, F. Sections médullaires incomplètes et locomotion chez le chat. *Bull. Acad. Nat. Med.* 167: 727–730, 1983.
85. Conway, B. A., H. Hultborn, and O. Kiehn. Proprioceptive input resets central locomotor rhythm in the spinal cat. *Exp. Brain Res.* 68: 643–656, 1987.
86. Cowley, K. C., and B. J. Schmidt. Some limitations of ventral root recordings for monitoring locomotion in the in vivo neonatal rat spinal cord preparation. *Neurosci. Lett.* 171: 142–146, 1994.
87. Cowley, K. C., and B. J. Schmidt. A comparison of motor patterns induced by *N*-methyl-D-aspartate, acetylcholine and serotonin in the in vitro neonatal rat spinal cord. *Neurosci. Lett.* 171: 147–150, 1994.
88. Crenna, P., and C. Frigo. Excitability of the soleus H-reflex arc during walking and stepping in man. *Exp. Brain Res.* 66: 49–60, 1987.
89. Dai, X., J. R. Douglas, J. I. Nagy, B. R. Noga, and L. M. Jordan. Localization of spinal neurons activated during treadmill locomotion using the c-fos immunohistochemical method. *Soc. Neurosci. Abstr.* 16: 889, 1990.
90. Dale, N., and A. Roberts. Excitatory amino acid receptors in *Xenopus* embryo spinal cord and their role in the activation of swimming. *J. Physiol. (Lond.)* 348: 527–543, 1984.
91. Degtyarenko, A. M., and T. V. Zavadskaya. Rearrangement of efferent activity of the locomotor generator under electrical activation of descending systems in immobilized cats. *Neurophysiology* 23: 113–119, 1991.
92. Delcomyn, F. Neural basis of rhythmic behavior in animals. *Science* 210: 492–498, 1980.
93. Deliagina, T. G., A. G. Feldman, I. M. Gelfand, and G. N. Orlovsky. On the role of central program and afferent inflow in the control of scratching movements in the cat. *Brain Res.* 100: 297–313, 1975.
94. Deliagina, T. G., G. N. Orlovsky, and G. A. Pavlova. The capacity for generation of rhythmic oscillations is distributed in the lumbosacral spinal cord of the cat. *Exp. Brain Res.* 53: 81–90, 1983.
95. Deliagina, T. G., G. N. Orlovsky, and C. Perret. Efferent activity during fictitious scratch reflex in the cat. *J. Neurophysiol.* 45: 595–604, 1981.
96. Dietz, V., G. Colombo, L. Jensen, and L. Baumgartner. Locomotor capacity of spinal cord in paraplegic patients. *Ann. Neurol.* 37: 574–582, 1995.
97. Dietz, V., J. Quintern, G. Boos, and W. Berger. Obstruction of the swing phase during gait: phase-dependent bilateral leg muscle coordination. *Brain Res.* 384: 166–169, 1986.
98. Dietz, V., J. Quintern, and M. Sillem. Stumbling reactions in man: significance of proprioceptive and pre-programmed mechanisms. *J. Physiol. (Lond.)* 386: 149–163, 1987.
99. Dietz, V., W. Zijlstra, and J. Duysens. Human neuronal interlimb coordination during split-belt locomotion. *Exp. Brain Res.* 101: 513–520, 1994.
100. Douglas, J. R., B. R. Noga, X. Dai, and L. M. Jordan. The effects of intrathecal administration of excitatory amino acid agonists and antagonists on the initiation of locomotion in the adult cat. *J. Neurosci.* 13: 990–1000, 1993.
101. Drew, T. Motor cortical cell discharge during voluntary gait modification. *Brain Res.* 457: 181–187, 1988.
102. Drew, T. The role of the motor cortex in the control of gait modification in the cat. In: *Neurobiological Basis of Human Locomotion*, edited by M. Shimamura, S. Grillner, and V. R. Edgerton. Tokyo: Japan Scientific Societies Press, 1991, p. 201–212.
103. Drew, T. Functional organization within the medullary reticular formation of the intact unanesthetized cat. III. Microstimulation during locomotion. *J. Neurophysiol.* 66: 919–938, 1991.
104. Drew, T. Motor cortical activity during voluntary gait modifications in the cat. I. Cells related to the forelimbs. *J. Neurophysiol.* 70: 179–199, 1993.
105. Drew, T., R. Dubuc, and S. Rossignol. Discharge patterns of reticulospinal and other reticular neurons in chronic, unrestrained cats walking on a treadmill. *J. Neurophysiol.* 55: 375–401, 1986.
106. Drew, T., and S. Rossignol. Phase-dependent responses evoked in limb muscles by stimulation of medullary reticular formation during locomotion in thalamic cats. *J. Neurophysiol.* 52: 653–675, 1984.
107. Drew, T., and S. Rossignol. A kinematic and electromyographic study of cutaneous reflexes evoked from the forelimb of unrestrained walking cats. *J. Neurophysiol.* 57: 1160–1184, 1987.
108. Drew, T., and S. Rossignol. Responses of the forelimb to perturbations applied during the swing phase of the step cycle. In: *Motor Control*, edited by G. N. Gantchev, B. Dimitrov, and P. Gatev. New York: Plenum Press, 1987, p. 171–175.
109. Drew, T., and S. Rossignol. Functional organisation within the medullary reticular formation of the intact unanaesthetized cat. I. Movements evoked by microstimulation. *J. Neurophysiol.* 64: 767–781, 1990.
110. Drew, T., and S. Rossignol. Functional organisation within the medullary reticular formation of the intact unanaesthetized cat. II. Electromyographic activity evoked by microstimulation. *J. Neurophysiol.* 64: 782–795, 1990.
111. Dubuc, R., J.-M. Cabelguen, and S. Rossignol. Rhythmic fluctuations of dorsal root potentials and antidromic discharges of single primary afferents during fictive locomotion in the cat. *J. Neurophysiol.* 60: 2014–2036, 1988.
112. Dubuc, R., S. Rossignol, and Y. Lamarre. The effects of 4-aminopyridine on the spinal cord: rhythmic discharges recorded from the peripheral nerves. *Brain Res.* 369: 243–259, 1986.
113. Duenas, S. H., G. E. Loeb, and W. B. Marks. Monosynaptic and dorsal root reflexes during locomotion in normal and thalamic cats. *J. Neurophysiol.* 63: 1467–1476, 1990.
114. Duenas, S. H., and P. Rudomin. Excitability changes of ankle extensor group Ia and Ib fibers during fictive locomotion in the cat. *Exp. Brain Res.* 228: 1–11, 1987.
115. Duysens, J. Reflex control of locomotion as revealed by stimulation of cutaneous afferents in spontaneously walking premammillary cats. *J. Neurophysiol.* 40: 737–751, 1977.
116. Duysens, J., and G. E. Loeb. Modulation of ipsi- and contralateral reflex responses in unrestrained walking cats. *J. Neurophysiol.* 44: 1024–1037, 1980.
117. Duysens, J., G. E. Loeb, and B. J. Weston. Crossed flexor reflex responses and their reversal in freely walking cats. *Brain Res.* 197: 538–542, 1980.
118. Duysens, J., and K. G. Pearson. The role of cutaneous afferents from the distal hindlimb in the regulation of the step cycle of thalamic cats. *Exp. Brain Res.* 24: 245–255, 1976.
119. Duysens, J., and K. G. Pearson. Inhibition of flexor burst generation by loading ankle extensor muscles in walking cats. *Brain Res.* 187: 321–332, 1980.

120. Duysens, J., and R. B. Stein. Reflexes induced by nerve stimulation in walking cats with implanted cuff electrodes. *Exp. Brain Res.* 32: 213–224, 1978.
121. Duysens, J., A. A. M. Tax, M. Trippel, and V. Dietz. Phase-dependent reversal of reflexly induced movements during human gait. *Exp. Brain Res.* 90: 404–414, 1992.
122. Duysens, J., A. A. M. Tax, M. Trippel, and V. Dietz. Increased amplitude of cutaneous reflexes during human running as compared to standing. *Brain Res.* 613: 230–238, 1993.
123. Edgerton, V. R., C. P. de Guzman, R. J. Gregor, R. R. Roy, J. A. Hodgson, and R. G. Lovely. Trainability of the spinal cord to generate hindlimb stepping patterns in adult spinalized cats. In: *Neurobiological Basis of Human Locomotion*, edited by M. Shimamura, S. Grillner, and V. R. Edgerton. Tokyo: Japan Scientific Societies Press, 1991, p. 411–423.
124. Edgerton, V. R., S. Grillner, A. Sjostrom, and P. Zangger. Central generation of locomotion in vertebrates. In: *Neural Control of Locomotion*, edited by R. Herman, S. Grillner, A. Sjostrom, and P. Zangger. New York: Plenum Press, 1976, p. 439–464.
125. Edgley, S. A., and E. Jankowska. Field potentials generated by group II muscle afferents in the middle lumbar segments of the cat spinal cord. *J. Physiol. (Lond.)* 385: 393–413, 1987.
126. Edgley, S. A., and E. Jankowska. An interneuronal relay for group I and II muscle afferents in the midlumbar segments of the cat spinal cord. *J. Physiol. (Lond.)* 389: 647–674, 1987.
127. Edgley, S. A., E. Jankowska, and S. Shefchyk. Evidence that mid-lumbar neurones in reflex pathways from group II afferents are involved in locomotion in the cat. *J. Physiol. (Lond.)* 403: 57–71, 1988.
128. Eidelberg E. Consequences of spinal cord lesions upon motor function, with special reference to locomotor activity. *Prog. Neurobiol.* 17: 185–202, 1981.
129. Eidelberg, E., J. L. Story, B. L. Meyer, and J. Nystel. Stepping by chronic spinal cats. *Exp. Brain. Res.* 40: 241–246, 1980.
130. Eidelberg, E., J. L. Story, J. G. Walden, and B. L. Meyer. Anatomical correlates of return of locomotor function after partial spinal cord lesions in cats. *Exp. Brain Res.* 42: 81–88, 1981.
131. Eidelberg, E., J. G. Walden, and L. H. Nguyen. Locomotor control in macaque monkeys. *Brain* 104: 647–663, 1981.
132. Eidelberg, E., and J. Yu. Effects of corticospinal lesions upon treadmill locomotion by cats. *Exp. Brain Res.* 43: 101–103, 1981.
133. Eilam, D., and G. Shefer. Reversal of interleg coupling in backward locomotion implies a prime role of the direction of locomotion. *J. Exp. Biol.* 173: 155–163, 1992.
134. El Manira, A., R. A. DiCaprio, D. Cattaert, and F. Clarac. Monosynaptic interjoint reflexes and their central modulation during fictive locomotion in crayfish. *Eur. J. Neurosci.* 3: 1219–1231, 1991.
135. Engberg, I., and A. Lundberg. An electromyographic analysis of muscular activity in the hindlimb of the cat during unrestrained locomotion. *Acta Physiol. Scand.* 75: 614–630, 1969.
136. English, A. W. Functional analysis of the shoulder girdle of cats during locomotion. *J. Morphol.* 156: 279–292, 1978.
137. English, A. W. An electromyographic analysis of forelimb muscles during overground stepping in the cat. *J. Exp. Biol.* 76: 105–122, 1978.
138. English, A. W. Interlimb coordination during stepping in the cat: effects of dorsal column section. *J. Neurophysiol.* 44: 270–279, 1980.
139. English, A. W. An electromyographic analysis of compartments in cat lateral gastrocnemius muscle during unrestrained locomotion. *J. Neurophysiol.* 52: 114–125, 1984.
140. English, A. W. Interlimb coordination during stepping in the cat. The role of the dorsal spinocerebellar tract. *Exp. Neurol.* 87: 96–108, 1985.
141. English, A. W., and O. I. Weeks. An anatomical and functional analysis of cat biceps femoris and semitendinosis muscles. *J. Morphol.* 191: 161–175, 1987.
142. Feldman, A. G., and G. N. Orlovsky. Activity of interneurons mediating reciprocal Ia inhibition during locomotion. *Brain Res.* 84: 181–194, 1975.
143. Fleshman, J. W., A. Lev-Tov, and R. E. Burke. Peripheral and central control of flexor digitorium longus and flexor hallucis longus motoneurons: the synaptic basis of functional diversity. *Exp. Brain Res.* 54: 133–149, 1984.
144. Floeter, M. K., G. N. Sholomenko, J.-P. Gossard, and R. E. Burke. Disynaptic excitation from the medial longitudinal fasciculus to lumbosacral motoneurons: modulation by repetitive activation, descending pathways, and locomotion. *Exp. Brain Res.* 92: 407–419, 1993.
145. Forssberg, H. Stumbling corrective reaction: a phase-dependent compensatory reaction during locomotion. *J. Neurophysiol.* 42: 936–953, 1979.
146. Forssberg, H., and S. Grillner. The locomotion of the acute spinal cat injected with clonidine i.v. *Brain Res.* 50: 184–186, 1973.
147. Forssberg, H., S. Grillner, and J. Halbertsma. The locomotion of the low spinal cat. I. Coordination within a hindlimb. *Acta Physiol. Scand.* 108: 269–281, 1980.
148. Forssberg, H., S. Grillner, J. Halbertsma, and S. Rossignol. The locomotion of the low spinal cat: II. Interlimb coordination. *Acta Physiol. Scand.* 108: 283–295, 1980.
149. Forssberg, H., S. Grillner, and S. Rossignol. Phasic gain control of reflexes from the dorsum of the paw during spinal locomotion. *Brain Res.* 132: 121–139, 1977.
150. Forssberg, H., S. Grillner, and A. Sjostrom. Tactile placing reactions in chronic spinal kittens. *Acta Physiol. Scand.* 92: 114–120, 1974.
151. Fukson, O. I., M. B. Berkinblit, and A. G. Feldman. The spinal frog takes into account the scheme of its body during the wiping reflex. *Science* 209: 1261–1263, 1980.
152. Fung, J., J. E. Stewart, and H. Barbeau. The combined effects of clonidine and cyproheptadine with interactive training on the modulation of locomotion in spinal cord injured subjects. *J. Neurol. Sci.* 100: 85–93, 1990.
153. Garcia-Rill, E. The basal ganglia and the locomotor regions. *Brain Res. Rev.* 11: 47–63, 1986.
154. Garcia-Rill, E., and R. D. Skinner. The mesencephalic locomotor region i. Activation of a medullary projection site. *Brain Res.* 411: 1–12, 1987.
155. Garcia-Rill, E., and R. D. Skinner. The mesencephalic locomotor region ii. Projections to reticulospinal neurons. *Brain Res.* 411: 13–20, 1987.
156. Garcia-Rill, E., R. D. Skinner, and J. A. Fitzgerald. Chemical activation of the mesencephalic locomotor region. *Brain Res.* 330: 43–54, 1985.
157. Garcia-Rill, E., R. D. Skinner, M. B. Jackson, and M. M. Smith. Connections of the mesencephalic locomotor region (MLR). I. Substantia nigra afferents. *Brain Res. Bull.* 10: 57–62, 1983.

158. Gauthier, L., and S. Rossignol. Contralateral hindlimb responses to cutaneous stimulation during locomotion in high decerebrate cats. *Brain Res.* 207: 303–320, 1981.
159. Gelfand, I. M., G. N. Orlovsky, and M. L. Shik. Locomotion and scratching in tetrapods. In: *Neural Control of Rhythmic Movements in Vertebrates*, edited by A. H. Cohen, S. Rossignol, and S. Grillner. New York: John Wiley & Sons, 1988, p. 167–199.
160. Getting, P. A. Comparative analysis of invertebrate central pattern generators. In: *Neural Control of Rhythmic Movements in Vertebrates*, edited by A. H. Cohen, S. Rossignol, and S. Grillner. New York: John Wiley & Sons, 1988, p. 101–127.
161. Giuliani, C. A., and J. L. Smith. Development and characteristics of airstepping in chronic spinal cats. *J. Neurosci.* 5: 1276–1282, 1985.
162. Godderz, W., M. Illert, and T. Yamaguchi. Efferent pattern of fictive locomotion in the cat forelimb: with special reference to radial motor nuclei. *Eur. J. Neurosci.* 2: 663–671, 1990.
163. Goldberg, M. R., and D. Robertson. Yohimbine: a pharmacological probe for study of the α_2-adrenoreceptor. *Pharmacol. Rev.* 35: 143–180, 1983.
164. Gorassini, M. A., A. Prochazka, G. W. Hiebert, and M. J. A. Gauthier. Corrective responses to loss of ground support during walking. I. Intact cats. *J. Neurophysiol.* 71: 603–609, 1994.
165. Gorska, T., T. Bem, and H. Majczynski. Locomotion in cats with ventral spinal lesions: support patterns and duration of support phases during unrestrained walking. *Acta Neurobiol. Exp.* 50: 191–200, 1990.
166. Gorska, T., T. Bem, H. Majczynski, and W. Zmyslowski. Unrestrained walking in cats with partial spinal lesions. *Brain Res. Bull.* 32: 241–249, 1993.
167. Gorska, T., H. Majczynski, T. Bem, and W. Zmyslowski. Hindlimb swing, stance and step relationships during unrestrained walking in cats with lateral funicular lesion. *Acta Neurobiol. Exp.* 53: 133–142, 1993.
168. Goslow, G. E., R. M. Reinking, and D. G. Stuart. The cat step cycle: hind limb joint angles and muscle lengths during unrestrained locomotion. *J. Morphol.* 141: 1–42, 1973.
169. Gossard, J.-P., R. M. Brownstone, I. Barajon, and H. Hultborn. Transmission in a locomotor-related group Ib pathway from hindlimb extensor muscles in the cat. *Exp. Brain Res.* 98: 213–228, 1994.
170. Gossard, J.-P., J.-M. Cabelguen, and S. Rossignol. Intra-axonal recordings of cutaneous primary afferents during fictive locomotion in the cat. *J. Neurophysiol.* 62: 1177–1188, 1989.
171. Gossard, J.-P., J.-M. Cabelguen, and S. Rossignol. Phase-dependent modulation of primary afferent depolarization in single cutaneous primary afferents evoked by peripheral stimulation during fictive locomotion in the cat. *Brain Res.* 537: 14–23, 1990.
172. Gossard, J.-P., J.-M. Cabelguen, and S. Rossignol. An intracellular study of muscle primary afferents during fictive locomotion in the cat. *J. Neurophysiol.* 65: 914–926, 1991.
173. Gossard, J.-P., and S. Rossignol. Phase-dependent modulation of dorsal root potentials evoked by peripheral nerve stimulation during fictive locomotion in the cat. *Brain Res.* 537: 1–13, 1990.
174. Grillner, S. Locomotion in the spinal cat. In: *Control of Posture and Locomotion. Adv. Behav. Biol.* 7, edited by R. B. Stein, K. G. Pearson, R. S. Smith, and J. B. Redford. New York: Plenum Press, 1973, p. 515–535.
175. Grillner, S. Control of locomotion in bipeds, tetrapods, and fish. In: *Handbook of Physiology, The Nervous System, Motor Control*, edited by V. B. Brooks. Bethesda, MD: Am. Physiol. Soc., 1981, p. 1179–1236.
176. Grillner, S. Neurobiological bases of rhythmic motor acts in vertebrate. *Science* 228: 143–149, 1985.
177. Grillner, S., and R. Dubuc. Control of locomotion in vertebrates: spinal and supraspinal mechanisms. In: *Functional Recovery in Neurological Disease*, edited by S. G. Waxman. New York: Raven Press, 1988, p. 425–453.
178. Grillner, S., and S. Rossignol. On the initiation of the swing phase of locomotion in chronic spinal cats. *Brain Res.* 146: 269–277, 1978.
179. Grillner, S., and M. L. Shik. On the descending control of the lumbosacral spinal cord from the mesencephalic locomotor region. *Acta Physiol. Scand.* 87: 320–333, 1973.
180. Grillner, S., P. S. G. Stein, D. G. Stuart, H. Forssberg, and R. M. Herman. *Neurobiology of Vertebrate Locomotion, Wenner-Gren International Symposium Series*. Hong Kong: Macmillan, 1986, p. 1–735.
181. Grillner, S., and P. Zangger. On the central generation of locomotion in the low spinal cat. *Exp. Brain. Res.* 34: 241–261, 1979.
182. Grillner, S., and P. Zangger. The effect of dorsal root transection on the efferent motor pattern in the cat's hindlimb during locomotion. *Acta Physiol. Scand.* 120: 393–405, 1984.
183. Guertin, P., M. Angel, M.-C. Perreault, and D. A. McCrea. Ankle extensor group I afferents excite extensors throughout the hindlimb during MLR-evoked fictive locomotion in the cat. *J. Physiol. (Lond.)* 487: 197–209, 1955.
184. Halbertsma, J. M. The stride cycle of the cat: the modelling of locomotion by computerized analysis of automatic recordings. *Acta Physiol. Scand. Suppl.* 521: 1–75, 1983.
185. Harris-Warrick, R. M. Chemical modulation of central pattern generators. In: *Neural Control of Rhythmic Movements in Vertebrates*, edited by A. H. Cohen, S. Rossignol, and S. Grillner. New York: John Wiley & Sons, 1988, p. 285–331.
186. Hart, B. L. Facilitation by strychnine of reflex walking in spinal dogs. *Physiol. Behav.* 6: 627–628, 1971.
187. Hasan, S. J., H. S. Keirstead, G. D. Muir, and J. D. Steeves. Axonal regeneration contributes to repair of injured brainstem-spinal neurons in embryonic chick. *J. Neurosci.* 13: 492–507, 1993.
188. Hasan, S. J., B. H. Nelson, J. I. Valenzuela, H. S. Keirstead, S. E. Shull, D. W. Ethel, and J. D. Steeves. Functional repair of transected spinal cord in embryonic chick. *Restorative Neurol. Neurosci.* 2: 137–154, 1991.
189. Helgren, M. E., and M. E. Goldberger. The recovery of postural reflexes and locomotion following low thoracic hemisection in adult cats involves compensation by undamaged primary afferent pathways. *Exp. Neurol.* 123: 17–34, 1993.
190. Hensbergen, E., and D. Kernell. Task-related differences in distribution of electromyographic activity within peroneus longus muscle of spontaneously moving cats. *Exp. Brain Res.* 89: 682–685, 1992.
191. Hishinuma, M., and T. Yamaguchi. Cervical interneurons oligosynaptically excited from primary afferents and rhythmically active during forelimb fictive locomotion in the cat. *Neurosci. Lett.* 111: 287–291, 1990.
192. Ho, S., and J. O'Donovan. Regionalization and intersegmental coordination of rhythm-generating networks in the spinal cord of the chick embryo. *J. Neurosci.* 13: 1354–1371, 1993.

193. Hochman, S., L. M. Jordan, and J. F. Macdonald. *N*-methyl-D-aspartate receptor-mediated voltage oscillations in neurons surrounding the central canal in slices of rat spinal cord. *J. Neurophysiol.* 72: 565–577, 1994.
194. Hochman, S., L. M. Jordan, and B. J. Schmidt. TTX-Resistant NMDA receptor-mediated voltage oscillations in mammalian lumbar motoneurons. *J. Neurophysiol.* 72: 1–4, 1994.
195. Hoffer, J. A., G. E. Loeb, N. Sugano, W. B. Marks, J. O'Donovan, and C. A. Pratt. Cat hindlimb motoneurons during locomotion: III. Functional segregation in sartorius. *J. Neurophysiol.* 57: 554–562, 1987.
196. Hoffer, J. A., N. Sugano, G. E. Loeb, W. B. Marks, M. O'Donovan, and C. A. J. Pratt. Cat hindlimb motoneurons during locomotion: II. Normal activity patterns. *J. Neurophysiol.* 57: 530–553, 1987.
197. Hoffmann, P., M. Illert, and E. Wiedemann. EMG recordings from the cat forelimb during unrestrained locomotion. *Neurosci. Lett.* 22(Suppl.): S126, 1985.
198. Hounsgaard, J., H. Hultborn, J. Jespersen, and O. Kiehn. Bistability of alpha-motoneurones in the decerebrate cat and in the acute spinal cat after intravenous 5-hydroxytryptophan. *J. Physiol. (Lond.)* 405: 345–367, 1988.
199. Hultborn, H., S. Meunier, C. Morin, and E. Pierrot-Deseilligny. Assessing changes in presynaptic inhibition of Ia fibres: a study in man and the cat. *J. Physiol. (Lond.)* 389: 729–756, 1987.
200. Hultborn, H., S. Meunier, E. Pierrot-Deseilligny, and M. Shindo. Changes in presynaptic inhibition of Ia fibres at the onset of voluntary contraction in man. *J. Physiol. (Lond.)* 389: 757–772, 1987.
201. Hultborn, H., N. Petersen, R. Brownstone, and J. Nielsen. Evidence of fictive spinal locomotion in the marmoset (*Callithrix jacchus*). *Soc. Neurosci. Abstr.* 19(225): 539, 1993.
202. Hutchison, D. L., R. R. Roy, S. Bodine-Fowler, J. A. Hodgson, and V. R. Edgerton. Electromyographic (EMG) amplitude patterns in the proximal and distal compartments of the cat semitendinosus during various motor tasks. *Brain Res.* 479: 56–64, 1989.
203. Jami, L., E. Pierrot-Deseilligny, and D. Zytnicki. *Muscle Afferents and Spinal Control of Movement.* Oxford: Pergamon Press, 1992, p. 1–470.
204. Jankowska, E., and S. Edgley. Interaction between pathways controlling posture and gait at the level of spinal interneurones in the cat. *Prog. Brain Res.* 97: 161–171, 1993.
205. Jankowska, E., and B. R. Noga. Contralaterally projecting lamina VIII interneurones in middle lumbar segments in the cat. *Brain Res.* 535: 327–330, 1990.
206. Jell, R. M., C. Elliott, and L. M. Jordan. Initiation of locomotion from the mesencephalic locomotor region effects of selective brain-stem lesions. *Brain Res.* 328: 121–128, 1985.
207. Jeneskog, T., and Y. Padel. An excitatory pathway through dorsal columns to rubrospinal cells in the cat. *J. Physiol. (Lond.)* 353: 355–373, 1984.
208. Jordan, L. M. Factors determining motoneuron rhythmicity during fictive locomotion. In: *Neural Origin of Rhythmic Movements, Soc. Exp. Biol. Symp., 37*, edited by A. Roberts and B. L. Roberts. Cambridge: Cambridge University Press, 1983, p. 423–444.
209. Jordan, L. M. Initiation of locomotion from the mammalian brainstem. In: *Neurobiology of Vertebrate Locomotion*, edited by S. Grillner, P. S. G. Stein, D. G. Stuart, and H. Forssberg. London: Macmillan, 1986, p. 21–37.
210. Jordan, L. M. Brainstem and spinal cord mechanisms for the initiation of locomotion. In: *Neurobiological Basis of Human Locomotion*, edited by M. Shimamura, S. Grillner, and V. R. Edgerton. Tokyo: Japan Scientific Societies Press, 1991, p. 3–20.
211. Jordan, L. M., R. M. Brownstone, and B. R. Noga. Control of functional systems in the brainstem and spinal cord. *Curr. Opin. Neurobiol.* 2: 794–801, 1992.
212. Jordan, L. M., C. A. Pratt, and J. E. Menzies. Locomotion evoked by brain stem stimulation: occurrence without phasic segmental afferent input. *Brain Res.* 177: 204–207, 1979.
213. Kanda, K., and H. Sato. Reflex responses of human thigh muscles to non-noxious sural stimulation during stepping. *Brain Res.* 288: 378–380, 1983.
214. Kato, M. Longitudinal myelotomy of lumbar spinal cord has little effect on coordinated locomotor activities of bilateral hindlimbs of the chronic cats. *Neurosci. Lett.* 93: 259–263, 1988.
215. Kato, M. Chronically isolated lumbar half spinal cord and locomotor activities of the hindlimb. In: *Neurobiological Basis of Human Locomotion*, edited by M. Shimamura, S. Grillner, and V. R. Edgerton. Tokyo: Japan Scientific Societies Press, 1991, p. 407–410.
216. Kato, M., S. Murakami, H. Hirayama, and K. Hikino. Recovery of postural control following chronic bilateral hemisections at different spinal cord levels in adult cats. *Exp. Neurol.* 90: 350–364, 1985.
217. Kato, M., S. Murakami, K. Yasuda, and H. Hirayama. Disruption of fore- and hindlimb coordination during overground locomotion in cats with bilateral serial hemisection of the spinal cord. *Neurosci. Res.* 2: 27–47, 1984.
218. Kazennikov, O. V., V. A. Selionov, and M. L. Shik. On the bulbospinal locomotor column in the cat. In: *Stance and Motion. Facts and Concepts*, edited by V. S. Gurfinkel, M. E. Ioffe, J. Massion, and J. P. Roll. New York: Plenum Press, 1987, p. 123–131.
219. Kjaerulff, O., I. Barajon, and O. Kiehn. Sulforhodamine-labelled cells in the neonatal rat spinal cord following chemically induced locomotor activity in vitro. *J. Physiol. (Lond.)* 478: 265–273, 1994.
220. Kniffki, K. D., E. D. Schomburg, and H. Steffens. Effects from fine muscle and cutaneous afferents on spinal locomotion in cats. *J. Physiol. (Lond.)* 319: 543–554, 1981.
221. Kriellaars, D. J., R. M. Brownstone, B. R. Noga, and L. M. Jordan. Mechanical entrainment of fictive locomotion in the decerebrate cat. *J. Neurophysiol.* 71: 1–13, 1994.
222. Kudo, N., and T. Yamada. *N*-Methyl-D,L-aspartate-induced locomotor activity in a spinal cord-hindlimb muscles preparation of the newborn rat studied in vitro. *Neurosci. Lett.* 75: 43–48, 1987.
223. Kuhta, P. C., and J. L. Smith. Scratch responses in normal cats: hindlimb kinematics and muscle synergies. *J. Neurophysiol.* 64: 1653–1667, 1990.
224. Kuhtz-Buschbeck, J. P., A. Boczek-Funcke, M. Illert, and C. Weinhardt. X-ray study of the cat hindlimb during treadmill locomotion. *Eur. J. Neurosci.* 6: 1187, 1994.
225. LaBella, L., A. Niechaj, and S. Rossignol. Low-threshold, short-latency cutaneous reflexes during fictive locomotion in the "semi-chronic" spinal cat. *Exp. Brain Res.* 91: 236–248, 1992.
226. LaBella, L. A., J. P. Kehler, and D. A. McCrea. A differential synaptic input to the motor nuclei of triceps surae from the caudal and lateral cutaneous sural nerves. *J. Neurophysiol.* 61: 291–301, 1989.

227. LaBella, L. A., and D. A. McCrea. Evidence for restricted central convergence of cutaneous afferents on an excitatory reflex pathway to medial gastrocnemius motoneurons. *J. Neurophysiol.* 64: 403–412, 1990.
228. Lai, Y. Y., and J. M. Siegel. Muscle tone suppression and stepping produced by stimulation of midbrain and rostral pontine reticular formation. *J. Neurosci.* 10: 2727–2734, 1990.
229. Lawrence, J. H., T. R. Nichols, and A. W. English. Cat hindlimb muscles exert substantial torques outside the sagittal plane. *J. Neurophysiol.* 69: 282–285, 1993.
230. Lennard, P. R., and J. W. Hermanson. Central reflex modulation during locomotion. *Trends Neurosci.* 8: 483–486, 1985.
231. Liddell, E. G., and C. G. Phillips. Pyramidal section in the cat. *Brain* 67: 1–9, 1944.
232. Loeb, G. E. The distal hindlimb musculature of the cat: interanimal variability of locomotor activity and cutaneous reflexes. *Exp. Brain Res.* 96: 125–140, 1993.
233. Loeb, G. E., W. B. Marks, and J. A. Hoffer. Cat hindlimb motoneurons during locomotion: IV. Participation in cutaneous reflexes. *J. Neurophysiol.* 57: 563–573, 1987.
234. Lovely, R. G., R. J. Gregor, R. R. Roy, and V. R. Edgerton. Effects of training on the recovery of full-weight-bearing stepping in the adult spinal cat. *Exp. Neurol.* 92: 421–435, 1986.
235. Lovely, R. G., R. J. Gregor, R. R. Roy, and V. R. Edgerton. Weight-bearing hindlimb stepping in treadmill-exercised adult spinal cat. *Brain Res.* 514: 206–218, 1990.
236. Lundberg, A. Half-centres revisited. In: *Regulatory Functions of the CNS. Principles of Motion and Organization. Adv. Physiol. Sci. Vol. 1*, edited by J. Szentagothai, M. Palkovits, and J. Hamori. Budapest: Pergamon Press, 1981, p. 155–167.
237. Lydic, R. Central pattern-generating neurons and the search for general principles. *FASEB J.* 3: 2457–2468, 1989.
238. Marple-Horvat, D. E., A. J. Amos, D. M. Armstrong, and J. M. Criado. Changes in the discharge patterns of cat motor cortex neurones during unexpected perturbations of ongoing locomotion. *J. Physiol. (Lond.)* 462: 87–113, 1993.
239. Matsukawa, K., H. Kamei, K. Minoda, and M. Udo. Interlimb coordination in cat locomotion investigated with perturbation. I. Behavioral and electromyographic study on symmetric limbs of decerebrate and awake walking cats. *Exp. Brain Res.* 46: 425–437, 1982.
240. McCrea, D., C. A. Pratt, and L. M. Jordan. Renshaw cell activity and recurrent effects on motoneurons during fictive locomotion. *J. Neurophysiol.* 44: 475–488, 1980.
241. Miller, S., and F. G. A. Van der Meche. Movements of the forelimbs of the cat during stepping on a treadmill. *Brain Res.* 91: 255–269, 1975.
242. Miller, S., and F. G. A. Van der Meche. Coordinated stepping of all four limbs in the high spinal cat. *Brain Res.* 109: 395–398, 1976.
243. Mori, S. Integration of posture and locomotion in acute decebrate cats and in awake, freely moving cats. *Prog. Neurobiol.* 28: 161–195, 1987.
244. Mori, S., K. Matsuyama, J. Kohyama, Y. Kobayashi, and K. Takakusaki. Neuronal constituents of postural and locomotor control systems and their interactions in cats. *Brain Dev.* 14: S109–S120, 1992.
245. Mori, S., T. Sakamoto, and K. Takakusaki. Interaction of posture and locomotion in cats: its automatic and volitional control aspects. In: *Neurobiological Basis of Human Locomotion*, edited by M. Shimamura, S. Grillner, and V. R. Edgerton. Tokyo: Japan Scientific Societies Press, 1991, p. 21–32.
246. Murphy, P. R., R. B. Stein, and J. Taylor. Phasic and tonic modulation of impulse rates in gamma-motoneurones during locomotion in premammillary cats. *J. Neurophysiol.* 52: 228–243, 1984.
247. Nathan, P. W. Effects on movement of surgical incisions into the human spinal cord. *Brain* 117: 337–346, 1994.
248. Noga, B. R., P. A. Fortier, D. J. Kriellaars, X. Dai, G. R. Detillieux, and L. M. Jordan. Field potential mapping of neurons in the lumbar spinal cord activated following stimulation of the mesencephalic locomotor region. *J. Neurosci.* 15: 2203–2217, 1995.
249. Noga, B. R., J. Kettler, and L. M. Jordan. Locomotion produced in mesencephalic cats by injections of putative transmitter substances and antagonists into the medial reticular formation and the pontomedullary locomotor strip. *J. Neurosci.* 8: 2074–2086, 1988.
250. Noga, B. R., D. J. Kriellaars, and L. M. Jordan. The effect of selective brainstem or spinal cord lesions on treadmill locomotion evoked by stimulation of the mesencephalic or pontomedullary locomotor regions. *J. Neurosci.* 11: 1691–1700, 1991.
251. Noga, B. R., S. J. Shefchyk, J. Jamal, and L. M. Jordan. The role of Renshaw cells in locomotion antagonism of their excitation from motor axon collaterals with intravenous mecamylamine. *Exp. Brain Res.* 66: 99–105, 1987.
252. O'Donovan, M. J., and A. Ritter. Optical recording and lesioning of spinal neurones during rhythmic activity in the chick embryo spinal cord. In: *Alpha and Gamma Motor Systems*, edited by A. Taylor, M. H. Gladden, and R. Durbaba. New York and London: Plenum Press, 1995, p. 557–563.
253. O'Donovan, M., E. Sernagor, G. Sholomenko, S. Ho, M. Antal, and W. Yee. Development of spinal motor networks in the chick embryo. *J. Exp. Zool.* 261: 261–273, 1992.
254. O'Donovan, M. J., M. J. Pinter, R. P. Dum, and R. E. Burke. Actions of FDL and FHL muscles in intact cats: functional dissociation between anatomical synergists. *J. Neurophysiol.* 47: 1126–1143, 1982.
255. Orlovsky, G. N. Activity of vestibulospinal neurons during locomotion. *Brain Res.* 46: 85–98, 1972.
256. Orlovsky, G. N. Activity of rubrospinal neurons during locomotion. *Brain Res.* 46: 99–112, 1972.
257. Orlovsky, G. N. The effect of different descending systems on flexor and extensor activity during locomotion. *Brain Res.* 40: 359–371, 1972.
258. Orlovsky, G. N. Cerebellum and locomotion. In: *Neurobiological Basis of Human Locomotion*, edited by M. Shimamura, S. Grillner, and V. R. Edgerton. Tokyo: Japan Scientific Societies Press, 1991, p. 187–199.
259. Orlovsky, G. N., and A. G. Feldman. Classification of lumbosacral neurons by their discharge pattern during evoked locomotion. *Neurophysiology* 4: 311–317, 1972.
260. Orlovsky, G. N., and A. G. Feldman. Role of afferent activity in the generation of stepping movements. *Neurophysiology* 4: 304–310, 1972.
261. Orsal, D., C. Perret, and J.-M. Cabelguen. Evidence of rhythmic inhibitory synaptic influences in hindlimb motoneurons during fictive locomotion in the thalamic cat. *Exp. Brain Res.* 64: 217–224, 1986.
262. Padel, Y., and J. L. Relova. A common somaesthetic pathway to red nucleus and motor cortex. *Behav. Brain Res.* 28: 153–157, 1988.
263. Palmer, C. I., W. B. Marks, and M. J. Bak. The responses of cat motor cortical units to electrical cutaneous stimula-

tion during locomotion and during lifting, falling and landing. *Exp. Brain Res.* 58: 102–116, 1985.
264. Patla, A. E., and M. Belanger. Task-dependent compensatory responses to perturbations applied during rhythmic movements in man. *J. Mot. Behav.* 19: 454–475, 1987.
265. Pearson, K. G. Common principles of motor control in vertebrates and invertebrates. *Annu. Rev. Neurosci.* 16: 265–297, 1993.
266. Pearson, K. G., and D. F. Collins. Reversal of the influence of group Ib afferents from plantaris on activity in medial gastrocnemius muscle during locomotor activity. *J. Neurophysiol.* 70: 1009–1017, 1993.
267. Pearson, K. G., W. Jiang, and J. M. Ramirez. The use of naloxone to facilitate the generation of the locomotor rhythm in spinal cats. *J. Neurosci. Meth.* 42: 75–81, 1992.
268. Pearson, K. G., J. M. Ramirez, and W. Jiang. Entrainment of the locomotor rhythm by group Ib afferents from ankle extensor muscles in spinal cats. *Exp. Brain Res.* 90: 557–566, 1992.
269. Pearson, K. G., and S. Rossignol. Fictive motor patterns in chronic spinal cats. *J. Neurophysiol.* 66: 1874–1887, 1991.
270. Perell, K. L., R. J. Gregor, J. A. Buford, and J. L. Smith. Adaptive control for backward quadrupedal walking. IV. Hindlimb kinetics during stance and swing. *J. Neurophysiol.* 70: 2226–2240, 1993.
271. Perreault, M.-C., M. J. Angel, P. Guertin, and D. A. McCrea. Effects of stimulation of hindlimb flexor group II muscle afferents during fictive locomotion. *J. Physiol. (Lond.)* 3598: 487: 211–220, 1995.
272. Perreault, M.-C., T. Drew, and S. Rossignol. Activity of medullary reticulospinal neurons during locomotion in the absence of phasic peripheral afferent feedback. *J. Neurophysiol.* 69: 2232–2247, 1993.
273. Perreault, M.-C., S. Rossignol, and T. Drew. Microstimulation of the medullary reticular formation during fictive locomotion. *J. Neurophysiol.* 71: 229–245, 1994.
274. Perret, C. Centrally generated pattern of motoneuron activity during locomotion in the cat. In: *Neural Origin of Rhythmic Movements. Soc. Exp. Biol. Symp., 37*, edited by A. Roberts and B. L. Roberts. Cambridge: Cambridge University Press, 1983, p. 405–422.
275. Perret, C., and J.-M. Cabelguen. Central and reflex participation in the timing of locomotor activations of a bifunctional muscle, the semi-tendinosus, in the cat. *Brain Res.* 106: 390–395, 1976.
276. Perret, C., and J.-M. Cabelguen. Main characteristics of the hindlimb locomotor cycle in the decorticate cat with special reference to bifunctional muscles. *Brain Res.* 187: 333–352, 1980.
277. Peterson, B. W., R. A. Maunz, N. G. Pitts, and R. G. Mackel. Patterns of projection and branching of reticulospinal neurons. *Exp. Brain. Res.* 23: 333–351, 1975.
278. Philippson, M. L'autonomie et la centralisation dans le système nerveux des animaux. *Trav. Lab. Physiol. Inst. Solvay. (Bruxelles.)* 7: 1–208, 1905.
279. Pierotti, D. J., R. R. Roy, R. J. Gregor, and V. R. Edgerton. Electromyographic activity of cat hindlimb flexors and extensors during locomotion at varying speeds and inclines. *Brain Res.* 481: 57–66, 1989.
280. Pilyavskii, A. I., I. A. Yakhnitsa, and N. V. Bulgakova. Antidromic dorsal root impulses during naturally occurring locomotion in rats. *Neurophysiology* 20: 417–422, 1989.
281. Pointis, D., and P. Borenstein. The mesencephalic locomotor region in cat: effects of local applications of diazepam and gamma-aminobutyric acid. *Neurosci. Lett.* 53: 297–302, 1985.
282. Pratt, C. A., C. M. Chanaud, and G. E. Loeb. Functionally complex muscles of the cat hindlimb. IV. Intramuscular distribution of movement command signals and cutaneous reflexes in broad, bifunctional thigh muscles. *Exp. Brain Res.* 85: 281–299, 1991.
283. Pratt, C. A., and L. M. Jordan. Ia inhibitory interneurons and Renshaw cells as contributors to the spinal mechanisms of fictive locomotion. *J. Neurophysiol.* 57: 56–71, 1987.
284. Pratt, C. A., and G. E. Loeb. Functionally complex muscles of the cat hindlimb. I. Patterns of activation across sartorius. *Exp. Brain Res.* 85: 243–256, 1991.
285. Prochazka, A. Sensorimotor gain control: a basic strategy of motor systems? *Prog. Neurobiol.* 33: 281–307, 1989.
286. Prochazka, A., K. H. Sontag, and P. Wand. Motor reactions to perturbations of gait proprioceptive and somesthetic involvement. *Neurosci. Lett.* 7: 35–39, 1978.
287. Rasmussen, K., J. Heym, and B. L. Jacobs. Activity of serotonin-containing neurons in nucleus centralis superior of freely moving cats. *Exp. Neurol.* 83: 302–317, 1984.
288. Rasmussen, K., D. A. Morilak, and B. L. Jacobs. Single unit activity of locus coeruleus neurons in the freely moving cat. I. During naturalistic behaviors and in response to simple and complex stimuli. *Brain Res.* 371: 324–334, 1986.
289. Rasmussen, S., A. K. Chan, and G. E. J. Goslow. The cat step cycle: electromyographic patterns for hindlimb muscles during posture and unrestrained locomotion. *J. Morphol.* 155: 253–270, 1978.
290. Roberts, A., and B. L. Roberts. *Neural Origin of Rhythmic Movements. Soc. Exp. Biol. Symp.*, 37, Cambridge: Cambridge University Press, 1983, p. 1–503.
291. Robertson, G. A., and P. S. Stein. Synaptic control of hindlimb motoneurones during three forms of the fictive scratch reflex in the turtle. *J. Physiol. (Lond.)* 404: 101–128, 1988.
292. Robinson, G. A., and M. E. Goldberger. The development and recovery of motor function in spinal cats. I. The infant lesion effect. *Exp. Brain Res.* 62: 373–386, 1986.
293. Robinson, G. A., and M. E. Goldberger. The development and recovery of motor function in spinal cats. II. Pharmacological enhancement of recovery. *Exp. Brain Res.* 62: 387–400, 1986.
294. Roby-Brami, A., and B. Bussel. Long-latency spinal reflex in man after flexor reflex afferent stimulation. *Brain* 110: 707–725, 1987.
295. Rossignol, S., and H. Barbeau. Pharmacology of locomotion: an account of studies in spinal cats and spinal cord injured subjects. *J. Am. Paraplegia Soc.* 16: 190–196, 1993.
296. Rossignol, S., H. Barbeau, and C. Julien. Locomotion of the adult chronic spinal cat and its modification by monoaminergic agonists and antagonists. In: *Development and Plasticity of the Mammalian Spinal Cord*, edited by M. Goldberger, A. Gorio, and M. Murray. Padova: Fidia Research Series III, Liviana Press, 1986, p. 323–345.
297. Rossignol, S., M. Belanger, H. Barbeau, and T. Drew. Assessment of locomotor functions in the adult chronic spinal cat. In: *Conference Proceedings: Criteria for Assessing Recovery of Function: Behavioral Methods*, edited by M. Brown and M. E. Goldberger. Springfield, NJ: A.P.A., 1989, p. 62–65.
298. Rossignol, S., and R. Dubuc. Spinal pattern generation. *Curr. Opin. Neurobiol.* 4: 894–902, 1994.

299. Rossignol, S., and L. Gauthier. An analysis of mechanisms controlling the reversal of crossed spinal reflexes. *Brain Res.* 182: 31–45, 1980.
300. Rossignol, S., C. Julien, L. Gauthier, and J. P. Lund. State-dependent responses during locomotion. In: *Muscle Receptors and Movement*, edited by A. Taylor and A. Prochazka. London: Macmillan, 1981, p. 389–402.
301. Rossignol, S., J. P. Lund, and T. Drew. The role of sensory inputs in regulating patterns of rhythmical movements in higher vertebrates. A comparison between locomotion, respiration and mastication. In: *Neural Control of Rhythmic Movements in Vertebrates*, edited by A. Cohen, S. Rossignol, and S. Grillner. New York: John Wiley & Sons, 1988, p. 201–283.
302. Rossignol, S., P. Saltiel, M.-C. Perreault, T. Drew, K. Pearson, and M. Belanger. Intralimb and interlimb coordination in the cat during real and fictive rhythmic motor programs. *Semin. Neurosci.* 5: 67–75, 1993.
303. Russell, D. F., and F. E. Zajac. Effects of stimulating Deiter's nucleus and medial longitudinal fasciculus on the timing of the fictive locomotor rhythm induced in cats by DOPA. *Brain Res.* 17: 588–592, 1979.
304. Schmidt, B. J., D. E. R. Meyers, J. L. Fleshman, M. Tokuriki, and R. E. Burke. Phasic modulation of short latency cutaneous excitation in flexor digitorum longus motoneurons during fictive locomotion. *Exp. Brain Res.* 71: 568–578, 1988.
305. Schmidt, B. J., D. E. R. Meyers, M. Tokuriki, and R. E. Burke. Modulation of short latency cutaneous excitation in flexor and extensor motoneurons during fictive locomotion in the cat. *Exp. Brain Res.* 77: 57–68, 1989.
306. Schomburg, E. D. Spinal sensorimotor systems and their supraspinal control. *Neurosci. Res.* 7: 265–340, 1990.
307. Schomburg, E. D. Modes of rhythmic motor patterns generated by the spinal cord in the cat. In: *Alpha and Gamma Motor Systems*, edited by A. Taylor, M. H. Gladden, and R. Durbaba. New York and London: Plenum Press, 1995, p. 564–571.
308. Schomburg, E. D., H.-B. Behrends, and H. Steffens. Changes in segmental and propriospinal reflex pathways during spinal locomotion. In: *Muscle Receptors and Movement*, edited by A. Taylor and A. Prochazka. London: Macmillan, 1981, p. 413–425.
309. Schouenborg, J., H. Weng,-R., and H. Holmberg. Modular organization of spinal nociceptive reflexes: a new hypothesis. *News Physiol. Sci.* 9: 261, 1994.
310. Selionov, V. A., and M. L. Shik. Medullary locomotor strip and column in the cat. *Neuroscience* 13: 1267–1278, 1984.
311. Sernagor, E., and M. J. O'Donovan. Whole-cell patch clamp recordings from rhythmically active motoneurons in the isolated spinal cord of the chick embryo. *Neurosci. Lett.* 128: 211–216, 1991.
312. Shefchyk, S., D. McCrea, D. Kriellaars, P. Fortier, and L. Jordan. Activity of interneurons within the L4 spinal segment of the cat during brainstem-evoked fictive locomotion. *Exp. Brain Res.* 80: 290–295, 1990.
313. Shefchyk, S. J., R. M. Jell, and L. M. Jordan. Reversible cooling of the brainstem reveals areas required for mesencephalic locomotor region evoked treadmill locomotion. *Exp. Brain Res.* 56: 257–262, 1984.
314. Shefchyk, S. J., and L. M. Jordan. Excitatory and inhibitory post-synaptic potentials in alpha-motoneurons produced during fictive locomotion by stimulation of the mesencephalic locomotor region. *J. Neurophysiol.* 53: 1345–1355, 1985.
315. Shefchyk, S. J., and L. M. Jordan. Motoneuron input-resistance changes during fictive locomotion produced by stimulation of the mesencephalic locomotor region. *J. Neurophysiol.* 54: 1101–1108, 1985.
316. Shefchyk, S. J., R. B. Stein, and L. M. Jordan. Synaptic transmission from muscle afferents during fictive locomotion in the mesencephalic cat. *J. Neurophysiol.* 51: 986–997, 1984.
317. Sherrington, C. S. Flexion-reflex of the limb, crossed extension-reflex, and reflex stepping and standing. *J. Physiol. (Lond.)* 40: 28–121, 1910.
318. Sherrington, C. S. Remarks on the reflex mechanism of the step. *Brain* 33: 1–25, 1910.
319. Shik, M. L. Action of the brainstem locomotor region on spinal stepping generators via propriospinal pathways. In: *Spinal Cord Reconstruction*, edited by C. C. Kao, R. P. Bunge, and P. J. Reier. New York: Raven Press, 1983, p. 421–434.
320. Shik, M. L., F. V. Severin, and G. N. Orlovsky. Control of walking and running by means of electrical stimulation of the mid-brain. *Biophysics* 11: 756–765, 1966.
321. Shimamura, M., V. R. Edgerton, and I. Kogure. Application of autoradiographic analysis of 2 deoxyglucose in the study of locomotion. *J. Neurosci. Methods* 21: 303–310, 1987.
322. Shimamura, M., S. Grillner, and V. R. Edgerton. *Neurobiological Basis of Human Locomotion.* Tokyo: Japan Scientific Societies Press, 1991, p. 1–447.
323. Shimamura, M., I. Kogure, and T. Fuwa. Role of joint afferents in relation to the initiation of forelimb stepping in thalamic cats. *Brain Res.* 297: 225–234, 1984.
324. Shimamura, M., I. Tanaka, and T. Fuwa. Comparison between spino-bulbo-spinal and propriospinal reflexes in thalamic cats during stepping. *Neurosci. Res.* 7: 358–368, 1990.
325. Shimanskii, Y. P., and K. V. Baev. Dependence of efferent activity parameters on limb position during fictitious scratching in decerebrate cats. *Neurophysiology* 15: 451–458, 1986.
326. Sjostrom, A., and P. Zangger. Muscle spindle control during locomotor movements generated by the deafferented spinal cord. *Acta Physiol. Scand.* 97: 281–291, 1976.
327. Smith, J. L., B. Betts, V. R. Edgerton, and R. F. Zernicke. Rapid ankle extension during paw shakes: selective recruitment of fast ankle extensors. *J. Neurophysiol.* 43: 612–620, 1980.
328. Smith, J. L., N. S. Bradley, M. C. Carter, C. A. Giuliani, G. Hoy, G. F. Koshland, and R. F. Zernicke. Rhythmical movements of the hindlimbs in spinal cat: considerations for a controlling network. In: *Development and Plasticity of the Mammalian Spinal Cord*, edited by M. E. Goldberger, A. Gorio, and M. Murray. Padova: Liviana Press, 1986, p. 347–362.
329. Smith, J. L., S. H. Chung, and R. F. Zernicke. Gait-related motor pattern and hindlimb kinetics for the cat trot and gallop. *Exp. Brain Res.* 94: 308–322, 1993.
330. Smith, J. L., M. G. Hoy, G. F. Koshland, D. M. Phillips, and R. F. Zernicke. Intralimb coordination of the paw-shake response: a novel mixed synergy. *J. Neurophysiol.* 54: 1271–1281, 1985.
331. Smith, J. L., L. A. Smith, R. F. Zernicke, and M. Hoy. Locomotion in exercised and non-exercised cats cordotomized at two or twelve weeks of age. *Exp. Neurol.* 76: 393–413, 1982.
332. Sqalli-Houssaini, Y., J. R. Cazalets, and F. Clarac. Oscillatory properties of the central pattern generator for loco-

motion in neonatal rats. *J. Neurophysiol.* 70: 803–813, 1993.

333. Sqalli-Houssaini, Y., J. R. Cazalets, F. Martini, and F. Clarac. Induction of fictive locomotion by sulphur-containing amino acids in an in vitro newborn preparation. *Eur. J. Neurosci.* 5: 1226–1232, 1993.
334. Steeves, J. D., and L. M. Jordan. Localization of a descending pathway in the spinal cord which is necessary for controlled treadmill locomotion. *Neurosci. Lett.* 20: 283–288, 1980.
335. Steeves, J. D., and L. M. Jordan. Autoradiographic demonstration of the projections from the mesencephalic locomotor region. *Brain Res.* 307: 263–276, 1984.
336. Steeves, J. D., B. J. Schmidt, B. J. Skovgaard, and L. M. Jordan. Effect of noradrenaline and 5-hydroxytryptamine depletion on locomotion in the cat. *Brain Res.* 185: 349–362, 1980.
337. Stein, P. S. The vertebrate scratch reflex. In: *Neural Origin of Rhythmic Movements. Soc. Exp. Biol. Symp.*, 37, edited by A. Roberts and B. L. Roberts. Cambridge: Cambridge University Press, 1983, p. 383–403.
338. Stein, P. S. Central pattern generators in the spinal cord. In: *Handbook of the Spinal Cord*, edited by R. A. Davidoff. New York: Marcel Dekker Inc., 1984, p. 647–672.
339. Stein, R. B. Reflex modulation during locomotion: functional significance. In: *Adaptability of Human Gait*, edited by A. E. Patla. North-Holland: Elsevier Science Publishers, 1991, p. 21–36.
340. Stein, R. B., and C. Capaday. The modulation of human reflexes during functional motor tasks. *Trends Neurosci.* 11: 328–332, 1988.
341. Taylor, A., and A. Prochazka. *Muscle Receptors and Movement.* London: Macmillan, 1981, p. 1–446.
342. Terakado, Y., and T. Yamaguchi. Last-order interneurons controlling activity of elbow flexor motoneurons during forelimb fictive locomotion in the cat. *Neurosci. Lett.* 111: 292–296, 1990.
343. Thelen, E., B. D. Ulrich, and D. Niles. Bilateral coordination in human infants: stepping on a split-belt treadmill. *J. Exp. Psychol.* 13: 405–410, 1987.
344. Tokuriki, M. Electromyographic and joint-mechanical studies in quadrupedal locomotion. I. Walk. *Jpn. J. Vet. Sci.* 35: 433–446, 1973.
345. Trulson, M. E., and B. L. Jacobs. Raphe unit activity in freely moving cats: correlation with level of behavioural arousal. *Brain Res.* 163: 135–150, 1979.
346. Udo, M., H. Kamei, K. Matsukawa, and K. Tanaka. Interlimb coordination in cat locomotion investigated with perturbation. II. Correlates in neuronal activity of Deiter's cells of decerebrate walking cats. *Exp. Brain Res.* 46: 438–447, 1982.
347. Viala, D., C. Buisseret-Delmas, and J. J. Portal. An attempt to localize the lumbar locomotor generator in the rabbit using 2-deoxy-[14C]glucose autoradiography. *Neurosci. Lett.* 86: 139–143, 1988.
348. Viala, D., and P. Buser. The effects of DOPA and 5-HTP on rhythmic efferent discharges in hindlimb nerves in the rabbit. *Brain Res.* 12: 437–443, 1969.
349. Viala, D., and P. Buser. Modalités d'obtention de rythmes locomoteurs chez le lapin spinal par traitements pharmacologiques (DOPA, 5-HTP, D-amphétamine). *Brain Res.* 35: 151–165, 1971.
350. Viala, D., and C. Vidal. Evidence for distinct spinal locomotion generators supplying respectively fore- and hindlimbs in the rabbit. *Brain Res.* 155: 182–186, 1978.
351. Viala, G., and P. Buser. Inhibition des activités spinales à caractère locomoteur par une modalité particulière de stimulation somatique chez le lapin. *Exp. Brain Res.* 21: 275–284, 1974.
352. Viala, G., D. Orsal, and P. Buser. Cutaneous fiber groups involved in the inhibition of fictive locomotion in the rabbit. *Exp. Brain Res.* 33: 257–267, 1978.
353. Vidal, C., D. Viala, and P. Buser. Central locomotor programming in the rabbit. *Brain Res.* 168: 57–73, 1979.
354. Vilensky, J. A., A. M. Moore, E. Eidelberg, and J. G. Walden. Recovery of locomotion in monkeys with spinal cord lesions. *J. Mot. Behav.* 24: 288–296, 1992.
355. Wallen, P., J. T. Buchanan, S. Grillner, R. H. Hill, J. Christenson, and T. Hokfelt. Effects of 5-hydroxytryptamine on the afterhyperpolarization, spike frequency regulation, and oscillatory membrane properties in lamprey spinal cord neurons. *J. Neurophysiol.* 61: 759–768, 1989.
356. Wallen, P., and S. Grillner. *N*-Methyl-D-aspartate receptor-induced, inherent oscillatory activity in neurons active during fictive locomotion in the lamprey. *J. Neurosci.* 7: 2745–2755, 1987.
357. Walmsley, B., J. A. Hodgson, and R. E. Burke. Forces produced by medial gastrocnemius and soleus muscles during locomotion in freely moving cats. *J. Neurophysiol.* 41: 1203–1216, 1978.
358. Wand, P., A. Prochazka, and K. H. Sontag. Neuromuscular responses to gait perturbations in freely moving cats. *Exp. Brain Res.* 38: 109–114, 1980.
359. Wernig, A., and S. Muller. Laufband locomotion with body weight support improved walking in persons with severe spinal cord injuries. *Paraplegia* 30: 229–238, 1992.
360. Whiting, W. C., R. J. Gregor, R. R. Roy, and V. R. Edgerton. A technique for estimating mechanical work of individual muscles in the cat during treadmill locomotion. *J. Biomech.* 17: 685–694, 1984.
361. Widajewicz, W., B. Kably, and T. Drew. Motor cortical activity during voluntary gait modifications in the cat. II. Cells related to the hindlimbs. *J. Neurophysiol.* 72: 2070–2089, 1994.
362. Windle, W. F., and A. M. Griffin. Observations on embryonic and fetal movements of the cat. *J. Comp. Neurol.* 52: 149–188, 1931.
363. Wisleder, D., R. F. Zernicke, and J. L. Smith. Speed-related changes in hindlimb intersegmental dynamics during the swing phase of cat locomotion. *Exp. Brain Res.* 79: 651–660, 1990.
364. Yakhnitsa, I. A., A. I. Pilyavsky, and N. V. Bulgokova. Presynaptic control of afferent input during real locomotion in rats. In: *Stance and Motion: "Facts and Concepts,"* edited by V. S. Gurfinkel, M. E. Ioffe, J. Massion, and J. P. Roll. New York: Plenum Press, 1988, p. 153–161.
365. Yamaguchi, T. Descending pathways eliciting forelimb stepping in the lateral funiculus: experimental studies with stimulation and lesion of the cervical cord in decerebrate cats. *Brain Res.* 379: 125–136, 1986.
366. Yamaguchi, T. Monopodal fictive locomotion evoked by cervical cord stimulation in decerebrate cats. *Neurosci. Lett.* 74: 69–74, 1987.
367. Yamaguchi, T. Cat forelimb stepping generator. In: *Neurobiological Basis of Human Locomotion*, edited by M. Shimamura, S. Grillner, and V. R. Edgerton. Tokyo: Japan Scientific Societies Press, 1991, p. 103–115.
368. Yamaguchi, T. Muscle activity during forelimb stepping in decerebrate cats. *Jpn. J. Physiol.* 42: 489–499, 1992.

369. Yamaguchi, T. Activity of cervical neurons during forelimb fictive locomotion in decerebrate cats. *Jpn. J. Physiol.* 42: 501–514, 1992.
370. Yang, J. F., and R. B. Stein. Phase-dependent reflex reversal in human leg muscles during walking. *J. Neurophysiol.* 63: 1109–1117, 1990.
371. Yang, J. F., R. B. Stein, and K. B. James. Contribution of peripheral afferents to the activation of the soleus muscle during walking in humans. *Exp. Brain Res.* 87: 679–687, 1991.
372. Young, R. P., S. H. Scott, and G. E. Loeb. An intrinsic mechanism to stabilize posture-joint-angle-dependent moment arms of the feline ankle muscles. *Neurosci. Lett.* 145: 137–140, 1992.
373. Zangger, P. The effect of 4-aminopyridine on the spinal locomotor rhythm induced by L-Dopa. *Brain Res.* 215: 211–223, 1981.
374. Zomlefer, M. R., J. Provencher, G. Blanchette, and S. Rossignol. Electromyographic study of lumbar back muscles during locomotion in acute high decerebrate and in low spinal cats. *Brain Res.* 290: 249–260, 1984.

6. The corticospinal system: a structural framework for the central control of movement

RICHARD P. DUM | *Departments of Neurosurgery and Physiology, SUNY Health Science Center at Syracuse, Syracuse, New York*

PETER L. STRICK | *Research Service, VA Medical Center, and Departments of Neurosurgery and Physiology, SUNY Health Science Center at Syracuse, Syracuse, New York*

CHAPTER CONTENTS

THE PROVISION OF A STRUCTURAL FRAMEWORK for examining how the central nervous system (CNS) of primates plans and executes voluntary movement serves as the objective of the chapter. Central motor commands to the spinal cord originate from multiple sites (134). The chapter will focus on the various regions of the cerebral cortex that contribute to the corticospinal system, which projects to motoneurons that activate muscles and to interneurons that are involved in spinal cord reflexes. This descending system provides the cerebral cortex with direct access to spinal cord mechanisms involved in generating motor output.

A dramatic shift has occurred in our ideas about the involvement of the cerebral cortex in motor control. Multiple cortical areas in the frontal lobe are now known to be involved in the generation and control of movement. Each of these cortical areas projects directly to the spinal cord and each receives a different pattern of cortical and subcortical input. Physiological studies indicate that each of these areas contains some neurons whose activity changes in relation to simple movements. In addition, there is evidence that each motor area contains neurons with unique relations to higher-order aspects of motor behavior. Thus, we believe that individual motor areas contribute specific attributes to the planning, execution, or control of voluntary movement. This chapter will describe the relevant anatomical and physiological evidence that has led to this new view of cortical motor function.

Due to the wide scope of this chapter, some issues will be considered only in general terms. We will concentrate on new perspectives that have resulted from contemporary primate studies, most of which have been published since the last edition of the *Handbook of Physiology, Section 1: The Nervous System* (28). For more detailed information on specific issues, the reader will be referred to pertinent reviews. The corticospinal system has been the subject of a recent book (190), and several recent reviews on this and related topics are available (e.g., 10, 38, 73, 94, 220, 236, 239).

HISTORICAL OVERVIEW

Classically, the primary motor cortex was viewed as the major, if not the sole, source of central command signals for the generation and control of movement. Other motor areas were thought to express their functions largely through interconnections with the primary motor cortex. This led to a hierarchical view of cortical organization in which the highest level was attributed to a region of the frontal lobe that was anterior to the primary motor cortex (M1) and termed the "premotor" cortex [Fig. 6.1; (e.g., 67)]. This cortical region was considered to be a center for the integration of complex skilled movements (32, 69, 109, 110). Lesions of premotor cortex in subhuman primates caused "a disorganization of more highly integrated voluntary movements producing a state akin to apraxia in man" (67; see also 109, 110). The output of the premotor cortex was believed to be sent to the primary motor cortex where the specific commands for movement were generated (e.g., 32, 68; for reviews, see 66, 94, 236,

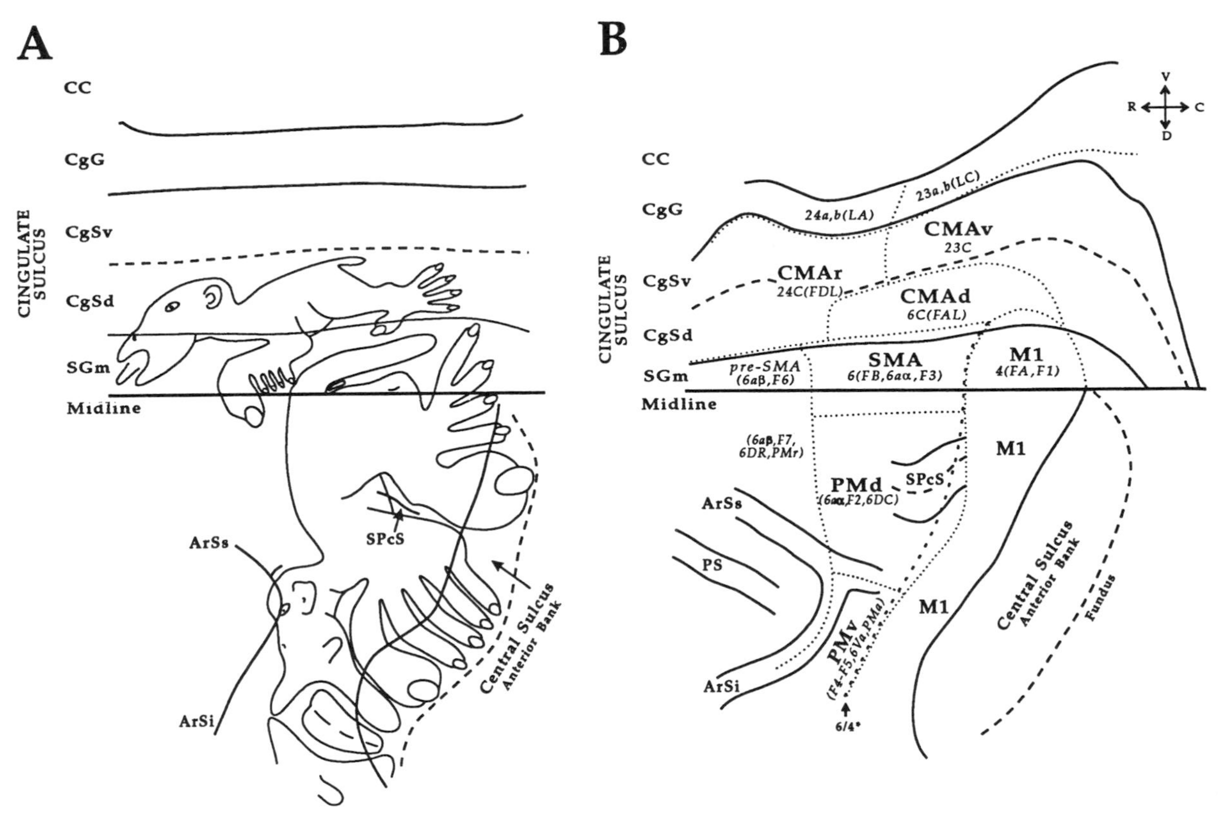

FIG. 6.1. Summary maps of the motor areas in the frontal lobe. *A*, Body representation in the frontal lobe based on surface stimulation. The medial wall is reflected upward to display the body map of the supplementary motor area (SMA) on the same figure as the body map of the precentral gyrus. According to Woolsey et al. (242), the SMA extends onto the dorsal bank of the cingulate sulcus. These authors did not explore the motor representation on either the ventral bank of the cingulate sulcus or the cingulate gyrus. [Adapted from Woolsey, et al. (242)]. *B*, An unfolded reconstruction of frontal lobe with the medial wall of the hemisphere reflected upward. The location of the arm representation in each motor area is indicated by the *lettered ellipses*. The boundaries between cytoarchitectonic areas are indicated by *dotted lines*. A *dashed line* indicates the fundus of the cingulate sulcus. [Adapted from He, Dum, and Strick (92, 93). Reprinted by permission of the Society for Neuroscience.] ArSi, arcuate sulcus, inferior limb; ArSs, arcuate sulcus, superior limb; CC, corpus callosum; CgG, cingulate gyrus; CgSd, cingulate sulcus, dorsal bank; CgSv, cingulate sulcus, ventral bank; CMAd, caudal cingulate motor area, dorsal bank; CMAv, caudal cingulate motor area, ventral bank; CMAr, rostral cingulate motor area; M1, primary motor cortex; PMd, dorsal premotor area; PMv, ventral premotor area; pre-SMA, pre-supplementary motor area; SPcS, superior precentral sulcus; SGm, superior frontal gyrus, medial wall; SMA, supplementary motor area.

239). Thus, the generation of motor commands was thought to proceed in a serial, hierarchical fashion.

CURRENT VIEWPOINT

In the past 15 years, our ideas about the organization and function of the cortical motor areas have undergone considerable revision. It is now clear that the cortical region originally designated as "premotor" is functionally heterogeneous and composed of multiple, spatially separate "premotor areas." In fact, the frontal lobe of monkeys contains at least six premotor areas that project directly to the primary motor cortex (for review, see 54, 55). Perhaps more importantly, each of the six premotor areas, like the primary motor cortex, projects directly to the spinal cord (e.g., 54, 55, 92, 93, 106, 148, 164, 173, 226). The number of corticospinal neurons in the premotor areas actually equals or exceeds the number in the primary motor cortex (55).

These findings raise serious questions about the utility of viewing the primary motor cortex as the "upper motoneuron" or "final common pathway" for the central control of movement (94, 134). They suggest that the premotor areas are, in some respects, at the same level of hierarchical organization as the primary motor cortex. Indeed, each premotor area appears to have the potential to influence the control of movement not only at the level of the primary motor cortex but also more directly at the level of the spinal cord (54, 55). Thus, each premotor area, along with the primary motor cortex, may represent a separate source of "central command signals" for the generation and control of movement. In the next section, we will describe the location and organization of each of these cortical motor areas.

FUNCTIONAL ANATOMY

Primary Motor Cortex

Motor Maps—Electrical Stimulation of the Cortical Surface. The primary motor cortex (M1) has long been defined physiologically as the cortical region where isolated movements of different body parts can be evoked at the lowest threshold of electrical stimulation (e.g., 136, 144, 156, 181, 242). We will only present a brief overview of M1 and its identification here (for more complete reviews, see 10, 94, 190). Although the precise anterior and posterior extent of M1 has been somewhat controversial, it is generally agreed that M1 occupies much of the anterior bank of the central sulcus and extends up onto the precentral gyrus (Fig. 6.1). This region corresponds to cytoarchitectonic area 4, which is distinguished by the presence of giant pyramidal shaped neurons in the fifth cortical layer (e.g., 27, 231, 232). Area 4 is differentiated from adjacent somatic sensory areas by the absence of a granular layer 4.

A single "motor map" of the body surface has been defined in M1 based on the movements evoked by electrically stimulating different sites within it [Fig. 6.1; (242; for review, see 94, 190)]. The face, arm, trunk, and leg are represented in a lateral to medial sequence along the central sulcus. In general, stimulation at caudal sites in M1 (in the anterior bank of the central sulcus) evokes contractions of distal limb musculature, whereas stimulation at rostral sites in M1 evokes contractions of more proximal body musculature.

Motor Maps—Intracortical Electrical Stimulation. The use of microelectrodes to stimulate and map the motor responses elicited from the cortex (e.g., 14) has modified our view of body representation in M1. Intracortical stimulation has confirmed the overall topography of face, arm, and leg representation as described above [Fig. 6.2; (6, 14, 51, 86, 99, 102, 104, 112, 136, 154, 172, 200, 218, 241)]. Murphy and his colleagues (136, 162) presented a modified view of how the limbs are mapped in area 4. In particular, they found that the representation of the proximal arm (elbow and shoulder) was located medial, rostral, and lateral to a central core of distal forelimb representation (fingers and wrist). At the borders of each representation, movements of adjacent joints were intermingled. They emphasized, as have subsequent studies using intracortical stimulation, that the same movement and/or contractions of muscles acting about the same joint can be evoked from multiple, spatially separate sites. In some studies (6, 51, 102, 104), even more complex patterns of muscle activation were observed. For example, Humphrey and Reed (104) found that intracortical stimulation in one region of M1 evoked reciprocal activation of wrist muscles, whereas stimulation at another region of M1 evoked co-contraction of the same muscles. It has been proposed that the overlap in the representation of different joints and the presence of multiple representations of a movement enables M1 to generate multiple synergies among muscles acting at the same or different joints (14, 51, 102, 136).

Representation of Movements or Muscles? There has been a longstanding controversy about whether movements or muscles are represented at given sites within the cortex (e.g., 185). The technique of intracortical stimulation, as applied in most mapping studies, cannot add much to this discussion for two

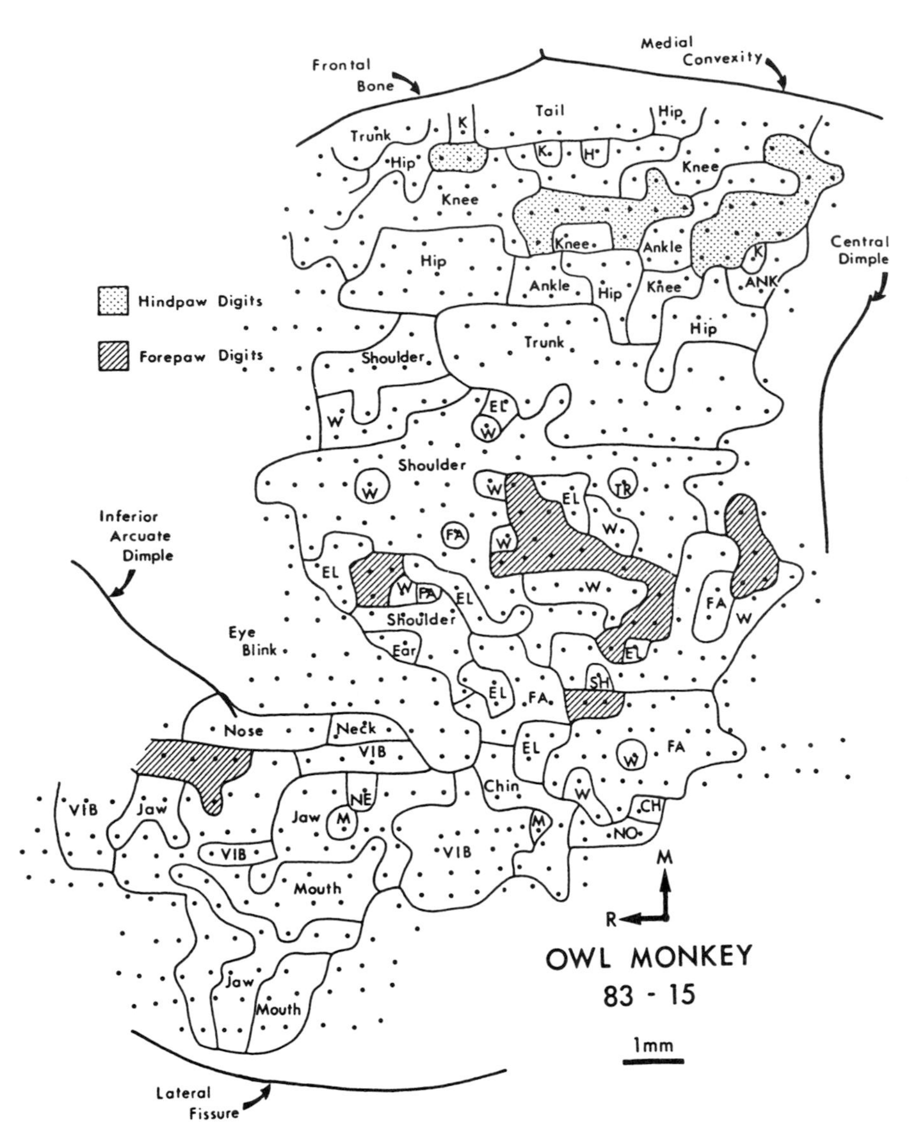

FIG. 6.2. Body map of the M1, lateral premotor cortex, and the SMA in an owl monkey as defined by intracortical stimulation. Electrode penetration sites that evoked movements at currents up to 30 μA are indicated by *dots*. The enclosed cortical regions indicate penetrations where movements of the same body part were evoked. K, knee; H, hip; ANK, ankle; W, wrist; EL, elbow; TR, trunk; FA, forearm; SH, shoulder; CH, chin; NO, nose; M, mouth; VIB, vibrissae; NE, neck. [From Gould, et al. (86), Copyright © 1986 by Wiley-Liss, Inc. Reprinted by permission of John Wiley & Sons, Inc.]

reasons. First, intracortical stimulation activates clusters of neurons rather than single neurons. Second, those applying this technique have used trains of stimuli that primarily lead to synaptic rather than direct activation of cortical neurons (11, 111; see also 141, 163).

Perhaps more relevant to the issue of muscle vs. movement representation are the anatomical and physiological studies that have examined the branching patterns of single corticospinal neurons. Physiological observations indicate that a significant fraction of corticospinal neurons (43%) project to multiple segments of spinal cord (208). Some of these corticospinal axons terminate in several motor nuclei in the spinal cord. In anatomical studies, Shinoda and co-workers (207) demonstrated that corticospinal axons can branch widely and terminate in up to four different motor nuclei (Fig. 6.3).

In general, these observations are consistent with the results of Fetz and his colleagues (39, 62; see also 29; for review, see 38), who used a novel application of the post spike–triggered averaging technique to study the branching patterns of single corticomotoneuronal (CM) cells (Fig. 6.4). They constructed averages of muscle activity triggered from the spikes of single CM cells. These averages demonstrated that a CM cell is typically connected to more than one muscle. In some cases, single CM cells could facilitate as many as six different muscles. Three major patterns of connectivity were observed: facilitation of agonists, facilitation of agonists with reciprocal suppression of antagonists, and pure suppression (Fig. 6.5). Facilitation was generally limited to muscles with synergistic actions, such as flexion or extension of a joint. Therefore, although CM cells generally facilitate more than one muscle, the "muscle field" of a single cell seems to be quite confined, facilitating only muscles that produce simple movements.

The branching of CM cells that facilitated intrinsic finger muscles tended to be more restricted (29) than

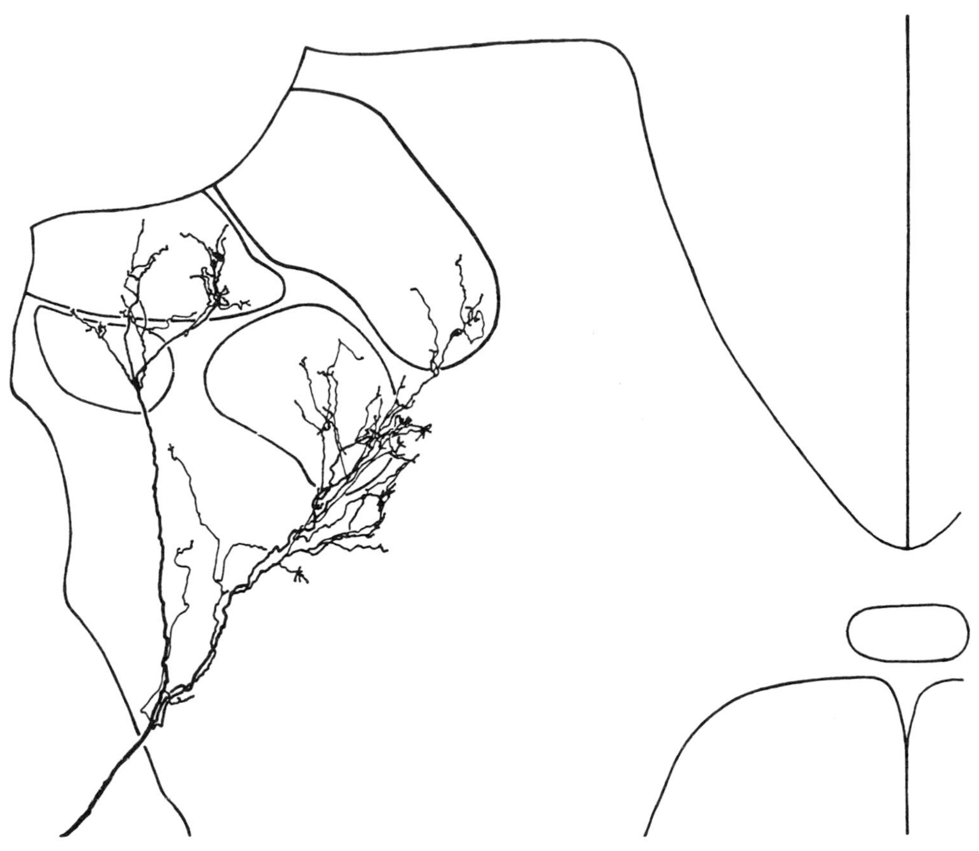

FIG. 6.3. Terminal distribution of a single corticospinal axon to several spinal motor nuclei. A single corticospinal axon originating from the "hand area" of the primary motor cortex of the monkey was reconstructed from 12 serial transverse sections at C7. Motoneurons in the two upper motor nuclei were identified by retrograde transport of HRP from the ulnar nerve. The branches of this corticospinal axon projected to at least four different motoneuron groups. Terminal boutons in close contact with the proximal dendrites of some HRP-filled motoneurons could be identified in three of them. [From Shinoda, Yokata, and Futami (207). Reprinted by permission of Elsevier Science, Ireland.]

those that facilitated wrist and extrinsic fingers muscles (62, 120). For 51% of the CM cells that innervated intrinsic hand muscles, Buys et al. (29) were able to detect facilitation in only a single muscle. Although sampling more muscles may have uncovered additional branches, this observation suggests that some CM cells are specialized to control individual finger movements.

Physiological studies of corticospinal branching patterns also observed that small clusters of neurons tended to send at least one of their branches to the same motoneuron pool (39, 208). This may explain why threshold stimulation of some cortical sites evoked contractions of a single muscle (e.g., 14). It raises the possibility that a framework for "muscle" representation exists at the level of small clusters of neurons. Needless to say, the longstanding controversy about representation in the motor cortex has not as yet been resolved.

Irrespective of what is represented, it has been proposed that the size of a body part in a motor map (and sensory maps as well) is influenced by the use of that body part (see 186). Thus, the map in M1 is thought to be plastic and capable of modification based on experience (52, 108, 171, 172, 199). There has also been considerable interest in synaptic plasticity in M1 and its potential relation to motor learning (10, 12). The issue of changes in M1 related to plasticity and motor learning is important but beyond the scope of the present review.

Physiological Specialization within M1. Another change in our view of M1 is the growing realization that this cortical area is not a homogeneous field. Based on a physiological analysis of the hand representation in a New World primate, the squirrel monkey, Strick and Preston (218, 219) proposed that M1 contains two maps of the hand (fingers and wrist) (Fig. 6.6). In the caudal hand representation, neurons were driven by peripheral input predominantly from cutaneous afferents. In contrast, neurons in the rostral hand representation were driven

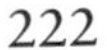

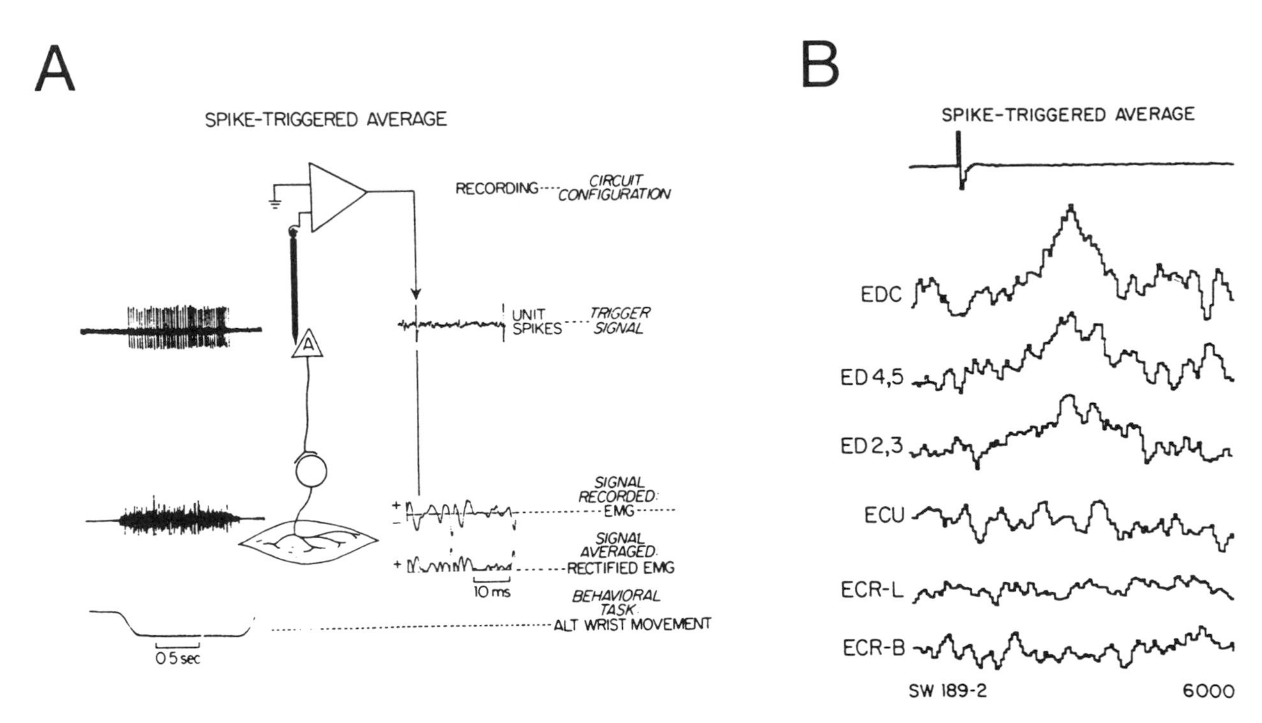

FIG. 6.4. Postspike facilitation by corticomotoneuronal cells. *A*, Summary of experimental technique for compiling spike-triggered averages. The microelectrode recorded activity of a task-related cell. Sample records show activity of an extension-related corticomotoneuronal cell, a wrist extensor muscle, and wrist position during an extension movement. Fast sweep shows unit spikes with raw EMG and full-wave rectified EMG. Full-wave rectified EMG activity was averaged over an interval from 5 ms before to 25 ms after the trigger event. [Adapted from Cheney and Fetz (39).] *B*, Postspike facilitation profiles evoked by a single corticomotoneuronal cell. This cell facilitated three of six wrist extensor muscles, with the strongest relationship being at the top. [Adapted from Cheney and Fetz (37). Reprinted by permission of the American Physiological Society.]

by peripheral input largely from muscle and/or joints. Motor maps and cytoarchitecture suggest the presence of multiple forelimb areas in another New World primate, the owl monkey, although the distribution of peripheral afferent input to these regions has not been examined [Fig. 6.2; (86, 212)].

Cutaneous and deep input also tend to innervate different portions of the forelimb representation in M1 of the macaque, an Old World primate. The caudal part of M1, located in the depths of the central sulcus, receives afferent input primarily from cutaneous sources. The rostral part of M1, located on the surface of the precentral gyrus, receives input largely from muscle and/or joints (137, 187). Hand movements can be evoked from both the rostral-surface and caudal-sulcus regions of M1 (200). Anatomical studies have shown that these rostral and caudal regions of M1 receive their densest input from different subdivisions of the ventrolateral thalamus (discussed later).

Inhomogeneities in M1 are not limited to the classical "arm area." A comparable sorting of peripheral afferent input has been seen in the hindlimb representation of the macaque M1, where the caudal portion receives predominantly cutaneous input and the rostral portion predominantly deep input (223). In addition, an analysis of the origin of corticospinal projections to different segments of the spinal cord suggests that another forelimb representation may exist along the mediolateral axis, at the junction of Woolsey's arm and leg areas (92). Thus, the internal organization of maps in M1 is clearly more complicated than previously thought. Strick and Preston (219) have suggested that these inhomogeneities represent functional specializations within M1 that have developed to deal with the specific demands of certain motor tasks. For example, the hand area of M1 that receives peripheral input largely from cutaneous receptors may be specialized to deal with tasks involving active palpation of objects. At this point, the functional consequences of the inhomogeneities within M1 remain to be determined.

Premotor Areas in the Frontal Lobe

Originally, the "premotor cortex" of primates was defined as the region of frontal agranular cortex

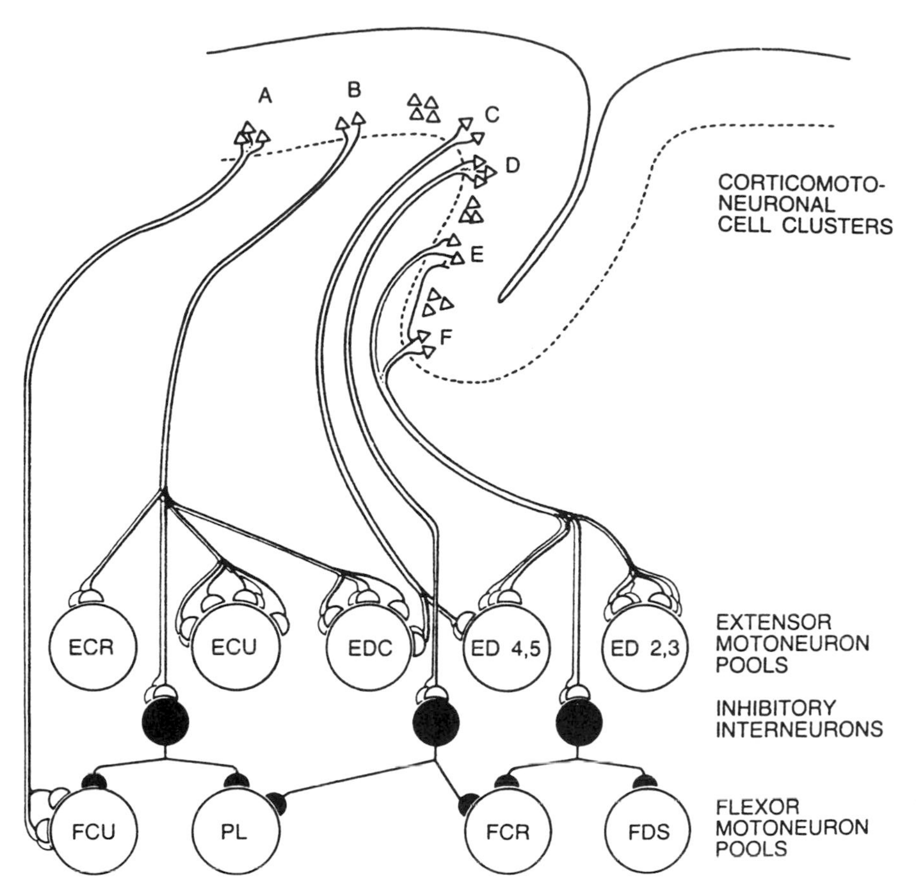

FIG. 6.5. Diagram of the simplest circuits that may mediate the basic pattern of a corticomotoneuronal cell's influence on wrist flexor and extensor motoneurons. Correlational evidence indicates that cells may facilitate agonist muscles with no effect on antagonist muscle (*A, C*); facilitate agonist muscles and simultaneously suppress antagonist muscles through a reciprocal inhibitory pathway (*B, E,* and *F*); or suppress certain muscles with no effect on their antagonists (*D*). Clustering and interconnection of cells with common targets is also suggested by these experiments. [From Cheney, Fetz, and Palmer (39). Reprinted by permission of the American Physiological Society.]

(area 6) that was located rostral to M1 (e.g., 67, 68). This region corresponds to area 6 on the lateral surface and the adjacent medial wall of the hemisphere (27, 231, 232). This cytoarchitectonic definition resulted in a premotor cortex that was functionally heterogeneous. For example, consistent and well-localized movements were evoked by surface electrical stimulation only in the part of area 6 that is located on the medial wall of the hemisphere. In fact, a complete "motor" map of the body could be defined in the medial part of the premotor cortex, and this region was termed the supplementary motor area (SMA) [Fig. 6.1; (182, 242)]. Further attempts to define the precise location and boundaries of premotor cortex using electrical stimulation of the cortical surface or cytoarchitectonic criteria have failed to produce a consensus. Thus, the location and even the existence of premotor cortex has been controversial (e.g., 17, 67, 101, 151, 239, 242).

Connections with M1. Our approach to the problem of determining the location of the premotor cortex has been operationally to define it as those regions in the frontal lobe that have direct projections to M1. According to this definition, premotor cortex is heterogeneous and is comprised of multiple, spatially separate areas [Figs. 6.1 and 6.7; (54, 55, 81, 213; see also 80, 126, 140, 143, 159, 161, 178)]. For example, the arm area of the primary motor cortex receives inputs from six cortical areas. Two of these regions are on the lateral surface of the hemisphere: the ventral premotor area (PMv) and the dorsal premotor area (PMd) (Fig. 6.1). The PMv includes a lateral portion of area 6 that is located ventral to the fundus of the arcuate spur, and it extends into the caudal bank of the inferior limb of the arcuate sulcus. The PMd lies in the portion of area 6 that is dorsal to the fundus of the arcuate spur and caudal to the genu of the arcuate sulcus. It includes

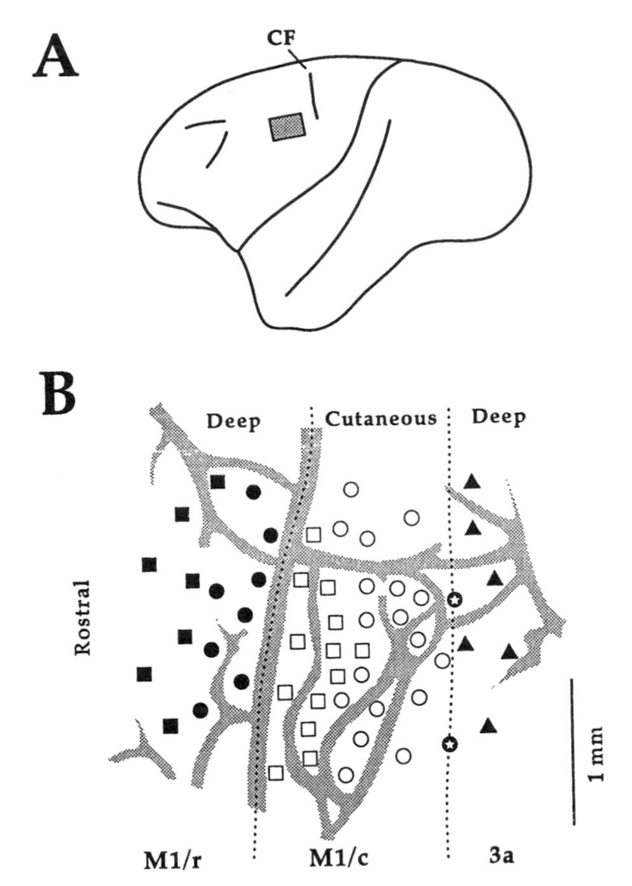

FIG. 6.6. Sensorimotor map in the primary motor cortex. *A*, The cortical region explored with intracortical stimulation is indicated on a lateral view of a squirrel monkey's brain. CF, central fissure. *B*, Map of the movements evoked by intracortical stimulation and the modality of the somatosensory input at the same sites within the arm representation of the primary motor cortex of a squirrel monkey. Microelectrode penetrations that encountered neurons receiving somatosensory input from "deep" receptors are indicated by *filled symbols*. Those sites that received peripheral input from "cutaneous" receptors are indicated by *open symbols*. *Circles* indicate penetrations where finger movements were evoked, and *squares* represent wrist movement sites. No movements were elicited at less than 30 μA at sites indicated by *triangles*. Major surface blood vessels are *shaded*. Histological analysis showed that the area 3a-4 border was located just rostral to the region containing *triangles*. *Dotted lines* indicate borders between physiologically defined cortical regions. M1/c, caudal region of the primary motor cortex; M1/r, rostral region of the primary motor cortex. [Adapted from Strick and Preston (219). Reprinted by permission of the American Physiological Society.]

the region within and adjacent to the superior precentral sulcus.

The other four premotor areas are on the medial wall of the hemisphere: the SMA, the rostral cingulate motor area (CMAr), the caudal cingulate motor area on the dorsal bank (CMAd), and the caudal cingulate motor area on the ventral bank (CMAv) (Figs. 6.1 and 6.7). The SMA is located within area 6 on the mesial surface of the superior frontal gyrus, and it is positioned just rostral to the hindlimb representation in M1. The CMAr lies within area 24c on the dorsal and ventral banks of the cingulate sulcus at levels anterior to the genu of the arcuate sulcus. The CMAd occupies area 6c largely on the dorsal bank of the cingulate sulcus at levels caudal to the genu of the arcuate. The CMAv lies just below the CMAd and is located in area 23c largely on the ventral bank of the cingulate sulcus. It should be apparent from this description that the anatomical organization of premotor cortex as a whole is more complicated than previously recognized (for reviews, see 68, 101, 220, 236, 239, 242).

Several investigators have attempted to determine the presence of body maps in the premotor areas based on their projections to different portions of M1. All the premotor areas, except for the PMv, are interconnected with the leg area of M1 (81, 149, 159, 160, 161, 213; see, however, 92). Surprisingly, only three of the premotor areas (the PMv, the SMA, and the CMAr) have representations of the face (81, 159, 160, 161, 213). Thus, according to this criterion, all body parts appear to be represented only in the SMA and the CMAr. Connections with M1 also have been used to examine the internal organization of arm representation in each premotor area; however, no clearly segregated topography was discovered (225). In this regard, an analysis of corticospinal projections to different segmental levels has been more informative (see below and 92, 93).

Corticospinal Origin. Although "area 6" sends as many axons to the spinal cord as M1 (198), the location of these corticospinal neurons in the premotor cortex was unclear. Indeed, an early attempt to locate these neurons in the SMA was unsuccessful (e.g., 48). As a consequence, the premotor areas were thought to influence the generation and control of movement largely through their direct connections with M1, projections to the origin of reticulospinal pathways, and their involvement in basal ganglia and cerebellar loops.

More recent studies have demonstrated that each of the premotor areas that innervate M1 also project directly to the spinal cord [Figs. 6.8 and 6.9; (54, 55, 92, 93; see also 21, 33, 53, 106, 121, 147, 148, 164, 173, 226)]. This includes the two premotor areas on the lateral surface of the hemisphere (PMv and PMd), as well as the four premotor areas on the medial wall (SMA, CMAr, CMAd, and CMAv). In fact, there is a striking correspondence between the distribution of corticospinal neurons in the premotor areas and the distribution of neurons in the premotor areas that project to M1 (compare Figs. 6.7 and

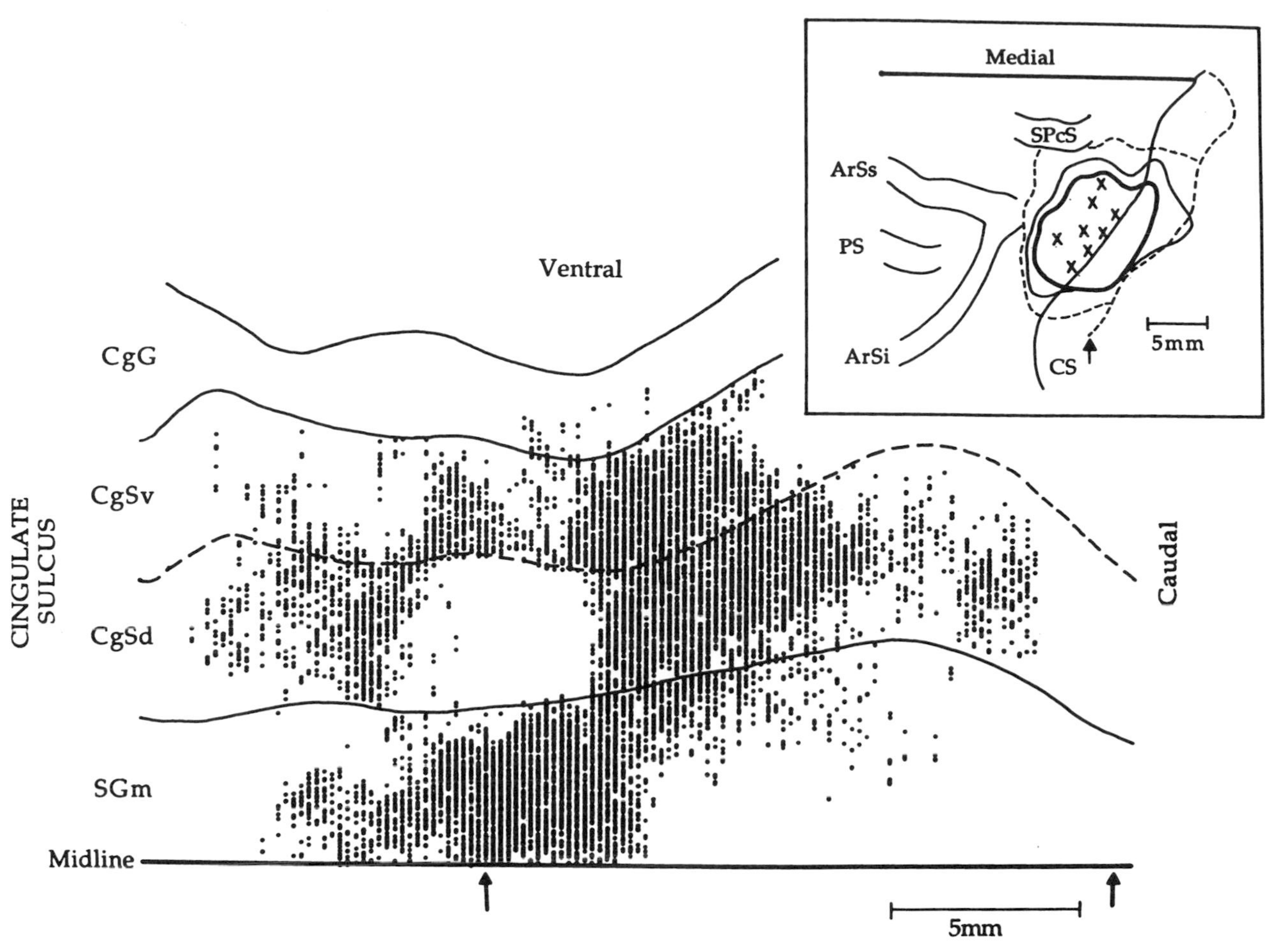

FIG. 6.7. Map of cortical neurons projecting from premotor areas on medial wall to arm region of primary motor cortex. WGA-HRP was injected into the arm region of the primary motor cortex. The spread of tracer is indicated on the flattened reconstruction of the frontal lobe (*inset at upper right*). Xs mark the site of needle penetration into the cortex. A *heavy line* encircles the densest region of reaction product, and a *lighter line* indicates the "halo" that surrounded it. The *dashed line* encircles the region of almost continuous cell labeling that surrounded the injection site. Every fourth section was used to reconstruct the distribution of labeled neurons (*dots*) on the medial wall. The genu of the arcuate sulcus (*left arrow*) and the junction of the central sulcus with the midline (*right arrow*) are indicated. ArSi, arcuate sulcus, inferior limb; ArSs, arcuate sulcus, superior limb; CgG, cingulate gyrus; CgSd, singulate sulcus, dorsal bank; CgSv, singulate sulcus, ventral bank; SPcS, superior precentral sulcus; SGm, superior frontal gyrus, medial wall. Note that neurons projecting to the arm region of the primary motor cortex are located in the same regions that project to cervical segments of the spinal cord (cf. Fig. 6.8). [From Dum and Strick (55). Reprinted by permission of the Society of Neuroscience.]

6.8). These observations indicate that all the premotor areas have the potential to influence the generation and control of movement directly at the level of the spinal cord, as well as at the level of the primary motor cortex.

The frontal lobe contains 60%–73% of the total number of corticospinal neurons (198, 226; Dum and Strick, unpublished observations). When considered together, the number of corticospinal neurons in the premotor areas equals or exceeds the number in M1 (55, 93; see also 226). Not surprisingly, the largest percentage of corticospinal neurons in the frontal lobe is located in M1 (43%). Among the premotor areas, the largest percentages are in the SMA (15%), PMd (15%), and CMAd (9%). The remaining premotor areas (PMv, CMAr, and CMAv) each have approximately 6%–7% of the total number of corticospinal neurons in the frontal lobe. In addition, the premotor areas collectively comprise more than 60% of the cortical area in the frontal lobe, which projects to the spinal cord (55). Furthermore, each of the premotor areas, like M1, contains local regions with a high density of corticospinal neurons [Fig. 6.8; (see also 55, 92, 93)]. The relative density of corticospinal neurons in two of the premotor areas, CMAd and CMAv, is indistinguishable from that in M1. The density of corticospinal neurons may be related to the ability of an area to generate

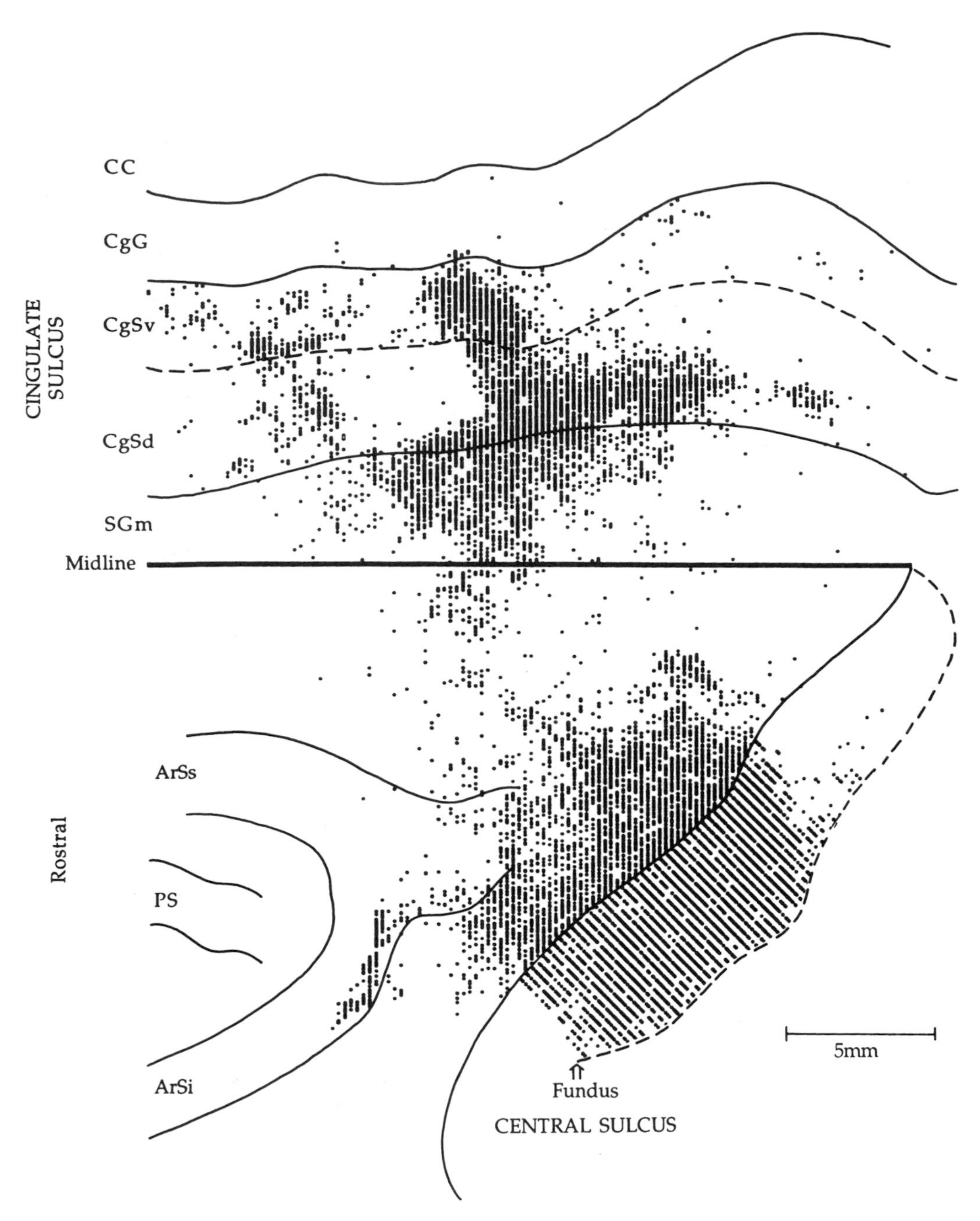

FIG. 6.8. Map of corticospinal neurons in the frontal lobe projecting to the cervical segments of the spinal cord. The WGA-HRP injection site included all segments located between the fourth cervical and the second thoracic segments. Each labeled cell is represented by a *dot*. Every fourth section was used to construct this map. ArSi, arcuate sulcus, inferior limb; ArSs, arcuate sulcus, superior limb; CgG, cingulate gyrus; CgSd, singulate sulcus, dorsal bank; CgSv, singulate sulcus, ventral bank; SPcS, superior precentral sulcus; SGm, superior frontal gyrus, medial wall. [From Dum and Strick (55). Reprinted by permission of the Society for Neuroscience.]

movement, either naturally or following electrical stimulation. Taken together, these observations lead to the conclusion that the premotor areas make a substantial contribution to the corticospinal system.

In general, corticospinal neurons have been subdivided into two categories—large cells with fast axonal conduction velocities and smaller cells with slower axonal conduction velocities. Most corticospinal neurons lie in the small size range (81%) (55, 103, 114, 164). The majority (79%) of the large corticospinal neurons is located in M1 (55). However, large corticospinal neurons are found in the PMv, PMd, SMA, and CMAd. The actual distribution of cell size for corticospinal neurons in the PMv and

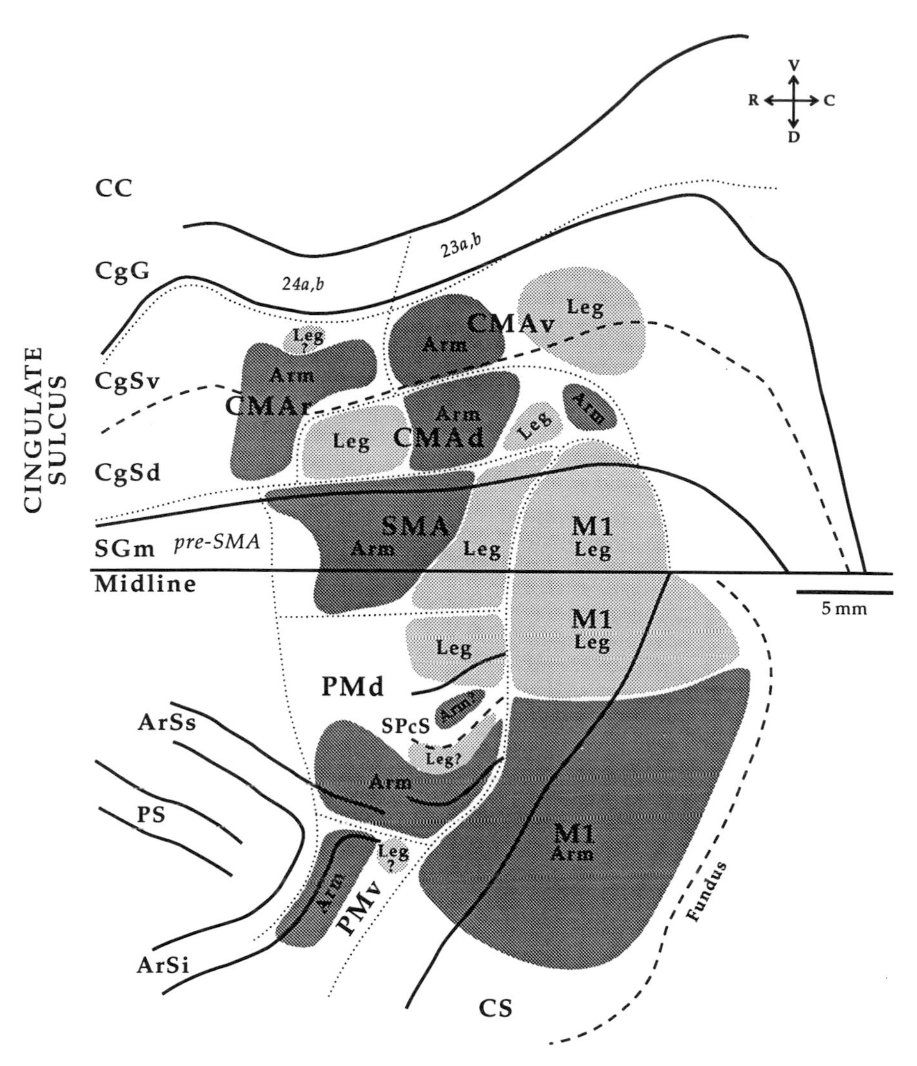

FIG. 6.9. Summary of "arm" and "leg" representation in each motor area in the frontal lobe. In this map, the arm representations are based on the location of neurons that project to upper and lower cervical segments. The leg representations are based on the location of neurons that project to lower lumbosacral segments. ArSi, arcuate sulcus, inferior limb; ArSs, arcuate sulcus, superior limb; CgG, cingulate gyrus; CgSd, singulate sulcus, dorsal bank; CgSv, singulate sulcus, ventral bank; SPcS, superior precentral sulcus; SGm, superior frontal gyrus, medial wall. [Adapted from He, Dum, and Strick (92, 93). Reprinted by permission of the Society for Neuroscience.]

PMd is not unlike that in M1 (55). Hence, even in this respect, some of the premotor areas have much in common with M1.

Body Maps—Anatomical Evidence. Anatomical and physiological studies reveal that single corticospinal neurons innervate a limited number of segments in the spinal cord (92, 208). Only 0.2% of the corticospinal neurons that project to cervical and lumbosacral segments branch and innervate both levels of the spinal cord (93). Similarly, only 5% of the corticospinal neurons that project to cervical levels branch and project to both upper and lower cervical segments (93). This limited branching has enabled an analysis of the origin of corticospinal projections to different segmental levels to reveal features of body maps in the premotor areas (92, 93). For example, all of the premotor areas, except for the PMv, project to cervical and to lumbosacral segments of the spinal cord (Fig. 6.9). In the PMv, a tiny patch of corticospinal neurons project to the thoracic but not the lumbar segments (92). In four of the premotor areas (PMd, SMA, CMAd, and CMAv), there is little overlap in the regions that project to cervical segments with those that project to lumbosacral segments. Since cervical segments are known to control arm movements (whereas lumbosacral segments are known to control leg movements) these anatomical findings suggest that these four premotor areas have separate arm and leg representations. Furthermore, the arm and leg representations in each of these premotor areas appear to be as distinct as those in M1. On the other hand, the few corticospinal neurons in the CMAr that project to lumbosacral levels overlap considerably with those projecting to cervical segments. This finding implies that the CMAr has a representation of the arm and leg, but these representations are not separate. These conclusions about arm and leg representations in the premotor areas are generally in accord with other anatomical and physiological mapping studies (81, 106, 144, 156, 159, 161, 213).

An analysis of corticospinal projections to upper and lower cervical segments has been used to examine the organization of proximal and distal representation within the premotor areas (92, 93). With some exceptions, lower cervical segments are primarily involved in the control of the distal forelimb movements, and upper cervical segments are largely involved in the control of the neck and proximal forelimb movements (for a discussion of the topographic organization of the spinal cord motor nuclei, see 92). All of the premotor areas except the PMv project to upper and to lower cervical segments. These results imply that each of these premotor areas has the potential to influence the control of both distal and proximal arm movements.

Although there is some overlap, the regions of each premotor area that project most densely to upper cervical segments are separate from the regions that project most densely to lower cervical segments. This is also the case for M1. Thus, the proximal and distal representations of the arm are as separate in the premotor areas as they are in M1. Some of the premotor areas are also like M1 in the relative amount of cortex allotted to projections to upper and lower cervical segments (92, 93). For example, the amount of M1 cortex occupied by corticospinal neurons that project to lower cervical segments is equal to that occupied by corticospinal neurons that project to upper cervical segments. This finding is consistent with the classical view that, even though the actual size of the hand is small, its representation in M1 is expanded relative to that of more proximal body parts. This expansion is thought to reflect the special involvement of M1 in the generation and control of highly skilled hand movements. Similarly, in the premotor areas on the medial wall, the amount of cortex occupied by neurons that project to lower cervical segments is either equal to (SMA) or greater than (CMAd, CMAv, and CMAr) that projecting to upper cervical segments. This implies that, for these premotor areas, the distal representation of the arm is as large as, if not larger than, the proximal representation of the arm. The opposite is true for the PMd and PMv, where the amount of cortex that projects to upper cervical segments is larger than that projecting to lower cervical segments. Viewed as a whole, these findings suggest that it is no longer appropriate to consider the premotor areas as simply concerned with body orientation and the control of proximal and axial body musculature. Instead, the premotor areas, particularly those on the medial wall, may play a prominent role in the generation and control of distal arm movements. Thus, the primary motor cortex does not appear to be the sole source of central commands for controlling all aspects of arm movement.

Body Maps—Physiological Evidence. Intracortical stimulation appears to be capable of evoking movements from each of the premotor areas. Most investigators report that the average threshold for evoking movement from stimulation in a premotor area is generally higher than that in M1, and that fewer "positive" sites are found in the premotor areas than in M1 (e.g., 144, 156, 233). Body maps of the premotor areas that are generated from the movements evoked by intracortical stimulation correspond in most respects to those defined by anatomical experiments. However, most of the premotor areas have not been mapped extensively with intracortical stimulation.

The topographical organization of the SMA is the most thoroughly determined of premotor areas (e.g., 144, 147, 156, 182, 242). The use of intracortical stimulation has permitted identification of distinct regions of face, arm, and leg representation (Fig. 6.10), but the internal organization of each representation has not been consistent among studies (144, 147, 156). This may be due to the fact that complex movements (three joints or noncontiguous joints) are evoked at some sites in the SMA, making determination of a body map difficult. The organization of arm representation within the SMA has been explored most extensively (144, 147, 156). Sites where movements of the distal forelimb were evoked tended to be located ventrally in the SMA, whereas sites where movements at more proximal joints were evoked tended to be located more dorsally. These observations correlate with the differential origin of corticospinal projections from the SMA to lower and upper cervical segments (93).

Just rostral to the SMA, on the mesial part of the superior frontal gyrus, is a region termed the pre-SMA [Figs. 6.1 and 6.9; (152; area F6 in 144; see also 2, 195)]. Intracortical stimulation here does not evoke movements (2, 152), except at some sites when longer trains of stimuli and higher currents are used (144). Arm movements are virtually the only

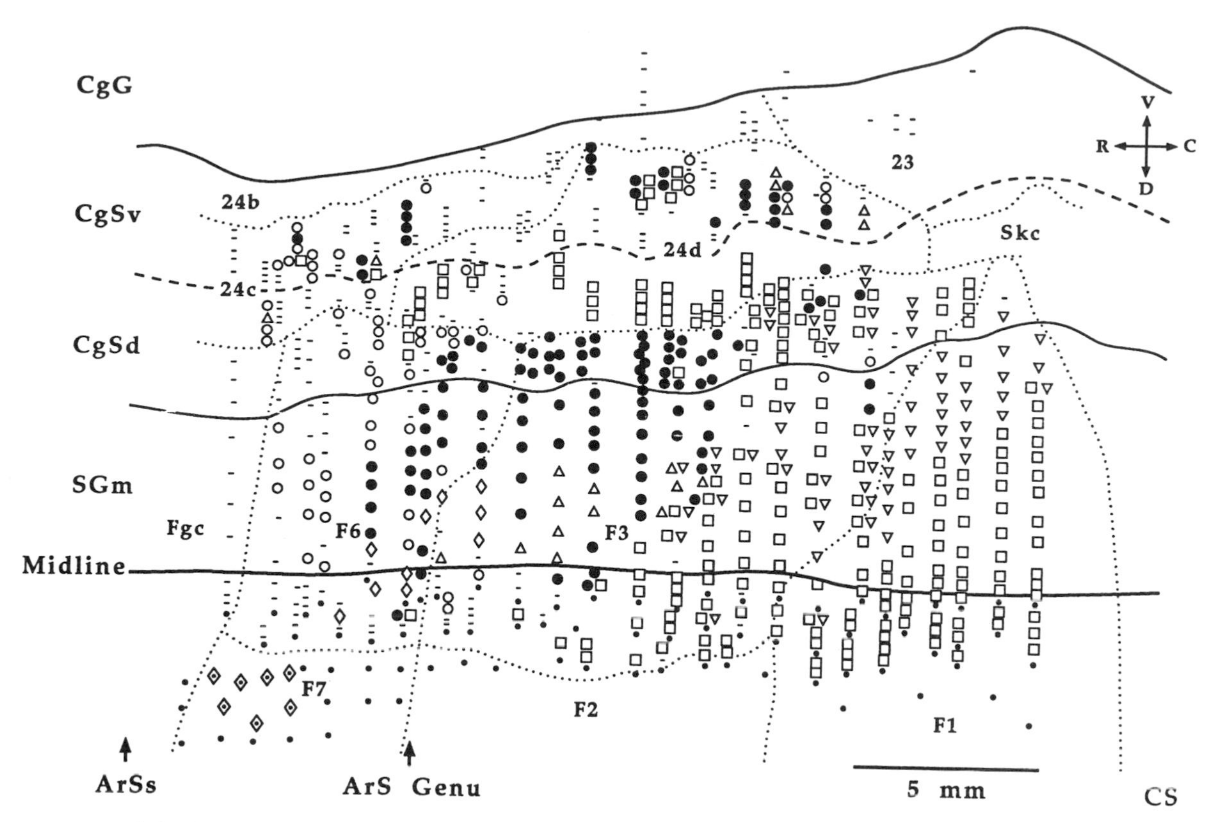

FIG. 6.10. Map of the body movements evoked by intracortical stimulation of the motor areas on the medial wall of the hemisphere of a macaque monkey. All movements were contralateral to the stimulated hemisphere. Key to movements—*diamonds*, face; *diamonds with dot*, eye; *filled circles*, arm; *open circles*, arm movements evoked with long train stimulation; *open squares*, leg; *open triangles*, neck and upper truck; *inverted triangles*, lower trunk and tail; *dash*, no response; *dot*, penetration site. ArSi, arcuate sulcus, inferior limb; ArSs, arcuate sulcus, superior limb; CgG, cingulate gyrus; CgSd, singulate sulcus, dorsal bank; CgSv, singulate sulcus, ventral bank; SPcS, superior precentral sulcus; SGm, superior frontal gyrus, medial wall. [Adapted from Luppino et al. (144). Copyright © 1991 by Wiley-Liss, Inc. Reprinted by permission of John Wiley & Sons, Inc.]

movement evoked from the pre-SMA, and these movements typically involved multiple joints, and often resembled natural movements. Movements evoked from the pre-SMA were usually slow, moving the arm from one position to another, rather than the brief, twitch-like contractions evoked from M1 or responsive sites in the premotor areas. The need for higher currents and longer stimulus trains is consistent with the fact that the pre-SMA lacks direct projections to the spinal cord (55, 93) and to M1 (55, 145).

In the cingulate motor areas, intracortical stimulation has evoked arm and leg movements [Fig. 6.10; (144; see also 156)]. These movements have characteristics similar to those evoked from the primary motor cortex except for a higher threshold. The locations of the arm and leg representations that were observed are, in general, consistent with the somatotopic maps generated from anatomical studies, although some differences exist [compare Fig. 6.9 to Fig. 6.10; (54, 55, 92, 93, 106, 159)]. Briefly, the region of the dorsal bank of the cingulate sulcus that is comparable to the CMAd contained a leg representation that was rostral to an arm representation (144; see also 156). A large arm representation was found in caudal portions of the ventral bank in a region comparable to the CMAv (Fig. 6.10). Unfortunately, physiological mapping has not explored the most caudal regions of the ventral bank, where anatomical studies have revealed a leg representation (159, 160). The more rostral region of the cingulate sulcus, corresponding to the CMAr, has been mapped by intracortical stimulation in only one animal (144). Stimulation there evoked arm movements intermingled with some leg movements (Fig. 6.10). The intermingling of these responses correlates with the anatomical observation that the origins of corticospinal projections to cervical and to lumbar segments overlap to some extent within the CMAr (93). Within the arm representation of each of the cingulate motor areas, both proximal and distal movements were evoked (144). However, no consistent pattern of proximal and distal arm representation was observed. A more detailed description of body maps in the cingulate motor areas is presented in Dum and Strick (56) and He et al. (93).

The PMv has been mapped with intracortical stimulation in only a single study (71). Movements of the distal forelimb were evoked from the rostral region of the PMv that is buried in the caudal bank of the arcuate sulcus. This region of the PMv projects only to upper cervical segments of the spinal cord and may evoke distal movements by influencing propriospinal neurons in these segments that project to lower cervical segments (for discussion, see 92).

There is no study that has specifically mapped the responses evoked by intracortical stimulation of the PMd. Indeed, in some physiological experiments, the border between M1 and the "premotor cortex" is defined as the point where intracortical stimulation is no longer capable of consistently evoking motor responses (e.g., 128, 233). However, several mapping studies of M1 also explored a caudal part of area 6, which is now considered part of the PMd (105, 136, 155). These studies showed that both proximal and distal movements could be evoked from this region.

Mapping studies in New World monkeys support the view that movements can be evoked from the PMd and PMv [Fig. 6.2; (51, 86, 212)]. Hand movements have been evoked from two regions on the lateral surface of the hemisphere that are rostral to the main arm area of M1. One of these sites is located medially and probably corresponds to the PMd, and the other is located more laterally and probably corresponds to the PMv. However, the homology among these cortical areas in New and Old World primates has not been definitively established.

In summary, it is now clear that intracortical stimulation in each premotor area is capable of evoking movements. This result raises an interesting question: Are the effects of stimulation mediated directly by corticospinal efferents from each premotor area or are they mediated by the corticocortical connection from each premotor area to M1 and corticospinal efferents from M1? This issue has not been thoroughly examined, although there is a short report concerning the pathways mediating responses evoked from the SMA (91). These authors used intracortical stimulation to define the arm and vibrissae representations in the SMA and M1 of the owl monkey. After ablation of M1, movements could still be elicited by stimulation of the SMA, and the current thresholds for evoking movement were in the normal range. These observations suggest that corticospinal efferents from the SMA are sufficient to mediate movements evoked by intracortical stimulation. This conclusion further emphasizes the parallel nature of the pathways originating from M1 and the SMA.

Corticospinal Terminations

Primary Motor Cortex. One measure of the function of a descending system is its pattern of termination within the different laminae of the spinal cord (for a complete discussion of this issue, see 134). The primary motor cortex of primates is known to have direct projections to lamina IX, where motoneurons are located; and to the intermediate zone of the spinal cord (laminae V–VIII), where the interneurons with direct projections to motoneurons are located [Figs. 6.11 and 6.12; (22, 36, 42, 133–135, 142, 191)]. The extent of projections from M1 to motor nuclei in the spinal cord varies in different primate species and appears to correlate with an animal's manual dexterity (22, 134). For instance, cebus monkeys have substantial direct projections from M1 to the spinal motor nuclei [Fig. 6.11*A*; (22)] and use a form of "precision grip" to pick up small objects and manipulate tools (7, 41, 235). In contrast, squirrel monkeys lack substantial direct projections to the motor nuclei [Fig. 6.11*B*; (22)] and pick up small objects with a "power grip" in which all the fingers work in unison to sweep up an object (41, 65). Thus, monosynaptic projections from the primary motor cortex to motoneurons in the ventral horn appear to provide part of the neural substrate for dexterous movements of the fingers (for references and review, see 22, 134).

Corticospinal projections also originate from regions of somatosensory and posterior parietal cortex. However, the efferents from these areas terminate largely in laminae of the dorsal horn, regions normally associated with the processing of somatic sensory information (e.g., 36, 42, 133, 134, 142, 191). In addition, physiological evidence suggests that the activity of these corticospinal efferents modulates the transmission of information in ascending somatosensory pathways (for references and review, see 186, 190). Thus, both anatomical and physiological evidence suggests that the pattern of a region's corticospinal terminations reflects its involvement in somatosensory processing or motor output.

Premotor Areas. Given the substantial number of corticospinal neurons in the premotor areas, how do efferents from each motor area terminate within the gray matter of the spinal cord? Do they terminate in a pattern similar to M1 efferents, reflecting a motor function or do they terminate in a pattern similar to efferents from the somatic sensory cortex, reflecting

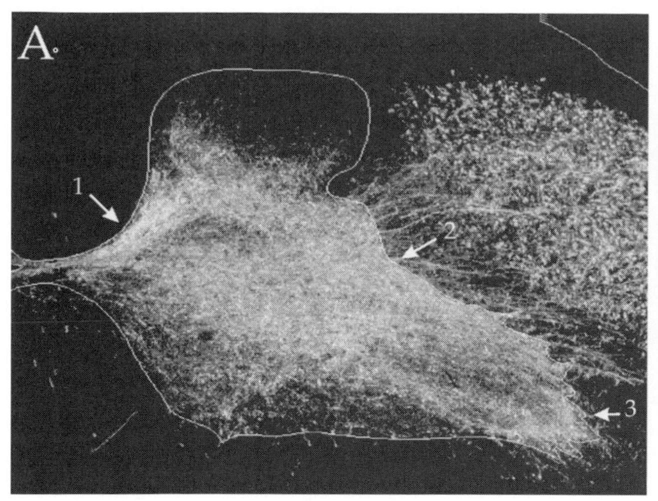

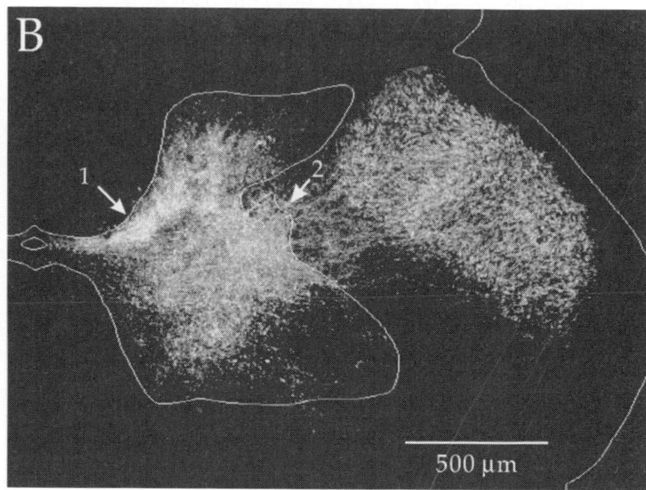

FIG. 6.11. Corticospinal terminations in cebus and squirrel monkeys. These images were "captured" using a digital imaging system and were taken under darkfield illumination with polarized light. *A*, Cebus monkey, C8. *B*, Squirrel monkey, C8. *Arrows* point to regions of dense termination at C8. Note that dense terminations are present in three regions in the cebus monkey, and only two in the squirrel monkey. [Adapted from Bortoff and Strick (22). Reprinted by permission of the Society for Neuroscience.]

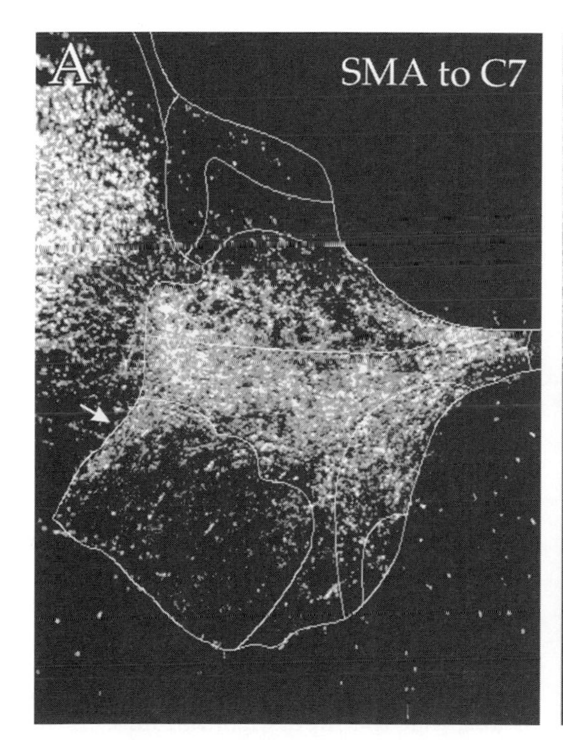

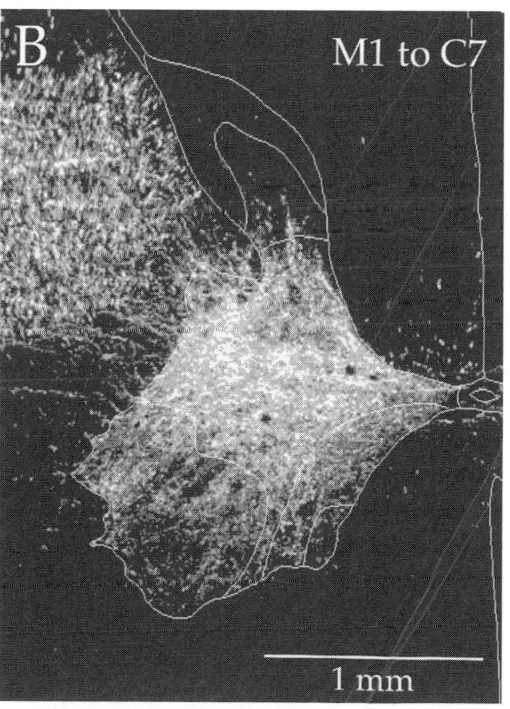

FIG. 6.12. Corticospinal terminations in C7 of a macaque monkey. These images were "captured" using a digital imaging system and were taken under darkfield illumination with polarized light. The outline of the gray matter and spinal laminae are indicated. *A*, SMA efferents terminate densely in intermediate zone of the gray matter of the cervical spinal cord. *Arrow* points to terminations in the dorsolateral part of lamina IX, which contains motoneurons. *B*, M1 efferents terminate in the same regions as do SMA efferents. Compared to SMA terminations, M1 terminations generally are more dense, are somewhat more extensive in lamina IX, and extend farther into the base of the dorsal horn (laminae V–VI).

an involvement in sensory processing? Unfortunately, this important issue has not been fully examined. Only brief and conflicting reports exist on the pattern of termination of corticospinal efferents from the SMA (48; also see abstracts in 24, 35, 57). We have recently examined SMA projections to the spinal cord using a sensitive technique for revealing patterns of termination. SMA efferents terminated densely in four regions of the gray matter of the cervical cord—a lateral portion of the intermediate zone (laminae V–VII), a medial portion of the intermediate zone (laminae VI–VII at the base of the dorsal columns), a ventromedial portion of the intermediate zone (laminae VII–VIII), and a dorsolateral part of the motor nuclei (lamina IX) (Fig. 6.12). The terminations in motor nuclei were found primarily in regions of lower cervical segments (C7–T1) known to contain motoneurons that innervate muscles of the fingers and wrist. In most respects, the pattern of SMA termination in the spinal cord was comparable to that of M1. Thus, the SMA appears to influence directly the same spinal circuitry as M1. Furthermore, these results indicate that the SMA has the potential to control hand movements directly through a pathway that is independent of M1.

INPUTS TO THE CORTICAL MOTOR AREAS

As noted earlier in this chapter, M1 has been viewed as the final stage in the processing of the central commands for motor output. Signals from the cerebellum, basal ganglia, and other cortical areas were thought to converge on M1, where they could influence the generation of descending commands. The recognition that multiple cortical areas project to the spinal cord has led to significant modifications of this view. We have suggested that each of the motor areas that projects to the spinal cord should be considered a nodal point for a functionally distinct efferent system that may differentially generate and/or control specific aspects of motor behavior (54). Obviously, an analysis of the inputs to these nodal points could provide some insight into the unique functional contributions of each motor area.

Identification of the inputs to M1 and the premotor areas is complicated by several factors. First, the location and boundaries of the premotor areas have only recently been identified and are still subject to modification. As a consequence, information about the cortical and subcortical inputs to some motor areas is either lacking or limited (e.g., CMAr, CMAd, and PMd). In addition, the boundaries of several premotor areas have changed considerably from their initial description. For example, the SMA proper is located more caudally than originally thought (55, 93, 144, 152). Thus, some experiments that were intended to examine inputs to the SMA actually studied the connections of a functionally distinct but rostrally adjacent region that is now termed the pre-SMA. Another major complicating factor is the general assumption that the pattern of input to one part of a motor area is representative of the pattern to other parts of that area. Given the unique involvement of certain body parts in specific motor tasks (e.g., orofacial musculature in vocalization), this is an unwarranted assumption. Indeed, we have noted above that the arm area of M1 is not a homogeneous field. Below we will describe the finding that different parts of the arm representation receive their most substantial input from separate regions of the ventrolateral thalamus (95, 150). Because of these and other complexities, the analysis of inputs to each of the cortical motor areas is still evolving. Thus, in the next sections, we will focus on the general principles of input organization for the arm representations of each cortical motor area. Our presentation is limited to what appear to be the major inputs to each area based on an analysis of the results from recent publications. Furthermore, our description is restricted to observations from experiments on laboratory primates capable of relatively independent movements of the fingers (i.e., macaques and cebus monkeys).

Inputs to Primary Motor Cortex

Parietal Cortex. The past 15 years has seen some evolution in our concepts about the pattern of cortical inputs to M1. It had been generally accepted that M1 received input from all of the cytoarchitectonic fields (areas 3a, 3b, 1, and 2) of the primary somatic sensory cortex (SI) and from the secondary somatic sensory cortex (SII) (e.g., 113, 178). On the other hand, regions of posterior parietal cortex (e.g., areas 5 and 7) were not thought to project directly to M1, but had substantial connections with the premotor areas in the frontal lobe, precerebellar nuclei, and basal ganglia circuits (5, 60, 122). It is now clear that the major source of input from the parietal lobe to M1 originates from a lateral portion of area 5 [Fig. 6.13 and Table 6.1; (e.g., 44, 54, 70, 80, 81, 140, 216)]. On the other hand, present evidence indicates that the inputs from SI and SII are less substantial than previously thought and have a more restricted origin [Table 6.1; (e.g., 44, 54, 70, 140, 229)]. Generally, SI fields, which are at an "early" stage in the processing of peripheral afferent information, have little (areas 3a and 1) or no (area 3b)

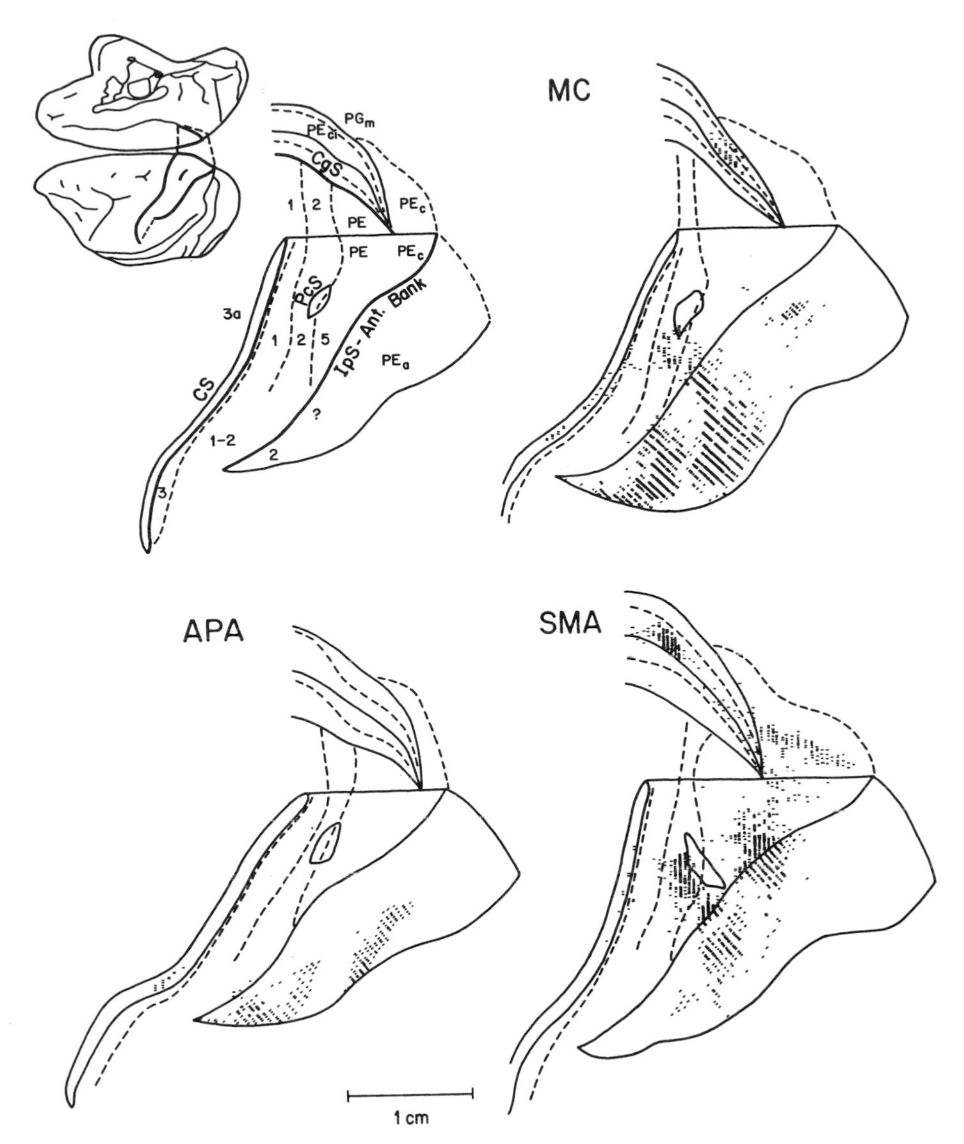

FIG. 6.13. Origin of parietal lobe projections from the postcentral cortex and the anterior bank of the intraparietal sulcus to the arm areas of the primary motor cortex (MC), the arcuate premotor area (APA; termed the PMv in this chapter), and the SMA. *Upper left*, The *dashed lines* on the small view of the brain indicate the region of parietal lobe that is enlarged in each of the other panels. The cytoarchitectonic areas are labeled with *numbers* or *small lettering* on the unfolded reconstruction of these regions. In the remaining panels, each *dash* represents a neuron labeled following tracer injection into the arm area of the designated cortical region. Note that MC receives dense input from a lateral region of area 5 (PEa) buried in the anterior bank of the intraparietal sulcus, and the SMA receives input from more medial regions of area 5. CgS, cingulate sulcus; IpS, intraparietal sulcus; PcS, postcentral sulcus. [From Dum and Strick (54). Copyright © 1991 by Wiley-Liss, Inc. Reprinted by permission by John Wiley & Sons, Inc.]

input to M1 (e.g., 44, 80, 100, 140). On the other hand, SI fields at a "later" stage of processing have a modest input to M1 (area 2). Direct projections from SII to M1 were present in most studies (44, 80, 81, 140) but were not substantial in others (54). M1 also appears to receive some input from area 7b and cortical field PEci on the medial wall of the hemisphere (54, 80, 81, 140). However, none of the inputs from these areas to M1 approaches the density and extent of input from area 5.

As noted earlier, neurons in M1 are known to receive cutaneous and deep input with short latency from the periphery. How this input gains access to M1 has been a longstanding controversy. Although M1 receives some input from primary and secondary somatosensory areas, removal of these areas along with the cerebellum leaves peripheral input to M1 largely intact (10, 13). On the other hand, section of the dorsal columns, a major pathway for input to the parietal cortex, abolishes the peripheral respon-

TABLE 6.1. *Parietal Lobe Connections to Motor Areas in the Frontal Lobe*

Area	M1	PMd	PMv	SMA	CMAd	CMAv	CMAr
3a, 3b, 1	+				+	+	
Area 2	++	+	+	++	+	++	
Med. 5	+			+++	+	++	
Lateral 5	+++	+++	+	+++	+++	+++	
7ips	+		+++				
7b rost			+++		++	+++	+++
7b caud	+	++		++		+++	+
SII	+?	+	+++	+?	+++		+++
Insula			+?	+?	+++	+	+++
PEci	+	+		++	++	+	++

The strength of parietal lobe input is normalized for each motor area (i.e., column comparisons are generally valid but row comparisons are not). Sparse inputs are not included. ? indicates that connections were present in some experiments but not in others.

siveness of M1 neurons (25). Some have argued that a pathway from the dorsal columns terminates in a thalamic region that projects directly to M1 (for references and discussion, see 10). However, there is no compelling anatomical evidence that such a pathway exists in the primate (227). Thus, the major route by which somatosensory information reaches M1 has not been firmly established. Although it is clear that parietal cortex is not a critical link in this pathway, results from recent studies suggest that the interconnections between SI and M1 are particularly important for the modifications in behavior that occur when an animal learns a new motor task under sensory guidance (10, 180).

Frontal Lobe. All of the premotor areas, by definition, project directly to M1 (54, 55, 81, 161, 213). On the other hand, M1 does not receive input from other regions of prefrontal or cingulate cortex proper. With one exception, the density of projections from the premotor areas to M1 matches the density of their projection to the spinal cord. For example, the CMAr has a relatively weak projection to the spinal cord and to M1 (55, 143). The PMv is, however, exceptional in possessing sparse projections to the spinal cord but dense projections to M1.

In general, the projections from the premotor areas to M1 are somatotopically organized (81, 149, 159–161, 213). However, some differences in the precise patterns of input from each premotor area to the arm representation in M1 exist. According to Tokuno and Tanji (225), the PMd projects predominantly to the proximal arm representation in M1, whereas the PMv projects primarily to the distal arm representation. All of the premotor areas on the medial wall project to the proximal and distal representations in M1. Different portions of the hand representation in M1 receive input from the CMAd and CMAv (97). The CMAd projects most densely to the portion of the hand representation that is buried in the anterior bank of the central sulcus. In contrast, the CMAv projects most densely to the portion of the hand representation located on the crest of the precentral gyrus. Efferents from the SMA appear to innervate both regions (Holsapple, Preston, and Strick, unpublished observations).

Basal Ganglia and Cerebellar Input. The cortical motor areas receive subcortical input from multiple sources including ventral and intralaminar nuclei of the thalamus, the nucleus basalis of Meynert, the amygdala, and brainstem cell groups like the locus coeruleus and raphe. Clearly, the most substantial source of subcortical input to the cortical motor areas arises from various portions of the ventrolateral thalamus. This region provides the major route by which the output of the cerebellum and basal ganglia gain access to the frontal lobe. This section will focus entirely on the anatomy of these subcortical systems.

Although there has been some disagreement, it is now generally accepted that the arm representation in M1 receives its densest input from two subdivisions of the ventrolateral thalamus: ventralis lateralis pars oralis (VLo) and ventralis lateralis posterior pars oralis (VPLo) [Fig. 6.14; (45, 150, 177, 201, 237, 238)]. VLo is a major site of termination of efferents from an output nucleus of the basal ganglia, the internal segment of the globus pallidus (GPi) (49, 107, 124, 127, 168). VPLo, in contrast, is a major site of termination of efferents from the deep cerebellar nuclei: the dentate, interpositus, and fastigial (8, 9, 20, 34, 107, 119, 123, 132, 183, 209). Consequently, the M1 arm representation is the target of both basal ganglia and cerebellar output [Fig. 6.14; (see also 167, 224)]. This conclusion has recently been confirmed by Hoover and Strick (98), who showed that neurons in both the dentate nucleus and the internal segment of the globus pallidus were labeled after retrograde transneuronal trans-

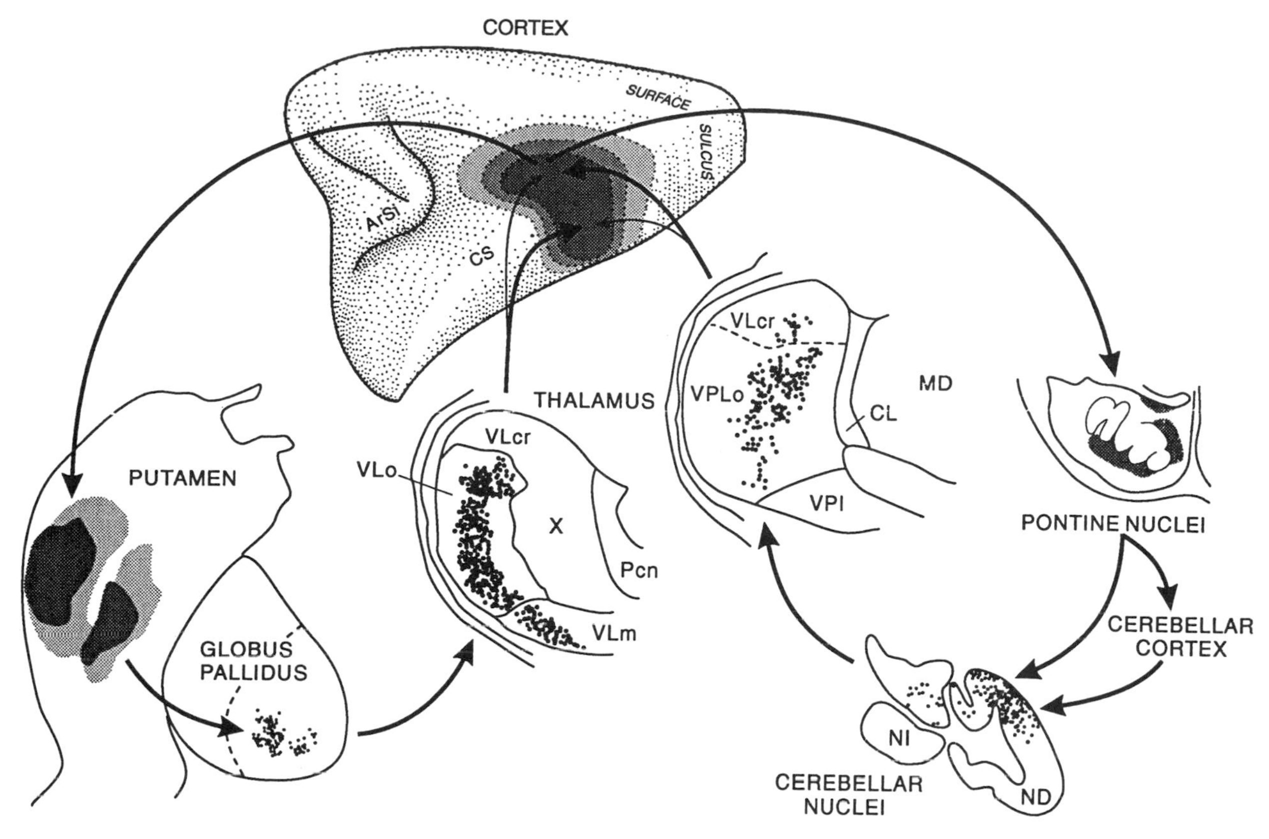

FIG. 6.14. Summary diagram of the "loops" between the primary motor cortex and two subcortical structures, the basal ganglia and the cerebellum. Coronal sections of the thalamus (*center*) show the location of neurons (*dots*) that project from the ventrolateral thalamus to the surface and sulcus of the primary motor cortex. The *shading* in the primary motor cortex indicates, from dark to light, the hand, elbow, and shoulder representations. [Adapted from Holsapple, Preston, and Strick (95). Reprinted by permission of the Society for Neuroscience.] The cortical efferent terminations in the putamen are *shaded* according to the intensity of anterograde labeling (see 215). The location of the labeled cells in the globus pallidus was determined by retrograde transneuronal transport of virus. [Adapted from Hoover and Strick (98), © 1993 American Association for the Advancement of Science. Reprinted by permission.] The *shading* in the diagram of the pontine nuclei indicate the location of terminations from the primary motor cortex. [Adapted from Brodal (26). Reprinted by permission of Oxford University Press.] The location of labeled neurons in the deep cerebellar nuclei was determined by retrograde transneuronal transport of virus. [Adapted from Strick, Hoover, and Mushiake (217). Reprinted by permission of Elsevier Science.] See text for further explanation.

port of herpes simplex virus type 1 from injection sites in the arm area of M1.

Different subdivisions of the ventrolateral thalamus innervate different portions of M1 (95, 150). Some have suggested that cerebellar input to M1 preferentially influences regions of distal representation, and basal ganglia input preferentially influences regions of proximal representation (150). A portion of the proximal arm representation in M1 does receive its most substantial input from VLo (Table 6.2). However, a sorting of pallidal and cerebellar pathways to proximal and distal cortical representations does not appear to fully describe the patterns of input to the hand representation in M1 [Fig. 6.14; (95)]. The portion of the hand representation located on the crest of the precentral gyrus receives its densest input from VPLo, a target of cerebellar efferents. In contrast, the portion of the hand representation located in the central sulcus receives its densest input from the VLo, a target of basal ganglia output. This finding indicates that pallidal output to M1 is not limited to influencing movements at proximal joints, but also is concerned with the

TABLE 6.2. *Major Thalamic Input to the Primary Motor Cortex*

Cortex	M1/Hand-Surface*	M1/Hand-Sulcus†	M1/Proximal‡
VL Thalamus Subcortical	VPLo Cerebellar	VLo Pallidal	VLo Pallidal

*Representation of the hand on the surface of the precentral gyrus. †Representation of the hand in the anterior bank of the central sulcus. ‡Representation of proximal arm musculature on the surface of the precentral gyrus.

control of distal arm movements (for discussion, see 95).

Inputs to the Premotor Areas

Interconnections among the Motor Areas. Although the inputs and outputs of individual premotor areas have been examined in a number of studies, no quantitative analysis of interconnections among the premotor areas exists. Hence, our comments will summarize the general features that emerge from the results of recent studies. Three specific features of the interconnections among the premotor areas deserve emphasis. First, the premotor areas on the medial wall of the hemisphere (SMA, CMAr, CMAd, and CMAv) are densely interconnected with one another. In contrast, the premotor areas on the lateral surface (PMd and PMv) do not appear to have substantial interconnections (17, 54, 129, 149, 159). Second, of all the premotor areas, the SMA is notable in the extent of its interconnections with the other premotor areas. Each of the other premotor areas has dense reciprocal connections with the SMA. Third, the extent to which the PMv and PMd project to the cingulate motor areas is uncertain. It appears that the lateral premotor areas project to these regions, but not densely. These patterns of connectivity further emphasize that the PMd and PMv are fundamentally distinct from each other and from the motor areas on the medial wall.

Parietal Cortex. Parietal lobe input to the motor areas appears to follow a general trend. The subdivisions of the primary somatosensory cortex that are involved in the initial stages of processing incoming cutaneous and proprioceptive information (i.e., areas 3a, 3b, 1) have only sparse connections with any of the premotor areas [Fig. 6.13 and Table 6.1; (e.g., 44, 54, 81, 126, 129, 145, 149, 159, 160; Holsapple and Strick, unpublished observations; Shima, Dum, and Tanji, unpublished observations)]. On the other hand, area 2, which is thought to be at an intermediate stage of somatosensory processing, has dense interconnections with the SMA and less intense projections to the other motor areas (e.g., 44, 54, 81, 126, 129, 145, 149, 159, 160; Holsapple and Strick, unpublished observations; Shima, Dum, and Tanji, unpublished observations). The densest and most widespread connections from the parietal lobe to the motor areas originate in the posterior parietal cortex, areas 5 and 7 [Table 6.1; (e.g., 44, 54, 70, 81, 126, 129, 145, 149, 159, 160, 205, 213; Holsapple and Strick, unpublished observations; Shima, Dum, and Tanji, unpublished observations)]. These two regions are thought to be at the highest level of somatosensory processing and are thought to participate in multisensory integration, spatial attention, affect, and motor control (e.g., 146). Every motor area in the frontal lobe is richly interconnected with parts of at least one, and possibly both, of these posterior parietal areas. However, the actual origin of projections from areas 5 and 7 to different motor areas frequently arises from separate locations. For example, the portion of area 7 that is buried in the intraparietal sulcus projects densely to the PMv, but not the PMd or any of the motor areas on the medial wall (54, 129, 149). The medial portion of area 5 in the intraparietal sulcus innervates several of the motor areas on the medial wall but does not appear to project to the PMv or the PMd (54, 56, 129, 149, 159; Holsapple and Strick, unpublished observations). The premotor areas also receive input from parietal fields buried in the lateral sulcus (e.g., SII and granular insular cortex) and from a field posteriorly in the cingulate sulcus (e.g., PEci). SII projects densely to the PMv, CMAd, and CMAr (15–17, 54, 56, 126, 184, 230). Projections from PEci appear to innervate all of the motor area on the medial wall (54, 145, 159; Holsapple and Strick, unpublished observations; Shima, Dum, and Tanji, unpublished observations). When viewed from the perspective of individual premotor areas, each motor field appears to receive a unique spectrum of inputs from the different parietal areas (Table 6.1).

Prefrontal Cortex. The only major input to the premotor areas from prefrontal cortex originates from the dorsolateral prefrontal cortex (Walker's area 46) (e.g., 19, 143, 160). The most substantial and extensive interconnections link the PMv and area 46 (143). Less substantial projections from area 46 reach the CMAr, CMAv, and SMA. The input from area 46 to the SMA and CMAv appears to be restricted to their proximal arm representations. These observations indicate that the output of prefrontal cortex targets specific premotor areas and even subregions within them. The projections of area 46 to the premotor areas provide the prefrontal cortex with relatively direct access to the primary motor cortex, spinal cord, and motor output. Thus, the influence of the prefrontal cortex upon the motor system may be widespread and applied at multiple nodes in the processing of motor behavior.

Goldman-Rakic and colleagues have argued that the prefrontal cortex is part of a widespread system that underlies spatially guided behavior (83, 84). The PMv receives input from many of the parietal lobe areas that innervate area 46, is densely interconnected with area 46 and, thus, appears to be part of the same neural system. The prefrontal cortex is

TABLE 6.3. *Major Thalamic Input to the Premotor Areas on the Lateral Surface*

Cortex	PMv/Distal*	PMv/Proximal†	PMd
VL Thalamus	"X"	VLo	VLo/rostral VLc
Subcortical	Cerebellar	Pallidal	Pallidal

*Representation of the distal arm musculature. †Representation of the proximal arm musculature.

thought to access and temporally store information about the location objects in extrapersonal space. This information may be relayed from area 46 to the PMv and used to guide motor output based on information stored in "working memory."

Limbic Cortex. No experimental evidence supports the existence of strong connections between "limbic" cortex in the cingulate gyrus and the motor areas in the frontal lobe (for review, see 56). Although one might suspect that the cingulate motor areas would be interconnected with the cingulate gyrus due to proximity, there is little support for such connections. It is important to recognize, however, that the pattern of cortical projections to the cingulate motor areas may require revision due to the present paucity of studies with tracer injections confined to a single cingulate area.

Basal Ganglia and Cerebellar Input. In the past, the premotor cortex, along with other cortical areas, was thought to provide a major source of input to the basal ganglia and cerebellum (for references and review, see 4, 28, 210). On the other hand, the outputs from the basal ganglia and cerebellum were thought to converge upon a single region of the thalamus, the ventrolateral nucleus. This nucleus was believed to project to a single cortical area, the primary motor cortex (e.g., 5, 122). According to this scheme, basal ganglia and cerebellar loops were viewed as a means of taking information from widespread regions of the cerebral cortex and "funneling" it to the primary motor cortex. These subcortical loops were largely "open" in the sense that much of the cortex providing information to the loop did not subsequently receive any output from the loop.

Recent findings have led to substantial modifications of this view (e.g., 4, 54, 85, 89, 90, 98, 201).

TABLE 6.4. *Major Thalamic Input to the Premotor Areas on the Medial Wall*

Cortex	SMA	CMAd	CMAv	CMAr
VL Thalamus	VLo	VLo	Caudal VLc	VApc
Subcortical	Pallidal	Pallidal	Cerebellar	Pallidal

Considerable evidence now exists that the outputs from the basal ganglia and cerebellum do not converge on the same region of the thalamus as shown in Figure 6.14. Instead, each subcortical system terminates in a distinct set of thalamic nuclei. For example, using Olszewski's (175) terminology, efferents from the globus pallidus terminate in ventralis anterior pars parvocellularis (VApc), ventralis lateralis pars oralis (VLo), and the rostral portion of ventralis lateralis pars caudalis (VLc). In contrast, efferents from the deep cerebellar nuclei terminate in ventralis posterior lateralis pars oralis (VPLo), the caudal part of ventralis lateralis pars caudalis (VLc), ventralis lateralis pars postrema (VLps), and area X. These thalamic nuclei project to multiple regions in the frontal lobe including M1 and the premotor areas. Thus, many of the frontal lobe regions that provide input to basal ganglia and cerebellar circuits have the potential to be the target of the output from these circuits. This creates the possibility that part of the structural framework of cortical interconnections with the basal ganglia and cerebellum takes the form of multiple "closed" loops rather than the single open-loop circuit previously conceived (215).

The exact details concerning which thalamic nuclei innervate specific cortical areas has not as yet been fully determined; however, it is clear that any single cortical area receives thalamic input from multiple nuclei in the ventrolateral thalamus. In general, one thalamic nucleus appears to provide the most substantial input to an individual premotor area. Even when two cortical motor areas receive input from the same thalamic nucleus, this input originates from largely separate regions within that nucleus. In other instances, different regions within a single motor area are innervated by distinct nuclei of the ventrolateral thalamus as illustrated for M1 in Figure 6.14. Similarly, the representation of the distal arm within the PMv receives its most substantial input from area X, a target of cerebellar efferents (150, 177, 201). In contrast, the proximal arm representation in the PMv receives its most substantial input from VLo, a target of pallidal efferents (150). As yet, no experiments have specifically addressed the origin of thalamic input to the PMv, but VLo and parts of VLc (pallidal targets) appear to be likely candidates (123).

Although few studies have examined the origin of thalamic input to the premotor areas on the medial wall of the hemisphere, the available data suggest a general pattern of connectivity. The major portion of the arm representation in the SMA is innervated by a pallidothalamocortical pathway via VLo (98, 201, 237). Pallidal input also appears to reach the CMAd via VLo (96) and the CMAr via VApc

(Shima, Dum, and Tanji, unpublished observations). The major thalamic input to the CMAv appears to be the caudal part of VLc, which is a target of cerebellar efferents (96). Thus, the cerebellum and basal ganglia gain access to the premotor areas on the medial wall and to those on the lateral surface. Furthermore, there are examples where cerebellar and pallidal input gains access to regions of distal representation, as well as examples where they gain access to regions of proximal representation.

One major difficulty concerning the identification of the cortical targets of basal ganglia and cerebellar output is that these conclusions are largely based on comparisons of data from separate experiments. For example, the pattern of thalamic labeling seen after an injection of retrograde tracer into the SMA (e.g., 201, 237, 238) has been compared to that observed following the injection of an anterograde tracer into the globus pallidus (e.g., 49). One of the many problems with comparisons of this sort is that variations in thalamic nomenclature and borders can lead to considerable controversy in defining patterns of overlap (for recent discussions on this issue, see 45, 95). One solution to this problem has been to inject multiple types of tracers into a single animal. A retrograde tracer is injected into a cortical area and an anterograde tracer into a subcortical site. Then, the material is examined to determine whether there is any overlap in the thalamus of labeling from the two tracers. Tokuno et al. (224) have used this approach to confirm that the arm area of the SMA is a target of pallidal projections.

Unfortunately, there are several problems with the use of double labeling to examine multisynaptic connections. The absence of overlap could result from injection sites that do not match (e.g., a cortical injection into the "arm" representation and subcortical injection into the leg representation). Discriminating between overlap and interdigitation of regions of labeling can be difficult. Furthermore, terminations near a group of labeled neurons may not actually synapse on them. To overcome some of these difficulties, several investigators have developed techniques that involve transneuronal transport of tracer substances. The most successful transneuronal tracer in primates is live herpes simplex virus type 1 (HSV-1) (e.g., 98, 214, 243). One strain of HSV-1 (McIntyre-B) is transported transneuronally in the retrograde direction from cortical injection sites (98, 243). Injections of this strain into the arm area of the primary motor cortex labeled "first-order" neurons in regions of the ventrolateral thalamus that project to the primary motor cortex. In addition, "second-order" neurons were labeled in regions of the dentate, interpositus, and globus pallidus that are known to project to the ventrolateral thalamus. Likewise, virus injections into other premotor areas, such as the arm areas of the PMv and SMA, revealed that they too are the target of outputs from the basal ganglia and cerebellum (98, 217). Furthermore, injections of HSV-1 into the arm areas of M1, PMv, and SMA resulted in labeled neurons in three separate regions in the globus pallidus [Fig. 6.15; (98)]. Similar results are seen in the dentate nucleus after virus injections into the arm areas of M1 and the PMv (217). Thus, virus transport has demonstrated that the basal ganglia and cerebellum contain distinct "output channels," with each channel targeting a different cortical motor area.

PHYSIOLOGICAL OVERVIEW

One goal of this chapter has been to provide an overview of the structural framework that is responsible for the central generation and control of voluntary movement. This framework has four significant features. First, the frontal lobe contains multiple, spatially separate motor areas. These include the primary motor cortex and six premotor areas. Each of the premotor areas projects not only to the primary motor cortex but also directly to the spinal cord. The patterns of termination of these corticospinal projections suggest that they innervate motoneurons and/or last-order interneurons that project to motoneurons. The spinal projections afford each cortical motor area the potential to influence the spinal machinery responsible for producing motor output. Thus, a critical new feature of the structural framework for the central control of movement is the presence of multiple cortical efferent systems, in addition to the primary motor cortex.

A second important feature is that all of the cortical motor areas receive input from subdivisions of the ventrolateral thalamus. These subdivisions are the site of termination of basal ganglia and cerebellar efferents. As a consequence, the premotor areas and M1 participate in multiple parallel loops with the basal ganglia and cerebellum by both projecting to and receiving input from these subcortical structures.

A third major feature is that each cortical motor area receives a unique pattern of cortical input. This arrangement creates the possibility that each area processes a unique mixture of sensory and cognitive information. The final important feature of this framework is the rich interconnections that exist among the cortical motor areas. The connections could serve many functions, including the coordination of output commands among the motor areas.

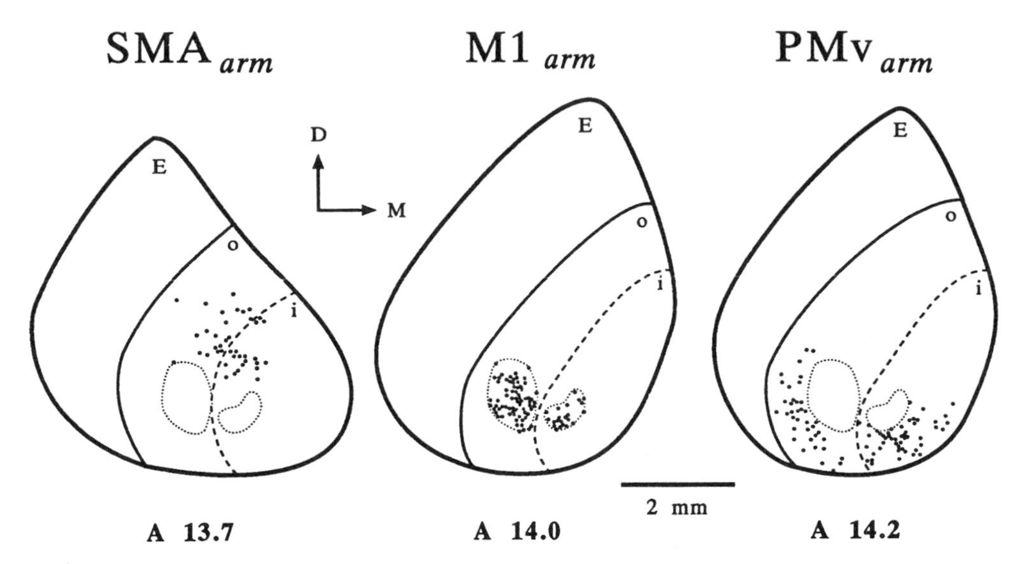

FIG. 6.15. Location of globus pallidus neurons that innervate thalamic nuclei projecting to the SMA, M1, and PMv. Neurons in the internal segment of the globus pallidus (GPi) were labeled by retrograde transneuronal transport of herpes simplex virus type 1 (HSV-1) following injections into the arm representations of the SMA, M1, or PMv of monkeys. The *dots* indicate the position of labeled cells observed in two or three coronal sections near the same stereotaxic level (A 14.0). For comparison, the *dotted line* indicates the region of the GPi containing neurons labeled from M1. The *thick solid line* indicates the outline of the globus pallidus. The *thin solid line* indicates the border between the internal and external (E) segments of GP. The *dashed line* indicates the border between the inner and outer portions of the GPi. i, inner portion of the GPi; o, outer portion of GPi; D, dorsal; M, medial. [Adapted from Hoover and Strick (98). © 1993 American Association for the Advancement of Science. Reprinted by permission.]

The unique set of cortical and subcortical inputs impinging on each motor area, as well as their independent access to the spinal cord, have led us to propose that each area is a nodal point in a functionally distinct efferent system (54). The direct projections of each premotor area to the spinal cord suggest that each area could independently contribute motor commands for the execution of movement. This aspect of the anatomical framework contrasts strikingly with the classic view that only the primary motor cortex had direct influence on the spinal mechanisms of motor control. Thus, the anatomical organization of the cortical motor areas suggests that each could function at multiple levels of motor processing, from higher level aspects of motor planning to the generation of motor output. In the remainder of this chapter, we will review some of the recent physiological evidence concerning the contributions of each efferent system to different aspects of motor behavior. Our review will focus on the premotor areas. Detailed descriptions of the response properties of neurons in M1 can be found in several recent reviews (38, 58, 73, 94, 190).

Before proceeding, we want to raise several notes of caution regarding the evaluation of results from the physiological studies in behaving animals. Because of the spatial arrangement of the cortical motor areas, no single study has been able to examine neuron activity in all of the motor areas. Second, several of the motor areas have only recently been discovered. As a consequence, few physiological studies have been performed in these areas. Third, studies of the premotor areas generally have not examined the activity of "identified" neurons. For example, we know a great deal about the activity of corticospinal neurons in M1, but know very little about the activity of this type of neuron in the premotor areas. Thus, an examination of the response properties of neurons in the premotor areas is still at an early stage.

Common Activation of the Motor Areas

Simple Motor Tasks. "Simple" movements are ones that are easy to perform, such as making and opening a fist, tapping a response key, and flexion/extension of the elbow or wrist. These motor responses are considered complex, however, when they become part of a behavioral paradigm with complicated contingencies (i.e., press the right key when you see the letters A, C, or E; press the left key when you see the letters B, D, or F). Many neurons in M1 are related to the performance of simple movements and alter their activity prior to movement onset (58, 94, 190). Even the addition of behavior contingencies often does not weaken the relation between movement and the activity of M1 neurons. Similarly, neurons related to simple movements have been found in all of the premotor areas. Some of these neurons discharge prior to the onset of movement [PMd (128, 130, 131, 174, 233), the PMv (128, 130, 131), the SMA (174, 221) and the cingulate motor areas (206)]. Activation in M1 and in the premotor areas, particularly those on the medial wall of the hemisphere, is seen in functional imaging studies during simple movements (e.g., 40, 87, 88, 192). Taken together these results suggest that multiple motor areas are involved in the generation of even the simplest motor commands.

Relation to Parameters of Movement. One of the striking features of neuron activity in M1 is its relation to different parameters of movement, such as direction and force. For example, many cortical neurons are reciprocally active for opposing directions of movement about a single joint, such as wrist flexion/extension (for references and review, see 58). A wider range of directional coding of M1 neurons (e.g., two- and three-dimensional space) has been examined in recent experiments by Georgopoulos and colleagues (30, 31, 77, 79, 117, 204). They found that the activity of M1 neurons was maximal for a "preferred" direction, but was broadly tuned about this axis (Fig. 6.16). Thus, single neurons in M1 did not provide unambiguous information about the direction of an upcoming movement. The preferred directions of individual cells were distributed uniformly among all possible directions. Because of their broad directional tuning, a large population of M1 neurons is active for any given direction of movement. Based on these findings, Georgopoulos and his colleagues (74) proposed that M1 neurons used a "population code" to determine movement direction. Each neuron in the population contributes a vector in its preferred direction. The magnitude of this vector is proportional to a cell's activity for the particular direction being examined. The population vector calculated in this manner accurately predicts the movement direction in two-dimensional [Fig. 6.17; (74, 78)] as well as in three-dimensional space (30, 31, 79). In fact, this population vector could

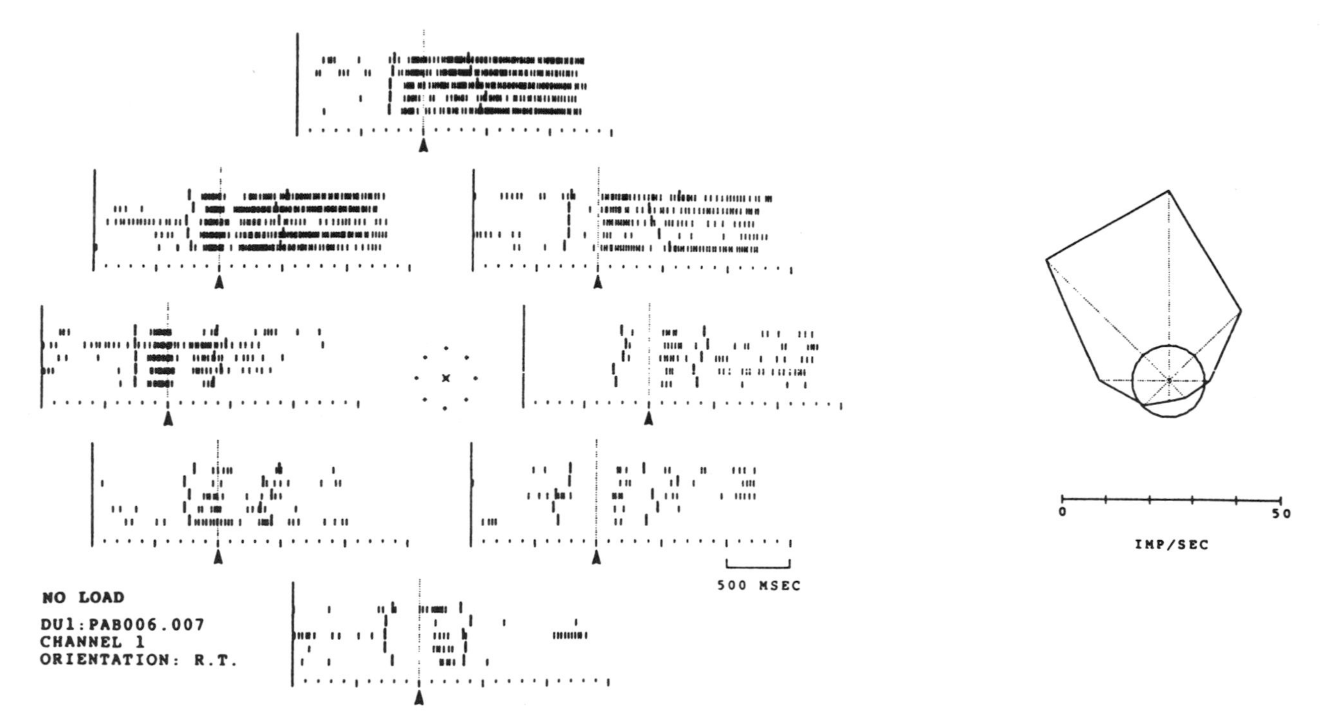

FIG. 6.16. The discharge pattern of a shoulder joint–related neuron in M1 of a monkey is shown for reaching movements in eight directions. Rasters of cell activity (*left*) are illustrated for eight radial directions of movement from the center hold zone (*x*). Rasters are aligned to the onset of movement (*arrowheads below dotted lines*). The appearance of the target light in each trial is indicated by the *heavy tick mark* to the left of the *arrow*, and the end of the movement is designated by the *heavy tick mark* to the right of the *arrow*. In the polar plot (*right*), the mean discharge of the cell during movement time (from the appearance of the target light to the end of movement) is indicated by the length of the axis corresponding to each direction of movement. This response may be compared to the cell's mean discharge during the control period (all center hold epochs averaged together), which is equal to the radius of the circle. The cell's preferred direction of discharge is toward the upper left and decreases continuously to reach a minimum in the downward direction. The cell's activity during the movement time period showed an excellent fit (R^2 = 0.94) to a sinusoidal curve. [From Kalaska et al. (117). Reprinted by permission of the Society for Neuroscience.]

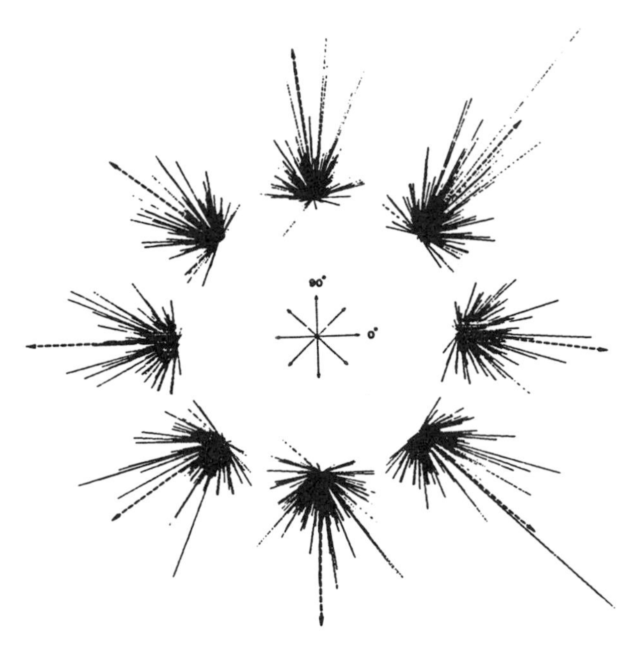

FIG. 6.17. Representation of movement direction by a neuronal population code. The directional vectors for neurons (*thin lines*) in M1 of a monkey are illustrated for each of eight directions of reaching movements (*diagram at center*). The population vector (*interrupted lines with arrows*) calculated from the individual cell vectors is closely aligned to its corresponding movement direction. The cell vectors producing each population vector are symmetrically distributed around it. [From Georgopoulos et al. (74). © 1983 Springer-Verlag. Reprinted by permission.]

predict movement direction during the preparatory period prior to movement onset (75) and during a constantly varying movement trajectory (202, 203). These results have led Georgopoulos to propose that M1 calculates kinematic parameters of movement (i.e., movement direction or hand path) and that the final conversion of these signals into specific joint torques or muscle activation patterns occurs in subcortical structures, primarily the spinal cord (72). The extent to which the directional tuning of M1 neurons is related to higher order processing of movement direction vs. other variables like muscle activity remains a current topic of debate (e.g., 166).

The presence of neurons with directionally tuned activity is not limited to M1 but is a ubiquitous property of cortical and subcortical regions that are anatomically linked to M1. These regions include the PMd (31, 130, 233), deep cerebellar nuclei (63), area 5 (116), area 2 (115), and possibly the basal ganglia (76). Judging from the latency at which neuronal activity increases in relation to movement onset, cortical areas appear to be activated in the following sequence: area 6, area 4, area 5, and area 2 (118). It is important to note that there is extensive overlap in activation latencies of cortical neurons in the different areas. This suggests that many of the processes for the planning, initiation, and execution of movement are occurring simultaneously in multiple cortical regions (see also 3).

Neuronal Relations to Muscle Force. It is well known that neurons in M1 modulate their firing rate in relation to various aspects of the tonic and/or dynamic aspects of the force produced at a joint (for references and review, see 58). The percentage of neurons in M1 displaying activity related to different static levels of force is highest among identified pyramidal tract neurons (59, 234) and appears to be a universal property of M1 neurons that connect directly with spinal cord motoneurons [corticomotoneuronal cells (37)]. Many M1 neurons display activity that does not simply parallel force or muscle activity. In fact, some corticomotoneuronal cells with activity well correlated to different levels of static force were inactive during ballistic movements (37).

There is little evidence for force coding of neuronal activity in the premotor areas. However, this issue has only been systematically examined in the PMv, where some neurons exhibit significant, positive relationships between firing rate and static torque (234). Although the overall proportion of neurons showing force-firing frequency relations was higher in M1, the proportions in M1 and the PMv were virtually the same when only pyramidal tract neurons were compared. M1 neurons tended to exhibit the greatest modulation of their activity in relation to low levels of static force and appear to be particularly important in the control of fine forces (59, 234). On the other hand, the activity of PMv neurons was correlated to the entire range of muscle force examined (234). Some neurons in the PMd and SMA also show patterns of activity related to static and/or dynamic changes in force (43, 130). These observations are consistent with the notion that the control of force output is the result of signals from the premotor areas as well as M1. Indeed, Alexander and Crutcher (3) have argued that the specification of movement parameters is a spatially distributed process that occurs simultaneously in motor and premotor areas.

Specialization of Motor Processing in the Motor Areas

One hypothesis to account for the relatively large number of motor areas in primates is that each motor area makes some unique contribution to the planning, preparation, initiation, and/or execution of movement (54). The results of recent physiological studies using a variety of behavioral paradigms provide support for this point of view. Below, we will describe results indicating that the cortical motor areas are differentially involved in such diverse aspects of motor behavior as motor preparation, visual guidance, internal generation, and movement sequences. In some instances, one specific motor area appears to be especially concerned with a particular task component (e.g., PMv and visually guided behavior). In others, the premotor areas as a group appear to differ from the primary motor cortex in their involvement in a specific task component (e.g., motor preparation).

Preparation for a Motor Response. Multiple studies have investigated the activity of neurons in the cortical motor areas during tasks that include an "instructed delay period" (Fig. 6.18). At the start of this period, an instruction is given that allows the subject to prepare part or all of their motor response. After a delay, a go signal is given that triggers the response. A gradual or sustained change in activity in the delay period after the onset of the instruction is potentially related to the motor set of the animal (*set-related*). Some set-related activity has been shown to correlate with parameters of movements like movement amplitude and direction. Other set-related activity appears to correlate with higher level aspects of motor planning such as the target or goal of a movement.

Some form of set-related activity has been observed in all the motor areas examined in the frontal lobe including M1 (2, 75, 193), and PMd (2, 128, 130, 193, 233, 240), the SMA (2, 174), and the pre-SMA (2, 152). Changes in activity during an instructed delay period appear to be much less frequent in the PMv. When such activity is present it appears to be related to the onset of a visual target that is the instructional stimulus (130; see, however, 82). The cingulate motor areas have not been examined for set-related activity (206).

Although each cortical motor area has some set-related activity, the proportion of these neurons appears to vary considerably among motor areas (e.g., 2, 174, 233). This issue is best examined when two or more motor areas are sampled in an animal performing a task that includes an instructed delay period. In such experiments, the PMd (128, 130, 193) and the SMA (2, 174) have a higher proportion of set-related neurons than M1. These findings suggest that the SMA and PMd are more concerned with motor preparation and planning than are M1 and the PMv.

Anticipation of Behavioral Events. Wise and colleagues have observed gradual changes in activity that precede the onset of an instructional stimulus (50, 153, 228). Such *anticipatory* activity is usually observed only when a fixed delay period is used between the start of a trial and the presentation of the stimulus. The onset of anticipatory activity can begin immediately after trial initiation to almost 5 s later (228). Usually the anticipatory activity does not reflect the direction of the upcoming movement, suggesting that it is not involved in the specification of movement parameters. The presence or absence of the anticipatory activity can be related to task conditions, being present when the stimulus has greater instructional significance (50). Anticipatory activity has only been examined in the PMd, and its presence in other areas remains to be examined.

Signal-Related Activity. Neurons in several of the premotor areas display a phasic response after the onset of an instructional stimulus. Such signal-related activity is rather ubiquitous in the premotor areas [e.g., SMA (174), the PMd (50), and the PM (82)], but is seldom found in M1. Signal-related activity could be a pure sensory response to the instructional stimulus or could depend on the significance of the stimulus. In the most careful examination of this question to date, di Pellegrino and Wise (50) determined that the most important parameter for signal-related activity in the PMd is the instructional significance of the stimulus and not its spatial, attentional or mnemonic attributes. These results are consistent with the proposal that the PMd is involved in forming associations between specific motor responses and arbitrary sensory stimuli (see later under Conditional Association).

Visual Guidance of Movement. In many circumstances, the location and physical characteristics of an object *visually* guides the selection of the appropriate motor response. For example, picking up a raisin or a coffee cup requires both accurate reaching to the object and the proper hand configuration to grasp it. Of the six premotor areas, the PMv is by general consensus thought to be particularly involved in this aspect of motor behavior. Mushiake et al. (165) trained monkeys to make a sequence of movements by pressing touch pads as they were illuminated or to perform the same sequence from memory. PMv neurons tended to be active during the visually triggered movement sequences, but not during memory-guided sequences.

After lesions that included the PMv, monkeys were unable to reach around a clear barrier to retrieve morsels of food (158). One interpretation of this result is that the PMv lesion left an animal unable to use information about the barrier to guide movements around it. Thus, the animal used other,

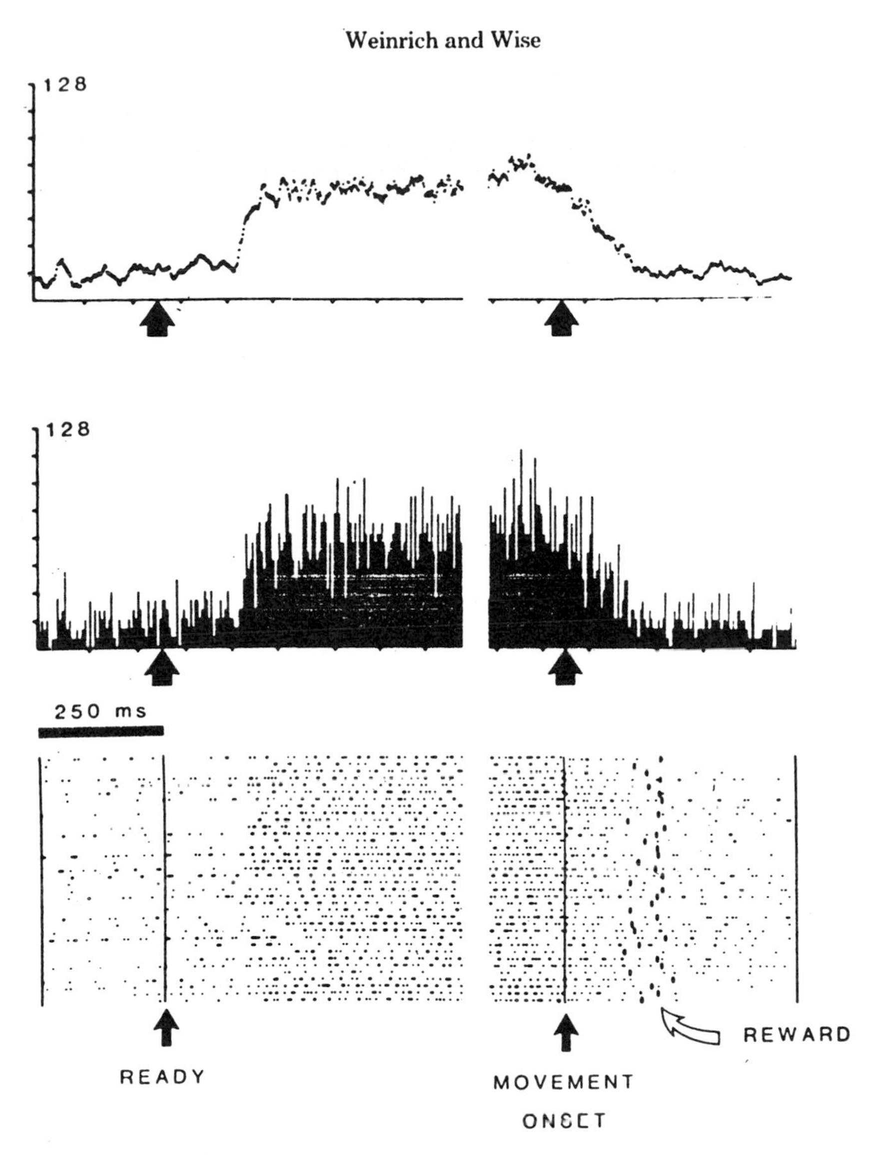

FIG. 6.18. A set-related neuron in the PMd of the monkey. This unit had a sustained increase in activity during an instructed delay period when the upcoming movement direction was to the left. Unit activity is aligned on the appearance of the visual instruction signal (*left*) and on movement onset (*right*). The unit's activity is shown as a reciprocal interval plot for the summed trials (*top*), in a histogram (*middle*), and as rasters (*bottom*). In the rasters, each *dot* represents an action potential and each *line* of the raster represents one movement trial. [Adapted from Weinrich and Wise (233). Reprinted by permission of the Society for Neuroscience.]

potentially subcortical mechanisms, which naturally guide movements to targets "like a magnet." Others have found that monkeys with unilateral PMv lesions neglect to use their contralateral hand and mouth for reaching and grasping (196).

The activity of neurons in the PMv is, in some instances, dependent on a linkage between the visual stimulus and the subsequent movement. Godschalk et al. (82) trained monkeys to reach through a hole in a plastic plate to retrieve visible food rewards placed at one of three locations (82). Most neurons changed their activity between the time when food became visible and the time when the monkey was allowed to reach for the reward. Once the animal began to move, however, the activity of many of these neurons returned to baseline levels. Just viewing the food reward was not sufficient to activate these neurons. Instead, changes in activity depended on the association between localizing the reward and preparing to reach for it.

Rizzolatti and his colleagues (194) have examined the activity of PMv neurons during a wide variety of behaviors such as reaching, grasping, and ingesting food items of different sizes and shapes. They found that PMv activity was often related to specific parts of a movement, such as the use of the hand in "precision grip" or in "whole-hand prehension" [Fig. 6.19; (194)]. They reported that many PMv neurons exhibited about the same activity for reaching and grasping a similar object with either arm. Based on this and other observations, they concluded that the PMv is involved in a relatively high level of motor processing. Rizzolatti et al. (194) proposed that different classes of PMv neurons "form a vocabulary of motor acts and that this vocabulary can be accessed by somatosensory and visual stimuli."

In a prior section (see earlier under INPUTS TO THE PREMOTOR AREAS), we presented an overview of the cortical inputs to the PMv. There we noted that it is the target of major inputs from portions of posterior parietal cortex (areas 5 and 7) and dorsolateral prefrontal cortex (area 46). Both of these cortical regions are involved in spatially guided behavior. They may provide information about the location of objects either from current data or from memory. Thus, both the anatomical and physiological data available support the concept that PMv is involved in important aspects of the visual guidance of limb movement, and perhaps the guidance of movement based on external spatial cues in general.

Conditional Associations. Visual symbols or auditory signals (language) are frequently used to instruct various movements. These conditional associations differ from strictly visually guided movements in that the inherent characteristics of the stimulus do not provide any clues as to the appropriate response. For instance, the color of a traffic signal does not intrinsically indicate whether to brake or accelerate. In such situations, we must learn an arbitrary association between a symbol and a motor act.

Passingham (179) proposed that the ability to perform tasks that required the association of a motor

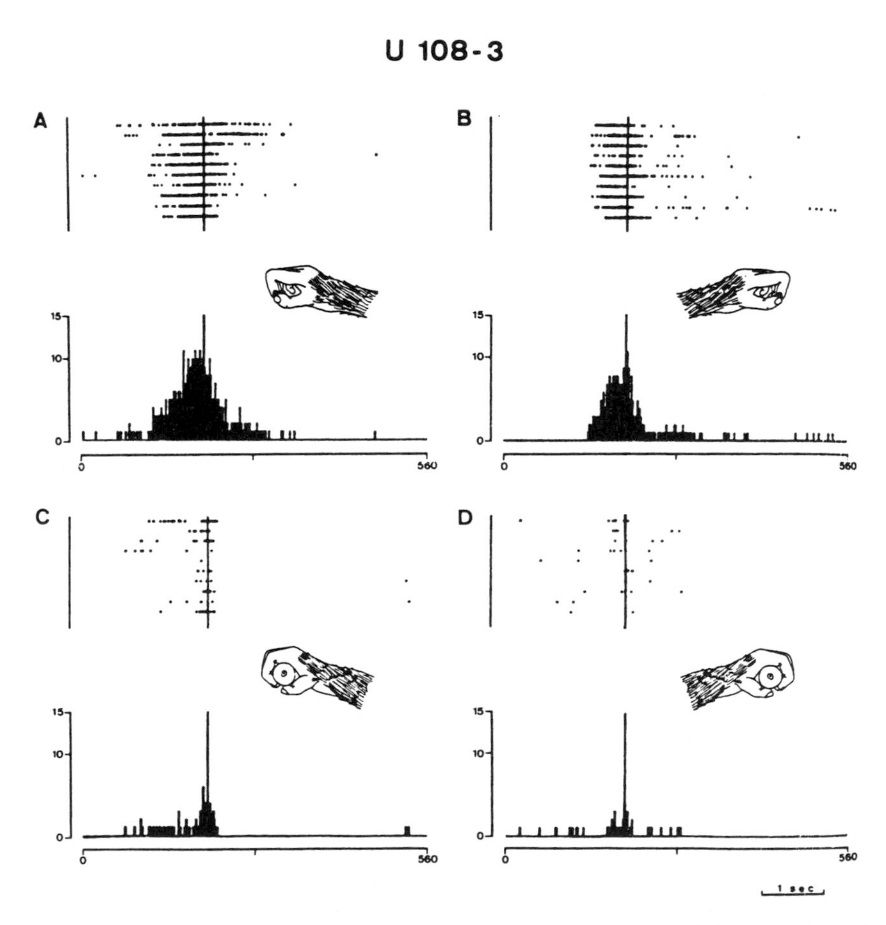

FIG. 6.19. Discharge of a PMv neuron during visually guided reaching and grasping. Individual rasters and histograms are aligned with the hand's contact with the object (*central vertical line*). This neuron was classified as a "grasping-with-the-hand" neuron. *A* and *B*, Neuronal discharge was related to grasping with a precision grip. Note that the discharge was nearly identical during testing of the contralateral (*A*) or ipsilateral hands (*B*). *C* and *D*, Neuronal discharge was weakly related to grasping a cylinder with whole-hand prehension. Bin width is 10 ms. [From Rizzolatti et al. (194). © 1988 Springer-Verlag. Reprinted by permission.]

response with a particular sensory stimulus depends on the lateral premotor cortex (PMv and PMd). Support for this proposal comes from an experiment that examined activity in the PMd during a task that required monkeys to learn associations between arbitrary visual stimuli and directions of limb movement (157). They found that neurons in the PMd began to exhibit consistent changes in activity during the instructed delay and/or movement execution periods as the monkey learned to associate a particular direction of movement with a specific symbol. The same neuron displayed little or no change in activity for movements in the identical direction when they were made following the presentation of a new symbol, until a new association was made. Such associations developed over several trials. Thus, neuron activity was not related to either the movement direction or the stimulus per se, but to the correct association of a visual stimulus and a particular movement (see also 50). Mitz and colleagues (157) concluded that the PMd was involved in the retrieval of sensorimotor associations, rather than in the learning of new associations, because the coupling of neuron activity to movement lagged behind correct performance of the task.

The conditional association paradigm has not been used in recording studies of other cortical motor areas in laboratory primates. A functional imaging study of human cortex during a conditional association task did not reveal differential activation in any of the premotor areas. However, based on the results from the lesion studies of Passingham (179), it is not unreasonable to speculate that the PMd, and the portion of area 6 rostral to it, are more involved in this type of motor task than the motor areas on the medial wall of the hemisphere.

Self-Paced Movements. Numerous investigators have tried to determine which cortical areas are involved in generating self-paced movements in humans. These movements are particularly interesting because they are internally triggered and are thought to represent the essence of volitional control. Self-paced movements are associated with distinct electrical potentials (e.g., readiness potentials) that can be recorded from the scalp of humans (see 125). The cortical localization of these potentials is controversial. For example, some studies have suggested that the readiness potential originates from the SMA (46, 138, 139), whereas others have concluded that it originates from the premotor cortex just rostral to M1 or even M1 itself (23, 169). Although the literature on this issue is too extensive to properly review here, a region on the mesial wall remains as a viable site for the source of the readiness potential and as a possible location for the initiation of self-paced movements.

Unfortunately, there has not been any systematic attempt to examine all of the premotor areas of monkeys and determine their potential differential involvement in self-paced movements. One study of this question, however, is particularly suggestive. Shima et al. (206) examined the activity of neurons in the cingulate motor areas in monkeys trained to perform simple key-press movements that were either self-paced or stimulus triggered. They found two foci of neurons that were related to their tasks. One focus was found in an anterior portion of the cingulate sulcus, in an area that included the CMAr. The other focus was located in a posterior portion of the sulcus, in a region that included both the CMAd and CMAv. The activity of neurons in the two foci were related to both simple motor tasks. Neurons in the anterior foci were notable because they had a more pronounced build-up of neuronal activity before self-paced movements than did neurons in the posterior region. Although evidence on other premotor areas is lacking, the results of Shima et al. suggest that the CMAr may be especially important in the volitional generation of movement. In this regard, strokes that involve the anterior cerebral artery lead to a syndrome termed "akinetic mutism," which is characterized by a profound absence of movement and speech (18, 61, 170).

Sequential Movements. The ability to perform sequences of movements is critical to many of the motor tasks we perform as part of our daily activities such as dressing, operating mechanical equipment, playing music, or participating in sports. Early functional imaging studies in humans promoted the hypothesis that the SMA was preferentially involved in the generation of movement sequences (176, 197). Roland and co-workers (197) reported that rCBF in the SMA increased during a remembered sequence of finger opposition movements, but not during simple finger movements. In contrast, rCBF in M1 was comparable in the two tasks. Furthermore, the SMA, but not M1, was activated when subjects *imagined* performing the movement sequence (see also 47, 192, 211). Subsequent imaging studies have questioned these results in two respects. First, studies using more sensitive imaging methods indicate that SMA activation is present, albeit small, during the performance of simple finger movements (40, 64, 88). Second, the area activated during the imagined performance of movement sequences appears to be the pre-SMA, and not the more caudally located SMA proper (e.g., 189, 211).

The differential involvement of the cortical motor areas of monkeys in sequential movements has just begun to be explored. Mushiake et al. (165) examined the activity of neurons in the SMA, PMd, and PMv in monkeys trained to perform sequences of reaching movements. The movement sequences were guided either by visual instructions or by remembered instructions. Neurons that were preferentially related to the performance of remembered sequences were predominantly located in the SMA and PMd. In fact, the SMA and PMd each contained some "sequence-specific" neurons that changed their activity only during the performance of one of several remembered sequences (Fig. 6.20). In contrast, neurons preferentially related to the performance of visually guided sequences were predominantly located in the PMv. Most neurons in M1 had similar changes in activity for both task conditions.

The design of the task employed by Mushiake et al. (165) required monkeys to perform a visually instructed sequence of reaching movements. Then, a visually instructed sequence was repeated enough times for the animal to perform it as a remembered sequence. Some neurons were active only during the transition period from the visually guided task to the remembered task. These "transition-specific" neurons were most numerous in the PMv. Such neurons might be particularly important for the acquisition of motor skills.

In a related experiment, Tanji and Shima (222) trained monkeys to perform three movements (push, pull, and turn) in different sequences. Neurons in M1 were related to the execution of a particular movement independent of its order in the sequence. On the other hand, the activity of some neurons in the SMA depended on the position of a particular movement in the sequence. Tanji and Shima (222) proposed that these cells contribute a signal necessary for specifying the serial order of movements within motor tasks.

Picard and Strick (188) have used the 2-deoxyglucose technique to map the metabolic activity on the

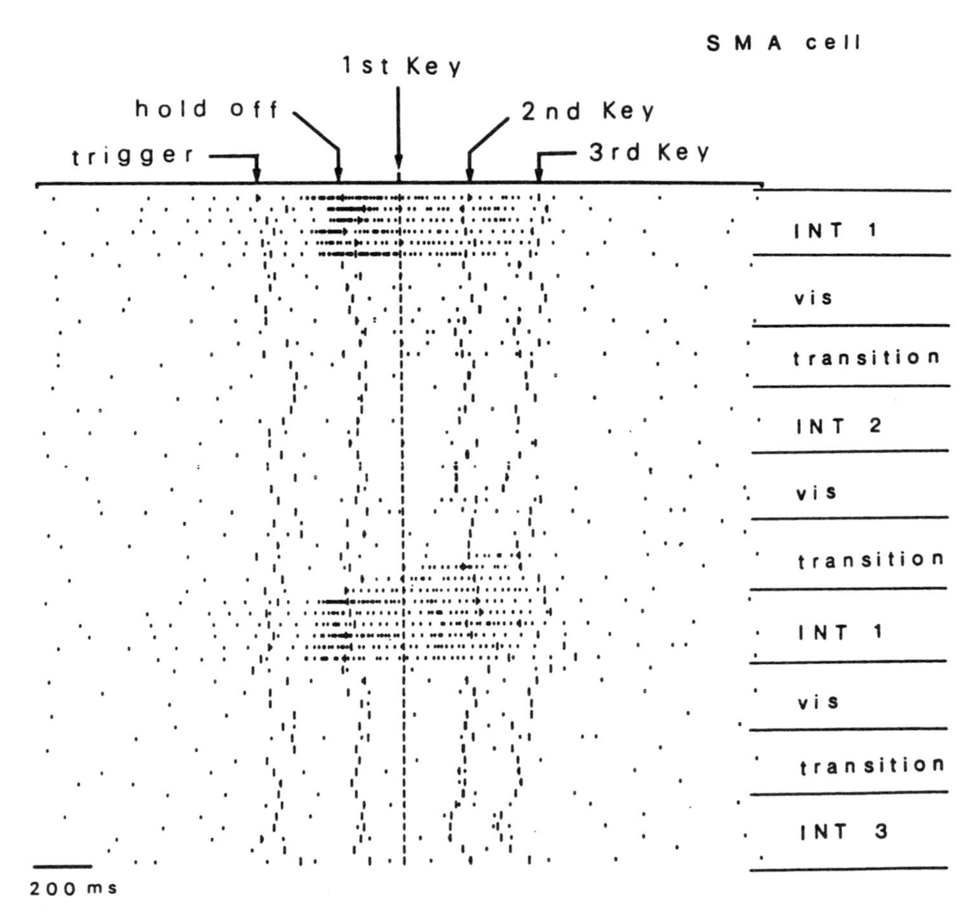

FIG. 6.20. A sequence-specific neuron recorded in the SMA of a macaque monkey. This neuron increased its activity only when the animal performed a remembered sequence of movements (*INT 1*). The neuron was not active during different remembered sequences (*INT 2* and *3*), visually guided sequences (*vis*) or the transitional phase (*transition*) between visually guided and remembered sequences. [Adapted from Mushiake, Inase, and Tanji (165). Reprinted by permission of the American Physiological Society.]

medial wall of the hemisphere in monkeys trained to perform remembered sequences of reaching movements. They found two sites of focal activation on the medial wall. One of these was located in the arm representation of the CMAd and the other was present in the pre-SMA. Activation in the other motor areas on the medial wall was either absent or less significant. These observations suggest that, of all the motor areas on the medial wall, the CMAd and the pre-SMA are preferentially involved in the internal guidance of sequential voluntary arm movements.

The absence of focal activation in the SMA in the study of Picard and Strick (188) is surprising, given the presence of sequence-specific neurons in this cortical area (165, 222). Several differences in the behavioral paradigms used in these studies may have contributed to these differences. For example, Picard and Strick overtrained their monkeys until the three elements of the movement sequence were performed as a stereotyped unit with invariant temporal characteristics. Mushiake et al. did not train their animals to the same level of performance. Tanji and Shima used a fundamentally different task in which each movement in the sequence was triggered by an external stimulus. Thus, it is possible that the involvement of specific cortical areas depends on both the specific requirements of the task and the level of the animal's training on it.

Further support for the importance of training comes from the observations of Aizawa et al. (1) on the SMA. Normally, the SMA contains many neurons that are related to the performance of a simple key-press task. However, Aizawa et al. found that few task-related neurons were present in the SMA of an animal that was overtrained for more than a year on this task. Next, they ablated M1. When the animal was sufficiently recovered from the effects of the lesion to perform the task, numerous movement-related neurons were again found in the SMA. This observation not only supports the notion that the participation of specific cortical areas shifts with the level of task acquisition, but also implies that the SMA participates in the recovery of motor function that follows damage to M1.

It is clear that the use of complex behavioral tasks, like sequential movements, reveals new features about the involvement of the cortical motor areas in specific aspects of motor behavior. Generally, one finds that the proportion of neurons that are preferentially related to a task varies among the motor areas. That particular categories of neurons (e.g., sequence-specific neurons) are seen in more than one motor area should not be surprising, given the dense interconnections among the motor areas. However, the concentration of neurons with unique characteristics in certain motor areas lends support to the concept that individual motor areas are specialized in terms of their functional involvement in specific aspects of motor behavior.

CONCLUSION

A major change has taken place in our ideas about the cortical control of movement. Anatomical and physiological investigations reveal that the central commands for movement do not emanate exclusively from M1. The frontal lobe contains multiple premotor areas in addition to the primary motor cortex. Each of the premotor areas projects directly to the spinal cord and each contains neurons with activity related to movement execution. The strong reciprocal connections among the cortical motor areas suggest that the programming and execution of movement is performed in a cooperative manner among these areas.

On the other hand, considerable evidence suggests that the premotor areas are not simply clones of the M1. Each premotor area receives a unique mix of corticocortical and subcortical inputs. This implies that each motor area is differentially involved in specific aspects of motor behavior. Physiological investigations support this conclusion. For example, some premotor areas appear to be particularly active during the preparation and generation of movement sequences, whereas others appear to be involved in the visual guidance of movement. However, it should be clear that we are only at the initial stage of examining the functional contributions of these cortical fields.

Our review indicates that the premotor areas influence motor processing at multiple levels. Development of an adequate model to explain the myriad of characteristics present in these motor areas remains a daunting challenge. Considerable effort will be required to decipher the unique functional contributions of each motor area and to understand their involvement in motor processes such as skill acquisition and retention, as well as movement planning and execution. The structural framework developed in this chapter should provide an important foundation for exploring these issues.

This work was supported by the VA Medical Research Service and Rehabilitation Research and Development Service, and by U.S. Public Health Service grant 24328 (PLS).

REFERENCES

1. Aizawa, H., M. Inase, H. Mushiake, K. Shima, and J. Tanji. Reorganization of activity in the supplementary motor area

associated with motor learning and functional recovery. *Exp. Brain Res.* 84: 668–671, 1991.
2. Alexander, G. E., and M. D. Crutcher. Preparation for movement: neural representations of intended direction in three motor areas of the monkey. *J. Neurophysiol.* 64: 133–150, 1990.
3. Alexander, G. E., and M. D. Crutcher. Neural representation of the target (goal) of visually guided arm movements in three motor areas of the monkey. *J. Neurophysiol.* 64: 164–178, 1990.
4. Alexander, G. E., M. R. DeLong, and P. L. Strick. Parallel organization of functionally segregated circuits linking basal ganglia and cortex. *Annu. Rev. Neurosci.* 9: 357–381, 1986.
5. Allen, G. I., and N. Tsukahara. Cerebrocerebellar communication systems. *Physiol. Rev.* 54: 957–1006, 1974.
6. Andersen, P., P. J. Hagan, C. G. Phillips, and T. P. Powell. Mapping by microstimulation of overlapping projections from area 4 to motor units of the baboon's hand. *Proc. R. Soc. Lond. B Biol. Sci.* 188: 31–36, 1975.
7. Antinucci, F., and E. Visalberghi. Tool use in *Cebus apella*: a case study. *Int. J. Primatol.* 7: 349–361, 1986.
8. Asanuma, C., W. T. Thach, and E. G. Jones. Distribution of cerebellar terminations and their relation to other afferent terminations in the ventral lateral thalamic region of the monkey. *Brain Res.* 286: 237–265, 1983.
9. Asanuma, C., W. T. Thach, and E. G. Jones. Anatomical evidence for segregated focal groupings of efferent cells and their terminal ramifications in the cerebellothalamic pathway of the monkey. *Brain Res.* 286: 267–297, 1983.
10. Asanuma, H. *The Motor Cortex*. New York: Raven Press, 1989.
11. Asanuma, H., A. Arnold, and P. Zarzecki. Further study on the excitation of pyramidal tract cells by intracortical microstimulation. *Exp. Brain Res.* 26: 443–461, 1976.
12. Asanuma, H., and A. Keller. Neurobiological basis of motor learning and memory. *Concepts Neurosci.* 2: 1–30, 1991.
13. Asanuma, H., and R. Mackel. Direct and indirect sensory input pathways to the motor cortex; its structure and function in relation to learning of motor skills. *Jpn. J. Physiol.* 39: 1–19, 1989.
14. Asanuma, H., and I. Rosen. Topographical organization of cortical efferent zones projecting to distal forelimb muscles in the monkey. *Exp. Brain Res.* 14: 243–256, 1972.
15. Baleydier, C., and F. Mauguiere. The duality of the cingulate gyrus in monkey: neuroanatomical study and functional hypothesis. *Brain* 103: 525–554, 1980.
16. Baleydier, C., and F. Mauguiere. Network organization of the connectivity between parietal area 7, posterior cingulate cortex and medial pulvinar nucleus: a double fluorescent tracer study in monkey. *Exp. Brain Res.* 66: 385–393, 1987.
17. Barbas, H., and D. N. Pandya. Architecture and frontal cortical connections of the premotor cortex (area 6) in the rhesus monkey. *J. Comp. Neurol.* 256: 211–228, 1987.
18. Barris, R. W., and H. R. Schuman. Bilateral anterior cingulate lesions. *Neurology* 3: 44–52, 1953.
19. Bates, J. F., and P. S. Goldman-Rakic. Prefrontal connections of medial motor areas in the rhesus monkey. *J. Comp. Neurol.* 336: 211–228, 1993.
20. Batton, R. R., A. I. Jayaraman, D. Ruggiero, and M. B. Carpenter. Fastigial efferent projections in the monkey: an autoradiographic study. *J. Comp. Neurol.* 174: 281–306, 1977.
21. Biber, M. P., L. W. Kneisley, and J. H. LaVail. Cortical neurons projecting to the cervical and lumbar enlargements of the spinal cord in young and adult rhesus monkeys. *Exp. Neurol.* 59: 492–508, 1978.
22. Bortoff, G. A., and P. L. Strick. Corticospinal terminations in two New-World primates: further evidence that corticomotoneuronal connections provide part of the neural substrate for manual dexterity. *J. Neurosci.* 13: 5105–5118, 1993.
23. Bötzel, K., H. Plendl, W. Paulus, and M. Scherg. Bereitschaftspotential: is there a contribution of the supplementary motor area? *Electroencephalogr. Clin. Neurophysiol.* 89: 187–196, 1993.
24. Brinkman, C. Supplementary motor area (SMA) and premotor area (PM) of the monkey's brain: distribution of degeneration in the spinal cord after unilateral lesions. *Neurosci. Lett.* 8: 36, 1982.
25. Brinkman, J., B. M. Bush, and R. Porter. Deficient influence of peripheral stimuli on precentral neurones in monkeys with dorsal column lesions. *J. Physiol. (Lond.)* 276: 27–48, 1978.
26. Brodal, P. The corticopontine projection in the rhesus monkey. Origin and principles of organization. *Brain* 101: 251–283, 1978.
27. Brodmann, K. *Vergleichende Lokalisationslehre der Grosshirnrinde in Ihren Prinzipien Dargestellt auf Grund des Zellenbaues*. Leipzig: Barth, 1909.
28. Brooks, V. B., and W. T. Thach. Cerebellar control of posture and movement. In: *Handbook of Physiology, The Nervous System, Motor Control*, edited by V. B. Brooks. Bethesda, MD: Am. Physiol. Soc., 1981, p. 877–946.
29. Buys, E. J., R. N. Lemon, G. W. Mantel, and R. B. Muir. Selective facilitation of different hand muscles by single corticospinal neurones in the conscious monkey. *J. Physiol. (Lond)*. 381: 529–549, 1986.
30. Caminiti, R., P. B. Johnson, and A. Urbano. Making arm movements within different parts of space: dynamic aspects in the primate motor cortex. *J. Neurosci.* 10: 2039–2058, 1990.
31. Caminiti, R., P. B. Johnson, C. Galli, S. Ferraina, and Y. Burnod. Making arm movements within different parts of space: the premotor and motor cortical representation of a coordinate system for reaching to visual targets. *J. Neurosci.* 11: 1182–1197, 1991.
32. Campbell, A. W. *Histological Studies on the Localization of Cerebral Function*. Cambridge: Cambridge University Press, 1905.
33. Catsman-Berrevoets, C. E., and H. G. J. M. Kuypers. Cells of origin of cortical projections to dorsal column nuclei, spinal cord and bulbar medial reticular formation in the rhesus monkey. *Neurosci. Lett.* 3: 245–252, 1976.
34. Chan-Palay, V. *Cerebellar Dentate Nucleus. Organization, Cytology and Transmitters*. Berlin: Springer-Verlag, 1977.
35. Cheema, S., B. L. Whitsel, and A. Rustioni. Corticospinal projections from pericentral and supplementary cortices in macaques as revealed by anterograde transport of horseradish peroxidase. *Neurosci. Lett.* 14: 62, 1983.
36. Cheema, S. S., A. Rustioni, and B. L. Whitsel. Light and electron microscopic evidence for a direct corticospinal projection to superficial laminae of the dorsal horn in cats and monkeys. *J. Comp. Neurol.* 225: 276–290, 1984.
37. Cheney, P. D., and E. E. Fetz. Functional classes of primate corticomotoneuronal cells and their relation to active force. *J. Neurophysiol.* 44: 773–791, 1980.

38. Cheney, P. D., E. E. Fetz, and K. Mewes. Neural mechanisms underlying corticospinal and rubrospinal control of limb movements. *Prog. Brain Res.* 87: 213–252, 1991.
39. Cheney, P. D., E. E. Fetz, and S. S. Palmer. Patterns of facilitation and suppression of antagonist forelimb muscles from motor cortex sites in the awake monkey. *J. Neurophysiol.* 53: 805–820, 1985.
40. Colebatch, J. G., M. P. Deiber, R. E. Passingham, K. J. Friston, and R. S. J. Frackowiak. Regional cerebral blood flow during voluntary arm and hand movements in human subjects. *J. Neurophysiol.* 65: 1392–1401, 1991.
41. Costello, M. B., and D. M. Fragaszy. Prehension in *Cebus* and *Saimiri*. I. Grip type and hand preference. *Am. J. Primatol.* 15: 235–245, 1988.
42. Coulter, J. D., and E. G. Jones. Differential distribution of corticospinal projections from individual cytoarchitectonic fields in the monkey. *Brain Res.* 129: 335–340, 1977.
43. Crutcher, M. D., and G. E. Alexander. Movement-related neuronal activity selectively coding either direction or muscle pattern in three motor areas of the monkey. *J. Neurophysiol.* 64: 151–163, 1990.
44. Darian-Smith, C., I. Darian-Smith, K. Burman, and N. Ratcliffe. Ipsilateral cortical projections to areas 3a, 3b, and 4 in the macaque monkey. *J. Comp. Neurol.* 335: 200–213, 1993.
45. Darian-Smith, C., I. Darian-Smith, and S. S. Cheema. Thalamic projections to sensorimotor cortex in the macaque monkey: use of multiple retrograde fluorescent tracers. *J. Comp. Neurol.* 299: 17–46, 1990.
46. Deecke, L., B. Groezinger, and H. H. Kornhuber. Voluntary finger movement in man: cerebral potentials and theory. *Biol. Cybern.* 23: 99–119, 1976.
47. Deiber, M. P., R. E. Passingham, J. G. Colebatch, K. J. Friston, and P. D. Nixon. Cortical areas and the selection of movement: a study with positron emission tomography. *Exp. Brain Res.* 84: 393–402, 1991.
48. DeVito, J. L., and O. A. Smith. Projections from the mesial frontal cortex (supplementary motor area) to the cerebral hemispheres and brainstem of the *Macaca mulatta*. *J. Comp. Neurol.* 111: 261–278, 1959.
49. DeVito, J. L., and M. E. Anderson. An autoradiographic study of efferent connections of the globus pallidus in *Macaca mulatta*. *Exp. Brain Res.* 46: 107–117, 1982.
50. di Pellegrino, G., and S. P. Wise. Visuospatial versus visuomotor activity in the premotor and prefrontal cortex of a primate. *J. Neurosci.* 13: 1227–1243, 1993.
51. Donoghue, J. P., S. Leibovic, and J. N. Sanes. Organization of the forelimb area in squirrel monkey motor cortex: representation of digit, wrist, and elbow muscles. *Exp. Brain Res.* 89: 1–19, 1992.
52. Donoghue, J. P., S. Suner, and J. N. Sanes. Dynamic organization of primary motor cortex output to target muscles in adult rats. II. Rapid reorganization following motor nerve lesions. *Exp. Brain Res.* 179: 492–503, 1990.
53. Dum, R. P., and P. L. Strick. Corticospinal projections from the motor areas in the frontal lobe. In: *Taniguichi Symposia on Brain Sciences No. 12: Neural Programming*, edited by M. Ito. Tokyo: Japan Scientific Societies Press, 1989, p. 49–63.
54. Dum, R. P., and P. L. Strick. Premotor areas: nodal points for parallel efferent systems involved in the central control of movement. In: *Motor Control: Concepts and Issues*, edited by D. R. Humphrey and H.-J. Freund. London: John Wiley & Sons, 1991, p. 383–397.
55. Dum, R. P., and P. L. Strick. The origin of corticospinal projections from the premotor areas in the frontal lobe. *J. Neurosci.* 11: 667–689, 1991.
56. Dum, R. P., and P. L. Strick. Cingulate motor areas. In: *Neurobiology of Cingulate Cortex and Limbic Thalamus*, edited by B. A. Vogt and M. Gabriel. Boston: Birkhauser, 1993, p. 415–441.
57. Dum, R. P., and P. L. Strick. Supplementary motor area (SMA) input to the cervical cord. *Soc. Neurosci. Abstr.* 19: 1210, 1993.
58. Evarts, E. V. Role of motor cortex in voluntary movements in primates. In: *Handbook of Physiology, The Nervous System, Motor Control*, edited by V. B. Brooks. Bethesda, MD: Am. Physiol. Soc., 1981, p. 1083–1120.
59. Evarts, E. V., C. Fromm, J. Kroller, and V. A. Jennings. Motor cortex control of finely graded forces. *J. Neurophysiol.* 49: 1199–1215, 1983.
60. Evarts, E. V., and W. T. Thach. Motor mechanisms of the CNS: cerebrocerebellar interrelations. *Annu. Rev. Physiol.* 31: 451–498, 1969.
61. Farris, A. A. Limbic system infarction. *Neurology* 19: 91–96, 1969.
62. Fetz, E. E., and P. D. Cheney. Postspike facilitation of forelimb muscle activity by primate corticomotoneuronal cells. *J. Neurophysiol.* 44: 751–772, 1980.
63. Fortier, P. A., J. F. Kalaska, and A. M. Smith. Cerebellar neuronal activity related to whole-arm reaching movements in the monkey. *J. Neurophysiol.* 62: 198–211, 1989.
64. Fox, P. T., J. M. Fox, M. E. Raichle, and R. M. Burde. The role of cerebral cortex in the generation of voluntary saccades in a positron emission tomographic study. *J. Neurophysiol.* 54: 348–369, 1985.
65. Fragaszy, D. M. Preliminary quantitative studies of prehension in squirrel monkeys (*Saimiri sciureus*). *Brain Behav. Evol.* 23: 81–92, 1983.
66. Freund, H.-J., and H. Hummelsheim. Lesions of premotor cortex in man. *Brain* 108: 697–733, 1985.
67. Fulton, J. F. Definition of the "motor" and "premotor" areas. *Brain* 58: 311–316, 1935.
68. Fulton, J. F. *Physiology of the Nervous System*. New York: Oxford University Press, 1949.
69. Fulton, J. F. and M. A. Kennard. A study of flaccid and spastic paralysis produced by lesions of the cerebral cortex in primates. *Assoc. Res. Nerv. Ment. Dis.* 13: 158–210, 1934.
70. Galyon, D. D., and P. L. Strick. Multiple and differential projections from the parietal lobe to the premotor areas of the primate. *Soc. Neurosci. Abstr.* 11: 1274, 1985.
71. Gentilucci, M., L. Fogassi, G. Luppino, M. Matelli, R. Camarda, and G. Rizzolatti. Functional organization of inferior area 6 in the macaque monkey. I. Somatotopy and the control of proximal movements. *Exp. Brain Res.* 71: 475–490, 1988.
72. Georgopoulos, A. P. Spatial coding of visually guided arm movements in primate motor cortex. *Can. J. Physiol. Pharmacol.* 66: 518–526, 1988.
73. Georgopoulos, A. Higher order motor control. *Annu. Rev. Neurosci.* 14: 361–377, 1991.
74. Georgopoulos, A. P., R. Caminiti, J. F. Kalaska, and J. T. Massey. Spatial coding of movement: a hypothesis concerning the coding of movement direction by motor cortical populations. *Exp. Brain Res.* 7(Suppl): 327–336, 1983.
75. Georgopoulos, A. P., M. D. Crutcher, and A. B. Schwartz. Cognitive spatial motor processes. III. Motor cortical prediction of movement direction during an instructed delay period. *Exp. Brain Res.* 75: 183–194, 1989.

76. Georgopoulos, A. P., M. R. DeLong, and M. D. Crutcher. Relations between parameters of step-tracking movements and single cell discharge in the globus pallidus and subthalamic nucleus of the behaving monkey. *J. Neurosci.* 3: 1586–1598, 1983.
77. Georgopoulos, A.P., J. F. Kalaska, R. Caminiti, and J. T. Massey. On the relations between the direction of two-dimensional arm movements and cell discharge in primate motor cortex. *J. Neurosci.* 2: 1527–1537, 1982.
78. Georgopoulos, A. P., J. F. Kalaska, M. D. Crutcher, R. Caminiti, and J. T. Massey. The representation of movement direction in the motor cortex: single cell and population studies. In: *Dynamic Aspects of Neocortical Function*, edited by G. M. Edelman, W. M. Cowan, and W. E. Gall. New York: John Wiley & Sons, 1984, p. 501–524.
79. Georgopoulos, A. P., R. E. Kettner, and A. B. Schwartz. Primate motor cortex and free arm movements to visual targets in three-dimensional space. II. Coding of the direction of movement by a neuronal population. *J. Neurosci.* 8: 2928–2937, 1988.
80. Ghosh, S., C. Brinkman, and R. Porter. A quantitative study of the distribution of neurons projecting to the precentral motor cortex in the monkey (*M. fascicularis*). *J. Comp. Neurol.* 259: 424–444, 1987.
81. Godschalk, M., R. N. Lemon, H. G. Kuypers, and H. K. Ronday. Cortical afferents and efferents of monkey postarcuate area: an anatomical and electrophysiological study. *Exp. Brain Res.* 56: 410–424, 1984.
82. Godschalk, M., R. N. Lemon, H. G. Kuypers, and J. van der Steen. The involvement of monkey premotor cortex neurones in preparation of visually cued arm movements. *Behav. Brain Res.* 18: 143–157, 1985.
83. Goldman-Rakic, P. S. Motor control function of the prefrontal cortex. In: *Motor Areas of the Cerebral Cortex (Ciba Foundation Symposium 132).* Chichester: John Wiley & Sons, 1987, p. 187–200.
84. Goldman-Rakic, P. S. Cellular and circuit basis of working memory in prefrontal cortex of nonhuman primates. *Prog. Brain Res.* 85: 325–335, 1990.
85. Goldman-Rakic, P. S., and L. D. Selemon. New frontiers in basal ganglia research. *Trends Neurosci.* 13: 241–244, 1990.
86. Gould, H. J., III, C. G. Cusick, T. P. Pons, and J. H. Kaas. The relationship of corpus callosum connections to electrical stimulation maps of motor, supplementary motor, and the frontal eye fields in owl monkeys. *J. Comp. Neurol.* 247: 297–325, 1986.
87. Grafton, S. T., R. P. Woods, J. C. Mazziotta, and M. E. Phelps. Somatotopic mapping of the primary motor cortex in humans: activation studies with cerebral blood flow and positron emission tomography. *J. Neurophysiol.* 66: 735–743, 1991.
88. Grafton, S. T., R. P. Woods, and J. C. Mazziotta. Within-arm somatotopy in human motor areas determined by positron emission tomography imaging of cerebral blood flow. *Exp. Brain Res.* 95: 172–176, 1993.
89. Graybiel, A. M. Neurotransmitters and neuromodulators in the basal ganglia. *Trends Neurosci.* 13: 244–254, 1990.
90. Graybiel, A. M., T. Aosaki, A. W. Flaherty, and M. Kimura. The basal ganglia and adaptive motor control. *Science* 265: 1826–1831, 1994.
91. Hahm, J., M. F. Huerta, P. L. Strick, I. Danielsson, and T. Pons. Parallel cortical pathways for the control of movement. *Soc. Neurosci. Abstr.* 18: 216, 1992.
92. He, S. Q., R. P. Dum, and P. L. Strick. Topographic organization of corticospinal projections from the frontal lobe: motor areas on the lateral surface of the hemisphere. *J. Neurosci.* 13: 952–980, 1993.
93. He, S. Q., R. P. Dum, and P. L. Strick. Topographic organization of corticospinal projections from the frontal lobe: motor areas on the medial surface of the hemisphere. *J. Neurosci.* 15: 3284–3306, 1995.
94. Hepp-Reymond, M. C. Functional organization of motor cortex and its participation in voluntary movements. In: *Comparative Primate Biology, Vol. 4: Neurosciences.* New York: Alan R. Liss, 1988, p. 501–624.
95. Holsapple, J. W., J. B. Preston, and P. L. Strick. The origin of thalamic inputs to the "hand" representation in the primary motor cortex. *J. Neurosci.* 11: 2644–2654, 1991.
96. Holsapple, J. W., and P. L. Strick. Premotor areas on the medial wall of the hemisphere: input from ventrolateral thalamus. *Soc. Neurosci. Abstr.* 15: 282, 1989.
97. Holsapple, J. W., and P. L. Strick. Pattern of projections from the premotor areas on the medial wall of the hemisphere to the primary motor cortex. *Soc. Neurosci. Abstr.* 17: 1020, 1991.
98. Hoover, J. E., and P. L. Strick. Multiple output channels in the basal ganglia. *Science* 259: 819–821, 1993.
99. Huang, C. S., M. A. Sirisko, H. Hiraba, G. M. Murray, and B. J. Sessle. Organization of the primate face motor cortex as revealed by intracortical microstimulation and electrophysiological identification of afferent inputs and corticobulbar projections. *J. Neurophysiol.* 59: 796–818, 1988.
100. Huerta, M. F. and T. P. Pons. Primary motor cortex receives input from area 3a in macaques. *Brain Res.* 537: 367–371, 1990.
101. Humphrey, D. R. On the cortical control of visually directed reaching: contribution by nonprecentral motor areas. In: *Posture and Movement*, edited by R. E. Talbot and D. R. Humphrey. New York: Raven Press, 1979, p. 51–112.
102. Humphrey, D. R. Representation of movements and muscles within the primate precentral motor cortex: historical and current perspectives. *Federation Proc.* 45: 2687–2699, 1986.
103. Humphrey, D. R., and W. S. Corrie. Properties of pyramidal tract neuron system within a functionally defined subregion of primate motor cortex. *J. Neurophysiol.* 41: 216–243, 1978.
104. Humphrey, D. R., and D. J. Reed. Separate cortical systems for control of joint movement and joint stiffness: reciprocal activation and coactivation of antagonist muscles. *Adv. Neurol.* 39: 347–372, 1983.
105. Huntley, G. W., and E. G. Jones. Relationship of intrinsic connections to forelimb movement representation in monkey motor cortex: a correlative anatomic and physiological study. *J. Neurophysiol.* 66: 390–413, 1991.
106. Hutchins, K. D., A. M. Martino, and P. L. Strick. Corticospinal projections from the medial wall of the hemisphere. *Exp. Brain Res.* 71: 667–672, 1988.
107. Ilinsky, I. A., and K. Kultas-Ilinsky. Sagittal cytoarchitectonic maps of the *Macaca mulatta* thalamus with a revised nomenclature of the motor-related nuclei validated by observations on their connectivity. *J. Comp. Neurol.* 262: 331–364, 1987.
108. Jacobs, K. M., and J. P. Donoghue. Reshaping the cortical motor map by unmasking latent intracortical connections. *Science* 251: 944–947, 1991.
109. Jacobsen, C. F. Influence of motor and premotor lesions upon retention of acquired skilled movements in monkey

and chimpanzees. *Assoc. Res. Nerv. Ment. Dis.* 13: 225–247, 1934.
110. Jacobsen, C. F. Functions of the frontal association areas in primates. *Arch. Neurol. Psychiatry* 33: 558–569, 1935.
111. Jankowska, E., Y. Padel, and R. Tanaka. The mode of activation of pyramidal tract cells by intracortical stimuli. *J. Physiol. (Lond.)* 249: 617–636, 1975.
112. Jankowska, E., Y. Padel, and R. Tanaka. Projections of pyramidal tract cells to alpha-motoneurones innervating hind-limb muscles in the monkey. *J. Physiol. (Lond.)* 249: 637–667, 1975.
113. Jones, E. G., and T. P. S. Powell. An anatomical study of converging sensory pathways within the cerebral cortex of the monkey. *Brain* 93: 793–820, 1970.
114. Jones, E. G., and S. P. Wise. Size, laminar and columnar distribution of efferent cells in the sensory-motor cortex of monkeys. *J. Comp. Neurol.* 175: 391–438, 1977.
115. Kalaska, J. F. The representation of arm movements in postcentral and parietal cortex. *Can. J. Physiol. Pharmacol.* 66: 455–463, 1988.
116. Kalaska, J. F., R. Caminiti, and A. P. Georgopoulos. Cortical mechanisms related to the direction of two-dimensional arm movements: relations in parietal area 5 and comparison with motor cortex. *Exp. Brain Res.* 51: 247–260, 1983.
117. Kalaska, J. F., D. A. D. Cohen, M. L. Hyde, and M. Prud'homme. A comparison of movement direction-related versus load direction-related activity in primate motor cortex, using a two-dimensional reaching task. *J. Neurosci.* 9: 2080–2102, 1989.
118. Kalaska, J. F., and D. J. Crammond. Cerebral cortical mechanisms of reaching movements. *Science* 255: 1517–1523, 1992.
119. Kalil, K. Projections of the cerebellar and dorsal column nuclei upon the thalamus of the rhesus monkey. *J. Comp. Neurol.* 195: 25–50, 1981.
120. Kasser, R. J., and P. D. Cheney. Characteristics of corticomotoneuronal postspike facilitation and reciprocal suppression of EMG activity in the monkey. *J. Neurophysiol.* 53: 959–978, 1985.
121. Keizer, K., and H. G. Kuypers. Distribution of corticospinal neurons with collaterals to the lower brain stem reticular formation in monkey (*Macaca fascicularis*). *Exp. Brain Res.* 74: 311–318, 1989.
122. Kemp, J. M., and T. P. Powell. The cortico-striate projection in the monkey. *Brain* 93: 525–546, 1970.
123. Kievit, J., and H. G. J. M. Kuypers. Organization of the thalamo-cortical connections to the frontal lobe in the rhesus monkey. *Exp. Brain Res.* 29: 299–322, 1977.
124. Kim, R., K. Nakano, A. Jayaraman, and M. B. Carpenter. Projections of the globus pallidus and adjacent structures: an autoradiographic study in the monkey. *J. Comp. Neurol.* 169: 263–289, 1976.
125. Kornhuber, H. H., L. Deecke, W. Lang, and A. Kornhuber. Will, volitional action, attention and cerebral potentials in man: Bereitschaftspotential, performance-related potentials, directed attention potential, EEG spectrum changes. In: *Volitional Actions, Advances in Psychology*, edited by W. Hershberger. New York: Elsevier Science Publishing, 1989, p. 107–169.
126. Künzle, H. Cortico-cortical efferents of primary motor and somatosensory regions of the cerebral cortex. *Neuroscience* 3: 25–39, 1978.
127. Kuo, J. S., and M. B. Carpenter. Organization of pallidothalamic projections in rhesus monkey. *J. Comp. Neurol.* 151: 201–236, 1973.
128. Kurata, K. Distribution of neurons with set- and movement-related activity before hand and foot movements in the premotor cortex of rhesus monkey. *Exp. Brain Res.* 77: 245–256, 1989.
129. Kurata, K. Corticocortical inputs to the dorsal and ventral aspects of the premotor cortex of macaque monkeys. *Neurosci. Res.* 12: 263–280, 1991.
130. Kurata, K. Premotor cortex of monkey: set- and movement-related activity reflecting amplitude and direction of wrist movements. *J. Neurophysiol.* 69: 187–200, 1993.
131. Kurata, K., and J. Tanji. Premotor cortex neurons in macaques: activity before distal and proximal forelimb movements. *J. Neurosci.* 6: 403–411, 1986.
132. Kusama, T., M. Mabuchi, and T. Sumino. Cerebellar projections to the thalamic nuclei in monkeys. *Proc. Jpn. Acad.* 47: 505–510, 1971.
133. Kuypers, H. G. J. M. Central cortical projections to motor and somato-sensory cell groups. *Brain* 83: 161–184, 1960.
134. Kuypers, H. G. J. M. Anatomy of the descending pathways. In: *Handbook of Physiology, The Nervous System, Motor Control*, edited by V. B. Brooks. Bethesda, MD: Am. Physiol. Soc., 1981, p. 567–666.
135. Kuypers, H. G. J. M., and J. Brinkman. Precentral projections of different parts of the spinal intermediate zone in the rhesus monkey. *Brain Res.* 24: 29–48, 1970.
136. Kwan, H. C., W. A. MacKay, J. T. Murphy, and Y. C. Wong. Spatial organization of precentral cortex in awake primates. II. Motor outputs. *J. Neurophysiol.* 41: 1120–1131, 1978.
137. Lamour, Y., V. A. Jennings, and H. Solis. Functional characteristics and segregation of cutaneous and non-cutaneous neurons in monkey precentral motor cortex (M1). *Soc. Neurosci. Abstr.* 6: 158, 1980.
138. Lang, W., M. Lang, F. Uhl, C. Koska, A. Kornhuber, and L. Deecke. Negative cortical DC shifts preceding and accompanying simultaneous and sequential finger movements. *Exp. Brain Res.* 71: 579–587, 1988.
139. Lang, W., D. Cheyne, R. Kristeva, R. Beisteiner, G. Lindinger, and L. Deecke. Three-dimensional localization of SMA activity preceding voluntary movement. *Exp. Brain Res.* 87: 688–695, 1991.
140. Leichnetz, G. R. Afferent and efferent connections of the dorsolateral precentral gyrus (area 4, hand/arm region) in the macaque monkey, with comparisons to area 8. *J. Comp. Neurol.* 254: 460–492, 1986.
141. Lemon, R. N., R. B. Muir, and G. W. Mantel. The effects upon the activity of hand and forearm muscles of intracortical stimulation in the vicinity of corticomotor neurones in the conscious monkey. *Exp. Brain Res.* 66: 621–637, 1987.
142. Liu, C. N., and W. W. Chambers. An experimental study of the cortico-spinal system in the monkey (*Macaca mulatta*). *J. Comp. Neurol.* 123: 257–284, 1964.
143. Lu, M.-T., J. B. Preston, and P. L. Strick. Interconnections between the prefrontal cortex and the premotor areas in the frontal lobe. *J. Comp. Neurol.* 341: 375–392, 1994.
144. Luppino, G., M. Matelli, R. M. Camarda, V. Gallese, and G. Rizzolatti. Multiple representations of body movements in mesial area 6 and adjacent cingulate cortex: an intracortical microstimulation study in the macaque monkey. *J. Comp. Neurol.* 311: 463–482, 1991.
145. Luppino, G., M. Matelli, R. Camarda, and G. Rizzolatti. Corticocortical connections of area F3 (SMA-proper) and area F6 (pre-SMA) in the macaque monkey. *J. Comp. Neurol.* 338: 114–140, 1993.

146. Lynch, J. C. The functional organization of posterior parietal association cortex. *Behav. Brain Sci.* 3: 485–534, 1980.
147. Macpherson, J. M., C. Marangoz, T. S. Miles, and M. Wiesendanger. Microstimulation of the supplementary motor area (SMA) in the awake monkey. *Exp. Brain Res.* 45: 410–416, 1982.
148. Martino, A. M., and P. L. Strick. Corticospinal projections originate from the arcuate premotor area. *Brain Res.* 404: 307–312, 1987.
149. Matelli, M., R. Camarda, M. Glickstein, and G. Rizzolatti. Afferent and efferent projections of the inferior area 6 in the macaque monkey. *J. Comp. Neurol.* 251: 281–298, 1986.
150. Matelli, M., G. Luppino, L. Fogassi, and G. Rizzolatti. Thalamic input to inferior area 6 and area 4 in the macaque monkey. *J. Comp. Neurol.* 280: 468–488, 1989.
151. Matelli, M., G. Luppino, and G. Rizzolatti. Patterns of cytochrome oxidase activity in the frontal agranular cortex of the macaque monkey. *Behav. Brain Res.* 18: 125–136, 1985.
152. Matsuzaka, Y., H. Aizawa, and J. Tanji. A motor area rostral to the supplementary motor area (presupplementary motor area) in the monkey: neuronal activity during a learned motor task. *J. Neurophysiol.* 68: 653–662, 1992.
153. Mauritz, K. H., and S. P. Wise. Premotor cortex of the rhesus monkey: neuronal activity in anticipation of predictable environmental events. *Exp. Brain Res.* 61: 229–244, 1986.
154. McGuinness, E., D. Sivertsen, and J. M. Allman. Organization of the face representation in macaque motor cortex. *J. Comp. Neurol.* 193: 591–608, 1980.
155. Mitz, A. R., and D. R. Humphrey. Intracortical stimulation in pyramidotomized monkeys. *Neurosci. Lett.* 64: 59–64, 1986.
156. Mitz, A. R., and S. P. Wise. The somatotopic organization of the supplementary motor area: intracortical microstimulation mapping. *J. Neurosci.* 7: 1010–1021, 1987.
157. Mitz, A. R., M. Godschalk, and S. P. Wise. Learning-dependent neuronal activity in the premotor cortex: activity during the acquisition of conditional motor associations. *J. Neurosci.* 11: 1855–1872, 1991.
158. Moll, L., and H. G. Kuypers. Premotor cortical ablations in monkeys: contralateral changes in visually guided reaching behavior. *Science* 198: 317–319, 1977.
159. Morecraft, R. J., and G. W. Van Hoesen. Cingulate input to the primary and supplementary motor cortices in the rhesus monkey: evidence for somatotopy in areas 24c and 23c. *J. Comp. Neurol.* 322: 471–489, 1992.
160. Morecraft, R. J., and G. W. Van Hoesen. Frontal granular cortex input to the cingulate (M3), supplementary (M2) and primary (M1) motor cortices in the rhesus monkey. *J. Comp. Neurol.* 337: 669–689, 1993.
161. Muakkassa, K. F., and P. L. Strick. Frontal lobe inputs to primate motor cortex: evidence for four somatotopically organized "premotor" areas. *Brain Res.* 177: 176–182, 1979.
162. Murphy, J. T., H. C. Kwan, W. A. MacKay, and Y. C. Wong. Spatial organization of precentral cortex in awake primates. III. Input-output coupling. *J. Neurophysiol.* 41: 1132–1139, 1978.
163. Murphy, J. T., H. C. Kwan, W. A. MacKay, and Y. C. Wong. Activity of primate precentral neurons during voluntary movements triggered by visual signals. *Brain Res.* 236: 429–449, 1982.
164. Murray, E. A., and J. D. Coulter. Organization of corticospinal neurons in the monkey. *J. Comp. Neurol.* 195: 339–365, 1981.
165. Mushiake, H., M. Inase, and J. Tanji. Neuronal activity in the primate premotor, supplementary, and precentral motor cortex during visually guided and internally determined sequential movements. *J. Neurophysiol.* 66: 705–718, 1991.
166. Mussa-Ivaldi, F. A. Do neurons in the motor cortex encode movement direction? An alternative hypothesis. *Neurosci. Lett.* 91: 106–111, 1988.
167. Nambu, A., S. Yoshida, and K. Jinnai. Movement-related activity of thalamic neurons with input from the globus pallidus and projection to the motor cortex in the monkey. *Exp. Brain Res.* 84: 279–284, 1991.
168. Nauta, W. J. H., and W. R. Mehler. Projections of the lentiform nucleus in the monkey. *Brain Res.* 1: 3–42, 1966.
169. Neshige, R., H. Lüders, and H. Shibasaki. Recording of movement-related potentials from scalp and cortex in man. *Brain* 111: 719–736, 1988.
170. Nielson, J. M., and L. J. Jacobs. Bilateral lesions of the anterior cingulate gyri. Report of a case. *Bull. Los Angeles Neurol. Soc.* 16: 231–234, 1951.
171. Nudo, R. J., W. M. Jenkins, and M. M. Merzenich. Repetitive microstimulation alters the cortical representation of movements in adult rats. *Somatosens. Mot. Res.* 7: 463–483, 1990.
172. Nudo, R. J., W. M. Jenkins, M. M., Merzenich, T. Prejean, and R. Grenda. Neurophysiological correlates of hand preference in primary motor cortex of adult squirrel monkeys. *J. Neurosci.* 121: 2918–2947, 1992.
173. Nudo, R. J., and R. B. Masterton. Descending pathways to the spinal cord. III. Sites of origin of the corticospinal tract. *J. Comp. Neurol.* 296: 559–583, 1990.
174. Okano, K., and J. Tanji. Neuronal activities in the primate motor fields of the agranular frontal cortex preceding visually triggered and self-paced movement. *Exp. Brain Res.* 66: 155–166, 1987.
175. Olszewski, J. *The Thalamus of the* Macaca mulatta. *An Atlas for Use with the Stereotaxic Instrument.* Basel: S. Karger AG, 1952.
176. Orgogozo, J. M., and B. Larsen. Activation of the supplementary motor area during voluntary movement in man suggests it works as a supramotor area. *Science* 206: 847–850, 1979.
177. Orioli, P., and P. L. Strick. Cerebellar connections with the motor cortex and the arcuate premotor area: an analysis employing retrograde transneuronal transport of WGA-HRP. *J. Comp. Neurol.* 28: 612–626, 1989.
178. Pandya, D. N., and H. G. Kuypers. Corticocortical connections on the rhesus monkeys. *Brain Res.* 13: 13–36, 1969.
179. Passingham, R. E. Premotor cortex and preparation for movement. *Exp. Brain Res.* 70: 590–596, 1988.
180. Pavlides, C., E. Miyashita, and H. Asanuma. Projection from the sensory to the motor cortex is important in learning motor skills in the monkey. *J. Neurophysiol.* 70: 733–741, 1993.
181. Penfield, W., and E. Boldrey. Somatic motor and sensory representation in the cerebral cortex of man as studied by electrical stimulation. *Brain* 60: 389–443, 1937.
182. Penfield, W., and K. Welch. Supplementary motor area of the cerebral cortex. *Arch. Neurol. Psychiatry* 66: 289–317, 1951.
183. Percheron, G. The thalamic territory of cerebellar afferents and the lateral region of the thalamus of the macaque in

stereotaxic ventricular coordinates. *J. Hirnforsch.* 18: 375–400, 1977.
184. Petrides, M., and D. N. Pandya. Projections to the frontal cortex from the posterior parietal region in the rhesus monkey. *J. Comp. Neurol.* 228: 105–116, 1984.
185. Phillips, C. G. Laying the ghost of "muscles versus movements." *Can. J. Neurol. Sci.* 2: 209–218, 1975.
186. Phillips, C. G., and R. Porter. *Corticospinal Neurons. Their Role in Movement. Monograph of the Physiological Society, no. 34.* London: Academic Press, 1977.
187. Picard, N., and A. M. Smith. Primary motor cortical activity related to the weight and texture of grasped objects in the monkey. *J. Neurophysiol.* 68: 1867–1881, 1992.
188. Picard, N., and P. L. Strick. 2-Deoxyglucose (2DG) uptake in the medial wall motor areas of behaving monkeys. *Soc. Neurosci. Abstr.* 20: 986, 1994.
189. Picard, N., and P. L. Strick. Motor areas of the medial wall: a review of location and functional activation. *Cereb. Cortex* 1995 (submitted).
190. Porter, R., and R. N. Lemon, *Corticospinal Function and Voluntary Movement.* Oxford: Oxford University Press, 1993, p. 428.
191. Ralston, D. D., and H. J. Ralston, III. The terminations of corticospinal tract axons in the macaque monkey. *J. Comp. Neurol.* 242: 325–337, 1985.
192. Rao, S. M., J. R. Binder, P. A. Bandettini, T. A. Hammeke, F. Z. Yetkin, A. Jesmanowicz, L. M. Lisk, G. M. Morris, W. M. Mueller, L. D. Estkowski, E. C. Wong, V. M. Haughton, and J. S. Hyde. Functional magnetic resonance imaging of complex human movements. *Neurology* 43: 2311–2318, 1993.
193. Riehle, A., and J. Requin. Monkey primate motor and premotor cortex: single-cell activity related to prior information about direction and extent of intended movement. *J. Neurophysiol.* 61: 534–549, 1989.
194. Rizzolatti, G., R. Camarda, L. Fogassi, M. Gentilucci, G. Luppino, and M. Matelli. Functional organization of inferior area 6 in the macaque monkey. II. Area F5 and the control of distal movements. *Exp. Brain Res.* 71: 491–507, 1988.
195. Rizzolatti, G., M. Gentilucci, R. M. Camarda, V. Gallese, G. Luppino, M. Matelli, and L. Fogassi. Neurons related to reaching-grasping arm movements in the area 6 (area 6a beta). *Exp. Brain Res.* 82: 337–350, 1990.
196. Rizzolatti, G., M. Matelli, and G. Pavesi. Deficits in attention and movement following the removal of postarcuate (area 6) and prearcuate (area 8) cortex in macaque monkeys. *Brain* 106: 655–673, 1983.
197. Roland, P. E., B. Larsen, N. A. Lassen, and E. Skinhoj. Supplementary motor area and other cortical areas in organization of voluntary movements in man. *J. Neurophysiol.* 43: 118–136, 1980.
198. Russell, J. R., and W. DeMeyer. The quantitative cortical origin of pyramidal axons of *Macaca mulatta. Neurology (Minneapolis)* 11: 96–108, 1961.
199. Sanes, J. N., S. Suner, and J. P. Donoghue. Dynamic organization of primary motor cortex output to target muscles in adult rats. I. Long-term pattern of reorganization following motor or mixed peripheral nerve lesions. *Exp. Brain Res.* 79: 479–491, 1990.
200. Sato, K. C., and J. Tanji. Digit-muscle responses evoked from multiple intracortical foci in monkey precentral motor cortex. *J. Neurophysiol.* 62: 959–970, 1989.
201. Schell, G. R., and P. L. Strick. The origin of thalamic inputs to the arcuate premotor and supplementary motor areas. *J. Neurosci.* 4: 539–560, 1984.
202. Schwartz, A. B. Motor cortical activity during drawing movements: single-unit activity during sinusoid tracing. *J. Neurophysiol.* 68: 528–541, 1992.
203. Schwartz, A. B. Motor cortical activity during drawing movements: population representation during sinusoid tracing. *J. Neurophysiol.* 70: 28–36, 1993.
204. Schwartz, A. B., R. E. Kettner, and A. P. Georgopoulos. Primate motor cortex and free arm movements to visual targets in three-dimensional space. I. Relations between single cell discharge and direction of movement. *J. Neurosci.* 8: 2913–2927, 1988.
205. Selemon, L. D., and P. S. Goldman-Rakic. Common cortical and subcortical targets of the dorsolateral prefrontal and posterior parietal cortices in the rhesus monkey: evidence for a distributed neural network subserving spatially guided behavior. *J. Neurosci.* 8: 4049–4068, 1988.
206. Shima, K., K. Aya, H. Mushiake, M. Inase, H. Aizawa, and J. Tanji. Two movement-related foci in the primate cingulate cortex observed in signal-triggered and self-paced forelimb movements. *J. Neurophysiol.* 65: 188–202, 1991.
207. Shinoda, Y., J. Yokota, and T. Futami. Divergent projection of individual corticospinal axons to motoneurons of multiple muscles in the monkey. *Neurosci. Lett.* 23: 7–12, 1981.
208. Shinoda, Y., P. Zarzecki, and H. Asanuma. Spinal branching of pyramidal tract neurons in the monkey. *Exp. Brain Res.* 34: 59–72, 1979.
209. Stanton, G. B. Topographical organization of ascending cerebellar projections from the dentate and interposed nuclei in *Macaca mulatta*: an anterograde degeneration study. *J. Comp. Neurol.* 190: 699–731, 1980.
210. Stein, J. F., and M. Glickstein. Role of the cerebellum in visual guidance of movement. *Physiol. Rev.* 72: 967–1017, 1992.
211. Stephan, K. M., G. R. Fink, R. E. Passingham, D. Silbersweig, A. O. Ceballos-Baumann, C. D. Firth, and R. S. J. Frackowiak. Functional anatomy of the mental representation of upper extremity movements in healthy subjects. *J. Neurophysiol.* 73: 373–386, 1995.
212. Stepniewska, I., T. M. Preuss, and J. H. Kaas. Architectonic, somatotopic organization, and ipsilateral cortical connections of the primary motor area (M1) of owl monkeys. *J. Comp. Neurol.* 330: 238–271, 1993.
213. Strick, P. L. How do the basal ganglia and cerebellum gain access to the cortical motor areas? *Behav. Brain Res.* 18: 107–123, 1985.
214. Strick, P. L., and J. P. Card. Transneuronal mapping of neural circuits with alpha herpesviruses. In: *Experimental Neuroanatomy: A Practical Approach*, edited by J. P. Bolam. Oxford: Oxford University Press, 1992, p. 81–101.
215. Strick, P. L., R. P. Dum, and N. Picard. Macro-organization of circuits connecting the basal ganglia with the cortical motor areas. In: *Models of Information Processing in the Basal Ganglia*, edited by J. Houk. Boston: MIT Press, 1995.
216. Strick, P. L., and C. C. Kim. Input to primate motor cortex from posterior parietal cortex (area 5). I. Demonstration by retrograde transport. *Brain Res.* 157: 325–330, 1978.
217. Strick, P. L., J. E. Hoover, and H. Mushiake. Evidence for "output channels" in the basal ganglia and cerebellum. In: *Role of the Cerebellum and Basal Ganglia in Voluntary Movement*, edited by N. Mano, I. Hamada, and M. R. DeLong. New York: Elsevier Science Publishing, 1993, p. 171–180.

218. Strick, P. L., and J. B. Preston. Two representations of the hand in area 4 of a primate. I. Motor output organization. *J. Neurophysiol.* 48: 139–149, 1982.
219. Strick, P. L., and J. B. Preston. Two representations of the hand in area 4 of a primate. II. Somatosensory input organization. *J. Neurophysiol.* 48: 150–159, 1982.
220. Tanji, J. The supplementary motor area in the cerebral cortex. *Neurosci. Res.* 19: 251–268, 1994.
221. Tanji, J., and K. Kurata. Neuronal activity in the cortical supplementary motor area related with distal and proximal forelimb movements. *Neurosci. Lett.* 12: 201–206, 1979.
222. Tanji, J., and K. Shima. Role for supplementary motor area cells in planning several movements ahead. *Nature* 371: 413–416, 1994.
223. Tanji, J., and S. P. Wise. Submodality distribution in sensorimotor cortex of the unanesthetized monkey. *J. Neurophysiol.* 45: 467–481, 1981.
224. Tokuno, H., M. Kimura, and J. Tanji. Pallidal inputs to thalamocortical neurons projecting to the supplementary motor area: an anterograde and retrograde double labeling study in the macaque monkey. *Exp. Brain Res.* 90: 635–638, 1992.
225. Tokuno, H., and J. Tanji. Input organization of distal and proximal forelimb areas in the monkey primary motor cortex: a retrograde double labeling study. *J. Comp. Neurol.* 333: 199–209, 1993.
226. Toyoshima, K., and H. Sakai. Exact cortical extent of the origin of the corticospinal tract (CST) and the quantitative contribution to the CST in different cytoarchitectonic areas. A study with horseradish peroxidase in the monkey. *J. Hirnforsch.* 23: 257–269, 1982.
227. Tracey, D. J., C. Asanuma, E. G. Jones, and R. Porter. Thalamic relay to motor cortex: afferent pathways from brain stem, cerebellum, and spinal cord in monkeys. *J. Neurophysiol.* 44: 532–554, 1980.
228. Vaadia, E., K. Kurata, and S. P. Wise. Neuronal activity preceding directional and nondirectional cues in the premotor cortex of rhesus monkeys. *Somatosens. Mot. Res.* 6: 207–230, 1988.
229. Vogt, B. A., and D. N. Pandya. Cortico-cortical connections of somatic sensory cortex (areas 3, 1, and 2) in the rhesus monkey. *J. Comp. Neurol.* 177: 179–191, 1978.
230. Vogt, B. A., and D. N. Pandya. Cingulate cortex of the rhesus monkey: II. Cortical afferents. *J. Comp. Neurol.* 262: 271–289, 1987.
231. Vogt, C., and O. Vogt. Allgemeinere Ergebnisse unserer Hirnforschung. *J. Psychol. Neurol. (Leipzig)* 25: 277–462, 1919.
232. von Bonin, G., and P. Bailey. *The Neocortex of* Macaca mulatta. Urbana, IL: University of Illinois Press, 1947.
233. Weinrich, M., and S. P. Wise. The premotor cortex of the monkey. *J. Neurosci.* 2: 1329–1345, 1982.
234. Werner, W., E. Bauswein, and C. Fromm. Static firing rates of premotor and primary motor cortical neurons associated with torque and joint position. *Exp. Brain Res.* 86: 293–302, 1991.
235. Westergaard, G. C., and D. M. Fragaszy. The manufacture and use of tools by capuchin monkeys (*Cebus apella*). *Zoo. Biol.* 4: 317–327, 1987.
236. Wiesendanger, M. Recent developments in studies of the supplementary motor area of primates. *Rev. Physiol. Biochem. Pharmacol.* 103: 1–59, 1986.
237. Wiesendanger, R., and M. Wiesendanger. The thalamic connections with medial area 6 (supplementary motor cortex) in the monkey (*Macaca fascicularis*). *Exp. Brain Res.* 59: 91–104, 1985.
238. Wiesendanger, R., and M. Wiesendanger. Cerebello-cortical linkage in the monkey as revealed by transcellular labeling with the lectin wheat germ agglutinin conjugated to the marker horseradish peroxidase. *Exp. Brain Res.* 59: 105–117, 1985.
239. Wise, S. P. The primate premotor cortex fifty years after Fulton. *Behav. Brain Res.* 18: 79–88, 1985.
240. Wise, S. P., and K.-H. Mauritz. Set-related neuronal activity in the premotor cortex of rhesus monkeys: effects of changes in motor set. *Proc. R. Soc. Lond. Biol. Sci.* 223: 331–354, 1985.
241. Wise, S. P., and J. Tanji. Supplementary and precentral motor cortex: contrast in responsiveness to peripheral input in the hindlimb area of the unanesthetized monkey. *J. Comp. Neurol.* 195: 433–451, 1981.
242. Woolsey, C. N., P. H. Settlage, D. R. Meyer, W. Sencer, T. P. Hamuy, and A. M. Travis. Patterns of localization in precentral and "supplementary" motor area and their relation to the concept of a premotor area. *Assoc. Res. Nerv. Ment. Dis.* 30: 238–264, 1952.
243. Zemanick, M. C., P. L. Strick, and R. D. Dix. Direction of transneuronal transport of herpes simplex virus 1 in the primate motor system is strain-dependent. *Proc. Natl. Acad. Sci. U. S. A.* 88: 8048–8051, 1991.

7. Postural orientation and equilibrium

FAY B. HORAK
JANE M. MACPHERSON | *R.S. Dow Neurological Sciences Institute, Legacy Good Samaritan Hospital & Medical Center, Portland, Oregon*

CHAPTER CONTENTS

THE POSTURAL CONTROL SYSTEM includes all the sensorimotor and musculoskeletal components involved in the control of two important behavioral goals, postural orientation and postural equilibrium. Postural orientation is the relative positioning of the body segments with respect to each other and to the environment, whereas postural equilibrium is the state in which all the forces acting on the body are balanced so that the body tends to stay in the desired position and orientation (static equilibrium) or to move in a controlled way (dynamic equilibrium). Postural control provides a stable body platform for the efficient execution of focal or goal-directed movements.

The most important change in the study of postural control over the last century has been in the theoretical framework for viewing posture. Whereas postural control was once regarded as the summation of parallel and hierarchical reflex pathways (167, 234), it is now viewed as the output of complex interactions among multiple neural systems underlying the behavioral goals of posture. Neural systems for sensory orientation, multijoint coordination, environmental adaptation, central set, and other functions interact with biomechanical constraints of the musculoskeletal system to accomplish task goals that require stability and particular orientation. Posture is no longer considered a static state but rather a dynamic interaction among many context- and task-specific, automatic neural behaviors.

Sensorimotor organization for postural orientation includes neural mechanisms for active control of joint stiffness as well as control of global variables such as trunk and head alignment. To understand the control of postural orientation requires knowing the relevant "reference frames" and their transformations by the nervous system (178). Information from the somatosensory, vestibular, and visual systems appears to be interpreted by the nervous system according to an internal representation of the body's motor and sensory dynamics, including expected sensory afferent input.

Sensorimotor coordination for dynamic equilibrium includes energy-efficient and computationally efficient movement strategies to control the many degrees of freedom of whole-body stabilization. New biomechanical models of posture suggest that much of the coordination and control of posture emerges from biomechanical constraints inherent in the musculoskeletal system and that the nervous system takes advantage of these constraints. Control of dynamic equilibrium includes automatic responses to unexpected disturbances as well as anticipatory postural adjustments accompanying voluntary, focal movements. Although postural coordination occurs by fast, automatic pathways, it can be significantly influenced by previous experience, practice, instruction, and long-term training.

The relative roles of the somatosensory, vestibular, and visual inputs for postural orientation and equilibrium can change, depending on the task and on the particular environmental context. The role of central nervous system (CNS) structures in postural control is not well understood. As with all motor tasks, the postural control process seems to be distributed throughout the CNS in a task- and context-dependent manner.

NEURAL CONTROL OF POSTURAL ORIENTATION AND EQUILIBRIUM

Behavioral Goals

The term "posture" encompasses several different aspects of motor coordination, such as controlling the position of the body's center of mass in a gravitoinertial environment; stabilizing body segments during voluntary movement; and maintaining specific positions of the body segments with respect to other segments, the environment, or both. Not all of these goals can always be accomplished in a particular task. For example, when an individual balances on a narrow surface by bending back and forth at the hips, he sacrifices the goal of upright orientation of the trunk in order to maintain equilibrium.

Postural orientation has two aspects: orienting the body to environmental variables such as earth vertical, and aligning various body parts in a specific orientation with respect to each other. Animals, including humans, tend to assume particular body postures that are characteristic for each task and that may function to control or optimize sensory inputs in addition to coordinating motor output. The orientation of the trunk may be one of the most important controlled variables, since this will determine the positioning of the limbs relative to objects with which we may wish to interact. The trunk and neck position combined determine the position of the head in space, which is important for the interpretation of sensory information from the head-based sensors. During complex motor tasks, most animals tend to stabilize their heads in space. As a result, the retina and the vestibular apparatus maintain a relatively constant orientation with respect to the environment; this may simplify the interpretation of visual and vestibular information. Body posture can be oriented to a variety of reference frames depending on the task and behavioral goals. The frame of reference can be visual, based on external cues in the surrounding environment; somatosensory, based on information from contact with external objects; or vestibular, based on gravitoinertial forces. Alternatively, the frame of reference may be an internal representation of body orientation or the environment, such as an estimated reference position from memory.

Postural equilibrium, or balance, is a critical component of most tasks. As in postural orientation, the control of the position and velocity of the *trunk in space* may be the main goal of the postural equilibrium system, since most of the mass of the body resides in the trunk. Although most studies of balance have focused on the ability to remain upright during stance, the control of dynamic equilibrium is also essential to the preparation and execution of voluntary movement. There are several sources of destabilizing influences on the body: external forces due to gravity and to interactions with the surrounding environment, as well as internal forces generated by the body's own movements. All forces, whether external or internal, ultimately act to accelerate the body at its center of mass. One role of the nervous system is to produce muscle forces that complement and coordinate all other forces acting on the body so as to control the position of the center of mass efficiently and thereby maintain equilibrium (59).

Biomechanical Principles

This section will discuss the physical principles of stability and balance, to provide a framework for understanding the control problems faced by the nervous system in regulating posture. An understanding of the biomechanics of posture is essential to an appreciation of how the nervous system achieves the sensorimotor coordination that results in postural control.

During stance, the forces acting on the body include the force due to gravity and the force exerted by the support surface(s). The center of mass (CoM) of the body, also called the center of gravity, is the point at which the entire mass of the body is balanced, and is the point at which the resultant of the external forces acts (269). There must be a force acting at the center of mass that is equal and opposite to the force of gravity for the body to be in equilibrium. In the quietly standing human, this second force is represented by the ground reaction force under the feet. In other words, the gravitational acceleration acting on the mass of the body generates a force that passes through the CoM and that is equal and opposite to the force exerted by the support surface against the feet. Since the body is segmented, the position of the CoM can change dramatically by changing body configuration (i.e., the relative position of the segments). Thus, the CoM may actually be located entirely outside the body, depending on postural orientation.

Although the body can assume a wide variety of segment configurations, the requirements of *static equilibrium* place a constraint on body posture; namely, the position of the horizontal projection of the body's CoM must lie within the base of support (Fig. 7.1). The support base is that region bounded by the points of contact between body segments and support surface. In free stance, the base of support is a quadrangle bounded by the heels and toes. Figure 7.1 illustrates a variety of support bases, such as feet, hands, and a tripedal support including one foot and two crutches. When the body is in contact with objects, the support base extends to include all support points such as the crutches in Figure 7.1C. In contrast, during movements such as locomotion, the projection of the CoM rarely lies within the base of support, but is continuously regulated to maintain *dynamic equilibrium*.

Stability in stance is a function of many factors. The standing quadruped is stable because the base of support bounded by the four feet is relatively large and the CoM of the animal is close to the ground relative to the dimensions of the support base. In contrast, the bipedal human is relatively unstable because the base of support is small and the CoM is high (at about the second lumbar vertebra). The larger the base of support, the larger the area in which the CoM can move without loss of equilibrium. Hayes (108) described static stability as the resistance to toppling due to external forces and outlined mechanical principles underlying stability: stability is proportional to (*1*) the area of the base support, (*2*) the distance from the line of gravity to the edge of the support base, (*3*) the inverse of the height of the CoM above the base of support, and (*4*) the weight of the body.

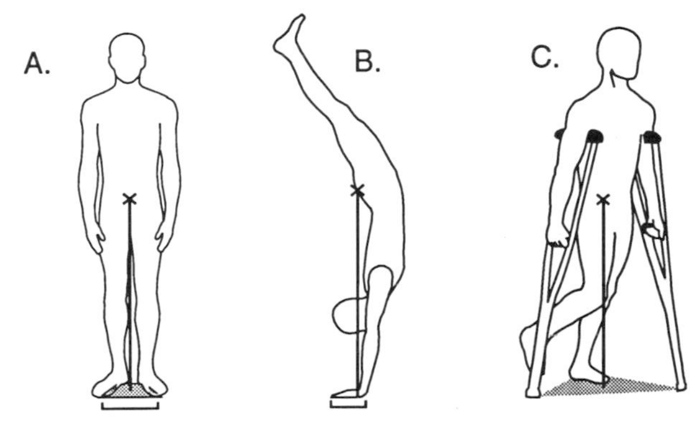

FIG. 7.1. Equilibrium in different postural orientations. The center of mass (CoM) of the body (indicated by the X) may lie inside (*A* and C) or outside (*B*) the body limits. The net ground reaction force takes origin within the base of support and must pass through the CoM if the body is in equilibrium.

Maintaining stability, even in quiet stance, is a *dynamic* and not a static task, since the body is never completely motionless. In the bipedal human, the center of mass is in continuous motion as the body sways. The continually varying muscle forces are reflected in the ground reaction force. The point of origin of the ground reaction force, termed the position of the center of pressure (CoP), traverses a complex trajectory on the support surface. Many investigators mistakenly equate the movements of the CoP with body sway; however, the center of pressure is *not* equivalent to the center of mass in the horizontal plane (see 269). CoP is related to force and reflects the *acceleration* of the body, whereas the projection of the CoM is a *position*. In order to determine the position of the CoM, both vertical and horizontal forces must be taken into account.

Many studies have analyzed the trajectory of the CoP in an attempt to quantify stability under the quasistatic conditions of normal body sway during stance. Various measures of CoP trajectory, such as the area of excursion, the deviation from the mean position, or the root mean square deviation have been examined but have not yielded much insight in terms of predicting instability or the likelihood of falling (e.g., 116). Other more recent approaches, using dynamical systems analysis (212) or models from statistical mechanics (41), indicate that the CoP trajectory cannot be characterized simply as a random process.

Maintaining equilibrium requires the exertion of force against the support surface in order to move the CoM into the region of stability. The transformation from muscle contraction to forces and then to movement of the CoM is mechanically complex, since the musculoskeletal system has a large number of degrees of freedom. Because the body segments are linked together by joints, contraction of any one muscle can cause acceleration at remote joints not crossed by that muscle due to inertial interactions (275). In postural adjustments, as in any other movement, there is not a simple relationship between muscle contraction, kinematics, or body segment movement, and kinetics, or forces generated at the joints and against the support surface (see Chapter 8).

In order for the nervous system to produce smoothly coordinated movements and maintain balance and equilibrium, it must estimate and anticipate the various forces acting on the body, such as gravitation, inertial coupling among body segments, frictional forces between body segments and the support surface, and so forth. It is active muscle forces *in combination with* all the external and indirect forces that give rise to movement. Coordination is achieved through the optimal blending of all these forces in a time-varying manner.

Postural Strategies

Postural adjustments for maintaining orientation and equilibrium arise from neural strategies that are formulated and implemented by complex sensorimotor control processes. The concept of a strategy has developed from accumulated evidence that postural adjustments are not merely the sum of simple reflexes but arise from a complex sensorimotor control system that is only beginning to be understood.

A postural strategy is a high-level plan formulated by the nervous system for achieving the overall goals of maintaining postural orientation and equilibrium. We believe that a strategy represents the dynamic reordering of the many postural variables that are controlled, into a new hierarchical organization. For any strategy, one or more postural goals, such as trunk orientation, gaze fixation, or energy expenditure, may take precedence over another set of goals, but this ordering will change depending on the task and the context. Many variables are controlled dynamically in the performance of postural adjustments, from the relatively simple variables of muscle length or force to the more global variables of body segment orientation or position of the CoM. Current studies of postural control attempt to determine which variables are being controlled and how that control is achieved.

There may be multiple strategies available to the postural control system for a given task, whether a postural adjustment to an unexpected disturbance or a voluntary movement. This stems from the idea that the musculoskeletal system has more degrees of freedom than are necessary to achieve the task goal, thereby allowing more than one solution in terms of the forces, movement patterns, and muscle activations. The neural strategy applies constraints to the musculoskeletal system by setting the hierarchical order of controlled variables, in order to achieve one particular solution for the postural task. We do not know how many different strategies may be available for any given task or condition, in part because it is difficult to separate the neural constraints from physical constraints such as the biomechanics of the joints and muscles.

The implementation of a postural strategy is described in terms of the kinematics, kinetics, and muscle synergies, but these do not define the strategy. In the implementation of a postural response, the nervous system commands the contraction and relaxation of muscles throughout the body. Forces developed by the muscles are transformed to joint torques and, ultimately, to forces applied against the support surface. The joint torques cause displacement of the body segments to maintain or restore postural orientation; the forces applied against the support surface move the body's CoM to maintain or restore postural equilibrium. For a given strategy, the precise details of the kinematics, kinetics, and muscle synergies are not fixed, but depend on many factors such as the initial conditions. A muscle synergy consists of the spatial pattern and temporal sequence of activation and relaxation of a group of muscles. Synergies themselves are highly variable, depending on factors such as the biomechanical conditions and the sensory context. Thus, any one strategy could be implemented by a variety of muscle synergies [see Macpherson (162) for a review of synergies].

In summary, postural adjustments for orientation and equilibrium arise from high-level neural strategies that are formulated and implemented by complex sensorimotor control processes. A strategy involves the dynamic reordering of the set of controlled postural variables such that each strategy is characterized by the precedence of one or more postural and movement goals.

POSTURAL ORIENTATION

The characteristic alignment of body segments unique to each species has several common features; alignment of head and trunk with respect to gravitoinertial and support surface references, and a characteristic intralimb geometry (e.g., semiflexed or extended posture). Each individual assumes a unique, stereotypical postural profile that represents an equilibrium among the many biomechanical and neural constraints for posture. This postural profile is rather stable, changing slowly, only in the face of changing biomechanical or neural constraints such as with aging, injury, or prolonged space flight (103, 155). Passive stiffness of connective tissue within and around muscle can account for most of antigravity stance in humans and large quadrupeds like elephants and giraffes, due to an alignment of limbs that minimizes the torque required to stabilize each joint; a greater degree of active muscle contraction is required in many small quadrupeds such as cats and dogs, whose limb segments are not aligned with the gravity vector (22, 92).

Stiffness and Tonic Muscle Activation

Muscle and joint stiffness plays a critical role in resisting displacement of the limbs due to external forces. Muscles with a high proportion of slow fiber types are most suited for the tonic contractions required for postural support, since they are the most fatigue resistant. When slow-twitch, postural muscles like soleus are tonically activated, their stiffness rises dramatically through an increase in the steepness and decrease in the threshold of the length/tension curve. In cats, the range of soleus muscle lengths observed in quiet standing and locomotion corresponds to the steepest part of the length/tension curve such that a given increment in muscle length results in the largest increase in force generation (96). In standing humans, soleus is stretched beyond its resting length and is tonically active to oppose the ankle flexor torque due to the gravitational force. The combination of passive stiffness and tonic muscle activity is a critical load-compensating mechanism that reduces sway in quiet stance and stabilizes body parts during movements. It allows significant development of force virtually instantaneously, and long before any peripherally or centrally driven signal could dynamically change muscle activation.

Although tonic muscle activity is certainly a factor in determining postural alignment, antigravity postures are not necessarily associated with a great deal of tonic muscle activation. In fact, there are many comfortably supported positions such as lying recumbent, sitting, and squatting that are associated with no recordable electromyographic (EMG) activity at all in humans (15). Erect stance in humans is often associated with tonic activity only in soleus and iliopsoas (deep hip flexor), and occasionally in the shoulder/neck (trapezius) and mandible; tibialis and the large hip and thigh muscles are largely silent in relaxed standing (138). The muscular effort required to maintain upright stance against gravity depends on the particular postural configuration and passive stiffness of joints and ligaments.

Controlling Postural Orientation

Recent years have brought great progress in our understanding of the mechanisms underlying postural control, due to changing theoretical approaches to the question of what is being controlled (19, 45, 93, 231). The decerebrate cat, which is characterized by tonic activation of extensor muscles and stereotyped, static reflexes, was long accepted as a good model for postural control (168, 240, 245). The problem with these or older studies is that posture was treated as a static state resulting from the sum of hardwired reflexes. It is now clear that posture is a dynamic interaction among a complex set of mechanisms organized around the control of functional goals such as orientation of the trunk and head to various frames of reference. New models and concepts for understanding complex, parallel systems like the nervous system consistently show that the whole is more than the sum of its parts; characterization of the behavior of a reduced preparation, such as the decerebrate cat, does not necessarily reveal the control mechanisms in the intact animal (85, 227).

In the study of postural orientation, we are searching for global variables that remain invariant in a task, thus simplifying the control process by limiting the degrees of freedom to be controlled. The strategies for orientation may change dramatically, depending upon the particular task and the individual's goals. For example, the two tasks of reading a book and carrying a full glass of water while walking quickly over irregular ground require two different postural strategies. When the individual is reading while walking, the relative motion between the arms and trunk is reduced by holding the elbows close to the trunk. When the individual is carrying the full glass while walking, the arms are in abduction and flexion, far from the trunk (67). The reading task requires a strategy in which the distal hand segment is stabilized with reference to vision, and thus, to trunk and head displacements, whereas the glass transport task requires stabilization of the hand with reference to gravity, so the arm movement must be freed from displacements of the trunk and head.

It has been suggested that the nervous system does not plan and control such strategies by determining each simple variable such as joint angular displacements or velocity, but by using a topological, or map-like, internal representation of movement in which a whole continuum of possible, equivalent strategies could accomplish the particular goal (1, 67). The variables of postural orientation such as alignment of the trunk (79, 188), limb geometry (146), and stabilization of the head or gaze (208, 222) are controlled in a task-specific manner, depending on the particular context, internal and external conditions, the subject's intentions, prior experience, practice, and the unconscious interpretation of sensory information (230).

Trunk Orientation. Studies of the perception of vertical under a variety of sensory conditions have led to the hypothesis that human subjects control the orientation of the trunk with respect to gravity (185–187, 189, 272). According to this hypothesis, signals from neck receptors, which code the orientation of the head relative to the trunk, are subtracted from vestibular otolith signals, which code head orientation relative to the gravity vector. The result is an error signal that is proportional to the deviation of the trunk from earth vertical. Mergner and colleagues (185) proposed that subjects use the trunk as a reference for three different perceptual tasks; namely, estimating the position of the head in space, head relative to trunk, and trunk in space, depending on the focus of attention. Indeed, humans can perceive very small amounts of passive trunk lateral flexion (<3 degrees) and trunk rotation (0.9 degrees), even when vestibular contributions have been ruled out (136, 256). The threshold for detection of rotation of the trunk is even lower than for rotation of the neck (185, 256). Mittelstaedt (190) proposed, based on both theoretical analysis and psychophysical experiments on patients with spinal cord lesions, that proprioceptive information from the lumbosacral area and internal organs is critical for perception of verticality.

Stabilization of the trunk and/or computation of the position of the trunk based on the estimated vertical may also be critical to using the trunk as an egocentric reference frame for arm and leg movements (195, 251, 272). During a leg elevation task, trained dancers spontaneously maintain the orientation of the trunk parallel to earth vertical, whereas untrained subjects do not, although in the untrained subjects the head is counter-rotated with respect to the trunk to maintain head orientation with respect to the environment (194). It is not clear whether this difference in trunk orientation is due to the specific training that dancers receive, or to differences in flexibility. Nevertheless, the amplitude of the leg movement appears to be computed with reference to the *trunk axis* rather than the external environment in both trained and untrained subjects (195). Thus, the trunk is an important reference frame in the internal representation of body geometry.

Gurfinkel and colleagues (105) systematically addressed the question of which component of vertical posture is regulated by examining postural muscle activity at the ankle during sinusoidal rotations of the support surface (0.2–2.2 Hz) in relation to ankle, trunk, and head position. They found that postural activation of soleus and gastrocnemius remained in phase with trunk angle relative to vertical at all frequencies of rotation but not with head angle relative to vertical, or ankle joint angle. In fact, external fixation of ankle angle or head tilt in space resulted in no significant change in ankle muscle activation during surface rotations, whereas fixation of the trunk in space abolished modulation of the ankle muscles at frequencies of rotation below 1 Hz (105). These results cannot be explained by the simple mechanisms of stretch reflexes or tonic neck and labyrinthine reflexes, and suggest that vertical trunk alignment may be a critically controlled variable for posture, at least for certain tasks.

Recent studies in intact cats suggest that the orientation of the trunk is an important controlled variable in quadrupeds as well as in humans, but that the trunk is stabilized with reference to the support surface rather than with reference to earth vertical. As shown in Figure 7.2, the trunk remains parallel to the support surface and both intralimb geometry and limb length are conserved during changes in forepaw–hindpaw separation (stance distance) or surface tilt in the cat (79, 146). Trunk and limb geometry are conserved even when the position of the center of mass is altered with a load (146), or when cat posture is dynamically perturbed (170; J. M. Macpherson, unpublished data).

The preferred stance posture of an intact cat can be defined by an optimal body geometry that mini-

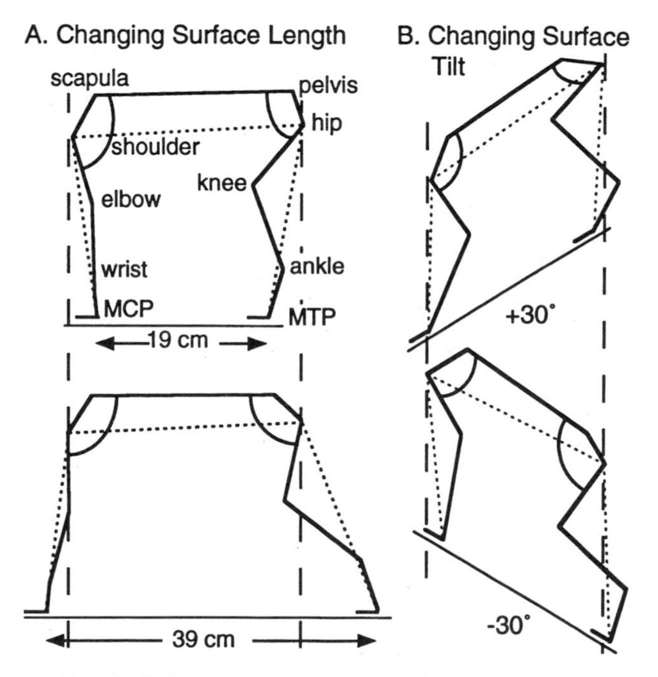

FIG. 7.2. Stick figures illustrating postural orientation in the cat. Changes in stance distance (*A*) or surface tilt (*B*) in the cat are accommodated primarily through pivoting of the limbs at the most proximal and distal joints. The trunk remains parallel to the support surface and intralimb geometry is relatively conserved. [*A* adapted from Fung and Macpherson (79), *B* adapted from Lacquaniti et al. (146).]

mizes energy consumption (79). The optical geometry was specified by the stance distance for which the sum of the squares of the intralimb joint torques was minimized. In the optimal body geometry, the trunk is oriented parallel to the surface and the forelimb axis (defined by a line joining shoulder and metacarpophalangeal joint) is parallel to earth vertical, whereas the hindlimb axis (from hip to metatarsophalangeal joint) is tilted inward. The ground reaction forces under fore- and hindlimbs are both tilted inward, resulting in compressive forces along the long axis of the vertebral column that help to stabilize the column and prevent the back from sagging.

Head Orientation. Orientation of the head with respect to earth vertical is another important postural variable that is stabilized during complex tasks such as walking, running, flying, and gymnastics. Figure 7.3 shows the relative stability of human and monkey head orientation during dynamic tasks by the constancy of the angle of the Frankfort plane, a line drawn through the auditory meatus and the orbit and approximating the plane of the horizontal semicircular canals. During locomotion, hopping, and running in place, humans appear to rotate the head

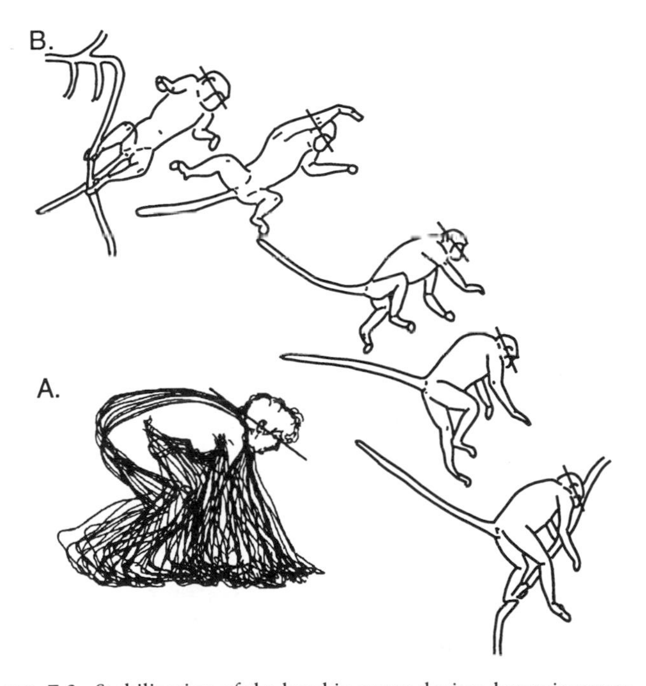

FIG. 7.3. Stabilization of the head in space during dynamic motor activities. *A*, Example of subject locomoting while maintaining the Frankfort plane at a constant angle with respect to vertical. Berthoz and Pozzo (21) created these drawings by tracing and superimposing time-lapse photos from Muybridge (196). *B*, Tracing from a cine film of a *Macaca mulatta* juvenile in the wild, leaping between branches. (Drawing courtesy of Dr. D. C. Dunbar.)

in the pitch plane in order to compensate for excessive vertical displacements of the head caused by motion of the legs, thus limiting the maximum Frankfort plane rotations to less than 20 degrees (222).

One of the underlying goals in the control of head position is stabilization of gaze (i.e., the intended direction of "looking" in spatial coordinates). Although head stabilization is not perfect, residual movements are small enough that the vestibulo-ocular reflex can compensate to maintain gaze stability (99). This hypothesis of gaze stabilization is consistent with studies showing that head stability does not diminish in the dark, but may be improved (11), and with studies showing that imagining a target in space in total darkness can improve head and trunk stability. During walking in the dark, the Frankfort plane is tipped nose down but with no change in stability (222).

Stabilization of the head in space may be more critical for some tasks and contexts than others, such as when somatosensory information is inadequate for postural orientation (208). The monkey jumping from one branch to another in Figure 7.3*B* is a good example of a task in which somatosensory information about contact surfaces is unavailable and the head tends to be stabilized in space while the body is changing orientation. Similarly, subjects attempting to balance on an unstable, rocking platform stabilize the head and trunk in space more so than when standing on a stable surface (224). There appears to be a threshold for movement above which the head becomes actively stabilized. For small body movements, head movement can be greater than trunk movement, whereas for large body movements, the head becomes better stabilized to earth vertical than the trunk (224). Head stability may also improve with practice as observed in comparing skilled and unskilled dancers or skaters (193).

Somatosensory information from the feet, legs, and trunk provides a stable frame of reference for postural orientation when the body is in contact with a stable surface, or when it moves at low velocities, and the head need not be stabilized (208). Gaze is stabilized during small, low-frequency head motions by vestibulo-ocular, cervico-ocular, and optokinetic mechanisms. In contrast, the head may be used as a frame of reference for orientation when subjects are not in contact with a surface or stand on compliant, unstable, or unpredictable surfaces and/or make large head and body movements. The head may need to be stabilized with respect to earth horizon when it is used as a frame of reference for postural stability.

Internal Representation of Postural Orientation

The vast repertoire of postural orientations, and their relationship to environmental and behavioral contexts, can best be understood by supposing that the nervous system integrates all available sensory information into a common "orientation interpretation center" based on an internal model of the body (144). Gurfinkel and colleagues (104) assert that this hypothetical internal model of postural orientation includes the representation of body configuration and dynamics, the perception of the borders between the body and extrapersonal space, the knowledge of sensory dynamics and expected sensory inputs, and the formation of task-dependent stationary reference systems. Convergence of inputs from multiple sensory modalities is required, since the control of postural muscle activity is based on variables such as position of the CoM, configuration and characteristics of the support surface, and contact forces between the body and the surface, variables that cannot be directly signaled by single receptor types. Convergence of sensory information is also needed because the interpretation of signals from receptors located at distal segments in a multilink chain, such as the head, requires knowledge of the state of the intermediate segments. The interpretation of afferent signals requires detailed knowledge of body dynamics and the current postural task conditions.

Mathematical models of spatial orientation have been developed that incorporate internal models of musculoskeletal and sensory dynamics to account for psychophysical and behavioral observations of orientation in complex environments (27, 184, 216). For example, Figure 7.4 shows a systems model using observer theory and suboptimal estimation to provide the nervous system with an estimate of gravitoinertial vertical as well as linear and angular self-motion (184). In this model, the CNS uses sensory information and the constraints of body biomechanics to create internal models of sensory and body dynamics. When a "desired orientation" is commanded, a copy of the control strategy is sent to the "internal model of body dynamics" to generate an "estimated orientation." This estimate is processed by the "internal model of sensory dynamics," yielding the "expected sensory afferent signals," which are compared to the actual sensory signals resulting from the movement. The difference between the actual and expected sensory afferent signal represents a "sensory conflict," or disorientation, which is minimized by changing the internal model to drive the "estimated orientation" toward the actual orientation. An external disturbance to posture changes sensory afferent signals and also drives the system to change the internal model of body dynamics as well as to implement a control strategy to reorient the body. It remains to be seen whether such models can predict postural orientation behavior as well as they predict eye movements and the conscious perception of orientation (184).

COORDINATION OF POSTURAL EQUILIBRIUM

Disturbances of postural equilibrium can result either from unexpected external forces, such as the sudden movement of the support surface, or as a conse-

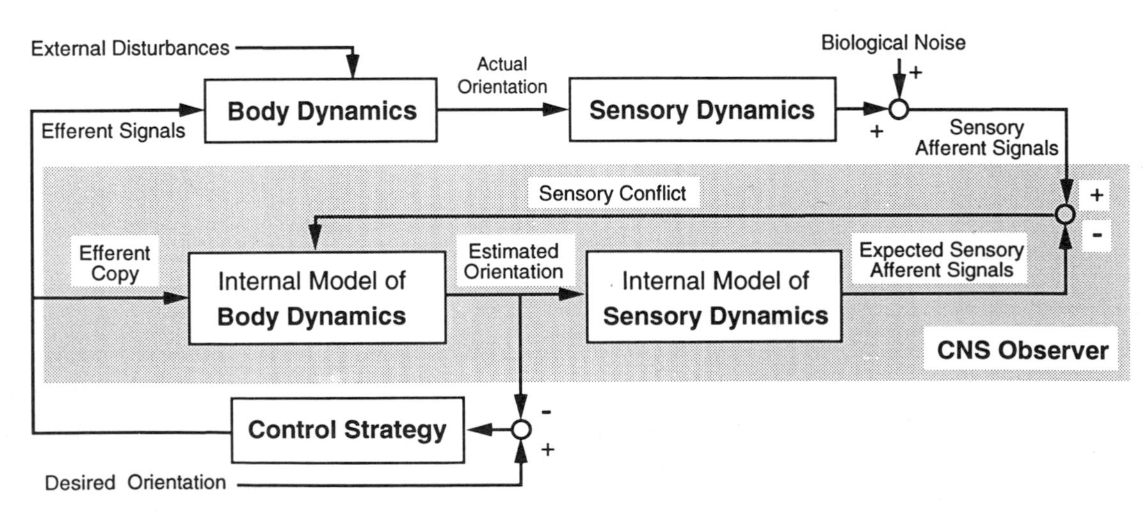

FIG. 7.4. Control system model for spatial orientation. See text for details. [Adapted from Merfeld et al. (184).]

quence of one's own voluntary movement. In the former case, sensory inputs provide information about the nature of the balance disturbance and are used to trigger the appropriate postural response. In the latter case, postural adjustments precede and accompany the focal movement in order to offset any destabilizing effects of the movement in an anticipatory or feedforward manner. Such a postural adjustment is an integral part of the movement and is necessary for achieving the task goals in a smoothly coordinated manner. Current models of the postural control system have contributed to our understanding of dynamic equilibrium.

Both trunk orientation and trunk position and velocity appear to have high priority for control in the neural strategies for postural orientation and equilibrium (131). Simple physical principles dictate that, to maintain equilibrium under static and dynamic conditions, the CoM of the body must be controlled. Whether or not the CoM is controlled *directly* by the nervous system is a matter of debate. There is no sensory receptor whose activity monitors the CoM, but it is possible that the CoM is derived computationally from sensory inputs from all the body segments. Alternatively, the position of the CoM could be approximated from trunk position, since most of the mass of the body is concentrated in the trunk.

Triggered Reactions to External Disturbances

Rapid, automatic postural responses are evoked whenever there is a disturbance applied to a body segment that tends to cause disequilibrium or changes in postural orientation. Any body segment and any group of muscles can be used in a postural role, depending on the task and the nature of the disturbance (175).

When the support surface under a quietly standing human or animal is suddenly moved, rapid and automatic postural reactions are evoked that oppose the perturbation and prevent loss of balance. The timing of the evoked EMG response is rapid, in the range of 70–100 ms in humans and 40–60 ms in cats from the initial acceleration of the surface. Indeed, these responses may be initiated before there is any significant displacement of the body's CoM (<5–10 mm). The equilibrium response is modified by a number of factors including the direction and velocity of the perturbation, initial position, prior experience, central set, and the nature of the ongoing motor task that was disturbed. The postural response is triggered by a subset of the sensory inflow resulting from the perturbation.

There is a continuum of strategies whereby the standing human can maintain balance in the face of a perturbation of the support surface. The ankle strategy (120, 203) is the most commonly used response during quiet stance. For example, when the body sways forward in response to a backward movement of the support, subjects will produce an extensor torque about the ankle joints that moves the CoP anteriorly, beyond the CoM. This force (CoP) reverses the direction of displacement of the CoM and drives it backward toward the original position, thus reducing sway. The sequential activation of ankle, knee, and hip extensors rotates the body about the ankle joints, with relatively little movement at the hip and knee (Figure 7.5). The ankle strategy maintains postural alignment while restoring the CoM, and is most useful for slow, small perturbations on a firm, even surface. The hip strategy (120, 207) consists of bending the trunk at the hip joints and, at the same time, counter-rotating at the neck and ankle joints by the sequential activation of the neck muscles, abdominals, and quadriceps (Figure 7.5). The hip strategy is useful for rapid or large amplitude perturbations and under conditions where it is difficult to produce much ankle torque (e.g., standing on a narrow beam or a compliant surface, or preleaning during stance). The ankle and hip strategies actually represent extremes of a response continuum. Subjects may combine hip and ankle strategies in any proportion, in which case there are several possible patterns of EMG activation (120, 207) in which the basic ankle and hip synergies are mixed (Fig. 7.5, *shaded area*).

Subjects may respond with a third strategy, stepping, for very large and/or fast perturbations, or when the goal of maintaining a vertical trunk orientation predominates (181). Stepping may also be observed with small perturbations that subjects have not experienced before, or when subjects receive no instruction about keeping the feet in place. These stepping responses can be initiated at the same latency as hip and ankle strategies.

The selection of a particular strategy depends not only on the characteristics of the perturbation, but also on the central set, which refers to the modification of automatic motor responses based on expectation of stimulus and task characteristics (see 228 for review). For example, when subjects are translated on a narrow beam, they use the hip strategy for maintaining equilibrium; when translated on a normal surface, they use the ankle strategy. However, when subjects switch from the beam to the normal surface, their first several trials show consider-

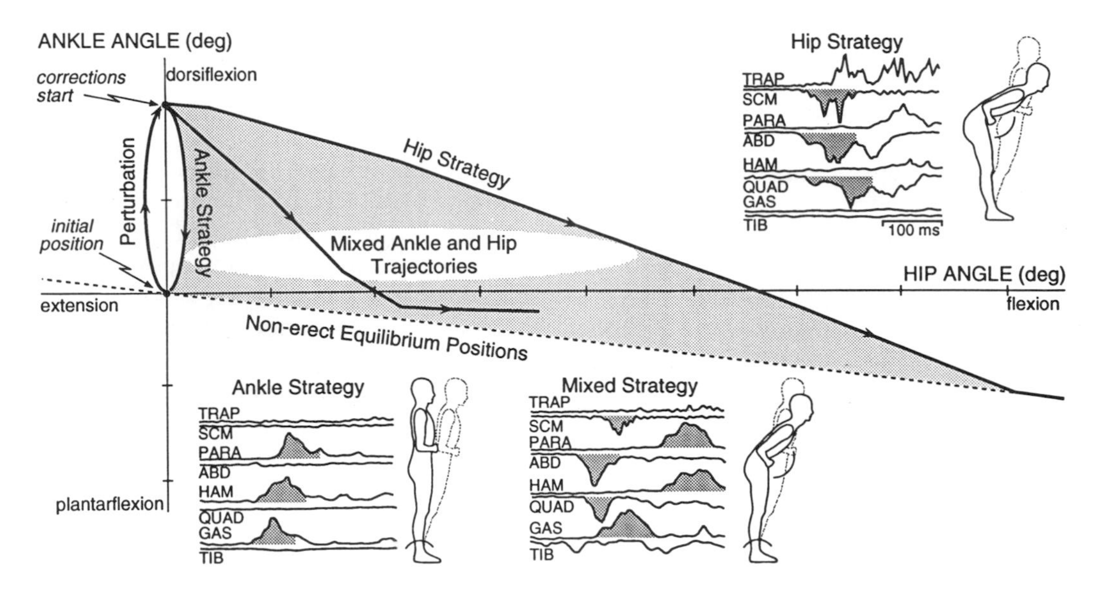

FIG. 7.5. Ankle-to-hip strategy continuum for dynamic equilibrium in standing humans. The plot of ankle angle vs. hip angle shows examples of trajectories in sagittal plane angle–angle space for the ankle, the hip, and mixed ankle and hip strategies. The initial, erect position is at the origin of the graph. The perturbation, a backward translation, induces forward sway primarily about the ankle joints to the dot on the upward-going ankle axis. The ankle strategy brings the subject back to the erect equilibrium position, whereas the hip strategy brings the subject to a nonerect equilibrium position. Mixed strategies can follow a trajectory anywhere within the *shaded region*. *Insets* show the patterns of EMG activity in the neck, trunk and leg for the various strategies. TRAP, trapezius; SCM, sternocleidomastoid; PARA, paraspinals; ABD, abdominals; HAM, hamstrings; QUAD, quadriceps; GAS, gastrocnemius; TIB, tibialis anterior. [Adapted from Horak and Nashner (120).]

able hip motion, and the change to the ankle strategy is not immediate (120). Thus, the prior experience on the beam alters central set to influence the response on the normal surface.

Each of the strategies described thus far has different priorities in the stabilization of various postural variables, a factor that could influence the choice of strategy. For example, the hip strategy permits faster movement of the CoM than does the ankle strategy; in contrast, the ankle strategy maintains vertical alignment of the legs and trunk, whereas the hip does not. In the ankle strategy, the head moves little and appears not to be actively stabilized (124, 141). In the hip strategy, the head is actively counterrotated in parallel with the hip rotation to stabilize gaze orientation with respect to the environment (208, 248). Modeling studies have shown that if the overriding postural goal is to return the CoM to the initial position following perturbation, then the hip strategy is more efficient than the ankle strategy, requiring less energy in terms of muscle activation (143). Nevertheless, the ankle strategy appears to be more commonly used and is the first line of defense in responding to postural perturbations. Thus, the choice of the ankle strategy may reflect the precedence of trunk verticality over energetics in this task.

Quadrupedal animals such as cats also use characteristic strategies to respond to perturbations of stance. Comparisons of cat and human postural responses have suggested that the neural strategies may be similar across species, whereas the implementation of the strategy depends on the postural configuration of stance (70, 165). When humans assume a quadrupedal posture similar to the cat, their postural responses are quite similar to those of the cat in both spatial and temporal patterns of EMG activation and in ground reaction force profiles. Similarly, when cats stand bipedally, their postural responses become significantly modified from the quadrupedal response. Thus, postural control in the cat provides a useful model for human postural control.

Studies in cats have examined the responses to translations in many directions in the horizontal plane and have extended our understanding of the organization of postural strategies and synergies. When the support surface under the cat is suddenly moved, the feet are carried along with the surface and the trunk remains behind due to inertia, with most of the joint angle changes occurring at hips and shoulders, and at the metacarpo- or metatarsophalangeal joints. The trunk remains aligned with the support surface and the intralimb geometry changes little as the trunk is propelled back to its original position with respect to the feet. No matter what direction the support surface is translated, the cat responds by exerting force in one of only two directions in the horizontal plane, the force constraint strategy (160), as illustrated in Figure 7.6*A*. This force pattern contributes to the stabilization of trunk orientation, particularly in the plane of lateral flexion.

The invariance in the ground reaction forces during translation is not the product of an invariant muscle synergy organization (36, 71, 161). Figure 7.6 shows examples of muscle activations (Fig. 7.6*B* and *C*) and the changes in torque at each of the joints (Fig. 7.6*D*) in response to horizontal translations in many directions. Each muscle shows a broad tuning in its recruitment during translation, with a maximum amplitude of activation for one characteristic direction, and decreasing amplitude as direction is increased or decreased (Fig. 7.6*C*). Note that some biarticular muscles show an activation pattern that overlaps the torque regions of both joints that are spanned by the muscle. For example, anterior sartorius is a hip flexor and knee extensor and it is recruited for directions in which there is a knee extensor torque *and* for directions in which there is a hip flexor torque (Fig. 7.6*C* and *D*). The probability of response of the muscle (percentage of trials in which a response is evoked) shows a pattern similar to the recruitment tuning curve (Fig. 7.6*B*). The falloff in probability with change in direction is not due to habituation or adaptation, since changing the direction of translation back to the preferred direction will immediately increase the amplitude and probability of response for the muscle. These character-

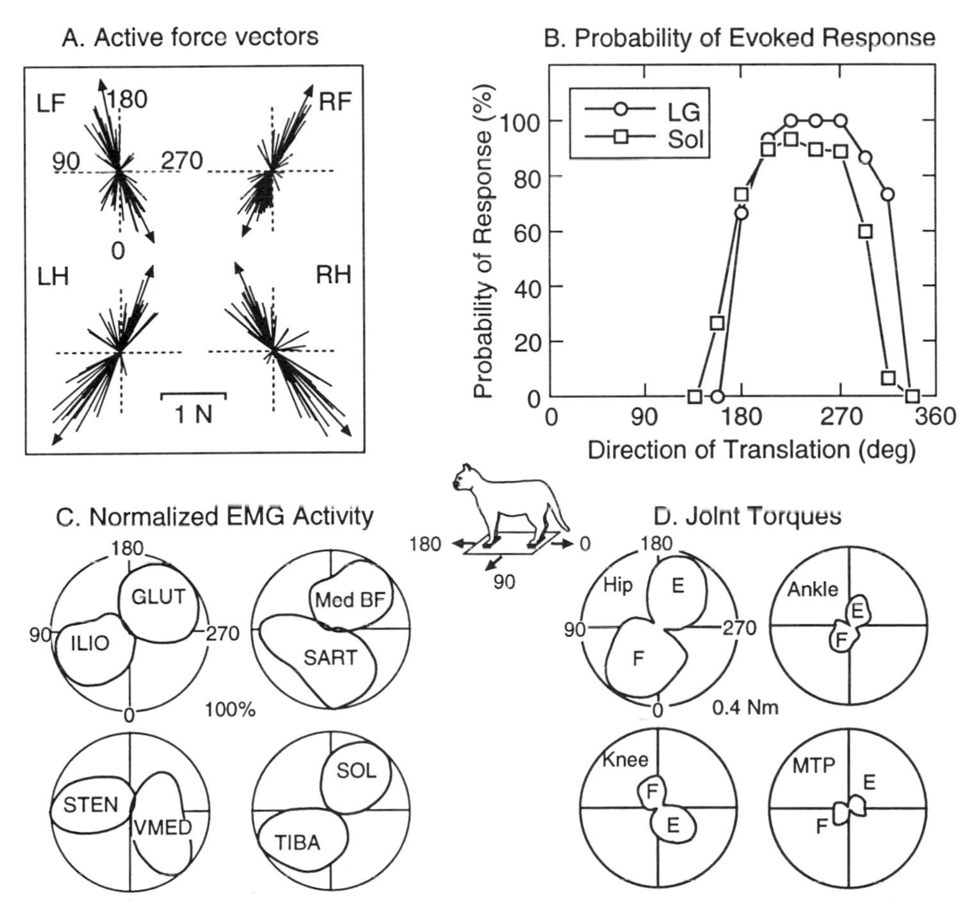

FIG. 7.6. Characteristics of postural responses of the cat to linear translation in many directions in the horizontal plane. *A*, Active horizontal plane force vectors exerted by each limb in response to 16 directions of translation. *Arrows* illustrate the mean vector directions for each cluster. LF, RF, left and right forelimb; LH, RH, left and right hindlimb. *Inset* shows coordinate system in degrees. *B*, Probability of response (% of responsive trials) for two selected muscles, lateral gastrocnemius (LG) and soleus (Sol) as a function of the direction of translation. Note the monotonic nature of the response profiles, and the fact that even for those directions that a muscle is activated, it may never be recruited for 100% of the trials (e.g., Sol). *C*, EMG tuning curves: activity evoked in several muscles during translation plotted in polar coordinates of direction of translation (degrees) vs. amplitude of normalized evoked activity. *D*, Peak change in torque during response to translation. The *circles* represent 0.4 Nm. F, flexor; E, extensor; GLUT, gluteus medius; ILIO, iliopsoas; Med BF, medial biceps femoris, SART, anterior sartorius; STEN, semitendinosus; VMED, vastus medialis; SOL, soleus; TIBA, tibialis anterior.

istics of muscle recruitment suggest that the muscle synergy that is recruited is unique for each direction of translation, even though the forces at the ground remain invariant. Muscle synergies are the implementation of a strategy and do not, in themselves, define the strategy.

Recent experiments in the cat (R. Jacobs and J. M. Macpherson, unpublished data) suggest that it is the force exerted at the ground, or the 'contact' force, that is the critical controlled variable during dynamic postural reactions. The contact force appears to be controlled by two parallel neural systems, one for force vector amplitude and the other for force vector direction. In response to translation in many directions, the thigh muscles subdivide into two functional groups according to the relationship of their evoked activity to the various forces and torques in the sagittal plane. The first group, consisting of monoarticular and some biarticular thigh muscles, shows an exponential relationship to the *amplitude* of the contact force and not to the torque at the spanned joint(s). A separate and distinct group of muscles, the biarticular rectus femoris, caudal semimembranosus, and middle biceps femoris, shows an exponential relationship to the difference in torque at knee and hip (Tknee-Thip) and *not* to the force amplitude. It can be shown that this second group of muscles is activated in relation to the *direction* of the contact force. This strategy of parallel control of the two components of the contact force, direction and amplitude, may simplify the control of the multisegmented limb. The specification of the appropriate contact force exerted by each of the four limbs will produce the necessary resultant force to propel the trunk (and CoM) back to its original position with respect to the feet and, thus, maintain postural equilibrium.

Postural reactions in response to external disturbances are essential for maintaining equilibrium, not only during stance but also during voluntary movement. During locomotion, the postural response to a disturbance of gait depends on the phase of the step cycle in both humans (18, 204) and cats (66). The pattern of EMG activation that is evoked is related to the nature of the postural imbalance (204). For humans walking on a treadmill (18), sudden acceleration of the belt pulls the stance limb backward with respect to the CoM and induces dorsiflexion of the ankle. The rapid response (~65 ms latency) consists of activation of gastrocnemius followed by hamstrings in the stance limb and tibialis anterior in the swing limb (18). The net effect is *shortening* of the step, involving both the stance phase of the perturbed limb and the swing of the contralateral limb. Sudden deceleration of the belt evokes postural responses in tibialis anterior of the stance limb with inhibition of the normally active gastrocnemius, along with activation of tibialis anterior of the swing limb. The net effect is a *prolongation* of the phase of the step cycle in which the perturbation occurs. For both directions of perturbation, normal locomotion is restored in the subsequent step cycle of both limbs (18), attesting to the effectiveness of the postural response.

Similar kinds of postural reactions have been observed during both treadmill and overground locomotion in cats. When cats experience sudden loss of support under the hindlimb during overground locomotion (the "trapdoor paradigm"), they exhibit characteristic postural responses that are tuned to the ongoing task (90). If the contralateral limb is bearing weight (stance phase), short-latency (30 ms) activation of flexor muscles is observed in the hindlimb that entered the hole; in contrast, if the contralateral limb is not bearing weight (swing phase), the hindlimb that entered the hole continues to extend while the swing phase of the contralateral limb is foreshortened (90). Thus, the postural response is appropriately modified to achieve the goals of restoring dynamic equilibrium and minimizing the disruption of the ongoing movement.

Task goals and previous instructions can significantly affect even the earliest component of automatic postural adjustments. For example, the early (100 ms) postural response to translation in human subjects can be modified by the instruction to "step as soon as the surface begins to move" (34), even though voluntary reaction time to a somatosensory cue is normally much longer than 100 ms. As seen in Figure 7.7, the postural response to backward translation involves bilateral activation of soleus and gastrocnemius. In contrast, the anticipatory postural adjustment preceding step initiation from the standing posture consists of inhibition in soleus and activation of tibialis. In the step, the CoM progresses forward and to the side of the stance limb whereas, in response to backward translation, the CoM is propelled backward to restore upright stance. When a step is triggered by a backward translation, the early activity evoked by the perturbation is significantly modified in a task-specific manner. Soleus and gastrocnemius activation is reduced bilaterally, but gastrocnemius is more reduced on the stance side. This asymmetry corresponds to the fact that initiation of step from quiet stance requires unilateral activation of the swing limb gastrocnemius for propulsion during heel-off (30, 31, 43). The preparatory postural adjustment for initiation of the step is also altered by the perturbation, such that subjects step more quickly when they are perturbed.

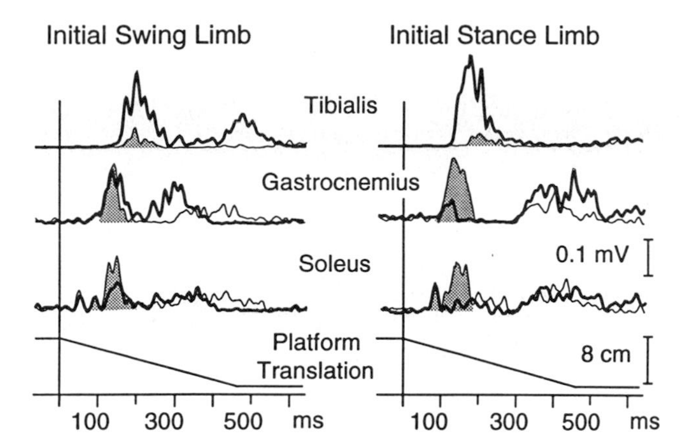

FIG. 7.7. Ankle muscle activation in the two lower limbs in response to backward translation of the support surface under two instructions, "remain standing" (*thin line, hatched fill*) and "step as soon as the perturbation is detected" (*thick line, no fill*). The response to translation alone consists of bilateral activation of soleus and gastrocnemius. When the instruction is to step, the postural response is significantly attenuated, particularly in the stance limb. [Adapted from Burleigh, Horak, and Malouin (34).]

Similarly, when subjects are exposed to a sudden surface tilt while initiating a push or pull on a handle, the postural response to the tilt is altered (271). Even the simple task of lowering the arm to touch a support bar influences the postural response evoked by rotation of the support surface. The postural response that is normally observed in tibialis following a toes-up rotation can be attenuated up to 50 ms prior to the relaxation of the deltoid, which initiates the arm-lowering task (242). The change in tibialis response is probably linked to the preparation of the voluntary movement, and not the arm movement or contact with the bar. These results demonstrate an interaction between the descending central program for voluntary movement and the postural program that is triggered by ascending information associated with a disturbance, even though the voluntary reaction time is considerably longer than the onset latency of the automatic postural response.

Anticipatory Postural Adjustments for Voluntary Movement

Posture is permissive to movement in that the various requirements of posture must be fulfilled in order for a movement to achieve its goal in a coordinated manner. A voluntary focal movement, such as raising an arm or taking a step, produces reaction forces that affect all the linked segments of the body and can destabilize the equilibrium of the CoM, producing loss of balance. Focal movements do not occur in isolation, but rather are accompanied by activity in many distant muscles that does not contribute directly to the focal movement itself. Such activity represents an active postural adjustment that either precedes the activation of the prime movers in a voluntary movement (16, 28, 68, 133, 174), or is simultaneous with the voluntary movement (44, 215). Through learning and adaptation, the nervous system anticipates the mechanical effects of a voluntary movement and adjusts the amplitude and timing of the accompanying postural component in order to minimize the disturbance to balance.

The anticipatory postural adjustment that accompanies a voluntary movement is an integral part of the motor program for that movement. As shown in Figure 7.8*A*, when a standing subject moves an arm rapidly, the first muscles to be activated are the leg muscles to stabilize the body against sway (16, 28,

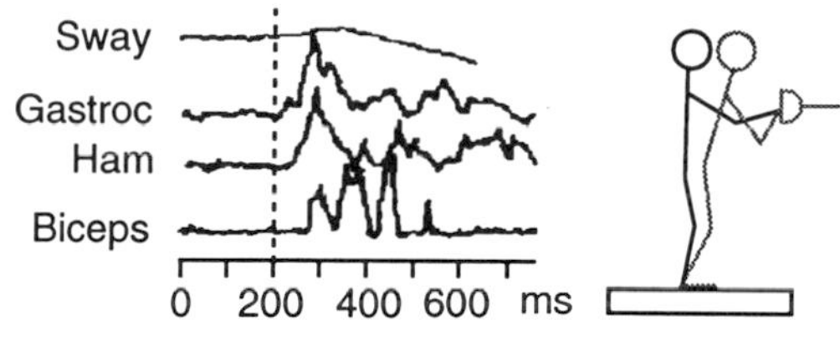

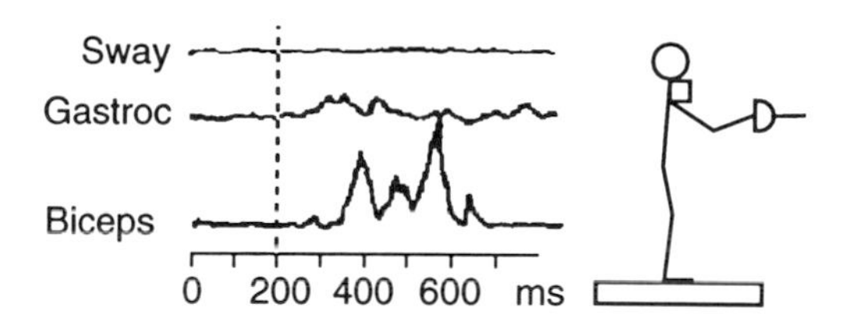

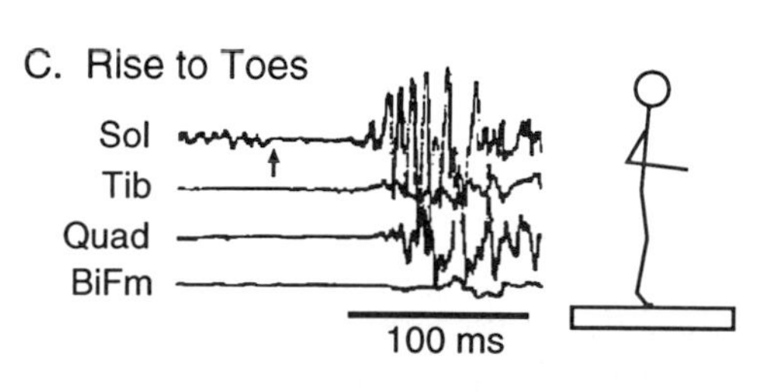

FIG. 7.8. *A*, The anticipatory postural response in the lower limb muscles, gastrocnemius (Gastroc) and hamstrings (Ham), precedes the onset of activity in biceps brachii (Biceps), the agonist for the arm-pull task. *B*, When the subject is firmly supported at the shoulder, the same arm-pull task illustrated in *A* does not elicit an anticipatory postural response in the leg muscles (compare gastrocnemius in *A* and *B*. *C*, In rocking forward on the toes, the first change in EMG is an inhibition of tonic activity in soleus (*arrow*), which allows the CoM to move forward toward the toes. This is followed by the focal response of activation of tibialis (Tib), soleus (Sol), and quadriceps (Quad). [*A* and *B* adapted from Cordo and Nashner (42), *C* adapted from Nardone and Schieppati (199).]

174). Similar yet task-specific postural responses are also observed during voluntary trunk movements (44, 215) and during the voluntary elevation of one leg in humans (194) and in cats (9, 68). Both activation of muscle and inhibition of ongoing contraction can contribute to the postural response. For example, the tonically active soleus is inhibited up to 150 ms prior to the activation of arm muscles in a bilateral arm-lifting task (28).

If the reaction time for the focal movement changes, so too does the latency of the anticipatory postural activity, such that the temporal relations are maintained between postural activity and focal activity (16). Furthermore the latency for activation of a muscle is shorter when that muscle serves a preparatory postural role than when it acts as a prime mover. In the arm-raising task, the anticipatory postural activation of biceps femoris and rectus femoris with respect to a tone signal is 50–100 ms earlier than the voluntary activation of those muscles when the instructed task is to move the leg (16). Similarly, the inactivation of soleus in a postural response is earlier than the voluntary relaxation of soleus from a tonically active state (199). The relative timing of the postural and focal muscle activity depends on the speed of the movement (152). Very slow movements may not show any significant postural activity, or there may be a slow, ramp-like increase in EMG activity following the onset of the focal movement (117).

The spatial pattern of EMG activity in the postural adjustment that accompanies voluntary movement is specific to the movement being performed, and is not merely a generalized co-contraction (16, 28, 42, 152, 174, 199). For example, activity of muscles in the two legs is asymmetric for a single arm raise, but symmetric when both arms are raised together because of the differences in the reaction forces related to the arm lift (16, 28). Anticipatory postural responses do not occur only in the legs, but are also seen in other body segments depending on the task. If a subject pulls on an object with the arm while steadying himself with the other arm the first muscles to be activated are those in the steadying arm (174). Rapid arm movements during ongoing locomotion on a treadmill are preceded by postural adjustments that are tuned not only to the direction of the arm movement (push or pull) but also to the phase of the step cycle, such that equilibrium is maintained with the least disruption of the ongoing locomotor activity (110, 206).

The presence of anticipatory postural activity depends on the task and on the conditions of support. As shown in Figure 7.8*B*, when the subject is stabilized by leaning against an external support, there is little or no anticipatory postural activity in the legs during a voluntary arm movement (42), since the destabilizing forces of the focal movement are passively opposed by the external support.

In the task of rising from a flat-footed stance to a stable posture standing on the toes, the initial postural response consists of inactivation of soleus (Figure 7.8*C*) and activation of tibialis anterior, causing a backward shift in the CoP, presumably to accelerate the CoM forward prior to rising up on the toes. In contrast, when subjects rise to the toes while holding on to a support with the arms, there is no preparatory activity in soleus and tibialis, nor is there a backward shift in CoP (199). Similarly, when subjects simply rise to the toes and immediately return to flat-footed stance, no preparatory postural activity is observed (37). If the rise to toes is initiated from a forward leaning position, again there is no anticipatory activation of tibialis (37). When the postural component is not present in this task, there is no advancing in time of the focal component, which led Nardone and Schieppati to hypothesize that these two components, postural and focal, are integral parts of the voluntary movement and that the postural component may be enhanced, reduced, or completely suppressed, depending on the context (199).

Postural adjustments are always correctly matched to the focal movement, suggesting that both these components of voluntary movement are integrated at the level of planning of the movement. For example, when subjects make an error in movement direction in a choice reaction time task, the postural response is always appropriate for the movement that is performed, rather than the movement that was commanded (42, 199).

The need to control the position of the body's CoM under both static and dynamic conditions can be considered as one of the overriding goals in many voluntary movements, and provides a reasonable explanation for much of the postural activity that accompanies focal movement. During a voluntary trunk movement involving flexion or extension at the hips, postural activity in the legs effectively produces a counterrotation at the ankles (44, 215). As a result, the CoM moves only about 1–2 cm even though the body configuration changes radically. Modeling studies showed that without the postural adjustment, the movement of the CoM would be as large as 12 cm (44).

Different postural strategies have been described for the voluntary lifting of one limb in the quadruped. When the limb is raised in response to an unexpected stimulus, the postural adjustment in cats and dogs consists of a diagonal weight support pattern in which the lifting limb and the diagonally opposite limb decrease vertical support and the other two limbs increase (68,80,133). In contrast, when the cat performs a reaction time lift to a tone signal, the weight shift occurs primarily onto the opposite limb of the same girdle, the nondiagonal support pattern. In the diagonal strategy the displacement of the CoM is minimized and the trunk orientation and alignment do not change; in the nondiagonal strategy the CoM is actively displaced and the trunk is flexed laterally (68). The nondiagonal strategy may be more energy efficient, but the diagonal strategy may allow a more rapid transition to locomotion.

Locomotion is a task in which several different variables of postural orientation and equilibrium are controlled simultaneously, including trunk orientation and position of the CoM. The trajectory of the CoM is controlled primarily by foot placement and travels along the medial border of the stance foot (246, 270). Although the CoM is rarely within the base of support during locomotion, its trajectory is controlled to maintain dynamic equilibrium. The trunk oscillates no more than 1–2 degrees in the sagittal plane through the active control of the hip musculature (258), whereas stabilization of the trunk in the mediolateral plane is achieved primarily through foot placement, but also through action of the pelvic and lateral spinal musculature (159).

Modeling of Postural Coordination

Computational models provide a powerful way to explore the biomechanical complexities of the musculoskeletal system and to examine possible control mechanisms. In the interplay between modeling and experimental approaches, experimental data are used to tune model parameters, and models generate predictions that are then tested experimentally. This multidisciplinary approach has the potential to make substantial contributions to our understanding of postural control.

Models have recently been developed to simulate the function of the individual muscles, the musculoskeletal geometry, and the segmental dynamics in postural control (14, 91, 109, 137). Muscle function is modeled using variations of Hill's model in which four parameters are used to describe the contraction characteristics of each muscle (274). Based on a given set of scaled muscle activations, the forces and motions of the limb model are computed (forward dynamics).

This approach was used to develop a model of human postural dynamics that reproduces the coordinative strategies that are used for a particular size and speed of postural sway initiated from any initial body position (142). The set of all biomechanically possible postural actions in the sagittal plane can be visualized by combining vectors representing acceleration of the ankle, knee, and hip resulting from the activation of each leg muscle, as shown in Figure 7.9*A*. Given the constraint of keeping the feet flat on the floor, the set of leg/trunk actions that is biomechanically possible is surprisingly limited, suggesting that the choices available to the nervous system are equally limited. The model pre-

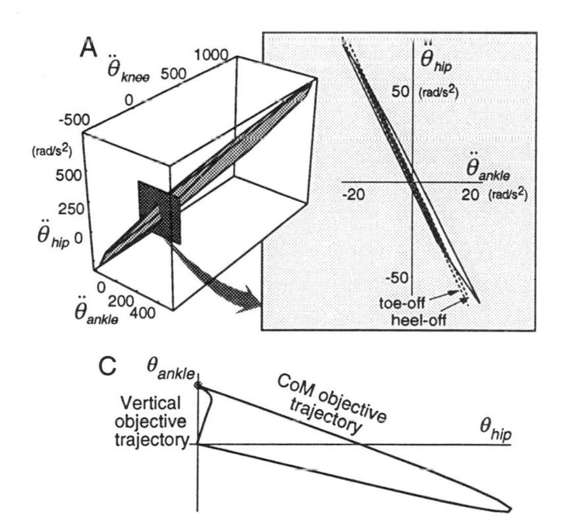

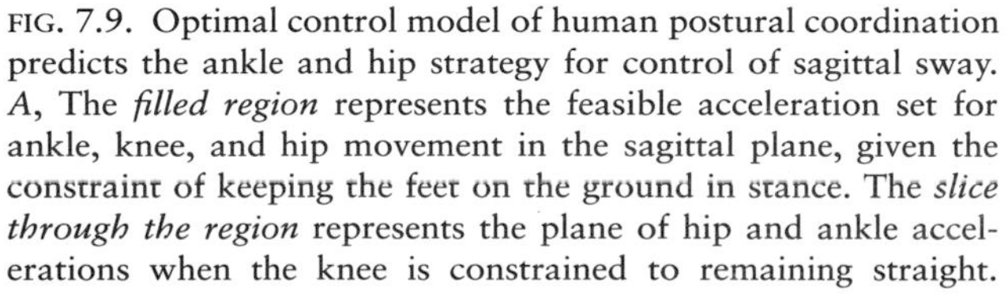

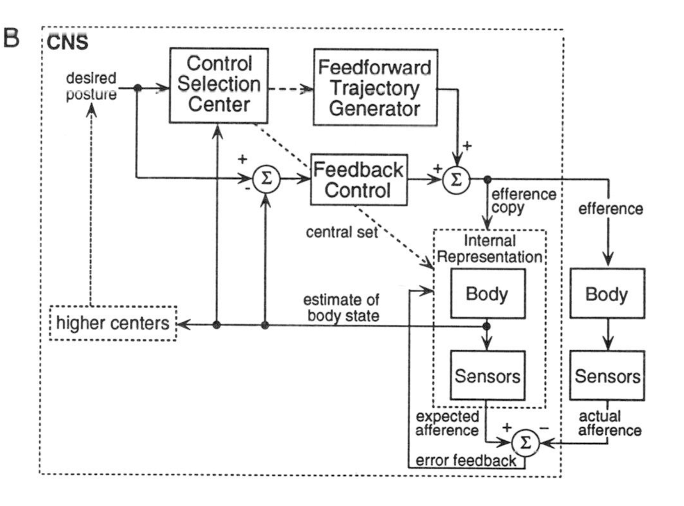

FIG. 7.9. Optimal control model of human postural coordination predicts the ankle and hip strategy for control of sagittal sway. *A*, The *filled region* represents the feasible acceleration set for ankle, knee, and hip movement in the sagittal plane, given the constraint of keeping the feet on the ground in stance. The *slice through the region* represents the plane of hip and ankle accelerations when the knee is constrained to remaining straight. There is only a narrow region in which the ankle strategy (*horizontal extent of shaded area*) may be used without the toes or heels lifting off. Note that the ankle acceleration scale has been expanded compared to the hip. *B*, Block diagram of the optimal control model (see text for details). *C*, Ankle/hip angle trajectories predicted by the model for two different cost functions. [Adapted from Kuo (142)].

dicts the experimental observations of a gradual transition from ankle to hip strategy as subjects change initial body tilt from upright stance to positions close to the limits of their toe or heel support (119). The model also shows that the hip strategy can result in maximal center-of-mass accelerations that are 20 times greater than those generated by the ankle strategy.

Kuo (142) models the postural controller as an optimizer (linear quadratic gaussian optimal controller) in which redundancy is resolved by minimizing various objective functions that penalize large-amplitude motor commands, and motions away from erect stance (Figure 7.9*B*). Unlike most linear control models, this one includes a "control selection center" that allows any combination of feedback and feedforward. The control selection center uses both the initial mechanical state and the desired state specified by "higher centers" to preselect the type of response necessary to counteract a postural disturbance and to choose the appropriate feedforward trajectories and feedback gains. This center also specifies an internal representation of the body and sensor dynamics through the mechanism of "central set" (27), thereby providing a prediction of expected afferent input. The difference between the expected input and the actual input is used to adjust the internal representation's estimate of body state, which is, in turn, used in feedback control.

According to this model, different body movement trajectories are predicted depending upon the variables (objectives) that are optimized (e.g., position of the CoM, head stability, or vertical alignment of the body). When the CoM must be returned to equilibrium with minimal energy expenditure, the model predicts that a hip strategy will always be observed in response to a simulated perturbation (Fig. 7.9*C*, CoM objective trajectory). In contrast, when a high priority is placed on vertical alignment of the trunk, the model predicts an ankle strategy (Fig. 7.9*C*, vertical objective trajectory).

Modeling, using modern control theories in combination with experimental data, provides a powerful approach for furthering our understanding of the control of postural orientation and equilibrium. A future goal is to expand such models to include the dynamics of multiple sensory input systems.

SENSORY CONTROL OF POSTURAL ORIENTATION AND EQUILIBRIUM

There are many common features in the sensory control of postural orientation and of dynamic equilibrium. Both use sensory information from multiple channels, including somatosensory (cutaneous and proprioceptive), vestibular, and visual. These sensory systems do *not* operate as independent, parallel channels that merely sum together at some point to result in a motor output. Rather, multiple sensory inputs are integrated and resolved by the postural control system to provide a coherent interpretation of the body's orientation and dynamic equilibrium. This information is then thought to be compared to an internal model of the body and any resulting error signal is used to generate motor commands in order to maintain the required postural variables at the desired level. This process occurs at the subconscious, involuntary level, producing automatic adjustments with short latencies.

Sensory Integration

The information coded by each sensory modality is unique, and each class of receptor operates optimally within a specific range of frequency and amplitude of body motion. Nevertheless, there is enough redundancy of sensory information that, in certain environments, balance can be maintained when information from one or more sensory channels is not available. Multiple channels of input are necessary in order to resolve ambiguities about postural orientation and body motion. Because the sensory receptors are part of the body itself, the interpretation of the afferent information within the reference frame of the surrounding world may not be singular and unique, thus leading to ambiguity. For example, the movement of an image across the retina (retinal slip) tells us that there is relative motion between the head and the surrounding visual environment, but vision alone cannot resolve what moved—the world or the self. Similarly, the otoliths, which detect linear forces acting on the head, cannot distinguish between static head tilt (force due to gravity) on a stationary body, and linear acceleration of the body relative to inertial space. The resolution of such ambiguities comes through the integration of information from multiple sources of input.

A dynamic weighting of sensory inputs may be necessary to optimize the control of postural stability. As mentioned previously, the main controlled variable for dynamic equilibrium may be the position and orientation of the trunk in space. How information about the trunk is derived from sensory inputs is task- and context-dependent. When the support surface is stable and firmly contacted, then proprioceptive and cutaneous information from the legs and feet may give the most reliable information about the trunk relative to the environment. In contrast, when the surface is unstable or contacted for only brief periods such as during rapid locomotion, then the combination of vestibular and neck proprioceptive information may provide the most veridical information about trunk orientation and velocity. Vestibular inputs detect acceleration of the head in a gravitoinertial reference frame, whereas the neck proprioceptors provide information about head relative to trunk. Thus, the combination of vestibular and neck inputs allows the system to derive trunk position and velocity relative to the environment.

The role of an individual sensory system in orientation and equilibrium can change depending upon the task, the availability of sensory information within a particular environment, and the movement strategies used in the task. After a lesion involving one sensory system, the nervous system may change the way the remaining senses are used through compensation and plasticity (171, 205). An example of the relative dependence of postural control on visual, vestibular, and somatosensory information comes from a study by Nashner and colleagues (25,205). They measured postural sway during erect stance while systematically manipulating one type of sensory information at a time: visual information by either eye closure or by stabilizing the visual surround with respect to body sway at the hip, called "sway referencing"; and somatosensory information by "sway referencing" the tilt of the support surface and, therefore, ankle joint angle. The role of vestibular input was examined by studying patients with various types of vestibular deficits. In the sway-referenced conditions, sensory information is not rendered absent but is "inaccurate" as a postural orientation reference.

In intact subjects, when visual *or* somatosensory inputs are altered, sway increases only slightly (conditions 2–4 in Fig. 7.10). When both visual *and* somatosensory inputs are altered, subjects rely primarily on vestibular inputs for orientation (conditions 5–6 in Fig. 7.10) and sway increases by 50%. As expected, patients with bilateral, profound loss of vestibular function fall when both somatosensory and visual information is either unavailable (condition 5) or unreliable (condition 6). Patients with well-compensated vestibular loss are able to stand without vision (conditions 2 and 3) or without reliable surface information (condition 4), suggesting that one sense alone is capable of preventing a fall in quiet stance (25, 205).

Sensory integration for postural control is not merely a summation of the individual channels, nor does it operate by consensus of the majority. The nervous system needs to extract and interpret the relevant sensory information to determine whether the body or the environment is still or in motion and to orient the body with respect to gravitoinertial forces and relevant surface and visual cues. Dynamic reweighting of sensory inputs, which depends upon the particular context, instruction, and practice enables humans and animals to maintain posture in changing sensory environments.

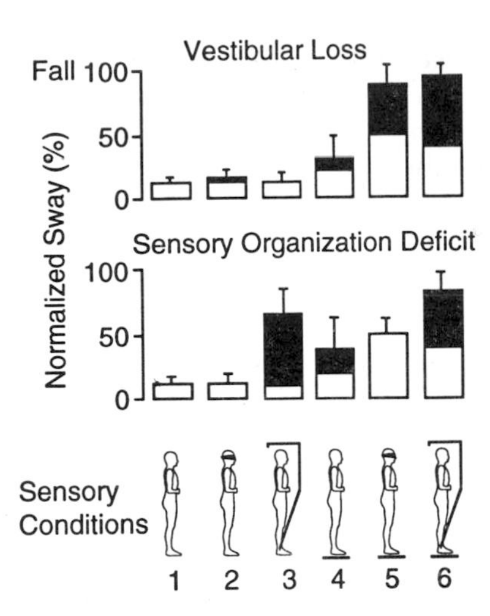

FIG. 7.10. Mean sway over 20 s of stance under six different sensory conditions in normal subjects (*open bars*) and in patients with vestibular loss (*top*), and a sensory organization deficit (*bottom*). Anterior/posterior peak-to-peak sway at the hips is normalized for each subject's height such that 100% represents a "fall." Sensory conditions include blindfolding (conditions 2 and 5), sway-referencing the visual surround (conditions 3 and 6), and sway-referencing the support surface (conditions 4, 5 and 6). [Adapted from Black et al. (25).]

Somatosensory System

Somatosensory afferents, which include mechanoreceptors in the skin, pressure receptors in deep tissues, muscle spindles, Golgi tendon organs, and joint receptors, provide critical information about postural orientation and equilibrium. Detailed descriptions of cutaneous mechanoreceptors and proprioceptors (spindles, tendon organs, joint receptors) and their characteristics and connections can be found in Chapters 3 and 4 of this volume. Somatosensors, because they are distributed throughout the body, are critical for determining the configuration of the body segments; in contrast, visual and vestibular receptors are located in a head that moves independently of the trunk and limbs, so *body* configuration and orientation information from head-based sensors is either limited or must be derived. Somatosensory receptors in the feet, legs, and trunk may be critically important for controlling the trunk, particularly under conditions where the subject maintains contact with a large, rigid, and stable support surface. Proprioceptive information from the neck is used in combination with vestibular information in order to derive trunk position and velocity. Blocking neck proprioceptive signals disrupts not only head stability but also body tone and postural stability (2,40). Somatosensory information informs the nervous system not only about the qualities of the support surface, such as compliance and slipperiness, but also about the forces that the body exerts against those surfaces.

Movement between the support surface and the feet generates shearing forces that can result in stretching and deformation of the skin and lead to activation of cutaneous and deep mechanoreceptors. Based on recordings from afferent fibers, Ferrington (76) found that the best stimulus for activating slowly adapting receptors in the paw pads of the cat was distortion of nerve endings rather than steady indentation or compression. Similarly, mechanoreceptors in human skin are exquisitely sensitive to stretch of the skin (72). Therefore, mechanoreceptors in the skin of the foot could fire in relation to shearing forces produced by a perturbation of stance, with the rate of firing providing information about velocity of the perturbation (94, 148). Direction could be coded by the sequence of activation of a population of mechanoreceptors in the foot (113). Both velocity (57) and direction (164) of a perturbation are represented in the initial burst of EMG activity, by the amplitude and spatial pattern of evoked activity, respectively.

Reduction of somatosensory information from the feet and ankle joints by cooling or by ischemic block at the ankles has no effect on unperturbed stance (55), even with absent or altered visual or vestibular inputs (121). However, body sway is increased during slow, small sinusoidal rotations of the support (55, 180). Local anesthetic block of the pedal afferents in dogs causes significant delays in the postural responses to fore-aft translation of the support surface (192). In contrast, anesthetization of the foot in humans does *not* alter the latency of postural response to a rapid rotation (55) or translation (121) of the support surface, although the postural strategy is altered. Instead of using the normal ankle strategy in response to translation, subjects without sensation from the feet incorporate a large degree of hip strategy in their response (121). Horak and colleagues concluded from these latter findings that somatosensory information from the feet is important in determining the feasible set of postural strategies that can be used under various conditions, and that information from the feet is needed in order for the ankle strategy to be used (121). It may be that loss of information about surface characteristics results in more dependence on vestibular inputs and that vestibular signals drive the hip strategy.

Muscle receptors in the leg provide important information for the postural control system. For low-amplitude sway that occurs primarily about the ankle joints, the length of the ankle muscles, soleus and tibialis anterior, will give a good approximation of the degree of body tilt and, therefore, the position of the trunk. Anesthetic block of afferent fibers through hypoxic ischemia from pressure cuffs applied at the thighs severely compromises balance in otherwise normal subjects. During quiet stance with eyes closed, ischemia of the legs results in a prominent oscillatory sway at around 1 Hz, resembling the sway of patients with tabes dorsalis in which the larger diameter-fibers are damaged (180). Stability is also greatly diminished during small, low-frequency sinusoidal rotations of the support surface (55).

The importance of muscle spindles for postural orientation has been demonstrated by the use of mechanical vibration (1–1.5 mm at 40–220 Hz) that selectively drives Ia afferents, and induces leaning and illusions of leaning in standing subjects (144). In the standing, blindfolded subject, vibration of gastrocnemius induces the illusion of muscle lengthening, which is interpreted subconsciously as forward body sway; this illusory sway is counteracted by a slow backward lean until activation of the tibialis is triggered to prevent a backward fall (see Chapter 4 in this *Handbook* for other vibration-induced illusions). Vibration results in muscle activity not only at local joints but also in remote muscle groups, to affect whole-body posture in freely standing subjects, depending on the interaction of the body with the support surface, and the relative configuration of the body parts (102, 236). For example, stretch of the neck extensors, trunk and leg flexors, or the extraocular muscles that lower the eyes is consistent with the sensation of backward sway; vibration of any of these muscles induces a forward body lean. These effects are additive—sway amplitude increases as more of these muscles are vibrated simultaneously (236).

The effect of vibration on postural orientation is influenced by the task requirements and the instructions to the subject (230). Figure 7.11*A* illustrates that when a standing subject receives vibration to the soleus (which induces an illusion of forward sway) during a task in which they are required to maintain a constant horizontal forearm position, not only do they sway backward but they also extend the elbow in order to keep the forearm oriented to perceived earth horizontal. When the subject is stabilized by external fixation and cannot sway back-

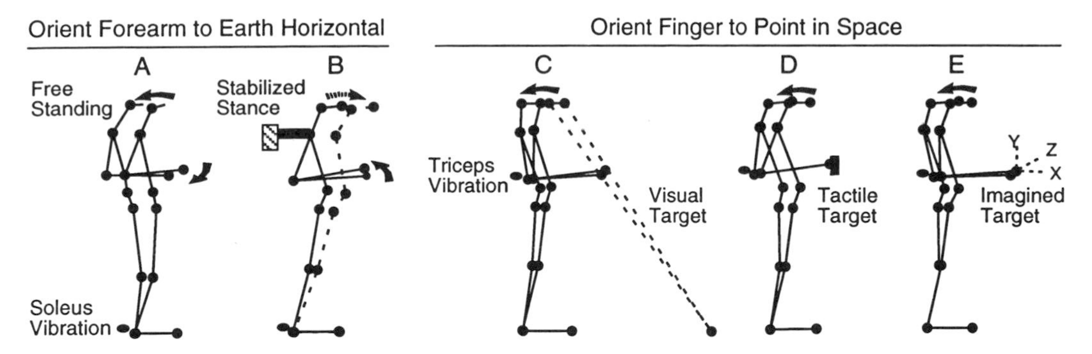

FIG. 7.11. Context-dependency of changes in postural orientation induced by vibration. *A* and *B*, Subjects are instructed to hold the forearm horizontal when freely standing (*A*) or stabilized at the trunk (*B*). *C* through *E*, Backward sway is induced by triceps brachii vibration when subjects are instructed to orient the finger to a visual target (*C*), a tactile target (*D*), or an imagined target in space (*E*). [Adapted from Quoniam et al. (230).]

ward, they perceive their body tilt to be in the opposite direction (i.e., forward) and they compensate by flexing the elbow (Fig. 7.11*B*). This suggests that the subjective orientation of the forearm is deduced from the subjective body verticality via a proprioceptive chain linking the external world to the forearm (230). Likewise, perceptual or cognitive factors can alter the effects of vibration on body posture. Normally, vibration of triceps brachii induces extension of the elbow. However, when subjects are required to anchor the tip of their index finger to a visual or tactile target in extrapersonal space, or even to an imagined target, vibration of triceps brachii induces a backward whole-body sway [Fig. 7.11*C*–*E*; (230)]. Proprioceptive information is interpreted by the postural control system in a flexible manner within the context of the behavioral requirements. This input helps define a postural reference frame for the body and its configuration, and interrelates body space with extrapersonal space.

New studies of postural orientation in unusual gravitoinertial environments suggest that somatosensory information alone may be sufficient for maintaining body orientation in stance. In order to remain standing in a large room that is rotating at constant velocity, subjects must orient to the tilted force field, which is the summation of gravitational and angular inertial vectors (77). Subjects without vestibular function are able to orient their bodies to the tilted force vector, even without a visual reference, suggesting that somatosensory information alone is sufficient (F. B. Horak, J. R. Lackner, and P. DiZio, unpublished observations).

Proprioceptive information is used not only for postural orientation but also for detecting perturbations of stance and triggering rapid responses to maintain postural equilibrium. Slowing and/or loss of conduction of proprioceptive information from the legs results in delays of 20–30 ms in postural responses to translation (130). The fact that certain muscles may be stretched by a postural disturbance does not, however, imply that postural responses are merely stretch reflexes mediated by spindle afferents. Horak and Moore (119) showed that when subjects are instructed to lean forward maximally at the ankles prior to a backward translation of the support surface, their postural response in the gastrocnemius muscle is smaller than that elicited from an erect position, even though the ankle extensors are prestretched in the leaning position. Subjects leaning close to their limit of stability use a hip strategy rather than ankle strategy in response to the perturbation (119).

Activation of a stretched muscle may actually be inappropriate for a postural response under certain conditions. For example, when the support surface under a standing subject is rapidly *rotated* to dorsiflex the foot, the soleus and gastrocnemius are stretched and rapid activation of the muscles is observed. This stretch response is destabilizing, since it enhances the backward sway induced by the perturbation. The postural response to stabilize sway following rotation consists of activation of the shortened tibialis anterior at 120 ms (6, 51, 89, 202). The stretch response in gastrocnemius is actually reduced in amplitude with repeated rotations (202). When a subject is *translated* backward with the same angular displacement and velocity at the ankle as in the toes-up rotation, the soleus and gastrocnemius are also stretched and activation of these muscles occurs at both short and medium latencies. No activation of the shortened tibialis is observed (198). Both rotation and translation stretch the ankle extensor muscles, but the postural response to the two perturbations is opposite, with flexors for rotation and extensors for translation.

Muscle stretch alone is not sufficient for triggering appropriate postural responses. When rotation and translation perturbations are calibrated to produce similar ankle rotation, soleus, which crosses only the ankle, undergoes the *same* amount of stretch during the two types of perturbation. In contrast, gastrocnemius, which crosses both ankle and knee, undergoes the same stretch as soleus during rotation, but a much smaller stretch during translation due to flexion of the knee (198). Gastrocnemius exhibits a strong postural activation for translation, when it is only slightly stretched, and no postural activation for rotation, when it undergoes a large stretch. Stretch signals from any one muscle are not sufficient to indicate unambiguously the nature of the postural disturbance. The population of inputs from stretched and shortened muscles is necessary to compute the effect of the disturbance on body CoM and to estimate the effect on postural orientation and equilibrium. It has also been hypothesized that the degree of activation of postural muscles is partly determined by the force or load on the limbs that is induced by the perturbation (59). This loading could be signaled by Golgi tendon organs and/or deep tissue and joint receptors.

Joint receptors could also provide information about angular displacement and, therefore, body sway. Evidence about the nature of the signal detected by joint afferents is conflicting, but the current consensus is that joint afferents alone do not give sufficient information about joint position, although they may signal joint movement and/or act as joint limit detectors and as nociceptors (179, 229). Alternatively, joint receptors could detect the direction and amplitude of loading due to external forces such as gravity by their sensitivity to compressive forces within the joint (32) and could thus contribute to the control of trunk position relative to the base of support (129).

Vestibular System

The vestibular receptors in the semicircular canals and macular otoliths are sensitive to angular and linear acceleration of the head, respectively. The otolith signal is a combination of all the linear accelerations acting on the head, including the constant acceleration due to gravity. Thus, the otoliths are stimulated as the head tilts with respect to gravity, such as during body sway. Otolith signals alone are probably not responsible for our sense of "verticality," since studies of orientation to perceived upright in subjects who are submerged under water show accuracy on the order of only ±20 degrees (211, 238), compared to ±1–2 degrees on land when somatosensory cues are available (188).

The semicircular canals, as angular accelerometers, are sensitive to higher frequencies of head motions than are the otoliths. The anterior and posterior canals, which detect pitch (rotation about the interaural axis) and roll (rotation about the naso-occipital axis) are especially important for detecting rapid postural sway such as occurs with rapid hip flexion or extension, but not for detecting low-frequency sway such as in quiet stance (201, 209). The threshold level for the vestibular detection of sway in the pitch plane is very close to the ±1 degree/s reported for the conscious perception of pitch motion (17, 219, 244).

The nervous system appears to use information about the position of the head in relation to the base of foot support to interpret and respond to vestibular error signals. The vestibular system can be artificially stimulated by low levels (0.2–6 mA) of galvanic current applied to the mastoid bone, probably activating the vestibular nerve and/or receptors directly (88). This stimulation elicits directionally specific alterations in stance posture such that subjects sway in the direction of the anode with a gain of about 1.2–1.7 degrees/mA up to but not exceeding their limits of stability (39). The direction of sway, however, also depends upon the position of the head or trunk in a way that corresponds to the spatial transformation of a vector from one frame of reference, the head, to another, the body (210, 259). For example (Fig. 7.12*A* and *B*), when the head, either alone or with the trunk, is rotated over the feet, the direction of body sway induced by positive galvanic current to the right ear changes from lateral to forward (111). If a trunk rotation is combined with a neck rotation in the opposite direction, thus keeping the face pointing forward, the sway direction is not changed from normal postural alignment (Fig. 7.12C), suggesting that a map of total-body proprioception is taken into account in interpretation of the galvanically induced vestibular sway signal (158).

The effects of vestibular stimulation are task- and context-dependent. The particular muscles activated by galvanic stimulation depends entirely upon the conditions of support. When subjects are standing freely, the largest effect of vestibular stimulation is on the gastrocnemius muscle. In contrast, if ankle muscles are not involved in postural orientation, such as when a subject is seated or externally supported in standing, there is no EMG response at the ankles (79, 253). The size of the galvanically induced sway is magnified when the support surface is compliant or unstable (78, 169, 210). Active or passive

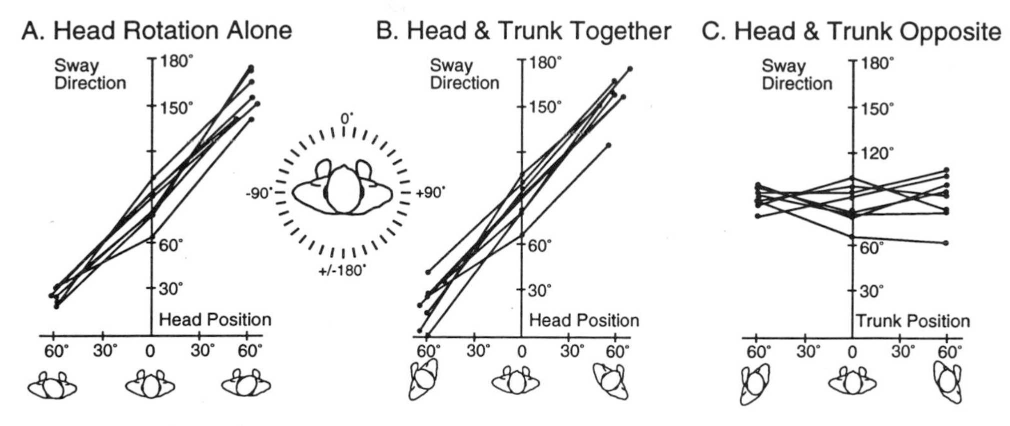

FIG. 7.12. Relationship between the head and trunk position and direction of body sway elicited by galvanic vestibular stimulation. *A*, Head rotation alone. *B*, Head and trunk rotated together. *C*, The face is kept forward by rotating the head and trunk in opposite directions. [Adapted from Lund and Broberg (158).]

body movements, particularly fast ones, also magnify the effects of galvanic vestibular stimulation, suggesting that vestibular information is more critical as an orientation reference in some tasks than in others (132, 249).

The direction of the vestibular response may depend upon a centrally integrated map of spatial perception and body configuration rather than a simple summation of vestibular and somatosensory inputs. When subjects are prevented from swaying, the galvanic stimulus produces illusory movement in a direction opposite to the sway that was evoked when standing freely, suggesting a shift in the internal representation of vertical (78, 221). When there is a mismatch between true and perceived head or body position, the direction of the response to vestibular stimulation corresponds to the spatial perception rather than the actual orientation of the head (106). For example, vibration of the right gluteus muscle induces an illusion of trunk and head rotation to the right. If vestibular stimulation is applied during this illusion, the direction of the postural response is similar to that observed when the head and trunk are actually turned to the right (104). Thus, vestibular information regarding body orientation appears to be interpreted with reference to an internal map of spatial perception that is influenced by context, other sources of sensory input, instructions, and expectations.

Vestibular afferents are responsible for triggering the response to sudden, unexpected falling. In both humans (95, 183, 265) and cats (263), an early activation is observed in extensor muscles (60–80 ms in humans) following a sudden drop of the body from a height (Fig. 7.13*A* and *B*). This early response is absent in patients without vestibular function and in cats whose otoliths have been destroyed (Fig. 7.13*B*). The early EMG response is thought to contribute to preparation for landing, and has been attributed to the otoliths (183, 263, but see 95).

In contrast, vestibular inputs are not required for the triggering of postural responses to movements of the support surface, especially when the subject is in contact with a stable, large surface (7, 53, 121, 166). Patients with bilateral loss of vestibular function show normal latencies and spatial patterning of EMG activation in leg and trunk muscles in response to translation [Fig. 7.13*C*, (121)] and rotation (7, 53) of the support surface. Similarly, even in the acute phase labyrinthectomized cats show no change in the timing and spatial pattern of EMGs evoked by translations in many directions in the horizontal plane (166).

Even though timing of postural responses is normal in bilateral vestibular loss, amplitude is not. Responses to surface translation are abnormally large (hypermetria) in both humans (115) and cats (166), as shown in Figure 7.13*D*. This hypermetria is an active overresponse, rather than an outcome of changes in passive stiffness (131). The underlying mechanism of vestibular hypermetria is not understood, but such overresponse is observed in cats for other behaviors such as head turning, jumping up from floor to chair (257), and jumping down (182). Vestibular patients can also exhibit smaller than normal responses (hypometria); for example, in response to surface rotations (8, 53, 140) and to sudden pushes on the trunk (35), again without changes in latency or spatial pattern of evoked EMG activity. Thus, vestibular inputs contribute to the magnitude of postural responses but are not critical for the trig-

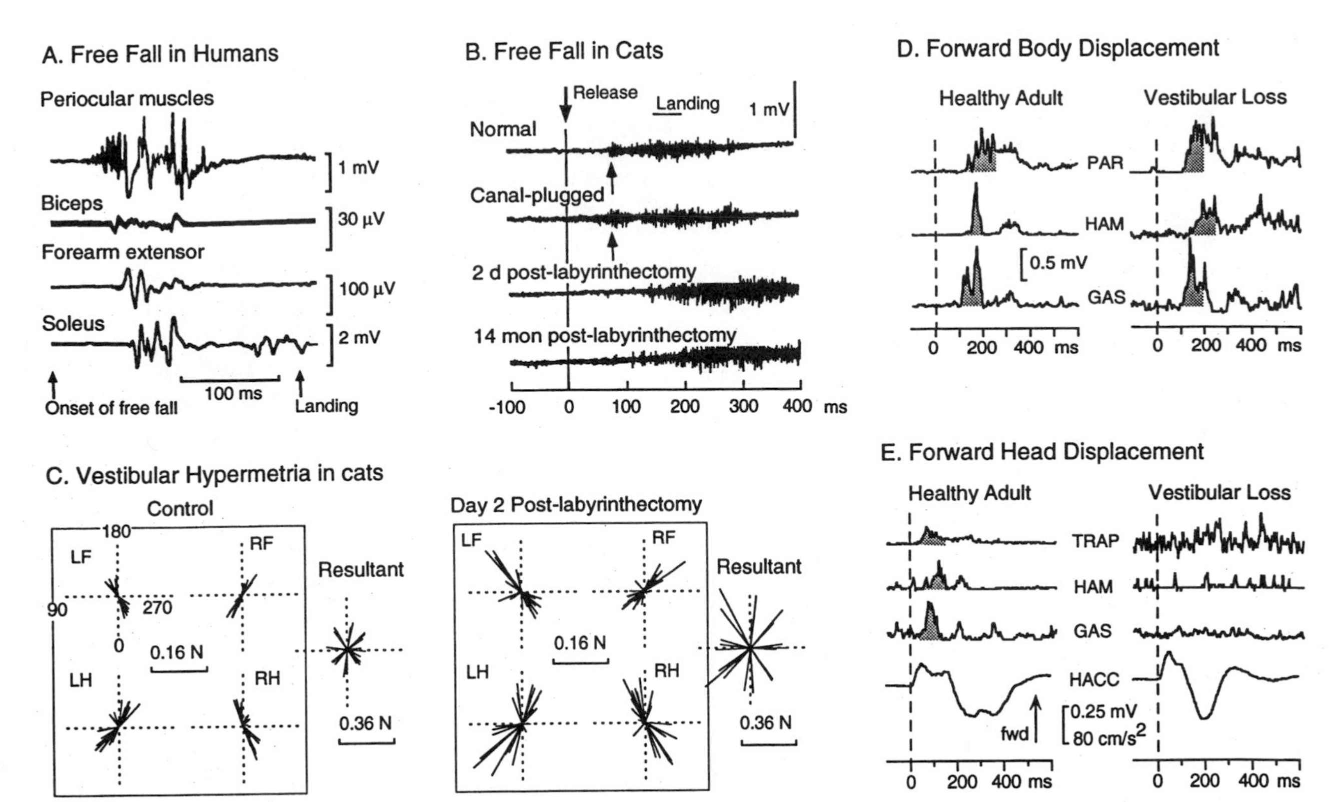

FIG. 7.13. *A*, Early activation of eye, arm, and leg muscles in a human subject during an unexpected drop from a height of 20 cm [Adapted from Greenwood and Hopkins (95).] *B*, Gastrocnemius activity in the cat during a sudden drop from a height of 45–50 cm onto a foam pad. Note that the early burst of activity (indicated by *arrow*) was unaffected by the inactivation of the semicircular canals through plugging, whereas this burst was absent following total bilateral labyrinthectomy, indicating that the early response is mediated by the otoliths. [Adapted from Watt (263).] *C*, Response to backward platform translation inducing forward body sway. Subjects with loss of vestibular function respond with a postural response that has similar timing but larger amplitude than that of healthy subjects. *Dashed line* indicates onset of platform movement. *D*, Active force response in the cat to translations in each of eight directions in the horizontal plane, before and after total bilateral labyrinthectomy. Note the increase in response amplitude after lesion, not only for each limb, but also for the resultant force vector (sum of the forces from each limb). Coordinate system as in Figure 7.6. [Adapted from Inglis and Macpherson (131).] *E*, Head acceleration (HACC) and EMG activity in a healthy subject and a patient with loss of vestibular function evoked by a perturbation to the head/neck at time 0. Note the absence of early neck and leg responses in the vestibular absent subject. TRAP, trapezius; HAM, hamstrings; GAS, gastrocnemius; PAR, paraspinals. [*C* and *E* adapted from Horak et al. (124).]

gering, spatial pattern, or velocity scaling of the initial postural response to surface perturbations.

Further argument against a strong vestibular component in postural responses to support surface perturbations comes from studies that compared displacement of the support to displacement of the head, which stimulates the vestibular system directly (61, 124, 125). Subjects' heads were subjected to sudden accelerations during stance, gait, and various balancing tasks through the use of a shoulder-mounted system of counterweights. Head acceleration evoked short-latency EMG activity not only in neck muscles but also in muscles throughout the trunk and lower limbs, as illustrated in Figure 7.13*E*. In contrast, patients lacking in vestibular function showed no evoked EMG activity in response to head perturbation (Fig. 7.13*E*). This suggests that vestibular inputs, and not neck proprioceptors may be responsible for the activity evoked by head perturbations (124, 128). However, caution is necessary in drawing conclusions based on subjects who have adapted to a lesion. It may be that vestibular-absent subjects adopt a strategy of suppressing neck afferent inputs, which would complicate conclusions about the role of neck afferents in intact subjects. Nevertheless, even large head perturbations in intact subjects resulted in EMG responses that were very small in amplitude compared to those elicited by support surface displacements. However, the response to a head perturbation increased during a balancing task in which subjects stood on a compliant platform (124) or on a see-saw (61). These results indicate that the gain of the vestibulospinal modulation is minimal when subjects stand on a firm surface, but increases when the surface is unstable.

Although vestibular information is not necessary for the triggering of a postural response to surface perturbations, such inputs may be necessary for the selection and use of movement strategies in which the head must be stabilized in space (121, 223). For example, although patients with loss of vestibular function respond normally with an ankle strategy to small translations on a large support surface, when these patients attempt to stand on a short surface they are not able to use the more appropriate hip strategy in response to translation, and rapidly lose their balance (121). In the hip strategy, the head and trunk counterrotate with respect to each other such that the head is actively stabilized with respect to the environment (208, 248). In this case, it is likely that the combination of vestibular and neck proprioceptive inputs provides more veridical information about trunk position than does somatosensory input from the legs and feet. This could account for the inability of vestibular-absent patients to control the position of the trunk in space while attempting to balance on a short surface. It appears that when vestibular inputs are lacking, the postural control system responds by limiting the repertoire of postural strategies, eliminating those for which the head must be actively stabilized and for which vestibular input is critical.

A major role of the vestibular system appears to be stabilizing the head in space and linking head movements with the responses needed to maintain balance (166, 254). For example, when a hip strategy is evoked by translation of the support surface, the earliest EMG activity is observed in neck muscles, followed by hip (208, 248). The neck muscle activity precedes any significant change in neck or hip angle, indicating that the counterrotation of the head with respect to the hip is part of the centrally organized response and not merely reactive. It may be that reliable vestibular information is necessary to coordinate this head movement and, moreover, that this information is expected by the nervous system in order to compare with an efference copy signal of the head movement command. Stabilization of the head in space may be necessary for the unambiguous interpretation of vestibular and neck proprioceptive information that is used in computing trunk position in space. Voluntary head movements exhibit the most striking deficit in acutely labyrinthectomized cats, appearing hypermetric and underdamped (166). Head turns to the side cause these cats to lose their balance immediately and fall over.

Body movements that destabilize the head probably have the greatest requirement for active mechanisms of head control and may be more difficult for subjects with loss of vestibular function to perform. Vestibular-deficient patients show larger than normal head accelerations and displacements with respect to the environment during complex motor activities such as standing on a tilting board, standing on one foot, and running in place (98, 223).

It has long been known that bilateral destruction of the vestibular apparatus produces profound effects on the motor system, and that these deficits are compensated to a certain extent over time (reviewed in 239). Unilateral vestibular lesion disrupts the normal alignment of the cervical vertebrae to earth vertical (262), but this abnormal posture recovers during the compensation process (47). Bilateral loss of vestibular function may be associated with a forward flexed head position as well as an active "locking" of the head on the trunk (248). Both humans and cats with acute bilateral loss of vestibular function show severe ataxia, weaving from side to side as the head is turned during gait (257). Recent studies suggest that patients with chronic, bilateral loss of vestibular function show more tonic background activity at the neck, trunk, and legs resulting in increased stiffness in responding to body or head displacements (124). Following the initial recovery period, however, loss of vestibular inputs has little effect on the ability to maintain quiet stance (166, 197) unless information from both somatosensory and visual systems is inadequate or erroneous (205).

In summary, vestibular information in conjunction with somatosensory information informs the nervous system about head position and motion to facilitate the appropriate postural orientation to gravitoinertial forces, allow smooth coordination of the head and trunk movements with reference to the environment, and select the appropriate magnitude of postural responses (reviewed in 123).

Visual System

Like somatosensory and vestibular information, the effect of vision on postural orientation and equilibrium depends on the task and context. The elimination of vision increases sway during stance, with the amount dependent upon the particular stance posture, the availability of accurate surface and vestibular information, central set, and cognitive factors such as fear of falling. Romberg (237) recognized that eye closure increased sway by 30% in feet-apart stance, 50% in tandem stance with one foot in front of the other, and even more in patients with central or peripheral neural disorders. In subjects who are instructed to sway as little as possible, or who fear falling, the excursion of the CoM may not increase significantly with eye closure (205). Stroboscopic illumination at frequencies of 3 Hz, which eliminates visual motion cues while maintaining stationary contours, also destabilizes posture, but not as much as eye closure (10). Vision stabilizes sway primarily at frequencies below 0.1 Hz (48).

Visual perception of motion relative to the environment is determined by the three-dimensional structure of the visual surround, as well as by the viewing conditions. Sway becomes greater as the distance between the eyes and the nearest visual marker increases, since distant objects produce a smaller angular displacement of the image on the retina compared to close objects. Visual objects must be less than 2.5 m from a subject in order to stabilize quiet stance (218). Factors such as visual acuity, level of illumination, and location and size of the stimulus within the visual field all affect how visual information stabilizes posture (153, 218).

A moving visual scene surrounding a stationary subject can induced a perceptual illusion of self-motion called "vection," and can affect body sway. The amplitude of the postural change is logarithmically proportional to image velocity and density of image pattern (154). Frequency analysis using sinusoidal movement of the visual surround has shown the strongest effect to be in the low-frequency range, below 0.2 Hz (20). The response to sinusoidal visual field inputs is nonlinear, since the gain decreases with increasing amplitude of the driving input (255). With linear visual field motion in the sagittal or transverse plane, body sway shows a phase lead for position at the low frequencies (<0.1–0.2 Hz), which gradually changes to an increasing phase lag at higher frequencies (26, 154, 255). Thus, both animals and humans track and anticipate predictable visual field motion as if to minimize the amount of relative displacement between the body and the environment, perhaps by minimizing retinal slip.

The peripheral retina was long thought to be primarily responsible for visually induced sway (153) but, recently, postural sway has been shown to be sensitive to radial flow in the fovea and laminar flow in the periphery but not vice versa, consistent with normal visual conditions (252). Although the sensation of self-motion is continuous during visual motion and can tilt the direction of apparent upright up to 40 degrees, healthy adults never sway beyond their limits of stability in response to visual cues alone if they are standing on a large, firm surface (50, 154).

Roll vection, which is induced by rotating a wide-angled visual image around the line of sight, causes the illusion of tilt in a direction opposite to the moving stimulus, as illustrated in Figure 7.14 (29, 50). Subjects compensate for this apparent body shift by tilting in the direction of the pattern of visual motion (154). The apparent displacement of both the visual and postural vertical can be explained as the result of a central recomputation of orientation of the gravity vector based on vision (82, 188). The threshold for the conscious perception of visual motion, however, is above the threshold for automatic postural realignment to visual motion cues, suggesting that the central representation of verticality for posture and perception are not necessarily identical. This is supported by a recent study showing that the direction of gaze affects postural responses to tilting rooms but not the perception of motion (84).

The influence of moving visual fields on postural stability depends on the characteristics not only of the visual environment, but also of support surface, including size of the base of support and its rigidity or compliance (10). Subjects standing quietly with a standard side-by-side foot separation are rarely destabilized by moving the visual field (except for children who are more visually dependent). In contrast, subjects standing in more difficult postures, such as the toe-to-heel Romberg stance or a one-footed stance, will often be destabilized by visual field movements, and forced to take a step in order to maintain balance (10, 53, 151). When the support surface is compliant, the sway induced by sinusoidal visual field rotation is four times larger than when the surface is fixed (219). Children under age 5 years, healthy adults standing on a balance beam, and some patients with vestibular disorders, how-

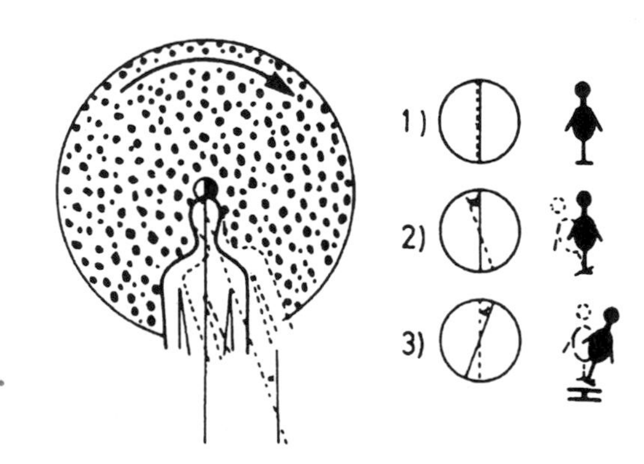

FIG. 7.14. Displacement of perceived vertical during rollvection induced by large disk rotating around subject's line of sight. Clockwise visual rotation causes an illusion of counterclockwise tilt of the observer's body (2) that is "corrected" by lateral body tilt in the same direction as the visual rotation (3). [Adapted from Brandt, Paulus, and Straube (29).]

ever, can fall when exposed to moving visual scenes, called a "visual push" (149, 151). When the visual surround is tilted, healthy subjects accurately perceive the room as tilting and the surface on which they are standing as stable, but patients with vestibular deficits often perceive the room as stable and the surface as tilting, and generally demonstrate larger body sway than normals (48).

Movement of the visual surround has a stronger influence when the support surface is also in motion, compared to conditions when the support is stationary. For example, when sway is induced by motion of the surround while the support surface is also in motion, sway is twice the amplitude of that induced by the same movement of the visual surround while the support is stationary (250). The gain of postural sway induced by predictable sinusoidal visual inputs in dogs was ten times higher when the surface was also in motion, compared to a stationary surface. These findings emphasize the fact that under conditions of visual conflict, the gain of visual information is enhanced and can dominate postural sway.

It was originally thought that visual inputs were too slow to have any effect on the rapid response to sudden perturbations of stance, since the sensation of motion induced by moving visual fields has a relatively long latency, on the order of 1 s, and the influence on body sway is also slow. Subsequent experiments have disproved this idea by showing that visual conflict situations can have a significant effect on short-latency, automatic postural responses. As shown in Figure 7.15, for example, when visual inputs are stabilized with respect to the head during a platform translation, the initial burst in gastrocnemius is significantly attenuated and forward sway increases (200, 261). A similar effect of visual stabilization was observed by other investigators on the short-latency otolith-mediated response to free-fall in both animals and humans (145, 265). In contrast, Figure 7.15 shows that merely closing the eyes during a postural perturbation has no effect on the early evoked response (261), suggesting that sensory context is an important factor in shaping the strategy for postural responses. Absence of vision under these conditions does not compromise postural performance, since other sensory channels provide sufficient information. In contrast, visual information that *conflicts* with that from other sensory channels can have a rapid and profound effect on postural responses.

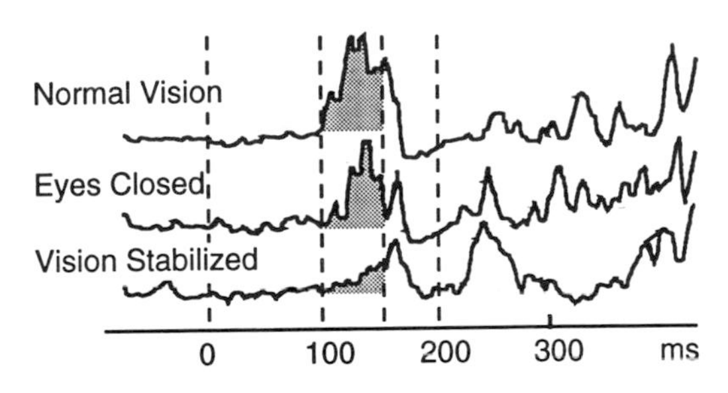

FIG. 7.15. Response of the gastrocnemius to forward sway induced by backward translation of the support surface. "Normal Vision" is the control response with eyes open. The "Eyes Closed" response shows no change in the evoked EMG activity with visual deprivation. "Vision Stabilized" is the response when the visual surround is stabilized with respect to the subject, showing a marked attenuation of the early burst of activity (at 100 ms). [Adapted from Vidal, Berthoz, and Millanvoye (261).]

Visual input plays an important role not only in the response to unexpected disturbances of balance but also in the anticipatory postural adjustments that accompany voluntary movements. In fact, the most significant role played by vision in both postural orientation and equilibrium may be in the feedforward control that is critical for avoiding obstacles and adapting to changing environmental conditions (64, 83, 150). Vision also becomes more critical for posture during development of motor abilities, the learning of a new skill, or when vestibular and/or somatosensory information is compromised (24, 171, 182, 217, 226, 273). When infants are just learning to sit or to stand independently and when adults are just learning a difficult balancing task such as standing on the hands, visual motion cues have a profound effect on balance (38, 247). It has been hypothesized that vision helps calibrate the proprioceptive system for novel tasks and conditions (82, 83).

In conclusion, the effect of visual information on the postural system is highly task- and context-dependent. The influence of vision on postural control is weighted up or down dynamically, depending on whether the visual input acts alone or in combination with perturbations of the support surface. In general, visual input dominates at low frequencies of body sway and when there is a conflict between vision and the other sensory inputs.

CENTRAL NEURAL CONTROL OF POSTURE

Spinal Cord and Brainstem

Although we now have some insight about the central structures and pathways used in the elaboration of voluntary movements, our knowledge of the central control of postural orientation and equilibrium is quite sparse. Current evidence suggests that spinal cord circuits alone are not capable of producing the organized equilibrium responses characteristic of the intact animal (225). It is well known that complex movements such as stepping and scratching are generated by the intrinsic circuitry of the spinal cord (reviewed in 97). Adult cats with a complete transection of the spinal cord at the thoracic level are capable of weight bearing and stepping with the hindlimbs (13, 156), but they cannot maintain lateral stability for any length of time. Spinal cats can balance for short periods of time, and can even remain standing during small, slow translations of the support surface, but they do not exhibit the complex patterns of evoked muscle activity characteristic of the intact cat (J. M. Macpherson, J. Fung, and R. Jacobs, unpublished observations). This primitive balance is probably maintained simply by the inherent stiffness of the muscles and ligaments and, perhaps, by local segmental reflex mechanisms (225). The basic circuits for stabilizing postural equilibrium are likely located at higher levels of the nervous system. This idea is supported by the evidence for complex integration of multimodal sensory inputs in the triggering of equilibrium responses.

The decerebrate cat, in which a transection is made at the level of the midbrain, can support its own weight due to the strong extensor tone in the limbs. However, this preparation requires stabilization and cannot correct for postural disturbances in the horizontal plane, suggesting that even brainstem–spinal cord circuits are insufficient for stability in stance. Nevertheless, some evidence exists for discrete postural centers in the brainstem. Electrical stimulation of the red nucleus in the standing cat evokes not only flexion of a limb, but also the corresponding postural adjustments in the other three limbs, suggesting that these processes are already linked at the level of the rubrospinal tract (232). Recent studies have identified regions in the pons and medulla that either facilitate or depress "postural tonus" in both decerebrate and intact, awake cats (157, 191). Muscle tone can be modulated in a continuous manner by electrically stimulating the brainstem at various sites in both decerebrate and awake cats during ongoing locomotion. Stimulation of the dorsal tegmental field reduces extensor muscle tone and makes an intact, freely moving animal sit and then lie down, whereas stimulation of the ventral tegmental field evokes the opposite effects and can induce a lying cat to stand up and walk. A critical level of "tone" is necessary for locomotion, since walking is suppressed when tone becomes too high or too low (191).

Stimulation of the dorsal tegmental field suppresses respiratory function as well as muscle tone, suggesting a coordination of both respiratory and postural motor function in this area (139). A colocalization of cardiovascular and postural function has also been seen in the dorsolateral pons and medial medulla in response to injections of cholinergic and glutamatergic agonists (147). The commingling of neuronal groups in the brainstem mediating cardiorespiratory function and postural tone provides a basis for the coordination of these functions during exercise.

Finally, the vestibular nuclear complex in the medulla and pons is an important center for the integration of vestibular, somatosensory, and visual information that is important for the control of postural orientation and equilibrium (267). Vestibulospinal pathways from this region, as well as reticulospinal pathways from the adjacent reticular formation, terminate on both motoneurons and interneurons that influence neck, axial, and limb musculature (reviewed in 268). The extent to which these and other descending tracts from brainstem structures influence and shape programs for postural orientation and equilibrium is not known.

Basal Ganglia

The critical role of the basal ganglia in postural control is demonstrated by the severely impaired postural alignment and the instability suffered by patients with basal ganglia pathology. The basal ganglia consist of many interconnected nuclei, with outputs to cortical and brainstem motor systems, tonic excitatory and inhibitory influences, and cholinergic and dopaminergic systems, each of which may participate in different sensorimotor mechanisms essential to maintaining equilibrium (3, 107, 172). Different basal ganglia pathways may be involved in descending connections to brainstem centers for locomotion in the subthalamus and mesencephalon, and for postural tone in the pontine reticular formation and locus coeruleus (5). Other basal ganglia loops from wide areas of cortex to sensorimotor and supplementary motor cortex may participate in every centrally initiated motor program, including postural programs for control of orientation and equilibrium (4).

The simplified schematic in Figure 7.16 illustrates how the basal ganglia could affect three separate postural pathways: tonic postural tone, centrally initiated postural adjustments, and externally triggered reactions. Basal ganglia projections to separate areas of the brainstem may affect background postural tone and adaptation of postural gain and set depending upon environmental context and initial con-

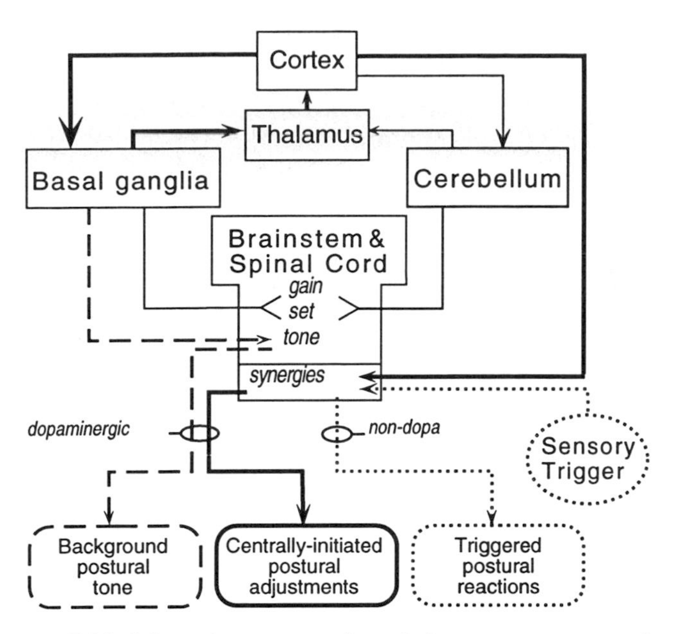

FIG. 7.16. Schematic representation of three separate postural systems for regulation of background postural tone, centrally initiated postural adjustments, and peripherally triggered postural reactions. Separate pathways show how basal ganglia disruption from parkinsonism could affect all three postural systems but dopamine replacement therapy improves only background postural tone and centrally initiated postural adjustments. [Adapted from Horak and Frank (114).]

ditions. Corticobasal ganglia loops affect centrally initiated postural adjustments preceding and accompanying volitional movement. Automatic postural responses triggered by external disturbances can be influenced by the basal ganglia control of brainstem centers for tone, gain, and set.

The basal ganglia have been considered essential for postural alignment and muscle tone since the time of Denny-Brown (46), who showed that bilateral lesions of the globus pallidus and/or substantia nigra result in a fixed, flexed posture of the head, trunk, and limbs. Parkinsonism, considered the best human model for examining basal ganglia postural disorders (174), is associated with excessive tonic activation of ankle, knee, and hip flexors during quiet stance. Dopamine replacement therapy decreases tonic muscle activity, particularly in the hyperactive flexors (34). Parkinsonian patients respond to slow, sinusoidal surface translations by modulation of large ankle flexor activity, whereas normal subjects use primarily ankle extensors (63). The flexed posture and tonic leg flexor activity of parkinsonian patients during stance is associated with a more posterior position of their center of body mass compared to intact subjects, which may be either the result or cause of the flexed posture (241). The enhanced tonic activation of muscles at rest may contribute to the increased inherent muscle stiffness of both the upper (264) and lower extremities of parkinsonian patients (60). Consequently, unexpected perturbations of stance result in less ankle, knee, and hip joint angular displacement as well as in slower displacement of the center of mass (63, 114). A higher resistance to muscle stretch in the rigid parkinsonian patient may help resist displacement evoked by external postural perturbations, but body center of mass can be maintained within only a small range by such passive forces without the addition of coordinated postural activity (122).

Although the latency of the initial postural response to surface displacement is normal in parkinsonian patients, their postural response includes excessive activation of antagonist muscles, not unlike that seen in healthy elderly subjects, but much exaggerated (60, 126, 243). The distal to proximal muscle activation pattern of the ankle synergy appears to be intact in parkinsonian subjects, but is confounded by the addition of hip synergy muscle activation, resulting in excessive coactivation. An intact postural synergy is consistent with Marsden's hypothesis (174) that overall motor plans are normal in parkinsonian patients but the execution and sequencing of those plans is impaired.

The basal ganglia appear critical for adapting postural strategies to changes in initial conditions and environmental support. Normally, the strategy for postural equilibrium changes rapidly when subjects stand on a different support configuration or support themselves with their hands, trunk, or by sitting. Unlike normal subjects, patients with Parkinson's disease use the same pattern of muscle activation to respond to surface displacements whether they stand on narrow or wide surfaces (122). Parkinsonian patients also do not suppress ankle muscle responses to surface tilts when supporting themselves with their arms (241) or when sitting (122, 243). Even when dopamine replacement improves their postural muscle activation patterns, parkinsonian patients show an inflexibility in their postural coordination consistent with a difficulty in modifying motor programs when required by task (173).

The basal ganglia do not appear to be essential for programming the postural adjustments accompanying voluntary movement, contrary to previous suggestions (176). Centrally initiated postural adjustments anticipatory to voluntary movement are of normal latency and pattern, but are reduced in magnitude in parkinsonian patients (235, 260). For example, anticipatory activation of tibialis anterior to move the CoM forward prior to rising onto the toes or to step initiation are very small in amplitude and duration in parkinsonian patients (114). The amplitude of activation of the prime movers, however, is also smaller than normal in parkinsonian patients, suggesting a general difficulty in energizing muscle activation and generating force for all centrally generated motor activity. Both anticipatory postural and focal muscle activation is significantly increased with dopamine replacement therapy, suggesting a common contribution of the basal ganglia to both components.

Low-force generation associated with slowness of movement or bradykinesia appears to be a major impediment to effective control of balance in parkinsonian patients. Insufficient agonist burst size in response to perturbations during stance has been shown for leg muscles (58) and may be resistant to dopamine replacement therapy (213). The inability to generate adequate force may be related to the very short duration and unfused character of the EMG activity combined with excessive antagonist activity (86). Basal ganglia influence on spinal circuitry, including decreased sensitivity of polysynaptic reflex pathways and increased recurrent and reciprocal inhibition, may contribute to decreased force generation, but central drive of basal ganglia output to motor cortex may also be important (33, 60, 214).

In summary, the basal ganglia participate in many aspects of sensorimotor integration critical for postural orientation and equilibrium such as regulation of tonic muscle activity, adaptation of motor patterns to context, and generation of adequate force for postural alignment and equilibrium responses. Based on studies with posturally impaired parkinsonian patients, however, the basal ganglia do not appear to be critical for orienting posture to different sensory cues, or for detecting disequilibrium and triggering a timely response.

Cerebellum

The cerebellum is thought to be critical for postural coordination and, like the basal ganglia, probably plays several different roles in control of posture involving sensorimotor integration (12). Lesions in different regions of the cerebellum produce very different effects on postural control (112). Lesions of the lateral hemispheres can produce profound disorders of timing for arm and hand coordination without significant effects on posture or gait (49). Lesion of the vestibulocerebellum results in impaired vertical orientation such that patients slowly drift away from upright posture, even with eyes open (56). The most profound deficits in dynamic postural control occur with damage to the anterior lobe of the cerebellum, which receives somatosensory inputs from throughout the body and projects to the spinal cord via the red nucleus and reticular formation (52, 135). Clinical signs of an anterior lobe lesion include severe ataxia of stance and gait with high-frequency anterior/posterior trunk oscillations and mild or absent motor deficits in the upper limbs (49, 52). The cause of the trunkal tremor in anterior lobe patients is not known but is likely related to difficulty controlling the magnitude rather than the timing of postural motor coordination.

Patients with lesions restricted to the cerebellum invariably show normal latencies of automatic postural responses evoked by unexpected perturbations of the support surface, suggesting that the initiation of these responses is independent of the cerebellum. In fact, the entire pattern of agonist and antagonist activation throughout the body in response to external postural perturbations is preserved in cerebellar patients, suggesting that the postural synergy is not selected or triggered by the cerebellum (118). In contrast, the duration and amplitude of automatic postural responses are much larger than normal in patients with anterior lobe disorders and may contribute to their large trunkal tremor and gait ataxia.

Both reactive and anticipatory postural adjustments are too large, or hypermetric, in anterior lobe patients (54, 118). The hypermetric postural responses result in disequilibrium because the patients overshoot their initial stance position when returning to upright. A recent study demonstrated that the postural hypermetria of cerebellar patients is not due to a general inability to modify response magnitude, since these patients can use somatosensory information to scale the amplitude of response according to the initial platform velocity (118). Moreover, these cerebellar patients compensate for the hypermetric responses by activating antagonist muscles later in the response (118, 127). Figure 7.17*A* shows an example where a hypermetric gastrocnemius burst, in response to a translation that induces forward sway, is counteracted by a large tibialis activation that is inversely scaled to translation amplitude.

The anterior lobe of the cerebellum appears critical for tuning the magnitude of postural responses through the mechanism of central set, in which prior experience with the stimulus is used to modify subsequent response amplitudes. When the amplitude of an impending postural response is predictable, intact subjects scale the magnitude of their postural response to the expected displacement amplitude; when amplitude is not predictable, subjects revert to a default amplitude of response, regardless of stimulus amplitude (Fig. 7.17*B*). Cerebellar patients with

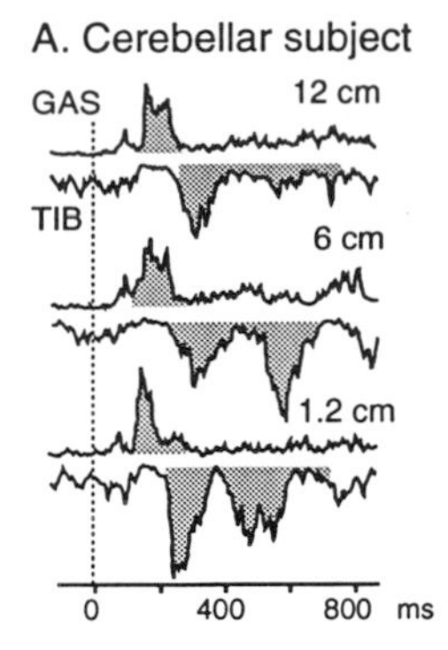

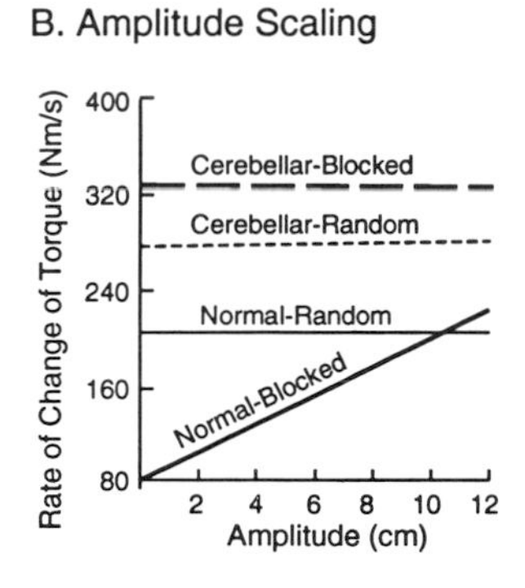

FIG. 7.17. *A*, Patient with anterior lobe cerebellar atrophy does not scale the initial gastrocnemius (GAS) response to varying amplitudes of platform displacement (indicated in centimeters), but uses later tibialis (TIB) antagonist activation to counteract the hypermetric GAS response. *B*, Mean regressions (N = 10 subjects) showing relationship between displacement amplitude and initial torque response in normal and cerebellar subjects. When trials are blocked in groups of like amplitudes, normal, but not cerebellar, subjects scale their initial response to the expected amplitude through the mechanism of central set. When trials are randomized for amplitude, no correlation is seen with initial response. [Adapted from Horak and Diener (118).]

anterior lobe signs always use the same amplitude of response, whether or not the stimulus amplitude is predictable, suggesting that they are unable to adjust their response based on prior experience (Fig. 7.17*B*). Unlike intact subjects, cerebellar patients are also unable to reduce, through practice, the magnitude of the destabilizing gastrocnemius activity that is evoked in response to a platform dorsiflexion (202). Together, these results are consistent with an important role for the cerebellum in a form of motor learning (i.e., adapting the magnitude of automatically triggered postural responses based on prior experience).

Cerebral Cortex

Although the motor areas of the cerebral cortex (see Chapter 6) are involved in the preparation for voluntary movement, their role in postural mechanisms and, in particular, in response to unexpected perturbations of stance is uncertain (178). Studies of forelimb placing in cats (177) have demonstrated that primary motor cortex (M1) is not necessary for the postural response that accompanies that movement. When placing was elicited in the limb ipsilateral to a motor cortex lesion, appropriate postural responses were observed not only in the ipsilateral hindlimb, but also in the contralateral fore- and hindlimbs. Similarly, the diagonal supporting response that is elicited by sudden loss of the support under one hindlimb was not modified by unilateral sensorimotor cortex ablation (69). In both cats (23) and dogs (134), the innate postural response to a conditioned limb lift persists following a similar cortical lesion.

The latency of the postural response to an unexpected perturbation is long enough that a loop through sensorimotor cortex could be involved, and this fact has been invoked as evidence of the participation of cortex in such responses. Indeed, the medium-latency response to unexpected perturbations has been referred to as a "transcortical reflex" (75, 220). However, latency alone does not provide sufficient proof of involvement of cortex. Studies have demonstrated that medium-latency responses can arise even from the isolated spinal cord, perhaps through reverberating loops within spinal interneuronal circuits (73, 74). Another approach has been to examine cerebral potentials evoked by a destabilizing perturbation. During locomotion, the early component of the evoked potential is reduced compared to the resting condition, suggesting that the rapidly conducting group I afferent inputs to cortex are gated out or diminished, and are therefore not important in triggering the postural response (62). If the slower conducting group II pathways are the primary source for triggering postural responses, then it is unlikely that transcortical routes are involved.

Although cortical involvement in the rapid response to unexpected perturbations of stance and gait is unlikely, it may be important in the anticipatory postural adjustments that accompany voluntary movement. For example, cells in motor cortex in the cat are modulated during modifications of gait to avoid obstacles (65). The extent to which these postural adjustments share the same mechanisms and processes as those elicited by unexpected perturbations is not known. Anticipatory postural adjustments may be either an integral and inseparable part of motor planning for voluntary movement, or a distinct process, organized in a parallel fashion and utilizing different circuits and mechanisms. For example, the supplementary motor area (SMA) (see Fig. 6.1) was thought to play a role in postural activity, since stimulation of this region produced complex and apparently coordinated movements of the forelimb in particular (87, 266). Similarly, stimulation of the dentate nucleus in the awake monkey activated complex synergies resulting in limb movement, presumably by activating cerebellothalamocortical circuits that are known to involve the SMA as well as motor cortex [(233); also see Chapter 6]. The extent to which these stimulus-evoked movements relate to functional postural mechanisms is not known.

The elaboration of a movement and the accompanying postural adjustment may be integrated, at least at the output level of the motor cortex. Electrical stimulation within the forelimb area of motor cortex in the standing cat results not only in flexion of the contralateral forelimb but also in a diagonal pattern of force change under the other three limbs (81, 232). The force change in the contralateral forelimb occurs at about the same time as the unloading that accompanies flexion in the ipsilateral forelimb. When the stimulation is applied in the hindlimb area of motor cortex to provoke hindlimb flexion, the postural adjustment in the forelimbs precedes any force change in the hindlimbs. Thus, stimulation of the limb area of motor cortex in an animal that is supporting itself in stance leads to a complex activation of muscles throughout the body that is appropriate for maintaining balance.

Studies of patients with various lesions in the frontal lobe provide some support for an involvement of secondary motor cortical areas in posture (100). Some patients with lesions in the inferior posterior region of frontal cortex exhibit oscillations in the CoP during quiet stance that are correlated with the rhythm of respiration. Such oscillations are not observed in intact subjects, which led Gurfinkel to speculate that subtle activation of hip and pelvic musculature normally accompanies respiration, and is timed to offset such oscillations and, furthermore, that the patients fail to produce these postural adjustments (101). Some patients with lesions in the medial posterior frontal lobe fail to activate their leg muscles as an anticipatory postural adjustment prior to an arm lift. From these results, Gurfinkel and Elner (100) concluded that the frontal lobe secondary motor areas do play some role in the elaboration of anticipatory postural adjustments that are necessary for the smooth and coordinated execution of movement.

CONCLUDING REMARKS

This chapter reviews the neural control of posture in terms of the two main functional goals of postural behavior: postural orientation, or alignment, and postural equilibrium, or balance. Posture is no longer considered simply as the summation of static reflexes but, rather, the complex interaction of sensorimotor processes and internal representations of those processes. Postural orientation involves active control of joint stiffness and such global variables as trunk and head alignment, based on the interpretation of convergent sensory information. Postural equilibrium involves coordination of efficient sensorimotor strategies to control the many degrees of freedom for stabilization of the body's center of mass during either unexpected or voluntary disturbances of stability. Inputs from somatosensory, vestibular, and visual systems are integrated in the control of orientation and equilibrium, and the relative weights placed upon each of these inputs is dependent upon the task goals and the environmental context. Many parts of the nervous system participate in the control of posture, but our understanding of this neural organization is sparse.

Future approaches to the study of posture should include neurophysiological, biomechanical, and psychophysical techniques in both animal and human models. Such a combination of approaches is most valuable when applied to the intact organism behaving in a variety of environments. Basic research is needed to clarify further the distinctions and interactions between control of posture and control of voluntary movement. More insight is needed on the basic variables controlled by the nervous system for postural orientation and equilibrium, how sensory information is used in that control, and the role of each region of the CNS. A better understanding of the capacity for adaptation and learning in the postural control system could have a significant impact on both training for elite athletic performance and rehabilitation for postural disorders.

We would like to thank Drs. Jean Massion and Victor Gurfinkel for their thought-provoking and helpful comments on this chapter, and Jill Knopf and Harriet Barshofsky for their excellent technical assistance. The authors were supported by National Institutes of Health grants AG06457 and DC01849 to FBH, NS29025 and DC01356 to JMM, and DC02072.

REFERENCES

1. Abbs, J. H., and K. J. Cole. Neural mechanisms of motor equivalence and goal achievement. In: *Higher Brain Functions. Recent Explorations of the Brain's Emergent Properties*, edited by S. P. Wise. New York: John Wiley & Sons, 1987, p. 15–43.
2. Abrahams, V. C. Neck muscle proprioception and motor control. In: *Proprioception, Posture and Emotion*, edited by D. Garlick. Kensington, Australia: University of New South Wales, 1982, p. 103–120.
3. Alexander, G. E., and M. D. Crutcher. Functional architecture of basal ganglia circuits: neural substrates of parallel processing. *Trends Neurosci.* 13: 266–271, 1990.
4. Alexander, G. E., M. R. Delong, and M. D. Crutcher. Do cortical and basal ganglionic motor areas use motor programs to control movement? *Behav. Brain Sci.* 15: 656–665, 1992.
5. Alexander, G. E., M. R. Delong, and P. L. Strick. Parallel organization of functionally segregated circuits linking

basal ganglia and cortex. *Annu. Rev. Neurosci.* 9: 357–382, 1986.

6. Allum, J. H. J. Organization of stabilizing reflex responses in tibialis anterior muscles following ankle flexion perturbations of standing man. *Brain Res.* 264: 297–301, 1983.
7. Allum, J. H. J., F. Honegger, and H. Schicks. Vestibular and proprioceptive modulation of postural synergies in normal subjects. *J. Vestib. Res.* 3: 59–85, 1993.
8. Allum, J. H. J., and C. R. Pfaltz. Visual and vestibular contributions to pitch sway stabilization in the ankle muscles of normals and patients with bilateral peripheral vestibular deficits. *Exp. Brain Res.* 58: 82–94, 1985.
9. Alstermark, B., and J. Wessberg. Timing of postural adjustment in relation to forelimb target-reaching in cats. *Acta Physiol. Scand.* 125: 337–340, 1985.
10. Amblard, B., and J. Cremieux. Role de l'information visuelle du mouvement dans le maintien de l'equilibre postural chez l'homme. *Agressolgie* 17C: 25–36, 1976.
11. Assaiante, C., and B. Amblard. Head stabilization in space while walking: effect of visual deprivation in children and adults. In: *Disorders of Posture and Gait*, edited by T. Brandt, W. Paulus, W. Bles, M. Dieterich, S. Krafczyk, and A. Straube. Stuttgart: Georg Thieme Verlag, 1990, p. 229–232.
12. Babinski, J. De l'asynergie cerebelleuse. *Rev. Neurol.* 7: 806–816, 1899.
13. Barbeau, H., and S. Rossignol. Recovery of locomotion after chronic spinalization in the adult cat. *Brain Res.* 412: 84–95, 1987.
14. Barin, K. Evaluation of a generalized model of human postural dynamics and control in the sagittal plane. *Biol. Cybern.* 61: 37–50, 1989.
15. Basmajian, J. V. *Muscles Alive. Their Functions Revealed by Electromyography*, 2nd ed. Baltimore, MD: Williams & Wilkins, 1967.
16. Belenkii, V. Y., V. S. Gurfinkel, and Y. I. Paltsev. Elements of control of voluntary movements. *Biophysics* 12: 154–161, 1967.
17. Benson, A. J., E. C. B. Hutt, and S. F. Brown. Thresholds for the perception of whole body angular movement about a vertical axis. *Aviat. Space Environ. Med.* 60: 205–213, 1989.
18. Berger, W., V. Dietz, and J. Quintern. Corrective reactions to stumbling in man: neuronal co-ordination of bilateral leg muscle activity during gait. *J. Physiol. (Lond.)* 357: 109–126, 1984.
19. Bernstein, N. *The Coordination and Regulation of Movements*. Oxford: Pergamon Press, 1967.
20. Berthoz, A., M. Lacour, J. F. Soechting, and P. P. Vidal. The role of vision in the control of posture during linear motion. In: *Reflex Control of Posture and Movement, Prog. Brain Res., Vol. 50*, edited by R. Granit, and O. Pompeiano. Amsterdam: Elsevier Science Publishers, 1979, p. 197–209.
21. Berthoz, A., and T. Pozzo. Intermittent head stabilization during postural and locomotory tasks in humans. In: *Posture and Gait: Development, Adaptation and Modulation*, edited by B. Amblard, A. Berthoz, and F. Clarc. Amsterdam: Excerpta Medica, 1988, p. 189–198.
22. Biewener, A. A. Scaling body support in mammals: limb posture and muscle mechanics. *Science* 245: 45–48, 1989.
23. Birjukova, E. V., M. Dufosse, A. A. Frolov, M. E. Ioffe, and J. Massion. Role of the sensorimotor cortex in postural adjustments accompanying a conditioned paw lift in the standing cat. *Exp. Brain Res.* 78: 588–596, 1989.
24. Black, F. O., and L. M. Nashner. Vestibulo-spinal control differs in patients with reduced versus distored vestibular function. *Acta Otolaryngol. Suppl.* 406: 110–114, 1984.
25. Black, F. O., C. L. Shupert, F. B. Horak, and L. M. Nashner. Abnormal postural control associated with peripheral vestibular disorders. *Prog. Brain Res.* 76: 263–275, 1988.
26. Bles, W., and G. Dewit. Study of the effects of optic stimuli on standing. *Agressologie* 17: 1–5, 1976.
27. Borah, J., L. R. Young, and R. E. Curry. Optimal estimator model for human spatial orientation. *Ann. N. Y. Acad. Sci.* 545: 51–73, 1988.
28. Bouisset, S., and M. Zattara. A sequence of postural movements precedes voluntary movement. *Neurosci. Lett.* 22: 263–270, 1981.
29. Brandt, T., W. Paulus, and A. Straube. Vision and posture. In: *Disorders of Posture and Gait*, edited by W. Bles and T. Brandt. Amsterdam: Elsevier, 1986, p. 157–175.
30. Breniere, Y., and M. C. Do. When and how does steady state gait movement induced from upright posture begin? *J. Biomech.* 19: 1035–1040, 1986.
31. Breniere, Y., and M. C. Do. Modifications posturales associees au lever du talon dans l'initiation du pas de la marche normale. *J. Biophys. Biomech.* 11: 161–167, 1987.
32. Burgess, P. R., J. Y. Wei, F. J. Clark, and J. Simon. Signaling of kinesthetic information by peripheral sensory receptors. *Annu. Rev. Neurosci.* 5: 171–187, 1982.
33. Burleigh, A. L., F. B. Horak, K. J. Burchiel, and J. G. Nutt. Effects of thalamic stimulation on tremor, balance, and step initiation: a single subject study. *Mov. Disord.* 8: 519–524, 1993.
34. Burleigh, A. L., F. B. Horak, and F. Malouin. Modification of postural responses and step initiation: evidence for goal directed postural interactions. *J. Neurophysiol.* 72: 2892–2902, 1994.
35. Bussel, B., R. Katz, E. Pierrot-Deseilligny, C. Bergego, and A. Hayat. Vestibular and proprioceptive influences on the postural reactions to a sudden body displacement in man. In: *Spinal and Supraspinal Mechanisms of Voluntary Motor Control and Locomotion*, edited by J. E. Desmedt. Basel: Karger, 1980, p. 310–322.
36. Chanaud, C. M., and J. M. Macpherson. Functionally complex muscles of the cat hindlimb. 3. Differential activation within biceps femoris during postural perturbations. *Exp. Brain Res.* 85: 271–280, 1991.
37. Clement, G., V. S. Gurfinkel, F. Lestienne, M. I. Lipshits, and K. E. Popov. Adaptation of postural control to weightlessness. *Exp. Brain Res.* 57: 61–72, 1984.
38. Clement, G., and D. Rezette. Motor behavior underlying the control of an upside-down vertical posture. *Exp. Brain Res.* 59: 428–484, 1985.
39. Coats, A. C. The sinusoidal galvanic body-sway response. *Acta Otolaryngol.* 74: 155–162, 1972.
40. Cohen, L. A. Role of eye and neck proprioceptive mechanisms in body orientation and motor coordination. *J. Neurophysiol.* 24: 1–11, 1961.
41. Collins, J. J., and C. J. Deluca. Open-hoop and closed-loop control of posture—a random-walk analysis of center-of-pressure trajectories. *Exp. Brain Res.* 95: 308–318, 1993.
42. Cordo, P. J., and L. M. Nashner. Properties of postural adjustments associated with rapid arm movements. *J. Neurophysiol.* 47: 287–302, 1982.
43. Crenna, P., and C. Frigo. A motor programme for the initiation of forward-oriented movements in humans. *J. Physiol. (Lond.)* 437: 635–653, 1991.

44. Crenna, P., C. Frigo, J. Massion, and A. Pedotti. Forward and backward axial synergies in man. *Exp. Brain Res.* 65: 538–548, 1987.
45. Das, P., and G. McCollum. Invariant structure in locomotion. *Neuroscience* 25: 1023–1034, 1988.
46. Denny-Brown, D. *The Basal Ganglia and Their Relation to Disorders of Movement.* London: Oxford University Press, 1962.
47. De Waele, C. W., Graf, P., and P. P. Vidal. A radiological analysis of the postural syndromes following hemilabyrinthectomy and selective canal and otolith lesions in the guinea pig. *Exp. Brain Res.* 77: 166–182, 1989.
48. Dichgans, J., and T. Brandt. Visual-vestibular interaction: effects on self-motion perception and postural control. In: *Handbook of Sensory Physiology, Vol. VIII: Perception,* edited by R. Held, H. Leibowitz, and H. Teuber. Berlin: Springer-Verlag, 1978, p. 756–804.
49. Dichgans, J., and H. C. Diener. Different forms of postural ataxia in patients with cerebellar diseases. In: *Disorders of Posture and Gait,* edited by W. Bles and T. Brandt. Amsterdam: Elsevier Science Publishers, 1986, p. 207–215.
50. Dichgans, J., R. Held, L. R. Young, and T. Brandt. Moving visual scenes influence the apparent direction of gravity. *Science* 178: 1217–1219, 1972.
51. Diener, H. C., F. Bootz, J. Dichgans, and W. Bruzek. Variability of postural "reflexes" in humans. *Exp. Brain Res.* 52: 423–428, 1983.
52. Diener, H. C., and J. Dichgans. Postural ataxia in late atrophy of the cerebellar anterior lobe and its differential diagnosis. In: *Vestibular and Visual Control on Posture and Locomotor Equilibrium,* edited by F. O. Black and M. Igarashi. Houston: Karger, 1985, p. 282–289.
53. Diener, H.-C., and J. Dichgans. On the role of vestibular, visual and somatosensory information for dynamic postural control in humans. *Prog. Brain Res.* 76: 253–262, 1988.
54. Diener, H. C., J. Dichgans, B. Guschlbauer, M. Bacher, H. Rapp, and P. Langenbach. Associated postural adjustments with body movement in normal subjects and patients with parkinsonism and cerebellar disease. *Rev. Neurol.* 146: 555–563, 1990.
55. Diener, H. C., J. Dichgans, B. Guschlbauer, and H. Mau. The significance of proprioception on postural stabilization as assessed by ischemia. *Brain Res.* 296: 103–109, 1984.
56. Diener, H. C., J. Dichgans, and K. H. Mauritz. What distinguishes the different kinds of postural ataxia in patients with cerebellar diseases? *Adv. Otorhinolaryngol.* 30: 285–287, 1983.
57. Diener, H. C., F. B. Horak, and L. M. Nashner. Influence of stimulus parameters on human postural responses. *J. Neurophysiol.* 59: 1888–1905, 1988.
58. Dietz, V. Pharmacological effects on posture and gait: significance of dopamine receptor antagonists in postural control. In: *Disorders of Posture and Gait,* edited by T. Brandt, W. Paulus, W. Bles, M. Dieterich, S. Krafcyzk, and A. Straube. Stuttgart: Georg Thieme Verlag, 1990, p. 340–345.
59. Dietz, V. Human neuronal control of automatic functional movements—interaction between central programs and afferent input. *Physiol. Rev.* 72: 33–69, 1992.
60. Dietz, V., W. Berger, and G. A. Horstmann. Posture in Parkinson's disease: impairment of reflexes and programming. *Ann. Neurol.* 24: 660–669, 1988.
61. Dietz, V., G. A. Horstmann, and W. Berger. Fast head tilt has only a minor effect on quick compensatory reactions during the regulation of stance and gait. *Exp. Brain Res.* 73: 470–476, 1988.
62. Dietz, V., J. Quintern, and W. Berger. Afferent control of human stance and gait—evidence for blocking of group-1 afferents during gait. *Exp. Brain Res.* 61: 153–163, 1985.
63. Dietz, V., W. Zijlstra, C. Assainte, M. Trippel, and W. Berger. Balance control in Parkinson's disease. *Gait Posture* 1: 77–84, 1993.
64. Drew, T. Visuomotor coordination in locomotion. *Curr. Opin. Neurobiol.* 1: 652–657, 1991.
65. Drew, T. Motor cortical activity during voluntary gait modifications in the cat. 1. Cells related to the forelimbs. *J. Neurophysiol.* 70: 179–199, 1993.
66. Drew, T., and S. Rossignol. A kinematic and electromyographic study of cutaneous reflexes evoked from the forelimb of unrestrained walking cats. *J. Neurophysiol.* 57: 1160–1184, 1987.
67. Droulez, J., and A. Berthoz. Servo-controlled (conservative) versus topological (projective) mode of sensory motor control. In: *Disorders of Posture and Gait,* edited by W. Bles and T. Brandt. Amsterdam: Elsevier Science Publishers, 1986, p. 83–97.
68. Dufosse, M., J. M. Macpherson, and J. Massion. Biomechanical and electromyographical comparison of two postural supporting mechanisms in the cat. *Exp. Brain Res.* 45: 38–44, 1982.
69. Dufosse, M., J. M. Macpherson, J. Massion, and E. Sybirska. The postural reaction to the drop of a hindlimb support in the standing cat remains following sensorimotor cortical ablation. *Neurosci. Lett.* 55: 297–304, 1985.
70. Dunbar, D. C., F. B. Horak, J. M. Macpherson, and D. S. Rushmer. Neural control of quadrupedal and bipedal stance: implications for the evolution of erect posture. *Am. J. Phys. Anthropol.* 69: 93–105, 1986.
71. Dunbar, D. C., and J. M. Macpherson. Activity of neuromuscular compartments in lateral gastrocnemius evoked by postural corrections during stance. *J. Neurophysiol.* 70: 2337–2349, 1993.
72. Edin, B. B. Quantitative analysis of static strain sensitivity in human mechanorecptors from hairy skin. *J. Neurophysiol.* 67: 1105–1113, 1992.
73. Eklund, G., K.-E. Hagbarth, J. V. Hagglund, and E. U. Wallin. Mechanical oscillations contributing to the segmentation of the reflex electromyogram response to stretching human muscles. *J. Physiol. (Lond.)* 326: 65–78, 1982.
74. Eklund, G., K.-E. Hagbarth, J. V. Hagglund, and E. U. Wallin. The "late" reflex responses to muscle stretch: the "resonance" hypothesis versus the "long-loop" hypothesis. *J. Physiol. (Lond.)* 306: 79–90, 1982.
75. Evarts, E. V. Motor cortex reflexes associated with learned movement. *Science* 179: 501–503, 1973.
76. Ferrington, D. G. Functional properties of slowly adapting mechanoreceptors in cat footpad skin. *Somatosens. Res.* 2: 249–262, 1985.
77. Fisk, J., J. R. Lackner, and P. Dizio. Gravitoinertial force level influences arm movement control. *J. Neurophysiol.* 69: 504–511, 1993.
78. Fitzpatrick, R., D. Burke, and S. C. Gandevia. Task-dependent reflex responses and movement illusions evoked by galvanic vestibular stimulation in standing humans. *J. Physiol. (Lond.)* 478: 363–372, 1994.
79. Fung, J., and J. M. Macpherson. Determinants of postural orientation in quadrupedal stance. *J. Neurosci.* 15: 1121–1131, 1995.

80. Gahery, Y., M. Ioffe, J. Massion, and A. Polit. The postural support of movement in cat and dog. *Acta Neurobiol. Exp.* 40: 741–756, 1980.
81. Gahery, Y., and A. Nieoullon. Postural and kinetic coordination following cortical stimuli which induce flexion movements in the cat's limbs. *Brain Res.* 149: 25–37, 1978.
82. Gibson, J. J. The relation between visual and postural determinants of the phenomenal vertical. *Psychol. Rev.* 59: 370–375, 1952.
83. Gibson, J. J. Visually controlled locomotion and visual orientation in animals. *Br. J. Psychol.* 493: 182–194, 1958.
84. Gielen, C. C. A. M., and W. N. J. C. Van Asten. Postural responses to simulated moving environments are not invariant for the direction gaze. *Exp. Brain Res.* 79: 167–174, 1990.
85. Gleick, J. *Chaos: Making a New Science*. New York: Viking Penguin, 1987.
86. Godaux, E., and D. Koulischer. Parkinsonian bradykinesia is due to depression in the rate of rise of muscle activity. *Ann. Neurol.* 31: 93–100, 1992.
87. Goldberg, G. Supplementary motor area structure and function: review and hypotheses. *Behav. Brain Sci.* 8: 567–616, 1986.
88. Goldberg, J. M., C. E. Smith, and C. Fernandez. Relation between discharge regularity and response to externally applied galvanic currents in vestibular nerve afferents of the squirrel monkey. *J Neurophysiol.* 51: 1236–1256, 1984.
89. Gollhofer, A., G. A. Horstmann, W. Berger, and V. Dietz. Compensation of translational and rotational perturbations in human posture: stabilization of the centre of gravity. *Neurosci. Lett.* 105: 73–78, 1989.
90. Gorassini, M. A., A. Prochazka, G. W. Hiebert, and M. J. A. Gauthier. Corrective responses to loss of ground support during walking. I. Intact cats. *J. Neurophysiol.* 7: 603–610, 1994.
91. Gordon, M. E., F. E. Zajac, G. Khang, and J. P. Loan. Intersegmental and mass center accelerations induced by lower extremity muscles: theory and methodology with emphasis on quasivertical standing postures. In: *Computational Methods in Bioengineering*, edited by R. L. Spilker and B. R. Simon. New York: American Society of Mechanical Engineers, 1988, p. 481–492.
92. Gray, J. Studies in the mechanics of the tetrapod skeleton. *J. Exp. Biol.* 20: 88–116, 1944.
93. Greene, P. H. Problems of organization of motor systems. *Prog. Theor. Biol.* 2: 303–338, 1972.
94. Greenspan, J. D. Influence of velocity and direction of surface-parallel cutaneous stimuli on responses of mechanoreceptors in feline hairy skin. *J. Neurophysiol.* 68: 876–889, 1992.
95. Greenwood, R., and A. Hopkins. Muscle responses during sudden falls in man. *J. Physiol. (Lond.)* 254: 507–518, 1976.
96. Grillner, S. The role of muscle stiffness in meeting the changing postural and locomotor requirements for force development by the ankle extensors. *Acta Physiol. Scand.* 86: 92–108, 1972.
97. Grillner, S. Locomotion in vertebrates: central mechanisms and reflex interaction. *Physiol. Rev.* 55: 247–304, 1975.
98. Grossman, G. E., and R. J. Leigh. Instability of gaze during locomotion in patients with deficient vestibular function. *Ann. Neurol.* 27: 528–532, 1990.
99. Grossman, G. E., R. J. Leigh, L. A. Abel, D. J. Lanska, and S. E. Thurston. Frequency and velocity of rotational head perturbations during locomotion. *Exp. Brain Res.* 70: 470–476, 1988.
100. Gurfinkel, V. S., and A. M. Elner. Contribution of the frontal lobe secondary motor area to organization of postural components in human voluntary movement. *Neurophysiology* 20: 5–10, 1988.
101. Gurfinkel, V., Y. M. Kots, E. I. Paltsev, and A. G. Feldman. The compensation of respiratory disturbances of the erect posture of man as an example of the organization of interarticular interaction. In: *Models of the Structural-Functional Organization of Certain Biological Systems*, edited by V. S. Gurfinkel, S. V. Formin, and M. L. Tsetlin. London: MIT Press, 1971, p. 382–395.
102. Gurfinkel, V. S., M. A. Lebedev, and Y. S. Levik. Effects of reversal in the human equilibrium regulation system. *Neurophysiology* 24: 297–304, 1992.
103. Gurfinkel, V. S., and Y. S. Levick. Perceptual and automatic aspects of the postural body scheme. In: *Brain and Space*, edited by J. Paillard. Oxford: Oxford University Press, 1991, p. 147–162.
104. Gurfinkel, V. S., Y. S. Levik, K. E. Popov, B. N. Smetanin, and V. Y. Shlikov. Body scheme in the control of postural activity. In: *Stance and Motion: Facts and Theories*, edited by V. S. Gurfinkel, M. E. Ioffe, J. Massion, and J. P. Roll. New York: Plenum Press, 1988, p. 185–193.
105. Gurfinkel, V. S., M. I. Lipshits, S. Mori, and K. E. Popov. Stabilization of body position as the main task of postural regulation. *Fiziol. Cheloveka* 7: 400–410, 1981.
106. Gurfinkel, V. S., K. E. Popov, B. N. Smetanin, and V. Y. Shlykov. Changes in the direction of vestibulomotor response in the course of adaptation to protracted static head turning in man. *Neurophysiology* 21: 159–164, 1989.
107. Hallett, M. Physiology of basal ganglia disorders: an overview. *Can. J. Neurol. Sci.* 20: 177–183, 1993.
108. Hayes, K. C. Biomechanics of postural control. *Exerc. Sports Sci. Rev.* 10: 363–391, 1982.
109. He, J., W. S. Levine, and G. E. Loeb. Feedback gains for correcting small perturbations to standing posture. *IEEE Trans. Autom. Contr.* AC-36: 322–332, 1991.
110. Hirschfeld, H., and H. Forssberg. Phase-dependent modulations of anticipatory postural activity during human locomotion. *J. Neurophysiol.* 66: 12–19, 1991.
111. Hlavacka, F., and C. Njiokiktjien. Postural responses evoked by sinusoidal galvanic stimulation of the labyrinth. *Acta Otolaryngol.* 99: 107–112, 1985.
112. Holmes, G. The cerebellum of man. *Brain* 62: 1–30, 1939.
113. Hongo, T., N. Kudo, E. Oguni, and K. Yoshida. Spatial patterns of reflex evoked by pressure stimulation of the foot pads in cats. *J. Physiol. (Lond.)* 420: 471–488, 1990.
114. Horak, F., and J. Frank. Three separate postural systems affected in parkinsonism. In: *Motor Control VII*, edited by D. G. Stuart, V. S. Gurfinkel, and M. Wiesendanger. Tucson: Motor Control Press (in press), 1995.
115. Horak, F. B. Comparison of cerebellar and vestibular loss on scaling of postural responses. In: *Disorders of Posture and Gait*, edited by T. Brandt, W. Paulus, W. Bles, M. Dieterich, S. Krafczyk, and A. Straube. Stuttgart: Georg Thieme Verlag, 1990, p. 370–373.
116. Horak, F. B. Effects of neurological disorders on postural movement strategies in the elderly. In: *Falls, Balance and Gait Disorders in the Elderly*, edited by B. Vellas, M. Toupet, L. Rubenstein, J. L. Albarede, and Y. Christen. Paris: Elsevier Science Publishers, 1992, p. 137–151.
117. Horak, F. B., and M. Anderson, P. Esselman, and K. Lynch. The effects of movement velocity, mass displaced and task certainty on associated postural adjustments made by nor-

mal and hemiplegic individuals. *J. Neurol. Neurosurg. Psychiatry* 47: 1020–1028, 1984.
118. Horak, F. B., and H. C. Diener. Cerebellar control of postural scaling and central set in stance. *J. Neurophysiol.* 72: 479–493, 1994.
119. Horak, F. B., and S. P. Moore. The effect of prior leaning on human postural responses. *Gait Posture* 1: 203–210, 1993.
120. Horak, F. B., and L. M. Nashner. Central programming of postural movements: adaptation to altered support-surface configurations. *J. Neurophysiol.* 55: 1369–1381, 1986.
121. Horak, F. B., L. M. Nashner, and H. C. Diener. Postural strategies associated with somatosensory and vestibular loss. *Exp. Brain Res.* 82: 167–177, 1990.
122. Horak, F. B., J. Nutt, and L. M. Nashner. Postural inflexibility in parkinsonian subjects. *J. Neurol. Sci.* 111: 46–58, 1992.
123. Horak, F. B., and C. L. Shupert. Role of the vestibular system in postural control. In: *Vestibular Rehabilitation*, edited by S. J. Herdman. Philadelphia: F. A. Davis Company, 1994, p. 22–46.
124. Horak, F. B., C. L. Shupert, V. Dietz, and G. Horstmann. Vestibular and somatosensory contributions to responses to head and body displacements in stance. *Exp. Brain Res.* 100: 93–106, 1994.
125. Horak, F. B., C. L. Shupert, V. Dietz, G. Horstmann, and F. O. Black. Vestibular somatosensory interaction in rapid responses to head perturbations. *Ann. N. Y. Acad. Sci.* 656: 854–856, 1992.
126. Horak, F. B., C. L. Shupert, and A. Mirka. Components of postural dyscontrol in the elderly: a review. *Neurobiol. Aging* 10: 727–738, 1989.
127. Hore, J., and T. Vilis. Loss of set in muscle responses to limb perturbations during cerebellar dysfunction. *J. Neurophysiol.* 51: 1137–1148, 1984.
128. Horstmann, G. A., and V. Dietz. The contribution of vestibular input to the stabilization of human posture: a new experimental approach. *Neurosci. Lett.* 95: 179–184, 1988.
129. Horstmann, G. A., and V. Dietz. A basic posture control mechanism: the stabilization of the centre of gravity. *EEG Clin. Neurophysiol.* 76: 165–176, 1990.
130. Inglis, J. T., F. B. Horak, C. L. Shupert, and C. Jones-Rycewicz. The importance of somatosensory information in triggering and scaling automatic postural responses in humans. *Exp. Brain Res.* 101: 159–164, 1994.
131. Inglis, J. T., and J. M. Macpherson. Bilateral labyrinthectomy in the cat: effects on the automatic postural response to translation. *J. Neurophysiol.* 73: 1181–1191, 1995.
132. Inglis, J. T., C. L. Shupert, F. Hlavacka, and F. B. Horak. The effect of galvanic vestibular stimulation on human postural responses during support surface translations. *J. Neurophysiol.* 73: 896–901, 1995.
133. Ioffe, M. E., and A. E. Andreyev. Inter-extremities coordination in local motor conditioned reactions of dog. *Zh. Vyssh. Nerv. Deiat. Im. I.P. Pavlova* 19: 557–565, 1969.
134. Ioffe, M. E., N. G. Ivanova, A. A. Frolov, and E. V. Birjukova. On the role of motor cortex in the learned rearrangement of postural coordinations. In: *Stance and Motion, Facts and Concepts*, edited by V. S. Gurfinkel, M. E. Ioffe, J. Massion, and J. P. Roll. New York: Plenum Press, 1988, p. 213–226.
135. Ito, M. *Cerebellum and Neural Control*. New York: Raven Press, 1984.
136. Jakobs, T., J. A. A. Miller, and A. B. Schultz. Trunk position sense in the frontal plane. *Exp. Neurol.* 90: 129–138, 1985.
137. Johansson, R., and M. Magnusson. Optimal coordination and control of posture and locomotion. *Math. Biosci.* 103: 203–244, 1991.
138. Joseph, J., and A. Nightingale. Electromyography of muscles of posture: leg muscles in males. *J. Physiol. (Lond.)* 117: 484–491, 1952.
139. Kawahara, K., and M. Suzuki. Descending inhibitory pathway responsible for simultaneous suppression of postural tone and respiration in decerebrate cats. *Brain Res.* 538: 303–309, 1991.
140. Keshner, E. A., J. H. J. Allum, and C. R. Pfaltz. Postural coactivation and adaptation in the sway stabilizing responses of normals and patients with bilateral vestibular deficit. *Exp. Brain Res.* 69: 77–92, 1987.
141. Keshner, E. A., M. H. Woollacott, and B. Debu. Neck, trunk and limb muscle responses during postural perturbations in humans. *Exp. Brain Res.* 71: 455–466, 1988.
142. Kuo, A. An optimal control model for analyzing human postural balance. *IEEE Trans. Biomed. Eng.* 42: 87–101, 1995.
143. Kuo, A. D., and F. E. Zajac. Human standing posture—multi-joint movement strategies based on biomechanical constraints. In: *Natural and Artificial Control of Hearing and Balance*, edited by J. H. J. Allum, D. J. Allum-Mecklenburg, F. P. Harris, and R. Probst. Amsterdam: Elsevier Science Publishers, 1993, p. 349–358.
144. Lackner, J. R., and M. levine. Changes in apparent body orientation and sensory localization induced by vibration of postural muscles: vibratory myesthetic illusions. *Aviat. Space Environ. Med.* 50: 346–354, 1979.
145. Lacour, M., and C. Xerri. Compensation of postural reactions to free-fall in the vestibular neurectomized monkey. Role of the visual motions cues. *Exp. Brain Res.* 40: 103–110, 1980.
146. Lacquaniti, F., M. Le Taillanter, L. Lopiano, and C. Maioli. The control of limb geometry in cat posture. *J. Physiol. (Lond.)* 426: 177–192, 1990.
147. Lai, Y. Y., and J. M. Siegel. Cardiovascular and muscle tone changes produced by microinjection of cholinergic and glutamatergic agonists in dorsolateral pons and medial medulla. *Brain Res.* 514: 27–36, 1990.
148. Lamotte, R. H., and M. A. Srinivasan. Tactile discrimination of shape: responses of slowly adapting mechanoreceptive afferents to a step stroked across the monkey fingerpad. *J. Neurosci.* 7: 1655–1671, 1987.
149. Lee, D. N., and E. Aronson. Visual proprioceptive control of standing in human infants. *Percep. Psychophys.* 15: 529–532, 1974.
150. Lee, D. N., and D. S. Young. Gearing action to the environment. In: *Generation and Modulation of Action Patterns, Exp. Brain Res. Vol. 15*, edited by H. Heuer and C. Fromm. Berlin: Springer-Verlag, 1986, p. 217–230.
151. Lee, S. N., and J. R. Lishman. Visual proprioceptive control of stance. *J. Hum. Mov. Studies* 1: 87–95, 1975.
152. Lee, W. A., T. S. Buchanan, and M. W. Rogers. Effects of arm acceleration and behavioral conditions on the organization of postural adjustments during arm flexion. *Exp. Brain Res.* 66: 257–270, 1987.
153. Leibowitz, H. W., C. A. Johnson, and E. Isabelle. Peripheral motion detection and refractive error. *Science* 177: 1207–1208, 1972.

154. Lestienne, F., J. Soechting, and A. Berthoz. Postural readjustments induced by linear motion of visual scenes. *Exp. Brain Res.* 28: 363–384, 1977.
155. Lestienne, F. G., and V. S. Gurfinkel. Postural control in weightlessness: a dual process underlying adaptation to an unusual environment. *Trends Neurosci.* 11: 359–362, 1988.
156. Lovely, R. G., R. J. Gregor, R. R. Roy, and V. R. Edgerton. Effects of training on the recovery of full-weight-bearing stepping in the adult spinal cat. *Exp. Neurol.* 92: 421–435, 1986.
157. Luccarini, P., Y. Gahery, and O. Pompeiano. Cholinoceptive pontine reticular structures modify the postural adjustments during the limb movement induced by cortical stimulation. *Arch. Ital. Biol.* 128: 19–45, 1990.
158. Lund, S., and C. Broberg. Effects of different head positions on postural sway in man induced by a reproducible vestibular error signal. *Acta Physiol. Scand.* 117: 307–309, 1983.
159. Mackinnon, C. D., and D. A. Winter. Control of whole body balance in the frontal plane during human walking. *J. Biomech.* 26: 633–644, 1993.
160. Macpherson, J. M. Strategies that simplify the control of quadrupedal stance. 1. Forces at the ground. *J. Neurophysiol.* 60: 204–217, 1988.
161. Macpherson, J. M. Strategies that simplify the control of quadrupedal stance. 2. Electromyographic activity. *J. Neurophysiol.* 60: 218–231, 1988.
162. Macpherson, J. M. How flexible are muscle synergies? In: *Motor Control: Concepts and Issues*, edited by D. R. Humphrey and H.-J. Freund. Chichester Ltd.: John Wiley & Sons, 1991, p. 33–47.
163. Macpherson, J. M. Changes in a postural strategy with inter-paw distance. *J. Neurophysiol.* 71: 931–940, 1994.
164. Macpherson, J. M. The force constraint strategy for stance is independent of prior experience. *Exp. Brain Res.* 101: 397–405, 1994.
165. Macpherson, J. M., F. B. Horak, and D. C. Dunbar. Stance dependence of automatic postural adjustment in humans. *Exp. Brain Res.* 78: 557–566, 1989.
166. Macpherson, J. M., and J. T. Inglis. Stance and balance following bilateral labyrinthectomy. In: *Natural and Artificial Control of Hearing and Balance*, edited by J. H. J. Allum, D. J. Allum-Mecklenburg, F. P. Harris, and R. Probst. New York: Elsevier Science Publishers, 1993, p. 219–228.
167. Magnus, R. *Body Posture* (English translation). New Delhi: Amerind Publishing Co., 1924.
168. Magnus, R. Some results of studies in the physiology of posture I. *Lancet* 211: 531–536, 1926.
169. Magnusson, M., H. Enbom, R. Johansson, and J. Wiklund. Significance of pressor input from the human feet in lateral postural control—the effect of hypothermia on galvanically induced body-sway. *Acta Otolaryngol.* 110: 321–327, 1990.
170. Maioli, C., and R. E. Poppele. Parallel processing of multisensory information concerning self-motion. *Exp. Brain Res.* 87: 119–125, 1991.
171. Marchand, A. R., and B. Amblard. Locomotion in adult cats with early vestibular deprivation: visual cue substitution. *Exp. Brain Res.* 54: 395–405, 1984.
172. Marsden, C. D. The mysterious motor function of the basal ganglia: the Robert Wartenberg lecture. *Neurology* 32: 514–539, 1982.
173. Marsden, C. D. Function of the basal ganglia as revealed by cognitive and motor disorders in Parkinson's disease. *Can. J. Neurol. Sci.* 11: 129–135, 1984.
174. Marsden, C. D., P. A. Merton, and H. B. Morton. Anticipatory postural responses in the human subject. *J. Physiol. (Lond.)* 275: 47P–48P, 1977.
175. Marsden, C. D., P. A. Merton, and H. B. Morton. Human postural responses. *Brain* 104: 513–534, 1981.
176. Martin, J. P. *The Basal Ganglia and Posture*. London: Pitman Medical Publishers, 1967.
177. Massion, J. Role of motor cortex in postural adjustments associated with movement. In: *Integration in the Nervous System*, edited by H. Asanuma and V. J. Wilson. Tokyo: Igaku-Shoin, 1979, p. 239–260.
178. Massion, J. Movement, posture and equilibrium: interaction and coordination. *Prog. Neurobiol.* 38: 35–56, 1992.
179. Matthews, P. B. C. Where does Sherrington's "muscular sense" originate? Muscles, joints, corollary discharges? *Annu. Rev. Neurosci.* 5: 189–218, 1982.
180. Mauritz, K.-H., and V. Dietz. Characteristics of postural instability induced by ischemic blocking of leg afferents. *Exp. Brain Res.* 38: 117–119, 1980.
181. McIlroy, W. E., and B. E. Maki. Changes in early automatic postural responses associated with the prior-planning and execution of a compensatory step. *Brain Res.* 631: 203–211, 1993.
182. McKinley, P. A., and J. L. Smith. Visual and vestibular contributions to prelanding EMG during jump-downs in cats. *Exp. Brain Res.* 52: 439–448, 1983.
183. Melvill Jones, G., and D. G. D. Watt. Muscular control of landing from unexpected falls in man. *J. Physiol. (Lond.)* 219: 729–737, 1971.
184. Merfeld, D. M., L. R. Young, C. M. Oman, and M. J. Shelhamer. A multidimensional model of the effect of gravity on the spatial orientation of the monkey. *J. Vestib. Res.* 3: 141–161, 1993.
185. Mergner, T., F. Hlavacka, and G. Schweigart. Interaction of vestibular and proprioceptive inputs. *J. Vestib. Res.* 3: 41–57, 1993.
186. Mergner, T., G. L. Nardi, W. Becker, and L. Deecke. The role of canal-neck interaction for the perception of horizontal trunk and head rotation. *Exp. Brain Res.* 49: 198–208, 1983.
187. Mergner, T., C. Siebold, G. Schweigart, and W. Becker. Human perception of horizontal trunk and head rotation in space during vestibular and neck stimulation. *Exp. Brain Res.* 85: 389–404, 1991.
188. Mittelstaedt, H. A new solution to the problem of the subjective vertical. *Naturwissenschaften* 70: 272–281, 1983.
189. Mittelstaedt, H. The role of the otoliths in the perception of the orientation of self and world to the vertical. *Zool. Jb. Physiol.* 95: 419–425, 1991.
190. Mittelstaedt, H., and E. Fricke. The relative effect of saccular and somatosensory information on spatial perception and control. *Adv. Otorhinolaryngol.* 42: 24–30, 1988.
191. Mori, S. Contribution of postural muscle tone to full expression of posture and locomotor movements: multi-faceted analyses of its setting brainstem–spinal cord mechanisms in the cat. *Jpn. J. Physiol.* 39: 785–809, 1989.
192. Mori, S., P. J. Reynolds, and J. M. Brookhart. Contribution of pedal afferents to postural control in the dog. *Am. J. Physiol.* 218: 726–734, 1970.
193. Mouchnino, L., R. Aurenty, J. Massion, and A. Pedotti. Coordinated control of posture and equilibrium during leg movement. In: *Disorders of Posture and Gait,* edited by T. Brandt, W. Paulus, W. Bles, M. Dieterich, S. Krafczyk, and

A. Straube. Stuttgart: Georg Thieme Verlag, 1990, p. 68–71.

194. Mouchino, L., R. Aurenty, J. Massion, and A. Pedotti. Coordination between equilibrium and head-trunk orientation during leg movement—a new strategy built up by training. *J. Neurophysiol.* 67: 1587–1598, 1992.
195. Mouchino, L., R. Aurenty, J. Massion, and A. Pedotti. Is the trunk a reference frame for calculating leg position? *Neuroreport* 4: 125–127, 1993.
196. Muybridge, E. *The Human Figure in Motion*. New York: Dover Publications, 1955.
197. Nakao, C., and J. M. Brookhart. Effects of labyrinthine and visual deprivation on postural stability. *Physiologist* 10: 259, 1967.
198. Nardone, A., A. Giordano, T. Corra, and M. Schieppati. Responses of leg muscles in humans displaced while standing. Effects of types of perturbation and of postural set. *Brain* 113: 65–84, 1990.
199. Nardone, A., and M. Schieppati. Postural adjustments associated with voluntary contraction of leg muscles in standing man. *Exp. Brain Res.* 69: 469–480, 1988.
200. Nashner, L., and A. Berthoz. Visual contribution to rapid motor responses during postural control. *Brain Res.* 150: 403–407, 1978.
201. Nashner, L. M. A vestibular posture control model. *Kybernetik* 10: 106–110, 1972.
202. Nashner, L. M. Adapting reflexes controlling the human posture. *Exp. Brain Res.* 26: 59–72, 1976.
203. Nashner, L. M. Fixed patterns of rapid postural responses among leg muscles during stance. *Exp. Brain Res.* 30: 13–24, 1977.
204. Nashner, L. M. Balance adjustment of humans perturbed while walking. *J. Neurophysiol.* 44: 650–664, 1980.
205. Nashner, L. M., F. O. Black, and C. Wall, III. Adaptation to altered support and visual conditions during stance: patients with vestibular deficits. *J. Neurosci.* 2: 536–544, 1982.
206. Nashner, L. M., and H. Forssberg. Phase-dependent organization of postural adjustments associated with arm movements while walking. *J. Neurophysiol.* 55: 1382–1394, 1986.
207. Nashner, L. M., and G. McCollum. The organization of human postural movements: a formal basis and experimental synthesis. *Behav. Brain Sci.* 8: 135–172, 1985.
208. Nashner, L. M., C. L. Shupert, and F. B. Horak. Head-trunk movement coordination in the standing posture. *Prog. Brain Res.* 76: 243–251, 1988.
209. Nashner, L. M., C. L. Shupert, F. B. Horak, and F. O. Black. Organization of posture control: an analysis of sensory and mechanical constraints. *Prog. Brain Res.* 80: 411–418, 1989.
210. Nashner, L. M., and P. Wilson. Influence of head position and proprioceptive cues on short latency postural reflexes evoked by galvanic stimulation of the human labyrinth. *Brain Res.* 67: 255–268, 1974.
211. Nelson, J. G. Effect of water immersion and body position upon perception of the gravitational vertical. *Aerospace Med.* 39: 806–811, 1968.
212. Newell, K. M., R. E. A. Van Emmerik, D. Lee, and R. L. Sprague. On postural stability and variability. *Gait Posture* 4: 225–230, 1993.
213. Nutt, J., F. Horak, and J. Frank. Scaling of postural responses in Parkinson's disease. In: *Posture and Gait: Control Mechanisms*, edited by M. Woollacott and F. Horak. Eugene, OR: University of Oregon Press, 1992, p. 4–7.
214. Obeso, J. A., P. Quesada, J. Artieda, and J. M. Martinez-Lage. Reciprocal inhibition in rigidity and dystonia. In: *Clinical Neurophysiology in Parkinsonism*, edited by P. J. Delwaide and A. Agnoli. New York: Elsevier Science Publishers, 1985, p. 9–18.
215. Oddsson, L., and A. Thorstensson. Fast voluntary trunk flexion movements in standing: motor patterns. *Acta Physiol. Scand.* 129: 93–106, 1987.
216. Oman, C. M. A hueristic mathematical model for the dynamics of sensory conflict and motion sickness. *Acta Otolaryngol.* 392: 1–44, 1982.
217. Paulus, W., A. Straube, and T. Brandt. Visual postural performance after loss of somatosensory and vestibular function. *J. Neurol. Neurosurg. Psychiatry* 50: 1542–1545, 1987.
218. Paulus, W. M., A. Straube, and T. Brandt. Visual stabilization of posture: physiological stimulus characteristics and clinical aspects. *Brain* 107: 1143–1164, 1984.
219. Peterka, R. J., and M. S. Benolken. Role of somatosensory and vestibular cues in attenuating visually-induced human postural sway. In: *Posture and Gait: Control Mechanisms*, edited by M. Woollacott and F. Horak. Eugene, OR: University of Oregon Books, 1992, p. 272–275.
220. Phillips, C. G. Motor apparatus of the baboon's hand. *Proc. Soc. Lond. B.* 173: 141–174, 1969.
221. Popov, K. E., B. N. Smetanin, V. S. Gurfinkel, M. P. Kudinova, and V. Y. Shlykov. Spatial perception and vestibulomotor responses in man. *Neurophysiology* 18: 548–553, 1986.
222. Pozzo, T., A. Berthoz, and L. Lefort. Head stabilization during various locomotor tasks in humans. I. Normal subjects. *Exp. Brain Res.* 82: 97–106, 1990.
223. Pozzo, T., A. Berthoz, L. Lefort, and E. Vitte. Head stabilization during various locomotor tasks in humans. 2. Patients with bilateral peripheral vestibular deficits. *Exp. Brain Res.* 85: 208–217, 1991.
224. Pozzo, T., Y. Levik, and A. Berthoz. Head stabilization in the frontal plane during complex equilibrium tasks in humans. In: *Posture and Gait: Control Mechanisms*, edited by M. Woollacott and F. Horak. Eugene: University of Oregon Books, 1992, p. 97–100.
225. Pratt, C. A., J. Fung, and J. M. Macpherson. Stance control in the chronic spinal cat. *J. Neurophysiol.* 71: 1981–1985, 1994.
226. Pratt, C. A., F. B. Horak, and R. M. Herndon. Differential effects of somatosensory and motor system deficits on postural dyscontrol in multiple sclerosis patients. In: *Posture and Gait: Control Mechanisms*, edited by M. Woollacott and F. Horak. Eugene, OR: University of Oregon Books, 1992, p. 118–121.
227. Procaccia, I. Universal properties of dynamically complex systems: the organization of chaos. *Nature* 333: 618–623, 1988.
228. Prochazka, A. Sensorimotor gain control: a basic strategy of motor systems? *Prog. Neurobiol.* 33: 281–307, 1989.
229. Proske, U., H.-G. Schaible, and R. F. Schmidt. Joint receptors and kinaesthesia. *Exp. Brain Res.* 72: 219–224, 1988.
230. Quoniam, C., J. P. Roll, A. Deat, and J. Massion. Proprioceptive induced interactions between segmental and whole body posture. In: *Disorders of Posture and Gait*, edited by T. Brandt, W. Paulus, W. Bles, M. Dieterich, S. Krafcyzk, and A. Straube. Stuttgart: Georg Thieme Verlag, 1990, p. 194–197.
231. Reed, E. S. An outline of a theory of action systems. *J. Mot. Behav.* 14: 98–134, 1982.

232. Regis, H., E. Trouche, and J. Massion. Movement and associated postural adjustment. In: *The Motor System: Neurophysiology and Muscle Mechanisms*, edited by M. Shahani. Amsterdam: Elsevier Science Publishers 1976, p. 349–361.
233. Rispal-Padel, L., F. Cicirata, and C. Pons. Contribution of the dentato-thalamic cortical system to control of motor synergy. *Neurosci. Lett.* 22: 137–144, 1981.
234. Roberts, T. D. M. *Neurophysiology of Postural Mechanisms*, 2nd Ed. London: Butterworth & Co. Ltd., 1978.
235. Rogers, M. W., C. G. Kukulka, and G. L. Soderberg. Postural adjustments preceding rapid arm movements in parkinsonian subjects. *Neurosci. Lett.* 75: 246–251, 1987.
236. Roll, J. P., J. P. Vedel, and R. Roll. Eye, head and skeletal muscle spindle feedback in the elaboration of body references. *Prog. Brain. Res.* 80: 113–123, 1989.
237. Romberg, M. H. *Lehrbuch der Mercenkrankheiten des Menschen*. Berlin: Duncker, 1851.
238. Ross, H. E., S. D. Crickmar, N. V. Sills, and E. P. Owen. Orientation to the vertical in free divers. *Aerospace Med.* 40: 728–732, 1969.
239. Schaefer, K.-P., and D. L. Meyer. Compensation of vestibular lesins. In: *Handbook of Sensory Physiology*, edited by H. H. Kornhuber. Berlin: Springer-Verlag, 1974, p. 463–490.
240. Schaltenbrand, G. The development of human motility and motor disturbances. *Arch. Neurol. Psychiatry*, 20: 720–730, 1928.
241. Schieppati, M., and A. Nardone. Free and supported stance in Parkinson's disease: the effect of posture and 'postural set' on leg muscle responses to perturbation, and its relation to the severity of the disease. *Brain* 114: 1227–1244, 1991.
242. Schieppati, M., A. Nardone, M. Grasso, and R. Siliotto. Time-course of amplitude changes of leg muscle responses to stance perturbation during a postural stabilization task in humans. *IUPS Abstr.* 3: 48, 1993.
243. Scholz, E., H. C. Diener, J. Noth, H. Friedmann, J. Dichgans, and M. Bacher. Medium and long latency EMG responses in leg muscles—Parkinson's disease. *J. Neurol. Neurosurg. Psychiatry* 50: 66–70, 1987.
244. Schweigart, G., S. Heimbrand, T. Mergner, and W. Becker. Perception of horizontal head and trunk rotation—modification of neck input following loss of vestibular function. *Exp. Brain Res.* 95: 533–546, 1993.
245. Sherrington, C. *The Integrative Action of the Nervous System*, 2nd Ed. New Haven, CT: Yale University Press, 1961.
246. Shimba, T. An estimation of center of gravity from force platform data. *J. Biomech.* 17: 53–60, 1984.
247. Shumway-Cook, A., and J. Woollacott. The growth of stability: postural control from a developmental perspective. *J. Mot. Behav.* 17: 131–147, 1985.
248. Shupert, C. L., F. O. Black, F. B. Horak, and L. M. Nashner. Coordination of the head and body in response to support surface translations in normals and patients with bilterally reduced vestibular function. In: *Posture and Gait: Development, Adaptation and Modulation*, edited by B. Amblard, A. Berthoz, and F. Clarac. New York: Elsevier Science Publishers, 1988, p. 281–289.
249. Smetanin, B. N., K. E. Popov, V. S. Gurfinkel, and V. Y. Shlykov. Effect of real and illusory movements on the human vestibulomotor reaction. *Neurophysiology* 20: 192–196, 1988.
250. Soechting, J. F., and A. Berthoz. Dynamic role of vision in the control of posture in man. *Exp. Brain Res.* 36: 551–561, 1979.
251. Soechting, J. F., and M. Flanders. Moving in three-dimensional space—frames of reference, vectors, and coordinate systems. *Annu. Rev. Neurosci.* 15: 167–191, 1992.
252. Stoffregen, T. A. Flow structure versus retinal location in the optical control of stance. *J. Exp. Psychol. Hum. Percept.* 11: 554–565, 1985.
253. Storper, I., and V. Honrubia. Is human galvanically induced triceps surae electromyogram a vestibulospinal reflex response? *Otolaryngol. Head Neck Surg.* 107: 527–536, 1992.
254. Takahashi, M., H. Hoshikawa, N. Tsujita, and I. Akiyama. Effect of labyrinthine dysfuntion upon head oscillation and gaze during stepping and running. *Acta Otolaryngol.* 106: 348–353, 1988.
255. Talbott, R. E. Postural reactions of dogs to sinusoidal motion in the peripheral visual field. *Am. J. Physiol.* 239 (*Regulatory Integrative Comp. Physiol.* 8): R71–R79, 1980.
256. Taylor, J. L., and D. I. McCloskey. Proprioceptive sensation in rotation of the trunk. *Exp. Brain Res.* 81: 413–416, 1990.
257. Thomson, D. B., J. T. Inglis, R. H. Schor, and J. M. Macpherson. Bilateral labyrinthectomy in the cat: motor behavior and quiet stance parameters. *Exp. Brain Res.* 85: 364–372, 1991.
258. Thorstensson, A., J. Nilsson, H. Carlson, and R. Zomlefer. Trunk movements in human locomotion. *Acta Physiol. Scand.* 121: 9–22, 1984.
259. Tokita, T., Y. Ito, and K. Takagi. Modulation by head and trunk positions of the vestibulo-spinal reflexes evoked by galvanic stimulation of the labyrinth. *Acta Otolaryngol.* 107: 327–332, 1989.
260. Traub, M. M., J. C. Rothwell, and C. D. Marsden. Anticipatory postural reflexes in Parkinson's disease and other akinetic-rigid syndromes and in cerebellar ataxia. *Brain* 103: 393–412, 1980.
261. Vidal, P. P., A. Berthoz, and M. Millanvoye. Difference between eye closure and visual stabilization in the control of posture in man. *Aviat. Space Environ. Med.* 53: 166–170, 1982.
262. Vidal, P. P., W. Graf, and A. Berthoz. The orientation of the cervical vertebral column in unrestrained awake animals. *Exp. Brain Res.* 61: 549–559, 1986.
263. Watt, D. G. D. Responses of cats to sudden falls: an otolith-originating reflex assisting landing. *J. Neurophysiol.* 39: 257–265, 1976.
264. Watts, R. L., W. W. Allen, W. Wiegan, and W. Young. Elastic properties of muscles measured at the elbow in man. II. Patients with parkinsonian rigidity. *J. Neurol. Neurosurg. Psychiatry* 49: 1177–1181, 1986.
265. Wicke, R. W., and C. M. Oman. Visual and graviceptive influences on lower leg EMG activity in humans during brief falls. *Exp. Brain Res.* 46: 324–330, 1982.
266. Wiesendanger, M., J. J. Seguin, and H. Kunzle. The suppelementary motor area—a control system for posture? In: *Control of Posture and Locomotion*, edited by R. B. Stein, K. B. Pearson, R. S. Smith, and J. B. Redford. New York: Plenum Press, 1973, p. 331–346.
267. Wilson, V. J., and G. Melvill Jones. *Mammalian Vestibular Physiology*. New York: Plenum Press, 1979.
268. Wilson, V. J., and B. W. Peterson. Vestibulospinal and reticulospinal systems. In: *Handbood of Physiology, The Nervous System, Motor Control*, edited by V. B. Brooks. Bethesda, MD: Am. Physiol. Soc., 1981, p. 667–702.
269. Winter, D. A. *Biomechanics and Motor Control of Human Movement*. New York: John Wiley & Sons, 1990, p. 277.

270. Winter, D. A., C. D. Mackinnon, G. K. Ruder, and C. Wieman. An integrated EMG/biomechanical model of upper body balance and posture during human gait. In: *Natural and Artificial Control of Hearing and Balance*, edited by J. H. J. Allum, D. J. Allum-Mecklenburg, F. P. Harris, and R. Probst. Amsterdam: Elsevier Science Publishers, 1993, p. 359–367.
271. Woollacott, M. H., M. Bonnet, and K. Yabe. Preparatory process for anticipatory postural adjustments—modulation of leg muscles reflex pathways during preparation for arm movements in standing man. *Exp. Brain Res.* 55: 263–271, 1984.
272. Young, L. R., C. M. Oman, D. G. Watt, K. E. Money, and B. K. Lichtenberg. Spatial orientation in weightlessnes and readaptation to earth's gravity. *Science* 225: 205–208, 1984.
273. Young, L. R., and M. Shelhamer. Microgravity enhances the relative contribution of visually-induced motion sensation. *Aviat. Space Environ. Med.* 61: 525–530, 1990.
274. Zajac, F. E. Muscle and tendon: properties, models, scaling, and application to biomechanics and motor control. *Crit. Rev. Biomed. Eng.* 17: 359–411, 1989.
275. Zajac, F. E., and M. E. Gordon. Determining muscle's force and action in multiarticular movement. *Exerc. Sport Sci. Rev.* 17: 187–230, 1989.

8. Biomechanical insights into neural control of movement

RONALD F. ZERNICKE | *Department of Surgery, University of Calgary, Calgary, Alberta, Canada*

JUDITH L. SMITH | *Department of Physiological Science, University of California, Los Angeles, Los Angeles, California*

CHAPTER CONTENTS

THE ACCELERATED INFUSION OF BIOMECHANICS TECHNIQUES into the study of neuromotor control has served, during the past few decades, as a catalyst for generating new insights into the control of movement. Today, when assessing the functional capacity of the neuromuscular system in animal or human models, it is common to use complementary biomechanical and electromyographic (EMG) techniques. In particular, quantifying the dynamics of limb movements has provided a window to examine the physical mechanisms underlying neuromotor control and has led to testable predictions for the neural control of limb movements.

In this chapter, we review recent progress in the overlapping areas of biomechanics and neuromotor control, and we highlight predictions about neural control that have emerged from the integration of these fields. Before delving into those predictions, however, we discuss basic elements of biomechanics and concepts of limb dynamics, concentrating on inverse dynamics models. Then, using the paw-shake response—rapid (10 Hz) cyclic actions of the cat's hindlimb—as an example, we explain how the application of inverse dynamics methods has generated testable predictions about the neural control of this stereotypic limb motion.

The remaining portions of the chapter focus on the role of dynamics in three areas: *(1)* control of different forms of walking and running in bipeds (human) and quadrupeds (cat), *(2)* control of arm movements for skilled tasks and changes in intersegmental dynamics that occur with the practice of complex arm movements, and *(3)* control of limb motions during human motor development with emphasis on changes in limb dynamics for spontaneous kicking and reaching motions during a period when the infant's limb growth is exuberant and limb mass and geometry change rapidly. By design, our chapter is not exhaustive in scope. Nevertheless, by focusing on limb-movement dynamics of animals and humans, we accent the usefulness of quantitative analyses for exploring the mechanisms of motor control and the insights physiologists and biomechanists may gain about neural control of limb motion.

ANALYTICAL TECHNIQUES AND TERMS

Biomechanics is the application of the principles and methods of mechanics to the study of biological systems (80). Variations on this generic definition include ". . . anything directly or indirectly pertaining to the effects of forces upon the form or motion of organic bodies or tissues" (42) and ". . . the science which investigates the effect of internal and external forces on human and animal bodies in movement and rest" (27). Although the scientific roots of biomechanics are deep (15, 16, 21, 33, 55, 125, 133, 134, 137, 171, 175, 203), the term "biomechanics" was coined by Bernstein as recently as 1923 (7).

In addition to giving a name to the field, Bernstein's ideas and research (8) have had a substantial impact on the integration of biomechanics, motor control, and motor development. In the context of human movement analyses, he was the first to articulate the concepts of *degrees of freedom, peripheral indeterminacy* (context-conditioned sensitivity), and *functional synergies* (coordinative structure) (108), which were discussed further by Turvey and colleagues (45, 196, 197).

Bernstein realized that understanding movement coordination is not accomplished by simply analyzing how individual muscles generate limb movements. Rather, during movements, the multiple, interconnected links of the human body are affected by external forces (e.g., gravity or contact forces), as well as motion-dependent forces generated by the moving body segments (inertial, centripetal, and Coriolis forces)—for example, movement of your hand will generate "motion-dependent" forces at your elbow and shoulder.

One of Bernstein's tenets is that movement patterns emerge through dynamic and symbiotic interactions between the organism and the environment; for example, during motor development, movement forms are not imposed on the organism by an autonomously maturing brain but are blended into the neuromuscular system via interactions with external feedback and forces (192). Movement regulation is a dynamic process in which adaptive and functional strategies (synergies) are developed to reduce the complexity of motor control (56).

Biomechanics Terminology

The same terms used in mechanics are also applied to *bio*mechanics. Mechanics is the branch of physics that deals with the *motions* or *states* of material bodies, and mechanics is typically divided into *kinematics* (dealing with different forms of motion) and *dynamics* (dealing with the physical causes for changes in motion). Dynamics is subdivided into two parts, *statics* and *kinetics*. Statics involves systems that are in equilibrium, forces acting on the body or system are balanced (55), and the body is at rest or moving at a constant velocity (zero acceleration). Kinetics deals with changes in motion caused by one or more unbalanced forces (204). When using biomechanical analyses to probe the control mechanisms underlying movement, it is important to recognize a basic difference between kinematics and dynamics. Kinematic variables describe or characterize the movement, the *effect*; whereas dynamics variables quantify the underlying *physical cause* of the movement.

In mechanics, kinematic variables include linear and angular position, velocity (time derivative of position), acceleration (time derivative of velocity), and jerk (time derivative of acceleration) of body segments or joints. During movements such as walking or reaching for an object, kinematic averages of joint angles or joint angular velocities can be synchronized temporally with EMG recordings of synergistic muscles to give a description of the movement.

Dynamics Variables

Here, we use *dynamics* in a more restricted, biomechanical sense, and not in the more global sense of "dynamical systems" (72, 111, 115, 116, 156, 191). Kelso, Haken, and others (72, 110) have written extensively about self-organizing patterns in nonequilibrium systems, synergetics, and qualitative dynamics and their application to biology and motor control. The reader is advised to review their work to gain a background in the global dynamics of complex biological systems.

In the more restricted biomechanical context, the primary variables of dynamics analyses include *force, torque*, and *power*. Force is a vector quantity and, thus, has magnitude and direction and is calculated as the product of the mass of a body (object) and its linear acceleration, Newton's second law, $F = m \cdot a$ (55, 120). In limb-movement kinetics, forces can either be internal or external. Internal forces can be generated either actively or passively by skeletal muscles, and passively by ligaments, tendons, periarticular structures, and friction in joints. External forces are applied to the body at contact points (e.g., ground forces on the foot during walking or the hand and pencil in contact with a writing surface), by objects being lifted or making contact with the body, or by passive sources such as wind resistance (204).

Because the human musculoskeletal system is a complex system of levers, body segments have a tendency to rotate about joint axes as internal or external forces are applied. The tendency to cause that rotation is quantified by determining the *torque* (also called a *moment* of force) applied to the segment. Torque (M) also is a vector, calculated as the applied force (F) times the perpendicular distance (r) between the line of action of the force and the joint axis of rotation, $M = r \times F$ (55).

By knowing the magnitude and sign of the muscular torque (M) being produced at a joint and that joint's angular velocity (ω), *joint muscle power* ($M \cdot \omega$) can be calculated (204). Joint muscle power reveals whether mechanical power is being generated or absorbed by the muscles crossing a joint. Power is *generated* at a joint when M and ω both are positive or both are negative. Power is *absorbed* at a joint when the product of M and ω is a negative value [$M \cdot (-\omega)$ *or* $(-M) \cdot \omega$]. For example, power generation will occur at the elbow if there is a flexor torque ($-M$) while the elbow is flexing (decreasing elbow angle produces $-\omega$), and power absorption will occur at the elbow if there is a flexor torque ($-M$) while the elbow is extending (increasing elbow angle produces ω). In a generic sense, muscle power generation is related to the shortening of an active muscle, and muscle power absorption is related to the lengthening of an active muscle.

When analyzing the dynamics of the human body, generally the segments of the body are approximated as rigid bodies or interconnected links (8, 35). Although deformations of soft tissues can occur during movement, soft-tissue deformations are usually negligible compared to the large excursions of the limb. Accepting that limitation, researchers then have a tractable problem, and rigid-body equations of motion can be used to quantify limb dynamics.

Single vs. Multiple Degrees of Freedom

In mechanics, "degrees of freedom" refer to the number of variables (coordinates) that are required to describe quantitatively a body segment's motion (137). For example, as your elbow flexes, only one degree of freedom (elbow angle) is needed to quantify the relative change occurring between the humerus and forearm. The forearm segment moving in a plane, however, requires three degrees of freedom to specify its motion: the (x, y) coordinates of any point on the rigid body and the orientation angle of the rigid body in the plane.

Natural limb motions of humans and other vertebrates occur in three dimensions and comprise multiple degrees of freedom, and as Soechting and Flanders (184) state, "certain concepts that seem clear in the context of simple movements become less so when one considers multijoint motions." (184, p. 391). With single degree of freedom motions (one-joint motions), the joint angular acceleration is directly proportional to the joint torque, and dynamics can be inferred directly from the kinematics. With the motions of the multijointed lower or upper extremity, however, this simple relation does not hold. While some contend that "there is something to be learned from reducing . . . motor control . . . to a single joint" (65, p. 245), others argue strongly that natural limb movements are not controlled at the single-joint level and, therefore, dynamics of multisegmental motions must be analyzed to understand more fully the planning and control of limb motions (95, 121, 184, 211).

In multijoint movements, the underlying physical cause (dynamics) of the motion cannot be discerned from the movement kinematics. Some of the reasons for this multijoint indeterminacy arises because biarticular muscles can produce different actions across the joints they span (211), and dynamic coupling occurs in multilinked segments (184). For example, the motion of the shoulder joint may depend not only on torques developed by shoulder muscles but also on accelerations and angular velocities of more distal segments, the forearm and hand (184). Knowing whether the shoulder (or any other joint) is moving or not (kinematic information) does not give us direct information about the underlying kinetics. Because the shoulder is flexing, for example, does not tell us whether there is a flexor muscle torque or an extensor muscle torque acting at the shoulder; the muscle torque (flexor) could be acting concentrically, or the muscle torque (extensor) could be acting eccentrically during the shoulder flexion. These are very different conditions of motor control and only a dynamics analysis will reveal those differences.

The nonintuitive relation between torque and motion was illustrated effectively by Soechting and Flanders [Fig. 8.1; (184)]. In their example of elbow and shoulder joint coordination during a person's sagittal-plane reach to a shoulder-level target, the anterior deltoid and biceps brachii (shoulder or elbow flexors) were active at the initiation of the motion. Consistent with the recorded EMG, there were active flexor torques at both the shoulder and elbow

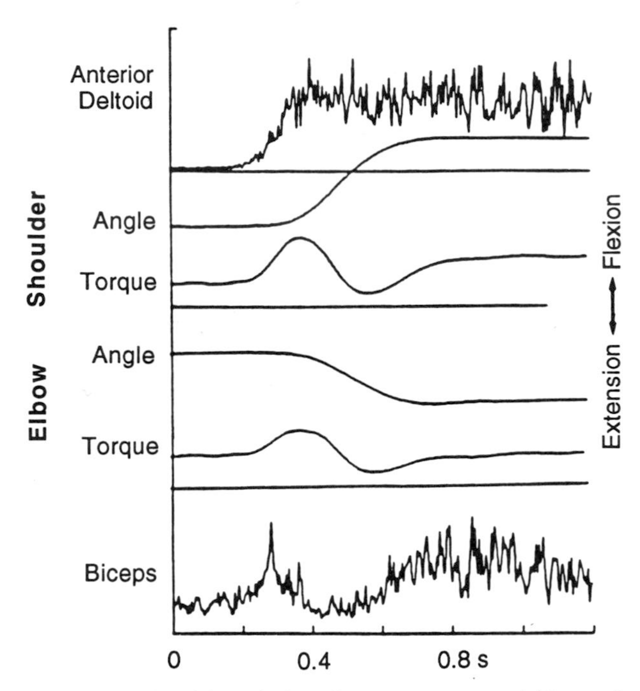

FIG. 8.1. Nonintuitive relations between torque and kinematics. Data are from a subject pointing forward, moving the hand in the sagittal plane to a target at shoulder level. The joint motions required were shoulder flexion (*upward angle trace*) and elbow extension (*downward angle trace*). While these opposite motions occurred, agonists for this action were shoulder flexors (e.g., anterior deltoid) *and* elbow flexors (e.g., biceps brachii), with shoulder and elbow joint torques that both had increased flexor influences. [Adapted from Fig. 11.3 of Soechting and Flanders (184).]

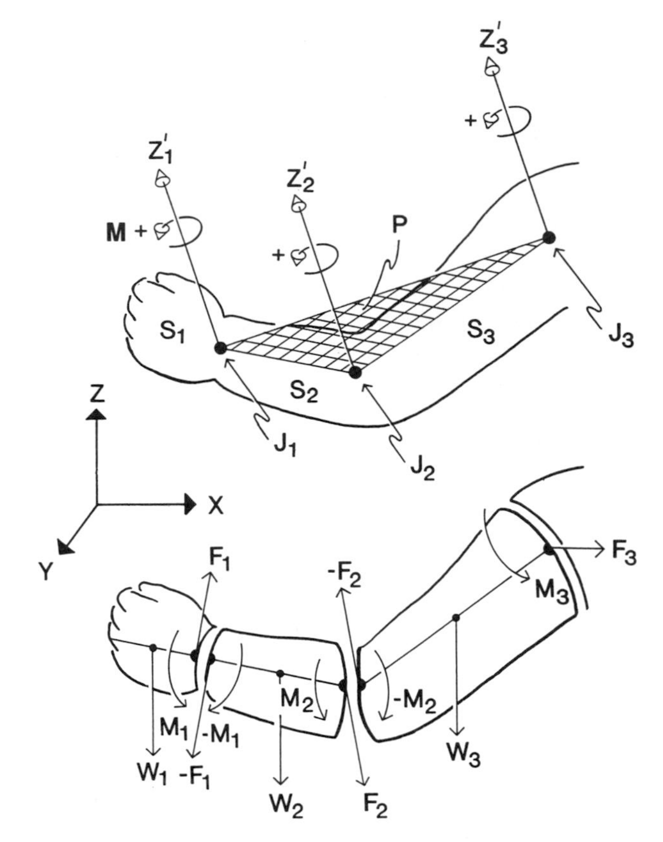

FIG. 8.2. Interpretive and free-body diagrams of a model of an infant's upper extremity. The upper diagram shows the limb positioned in an inertial (x-y-z) coordinate system. A positive torque is defined (M). The upper extremity is modeled as three interconnected rigid segments (S_1 hand, S_2 forearm, and S_3 upper arm) with frictionless joints (J_1 wrist, J_2 elbow, and J_3 shoulder). At each instant in time during a reach, a moving local plane (P) is calculated so that the plane contains the x-y-z coordinates of each of the three joint centers (J_1, J_2, J_3). The planar torques at the wrist, elbow, and shoulder are calculated with respect to the respective joint axes (Z_1', Z_2', Z_3') that pass through each joint center and are perpendicular to the moving local plane (P). In the lower portion of the figure is a free-body diagram of the upper extremity. Depicted are forces related to the hand, forearm, and upper arm segment weights (W_1, W_2, W_3) acting at their respective center of mass, and the wrist, elbow, and shoulder joint reaction forces (F_1, F_2, F_3) and torques (M_1, M_2, M_3). [Adapted from Fig. 1 of Zernicke and Schneider (214).]

joints; nevertheless, the shoulder *flexed* while the elbow *extended* during the reaching action.

Free-Body Diagram

In a rigid-body analysis of limb dynamics, a *free-body diagram* is first constructed, isolating the segment (link) of interest with all external applied forces drawn on the diagram (120). As an example, in the upper portion of Figure 8.2, we show a schematic of an infant's upper extremity, consisting of three segments connected by "frictionless" joints. The mathematical details and equations of motion for this three-segment model have been published (168) and, thus, here we provide a basic description of the elements of the model.

The three-segment upper extremity moves in an inertial reference frame that is oriented with respect to gravity, acting in the vertical direction (Fig. 8.2). We record the three-dimensional coordinates of the wrist, elbow, and shoulder and at each instant in time compute a "moving-local plane" (P) that always contains the coordinates of the wrist, elbow, and shoulder. In the moving-local plane, free-body diagrams are constructed, as illustrated in the lower portion of Figure 8.2. For each of the three segments, there is a force (F) related to each segment's weight acting through each segment's center of mass, and at each joint, there are equal and opposite joint reaction forces. For example, at the wrist joint, F_1 is the joint reaction force of the hand acting on the distal end of the forearm segment, while $-F_1$ is the equal and opposite effect of the forearm acting on the hand. The torques are computed with respect to axes that pass through the three joints and are perpendicular to the moving-local plane. The advantage of computing the torques in a moving-local plane is that a planar (two-dimensional) dynamics analysis can be used to gain insights into motor control without resorting to the complexity of a full-fledged three-dimensional dynamics analysis.

If a body is in *static equilibrium*, then all forces and torques acting on the body are balanced (e.g., $\Sigma F = 0$ and $\Sigma M = 0$), and the body either does not move or does not experience a change in velocity. If a body experiences a change in its velocity (accelerates) as a result of an applied force or forces, the *net effect* of the applied forces equals the product of segmental mass and linear acceleration ($\Sigma F = m \cdot a$; Newton's second law). The analogous situation for torques is $\Sigma M = I \cdot \alpha$; where, I is the segmental moment of inertia, and α is the segmental angular acceleration. Using D'Alembert's principle for *dynamic equilibrium* (33), Newton's equation can be written as $\Sigma F + (-m \cdot a) = 0$, where $(-m \cdot a)$ is an *inertial* force that balances the external forces, ΣF. The analogous relation for dynamic equilibrium for the torques is $\Sigma M + (-I \cdot \alpha) = 0$. If all but one of the unknowns in each of these basic equations of motion can be measured or approximated, then the dynamics of the system can be uniquely quantified, as explained next.

Dynamics Techniques

Zajac and Gordon (211) provide a cogent overview of dynamics methods that have been useful in motor control studies. They accent basic differences between *direct* and *inverse* dynamics techniques: *(1)* with direct dynamics, the motive forces or torques are known while the resulting system kinematics are observed or calculated, whereas *(2)* with inverse dynamics, the resulting motion is known while the underlying forces and torques are calculated.

Direct Dynamics. In a direct dynamics solution, the *inputs* to the system are the active and passive *internal* forces and torques (e.g., muscle and ligament forces), as well as *external* applied forces (e.g., ground reaction forces in walking), and the *output* is the motion of the body. Zajac and Gordon (211) call this the "natural" flow of events, because this is how the body typically generates movement. Obtaining accurate estimates of these internal forces and torques, however, can be problematic.

In direct dynamics analyses, measuring external reaction (contact) forces, generally, can be reliable and accurate. A force platform will measure the contact forces between a body part and the surface of the platform. Routinely, force platforms have been used in gait studies, with either humans (32, 137, 204) or animals [(53, 124); also see Fig. 8.3].

Compared to measuring external contact forces, measuring internal muscle or joint forces is technically more difficult. Nevertheless, several investigators have successfully obtained estimates of muscle forces from tendon force transducers or EMG signals. Tendon force transducers, either oval-shaped or E-shaped, have been used for studies of human (67) and animal locomotion (53, 68, 82, 86, 90, 174, 202). Strain gauges are attached to the metal element of the implanted transducer. As tensile forces are transmitted along a tendon passing through the transducer, the metal element deforms, and the resulting strains are proportional to the tendon forces. Thus, the tendon force can provide an estimate of the muscle force, as Fowler et al. (53) recently showed for cat walking (Fig. 8.3; see later under Stance Dynamics for Different Forms of Cat Walking).

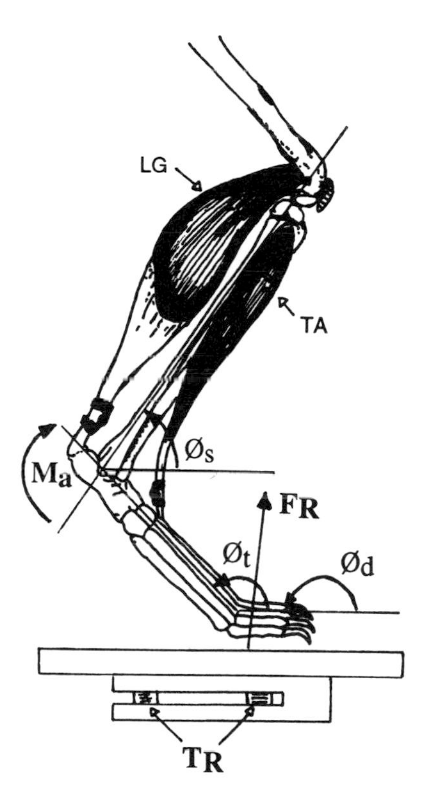

FIG. 8.3. Anatomical drawing of the cat hindlimb with a schematic of a force platform beneath it. E-shaped tendon transducers are shown on the lateral gastrocnemius (LG) and tibialis anterior (TA) tendons. F_R is the resultant ground reaction force vector acting on the plantar surface of the paw. Each force platform contains two piezoelectric transducers (T_R). Digit ($\emptyset_d$), tarsal ($\emptyset_t$), and shank ($\emptyset_S$) segment angles are calculated from the right horizontal. M_a is the muscle torque acting about the ankle joint. [Redrawn from Fig. 1(a) of Fowler et al. (53).]

Zajac and colleagues (87, 99, 210, 211) also note that a Hill-type model of muscle dynamics may be used in conjunction with a muscle's EMG signal to estimate the time-history of skeletal muscle force production. In such models, muscle force is estimated from the muscle fiber length–velocity relation and neural excitation (EMG signal), while factoring in tendon properties (211). Using EMG signals to estimate muscle forces has produced important insights into the neuromotor control of human locomotion (88, 89, 140, 151) and jumping (14).

Inverse Dynamics. The method of inverse dynamics is used to estimate the underlying forces and torques, when the kinematics of the motion and the inertial characteristics of the body are known. Typically, body segments of human and other animals can be approximated as a set of interconnected rigid links (35, 78, 100, 101, 124, 137, 204). Depending on the complexity of the analysis, a body can be represented as a few or many rigid-body segments.

To conduct an inverse dynamics analysis, one can find the mathematical derivations of rigid-body equations of motion detailed in several reports (17, 100–102, 137, 165, 166, 168, 204, 207, 211). The inverse dynamics approach has provided a window for examining the control of torques that influence limb trajectories during pointing and reaching tasks (5, 117, 214), human walking (17, 128, 158, 204, 215), running (123, 149, 151, 215), kicking (157, 213), sitting (186), and cycling (66, 136), as well as cat locomotion (53, 100, 146, 207), jumping (118), and the paw-shake response (101, 102, 182).

Optimization. Although the inverse dynamics method can quantify the generalized muscle torque at a joint, the calculated "muscle" torque includes forces arising not only from active muscle contractions, but also from passive deformations of muscles, tendons, ligaments, and other periarticular tissues. The muscle torque is a composite variable, and extracting active vs. passive contributions to the generalized muscle torque is a continuing quest.

Furthermore, relating the generalized muscle torque to the forces in the individual muscles that span a joint is neither a simple nor straightforward task, because the number of muscles exceeds the number of joints being analyzed (211). Recall that when analyzing the body as a system of mechanical links, if the number of system equations is not equal to the number of unknowns, the mathematical problem becomes *indeterminate*. With this inequality, if the number of equations is greater than the unknowns, the problem is *overdetermined* and, generally, no unique solution is feasible. Conversely, if the number of unknowns is greater than the number of equations, the problem is *underdetermined*, and an infinite number of solutions is possible (137). In biomechanics, the usual situation is that there are many more unknowns than there are system equations. Some investigators achieved a solution to this problem by making rational assumptions to either decrease the number of system unknowns (130, 143) or increase the number of system equations (151). Others, however, approached this problem by employing static or dynamic optimization techniques.

Static optimization methods have been used to solve the problem of distributing muscle torques among individual muscles during human locomotion (29, 30, 37, 142, 145, 170). A fundamental assumption of any optimization technique is that, within well-defined boundaries, there exists an "optimal" solution to the stated problem. In this context, an optimization problem can be defined by three quantities: cost function, design variables, and constraint functions. The *cost function* is what is "optimized" in the solution. In the optimization process, *design variables* (e.g., individual muscle forces) are systematically changed until the cost function is minimized, and all *constraint functions* are satisfied (e.g., muscular forces must be zero or positive) (137). Finding an effective and valid cost function, however, is an elusive and continuing challenge. For example, various cost functions have been proposed to optimize musculoskeletal function during locomotion, including minimization of: muscle forces (170), [muscle stress]^3 (30), or [muscle force/moment]^3 (81).

In contrast to static optimization, which only calculates the inputs at one instant in time (independent of past or future system states), a *dynamic optimization* algorithm incorporates ". . . a model of the system dynamics to find the inputs (e.g., EMGs), and all the outputs (e.g., forces), that maximize the performance of the whole task as defined by some single criterion." (211, p. 193). Although tractable, dynamic optimizations are computationally daunting, and (as with the cost function) finding a suitable "performance criterion" has also proven elusive. Nevertheless, the tantalizing power of dynamic optimization resides in the scope of the modeling; in addition to a model of the system dynamics, there is a model of what the movement task is trying to achieve (the performance criterion) (78, 118, 212). Although dynamic optimization has been employed to analyze jumping (77, 118), walking (25, 34), kicking (79), and arm movements (139), Zajac and Gordon (211) concluded that the full potential of the method remains to be realized.

INSIGHTS FROM INVERSE DYNAMICS

Equations of Motion

While the methods of inverse dynamics are not as mathematically complex or as potentially powerful as dynamic optimization methods, inverse dynamics techniques have, nonetheless, enabled researchers to understand more fully the biomechanical substrate of motor control and learning. Here, we provide a primer of inverse dynamics methods and illustrate how they have led to insights and predictions about neural control, using the cat paw-shake response as an example.

Inverse-dynamics equations of motion can be formulated in several ways, but the form we have used allows quantification not only of how muscles and gravity influence limb motion but also of how the motion of one segment affects other segments (limb intersegmental dynamics), which can be particularly significant in freely moving (unconstrained) limbs (100, 101, 184, 211). At each of the joints of the linked segments, we can partition the torques into five categories: net joint torque, gravitational torque, motion-dependent torques, contact torques, and generalized muscle torque (53, 100–102, 146, 165, 166, 168, 182, 192, 207, 214, 215). Using Newtonian equations, the net, gravitational, and motion-dependent torques are calculated directly from limb kinematics and anthropometric data. Contact torques arise whenever external forces influence limb motion, and a force transducer is typically used to quantify this component. The single unknown (generalized muscle torque) in the equation is calculated as a *residual* term, and the sum of the generalized muscle torque and the other torque components must equal the net joint torque ($\Sigma M = I \cdot \alpha$). These relations can be expressed as:

$$\begin{aligned} \textit{Net joint torque} &= \textit{gravitational torque} \\ &+ \textit{motion-dependent torques} \\ &+ \textit{contact torques} \\ &+ \textit{generalized muscle torque} \end{aligned} \quad (1)$$

where,

1. *Net joint torque* is the product of the segmental moment of inertia and segmental angular acceleration ($I \cdot \alpha$); it is the sum of all positive and negative torque components (gravitational, motion-dependent, contact, and muscle) acting at a joint.
2. *Gravitational torque* arises from gravity acting at the center of mass of each segment.
3. *Motion-dependent torques* are due to the motion of the segments in a linked system. These torques arise from mechanical interactions among segments, such as inertial forces proportional to segmental accelerations or centripetal forces proportional to the square of segmental velocities. For example, in the equations of motion for the arm, motion-dependent torques are related to: *(1)* shoulder linear accelerations; *(2)* upper arm, forearm, and hand angular accelerations; and *(3)* upper arm, forearm, and hand angular velocities. These components can be examined individually or summed and examined as the *total motion-dependent torque* (215). These torques quantify the limb intersegmental dynamics and are the "reactive phenomena" described by Bernstein when he said that ". . . the secret of coordination lies not only in not wasting superfluous force in extinguishing reactive phenomena but, on the contrary, in employing the latter in such a way as to employ active muscle forces only in the capacity of complementary forces." (8, p. 109)—these are the torque components that the mover should *exploit rather than resist.*
4. *Contact torques* are generated at joints as a consequence of external forces acting on limb segments. For example, during walking, ground reaction forces can produce torques at the ankle, knee, and hip joints of the lower extremity. With a freely moving and unconstrained limb (as in the swing phase of walking), the contact torque term in equation 1 will be zero.
5. *A generalized muscle torque* includes forces arising from active muscle contractions and from passive deformations of muscles, tendons, ligaments, and other periarticular tissues. Because the effects of active muscular forces are embedded within this component, the generalized muscle torque comprises the actively controlled elements of motor patterns; information about this torque component is important for revealing changes in the control of intralimb coordination.

In reviewing studies that quantify limb dynamics, differences in terms must be carefully noted. As mentioned earlier, the methods of *inverse dynamics* permit several, equally valid forms of rigid-body equations motion. Why a particular mathematical formulation is chosen by a research group, generally, relates to the specific questions the investigators hope to answer. Different names can refer to similar (or the same) mathematical quantities and, currently, there is no standard nomenclature in this area. For example, although we use D'Alembert's principle for calculating dynamic equilibrium, functionally, we prefer to think of ($I \cdot \alpha$) as the *net effect* of the torques applied to a segment ($\Sigma M = I \cdot \alpha$). We calculate *net joint torque* as the product of *segmental* angular acceleration (α) and *segmental* moment of inertia (I) (cf. equation 1), as has been done by numerous researchers (17, 10, 124, 143, 204). Ghez and co-workers (28, 58, 162) retain the basic D'Alembert form [$\Sigma M + (-I \cdot \alpha) = 0$] and calculate a term they call *self torque* ($-I \cdot \alpha$). Although *net joint torque* ($I \cdot \alpha$) appears to be the inverse of *self torque* ($-I \cdot \alpha$), this is not true, because the *self torque* represents the *joint* angular acceleration multiplied by the *effective inertia carried by the joint* as a part of a linked system (see later under Disrupted Proprioception Affects Limb Dynamics for details). Also, *generalized muscle torque* (28, 53, 58, 100–102, 146, 162, 165, 166, 168, 183, 207, 214, 215) is the same term some call *joint torque* (98, 185, 204), and while we use the term *motion-dependent torques*, others refer to *interaction torques* (28, 58, 162). Regardless of these differences in terms and formulation details, the fundamental approach to using inverse dynamics for answering questions about motor control is similar among investigators.

One other difference in inverse dynamics formations should be pointed out, because it may cause confusion in evaluating results. Must motion-dependent torques always be included in equation 1, or can they be neglected? The answer to that question depends on the movement studied. In unconstrained limb movements, motion-dependent torques can be significant, particularly if the movements are rapid (101, 162, 184, 211). Thus, motion-dependent torques must be calculated explicitly. In other movement circumstances, motion-dependent torques can be neglected with impunity (17), because they are insignificant compared to other forces. During the stance phase of walking, for example, the lower-limb inertial and centripetal forces are very small compared to the large forces supporting the weight of the body (53, 146, 204). The legitimacy of neglecting motion-dependent torques for stance was recently confirmed by Fowler and co-workers (53), who used a rigid-body dynamics formulation that neglected the limb's motion-dependent torques. In spite of this, they reported an excellent agreement between directly measured ankle muscle forces and ankle muscle forces estimated from inverse dynamics methods. (For more details see Stance Dynamics for Different Forms of Cat Walking and Fig. 8.18 of that section.)

Anthropometric Data

To use inverse dynamics to calculate joint forces and torques, accurate estimates are needed of segmental masses (m), center-of-mass locations, and segmental moments of inertia (I). In Manter's pioneering study (124), using force platforms and inverse dynamics to quantify the dynamics of cat locomotion, mass parameter data were reported for one cat. Hoy and Zernicke (100), later, took similar detailed anatomical measurements, determined mass parameters for a group of cats, and developed regression equations to predict the segment mass and inertial parameters of comparable cats. Their regression equations can accurately estimate (average multiple $R = 0.96$) cat fore- and hindlimb segmental moments of inertia, when only the total body mass, segment mass, and segment length are known.

For human adults, body segment parameters can be approximated by using published values (36), regression equations (24, 26, 209), or mathematical models (75, 76). With the Hatze model, for example, the human body is approximated by 17 segments with various geometric shapes. With standard anthropometric instrumentation, 242 measurements are taken to calculate the volumes of the 17 body segments, and body density values determined from cadaver studies (36) are used to calculate the mass, center-of-mass location, and moment of inertia of each body segment.

Although data have been published for children (106), until recently, no body segment parameter data existed for infants. The absence of such data precluded inverse dynamics analyses for infants. Schneider and colleagues (166), however, took anthropometric data from 18 infants and modified Hatze's three-dimensional model (75, 76) to make it applicable for infants (166). Using the modified model, with measurements from 44 infants for upper limbs and from 70 infants for lower limbs, the anthropometric inertial parameters (masses, center-of-mass locations, and transverse moments of inertia) for infant upper and lower limb segments were determined and used to formulate regression equations that predict limb anthropometric inertial parameters for use in equations of motion to analyze the limb dynamics of human infants (169). With these equations, researchers can calculate estimates of body segment parameters for use in dynamics analyses by knowing an infant's age, body mass, and the length and circumference of the segment of interest.

Predictions Using an Inverse Dynamics Model

As noted in the preceding section, the basic elements of inverse dynamics (rigid-body equations of motion and inertial parameters) are readily available for quantifying human and animal motion. But how can inverse dynamics techniques and a knowledge of limb dynamics provide insights into neural control mechanisms? One example of the utility of inverse dynamics for answering questions about neuromotor control emerges from a series of studies of the cat paw-shake response (53, 74, 101, 102, 112–114, 182).

The paw-shake response is a rapid and stereotypic pattern of cyclic hip, knee, and ankle motions that a cat uses to remove an irritant, such as water or tape, from its paw. This behavior is easily elicited in normal cats and cats that have recovered from spinal-cord surgical transection at a low thoracic level (182). Since the paw-shaking motor patterns are similar in normal and spinalized cats, here, we focus on the hindlimb dynamics of spinalized cats to emphasize the motor and integrative capacity of the lumbrosacral spinal cord in the absence of supraspinal influences (182).

To evoke a paw shake, a spinalized cat is held vertically, and tape is wrapped around the paw (Fig. 8.4*A*). The entire response consists of 8–12 cycles, in which the middle cycles may show steady-state oscillations (Fig. 8.4C). Each steady-state cycle (78–91 ms in duration) reveals an intriguing interplay of ankle and knee kinematics and dynamics. For example, the conjoint motions of the ankle and knee are evident in a representative steady-state cycle (Fig. 8.4*D*). At cycle onset (maximum ankle extension, see Fig. 8.4*A*, position 1), the ankle and knee joint motions are out of phase—the knee extends while the ankle flexes (Fig. 8.4*D*, *diagonal line a–b*). During this combined motion of the ankle and knee, an active lateral gastrocnemius muscle–tendon unit is forcibly stretched (ankle flexing, knee extending). In the remainder of the cycle, knee and ankle motions are sequential—first the knee flexes as the active vastus lateralis muscle–tendon unit is stretched (Fig. 8.4*D*, *vertical line b–c*) and then the ankle extends as the active tibialis anterior muscle–tendon unit is stretched (Fig. 8.4*D*, *horizontal line c–a*).

Throughout each steady-state cycle, a net ankle joint torque slows and reverses ankle motion (Fig. 8.5). During flexion, the net torque decreases its tendency to flex the ankle and achieves a maximum extensor effect prior to peak ankle flexion. While the ankle extends, the tendency of the net torque to extend the ankle decreases, and a maximum flexor effect is achieved prior to peak ankle extension. At the ankle joint the generalized muscle torque has a dominant effect on the net torque, as the influences of the component torques (gravity and motion-dependent torques) are minor (Fig. 8.5). Thus, the ankle muscle torque determines the ankle joint motion during the paw-shake cycle.

At the knee joint, however, motion-dependent torques are large and contribute substantially to the net knee torque. Torques related to paw angular acceleration dominate the motion-dependent torque

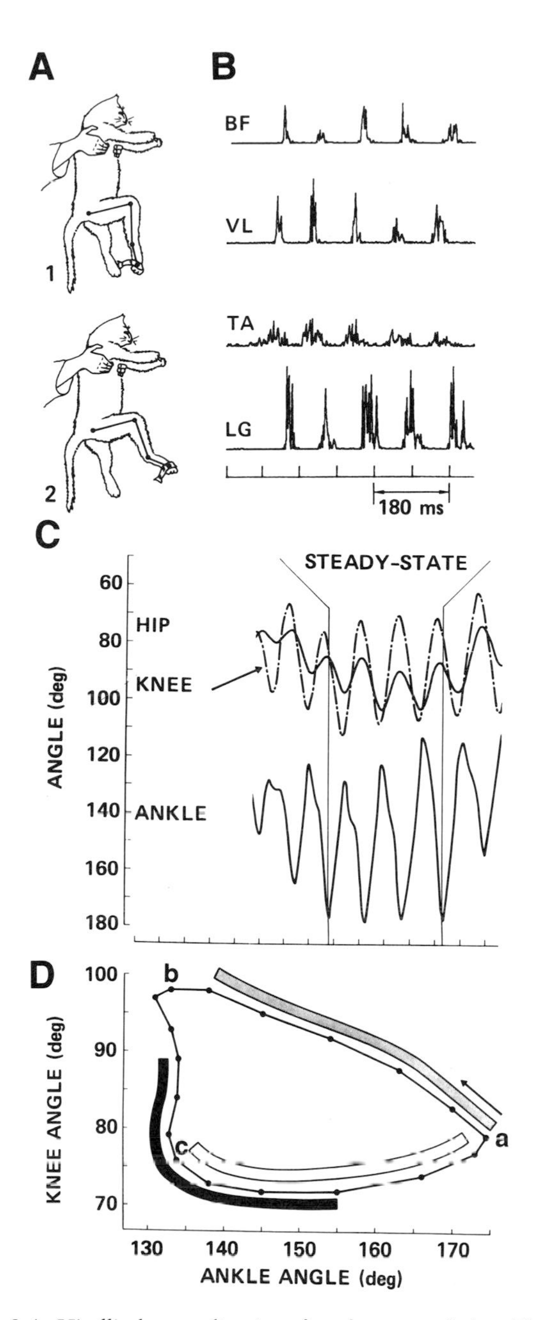

FIG. 8.4. Hindlimb coordination for the paw shake. The response is tested with the spinalized cat held vertically; tape is wrapped around the paw (*A*). Positions at the start of a cycle (*A1*, peak ankle extension) and mid-cycle (*A2*, peak ankle flexion) are shown. Hindlimb segments (thigh, leg, paw) are outlined; each joint (hip, knee, ankle) is marked by a *dot*. In *B*, EMG records of four cycles are from an ankle extensor (LG) and flexor (TA); knee extensor (VL) and hip extensor–knee flexor (BF). Kinematics for four steady-state cycles are shown in C; 50 ms intervals mark the abscissa. An angle–angle plot in *D* illustrates knee-ankle coordination for steady-state cycles. Each cycle begins at peak ankle extension (*a*) and proceeds in a counterclockwise direction. First the knee extends and ankle flexes. Peak knee extension (*b*) precedes peak ankle flexion. Next, the knee flexes and later the ankle extends (*c*). Dots on the curve mark time intervals of 5 ms. *Bars* indicate timing of EMG bursts for LG and BF (*stippled*), VL (*shaded*), and TA (*unshaded*). [Adapted from Figs. 2 and 3 of Smith and Zernicke (182).]

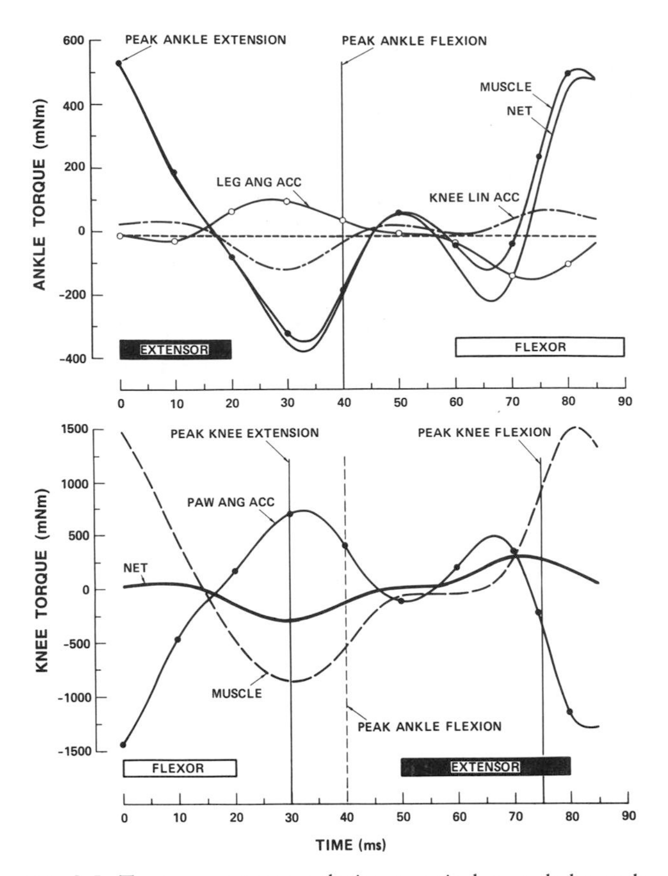

FIG. 8.5. Torque components during a typical paw-shake cycle. The net, muscle, and motion-dependent torques are shown for the ankle (*top*) and knee (*bottom*) joints. The gravitational torque was negligible at both joints and is not illustrated. At the ankle, the main motion-related torques (leg angular acceleration and knee linear acceleration) counterbalance each other, and the muscle torque dominated the net torque. Positive values represent flexor torques. At the knee, paw angular acceleration (the main inertial torque) is counterbalanced by muscle torque, and net torque is negligible. Positive values represent extensor torques. *Bars* show the timing of EMG bursts for extensor and flexor muscles at the ankle and knee. Records are aligned by cycle time; *vertical lines* mark kinematic events. [Adapted from Figs. 5A and 7A of Hoy et al. (102).]

components at the knee, but the effect of this motion-dependent torque is counteracted by the knee muscle torque, associated with recruitment of knee flexor muscles (Fig. 8.5). When the knee is fully extended during the cycle, the knee muscle torque is flexor to counterbalance the extensor torque associated with paw angular acceleration. Throughout the remainder of the cycle there continues to be a "mirror" or reciprocal interplay of the paw angular acceleration and muscle torques at the knee.

Thus, a key finding from these paw-shake dynamics analyses is that ankle muscles produce torques to control the paw dynamics directly, but the knee muscles produce torques to control the motion-dependent torques between the paw and lower leg (101, 102, 183). Before these inverse dynamics analyses, no data suggested that the motions at the ankle and knee were controlled differentially during paw shaking (183).

Armed with this information about paw-shake limb dynamics, predictions were made about the neural mechanisms responsible for controlling the movement. One obvious prediction was that motion-dependent feedback associated with paw angular acceleration is useful in setting the onset and recruitment level of knee muscles during the paw-shake cycle (101, 102, 183). Thus, in response to feedback disruption, the muscle recruitment pattern at the knee should be altered, but the muscle recruitment pattern at the ankle should be unaltered. To test that prediction, several experiments were conducted in which motion-dependent feedback from the hindlimb was altered (74, 113, 114). When, for example, a paw shake was elicited with the ankle and knee joints immobilized by a plaster cast, there was disruption of the knee extensor EMG pattern, but the flexor-extensor EMG patterns at the ankle were unaffected (Fig. 8.6*A*).

As another way of changing the normal feedback to the knee joint, Hart et al. (74) increased the mass of the paw by twofold. This substantial increase in paw mass (and altered paw moment of inertia) would have significant effects on the paw angular acceleration torques being generated at the knee. As illustrated in Figure 8.6*B*, the added mass on the cat's paw severely disrupted the vastus lateralis (knee extensor) EMG pattern, while the EMGs of the ankle flexor and extensor were unaltered from normal paw shaking. Thus, in the paw shake, there appears to be a differential neural control strategy for the ankle and knee joints. Results of the limb-casting and paw-weighting studies also suggest that lumbosacral networks responsible for the activity patterns of the ankle muscles may be preprogrammed and insensitive to proprioceptive perturbations.

CONTROL OF DIFFERENT LOCOMOTION FORMS

In contrast to the novel paw-shake response, locomotion provides a more generic example of the motor control insights to be gained from dynamics analyses. Interest in the biomechanics of locomotion and the role of dynamics in controlling or regulating various aspects of the step cycle originated with the pioneering research of Manter (124) for quadrupeds; and Fenn (44), Bresler and Frankel (17), Inman (104), and Bernstein (8) for humans. In this section, we will not recapitulate the wealth of biomechanical data on locomotion (for reviews, see 104, 105, 141,

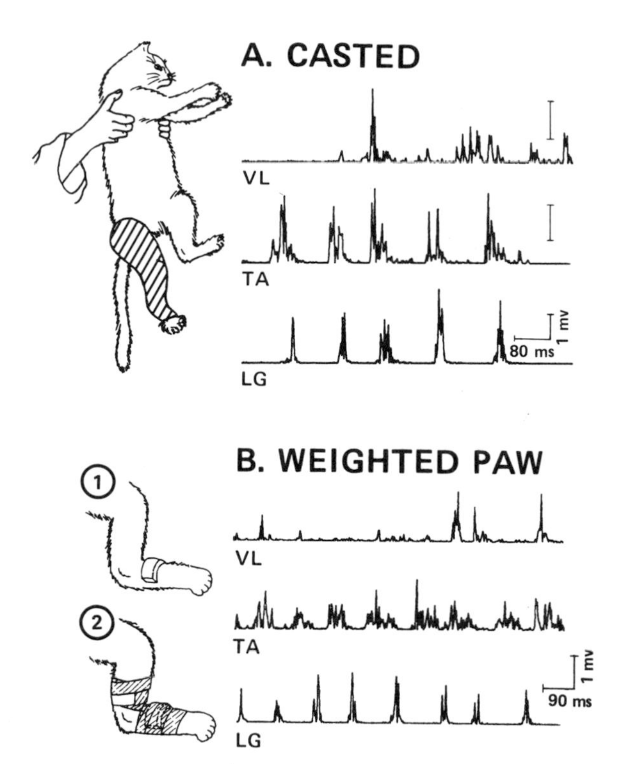

FIG. 8.6. Disruption of knee extensor activity during paw-shake responses elicited under two conditions. The EMG record in *A* shows a paw-shake response with knee and ankle joint immobilized by a plaster cast, while the record in *B* shows a response with a flexible piece of lead (46 g) secured to the paw (*B1*) by self-adhesive, elastic tape (*B2*). Under these conditions, the knee extensor (VL) activity was disrupted, but burst durations of ankle flexor (TA) and extensor (LG) muscles and their reciprocal activity were not perturbed. [Adapted from Fig. 6 of Smith and Zernicke (182).]

204), but we will focus on recent studies in which the application of inverse dynamics techniques generated predictions for neural control.

The two phases of the step cycle, swing and stance, are treated separately, and for both, data from the human lower limb and cat hindlimb illustrate basic concepts and insights for neural control. For the swing phase, data from dynamics analyses of the knee joint are presented to demonstrate basic principles, and to avoid unnecessary repetition, little attention is given to analogous data sets for the hip and ankle joints. For both swing and stance, the dynamics of forward walking are used as the foundation for understanding changes that occur with speed, gait, and different forms of walking, including backward and slope walking.

Swing-Phase Dynamics

Knee-Joint Dynamics during Swing for the Walk. At moderate walking speeds, the human knee joint undergoes a small range of flexion (15–24 degrees) to lift the foot during the flexion (F) phase of swing (Fig. 8.7*A*). Soon after knee flexion peaks (~120 degrees), knee extension is initiated. At the end of extension, the E phase [called E_1 by Philippson (148)], the knee joint is maximally extended (~180 degrees) for heel strike (138, 199, 215). Thus, the range of knee flexion is markedly less than for extension, and the F–E_1 transition occurs early in swing to bring the foot forward for heel contact (Fig. 8.7*A*).

The knee torque components associated with swing are illustrated in Figure 8.7*A*. Knee flexion at the onset of swing is due to the sum of the motion-dependent torques, of which a major component is leg angular acceleration. This inertial flexor torque is counterbalanced by the tendency of gravity and an extensor muscle torque (small in magnitude) to extend the knee. At midswing, the sum of the motion-dependent torque components becomes extensor and is counterbalanced largely by a flexor muscle torque.

From the kinetic data, we can predict that although contraction of knee flexor muscles is not needed to flex the knee at the onset of swing, contraction may be required at the end of swing to decelerate knee extension produced by the inertial motion-dependent torque component. Consistent with these predictions, EMG studies (138, 193, 205) show that knee flexor muscles, such as the hamstrings, are typically active only at the end of swing (see St-Sm in Fig. 8.8). Since knee extensor muscles, such as the vastii or rectus femoris, are also inactive at the onset of swing for a slow walk and slow run (see VL, VM, and RF at 1.4 m · s^{-1} in Fig. 8.8), it is possible that the small extensor muscle torque at the onset of swing is due largely to passive deformation of the periarticular and muscle tissues about the knee joint.

For the cat hindlimb, knee-joint kinematics and kinetics during swing are similar to those of the human lower limb, except for the torque components at the onset of swing. At moderate walking speeds, the cat's knee joint flexes about 25 degrees to lift the paw and then extends about 45 degrees to bring the paw forward for contact, with the F–E_1 transition occurring early in swing [Fig. 8.9; (20, 73, 207)]. At the onset of swing, a flexor muscle torque and the sum of the motion-dependent torques oppose an extensor gravity torque to create a net flexor torque (Fig. 8.10). In contrast to the human knee joint, power is generated at this phase, as the cat's knee flexes in conjunction with a flexor muscle torque (146). Recruitment of knee flexor muscles, such as the semitendinosus at the onset of swing [see ST in Fig. 8.9; (18, 39)] and posterior compartment of the

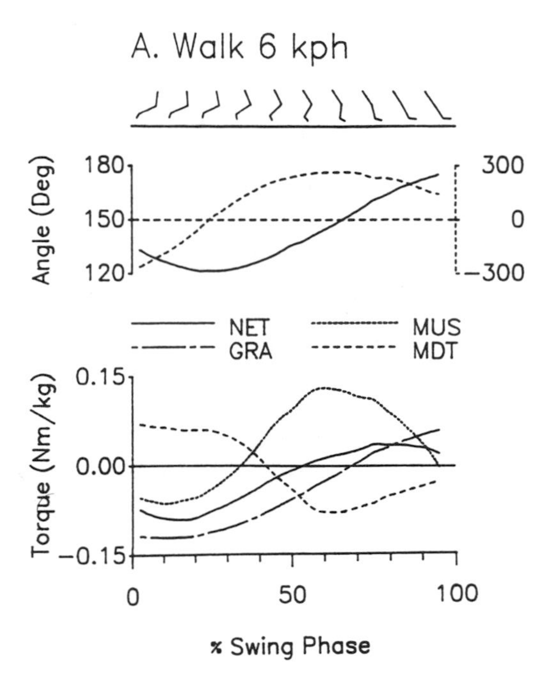

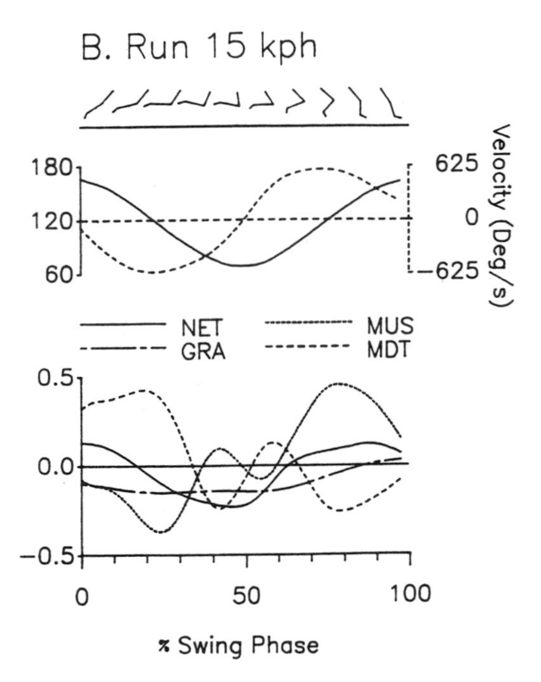

FIG. 8.7. Swing-phase kinematics and kinetics of the human knee joint for walking (1.67 m · s^{-1}) and running (4.16 m · s^{-1}). At the top of each panel, the position of the leg is shown at various stages of swing, from toe-off to heel contact. Upper plots show the angular displacement (*solid line*) and velocity (*dashed line*) for the knee joint. Middle plots illustrate the NET torque at the knee, and its three main components: NET = gravity (GRA) + muscle (MUS) + summed motion-dependent torque (MDT). Positive values represent flexor torques; negative values represent extensor torques. Data are normalized to the percentage of swing, and torque data are normalized to subject mass (Nm/kg). [Unpublished data from Zernicke et al. (215).]

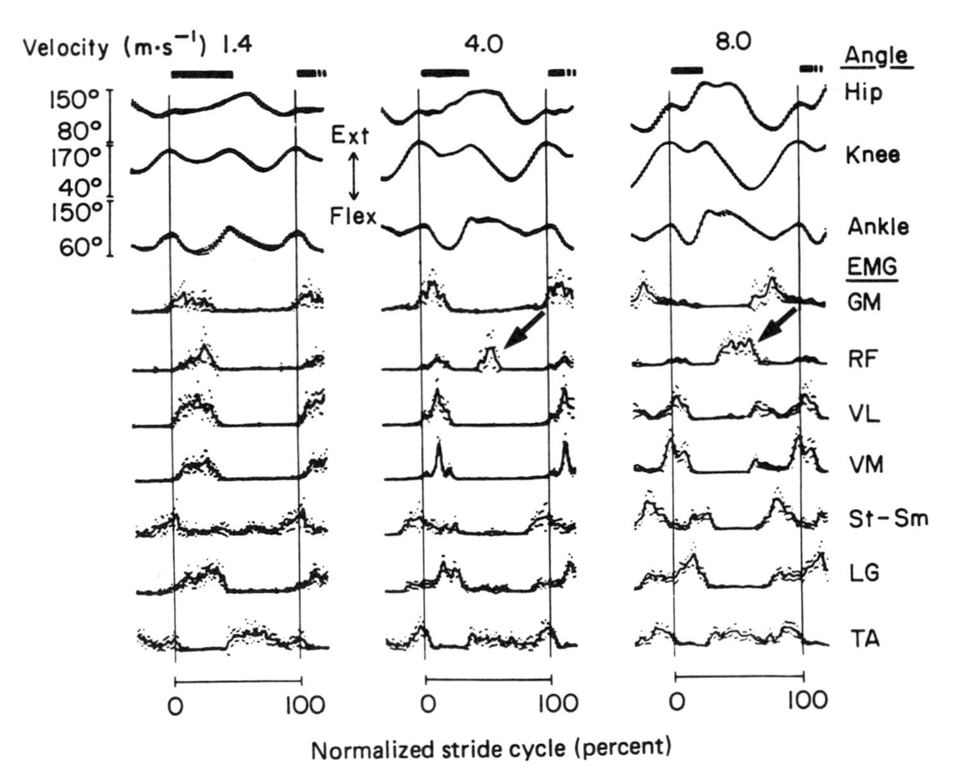

FIG. 8.8. Angular displacements and EMG for three speeds (human). Displacement data are normalized to percentage of step cycle, 0% = heel strike (stance onset) and 100% = toe-off (swing onset). Stance is indicated by a *bar* at the top of each record. GM, gluteus maximus (hip extensor); RF, rectus femoris (hip flexor, knee extensor; see text for explanation of *arrows*); VL, vastus lateralis (knee extensor); St-Sm, semitendinosus–semimembranous (hip extensor, knee flexor); LG, lateral gastrocnemius (knee flexor, ankle extensor); TA, tibialis anterior (ankle flexor). [Adapted from Fig. 11 of Nilsson et al. (138).]

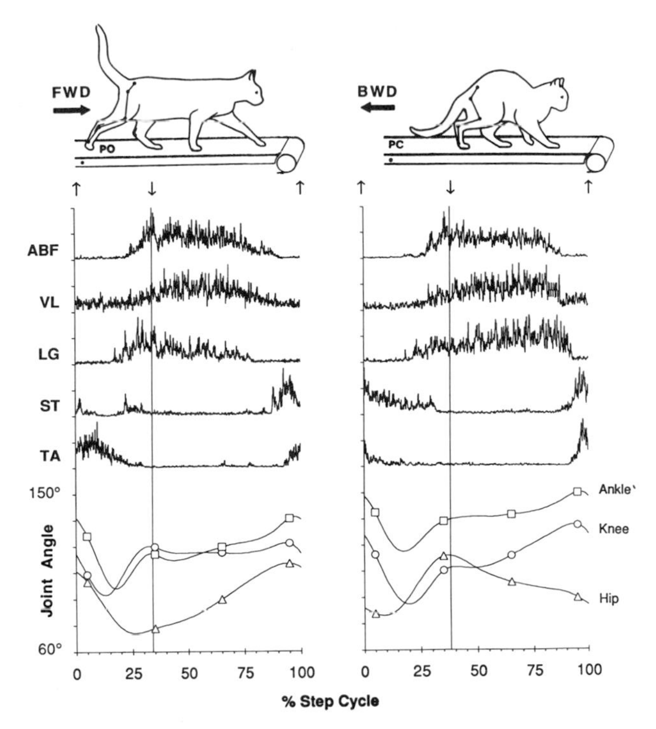

FIG. 8.9. Two forms of walking for the cat. The cat's position at paw-off (onset of swing) is illustrated for forward (FWD) walking, and the cat's position at paw contact (onset of stance) is shown for backward (BWD) walking. [Adapted from Fig. 1 of Smith et al. (178).] Typical EMG records and angular displacement for the hip, knee, and ankle are also illustrated for both forms of walking. ABF, anterior biceps femoris (hip extensor); VL, vastus lateralis (knee extensor); LG, lateral gastrocnemius (knee flexor, ankle extensor); ST, (hip extensor, knee flexor); TA, ankle flexor. *Arrows* at the top mark paw-off (*up arrow*) and paw contact (*down arrow*). [Adapted from Fig. 1 of Perell et al. (142).]

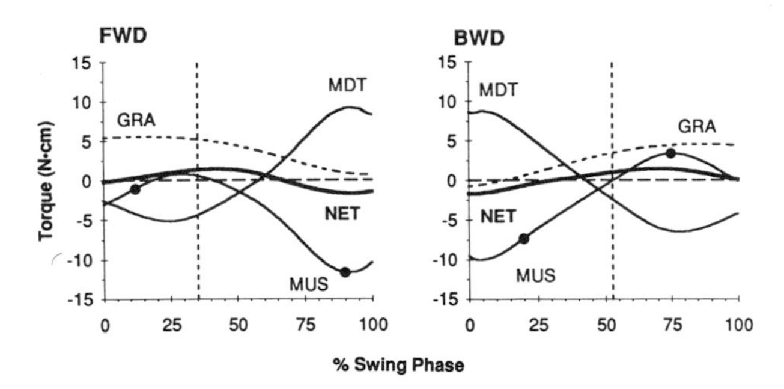

FIG. 8.10. Average swing-phase kinetics at a cat knee joint for several forward (FWD) and backward (BWD) steps at 0.6 m · s^{-1}. Positive values represent extensor torques, and negative values represent flexor torques; the *dashed horizontal line* indicates zero torque. *Dotted vertical lines* indicate the reversal from flexion to extension ($F-E_1$) at the knee joint. Torque components are: net torque (NET), gravitational torque (GRA), sum of the motion-dependent (MDT), and the muscle (MUS). [Adapted from Fig. 2 of Perell et al. (146).]

biceps femoris (23, 41), is consistent with the existence of a flexor muscle torque and power generation.

At the end of swing, the magnitude of the flexor muscle torque increases sharply at the knee joints of cats and humans, and power is absorbed as the knee extends in conjunction with a flexor muscle torque. During this terminal phase of swing, an inertial torque due to leg angular acceleration tends to extend the knee, and a flexor muscle torque counteracts this inertial torque. Activity of hamstring muscles at the end of the swing phase for humans (see St-Sm of Fig. 8.8) and cats (see ST in Fig. 8.9) during walking is consistent with the inverse dynamics finding of a flexor muscle torque at the knee. In slow-walking cats, however, there may be no knee flexor activity at the end of swing (6, 73, 179). During these steps, the flexor muscle torque at the knee is small, and Smith and Zernicke (183) hypothesized that the elastic recoil of stretching musculotendinous tissues of hamstring muscles (passive forces) is sufficient to decelerate knee extension at the end of swing. As walking speed increases, however, active forces are needed to combine with passive forces to decelerate knee extension at the end of swing.

Speed- and Gait-Related Changes in Swing Dynamics. Limb dynamics are speed related, and knowledge of these changes provides insight into the neural control of locomotion. As speed increases, humans switch from a walk to a run (195), the knee joint undergoes a greater range of motion, and angular velocities increase during swing (Fig. 8.7*B*). While profiles of the major torque components at the knee are similar for the walk and run, two speed-related changes are evident. First, the muscle torque and most motion-dependent torques are appreciably larger in magnitude, and second, there is a sizable extensor muscle torque during the first half of swing for the run that is not typical of the walk (Fig. 8.7).

Knowledge of speed-related differences about knee joint kinetics provides insight for understanding the EMG data reported by Nilsson and coworkers (138). They found that EMG amplitude (peak and integrated values) increased with speed, and during swing this was particularly notable for rectus femoris at the onset of swing. At slower speeds, the rectus femoris (knee extensor, hip flexor) exhibits a stance-related burst and is inactive during swing (see RF at 1.4 m · s^{-1} in Fig. 8.8). At faster walking speeds and running, however, a second burst becomes prominent at the onset of swing, and the magnitude and duration of this burst increase with speed (see *arrows* at 4 and 8 m · s^{-1} in Fig. 8.8). The additional rectus femoris burst at the onset of swing coincides with the need to counterbalance a large knee extensor torque related to leg angular acceleration, as well as the need for an increased flexor muscle torque at the hip.

Although the magnitude of the extensor muscle torque at the knee increases with speed at the onset of swing, uniarticular knee extensors, such as the vastii, are not recruited and do not actively contribute to this torque component (see VL and VM in Fig. 8.8). The burden of actively contributing to the muscle torque at the knee depends, therefore, on the recruitment of bifunctional muscles. Smith et al. (179) also found that recruitment patterns of bifunctional muscle were more responsive to speed-related changes in limb dynamics during swing than uniarticular muscles. Their example, described below, is drawn from speed- and gait-related changes at the cat's knee joint during swing.

The cat has three speed-related gaits (see 12, 69, 83, 84 and Chapter 5 in this *Handbook* for a full account of gaits). Compared to the slow walk, the range of knee flexion doubles (25 degrees vs. 50 degrees) during a slow gallop, and peak velocity of knee flexion increases linearly with speed (207). The range of knee extension increases more modestly; nonetheless, there is a linear increase in knee extension velocity with speed increases (207). Knee joint dynamics during swing are similar for the walk and trot, except that the muscle torque components and sum of the motion-dependent torques have larger magnitudes in the trot (207). At the trot-gallop transition, however, knee-joint dynamics reflect gait differences that are independent of speed. Smith et al. (179) obtained kinetic data from fast trotting steps and slow galloping steps recorded at 2.25 m · s^{-1}. For the trot, there was a robust *flexor* muscle torque at the knee during the onset of swing, but for the gallop, there was an *extensor* muscle torque at the onset (Fig. 8.11). Consequently, power was generated at the knee at the onset of the trot swing but absorbed at that same phase for the gallop.

Gait-related changes in the cat's knee-joint dynamics at the onset of swing are related to a precipitous increase in the magnitude of a flexor torque due to hip linear acceleration (100, 179, 207). During galloping, this motion-related torque tends to flex the knee at the onset of swing; this tendency increases in magnitude with gallop speed and is countered by an extensor muscle torque (207). The increased torque component due to hip linear acceleration is probably linked to increased extension of the lower spine that occurs at the end of stance and is sustained during the first part of swing (40, 63), in contrast to trunk muscle actions in human locomotion (194).

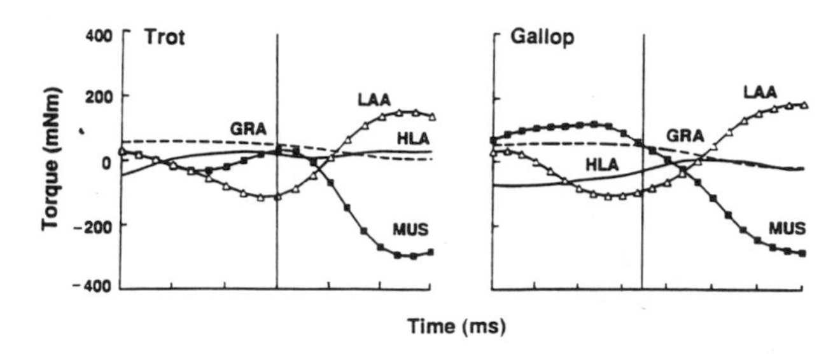

FIG. 8.11. Average swing-phase kinetics for the cat knee joint for several trot and gallop steps at 2.25 m · s^{-1}. *Vertical line* marks the F-E_1 transition. Torque components are: net torque (NET), gravitational torque (GRA), sum of motion dependent (MDT), and the muscle (MUS); here, motion-dependent torque components include leg angular acceleration (LAA) and hip linear acceleration (HLA). Positive values represent extensor torques, and negative values represent flexor torques. Time marks indicate 30 ms intervals. [Adapted from Fig. 9 of Smith et al. (179).]

Based on knee-joint dynamics data, Smith and colleagues (179) made predictions about the recruitment of knee flexor and extensor muscles during the swing phase of the gallop. First, they predicted there was no need for knee-flexor activity at the onset of swing, and second, they predicted a need for knee-extensor activity at the onset of swing. Regarding the first prediction, they (179) found that the flexor-related activity of the semitendinosus (a knee flexor) was virtually absent at the onset of swing for high gallop speeds and greatly reduced at slow gallop speeds (see STpo in Fig. 8.12). During the trot, however, knee flexor activity was robust, and increases in the duration and amplitude of flexor EMG were associated with increases in the duration and magnitude of the flexor muscle torque at the knee.

With the prediction for knee extensor activity at the onset of swing, Smith et al. (179) found that uniarticular knee extensors, such as the vastus lateralis, were not recruited. The recruitment of cat uniarticular extensor muscles, in fact, appears to be tightly linked to a stance-related synergy that is preset by the spinal pattern generator for locomotion (see later under Insights for Neural Control of Locomotion). Recruitment of bifunctional muscles, in contrast, appears to be mutable and responsive to changes in hindlimb dynamics. The cat's rectus femoris, a bifunctional muscle with hip flexor and knee extensor functions, provides a good example. The rectus femoris is usually active only at midstance during the walk and trot, but the rectus femoris may be continuously active from midstance to the end of the F phase of swing during the gallop (39, 159). If active at the onset of the gallop swing, the rectus femoris muscle will contribute actively to the extensor muscle torque at the knee joint.

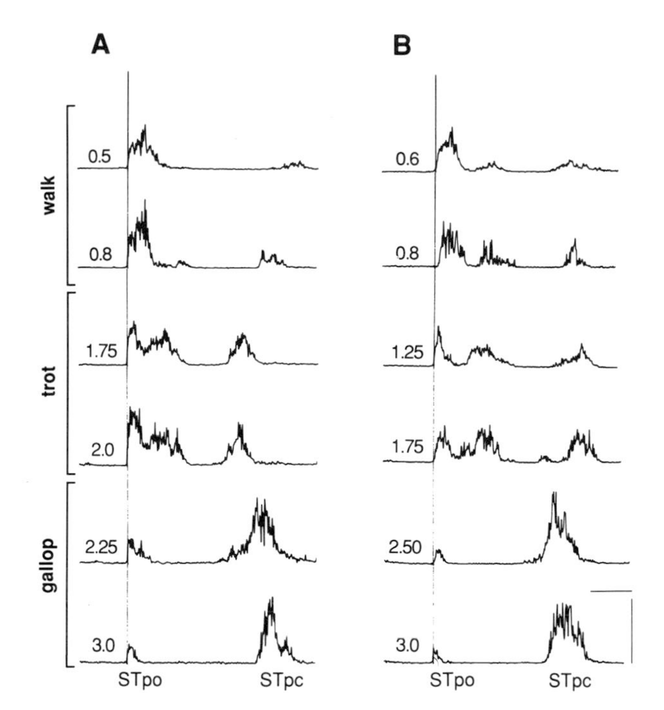

FIG. 8.12. Rectified-averaged EMG records from the semitendinosus (ST) for two speeds of walking, trotting, and galloping of two cats (*A* and *B*). The time-averaged records were triggered from the onset of the flexor-related burst at paw-off (STpo), marked by *vertical lines*. A total of 62 steps were averaged for cat *A* and 64 steps for cat *B*. Scale bars: horizontal, 80 ms; vertical, 1.0 mV for cat *A* and 0.5 mV for cat *B*. [Taken from Fig. 2 of Smith et al. (179) with publisher's permission.]

The two compartments of the cat's sartorius muscles offer another example of the bifunctional-mutability principle. The anterior compartment is bifunctional (hip flexor, knee extensor), but the medial compartment is unifunctional (hip and knee flexor). Both are active at the onset of swing for the walk and trot [see SAa and SAm of Fig. 8.13*A*; (91, 153–155, 159)]. While the EMG amplitude of the anterior sartorius EMG increases at the onset of the gallop swing, the EMG amplitude of the medial sartorius does not (C. A. Pratt and J. L. Smith, unpublished data). This recruitment difference is consistent with knee joint dynamics associated with the gallop swing.

Effects of Walking Forms on Swing-Phase Dynamics. Walking can take several forms that require a change of direction, such as backward or lateral walking, and changes in level, such as up-slope or down-slope walking. To illustrate how knowledge of changes in swing-phase dynamics provides insights for the neural control of walking, we compare kinematic and kinetic data for forward and backward walking, as well as the EMG for selected muscles.

During human backward walking, flexion at the knee joint lifts the foot at the onset of swing, and then the knee joint extends to position the toe for contact [Fig. 8.14; (193, 199, 205)]. The range of flexion exceeds that of extension, and the F–E_1 transition occurs late in swing. During most of the swing phase for backward walking, power is generated, and knee flexion coincides with a flexor muscle torque (Fig. 8.14). The presence of a long-lasting knee flexor torque is consistent with EMG data showing knee flexor activity (e.g., hamstring muscles) during the first half of backward swing (193). Thus, hamstring muscles are active at the end of forward swing to decelerate knee extension (power absorption) and during the first half of backward swing to accelerate knee flexion (power generation).

During backward walking, the cat's knee joint experiences a greater range of flexion, and the F–E_1

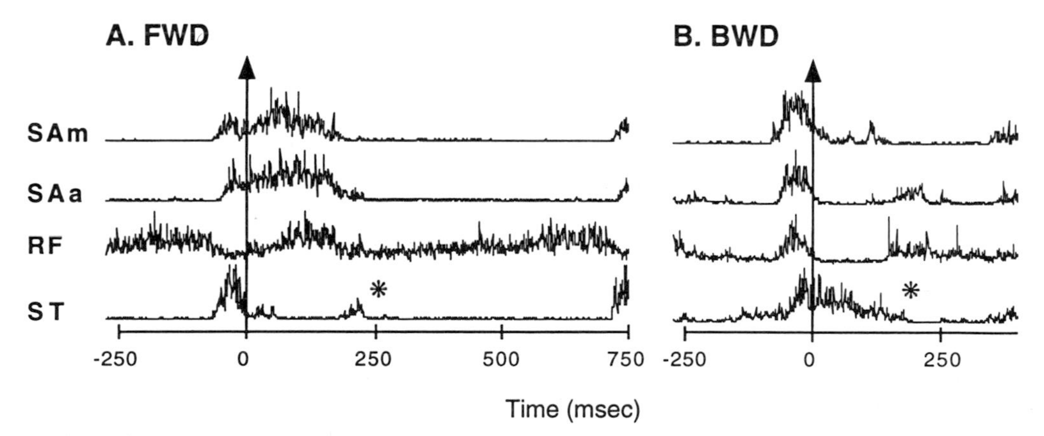

FIG. 8.13. Averaged-rectified EMG data of four biarticular muscles for several forward (*A*) and backward (*B*) treadmill steps (cat). Muscles are: medial and anterior sartorius (SAm, SAa), rectus femoris (RF), and the semitendinosus (ST). EMG data were averaged at paw-off (*arrow*). Asterisks (*) indicate paw contact. With calibration settings in *B* taken as 1, settings in *A* are 1.25 for SAm, 1.5 for SAa, 2.25 for RF, and 2.75 for ST. [Adapted from Fig. 3 of Pratt et al. (154).]

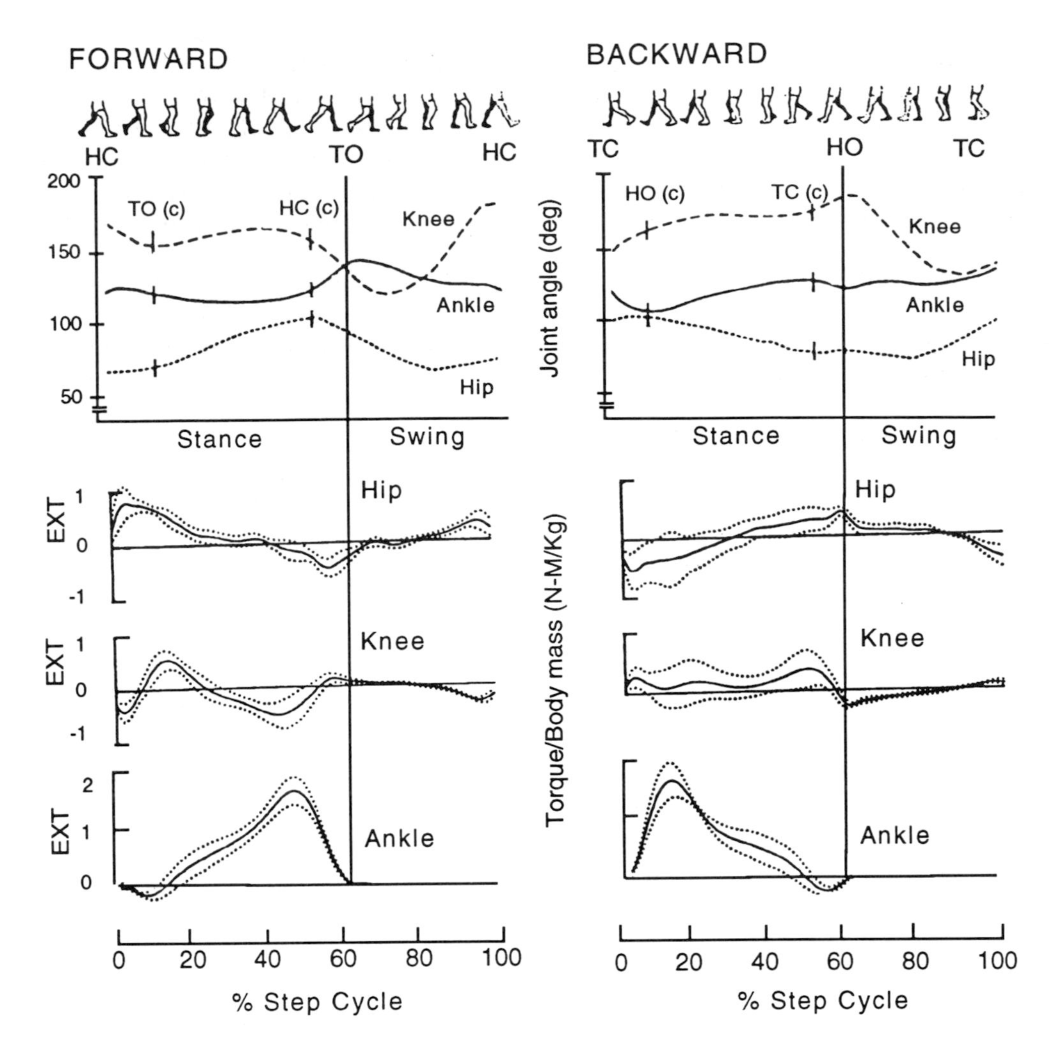

FIG. 8.14. Kinematics and muscle torque data for the normalized step cycle of two walking forms. Figurines at the top depict both behaviors. Angular displacement plots are redrawn from Vilensky et al. (199). All data are normalized to percentage of step cycle, starting at the onset of stance with heel contact (HC) for forward walking and toe contact (TC) for backward walking. Swing onset is marked by a *vertical line* at toe-off (TO) for forward walking and heel-off (HO) for backward walking. Stance and swing onsets are also indicated for the contralateral (*c*) leg. Kinetic data, normalized to body mass (N · m/kg), are redrawn from Winter et al. (204). Positive torque values indicate extensor muscle torques (EXT); *dotted lines* represent the coefficient of variation for the torque data.

transition occurs late in swing (Fig. 8.9). The profile of knee dynamics for the swing phase of backward walking is nearly a mirror image of the swing-phase profile of forward walking, with one important difference. For forward walking, the muscle torques at the onset and end of swing are flexor, but for backward walking, the muscle torque at the end of swing is extensor (Fig. 8.10). The kinetic data are consistent with EMG records showing that knee flexor activity is continuous during most of the swing phase of backward walking (see ST in Fig. 8.9). At the end of swing, however, an extensor muscle torque counters the tendency of motion-dependent torques to continue flexing the knee. The vastii muscles are active just prior to paw contact (see VL in Fig. 8.9*B*), and the rectus femoris and anterior sartorius have a small burst around paw contact (see SAa and RF in Fig. 8.13*B*).

Smith and co-workers (176, 178) recently initiated studies to compare knee-joint dynamics during the swing phase for up- and down-slope walking at moderate (25%–50%) and steep (>75%) grades. During the swing phase of up-slope walking, the duration of flexion is prolonged, and the range of flexion is increased to raise the paw for contact at a higher level (Figure 8.15). Preliminary kinetic data indicate that prolonged knee flexion during this phase of up-slope walking coincides with flexor torque components related to hip linear acceleration and thigh angular acceleration (176). Accordingly, the kinetic profile at the knee joint for up-slope walking appears similar to that for slow galloping.

These preliminary findings generated a prediction (being tested by Smith and colleagues) that muscles with knee-flexor action will not be active during knee flexion. Instead, biarticular muscles with knee-extensor action are expected to be active to decelerate the rate of knee flexion during the F phase of swing for up-slope walking.

During down-slope walking, knee-flexion range and duration are reduced, while knee-extension range and duration are increased to lower the paw for contact (Fig. 8.15). Preliminary EMG data (178) reveal an increase in semitendinosus paw-off burst with steeper downhill slopes. Muscle tension at any level of activation, however, is related to the well-studied length–tension properties [discussed by Goslow et al. (63)], and during down-slope walking, the knee is still flexed at the end of stance—particularly on steep slopes. The cat's hamstrings, therefore, may be in a shortened state and require greater recruitment to meet the demands for contractile tension.

Stance-Phase Dynamics

During the stance phase of walking, the inertial and centripetal forces affecting the supporting limb are small compared to the much larger forces supporting the weight of the body. Thus, motion-dependent torques are comparatively small and can be omitted in inverse dynamics calculations (54, 146, 206). Consequently, as noted in equation 1, the net joint torque at any weight-bearing joint is the sum of the muscle torque, contact torques (generated from ground-reaction forces), and gravity-related torques. In this section, we consider kinetic data based primarily on inverse dynamics calculations that provide insights into the control of stance during different forms of locomotion.

Stance-Phase Kinetics for Human Walking. Stance is initiated with heel contact and ends with toe-off (Fig. 8.16*A*). Just after heel contact, the knee joint "yields" (flexes), and the yield is followed by a plateau during which the knee joint undergoes only a small range of motion (195). Knee flexion is initiated before toe-off (Fig. 8.14). During the first half of stance, the horizontal ground-reaction force provides a braking action, and during the second half of stance, a propulsive force is generated (Fig. 8.16*B*). The vertical ground reaction force has two peaks—the first occurs when the contralateral toe is lifted (one limb is fully weight bearing), and the second occurs when the contralateral heel makes contact [Fig. 8.16*B*; (104)].

Uniarticular knee extensors (e.g., vastii muscles), usually recruited just after heel contact, are active during the first half of stance and then are inactive for the remainder of stance [see VL and VM of Fig. 8.8; (138, 193, 205)]. These EMG data are consistent with the stance-phase kinetics for the knee joint (Fig. 8.12). Early in stance an extensor muscle torque develops, and power is typically absorbed as the knee yields (205). Near midstance, a flexor muscle torque develops and peaks just before stance ends. At the end of stance, therefore, power is generated (205) as flexion coincides with a flexor muscle torque at the knee. Major knee flexor muscles (e.g., hamstrings), however, are relatively inactive during the last half of stance (see St-Sm of Fig. 8.8). Given these data, which muscles contribute to the flexor muscle torque and the power generation at the knee? The gastrocnemius, a biarticular muscle with knee-flexor and ankle-extensor actions, is a prime candidate, as it is active throughout stance, often reaching peak activity at the end of stance (see LG of Fig. 8.8).

During backward walking, stance contact is made with the toe, and swing is initiated when the heel is lifted from the walking surface. At toe contact, the knee begins to extend and, although extension continues throughout stance, there is often a plateau in which knee extension is minimal (Fig. 8.14). During the stance phase of backward walking, an extensor muscle torque persists, consistent with knee-extensor activity that begins at the onset of stance and ends just before heel-off (193, 205). Also, the rectus femoris (a knee extensor) is active most of stance for backward walking but not for stance of forward walking (193, 205). Rectus femoris EMG is particularly large in amplitude during the first half of backward stance (193), and the contraction likely contributes to a flexor muscle torque at the hip and an extensor muscle torque at the knee (Fig. 8.14).

Stance-Phase Kinetics for Cat Walking. For the cat, stance is initiated when the plantar pads of the hind paw contact the ground and ends when the pads are lifted from the ground. The paw remains digitigrade during stance (Fig. 8.16*C*). Horizontal ground-reaction forces provide a brief braking force during the first third of stance, and a propulsive force occurs during the remainder of stance [Fig. 8.16*D*; (53, 124, 146)]. The vertical ground-reaction force peaks during the first third of stance (Fig. 8.16*D*), and the peak usually coincides with the end of the yield.

Stance kinematics for the cat's knee joint can be divided into three epochs: *(1)* at onset the knee flexes [yield or E_2 phase; (148)]; *(2)* during midstance, there is often a plateau period with minimal knee motion (usually extension); and *(3)* at the end, the

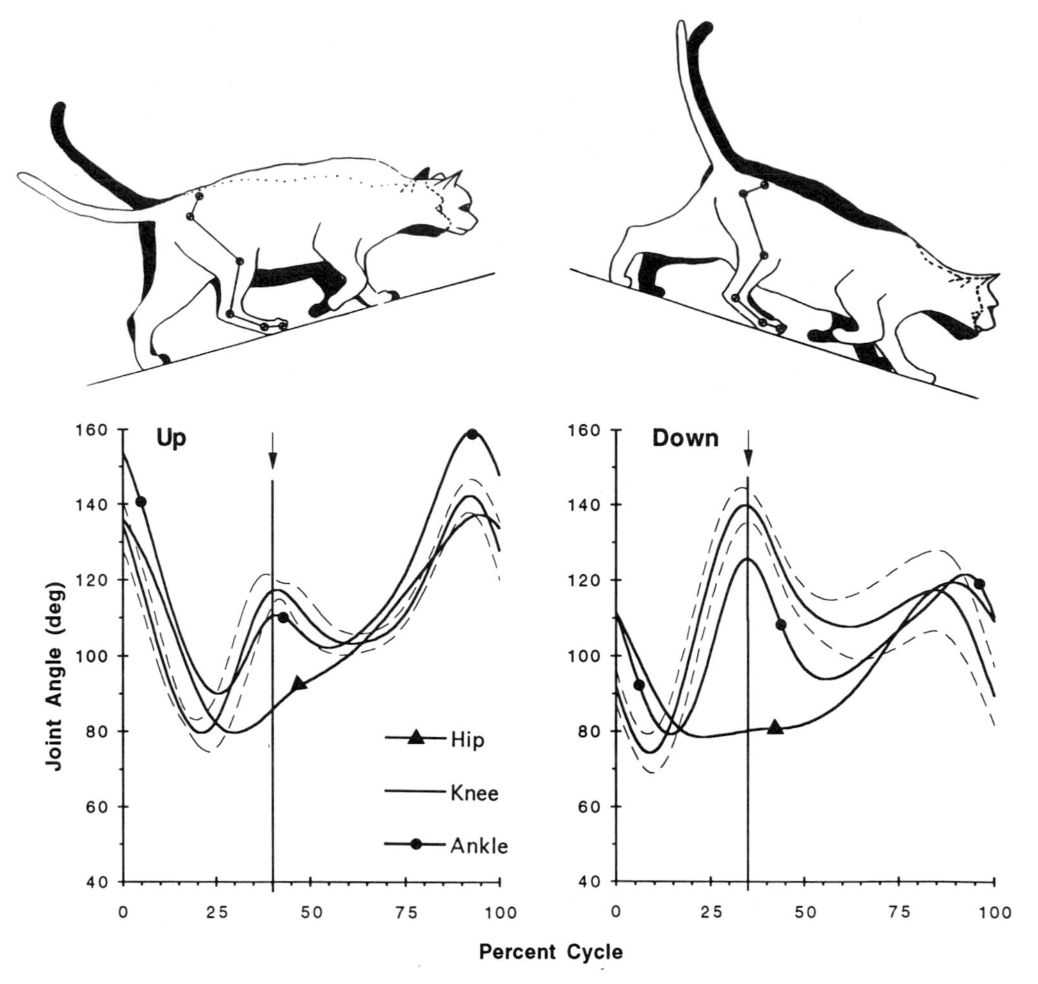

FIG. 8.15. Kinematics of the cat's hindlimb for up- and downslope walking; slope at a 33% grade. Drawings above the graphs illustrate the cat's posture at contact for the left hind paw. The two shadowed figures show the cat's posture at the same instance for level walking. Within the graphs, the *dashed lines* represent the standard deviation of the angular displacement data for the knee joint. Data are graphed from the onset of swing and normalized to percentage of cycle. *Vertical lines* indicate the onset of stance at paw contact. [Unpublished data from Smith et al. (176) and Smith and Carlson-Kuhta (178).]

knee extends more rapidly, reaching peak extension just before paw-off. The last two epochs are usually called the E_3 phase (148). Extensor muscles (e.g., vastii) are active during the E_2 phase and most of the E_3 phase, except for the last 80–100 ms (Fig. 8.9). Knee extensor activity is consistent with an extensor muscle torque at the knee joint for all but the initial segment of stance (Fig. 8.17*A*). During the first half of stance, power is absorbed as the knee flexes, but power is generated as the knee extends during the second half of stance (146).

The generalized muscle torque at the ankle is extensor during most of stance in forward walking for humans (Fig. 8.14) and cats (Fig. 8.17*A*). In a recent study, Fowler et al. (53) estimated the contribution of four ankle muscles to the generalized extensor muscle torque calculated for the ankle joint by inverse dynamics techniques (Fig. 8.16). Individual forces for four primary ankle extensor muscles were measured during stance from buckle-tendon transducers. The muscle torque for each muscle was determined as the product of the tendon-force values and each muscle's moment arm estimate (119). Soleus and plantaris muscles contributed to the extensor ankle torque throughout stance, while gastrocnemius contributed only during the first third of stance [Fig. 8.18; (53)]. The sum of the individual muscle torques (calculated from measured tendon forces and moment arm lengths) was similar to the generalized muscle torque calculated by the inverse dynamics method. This direct comparison is rare, and cross-validates both methods.

Stance Dynamics for Different Forms of Cat Walking. Compared to level walking, when a cat walks up an incline (Fig. 8.15), greater propulsive forces are needed for vertical lift, propulsive impulse is increased, and breaking impulse is decreased (53). The decrease in braking impulse at the onset of stance is consistent with the cat placing its paw more caudal to the hip joint at contact during up-slope walking than during level walking (177). Compared to level walking, peak ankle-extensor torque increases in up-slope walking and contractile forces increase in the gastrocnemius and plantaris but not soleus (53, 82). Preliminary EMG data, presented by Smith and Carlson-Kuhta (178), indicate that magnitudes of hip-, knee-, and ankle-extensor EMG increase with slope. Thus, hip- and knee-extensor muscle torques likely increase at steeper slopes. Also, during up-slope walking, the cat's posterior bifunctional muscles (e.g., semitendinosus) become active during stance (178), suggesting their recruitment (as hip extensors) is necessary to complement the recruitment of uniarticular hip extensors, typically recruited without the hamstrings during level walking.

No kinetic data for down-slope stance is published. Recently, Smith and Carlson-Kuhta (178) reported that flexor activity at the hip and ankle joints replaces extensor activity during stance when the cat walks down-slope (17°–45°). Hip flexor activity, for example, begins at paw contact and persists most of stance. Why are flexors active? Perhaps joint power is absorbed as extension is due to external contact forces at the hip joint and countered by a flexor muscle torque that slows the rate of hip extension.

An analysis of stance-phase dynamics for backward walking was recently presented by Perell and co-workers (146). During stance, a cat's hip joint flexes causing the body to move backwards over the weight-bearing limb (Fig. 8.9). As the hip flexes, the knee and ankle extend, and little or no yield occurs. The horizontal ground-reaction force provides a braking (forward-directed) impulse for 50%–60% of the stance phase for backward walking; thereafter, a small propulsive (backward) impulse develops (see Fig. 5 in 146).

Muscle torques for the stance phase of backward walking are largely extensor at the hip joint (Fig. 8.17*B*), and power is absorbed as uniarticular hip extensors (e.g., anterior biceps femoris; see ABF of Fig. 8.9) undergo active lengthening. In contrast, the ankle generates power, as uniarticular ankle extensors (e.g., soleus) experience active contraction. The knee muscle torque has a biphasic profile, with a shift from an extensor to a flexor torque at mid-stance (Fig. 8.17*B*). During the first 40% of backward stance, the knee joint generates power as an extensor torque coincides with knee extension, and

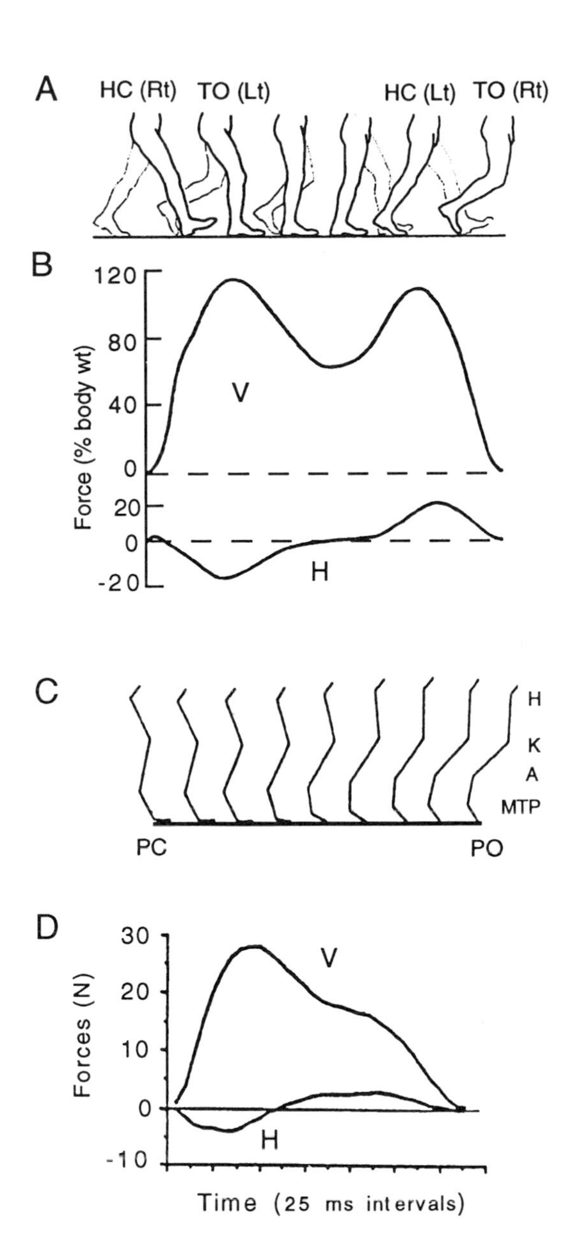

FIG. 8.16. Stance-phase kinetics for walking in human and cat. The human leg (*A*) and cat hindlimb (*C*; joints are labeled: H, hip; K, knee; A, ankle; MPT, metatarsophalangeal) are illustrated for stance, beginning with heel contact (HC) and ending with toe-off (TO) in *A* and beginning with paw contact (PC) and ending with paw-off (PC) in *C*. In *B* and *D*, vertical (V) and horizontal (H) ground reaction force components are illustrated. Negative components for H are braking and positive are propulsive forces. [Force data in *B* are expressed in percentage of body weight and redrawn from Inman (104), and force data in *D* are absolute values (Newton, N) for a 49 N cat and redrawn from Fowler et al. (53).]

power is absorbed during the rest of stance as a flexor muscle torque coincides with knee extension.

The presence of a flexor torque and the anterior orientation of the ground-reaction force with respect to the knee joint suggest that contractile or passive forces are needed to prevent knee hyperextension at the end of stance. This prediction led to a better understanding of EMG data reported for the gastrocnemius during stance (18). The gastrocnemius can contribute to a flexor muscle torque at the knee and to an extensor muscle torque at the ankle. During stance for forward walking, this dual action is not required, and recruitment ceases or is greatly reduced by the first half of stance (Fig. 8.9). Interestingly, the muscle torque profile at the cat knee for backward walking (Fig. 8.17*B*) is similar to that for the human knee during forward walking (Fig. 8.14).

During the last half of the stance phase for backward walking, a power transfer is possible from the knee to the ankle (via active gastrocnemius muscles), because power is absorbed at the knee and generated at the ankle. Power can transform from a joint absorbing power to a joint generating power only if a biarticular muscle is active and joint torques are consistent with the muscle's action (103).

Insights for Neural Control of Locomotion

Mammalian locomotion is thought to be controlled by a tripartite neural system. At the core of this system is the central pattern generator (CPG) (see Chapter 5), which issues a basic locomotor-like pattern. The CPG is modulated by input from supraspinal centers and motion-related feedback from the limbs (see Chapter 3). The relative importance of each component in determining the program details is controversial (71, 122, 147).

Buford and Smith (18, 19) argue that a single CPG provides the basic motor signals common to all forms of locomotion. Unique details necessary for different forms of locomotion, in contrast, depend on interactions among the tripartite system (CPG, feedback, and supraspinal input). Smith and colleagues have identified cat hindlimb muscles that exhibit relatively immutable motor patterns during different forms of locomotion (19, 154, 176, 177, 179). Muscles in this category are typically uniarticular muscles or biarticular muscles that have the same function at both joints, such as the medial sartorius (hip and knee flexor). These muscles function either as extensors with stance-related activity or as flexors with swing-related activity.

These reciprocal synergies could be controlled by a CPG similar to those described by Lundberg (122) and Grillner (69), and the CPG command to muscles associated with each synergy could be relatively immutable and independent of gait or walking form. Hip extensor recruitment, for example, may be set at the same level by the CPG for forward and backward walking. Force output is sufficient to effect a shortening contraction during stance of forward walking, and the hip joint extends. Force output during the stance phase of backward walking, in contrast, is not adequate to effect a shortening contraction and the hip flexes as hip flexors undergo a lengthening contraction. In this manner, CPG output to hip extensors may be independent of the direction of walking, and external contact forces (different for each walking form) determine whether the hip flexes or extends. Grillner (69) predicted, on the basis of joint displacement data, that hip flexor muscles would be active during the stance phase of backward walking (with knee and ankle extensors). This intuitive but incorrect prediction was made before the availability of stance-related kinetic data.

The nervous system is capable of modulating the duration and intensity of the motor commands. During locomotion, force modulation can be governed by descending centers responsible for changing the excitability of CPG units; additionally, motion-related feedback from the hindlimbs can modulate the CPG network. In some cases, gain setting may

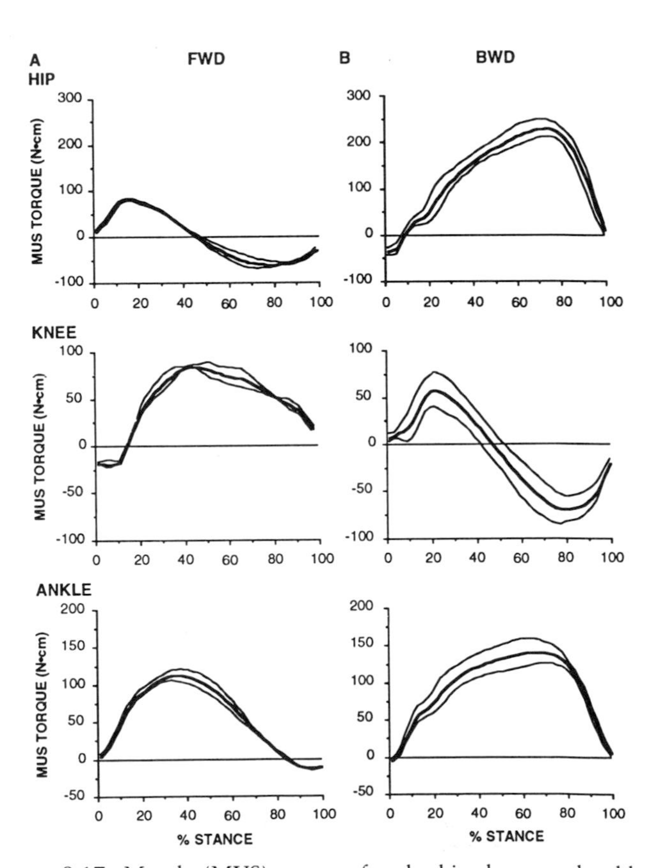

FIG. 8.17. Muscle (MUS) torques for the hip, knee, and ankle joints for the cat hindlimb during stance of forward (*A*) and backward (*B*) treadmill walking. Mean (*solid line*) and standard deviations (*dashed lines*) are data from four steps of one cat. For all plots, extensor torques are positive, and flexor torques are negative values. [Adapted from Fig. 7 of Perell et al. (146).]

be an appropriate mechanism to produce the needed increase in motor-unit recruitment and force. For example, the force output of the gastrocnemius is related in a linear fashion to the speed of locomotion (180, 202). For other muscles such as the soleus, however, EMG amplitude and force output are relatively immutable and unrelated to speed or gait (202).

While motor patterns of unifunctional muscles are independent of gait and locomotor form, motor patterns of bifunctional muscles are linked to limb dynamics. For example, the semitendinosus (hip flexor and knee extensor) has two bursts of activity during forward walking, one at the end of stance and one at the end of swing. It has only one brief burst at the end of swing during the fast gallop and a single prolonged burst during the swing phase of backward walking. For up-slope walking, however, the semitendinosus has a prolonged single burst that is stance related (176, 178). The semitendinosus, therefore, switches synergies and exhibits swing- or stance-related activity depending on the form of walking and the limb dynamics.

The diverse patterns associated with semitendinosus recruitment in the intact preparation do not appear to be programmed centrally. Although motor patterns for the semitendinosus are not the same for all "fictive" preparations (see Chapter 5), the patterns described in the current literature lack specific details that are characteristic of normal locomotion

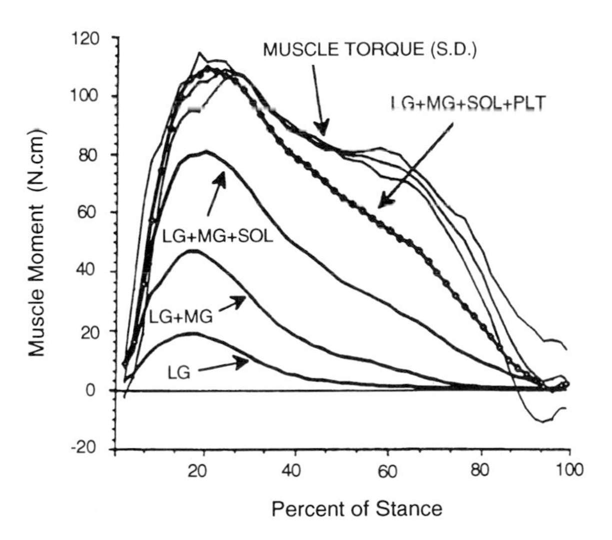

FIG. 8.18. The average muscle torque at the ankle and standard deviation curves calculated from the stance phase of three step cycles from walking cats. Lateral gastrocnemius (LG) and medial gastrocnemius (MG) muscle torques were calculated from one of these step cycles. Plantaris (PLT) and soleus (SOL) moments were calculated from two steps cycles from another cat. With these conditions in mind, the data demonstrate how each ankle extensor muscle contributes to a muscle torque of this magnitude during stance. [Adapted from Fig. 7 of Fowler et al. (53).]

(also see 3, 71, 144, 147). What factors are responsible for the details? Certainly some modulation by motion-dependent feedback is necessary, and also input from descending brainstem centers could preset the CPG so that feedback is gated.

Posture, for example, may be set by brainstem centers [(reviewed in 129); also see Chapter 7], and postural needs for various walking forms are different. Goal-dependent input from supraspinal centers may bias the spinal CPG, and motion-related feedback may be differentially gated on this basis. During forward stance, for example, a specific range of hip extension and unloading of ankle extensors are crucial for switching from an extensor to a flexor synergy (3, 38, 70). The same feedback during backward walking, however, is inappropriate because the hip is flexed at the end of stance, and ankle extensors (particularly gastrocnemius) show increased loading until the end of stance. It remains to be revealed which proprioceptive cues are used during backward walking to facilitate this switch.

By studying different forms of locomotion, neuroscientists together with biomechanists are beginning to understand the requirements for both common and unique motor patterns that must be handled by the nervous system. The locomotor CPG may provide a common (immutable) motor output, but the unique (mutable) motor output is probably adapted from the "generalized" central pattern by the modifying actions of supraspinal tracts and motion-related feedback from the limbs. Biomechanics, especially limb dynamics data, has been and will continue to be important for revealing these insights.

ROLE OF DYNAMICS IN THE CONTROL OF ARM MOVEMENTS

Analysis of isolated, single-joint movements can provide insight into the rudiments of motor programs (64, 65), but, as we have shown for locomotion, the control of natural limb motions involves the intricate coordination and timing of multiple joints, body segments, and muscles (95, 121, 184). Even a simple action, such as moving your arm from your side to knock on a door, is a three-dimensional, multijoint movement task, involving a daunting array of skeletal and neuromuscular elements. Typically, we take little heed of this complexity, and each day we blithely produce well-coordinated movements and adapt to a myriad of movement contexts.

In this section, we focus on the role of limb dynamics in the control of arm movements. We chose arm movements because: *(1)* arm movements are multiarticular; *(2)* many of the models and theories of the planning and execution of movements focus on arm motions; and *(3)* posture, proprioception, and dynamics can have significant effects on arm motor control. As we stated, the emphasis here is on arm-movement *dynamics*; we do not concentrate on movement *planning*, as this is discussed extensively elsewhere (31, 46, 49, 95, 127, 160, 172, 184).

Limb Postural Dynamics

The physical attributes of a limb provide a structural framework on which movement dynamics is superimposed. Because limbs are comprised of interconnected viscoelastic masses, movement control must account for limb-segment position and inertia, as well as joint stiffness and viscosity. In the past decade, there has been a burst of interest in how these physical attributes (*postural dynamics*) of a limb are modulated or controlled during motion (95). Elsewhere (9–11, 43, 46, 48, 93, 127, 131, 172, 173) you will find detailed discussions of the relation between movement control and the elastic properties of the motor system (e.g., end-point position, stiffness, and postural modules); therefore, here we only sample a few of the salient issues related to limb postural dynamics.

As Hogan, Bizzi, Mussa-Ivaldi, and colleagues (93, 94, 95, 132) have shown, by reorienting a limb's segments, the central nervous system can modulate the "effective inertial behavior" of arm segments by changing the limb's mechanical impedance (e.g., stiffness and viscosity). For example, end-point inertia (resistance to motion) of the upper extremity can be altered by changing the configuration of the hand, forearm, and upper arm (Fig. 8.19). Hogan depicts the effective inertial behavior of the limb's end-point as an ellipse (Fig.8.19*B*), with *arrows* representing the force vectors required to accelerate the end-point (94, 95). Even without movement of the end-point location, the reorientation of a limb's segments produces large changes in the "inertial response of the limb," changing the effort necessary to change the limb's position (Fig. 8.19*C–E*). If an anterior-to-posterior force (toward the shoulder) was applied to the hand in Fig. 8.19*D*, the force would be resisted by a combined inertia of the hand, forearm, and upper arm (ellipse major axis; a large resistance to motion, yielding a small acceleration). If, however, the same force magnitude was applied to the hand from a left-to-right direction, then the perturbing force would be resisted mainly by the hand moment of inertia (ellipse minor axis; thus a much smaller resistance to motion and a large acceleration).

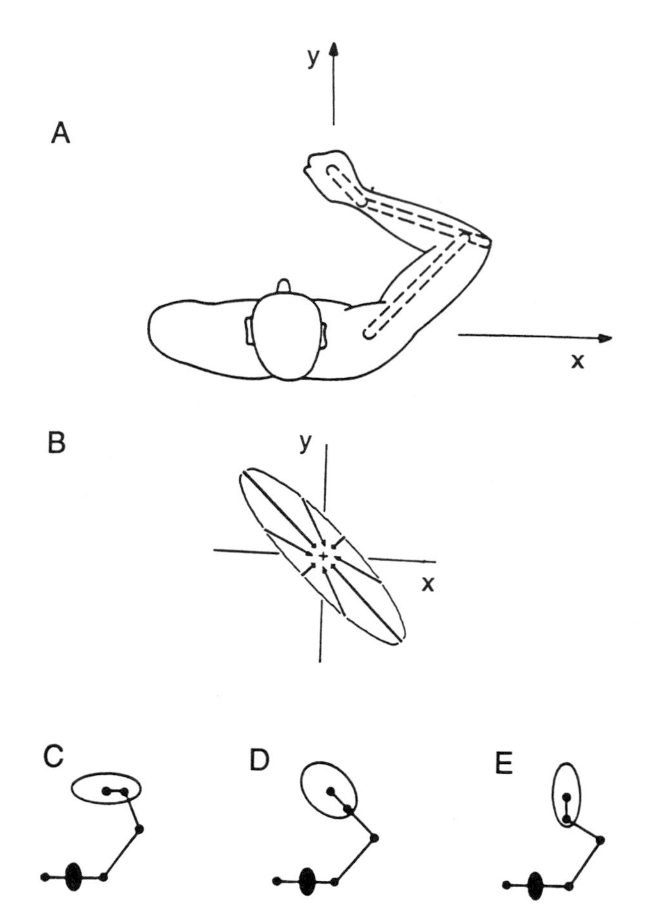

FIG. 8.19. A planar, three-segment model of the arm (*A*). The directional property of the *effective inertial behavior* of the upper limb's end-point is represented as an *ellipse* (*B*). Force vectors required to accelerate the end-point are shown as *arrows*, and the vector from the *head of the arrow* to the origin of the coordinate frame represents the corresponding acceleration. Changes in the effective end-point inertia of the limb that are achieved by changing the limb configuration (while the end-point remains stationary) are shown as *ellipses C, D*, and *E*. [Adapted from Fig. 11 of Hogan et al. (95).]

Obvious examples of posture-related dynamic behavior of limbs are evident as a moving limb makes contact with a stationary object (e.g., the chalk in your hand when contacting a chalkboard). If you jumped down from a 1 m wall onto a sidewalk, your "limb dynamics" and the motor-control task would be markedly different if you landed with extended knees vs. with flexed knees. These "contact" situations, however, are not the only circumstances in which limb postural dynamics can play a role in motor behavior; a limb's physical attributes (postural dynamics) can also affect a freely moving limb.

Hogan and colleagues suggest that changing the configuration of a limb may be a fundamental mechanism for modulating the directional aspects of limb stiffness, viscosity, and inertia (95). Also, Gordon and colleagues found that systematic errors in reaching behaviors are related to the effective inertial behavior of the arm (61, 62). While reaching for targets placed at a variety of distances and locations, subjects apparently programmed the magnitude of the initial force to accelerate the hand, but did not always compensate for the direction-dependent differences in inertial resistance (62). Normal subjects compensated for differences in acceleration by varying movement time. There was a remarkably strong correspondence between the accelerations and the limb's anisotropic inertial field (e.g., Fig. 8.19) described by Hogan and colleagues (94, 95). This compensation, however, did not occur in deafferentated patients performing these movements without vision, but was evident for brief periods after the patients saw their limb (57, 60). These results suggest that compensation can occur through feedforward mechanisms and that information about limb properties may serve to update an internal model of limb mechanical properties.

Although emphasized only more recently, the endemic postural dynamics of a limb provides the physical framework for movement. Thus, to understand the underlying mechanisms of limb motor control, it is important to recognize that a limb's movement dynamics must be mapped onto the viscoelastic and inertial attributes of the limb.

Intersegmental Dynamics Change with Practice

To highlight how movement dynamics, per se, can influence motor control, Schneider and colleagues (165) tested Bernstein's (8) suggestion that practice alters coordination among muscle, gravitational, and motion-dependent joint torques. These issues were examined because they are not emphasized in "motor learning" studies, and "motor control" studies do not emphasize practice-related changes in movement control. Although the motor-learning studies have delved into motor-skill acquisition (2), motor performance is typically reported as an outcome measure, such as movement time; those data add comparatively little to our understanding of how movement *control* changes during practice. The studies (85, 126, 201) reporting changes in movement patterns during practice typically involve simple tasks that are inadequate for answering questions about the control of multisegmented limbs moving in three-dimensional gravitational space.

Motor control research, conversely, has been directed mainly toward understanding the mechanisms of movement control, as in the formation of arm and hand trajectories in humans (1, 5, 117) or robotic systems (4, 97), in kinematic (200) or EMG invariances (59), and in principles of optimization (50, 93, 135). Until recently, these studies have focused on constrained movements analyzed in terms of kinematics, with little information available about spatial movement dynamics (4, 98). In the studies we describe here, only a brief overview of methods is provided, as details are provided elsewhere (165, 167, 168).

A Paradigm of Rapid Reversals. Subjects were asked to perform maximal-speed arm movements. Each subject was seated in front of a clear Plexiglas sheet on which arrows marked the location of upper and lower target light beams (Fig. 8.20). Subjects sat on a straight-backed chair with the pelvis and torso restrained in the chair by lap and shoulder belts. Instructed to "go as fast as possible," subjects started at the lower light beam, rounded a barrier that was placed midway between the two targets, broke the upper light beam, again rounded the barrier, and stopped in the lower light beam. Accuracy was not an issue, but they were required to interrupt the upper light beam and stop in the lower light beam.

In a study by Schneider and colleagues (165), adult volunteers each performed 100 practice trials, while in a follow-up study (214) other subjects per-

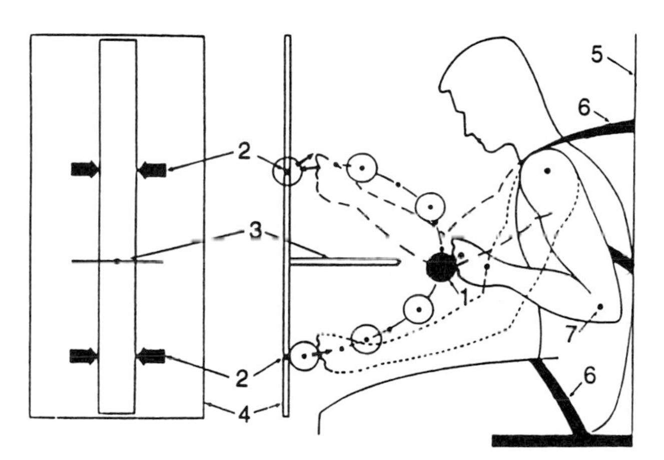

FIG. 8.20. A frontal (left side) and lateral view (right side) of experimental set-up and subject position. Numbers denote the following: (*1*) circular black-metal plate connected by a stem to a wooden-dowel handle that subjects grasped; (*2*) light beams (photoelectric cells plus infrared LEDs) attached to the Plexiglas sheet with *black arrows* indicating the targets' positions; (*3*) T-shaped barrier that subjects circumnavigated; (*4*) suspended, clear Plexiglas sheet with center slit; (*5*) straight-backed chair; (*6*) seat belts; and (*7*) markers attached at the glenohumeral, elbow, wrist, and third metacarpophalangeal joints, and the center of the circular metal plate. Subjects started and ended the movement with the circular plate held steady in the lower light beam. The upper light beam only had to be interrupted by the metal plate as subjects reversed their upward motion to begin the downward phase of the task. [Adapted from Fig. 1 of Schneider and Zernicke (167).]

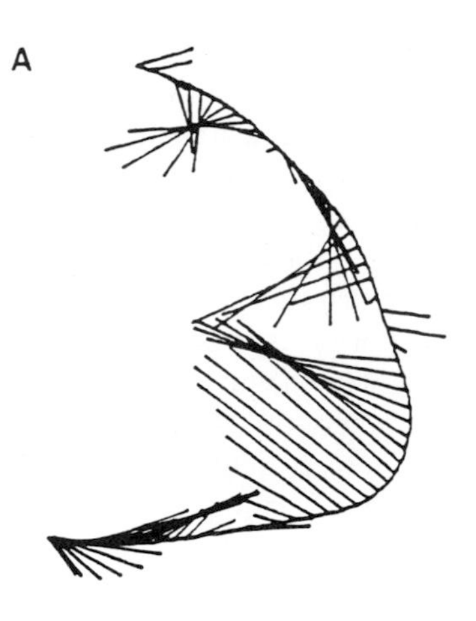

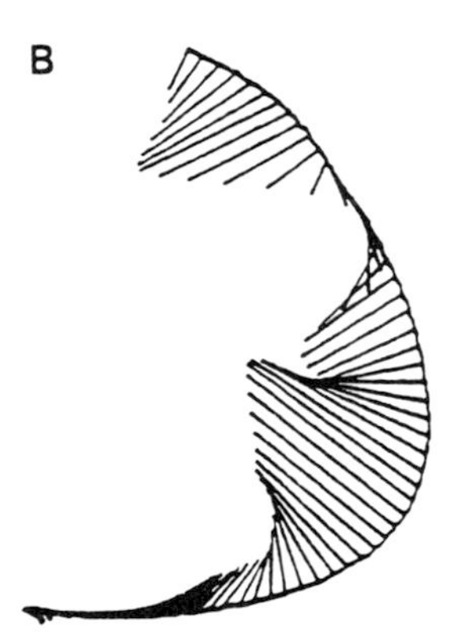

FIG. 8.21. Exemplar hand paths for the upward phase, with acceleration vectors (sagittal plane) for a before-practice (*A*) and an after-practice movement (*B*). The "before-practice" trial was the slowest time, although subjects were attempting to go "as fast as possible." The movement time for each of the trials was the same, as subjects—after practicing the task—repeated the movement at the less than maximal speed. The hand path is the *continuous curved line*, whereas at successive and equal points in time, the linear acceleration vectors (denoting magnitude and direction) are shown as *straight lines* originating from the hand path. To scale the dimensions of the acceleration vectors to the dimensions of the hand path, the magnitudes of the acceleration vectors were multiplied by 0.005. [Taken from Fig. 4 of Schneider and Zernicke (168), with publisher's permission.]

formed 120 practice trials, returned 1 day later, and performed another 20 trials to assess skill retention. After completion of the practice trials in the follow-up study, subjects repeated the movement task across a range of movement times, from very slow to fast. The arm kinematics were quantified, and EMGs for biceps brachii, triceps brachii, anterior deltoid, and posterior deltoid were recorded. Three-dimensional movement kinematics and planar limb dynamics were analyzed.

During practice trials, movement times decreased significantly. From the slowest to the fastest trial, an average 36% decrease in movement time was achieved, with the slowest trial equaling about 1,000 ms and the fastest trial about 600 ms. The major decrease occurred in the first 25 practice trials, as an exponential decrease in movement time occurred with practice.

As subjects became faster during practice, hand paths became more parabolic in shape, with the apex near the barrier (Fig. 8.21). The path changed from a motion in which the hand was pulled out of the lower target (Fig. 8.21*A*), moved nearly straight up to clear the barrier, and moved into the upper target to a path (Fig. 8.21*B*) that appeared more rounded and smooth. When the hand linear-acceleration vectors (straight lines originating from the curved line; Fig. 8.21) were superimposed on the hand path and the before-and-after practice patterns compared, it was evident that at the beginning of practice the acceleration vectors fluctuated, indicating frequent changes in acceleration magnitude and direction.

These studies also helped probe a component of movement optimization. It has been proposed that skilled movements can be acquired through practice that is directed toward achieving an objective, such as movement accuracy (135). In addition to task-specific goals, however, more global movement objectives have been proposed, including, *efficiency* (8), *economy* and *effectiveness* (22), *minimum cost* (31), *minimum torque change* (198), *or smoothness* (135). To understand how movement control may be related to these objectives requires quantification of a physical movement characteristic.

Intuitively, many agree that "jerky" movements are the opposite of "smooth" movements. This movement "smoothness" can be quantified as *jerk* (47, 50, 51, 93, 135). The jerk-time function is the third time derivative of a displacement-time function, and Nelson (135) showed that total *jerk-cost* can be calculated as *mean-squared jerk*. Flash and Hogan (94, 96) suggest that the "minimization of mean-squared jerk is a mathematical model of one movement objective, the production of smooth graceful movements." If one goal of motor coordination is to produce the smoothest movement, *jerk-cost* should be less for practiced movements than for unpracticed movements. This was examined by analyzing modulations in jerk-cost during practice of a motor task and after the task was well-practiced (167).

With practice of the time-minimized motion (Fig. 8.21), although the acceleration vectors increased in magnitude, the vectors became more consistent in direction. The movement looked "smoother," and this observation was confirmed when jerk-cost was calculated. Total jerk-cost was significantly less for identical-duration movements in the after-practice vs. before-practice trials. The jerk-cost components (representing the magnitudinal and directional changes in hand acceleration vector) were of similar magnitudes, and both components were substantially less in the after-practice vs. the before-practice trials (167).

Practice-Related Changes in Intersegmental Dynamics. How can movement dynamics change to produce the alterations in movement kinematics? To answer that question, Zernicke and Schneider (214) focused on the reversal at the upper target, because the prominent changes in kinematics occurred in that region of the motion. Representative intersegmental dynamics for the reversal region at the shoulder joint are provided in Figure 8.22.

As the hand approached the upper target, the shoulder joint flexed, and shoulder extension started as the hand left the upper target. In Figure 8.22, shoulder torques are compared for *before* (Fig. 8.22*A*; trial 1) vs. *after* practice (Fig. 8.22*B*; trial 100). At the shoulder joint, positive torques tended to extend the shoulder, and negative torques tended to flex the shoulder. In the initial practice trials, during the reversal, the dominant motion-dependent torque component was related to upper-arm-angular acceleration that tended to flex the shoulder joint. This small flexor torque was counteracted by an extensor torque produced by gravity, together with a small muscle torque. The shoulder torques, basically, were balanced, as a small muscle extensor torque assisted gravity in counteracting the motion-dependent torque component due to upper-arm-angular acceleration.

By the end of practice (Fig. 8.22*B*), however, a marked increase in the upper-arm-angular acceleration torque had developed—still acting to flex the shoulder (note the large magnitude differences in the ordinate axes of before- vs. after-practice graphs). Because the limb position at the reversal was similar at the start and end of practice, the absolute magnitude of the gravitational torque remained unchanged, and its relative importance was, therefore, greatly diminished by the end of practice. After practice, gravity had little effect in reversing shoulder motion, and a large extensor torque was generated by the shoulder muscles to counteract the large motion-dependent, flexor inertial torque—related to upper arm acceleration, needed to produce the requisite net extensor torque for reversing the motion. To compensate for an increased flexor torque (associated with an increased acceleration of the limb) at the shoulder, the muscle torque had to increase significantly.

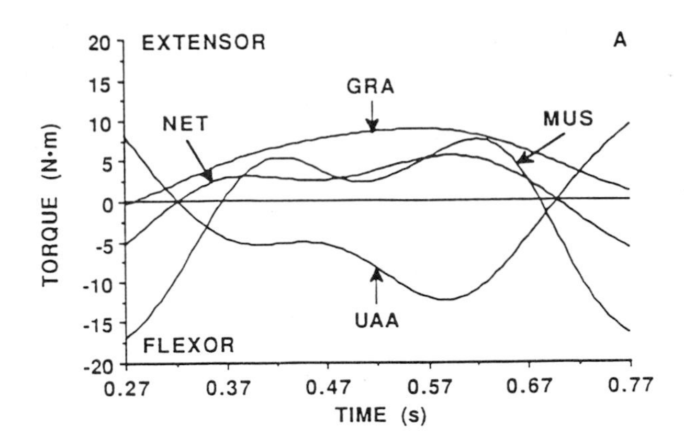

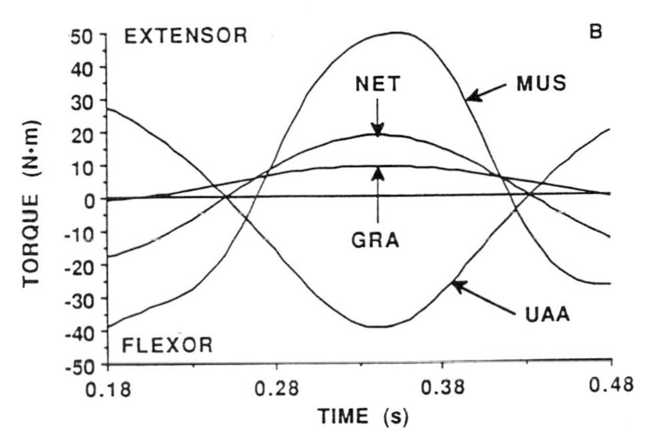

FIG. 8.22. Shoulder-joint torques for a before-practice (*A*) and after-practice (*B*) movement during the reversal in the upper target. Positive torques tend to cause shoulder extension, and negative torques tend to cause shoulder flexion (lifting the arm). There is a difference of more than twofold in the ordinates of *A* and *B*. The torque components illustrated are: NET, net joint torque; MUS, muscle torque; GRA, gravitational torque; UAA, inertial torque related to upper arm angular acceleration. [Taken from Fig. 4 of Zernicke and Schneider (214), with publisher's permission.]

Biceps brachii and triceps brachii EMG activities showed tonic activity during early practice, while the anterior and posterior deltoid EMGs were phasic. In early practice, the anterior deltoid shortened to flex the shoulder to move the hand toward the upper target, and the posterior deltoid actively slowed shoulder flexion as the hand entered the upper target. In slower trials, co-contraction occurred in anterior and posterior deltoid as the hand reversed its direction at the upper target. In the faster trials, however, the posterior deltoid was recruited significantly earlier in the motion as the hand approached the upper target. Thus, the phasic recruitment of the posterior deltoid may have slowed the rate of shoulder flexion and put the posterior deltoid muscle–tendon unit on stretch to enhance the speed of shoulder extension when the hand left the upper target.

Inverse dynamics analysis suggested that, after practice, muscle torques were used to counteract more effectively and to complement motion-dependent torques and that practice altered the coordination among muscular and motion-dependent torques. EMG results further suggested that the recruitment of muscles during active lengthening exploited the passive mechanical (viscoelastic) properties of the muscle and tendon (167). These findings reinforce the concept that intersegmental dynamics can play an important role for the control of limb trajectories, as noted by Ghez and colleagues (28, 58, 162), Hollerbach and Flash (98), and Soechting and Flanders (184). These experiments also indicate that significant changes in dynamics can occur during the practice of a motor task.

Consistent with Bernstein's concepts of coordination (8), the results of Schneider and co-workers showed that muscle forces can counteract and complement motion-dependent torques and that practice can alter the coordination among muscular, gravitational, and motion-dependent torques. For example, the torque patterns at the shoulder joint during the movement reversal indicated—already at the beginning of practice—that passive torques played some role in the control of the movement. Nevertheless, with this complex, multijointed movement, practice was needed to coordinate the active and passive forces of the moving arm so that subjects could use muscle torques effectively as complementary forces. This is an important feature of skilled movement acquisition, in that the person not only avoids "wasting superfluous force" (8), but exploits the passive forces to enhance coordination. Each subject's motor problem involved "supplementing" the passive properties of the moving limb—in effect minimizing the discrepancy between the initial dynamics profile and the optimized limb dynamics.

Bernstein indicated that practice is the process of solving a motor problem using techniques perfected from repetition to repetition, resulting in a "reorganization" of the motor program. This reorganization of the limb dynamics and motor program may involve the processing of afferent feedback, as highlighted by the disrupted limb dynamics in patients with proprioceptive deficits.

Disrupted Proprioception Affects Limb Dynamics. Deafferentation does not eliminate volitional movements, but it is generally recognized that proprioceptive feedback plays a significant role in the control of movement (52, 60, 152, 163, 164; also see Chapters 3 and 5). For example, individuals with large-fiber sensory neuropathies who have intact muscle strength but loss of joint position, vibration, and discriminative-touch sensation have marked deficits in their ability to correct position error and limb movements when they are not able to see their arm (57, 60, 162–164). Such individuals have "deafferentated" upper limbs with regard to kinesthesia and touch. Although they experience problems in controlling single-joint arm movements without vision (52, 161, 164), control problems are exacerbated for multijoint arm movements that include rapid reversals (58, 163). Ghez and co-workers (58, 162) hypothesized that the substantial reversal errors result from the lack of proprioception "normally important for controlling intersegmental dynamics."

To test this hypothesis, Ghez and co-workers (58, 162) examined six arm motions in which motion-dependent torques at the elbow joint systematically increased. The template-tracing task designed for this purpose is complex and bears explanation here. The subject's arm was supported in the horizontal plane by a low-inertia brace equipped with ball-bearing joints and potentiometers under the elbow and shoulder joints. A magnetic pen attached to the brace above a digitizing tablet allowed the subject's hand path to be monitored and displayed on a front screen. Template lines that radiated in six different directions from a common point were also displayed on the screen. The lengths of the template lines were designed to keep elbow joint angular excursions the same for all target directions, while shoulder joint angular excursions increased systematically across the six directions. Subjects were told to trace the template line (to and fro) accurately at a comfortable speed (within 2.5 s) and to keep their handpaths straight. To prevent visual guidance of the task, vision of the subject's arm was blocked, and the screen cursor was blanked at motion onset. On every third trial, however, knowledge of results was given by a screen display of the subject's hand path marked against the template.

The upper portion of Fig. 8.23*A* illustrates the hand path for two template directions, as well as the angular excursions of the elbow and shoulder joints for a control subject. For the 0-degree target direction (template line to the subject's right in the 3-o'clock direction), angular motions at the shoulder joint were minimal; in contrast, shoulder motions were substantial for the 125-degree direction (template line extended forward in the 11-o'clock direction). Elbow joint kinematics, consistent with the design, were similar for both target directions, and the hand paths to both targets were straight with a tight reversal. The upper portion of Figure 8.23*B* illustrates the same tasks for a subject with a deafferentated limb. For the 0-degree direction, the hand path was relatively straight (though hypermetric) with a sharp reversal, similar to the control subject's reversal. For the 125-degree direction, however, the abnormal hand path had a very wide reversal caused by a marked increase in elbow joint flexion.

Analysis of the elbow joint torques revealed that deafferentated subjects were unable to compensate for large motion-dependent torques that developed at the elbow joint during the 125-degree reversal. For the 0-degree direction, motion-dependent torques at the elbow joint (called *interaction* torque by Ghez and co-workers; see "Inter" in Fig. 8.23) were negligible because the shoulder joint excursion was minimal. At the reversal, the profile of the muscle torque was a mirror image of the *self*-torque ($-I \cdot \alpha$). When the muscle torque is opposite in sign to the *self*-torque, its action serves to accelerate the angular motion of the joint (162), and flexor muscle contraction in Fig. 8.23*A* (see biceps EMG) appears well timed to effect elbow joint acceleration for the reversal.

For the control subject, a large interactive torque developed at the elbow joint due to the complementary shoulder joint excursions at the 125-degree reversal, while the *self*-torque at the elbow joint was the same (in magnitude and sign) for the 0- and 125-degree reversals. For the 125-degree reversal, the elbow joint muscle torque was extensor rather than flexor and in the same direction as the *self*-torque, suggesting that its action countered the acceleration caused by the interaction torque. These kinetic data were consistent with the prolonged triceps EMG (Fig. 8.23*A*) and suggest that a lengthening contraction of elbow extensors opposed the flexor interaction torque at the elbow joint to maintain a tight hand-path reversal for control subjects. The motion-dependent torque at the elbow joint of the deafferentated subject, in contrast, was not initially countered by an appropriate muscle torque. A flexor muscle torque actually accentuated the interaction torque, and elbow flexion was exaggerated at the onset of the 125-degree reversal (Fig. 8.23*B*).

These findings by Ghez and co-workers (58, 162) show that deafferentated subjects could not maintain elbow kinematics independent of the mechanical effects of the shoulder motion. They hypothesize that proprioceptive feedback is important for controlling intersegmental dynamics and envision that the control occurs through a feedforward mechanism (see Chapter 3) in which descending commands are used to update an internal model of the limb. In support of the feedforward hypothesis, Ghez et al. (57, 58) reported that deafferentated subjects were able to improve their performance on the template-tracing task after vision of the screen cursor or of their arm performing the movements. Also, practice with vision in one target direction improved accuracy in other directions during subsequent trials, suggesting that subjects were learning a general rule rather than the production of a specific motor response. The marked improvement produced by vision of the limb, however, degraded within a few minutes after vision was blocked, suggesting that internal models of the limb dynamics require continuous updating.

CHANGES IN LIMB DYNAMICS DURING DEVELOPMENT

Rapid developments are occurring in the combined areas of biomechanics and neuromotor development. There is a strong emphasis on integrative research to better understand the mechanisms responsible for the acquisition and control of movements during development. Thelen and colleagues (192) suggest that the recent applications of dynamical systems analysis, inverse dynamics methods, and motor-control principles to the study of infant and child motor behavior have sparked this rising interest in motor development (13, 92, 110, 150, 183, 187, 189, 191, 192, 208, 214). Pick (150) states that trying to understand the "control of action" (8) has become a prime focus for current motor-development research.

In an effort to bring methods of inverse dynamics to bear on questions related to developmental motor control, during the past several years Esther Thelen and colleagues have collaborated on extensive cross-sectional and longitudinal projects, charting how limb movements of infants change during the first year of life (107, 166, 188, 192, 214). It is apparent that during the first of year of life human infants undergo dramatic changes in motor control. They must acquire motor skills as their body segments change rapidly in mass and geometry, and as the nervous system undergoes rapid development. While body segments change markedly in size, infants must coordinate a daunting array of muscular and interactive forces to learn to control limb movements. Inverse dynamics techniques, therefore, can provide a window to view the role of limb dynamics as infants acquire and refine motor patterns—in both lower and upper limbs. In the following, we review recent findings on the dynamics of spontaneous kick-

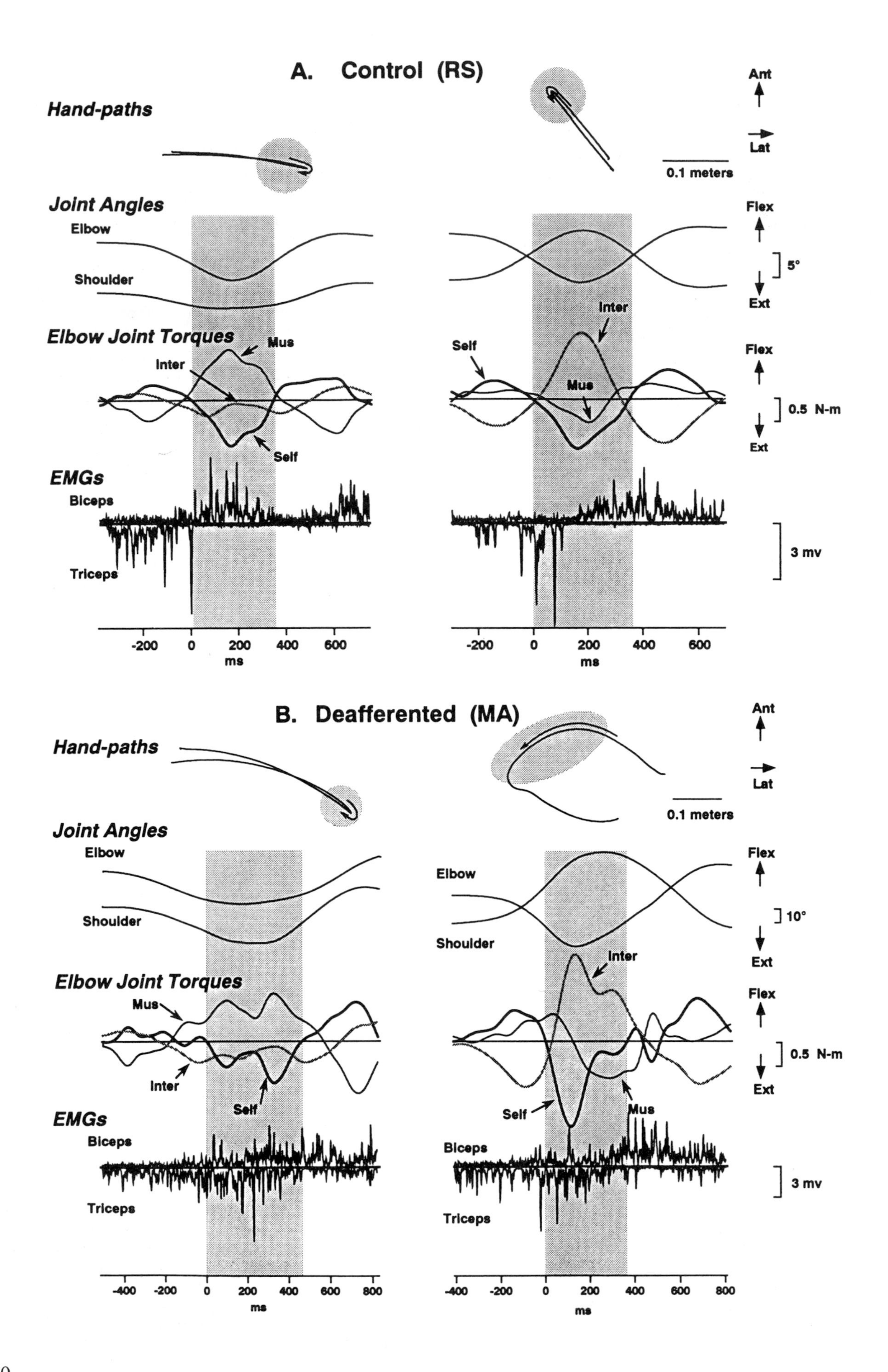
A. Control (RS)
Hand-paths
Ant
Lat
0.1 meters
Joint Angles
Elbow
Shoulder
Flex
5°
Ext
Elbow Joint Torques
Mus
Inter
Self
Flex
0.5 N-m
Ext
EMGs
Biceps
Triceps
3 mv
-200
0
200
400
600
ms
B. Deafferented (MA)
Hand-paths
Ant
Lat
0.1 meters
Joint Angles
Elbow
Shoulder
Flex
10°
Ext
Elbow Joint Torques
Mus
Inter
Self
Flex
0.5 N-m
Ext
EMGs
Biceps
Triceps
3 mv
-400
-200
0
200
400
600
800
ms

ing behaviors and the acquisition of reaching within the first year of life (107, 166, 188, 192, 214).

Spontaneous Kicking Behaviors

For 3-month-old infants, lower extremity dynamics have been quantified during spontaneous kicks of varying intensity, ranging from nonvigorous to vigorous (166, 188). When behaviorally aroused, infants in a supine position readily produce kicking actions of coordinated flexion-extension cycles of the hip, knee, and ankle joints that are frequently forceful and rapid (cycle durations of 600–800 ms). Thelen and Fisher (190) note that although most infants perform these kicks, the kicks do not appear to be goal directed. These spontaneous limb actions are typically unconstrained, and significant motion-dependent torques can develop, depending on the speed or "vigor" of the kicking action (166). Furthermore, the supine infant must contend with gravitational effects, which change as the limb is flexed and extended.

In nonvigorous kicks, the reversal at the hip joint was primarily a result of gravity acting on the limb and being opposed by a hip-muscle flexor torque and flexor torques generated by forces between the segments of the limb (motion-dependent torques). At the hip reversal in vigorous kicks, however, an extensor muscle torque was needed to counteract the flexor effect of the motion-dependent torque, and (in very vigorous kicks) the hip-flexor effect of gravity. The greatest muscular torques were needed at the start and end of the kicking motion—first to overcome the limb inertia and counteract gravity and later to slow and stop the downward motion of the end of the kick. With the changes in motion-dependent torques, the muscle torques changed to produce the net torque needed to complete the action. As a consequence, smooth trajectories resulted from the interplay of the gravitational, muscular, and motion-dependent torques (166).

To examine the sensitivity of these dynamics to the gravitational field, the spontaneous kicking of 3-month-old infants was quantified as they kicked with three different torso orientations—supine, 45 degrees, and vertical (107). As with supine kicking, in the 45-degree and vertical orientations, infants easily performed spontaneous kicking, with various ranges of motion and vigor and with either single or multiple kicking actions. In the more upright postures, gravitational resistance at the hip was four to ten times greater than the resistance met in the supine posture, necessitating much larger hip muscle torques to generate hip flexion. Regardless of torso orientation, however, the reversal of the hip-joint motion was produced by the gravitational torque component—with one exception. That exception, as mentioned previously (166), was in a supine, vigorous kick with a large hip-joint range of motion. In that case, the reversal at the hip was produced not by the hip-flexor torque modulating the gravitational extensor torque, but by an active hip extensor muscle torque.

In the vertical posture, infants had a substantially reduced hip-joint range of motion and tighter coupling between hip and knee flexion-extension motions. In the supine and 45-degree postures, the gravitational torques were resisted by hip flexors and knee extensors, and obviously as the body became more upright, the effects of the gravitational torques diminished. While in the vertical posture, the effect of the gravitational torque at the knee was either flexor or extensor, depending on the limb configuration and nature of the kick.

These studies indicate that the nascent motor system can adjust to changes in the external force environment without the benefit of training or intentionality (107). With these spontaneous kicking actions, a 3-month-old infant already has the facultative capacity to adjust muscular torques to counteract the effects of motion-dependent torques.

Acquisition of Reaching

The ability to reach for an object is a significant motor milestone that usually emerges in months 3–5 of an infant's first year (188). The word "emerges" is used in a specific context, as apparently the goal-directed reaching develops from an ongoing background of other movements of the arms. In the case

FIG. 8.23. Hand paths, dynamics, and EMG for arm movements in two directions for a control (*A*) and deafferentated (*B*) subject. See text for description of the template-tracing task. Ensemble averages for joint angles (*top*), elbow joint torque components (*middle*), and EMG records (*bottom*) are illustrated for movements made along the 0-degree template (*left*) and the 125-degree template (*right*). Torque components include an interaction torque (*Inter*; same as the motion-dependent torque of equation 1), a generalized muscle torque (*Mus*; same as the generalized muscle torque of equation 1), and a *self*-torque [$Self = (-I \cdot \alpha)$]; see Sainburg et al. (162) for a comparison of the *self*-torque and the *net* joint torque in equation 1. Data for each record are averaged across five trials and aligned to the zero cross (abscissa) in elbow joint flexor acceleration. Shading highlights the interval of flexor acceleration, encompassing the hand-path reversal. [Adapted from Figs. 7 and 8 of Sainburg et al. (162).]

of the infants in the Thelen longitudinal study (188, 214), kinematic, EMG, and dynamic details are being quantified to determine how infants learned to solve the problem of reaching an object. With these data, the following questions will be addressed: *(1)* How do the dynamics of upper extremity movements change during the first year of life? *(2)* How are the undirected, erratic limb movements of very young infants later molded into well-coordinated, precise reaching movements? and *(3)* As infants harness the dynamics of their upper extremity during reaching, do they learn to exploit the motion-dependent torques of their limbs—similar to adults learning a new motor task?

These are only a few of the numerous questions that can be investigated as methods of inverse dynamics are used to examine the mechanisms underlying changes in motor control during development. Thelen and collaborators (188, 214) are continuing to address these questions with data from four normal, full-term infants (one girl and three boys). Each of these infants was studied twice weekly from 3 weeks of age to 30 weeks and twice every 2 weeks thereafter until 52 weeks of age—as they gained dexterity in a standard task of reaching to a toy. During the first of the two weekly sessions, the infants were videotaped in a naturalistic play session with parents to assess their natural motor progress, unencumbered with the experimental equipment. The other session each week consisted of the gathering of EMG, three-dimensional kinematic, and anthropometric data to be used in dynamics analyses (188, 214).

For all reaching trials, infants were seated in an armless, inclined (30 degrees from the vertical) infant seat, with their torsos secured to the backrest with a snug but comfortable broad band. Data were collected in 14 s epochs to increase the likelihood of capturing salient arm movements. The study design comprised three conditions: baseline, social, and toy trials. A *baseline* trial was collected at the beginning and end of each session. In the baseline trials, the parent was in the view of the infant, but not actively engaging them, and no toy was present. A *social* trial was one in which the parent interacted with the infant, and a *toy* trial involved presenting small, graspable toys to the infant at midline, shoulder height. The data discussed here are based principally on a contrast of "active" infants vs. "quiet" infants. Because the focus in this chapter is on limb dynamics, we do not emphasize kinematic details but rather the changes in torque components as infants learned to reach.

Controlling Torque Components. The infants first reached the toy at ages ranging from weeks 12 to 22. For example, one active infant (Nathan) performed arm-extended reaches at week 12 that hit the toy as part of spontaneous, undirected "flapping" movements (188, 214). Through week 22, most of Nathan's reaches or attempted reaches had hand trajectories with frequent reversals of direction and with hand paths apparently not directed at the toy. In weeks 26 through 42, there were more sequentially organized hand paths and a plateau in the number of hand-path reversals (188); the nature of his hand path was to first move his hand away from his side and then move, rather directly, upward and to the midline to reach the toy. During the last few weeks of the first year, Nathan's hand movements tended to be more smooth and directed upward, forward, and toward the midline to the toy (188).

During early reaches, coordination between Nathan's elbow and shoulder joint actions was erratic and quite variable. Later, as he gradually began to move more directly to the toy, a more consistent pattern emerged—first elbow flexion, followed by shoulder flexion, with the maximum velocities of elbow extension and shoulder flexion happening close in time as the hand moved toward the toy.

In early reaching movements (weeks 5–22), Nathan principally used flexor muscle torques at both the shoulder and elbow joints to counteract the gravitational extensor torque. Later (weeks 26–38), sequential motions of the hand were linked to modulation of flexor muscle torques at the elbow and shoulder; an increase in flexor muscle torque at the shoulder was followed by an increase in flexor muscle torque at the elbow. The muscular torques at the shoulder and elbow became more tightly coupled during weeks 48–51, with the shoulder muscle torques of greater magnitude than the elbow.

In sum, Nathan learned to control the excessive motion-dependent torques of the early reaches, thereby producing a smoother reaching pattern at the older age. At 17 weeks of age, for example, Nathan had to use a large shoulder muscle moment to offset the large, erratic motion-dependent torques (Fig. 8.24*A*). In contrast, Figure 8.24*B* shows how the motion-dependent torques are reduced in magnitude and are modulated during the interplay between muscular and gravitational torques as Nathan moved to the toy at 51 weeks of age.

The motion-dependent torques, associated with inertial and centripetal forces, were excessive and poorly controlled in the early reaches. As Nathan gained skill in reaching, he was able to damp the extraneous, unproductive motion-dependent torques, while learning to use appropriately timed

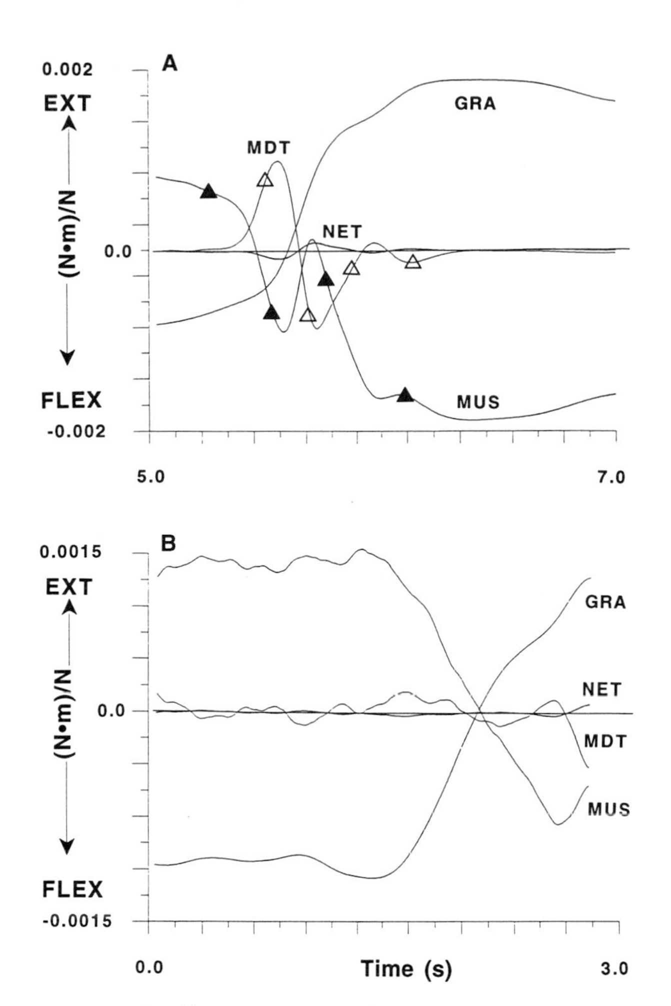

FIG. 8.24. Shoulder joint torques for representative reaches at week 17 (*A*) and week 51 (*B*). Absolute times within a 14 s epoch are given; the two reaches occurred at 5.5 s (*A*) and 2–3 s (*B*). Positive torques tend to cause shoulder extension, and negative torques tend to produce shoulder flexion. The torque components are: NET, net joint torque; MUS, generalized muscle torque; GRA, gravitational torque; MDT, sum of all motion-dependent torques. Torques are normalized to infant's body weight (N) at the different ages. [Adapted from Fig. 9 of Zernicke and Schneider (214).]

motion-dependent torques to complement muscle torques. Inertial torques related to upper-arm and forearm angular accelerations and linear acceleration of the shoulder joint were the most prominent intersegmental torques throughout the first year of reaching development. During weeks 50–51, in particular, Nathan's inertial motion-dependent torques (upper-arm and forearm angular accelerations) at both the shoulder and elbow were generally in phase. As the hand approached the toy, shoulder and elbow flexor muscle torques were modulated in response to the varying flexor or extensor effects of these interactive torques.

The more precisely coordinated arm movements observed in Nathan's last month were related to a more effective use of motion-dependent torques and forces, with less dependence on muscular torques alone to generate his limb movements. As the segmental, motion-dependent torque became more in phase, Nathan learned to use muscular torques to modulate the effects of the motion-dependent torques as he approached the toy (169, 214).

Contrasting Strategies. In contrast to the more active infants (typical of Nathan), the quieter infants had distinctly different strategies for reaching the target. While active infants achieved their first reaches between weeks 12–15, quieter infants achieved their first reaches at weeks 21–22. At the time of their first reaches, the quieter infants were more likely to accomplish their reaches as unimanual actions. *Reach onset* was the first week in which the infants consistently touched the toy by flexing and abducting the shoulder up and away from the body and extending the elbow, while looking at the toy (188).

As one of the two active infants, Gabriel initiated his reaches from a background of rhythmic, rapid arm motions. By stiffening his limbs, through muscle co-contraction, he was able to slow his speed and dampen his extraneous motion-dependent forces. Nathan, the other active infant, also produced varied and complex flapping movements of his arms. He, like Gabriel, appeared to be swiping at the toy, but as noted previously, Nathan learned to dampen and counterbalance the excessive motion-dependent torques as he continued to refine his reaching technique. In contrast to the active infants, the quiet infants switched from low-energy coactivation strategies to one with increased energy (coming primarily from the shoulder).

An interesting consequence of the "active" vs. "quiet" approach to reaching the toy is revealed in Figure 8.25. At the onset of reaching, Nathan (active infant) had rather erratic hand motions in the approach to the toy. In contrast, Justin (quiet infant) after being successful in his reach, had an *increase* in erratic movements in the next 2 weeks. Occasionally, when Justin increased the energy and speed of the reaching action, he found that he had not practiced with the larger motion-dependent torques that were now being generated. Thus, Justin had to learn to control these new torques, and later, he too was able to dampen the motion-dependent torques and smoothly move to grasp the toy.

CONCLUDING REMARKS

During everyday activities such as walking, running, or reaching, limb motions are generated from inter-

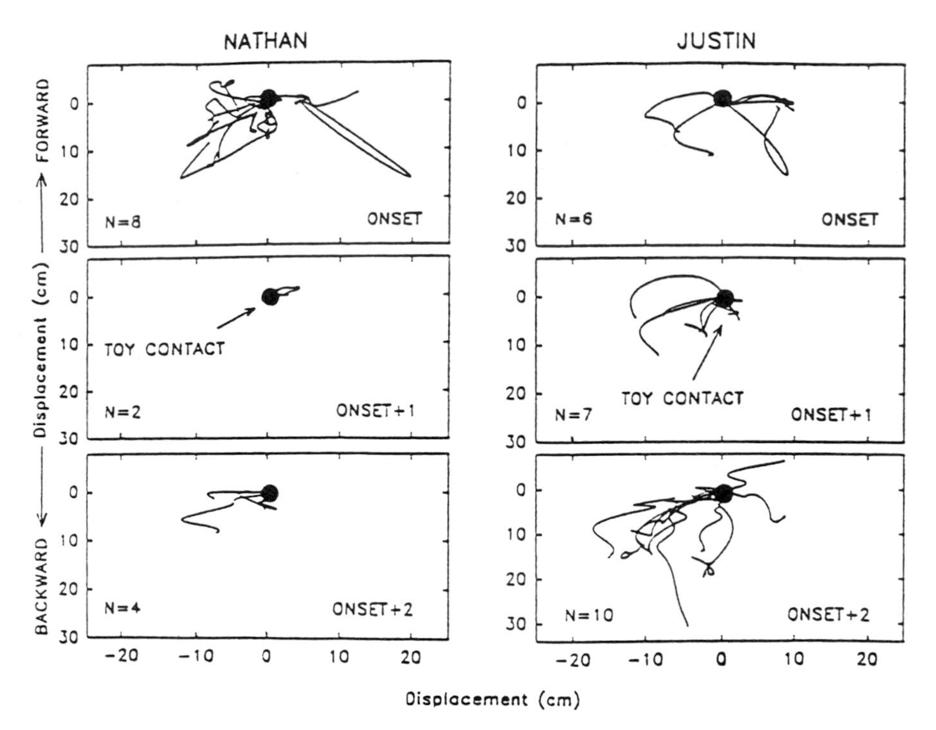

FIG. 8.25. Hand trajectories of all analyzable trials at *reach onset* (top record of each panel), *onset plus 1 week* (middle record), *onset plus 2 weeks*, (bottom record) during which the "active infant" (Nathan) and the "quiet infant" (Justin) contacted the toy (*black dot*). Only the trajectory of the hand contacting the toy is illustrated. Your perspective is from a top view (as though you were directly above each infant, looking down on his head as he faced the toy directly in front of him). Trajectories were normalized to the space-time coordinates of the toy contact and are plotted for the last 3 s prior to hand-toy contact. [Adapted from Figs. 15 and 22 of Thelen et al. (188).]

actions among segmental linkages, tissue viscoelastic behaviors, contractions of skeletal muscles, and neural efferent and afferent signals. Each of these contributing elements is profoundly complex, and as a coordinated system, understanding the neural control of limb movements is an enormous challenge. Quantifying limb dynamics, however, provides a powerful tool in our armamentarium for revealing the mechanisms of neuromotor control.

Dynamical analyses reveal that muscle contractions can function directly to control limb dynamics or to counteract interactive torques arising from mechanical interactions between limb segments. During development and learning, intersegmental dynamics of the limb may change as the nervous system exploits them to achieve efficient and coordinated limb motions. Biomechanists and motor control theorists focus on quantifying these changes and understanding elements of motion efficiency. Neuroscientists generally focus on how (and where) effective motor patterns are programmed to exploit these intersegmental dynamics and how (or if) motion-related feedback is used by the nervous system to monitor internal (as well as external) forces that accompany limb motions.

Movement regulation is a dynamic process in which adaptive and functional strategies are developed to reduce the complexity of motor control. By combining efforts, scientists interested in the control of movement will meet the challenge. While some important neural control insights have already been made using dynamics analyses, with advances in dynamics models and the application of these techniques to a wider range of questions, the future holds even brighter prospects for advancing our knowledge of neural control through dynamics analyses.

We are indebted to Elizabeth Mortimer Roberts at the University of Wisconsin, who mentored both of us as doctoral students in areas of neural control and limb dynamics. We are also grateful for the many contributions of a number of our doctoral students, postdoctoral fellows, and visiting scholars, who assisted us in exploring aspects of limb dynamics and predictions related to the neural control of limb movement at the University of California, Los Angeles. These include John Buford, Patricia Carlson-Kuhta, Melissa Gross (Hoy), Gail Koshland, Patricia McKinley, Karen Perell, and Klaus Schneider, as well as our faculty colleague, Robert Gregor. We thank Claude Ghez and his Columbia University colleagues, Robert Sainburg, Scott Cooper, and James Gordon, for sending preprints of their recent papers, providing Figure 8.23, and assisting us in understanding their joint-torque formulations. In the area of neuromotor development, we wish to acknowledge the collaboration with Esther Thelen and her colleagues at the University of Indiana. We appreciate the insightful reviews of earlier chapter drafts by many of those listed in this acknowledgment and thank Arthur Prochazka for suggesting the title. We also thank Oliver Wang for preparing many of the figures adapted for this chapter. Work on this chapter was made possible by a grant from the Alberta Heritage Foundation for Medical Research to RFZ (14542) and a grant from the National Institute of Neurological Disorders and Stroke to JLS (NS 19864).

REFERENCES

1. Abend, W., E. Bizzi, and P. Morasso. Human arm trajectory formation. *Brain* 105: 331–348, 1982.
2. Adams, J. A. Historical review and appraisal of research on the learning, retention, and transfer of human motor skills. *Psychol. Bull.* 101: 41–74, 1987.
3. Andersson, O., and S. Grillner. Peripheral control of the cat's step cycle I. Phase dependent effects of ramp-movements of the hip during "fictive locomotion." *Acta Physiol. Scand.* 113: 89–101, 1981.
4. Atkeson, C. G. Learning arm kinematics and dynamics. *Annu. Rev. Neurosci.* 12: 157–183, 1989.
5. Atkeson, C. G., and J. M. Hollerbach. Kinematic features of unrestrained vertical arm movements. *J. Neurosci.* 5: 2318–2330, 1985.
6. Barbeau, H., C. Julien, and S. Rossignol. The effects of clonidine and yohimbine on locomotion and cutaneous reflexes in the adult spinal cat. *Brain Res.* 437: 83–96, 1987.
7. Bernstein, N. Studies of the biomechanics of the stroke by means of photo-registration. Research of the Central Institute of Work: Moscow: N1: 19–79, 1923 (in Russian).
8. Bernstein, N. *Co-ordination and Regulation of Movements.* New York: Pergamon Press, 1967.
9. Bizzi, E., and W. K. Abend. Control of multijoint movement. In: *Comparative Neurobiology, Modes of Communication in the Nervous System*, edited by F. Strumwasser and M. Dohen, New York: John Wiley & Sons, 1985, p. 255–277.
10. Bizzi, E., W. Chapple, and N. Hogan. Mechanical properties of muscles: implications for motor control. *Trends Neurosci.* 5: 395–398, 1982.
11. Bizzi, E., F. A. Mussa-Ivaldi, and S. Giszter. Computations underlying the execution of movement: a biological perspective. *Science* 253: 287–291, 1991.
12. Blaszczcyk, J., and G. E. Loeb. Why cats pace on the treadmill. *Physiol. Behav.* 53: 501–507, 1993.
13. Bloch, H., and B. I. Bertenthal. *Sensory-Motor Organizations and Development in Infancy and Early Childhood.* Dordrecht, Netherlands: Kluwer Academic Publishers, 1990.
14. Bobbert, M. F., P. A. Huijing, and G. J. van Ingen Schenau. A model of the human triceps surae muscle-tendon complex applied to jumping. *J. Biomech.* 19: 887–898, 1986.
15. Borelli, G. A. *De Motu Animalium.* Editio Altera Correctior emendatior, Lugduni Nin Batavis, J. de Vivie, C. Bouteseyn, D. a Gaebuck, and P. Vander AA., 1685 (later edition).
16. Braune, C. W., and O. Fischer. Ueber den Schwerpunkt des menschlichen Koerpers mit Ruecksicht auf die ausruestung des deutschen Infanteristen. *Abhandlungen der Mathematisch-physikalischen Classe der Koenigl. Saechisschen Gesellschaft der Wissenschaften*, 15: 561–572, 1889.
17. Bresler, B., and J. P. Frankel. The forces and moments in the leg during level walking. *Trans. Am. Soc. Mech. Eng. (J. Biomech. Eng.)* 72: 27–36, 1950.
18. Buford, J. A., and J. L. Smith. Adaptive control for backward quadrupedal walking. II. Hindlimb muscle synergies. *J. Neurophysiol.* 64: 756–766, 1990.
19. Buford, J. A., and J. L. Smith. Adaptive control for backward quadrupedal walking. III. Stumbling corrective responses and cutaneous reflex sensitivity. *J. Neurophysiol.* 70: 1102–1114, 1993.
20. Buford, J. A., R. F. Zernicke, and J. L. Smith. Adaptive control for backward quadrupedal walking. I. Posture and hindlimb kinematics. *J. Neurophysiol.* 64: 745–755, 1990.
21. Cajori, F. (Ed.) *Sir Isaac Newton's Mathematical Principles of Natural Philsophy and His System of the World.* (A. Mottee, translation). Berkeley: University of California Press. (originally published, 1729), 1946.
22. Cavanagh, P. R., and R. Kram. The efficiency of human movement—a statement of the problem. *Med. Sci. Sports Exerc.* 17: 304–308, 1985.
23. Chanaud, C. M., C. A. Pratt, and G. E. Loeb. Functionally complex muscles of the cat hindlimb. V. The role of histochemical fiber type regionalization and mechanical heterogeneity in differential muscle activation. *Exp. Brain Res.* 85: 300–313, 1991.
24. Chandler, R. F., C. E. Clauser, J. T. McConville, H. M. Reynolds, and J. W. Young. *Investigation of the Inertial Properties of the Human Body.* (Technical Report DOT HS-801 430) Wright-Patterson Air Force Base: Ohio, 1975.
25. Chow, C. K., and D. H. Jacobson. Studies of human locomotion via optimal programming. *Math. Biosci.* 10: 239–306, 1971.
26. Clauser, C. E., J. T. McConville, and J. W. Young. *Weight, Volume and Center of Mass of Segments of the Human Body.* (AMRL Technical Report) Wright-Patterson Air Force Base, Ohio, 1969.
27. Contini, R. Preface. *Hum. Factors* 5: 423–425, 1963.
28. Cooper, S. E., J. H. Martin, and C. Ghez. Differential effects of localized inactivation of deep cerebellar nuclei on reaching in the cat. *Soc. Neurosci. Abstr.* 19: 1278, 1993.
29. Crowninshield, R. D. Use of optimization techniques to predict muscle forces. *J. Biomech. Eng.* 100: 88–92, 1978.
30. Crowninshield, R. D., and R. A. Brand. A physiologically based criterion of muscle force prediction in locomotion. *J. Biomech.* 14: 793–801, 1981.
31. Cruse, H., M. Bruewer, and J. Dean. Control of three- and four-joint arm movement: strategies for a manipulator with redundant degrees of freedom. *J. Mot. Behav.* 25: 131–139, 1993.
32. Cunningham, D. M., and G. W. Brown. Two devices for measuring the forces acting on the human body during walking. *Proc. Soc. Exp. Stress Analysis* 9: 75–90, 1952.
33. D'Alembert, J. L. *Traite de dynamique.* Paris: David, 1758.
34. Davy, D. T., and M. L. Audu. A dynamic optimization technique for predicting muscle forces in the swing phase of gait. *J. Biomech.* 20: 187–201, 1987.
35. Dempster, W. T. Free body diagrams as an approach to the mechanics of human posture and motion. In: *Biomechanical Studies of the Musculo-Skeletal System*, edited by F. G. Evans. Springfield, IL: Charles C Thomas, 1961, p. 81–135.
36. Dempster, W. T. *Space Requirements of the Seated Operator: Geometrical, Kinematic and Mechanical Aspects of the Body with Special Reference to the Limbs.* (WADC Technical Report No. 55–159). Wright-Patterson Air Force Base: Ohio, 1955.

37. Dul, J., G. E. Johnson, R. Shiavi, and M. A. Townsend. Muscular synergism—II. A minimum-fatigue criterion for load sharing between synergistic muscles. *J. Biomech.* 17: 675–684, 1984.
38. Duysens, J., and K. G. Pearson. Inhibition of flexor burst generation by loading ankle extensor muscles in walking cats. *Brain Res.* 187: 321–332, 1980.
39. Engberg, I., and A. Lundberg. An electromyographic analysis of muscular activity in the hindlimb of the cat during unrestrained locomotion. *Acta Physiol. Scand.* 75: 614–630, 1969.
40. English, A. The functions of the lumbar spine during stepping in the cat. *J. Morphol.* 165: 55–66, 1980.
41. English, A. W., and O. Weeks. An anatomical and functional analysis of cat biceps femoris and semitendinosus muscles. *J. Morphol.* 191: 161–175, 1987.
42. Evans, F. G. Biomechanical implications of anatomy. In: *Selected Topics on Biomechanics*, edited by J. M. Cooper. Chicago: Athletic Institute, 1971, p. 3–30.
43. Feldman, A. G. Once more on the equilibrium-point hypothesis (λ model) for motor control. *J. Mot. Behav.* 18: 17–54, 1986.
44. Fenn, W. O. Work against gravity and work due to velocity changes in running. *Am. J. Physiol.* 93: 433–462, 1930.
45. Fitch, H. L., B. Tuller, and M. T. Turvey. The Bernstein perspective: III. Tuning of coordinative structures with special reference to perception. In: *Human Behavior: An Introduction*, edited by J. A. S. Kelso. Hillsdale, NJ: Lawrence Erlbaum Associates, 1982, p. 271–282.
46. Flanagan, J. R., D. J. Ostry, and A. G. Feldman. Control of trajectory modifications in target-directed reaching. *J. Mot. Behav.* 25: 140–152, 1993.
47. Flash, T. *Organizing principles underlying the formation of hand trajectories.* Ph.D. thesis, Cambridge, MA: Massachusetts Institute of Technology, 1983.
48. Flash, T. The control of hand equilibrium trajectories in multi-joint arm movement. *Biol. Cybern.* 57: 257–274, 1987.
49. Flash, T., and E. Hennis. Arm trajectory modification during reaching towards visual target. *J. Cognit. Neurosci.* 3: 220–230, 1991.
50. Flash, T., and N. Hogan. Evidence for an optimization strategy in arm trajectory formation. *Soc. Neurosci. Abstr.* 8: 282, 1982.
51. Flash, T., and N. Hogan. The coordination of arm movements: an experimentally confirmed mathematical model. *J. Neurosci.* 5: 1688–1703, 1985.
52. Forget, R., and Y. Lamarre. Rapid elbow flexion in the absence of proprioceptive and cutaneous feedback. *Hum. Neurobiol.* 6: 27–37, 1987.
53. Fowler, E. G., R. J. Gregor, J. A. Hodgson, and R. R. Roy. Relationship between ankle muscle and joint kinetics during the stance phase of locomotion in the cat. *J. Biomech.* 26: 465–483, 1993.
54. Fowler, E. G., R. J. Gregor, and R. R. Roy. Differential kinetics of fast and slow ankle extensors during the paws-shake in the cat. *Exp. Neurol.* 99: 219–224, 1988.
55. Fung, Y. C. *Biomechanics: Motion, Stress, and Growth.* New York: Springer-Verlag, 1990.
56. Gelfand, I. M., V. S. Gurfinkel, M. L. Tsetlin, and M. L. Shik. Some problems in the analysis of movements. In: *Models of the Structural-Functional Organization of Certain Biological Systems*, edited by I. M. Gelfand, V. S. Gurfinkel, M. L. Tsetlin, and M. L. Shik. Cambridge, MA: MIT Press, 1971.
57. Ghez, C., J. Gordon, and M. F. Ghilardi. Impairments of reaching movements in patients without proprioception. II. Effects of visual information on accuracy. *J. Neurophysiol.* (in press).
58. Ghez, C., and R. Sainburg. Proprioceptive control of interjoint coordination. *Can. J. Physiol. Pharmacol.* (in press).
59. Gielen, C. C. A. M., K. van den Oosten, and G. ter Gunne. Relation between EMG activation patterns and kinematic properties of aimed arm movements. *J. Mot. Behav.* 17: 421–442, 1985.
60. Gordon, J., M. F. Ghilardi, and C. Ghez. Impairments of reaching movements in patients without proprioception. I. Spatial errors. *J. Neurophysiol.* (in press).
61. Gordon, J., M. F. Ghilardi, and C. Ghez. Accuracy of planar reaching movement. I. Independence of direction and extent variability. *Exp. Brain Res.* 99: 97–111, 1994.
62. Gordon, J., M. F. Ghilardi, S. E. Cooper, and C. Ghez. Accuracy of planar reaching movement. II. Systematic extent errors resulting from inertial anisotropy. *Exp. Brain Res.* 99: 112–130, 1994.
63. Goslow, G. E., R. M. Reinking, and D. G. Stuart. The cat step cycle: hind limb joint angles and muscle lengths during unrestrained locomotion. *J. Morphol.* 141: 1–41, 1973.
64. Gottlieb, G. L. A computational model of the simplest motor program. *J. Mot. Behav.* 25: 153–161, 1993.
65. Gottlieb, G. L., D. M. Corcos, and G. C. Agarwal. Strategies for the control of voluntary movements with one mechanical degree of freedom. *Behav. Brain Sci.* 12: 189–224, 1990.
66. Gregor, R. J., P. R. Cavanagh, and M. LaFortune. Knee flexor moments during propulsion in cycling: a creative solution to Lombard's Paradox. *J. Biomech.* 18: 307–316, 1985.
67. Gregor, R. J., P. V. Komi, R. C. Browning, and M. A. Jarvinen. Comparison of the triceps surae and residual muscle moments at the ankle during cycling. *J. Biomech.* 24: 287–297, 1991.
68. Gregor, R. J., R. R. Roy, W. C. Whiting, R. G. Lovely, J. Hodgson, and V. R. Edgerton. Mechanical output of the cat soleus during treadmill locomotion: *In vivo* vs. *in situ* characteristics. *J. Biomech.* 21: 721–732, 1988.
69. Grillner, S. Control of locomotion in bipeds, tetrapods, and fish. In: *Handbook of Physiology, The Nervous System, Motor Control*, edited by V. B. Brooks. Bethesda, MD: Am. Physiol. Soc., 1981, p. 1179–1236.
70. Grillner, S., and S. Rossignol. On the initiation of the swing phase of locomotion in chronic spinal cat. *Brain Res.* 146: 269–277, 1978.
71. Grillner, S., and P. Zangger. On the central generation of locomotion in the low spinal cat. *Exp. Brain Res.* 34: 241–261, 1979.
72. Haken, H. *Synergetics: An Introduction.* Heidelberg: Springer-Verlag, 1977.
73. Halbertsma, J. M. The stride cycle of the cat: the modeling of locomotion by computerized analysis of automatic recordings. *Acta Physiol. Scand. Suppl.* 521: 1–75, 1983.
74. Hart, T. J., E. M. Cox, M. G. Hoy, J. L. Smith, and R. F. Zernicke. Intralimb kinetics of perturbed paw-shake response. In: *Biomechanics X-A*, edited by B. Jonsson. Champaign, IL: Human Kinetics Publishers, 1987, p. 471–478.
75. Hatze, H. *A Model for the Computational Determination of Parameter Values of Anthropomorphic Segments.* NRIMS Technical Report TWISK 79, Pretoria, South Africa, 1979.

76. Hatze, H. A mathematical model for the computational determination of parameter values of anthropomorphic segments. *J. Biomech.* 13: 833–843, 1980.
77. Hatze, H. A comprehensive model for human motion simulation and its application to the take-off phase of the long jump. *J. Biomech.* 14: 135–142, 1981.
78. Hatze, H. Quantitative analysis, synthesis and optimization of human motion. *Hum. Mov. Sci.* 3: 5–25, 1984.
79. Hatze, H. The complete optimization of a human motion. *Math. Biosci.* 28: 99–135, 1976.
80. Hatze, H. Was ist Biomechanik (What is biomechanics)? *Leibesuebungen Leibeserziehung.* 25: 33–34, 1971.
81. Herzog, W., and T. R. Leonard. Validation of optimization models that estimate the forces exerted by synergistic models. *J. Biomech.* 24: 31–39, 1991.
82. Herzog, W., T. R. Leonard, and A. C. S. Guimaraes. Forces in gastrocnemius, soleus, and plantaris tendons of the freely moving cat. *J. Biomech.* 26: 945–953, 1993.
83. Hildebrand, M. Analysis of asymmetrical gaits. *J. Mammal.* 58: 131–156, 1977.
84. Hildebrand, M. The adaptive significance of tetrapod gait selection. *Am. Zool.* 20: 255–267, 1980.
85. Hobart, D. J., D. L. Kelley, and L. S. Bradley. Modifications occurring during acquisition of a novel throwing task. *Am. J. Phys. Med.* 54: 1–24, 1975.
86. Hodgson, J. A. The relationship between soleus and gastrocnemius muscle activity in conscious cats: a model for motor unit recruitment. *J. Physiol. (Lond.)* 337: 553–562, 1983.
87. Hof, A. L., and J. W. van den Berg. EMG force processing. I. An electrical analogue of the Hill muscle model. *J. Biomech.* 14: 747–758, 1981.
88. Hof, A. L., B. A. Geelen, and J. W. van den Berg. Calf muscle moment, work and efficiency in level walking: role of series elasticity. *J. Biomech.* 16: 523–537, 1983.
89. Hof, A. L., C. N. A. Pronk, and J. A. van Best. Comparison between EMG to force processing and kinetic analysis for the calf muscle moment in walking and stepping. *J. Biomech.* 20: 167–178, 1987.
90. Hoffer, J. A., A. A. Caputi, I. E. Pose, and R. I. Griffiths. Roles of muscle activity and load on the relationship between muscle spindle length and whole muscle length in the freely walking cat. *Prog. Brain Res.* 80: 75–85, 1989.
91. Hoffer, J. A., G. E. Loeb, N. Sugano, W. B. Marks, M. J. O'Donovan, and C. A. Pratt. Cat hindlimb motoneurons during locomotion. III. Functional segregation in sartorius. *J. Neurophysiol.* 57: 554–773, 1987.
92. Hofsten, C. von. Structuring of early reaching movements: a longitudinal study. *J. Mot. Behav.* 23: 280–292, 1991.
93. Hogan, N. An organizing principle for a class of voluntary movements. *J. Neurosci.* 4: 2745–2754, 1984.
94. Hogan, N. The mechanics of multi-joint posture and movement control. *Biol. Cybern.* 52: 315–331, 1985.
95. Hogan, N., E. Bizzi, F. A. Mussa-Ivaldi, and T. Flash. Controlling multijoint behavior. *Exerc. Sport Sci. Rev.* 15: 153–190, 1989.
96. Hogan, N., and T. Flash. Moving gracefully: quantitative theories of motor coordination. *Trends Neurosci.* 10: 170–174, 1987.
97. Hollerbach, J. M. Computers, brains, and the control of movement. *Trends Neurosci.* 5: 189–192, 1982.
98. Hollerbach, J. M., and T. Flash. Dynamic interactions between limb segments during planar arm movement. *Biol. Cybern.* 44: 67–77, 1982.
99. Hoy, M. G., F. E. Zajac, and M. E. Gordon. A musculoskeletal model of the human lower extremity: the effect of muscle, tendon, and moment arm on the moment-angle relationship of musculotendon actuators at the hip, knee, and ankle. *J. Biomech.* 23: 157–169, 1990.
100. Hoy, M. G., and R. F. Zernicke. Modulation of limb dynamics in the swing phase of locomotion. *J. Biomech.* 18: 49–60, 1985.
101. Hoy, M. G., and R. F. Zernicke. The role of intersegmental dynamics during rapid limb oscillations. *J. Biomech.* 19: 867–877, 1986.
102. Hoy, M. G., R. F. Zernicke, and J. L. Smith. Contrasting roles of inertial and muscular moments at ankle and knee during paw-shake response. *J. Neurophysiol.* 54: 1282–1294, 1985.
103. Ingen Schenau, G. J. van. From rotation to translation: constraints of multi-joint movements and the unique action of bi-articular muscles. *Hum. Mov. Sci.* 8: 301–337, 1989.
104. Inman, V. T. Human locomotion. *Can. Med. Assoc. J.* 94: 1047–1054, 1966.
105. Jayes, A., and R. M. Alexander. Mechanics of locomotion of dogs (*Canis familiaris*) and sheep (*Ovis aries*). *J. Zool. Lond.* 185: 289–308, 1978.
106. Jensen, R. K. Body segment mass, radius and radius of gyration proportions of children. *J. Biomech.* 19: 359–368, 1986.
107. Jensen, J. L., B. D. Ulrich, E. Thelen, K. Schneider, and R. F. Zernicke. Adaptive dynamics of the leg movement patterns of human infants: I. The effects of posture on spontaneous kicking. *J. Mot. Behav.* 26: 303–312, 1994.
108. Kelso, J. A. S. (Ed.) *Human Behavior: An Introduction.* Hillsdale, NJ: Lawrence Erlbaum Associates, 1982.
109. Kelso, J. A. S., and J. Clark. *The Development of Movement Control and Coordination.* New York: John Wiley & Sons, 1982.
110. Kelso, J. A. S., M. Ding, and G. Schoener. Dynamic pattern formation: a primer. In: *A Dynamic Systems Approach to Development: Applications*, edited by L. B. Smith and E. Thelen, Cambridge, MA: MIT Press, 1993, p. 13–50.
111. Kelso, J. A. S., B. Tuller, and K. S. Harris. A "dynamic pattern" perspective on the control and coordination of movement. In: *The Production of Speech*, edited by P. MacNeilage. New York: Springer-Verlag, 1983, p. 137–173.
112. Koshland, G. F., M. G. Hoy, J. L. Smith, and R. F. Zernicke. Coupled and uncoupled limb oscillations during paw-shake response. *Exp. Brain Res.* 83: 587–597, 1991.
113. Koshland, G. F., and J. L. Smith. Mutable and immutable features of paw-shake responses after hindlimb deafferentation in the cat. *J. Neurophysiol.* 62: 162–173, 1989.
114. Koshland, G. F., and J. L. Smith. Paw-shake responses with joint immobilization: EMG changes with atypical feedback. *Exp. Brain Res.* 77: 361–373, 1989.
115. Kugler, P., J. A. S. Kelso, and M. T. Turvey. On the control and co-ordination of naturally developing systems. In: *The Development of Movement Control and Co-ordination*, edited by J. A. S. Kelso and J. E. Clark. New York: John Wiley & Sons, 1982, p. 5–78.
116. Kugler, P. N., and M. T. Turvey. *Information, Natural Law, and the Self-Assembly of Rhythmic Movement.* Hillsdale, NJ: Lawrence Erlbaum Associates, 1987.
117. Lacquaniti, F., and J. F. Soechting. Coordination of arm and wrist motion during a reaching task. *J. Neurosci.* 2: 399–408, 1982.
118. Levine, W. S., F. E. Zajac, M. R. Belzer, and M. R. Zomlefer. Ankle controls that produce a maximal vertical jump when other joints are locked. *IEEE Trans. Auto. Control* AC-28: 1008–1016, 1983.

119. Lieber, R. L., and J. L. Boakes. Sarcomere length and joint kinematics during torque production in the frog hindlimb. *Am. J. Physiol.* 254 (*Cell Physiol.* 23): C759–C768, 1988.
120. Likins, P. W. *Elements of Engineering Mechanics*. New York: McGraw-Hill, 1973.
121. Loeb, G. E. Strategies for the control of studies of voluntary movements with one degree of freedom. *Behav. Brain Sci.* 12: 227, 1990.
122. Lundberg, A. Half-centres revisited. In: *Adv. Physiol. Sci. Organization Principles*, edited by J. Szentagotheu, M. Palkovitis, and J. Hamori. Budapest: Pergamon Akademiai Kiado, 1981, p. 155–167.
123. Mann, R. A. Biomechanics of walking, running, and sprinting. *Am. J. Sports Med.* 8: 345–350, 1980.
124. Manter, J. T. The dynamics of quadrupedal walking. *J. Exp. Biol.* 15: 522–540, 1938.
125. Marey, E. J. *Mouvement*. Paris: B. Masson, 1984.
126. Marteniuk, R. G., and S. K. E. Romanow. Human movement organization and learning as revealed by variability of movement, use of kinematic information, and Fourier analysis. In: *Memory and Control of Action*, edited by R. A. Magill. New York: Elsevier North-Holland, 1983.
127. McIntyre, J., and E. Bizzi. Servo hypotheses for the biological control of movement. *J. Mot. Behav.* 25: 193–202, 1993.
128. Mena, D., J. M. Mansour, and S. R. Simon. Analysis and synthesis of human swing leg motion during gait and its clinical application. *J. Biomech.* 14: 823–832, 1981.
129. Mori, S. Integration of posture and locomotion in acute decerebrate cats and in awake freely moving cats. *Prog. Neurobiol.* 28: 161–195, 1987.
130. Morrison, J. B. Bioengineering analysis of force actions transmitted by the knee joint. *Biomed. Eng.* 3: 164–170, 1968.
131. Mussa-Ivaldi, F. A., and S. Giszter. Vector field approximation: a computational paradigm for motor control and learning. *Biol. Cybern.* 67: 491–500, 1993.
132. Mussa-Ivaldi, F. A., N. Hogan, and E. Bizzi. Neural and geometric factors subserving arm posture. *J. Neurosci.* 5: 2732–2743, 1985.
133. Muybridge, E. *The Human Figure in Motion*. New York: Dover, 1955.
134. Muybridge, E. *Animals in Motion*. New York: Dover, 1957.
135. Nelson, W. Physical principles for economies of skilled movements. *Biol. Cybern.* 46: 135–147, 1983.
136. Newmiller, J., M. L. Hull, and F. E. Zajac. A mechanically decoupled two force component bicycle pedal dynamometer. *J. Biomech.* 21: 375–386, 1988.
137. Nigg, B. M., and W. Herzog. *Biomechanics of the Musculoskeletal System*. Sussex, England: Wiley, 1994.
138. Nilsson, J., A. Thorstensson, and J. Halbertsma. Changes in leg movements and muscle activity with speed of locomotion and mode of progression in humans. *Acta Physiol. Scand.* 123: 457–475, 1985.
139. Oguztoereli, M. N., and R. B. Stein. Optimal control of antagonistic muscles. *Biol. Cybern.* 48: 91–99, 1983.
140. Olney, S. J., and D. A. Winter. Prediction of knee and ankle moments of force in walking from EMG and kinematic data. *J. Biomech.* 18: 9–20, 1985.
141. Pandy, M. G., V. Kumar, N. Berme, and K. J. Waldron. The dynamics of quadrupedal locomotion. *J. Biomech. Eng.* 110: 230–237, 1988.
142. Patriarco, A. G., R. W. Mann, S. R. Simon, and J. M. Mansour. An evaluation of the approaches of optimization models in the prediction of muscle forces during human gait. *J. Biomech.* 14: 513–525, 1981.
143. Paul, J. P. Biomechanics of the hip joint and its clinical relevance. *Proc. R. Soc. Med.* 59: 943–948, 1966.
144. Pearson, K. G., and S. Rossignol. Fictive motor patterns in chronic spinal cats. *J. Neurophysiol.* 66: 1874–1887, 1991.
145. Pedotti, A., V. V. Krishnan, and L. Stark. Optimization of muscle-force sequencing in human locomotion. *Math. Biosci.* 38: 57–76, 1977.
146. Perell, K. L., R. J. Gregor, J. A. Buford, and J. L. Smith. Adaptive control for backward quadrupedal walking. VI. Hindlimb kinetics during stance and swing. *J. Neurophysiol.* 70: 2226–2240, 1993.
147. Perret, C., and J-M. Cabelguen. Main characteristics of the hindlimb locomotor cycle in the decorticate cat with special reference to bifunctional muscles. *Brain Res.* 187: 333–352, 1980.
148. Philippson, M. L'autonomie et la centralisation dans les systeme nerveux des animaux. *Trav. Lab. Physiol. Inst. Solvay (Bruxelles)* 7: 1–208, 1905.
149. Phillips, S. J., E. M. Roberts, and T. C. Huang. Quantification of intersegmental reactions during rapid swing motion. *J. Biomech.* 16: 411–418, 1983.
150. Pick, H. L. Motor development: the control of action. *Dev. Psychobiol.* 25: 867–870, 1989.
151. Pierrynowski, M. R., and J. B. Morrison. Estimating the muscle forces generated in the human lower extremity when walking: a physiological solution. *Math. Biosci.* 75: 69–102, 1985.
152. Polit, A., and E. Bizzi. Characteristics of motor programs underlying arm movements in monkey. *J. Neurophysiol.* 42: 183–194, 1979.
153. Pratt, C. A., J. A. Buford, and J. L. Smith. Mutable activation of bifunctional thigh muscles during forward and backward walking. *Soc. Neurosci. Abstr.* 18: 1555, 1992.
154. Pratt, C. A., J. A. Buford, and J. L. Smith. Adaptive control for backward quadrupedal walking: V. Mutable activation of bifunctional thigh muscles. *J. Neurophysiol.* (in press), 1995.
155. Pratt, C. A., and G. E. Loeb. Functionally complex muscles of the cat hindlimb. I. Patterns of activation across sartorius. *Exp. Brain Res.* 85: 243–256, 1991.
156. Prigogine, I. *From Being to Becoming*. San Francisco: Freeman, 1980.
157. Putnam, C. A. Interaction between segments during a kicking motion. In: *Biomechanics VIII-B*, edited by H. Matsui and K. Kobayashi. Champaign, IL: Human Kinetics Publishers, 1983, p. 688–694.
158. Putnam, C. A. A segment interaction analysis of proximal-to-distal sequential segment motion patterns. *Med. Sci. Sports Exerc.* 23: 130–144, 1991.
159. Rassmussen, S., A. K. Chan, and G. E. Goslow. The cat step cycle: electromyographic patterns of muscles during posture and unrestrained locomotion. *J. Morphol.* 155: 253–270, 1978.
160. Rosenbaum, D. A., S. E. Engelbrecht, M. M. Bushe, and L. D. Loukopoulos. Knowledge model for selecting and producing reaching movements. *J. Mot. Behav.* 25: 217–227, 1993.
161. Rothwell, J. C., M. M. Traub, B. L. Day, J. A. Obeso, P. K. Thomas, and C. D. Marsden. Manual motor performance in a deafferented man. *Brain* 105: 515–542, 1982.
162. Sainburg, R. F., M. F. Ghilardi, H. Poizner, and C. Ghez. The control of limb dynamics in normal subjects and pa-

tients without proprioception. *J. Neurophysiol.* 73: 820–835, 1995.
163. Sainburg, R. L., H. Poizner, and C. Ghez. Loss of proprioception produces deficits in interjoint coordination. *J. Neurophysiol.* 70: 2136–2147, 1993.
164. Sanes, J. N., K. H. Mauritz, M. C. Dalakas, and E. V. Evarts. Motor control in humans with large-fiber sensory neuropathy. *Hum. Neurobiol.* 4: 101–114, 1985.
165. Schneider, K., R. F. Zernicke, R. A. Schmidt, and T. J. Hart. Changes in limb dynamics during the practice of rapid arm movements. *J. Biomech.* 22: 805–817, 1989.
166. Schneider, K., R. F. Zernicke, B. D. Ulrich, J. J. Jensen, and E. Thelen. Understanding movement control in infants through the analysis of limb intersegmental dynamics. *J. Mot. Behav.* 22: 493–520, 1990.
167. Schneider, K., and R. F. Zernicke. Jerk-cost modulations during the practice of rapid arm movements. *Biol. Cybern.* 60: 221–230, 1989.
168. Schneider, K., and R. F. Zernicke. A FORTRAN package for the planar analysis of limb intersegmental dynamics from spatial coordinate-time data. *Adv. Eng. Software* 12: 123–128, 1990.
169. Schneider, K., and R. F. Zernicke. Mass, center of mass, and moment of inertia estimates for infant limb segments. *J. Biomech.* 25: 145–148, 1992.
170. Seireg, A., and R. J. Arvikar. The prediction of muscular load sharing and joint forces in the lower extremities during walking. *J. Biomech.* 8: 89–102, 1975.
171. Serret, M. J.-A. *Oevres de Lagrange* (Vols. 11 and 12). Paris: Guther-Villars, 1888–1889.
172. Shadmehr, R. Control of equilibrium position and stiffness through postural modules. *J. Mot. Behav.* 25: 228–241, 1993.
173. Shadmehr, R., F. A. Mussa-Ivaldi, and E. Bizzi. Postural force fields and their role in generation of multi-joint movements. *J. Neurosci.* 13: 45–62, 1993.
174. Sherif, F. M., R. J. Gregor, L. M. Lui, R. R. Roy, and C. L. Hager. Correlation of myoelectric activity and muscle force during selected cat treadmill locomotion. *J. Biomech.* 16: 691–701, 1983.
175. Singer, C. (Ed.) *A Short History of Scientific Ideas to 1900.* New York: Oxford University Press, 1959.
176. Smith, J. L., J. A. Buford, C. Chen, T. V. Trank, O. Wang, and H. S. Wijesinghe. Multifunctional CPG for the control of different forms of cat locomotion. *Physiologist* 36: A–22, 1993.
177. Smith, J. L., J. A. Buford, and R. F. Zernicke. Constraints during backward walking in the quadruped. In: *Posture and Gait: Development, Adaptation and Modulation*, edited by B. Amblard, A. Berthoz, and F. Clarac. Amsterdam: Elsevier Science Publishers, B. V., 1988, p. 391–400.
178. Smith, J. L., and Carlson-Kuhta, P. Unexpected motor patterns for hindlimb muscles during slope walking in the cat. *J. Neurophysiol.* 74: 2211–2215, 1995.
179. Smith, J. L., S. H. Chung, and R. F. Zernicke. Gait-related motor patterns and hindlimb kinetics for the cat trot and gallop. *Exp. Brain Res.* 94: 308–322, 1993.
180. Smith, J. L., V. R. Edgerton, B. Betts, and T. C. Collatos. EMG of slow and fast extensors of the cat during posture, locomotion, and jumping. *J. Neurophysiol.* 40: 503–513, 1977.
181. Smith, J. L., M. G. Hoy, G. F. Koshland, D. M. Phillips, and R. F. Zernicke. Intralimb coordination of the paw-shake response: a novel mixed synergy. *J. Neurophysiol.* 54: 1271–1281, 1985.
182. Smith, J. L., and R. F. Zernicke. Predictions for neural control based on limb dynamics. *Trends Neurosci.* 10: 123–128, 1987.
183. Smith, L. B., and E. Thelen. *A Dynamic Systems Approach to Development: Applications.* Cambridge, MA: MIT Press, 1993.
184. Soechting, J. F., and M. Flanders. Arm movements in three-dimensional space: Computation, theory, and observation. *Exerc. Sport Sci. Rev.* 19: 389–418, 1991.
185. Soechting, J. F., and F. Lacquaniti. Invariant characteristics of a pointing movement in man. *J. Neurosci.* 1: 710–720, 1981.
186. Son, K., J. A. Ashton-Miller, and A. B. Schultz. The mechanical role of the trunk and lower extremities in a seated weight-moving task in the sagittal plane. *J. Biomech. Eng.* 110: 97–103, 1988.
187. Thelen, E. The (re)discovery of motor development: learning new things from an old field. *Dev. Psychol.* 25: 946–949, 1989.
188. Thelen, E., D. Corbetta, K. Kamm, J. P. Spencer, K. Schneider, and R. F. Zernicke. The transition to reaching: mapping intention and intrinsic dynamics. *Child Dev.* 64: 1058–1098, 1993.
189. Thelen, E., and D. M. Fisher. From spontaneous to intentional behavior: kinematic analysis of movement changes during very early learning. *Child Dev.* 54: 129–140, 1983.
190. Thelen, E., and D. M. Fisher. The organization of spontaneous leg movement in newborn infants. *J. Mot. Behav.* 15: 353–377, 1983.
191. Thelen, E., J. A. S. Kelso, and A. Fogel. Self-organizing systems and infant motor development. *Dev. Rev.* 7: 39–65, 1987.
192. Thelen, E., R. F. Zernicke, K. Schneider, J. L. Jensen, K. Kamm, and D. Corbetta. The role of intersegmental dynamics in infant neuromotor development. In: *Tutorials in Motor Behavior II*, edited by G. E. Stelmach and J. Requin. Amsterdam: Elsevier Science Publishers, B. V., 1992, p. 533–548.
193. Thorstensson, A. How is the normal locomotor program modified to produce backward walking? *Exp. Brain Res.* 61: 664–668, 1986.
194. Thorstensson, A., H. Carlson, M. R. Zomlefer, and J. Nilsson. Lumbar back muscle in relation to trunk movements during locomotion in man. *Acta Physiol. Scand.* 116: 13–20, 1982.
195. Thorstensson, A., and H. Roberthson. Adaptations to changing speed in human locomotion: speed of transition between walking and running. *Acta Physiol. Scand.* 131: 221–214, 1987.
196. Tuller, B., H. L. Fitch, and M. T. Turvey. The Bernstein perspective: II. The concept of muscle linkage or coordinative structure. In: *Human Behavior: An Introduction*, edited by J. A. S. Kelso. Hillsdale, NJ: Lawrence Erlbaum Associates, 1982, p. 253–270.
197. Turvey, M. T., H. L. Fitch, and B. Tuller. The Bernstein perspective: I. The problems of degrees of freedom and context-conditioned variability. In: *Human Behavior: An Introduction*, edited by J. A. S. Kelso. Hillsdale, NJ: Lawrence Erlbaum Associates, 1982, p. 239–252.
198. Uno, Y., M. Kawato, and R. Suzuki. Formation and control of optimal trajectory in human multijoint arm movements: minimum torque-change model. *Biol. Cybern.* 61: 89–101, 1989.
199. Vilensky, J. A., E. Bankiewicz, and G. Gehlsen. A kinematic comparison of backward and forward walking in humans. *J. Hum. Mov. Studies* 13: 29–50, 1987.

200. Viviani, P., and M. Cenzato. Segmentation and coupling in complex movements. *J. Exp. Psychol. Hum. Percept. Perform.* 11: 828–845, 1985.
201. Vorro, J. R. Stroboscopic study of motion changes that accompany modifications and improvements in a throwing performance. *Res. Q.* 44: 216–226, 1973.
202. Walmsley, B., J. A. Hodgson, and R. E. Burke. Forces produced by medial gastrocnemius muscles in cats. *J. Neurophysiol.* 41: 1203–1216, 1978.
203. Weber, W., and E. Weber. *Die Mechanik der Menschlichen Gehwerkzeuge (Mechanics of Human Gait).* Goettingen: Dieterichschen Buchbandlung, 1836.
204. Winter, D. A. *Biomechanics and Motor Control of Human Movement*, 2nd Ed. New York: John Wiley & Sons, 1990.
205. Winter, D. A., N. Puck, and J. F. Yang. Backward walking: a simple reversal of forward walking? *J. Mot. Behav.* 21: 291–305, 1989.
206. Winter, D., and D. G. E. Robertson. Joint torque and energy patterns in normal gait. *Biol. Cybern.* 29: 137–142, 1978.
207. Wisleder, D., R. F. Zernicke, and J. L. Smith. Speed-related effects on intersegmental dynamics during the swing phase of cat locomotion. *Exp. Brain Res.* 79: 651–660, 1990.
208. Woollacott, M., and A. Shumway-Cook. *The Development of Posture and Gait across the Lifespan.* Columbia, SC: University of South Carolina Press, 1989.
209. Yeadon, M. R., and M. Morlock. The appropriate use of regression equations for the estimation of segmental inertial parameters. *J. Biomech.* 22: 683–689, 1989.
210. Zajac, F. E. Muscle and tendon: properties, models, scaling, and application to biomechanics and motor control. *Crit. Rev. Biomed. Eng.* 17: 359–411, 1989.
211. Zajac, F. E., and M. E. Gordon. Determining muscle's force and action in multiarticular movement. *Exerc. Sport Sci. Rev.* 17: 187–230, 1989.
212. Zajac, F. E., and W. S. Levine. Novel experimental and theoretical approaches to study the neural control of locomotion and jumping. In: *Posture and Movement: Perspective for Integrating Sensory and Motor Research on the Mammalian Nervous System*, edited by R. Talbott and D. Humphrey. New York: Raven Press, 1979, p. 259–279.
213. Zernicke, R. F., and E. M. Roberts. Lower extremity forces and torques during systematic variation of non-weightbearing motion. *Med. Sci. Sports* 10: 21–26, 1978.
214. Zernicke, R. F., and K. Schneider. Biomechanics and developmental neuromotor control. *Child Dev.* 64: 982–1004, 1993.
215. Zernicke, R. F., K. Schneider, and J. A. Buford. Intersegmental dynamics during gait: implications for control. In: *Adaptability of Human Gait*, edited by A. E. Patla. North Holland, Elsevier Science Publishers, 1991, p. 187–202.

II

Control of Respiratory and Cardiovascular Systems

Associate Editors Jerome A. Dempsey, John M. Johnson, and Peter D. Wagner

9. Central neural control of respiration and circulation during exercise

TONY G. WALDROP | *Department of Molecular and Integrative Physiology, University of Illinois, Urbana, Illinois*

FREDERIC L. ELDRIDGE | *Departments of Medicine and Physiology, University of North Carolina, Chapel Hill, North Carolina*

GARY A. IWAMOTO | *Department of Veterinary Biosciences, University of Illinois, Urbana, Illinois*

JERE H. MITCHELL | *Department of Internal Medicine, University of Texas Southwestern Medical School, Dallas, Texas*

CHAPTER CONTENTS

VIRTUALLY ALL INDIVIDUALS PARTICIPATE IN PHYSICAL ACTIVITY (i.e., exercise) to a greater or lesser degree on a daily basis. One might assume that control of such a basic activity would be well understood. Despite over a century of investigation, however, there is still intense debate over the major mechanisms responsible for controlling the respiratory and cardiovascular systems during exercise. This incomplete understanding of the regulation of ventilation in exercise has been described by Grodins (109) as "exercise hyperpnea, the ultra secret." Published in 1981, this statement included the assertion that "where we stand now is where we were before" (i.e., 1960). The same lack of understanding characterized our knowledge of regulation of the cardiovascular system during exercise. However, recent studies have helped unravel this puzzle (73). The increased understanding of the central neural control of respiratory and autonomic function will be covered in this chapter. The next chapter will focus on reflex control during exercise.

When exercise occurs, the utilization of oxygen (O_2) and oxidizable substrate and the production of carbon dioxide increase in the working muscle. Simple considerations tell us that the rates of oxygen delivery and removal of carbon dioxide (CO_2) must increase if appropriate levels of arterial and tissue gases are to be maintained and if a progressive bodily deficit of O_2 and a surplus of CO_2 are to be avoided. In the case of respiration, the increased requirements for O_2 uptake and disposal of CO_2 at the lung must be met by increased effective ventilation (i.e., alveolar or non–dead space ventilation). In the case of circulation, increased delivery of O_2 and return of CO_2 must be accomplished by an increase in cardiac output, although part of this need can be met by a widening of the arteriovenous differences in the concentrations of these gases (188). In the steady state of mild to moderate exercise, the increase in ventilation and the cardiovascular changes tend to parallel the intensity of the exercise, expressed as workload or change in metabolic rate (Figs. 9.1 and 9.2).

Not only do the respiratory and circulatory changes begin to occur very rapidly after the onset of exercise but they are quantitatively so well matched to the workload, or metabolic rate, that in the steady state of mild to moderate exercise the two main traditional chemical stimuli, arterial P_{CO_2} and P_{O_2}, remain relatively constant[1] at their resting levels (isocapnic hyperpnea) in human beings (Fig. 9.1). This was noted as early as 1886 by Zuntz and Geppert (277). Even during the transients at onset and endset of exercise, the ventilatory and circulatory responses are matched to CO_2 production and return well enough so that there is only a modest brief hypocapnia within the first minute after onset and a brief increase of P_{CO_2} within the first minute after offset. One of the most difficult and longstanding problems in exercise physiology has been to understand the mechanisms that underlie these responses.

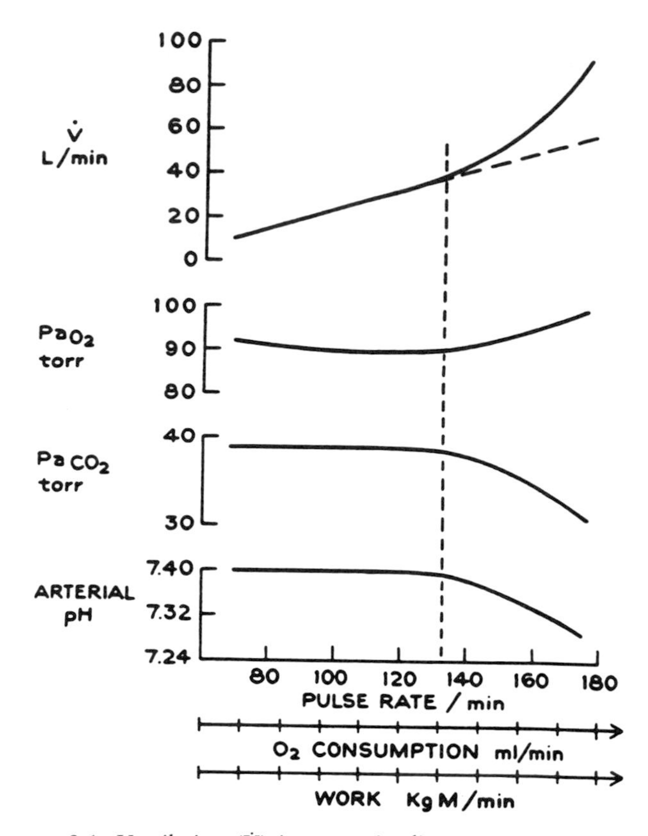

FIG. 9.1. Ventilation (V̇) increases in direct proportion to the workload during mild and moderate rhythmic exercise in humans such that arterial P_{O_2}, P_{CO_2}, and pH remain constant. [From Waldrop (254).]

[1]During heavy exercise, above about 60% of maximum level of performance, ventilation becomes excessive relative to metabolic rate, and hypocapnia develops. In this special case, the excessive breathing appears to be due to stimuli that are in addition to those normally operating during mild to moderate exercise. These stimuli probably include the effects of metabolic acidosis, increasing potassium concentration on the carotid bodies, increased neural input from muscular receptors, and increasing input to the medullary controller by central mechanisms (central command) [see Eldridge and Waldrop (73) for discussion]. Most of the discussion in the present review will be related to mild and moderate exercise where the excessive breathing does not normally occur in humans.

RESPIRATION

Historically, there have been three main groups of hypotheses regarding the hyperpnea of exercise. The first two, involving peripheral control, hold that the stimulation of breathing is achieved through sensory feedback after the onset of exercise.

One group of feedback mechanisms involves sources traditionally related to respiration. Because the steady-state hyperpnea is more or less proportional to the increased metabolic rate, many investigators have concluded that chemical factors, variously proposed to be acting in brainstem, carotid bodies, or lungs, must be the basis of the stimulation. However, arterial levels of CO_2 and O_2 do not change much during human exercise (Fig. 9.1), and

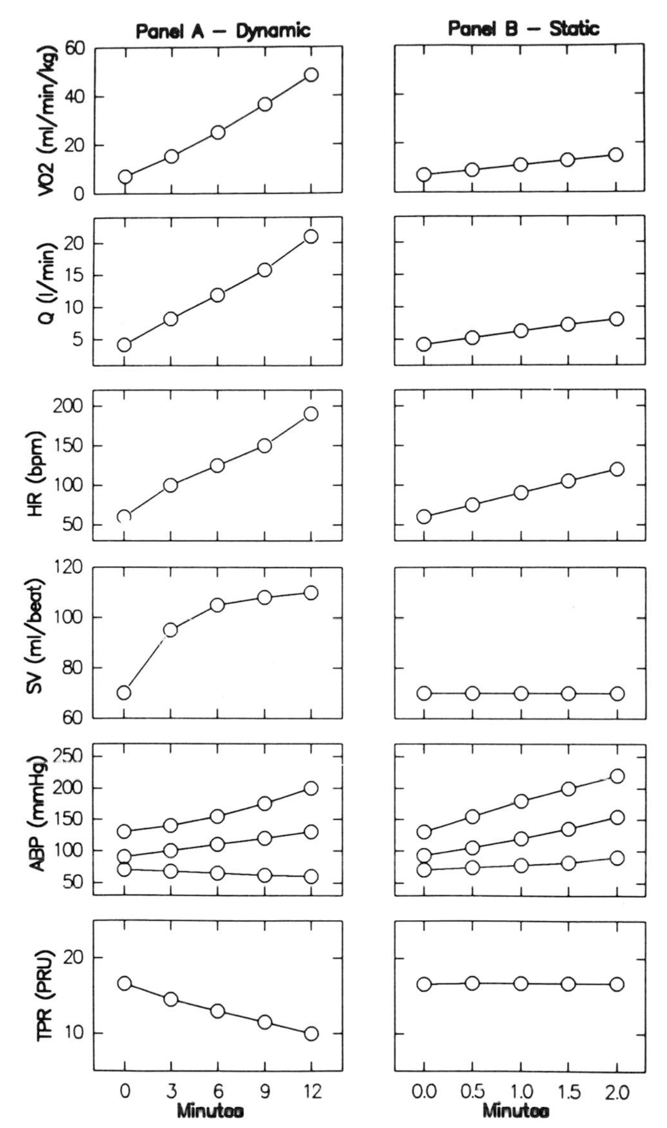

FIG. 9.2. Examples of cardiovascular responses to *(A)* dynamic and *(B)* static exercise. The dynamic exercise was progressively increased to $\dot{V}O_2$max; the static exercise was sustained at 30% of maximal voluntary contraction. Q, cardiac output; HR, heart rate; SV, stroke volume; ABP, systolic *(top line)*, mean *(middle line)*, and diastolic *(bottom line)* arterial blood pressure; TPR, total peripheral resistance. [From Mitchell and Raven (182).]

P_{CO_2} goes down in animals.[2] Furthermore, the increase in ventilation after the onset of exercise occurs too rapidly to be explained by slowly developing chemical factors in arterial and venous blood (147). Thus, it is necessary to postulate other mechanisms.

[2]It must be pointed out that the concept of isocapnic hyperpnea applies mainly to human exercise because in most animal species, including ponies (197), goats (228), rats (88), swine (113), dogs (113), lizards (179), birds (142), and cats (51, 71), arterial P_{CO_2} falls with the onset of exercise and remains decreased during continuing exercise.

The second group involves feedback from nonrespiratory related sources. These include reflexes from the heart, changes in temperature and cardiac output and, more importantly, activation of mechanical or chemical receptors in the working muscle (135, 169). The latter neurally mediated mechanism would be one that could explain the rapid increase of breathing at the onset of exercise.

The third main hypothesis is that of a feedforward control mechanism; it postulates that areas in the suprapontine brain produce a command signal capable of driving not only the locomotion during exercise but also the respiratory system (277). Such a parallel central command mechanism could lead to neurally driven hyperpnea, which would occur very quickly after onset of exercise and lead to a roughly proportional response in both systems.

One of the earliest lists of hypotheses offered by Zuntz and Geppert (277) in 1886 includes most of the categories still considered to be important. These investigators wrote that the hyperpnea could not be accounted for by arterial gas levels in neural centers—they were, of course, unaware of the respiratory function of the carotid bodies—and suggested the following possibilities: *(1)* that exercise introduces into the blood an identified substance that acts on respiratory centers (the substance X hypothesis); *(2)* that blood changed by muscular activity excites nerve endings in the lungs (the venous chemoreceptor hypothesis); *(3)* that neural receptors in exercising muscle are excited and stimulate breathing by direct neural mechanisms (the peripheral neurogenic hypothesis); and finally *(4)* that voluntary activation of muscles for locomotion and exercise simultaneously co-stimulates the respiratory centers involuntarily (the central command or feedforward hypothesis).

Despite subsequent studies of various mechanisms, there is still incomplete understanding and quantitation of many and certainly not full agreement regarding their relative importance in the actual integrated response. Eldridge and Waldrop (73) recently presented a review of material on the question. Despite the uncertainties, these authors came to some conclusions about the relative importance of various mechanisms and presented their views of the dynamic response of breathing to exercise. They included the following: *(1)* the rapid increase of ventilation following onset of exercise (phase 1) involves primarily central command drive (feedforward), perhaps augmented by feedback from muscular afferents (peripheral neurogenic); *(2)* the subsequent slowly rising ventilation over the next 3–4 minutes (phase 2) involves continuation of the command drive and afferent feedback from muscles, plus a rising component of neural drive associated with short-term potentiation of respiratory neurons (the so-called afterdischarge mechanism) and a component of stimulation from rising arterial [K+] acting on the carotid bodies (possibly the substance X mechanism); *(3)* the steady-state (phase 3) involves all of these mechanisms that have reached stable levels; and *(4)* throughout phases 2 and 3, feedback of respiratory variables acts to stabilize or "fine-tune" breathing at the level primarily dictated by the nonrespiratory mechanisms.

It can be seen that the major mechanisms proposed in this scheme of Eldridge and Waldrop (73) are basically the same as those proposed by Zuntz and Geppert (277) over a century before, with one exception. That exception is the proposed involvement of the mechanism of short-term potentiation of respiratory neuronal pathways in the medulla.

CIRCULATION

The categories of mechanisms proposed for the rapid and sustained increase of circulation are similar to those of breathing, with the possible exception of chemosensory feedback involving CO_2 and O_2. A central command mechanism was proposed in 1893 by Johansson (133) to explain the rapid changes of circulation that accompany exercise. In addition, there is certainly neural feedback from contracting muscles. A review of these mechanisms responsible for cardiovascular control during exercise was published recently (181). A major focus of this chapter will be upon the central command control of circulation during exercise. The peripheral feedback control of circulation during exercise will be the focus of the next chapter.

The purpose of this chapter is not to look at the entirety of the mechanisms proposed to produce the respiratory and circulatory responses to exercise but rather to examine specifically *(1)* those emanating from the brain rostral to the main respiratory and circulatory control areas in the medulla (i.e., the central command mechanism), and *(2)* the proposed contribution of short-term potentiation of medullary neurons to the respiratory and circulatory responses.

Both this chapter and the following one will point out that neural control during exercise involves a large number of central nervous system (CNS) sites ranging from possible cortical areas to the lumbar and sacral portions of the spinal cord. Obviously, considerable integration of activity must occur not only because of the different neural mechanisms active during exercise but also due to the large number of CNS sites involved. This integration among mechanisms involved in exercise regulation as well as integration of other cardiorespiratory reflexes with central command will also be discussed in this chapter.

CENTRAL COMMAND MECHANISMS

Central Drive of Locomotion

A discussion of the central command control of the cardiorespiratory systems during exercise must take into account the sites involved with locomotion and other types of somatomotor activity. Locomotion is an important comparison because, like the respiratory apparatus and sympathetic outflow, it relies on activity in supraspinal regions that are linked together functionally and impinge on brainstem and spinal circuitry. Moreover, much evidence has implicated several identified locomotor sites with cardiorespiratory regulation.

Sites which when activated elicit locomotion will be the primary focus of this presentation. Recent evidence suggests that motoneuron recruitment patterns and firing rates produced by brainstem locomotor area stimulation are consistent with those occurring during voluntary locomotion in the normal animal (238, 239).

Locomotor Pattern Generator

It is clear that the central pattern generator (CPG) for locomotion is self-contained at the level of the mammalian spinal cord. This idea has its origins in the experiments of Graham-Brown (105–107) early in this century, which were the first to suggest that spinal "half-centres" existed that contained the entire pattern of motor activity necessary for largely coordinated locomotion, including both the swing and stance phases. In these early experiments, the activity developed in a sequence of events in the hindlimbs after transection of the thoracic spinal cord. The locomotor patterns were not dependent on afferent input and thus were apparently not reflex action. In more recent experiments, Miller and Meche (174) showed that coordinated hindlimb and forelimb locomotion could be obtained from the high spinal cat. Thus, it is clear that the actual pattern generator for locomotion is contained within the spinal cord.

Supraspinal Locomotor Sites

A number of supraspinal sites are known to impinge either directly or indirectly upon the spinal locomotor rhythm generator. Many of these sites are also known to exert an influence upon the cardiovascular and respiratory systems.

Cerebral Cortex. There can be no doubt that exercise is usually a form of *voluntary movement*. Therefore, voluntary locomotion must be dependent, in the intact animal, to some degree on motor activity influenced by the motor cortex. Fritsch and Hitzig (93) were the first to report that stimulation of the motor cortex produces movement. Movements obtained by stimulation of the primary motor cortex can be described as simple muscle contractions which, at low threshold, affect the distal limb musculature.

Other cortical areas, in addition to the primary motor cortex, are involved in locomotion. Premotor and supplementary motor cortex have reciprocal connections with each other and the primary motor cortex. The premotor cortex has been implicated in preparation for movement while the supplementary motor area produces complex patterns of movement on stimulation. The premotor cortex projects primarily to medullary reticular formation, one of the areas involved in reticulospinal outflow controlling cardiorespiratory activity.

Diencephalon. Numerous studies have demonstrated that stimulation in the diencephalon elicits locomotion. However, the exact anatomical definition of the effective site has been inconsistent; effective areas have been reported in an area extending from the subthalamus to the caudal hypothalamus just dorsal to the mammillary bodies. Orlovskii (195) and Eldridge et al. (71) have shown the area in schematic diagrams as a sphere located at Horsley-Clarke coordinates A8–10, L1–2 and H–2–4 (Fig. 9.3) in the cat. Recent work with electrical and chemical stimulation suggests that the area may project a bit more rostrally to Horsley-Clarke A11 and certainly extends medially to the area bounded by a line connecting the mamillothalamic tract and the column of the fornix as well as medially to the third ventricle (257). Anatomical brain sites within this region include the posterior hypothalamic area, dorsal hypothalamic area, and portions of the lateral hypothalamic area. This locomotor region has been referred to as the hypothalamic locomotor region by Waldrop et al. (257) and Orlovskii (195). These hypothalamic areas have long been known to be involved in cardiorespiratory regulation.

A subthalamic locomotor region was described by Waller (266) and later by Grossman (110). This region includes more lateral aspects of the hypothalamus as well as the zona incerta, the subthalamic nucleus, and the fields of Forel. Smith et al. (229) found that electrical stimulation in this area produces locomotion similar to that observed in conscious dogs running on a treadmill.

Connections of diencephalic locomotor areas have been examined by several investigators. Both Mel'nivoka (172) and Orlovskii (196) have recorded extracellular activity of neurons that are excited by electrical stimulation of the hypothalamic locomotor region in anesthetized cats. Neurons located in the mesencephalic locomotor region and throughout the reticular formation of the pons and medulla were activated by stimulation of the hypothalamic locomotor region. These findings are in agreement with the work of Baev et al. (17), who used retrograde transport of horseradish peroxidase (HRP) to determine efferent projections of the hypothalamic locomotor region (HLR). They concluded that the major projections of the HLR were to the mesencephalic locomotor region including the cuneiform nucleus

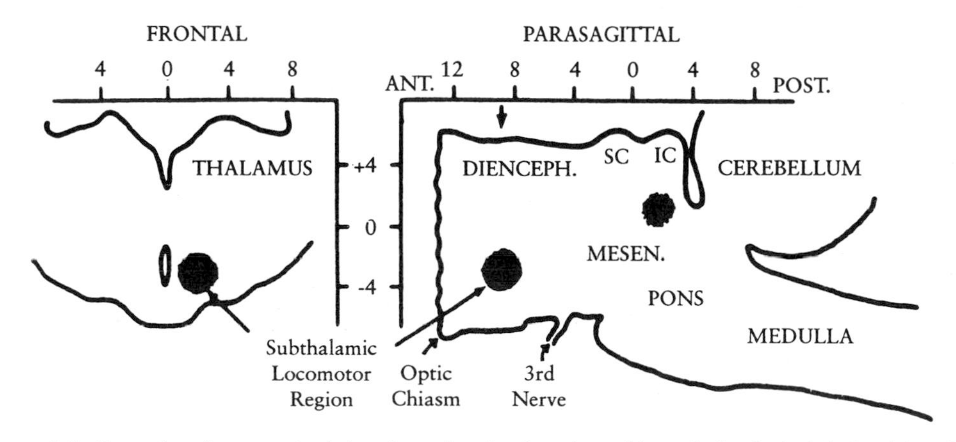

FIG. 9.3. Frontal and parasagittal drawings showing location of hypothalamic (subthalamic) and mesencephalic locomotor regions in the cat. [Adapted from Eldridge et al. (72).]

and locus coeruleus and the medial reticular formation of the ipsilateral brainstem. Evidence was also found for direct projections from the hypothalamus to the cervical and lumbar regions of the spinal cord. Similar findings have also been reported in the monkey, rat, and cat by Saper and colleagues (215). These findings have been expanded in a study by Luiten et al. (161) who demonstrated that neurons in the paraventricular hypothalamus project to sites in the medulla and spinal cord that are involved in autonomic regulation.

Experiments by Baev et al. (16) demonstrated projections to the HLR from areas known to be involved in the regulation of motor activity. Projections from areas 4 and 6 of the motor cortex and the endopeduncular nucleus to the HLR were identified using retrograde tracing techniques. Projections to the HLR from brainstem sites have been investigated by injecting HRP into areas of the hypothalamus which, when stimulated, elicit locomotion in anesthetized cats (27). Retrograde transport occurred to a number of pontine and medullary sites, including the raphe nuclei, the reticular formation, and parabrachial nucleus, which are known to be involved in cardiovascular regulation.

Mesencephalon. A midbrain locomotor region has been extensively studied and is referred to as the mesencephalic locomotor region (MLR) (Fig. 9.3). Shik, Severin, and Orlovskii (224) and Garcia-Rill, and colleagues (99, 100, 227) have shown that electrical stimulation in the caudal portion of the nucleus cuneiformis including the pedunculopontine nucleus evokes locomotion in a mesencephalic cat preparation. Similar results were obtained with chemical stimulation of the MLR (100). The mesencephalic locomotor region is reciprocally connected with the locomotor regions in the diencephalon; however, lesion of the MLR does not prevent locomotion produced by stimulation in the hypothalamic locomotor region (223). The MLR also sends connections to the pontomedullary locomotor strip (99).

Locomotor Strip in the Pons and Medulla. Shik and Yagosditsyn (225, 226) and Mori et al. (186) used electrical stimulation to show that a locomotor area extends from the region of the MLR in a continuous strip through the pons and medulla. This strip in the cat lies approximately 4 mm from the midline, extends caudally from the MLR to approximately P18, and is at the approximate level of the nucleus of the trigeminal.

Shik and Yagosditsyn (225, 226) have concluded that the pontomedullary locomotor strip is a group of highly interconnected cells through which signals from the MLR are passed down to the spinal cord. Afferent connections of the locomotor strip include the spinal trigeminal nucleus, lateral parabrachial nucleus, the nucleus tractus solitarius and reticular formation. Many of these areas projecting to the locomotor strip are known brainstem cardiovascular and respiratory regions (78, 101).

CENTRAL COMMAND CONTROL OF RESPIRATION AND CIRCULATION IN ANIMALS

A wide range of preparations have been utilized for examining the role of central command in regulating the cardiorespiratory system during exercise. Awake human and animal studies have the advantage of permitting the study of true exercise. However, a disadvantage of these experiments is that few, if any, invasive procedures can be performed and, as a result, it is difficult to isolate a mechanism of regulation. Instead, many of the studies in humans become more correlative than mechanistic. Anesthetized or decerebrate animal preparations, therefore, have provided more detail about the central command control of respiration and circulation. A potential drawback of these studies, however, is that evoked activity rather than voluntary exercise is involved. These studies rest on the assumption that the same control mechanisms are active during evoked and voluntary exercise. Thus, it is necessary to compare results from these anesthetized preparations with studies performed in awake animals and humans. Therefore, this chapter will examine results obtained from both anesthetized preparations as well as awake animals and humans to present an integrated view of the role of central command in exercise regulation.

The concept of a central neural mechanism involved in cardiovascular regulation was first proposed in 1893 by Johansson (133), who suggested that motor impulses to muscles were also able to excite the centers controlling the heart. This hypothesis was postulated by Zuntz and Geppert (277) as well as by Krogh and Lindhard (147) to include control of the respiratory system during exercise. These investigators suggested from studies performed in human subjects that motor signals "irradiated" onto cardiovascular and respiratory control neurons in the brainstem. The central mechanism described by Krogh and Lindhard (147) has long been referred to as "cortical irradiation." Subsequently, this has been termed "central command" (104). Thus, the cardiorespiratory response is caused by a direct action of the central command descending from higher centers on the cardiovascular and respiratory control areas that in turn regulate the sympathetic and parasympathetic efferent activity to the heart and blood vessels as well as respiratory outflow to respiratory muscles.

The concept of central command ("cortical irradiation") involves a parallel, simultaneous excitation of neuronal circuits controlling the locomotor and cardiorespiratory systems, thus serving as a feedforward control mechanism. It is thought that the neural signal that descends from suprapontine control areas in the rostral brain to spinal locomotor neurons also projects to cardiovascular and respiratory areas in the medulla. Therefore, cardiovascular and respiratory function is increased simultaneously with the onset of exercise and is maintained throughout the exercise period. This feedforward mechanism has the potential to generate cardiorespiratory responses to exercise without requiring feedback from a reflex neural mechanism.

Central command must act ultimately through medullary neurons that are involved in controlling sympathetic and parasympathetic nerve activity. It is not known if central command acts directly on the circuits responsible for generation of autonomic nervous system activity in the brainstem, on the outflow neurons in the ventrolateral medulla, or on interneurons. However, it is probable that neurons in the ventrolateral medulla are involved. Numerous studies have demonstrated that neurons in the ventrolateral medulla have a sympathetic nerve-related discharge, receive baroreceptor input, and project to the intermediolateral spinal cord (101, 111, 116). Since a rise in sympathetic nerve discharge is elicited by increases in central command, this medullospinal projection must be activated during exercise. In fact, it has been shown that stimulation of locomotor regions in the hypothalamus thought to be involved in central command activates neurons in the ventrolateral medulla (191).

Cerebral Cortex

An early test of the central command hypothesis was to examine cardiorespiratory responses to electrical stimulation of motor cortex regions that evoke movement of limb muscles. Thus, investigators sought in this type of experiment to determine if increased descending motor drive produced a corresponding drive to cardiorespiratory control areas. Clarke, Smith, and Shearn (37) measured limb blood flow in anesthetized monkeys during electrical stimulation in the primary motor cortex. Sites were located which when stimulated evoke movement of one limb. Further limb movement was then prevented by sectioning of motor nerves below the level of autonomic outflow or by muscular paralysis. Stimulation produced a 10%–50% increase in blood flow to the same limb that had previously contracted. However, little or no change in arterial pressure or heart rate occurred during stimulation. This latter finding differed from the results reported by Green and Hoff (108). These investigators found that a rise in arterial pressure was elicited by stimulation of the motor cortex in both the monkey and cat anesthetized with ether and paralyzed with curare. In addition, a concomitant decrease in renal blood flow and an increase in limb blood flow occurred during stimulation. The changes in limb flow persisted after adrenalectomy but were absent after sectioning of the nerve supply to the limb. It was concluded that "there are certain nervous pathways, originating in the motor cortex, excitation of which results in a redistribution of blood, decreasing the supply to the abdominal viscera and increasing that to those parts which would be made active by the simultaneous excitation of the motor efferent pathways from the same areas of the cortex" (108). Even though these investigators were not examining the control of the cardiovascular system during exercise, this statement is an elegant definition of cortical irradiation as proposed by Krogh and Lindhard (147).

Similar experiments have been performed by other investigators who usually reported small increases in heart rate and blood pressure from stimulation of the motor cortex of mammals (74, 123, 265). However, Hilton, Spyer, and Timms (118) have noted that some of the responses to electrical stimulation of the motor cortex can be explained by factors other than a neurogenically mediated drive to the cardiovascular systems from the motor cortex. For example, it was shown that blood flow changes in limb muscles are often secondary to the muscular contraction elicited by cortical stimulation. Moreover, one must take care that the stimulation does not spread to meningeal afferent fibers or to the hypothalamus. Hilton et al. (118) did not observe any cardiovascular responses to cortical stimulation after careful controls were made for these two criticisms. Thus, it appears that little or no parallel activation of the cardiovascular system derives from impulses originating from the motor cortex.

Hypothalamic Locomotor Region

Other sites in the brain besides the motor cortex are now known to be involved in the production of locomotion and other types of muscular work. Waller

(266) showed that electrical stimulation in the lateral hypothalamus and adjacent areas, including the fields of Forel, in lightly anesthetized cats produces rhythmic movements similar to those seen during normal walking or running. These findings were subsequently corroborated and expanded by Grossman (110) and by Orlovskii and colleagues (196, 223, 224), who called this area the "subthalamic locomotor region." It was also shown that unanesthetized decorticate cats will run spontaneously, indicating that the motor cortex is not requisite for the generation of descending motor signals.

The actual neuroanatomical substrate for the so-called subthalamic locomotor region probably includes areas in the hypothalamus as well as structures lateral to the hypothalamus including the fields of Forel. However, the discrete region which when stimulated can produce both coordinated locomotion and appropriate cardiorespiratory responses is comprised of parts of the posterior and dorsal hypothalamic areas (17, 257). Therefore, it seems most appropriate to designate this area as the hypothalamic locomotor region. The hypothalamic locomotor region is most likely a part of the "defence area" described by Hilton and colleagues (1, 115, 117).

Rushmer and colleagues (210, 229) were the first to question if stimulation of the diencephalon produces a parallel activation of cardiorespiratory activity. They demonstrated that electrical stimulation of the H1 and H2 fields of Forel produced running movements that were accompanied by changes in cardiovascular function similar to those observed in dogs running voluntarily on a treadmill. Since the cardiovascular responses to diencephalic stimulation persisted after muscular paralysis, descending motor signals must have been responsible for parallel activation of the locomotor and cardiovascular systems. Similar results were obtained by Marshall and Timms (165) from studies performed in anesthetized cats.

A more complete characterization of this area has been conducted by Eldridge and co-workers (71, 72, 177), who studied anesthetized brain-intact and unanesthetized decorticate cats (Fig. 9.4). These investigators demonstrated that electrical stimulation in the hypothalamic locomotor region produces locomotion accompanied by proportional increases in respiration and arterial pressure. Moreover, stimulation in paralyzed animals produces "fictive locomotion" (recorded as motor nerve activity) and increases in phrenic nerve activity and arterial pressure (Fig. 9.5). Furthermore, it was demonstrated that these responses persist even after preventing changes in feedback from peripheral chemoreceptors, baroreceptors, lung receptors, and central chemoreceptors. It was also noted that spontaneous bursts of actual and fictive locomotion with concomitant increases in respiratory activity and arterial pressure occur in the unanesthetized decorticate cats, indicating that cortical regions are not necessary for parallel activation of cardiorespiratory and locomotor activity. Thus, it was concluded that command signals emanating from the hypothalamus are the major cause for the changes in respiration and circulation that occur during exercise. This conclusion suggests that activation of neurons in this hypothalamic region provides a model for central command and simulates the central neural mechanism that controls the cardiorespiratory systems during exercise.

In addition to the cardiorespiratory responses reported by Eldridge co-workers (71, 72), Waldrop et al. (259) have demonstrated that electrical stimulation of the hypothalamic locomotor region in anesthetized cats produces increases in ventricular pressure and contractility and a redistribution of blood flow similar to that seen during voluntary exercise in awake cats [Fig. 9.6; (48)]. These changes, which were measured using the radioactive microsphere technique, include increased blood flow to the heart, diaphragm, and limb skeletal muscles and a concomitant decrease in flow to the kidneys (Fig 9.7). In addition, the vascular resistance of the intestines, gallbladder, and stomach increased during stimulation. These blood flow changes are similar to those reported by other investigators who stimulated in areas including (probably) the hypothalamic locomotor region (36, 86).

A problem with all of the above studies, which used electrical stimulation of the hypothalamic locomotor region, is that both cell bodies and fibers of passage were stimulated. Therefore, the observed responses could have resulted from stimulation of axons whose cell bodies were located distant to the hypothalamic locomotor region. Eldridge et al. (71) addressed this possibility by injecting a γ-aminobutyric acid (GABA) receptor antagonist, which is thought to affect only receptors on cell bodies. Injection of the antagonist into the hypothalamic locomotor region elicited all the responses seen with electrical stimulation, suggesting that the observed responses are due to stimulation of cell bodies alone in the hypothalamic locomotor region. However, relatively large volumes (2–5 μl) were injected in this study; thus, the responses could have resulted from spread of the antagonist to sites outside of the hypothalamic locomotor region. Waldrop et al. (257) and Bauer et al. (22) have subsequently reported that microinjections (100–500 nl) of GABA antagonists into the posterior hypothalamus produce increases in arterial pressure, heart rate, and minute ventila-

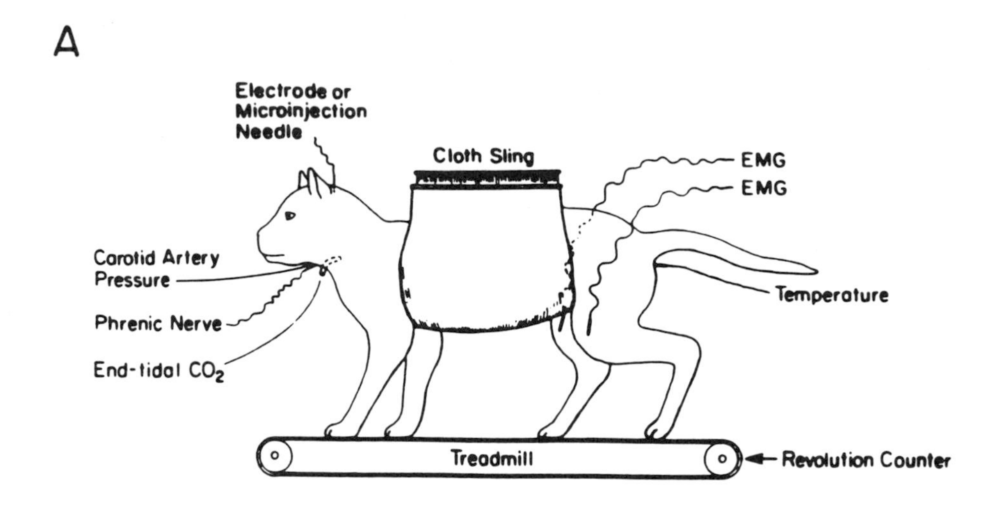

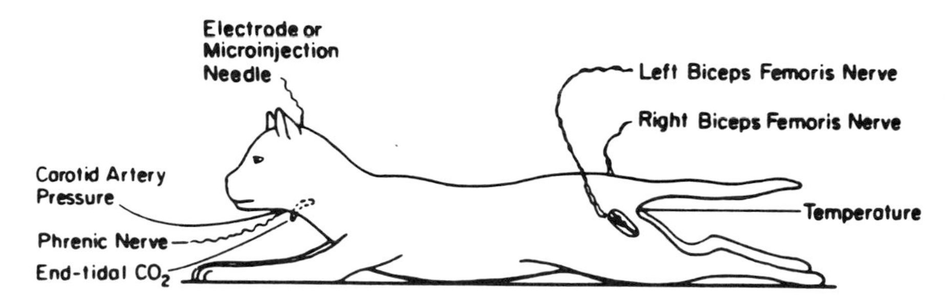

FIG. 9.4. Animal preparations utilized for studying exercise in the unanesthetized decorticate cat *(A)* and fictive locomotion in the paralyzed ventilated cat *(B)*. [Adapted from Eldridge et al. (71).]

tion that are accompanied by locomotor movements of the limbs of both cats and rats (Figs. 9.8 and 9.9). Moreover, these responses were reversed by microinjections of a GABA agonist. Similar responses have been obtained by DiMicco and colleagues (52, 272). In addition, Stremel and Joshua (235) have shown that microinjection of a GABA antagonist into the posterior hypothalamus elicits splanchnic microvascular constriction. All these results indicate that stimulation of cell bodies alone in the hypothalamic locomotor region produces all the cardiorespiratory and locomotor responses evoked by electrical stimulation and that a GABAergic mechanism exerts a tonic depressive influence over the cardiorespiratory and locomotor systems by an action in the posterior hypothalamus. Moreover, it is possible that a lifting (or disinhibition) of the GABAergic inhibition exerted upon the posterior hypothalamus is responsible for locomotion and the cardiorespiratory responses to exercise (263). The site of origin for the neurons that produce the GABAergic inhibition is not known; however, a number of brainstem and more rostral sites are known to project to the hypothalamic locomotor region.

The hypothalamic locomotor region has also been shown to be involved in controlling sympathetic outflow. Studies by Pitts and colleagues (202, 203) demonstrated that electrical stimulation of the posterior hypothalamus elicits increases in sympathetic nerve activity that can be correlated with changes in arterial pressure. These earlier findings have been extended by a number of investigators including Dean and Coote (44), who found that the cardiorespiratory responses to posterior hypothalamic stimulation were accompanied by appropriate changes in sympathetic outflow to the kidney and limb skeletal

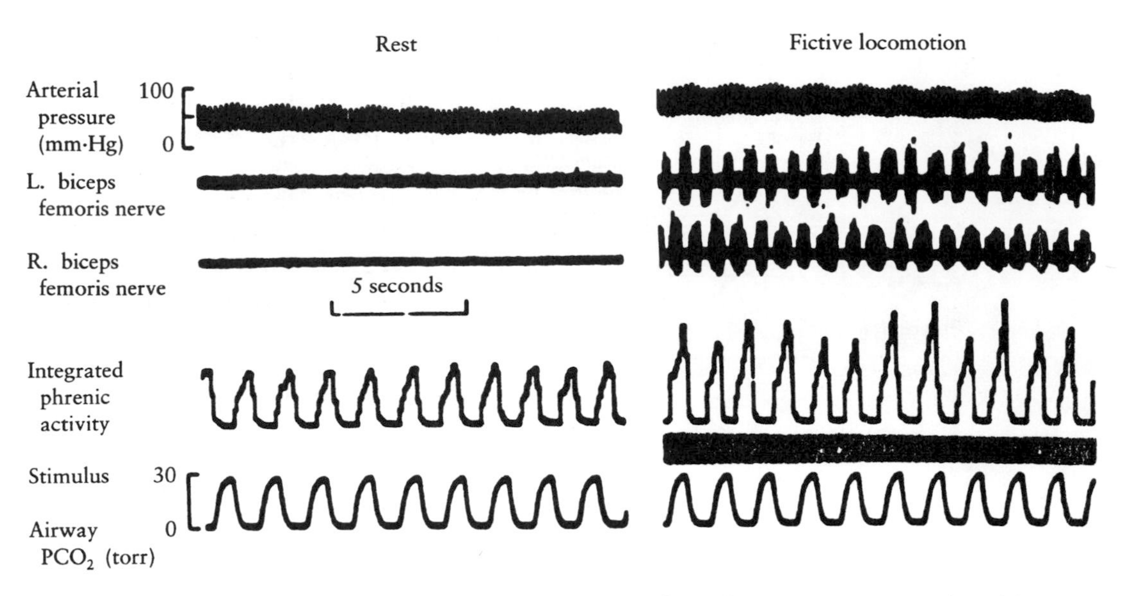

FIG. 9.5. Example of the respiratory, cardiovascular, and fictive locomotor responses elicited by stimulation in the hypothalamic locomotor region of a paralyzed cat. [From Eldridge et al. (71).]

muscle of anesthetized cats. Recent experiments have shown that microinjection of a GABA antagonist into the hypothalamic locomotor region elicits increases in both phasic and tonic discharge in cervical sympathetic nerve activity that correlate with concomitant heart rate and arterial pressure responses [Fig. 9.10; (256, 272)]. Moreover, it has been shown that unit activity recorded from posterior hypothalamic neurons correlates with sympathetic discharge recorded from the inferior cardiac nerve (19, 50, 244). Lesions of this and surrounding diencephalic areas produce a fall in sympathetic nerve discharge (128, 129). These findings taken together support the possibility that areas in the posterior hypothalamus can modulate sympathetic nerve activity in a manner consistent with the alterations seen during exercise.

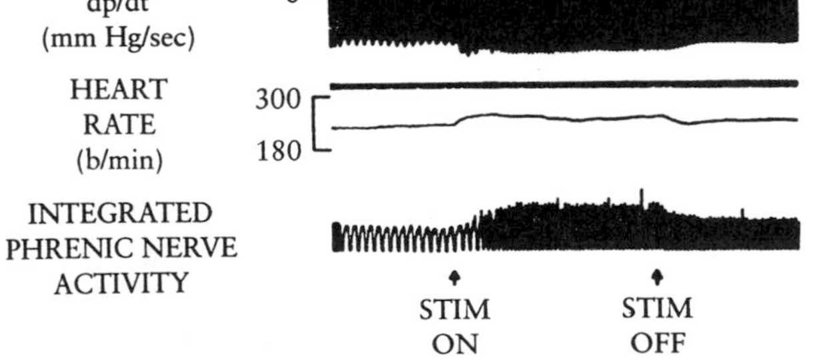

FIG. 9.6. Hemodynamic and respiratory responses to electrical stimulation of the hypothalamic (subthalamic) locomotor region. [From Waldrop et al. (259).]

The effects upon the cardiovascular responses to voluntary exercise of destroying diencephalic locomotor areas have been examined in several studies. In experiments from Rushmer's (210) laboratory, bilateral lesions were placed in the fields of Forel of dogs that had been instrumented for chronic cardiovascular monitoring. No cardiovascular responses to treadmill exercise were observed in one of the dogs with the bilateral lesions. However, this experiment has been reported only in a textbook by Rushmer and the data from only one of the dogs were given. Similar experiments have been conducted subsequently in baboons performing isometric exercise (120). This preliminary study reported that in only two of the five baboons studied were the cardiovascular responses to isometric exercise reduced following diencephalic lesions. In a recent experiment, Ordway et al. (194) examined the effects of lesioning the hypothalamic locomotor region upon the cardiovascular responses of dogs running upon a treadmill. Bilateral lesions did not compromise the cardiovascular responses to exercise in any of the dogs studied. Thus, at present, evidence suggests that conscious animals deprived of the locomotor areas in and adjacent to the posterior hypothalamus display

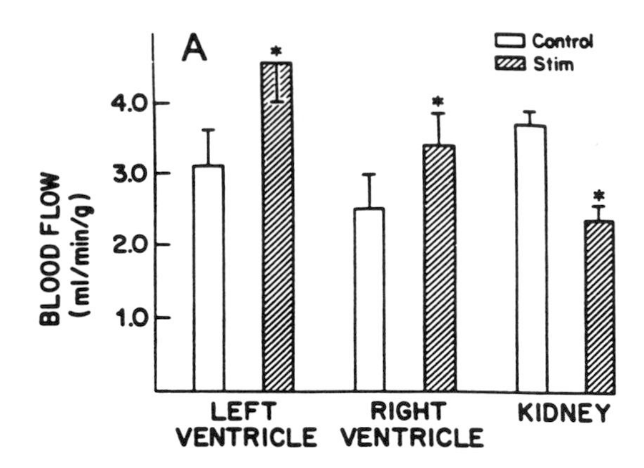

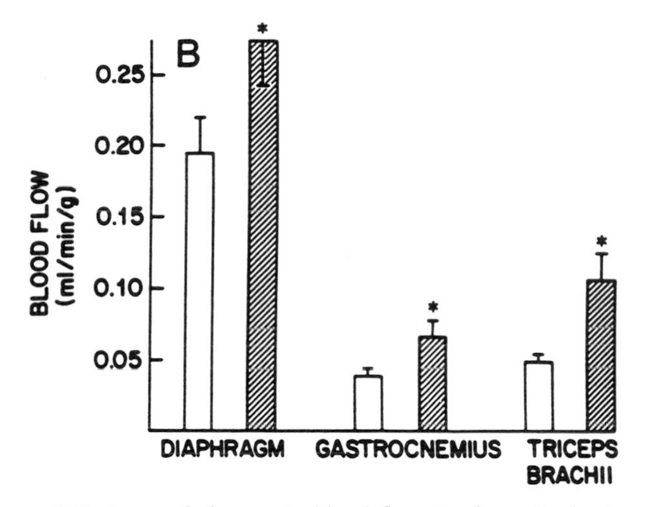

FIG. 9.7. Averaged changes in blood flow (as determined using the radioactive microsphere technique) to the heart, kidneys, diaphragm, and selected limb muscles of anesthetized cats during stimulation of the hypothalamic locomotor region. [From Waldrop et al. (259).]

normal cardiovascular responses to dynamic exercise. The possibility exists that other areas in the brain assume the functions of this area when animals are deprived of structures that normally modulate cardiovascular responses to exercise.

The above physiological studies support the idea that the hypothalamic locomotor region is involved in central command. In addition, the connectivity of the hypothalamic locomotor and surrounding regions provides anatomical support for a role of this region in cardiorespiratory regulation (125, 153, 160, 267). Hilton et al. (116) used electrical stimulation to trace a pathway from the posterior hypothalamus to a superficial site in the ventrolateral medulla. Stimulation of a narrow strip down to the medulla elicited the cardiorespiratory responses produced by activation of posterior hypothalamic neurons. In addition, bilateral lesions and application of glycine to the ventral lateral medulla abolished the responses to hypothalamic stimulation. This area of the medulla has been shown to be a site of outflow of sympathetic discharge to the spinal cord (101, 111). Thus, it appears that the cardiovascular responses evoked by stimulation of the hypothalamic locomotor region depend upon a descending pathway to an area of the medulla involved in regulation of sympathetic activity. It should be pointed out that this descending pathway lies ventral to the brainstem locomotor strip.

A precise characterization of the descending projections of the caudal hypothalamus and surrounding regions was performed recently by Barman (18). Antidromic activation and computer averaging techniques were utilized to determine projections of hypothalamic neurons whose basal discharge was related to sympathetic nerve activity. The major projection of these "sympathetic" hypothalamic neurons was to the periaqueductal gray, the ventrolateral medulla, and the lateral tegmental fields in the medulla. All of these areas are known to be involved in cardiovascular regulation. Moreover, Saper and colleagues (215) have shown that a number of brainstem sites that regulate autonomic function have reciprocal connections with the posterior hypothalamus.

Thus, considerable evidence supports the hypothesis that the hypothalamic locomotor region is involved in the central neural mechanism regulating the cardiovascular system during exercise. Activation of this region elicits locomotion and adjusts cardiovascular activity in a manner appropriate for the work (exercise) being performed. In addition, this hypothalamic area has both the afferent and efferent connections necessary for regulating motor activity and controlling the cardiovascular system during exercise.

Mesencephalic Locomotor Region

Several laboratories have demonstrated that either electrical or chemical stimulation of an area in the mesencephalon, MLR, produces locomotion in both rats and cats (99, 100, 227, 232, 233). This region has connections with the hypothalamic locomotor region and other areas known to be involved in the control of locomotion and cardiorespiratory activity (99, 232). Electrical stimulation of this area has also been shown to produce increases in arterial pressure and heart rate in anesthetized cats (71). Bedford et al. (24) recently used a decerebrate rat preparation to further investigate the role of the mesencephalic locomotor region. Electrical stimulation of this area elicited locomotion and produced increases in heart

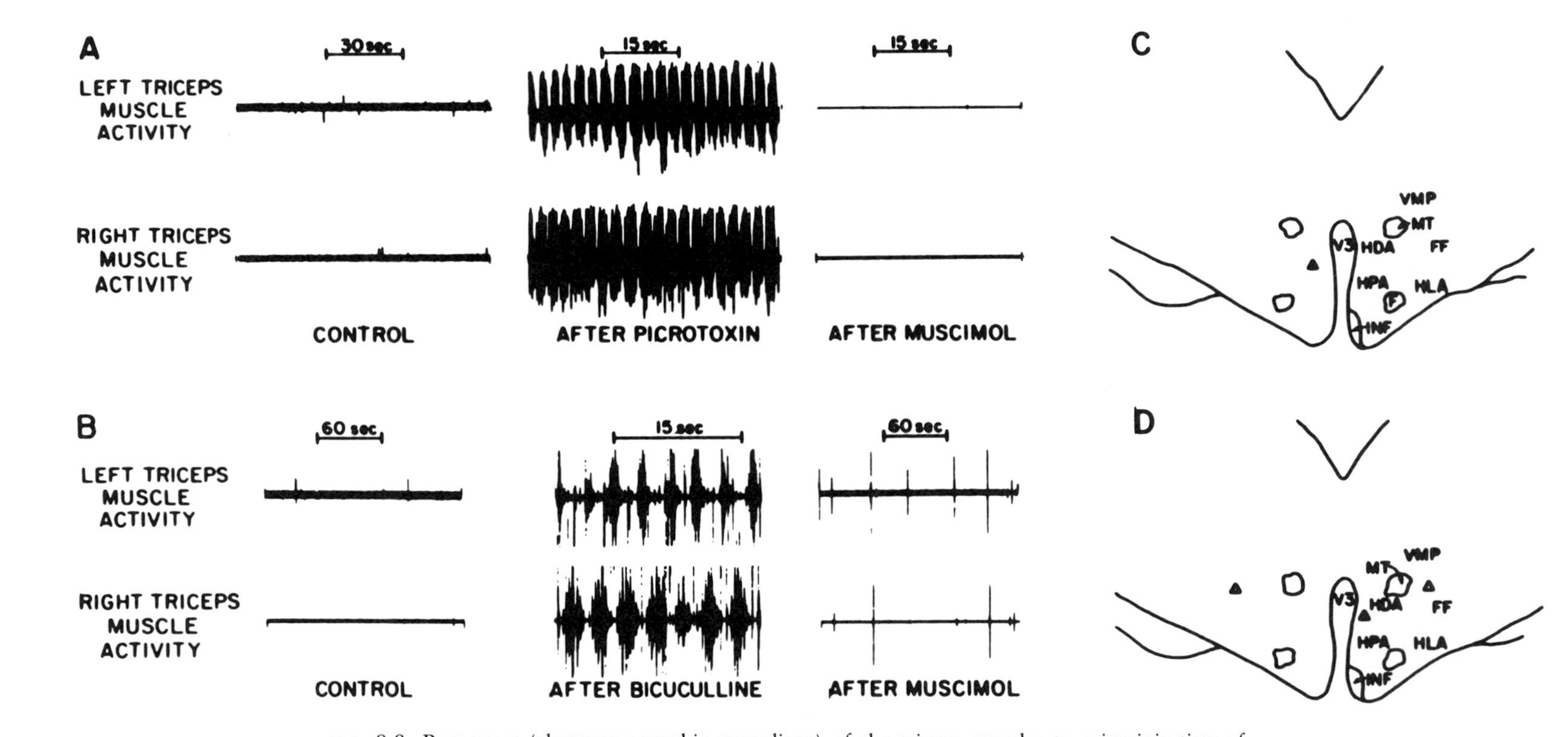

FIG. 9.8. Responses (electromyographic recordings) of the triceps muscles to microinjection of GABA antagonists (*A*, picrotoxin; *B*, bicuculline) and a GABA agonist (muscimol) into the hypothalamic locomotor region of an anesthetized cat. Both antagonists produced rhythmic, alternating bursts of left and right triceps activity that were reversed by the GABA agonist. Location of the injections are denoted by *filled triangles* in *C* and *D*. [From Waldrop et al. (257).]

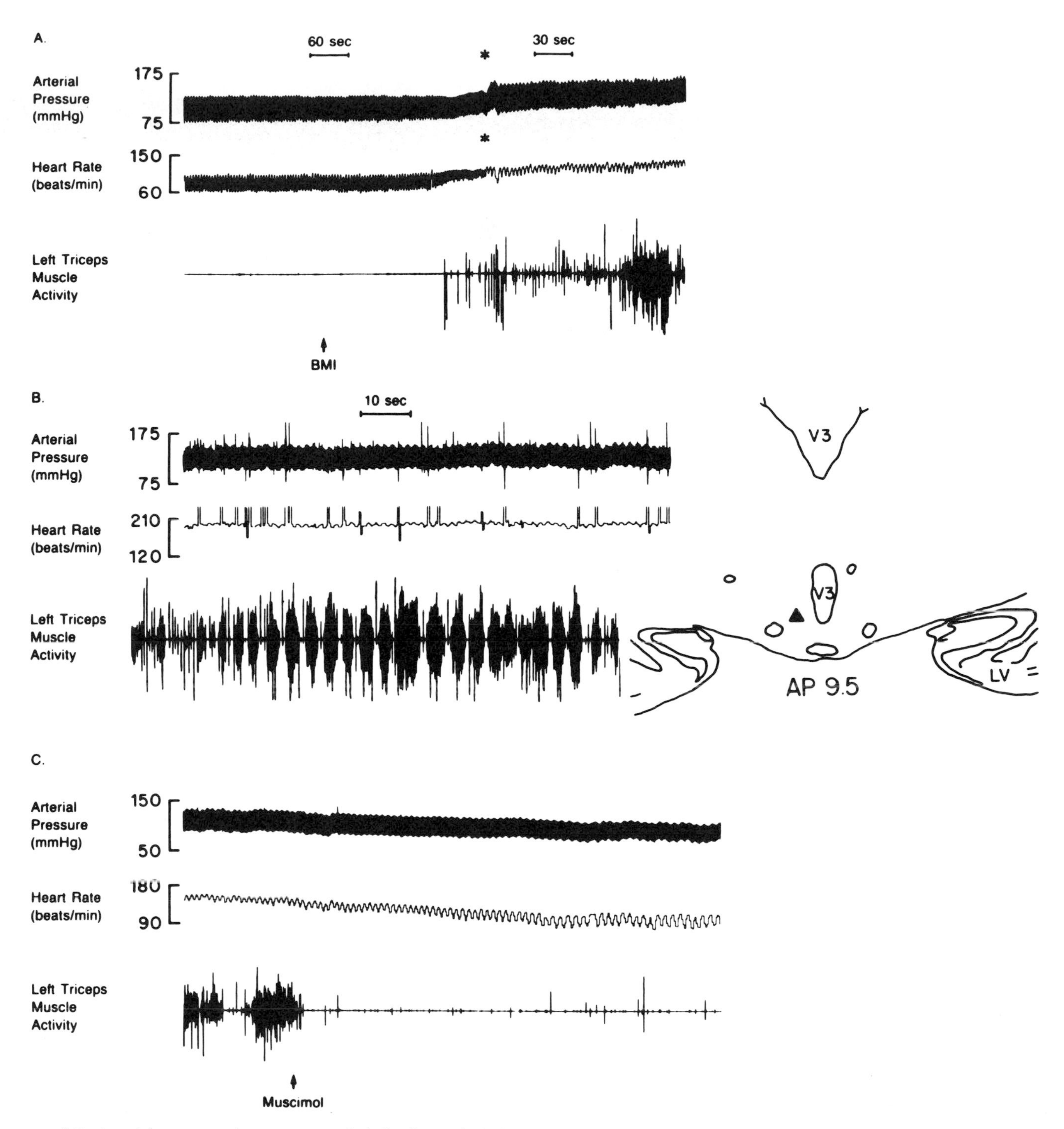

FIG. 9.9. Arterial pressure, heart rate, and skeletal muscle (triceps) responses to microinjection of a GABA antagonist [bicuculline methiodide (BMI)] into the hypothalamic locomotor region of an anesthetized cat. The responses evoked by the GABA antagonist were reversed by microinjection of a GABA agonist (muscimol) into the same hypothalamic site. The injection site is denoted by a *filled triangle* on the line drawing. [From Waldrop et al. (257).]

rate and blood pressure. These cardiovascular changes could still be evoked during muscular paralysis, indicating that activation of muscle receptors was not requisite for the observed responses. In addition, it was demonstrated that the locomotor and cardiovascular responses could be produced by stimulation of cell bodies alone in the MLR. These findings indicate that this locomotor region may also be involved in the central control of cardiovascular function during dynamic exercise.

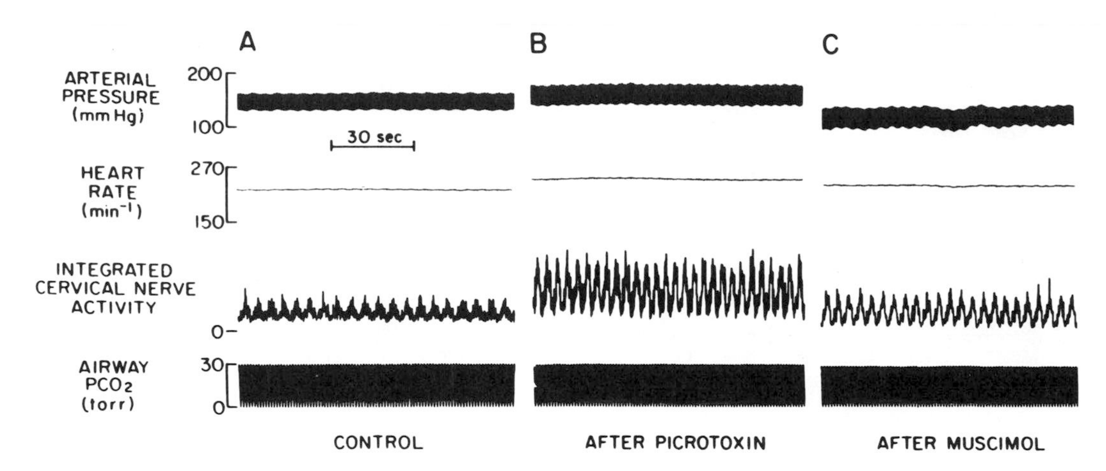

FIG. 9.10. Arterial pressure, heart rate, and sympathetic nerve (cervical nerve activity) responses to microinjection of a GABA antagonist (picrotoxin) into the hypothalamic locomotor region of an anesthetized cat. The increased activity *(B)* elicited by the injection was reversed by microinjection of a GABA agonist [muscimol, *(C)*]. [From Waldrop and Bauer (256).]

Amygdala

The amygdala is another area that may modulate cardiovascular responses during exercise. Electrical and chemical stimulation of this region elicits cardiovascular responses and motor activity (119, 166). In addition, Langhorst and colleagues (149) have shown an association of amygdala neuronal discharge with motor activity, respiration, and arterial pressure. The precise role of this area in exercise regulation demands further investigation.

Awake, Exercising Animal Studies

Several studies have provided strong support for central command in awake animals during exercise. In one study, baboons used a forearm to do static exercise under normal conditions and during partial neuromuscular blockade (120). The hypothesis in this study was that more motor units (i.e., greater central command) would be required to perform the same work during partial muscular blockade. An augmented pressor response to a similar workload occurred during the partial blockade conditions. Thus, it was concluded that the magnitude of arterial pressure responses to exercise is related to the central command signal.

Two recent studies have recorded renal sympathetic nerve activity in awake, exercising animals. Matsukawa et al. (167) examined cardiovascular responses in cats that had been trained to perform static exercise with a forelimb. Increases in cardiovascular and sympathetic activity were observed immediately upon the beginning of exercise (Fig. 9.11). The authors of this study concluded that this rapid response was due to central command. A similar study was performed recently with rabbits trained to run on a treadmill (193). Very rapid increases in renal sympathetic nerve activity were also observed in these animals during dynamic exercise. Both these studies indicate that the changes occurring at the onset of exercise are due to neural mechanisms but do not permit one to conclude that central command rather than peripheral feedback is the responsible mechanism.

SHORT-TERM POTENTIATION

It is well known that activation of a synapse and firing of a neuron leave behind an altered state of that neuron. Such changes represent a sort of memory of the preceding event and indicate plasticity of neuronal function. Two main types of memories exist. One develops fairly rapidly and is of relatively short duration, lasting milliseconds to minutes, and has been termed *short-term memory.* It can be facilitatory or inhibitory in effect. It is thought to be related to firing-evoked changes of the presynaptic terminal. The other, long-term memory, develops more slowly and is of relatively long duration, hours to days; it has been termed *long-term potentiation* (LTP) when facilitatory and *long-term depression* (LTD) when inhibitory. The mechanisms include activation of second-messenger systems and changes of neuronal gene expression that lead to changes in postsynaptic receptors, but there is evidence that presynaptic receptors can be involved as well (75). The latter investigators showed that some neurons exhibit both short- and long-term facilitatory memories but that they are not necessarily activated at the same time.

A short-term memory was probably shown first by Sherrington (222), who found that following a

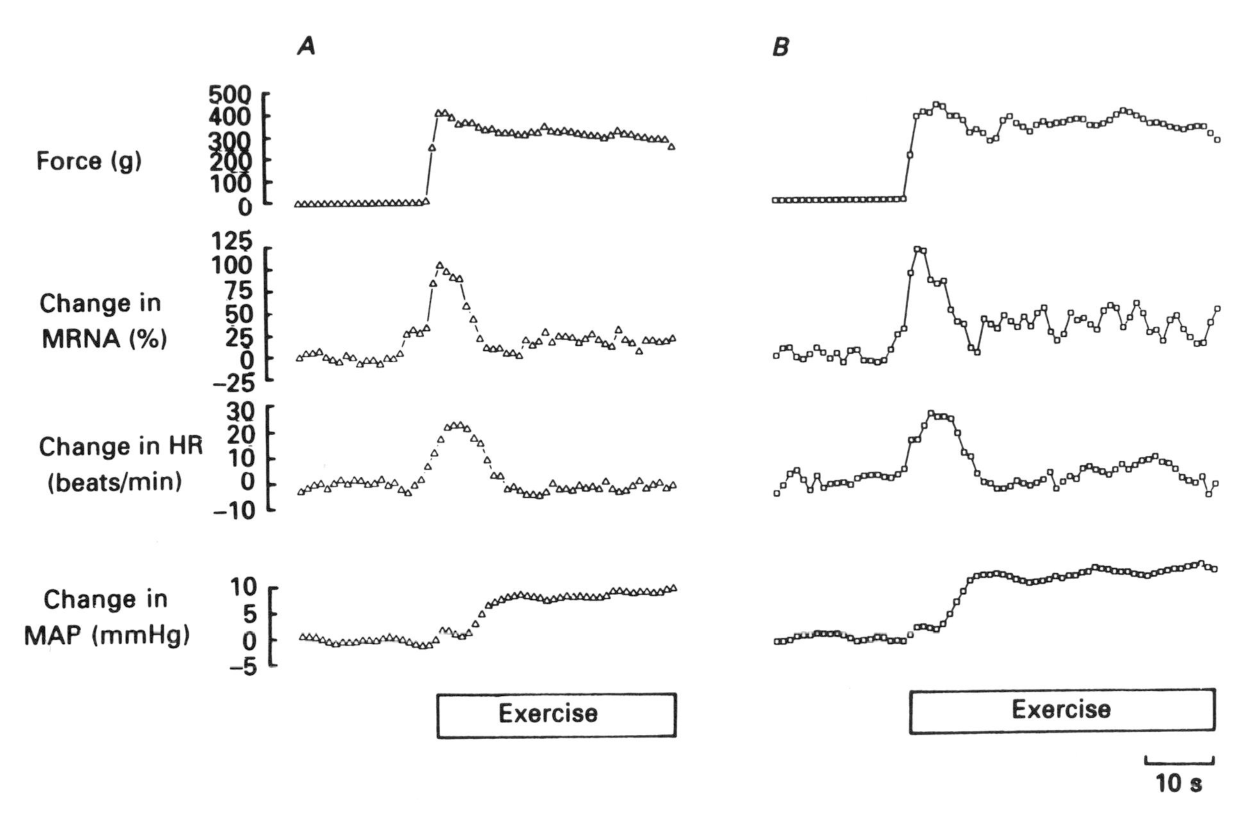

FIG. 9.11. Averaged changes in force, mean renal sympathetic nerve activity (MRNA), heart rate (HR), and mean arterial blood pressure (MAP) during two bouts of static exercise performed by a conscious cat. [From Matsukawa et al. (167).]

brief stimulation of the afferent side of a reflex arc in the spinal cord there was a prolonged but declining activation of motor activity that long outlasted the exhibition of the stimulus. He termed this an "afterdischarge." Such short-lasting processes have now been shown to occur in a wide variety of neuronal systems. They are present in hippocampal neurons (170), during sympathetic ganglion activity (150), in motoneuron reflex activity following stimulation of suprabulbar reticular formation (146), in the neuromuscular junction of the frog (163), in the rat diaphragm (94), during shivering (28), and following induced locomotion (71) in the cat. Thus, the memories appear to be ubiquitous in the nervous system and not limited to the respiratory control system.

Studies in the various systems, including hippocampal neurons in brain slices (170) and preparations of neuromuscular junctions (162, 209, 270) indicate that the short-term memories are related to changes in the presynaptic membrane during repetitive firing. These changes lead to gradually increasing neurotransmitter release and thus greater effects on the postsynaptic neuron's firing, even though stimulation of the presynaptic neuron remains constant. Magleby (162) has suggested that there may be as many as four different processes involved in the short-term memory: *facilitation* of transmitter release, which has two components with decay time constants (τ) of 50 and 300 ms; *augmentation*, with a decay τ of about 7 s; and *potentiation*, with decay τ values on the order of tens of seconds to minutes. The time course of development of the changes may be different than the decay and appears to be more related to the number of firings of the terminal than to the absolute duration of the stimulus. Both are probably exponential in form.

Several possible mechanisms have been proposed. One is that firing-induced membrane changes lead to the gradual accumulation of Ca^{2+} in the presynaptic terminal and thus to the increased transmitter release. The slow exponential decline (afterdischarge) would be related to removal of this excess Ca^{2+} (46, 162, 276). Ca^{2+} entry into nerve terminals in response to an action potential is known to be rapid (138), and its accumulation might be expected to be more rapid than its extrusion which, in contrast, can take several minutes (46). A second possibility is that the firing-induced changes of excitability of the terminal involve a decrease in membrane conductance to K^+ induced by cyclic adenosine monophosphate (AMP) (134). Finally, it has been shown that a calcium-dependent phosphorylation of a synaptic vesicle protein can potentiate transmitter release (158).

Respiration

The respiratory response to stimuli that facilitate respiration has two distinct components. The first, a rapid increase, occurs with the onset of the stimulus and accounts for about half of the full response (59). This rapid increase has been attributed to a relatively direct effect of the stimulus on medullary respiratory neurons (66). The second component is a slower increase of respiratory activity that follows the onset of the stimulus, gradually increases as the stimulus continues, and eventually reaches a steady-state plateau. Upon cessation of the stimulus, there is a rapid decrease of respiratory activity, thought to be the result of removal of the direct effect (66), but the level remains higher than the control. This increased respiration then exponentially declines (an afterdischarge) to the control level over a period of 4–5 min. It has been proposed that these slower changes are due not to direct effects of the stimulus, but to the activation and decay of a short-lasting memory (253).

Terms used to identify the phenomenon have included *afterdischarge*, *habituation* (136), *persistence* (236), *inertia* (56), *"fly-wheel effect"* (10), *neuronal plasticity* (137), and *short-term memory* (70). Although in the past most attention has been paid to the poststimulus phenomenon (the afterdischarge), it should be clear that the latter represents the gradual decay of a process that developed during the period of increased neuronal activity caused by the stimulation. Of the short-term memories, only that of potentiation has time courses of development (seconds) and decay (minutes) that would fit the findings for respiration, so it has been suggested that the most appropriate term is *short-term potentiation* (STP) of the neuronal activity associated with respiration (253). Since the ventilatory response to exercise is facilitatory and evolves over a relatively short time, about 4–5 min, and the return to resting level takes a similar amount of time, it is reasonable to think that the short-term memory, potentiation, could be one of the participants in the response. The discussion will therefore focus on the STP, although it should be noted that an element of long-term memory cannot be ruled out.

Studies in Animals. Gesell and his colleagues (103) first demonstrated in dogs that the hyperpnea resulting from stimulation of a carotid sinus nerve persisted for almost a minute after end of the stimulus, despite hypocapnia and blood alkalemia caused by the hyperpnea. Because the phenomenon appeared to be similar to that described by Sherrington (222), they called their finding a respiratory afterdischarge. Dutton et al. (55) also found that rapid removal of stimulus input from the carotid bodies, by means of quasi–square-wave changes in P_{CO_2} to separately perfused carotid arteries of dogs with constant systemic P_{CO_2}, led to a "nearly exponential" slow return toward the control level. The recovery was incomplete at 20 s, which was as long as it was studied. Intermittent square-wave increases in P_{CO_2} (3 s on, 3 s off) at the carotid bodies caused almost as much increase in ventilation as did continuous stimulation (56). These authors concluded that there must be a central integrating mechanism, or "inertial" force, responsible for the slow recovery after a stimulus and for maintaining ventilatory output in the presence of intermittent input.

Evidence for this mechanism was also found when active, neurally generated hyperventilation produced by carotid sinus nerve or leg muscle stimulation in spontaneously breathing, anesthetized (58) or decerebrate cats (60) was compared with passive or mechanically generated hyperventilation with equal degrees of hypocapnia. Passive hyperventilation was always followed by apnea, whereas neurally generated hyperventilation was followed by hyperpnea that declined slowly to the control level despite the presence of continuing hypocapnia. It was proposed that the latter must be due to a central neural mechanism that was not activated during the passive hyperventilation.

Studies using phrenic nerve activity in paralyzed animals, in which arterial P_{CO_2} and P_{O_2} can be kept constant and in which a role for other chemical and mechanical feedback mechanisms can be eliminated by ablation of buffer nerves, have provided the clearest demonstrations of features of the phenomenon of respiratory STP and the afterdischarge. A typical example (Fig. 9.12) shows the respiratory responses to a continuous stimulation of a carotid sinus nerve. There is an immediate response to the stimulus, then a gradual increase to a stable level. With cessation of the stimulus there is an immediate fall of respiratory activity but to a higher level than control. This is then followed over some minutes by a gradual decrease of activity to the original level.

That there are two clear components to the response is shown by four types of evidence:

1. One study (Fig. 9.13) was performed in an animal that had fortuitously developed apneustic

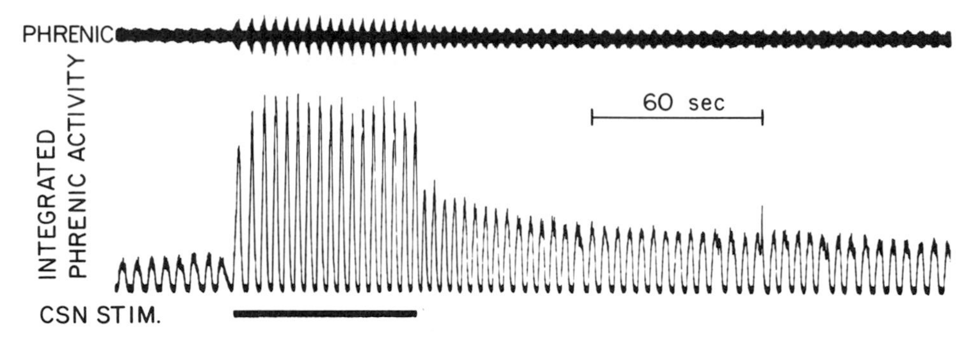

FIG. 9.12. Recording of phrenic nerve and integrated phrenic activity during control *(left)*, during stimulation *(bar)* of a carotid sinus nerve, and during recovery in a paralyzed, vagotomized cat with partial pressures of CO_2 and O_2 kept constant by means of a servocontrolled ventilator. It shows the rapid increase of respiration at stimulus onset, further increase to a steady-state within two breaths, and a rapid decrease on stimulus cessation followed by a slow recovery process (afterdischarge).

breathing. It can be seen that the slowly rising potentiation during stimulation of calf muscles (*bar*) and its decay during recovery is independent of the actual breaths, and modulates the amplitude of respiratory activity even during the prolonged inspirations. This figure demonstrates the relatively rapid development of STP compared to its much slower decay.

2. The difference is also shown in a second study (66) wherein the responses to continuous stimulation of a carotid sinus nerve (Fig. 9.14*A*) were compared to expiratory-only (Fig. 9.14*B*) and to alternate breath stimulations (Fig. 9.14*C*). With expiratory-only stimulations, the direct inspiratory effect is absent and only the increasing STP is seen. With alternate breath stimulation, the direct effect plus the increasing STP is seen in the stimulated breaths but only the rising STP is seen in the unstimulated breaths. With all three types of stimulation, the magnitude of potentiation is similar and its decay is the same.

3. The third study demonstrated a lack of effect of vagal pulmonary stretch receptor fiber input, even to the point of complete inhibition of respiration during the stimulation, on the subsequent course of the afterdischarge (65). Furthermore, vagally mediated, complete suppression of inspiratory activity during a period of facilitatory carotid sinus nerve stimulation did not prevent activation of the mechanism that leads to the STP (Fig 9.15).

4. Finally, it has been shown that the potentiation can be demonstrated by indirect means even when the level of central respiratory neural drive is subthreshold for generation of rhythmic respiratory activity (62).

Respiratory STP is activated by a wide variety of inputs that have facilitatory effects on respiration. They include stimulations of the carotid body (55, 103), carotid sinus nerve (59, 250), vagal fibers of rapidly adapting receptors (136), and peripheral muscles (59) or nerves in the extremities (130, 220,

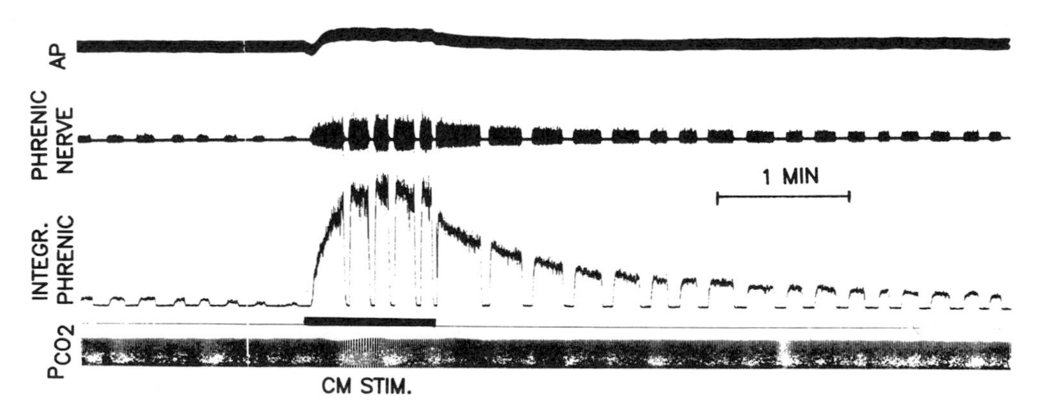

FIG. 9.13. Example of development and recovery of respiratory short-term potentiation with stimulation of calf muscles (CM) in paralyzed, vagotomized cat with controlled P_{CO_2}. The animal had fortuitously developed apneustic breathing. The potentiation develops and decays according to its usual time course and is independent of the actual respirations.

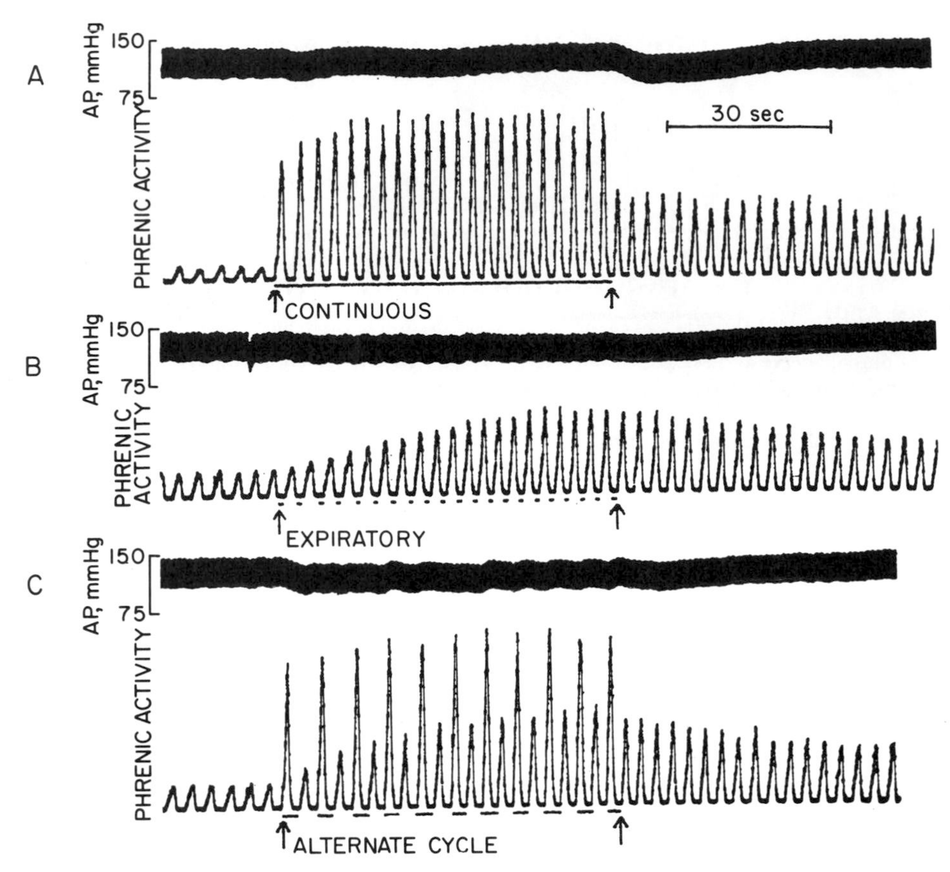

FIG. 9.14. Effects of different modes of stimulating carotid sinus nerve on respiratory (phrenic) responses and recovery in paralyzed, vagotomized cat. *A*, Continuous stimulation. *B*, Expiratory-only stimulation. *C*, Alternate-cycle stimulation. Stimulated breaths of alternate-cycle experiment are similar to those of continuous stimulation, and nonstimulated breaths are similar to those of expiratory stimulation. Despite differences in direct effects of stimulus, the amount of potentiation and the decay (afterdischarge) patterns are similar in all three experiments. Slowly rising activity during expiratory-only stimulations represents increasing activation of potentiation. AP, arterial pressure. [From Eldridge and Gill-Kumar (66).]

258). It is also activated during electrical stimulation of ventral medulla (159) and with CO_2 stimulation of medullary chemoreceptors (69, 249), and an afterdischarge can be demonstrated following removal of presumed chemoreceptor input by rapid cooling of the intermediate areas of ventral medulla (67, 176, 217). The slowly decaying potentiation also appears after stimulation of mesencephalic reticular formation and rostral pons (32, 130, 136), and STP is activated during both actual and fictive locomotion evoked by hypothalamic stimulation in decorticate cats (71). It should also be pointed out that voluntary hyperventilation in humans, presumably driven from the cerebral cortex, also activates the STP (see later under Voluntary Hyperventilation.)

There are a number of studies of procedures that do not affect the potentiation. Anesthesia does not prevent the activation of the process (59), nor does the level of anesthesia appear to affect the development or form of the afterdischarge (250). Various ablative procedures have little or no effect on its development. They include decerebration (60), decerebellation (61), spinal cord transection at C7–T1 and severing peripheral buffer nerves (59). The findings indicate that the mechanism for STP lies in the medulla and pons. Although the potentiation can be readily demonstrated in single inspiratory and expiratory neurons in the medulla, where its characteristics are similar to those found in the phrenic nerve [see Fig. 8 in ref. (73)], the potentiation (as shown above in Figs. 9.13 and 9.15) is not dependent upon actual firing of respiratory neurons and therefore must be generated ahead of them.

Magnitude. The magnitude of the potentiation has only been roughly quantified. When the measurement is made at low baseline levels of respiratory activity, the potentiation is of a magnitude similar to the rapid changes at onset and offset of a stimulus. Examples are shown in Figures 9.12 and 9.14 where the potentiation almost doubles the direct effect of the stimulation. However, the potentiating mechanism develops progressive saturation (59, 68, 250).

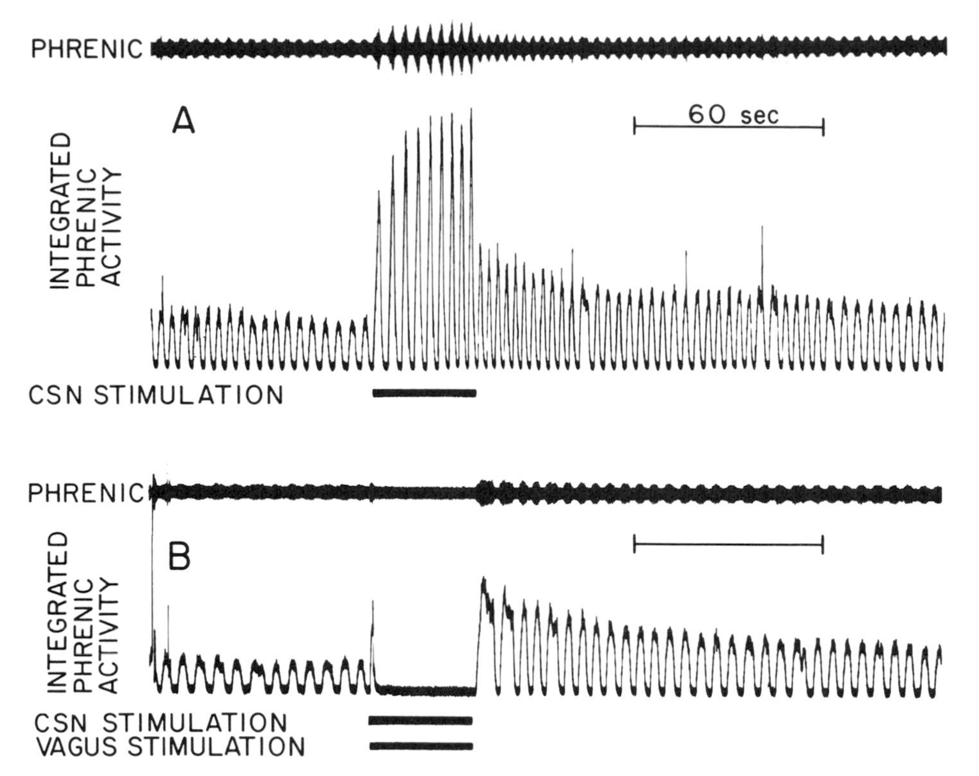

FIG. 9.15. Experiments showing that complete suppression of inspiratory activity during carotid sinus nerve (CSN) stimulation does not prevent potentiation in paralyzed, vagotomized cat. *A*, Control experiment showing baseline activity at left, effect of CSN stimulation of 30 s, and recovery. *B*, Baseline activity at left, effect of combined CSN and vagal stimulation, and recovery. Although inspirations are completely inhibited by vagal effects during combined stimulation, poststimulation respiratory activity is augmented, just as in control experiment, and decays with approximately the same time course. [From Eldridge and Gill-Kumar (65).]

Thus, as baseline level of respiratory activity increases, the component of potentiation also increases and becomes an ongoing part of that level. With additional stimulation, the remaining available potentiation therefore becomes progressively smaller, even to the point of disappearing (i.e., no apparent afterdischarge) at very high baseline levels of respiratory activity (68). If the baseline level of respiratory activity is below the threshold for rhythmic respiration (the apneic threshold), the potentiation and afterdischarge will have the appearance of being attenuated (62), but may not be truly so because some of it is subthreshold.

Time courses. The time courses of development of STP and its decay have been best defined by studies in the paralyzed animal preparation. Both the onset and offset functions appear to be exponential in form. The only systematic study of the development of respiratory STP was in cats and revealed an average τ of about 9 s (253). The average of the decay function in these cats was 46 s. Other studies in animals, including cats and piglets, have shown decay functions with τ ranging from 40–60 s (59, 66, 151).

Most studies involving activation of the potentiation by some respiratory stimulus in spontaneously breathing anesthetized or awake animals are unsatisfactory for determination of a decay time constant because, as pointed out by Engwall et al. (76), the magnitude and duration of the apparent afterdischarge are greatly attenuated if P_{CO_2} is allowed to decrease even slightly during the stimulus. The hypocapnia thus modifies poststimulus breathing by its effects on respiratory drive rather than by any clear effect on the potentiation and its decay.

Engwall et al. (76, 77) did attempt to measure the time course of the afterdischarge in awake goats that had been kept isocapnic during hypoxic stimulation of a carotid body. They found definite evidence of STP, as reflected by the presence of an afterdischarge, but the decay τ values were shorter (in the 17–30 s range) than those reported in paralyzed animals. There are two reasons to believe that the short τ values do not reflect those of the potentiation itself: *(1)* isocapnia was maintained only during the period of stimulation and not during recovery when the afterdischarge was occurring—the resulting hypocapnia may have led to an attenuation of the apparent afterdischarge that would not necessarily reflect the decay of the potentiation, and *(2)* the time constant was calculated by finding the time from end of stimulation to the time at which 63% of the decrease between end-stimulated breathing value and control had occurred. However, if the initial rapid fall of respiration on withdrawal of a stimulus (see Fig. 9.12) represents a direct effect and is separate from the potentiation (66), then only the slow portion of the decrease (the decay of potentiation) should be used for calculation of τ.

The effect on the calculated time constant including the stimulated breathing level is demonstrated in the idealized semilog graph of Figure 9.16, where the decay τ of the potentiation is known to be 50 s. If it is assumed that the potentiation represents half (or 50 units) of the total stimulated level, then the time constant (at 37% of 50 units) will be the appropriate 50 s (point A). If, on the other hand, the analysis includes all of the stimulated level (100 units), then 63% of the fall (37% of 100 units) will occur at 15.3 s (point B), a calculated τ that is incorrectly short.

Factors that may affect short-term potentiation. As noted above, there are factors, such as transient P_{CO_2} changes, varying baseline levels of breathing and saturation of output, and vagal pulmonary stretch receptor input that can modify the patterns

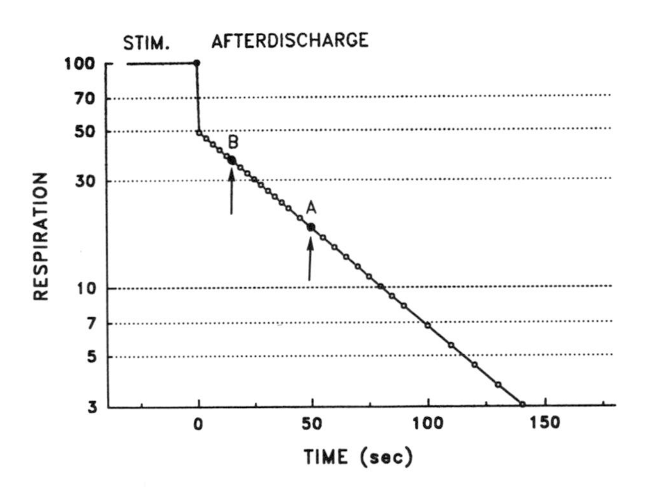

FIG. 9.16. Semilogarithmic plot of respiratory activity (units) vs. time during a stimulation (STIM.) and decay of potentiation (AFTERDISCHARGE) to show potential error in measurement of its time constant (τ). The true τ of the decay is 50 s. If the τ is measured as the 63% decay from the true starting level of 50 units, it will give the correct value of 50 s *(point A)*. However, some of the total decrease, the loss of the direct effect of the stimulus, is not part of the exponential function. Thus, if the τ is measured as a 63% decay from the end-stimulation level of 100 units, then an incorrect τ of only 15.3 s *(point B)*will be calculated.

of breathing during an afterdischarge. Are there any that truly affect the development and decay of potentiation? No specific blocking agent has been found. A study in unanesthetized, paralyzed cats that were decerebrated found longer than usual τ values for the afterdischarge (60). Since the suprapontine brain is not necessary for respiratory STP, the mechanism for the finding is not clear, although it is possible that decerebration allowed an unrecognized component of LTP to be included in the response.

It has been proposed that the periodic breathing (Cheyne-Stokes) associated with diffuse disease of the brain may be related to a defect in the potentiating mechanism (275). Why such diffuse disease should affect a presynaptic potentiating mechanism is not clear and there is no direct evidence that it does, although such patients do have loss of posthyperventilation hyperpnea and even apnea (204).

There is one factor that has been reported to affect the duration of the afterdischarge. In paralyzed cats whose brains were being made progressively hypoxic by means of carbon monoxide, it was found that the afterdischarge became progressively shorter as hypoxia worsened (173). Engwall et al. (77), on the other hand, did not find an effect on the afterdischarge from brain hypoxia (Pa_{O_2} ~40 mm Hg). It is difficult to see why a presynaptic process should be affected by hypoxia. However, it is possible that it activated another process, such as increases of the depressive neurotransmitters GABA or adenosine that affect neurons postsynaptically. In this case, the appearance of the afterdischarge might be affected by this secondary mechanism even though the potentiating mechanism itself is unchanged.

Other proposed mechanisms. Eldridge (59) originally suggested that the respiratory afterdischarge might be related to "reverberation" of neural activity in nonrespiratory neurons in the reticular formation. However, recent work from one of our laboratories (F.L.E.) has been unable to demonstrate appropriate increases and decays of firing in nonrespiratory neurons in medulla, pons, mesencephalon, or diencephalon that would support this hypothesis (252). A second possibility, that the potentiation involves one of the relatively long-acting central neurotransmitters, was ruled out for serotonin, dopamine, and norepinephrine (175), and β-adrenergic agents, isoproterenol, and metaprolol, have no effect (84). The third possibility concerns the extracellular environment of respiratory neurons. A rise of extracellular fluid [K^+], which occurs during respiratory neuronal firing (207), could further depolarize neurons and cause more firing (237). However, the rise of [K^+] around respiratory neurons is quite small and the time course of reuptake relatively rapid, making it improbable that there would be a correlation with the prolonged decay phase of the potentiation. The most likely mechanism thus remains that of short-term potentiation.

Studies in Humans. The existence of a short-term respiratory memory in human beings has been shown in several ways. Studies of the variability of tidal volume and respiratory frequency indicate that the changes occurring with time are not random (25, 26, 205). Also, the depth and duration of the breathing cycle are not independent of the preceding cycles, findings which led to a conclusion that there is a respiratory control mechanism that acts as a short-term memory (26).

Voluntary hyperventilation. The second type of evidence comes from studies of breathing after voluntary hyperventilation. It is well known that posthyperventilation apnea develops in both anesthetized and awake human beings, as in animals, after passive (i.e., mechanically generated) hyperventilation. Here the apnea can be attributed solely to decrease in chemoreceptor-mediated (CO_2) input to the respiratory controller. Workers early in the century (112, 114, 187) also reported apnea immediately after voluntary hyperventilation; they attributed the apnea to loss of chemical (CO_2) stimulation of central chemoreceptors. However, many subsequent studies, beginning with Boothby (29), have noted that voluntary hyperventilation of short duration ($\leq$ 1 min) usually does not lead to apnea in the immediate posthyperventilation period, despite the hypocapnia that develops (8, 81, 178, 204, 240). Instead there is often an hyperpnea with no or rare apneas (29, 81, 178, 240), an hyperpnea that declines fairly rapidly to or somewhat below control. The findings are consistent with the development of potentiation during the hyperventilation, and its subsequent decay, and shows that cortical input to the respiratory controller acts in the same way as do other neural inputs that activate the STP in animals.

It is difficult to perform a satisfactory quantitative analysis of the afterdischarge in this setting for two reasons. First, because some of the neural activity emanating from the cortex probably bypasses the medullary respiratory controller and acts directly on cervical and thoracic spinal respiratory motoneurons via paucisynaptic pathways (7, 40, 98, 157), the controller may not be engaged as much, relative to the increase of ventilation, as by other kinds of respiratory stimulation whose effects are mainly in the medulla. Thus, the potentiation, relative to the ventilatory response, may also be less.

Second, and more important, the hypocapnia resulting from hyperventilation leads to a secondary decrease of respiratory stimulation during the recovery period, which will interfere with the ventilatory expression of the decaying potentiation and thus produce an apparently short afterdischarge, hypopnea, and even apnea. Meah and Gardner (171) have recently restudied the problem; they used longer periods of hyperventilation (3 and 6 min), during which body stores of CO_2 would have been more depleted than in the short hyperventilations of most of the studies noted above, and followed recovery for a longer time. Apneas were rarely found in the immediate (first minute) posthyperventilation period, consistent with a respiratory afterdischarge, but after that apneas gradually increased in number and length. The investigators showed that the apneas were related to a reduction of CO_2, measured as end-tidal P_{CO_2}. In an attempt to circumvent the problem of hypocapnia, hyperventilation and recovery were studied under isocapnic conditions, using a computer-controlled system to keep end-tidal P_{CO_2} constant (236). These workers found that no apneas occurred and an afterdischarge was usually present. The average τ of the afterdischarge was 22 s, shorter than that found in paralyzed animals. It was hoped that end-tidal isocapnia meant that arterial and central P_{CO_2} were also isocapnic; however, there is a likelihood that both of the latter were actually less than end-tidal value (15). Thus, hypocapnia may still have affected the apparent afterdischarge, although not necessarily the potentiation.

Hypoxic stimulation. Several recent studies have confirmed, by the use of respiratory stimuli other than voluntary hyperventilation, that potentiation and an afterdischarge do occur in human beings. All of these studies used hypoxic hypoxia to stimulate breathing through its effect on the carotid bodies (5, 15, 87, 102). The actual experimental designs varied.

One type of study involved only short exposures (15–90 s) to hypoxia. Georgopoulos et al. (102) studied normal conscious humans. Following abrupt hyperoxic termination of the hypoxia (8.5% $F_{I_{O_2}}$ for 35–50 s) there was, despite the existing hypocapnia and hyperoxia during the posthypoxic recovery transient, a gradual ventilatory decline to baseline without an apparent undershoot. The same laboratory reperformed the experiment (5) in normal elderly subjects (average age 62 years) and obtained similar results. Prolonging the period of hypoxia to 90 s had no effect on the findings.

Fregosi (87) investigated normal subjects during mild exercise, using 10% $F_{I_{O_2}}$ or four to five breaths of N_2; he also found evidence of an exponential decay (τ about 28 s) of short-term potentiation with both types of stimulation, again despite hypocapnia and hyperoxia during the recovery period.

Badr et al. (15) studied poststimulus potentiation after a minute of hypoxia (8% $F_{I_{O_2}}$) in subjects during non–rapid eye movement (NREM) sleep. Hyperoxic termination of the hyperpnea was associated with declining hyperpnea for four to six breaths when end-tidal P_{CO_2} was kept constant. On the other hand, when end-tidal hypocapnia was allowed to develop during the hypoxically evoked hyperventilation, there was poststimulus hypoventilation for 45 s. The authors concluded that poststimulation hyperpnea, consistent with potentiation and its decay, occurs in NREM sleep as long as the hypoxic stimulation is brief and arterial P_{CO_2} is maintained constant. However, if hypocapnia develops, the loss of central and peripheral chemoreceptor stimuli to the controller may mask or counterbalance the excitatory effects of potentiation, with hypoventilation the result.

Thus, all of these studies yielded evidence for development of short-term potentiation of respiration during a period of hypoxic stimulation. Again, quantitation of the process in terms of magnitude or time course is difficult in this setting because of changes of other respiratory factors such as arterial (and probably central) P_{CO_2}, which decreases even when end-tidal P_{CO_2} is kept constant (15), and hypoxic changes of medullary blood flow, which might reduce medullary P_{CO_2}.

In contrast to the results after brief hypoxic stimulations, several studies have shown that more prolonged hypoxia (5–25 min) leads to an apparent absence of the afterdischarge, with poststimulus hypopnea and sometimes apnea, even if the subject is kept end-tidally isocapnic (15, 102). Badr et al. (15) suggested that the afterdischarge was either abolished or overriden after these hypoxic exposures. Does this mean that prolonged hypoxia in humans impairs the mechanism that causes the potentiation? The answer has to be "not necessarily," because what appears in ventilation may be a result of the potentiation and another depressive factor occurring at the same time. We pointed out earlier that it is difficult on theoretical grounds to see why hypoxia should affect directly a presynaptic mechanism that leads to the potentiation. Other possible reasons for the loss of afterdischarge, in contrast to the potentiation, include:

1. There may be mild arterial hypocapnia despite end-tidal isocapnia (15).
2. Increased medullary blood flow resulting from the hypoxia might reduce medullary P_{CO_2}/H^+, so that the recovery period is affected and the afterdischarge masked.
3. It is unlikely that direct hypoxic depression of neurons (hypoxic depolarization) is occurring with the levels of hypoxia in these experiments. However, sustained hypoxia could easily lead to neural inhibition (hyperpolarization) due to short-lasting accumulations of inhibitory neurochemicals such as adenosine or GABA, and to longer lasting effects (LTD) brought on via activation of second-messenger systems by such agents (64).

In a careful analysis, Badr et al. (15) considered these possibilities in detail and concluded that no single mechanism can explain the hypoxic posthyperventilation apnea, which must therefore be due to complex interactions of all.

Functional Significance of Short-Term Potentiation. Respiratory short-term potentiation appears to be an intrinsic response of neurons in the respiratory control system to their own increased activity. It is clearly not stimulus specific. In the past, full ventilatory responses to neural stimuli were assumed to be accomplished rapidly; the existence of the potentiating mechanism makes this assumption incorrect, both during and after a stimulus. Because the potentiation acts as a self-amplifying mechanism, the ultimate respiratory response to any stimulus will be greater than the direct effect of the stimulus alone. This combined with the slowness of the changes leads to an ability to integrate and smooth out the effects of changes of stimuli, thereby preventing large and rapid changes of ventilation that might otherwise result. The potentiation thus appears to be an important factor in maintaining the stability of breathing. It is important in helping to prevent the occurrence of posthyperventilation apnea (240), and it has been suggested that periodic breathing would be more likely to occur if the mechanism were defective (275).

Role in the Respiratory Response to Exercise. Because the respiratory STP occurs with all facilitatory respiratory stimuli in animals and man, it has been proposed that it must be a component of the response to exercise (59). In their analysis of the mechanisms of exercise hyperpnea, Eldridge and Waldrop (73) suggested that the potentiation "must make a sizable contribution to the ventilatory response" and that "its time course can explain much of the slow increase of ventilation after the onset of exercise" (i.e., the phase II increase to steady-state at 4–5 min) and "most of the slow decrease during recovery" [i.e., the slow decrease (phase IIR) to near steady-state that occurs at about 5 min].

There are three main questions to be asked about this hypothesis:

1. Does STP occur during exercise? The most that can be said is that a respiratory afterdischarge does occur after both actual locomotion (exercise) in nonparalyzed animals and after fictive locomotion in paralyzed animals (71). Thus, it probably occurs during exercise in humans.

2. Does STP contribute to the magnitude of the respiratory response to exercise? Probably yes, but since no way of solely blocking the potentiating mechanism in intact subjects has been found, there is no way to test the question experimentally. Thus, the only basis for the conclusion is the experimental findings in animals that the potentiation accounts for about half of the overall respiratory response to any of a large number of stimuli, including those that can plausibly occur during exercise. Also, the model shown in Figure 9.18 suggests that the magnitude is affected (see below).

3. Does STP affect the dynamics of the response, and especially does it account for the slowly rising (phase II) ventilation after onset of exercise and the slowly falling ventilation during recovery (phase IIR)? First, it cannot possibly be responsible for the gradually increasing component during most of the phase II period. The reason lies in the STP's onset τ of about 10 s which means that 90% of the potentiation will have developed by 23 s (Fig. 9.17). Thus, most of the increase of ventilation that occurs after that time must be due to other mechanisms. Second, because the τ of the potentiation's decay is about 50 s, it is likely that it plays a greater role in the early part of the phase IIR decrease of respiration (Fig. 9.17), but the decay will still be greater than 90% complete at 2 min, so again other mechanisms must be invoked to explain the further decrease actually found in exercising subjects.

On the other hand, STP probably does affect the early dynamics of the responses. This question has been approached by means of a computer-based mathematical model[3] of the respiratory control system developed by one of the authors (F.L.E.). In addition to the traditional feedback mechanisms involving CO_2 and O_2, the model includes those features postulated by Eldridge and Waldrop (73) to be important in exercise hyperpnea; they include the rapidly acting neural mechanisms (central command and input from muscles), short-term potentiation with an onset τ of 10 s and offset τ of 50 s, and serum $[K^+]$ rising during exercise (τ of 45 s) and falling during recovery [τ of 30 s (38)]. Figure 9.18*A* represents the findings at rest ($\dot{V}O_2$ of 0.25 liter/min), during exercise ($\dot{V}O_2$ of 1.0 liter/min) for 6 min, and during recovery in the intact model that has all of the features noted above. It shows ventilation (liter per minute) and end-tidal, mean arterial, and medullary PCO_2 (mm Hg), which were calculated continuously while running the model. It can be seen that the pattern of the ventilatory response is much like the well-known studies of Dejours (45) and diagram of Whipp (271); there are transient changes of arterial and medullary PCO_2, but they have the same value at 6 min of exercise as they did at rest.

Fig. 9.18*B* shows the same rate of exercise in the model which, except for a removal of the short-term potentiation, has been set up so that all parameters are the same. The differences of the findings from those of the model with STP intact (Fig. 9.18*A*) are two: *(1)* at 6 min of exercise there is a slightly lower ventilation (18.5 vs. 18.8 liter/min) and slightly higher arterial (41.0 vs. 39.8 mm Hg) and medullary (46.9 vs. 45.5 mm Hg) PCO_2 values, suggesting that the loss of STP does affect the magnitude of the respiratory response; and *(2)* without STP there is a quite marked oscillation of ventilation after the onset and again after the offset of exercise; these do not occur in the intact model and reflect the loss of the damping effect of the potentiation. The model thus supports the idea that STP does have an im-

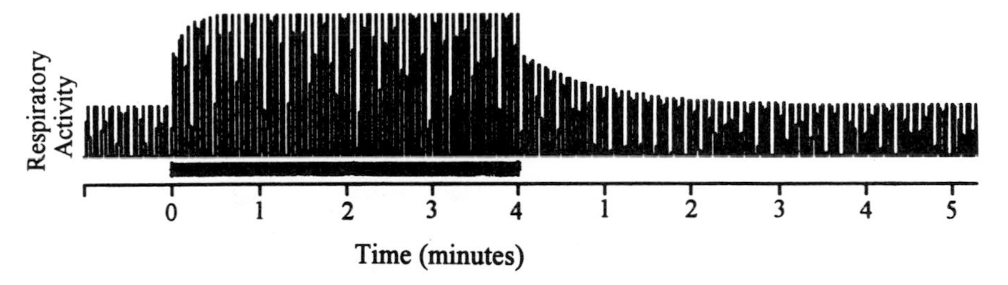

FIG. 9.17. Computer-generated neural inspiratory (phrenic equivalent) activity in a model that incorporates short-term potentiation (onset τ, 10 s; offset τ, 50 s) and that mimicks constant blood gases and has no other feedback. Control at left, then a 4 min facilitatory stimulus *(bar)*, and then 5 min of recovery. The STP has almost no effect on the pattern after the first 30 s of stimulation and little effect on the recovery after 2 min. (The irregular patterns in the tracing are pixel effects from the computer screen and have no physiological meaning.)

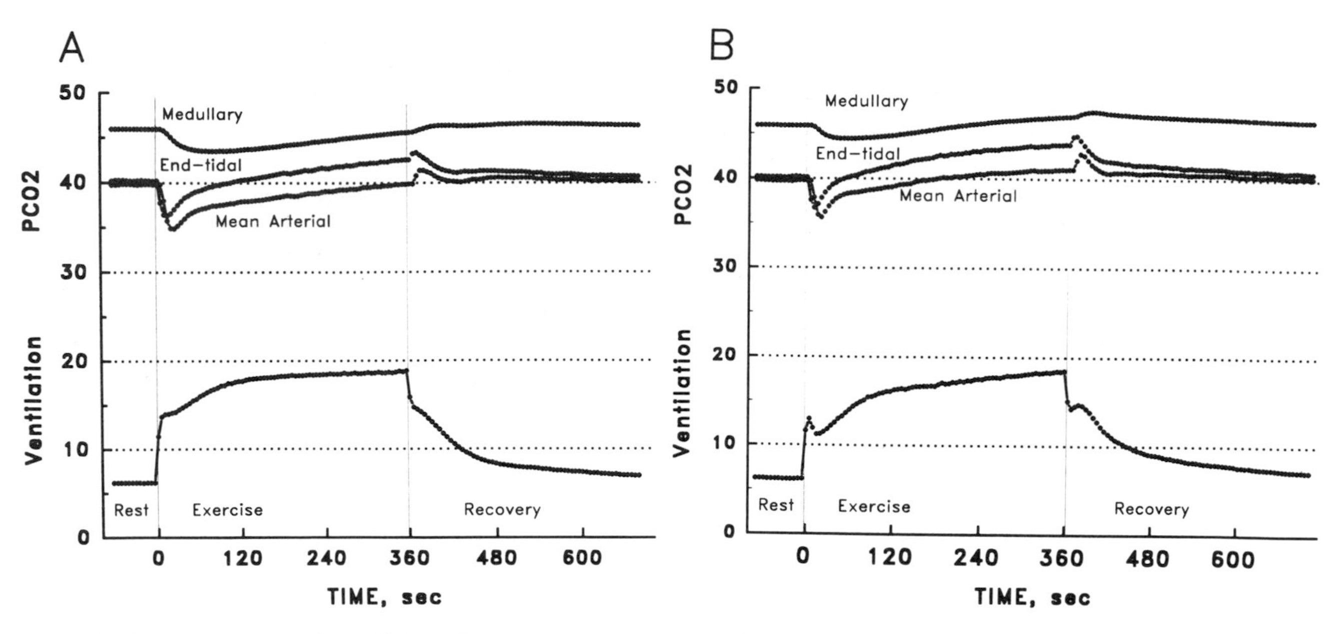

FIG. 9.18. Computer-generated ventilation (liters per minute) and arterial, end-tidal, and medullary P_{CO_2} during rest (V_{O_2} = 0.25 liter/min), 6 min of exercise ($\dot{V}_{O_2}$ = 1.0 liter/min), and recovery (see text and footnote for details of model). In panel *A* the model includes the usual short-term potentiating (STP) mechanism (τ on = 10 s; τ off = 50 s); it yields a typical and normal ventilatory response to exercise. In panel *B* the STP has been removed, with the result that ventilation at the end of the 6 min of exercise is slightly less than in the model with STP, all P_{CO_2} values are slightly higher, and there are increased oscillations of ventilation after both onset and cessation of exercise.

portant role in the dynamics of the respiratory response, preventing inappropriate over- and undershoots of ventilation at the times of transition from rest to exercise and vice versa.

CENTRAL COMMAND CONTROL OF RESPIRATION AND CIRCULATION IN HUMANS

Respiration

Exercise can be divided into two different forms that evoke specific respiratory responses (254). Both static (isometric) and dynamic (rhythmic) exercise are encountered by most individuals on a daily basis. Static exercise is defined as muscular contraction that is characterized by a change in developed tension accompanied by small changes in the length of the contracting muscles. Lifting or pushing heavy objects are types of static exercise. Dynamic exercise involves muscular contraction consisting primarily of changes in the length of the muscle with only minor changes in the tension of the active muscles. The respiratory responses to both types of exercise have been extensively documented.

Static Exercise. The respiratory response to static exercise has been well characterized by several investigators who have shown that the rate of development and magnitude of the response is related to the amount of developed tension. Myhre and Andersen (190) examined the respiratory responses to sustained handgrip exercise at four different levels of tension development. A similar pattern of respiratory changes was evoked by the different levels of contraction. An initial rapid increase in ventilation was observed that often preceded the beginning of the contraction (Fig. 9.19). A gradual increase followed the initial response, with a larger increase occurring in the final minute of the 5-min contraction.

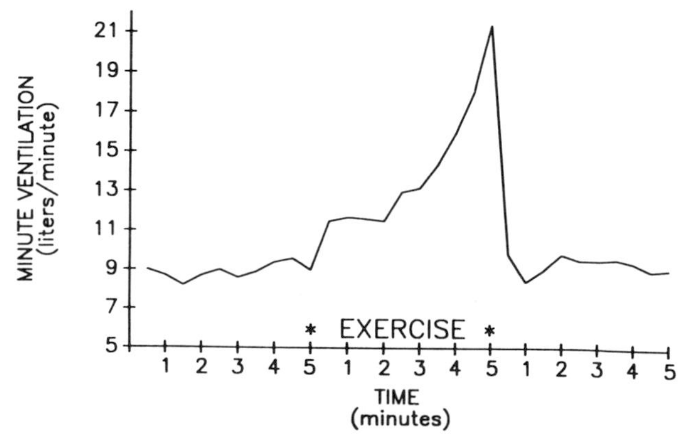

FIG. 9.19. Schematic representation of the ventilatory response to static (handgrip) exercise. *Asterisks* denote the onset and end of the exercise bout. [From Waldrop (255).]

A large, rapid fall in ventilation occurred at the end of the contraction, followed by a more gradual return to baseline. The increased ventilation during the handgrip exercise is due to an increased tidal volume, with no significant increase in respiratory frequency (189).

Muza et al. (189) have shown that the respiratory response to static handgrip exercise is a hyperventilation as evidenced by a fall in end-tidal P_{CO_2}. In one group of subjects, end-tidal P_{CO_2} was maintained constant during the exercise to examine the role that changes in chemoreceptor input has on the respiratory response to static exercise. The magnitude and pattern of the response to hand-grip exercise was not altered during this isocapnic protocol, indicating that chemoreceptor input does not play a major role in modulating the respiratory responses to exercise. Subjects were also asked to rate the estimated effort required for the contractions performed at different tension levels. Both the time course and magnitude of the perceived effort was directly proportional to the magnitude of the ventilatory response. Muza et al. (189) concluded that this correlation is consistent with mediation of the respiratory response by a central command mechanism.

Wiley and Lind (273) also examined the respiratory response to static exercise in human subjects who performed sustained static contractions with both the forearm and leg. A similar hyperventilatory response was observed in their study as was seen with handgrip exercise alone; however, simultaneous contractions of both the arm and leg did not produce an additive respiratory response. Additional studies were performed to consider potential mechanisms responsible for the observed responses. First, the responses to static contraction with and without vascular occlusion were compared. Since the magnitude and pattern of the changes in ventilation did not differ between the two protocols, stimulation of muscle or other chemoreceptors by metabolites released from the contracting muscles was excluded. The possibility of the responses being due to pain was also considered unlikely, since the perceived feelings during the unoccluded handgrip were only minor discomfort. However, feelings of intense pain were reported for the contractions during vascular occlusion. Thus, it was concluded that either a reflex originating from activation of mechanically sensitive receptors in the contracting muscles or joints or "central nervous drive" were responsible for the observed respiratory and cardiovascular responses (273).

Duncan et al. (54) studied two patients with sensory deficits during handgrip exercise. Both patients had sensory neuropathies resulting in a loss of forearm sensation; one patient had an almost complete left hemisection at the fifth cervical segment due to injuries suffered in an automobile accident. He had normal motor function of the forearm on the affected side but had no sense of pain, temperature, or touch. The other patient had a congenital sensory neuropathy that resulted in a complete loss of pain and cutaneous sensations in the arms. Handgrip exercise was accompanied by small but significant increases in ventilation in both subjects. The sensory disorders preclude either pain or afferent feedback from exercise-sensitive receptors in the active muscle as explanations for the increases in breathing during the static exercise. Therefore, descending central drive appears to be the mediator of the exercise responses in these patients.

Goodwin, McCloskey, and Mitchell (104) designed experiments to test specifically for the role of central command during static exercise. In their studies, vibration was applied to an agonist muscle performing a static contraction to elicit reflex contractions via activation of muscle spindles. The hypothesis was that this would result in a reduction in central command, since less descending drive would be required to maintain a constant tension (Fig. 9.20*A*). Associated with the vibration-associated decrease in central command was a smaller respiratory response as compared to a static contraction without accompanying muscle vibration (Fig. 9.21*A*). An additional protocol involved vibration applied to a muscle antagonist to that muscle statically contracting, thereby evoking a reflex inhibition of the active muscle (Fig. 9.20*B*). As a result, increased central command was needed to maintain a constant muscle tension during the exercise bout. Associated with this protocol was an increased respiratory response (Fig. 9.21*B*). Thus, ventilatory responses changed proportional to the changes in central command.

A recent study by Gandevia et al. (97) provides indirect support for a major role of central command in mediating the ventilatory responses to static exercise. Subjects were studied before and after complete motor paralysis as induced by an exceedingly large dose of atracurium (i.e., five times greater than is used normally during surgical procedures). The completeness of blockade was validated by the loss of electromyographic (EMG) responses to transcutaneous stimulation of the phrenic nerve and tibial nerves. No direct measure of respiratory drive was possible in these totally paralyzed subjects, who were ventilated throughout the period of paralysis. However, all subjects had a sense of increased ventilation during fictive contractions of forearm muscles. Obviously, the only mechanisms that could explain the perceived ventilatory response would be central command.

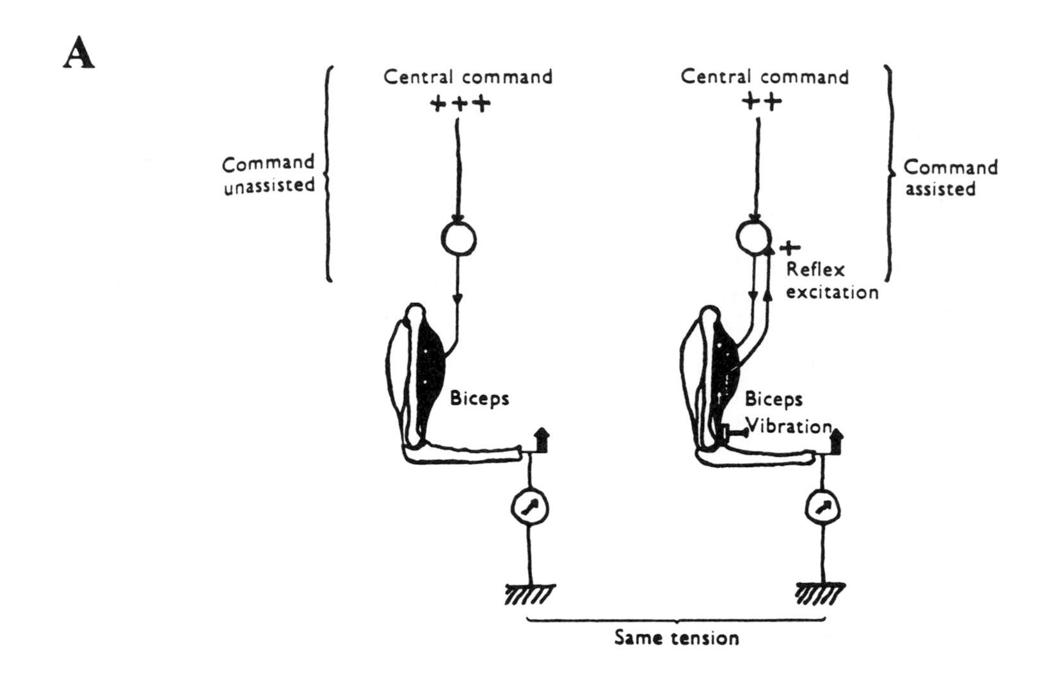

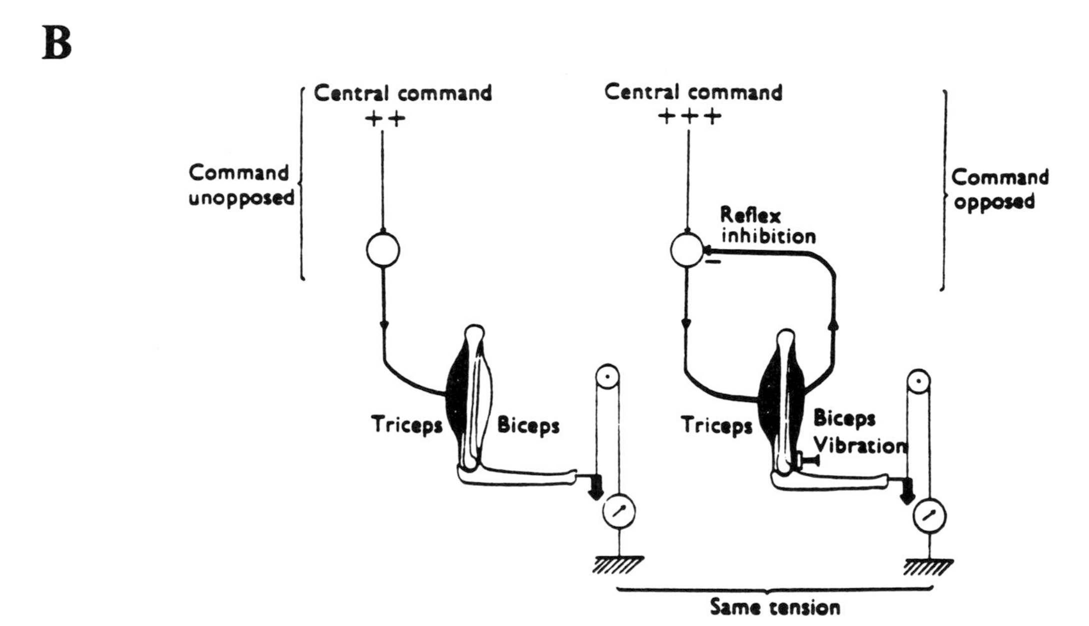

FIG. 9.20. *A*, Experimental design for reducing the magnitude of central command required to achieve a muscle tension. The drawing shows how vibration is used to activate primary afferents from the contracting muscles, thereby contributing reflex excitation of the motoneurons innervating the muscle. The same amount of force can be generated as was true without the reflex excitation (on the left) but with a reduced central command component. *B*, Experimental design for increasing the magnitude of central command required to achieve a muscle tension. The drawing shows how vibration is used to activate primary afferents from a muscle (biceps) antagonist to the contracting muscles, thereby contributing reflex inhibition of the motoneurons innervating the contracting muscle. An increased central command component is required in order for the same amount of force to be generated as was true without the reflex inhibition (on the left). [Adapted from Goodwin et al. (104).]

Dynamic Exercise. The respiratory responses associated with dynamic exercise have long been known from the pioneering work of Krogh and Lindhard (147) in 1913. They demonstrated that there is an increase in ventilation immediately at the onset of exercise on a cycle ergometer. Subsequent studies have shown that this initial rapid increase in breathing is followed by a more gradual increase in breathing over the first 2–5 min of dynamic exercise (Fig. 9.22). The secondary rise in ventilation reaches

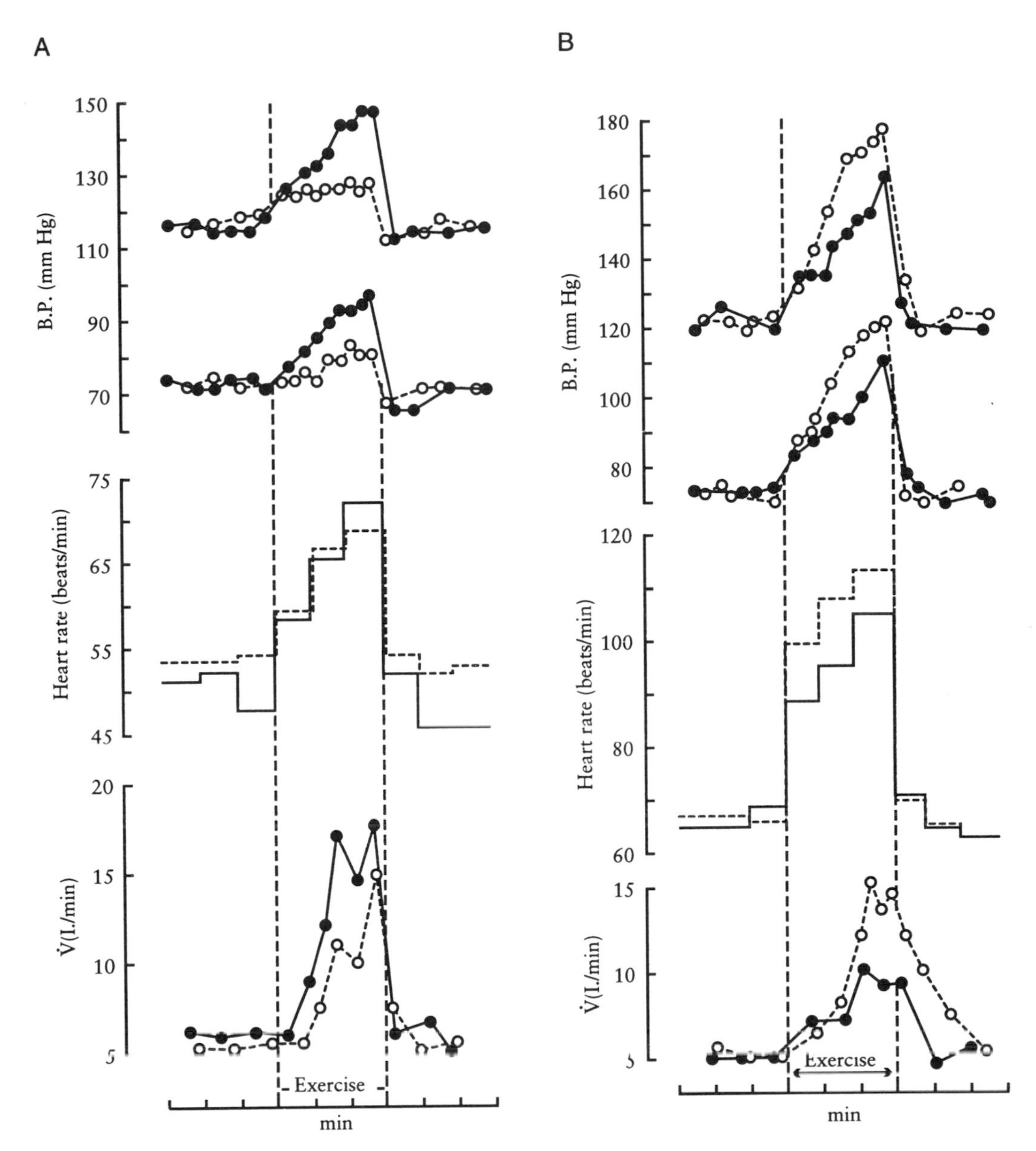

FIG. 9.21. *A*, Reduction of central command. The blood pressure, heart rate, and ventilatory responses during a normal contraction are shown by the *filled circles* and *continuous lines*; the responses when vibration was used to reduce central command are shown by *open circles* and *interrupted lines*. *B*, Augmentation of central command. The blood pressure, heart rate, and ventilatory responses during a normal contraction are shown by the *filled circles* and *continuous lines*; the responses when vibration was used to increase central command are shown by *open circles* and *interrupted lines*. [Adapted from Goodwin et al. (104).]

a plateau level that is maintained throughout the duration of the exercise bout. At the end of the exercise bout, there is an abrupt fall in ventilation followed by a gradual return to the baseline ventilation. Some debate exists over how well arterial P_{CO_2} is regulated during dynamic exercise in humans. Most frequently it is stated that isocapnia persists throughout bouts of mild or moderate exercise (268). However, several investigators have observed a small fall in arterial P_{CO_2} at the onset of dynamic exercise in humans (9, 35, 43, 85). It has been argued from a review of the literature that hyperventilation is more common during treadmill exercise than is the case for exercise on a cycle ergometer.

Krogh and Lindhard (147) considered several mechanisms responsible for the increases in respiration that occur during rhythmic exercise. Their consideration of mechanisms was based upon those suggested by Johansson (133) in 1893 for the regulation of heart rate during exercise. Krogh and Lindhard (147) concluded that "motor impulses irradiate to centres governing the respiration" (i.e., cortical

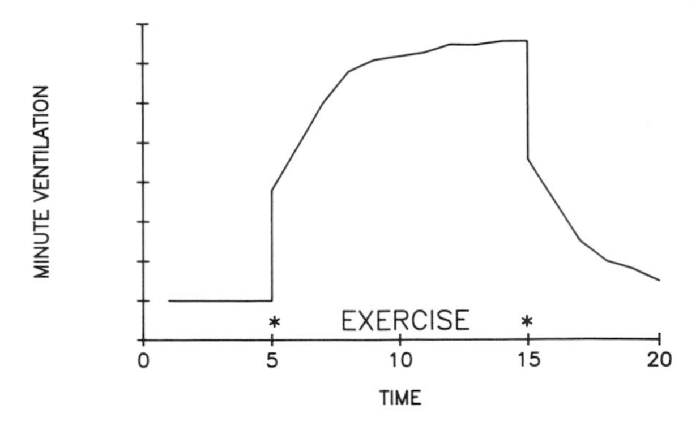

FIG. 9.22. Schematic representation of the ventilatory response to static (handgrip) exercise. *Asterisks* denote the onset and end of the exercise bout. [From Waldrop (254).]

irradiation). They argued that this cortical irradiation resulted in an increased sensitivity of brainstem respiratory neurons to hydrogen ions.

The concept of cortical irradiation or central command as first proposed by Johansson and refined by Krogh and Lindhard (147) has led to over a century of investigation into the mechanisms responsible for regulating respiration during exercise. Even though these early experiments provided no direct evidence for central command and based their conclusions on false assumptions, their concepts remain strong. A number of studies performed on humans have tested the hypothesis that central command is a major determinant of the respiratory responses to exercise. There has not been a concensus from these studies as to the importance of central command; this lack of agreement likely results from the fact that it is impossible to control for all possible confounding variables in noninvasive human studies. Dempsey et al. (47) have stated this problem well in a prior review: "Attempts to answer these questions in the intact, exercising model, in which [all] of the potential primary stimuli are operative, yields only correlative data, while abundant and impressive, clearly fail to separate cause and effect." Nonetheless, several studies have provided strong support for the involvement of central command.

Asmussen and colleagues (10–14) performed an extensive series of experiments with humans exercising on a cycle ergometer. Even though these investigators concluded that a peripheral reflex provided the major source of respiratory stimulation during exercise, an examination of their work provides strong support for the central command mechanism. In one set of experiments, the respiratory responses associated with dynamic exercise were examined before and during occlusion of blood flow to the legs produced by inflation of blood pressure cuffs (12). Pulmonary ventilation as well as heart rate and arterial pressure increased to a greater extent during the exercise period with occlusion of blood flow even though the work rate remained constant. Asmussen and Nielsen (12) found by recording surface EMG activity that an increased number of motor units had to be activated in order to maintain tension during the occluded exercise. Thus, it is obvious that there was an increased central nervous system drive (i.e., central command) active during the exercise with occluded blood supply. Therefore, the enhanced ventilatory response may be explained by the increase in central command. Further support for this conclusion is that the subjects felt as if "the work was becoming heavier and heavier" during the occluded state.

Another study by Asmussen et al. (11) used curare to partially paralyze the active muscles during exercise on a cycle ergometer. Since curare is known to block motor end-plates, there had to be an increased descending drive to activate additional motor units to maintain a constant work. Associated with the increased motor activation was an increase in ventilation as was the case for the occlusion studies described above. Galbo et al. (95) have recently duplicated these findings with partial neuromuscular blockade (i.e., larger ventilatory responses for a given workload during paralysis). Both the curarization and occlusion studies argue strongly in support of central command as the major mediator of respiratory responses during dynamic exercise. However, it should be noted that Asmussen and colleagues (11) concluded that gamma loop activation of motor units during these two protocols would lead to increased afferent feedback to the reticular formation (i.e., a feedback signal as the mediator of the respiratory responses). This explanation seems less likely with the increased knowledge about the gamma loop that has been obtained since the work of Asmussen. Moreover, the afferents (groups I and II) that would be stimulated by such a postulated mechanism have been shown to not affect respiratory drive. It is interesting that Asmussen ultimately accepted the idea of central command over the gamma loop hypothesis in a review he wrote years after his initial studies were performed (10).

Innes et al. (132) studied three groups of subjects with unilateral leg weakness to test the hypothesis that respiratory responses to a given work rate would require more descending central command when the exercise was performed with the weak leg as compared to the normal leg. Three groups of subjects with unilateral leg weakness were studied: *(1)* patients recovering from orthopedic problems who had no sensory impairment in their weak leg, *(2)* two patients with neurological disorders, and *(3)* eight normal subjects in which leg weakness was induced by percutaneous local anesthetic blockade of the femoral nerve. For all groups, the ventilatory response at a given workload with exercise of the weak leg was greater than that with normal leg. Since the exercise V_{O_2} did not differ between the two protocols, exercise with the weak leg elicited a ventilatory response out of proportion to the metabolic rate. The authors of this study concluded that the ventilatory response to dynamic exercise is influenced by central neural drive.

Several studies have compared ventilatory responses to voluntary exercise with those elicited during muscular contraction produced by electrical stimulation of leg muscles (2–4, 14, 31, 230). Asmussen et al. (14) used this protocol in 1943 to test the hypothesis that no central command would be present during dynamic exercise elicited by electrical stimulation of the muscle. They found that electrically induced contractions produced the same respiratory response as that observed with voluntary contractions for a given workload. Therefore, it was concluded that the ventilatory response during exercise arose "reflexly from the working muscles." These results were later confirmed by similar studies performed by Adams et al. (2), who found a tight correlation between ventilation and workload during both voluntary and electrically induced contractions. In addition, similar results have been obtained in subjects during voluntary and electrically induced static contractions. An expansion of these experiments was reported in a recent study (230). Subjects were studied during voluntary exercise (central command and muscle reflex active), during muscle stimulation (absence of central command *assumed*), and during muscle stimulation with epidural anesthesia (absence of both central command and muscle reflex *assumed*). The ventilatory responses to dynamic leg exercise did not differ during the three protocols; thus, it was concluded that humoral mechanisms may play a role in regulating exercise ventilation.

These experiments with muscle contraction evoked by electrical stimulation have been used to argue against a major role for central command in exercise regulation. However, a number of factors have to be considered that weaken this argument. First, it is very likely that redundant mechanisms exist for regulating ventilation during exercise (211, 262). Absence of one mechanism, as may be the case with the muscle stimulation experiments, may enhance the role of other mechanisms such as the muscle reflex and humoral involvement such as potassium stimulation of carotid body (73). This redundancy phenomenon was stated extremely well by Yamamoto (274), who wrote: "You may have sufficient mechanisms; each of which in a given, isolated circumstance explains the whole phenomenon. When they act simultaneously they mask each other." This statement is especially appropriate in human studies, where it is extremely difficult to ever study only one mechanism in isolation. A second concern with the muscle stimulation experiments is that electrical activation would likely produce both contractions and direct activation of muscle afferents. Therefore, a portion of the respiratory responses could have resulted from electrical stimulation of group III and IV afferents that are involved in the muscle reflex (73). Another concern is the likelihood that central command is present during contraction produced by muscle stimulation. The subjects had a sensation of the muscle contracting that may have triggered descending drive to supplement the contractions. Moreover, feedback from contracting muscles is known to activate hypothalamic neurons involved in the central command mechanism (264). Thus, both central command and the muscle reflex would have been active immediately after the onset of the contractions. Therefore, the conclusions drawn from the muscle stimulation experiments should be considered with a great deal of skepticism.

Another approach to examining the role of central command was utilized by Fernandes et al. (79), who used epidural anesthesia to block afferent feedback from contracting muscles. In this protocol, the ventilatory responses to exercise could be evaluated with central command present but in the absence of the muscle reflex. The ventilatory response was examined in men who exercised at several different workloads including an intensity that produced exhaustion. In all cases, blockade of muscle afferents did not alter the ventilatory response to exercise. Thus, central command alone was able to elicit the full response to exercise.

The original theory for cortical irradiation proposed by Krogh and Lindhard (147) was a centrally induced increase in CO_2 sensitivity of respiratory neurons resulting in the increased ventilation during exercise. This theory has been examined by several investigators who have provided little support for the hypothesis. It has been shown that there is not a change in the central chemoreceptor threshold during exercise; furthermore, any change in sensitivity of inhaled CO_2 noted during exercise is too small to explain the exercise-associated ventilatory changes observed in humans (3, 34, 41, 53, 139, 269). Strong evidence against the involvement of CO_2 sensitivity in the central command mechanism was presented recently by Shea et al. (221), who studied children with congenital central hypoventilation syndrome. Even though these subjects had a greatly blunted ventilatory response to inhaled CO_2, their respiratory responses during treadmill exercise did not differ from normal subjects. Thus, these experiments argue against the involvement of both central and peripheral chemoreceptors or changes in CO_2 sensitivity in exercise hyperpnea. Therefore, central command probably acts through a direct activation of neurons involved in respiratory control and not through an alteration of CO_2 sensitivity.

Fink et al. (82) have recently concluded that changes in cortical activity are involved in the central command mechanism during dynamic leg exercise in humans. In a technically demanding experiment, cerebral blood flow measurements were performed with positron emission tomography (PET) coupled with morphological data obtained with magnetic resonance imaging (MRI) to localize brain areas active during exercise. Several cortical and subcortical areas, including the areas of the motor cortex responsible for activation of inspiratory muscles, displayed increased activity during the exercise bout compared to control conditions. These authors concluded that exercise hyperpnea could involve a feedforward mechanism emanating from neurons in the motor cortex.

Circulation

Several different experimental strategies have been employed in an attempt to study the contributions of the central neural mechanism in determining the cardiovascular response to both static and dynamic exercise. In some of these experimental designs "central command" has been enhanced, diminished, or eliminated and in others the reflex neural mechanism has been decreased or abolished.

Studies Utilizing Neuromuscular Blockade

Hemodynamic studies. One strategy to enhance the contribution of central command is to study the cardiovascular response to static or to dynamic exercise before and after the muscles are weakened by partial curarization. The rationale for this intervention is that during partial neuromuscular blockade more motor command is required for the weakened muscles to generate the same amount of force during static exercise or to perform the same amount of work during dynamic exercise. It is hypothesized that the greater motor command would also enhance the hemodynamic response by a parallel increased activation of the cardiovascular control areas in the medulla.

Freyschuss (90) studied the heart rate and blood pressure responses to static handgrip exercise before and after paralysis of the muscle groups involved by injection of succinylcholine into the brachial artery. When static contractions were attempted at 70% of the maximal voluntary contraction (MVC), the heart rate and blood pressure responses to intended contractions after paralysis were 64% and 55%, respectively, of the changes observed during an actual contraction at 70% MVC. McCloskey (168) performed similar experiments after the local intravenous injection of curare into the forearm and found that the increase in arterial systolic and diastolic pressure was greater than in the control study when the same force was developed during handgrip. Leonard et al. (152) have also studied the heart rate and arterial blood pressure response to static leg extension in subjects before and after intravenous neuromuscular blockade with tubocurarine (Fig. 9.23). An amount of tubocurarine was administered that reduced the MVC to about 50% of the control value. When the same absolute force was maintained (10% of the initial MVC) and central command was enhanced, the increases in heart rate and arterial blood pressure were greater during neuromuscular blockade than during the control study (Fig. 9.23, *left*). However, when the same relative force was maintained (30% of the MVC immediately prior to the static exercise) and central command presumably was unchanged, the increases in heart rate and arterial blood pressure were the same during the two studies (Fig. 9.23, *right*). This study demonstrated the importance of central command in determining the magnitude of the cardiovascular response to static exercise.

Hobbs and Gandevia (121) recorded heart rate and arterial blood pressure responses in normal subjects who attempted to contract arm muscles paralyzed by the local infusion of lidocaine and anoxia and in paraplegic patients who attempted to contract their paralyzed leg. They found significant increases in heart rate and arterial blood pressure during attempted contractions with acutely paralyzed muscles in normal subjects; however, no cardiovascular responses were elicited in patients when they attempted to contract their chronically paralyzed legs. This study suggested that the central neural mechanism can cause a cardiovascular response in the absence of afferent feedback from the contracting muscles, but that spinal cord integrity appears to be necessary for the motor signal to cause the cardiovascular response. It has also been shown that the blood pressure and heart rate responses are greater when the intensity of central command is greater (96, 183). In the study of Mitchell et al. (183), subjects performed static handgrip at 15% MVC before and after two levels of neuromuscular blockade. During the control study, there was no increase in

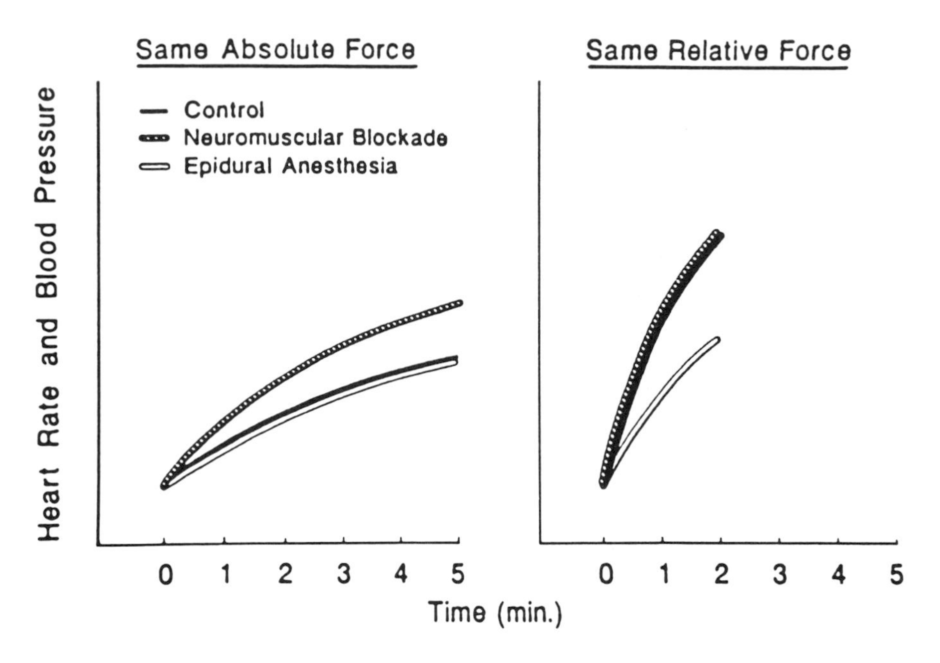

FIG. 9.23. Effect on heart rate and blood pressure responses to static exercise of neuromuscular blockade and of epidural anesthesia. *Left*, Comparison of each intervention to control at the same absolute force. *Right*, Comparison at the same relative force. [From Mitchell et al. (184).]

heart rate and a small increase in blood pressure. When the subjects maintained the same force at the lower level of neuromuscular blockade, there was an increase in heart rate and a greater increase in blood pressure than during the control study. At the higher level of neuromuscular blockade the subjects were unable to maintain the force and there was a greater increase in heart rate and blood pressure than during the lower level of curare. In the study by Gandevia and Hobbs (96), central command and the reflex from metaboreceptors in the same subjects were studied by utilizing local neuromuscular blockade and the postexercise ischemia response. They found that the cardiovascular responses were greater with increased central command and with increased metaboreceptor activity. Furthermore, these two mechanisms did not produce the same pattern of cardiovascular responses.

Recently, Gandevia et al. (97) reported the cardiovascular responses to attempted muscle contractions in totally paralyzed subjects. They found that during complete paralysis the heart rate and blood pressure responses to maximal attempted static handgrip contraction were of the same magnitude as the cardiovascular responses to actual maximal contraction, which were maintained for 45 s before paralysis. In addition, the cardiovascular responses during paralysis were the same when the subject attempted contraction of the hand or of all the muscles of the body. It is also of interest that graded levels of attempted contraction in one subject (increased levels of central command) caused graded increases in heart rate and blood pressure (Fig. 9.24). Thus, the cardiovascular responses correlated with the degree of intended effort even when the subject was totally paralyzed and could not produce any muscle force.

Studies during dynamic exercise by Ochwadt et al. (192) and Asmussen et al. (11) reported that the increases in heart rate and blood pressure were greater at the same work rate when the strength of the ex-

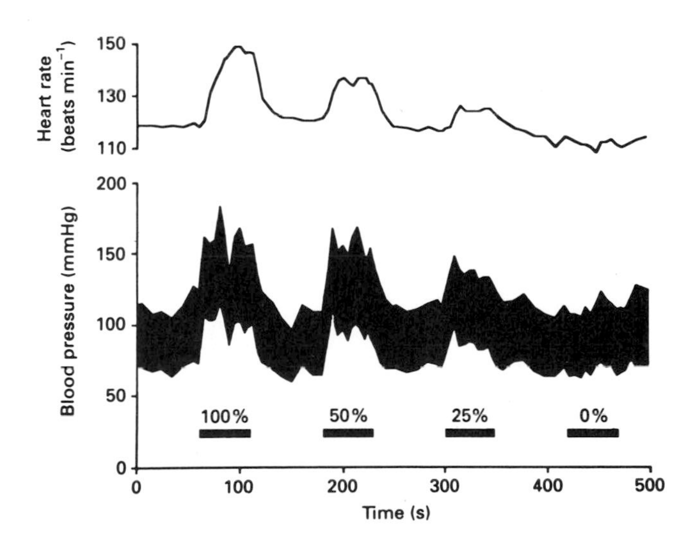

FIG. 9.24. Effect of intended contraction on heart rate and blood pressure in a totally paralyzed subject. *Bars* indicate the time when contractions were attempted with values for percentage of MVC. [From Gandevia et al. (97).]

ercising muscles was reduced by partial curarization. Thus, in these studies, the cardiovascular response was related to the greater motor command required for a given work rate. Galbo, Kjær, and Secher (95) also found a greater heart rate and blood pressure response at a given work rate after partial curarization; however, no difference was found when these variables were related to oxygen consumption. In their study, a graded maximal exercise test was performed on a cycle ergometer both before and after neuromuscular blockade (Fig. 9.25). During a high level of neuromuscular blockade, the heart rate and blood pressure responses were much lower during maximal effort than they were during the control study. When the work rate increased during maximal effort as the muscles became stronger while the neuromuscular blockade waned, heart rate and blood pressure increased (Fig. 9.25). Thus, during dynamic exercise, the cardiovascular response was determined by the activity of the working muscle as measured by the oxygen consumption and not by the intended effort (central command). Therefore, the reflex mechanism was determining the cardiovascular response during dynamic exercise.

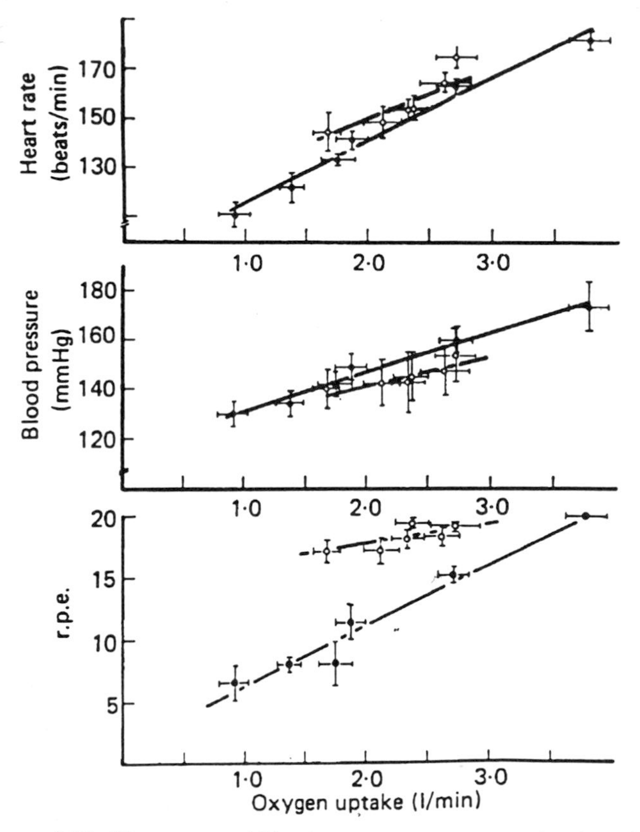

FIG. 9.25. Heart rate and blood pressure responses and rating of perceived exertion (r.p.e. units on scale of 6–20) during progressive exercise to maximal. *Filled circles* represent exercise during the control study and *open circles* represent maximal effort as the neuromuscular blockade decreased. Values are means ± SEM. [From Galbo et al. (95).]

Microneurographic studies. Microneurographic recordings of postsynaptic sympathetic efferent activity (SNA) to resting muscle and to skin is an important technique that has been used to study the responses during both static and dynamic exercise (164, 212, 214, 243, 246, 247, 251). This technique has been utilized to study muscle SNA during static handgrip contractions and during postexercise circulatory arrest for 2 min each (164, 251). Muscle SNA does not begin to increase until about 1 min after the exercise is initiated and then progressively increases during the second minute. During postexercise circulatory arrest, the muscle SNA increases further and remains elevated until the circulation is restored. Since muscle SNA is higher following exercise than it is during actual handgrip contraction when central command is present, it was suggested that central command may inhibit muscle SNA (164).

The effects of central command on muscle SNA during static exercise were further investigated by Victor et al. (245), who performed studies before and after neuromuscular blockade. Static handgrip of 15% MVC caused no increase in resting muscle SNA; however, a handgrip at 30% MVC caused a marked increase above the control level. After neuromuscular blockade, an attempted static contraction that developed no force caused a small increase, and not a decrease in muscle SNA. Thus, central command does not inhibit but causes a slight increase in sympathetic nerve activity during sustained static handgrip contraction.

Central command has a much greater influence on muscle SNA during intermittent static exercise (248). When muscle SNA was recorded during intermittent static handgrip contractions (contract 3 s, relax 9 s) for 4 min, there was a synchronization of muscle SNA at 75% MVC but not at 25% or 50% MVC before neuromuscular blockade (Fig. 9.26). Muscle SNA was about six times higher during the contraction periods than during the relaxation periods. After partial neuromuscular blockade, this synchronization was present at a force that represented 25% MVC before the blockade (Fig. 9.26). Thus, during intense static exercise, central command causes synchronization of motor activity and of sympathetic activity to resting skeletal muscle.

Studies Using Fatiguing Muscle Contractions

Hemodynamic studies. Another strategy to determine the contribution of the central neural mechanism is to study fatiguing muscle contractions. Lind et al. (156) demonstrated that with fatiguing ten-

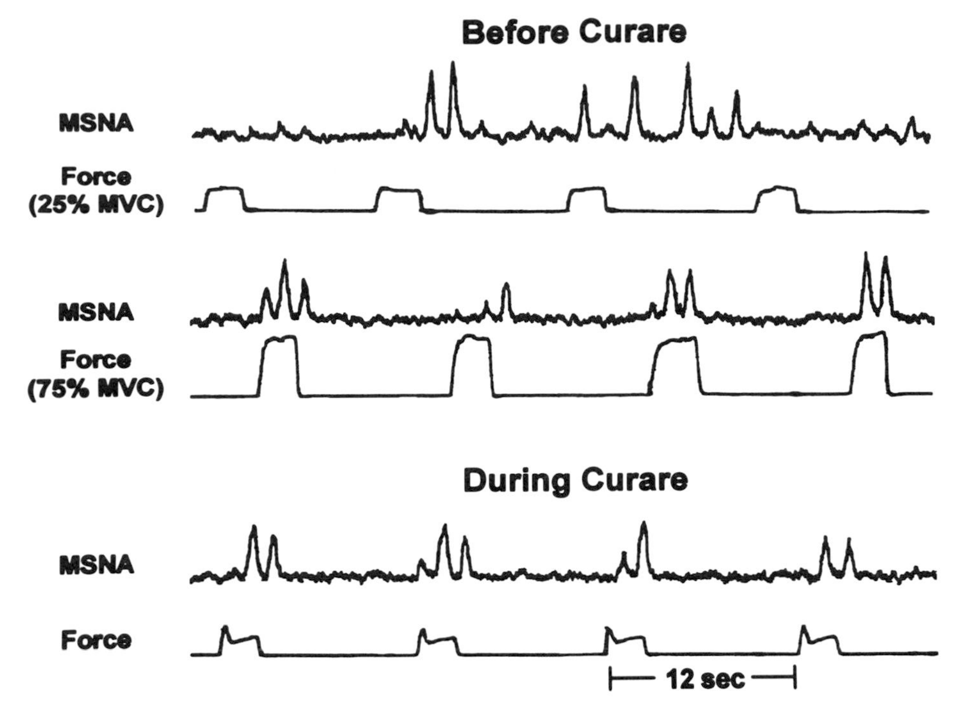

FIG. 9.26. Muscle sympathetic nerve activity (MSNA) and force. % MVC, percentage of maximal voluntary contraction. A study from one subject before and during partial neuromuscular blockade with curare. [From Victor et al. (248).]

sions, heart rate and blood pressure progressively increased thoughout the contractions. Also, the amplitude of the surface EMG progressively increases during fatiguing isometric contractions (155).

Goodwin, McCloskey, and Mitchell (104) have shown that repeated contractions for 2 min of the biceps at 40% MVC produced greater increases in arterial systolic pressure as fatigue occurred and the effort was greater. Eklund and Kaijser (57) also showed that heart rate and mean arterial blood pressure continuously increased with a fatiguing handgrip contraction. Schibye et al. (216) recorded arterial blood pressure and heart rate while monitoring the EMG activity of the contracting muscle. These investigators made the assumption that the rectified, smoothed EMG activity could be used as an index of descending motor drive to the muscles and, thus, an indication of central command. When subjects maintained a constant force of static contraction (knee extension) at 20% MVC, arterial blood pressure and heart rate increased at the onset of the contraction and continued to increase gradually throughout the contraction in direct proportion to the parallel increases in EMG activity. The increase in EMG activity was assumed to result from greater numbers of motor units being activated in order to maintain a constant force as the muscle fatigued. Thus, heart rate and arterial blood pressure rose as the contraction continued in direct proportion to increasing central motor command.

Microneurographic studies. Seals and Enoka (219) have measured EMG activity in the forearm along with muscle sympathetic nerve activity to the leg during fatiguing handgrip contractions. They found that the sympathetic nerve activity to a resting muscle was directly related to muscle fatigue as indicated by the EMG. It has also been shown that muscle sympathetic nerve activity is related to the rating of subjective fatigue sensation (213). When a static handgrip contraction was maintained at 25% MVC until exhaustion, the sensation of fatigue effort showed a minimal value. At this level of effort, central command may contribute to the regulation of sympathetic nerve activity to resting muscle (246, 248).

Central command has been shown to activate skin sympathetic nerve activity during static exercise (214, 251). In the study by Vissing et al. (251), static handgrip at 30% MVC was performed for 2 min followed by postexercise circulatory occlusion for 2 more min. With the onset of static handgrip there was an immediate increase in skin SNA followed by a progressive increase while the contraction was maintained. During postexercise circulatory arrest, the skin SNA returned to normal. Furthermore, they studied the effect of muscular fatigue on the skin

SNA response to static handgrip (Fig. 9.27). They hypothesized that fatigue would increase the level of central command required to maintain a given muscle force and result in a greater increase in sympathetic SNA. With three sequential static handgrip contractions, there was an increase in the rating of perceived effort to maintain the same level of force. Also, skin SNA increased along with the level of effort. They concluded from this study that central command can be an important stimulus to sympathetic outflow. Seals (218) also studied handgrip contraction at 20%, 40%, and 60% MVC sustained to exhaustion. He found that skin SNA was independent of force above a threshold level. However, he did not find a connection between the perceived effort and skin SNA.

Activation of Group Ia Afferents in Skeletal Muscle. Another strategy to investigate the cardiovascular response during static exercise is to vibrate the tendon of a contracting muscle or the antagonist muscle, which either enhances or diminishes central command. Goodwin, McCloskey, and Mitchell (104) studied the cardiovascular responses to static exercise while varying the amount of central motor command required to maintain a given level of developed force. High-frequency vibration was applied to either the contracting muscle or an antagonist muscle in order to increase afferent discharge from the muscle spindle primary endings (Ia afferents) (Fig. 9.20). Activation of the Ia afferents in a contracting muscle produces an increase in the motor drive to that muscle by a spinal reflex such that less central command is required to produce a given level of force. More central command is required, however, if the Ia afferents are activated in an antagonistic muscle, thereby producing a decrease in motor drive to the contracting muscle by a spinal reflex. When the subjects performed static exercise, their arterial blood pressure and heart rate increased; however, the increases were less when central command was reduced by vibration of the contracting muscle and more when central command was increased by vibration of the antagonist muscle (Fig. 9.21). This study suggests there were parallel changes in the drive to the cardiovascular control areas from the descending motor signals that control muscular contraction.

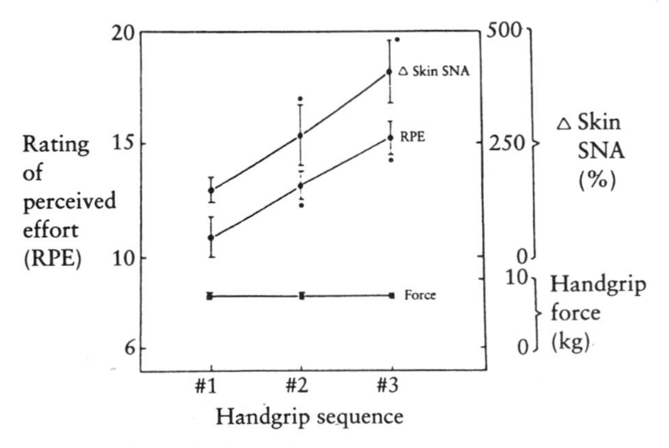

FIG. 9.27. Effect of muscle fatigue on rating of perceived effort (RPE) and peak increase in skin sympathetic nerve activity [Skin SNA (%)] of the same handgrip force (kg). Data are mean ± SEM. *Asterisks* denote significant differences from previous handgrip contraction ($P<0.05$). [From Vissing et al. (251).]

Studies Using Direct Electrical Activation of Skeletal Muscle. A strategy to eliminate central command has been to induce either static or dynamic exercise by direct electrical stimulation of skeletal muscle. Hollander and his co-workers (30, 124, 200) have found that static exercise induced by direct electrical stimulation of skeletal muscle causes an immediate increase in heart rate that was the same as that obtained during voluntary contraction of the same muscle. The rapid increase in heart rate with induced exercise suggested that the reflex was activated by muscle mechanoreceptors rather than muscle metaboreceptors (124). Also, the rapid fall in heart rate during postexercise circulatory arrest suggests that metaboreceptors are not involved in the heart rate changes during exercise.

Hultman and Sjöholm (131) studied the heart rate and arterial blood pressure response to voluntary and electrically induced static leg extension in man. They found that the cardiovascular response was identical under both conditions. They concluded that during static leg exercise the reflex mechanism alone can produce the normal cardiovascular response. More recently, Friedman et al. (92) have performed a similar study with cardiac output measurements and found the same increases in cardiac output, stroke volume, and peripheral vascular resistance during voluntary and electrically induced static leg exercise at 20% maximal voluntary contraction for 5 min.

Direct electrical activation of skeletal muscle has also been used to induce dynamic exercise. In 1917 Krogh and Lindhard (148) showed that during both voluntary and induced dynamic exercise the heart rate and circulation rate are linear functions of the oxygen consumption. This finding has been confirmed by many investigators (4, 13, 143, 234). Strange et al. (234) studied the hemodynamic responses during voluntary and electrically induced dynamic leg kicking (Fig. 9.28). Mean arterial pressure was slightly higher during electrically induced than during voluntary dynamic exercise. However,

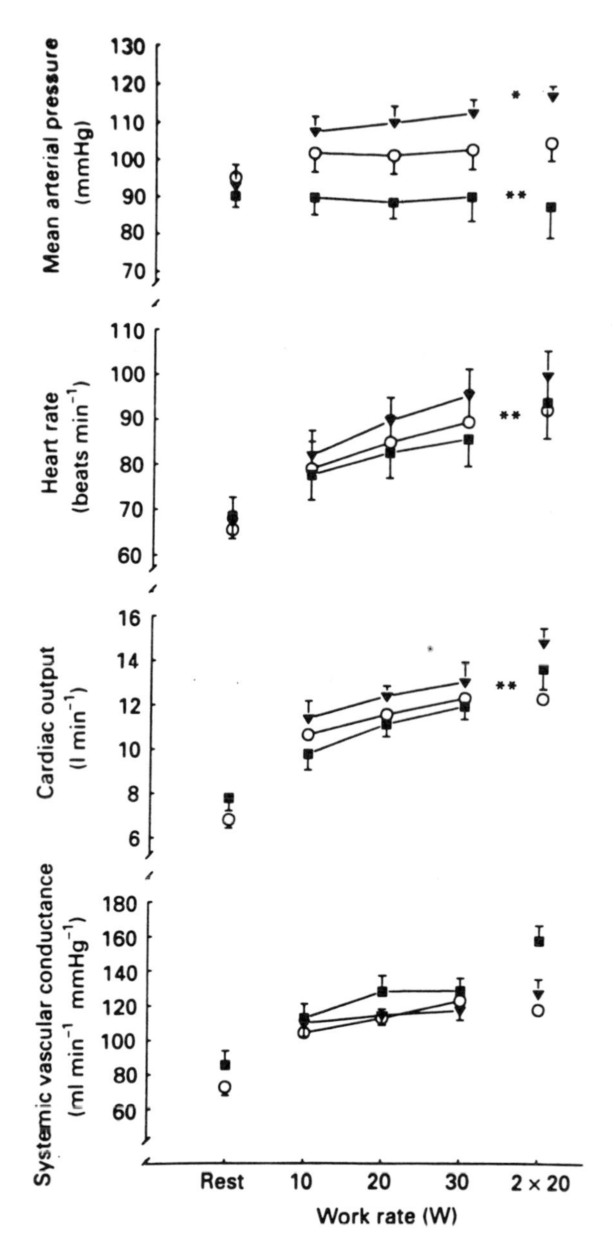

FIG. 9.28. Hemodynamic values at rest and during work rates of 10, 20, and 30 watts (W) performed with one leg and 2 X 20 W performed with two legs. *Open circles* represent voluntary dynamic exercise, *filled triangles* represent electrically induced exercise, and *filled rectangles* represent electrically induced exercise during epidural anesthesia. Values are mean ± SEM. Asterisk denotes differences between voluntary and electrically induced exercise before epidural anesthesia. *Double asterisks* denote differences between electrically induced exercise with and without epidural anesthesia. [From Strange et al. (234).]

there was no difference between heart rate, cardiac output, and systemic vascular conductance. Also in their study, the leg oxygen consumption was higher during induced exercise than during voluntary exercise at a given work rate, which suggests a more inefficient type contraction during electrical stimulation.

Studies with Epidural Anesthesia. Another strategy that has been used to study the role of central command during static and dynamic exercise is epidural anesthesia (80, 145). Mitchell et al. (183) and Kjaer et al. (144) studied the cardiovascular response to static leg extension before and after epidural anesthesia. Epidural anesthesia not only reduced the MVC to 50% by motoneuron blockade but, in addition, caused a block of sensory feedback from the contracting muscles. In the study by Mitchell et al. (183), the increases in heart rate and arterial blood pressure were the same when the same absolute force was maintained and central command was enhanced (Fig. 9.23, *left*). However, the increases in heart rate and arterial blood pressure were less during epidural anesthesia than during the control study when the same relative force was maintained and central command was presumably the same (Fig. 9.23, *right*). This study demonstrated the importance of the reflex mechanism in determining the magnitude of the cardiovascular response to static exercise. This conclusion is opposite to that suggested by the studies with neuromuscular blockade (152).

A further understanding of the roles of the central neural and the reflex mechanisms in determining the cardiovascular response during static exercise can be obtained by comparing the results of the study with epidural anesthesia by Mitchell et al. (183) and the study with neuromuscular blockade by Leonard et al. [Fig. 9.23 (152)]. During neuromuscular blockade, the effect of an increased central command when the same absolute force is developed is not counterbalanced by an attenuated afferent feedback from the contracting muscles and the increases in heart rate and arterial blood pressure are greater than during the control study. In addition, during neuromuscular blockade the effect of the same central command when the same relative force is developed is not diminished by a decrease in afferent feedback from the contracting muscle and the cardiovascular responses are the same during the two conditions. However, during epidural anesthesia the effect of an increased central command when the same absolute force is developed is counterbalanced by an attenuated afferent feedback from the contracting muscles and the increase in the cardiovascular responses are the same under the two conditions. Also, during epidural anesthesia the effect of the same central command when the same relative force is developed is diminished by the decrease in afferent feedback from the contracting muscle and the cardiovascular response is less during epidural anesthesia. Considered together, the results of these two studies are complementary and support the concept that both a central and a reflex neural mechanism can play important roles in regulating the cardiovascular response to static exercise in man.

Studies during dynamic exercise by Hornbein, Sørensen, and Parks (127) reported that the blood pressure response was not affected by an epidural block, but the extent of the blockade of small sensory fibers was not reported. Later, Freund et al. (89) demonstrated that the heart rate and blood pressure responses to mild dynamic exercise were normal in subjects after epidural anesthesia that abolished the maintenance of blood pressure during postexercise circulatory occlusion. They concluded that the cardiovascular response to mild dynamic exercise is normal when the exercise reflex is not functioning. However, Fernandes et al. (79) found that even though the heart rate response to submaximal and maximal dynamic exercise was not affected by epidural anesthesia, the blood pressure response was markedly attenuated. The study by Fernandes et al. (79) suggests that central command was not able to maintain blood pressure during dynamic exercise.

More recent studies have used epidural anesthesia to further investigate neural control of the cardiovascular system during dynamic exercise. Friedman et al. (91) found that epidural anesthesia with 1% lidocaine blocked the blood pressure response to cold pressor test, eliminated laser-induced evoked potentials, and increased the pain threshold of the foot. In these subjects, during epidural anesthesia, the blood pressure, heart rate, and cardiac output responses during dynamic exercise were the same as during the control study. Also, blood pressure remained elevated to the same level during postexercise ischemia as during the control study. This implies that a partial blockade of group III and IV muscle afferents can decrease the mean arterial pressure response to the cold pressor test and increase the pain threshold, but that a complete or almost complete block of these afferent fibers is necessary to decrease the blood pressure response to dynamic exercise and to postexercise circulatory occlusion.

The cardiovascular response has also been studied during electrically induced dynamic exercise before and after complete epidural anesthesia (143, 234). Some of the findings in the study by Strange et al. (234) are shown in Figure 9.28. The increase in mean arterial pressure during electrically induced exercise was abolished by epidural anesthesia. Also, the increases in heart rate and cardiac output were less during electrically stimulated dynamic exercise with epidural anesthesia than during stimulated exercise without epidural anesthesia. However, there was no difference in the response of systemic vascular resistance during these two exercise protocols. Kjær et al. (143) found similar results at work levels of higher intensity during electrically stimulated leg cycling in normal subjects after epidural anesthesia.

Studies of Patients with Sensory and Motor Disorders

Sensory disorders. Patients who have various types of afferent sensory disorders have also been used to separate the central from the reflex neural mechanism during static exercise. Alam and Smirk (6) studied a patient with a spinal cord lesion who had no sensation but almost normal motor function of the right lower leg and both normal sensation and motor function of the left leg. Thus, it was possible to compare cardiovascular responses to equal intensities of dynamic exercise performed with the normal leg and with the leg lacking feedback from the contracting muscle. Dynamic exercise of either leg during arrested flow elicited the same increases in arterial blood pressure and heart rate. However, arterial blood pressure only remained elevated after exercise with occluded circulation in the normal leg. Since no feedback from muscle receptors or release of muscle metabolites into the general circulation could have occurred during exercise of the leg with no sensation, the cardiovascular response must have resulted from activation of the cardiovascular control areas by a central neural mechanism. Similar results were obtained during static exercise by Duncan, Johnson, and Lambie (54) in studies on two patients with sensory disorders of forearm afferent nerves. Both patients had normal motor function, but one had a partial Brown-Séquard lesion of the cervical spinal cord and the other had a hereditary sensory neuropathy. Static exercise performed both with and without arterial occlusion of the affected arm evoked increases in arterial blood pressure and heart rate in both patients. These two studies (6, 54) demonstrate that cardiovascular responses to static exercise can occur without afferent input from the contracting muscles or from unidentified humoral receptors located outside the contracting muscles.

Contradictory findings, however, were reported by Lind et al. (154), who studied a patient with syringomyelia affecting the forearm sensory nerves in one arm. An increase in arterial blood pressure was observed during static handgrip with the normal arm, but no increase in pressure occurred when the affected arm performed static handgrip. They concluded that the cardiovascular response to static exercise was dependent on the reflex neural mechanism.

Motor disorders. Patients with various types of motor disorders causing one-legged weakness have also been used to determine the effects of an enhanced central command on the cardiovascular response during both static and dynamic exercise (132, 185). Mitchell et al. (185) studied soccer players who had injured one leg that was immobilized in a cast and who continued to train with the normal leg. When the cast was removed, the previously injured leg was smaller and had an MVC that was 60% that of the normal leg. When each leg sustained the same absolute force, the arterial systolic pressure was the same; when each leg sustained the same relative force, the arterial systolic pressure was higher with the normal leg than with the weak leg. Also, the smooth, rectified EMG was the same in each leg when the absolute force development was the same but was higher in the normal leg than in the weak leg when the same relative force was developed. This study suggests that the cardiovascular response is the same when the same number of motor units are active.

Innes et al. (132) studied a group of subjects with painless unilateral leg weakness caused by either immobilization, a neurological disorder, or a peripheral anesthetic block. The subjects performed one-legged cycling at the same work rate (O_2 consumption) with both the weak and the strong leg (Fig. 9.29). In the normal subject, the cardiovascular responses were the same from each leg during one-legged cycling. In the subjects with unilateral leg weakness, the heart rate and blood pressure were higher and the cardiac output and stroke volume were the same during cycling with the weak leg as compared to the strong leg. This study suggests that central command is important in determining the heart rate and blood pressure response to dynamic exercise.

INTERACTIONS BETWEEN CENTRAL COMMAND AND PERIPHERAL FEEDBACK

Both central command and feedback originating from contracting muscles are known to produce increases in cardiovascular function. Moreover, both of these mechanisms are probably active in generating the appropriate responses to exercise during voluntary exercise. Mitchell (180) has pointed out that these are redundant control mechanisms operative during exercise and that neural occlusion occurs. Evidence supporting neural occlusion in the cardiovascular responses to exercise has been presented to support this contention. Waldrop et al. (262) demonstrated that putative central command and reflexes evoked by muscular contraction exert smaller cardiorespiratory effects when activated simultaneously than when activated individually. These findings have been corroborated by Rybicki et al. (211), who also showed that the reduced responses during simultaneous activation of both the central and reflex mechanisms does not result from saturation of the involved neuronal circuitry.

Since both central command and peripheral feedback are likely to be active simultaneously during exercise, central neural sites must exist that integrate information from both of these mechanisms in order to provide the appropriate cardiovascular responses to exercise. Only a few studies have sought to locate such central nervous system areas. One site that has been considered is the hypothalmic locomotor region (HLR). Bilateral lesions of the HLR in anesthetized cats attenuate the heart rate response to muscular

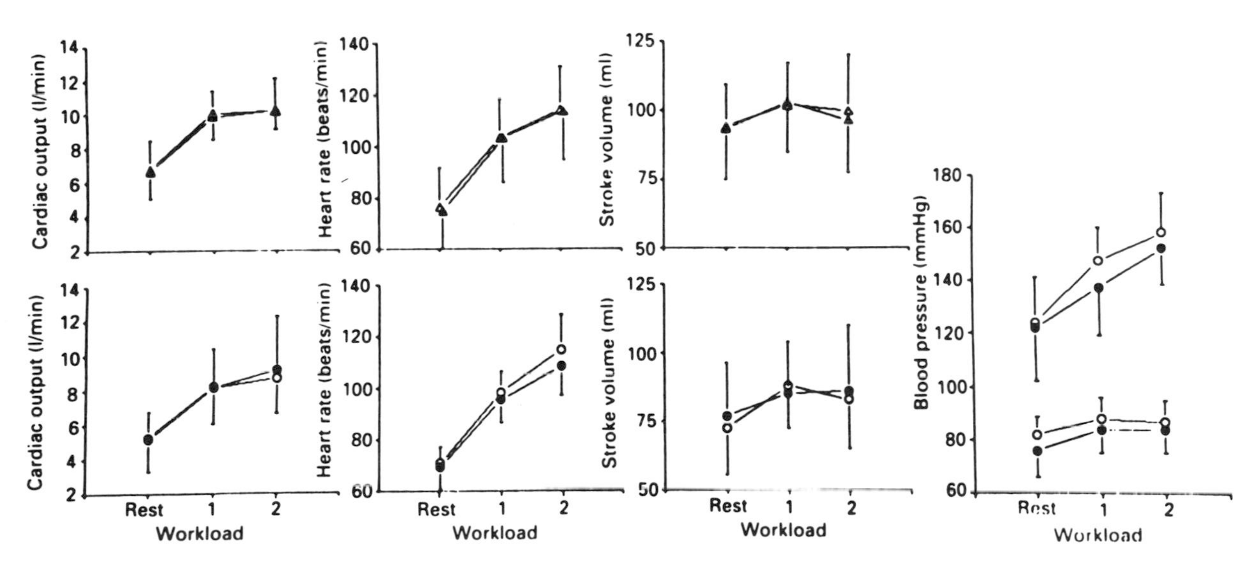

FIG. 9.29. Cardiac output, heart rate, stroke volume, and blood pressure at rest and during one-legged exercise at two workloads. Upper three panels in normal subjects with no weakness. (Δ, right leg; ▲, left leg). Lower four panels in subjects with one weak leg (●, normal leg; ○, weak leg). Values are means (± SD). [From Innes et al. (132).]

contraction (261). In addition, Waldrop and Stremel (264) have shown that the majority of neurons recorded from in the hypothalamic locomotor region are stimulated by muscular contraction (Fig. 9.30). Since the HLR is thought to play a role in the central command mechanisms, these results suggest that this hypothalamic region may serve as an integrative region for cardiovascular control during exercise.

Nolan et al. (191) have provided electrophysiological support that peripheral feedback from contracting muscles and descending central command converge on neurons in the ventrolateral medulla. Both this study and prior results demonstrated that many neurons in the ventrolateral medulla increase their discharge during static muscular contraction elicited by ventral root stimulation in anesthetized cats (20, 23, 191). Approximately 50% of the contraction-sensitive neurons were also stimulated by activation of simulated central command (caudal hypothalamic stimulation). Moreover, computer analyses revealed that these neurons had a basal discharge frequency related to cardiovascular and/or respiratory rhythms, indicating an involvement in cardiorespiratory function. A previous study demonstrated that an excitatory amino acid synapse in this medullary region is involved in the mediation of the pressor reflex elicited by static muscular contraction (21). In sum, these findings suggest that integration of central command and peripheral feedback occurs in the ventrolateral medulla.

It is likely that integration of mechanisms providing drive to the cardiorespiratory systems during ex-

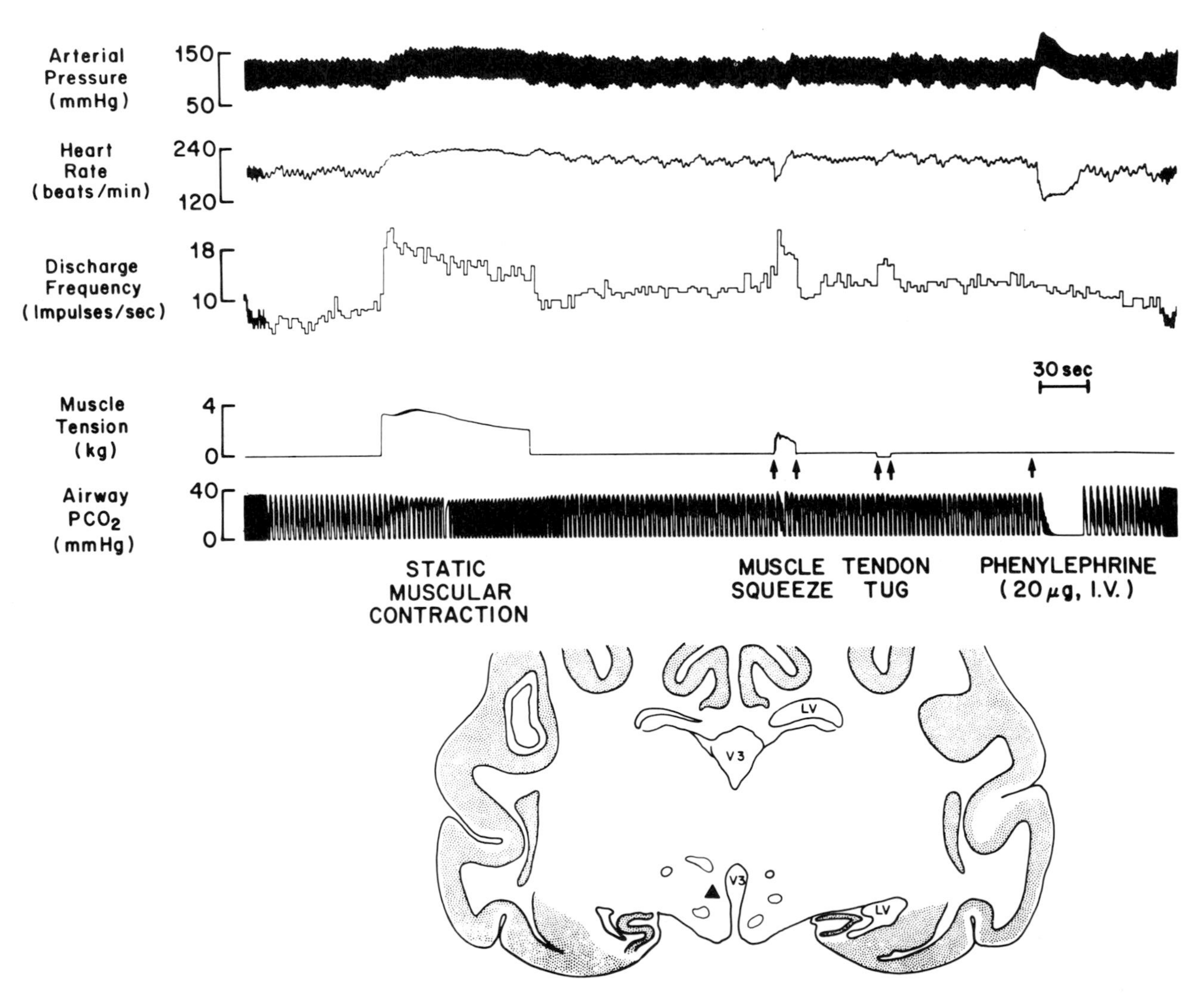

FIG. 9.30. Effects of static muscular contraction (elicited by ventral root stimulation) upon arterial pressure, heart rate, and the discharge frequency of a posterior hypothalamic neuron of an anesthetized cat. Note that contraction and other mechanical stimulation of the gastrocnemius muscles increased the discharge frequency of this neuron. Baroreceptor stimulation produced by a phenylephrine-induced increase in arterial pressure had no significant effect upon this neuron. Location of the neuron is indicated by the *filled triangle* in the line drawing at bottom. [From Waldrop and Stremel (264).]

ercise exists at many areas in the CNS, ranging from the cerebral cortex to the spinal cord. For example, Waldrop and Iwamoto (260) have recently provided support for muscle afferent input impinging upon insular cortex neurons. Moreover, studies have indicated that the pressor reflex elicited by exercise can be modulated by spinal mechanisms (181). These levels of integration demonstrate the complexity of control mechanisms responsible for providing appropriate changes in breathing and cardiovascular activity during exercise. Future studies are needed to further clarify the integration that is demanded during exercise.

INTERACTION OF CENTRAL COMMAND WITH CARDIORESPIRATORY REFLEXES

Baroreceptor Reflex

It has been reported that the baroreceptor reflex does not produce as much slowing of the heart rate during exercise as is the case during rest (42, 122). Evidence exists suggesting that the central command mechanism may be responsible for at least a portion of this modulation of the baroreceptor reflex during exercise. Electrical stimulation of the portion of the posterior hypothalamus that corresponds to the hypothalamic locomotor region has been reported by several investigators to blunt the baroreceptor mechanism in anesthetized cats (39, 231). However, these studies utilizing electrical stimulation are difficult to interpret, since both cell bodies as well as fibers of passage were stimulated. This criticism has been addressed in a recent study in which chemicals were injected into the hypothalamus that affect cell bodies without an effect upon axons. Microinjection of GABA antagonists into the posterior hypothalamus reduces baroreflex-mediated respiratory inhibition and bradycardia in both cats and rats (22, 49). The microinjections also produced increases in arterial pressure and heart rate that were accompanied by locomotor movements in those animals that were studied nonparalyzed. Thus, it appears that activation of the posterior hypothalamic neurons that produce locomotor movements and cardiorespiratory responses appropriate for exercise also exert a depressive effect upon the baroreceptor reflex. Therefore, the modulation of the baroreceptor reflex that occurs during exercise may result from activity of posterior hypothalamic neurons. Moreover, the cardiovascular responses to exercise and the associated modulation of the baroreceptor reflex appear to involve a GABAergic mechanism in the posterior hypothalamus.

Hering-Breuer Reflex

An early study by Redgate (206) found that microinjection of an anesthetic into the caudal hypothalamus enhances the respiratory inhibition produced by the Hering-Breuer reflex. Moreover, it has been shown that the Hering-Breuer reflex is inhibited during locomotion induced by stimulating the caudal hypothalamus (208). It is also interesting that vagotomy abolishes spontaneous locomotion that occurs in unanesthetized decerebrate cats (71); a recent study demonstrated that stimulation of vagal afferents inhibits locomotion (201). Thus, the possibility exists that the Hering-Breuer reflex or other vagally mediated mechanisms may play an important role in the central command regulation of locomotor and respiratory activity during exercise.

Chemoreceptor Reflexes

Neurons in the hypothalamic locomotor region are also thought to modulate the respiratory responses to hypercapnia. Microinjection of GABA antagonists or synthesis inhibitors into this area accentuates the respiratory response to inhalation of CO_2 (199, 255). However, the arterial pressure responses to hypercapnia and hypoxia do not appear to be affected by activation of the hypothalamic locomotor region (199, 255). Recent findings indicate that an excitatory amino acid synapse in the caudal hypothalamus modulates the respiratory response to hypoxia (126). Electrical stimulation of this hypothalamic area inhibits the bradycardia elicited by stimulation of the peripheral chemoreceptors in anesthetized cats (242). It has also been shown that electrical stimulation of the carotid sinus nerve excites neurons in the posterior hypothalamus (33, 241). A recent study has shown that the majority of hypothalamic neurons that respond to hypoxia and hypercapnia have a resting discharge related to sympathetic nerve activity and/or the cardiac cycle (50). It is not known if the same neurons that respond to hypoxia and hypercapnia are the ones involved in locomotor and/or central command activities. However, it is possible that integration of these reflexes occurs in the hypothalamus during exercise.

CONCLUSIONS

Studies in both animals and humans have convincingly demonstrated that a central command mechanism plays an important role in determining the cardiorespiratory responses to dynamic and static exercise. This central neural mechanism is related to the neural activity responsible for the recruitment of motor units and initiates the cardiorespiratory response by causing the immediate changes in the level of efferent activity of the sympathetic and parasympathetic nervous systems to the heart and blood vessels as well as outflow to respiratory muscles. Other drives, including a peripheral feedback reflex originating in contracting skeletal muscles, act in concert with central command to provide a matching of cardiorespiratory drive to the intensity of exercise. Short-term potentiation is important in the dynamics and magnitude of the respiratory response to exercise. This mechanism likely prevents over- and undershoots of ventilation at the transitions from rest to exercise and vice versa.

The relative importance of central command and the peripheral feedback reflex in determining cardiorespiratory responses to exercise likely depends upon the type of exercise (static or dynamic), the intensity of the exercise, the time after onset of the exercise (e.g., immediate, steady state, exhaustion), and the effectiveness of cardiorespiratory adjustments to meet the increased metabolic demands of the contracting muscles. Therefore, to argue which of these two control mechanisms is the more important does not appear to be a very useful endeavor. However, it is important to determine how these two mechanisms are integrated during exercise to cause the appropriate cardiorespiratory responses for the intensity of the muscular effort. Even though many questions remain unanswered concerning how this is accomplished, it appears that the two neural mechanisms are somewhat redundant rather than additive, and that they impinge upon the same regulatory neurons in the medulla, and, possibly, other sites, where integration occurs. In addition, other neural impulses, in addition to the central and reflex mechanisms, are transmitted during exercise to control areas in the CNS.

Many of the attempts to determine the importance of central command or the peripheral reflex have involved trying to examine the responses to activation of only one of these in isolation. It has been difficult, if not impossible, to devise an experiment in which only one of these mechanisms is active. In addition, this type of evaluation is not the most desirable, since it also tries to remove other reflexes and mechanisms that are not the primary mediators of the exercise response but no doubt interact with central command and the peripheral reflex originating in contracting skeletal muscles.

A more desirable way to examine the importance of central command would be to examine the observed responses to exercise in the situation where all other mechanisms remained active but central command was removed. Even though this has been attempted in animal and human experiments, it has proven difficult to be sure that central command has really been removed from the experiment. However, one of the authors (F.L.E.) has recently developed a computer model of the respiratory control system that permits one to do this simulated experiment (see footnote 3 for details). It is possible to use this model to examine the relative importance of central command in regulating the respiratory response to dynamic exercise.

Figure 9.31*A* shows the respiratory response to dynamic exercise as generated by this computer model. Notice that this very closely mimics the respiratory response observed in exercising humans (compare with Figure 9.22). In Fig. 9.31*B*, only the central command component has been removed. Note that even though the ventilation at 6 min is only slightly less than normal, the fast, initial response to exercise is missing and the response is dependent upon the rising P_{CO_2}. Thus, central command is required for the initial response to exercise and for providing drive throughout the exercise period such that CO_2 is maintained constant. In addition, several other mechanisms interact with central command to produce the appropriate respiratory (and cardiovascular responses) to exercise.

A complete understanding of the neural control of respiration and circulation during exercise is very difficult because of the complexity and redundancy of the control systems. Even though our knowledge has greatly increased in recent years, many questions remain unanswered. It is hoped that future research will answer these questions; however, as new knowledge is acquired, more questions will likely evolve.

Work from the authors' laboratories was supported by HLO6296 (J.H.M., T.G.W., G.A.I.), HL38726 (T.G.W.), AHA Established Investigator Award (T.G.W.), HL37400 (G.A.I.), and USPHS Merit Award HL17689 (F.L.E.).

[3]The model uses the Fitzhugh-Bonhoffer-Bon der Pol equations (63, 83), which produce a continuous limit-cycle, to represent the central pattern generator. The output of the generator activates both inspiratory and expiratory respiratory muscles, which in turn produce pressures that act against elastic recoil and airway resistance to produce a tidal volume. Standard mass balance equations are used for CO_2 and O_2 exchange (140, 141): dead space is set at 0.15 liter; V_{O_2} is 0.25 liter/min at rest; cardiac output is 5.0 liter/min at rest. There is a separate set of equations and parameters for medullary metabolic rate and circulation so that medullary P_{CO_2} can be calculated. During exercise, both cardiac output and arteriovenous O_2 and CO_2 differences increase appropriately.

Feedback occurs via carotid bodies, with multiplicative interaction between P_{O_2} and P_{CO_2}, and via central chemoreceptors responding to medullary P_{CO_2}. Short-term potentiation (onset τ is 10 s and offset τ is 50 s) is continuously determined and added as an input to the controller. During exercise, an input equivalent to the central command signal is added, and arterial $[K^+]$ increasing from its resting value during the course of exercise is given a stimulatory effect on the carotid bodies (198).

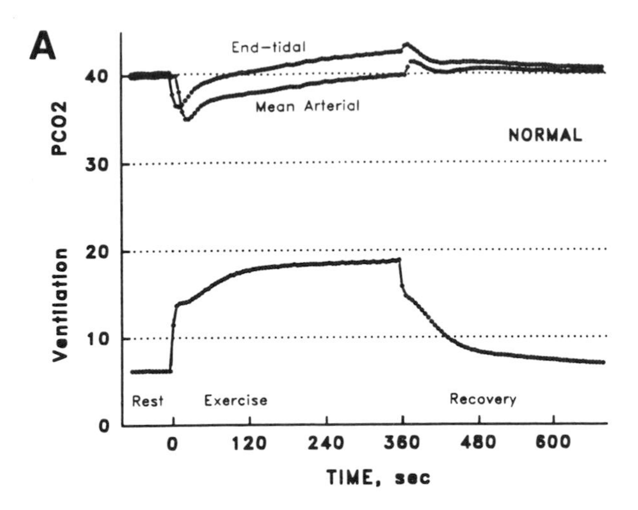

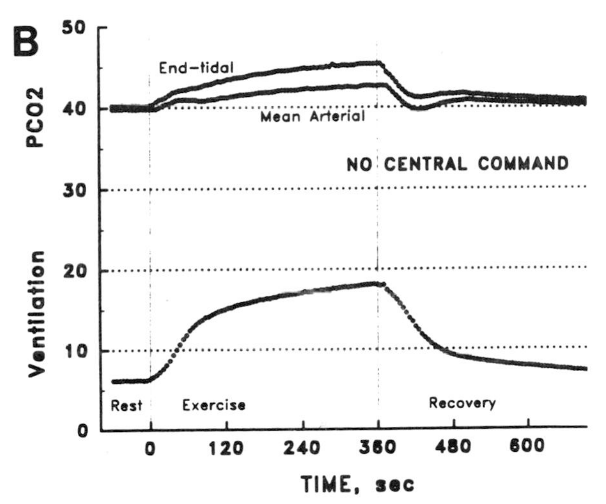

FIG. 9.31. Computer-generated ventilatory and P_{CO_2} responses to dynamic exercise. Panel *A* shows the normal responses with all mechanisms present. In panel *B*, only the central command component has been deleted. Notice the loss of the initial fast respiratory component but with the peak response differing little from that observed in panel *A*. The respiratory response is now dependent upon the rising P_{CO_2}. Details of the computer model are described in the text.

REFERENCES

1. Abrahams, V. C., S. M. Hilton, and A. W. Zbrozyna. Active muscle vasodilation produced by stimulation of the brain stem: its significance in the defence reaction. *J. Physiol. (Lond.)* 154: 491–513, 1960.
2. Adams, L., H. Frankel, J. Garlick, A. Guz, K. Murphy, and S. J. G. Semple. The role of spinal cord transmission in the ventilatory response to exercise in man. *J. Physiol. (Lond.)* 355: 85–97, 1984.
3. Adams, L., J. Garlick, A. Guz, K. Murphy, and S. J. G. Semple. Is the voluntary control of exercise in man necessary for the ventilatory response? *J. Physiol. (Lond.).* 355: 71–83, 1984.
4. Adams, L., A. Guz, J. A. Innes, and K. Murphy. The early circulatory and ventilatory response to voluntary and electrically induced exercise in man. *J. Physiol. (Lond.)* 383: 19–30, 1987.
5. Ahmed, M., G. G. Giesbrecht, C. Serrette, D. Georgopoulos, and N. R. Anthonisen. Respiratory short-term potentiation (after-discharge) in elderly humans. *Respir. Physiol.* 93: 163–173, 1993.
6. Alam, M., and F. H. Smirk. Unilateral loss of a blood pressure raising, pulse accelerating, reflex from voluntary muscle due to a lesion of the spinal cord. *Clin. Sci.* 3: 247–258, 1938.
7. Aminoff, M. J., and T. A. Sears. Spinal integration of segmental, cortical and breathing inputs to thoracic respiratory motoneurons. *J. Physiol. (Lond.)* 215: 557–575, 1971.
8. Ashbridge, K. M., S. Jennett, and J. B. North. The absence of post-hyperventilation in the wakeful state. *J. Physiol. (Lond.)* 230: 52P, 1973.
9. Asmussen, E. Ventilation at transition from rest to exercise. *Acta Physiol. Scand.* 89: 68–78, 1973.
10. Asmussen, E. Control of ventilation in exercise. *Exerc. Sport Sci. Rev.* 11: 24–54, 1983.
11. Asmussen, E., S. H. Johansen, M. Jorgensen, and M. Nielsen. On the nervous factors controlling respiration and circulation during exercise. Experiments with curarization. *Acta Physiol. Scand.* 63: 343–350, 1965.
12. Asmussen, E., and M. Nielsen. Experiments on nervous factors controlling respiration and circulation during exercise employing blocking of the blood flow. *Acta Physiol. Scand.* 60: 103–111, 1964.
13. Asmussen, E., M. Nielsen, and G. Wieth-Pedersen. Cortical or reflex control of respiration during muscular work? *Acta Physiol. Scand.* 6: 168–175, 1943.
14. Asmussen, E., M. Nielsen, and G. Wieth-Pedersen. On the regulation of the circulation during muscular work. *Acta Physiol. Scand.* 6: 353–358, 1943.
15. Badr, M. F., J. B. Skatrud, and J. A. Dempsey. Determinants of poststimulus potentiation in humans during NREM sleep. *J. Appl. Physiol.* 73: 1958–1971, 1992.
16. Baev, K. V., V. K. Berezovskii, T. T. Kebkalo, and L. A. Savos'kina. Forebrain projections to the hypothalamic locomotor region in cats. *Neirofiziologiya* 17: 255–263, 1985.
17. Baev, K. V., V. K. Berezovskii, T. T. Kebkalo, and L. A. Savos'kina. Projections of neurons of the hypothalamic locomotor region to some brainstem and spinal cord structures in the cat. *Neirofiziologiya* 17: 817–823, 1985.
18. Barman, S. M. Descending projections of hypothalamic neurons with sympathetic nerve-related activity. *J. Neurophysiol.* 64: 1019–1032, 1990.
19. Barman, S. M., and G. L. Gebber. Hypothalamic neurons with activity patterns related to sympathetic nerve discharge. *Am. J. Physiol.* 242 (*Regulatory Integrative Comp. Physiol.* 11): R34–R43, 1982.
20. Bauer, R. M., G. A. Iwamoto, and T. G. Waldrop. Discharge patterns of ventrolateral medullary neurons during muscular contraction. *Am. J. Physiol.* 259 (*Regulatory Integrative Comp. Physiol.* 28): R606–R611, 1990.
21. Bauer, R. M., G. A. Iwamoto, and T. G. Waldrop. Ventrolateral medullary neurons modulate pressor reflex to muscular contraction. *Am. J. Physiol.* 257 (*Regulatory Integrative Comp. Physiol.* 26): R1154–R1161, 1989.
22. Bauer, R. M., M. B. Vela, T. Simon, and T. G. Waldrop. A GABAergic mechanism in the posterior hypothalamus modulates baroreflex bradycardia. *Brain Res. Bull.* 20: 633–641, 1988.
23. Bauer, R. M., T. G. Waldrop, G. A. Iwamoto, and M. A. Holzwarth. Properties of ventrolateral medullary neurons

that respond to muscular contraction. *Brain Res. Bull.* 28: 167–178, 1992.
24. Bedford, T. G., P. K. Loi, and C. C. Crandall. A model of dynamic exercise—the decerebrate rat locomotor preparation. *J. Appl. Physiol.* 72: 121–127, 1992.
25. Benchitrit, G., and T. Pham Dinh. Analyse d'une étude statistique de las ventilation cycle par cycle chez l'homme aur repos. *Biom. Humaine* 8: 7–19, 1973.
26. Benchitrit, G., and T. Pham Dinh. Un essai d'analyse statistique de séries de données respiratoires. *Rev. Stat. Appl.* 12: 51–68, 1974.
27. Berezovskii, V. K., T. G. Kebkalo, and L. A. Savos'kina. Afferent brainstem projections to the hypothalamic locomotor region of the cat brain. *Neurophysiology* 16: 279–286, 1984.
28. Birzis, L., and A. Hemingway. Shivering as a result of brain stimulation. *J. Neurophysiol.* 20: 91–99, 1957.
29. Boothby, W. M. Absence of apnoea after forced breathing. *J. Physiol. (Lond.)* 45: 328–333, 1912.
30. Borst, C., A. P. Hollander, and L. N. Bouman. Cardiac acceleration elicited by voluntary muscle contractions of minimal duration. *J. Appl. Physiol.* 32: 70–77, 1972.
31. Brice, A. G., H. V. Forster, L. G. Pan, A. Funahashi, T. F. Lowry, C. L. Murphy, and M. D. Hoffman. Ventilatory and Pa_{CO_2} responses to voluntary and electrically induced leg exercise. *J. Appl. Physiol.* 64: 218–225, 1988.
32. Budzinska, K. Respiratory cycle as an index of CNS excitability. Warsaw: University of Warsaw, Ph.D. thesis, 1978.
33. Calaresu, F. R., and J. Ciriello. Projections to the hypothalamus from buffer nerves and nucleus tractus solitarius in the cat. *Am. J. Physiol.* 239 (*Regulatory Integrative Comp. Physiol.* 8): R130–R136, 1980.
34. Casey, K., J. Duffin, and G. V. McAvoy. The effect of exercise on the central-chemoreceptor threshold in man. *J. Physiol. (Lond.)* 383: 9–18, 1987.
35. Cerretelli, P., R. Sikand, and L. E. Fahri. Readjustments in cardiac output and gas exchange during onset of exercise and recovery. *J. Appl. Physiol.* 21: 1345–1350, 1966.
36. Clarke, N. P., and R. F. Rushmer. Tissue uptake of ^{86}Rb with electrical stimulation of hypothalamus and midbrain. *Am. J. Physiol.* 213: 1439–1444, 1967.
37. Clarke, N. P., O. A. Smith, and D. W. Shearn. Topographical representation of vascular smooth muscle of limbs in primate motor cortex. *Am. J. Physiol.* 214: 122–129, 1968.
38. Conway, J., D. J. Patterson, E. S. Peterson, and P. A. Robbins. Changes in arterial potassium and ventilation in response to exercise in humans. *J. Physiol. (Lond.)* 399: 36P, 1988.
39. Coote, J. H., S. M. Hilton, and J. F. Perez-Gonzalez. Inhibition of the baroreceptor reflex on stimulation in the brain stem defence centre. *J. Physiol. (Lond.)* 288: 549–560, 1979.
40. Corfield, D. R., K. Murphy, and A. Guz. Does cortical activation of the human diaphragm act via brainstem respiratory centres? *J. Physiol. (Lond.)* 467: 17P, 1993.
41. Cunningham, D. J. C., B. B. Lloyd, and J. M. Patrick. The relation between ventilation and end-tidal P_{CO_2} in man during moderate exercise with and without CO_2 inhalation. *J. Physiol. (Lond.)* 169: 104–106, 1963.
42. Cunningham, D. J. C., E. S. Petersen, R. Peto, T. G. Pickering, and P. Sleight. Comparison of the effect of different types of exercise on the baroreflex regulation of heart rate. *Acta Physiol. Scand.* 86: 444–455, 1972.
43. D'Angelo, E., and G. Torelli. Neural stimuli increasing respiration during different types of exercise. *J. Appl. Physiol.* 30: 116–121, 1971.
44. Dean, C., and J. H. Coote. Discharge patterns in postganglionic neurones to skeletal muscle and kidney during activation of the hypothalamic defence areas in the cat. *Brain Res.* 377: 271–278, 1986.
45. Dejours, P. Control of respiration in muscular exercise. In: *Handbook of Physiology, Respiration*, edited by W. O. Fenn and H. Rahn. Washington, DC: Am. Physiol. Soc., 1964, p. 631–648.
46. Delaney, K. R., R. S. Zucker, and D. W. Tank. Calcium in motor nerve terminals associated with post-tetanic potentiation. *J. Neurosci.* 9: 3558–3567, 1989.
47. Dempsey, J. A., E. H. Vidruk, and S. M. Mastenbrook. Pulmonary control systems in exercise. *Federation Proc.* 39: 1498–1505, 1980.
48. Diepstra, G., W. Gonyea, and J. H. Mitchell. Distribution of cardiac output during static exercise in the conscious cat. *J. Appl. Physiol.* 52: 642–646, 1982.
49. Dillon, G. H., C. A. Shonis, and T. G. Waldrop. Hypothalamic GABAergic modulation of respiratory responses to baroreceptor stimulation. *Respir. Physiol.* 85: 289–304, 1991.
50. Dillon, G. H., and T. G. Waldrop. Responses of feline caudal hypothalamic cardiorespiratory neurons to hypoxia and hypercapnia. *Exp. Brain Res.* 96: 260–272, 1993.
51. Dimarco, A. F., J. R. Romaniuk, C. von Euler, and Y. Yamamoto. Immediate changes in ventilation and respiratory pattern with onset and offset of locomotion in the cat. *J. Physiol. (Lond.)* 343: 1–16, 1983.
52. DiMicco, J. A., V. M. Abshire, K. D. Hankins, R. H. B. Sample, and J. H. Wible. Microinjection of GABA antagonists into the posterior hypothalamus elevates heart rate in anesthetized rats. *Neuropharmacology* 25: 1063–1066, 1986.
53. Duffin, J., R. R. Gechbache, R. C. Goode, and S. A. Chung. The ventilatory response to carbon dioxide in hyperoxic exercise. *Respir. Physiol.* 40: 93–105, 1980.
54. Duncan, G., R. H. Johnson, and D. G. Lambie. Role of sensory nerves in the cardiovascular and respiratory changes with isometric forearm exercise in man. *Clin. Sci.* 60: 145–155, 1981.
55. Dutton, R. E., W. A. Hodson, D. G. Davies, and A. Fenner. Effect of rate of rise of carotid body P_{CO_2} on the time course of ventilation. *Respir. Physiol.* 3: 367–379, 1967.
56. Dutton, R. E., R. S. Fitzgerald, and N. Gross. Ventilatory response to square-wave forcing of carbon dioxide at the carotid bodies. *Respir. Physiol.* 4: 101–108, 1968.
57. Eklund, B., and L. Kaijser. Blood flow in the resting forearm during prolonged contralateral isometric handgrip and muscle effort. *J. Physiol. (Lond.)* 227: 359–366, 1978.
58. Eldridge, F. L. Posthyperventilation breathing: different effects of active and passive hyperventilation. *J. Appl. Physiol.* 34: 422–430, 1973.
59. Eldridge, F. L. Central neural respiratory stimulatory effect of active respiration. *J. Appl. Physiol.* 37: 723–735, 1974.
60. Eldridge, F. L. Central neural stimulation of respiration in unanesthetized decerebrate cats. *J. Appl. Physiol.* 40: 23–28, 1976.
61. Eldridge, F. L. Maintenance of respiration by central neural feedback mechanisms. *Federation Proc.* 36: 2400–2404, 1977.
62. Eldridge, F. L. Subthreshold central neural respiratory activity and afterdischarge. *Respir. Physiol.* 39: 327–343, 1980.

63. Eldridge, F. L. Phase resetting of respiratory rhythm—experiments in animals and models. In: *Springer Series in Synergetics, Vol. 55. Rhythms in Physiological Systems*, edited by H. Haken and H. P. Koepchen. Berlin: Springer-Verlag, 1991, p. 165–175.
64. Eldridge, F. L. Overview: role of neurochemicals and hormones. In: *Control of Breathing and its Modeling Perspective*, edited by Y. Honda, et al. New York: Plenum Press, 1992, p. 187–196.
65. Eldridge, F. L., and P. Gill-Kumar. Lack of effect of vagal afferent input on central neural respiratory afterdischarge. *J. Appl. Physiol.* 45: 339–344, 1978.
66. Eldridge, F. L., and P. Gill-Kumar. Central neural respiratory drive and afterdischarge. *Respir. Physiol.* 40: 49–63, 1980.
67. Eldridge, F. L., and P. Gill-Kumar. Central neural drive mechanisms and respiratory afterdischarge—the "T-pool" concept. In: *Central Nervous Control Mechanisms in Breathing*, edited by C. von Euler and H. Lagercrantz. Oxford: Pergamon Press, 1980, p. 101–113.
68. Eldridge, F. L., P. Gill-Kumar, and D. E. Millhorn. Input-output relationships of central neural circuits involved in respiration in cats. *J. Physiol. (Lond.)* 311: 81–95, 1981.
69. Eldridge, F. L., J. P. Kiley, and D. Paydarfar. Dynamics of medullary hydrogen ion and respiratory responses to square-wave change of arterial carbon dioxide in cats. *J. Physiol. (Lond.)* 383: 627–642, 1987.
70. Eldridge, F. L., and D. E. Millhorn. Oscillation, gating, and memory in the respiratory control system. In: *Handbook of Physiology, The Respiratory System, Control of Breathing*, edited by N. S. Cherniack and J. G. Widdicombe. Bethesda, MD: Am. Physiol. Soc., 1986, p. 93–114.
71. Eldridge, F. L., D. E. Millhorn, J. P. Kiley, and T. G. Waldrop. Stimulation by central command of locomotion, respiration and circulation during exercise. *Respir. Physiol.* 59: 313–337, 1985.
72. Eldridge, F. L., D. E. Millhorn, and T. G. Waldrop. Exercise hyperpnea and locomotion: parallel activation from the hypothalamus. *Science* 211: 844–846, 1981.
73. Eldridge, F. L., and T. G. Waldrop. Neural control of breathing during exercise. In: *Exercise: Pulmonary Physiology and Pathophysiology*, edited by B. Whipp and K. Wasserman. New York: Marcel Dekker, Inc., 1991, p. 309–370.
74. Eliasson, S., P. Lindgren, and B. Uvnas. Representation in the hypothalamus and the motor cortex in the dog of the sympathetic vasodilator outflow to the skeletal muscles. *Acta Physiol. Scand.* 27: 18–27, 1952.
75. Emptage, N. J., and T. J. Carew. Long-term synaptic facilitation in the absence of short-term facilitation in *Aplysia* neurons. *Science* 262: 253–256, 1993.
76. Engwall, M. J. A., L. Daristotle, W. Z. Niu, J. A. Dempsey, and G. E. Bisgard. Ventilatory afterdischarge in the awake goat. *J. Appl. Physiol.* 71: 1511–1517, 1991.
77. Engwall, M. J. A., C. A. Smith, J. A. Dempsey, and G. E. Bisgard. Ventilatory afterdischarge and central respiratory drive interactions in the awake goat. *J. Appl. Physiol.* 76: 416–423, 1994.
78. Euler, C. von. Brain stem mechanisms for generation and control of breathing pattern. In: *Handbook of Physiology, The Respiratory System, Control of Breathing*, edited by N. S. Cherniack and J. G. Widdicombe. Bethesda, MD: Am. Physiol. Soc., 1986, p. 1–67.
79. Fernandes, A., H. Galbo, M. Kjaer, J. H. Mitchell, N. H. Secher, and S. N. Thomas. Cardiovascular and ventilatory responses to dynamic exercise during epidural anaesthesia in man. *J. Physiol. (Lond.)* 420: 281–293, 1990.
80. Fernandes, A., H. Galbo, M. Kjær, N. H. Secher, F. W. Bach, H. Galbo, D. R. Reeves, Jr., and J. H. Mitchell. Hormonal, metabolic, and cardiovascular responses to static exercise in humans: influence of epidural anesthesia. *Am. J. Physiol.* 261 (*Endocrinol. Metab.* 24): E214–E220, 1991.
81. Fink, B. R. Influence of cerebral activity in wakefulness on regulation of breathing. *J. Appl. Physiol.* 16: 15–20, 1961.
82. Fink, G. R., L. Adams, J. D. G. Watson, J. A. Innes, B. Wuyam, I. Kobayashi, D. R. Corfield, K. Murphy, R. S. J. Frackowiak, T. Jones, and A. Guz. Motor cortical activation in exercise-induced hyperpnoea in man: evidence for involvement of supra-brainstem structures in control of breathing. *J. Physiol. (Lond.)* 473: 58P, 1993.
83. Fitzhugh, R. Impulses and physiological states in theoretical models of nerve membrane. *Biophys. J.* 1: 445–466, 1961.
84. Folgering, H. Beta-adrenergic drugs do not affect phrenic nerve afterdischarge. *Pflugers Arch.* 391: 355–356, 1981.
85. Fordyce, W. E., F. M. Bennett, S. K. Edelman, and F. S. Grodins. Evidence in man for a fast neural mechanism during the early phases of exercise hyperpnea. *Respir. Physiol.* 48: 27–43, 1982.
86. Forsyth, R. P. Hypothalamic control of the distribution of cardiac output in the unanesthetized rhesus monkey. *Circ. Res.* 26: 783–794, 1970.
87. Fregosi, R. F. Short-term potentiation of breathing in humans. *J. Appl. Physiol.* 71: 892–899, 1991.
88. Fregosi, R. F., and J. A. Dempsey. Arterial blood acid-base regulation during exercise in rats. *J. Appl. Physiol.* 57: 396–402, 1984.
89. Freund, P. R., L. B. Rowell, T. M. Murphy, S. F. Hobbs, and S. H. Butler. Blockade of the pressor response to muscle ischemia by sensory nerve block in man. *Am. J. Physiol.* 237 (*Heart Circ. Physiol.* 6): H433–H439, 1979.
90. Freyschuss, V. Cardiovascular adjustments to somatomotor activation. *Acta Physiol. Scand. Suppl.* 342: 1–63, 1970.
91. Friedman, D. B., J. Brennum, F. Sztuk, O. B. Hansen, P. S. Clifford, F. W. Bach, L. Arendt-Nielsen, J. H. Mitchell, and N. H. Secher. The effect of epidural anaesthesia with 1% lidocaine on the pressor response to dynamic exercise in humans. *J. Physiol.* 470: 681–691, 1993.
92. Friedman, D. B., C. Peel, and J. H. Mitchell. Cardiovascular responses to voluntary and nonvoluntary static exercise in humans. *J. Appl. Physiol.* 73: 1982–1985, 1992.
93. Fritsch, G., and J. E. Hitzig. Uber die elektrische Erregbarkeit des Grooshirns. *Archives fur anatome, physiologie und wissenschaftliche Medizin,* 1870, p. 300–332.
94. Gage, P. W., and J. I. Hubbard. An investigation of the post-tetanic potentiation of end-plate potentials at a mammalian neuromuscular junction. *J. Physiol. (Lond.)* 184: 353–375, 1966.
95. Galbo, H., M. Kjaer, and N. H. Secher. Cardiovascular, ventilatory and catecholamine responses to maximal dynamic exercise in partially curarised man. *J. Physiol. (Lond.)* 389: 557–568, 1987.
96. Gandevia, S. C., and S. F. Hobbs. Cardiovascular responses to static exercise in man: central and reflex contributions. *J. Physiol. (Lond.)* 430: 105–117, 1990.
97. Gandevia, S. C., K. Killiam, D. K. McKenzie, M. Crawford, G. M. Allen, R. B. Gorman, and J. P. Hales. Respiratory sensations, cardiovascular control, kinaesthesia and transcranial stimulation during paralysis in humans. *J. Physiol. (Lond.)* 470: 85–107, 1993.

98. Gandevia, S. C., and J. C. Rothwell. Activation of the human diaphragm from the motor cortex. *J. Physiol. (Lond.)* 384: 109–118, 1987.
99. Garcia-Rill, E. The basal ganglia and the locomotor regions. *Brain Res. Rev.* 11: 47–63, 1986.
100. Garcia-Rill, E., R. D. Skinner, and J. A. Fitzgerald. Chemical activation of the mesencephalic locomotor region. *Brain Res.* 330: 43–54, 1985.
101. Gebber, G. L. Central determinants of sympathetic nerve discharge. In: *Central Regulation of Autonomic Functions,* edited by A. D. Loewy and K. M. Spyer. New York: Oxford University Press, 1990, p. 126–144.
102. Georgopoulos, D., Z. Bshouty, M. Younes, and N. R. Anthonisen. Hypoxic exposure and activation of the afterdischarge mechanism in conscious humans. *J. Appl. Physiol.* 69: 1159–1164, 1990.
103. Gesell, R., C. R. Brassfield, and M. A. Hamilton. An acid-neurohumoral mechanism of nerve cell activation. *Am. J. Physiol.* 136: 604–608, 1942.
104. Goodwin, G. M., D. I. McCloskey, and J. H. Mitchell. Cardiovascular and respiratory responses to changes in central command during isometric exercise at constant muscle tension. *J. Physiol. (Lond.)* 226: 173–190, 1972.
105. Graham Brown, T. The intrinsic factors in the act of progression in the mammal. *Proc. R. Soc. Lond.* 84B: 308–319, 1911.
106. Graham Brown, T. The phenomenon of "narcosis progression" in mammals. *Proc. R. Soc. Lond.* 86B: 140–164, 1913.
107. Graham Brown, T. On the nature of the fundamental activity of the nervous centres; together with an analysis of the conditioning of rhythmic activity in progression, and a theory of the evolution of function in the nervous system. *J. Physiol. (Lond.)* 48: 18–46, 1914.
108. Green, H. D., and E. C. Hoff. Effects of faradic stimulation of the cerebral cortex on limb and renal volumes in the cat and monkey. *Am. J. Physiol.* 118: 641–658, 1937.
109. Grodins, F. S. Exercise hyperpnea. The ultra secret. *Adv. Physiol. Sci.* 10: 243–251, 1981.
110. Grossman, R. G. Effects of stimulation of non-specific thalamic system on locomotor movements in cat. *J. Neurophysiol.* 21: 85–93, 1958.
111. Guyenet, P. G. Role of the ventral medulla oblongat in blood pressure regulation. In: *Central Regulation of Autonomic Functions,* edited by A. D. Loewy and K. M. Spyer. New York: Oxford University Press, 1990, p. 145–167.
112. Haldane, J. S., and J. G. Preistly. The regulation of lung ventilation. *J. Physiol. (Lond.)* 32: 225–266, 1905.
113. Hastings, A. B., F. C. White, T. M. Sanders, and C. M. Bloor. Comparative physiological responses to exercise stress. *J. Appl. Physiol.* 52: 1077–1083, 1982.
114. Henderson, Y. Acapnia and shock. IV. Fatal apnoea after excessive respiration. *Am. J. Physiol.* 25: 310–333, 1910.
115. Hilton, S. M. Central nervous origin of vasomotor tone. *Adv. Physiol. Sci.* 8: 1–12, 1981.
116. Hilton, S. M., J. M. Marshall, and R. J. Timms. Ventral medullary relay neurons in the pathway from the defence areas of the cat and their effect on blood pressure. *J. Physiol. (Lond.)* 345: 149–166, 1983.
117. Hilton, S. M., and W. S. Redfern. A search for brain stem cell groups integrating the defence reaction. *J. Physiol. (Lond.)* 378: 213–228, 1986.
118. Hilton, S. M., K. M. Spyer, and R. J. Timms. The origin of the hind limb vasodilatation evoked by stimulation of the motor cortex in the cat. *J. Physiol. (Lond.)* 287: 545–557, 1979.
119. Hilton, S. M., and A. W. Zbrozyna. Amygdaloid region for defence reactions and its efferent pathway to the brain stem. *J. Physiol. (Lond.)* 165: 160–173, 1963.
120. Hobbs, S. F. Central command during exercise: parallel activation of the cardiovascular and motor systems by descending command signals. In: *Circulation, Neurobiology and Behavior*, edited by O. A. Smith, R. A. Galosy, and S. M. Weiss. Amsterdam: Elsevier Science Publishers, 1982, p. 217–231.
121. Hobbs, S. F., and S. C. Gandevia. Cardiovascular responses and the sense of effort during attempts to contract paralyzed muscles: role of the spinal cord. *Neurosci. Lett.* 57: 85–90, 1985.
122. Hobbs, S. F., and D. I. McCloskey. Effect of spontaneous exercise on reflex slowing of the heart in decerebrate cats. *J. Auton. Nerv. Syst.* 17: 303–312, 1986.
123. Hoff, E. C., J. F. Kell, Jr., and M. N. Carroll, Jr. Effects of cortical stimulation and lesions on cardiovascular function. *Physiol. Rev.* 43: 68–114, 1963.
124. Hollander, A. P., and L. N. Bouman. Cardiac acceleration in man elicited by a muscle-heart reflex. *J. Appl. Physiol.* 38: 272–278, 1975.
125. Holstege, G. Some anatomical observations on the projections from the hypothalamus to brainstem and spinal cord: an HRP and autoradiographic tracing study in the cat. *J. Comp. Neurol.* 260: 98–126, 1987.
126. Horn, E. M., and T. G. Waldrop. Modulation of the respiratory responses to hypoxia and hypercapnia by synaptic input onto caudal hypothalamic neurons. *Brain Res.* 664: 25–33, 1994.
127. Hornbein, T. F., S. C. Sφrensen, and C. R. Parks. Role of muscle spindles in lower extremities in breathing during bicycle exercise. *J. Appl. Physiol.* 27: 476–479, 1969.
128. Huang, Z. -S., G. L. Gebber, S. M. Barman, and K. J. Varner. Forebrain contribution to sympathetic nerve discharge in anesthetized cats. *Am. J. Physiol.* 252 (*Regulatory Integrative Comp. Physiol.* 21): R645–R652, 1987.
129. Huang, Z. -S., K. J. Varner, S. M. Barman, and G. L. Gebber. Diencephalic regions contributing to sympathetic nerve discharge in anesthetized cats. *Am. J. Physiol.* 254 (*Regulatory Integrative Comp. Physiol.* 23): R249–R256, 1986.
130. Hugelin, A., and M. I. Cohen. The reticular activating system and respiratory regulation in the cat. *Ann. N. Y. Acad. Sci.* 109: 586–603, 1963.
131. Hultman, E., and H. Sjoholm. Blood pressure and heart rate response to voluntary and non-voluntary static exercise in man. *Acta Physiol. Scand.* 115: 499–501, 1982.
132. Innes, J. A., S. C. De Cort, P. J. Evans, and A. Guz. Central command influences cardiorespiratory response to dynamic exercise in humans with unilateral weakness. *J. Physiol. (Lond.)* 448: 551–563, 1992.
133. Johansson, J. E. Uber die Einwirkung der Musdeltatigkeit auf die Atmun und die Herztatigkeit. *Skand. Arch. Physiol.* 5: 20–66, 1893.
134. Kaczmarek, L. K., and F. Strumwasser. The expression of long lasting afterdischarge in peptidergic neurons of *Aplysia* bag cell neurons. *J. Neurosci.* 1: 626–634, 1981.
135. Kao, F. F. An experimental study of the pathways involved in exercise hyperpnea employing cross-circulation techniques. In: *The Regulation of Human Respiration,* edited by D. J. C. Cunningham and B. B. Lloyd. Philadelphia: F. A. Davis Company, 1963, p. 461–502.
136. Karczewski, W. A., K. Budzinska, H. Gromysz, R. Herczynski, and J. R. Romaniuk. Some responses of the res-

piratory complex to stimulation of its vagal and mesencephalic inputs. In: *Respiratory Centres and Afferent Systems*, edited by B. Duron. Paris: INSERM, 1976, p. 107–115.

137. Karczewski, W. A., and J. R. Romaniuk. Neural control of breathing and central nervous system plasticity. *Acta Physiol. Pol. Suppl.* 20: 1–10, 1980.
138. Katz, B., and R. Miledi. The role of calcium in neuromuscular facilitation. *J. Physiol. (Lond.)* 195: 481–492, 1968.
139. Kelly, M. A., M. D. Laufe, R. P. Millman, and D. D. Peterson. Ventilatory response to hypercapnia before and after athletic training. *Respir. Physiol.* 55: 393–400, 1984.
140. Khoo, M. C. K., A. Gottschalk, and A. I. Pack. Sleep-induced periodic breathing and apnea: a theoretical study. *J. Appl. Physiol.* 70: 2014–2024, 1991.
141. Khoo, M. C. K., R. E. Kronauer, K. P. Strohl, and A. S. Slutsky. Factors inducing periodic breathing: a general model. *J. Appl. Physiol.* 53: 644–659, 1982.
142. Kiley, J. P., W. D. Kuhlman, and M. R. Fedde. Respiratory and cardiovascular responses to exercise in the duck. *J. Appl. Physiol.* 47: 112–136, 1979.
143. Kjær, M., G. Perko, N. H. Secher, R. Boushel, N. Beyer, S. Pollack, A. Horn, A. Fernandes, T. Mohr, S. F. Lewis, and H. Galbo. Cardiovascular and ventilatory responses to electrically induced cycling with complete epidural anaesthesia in humans. *Acta Physiol. Scand.* 151: 191–207, 1994.
144. Kjær M., N. H. Secher, F. W. Bach, H. Galbo, D. R. Reeves, Jr., and J. H. Mitchell. Hormonal, metabolic, and cardiovascular responses to static exercise in humans: influence of epidural anesthesia. *Am. J. Physiol.* 261 (*Endocrinol. Metab.* 24): E214–E220, 1991.
145. Kjær, M., N. H. Secher, F. W. Bach, S. Sheikh, and H. Galbo. Hormonal and metabolic responses to dynamic exercise in man: effect of sensory nervous blockade. *Am. J. Physiol.* 257 (*Endocrinol. Metab.* 20): E95–E101, 1989.
146. Kleyntjens, F., K. Koizumi, and C. McC. Brooks. Stimulation of suprabulbar reticular formation. *Arch. Neurol. Psychiatry* 73: 425–438, 1955.
147. Krogh, A., and J. Lindhard. The regulation of respiration and circulation during the initial stages of muscular work. *J. Physiol. (Lond.)* 47: 112–136, 1913.
148. Krogh, A., and J. Lindhard. A comparison between voluntary and electrically induced muscular work in man. *J. Physiol. (Lond.)* 51: 182–201, 1917.
149. Langhorst, P., M. Lambertz, G. Schultz, and G. Stock. Role played by amygdala complex and common brainstem system in integration of somatomotor and autonomic components of behavior. In: *Organization of the Autonomic Nervous System: Central and Peripheral Autonomic Mechanisms*. New York: Alan R. Liss, Inc., 1987, p. 347–361.
150. Larabee, M. G., and D. W. Bronk. Prolonged facilitation of synaptic excitation in sympathetic ganglia. *J. Neurophysiol.* 10: 139–154, 1947.
151. Lawson, E. E., and W. A. Long. Central neural respiratory response to carotid sinus nerve stimulation in newborns. *J. Appl. Physiol.* 56: 1614–1620, 1984.
152. Leonard, B., J. H. Mitchell, M. Mizuno, N. Rube, B. Saltin, and N. H. Secher. Partial neuromuscular blockade and cardiovascular responses to static exercise in man. *J. Physiol. (Lond.)* 359: 365–379, 1985.
153. Li, P., and T. A. Lovick. Excitatory projections from hypothalamic and midbrain defense regions to nucleus paragigantocellularis lateralis in the rat. *Exp. Neurol.* 89: 543–553, 1985.
154. Lind, A. R., G. W. McNicol, R. A. Bruce, H. R. MacDonald, and K. W. Donald. The cardiovascular responses to sustained contractions of a patient with unilateral syringomyelia. *Clin. Sci.* 35: 45–53, 1968.
155. Lind, A. R., and J. S. Petrofsky. Amplitude of the surface electrocardiogram during fatiguing isometric contractions. *Muscle Nerve* 2: 257–264, 1979.
156. Lind, A. R., S. R. Taylor, P. W. Humphreys, B. M. Kennelly, and D. W. Donald. Circulatory effects of sustained muscle contraction. *Clin. Sci.* 27: 229–244, 1964.
157. Lipski, J., A. Bektas, and R. Porter. Short latency inputs to phrenic motoneurones from the sensorimotor cortex in the cat. *Exp. Brain Res.* 61: 280–290, 1986.
158. Llinas, R., T. L. McGuinnes, C. S. Leonard, M. Sugimori, and P. Greengard. Intraterminal injection of synapsin I or calcium/calmodulin-dependent protein kinase II alters neurotransmitter release at the squid giant synapse. *Proc. Natl. Acad. Sci., U. S. A.* 82: 3035–3039, 1985.
159. Loeschcke, H. H., J. DeLattre, M. E. Schlafke, and C. O. Trouth. Effects on respiration and circulation of electrically stimulating the ventral surface of the medulla oblongata. *Respir. Physiol.* 10: 184–197, 1970.
160. Lovick, T. A. Projections from the diencephalon and mesencephalon to nucleus paragigantocellularis lateralis in the cat. *Neuroscience* 14: 853–861, 1985.
161. Luiten, P. G. M., G. J. Ter Horst, H. Karst, and A.B. Steffens. The course of paraventricular hypothalamic efferents to autonomic structures in medulla and spinal cord. *Brain Res.* 329: 374–378, 1985.
162. Magleby, K. L. Synaptic transmission, facilitation, augmentation, potentiation, depression. In: *Encyclopedia of Neuroscience*, edited by G. Edelman. Boston: Birkhauser, 1987, p. 1170–1174.
163. Magleby, K. L., and J. E. Zengel. A quantitative description of stimulation-induced changes in transmitter release at the frog neuromuscular junction. *J. Gen. Physiol.* 80: 613–638, 1982.
164. Mark, A. L., R. G. Victor, C. Nerhed, and B. G. Wallin. Microneurographic studies of the mechanisms of sympathetic nerve responses to static exercise in humans. *Circ. Res.* 57: 461–469, 1985.
165. Marshall, J. M., and R. J. Timms. Experiments on the role of the subthalamus in the generation of the cardiovascular changes during locomotion in the cat. *J. Physiol. (Lond.)* 301: 92–93P, 1980.
166. Maskati, H. A. A., and A. W. Zbrozyna. Cardiovascular and motor components of the defense reaction elicited in rats by electrical and chemical stimulation in amygdala. *J. Auton. Nerv. Syst.* 28: 127–132, 1989.
167. Matsukawa, K., J. H. Mitchell, P. T. Wall, and L. B. Wilson. The effect of static exercise on renal sympathetic nerve activity in conscious cats. *J. Physiol. (Lond.)* 434: 453–467, 1991.
168. McCloskey, D. I. Centrally-generated commands and cardiovascular control in man. *Clin. Exp. Hypertens.* 3: 369–378, 1981.
169. McCloskey, D. I., and J. H. Mitchell. Reflex cardiovascular and respiratory responses originating in exercising muscle. *J. Physiol. (Lond.)* 224: 173–186, 1972.
170. McNaughton, B. L. Long-term synaptic enhancement and short-term potentiation in rat fascia dentata act through different mechanisms. *J. Physiol. (Lond.)* 324: 249–262, 1982.
171. Meah, M. S., and W. N. Gardner. Post-hyperventilation apnoea in conscious humans. *J. Physiol. (Lond.)* 477: 527–538, 1994.

172. Mel'nikova, Z. L. Connections of the subthalamic and mesencephalic "locomotor regions" in rats. *Neirofiziologiya* 9: 275–280, 1977.
173. Melton, J. E., Q. P. Yu, J. A. Neubauer, and N. H. Edelman. Modulation of respiratory responses to carotid sinus nerve stimulation by brain hypoxia. *J. Appl. Physiol.* 73: 2166–2171, 1992.
174. Miller, S., and F. G. A. van der Meche. Coordinated stepping of all four limbs in the high spinal cat. *Brain Res.* 109: 395–398, 1976.
175. Millhorn, D. E., F. L. Eldridge, and T. G. Waldrop. Pharmacologic study of respiratory afterdischarge. *J. Appl. Physiol.* 50: 239–244, 1981.
176. Millhorn, D. E., F. L. Eldridge, and T. G. Waldrop. Effects of medullary area I(s) cooling on respiratory response to chemoreceptor input. *Respir. Physiol.* 49: 23–39, 1982.
177. Millhorn, D. E., F. L. Eldridge, T. G. Waldrop, and J. P. Kiley. Diencephalic regulation of respiration and arterial pressure during actual and fictive locomotion in cat. *Circ. Res.* 61 (Suppl. I): I-53–I-59, 1987.
178. Mills, J. N. Hyperpnea induced by forced breathing. *J. Physiol. (Lond.)* 105: 95–116, 1946.
179. Mitchell, G. S., T. T. Gleeson, and A. F. Bennett. Ventilation and acid base balance during graded activity in lizards. *Am. J. Physiol.* 238 (*Regulatory Integrative Comp. Physiol.* 7): R27–R37, 1981.
180. Mitchell, J. H. Cardiovascular control during exercise: central and reflex neural mechanisms. *Am. J. Cardiol.* 55: 33D–41D, 1985.
181. Mitchell, J. H. Neural control of the circulation during exercise. *Med. Sci. Sports Exer.* 22: 141–154, 1990.
182. Mitchell, J. H., and P. B. Raven. Cardiovascular response and adaptation to exercise. In: *Physical Activity, Fitness and Health: International Proceedings and Consensus Statement*, edited by C. Bouchard, R. Shephard, and T. Stephens. Champaign, IL: Human Kinetics Publishers, 1994, p. 286–298.
183. Mitchell, J. H., D. R. Reeves, Jr., H. B. Rogers, and N. H. Secher. Epidural anaesthesia and cardiovascular responses to static exercise in man. *J. Physiol. (Lond.)* 417: 13–24, 1989.
184. Mitchell, J. H., D. R. Reeves, Jr., H. B. Rogers, N. H. Secher, and R. G. Victor. Autonomic blockade and the cardiovascular responses to static exercise in partially curarized man. *J. Physiol. (Lond.)* 413: 433–335, 1989.
185. Mitchell, J. H., B. Schibye, F. C. Payne, III, and B. Saltin. Response of arterial blood pressure to static exercise in relation to muscle mass, force development, and electromyographic activity. *Circ. Res.* 48 (Suppl. I): I-70–I-75, 1981.
186. Mori, S., H. Nishimura, C. Kurakami, T. Yamamura, and M. Aoki. Lower brainstem "locomotor region" in the mesencephalic cat. In: *Integrative Control Function of the Brain,* edited by M. Ito. Tokyo: Kodansha Press, 1978.
187. Mosso, A. La physiologie de l'apnée etudiée chez l'homme. *Arch. Ital. Biol.* 40: 1–30, 1903.
188. Murray, J. F. *The Normal Lung*. Philadelphia: W. B. Saunders Company, 1976.
189. Muza, S. R., L. -Y Lee, R. L. Wiley, S. McDonald, and F. W. Zechman. Ventilatory responses to static handgrip exercise. *J. Appl. Physiol.* 54: 1457–1462, 1983.
190. Myhre, K., and K. L. Andersen. Respiratory responses to static muscular contraction. *Respir. Physiol.* 12: 77–89, 1971.
191. Nolan, P. C., J. A. Pawelczyk, and T. G. Waldrop. Neurons in the ventrolateral medulla receive input from descending "central command" and feedback from contracting muscles. *Physiologist* 35: 240, 1992.
192. Ochwadt, B., E. Bücherl, H. Kreuzer, and H. H. Loeschcke. Beeinflussing der Atemsteigerung bei Muskelarbeit durch partiellen neuromuscularen Block (Tubocurarine). *Pflugers Arch.* 269: 613–621, 1959.
193. O'Hagan, K. P., L. B. Bell, S. W. Mittelstadt, and P. S. Clifford. Effect of dynamic exercise on renal sympathetic nerve activity in conscious rabbits. *J. Appl. Physiol.* 74: 2099–2104, 1993.
194. Ordway, G. A., T. G. Waldrop, G. A. Iwamoto, and B. J. Gentile. Hypothalamic influences on cardiovascular response of beagles to dynamic exercise. *Am. J. Physiol.* 257 (*Heart Circ. Physiol.* 28): H1247–H1253, 1989.
195. Orlovskii, G. N. Spontaneous and induced locomotion of the thalamic cat. *Biophysics* (USSR—English translation) 14: 1154–1162, 1969.
196. Orlovskii, G. N. Connexions of the reticulo-spinal neurones with the "locomotor sections" of the brain stem. *Biofizika* 15: 171–177, 1970.
197. Pan, L. G., H. V. Forster, G. E. Bisgard, R. P. Kaminski, S. M. Dorsey, and M. A. Busch. Hyperventilation in ponies at the onset and during steady-state exercise. *J. Appl. Physiol.* 54: 1394–1402, 1983.
198. Patterson, D. J. Potassium and ventilation in exercise. *J. Appl. Physiol.* 72: 811–820, 1992.
199. Peano, C. A., C. A. Shonis, G. H. Dillon, and T. G. Waldrop. Hypothalamic GABAergic mechanism involved in the respiratory response to hypercapnia. *Brain Res. Bull.* 28: 107–113, 1992.
200. Petro, J. K., A. P. Hollander, and L. N. Bouman. Instantaneous cardiac acceleration in man induced by a voluntary muscle contraction. *J. Appl. Physiol.* 29: 794–798, 1970.
201. Pickar, J. G., J. M. Hill, and M. P. Kaufman. Stimulation of vagal afferents inhibits locomotion in mesencephalic cats. *J. Appl. Physiol.* 74: 103–110, 1993.
202. Pitt, R. F., and D. W. Bronk. Excitability cycle of the hypothalamus-sympathetic neurone system. *Am. J. Physiol.* 135: 504–525, 1942.
203. Pitts, R. F., M. G. Larrabee, and D. W. Bronk. An analysis of hypothalamic cardiovascular control. *Am. J. Physiol.* 134: 359–383, 1941.
204. Plum, F., H. W. Brown, and E. Snoep. The neurological significance of posthyperventilation apnea. *JAMA*, 181: 1050–1055, 1962.
205. Priban, I. P. An analysis of some short-term patterns of breathing in man at rest. *J. Physiol. (Lond.)* 166: 425–434, 1963.
206. Redgate, E. S. Hypothalamic influence on respiration. *Ann. N. Y. Acad. Sci.* 109: 606–618, 1963.
207. Richter, D. W., H. Camerer, and U. Sonnhof. Changes in extracellular potassium during the spontaneous activity of medullary respiratory neurones. *Pflugers Arch.* 376: 139–149, 1978.
208. Romaniuk, J. R., S. Kasicki, and U. Borecka. The Breuer-Hering reflex at rest and during electrically induced locomotion in the decerebrate cat. *Acta Neurobiol. Exp.* 46: 141–151, 1986.
209. Rosenthal, J. Post-tetanic potentiation at the neuromuscular junction of the frog. *J. Physiol. (Lond.)* 203: 121–133, 1969.
210. Rushmer, R. F. *Structure and Function of the Cardiovascular System.* Philadelphia: W. B. Saunders Company, 1972, p. 94–97, 142–144, 220–243.
211. Rybicki, K. J., R. W. Stremel, G. A. Iwamoto, J. H. Mitchell, and M. P. Kaufman. Occlusion of pressor responses to

posterior diencephalic stimulation and static muscular contraction. *Brain Res. Bull.* 22: 306–312, 1989.
212. Saito, M., H. Abe, S. Iwase, and T. Mano. Responses in muscle sympathetic nerve activity in sustained and rhythmic muscle contraction. *Environ. Med.* 33: 33–41, 1989.
213. Saito, M., T. Mano, and S. Iwase. Sympathetic nerve activity related to local fatigue sensation during static contraction. *J. Appl. Physiol.* 67: 980–984, 1989.
214. Saito, M., M. Nato, and T. Mano. Different responses in skin and muscle sympathetic nerve activity to static muscle contraction. *J. Appl. Physiol.* 69: 2085–2090, 1990.
215. Saper, C. B., A. D. Loewy, L. W. Swanson, and W. M. Cowan. Direct hypothalamo-autonomic connections. *Brain Res.* 117: 305–312, 1976.
216. Schibye, B., J. H. Mitchell, F. C. Payne, and B. Saltin. Blood pressure and heart rate response to static exercise in relation to electromyographic activity and force development. *Acta Physiol. Scand.* 113: 61–66, 1981.
217. Schlafke, M. E., and H. H. Loeschcke. Lokalization einer an de regulation von Atmung und Kreislauf betieligten Gebietes an de ventralen Oberflack der Medulla Oblongata durch Kalte blockage. *Pflugers Arch.* 297: 205–220, 1967.
218. Seals, D. R. Influence of force on muscle and skin sympathetic nerve activity during sustained isometric contractions in humans. *J. Physiol. (Lond.)* 462: 147–159, 1993.
219. Seals, D. R., and R. M. Enoka. Sympathetic activation is associated with increases in EMG during fatiguing exercise. *J. Appl. Physiol.* 66: 88–95, 1989.
220. Senapati, J. M. Effect of stimulation of muscle afferents on ventilations of dogs. *J. Appl. Physiol.* 21: 242–246, 1966.
221. Shea, S. A., L. P. Andres, D. C. Shannon, and R. B. Banzett. Ventilatory responses to exercise in humans lacking ventilatory chemosensitivity. *J. Physiol. (Lond.)* 468: 623–640, 1993.
222. Sherrington, C. Lecture II. Co-ordination in the simple reflex. In: *The Integrative Action of the Nervous System*, 2nd ed. New Haven, CT: Yale University Press, 1947, p. 36–69.
223. Shik, M. L., and G. N. Orlovskii. Neurophysiology of locomotor automatism. *Physiol. Rev.* 56: 465–501, 1976.
224. Shik, M. L., F. V. Severin, and G. N. Orlovskii. Control of walking and running by means of electrical stimulation of the midbrain. *Biofizika* 11: 659–666, 1966.
225. Shik, M. L., and A. S. Yagosditsyn. The pontobulbar locomotor strip. *Neurophysiology* 9: 72–74, 1977.
226. Shik, M. L., and A. S. Yagosditsyn. Unit responses in the locomotor strip of the cat hindbrain to microstimulation. *Neurophysiology* 10: 373–379, 1978.
227. Skinner, R. D., and E. Garcia-Rill. The mesencephalic locomotor region (MLR) in the rat. *Brain Res.* 323: 385–389, 1984.
228. Smith, C. A., G. S. Mitchell, L. C. Jameson, T. I. Musch, and J. A. Dempsey. Ventilatory response of goats to treadmill exercise: grade effects. *Respir. Physiol.* 54: 331–341, 1983.
229. Smith, O. A., Jr., R. E. Rushmer, and E. P. Lasher. Similarity of cardiovascular responses to exercise and to diencephalic stimulation. *Am. J. Physiol.* 198: 1139–1142, 1960.
230. Splengler, C. M., D. von Ow, and U. Boutellier. The role of central command in ventilatory control during static exercise. *Eur. J. Appl. Physiol.* 68: 162–169, 1994.
231. Spyer, K. M. Neural organisation and control of the baroreceptor reflex. *Rev. Physiol. Biochem. Pharmacol.* 88: 23–124, 1981.
232. Steeves, J. D., and L. M. Jordan. Autoradiographic demonstration of the projections from the mesencephalic locomotor region. *Brain Res.* 307: 263–276, 1984.
233. Steeves, J. D., L. M. Jordan, and N. Lake. The close proximity of catecholamine-containing cells to the mesencephalic locomotor region (MLR). *Brain Res.* 100: 663–670, 1973.
234. Strange, S., N. H. Secher, J. A. Pawelczyk, J. Karpakka, N. J. Christensen, J. H. Mitchell, and B. Saltin. Neural control of cardiovascular responses and of ventilation during dynamic exercise in man. *J. Physiol. (Lond.)* 470: 693–704, 1993.
235. Stremel, R. W., and I. G. Joshua. Disinhibition of posterior hypothalamic neurons elicit splanchnic microvascular constriction. *Soc. Neurosci. Abstr.* 19: 958, 1993.
236. Swanson, G. D., D. S. Ward, and J. W. Bellville. Posthyperventilation isocapnic hyperpnea. *J. Appl. Physiol.* 40: 592–596, 1976.
237. Sykova, E. Activity-related fluctuations in extracellular ion concentrations in the central nervous system. *News Physiol. Sci.* 1: 57–61, 1986.
238. Tansey, K. E., A. K. Yee, and B. R. Botterman. Force modulation due to firing rate variation in single motor units during centrally evoked muscle contractions. *Soc. Neurosci. Abstr.* 16: 115, 1990.
239. Tansey, K. E., and B. R. Botterman. Recruitment order and discharge patterns among pairs of motor units evoked by brainstem stimulation. *Soc. Neurosci. Abstr.* 15: 919, 1989.
240. Tawadrous, F. D., and F. L. Eldridge. Posthyperventilation breathing patterns after active hyperventilation in man. *J. Appl. Physiol.* 37: 353–356, 1974.
241. Thomas, M. R., and F. R. Calaresu. Responses of single units in the medial hypothalamus to electrical stimulation of the carotid sinus nerve in the cat. *Brain Res.* 44: 49–62, 1972.
242. Thomas, M. R., and F. R. Calaresu. Hypothalamic inhibition of chemoreceptor-induced bradycardia in the cat. *Am. J. Physiol.* 225: 201–208, 1973.
243. Valbo, A. B., R. -E. Hagbarth, H. E. Torebjörk, and B. G. Wallin. Somatosensory proprioceptive and sympathetic activity in human peripheral nerves. *Physiol. Rev.* 59: 919–957, 1979.
244. Varner, K. J., S. M. Barman, and G. L. Gebber. Cat diencephalic neurons with sympathetic nerve-related activity. *Am. J. Physiol.* 254 (*Regulatory Integrative Comp. Physiol.* 23): R257–R267, 1988.
245. Victor, R. G., S. L. Pryor, N. H. Secher, and J. H. Mitchell. Effects of partial neuromuscular blockade on sympathetic nerve responses to static exercise in humans. *Circ. Res.* 65: 468–476, 1989.
246. Victor, R. G., and D. R. Seals. Reflex stimulation of sympathetic outflow during rhythmic exercise in humans. *Am. J. Physiol.* 257 (*Heart Circ. Physiol.* 26): H2017–H2024, 1989.
247. Victor, R. G., D. R. Seals, and A. L. Mark. Differential control of heart rate and sympathetic nerve activity during dynamic exercise. Insight from intraneural recordings in humans. *J. Clin. Invest.* 79: 508–516, 1987.
248. Victor, R. G., N. H. Secher, T. Lyson, and J. H. Mitchell. Central command increases muscle sympathetic nerve activity during intense intermittent isometric exercise in humans. *Circ. Res.* 76: 127–131, 1995.
249. Vis, A. *Dynamic aspects of the regulation of breathing*. Nijmegen: The Netherlands, Katholieke University, Ph.D. thesis, 1981.

250. Vis, A., and H. Folgering. Phrenic nerve afterdischarge after electrical stimulation of the carotid sinus nerve in cats. *Respir. Physiol.* 45: 217–227, 1981.
251. Vissing, S. F., U. Scherrer, and R. G. Victor. Stimulation of skin sympathetic nerve discharge by central command. Differential control of sympathetic outflow to skin and skeletal muscle during static exercise. *Circ. Res.* 69: 228–238, 1991.
252. Wagner, P. G. *Further characterization of the central nervous system mechanism involved in the generation of a respiratory afterdischarge*. Chapel Hill, NC: University of North Carolina at Chapel Hill, Ph.D. thesis, 1990.
253. Wagner, P. G., and F. L. Eldridge. Development of short-term potentiation of respiration. *Respir. Physiol.* 83: 129–140, 1991.
254. Waldrop, T. G. Respiratory responses and adaptations to exercise. In: *Scientific Foundations of Sports Medicine*, edited by C. C. Teitz. Toronto: B. C. Decker, Inc., 1989, p. 59–76.
255. Waldrop, T. G. Posterior hypothalamic modulation of the respiratory response to CO_2 in cats. *Pflugers Arch.* 418: 7–13, 1991.
256. Waldrop, T. G., and R. M. Bauer. Modulation of sympathetic discharge by a hypothalamic GABAergic mechanism. *Neuropharmacology* 28: 263–269, 1989.
257. Waldrop, T. G., R. M. Bauer, and G. A. Iwamoto. Microinjection of GABA antagonists into the posterior hypothalamus elicits locomotor activity and a cardiorespiratory activation. *Brain Res.* 444: 84–94, 1988.
258. Waldrop, T. G., F. L. Eldridge, and D. E. Millhorn. Prolonged post-stimulus inhibition of breathing following stimulation of afferents from muscle. *Respir. Physiol.* 50: 239–254, 1982.
259. Waldrop, T. G., M. C. Henderson, G. A. Iwamoto, and J. H. Mitchell. Regional blood flow responses to stimulation of the subthalamic locomotor region. *Respir. Physiol.* 64: 93–102, 1986.
260. Waldrop, T. G., and G. A. Iwamoto. Neurons in the insular cortex are responsive to muscular contraction and have sympathetic and/or cardiac-related discharge. *Soc. Neurosci. Abstr.* 20: 1370, 1994.
261. Waldrop, T. G., D. C. Mullins, and M. C. Henderson. Effects of hypothalamic lesions on the cardiorespiratory responses to muscular contraction. *Respir. Physiol.* 66: 215–224, 1986.
262. Waldrop, T. G., D. C. Mullins, and D. E. Millhorn. Control of respiration by the hypothalamus and by feedback from contracting muscles in cats. *Respir. Physiol.* 64: 317–328, 1986.
263. Waldrop, T. G., and J. P. Porter. Hypothalamic involvement in respiratory and cardiovascular regulation. In: *Regulation of Breathing*, edited by J. A. Dempsey and A. I. Pack. New York: Marcel Dekker, Inc., 1995, p. 315–364.
264. Waldrop, T. G., and R. W. Stremel. Muscular contraction stimulates posterior hypothalamic neurons. *Am. J. Physiol.* 256 (*Regulatory Integrative Comp. Physiol.* 25): R348–R356, 1989.
265. Wall, P. D., and K. H. Pribram. Trigeminal neurotomy and blood pressure responses from stimulation of lateral cerebral cortex of *Macaca mulatta*. *J. Neurophysiol.* 13: 409–412, 1950.
266. Waller, W. H. Progression movements elicited by subthalamic stimulation. *J. Neurophysiol.* 3: 300–307, 1940.
267. Wang, S. C., and S. W. Ranson. Descending pathways from the hypothalamus to the medulla and spinal cord. Observations on blood pressure and bladder responses. *J. Comp. Neurol.* 71: 457–472, 1939.
268. Wasserman, K., B. J. Whipp, and R. Casaburi. Respiratory control during exercise. In: *Handbook of Physiology, The Respiratory System, Control of Breathing*, edited by N. S. Cherniack and J. G. Widdicombe. Bethesda, MD: Am. Physiol. Soc., 1986, p. 595–619.
269. Weil, J. V., E. Byrne-Quinn, I. E. Sodal, J. S. Line, R. E. McCollough, and G. F. Filley. Augmentation of chemosensitivity during mild exercise in normal man. *J. Appl. Physiol.* 33: 813–819, 1972.
270. Weinrich, D. Ionic mechanism of post-tetanic potentiation at the neuromuscular junction of the frog. *J. Physiol. (Lond.)* 212: 431–446, 1971.
271. Whipp, B. J. The control of exercise hyperpnea. In: *Regulation of Breathing, Part I*. New York: Marcel Dekker, Inc., 1981, p. 1069–1139.
272. Wible, J. H., F. C. Luft, and J. A. DiMicco. Hypothalamic GABA suppresses sympathetic outflow to the cardiovascular system. *Am. J. Physiol.* 254 (*Regulatory Integrative Comp. Physiol.* 22): R680–R687, 1988.
273. Wiley, R. L., and A. R. Lind. Respiratory responses to sustained static muscular contractions in humans. *Clin. Sci.* 4: 221–234, 1971.
274. Yamamoto, W. S. Looking at the regulation of ventilation as a signalling process. In: *Muscular Exercise and the Lung*, edited by J. A. Dempsey and C. E. Reed. Madison, WI: University of Wisconsin Press, 1977, p. 137–149.
275. Younes, M. The physiological basis of central apnea and periodic breathing. *Curr. Pulmonol.* 10: 265–326, 1989.
276. Zucker, R. S. Short-term synaptic plasticity. *Annu. Rev. Neurosci.* 12: 13–31, 1989.
277. Zuntz, N., and J. Geppert. Uber die Natur der normalen Atemreize und den Ort ihrer Wirkung. *Arch. Ges. Physiol.* 38: 337–338, 1886.

10. Reflexes controlling circulatory, ventilatory and airway responses to exercise

MARC P. KAUFMAN | *Division of Cardiovascular Medicine, Departments of Internal Medicine and Human Physiology, University of California, Davis, Davis, California*

HUBERT V. FORSTER | *Department of Physiology, Medical College of Wisconsin, Milwaukee, Wisconsin*

CHAPTER CONTENTS

EXERCISE HAS MARKED EFFECTS on the cardiovascular and respiratory systems. For example, both dynamic and static exercise increase ventilation and heart rate, the latter effect being caused by vagal withdrawal as well as by sympathetic activation. Moreover, static and heavy dynamic exercise increase arterial pressure. The precise nature of the mechanisms responsible for these autonomic and ventilatory effects is unclear, but a reflex arising from exercising muscles as well as reflexes arising from the heart, great vessels, and carotid bodies are important candidates. The purpose of this chapter is to define how these reflex mechanisms contribute to the exercise-induced activation of the autonomic and ventilatory systems. Central command, a feedforward mechanism, is another important candidate, and its role in causing the cardiovascular and respiratory responses to exercise is addressed in Chapter 9.

The first part of this chapter will focus on how reflexes from skeletal muscle, the heart, and great vessels, as well as the carotid bodies, affect the cardiovascular system during exercise. Particular attention will be paid to defining the components of the reflex arc arising from contracting limb muscles. These components have not been described previously in detail. Description of this reflex arc will include the discharge properties of the primary afferents arising from contracting muscle, the central neural pathways, their neurotransmitters, as well as their end-organ effects.

The second part of this chapter will focus on how reflexes from skeletal muscle, the heart, the lungs, and the carotid bodies affect the respiratory system during exercise. The second part also contains some discussion about ventilatory load compensation, short-term modulation, and the mediation of exercise hyperpnea by multiple mechanisms. The chapter finishes with some speculation about the importance of these reflexes in causing the autonomic and ventilatory responses to exercise.

REFLEX CARDIOVASCULAR RESPONSES TO MUSCULAR CONTRACTION IN ANESTHETIZED AND DECEREBRATE ANIMALS

Sensory Innervation of Skeletal Muscle

Hindlimb as well as forelimb skeletal muscle is innervated by five types of sensory nerves. These have been labeled groups I through IV, with the first group having two subtypes, Ia and Ib. The classification scheme is based on the diameter and the degree of myelination of the sensory (i.e., afferent) fibers, both of which are important determinants of axonal conduction velocity (55, 221). Specifically, the thicker the fiber and the more myelin surrounding it, the faster the fiber conducts impulses.

In cats, group Ia and Ib muscle afferents are thickly myelinated and conduct impulses between 72 and 120 m/s. The receptors of group Ia afferents are primary muscle spindles and those of group Ib afferents are Golgi tendon organs. Primary spindle afferents (i.e., group Ia) are situated "in parallel" with the skeletal muscle fibers that they innervate. Consequently, the discharge of primary spindle afferents is stimulated by stretch (i.e., lengthening) of the muscle but is inhibited by contraction (i.e., shortening). Golgi tendon organs, on the other hand, are situated in series with the muscle fibers they innervate; consequently, these afferents are stimulated by both muscle stretch and contraction.

Group II afferents, also known as secondary spindles, are myelinated and in cats conduct impulses between 31 and 71 m/s. The receptors of these afferents (i.e., the spindles), like their group Ia counterparts, are situated "in parallel" with the muscle fibers that they innervate. Although secondary spindle afferents (i.e., group II) are stimulated by muscle stretch, they are not capable of signaling the rate at which this occurs. In contrast, primary spindle afferents (i.e., group Ia) are capable of signaling the rate of stretch; consequently, they are said to be "dynamically sensitive." Skeletal muscle is also supplied to nonspindle group II afferents, which are sensitive to mechanical distortion of their receptive fields, but not to muscle stretch.

Group III afferents, also known as Aδ fibers, are thinly myelinated and conduct impulses between 2.5 and 30 m/s. Their receptors are free nerve endings. Group IV afferents, also known as C-fibers, are unmyelinated and conduct impulses at less than 2.5 m/s. Like their group III counterparts, the receptors of group IV afferents are free nerve endings. Nevertheless, the endings innervating both group III and IV afferents are almost entirely surrounded by Schwann cells. A small portion of the ending is bare, and this area is thought to be the site of action for the stimuli that activate these group III and IV afferents. Moreover, the bare areas of the nerve ending have been shown to contain mitochondria and other structures suggesting that these areas are indeed the receptive part of the sensory neuron (8).

Serial reconstruction of electron micrographs has revealed the locations of the endings of group III and IV afferents in the calcaneal (i.e., Achilles) tendon of the cat (8). Five locations were found for the endings of group III afferents. Two of these locations were in vessels (venules and lymph), two were in the connective tissue of the peritenonium externum and internum, and the other was in the endoneurium. The locations of the endings of group IV afferents displayed a marked topographic relationship to the blood and lymphatic vessels of the tendon. Moreover, group IV endings, but not group III, contain granulated vesicles, the content of which is unknown. These granulated vesicles may contain neuropeptides, whose release via the "axon reflex" evokes vasodilation. Obviously, the location of the group IV endings in blood vessels is ideal to cause this dilation. In addition, preliminary description of the locations of the endings of group III and IV afferents in the triceps surae muscles of the cat appear to parallel closely the locations of these endings in the calcaneal tendon (477). In both the tendon and the muscles, the diameters of the group III endings were found to be larger than those of the group IV endings. Also, group III endings had more mitochondria and had a more distinct receptor matrix than did group IV endings (8, 477).

Reflex Autonomic Responses to Stimulation of Muscle Afferents in Anesthetized Animals

Four types of stimuli have been used to investigate the reflex autonomic responses to stimulation of sensory nerves with endings in skeletal muscle of anesthetized animals. These stimuli are electrical pulses applied to muscle nerves, injection of chemicals into the arterial supply of skeletal muscle, contraction of hindlimb muscle, and mechanical stimulation of hindlimb muscle. The use of each type of stimulus poses certain limitations upon the interpretation of one's findings; these limitations will be discussed. Nevertheless, the use of each type of stimulus has revealed important information about the reflex control of the autonomic nervous system by sensory nerves in skeletal muscle. This information has led consistently to the conclusion that stimulation of thinly myelinated (i.e. group III) and unmyelinated (i.e., group IV) muscle afferents reflexly increases cardiovascular and ventilatory function, whereas stimulation of thickly myelinated (i.e., group Ia, Ib and II) muscle afferents has little or no effect.

Electrical Stimulation of Muscle Nerves. Electrical stimulation of muscle nerves has been an appealing technique because it is simple to use and provides an easily quantified stimulus, the timing of which can be controlled precisely. Furthermore, this technique takes advantage of the well-known fact that the thickest fibers (i.e., group I) have the lowest threshold for activation by electrical pulses. Moreover, the response has a sudden onset, is repeatable, and is usually large in magnitude. In addition and most importantly, measurement of the compound action potential that is evoked by an electrical pulse enables the investigator to reach a conclusion about the fiber types that were activated by the stimulus. Despite this impressive advantage, the use of electrical stimulation has severe drawbacks. Probably the most significant one is that applying electrical pulses to a nerve even at low frequencies rarely simulates the discharge patterns of afferent fibers stimulated by physiological or pathophysiological conditions. Furthermore, electrical stimulation of a nerve does not distinguish between axons signaling different modalities of sensation. Moreover, the frequency of the electrical pulses applied to a nerve often is in excess of the frequency generated by naturally occurring stimuli. Finally, measurements of the compound action potential, which indicate the synchronous discharge of action potentials by many fibers, may not reveal the activation of a small number of other fibers, which in fact may be the initiators of any observed reflex autonomic effect.

Electrical stimulation of rapidly conducting group III muscle afferents has been shown to decrease reflexly arterial pressure and heart rate (235, 288, 337, 440) but to increase reflexly ventilation (427). The definition of rapidly conducting group III afferents is not precise, but examination of the evidence suggests that it encompasses muscle afferents conducting between 20 and 30 m/s, with the low end extending possibly to 17 m/s (95). On the other hand, electrical stimulation of slowly conducting (i.e., 2.5 to 17–20 m/s) group III and IV afferents consistently increases autonomic function. These reflex effects have been shown to include arterial pressure, cardiac rate, cardiac contractility, ventilation, and sympathetic discharge (172, 194, 235, 245, 337, 407, 416, 427).

Although there is widespread agreement that autonomic and ventilatory functions are increased reflexly by stimulation of muscle nerves at current intensities that are sufficient to recruit group III and IV afferents, there is considerable controversy about whether autonomic and ventilatory function is also increased reflexly by electrical stimulation of muscle nerves at current intensities that recruit only group I and II afferents. For example, there are a substantial number of reports that electrical stimulation of group I and II muscle afferents reflexly increases arterial pressure, heart rate, and breathing in anesthetized animals (45, 67, 68, 271, 361, 427). In contrast, others find that stimulation of group I and II afferents has no effect on these variables (235, 282, 337, 385, 407, 414, 440, 459, 461, 462).

This controversy might be resolved by an examination of the types of afferent fibers recruited by the electrical pulses. Two methods have been used to identify the fiber types recruited by the electrical stimuli. The first was the measurement of compound action potentials, and the second was the measurement of the stimulus current as a multiple of motor threshold (i.e., the minimal current needed to evoke a muscle twitch). We speculate that neither method revealed that a small number of group III afferents were recruited by electrical pulses that were believed to activate only group I and II afferents. This speculation might be supported by the fact that many of the studies that claimed to activate electrically only group I and II afferents used a 100 μs pulse width, a duration that is capable also of activating group III afferents (508). In fact, the probability of selectively activating group I and II afferents is greater if pulse widths of 50 μs or less are used than if pulse widths of 100 μs are used. In fact, group I and II afferents can be activated with pulse widths as low as 25 μs. On the other hand, the possibility exists that stimulation of group I and II afferents evokes cardiovascular and respiratory reflexes. If this is in fact the case, the evidence from anesthetized animals suggests that the reflex increases are quite modest compared to those evoked by stimulation of group III and IV afferents.

Whereas the cardiovascular and ventilatory responses to electrical stimulation of group III and IV muscle afferents are well known, the responses of the conducting airways to this stimulation have only been described recently. For example, stimulation of rapidly conducting group III, slowly conducting group III, and group IV muscle afferents relaxes reflexly airway smooth muscle in both anesthetized dogs (367, 407) and cats (455). The efferent arm of this reflex arc in anesthetized dogs consists of cholinergic (i.e., vagal) withdrawal to airway smooth muscle. Excitation of β-adrenergic pathways to the airway played no role in this effect (407). The efferent arm of the reflex airway dilation evoked by stimulation of group III and IV afferents in anesthetized cats is unknown. One candidate is the nonadrenergic noncholinergic pathway, which exists in cats, monkeys, and humans, but not in dogs (406). Cholinergic pathways also appear to be responsible for the airway dilation evoked by dynamic exercise in humans (242, 486), but the neural mechanism causing this dilation in humans is unknown. Three candidates are the muscle reflex, the central command, and the Hering-Breuer reflex.

Electrical stimulation of group III and IV hindlimb afferents has also been shown to have reflex effects on the upper airways, structures whose caliber is under the control of skeletal rather than smooth muscle. Stimulation of these thin fiber afferents has been shown to increase the electromyographic (EMG) discharge of dilator muscles of the upper airway (194, 455). These studies revealed no evidence that electrical stimulation of group I and II afferents had any reflex effect on the activity of skeletal muscles controlling the caliber of the upper airway.

Injection of Chemicals. Injection of certain chemicals into the arterial supply of hindlimb skeletal muscle has reflex effects on the cardiovascular and respiratory systems that are highly similar to those evoked by electrical stimulation of hindlimb group III and IV afferents. The chemicals used to evoke these reflex effects are sometimes algesic and are often metabolic by-products of muscular contraction. The latter is an obvious reason why chemicals have been used to evoke reflex autonomic responses.

The reflex effect evoked by injection of chemicals into the arterial supply of the hindlimb muscles of anesthetized animals includes increases in mean arterial pressure, cardiac rate, cardiac contractility, cardiac output, breathing frequency, tidal volume, and airway dilation. The chemicals used to evoke these reflex effects have been potassium (297, 408, 415, 458, 501), capsaicin (87, 99, 256, 491), bradykinin (256, 369, 415, 447, 458, 460), lactic acid (445, 467), citrate (460), and diprotonated sodium phosphate (438, 460). These reflex effects have been obtained in several species, including cats, rabbits, and dogs. Injection of these chemicals into the arterial supply of hindlimb skeletal muscle can be extremely painful; therefore, these experiments cannot be done without either anesthesia or decerebration. Intra-arterial injection of serotonin (415, 458), adenosine, vasopressin, angiotensin, epinephrine, norepinephrine, oxytocin, and nicotine (458) have been reported to evoke no reflex autonomic effects. Likewise, intra-arterial injection of lactate at a neutral pH has been found to evoke no reflex effects (401).

The origin of the reflex evoked by lactic acid in rats is unclear. Thimm et al. (467) reported that injection of lactic acid into the arterial supply of the rat's hindlimb reflexly increased heart rate. Gregory et al. (182) confirmed this finding. Nevertheless, Gregory et al. (182) found that cutting the nerves supplying the hindlimb muscles of rats had no effect on the heart rate increase evoked by intra-arterial injection of lactic acid, whereas cutting the nerves supplying the hindlimb skin abolished or greatly attenuated the increase.

The chemicals named above stimulate group III and IV muscle afferents. In addition, injection of these chemicals has little or no direct effect on the discharge of group I or II muscle afferents (i.e., spindles or Golgi tendon organs). However, these chemicals can indirectly increase the discharge of these thickly myelinated afferents by reflexly activating γ-motoneurons (see below). One chemical that does stimulate muscle spindles (i.e., group Ia and II) and to a lesser extent Golgi tendon organs (i.e., group Ib) is succinylcholine (124, 175, 481). Injection of succinylcholine into the arterial supply of hindlimb muscle in anesthetized cats has no effect on ventilation, arterial pressure, or heart rate (481). Moreover, injection of succinylcholine into the arterial supply of hindlimb skeletal muscle does not stimulate group III and IV afferents if the muscle is not allowed to fasciculate (481). These findings provide support for the hypothesis that stimulation of group I and II hindlimb muscle afferents have little or no effect on cardiovascular or ventilatory function.

The use of chemical injections to evoke these reflex autonomic effects has one important advantage and two important disadvantages. The advantage is that metabolic products of muscular contraction can be screened for their ability to evoke autonomic effects similar to those evoked by exercise. This advantage, when combined with knowledge of the concentration of the injected metabolite in the interstitium of the skeletal muscle, is a powerful strategy with which an investigator can assess the contribution of a substance to the reflex pressor response to exercise. One disadvantage is that interstitial concentrations of most injected metabolites cannot yet be measured with current technology.

This makes it impossible to know if the injected metabolite is capable of evoking a reflex at concentrations caused by muscular contraction. For example, although static contraction increases intramuscular concentrations of bradykinin and arachidonic acid (395, 446), the inability to measure on line interstitial concentrations of these substances or their metabolites has left uncertain their roles in causing the exercise pressor reflex.

The second disadvantage of injections of metabolites into the arterial supply of hindlimb muscle is that a concentration gradient is established. This gradient is high in the arterial wall and low in the interstitium of the skeletal muscle. Hence, reflex effects can be evoked by the stimulation of sensory nerve endings in the arteriolar walls, where the concentration of the injected metabolite is probably much higher than that occurring during muscular contraction. A gradient of precisely this nature may have occurred in the studies examining the role of potassium in evoking the exercise pressor reflex (409).

To make a case that any particular metabolite plays an important role in causing the exercise pressor reflex, an investigator must be able to show that exogenous injection of it causes autonomic effects highly similar to those evoked by exercise. The need to provide this information clearly outweighs the two disadvantages cited above. Nevertheless, these disadvantages must always be considered when interpreting the data.

Contraction of Hindlimb Skeletal Muscle. Contraction has been the third method used to investigate the reflex autonomic responses to stimulation of sensory nerves with endings in hindlimb skeletal muscle. In anesthetized animals, contraction of hindlimb muscles is often accomplished by electrical stimulation of the peripheral cut ends of the lower lumbar and upper sacral ventral roots, which contain the axons of α- and γ-motoneurons. Contraction of these muscles has also been accomplished by electrical stimulation of the intact nerves, with the electrode usually being placed at the point of entry of the nerve into the muscle.

There is overwhelming evidence that static (i.e., tetanic) contraction of hindlimb muscles reflexly increases arterial pressure, heart rate, and minute volume of ventilation in anesthetized cats (94, 234, 311), dogs (79, 98, 141, 459, 468), and rabbits (462), but not in rats (365, 475). The above-mentioned increases in arterial pressure, heart rate and ventilation are the three best known components of the exercise pressor reflex but in reality are only part of a large constellation of reflexes evoked by to static muscular contraction in anesthetized animals. This constellation of reflexes includes increases in cardiac output (98, 119), relaxation of airway smooth muscle (257, 260, 300), increases in cardiac contractility (141, 338), and increases in the electrical activity of skeletal muscles whose contraction dilates the upper airways (412). Moreover, static contraction in anesthetized dogs decreases reflexly blood flow to the kidney, but has no effect on flow to the brain, heart, liver and spleen (78, 98). Finally, static contraction increases reflexly α-adrenergic tone to the coronary arteries, but the constrictor effect is masked by a metabolic vasodilation evoked in turn by the contraction-induced increases in cardiac rate and contractility (20).

McCloskey and Mitchell (311) showed that the afferent arm of the reflex arc causing the pressor response to static contraction of hindlimb muscles of cats was comprised of group III (Aδ) and IV (C) fibers. These investigators found that application of lidocaine to the dorsal roots, a maneuver that blocked impulse conduction in group III and IV afferents but not in group I and II fibers, prevented the increase in heart rate and blood pressure seen during contraction (Fig. 10.1). By contrast, application of

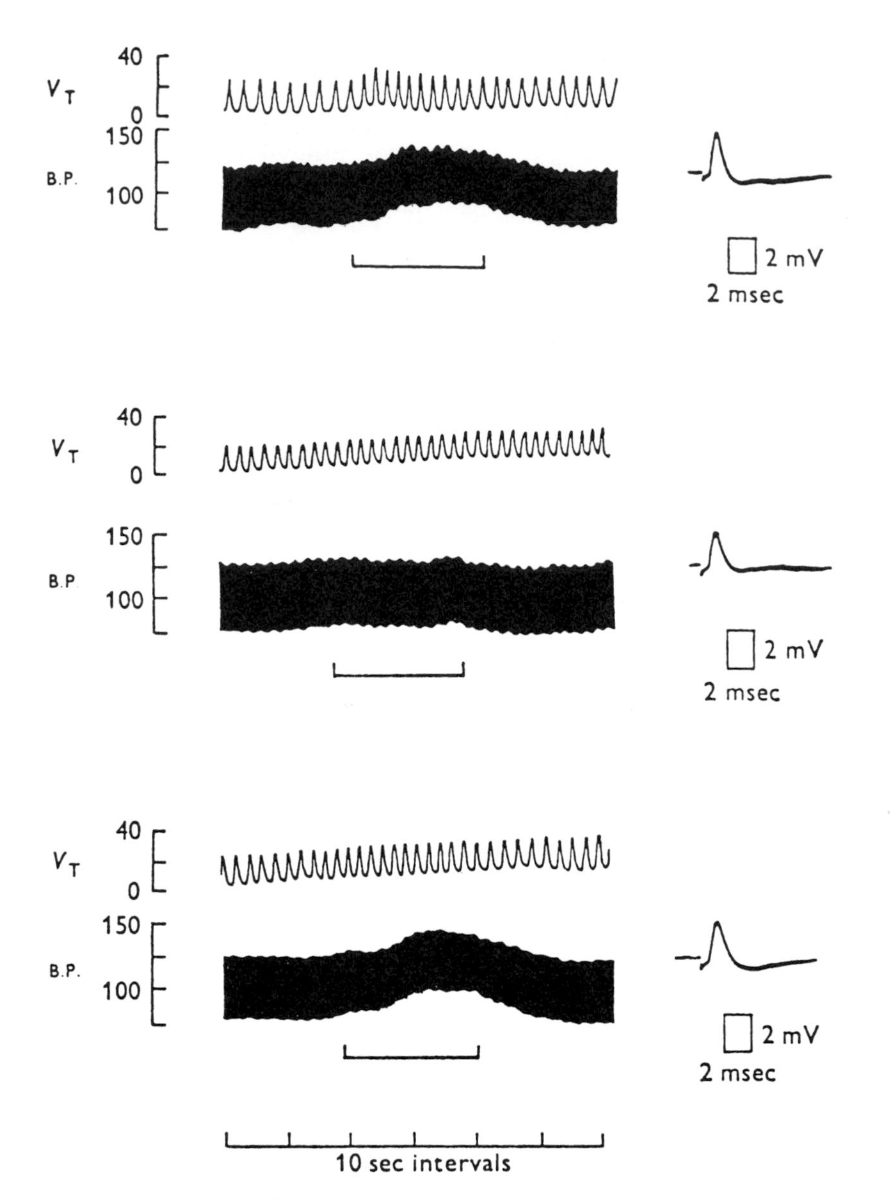

FIG. 10.1. Records of tidal volume, arterial blood pressure, and dorsal root compound action potential from three periods of static hindlimb contraction in a chloralos-anesthetized cat. From above downward are shown a control period of exercise; a period of exercise that commenced 3½ min after application of a few drops of 0.125% lidocaine solution to the dorsal roots. Note that this period of contraction produced no pressor or ventilatory response, although the A-wave of the compound action potential was little, if at all, reduced; and in the bottom set of records, a further control period of exercise begun some minutes after the lidocaine had been washed away with warm saline. [Reprinted with permission from McCloskey and Mitchell (311).].

direct anodal current to the dorsal roots, a maneuver that blocked impulse conduction in group I and II afferents but not in group III and IV afferents, had no effect on these responses to induced muscle contractions. Tibes (468) subsequently confirmed in dogs these findings of McCloskey and Mitchell (311) in cats. Using cold to block impulse conduction in afferent fibers supplying hindlimb muscles, Tibes (468) found that group III and IV afferents were responsible for the reflex increases in arterial pressure, heart rate, and ventilation evoked by dynamic contraction.

In anesthetized preparations, repetitive twitch contractions of the hindlimb muscles has been found to decrease arterial pressure, an effect which is the opposite to that evoked by static contractions. The mechanism causing this decrease may be dependent on the species being studied. In chloralose-anesthetized cats, repetitive twitch contraction (5 Hz) induced by electrical stimulation of the ventral roots decreased arterial pressure in about half the preparations tested. Section of the dorsal roots innervating the contracting muscles had no effect on this depressor effect and, therefore, it was attributed to metabolic vasodilation in the working hindlimb. When repetitive twitch contraction did evoke a pressor response, the increases were abolished by cutting the dorsal roots (261). The increase in arterial pressure, therefore, was reflex in origin. Subsequently, repetitive twitch contraction of the hindlimb muscles in decerebrate unanesthetized cats was shown to evoke a reflex pressor response in every cat tested (234).

The mechanism causing the depressor response to repetitive twitch contraction in anesthetized rabbits and dogs appears to be different from that causing this depressor response in anesthetized cats. Repetitive twitch contractions (3 Hz), induced by electrical stimulation of the hindlimb nerves of anesthetized rabbits and dogs decreased arterial pressure and heart rate, and increased ventilation (459, 462). These effects were reflex in origin and were initiated by muscular contraction. Likewise, Clement (77) reported that in anesthetized dogs repetitive twitch contractions (5 Hz), induced by electrical stimulation of the ventral roots, also reflexly decreased arterial pressure. The sensory nerves responsible for evoking these contraction-induced depressor reflexes are not known, but it is reasonable to speculate that they might be the thickly myelinated group III fibers, whose electrical stimulation reflexly decreases arterial pressure and heart rate.

The expression as well as the magnitude of the reflex pressor response to muscular contraction depends on several factors. For example, the greater the tension developed by the contracting muscles, the greater the pressor reflex (94, 226). Likewise, the greater the muscle mass contracted, the greater the pressor reflex (226, 311, 312).

The role played by red (i.e., oxidative) and white (i.e., glycolytic) muscle fibers in evoking the pressor reflex to muscular contraction remains to be fully explored. When they used decerebrate-unanesthetized cats, Iwamoto and Botterman (226) found that contraction of the soleus muscle evoked a small pressor response and that contraction of the gastrocnemius muscles evoked a large pressor response. The difference in the magnitude of the pressor reflex responses to contraction in the decerebrate-unanesthetized cat was attributed to a difference in the mass of the two muscles, the soleus weighing 4 g and the gastrocnemius muscles weighing about 22 g. The obvious implication of muscle mass is that small muscles contain fewer sensory nerves than do large muscles (410). Iwamoto and Botterman (226) showed convincingly that oxidative muscles are capable of evoking reflex autonomic effects. Moreover, they have also shown that the excitability level (i.e., type and depth of anesthesia) of the central nervous system (CNS) plays an important role in determining the magnitude of the reflex. This excitability level, which is higher in the decerebrate-unanesthetized cat than in the chloralose-anesthetized cat, facilitates a reflex response to contraction of a small muscle such as the soleus. Despite these important findings, the hypothesis that contraction of white muscle produces a larger reflex autonomic response than does contraction of an equal mass of red muscle needs to be tested. If this hypothesis was verified, it would support the concept that muscle metabolism plays an important role in evoking the exercise pressor reflex.

The exercise pressor reflex is believed to be, at least in part, the result of a mismatch between blood supply and demand in the contracting muscles. If this is in fact the case, then contraction under ischemic conditions should evoke a larger reflex than should contraction under freely perfused conditions. Occlusion of the arterial and venous supply of hindlimb skeletal muscle in anesthetized cats enhances the reflex cardiovascular responses to static contraction (94, 311, 378, 448). Occlusion also enhances the reflex airway dilation evoked by static contraction in anesthetized dogs (366).

In addition to metabolic factors caused by a mismatch between blood supply and demand in contracting muscles, the exercise pressor reflex may be elicited partly by mechanical deformation of the receptive fields of thin fiber afferents. Static contraction of the hindlimb muscles of anesthetized cats and rats, for example, increases reflexly renal, coronary, and adrenal sympathetic nerve activity with a latency of less than 1 s (305, 306, 472, 475). This rapid reflex effect appears to be best explained by a mechanical stimulus rather than by a metabolic one because the latter should take time to develop. In addition, intermittent tetanic contraction synchronizes renal nerve discharge, a reflex response that appears to be elicited by a mechanical stimulus (Fig. 10.2) (472).

In cats and dogs anesthetized with α-chloralose, muscular contraction reflexly increases heart rate, but the magnitude of the effect is small and its onset is slow, often requiring 5–10 s to appear (94, 311, 338). Moreover, the reflex heart rate increase is prevented by β-adrenergic blockade (338), but not by cholinergic blockade (94). These findings have led to the conclusion that the muscle reflex increases heart rate by sympathetic activation but not by vagal withdrawal.

The latter aspect of this conclusion has been challenged recently in an elegant study by McMahon and McWilliam (316). These investigators found that brief (i.e., 5 s) static contraction of the hindlimb

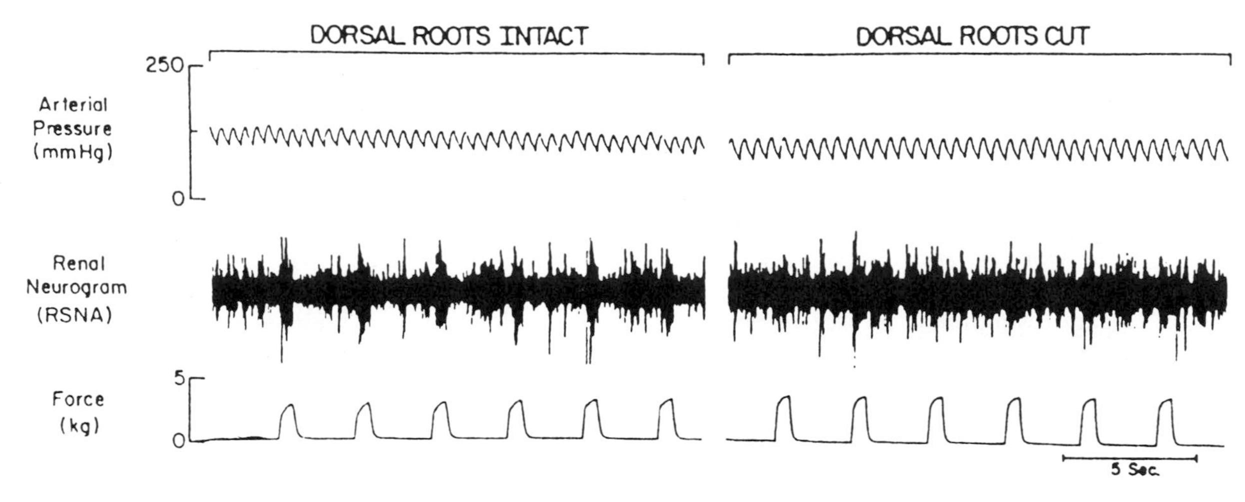

FIG. 10.2. Recordings of renal sympathetic nerve activity (RSNA) in a chloralose-anesthetized cat showing changes in RSNA evoked by intermittent tetanic contractions of the triceps surae. This maneuver synchronized the sympathetic activity such that each increase in muscle tension caused a large burst of RSNA before but not after dorsal root section. [Reprinted with permission from Victor et al. (472).]

muscles of decerebrate unanesthetized cats reflexly increased heart rate within 700 ms of the onset of muscular activity. The magnitude of the contraction-induced increase in heart rate was greater when pressure in the carotid sinus was high than when pressure was low. Moreover, cholinergic blockade with atropine prevented the rapid cardiac acceleration reflexly evoked by static contraction.

The findings reported by McMahon and McWilliam (316) have provided strong evidence that the muscle reflex can increase heart rate by withdrawal of vagal tone to the sinoatrial (S-A) node. In addition, the rapidity of the vagal withdrawal suggests that it was caused by the stimulation of group III mechanoreceptors (see below) in the contracting muscle. Furthermore, the findings of McMahon and McWilliam (316) raise the possibility that chloralose anesthesia suppresses baseline vagal tone to the S-A node and results in a blunted heart rate response to muscular contraction. This possibility is strongly supported by the finding that unanesthetized decerebrate cats display a much larger reflex tachycardic response to static contraction than do the same cats after they have been anesthetized with chloralose (234).

Mechanical Stimulation of Hindlimb Muscle. Two methods of mechanical stimulation have been used to evoke reflex autonomic effects from hindlimb skeletal muscle in anesthetized animals. The first has been the application of pressure to the muscles and the second has been tendon stretch. The purpose of either method of stimulation has been to stimulate mechanically sensitive afferents in skeletal muscle at rest. The application of pressure to the triceps surae muscles of anesthetized cats has been shown to increase reflexly both ventilation (130, 208, 245, 427) and arterial pressure, but to have no effect on heart rate (445). The pressor response to the application of pressure was quite modest (445) and may have been blunted by the use of chloralose anesthesia. Tendon stretch, the second method, has also been shown to increase reflexly ventilation (130, 245), as well as mean arterial pressure, heart rate, and cardiac contractility (445). For the cats' calcaneal tendon, the stretch threshold to evoke a pressor response appears to be a passive developed tension of 500 g. Calcaneal tendon stretch that develops passive tensions of 300 g or less evokes reflex depressor responses (440, 445), effects presumably caused by the stimulation of thickly myelinated group III muscle afferents. Both methods of stimulation (i.e., pressure and stretch) demonstrate that activation of mechanoreceptors in hindlimb skeletal muscle are capable of evoking autonomic reflex responses similar to those evoked by muscular contraction.

Discharge Properties of Group III and IV Muscle Afferents

Almost all of our knowledge about the discharge properties of group III and IV muscle afferents, the sensory nerves whose activation by contraction is responsible for the exercise pressor reflex (311), has been obtained from experiments on animals. Recently, however, group III and IV afferents, conducting between 0.6 and 13.5 m/s, have been shown to innervate human skeletal muscle (302, 434). One of the first to investigate the discharge properties of these afferents was Paintal (368), who found that group III endings located in the hindlimb muscles of dogs responded to punctate pressure. Since then, several laboratories have independently reached similar conclusions about the discharge properties of these thinly myelinated afferents. These are: (1) that about half respond to twitch contraction, be it intermittent tetanic or maintained tetanic (static) contraction (132, 255, 330, 368); (2) that about half respond to intra-arterial injection of bradykinin, a potent algesic agent (255, 283, 323); (3) that many are discharged by non-noxious punctate pressure applied to their receptive fields (195, 255, 263, 283, 330, 368); and (4) that their response to tendon stretch is variable, with some investigators finding a frequent effect (1), others finding a moderate effect (195, 255, 258, 330), and still another finding an infrequent effect (368).

Group III Afferents. Group III muscle afferents are believed to possess polymodal discharge properties (283) because they respond to both chemical and mechanical stimuli. This belief, however, is controversial because it is based on the responses of group III afferents to large and possibly unphysiological doses of bradykinin (see 326). Nevertheless, the mechanical sensitivity of these afferents might be their most relevant discharge property when assessing their contribution to evoking reflex autonomic adjustments to exercise. For example, they respond vigorously at the onset of tetanic contraction, with the first impulse often being discharged within 200 ms of the start of this maneuver (Fig. 10.3) (255). Moreover, these afferents increase their responses to tetanic contractions as the tension developed by the working muscle increases (195, 255, 330). In addition, they usually decrease their discharge rate during tetanic contraction as the tension developed by the working muscle decreases (195, 255). Finally, group III afferents are capable of synchronizing their discharge with a constantly oscillating stimulus, be it either 5 Hz twitch contraction (263) or intermittent tetanic contraction (330).

Despite their obvious mechanical sensitivity, group III afferents might also respond to the metabolic products of muscular contraction. For example, they are stimulated by bradykinin (255, 283, 323), potassium (207, 283, 323, 409, 466), arachidonic acid (399) and lactic acid (399, 436, 466). Of these metabolites, only potassium (409) and lactic acid (436, 466) have been shown, as of yet, to stim-

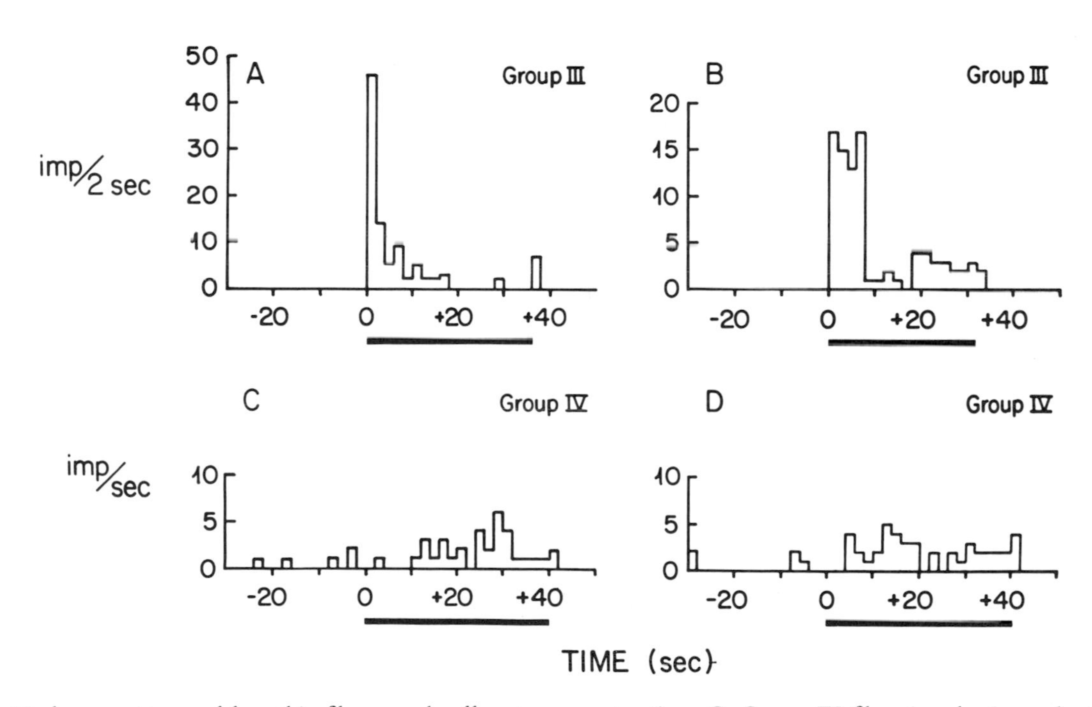

FIG. 10.3. Discharge patterns of four thin fiber muscle afferents that responded to static contraction. Contraction period depicted by *black bar*. *A*, Group III fiber (conduction velocity 17.8 m/s) discharged vigorously at onset of contraction, but then its firing rate decreased even though muscle continued to contract. *B*, Group III fiber (conduction velocity 9.6 m/s) discharged vigorously at start of contraction, adapted, and then fired again during contraction. *C*, Group IV fiber (conduction velocity 1.3 m/s) started to fire 10 s after onset of contraction and then gradually increased its firing rate during contraction period. Note that firing of fiber slowed even though muscle continued to contract. *D*, Group IV fiber (conduction velocity 1.1 m/s) fired irregularly 4 s after onset of static contraction. [Reprinted with permission from Kaufman et al. (255).]

ulate group III afferents in concentrations that may approximate those occurring in a contracting muscle. Sensitivity to metabolic products of contraction might explain why some group III afferents display a secondary response to static contraction at a time when the working muscle is fatiguing (255). In addition, histamine and serotonin stimulate group III afferents, but the required doses were quite high and the percentage of afferents stimulated was small (323). Also, it is unclear whether concentrations of histamine and serotonin increase above resting levels when skeletal muscle is contracted.

Group IV Afferents. In many respects, group IV muscle afferents possess different discharge properties than do group III muscle afferents. Although both respond to muscular contraction, group IV afferents often do not discharge vigorously at the onset of contraction as do group III afferents. Instead, group IV afferents usually display obvious responses to contraction with latencies of 5–30 s (Fig. 10.4) (255, 330). Nevertheless, group IV afferents sometimes generate one to two impulses at the onset of contraction, a response suggesting that they might possess a minimal mechanical sensitivity. Moreover, about half of the group IV afferents respond more to a static contraction while the muscles are ischemic than to a static contraction of equal magnitude while the muscles are freely perfused (Fig. 10.5) (46, 244, 262, 330). By contrast, only about 10–12% of the group III afferents respond more to an "ischemic" contraction than to a "freely perfused" one (262, 330). Therefore, group IV afferents appear to be primarily responsible for the amplification by ischemia of the reflex pressor responses to static contraction. In addition, group IV afferents are much less sensitive than are group III afferents to either probing their receptive fields or to tendon stretch. Most often, group IV afferents require noxious pinching of their receptive fields to discharge them, and frequently they do not respond to even noxious tendon stretch (255, 258, 268, 330).

Group IV afferents are stimulated by the same substances that have been shown to stimulate group III afferents. Hence, intra-arterial injection of bradykinin (255, 323, 329), potassium (207, 258, 323), lactic acid (174, 399, 466) and arachidonic acid (Fig. 10.6) (399) stimulate at least half of the group IV afferents tested. In addition, prostaglandin E_2 stimulates about half of the group IV afferents tested (324); the responses of group III afferents to this substance are unknown as of yet. Histamine and serotonin stimulated only a few group IV afferents and the threshold doses appeared to be quite high (268, 323).

Role Played by Metabolites in Stimulating Group III and IV Afferents. Metabolic products of muscular contraction are likely to play two important roles in causing the responses of group III and IV afferents to exercise. The first role is to signal that blood supply and demand are mismatched (i.e., ischemia). One cause of this signal could be insufficient washout of metabolites in the exercising muscles. A second cause could be the generation of a metabolite that was not generated when there was no mismatch. A third is that the metabolic error signal is multifactorial, and that only the right combination of metabolites, injected exogenously, will reveal which afferents are signaling that a mismatch exists. With regard to the first role, the metabolic substance signaling a mismatch is not known. Some candidates include lactic acid, bradykinin, and cyclooxygenase products of arachidonic acid. Exogenous injection of these substances stimulated equal proportions of group III and IV afferents, whereas ischemia increased the responses to contraction of a higher proportion of group IV afferents than group III afferents (262, 330). Therefore, the possibility exists that none of these products of contraction provide the "metabolic error signal." Alternatively, the doses of these substances, which were injected intra-arterially, may have produced concentrations in the muscle that greatly exceeded those produced by contraction. Thus, exogenous intra-arterial injections of low concentrations of these metabolites need to be tested.

The second role played by metabolic products of muscular contraction might be to stimulate afferents that are sensitive to neither ischemic metabolites nor mechanical distortion of their receptive fields. With regard to this second role played by metabolic products of contraction in stimulating afferents during exercise, potassium might be one candidate to activate the group III and IV endings that are neither mechanically nor ischemically sensitive. Potassium, however, is probably not a metabolite that signals a mismatch between blood supply and demand in a muscle contracting under ischemic conditions because the afferents respond transiently to it even though its concentration remained elevated for several minutes (409). This transient effect contrasts with the maintained reflex responses to postexercise ischemia in humans (6, 303).

Hypoxia is one possible consequence of a mismatch between blood supply and demand in exercising skeletal muscle. So far, the evidence that hypoxia is the signal for this mismatch is weak. For example, with the triceps surae muscle at rest, ventilation of the lungs of barbiturate-anesthetized cats with 5% oxygen in nitrogen for 3–4 min, a maneu-

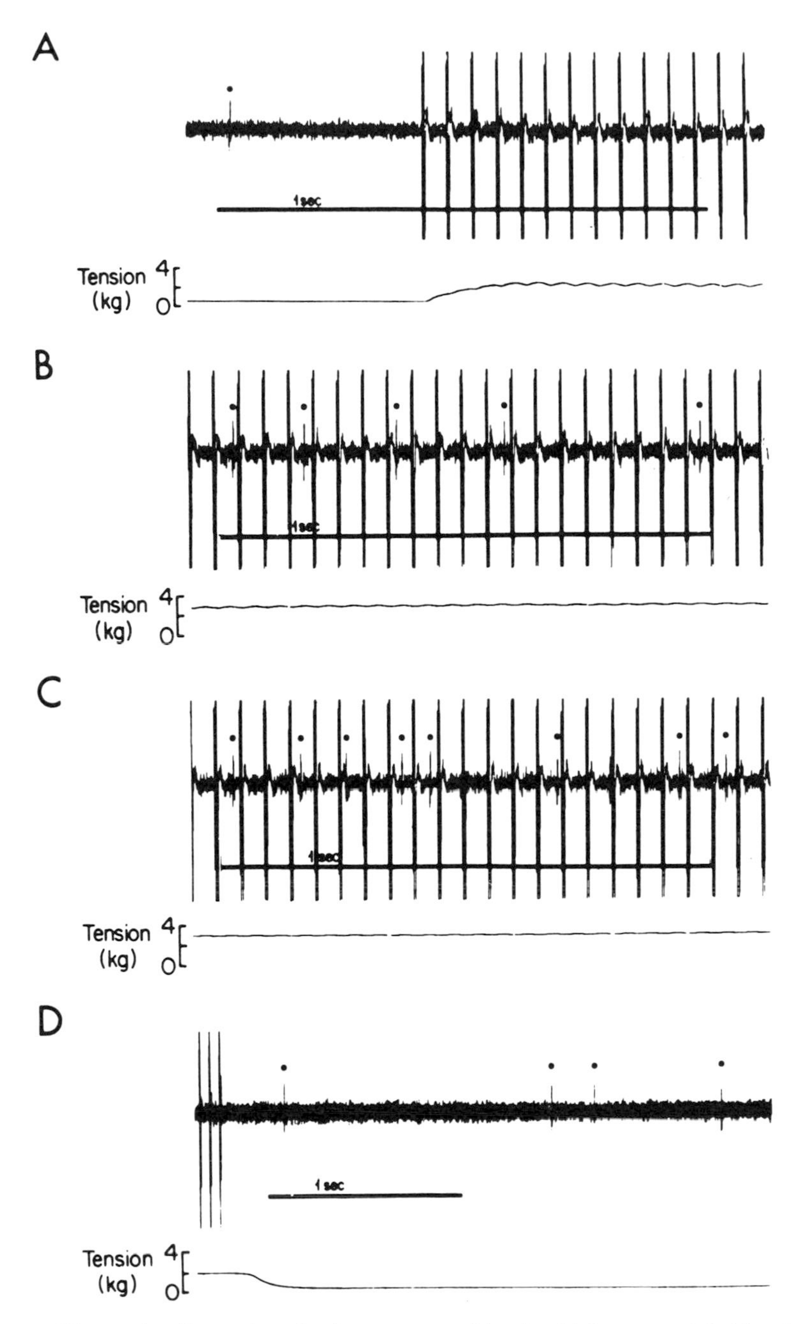

FIG. 10.4. Stimulation of group IV muscle afferent (conduction velocity 0.5 m/s) by contraction of gastrocnemius muscle, induced by ventral root stimulation. *Filled circle* (•) has been placed over each impulse discharge by group IV afferent. *A*, At onset of muscular contraction, group IV fiber did not fire. *B*, 8 s after end of *A*, group IV fiber has increased its firing rate over control level, which averaged 0.6 imp/s. *C*, 21 s after end of *B*, fiber is firing at greater rate than in *B*. *D*, After the contraction period, which lasted 45 s, fiber discharged. Horizontal bar in *A*–*D* represents 1 s. Note that chart recorder speed was slower in *D* than in *A*–*C*. [Reprinted with permission from Kaufman et al. (255).]

ver that reduced the arterial Po_2 to 22 mm Hg, had only a trivial stimulatory effect on the activity of group IV afferents and had no effect on the activity of group III afferents. Most importantly, hypoxic ventilation of the lungs for this period of time did not increase the concentration of lactate or hydrogen ions in the femoral venous blood. In addition, static contraction of the triceps surae muscles during hypoxic ventilation did not stimulate group III and IV afferents to a greater extent than did static contraction during normoxic ventilation (206).

Sensitization of Group III and IV Afferents. The responses of group III and IV afferents to muscular

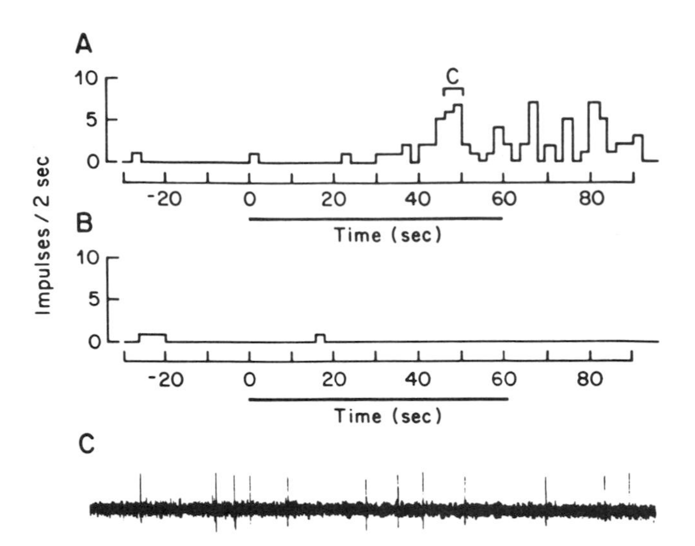

FIG. 10.5. Effect of ischemia on response to static contraction of a group IV afferent (conduction velocity 0.8 m/s) whose receptive field was in triceps surae. *A*, Stimulation of afferent by ischemic static contraction (represented by *bar*). Note maintained stimulation of afferent after end of contraction. *B*, Nonischemic contraction (represented by *bar*) had no effect on afferent. *C*, Recording of impulse activity of group IV afferent during period of time, depicted by bracket with C over it in *A*. [Reprinted with permission from Kaufman et al. (262)]

contraction is altered by changes in the chemical milieu of the interstitial space. For example, intra-arterial injection of bradykinin increased the responses of both group III and IV afferents to intermittent tetanic contraction of the triceps surae muscles (327). Likewise, intra-arterial injections of arachidonic acid increased the responses of group III but not those of group IV afferents to static contraction (398, 400). Manipulations of the chemical milieu of the interstitium of the triceps surae muscle that decrease the concentrations of various metabolites also have an effect on the afferents' response to contraction. Hence, indomethacin and aspirin, substances that decrease the muscle's ability to synthesize prostaglandins and thromboxanes, decreased the responses of group III and IV afferents to static contraction of the triceps surae muscles (398, 400). Likewise, sodium dichloroacetate, a compound that decreases the concentrations of lactic acid in the muscle, decreased the responses of group III afferents to static contraction of the triceps surae muscles (436). Specifically, dichloroacetate decreased the sensitivity of the group III afferents to the first 10 s of static contraction. One interpretation of this finding is that the concentration of lactic acid in muscle determines, in part, the mechanical sensitivity of the group III afferents with which it is innervated. The effect of dichloroacetate on the responses of group IV afferents to contraction is not known.

The finding that the concentrations of bradykinin and cyclooxygenase products of arachidonic acid in skeletal muscle increase the sensitivity of group III and IV afferents to contraction has an important implication for the interpretation of experimental results. Both inflammation and trauma increase the concentrations of these substances in skeletal mucle. Consequently, the degree of inflammation and trauma to skeletal muscle needs to be considered when determining the effects of muscular contraction on the discharge of group III and IV afferents. Consideration of this possibility is critical in skeletal muscle preparations that have undergone extensive surgery or have been manipulated manually to stimulate the receptive fields of group III and IV afferents. In addition, the effects of anti-inflammatory agents, such as dexamethasone and aspirin-like drugs, on the responsiveness of these thin fiber afferents to contraction also needs to be considered carefully. Dexamethasone, for example, is frequently given to reduce brain swelling after decerebration.

Muscular Contraction vs. Exercise. Muscular contraction, induced by electrical stimulation of the axons of α-motoneurons in either the ventral roots or the peripheral nerves, has been an extremely useful tool with which to study the mechanical and metabolic sensitivities of group III and IV muscle afferents. Nevertheless, electrical stimulation recruits α-motoneurons in an order opposite to that occurring during reflex or physiological activation (198). Specifically, electrical stimulation recruits the fastest conducting (i.e., thickest) α-motoneurons first, whereas exercise, be it static or dynamic, recruits the slowest conducting (i.e., thinnest) α-motoneurons first (210). Moreover, electrical stimulation discharges α-motoneurons synchronously, whereas exercise discharges them asynchronously (209, 211, 494).

In light of these findings, muscular contraction, induced by electrical stimulation of α-motoneurons should not be considered the same as exercise. Differences between the recruitment orders and discharge patterns of α-motoneurons during "muscular contraction" and during "exercise" might result in the stimulation of different populations of group III and IV muscle afferents. For example, different α-motoneuron recruitment orders and discharge patterns could, conceivably, cause different mechanical stresses on the receptive fields of mechanoreceptors as well as cause different patterns of blood flow through the working muscle. This latter effect, in turn, could cause differences between metaboreceptor responses to muscular contraction and those to exercise.

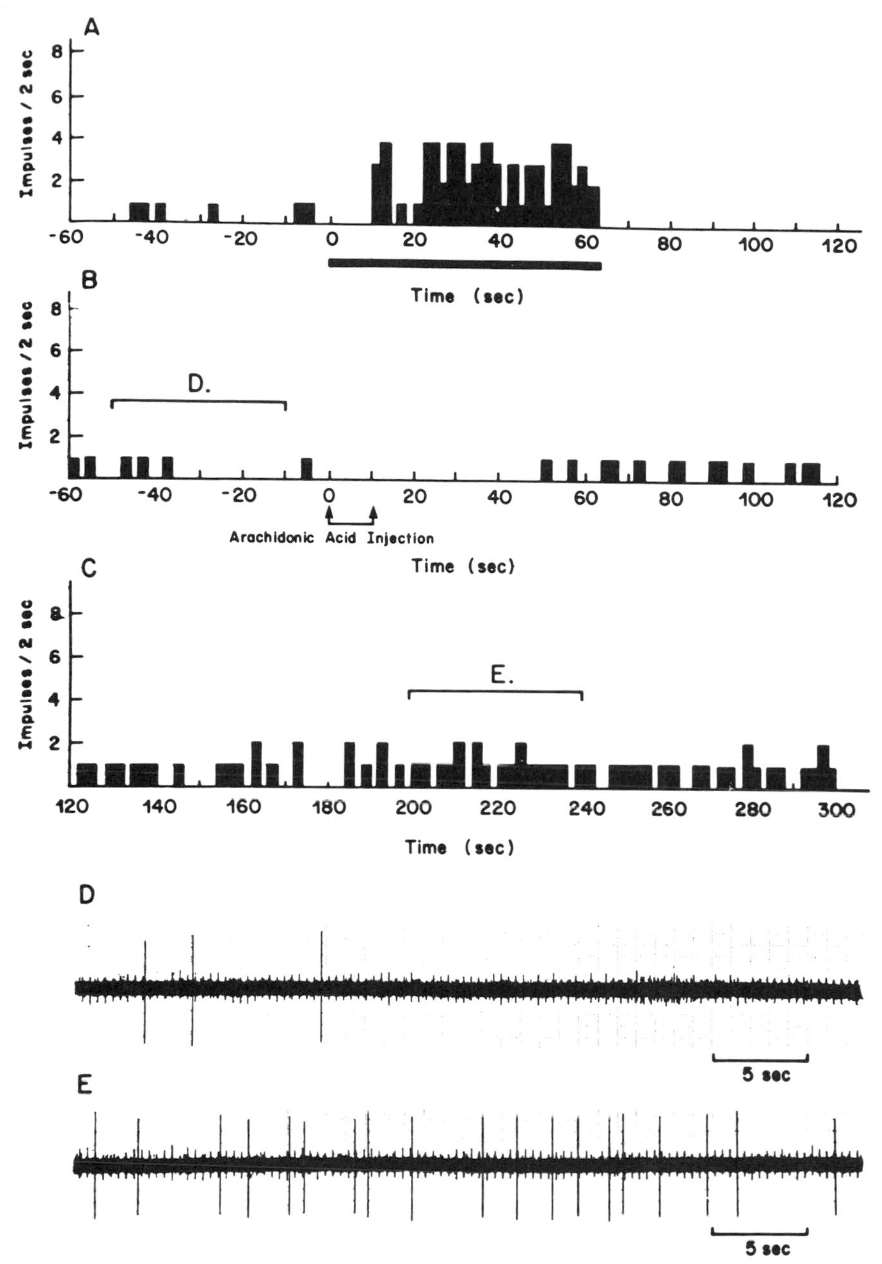

FIG. 10.6. Effects of static contraction (*A*) and arachidonic acid (1 mg in 1 ml) injection into femoral artery (*B* and *C*) on discharge of a group IV afferent (conduction velocity 1.1 m/s). ■, Contraction period in *A*. Note that *B* and *C* are continuous in time. *D*, Recording of the impulse activity of afferent during period of time depicted by *bracket* with *D* over it in *B*. *E*, Recording of impulse activity of afferent during period of time depicted by the *bracket* with *E* over it in *C*. [Reprinted with permission from Rotto and Kaufman (399).]

The difficulties in equating muscle contraction with exercise made it imperative to determine the effect, "if any," of a true form of exercise on the discharge of thin fiber muscle afferents. So far, more than half of the group III afferents tested have been shown to be stimulated by dynamic exercise. Specifically, using decerebrate unanesthetized cats made to walk on a treadmill, Pickar et al. (384) found that group III afferents with endings in the triceps surae muscles discharged in synchrony with the contraction phase of the step cycle (Fig. 10.7). Pickar et al. also found that the threshold tension required to stimulate these group III afferents during exercise was quite low. The simplest interpretation of these findings is that low-intensity dynamic exercise stimulates mechanically sensitive group III muscle afferents. As of yet, the effect of a true form of dynamic exercise on the discharge of group IV muscle affer-

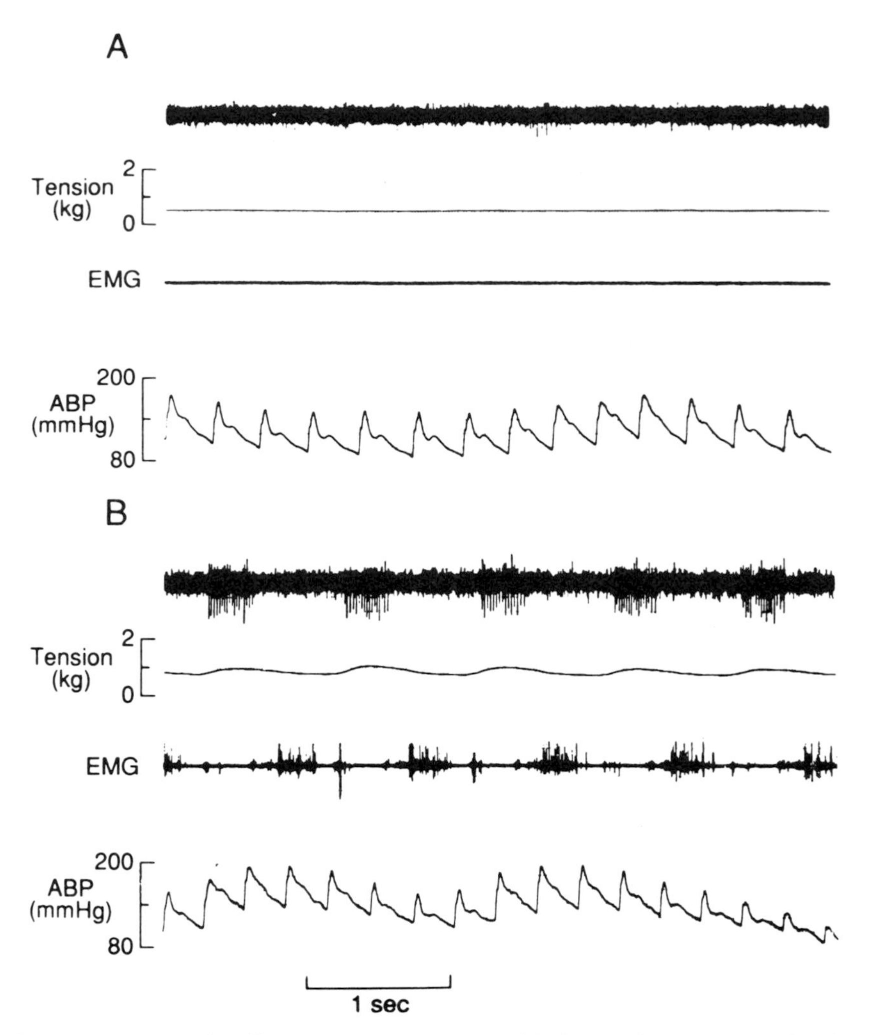

FIG. 10.7. Response of a group III muscle afferent in triceps surae muscles to dynamic exercise. Afferent (conduction velocity 11.7 m/s) was strongly sensitive to exercise. *A*: Control period before and *B*, 5-step cycles during walking evoked by stimulation of MLR. [Reprinted with permission from Pickar, Hill, and Kaufman (383).]

ents has not been examined. Likewise, the effect of static exercise on the discharge of group III and IV afferents has not been examined.

The Site of the First Synapse—The Dorsal Horn

Anatomical and Electrophysiological Evidence. Group III and IV muscle afferents with endings in hindlimb muscle enter the spinal cord by the dorsal roots and make their synapse in the dorsal horn of the gray matter. A small number of group IV afferents send their axons into the ventral roots, a finding in exception to the law of Bell and Magendie. This law states that the dorsal roots are comprised solely of sensory fibers and the ventral roots are comprised solely of motor fibers. Convincing evidence has been presented that these group IV fibers reverse their course in the ventral roots and enter the dorsal horn via the dorsal roots (22, 394, 432). In addition, most of these unmyelinated (i.e., group IV) fibers, which make a U-turn in the ventral roots, innervate the viscera and skin (82). One can easily avoid activating these "ventral root C-fibers" when electrically stimulating the ventral roots to contract hindlimb muscle by keeping the current intensity of the electrical pulses at or below three times motor threshold; unmyelinated (i.e., C-fiber) axons require much higher currents to activate them than do the axons of α-motoneurons, which are maximally recruited by current intensities of three times motor threshold.

Light and Perl (293) were among the first investigators to use horseradish peroxidase (HRP) to trace the termination of thin fiber sensory nerves in the dorsal horn of the spinal cord. When they used light microscopy, Light and Pearl found labeling from the terminals of thinly myelinated (i.e., Aδ-fiber) afferents in Rexed's lamina I (i.e., the marginal zone) and in the inner portion of lamina II (i.e., the substantia gelatinosa). In addition, labeling from the terminals of presumed unmyelinated (i.e., C-fiber) afferents was found in both the inner and outer portions of lamina II. The terminal labeling described by Light and Perl (293) arose from the application of HRP to the cut central ends of the cervical, lumbar, and sacral dorsal roots of cats, rats, and monkeys. This labeling, therefore, represented the termination of afferent fibers innervating a variety of structures including, muscle, skin, joints, and bone.

Subsequently, Craig and Mense (97) and Mense and Craig (325) applied wheat germ agglutin conjugated to HRP (WGA-HRP) to the gastrocnemius and soleus nerves of cats. The application of WGA-HRP to these nerves was an attempt to limit terminal labeling in the dorsal horn to only muscle afferents. Terminal labeling was found with light microscopy in laminae I and V; it was not found in significant amounts in laminae II–IV (97, 325). The terminal labeling in laminae I and V was attributed to thin fiber muscle afferents, because WGA-HRP is believed to label predominantely C-fiber (i.e., group IV) terminals in the dorsal horn (456).

These reports have been confirmed and extended by studies in which the cell bodies of group III gastrocnemius afferents were impaled and filled with HRP. Terminal labeling in these filled dorsal root ganglion cells was found in laminae I and V (328). Impaling and filling small cells such as those supplying the axons of group III and IV afferents is extremely difficult, and consequently it has not been done for group IV afferents, the cell bodies of which are smaller in size than those of group III afferents.

Electrophysiological studies have also provided important information about the location of the synapses made by group III and IV afferents in the dorsal horn. Thus, group III afferents, when stimulated electrically, excited cells in laminae I, II, V, and VI (212, 386). Furthermore, group III and IV muscle afferents, when stimulated by algesic substances, excited spinothalamic cells, whose dendrites were located in laminae II–VI, but were not located in lamina I (149). Moreover, stimulation of free nerve endings (i.e., group III, IV, and nonspindle group II) in hindlimb skeletal muscle by tetanic contraction, muscle stretch, and non-noxious probing stimulated cells in laminae V–VII of decerebrate-spinal cats (76). Electrophysiological findings, though valuable, must be interpreted cautiously because of the difficulty involved in determining the number of synapses between the stimulus and the dorsal horn cell responsive to it. This is especially true when dealing with slowly conducting afferents. Delays between the onset of a stimulus and the appearance of a spike in the dorsal horn might be due to transmission across many synapses.

Electrophysiological experiments have provided two other important findings. The first is that cold block of descending input from central neural structures above the lumbar spinal cord increased the number of receptive fields of dorsal horn cells receiving hindlimb input. The second is that cold block increased the mechanical responsiveness of those cells to a given stimulus (212). The most likely interpretation of these findings is that the dorsal horn receives from higher central neural structures a tonic inhibitory input that functions to gate or dampen group III and IV afferent input. This might be one mechanism whereby central command, arising from the hypothalamic locomotor region (131), might gate the muscle reflex. In addition, this mechanism might provide a neurophysiological basis for "redundancy." However, with respect to the autonomic responses to exercise, as of yet, there is no evidence that such gating occurs in the dorsal horn.

Neurotransmitters and Neuromodulators in the Dorsal Horn. Thin fiber muscle afferents (i.e., groups III and IV) are thought to release onto cells in the dorsal horn a neurotransmitter, which acts rapidly, as well as a neuromodulator, which acts slowly. The nature of the neurotransmitter is not firmly established, but glutamate is one substance that is a strong candidate. The neuromodulator might be substance P, an 11 amino acid peptide, but others such as somatostatin and calcitonin gene-related peptide (CGRP) might also function in this role.

Glutamate, an excitatory amino acid, has been known for some time to be contained by primary afferents synapsing in the dorsal horn (173, 236). More recently, glutamate was found in electron microscopic studies to be contained in scalloped terminals that were dark and which possessed agranular vesicles. These terminals, which were found in laminae I and II, were believed to be the endings of thinly myelinated (i.e., group III) and unmyelinated (i.e., group IV) primary afferent fibers (111). Moreover, substance P was often co-localized with glutamate in the spinal terminals of these group III and IV afferents (111).

Other findings point to a possible role for glutamate in the spinal neurotransmission of sensory input from the hindlimb. In addition to being contained in the terminals of group III and IV afferents, glutamate was found to be released in the dorsal horn when thin fiber somatic afferents were activated (246, 396). Moreover, glutamate can activate spinal neurons (106, 422, 423).

The role of glutamate in the spinal transmission of sensory input from the hindlimb has also been investigated. Yoshimura and Jessell (513), who used a rat spinal cord preparation in vitro, found that CNQX was much more effective than APV in attenuating the amplitude of the evoked presynaptic potentials (EPSPs) in cells in lamina II that were elicited by electrical stimulation of group III and IV afferent fibers in the dorsal roots. Because CNQX blocks non-N-ethyl-D-aspartate (non-NMDA) receptors (i.e., kainate and quisqualate) and APV blocks NMDA receptors, Yoshimura and Jessell (513) concluded that the former play an important postsynaptic role in the neurotransmission of afferent input into the spinal cord. In addition, these investigators showed that two non-NMDA receptor agonists, AMPA and kainate, which are not substrates for the high affinity L-glutamate reuptake system, depolarized glutamate-insensitive cells in the substantia gelatinosa (i.e., lamina II) of the dorsal horn. Moreover, CNQX administration attenuated the depolarizations evoked by AMPA and kainate. Yoshimura and Jessell (513) interpreted their findings to mean that a lack of sensitivity of dorsal horn cells to glutamate, such as that reported by Schneider and Perl (423), might be caused by rapid reuptake of this excitatory amino acid.

The in vitro spinal cord preparation has provided important insights into neurotransmission in the dorsal horn. Nevertheless, extension of the observations made for neurotransmission in the in vitro spinal preparation to neurotransmission of group III and IV afferent input to the spinal cord of an exercising mammal is risky. The most important limitation of the in vitro model is the necessity to activate thin fiber afferents by electrical stimulation of the dorsal roots. This stimulation offers no specificity over the origin of the sensory endings innervating the fibers being activated. Moreover, it offers no specificity over the sensory modality transduced by the fibers being activated. Finally, most observations in the in vitro model have been made in tissue obtained from rodents, a species that probably do not possess an exercise pressor reflex (365, 475).

Considerable evidence has accumulated to suggest that tachykinins, such as substance P and neurokinin A and B, function as neuromodulators in the dorsal horn. This is the site of the first synapse in the muscle reflex arc that contributes to the autonomic adjustments to exercise. For example, electrical stimulation of group III and IV afferent fibers in the sciatic nerve releases substance P in the dorsal horn (169). Likewise, static contraction of hindlimb muscles releases substance P and neurokinin A in the dorsal horn (123, 506). Moreover, section of the dorsal roots attenuates greatly the contraction-induced release of substance P in the dorsal horn (506).

There is also anatomical and electrophysiological evidence suggesting that substance P has a neuromodulator role in the dorsal horn. Thus, substance P has been found in the spinal terminals of presumed group III and IV axons traveling in the dorsal roots (66, 111, 213, 356). In addition, substance P has been shown in extracellular recording studies to stimulate dorsal horn cells receiving noxious input (199, 392). Intracellular recording studies have shown that application of substance P to dorsal horn cells causes a slow depolarization, an effect which is consistent with a neuromodulator role for this peptide in the spinal cord (168, 344). Substance P and CGRP also enhances the electrically evoked release of glutamate from thin fiber afferents in the lumbar dorsal roots (246). Likewise, substance P enhances the release of glutamate in the dorsal horn that was evoked by a noxious stimulus applied to the paw (442).

Somatostatin and calcitonin-gene related peptide (CGRP) are two other neuromodulator candidates in the dorsal horn. Hokfelt et al. (213) reported that in rats somatostatin was found in different spinal terminals than those in which substance P was found. In contrast, Cameron et al. (66) reported that in rats somatostatin and substance P were located in the same spinal terminals. Somatostatin is rarely found in the spinal terminals of muscle afferents in rats, but this peptide is frequently found in the terminals of skin afferents (356). Note again that contraction of hindlimb skeletal muscle in rats does not evoke a pressor reflex response (365, 475), whereas contraction in humans, dogs, cats, and rabbits does (see above). It would be interesting to determine whether the spinal terminals of muscle afferents contain somatostatin in species exhibiting an "exercise pressor reflex."

Klein et al. (267) found that electrically induced activity of Aδ and C-fibers in the sciatic nerve of rats depleted CGRP in the superficial dorsal horn (i.e., laminae I and II). Moreover, electrically induced activity in A_α and A_β fibers (i.e., groups I and II) did not deplete CGRP in the dorsal horn. These findings are consistent with a neuromodulator role for CGRP when it is released by the spinal terminals of group III and IV afferents. In addition, CGRP has been colocated immunohistochemically with substance P in the spinal terminals of thin fiber afferents in laminae I, II, and V of the dorsal horn of rats (500).

Role of Spinal Neurotransmitters and Neuromodulators in the Exercise Pressor Reflex

Recent evidence indicates that excitatory amino acids, such as glutamate and aspartate, play an important role in the spinal transmission of the exercise pressor reflex. In chloralose-anesthetized cats, Hill et al. (205) found that intrathecal lumbosacral injection of CNQX, a non-NMDA receptor antagonist, significantly attenuated the pressor and tachycardic components of the exercise pressor reflex. In contrast, intrathecal lumbosacral injection of CPP and AP5, two NMDA receptor antagonists, had no effect on these two components of the reflex. In the same cats, however, intrathecal thoracic injection of AP5 significantly attenuated the pressor response to electrical stimulation of the rostral medulla (205). These findings were interpreted to mean that non-NMDA receptors, but not NMDA receptors, play an important role in the spinal neurotransmission of the exercise pressor reflex arc. This interpretation must be viewed with caution, however, because recent electrophysiological evidence has shown that chloralose anesthesia impairs NMDA receptor function in the dorsal horn of the lumbar spinal cord of cats (391). Subsequent studies in decerebrate unanesthetized cats have revealed that NMDA receptor blockade with AP5, injected intrathecally, had no effect on the initial phase of the pressors ventilatory and tachycardic responses to contraction, but did attenuate the secondary phases (i.e. after 15 seconds) of these responses (Adreani et al., unpublished observations).

There is substantial evidence that substance P plays a modulator role in the spinal transmission of the exercise pressor reflex arc. In chloralose-anesthetized cats, intrathecal injections of either a peptide antagonist to substance P or an antibody to substance P decreased by half the reflex pressor response to static contraction of the triceps surae muscles (204, 254, 259). In a subsequent study, injection of this peptide antagonist into the spinal gray matter attenuated the reflex pressor response to static contraction of the triceps surae muscles, but had no effect on the reflex pressor response to stretching the calcaneal (i.e., achilles) tendon (507). This latter finding suggested that stretch-activated mechanoreceptors in contracting skeletal muscle did not release substance P as their neurotransmitter/neuromodulator.

The peptide antagonist to substance P used in the above studies was D-Pro^2, D-Phe^7, D-Trp^9-substance P (204, 254, 507). This antagonist blocks two of the three neurokinin receptors (i.e., NK-1 and NK-2) known to be present in the spinal cord. In addition, this substance P antagonist has local anesthetic effects (252). Recently, antagonists with activities specific for either the NK-1 or NK-2 receptor have been developed. When they used three selective tachykinin receptor antagonists, Hill et al. (204) demonstrated that blockade of the NK-1 receptor with CP-96345 attenuated both the reflex ventilatory and pressor responses to static contraction. Moreover, Hill et al. (204) found that blockade of either the NK-2 receptor or the NK-3 receptor had no effect on these reflex responses. These findings led Hill et al. (204) to conclude that although both substance P and neurokinin A are released in the dorsal horn by the group III and IV afferents stimulated by muscular contraction, these neuropeptides exert their reflex actions on autonomic function by activating NK-1 receptors.

Despite the fact that impressive evidence supports a role for substance P as a neuromodulator in the first synapse of the reflex arc evoking the pressor response to muscular contraction, a note of caution is in order. Microinjection of substance P into the dorsal horn does not increase arterial pressure or heart rate (507). This finding is disturbing because exogenous administration of substance P into its anticipated site of action (i.e., the dorsal horn) should evoke cardiovascular effects similar to those evoked reflexly by muscular contraction. A possible explanation for this disturbing finding might be that substance P, a slow-acting neuromodulator, must be co-released in the dorsal horn with glutamate, a fast-acting neurotransmitter, to evoke its autonomic effects.

Somatostatin is another neuromodulator candidate in the dorsal horn. It has been localized in the spinal terminals of the thin fiber afferents traveling in the dorsal roots. Like substance P, evidence exists that somatostatin participates in the spinal transmission of the exercise pressor reflex. Intrathecal or microinjection into the spinal gray matter of a peptide antagonist to somatostatin has been shown to attenuate the reflex pressor response to static contraction of the hindlimb muscles of chloralose anesthetized cats (313, 507). In addition, microinjection of the somatostatin antagonist did not affect the reflex pressor response to stretching the calcaneal tendon (507). Finally, microinjection of somatostatin into the dorsal horn of chloralose-anesthetized cats did not evoke a pressor response (507).

The evidence supporting a neuromodulator role for somatostatin and substance P in the spinal transmission of the exercise pressor reflex must be viewed cautiously. First, one must keep in mind that the efficacy of the blockade of these neuropeptides by their antagonists has not been established within the context of this reflex. In other words, the fact that microinjection of either somatostatin or substance P into the dorsal horn failed to evoke a pressor response prevents the investigator from demonstrating that the antagonist was effective. Second, these findings provide no information that attenuation of the pressor response to static contraction occurred because the first synapse of this reflex arc was antagonized.

CGRP is another potential neuromodulator in the spinal transmission of the exercise pressor reflex. CGRP has been co-localized with substance P in the spinal terminals of these unmyelinated afferents (356, 500). Nevertheless, the role played by CGRP in the spinal transmission of the reflex pressor to muscular contraction is not known.

Norepinephrine (107) and met-enkephalin (332) have been found in the terminals of axons whose cell bodies are located in the dorsal horn of the spinal cord. Likewise, serotonin (243) has been found in the dorsal horn, but it comes from the axon terminals whose cell bodies are located in the medullary and pontine raphe. Individual intrathecal injection of either α-adrenergic, opioid, or serotonergic agonists attenuated the reflex pressor and ventilatory responses to static hindlimb contraction in chloralose-anesthetized cats. On the other hand, individual intrathecal injection of antagonists to these substances did not potentiate the reflex pressor or ventilatory responses to contraction (201–203). The simplest interpretation of these findings is that endogenous release of serotonin, met-enkephalin, and norepinephrine play no role in buffering the reflex autonomic responses to muscular contraction in anesthetized animals.

Vasopressin has also been found in the dorsal horn of the spinal cord. There are two sources of vasopressin. The first is the paraventricular and supraoptic nuclei of the hypothalamus (244). These cell bodies project their axons to the dorsal horn. The second source is the primary afferents, whose cells bodies are located in the dorsal root ganglia (331). Intrathecal injection of a V_1 receptor antagonist to vaspressin potentiates the reflex pressor response to static contraction in chloralose anesthetized cats, whereas intrathecal injection of the agonist (i.e., vasopressin) attenuates the response (449). These findings suggest that endogenous release of vasopressin in the spinal cord buffers the reflex autonomic responses to contraction of hindlimb muscles.

Pathways Ascending from the Dorsal Horn

Supraspinal pathways are essential for the full expression of the exercise pressor reflex in decerebrate unanesthetized cats. For example, transection of the cervical spinal cord at the C1 level eliminated all but a small portion (i.e., 6 mm Hg) of this reflex (234). On the other hand, transection of the medulla 5 mm rostral to the obex had only a small effect on the magnitude of the exercise pressor reflex (234). Pathways rostral to the inferior colliculi, the site of the decerebrate transection, do not appear essential to express the exercise pressor reflex. Midcollicular decerebration had no effect on the reflex in chloralose anesthetized cats (234). Furthermore, removal of the cerebellum had no effect on this reflex in the decerebrate unanesthetized cat (234).

These findings strongly suggest that an intact medulla is needed to express the exercise pressor reflex (234). The precise pathway from the dorsal horn of the lumosacral spinal cord to the medulla is unknown, but the dorsolateral sulcus region of the cord appears to be involved. Lesions of this region attenuated the reflex pressor response evoked by muscular contraction in anesthetized dogs (277). An alternative spinal pathway may also be involved because, in decerebrate cats, the reflex pressor response to contraction persists in an attenuated but substantial form after bilateral lesioning of the dorsolateral sulcus region (227). Although the location of this alternative pathway is unknown, the ventral spinal cord is a likely candidate.

The pathway of the exercise pressor reflex arc ascending from the lumbosacral dorsal horn has also been investigated in conscious dogs performing hindlimb treadmill exercise. Kozelka et al. (276) found that bilateral lesions of the dorsolateral sulcus region had no effect on the modest pressor-tachycardic responses to exercise when the hindlimbs were freely perfused. However, these lesions significantly attenuated the large pressor-tachycardic responses to exercise when the hindlimbs were ischemic.

The Ventrolateral Medulla

There is substantial evidence indicating that the ventrolateral medulla is an important pathway in the reflex arc controlling autonomic function when hindlimb skeletal muscle is contracted. The ventrolateral medulla is usually divided into a caudal and a rostral component by investigators interested in autonomic function. In the cat, the caudal ventrolateral medulla (CVLM) extends 1.5–2 mm dorsally from the ventral surface, and rostrocaudally from the caudal pole of the lateral reticular nucleus to the rostral pole of this nucleus (74). Ciriello and Calaresu (72) offered the first clue that the CVLM might be part of the central neural circuitry of the "exercise pressor reflex" arc. They showed that bilateral electrolytic lesions of the lateral reticular nucleus abolished the reflex pressor response to electrical stimulation of cat sciatic nerve. Subsequently, Iwamoto et al. (230) reported that bilateral electrolytic lesions of the lateral reticular nucleus abolished the reflex pressor response to static contraction of cat hindlimb muscles.

Despite these findings, a role for the CVLM in the pathway evoking the exercise pressor reflex has been controversial. This controversy originated with the studies performed by Ciriello and Calaresu (72) and Iwamoto et al. (230), which were done before the advent of chemical lesioning techniques, and therefore could not distinguish between the destruction of cell bodies and the destruction of axons. Subsequently, Stornetta et al. (451) reported that in rats bilateral microinjections into the CVLM of kainic acid, which destroys cell bodies but not fibers of passage, had no effect on the reflex pressor response to electrical stimulation of the sciatic nerve. Stornetta et al. (451) also found that bilateral electrolytic lesions of the CVLM abolished the reflex pressor response to electrical stimulation of the sciatic nerve. Stornetta et al. (451) concluded that the electrolytic lesions of the CVLM that abolished the reflex pressor response to static contraction (230) were caused by the destruction of fibers of passage and not by the destruction of cell bodies and dendrites.

In contrast, Bauer et al. (33) showed that bilateral microinjections of kynurenic acid into the CVLM (as well as into the rostral VLM) significantly and reversibly attenuated the reflex pressor response to static contraction of the hindlimb muscles in chloralose anesthetized cats. Kynurenic acid is a broad-spectrum inotropic excitatory amino acid antagonist that blocks receptors on cell bodies and dendrites, but not on axons. The difference between the finding reported by Bauer et al. (33) and that reported by Stornetta et al. (451) might be explained by either one of two factors. First, Bauer et al. (33) microinjected by kynurenic acid into the CVLM, but not into the lateral reticular nucleus. By contrast, Stornetta et al. (451) microinjected kainic acid into this nucleus. Second, the difference might be explained by the fact that Bauer et al. (33) used cats, a species that has an exercise pressor reflex, and that Stornetta et al. (451) used rats, a species that probably does not.

Species differences between cats and rats raise two other points. First, electrical stimulation of muscle nerves in cats reflexly increases arterial pressure in cats (see above) but decreases arterial pressure in rats (451). Second, the sympathetic reflex arising from electrical stimulation of the sciatic nerve in cats is due in large part to the activation of C-fibers (421), whereas the sympathetic reflex arising from electrical stimulation of this nerve in rats is due in large part to the activation of Aδ fibers; C-fibers appear to play only a small role in causing this reflex (343). These differences between cats and rats make any comparison between the finding reported by Ciriello and Calaresu (72) in cats and the finding reported by Stornetta et al. (451) in rats tenuous.

The second source of controversy over the role of the CVLM in the exercise pressor reflex arc has been that stimulation of this area most frequently evoked a depressor effect (54, 502). However, several reports have indicated that chemical stimulation of cell bodies in the caudal-most portion of the CVLM can generate a pressor effect in both cats (228) and rats (54, 171). Nevertheless, the CVLM sites, which when chemically stimulated evoke a pressor response, do not appear to be the same as the sites, which when microinjected with kynurenic acid, attenuated the exercise pressor reflex (33). The former appear caudal to the latter.

Two other lines of evidence support the notion that the CVLM plays a role in the exercise pressor reflex arc. First, static contraction of the anesthetized cat hindlimb muscles increased the metabolic activity of CVLM cells (233). Many of the cell bodies shown to increase their metabolic activity, as determined by the uptake of radioactive glucose (233), were in that part of the CVLM that, when microinjected with kynurenic acid, significantly attenuated the exercise pressor reflex (33).

The second line evidence supporting a role for the CVLM in the exercise pressor reflex arc involves studies that recorded the extracellular discharge of cells in this area. Static contraction of hindlimb muscles altered the discharge of cells in the CVLM (229). This discharge displayed an initial segment-somatodendritic component, which is indicative of the recording arising from a cell body and not an axon. Moreover, the discharge of these CVLM cells was markedly affected by femoral arterial injection of capsaicin (229), which is a potent stimulant of group IV muscle afferents (253, 255). These studies were confirmed and extended by Bauer et al. (34, 36), who used spike-triggered averaging to show that many of the CVLM cells responding to contraction displayed a discharge that was temporally correlated to either the cardiac cycle or to sympathetic nerve activity.

In chloralose-anesthetized cats, static contraction of hindlimb muscles was found to evoke two patterns of stimulation from CVLM cells. The first was a sudden burst of impulses beginning 0.5–3.0 s after the onset of contraction, whereas the second was a delayed increase in activity beginning 10–20 s after the onset of contraction (34, 36, 229). These discharge patterns appears quite similar to the discharge patterns of group III and IV muscle afferents, respectively, which responded to static contraction of the triceps surae muscles (255). Moreover, some of these CVLM cells projected their axons to the intermediolateral horn of the thoracic spinal cord, the site of origin of the cell bodies of sympathetic preganglionic fibers (36).

The nucleus ambiguus of the medulla in cats and many other species contains the cells of origin of vagal preganglionic fibers, whose inhibition causes the heart to increase its rate and the airways to dilate (307, 308). Static contraction of the hindlimb muscles in cats has been shown to inhibit the discharge of cells in or near the nucleus ambiguus (229). These cells, however, were not identified as projecting their axons into the vagus nerve; therefore, their function was not known.

The rostral ventrolateral medulla (RVLM) is another bulbar site that may be part of the exercise pressor reflex arc. Rostrocaudally, the RVLM begins in cats at the rostral pole of the lateral reticular nucleus and ends just ventral to the retrofacial nucleus (74). In contrast to the CVLM, a large number of RVLM cells have been shown to project their axons to the intermediolateral horn of the cord (61, 397).

RVLM cells whose discharge is temporally correlated with sympathetic activity have been shown to receive input from contracting hindlimb skeletal muscle (34, 36). Furthermore, bilateral microinjection of kynurenic acid into the RVLM has been shown to attenuate in a reversible manner the exercise pressor reflex (33). Kynurenic acid is a broad-spectrum antagonist to excitatory amino receptors and it does not distinguish NMDA from non-NMDA receptors. Recently, however, bilateral microinjections of a non-NMDA receptor antagonist into the RVLM of the rat significantly attenuated, if not abolished, the pressor response to electrical stimulation of the sciatic nerve (265). This finding raises the possibility, as yet untested, that non-NMDA receptors in the RVLM participate in the neurotransmission of the exercise pressor reflex arc.

The role of the VLM, be it either rostral or caudal, in the ventilatory component of the exercise pressor reflex is unclear. Bilateral microinjections of kynurenic acid into either the CVLM or the RVLM had no effect on the ventilatory response to static contraction in chloralose-anesthetized cats, although these microinjections did attenuate the pressor response (33). One explanation for the finding that kynurenic microinjection had no effect on the ventilatory response to contraction might be that excitatory amino acid receptors do not participate in this component of the exercise pressor reflex. Alternatively, another reflex, such as that arising from the carotid body, might have compensated for the loss of the exercise pressor reflex.

The caudal ventrolateral medulla appears to play a critical role in the reflex airway dilation evoked by static contraction in chloralose-anesthetized dogs. For example, microinjection into the CVLM of either cobalt chloride, which prevents presynaptic release of neurotransmitter (279), or ibotenic acid, an excitotoxin (425), greatly attenuated the reflex airway dilation evoked by either static contraction of both gastrocnemius muscles or electrical stimulation of the sciatic nerve (367). Likewise, bilateral microinjection into the CVLM of an NMDA receptor antagonist also attenuated the reflex airway dilation evoked by either of these maneuvers (443). Bilateral microinjection into the CVLM of a non-NMDA receptor antagonist had no effect on the airway dilation evoked by either maneuver (443). In these experiments, bilateral microinjection into the CVLM of cobalt chloride, ibotenic acid, and excitatory amino acid receptor antagonists had no significant effect on the pressor reflex response to contraction or to sciatic nerve stimulation (367, 443). This lack of effect might be explained by the finding that in chloralose-anesthetized dogs, chemical stimulation of CVLM sites that cause airway dilation either have no effect on arterial pressure or decrease it (91, 193). This finding as well as the fact that blockade of these sites had no effect on the pressor response to static muscular contraction suggests that bronchodilator sites in the CVLM are not part of the neural circuitry causing the reflex cardiovascular responses to contraction of hindlimb muscles in anesthetized dogs.

Groups of cell bodies containing catecholamines are found in the ventrolateral medulla of many species. Specifically, norepinephrine-containing cells are found in the CVLM, and epinephrine-containing cells are found in the RVLM (73, 232, 405). The relationship between these catcholamine-containing cells in either the RVLM or the CVLM and any of the neural pathways comprising the autonomic components of the exercise pressor reflex is unclear.

The controversy about whether the CVLM and/or the RVLM participate in the exercise pressor reflex arc appears to be resolvable experimentally. Until that is accomplished, the following working hypothesis might prove to be useful. This is that the medullary circuitry necessary to express the exercise pressor reflex is widely distributed and involves neuronal pools found in both the CVLM and the RVLM. The experimental analysis of this medullary circuitry must be specific to the particular component of the exercise pressor reflex being investigated. Great care should be taken when attempting to generalize about the central neural pathway used to express different components of this reflex. Finally, it would be useful to know whether cells in either the CVLM or the RVLM project their axons to either the intermediolateral horn, the phrenic nucleus, or the vagal motor nuclei (i.e., nucleus ambiguus and dorsal motor nucleus). These projections might offer important insights about the function of these VLM cells. It would also be useful to know whether these cells contain catecholamines.

Other Central Neural Structures

Serial sectioning of the neuraxis has revealed that central neural structures rostral to the medulla are not needed to express most of the blood pressure component of the exercise pressor reflex (234). Nevertheless, serial sectioning experiments must be interpreted cautiously because the technique removes simultaneously multiple structures and fiber tracts. Consequently, the use of serial sectioning leaves open the possibility that counterbalancing influences have been removed from the neuraxis.

The role played in the exercise pressor reflex arc by the posterior hypothalamic region, which has been suggested to contain the anatomical locus for central command (131), is complicated. Bilateral lesions of this region in chloralose-anesthetized cats had no effect either on the increase in minute ventilation or the increase in arterial pressure that was evoked by static contraction of the hindlimb muscles (480). Nevertheless, these lesions increased the heart rate and breathing frequency responses to contraction. The finding that static contraction of the hindlimb muscles increased the discharge rate of neurons in the posterior hypothalamic locomotor region (482) might provide an electrophysiological basis for this region playing a small role in the exercise pressor reflex arc.

The exercise pressor reflex arc may include the supraoptic nucleus of the hypothalamus. Supraoptic cells projecting axons to the neurohypophysis of anesthetized cats are stimulated by contraction of the triceps surae muscles. Moreover, these cells were shown to be stimulated by activation of group III and IV afferents, but not by activation of group I and II afferents (247). One interpretation of these findings is that vasopressin secretion is another component of the constellation of responses comprising the exercise pressor reflex.

The midbrain and pons have also been examined for their participation in the exercise pressor reflex arc. In chloralose-anesthetized cats, bilateral lesions of the dorsal periaqueductal gray of the midbrain attenuated the pressor response to fatiguing contractions of the hindlimb muscles (503). In contrast, bilateral lesions of the dorsal raphe nuclei of the pons (503) or the nucleus reticularis gigantocellularis, which is found at the pontomedullary border (393) had no effect on the exercise pressor reflex.

In summary, an intact ventrolateral medulla appears to be necessary to express fully the autonomic components of the exercise pressor reflex. Central neural structures rostral to the VLM probably are not needed to express most of the reflex. Nevertheless, these rostral structures may play a modulating role that can affect the pattern or "topography" of a reflex response to muscular contraction. Finally, recognition that the specific circumstances of the experiment can influence its outcome is important. In other words, either anesthesia or decerebration may affect how various structures in the brain participate in the exercise pressor reflex arc.

Final Common Pathways

There are many reflex autonomic responses to stimulation of hindlimb muscles afferents. This portion of the chapter will address only the outflows that innervate the heart, the diaphragm, the conducting airways, and the arterioles. The final common pathway to the respiratory muscles will be discussed only briefly because the locations of the cells of origin of the motor axons innervating these muscles are too well known to require discussion here. Also, the connections between the cells of origin of the motor axons innervating the muscles of respiration and the rest of the reflex arc controlling breathing during hindlimb muscular contraction are unknown.

Until recently, the muscle reflex was thought to have little, if any, effect on vagal efferent activity to the heart. As a result, little effort was expended in determining the pathways from the contracting hindlimb muscles to the vagal outflow arising from the medulla. Now that evidence has been presented that chloralose anesthesia in cats masked the vagal withdrawal evoked reflexly by static muscular contraction (316), this neural pathway should be investigated.

In cats, the region of the nucleus ambiguus contains the cells of origin of vagal preganglionic fibers, which when stimulated cause the heart to slow its rate (44, 307). These cardiomotor vagal fibers conduct impulses in the B-fiber range (i.e., 3–15 m/s), and discharge with an expiratory, and usually a pulse synchronous rhythm (284, 307). In cats, the dorsal motor nucleus contains the cells of origin of a second group of vagal preganglionic fibers (44). The function of these fibers, which conduct impulses in the C-fiber range (i.e., < 2.5 m/s) is unknown

(146), but one possibility is that they might, when stimulated, decrease cardiac contractility (167). Alternatively, these vagal C-fibers might function to dilate the coronary arteries (139). In any event, these C-fibers do not appear to cause cardiac slowing in cats.

In contrast to cats, stimulation of vagal C-fibers in rats (352) and rabbits (147) does cause cardiac slowing. In rabbits, this slowing is blocked by atropine but not by hexamethonium, a finding that raises the possibility that a noncholinergic nonadrenergic transmitter is functioning at the ganglion (i.e., is released by the preganglionic fiber). Alternatively, an axon reflex that releases acetylcholine might be operative (147). If the former possibility is true, then the cells of origin of these vagal preganglionic C-fibers is the dorsal motor nucleus (238, 353). If the latter is true, then the cells of the sensory axons would be located in the nodose or possibly the jugular ganglia.

Stimulation of vagal preganglionic B-fibers in rats and rabbits also causes cardiac slowing. The cells of origin for these B-fibers in rats are located solely in the region of the nucleus ambiguus (353), whereas the cells of origin for these B-fibers in rabbits are located both in the region of the nucleus ambiguus and the dorsal motor nucleus (238). The cells of origin for vagal efferent fibers projecting to the heart in dogs are located in both the nucleus ambiguus and the dorsal motor nucleus (44, 216). The function of these anatomically identified cell bodies is not known.

The region of the nucleus ambiguus is believed to contain the cells of origin of the vagal preganglionic fibers whose stimulation causes airway smooth muscle to constrict. In cats, cells in the region of the nucleus ambiguus have been shown to be antidromically invaded from the pulmonary branches of the vagus nerve. Moreover, the calculated conduction velocities of the axons of these antidromically invaded cells were in the B-fiber range (308). These conduction velocities were consistent with those reported by Widdicombe (498) for vagal efferent fibers whose activation caused airway smooth muscle to constrict. Widdicombe (498) also reported that these vagal efferent fibers discharged spontaneously with an inspiratory rhythm. This finding was confirmed and extended by McAllen and Spyer (308), who recorded the spontaneous activity of cells in the region of the nucleus ambiguus that were antidromically invaded from the pulmonary branches of the vagus nerve.

Cells in the dorsal motor nucleus of cats were shown subsequently to be invaded antidromically from the pulmonary branches of the vagus nerve. The conduction velocities of their axons, however, were shown to be in the C-fiber range (146). These cells, consequently, were thought not to constrict airway smooth muscle. Instead, they might cause mucous secretion or dilation of the vasculature of the airway.

Recently, axon terminals containing γ-aminobutyric acid (GABA) have been shown to synapse onto the dendrites and cell bodies of vagal motoneurons in cats. Some of these motoneurons, which had their cell bodies in the region of the nucleus ambiguus, projected their axons to the cardiac branch of the vagus nerve (301). These findings raise the possibility that a GABAergic synapse onto vagal motoneurons supplying the heart and conducting airways is responsible for the reflex cardiac acceleration and airway dilation evoked by muscular contraction.

The sympathetic outflow to the heart, blood vessels, and adrenal gland arises from the intermediolateral (IML) horn of the thoracic and upper lumbar spinal cord. Experiments performed on anesthetized dogs and cats have shown beyond a doubt that sympathetic tone to these organs is increased reflexly by static contraction of the hindlimb muscles (20, 79, 98, 338, 475, 478). With regard to the exercise pressor reflex arc, the central neural pathway from the ventrolateral medulla to the IML has been partly uncovered. For example, cells in the RVLM receiving input from contracting skeletal muscle and discharging in synchrony with the sympathetic outflow project their axons to the IML (34, 36). The nature of the neurotransmitter released by the axons of RVLM neurons onto sympathetic preganglionic neurons in the IML is unknown, but excitatory amino acids probably play an important role (35); postsynaptically these amino acids may bind to an NMDA receptor in the IML (39). Substance P, acting either as a neurotransmitter or as a neuromodulator, is another candidate (196).

The phrenic motor nucleus of the cervical spinal cord contains the cells of origin of the α-motoneurons, whose discharge causes the diaphragm to contract. The phrenic motoneuron pool contains few γ-motoneurons, a feature that distinguishes it from motoneuron pools innervating limb skeletal muscles. In rats, axons arising from cells in the ventral respiratory group have been shown to synapse on phrenic motoneurons (133). Moreover, the phrenic motor nucleus in rats has been shown to receive a serotonergic, noradrenergic, and GABAergic innervation (516). In addition, the phrenic motor nucleus receives in rats inspiratory drive from a bulbospinal projection that uses an excitatory amino acid as a neurotransmitter (298, 315). The role played by any of these potential neurotransmitters in the phrenic motor nucleus when ventilation is increased by the "exercise pressor reflex" is unknown.

Interaction Between the Arterial Baroreflex and the Exercise Pressor Reflex in Anesthetized and Decerebrate Animals

The advantage of using an anesthetized or decerebrate preparation over a conscious preparation is that one can eliminate central command, thereby allowing one to examine the interaction between the arterial baroreflex and the exercise pressor reflex. Experiments using a paradigm in which the baroreflex is assessed both at rest and during static contraction of the hindlimb muscles have yielded conflicting results. Previously, stimulation of the arterial baroreceptors while the hindlimb muscles were statically contracting evoked the same decreases in heart rate as did the same stimulation of the baroreceptors while the hindlimb muscles were at rest. This finding has been reported in both anesthetized dogs (453) and decerebrate unanesthetized cats (93). Recently, however, inhibition of the cardiac vagal component of the carotid baroreflex while the hindlimb muscles were statically contracted has been reported in decerebrate cats (Fig. 10.8) (320). In addition, electrophysiological evidence has been presented showing that hindlimb muscular contraction inhibited the evoked activity of nucleus tractus solitarius cells that received baroreceptor input. Moreover, the inhibition of this evoked activity was thought to be caused by the release of GABA in the nucleus tractus solitarius (317).

Hindlimb somatic afferents, when activated electrically, attenuate the cardiac component of the arterial baroreflex in several species. These species include cats (93, 319, 390) dogs (275, 281) and rats (351). McWilliam and Yang (319) have shown that electrical stimulation of rapidly conducting (i.e., group I and II) somatic afferents did not attenuate the baroreflex, whereas stimulation of slowly conducting (i.e., group III and IV) somatic afferents did attenuate this reflex. Moreover, McWilliam and Yang (319) showed that the attenuation of the baroreflex occurred with rates of stimulation as low as 5 Hz, a frequency that is within the range discharged by group III muscle afferents during static contraction. Nevertheless, studies showing that electrical stimulation of somatic afferents attenuated the baroreflex must be interpreted cautiously because afferents innervating skin, joints, and bone, as well as hindlimb skeletal muscle, can be activated.

Experiments in anesthetized animals that compared the magnitude of the exercise pressor reflex before barodenervation with that after barodenervation, have yielded results consistent with those reported in humans (420) and conscious dogs (278,

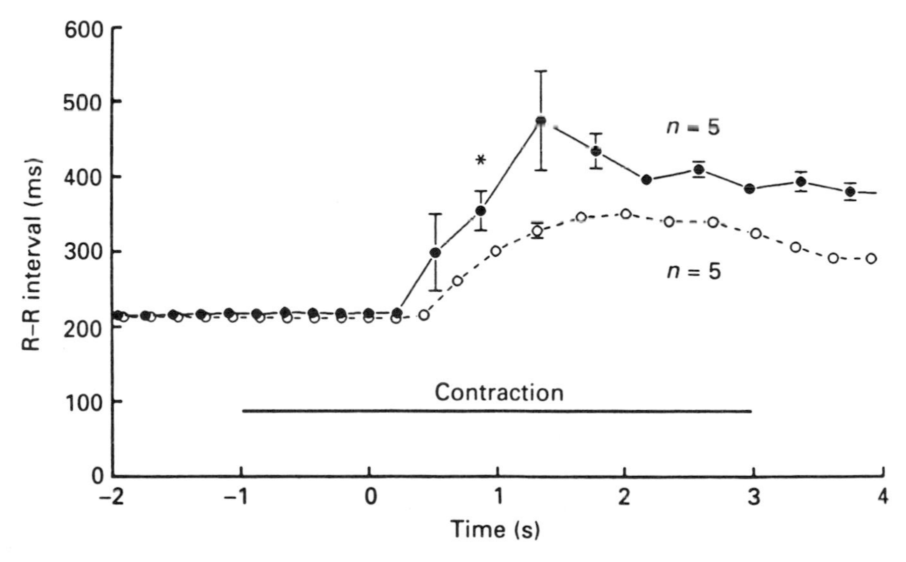

FIG. 10.8. Mean (± SEM) R-R intervals from one decerebrate cat in response to an increase in carotid sinus pressure at time zero, at rest (●——●), and during hindlimb contraction elicited by ventral root stimulation at 50 Hz (○——○). Baroreceptor responses at rest and during contraction were tested in an alternating sequence. The third R-R interval (marked by *asterisk*) and subsequent R-R intervals after sinus pressure elevation were significantly longer at rest than during contraction ($P<0.05$). No error bar is visible if smaller than the symbol. The period of contraction is denoted by the bar. Neither the initial nor the final carotid sinus pressure were significantly different in the resting and contracting situations; similarly, systolic and diastolic arterial pressures and R-R intervals immediately before sinus pressure elevation, were not significantly different in the two situations. [Reprinted with permission from McWilliam, Yang, and Chien (320).]

322, 430, 483). Specifically, Waldrop and Mitchell (479) found that section of the aortic, vagus, and carotid sinus nerves in chloralose-anesthetized cats increased the reflex pressor response to static contraction of the hindlimb muscles. Denervation of the arterial and cardiac baroreceptors, however, was found to have no effect on the contraction-induced regional distribution of the cardiac output.

Unfortunately, the interaction between cardiopulmonary reflexes and the exercise pressor reflex has not been investigated in decerebrate or anesthetized animals. Some preliminary information, however, has been obtained from experiments in which the sciatic nerve of chloralose-anesthetized dogs was stimulated electrically at current intensities sufficient to activate C-fibers (465). This study showed that the renal vasoconstrictor response to sciatic nerve stimulation was decreased by expansion of the blood volume (which, in turn, was presumed to stimulate cardiopulmonary receptors). Moreover, the renal vasoconstrictor response to sciatic nerve stimulation was restored by bilateral vagotomy (465).

EVIDENCE FOR THE EXERCISE PRESSOR REFLEX IN HUMANS AND CONSCIOUS ANIMALS

Feedback from Contracting Limb Skeletal Muscle in Humans and Conscious Animals

Zuntz and Geppart proposed (517) that a reflex arising from the accumulation of metabolites in exercising muscles activated the cardiovascular and respiratory systems. Alam and Smirk (6) were the first to provide experimental evidence that a reflex arising from exercising skeletal muscle increased arterial blood pressure in humans. Specifically, they demonstrated that the pressor response to dynamic exercise of the calf muscles persisted after the end of the exercise period if the circulation to the legs was arrested. Alan and Smirk (6) hypothesized that this pressor response, an effect that has been replicated many times for both dynamic and static exercise (53, 136, 160, 165, 303, 339, 402, 411, 435, 437, 470, 473, 474) was a reflex that arose from the trapping of metabolic by-products of contraction in the previously exercising limb muscles. Presumably, these metabolites stimulated sensory nerve endings in the previously exercising muscles.

The postexercise pressor effect that is sustained by arresting the circulation to the working limb has been termed the "muscle chemoreflex" (404) and has been shown to be directly proportional to the mass of muscle being exercised (159). The magnitude of the muscle chemoreflex is also directly proportional to the intensity of the exercise (6, 402, 473). Another component of the muscle chemoreflex is an increase in sympathetic nerve discharge to nonexercising skeletal muscle (303, 435, 470, 473). The magnitude of this discharge has been shown to be correlated directly to vascular resistance in hindlimb skeletal muscle (426). In addition, the muscle chemoreflex has a cardiac component, but its presence appears to depend directly on the mass of the exercising skeletal muscle; that is, circulatory arrest of large muscle masses such as both legs evoked a postexercise increase in heart rate, whereas arrest of a small mass such as the hand and forearm did not (7, 53, 160). Recently, O'Leary has shown in conscious dogs that the efferent arm of the cardiac component of the muscle chemoreflex is comprised of sympathetic activation and not vagal withdrawal (360). In contrast to the cardiovascular and muscle sympathetic nerve components described above, the muscle chemoreflex evoked by postexercise circulatory arrest does not appear to have a ventilatory component (160, 402). Likewise, this chemoreflex does not appear to have a skin sympathetic component (411, 476).

The hypothesis that the muscle chemoreflex plays a role in causing the autonomic adjustments to exercise assumes that the sensory nerve endings stimulated by postexercise circulatory occlusion are also stimulated by exercise. The value of the muscle chemoreflex, which is measured after the end of the exercise period, is that it enables the investigator to measure the contribution of muscle metabolites (and the sensory endings stimulated by them) to the autonomic responses to exercise. Because the muscles are at rest, this measurement is not confounded by the contribution of either central command or mechanoreflexes arising from skeletal muscle. Consequently, assessment of the magnitude of the muscle chemoreflex is a valuable experimental tool that has been quite useful in increasing our understanding of the mechanisms causing the autonomic adjustments to exercise. Nevertheless, investigators, when interpreting muscle chemoreflex data, need to consider the possibility that the discharge frequencies of metaboreceptors responding to postexercise circulatory occlusion might be less than those of metaboreceptors responding to ischemic exercise. Investigators also need to consider that the number of metaboreceptors discharging during postexercise ischemia might be less than the number of metaboreceptors discharging during ischemic exercise (262).

Until recently, the physiological significance of the muscle chemoreflex was in doubt because it was measured only when skeletal muscles were not contracting. In an elegant study, Joyner and Wieling

(240) demonstrated that the muscle chemoreflex had a tonic effect on sympathetic discharge when humans performed high intensity handgrip rhythmic exercise. Specifically, Joyner and Wieling (240) found that increasing blood flow to the forearm significantly attenuated the muscle sympathetic nerve response to handgrip (Fig. 10.9). Moreover, the increase in forearm blood flow, accomplished by surrounding the limb with negative pressure, also significantly attenuated the pressor and muscle sympathetic nerve responses to postexercise ischemia. Joyner and Wieling (240) also found that increasing blood flow to the forearm had no effect on the tachycardic response to either handgrip or to postexercise ischemia.

The muscle chemoreflex in humans can also be demonstrated to function during exercise as well as afterwards if blood flow to the working limb is reduced by positive pressure (Fig. 10.10) (127). This maneuver has been used to determine the "threshold" level of exercise needed to evoke the muscle chemoreflex. In humans, this threshold for reflexly increasing blood pressure appears to be low when large muscle masses, such as both legs, are exercised (403). In other words, the muscle chemoreflex is active during mild exercise in humans, such that small decreases in muscle blood flow cause a greater rise in mean arterial pressure than can be attributed to the mechanical effects of positive pressure on arterial pressure (403). On the other hand, the threshold for the muscle chemoreflex in humans appears to require moderate to high levels of exercise when a small muscle mass, such as one hand and forearm, are exercised (239). In addition, reductions in leg blood flow with positive pressure can increase the ventilatory response to dynamic exercise (i.e., bicycling) (127, 505). This increase in ventilation has also been attributed to the muscle chemoreflex.

The threshold for the muscle chemoreflex in dogs exercising on a treadmill has also been described. During mild dynamic exercise, blood flow–dependent metabolic signals arising from the working muscles are not thought to be the primary stimulus that increases autonomic function. However, at moderate to heavy levels of dynamic exercise, metabolic stimuli evoking the muscle chemoreflex are likely to play an important role in causing these autonomic effects (509). Moreover, the metabolic stimulus evoking the muscle chemoreflex at moderate to heavy levels of dynamic exercise is believed to be generated when oxygen delivery to the working muscles decreases below some critical level (431).

Involuntary contraction of skeletal muscle induced by percutaneous electrical stimulation has been a second method that has been used to evoke autonomic reflexes in humans. The utility of this method lies in its ability to avoid the confounding effects of central command; however, it is not able to distinguish easily mechanoreceptor- from metaboreceptor-induced reflex effects. In addition, electrical stimulation may activate afferent fibers directly. Moreover, because the electrical stimulation is thought to activate motoneurons rather than muscle fibers, the recruitment order and firing frequency of motor units activated by electrical stimulation is different than

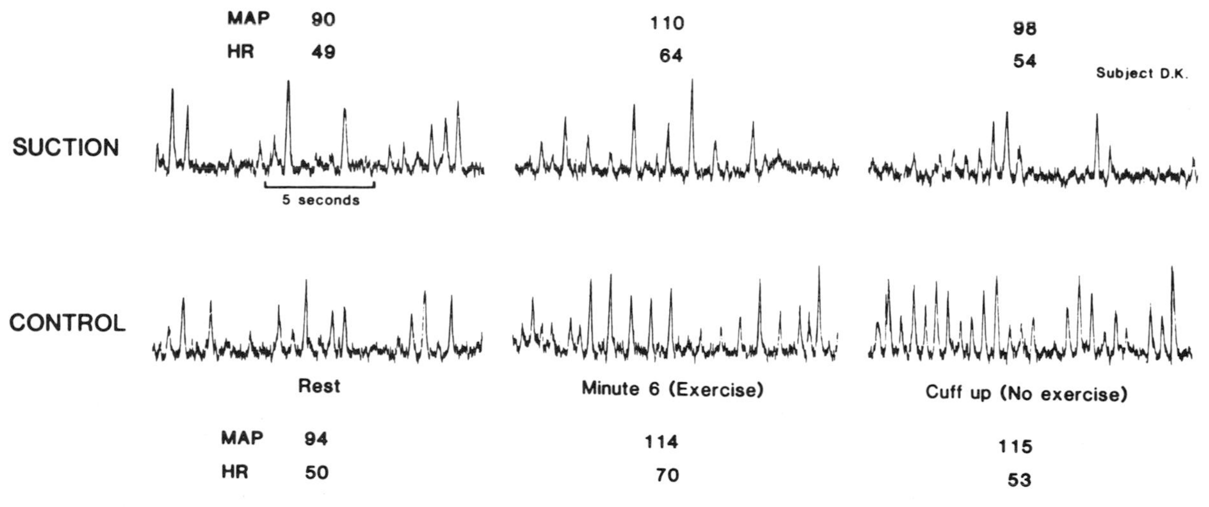

FIG. 10.9. Individual microneurographic record of MSNA, MAP, and HR (beats per minute) responses to 6 min of rhythmic handgrip to 50% of maximum voluntary contraction. In this subject, MSNA increased during 6 min of exercise, and this increase was maintained after exercise when arm cuff was inflated. MAP responses to exercise were similar during exercise in two trials, but MAP was lower during postexercise ischemia (cuff up) after suction. HR responses were similar throughout. [Reprinted with permission from Joyner and Wieling (240).]

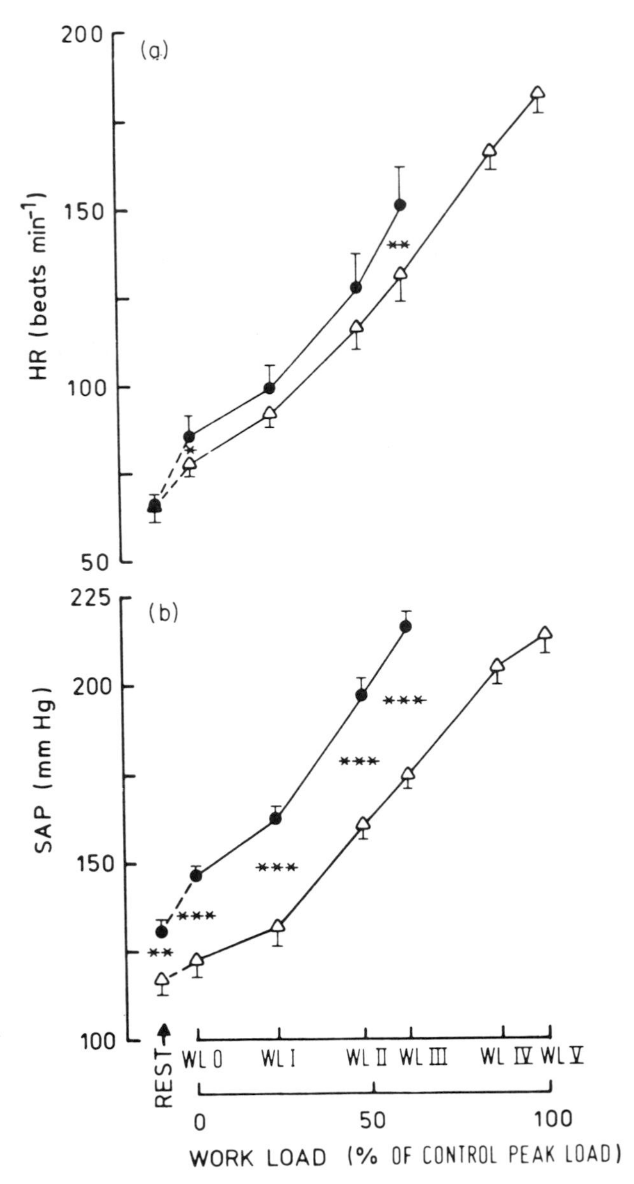

FIG. 10.10. Heart rate (a) and systolic arterial pressure (b) at rest and as functions of external workload in the leg positive pressure (●) and control (△) conditions, all data referring to steady state. On the abscissa, workloads are given as a percentage of the peak load attained in the control condition, with WL 0-V representing 0%, 23%, 48%, 61%, 87%, and 100% of this load and WL III indicating the highest load that could be managed in the leg positive-pressure condition. Values are means; (*a*) n = 7, (*b*) n = 8. *Vertical bars:* I SEM. *$P<0.05$, **$P<0.01$, ***$P<0.001$. [Reprinted with permission from Eiken and Bjurstedt (127).]

the recruitment order and frequency activated voluntarily by central command.

Despite these limitations, the use of electrical stimulation to involuntarily contract skeletal muscles in humans has shown repeatedly that mean arterial pressure, sympathetic discharge to both skin and nonexercising muscle, heart rate, cardiac output, and ventilation increased (2, 14, 109, 214, 220, 231, 303, 411, 452). Some components of this constellation of responses to involuntary contraction may be a reflex arising either from the working muscles or from the direct activation of afferent fibers. Alternatively, a metabolic by-product of involuntary muscular contraction may have circulated to another region, such as the lungs or carotid bodies, to evoke these responses. This alternative explanation does not appear to be the case for the pressor response to involuntary contraction because it was abolished by epidural blockade with either lidocaine or bupivicaine (452). On the other hand, the increases in both heart rate and cardiac output, as well as ventilation, that were evoked by involuntary contraction were attenuated but not abolished, by epidural blockade (452). While the attenuation of these effects was statistically significant, it was a small part of the overall effect.

The third method used to demonstrate that feedback from exercising skeletal muscle reflexly alters autonomic function has also employed epidural blockade. This method has compared the autonomic responses to leg exercise (performed voluntarily) before blockade with those performed voluntarily after blockade. One advantage of this method of study is that any autonomic resonse that is attenuated or abolished by epidural blockade can be attributed to a reflex mechanism arising from the exercising muscle. Reaching such a conclusion requires one to demonstrate that the epidural blockade has not impaired the sympathetic outflow (i.e., the motor pathway of the reflex arc). This demonstration can be done by showing that the epidural blockade has not attenuated the pressor reflex that arises by placing ice either on the forehead or on the hand (i.e., "the cold pressor test"). One disadvantage of this method is that any autonomic response that remains unchanged by epidural blockade cannot with any certainty be interpreted as not being caused by a reflex arising from the exercising muscle. For example, a redundant mechanism, such as central command, might compensate for an attenuated muscle reflex.

Epidural blockade has been shown to attenuate greatly, if not abolish, the pressor response to dynamic exercise of a large muscle mass, such as both legs (140, 160, 266, 452). Moreover, when epidural blockade has been shown to diminish the pressor response to exercise, it has also been shown to diminish the pressor response to postexercise circulatory arrest (140). Likewise, when epidural blockade has been shown to have no effect on the pressor response to dynamic exercise, it has been shown to have no effect on the pressor response to postexercise circulatory arrest (i.e., the muscle chemoreflex) (161). These findings are consistent with the previously stated assumption that the sensory nerve endings in skeletal muscle that are stimulated by the muscle chemoreflex are also stimulated by exercise.

In contrast to the pressor response, the heart rate and ventilatory responses to dynamic exercise are not affected by epidural blockade (140). It seems reasonable to speculate that a reflex arising from skeletal muscle does not cause the increases in heart rate and ventilation that are evoked by dynamic exercise. A redundant mechanism might explain why the heart rate and ventilatory responses to dynamic exercise are still present after epidural blockade. If this is in fact the case, then one must also explain why this redundant mechanism would compensate for the heart rate and ventilatory components but not for the pressor component of the response constellation to dynamic exercise.

Blockade of sensory nerve discharge attenuates the cardiovascular responses to static exercise as well as those to dynamic exercise. For example, axillary blockade prevented the increase in heart rate evoked by brief (i.e., 4 s) maximal voluntary static handgrip; this blockade, surprisingly, did not significantly attenuate the pressor response to maximal static handgrip (289). In addition, epidural blockade attenuated significantly the pressor-tachycardic responses to prolonged (i.e., 2 min) extension of one leg (339).

Neuromuscular blockade with curare-like agents has been the fourth method used to determine the contribution of a reflex originating in contracting muscle to the autonomic adjustments to exercise in humans. Galbo et al. (163) examined the cardiovascular and ventilatory responses to bicycle exercise before and during partial neuromuscular blockade induced by curare. These investigators found that when central command was maintained at its maximum level, increases in exercise-induced oxygen uptake, which occurred as the paralyzing effect of the curare wore off, evoked large increases in mean arterial pressure, heart rate, and ventilation. Galbo et al. (163) interpreted these findings as providing support for a role for a peripheral factor such as a muscle reflex in causing the autonomic adjustments to dynamic exercise. Specifically, these investigators thought that this reflex arose from the stimulation of metaboreceptors in the exercising muscles.

Subsequently, Victor et al. (471) examined the effect of neuromuscular blockade induced by curare on the autonomic responses to static handgrip exercise. They found that attempted exercise while the subjects were paralyzed partially by curare yielded increases in mean arterial pressure and sympathetic nerve activity to nonexercising muscles that were trivial compared with the increase in these variables that were evoked by actual handgrip performed before curare (Fig. 10.11). In contrast to the increase in arterial pressure, the vagally mediated heart rate increase evoked by attempted handgrip was no different than that evoked by actual handgrip.

The work by Victor et al. (471) had an important impact on the field because it provided strong evidence that during exercise a reflex arising from contracting muscle controlled the increases in arterial pressure and in sympathetic discharge to the vasculature of skeletal muscle, whereas central command controlled the increase in heart rate due to vagal withdrawal. This evidence becomes all the more impressive when one considers the fact that the small increases in arterial pressure and muscle sympathetic nerve activity evoked by attempted contraction in the study by Victor et al. (471) occurred at a time

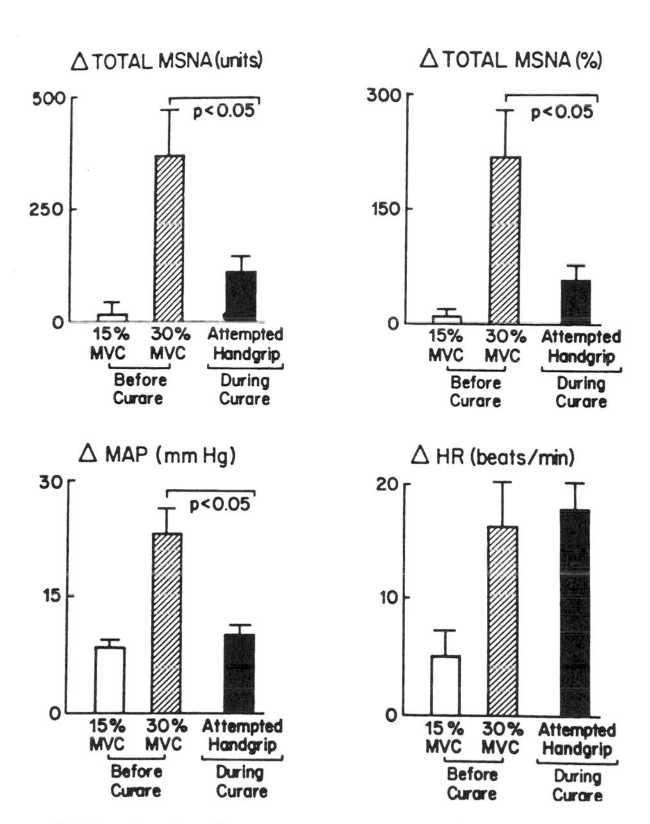

FIG. 10.11. Graphs of peak increases in total muscle sympathetic nerve activity (MSNA), mean arterial pressure (MAP), and heart rate (HR) caused by static handgrip at 15% MVC (*open bars*) and at 30% MVC (*hatched bars*) before curare infusion and by attempted handgrip during a high dose of curare (*solid bars*). During curare infusion, subjects used near-maximal effort to attempt sustained handgrip but generated almost no force. Without sustained contraction, the intent to exercise alone (i.e., central command) caused much smaller increases in MSNA and arterial pressure than normally caused by an actual static handgrip at 30% MVC even though the effort was greater with the attempted than with the actual contraction. In contrast, heart rate increased as much with the attempted handgrip as with the actual handgrip at 30% MVC. Entries are mean ±SEM for eight subjects. [Reprinted with permission from Victor et al. (471).]

when central command was near maximal. Recently, Gandevia et al. (166) have claimed that the pressor response to attempted handgrip exercise in totally paralyzed subjects is no different than that in response to actual handgrip performed with maximal effort. Gandevia et al. (166) did not measure muscle sympathetic nerve activity in their experiments. Obviously, the report by Gandevia et al. (166) conflicts with the report by Victor et al. (471), and we can offer no explanation for this discrepancy.

In summary, substantial evidence exists that a reflex arising from contracting skeletal muscles contributes to the autonomic adjustments to exercise in humans and conscious animals. This reflex mechanism appears to make an especially important contribution to the exercise-induced increases in sympathetic discharge that function to constrict the vasculature of nonexercising skeletal muscle. Although the muscle reflex can increase heart rate (see 420), cardiac output, and ventilation during exercise, there appears to be little doubt that other mechanisms can substitute for it.

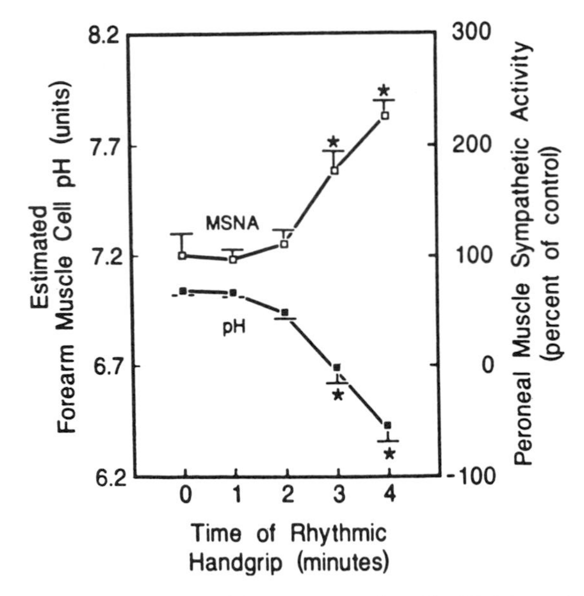

FIG. 10.12. Responses of forearm muscle cell pH (■) as determined by ³P-NMR and of peroneal muscle sympathetic nerve activity (□) during 4 min of rhythmic handgrip (2 min at 30% MVC followed by 2 min at 50% MVC). Data represent mean ±SE for seven subjects (*P<0.05 vs. control). [Reprinted with permission from Victor et al. (470).]

The Nature of the Stimulus Evoking the Exercise Pressor Reflex

The stimulus that evokes the exercise pressor reflex is either mechanical or metabolic in nature. From a teleological point of view, many physiologists believe that the purpose of the stimulus arising from exercising muscle is to signal the CNS that there is a mismatch between blood supply and demand in the exercising muscle. This belief has caused most investigators to focus their attention on unmasking the nature of the metabolic stimulus. On the other hand, there is also evidence that mechanical distortion of receptive fields, induced by muscular contraction, can also function as a stimulus for the exercise pressor reflex.

Metabolic Stimuli. Recently, two reports appearing almost simultaneously have been seminal in advancing our understanding about the nature of the metabolic stimulus evoking the exercise pressor reflex. Using ^{31}P nuclear magnetic resonance (NMR) spectroscopy, both reports have shown that the time course and magnitude of three components of the exercise pressor reflex were associated directly with the intracellular concentration of hydrogen ions in the contracting muscles (435, 470). The three components of the reflex were mean arterial pressure, vascular resistance to the calf muscles and sympathetic nerve activity to nonexercising muscles (Figs. 10.12 and 10.13). In addition, neither report indicated an association between the exercise-induced

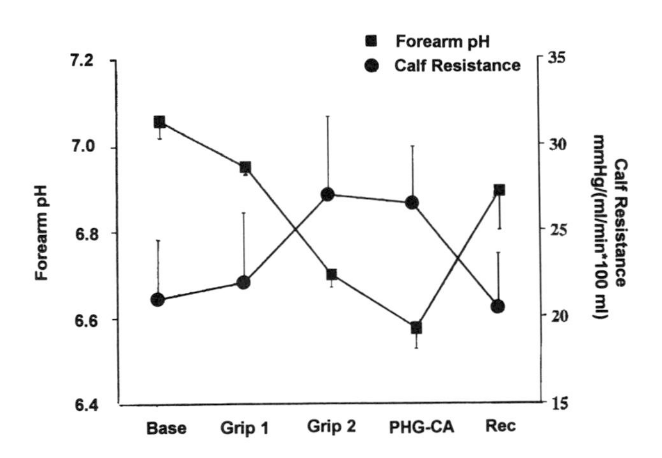

FIG. 10.13. Changes in forearm muscle pH and calf vascular resistance during static forearm exercise at 30% MVC. Base = 5 min of baseline data. Grip 1 and 2 represent each minute of static exercise; PHG-CA, posthandgrip circulatory arrest, and represents the mean value of 3 min of data; Rec, recovery and represents data during the third minute of recovery. Measurements were made during exercise of dominant and non-dominant forearms of six individuals. *Bars* represent ± SEM. This figure demonstrates the roughly inverse relationship between changes in pH and calf vascular resistance during forearm exercise. [Reprinted with permission from Sinoway et al. (435).]

changes in intracellular concentrations of adenosine diphosphate, inorganic phosphate, and phosphocreatine and the autonomic components of the reflex. An additional finding reported in both studies was that circulatory occlusion of the working muscles, initiated at the end of the exercise bout, maintained the elevated intracellular hydrogen ion concentration in these muscles. Likewise, circulatory occlusion maintained a substantial part of the increase in mean arterial pressure, calf vascular resistance, and muscle sympathetic nerve activity. In contrast, the increase in heart rate that was evoked during exercise was not maintained during postexercise circulatory occlusion (435, 470).

The reports by Victor et al. (470) and Sinoway et al. (435) demonstrated a correlative relationship between two variables; namely, the exercise pressor reflex and the intracellular concentration of hydrogen ions in working skeletal muscle. Once this relationship was established, both groups of investigators tested the hypothesis that decreasing the ability of exercising skeletal muscle to produce hydrogen ions blunted the pressor reflex. This was demonstrated in different ways, but the results of each supported the hypothesis being tested.

In the first report, Pryor et al. (389), compared the cardiovascular and muscle sympathetic nerve responses to static handgrip in subjects with McArdle's disease with the cardiovascular and muscle sympathetic nerve responses to handgrip in normal subjects. In this disease, skeletal muscle is deficient in the myophosphorylase enzyme and therefore converts little if any glycogen to glucose. Consequently, the skeletal muscle of patients with McArdle's disease produces little, if any, lactic acid when it contracts. The increases in arterial pressure and in sympathetic nerve activity evoked by static handgrip in normal subjects were significantly greater than those evoked by handgrip in subjects with McArdle's disease. In contrast, the increase in heart rate evoked by handgrip in normal subjects was no different than that evoked by handgrip in subjects with McArdle's disease. Furthermore, Pryor et al. (389) found that McArdle's subjects did not differ from normal subjects in their ability to generate sympathetic reflex responses either to placing the hand in ice water or to a Valsalva maneuver (Fig. 10.14). The findings by Pryor et al. (389) supported the hypothesis that the production of hydrogen ions by working muscle in humans causes the reflex increases in arterial pressure and muscle sympathetic nerve activity that are evoked by exercise. In contrast, Pryor et al. (389) thought that the production of hydrogen ions by working muscle was not responsible for the increase in heart rate evoked by exercise.

The second demonstration that the production of hydrogen ions by the working muscle plays an important role in evoking the exercise pressor reflex was done by Ettinger et al. (136). These investigators examined the autonomic responses to static handgrip exercise before and after intravenous administration of dichloroacetate, a compound that increases the activity of pyruvate dehydrogenase. Dichloroacetate decreased both the pressor and mus-

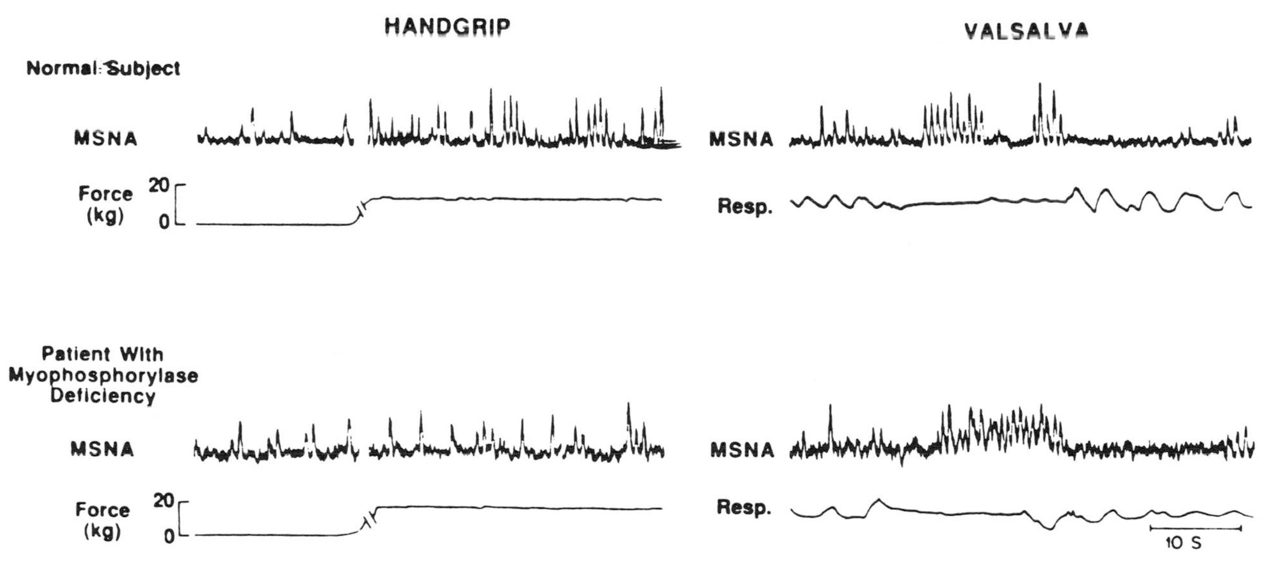

FIG. 10.14. Original records of MSNA in two subjects showing peak responses during static handgrip at 30% MVC and during phases 2 and 3 of a Valsalva maneuver. Whereas MSNA responses evoked by static handgrip were markedly attenuated in the patient with myophosphorylase deficiency, increases in MSNA evoked by the Valsalva maneuver were comparable in the normal subject and patient. [Reprinted with permission from Pryor et al. (389).]

cle sympathetic nerve responses to static exercise, but had no effect on the tachycardic response to exercise; it also attenuated the concentrations of lactate and hydrogen ions in the venous outflow from the exercising muscle. Moreover, dichloroacetate decreased the pressor and muscle sympathetic nerve responses to postexercise circulatory arrest. At the same time, dichloroacetate attenuated the autonomic responses to handgrip.

Glycogen depletion, accomplished by a 24 hr fast and prior high-intensity exercise, has also been used to decrease lactic acid production during bicycling (439). Glycogen depletion, which was verified by muscle biopsy, attenuated both the increase in venous lactate concentrations and the pressor response to exercise. Moreover, depletion attenuated the decrease in forearm vascular conductance during postexercise circulatory arrest (i.e., the muscle chemoreflex).

The relationship between intracellular hydrogen ion concentration in contracting muscle and muscle sympathetic nerve activity appears strong when one examines a single bout of exercise (136, 389, 435, 470). This relationship, however, breaks down when one correlates intracellular pH and MSNA over a series of contractions and rest periods (438). This correlation revealed that intracellular diprotonated phosphate concentrations predicted muscle sympathetic nerve activity far better than did intracellular hydrogen ion concentrations (438).

There is additional evidence showing that the relationship between intracellular muscle pH and muscle sympathetic nerve activity breaks down. For example, Sinoway et al. (437) showed that physical conditioning of forearm muscles attenuated the reflex increase in sympathetic nerve activity evoked by exercise and by postexercise circulatory arrest. The reflex was attenuated despite the fact that the hydrogen ion concentrations of the exercising muscles in the conditioned arms were no different than those of the exercising muscles in the nonconditioned arms. The cause of the conditioning-induced attenuation of the exercise pressor reflex is unknown. One possibility is that conditioning attenuated the production of another metabolite.

Recent evidence points to two candidates, adenosine (96) and cyclooxygenase metabolites of arachidonic acid (145). Specifically, intra-arterial injection of theophylline, which blocked adenosine receptors in the contracting forearm, attenuated the pressor response to forearm exercise. Likewise, intravenous injection of ketoprofen, which blocked the activity of cyclooxygenase, also attenuated this response (145). The effect of theophylline in humans is somewhat surprising because in anesthetized animals, injection of adenosine into the arterial supply of hindlimb skeletal muscle had no effect on the cardiovascular and respiratory systems (458); moreover, it had only small effects on group III and IV afferent discharge (399). A species difference may explain this disparity. Likewise, the effect of ketoprofen is also surprising because previous use of single-dose oral cyclooxygenase blockade in humans had no effect on the autonomic responses to static handgrip (110). This disparity might be explained by the fact that in the study using oral cyclooxygenase blockade (i.e., Davy et al. [110]) no evidence was presented that prostaglandin levels in the blood were decreased. In contrast, in the study in which intravenous ketoprofen was used (i.e., Fontana et al. [145]), venous thromboxane B_2 levels were decreased to almost zero.

Mechanical Stimuli. Mechanical distortion of receptive fields of sensory nerve endings in contracting muscle is a second factor that might evoke the exercise pressor reflex in humans. One of the first studies to raise this possibility was done by Hollander and Bouman (214), who reported that heart rate increased 550 ms after the onset of an electrically evoked muscle contraction. The heart rate increase was caused by vagal withdrawal and, because of its short latency, was attributed to a reflex arising from mechanoreceptors in the contracting muscle. Although the importance and existence of this "muscle-heart reflex" in humans has been challenged (231), recent evidence in cats has provided strong support for it (see below) (316). Nevertheless, the muscle-heart reflex is not necessary for the vagally mediated increase in heart rate that occurs at the onset of exercise; this increase has been shown to be evoked by attempted exercise in subjects paralyzed with curare-like drugs (165, 290).

Passive movement of the legs as well as compression of limbs have been two other methods used to demonstrate that mechanoreceptor stimulation reflexly affects the autonomic nervous system. Passive movement of the legs was achieved by strapping subjects' feet to the pedals of a stationary tandem bicycle, which in turn was cycled by a staff member (351). Passive cycling of the legs significantly increased heart rate above baseline within 1 s of the onset of limb movement. In fact, this increase and its time course did not differ significantly from that evoked in staff members by active cycling. Moreover, passive cycling provoked no measurable EMG activity in the legs of the subjects, a finding that suggests that central command was not activated in these individuals. Passive cycling was concluded to increase reflexly heart rate by stimulating mechanoreceptors in the joints and muscles of the legs. Unfortunately, other variables such as ventilation, arterial pressure, and oxygen consumption were not measured in this cleverly designed study.

Compression of both legs, which was achieved by inflation of a medical antishock trouser (MAST) device, has been shown to increase reflexly mean arterial pressure and heart rate (162, 504), whereas compression of one arm had no effect on these variables (310). The mass of tissue stimulated might explain this difference. Nevertheless, forearm exercise with compression was found to evoke greater increases in mean arterial pressure and muscle sympathetic nerve activity than did forearm exercise without compression (310). This increase in responsiveness was thought to be caused by a compression-induced mechanoreceptor sensitization, an effect that could not be measured until the forearm muscles exercised.

Experiments in which either passive cycling or limb compression was used have advanced the hypothesis that mechanoreceptors contribute to the reflex control of the autonomic nervous system during exercise. Nevertheless, the interpretation of the experimental findings must be guarded because the stimulus causing mechanoreceptor stimulation was not selective. In other words, passive cycling may have stimulated mechanoreceptors in both muscles and joints. Likewise, limb compression may have stimulated mechanoreceptors in both muscles and skin and perhaps in the joints as well.

Limb congestion, induced by venous occlusion, has been a second method used to demonstrate that mechanoreceptors in contracting muscle can evoke autonomic reflex effects. McClain et al. (309) found that venous congestion augmented the increase in arterial pressure, heart rate, and muscle sympathetic nerve activity that was evoked by either voluntary or involuntary (i.e., electrically induced) handgrip. ^{31}P NMR revealed that venous congestion had no effect on the hydrogen ion or diprotonated phosphate ion concentrations in the contracting muscles. Hence, differences in metaboreceptor stimulation were thought unlikely to account for these results. Moreover, venous congestion had no effect on the increase in skin sympathetic nerve activity that was evoked by exercise performed voluntarily. Such an increase in activity is believed to be caused mostly by central command (411, 476). McClain et al. (309) concluded that the most probable explanation for their findings was that venous congestion increased interstitial pressure in the forearm muscles, and that this increase in pressure, in turn, sensitized mechanoreceptors.

In summary, there is substantial evidence that a reflex arising from contracting muscle plays a significant role in causing the autonomic adjustments to exercise. In addition, the stimuli evoking this reflex are unknown, but the available evidence strongly supports the hypothesis that metabolites produced by a mismatch between blood supply and demand in the exercising muscle are involved. Moreover, this metabolite might be either lactic acid or some other factor generated by inadequate oxygen delivery to exercising muscle.

In healthy humans, the evidence that mechanoreceptors are responsible for causing the exercise pressor reflex is less plentiful than is the evidence that metaboreceptors are responsible for causing this reflex. Two factors render the human "a difficult preparation" in which to obtain evidence that mechanoreceptor stimulation causes part of the exercise pressor reflex. First, the involuntary (i.e., electrically induced) contractions used to evoke a mechanoreceptor reflex have been kept small (i.e., 10–20% of the maximal voluntary contraction) in order to avoid activation of nociceptive afferents. Consequently, the tension developed by the contracting muscles may have been below the threshold needed to activate mechanoreceptors. Second, attempts to demonstrate a "mechanoreceptor reflex" in humans have focused on sympathetic nerve activity innervating one vascular bed, namely nonexercising limb muscles (e.g., 303). Although these attempts have been unsuccessful, the possibility remains that mechanoreceptor stimulation may increase the activity of sympathetic nerves innervating the viscera. For example, mechanoreceptor stimulation has been shown to increase reflexly sympathetic discharge to the kidney and heart in anesthetized animals (306, 472).

CONTRIBUTION OF PERIPHERAL AFFERENTS TO THE EXERCISE HYPERPNEA

Afferents from the Exercising Limbs

Detail was provided in the preceding section on the receptor mechanisms in exercising limbs and the reflex pathway through which these receptors influence circulatory control during exercise. This section will summarize major findings on the influence of limb afferents on breathing during exercise.

Because of the importance of the chemical and mechanical conditions in contracting muscle to exercise performance, it seems reasonable to postulate that these conditions have some influence on the exercise hyperpnea. Moreover, a neural signal from the muscles could account for the rapid onset of the hyperpnea (13, 112, 280) and the signal could be proportional to metabolic rate thereby accounting for the matching of ventilation to oxygen consumption during submaximal exercise (112, 117, 496). In addition, passive movement of the legs slightly increases ventilation in spinal cord-intact humans (90, 192, 342) but not in T5–T12 paraplegics (342). Accordingly, numerous studies have been conducted on many different species utilizing widely varying techniques to gain insight into the role of limb afferents in the exercise hyperpnea.

Electrically Induced Muscle Contractions in Anesthetized Animals. A series of studies by Kao et al. (248–251) provide strong support for peripheral neurogenic mediation of the exercise hyperpnea. The key feature of these studies was the apparent isolation of muscle afferents from not only central command but also humoral (blood-borne) stimuli. Muscle contraction of the hindlimbs of a dog were electrically induced (neural dog). The blood perfusing these muscles was provided by a second dog (humoral dog) through anastomosis of the abdominal arteries and veins of the exercising and nonexercising dogs. At the onset of muscle contraction, ventilation increased in the neural dog, but it did not in the humoral dog, until its Pa_{O_2} decreased and Pa_{CO_2} increased (Fig. 10.15). The hyperpnea in the neural dog was eliminated by ablation of the lateral spinal columns or by transection of the spinal cord. The hyperpnea in the humoral dog was quantitatively consistent with ventilatory responsiveness to the observed changes in arterial blood gases. Kao et

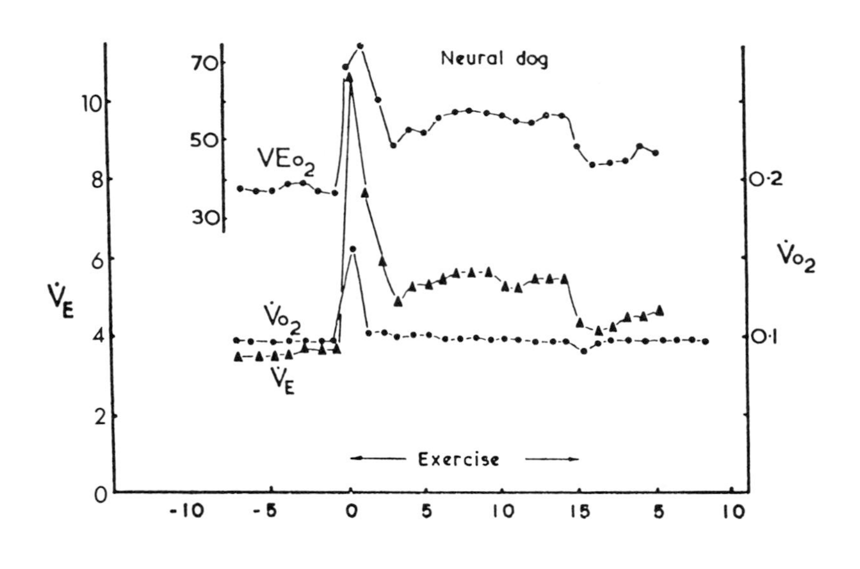

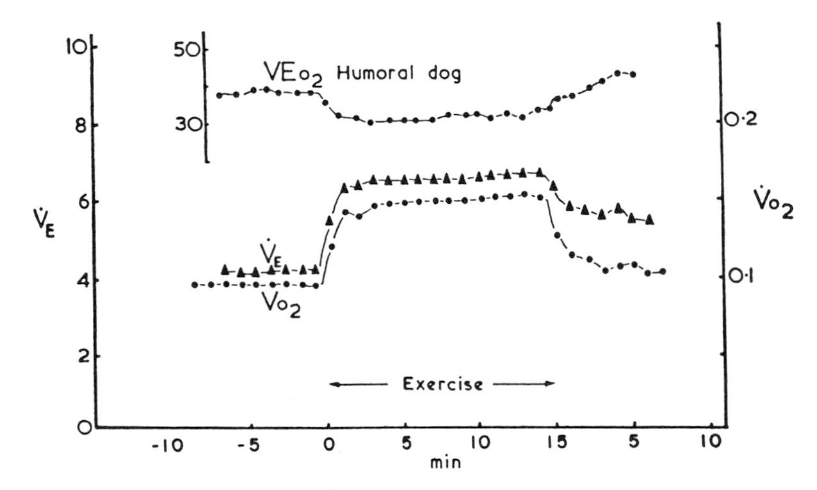

FIG. 10.15. The time course of pulmonary ventilation ($\dot{V}_E$), oxygen consumption ($\dot{V}O_2$) and the $\dot{V}_E$–$\dot{V}O_2$ and ($\dot{V}_EO_2$) in a neural dog when the hindlimb muscles were induced electrically to contract and the venous blood from the hindlimbs was diverted to a humoral dog. [Reprinted with permission from Kao (248).]

al. (248) thus concluded "there is certainly a peripheral neurogenic drive which must be considered as the, or one of the mechanisms of exercise hyperpnea."

Investigators other than Kao et al. have found that electrically induced muscle contractions in anesthetized animals increases ventilation. Comroe and Schmidt (90) electrically induced exercise by stimulation of ventral roots in anesthetized dogs. Ventilation increased with muscle contraction, and this hyperpnea was eliminated by spinal cord transection. Mitchell et al. (311, 338) in two studies electrically stimulated ventral roots L7–S1 to cause isometric contractions of the hindlimbs of anesthetized cats. A hyperpnea accompanied the contractions but the hyperpnea was absent when dorsal roots were cut to eliminate afferent feedback from the muscles. The authors concluded that in this preparation the hyperpnea during contraction was mediated by muscle afferents. Bennett (41) induced exercise by stimulation of the peripheral ends of severed sciatic nerves of anesthetized dogs. Ventilation did not increase sufficiently during exercise to maintain Pa_{CO_2} homeostasis; thus, Bennett concluded that afferents from the muscles that were not intact in this preparation may play a role in the normal ventilatory response in intact animals. Tibes (468) also induced hindlimb contraction in anesthetized dogs by stimulation of the sciatic nerves. Contraction resulted in an increase in ventilation that was abolished by cold block of afferents from the contracting muscles. Afferents in nonmyelinated or small myelinated group III and IV fibers were of most importance. Slightly different studies were completed by Senapati (427) but the results are consistent with the above. He electrically stimulated the central end of the lateral gastrocnemius-soleus nerve at intensities to activate only group I and II fibers or at higher intensities to activate group III afferents. He found that ventilation increased with stimulation and the greatest increase occurred when group III fibers were activated. Applying pressure to the muscle and stretching the muscles also increased ventilation. The results of these studies support the conclusion of Kao that muscle afferents could contribute to the exercise hyperpnea.

Other investigators' findings and conclusions differ from the above. Comroe and Schmidt (90) electrically induced exercise in the hindlimb of anesthetized cats. A hyperpnea during contraction was not altered by spinal cord transection. In dogs and cats, Lamb (287) electrically stimulated sciatic nerves to elicit muscle contractions that increased metabolic rate and ventilation threefold and thereby maintained blood gas homeostasis. These responses were not altered after lumbar spinal cord transection. Similarly, Cross et al. (101) compared responses to electrically induced contractions of anesthetized dogs before and after cord transection. The results are perplexing because ventilation and metabolic rate increased proportionately the same both before and after cord transection but Pa_{CO_2} was higher during muscle contraction after cord transection. Nevertheless, this group concluded the spinal cord was not needed for a normal ventilatory response to electrically induced work. Levine (291) electrically induced muscle contraction of the hindlimbs of anesthetized dogs after spinal transection at L2. Contractions increased both ventilation and metabolic rate about 170% without any change in arterial blood gases and pH. He concluded that "muscular exercise can stimulate $\dot{V}_E$ via humoral factors." Weissman et al. (493) induced hindlimb muscle contraction in anesthetized cats by bilateral electrical stimulation of ventral roots L7, S1, and S2. Breathing did not increase immediately with initiation of contractions but did progressively increase to maintain Pa_{CO_2} at or near control levels. Sectioning the spinal cord at L1–L2 did not alter the ventilatory responses and Pa_{CO_2} homeostasis. These authors conclude that "reflex discharge of afferent nerves from the exercising limbs was not requisite for the matching of ventilation to metabolic demand during exercise."

It is not possible to conclude from the results of the studies on electrically induced muscle contractions in nonhuman anesthetized mammals whether an intact spinal cord is requisite for the induced hyperpnea. The cause of the discrepant findings is not known, but it might stem from the unphysiologic nature of the preparations or from the anesthetic regimen employed. Moreover, an inherent problem with these studies is that the changes in ventilation and metabolic rate are very small. As a result, it is questionable whether the protocols and measurement techniques are sufficiently stringent to provide the resolution needed to distinguish between alternative hypothesis.

Muscle Chemoreflex in Anesthetized Animals. The postulate of muscle chemoreceptors contributing to the exercise hyperpnea is suggested by data already summarized that a muscle chemoreflex influences arterial blood pressure regulation during exercise. This hypothesis has been tested in anesthetized animals by venous occlusion during electrically induced muscle contractions. The rationale for venous occlusion is that it would create ischemia in the muscles; thus, if a muscle chemoreflex contributes to the exercise hyperpnea, ventilation should increase during venous occlusion. During electrically induced muscle contractions, Comroe and Schmidt (90) found in cats that venous occlusion attenuated the contraction-induced hyperpnea, while in dogs they found that occlusion did not alter the hyperpnea. Accordingly, in both species the findings do not support the hypothesis.

The hypothesis has also been tested in anesthetized animals by: (1) perfusion of isolated legs with hypercapnic, acidotic, and hypoxemic blood or with venous blood collected previously from exercising legs, and (2) intra-arterial injections of chemical agents known to change during exercise. Data from at least seven different studies (90, 112, 113, 225, 341, 401, 402) do not support the hypothesis. In other words, none of these conditions that altered chemical status in muscles resulted in an increase in breathing. In contrast, then, to the studies on arterial blood pressure regulation, these studies on anesthetized animals do not support the hypothesis of a muscle chemoreflex contributing to the exercise hyperpnea.

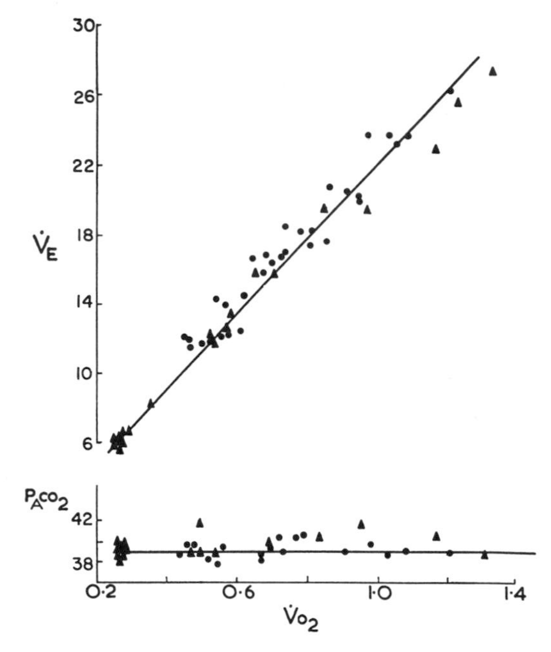

FIG. 10.16. The relationship between pulmonary ventilation ($\dot{V}_E$) and alveolar P_{CO_2} (P_{ACO_2}) to oxygen consumption ($\dot{V}O_2$) during voluntary (Δ) and electrically induced muscle contraction (●) in a single awake human subject. [Reprinted with permission from Asmussen and Nielsen (18).]

Electrically Induced Muscle Contractions in Awake Humans. Electrically induced muscle contractions in awake humans has been repeatedly used to gain insight into the mechanisms causing the exercise hyperpnea. Adams et al. (2), Asmussen, et al. (19), and Brice et al. (60) all compared the ventilatory responses of spinal cord-intact humans performing work voluntarily with work electrically induced. Investigators in these studies found the responses virtually identical including the relationship between ventilation and metabolic rate (Fig. 10.16) and the temporal pattern of arterial blood gases, $\dot{V}_E$, f, V_T, T_I and T_E. Investigators in these studies devised means that suggest central command was indeed bypassed; thus, these data provide evidence that limb afferents potentially could mediate the exercise hyperpnea. However, other investigators (3, 19, 59, 62) have found that the hyperpnea during electrically induced muscle contraction in paraplegic humans is indistinguishable from the hyperpnea during electrically induced muscle contraction in spinal cord-intact humans. These data appear inconsistent with mediation of the hyperpnea by spinal afferents and suggest that a humoral mechanism mediates the hyperpnea. However, data from a venous occlusion study in paraplegics are inconsistent with humoral mediation of this hyperpnea in paraplegics (62). Muscle contraction of the legs of paraplegics was electrically induced. Once in a steady state, cuffs around the contracting muscles were inflated to attenuate venous return from the muscles. Oxygen consumption, Pa_{CO_2}, and ventilation all decreased with venous occlusion, but the decrease in Pa_{CO_2} preceded the decrease in ventilation by several seconds. Moreover, the decrease in ventilation was predictable from the decrease in Pa_{CO_2} and the normal CO_2 responsiveness of humans. The cause of hyperpnea in these paraplegics is thus not apparent. The importance of these data might be that they indicate that electrically induced exercise in paraplegics, spinal cord–intact humans, and in anesthetized animals is not a suitable model for study of the mechanism mediating the exercise hyperpnea under physiologic conditions.

Muscle Chemoreflex in Awake Humans. Asmussen et al. (14, 18) tested the hypothesis of a muscle chemoreflex by studying humans exercising on a bicycle with and without occluding venous return from the muscles. Venous occlusion reduced oxygen consumption by 20–50% indicating that blood and metabolites were being trapped in the muscles. In their initial study (14), ventilation did not change with occlusion, thus, with the reduced flow of CO_2 to the lungs, alveolar P_{CO_2} decreased. In their second study (18), Pa_{CO_2} was maintained constant during occlusion by the addition of CO_2 to the inspirate. In this study, ventilation increased during occlusion. Barmen et al. (30) completed a study similar to that of

Asmussen et al. They found that venous occlusion slightly reduced the hyperpnea during treadmill exercise, with a rebound increased hyperpnea once occlusion was eliminated. They did not monitor Pa_{CO_2}; thus, the reduced hyperpnea during occlusion may have been due to reduced stimulation at carotid and brain chemoreceptors. Asmussen et al. (18) concluded that the increased ventilation during occlusion is "neurogenic caused by the increasing anaerobiosis in the blocked muscles. The nervous impulses involved may be elicited from muscle chemoreceptors or they may stem from mechanoreceptors being activated through an observed recruitment of new motor units necessitated by the anaerobiosis."

A major concern with venous occlusion during exercise in awake humans is the associated discomfort and/or psychological effects of the occlusion process. Asmussen et al. felt, though, that their subjects did not experience undue pain and were virtually oblivious to the occlusion. Nevertheless, it should be emphasized that numerous factors other than the chemical status in the muscles can be altered during venous occlusion and these potential alterations should be considered in interpreting the data.

Because of the complications involved with venous occlusion, two investigative groups (127, 505) have tested the muscle chemoreflex hypothesis in awake humans using a slightly different technique. The legs of subjects were enclosed in a chamber. During supine cycle ergometry, perfusion of the legs was reduced by about 20% by increasing the pressure in the chamber up to 50 mm Hg. Increasing the pressure resulted in ventilation increasing above and end tidal CO_2 decreasing below exercising without increased pressure (Fig. 10.17). The authors thus concluded that the augmented ventilation could be due to "accumulation of intramuscular metabolites at the working limb and/or a direct effect of increased intramuscular tissue pressure." However, lactacidosis was also evident in the blood and the subjects perceived greater fatigue during exercise with reduced leg perfusion. Accordingly, as with the venous occlusion studies, factors other than potential muscle chemoreceptors may have contributed to the augmented ventilation under these conditions.

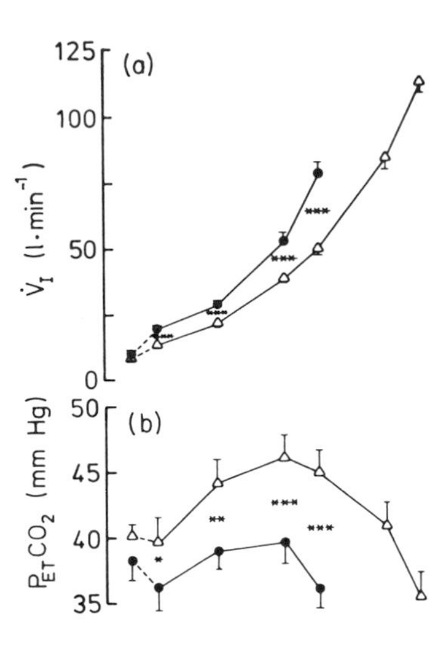

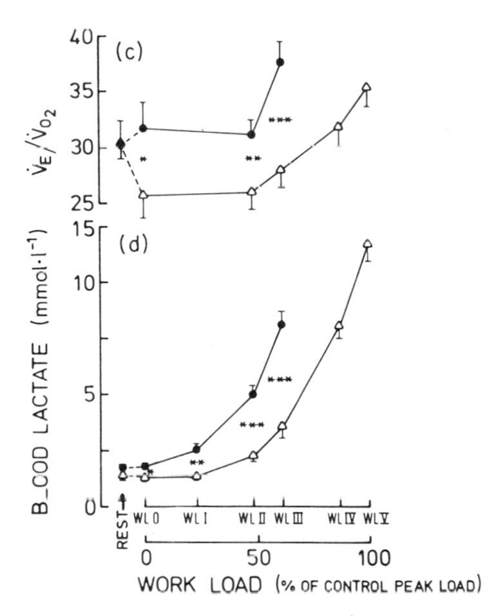

FIG. 10.17. The pulmonary ventilation ($\dot{V}_I$) end tidal CO_2 (P_{ETCO_2}), the ratio of $\dot{V}_I$ to metabolic rate ($\dot{V}O_2$), and blood lactate during several intensities of bicycle exercise in human subjects. *Open triangles* represent data with unobstructed leg blood flow and *closed circles* represent data when blood flow to the legs was reduced about 20% by increasing pressure around the legs to 50 mm Hg. [Reprinted with permission from Williamson et al. (505).]

Anesthetic Block of Muscle Afferents in Awake Humans. Three different studies (140, 217, 452) have attempted to gain insight into the exercise hyperpnea using anesthetic block of muscle afferents during normal exercise. Hornbien et al. (217) selectively blocked γ-efferent fibers using 15–20 ml of lidocaine injected into the lumbar peridural space. They demonstrated that small γ-efferent fibers were blocked, while larger α-fibers were spared. They found no effect on ventilation of γ-efferent blockade during the onset, steady state, or cessation of exercise at a $\dot{V}O_2$ of about 2 ℓ pd min^{-1}. They concluded that muscle spindle afferents do not contribute to the exercise hyperpnea. Fernandes et al. (140) injected bupivacaine at the L3–L4 vertebral interspace in humans and verified leg afferent neural blockade by cutaneous sensory analgesia below T10-T11. When the subjects exercised after epidural anesthesia, arterial blood pressure was reduced from control experiments but ventilation and heart rate were not altered. The authors concluded that muscle afferents may not be necessary to elicit a normal ventilatory response to exercise. The hypotension with epidural block complicates interpretation of the ventilatory data because hypotension is associated with increased breathing (64, 358). The potential exists that a reduced stimulus to ventilation by attenuation of muscle afferents was offset by increased stimulus to ventilation by the hypotension. Strange et al. (452) studied the effect of epidural anesthesia on the ventilatory response to electrically induced dynamic knee extension. Neural blockade was verified by cutaneous sensory anesthesia below T8–T10 and complete paralysis of both legs. Muscle contraction caused a doubling of metabolic rate and ventilation and a 2–3 mm Hg decrease in Pa_{CO_2} both with and without leg paralysis. Mean arterial blood pressure increased during muscle contraction without anesthesia, but it remained at control levels with anesthesia. The authors concluded that neural reflex mechanisms are not essential for the ventilatory response to dynamic muscle contractions. The results of these studies on anesthetic block of muscle afferents suggest that the ventilatory response to muscle contraction is not critically dependent on muscle afferents. These findings are thus consistent with a normal ventilatory response to electrically induced muscle contractions in paraplegic humans.

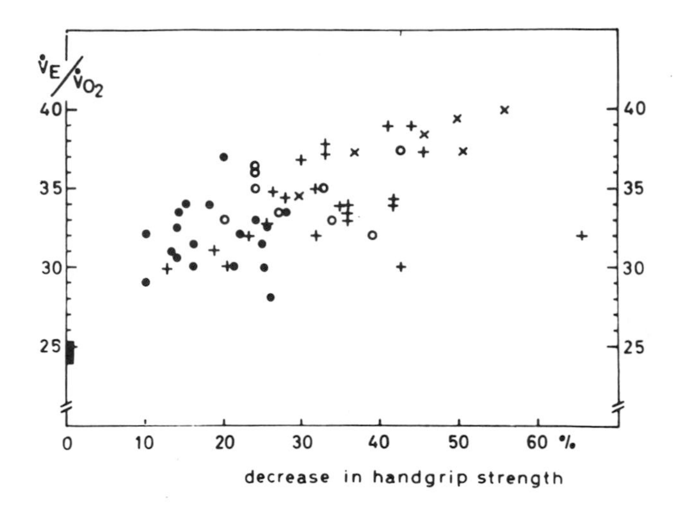

FIG. 10.18. The relationship between the ratio of pulmonary ventilation to metabolic rate ($\dot{V}_E/\dot{V}O_2$) and the reduction in handgrip strength during neuromuscular blockade by tubocurarine. Note that as the degree of block increased the $\dot{V}_E/\dot{V}_2$ ratio increased. [Reprinted with permission from Asmussen (12).]

Neuromuscular Blockade in Awake Humans. Neuromuscular blockade with curare-like agents has been another method used to determine the contribution of a reflex originating in contracting muscle to the ventilatory adjustments to exercise in humans. Asmussen (12) and Galbo et al. (163) examined the cardiovascular and ventilatory responses to bicycle exercise before and during partial neuromuscular blockade induced by curare. The two investigative groups used different paradigms but the major finding was the same; curare increased the ratio of ventilation to metabolic rate (Fig. 10.18). Asmussen (12) postulated that the mechanism of this increase was similar to the increase during venous occlusion. In both cases, individual motor units lose contractile power; therefore, activation of motor units must be increased to maintain a constant work rate. They further postulated that muscle activation occurs through the γ-loop and that it is the increased γ-afferents that accounts for the augmented hyperpnea during curare block and venous occlusion. Galbo et al. (163) also concluded that these findings provide support for a role for a peripheral factor such as a muscle reflex in causing the ventilatory adjustments to dynamic exercise. Specifically, these investigators thought that this reflex arose from the stimulation of metaboreceptors in the exercising muscles.

Lesioning Spinal Afferents in Awake Ponies. In many of the aforementioned studies, the techniques used may not have provided the type of muscle contraction that occurs during voluntary dynamic exercise. This consideration led to a recent study in which ponies performed normal treadmill exercises before and 3–4 weeks after attenuating spinal afferents through surgical lesions of dorsal lateral spinal pathways (375) at the first lumbar level. Prior to surgery, mild and moderate treadmill walking reduced Pa_{CO_2} by 2.7 and 4.1 mm Hg during the first 30 s at the 2 respective work rates (Fig. 10.19). This is the normal response of most mammals. One month following surgery, the exercise hypocapnia was attenuated to only 1.5 and 2.3 mm Hg. During steady-state walking, the hypocapnia was also attenuated after partial spinal lesion, but it was not altered during treadmill running. The hypocapnia during treadmill walking was reduced primarily by a lowered breathing frequency. This attenuation of the hypocapnia and hyperpnea during treadmill walking suggests that spinal afferent information may play some role in the exercise hyperpnea in awake ponies. These data probably underestimate this contribution for two reasons. *First*, afferent innervation of the forelimbs remained intact and it could not be determined whether hindlimb afferents were totally eliminated. *Second*, learning (444) or long-term modu-

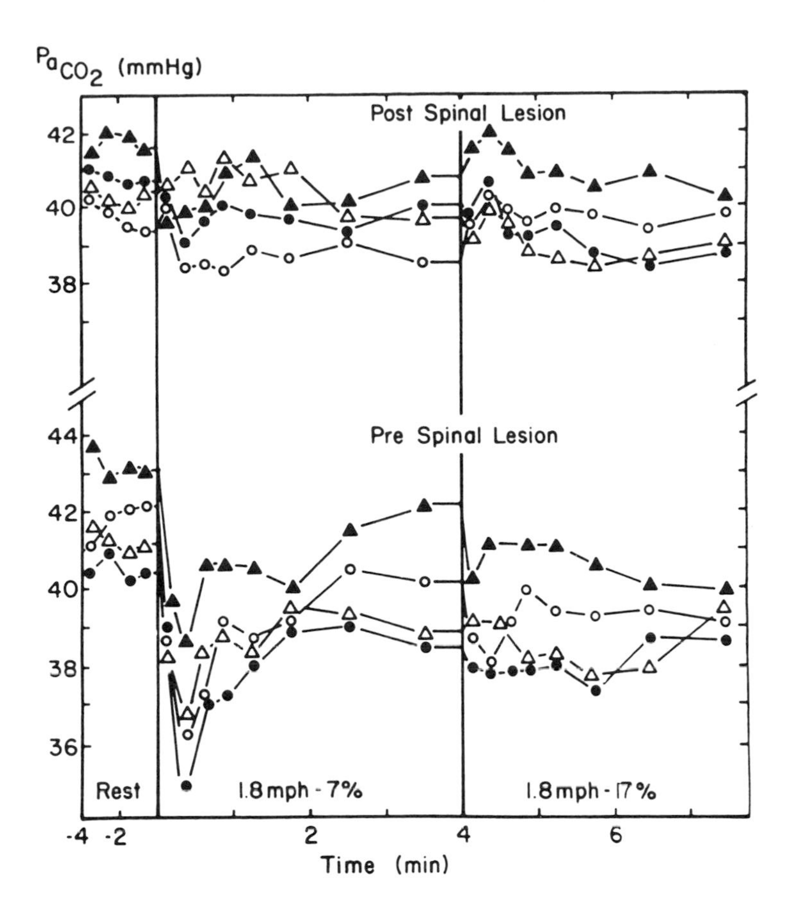

FIG. 10.19. $PaCO_2$ response to two levels of treadmill exercise repeated in one pony on several different days before and 3 weeks after partial lesioning the dorsal lateral spinal columns at the L2 level. The different symbols represent separate days. Note the attenuated exercise hypocapnia following spinal lesioning. [Reprinted with permission from Pan et al. (375).]

lation (334, 335) may have occurred during the 1 month of recovery from the lesions. Most of the ponies were virtually incapable of walking for days after lesioning due to sensory loss or motor weakness, but eventually they recovered to the extent that they walked almost normally. Measurements soon after lesioning in some ponies suggested a greater attenuation of ventilation than observed 1 month post lesioning. Since learning or long-term modulation within the ventilatory control system appears to occur in goats after thoracic dorsal rhizotomy (334, 335) it is conceivable these changes also occurred after lumbar spinal lesions. Accordingly, spinal afferents may contribute more to the exercise hyperpnea than indicated after the spinal lesions in ponies.

Entrainment of Breathing Frequency with Stride Frequency. Several mammals, including humans, demonstrate entrainment or a coupling of breathing frequency with limb movement frequency (11, 38, 40, 57, 114, 116, 158, 191, 318). The entrainment in quadrupeds occurs during trotting, cantering, and galloping (11, 38, 57, 114). The physiological benefits and implications have been detailed elsewhere (114). The mechanism of this coupling has not been established. One possible mechanism is through spinal afferents. Indeed, studies on humans have shown that breathing frequency is higher during treadmill running than walking at equivalent metabolic rates (114, 191). The fact that breathing frequency was attenuated by partial spinal lesions in ponies (375) provides additional evidence that breathing frequency and possibly entrainment is influenced by spinal afferents.

Summary and Conclusions of Contribution by Afferents from Exercising Limbs to the Exercise Hyperpnea. There are limitations in each of the studies that have been conducted to test the hypothesis that muscle afferents mediate or contribute to the exercise hyperpnea. A consequence of these limitations is that the individual and combined results do not provide convincing evidence that muscle afferents mediate or contribute to exercise hyperpnea. On the other hand, in spite of the limitations, results of several of the studies suggest that muscle afferents may have some role in the exercise hyperpnea. In other words, there is enough suggestive evidence to warrant additional studies on this topic.

The Carotid Chemoreceptor Afferents

Basic Structure and Function. The carotid bodies are small bilateral organs located near the bifurcations of the common carotid arteries (285, 355). They consist of type I or glomus cells that are innervated by fibers of the carotid sinus nerve (a branch of the ninth cranial nerve). The cell-nerve complex is surrounded by processes of type II cells that serve a glial-like function. The type I cell cytoplasm has numerous organelles and a morphological relationship with the nerve ending consistent with the structure of a chemical reciprocal synapse. The major natural stimuli are hypoxemia, hypercapnia, acidosis, and hyperkalemia. The exact chemosensory mechanism by which each of these stimuli is detected remains controversial, but current evidence suggests these stimuli induce an increase in cytoplasmic [Ca^{2+}] in the type I cell that results in neurotransmitter release from the cell that initiates the postsynaptic events at the nerve ending leading to a propagated action potential in the sinus nerve.

At normal levels of the natural stimuli, there is a low-level, irregular sensory discharge pattern by the carotid chemoreceptors (285, 355). The discharge response curve to hypoxia is hyperbolic, with a sharp increase in discharge at a Pa_{O_2} of about 40–50 mm Hg. The response to CO_2/H^+ is linear over the physiologic range with a definable threshold stimulus, that is, a level of CO_2/H^+ below which a further decrease in stimulus does not reduce the rate of discharge. The chemosensory elements respond quickly to changes in stimuli as indicated by changes in sinus nerve activity with breath-to-breath oscillations in stimulus levels (27, 52). The changes in breathing with changes in stimulus levels resemble the characteristics of the chemoreceptors. The basal level of chemoreceptor activity contributes to the eupneic level of breathing as demonstrated by the hypoventilation that occurs as a result of carotid body denervation (50, 156, 371).

Role in Hyperpnea of Submaximal Exercise. It has been known for years that in humans, alveolar and arterial P_{CO_2} and P_{O_2} differ minimally between rest and the steady state of mild and moderate exercise (12, 31, 112, 114, 121, 359, 514). In addition, even when exercise intensity is rapidly changed, there is only a 1–3 mm Hg change in Pa_{CO_2} and Pa_{O_2}, and a 0.01–0.02 change in arterial pH (158, 345). In virtually all nonhuman species studied, the magnitude of these transient changes is more than in humans, and in the steady state of exercise there is clearly a workload dependent arterial hypocapnia and alkalosis (50, 58, 80, 142, 143, 150, 371–375). In other words, P_{O_2}, P_{CO_2} and H^+ stimulus level at the carotid chemoreceptors clearly do not increase in a manner expected to account for the hyperpnea of exercise. In fact, each stimulus changes slightly in the direction opposite to that required to explain the hyperpnea. Nevertheless, it has been hypothesized that by various mechanisms the carotid chemoreceptors contribute to and/or account for the exercise hyperpnea.

Increased gain of chemoreceptors. Carotid chemoreceptors have been postulated to mediate the hyperpnea as a result of increased gain of these chemoreceptors. Gain is defined in this context as an increased receptor output for the same stimulus level. It follows then that the increased output would mediate the hyperpnea. Support for this postulate came from findings that carotid chemoreceptor firing rate was increased in anesthetized cats during passive rhythmic movements of the hindlimbs (47). This increased activity was abolished by section of the cervical sympathetic nerve or the postglanglionic branch to the carotid body or by section of the femoral and sciatic nerves. Evidence against this postulate was provided when stimulation of breathing by electrically induced muscular contraction of hindlimb muscles of cats had no effect on afferent discharge from the carotid chemoreceptors (47). Moreover, others (128) blocked carotid sympathetic innervation in humans by injection of lidocaine into the stellate ganglia bilaterally and found no significant change in $\dot{V}_E$ or blood gases during 9 min of submaximal exercise. These data do not rule out increased chemoreceptor gain during exercise because factors unrelated to sympathetic innervation could increase carotid chemoreceptor activity and ventilatory responsiveness (88, 103). If chemoreceptor gain does increase during exercise, then the ventilatory responses to elevated CO_2/H^+ and to lowered O_2 should be greater during exercise than at rest. However, there is no clear indication that ventilatory responsiveness to CO_2/H^+ is increased during exercise (12, 16, 75, 104, 122, 264, 340, 388, 492). Moreover, even though the ventilatory response to hypoxia is greater during exercise than at rest (12, 492), there is no clear evidence that small (<5 mm Hg) increases or decreases around the normal level of Pa_{O_2} during exercise has an affect on $\dot{V}_E$ (unpublished). Accordingly, we conclude that the hyperpnea of exercise is not mediated by changes in carotid chemoreceptor gain.

Increased breath-to-breath oscillations in chemoreceptor activity. Within-breath changes in Pa_{CO_2}, Pa_{O_2}, and arterial pH have been hypothesized to provide a signal for the hyperpnea of exercise (25, 170, 457, 464, 510). This hypothesis is based on findings that (1) the within-breath changes in blood gases are altered by exercise (102), (2) at rest and during exercise carotid chemoreceptor activity oscillates in the same manner as blood gases (27, 52), (3) changes in these oscillations have been found to increase breathing (51, 176, 417), and (4) increasing lung CO_2 delivery by 2.6-fold locked respiratory rhythm to the peak of arterial CO_2 oscillation (457). However, the magnitude of ventilatory changes secondary to changes in oscillation are small (355, 417). Indeed, results of a recent study of ventilatory dynamics and oscillation during exercise by humans led to the conclusion that oscillation in blood gases during exercise contributes minimally to the exercise hyperpnea (484).

Integral control during exercise. A third hypothesis is that the respiratory center functions as an integral controller during exercise (487). It was proposed that integral control functioned as follows. A transient hypercapnia at the onset of exercise increases carotid chemoreceptor activity, which increases breathing to restore Pa_{CO_2} to normal. Breathing then remains elevated until there is a transient hypocapnia at the termination of exercise. This theory is not supported by data showing that the predominant change in Pa_{CO_2} at the onset of exercise is a slight hypocapnia. This hypothesis is thus rejected.

Increased plasma $[K^+]$ during exercise. The most recent postulate is that carotid chemoreceptors contribute to the exercise hyperpnea through an effect on chemoreceptor activity of exercise hyperkalemia (376). In anesthetized cats, intravenous injection of K^+ increases carotid chemoreceptor discharge rate and ventilation, and this hyperpnea is abolished by bilateral carotid and aortic chemodenervation (26, 294). For both humans and ponies, plasma $[K^+]$ (during all levels of exercise) is linearly related to CO_2 production and during submaximal exercise ventilation is linearly related to plasma $[K^+]$ (92, 153, 295, 314, 376). On the other hand, lowering of plasma $[K^+]$ in chronically hyperkalemic humans does not alter ventilation (120). Finally, intravenous infusion of K^+ in awake goats to increase plasma $[K^+]$ equivalent to moderate exercise had only a small affect on $\dot{V}_E$ (485). The evidence in support of K^+ at the carotid chemoreceptors contributing to the exercise hyperpnea remains largely circumstantial.

Carotid chemoreceptor denervation studies. The studies of Wasserman et al. (490) and Honda et al. (215) on asthmatics with their carotid chemoreceptors resected (CCR) are often cited as providing evidence that these chemoreceptors contribute to the exercise hyperpnea. The time constant of $\dot{V}_E$ in response to exercise is greater in CCR asthmatics than in age-matched control subjects. There is thus a transient hypercapnia in CCR asthmatics but not in the control subjects (Fig. 10.20). Wasserman et al. subsequently found that any condition that increased carotid chemoreceptor activity decreased the time constant of ventilation in response to exercise (183, 362) whereas conditions that decreased chemoreceptor activity increased the time constant (70). Consequently, Wasserman et al. concluded that the carotid chemoreceptors "are responsible, in part, for the rate of increase in $\dot{V}_E$ to steady-state exercise" (490).

The preceding studies by Wasserman et al. and Honda et al., however, raise two major concerns. First, the changes in plasma $[H^+]$ and Pa_{O_2} that were found to affect the kinetics of ventilation to exercise can also affect breathing by mechanisms other than those originating from carotid chemoreceptors (48). For example, brain $[H^+]$ and presumably intracranial chemoreceptor stimulation change very quickly with changes in plasma $[H^+]$ (464). These changes could mediate the changes in kinetics of ventilation to exercise caused by metabolic acidosis and alkalosis. In addition, changes in Pa_{O_2} affect breathing through mechanisms in the brain (48). Some of these mechanisms increase breathing, whereas others depress breathing. The altered change in kinetics of ventilation to exercise cannot, therefore, be simply ascribed to altered carotid chemoreceptor activity. Second, it was assumed that the chemoreceptor resection rather than the asthma caused the abnormal response in CCR asthmatics. However, it was not established that the CCR asthmatics had normal pulmonary mechanics during exercise. Thus, the exercise hypercapnia could have stemmed from altered pulmonary mechanics or some other factor related to asthma. Increased external airway resistance in nonasthmatic humans and in nonhuman species causes hypercapnia during exercise (150, 154, 515) and this hypercapnia is accentuated when carotid chemoreceptor activity is attenuated by hyperoxia. Moreover, it was recently found that asthmatics with intact carotid chemoreceptors were hypercapnic during exercise and this hypercapnia was accentuated by hyperoxia (150). During hyperoxia, Pa_{CO_2} increased by 5 mm Hg between rest and moderate exercise in these chemoreceptor intact asthmatics dur-

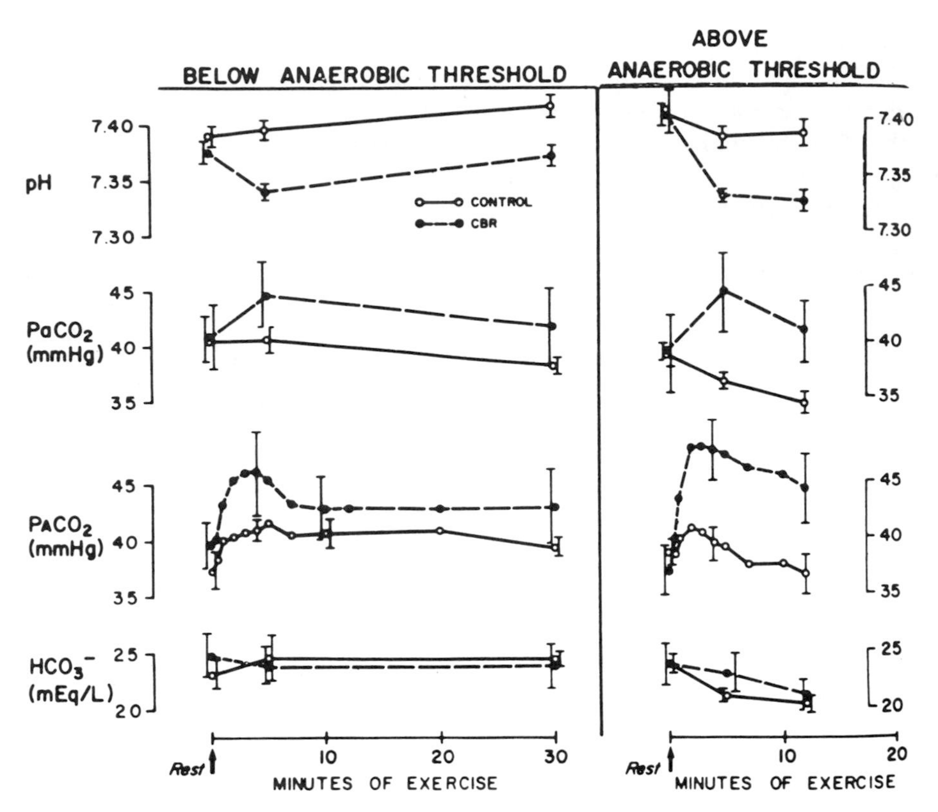

FIG. 10.20. Average arterial and end-tidal CO_2 tensions (Pa_{CO_2} and PA_{CO_2}) respectively, arterial pH, and bicarbonate for control and carotid chemoreceptor–resected (CBR) asthmatics below (*left*) and above (*right*) the anaerobic threshold. [Reprinted with permission from Wasserman et al. (490).]

ing exercise. Inasmuch as this increase is nearly identical to the exercise-induced increase in Pa_{CO_2} in the CCR asthmatics, these patients appear not to be an appropriate model for assessing the role of the carotid chemoreceptors in the exercise hyperpnea. Because attenuation of carotid chemoreceptor activity by hyperoxia during exercise accentuates the arterial hypercapnia of exercise during ventilatory loading (150), asthma (150), and in patients with chronic obstructive pulmonary disease (349), it appears that the role of the carotid chemoreceptors during exercise is to "fine tune" alveolar ventilation in order to minimize disruptions in arterial blood gases and pH.

The above conclusion is supported by data on nonhuman mammals. The hyperventilation during the first 30 s of a change in metabolic rate is greater in CCR dogs (142), goats (50), and ponies (155, 156, 371), than it is in chemoreceptor-intact animals (Fig. 10.21). An accentuated hyperventilation is also observed in normal ponies when chemoreceptor activity is attenuated through hyperoxia (156). Moreover, partial spinal lesioning, referred to earlier, results in hypoventilation in some ponies during exercise, and this hypoventilation is accentuated after CCR (374). It is evident, therefore, that these chemoreceptors minimize bidirectionally any deviation from the normal Pa_{CO_2}. Accordingly, it appears the role of the carotid chemoreceptors during exercise in nonhuman and in human species is to "fine tune" $\dot{V}_A$ to meet the metabolic needs for gas exchange.

Summary and conclusions of role during submaximal exercise. In summary, the breath-by-breath changes in blood gases and the elevated plasma [K^+] during submaximal exercise might potentially alter the input from the carotid chemoreceptors to the medullary controllers of ventilation. However, the magnitude of these potential affects and the effects of attenuation of chemoreceptor activity by hyperoxia and surgical denervation suggest that these chemoreceptors do not provide a "primary" drive for the exercise hyperpnea. Rather, many data are consistent with the concept that the chemoreceptors provide a fine tuning of alveolar ventilation during exercise.

Role in Hyperventilation During Heavy Exercise

Rationale for hypothesis and supportive data. In humans there is a good correlation between plasma

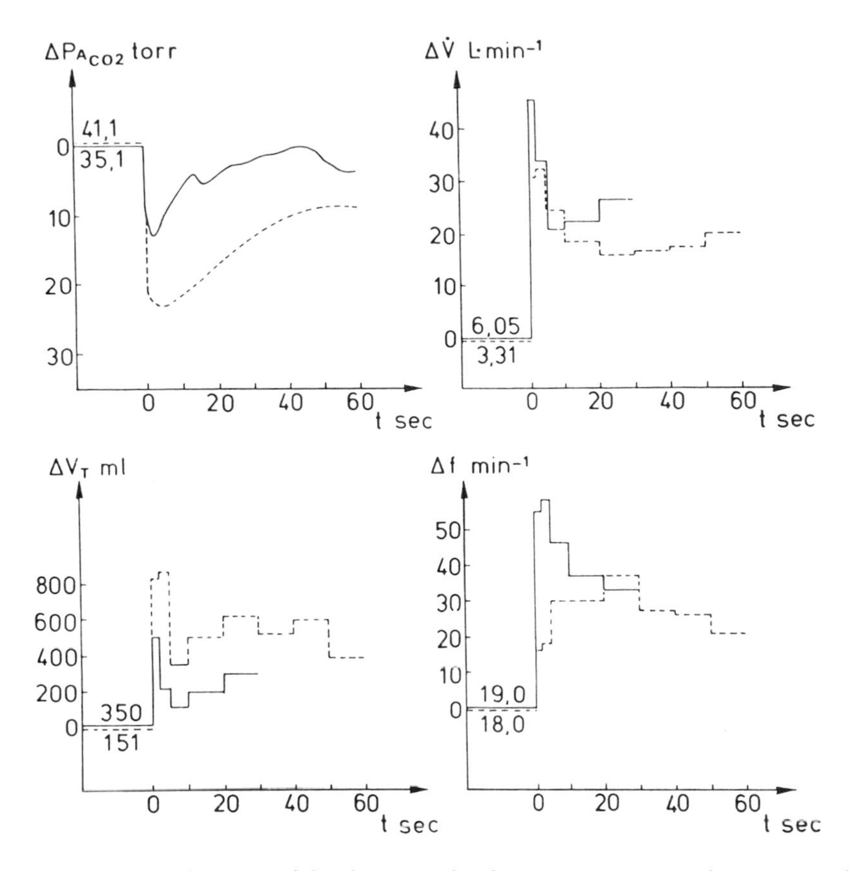

FIG. 10.21. The temporal pattern of the change in alveolar P_{CO_2} ($\Delta P_{A_{CO_2}}$), pulmonary ventilation ($\Delta \dot{V}_I$), tidal volume (ΔV_T), and breathing frequency (Δf) in a dog before (*full lines*) and after carotid chemodenervation (*dashed line*). [Reprinted with permission from Flandrois, Lacour, and Eclache (142).]

$[H^+]$ and exercise-induced hyperventilation (115, 117, 496). At low work rates, hyperventilation is minimal and plasma pH is near normal, but between 60–80% of maximal $\dot{V}O_2$, hyperventilation is accentuated and at the same time a lactacidosis becomes apparent. Both hyperventilation and plasma lactacidosis progressively increase as work intensity rises beyond 70% of maximum. This correlation provides much of the basis for the theory that heavy exercise hyperventilation is mediated by increased H^+ stimulating carotid chemoreceptors (15, 112, 350, 496). Theoretically, several other changes may also increase carotid chemoreceptor activity during heavy exercise. For example, plasma $[K^+]$ (376, 377) and catecholamine concentration (137, 189) both increase and these acting alone and/or synergistically with P_{O_2} and H^+ should increase chemoreceptor activity (12, 16, 65, 105, 144, 376, 492).

Increasing P_{O_2} by raising PI_{O_2} during heavy exercise decreases $\dot{V}_E$ and plasma [lactate] and increases Pa_{CO_2} and arterial pH (15, 17, 29). Hyperoxia presumably reduces stimulation of carotid chemoreceptors by lowering both plasma $[H^+]$ and increasing Pa_{O_2}. In addition, hyperoxia reduces the synergism between the P_{O_2}i2 and the exercise stimuli and between the P_{O_2} and both H^+ and K^+ stimuli at the carotid chemoreceptor. There are thus several potential ways by which hyperoxia can reduce chemoreceptor activity. Other evidence suggests though that the reduced ventilation with hyperoxia might not be solely chemoreceptor mediated. Specifically, when Pa_{O_2} is increased from 90 to 200 mm Hg, the decrease in breathing is the same as when Pa_{O_2} is increased from 200 to 600 mm Hg (17, 29). It is doubtful that O_2 stimulation of the chemoreceptors decreases equally between 90 to 200 mm Hg and between 200 and 600 mm Hg. Furthermore, increasing Pa_{O_2} improves tissue oxygenation, reduces blood lactate, and generally has effects opposite to that of the muscle ischemia that occurs with venous occlusion. In other words, just as with venous occlusion, hyperoxia causes multiple effects in the exercising muscles and elsewhere in the body including the brain. Many of these changes potentially contribute to the change in breathing when increasing Pa_{O_2} during heavy exercise.

The CCR asthmatics previously mentioned did not hyperventilate during heavy exercise (490); their Pa_{CO_2} increased above rest during heavy exercise (Fig. 10.20). These findings are often cited to support the theory that the carotid chemoreceptors mediate the hyperventilation during heavy exercise. However, these CCR asthmatics were hypercapnic and acidotic even during mild exercise, and recent data suggest that asthma and not CCR is the primary cause of their abnormal ventilatory response to submaximal exercise (150).

Data inconsistent with carotid chemoreceptor mediation of hyperventilation. Other data from human studies are inconsistent with H^+ mediation of hyperventilation during heavy exercise. First, lactic acid production during heavy exercise has been attenuated by dietary manipulation, but the hyperventilation was unaffected (179, 188, 219). Second, patients with McArdle's syndrome are incapable of producing lactic acid, yet they hyperventilate during heavy exercise (187, 377). These studies suggest a dissociation between hyperventilation and acidosis during heavy exercise. McArdle's syndrome is a questionable model for these studies because these subjects hyperventilate even during submaximal exercise. Apparently, some factor not present in normal subjects causes hyperventilation at all workloads in these patients. Thus, this model has not provided clear insights into the mechanism of hyperventilation during heavy exercise.

Hyperventilation during heavy exercise is not accentuated in ponies with intact carotid chemoreceptors (373). Rather, exercise hypocapnia is linearly related to work rate irrespective of arterial pH, which is alkaline below about 60% of maximum $\dot{V}O_2$ and then becomes progressively acidotic above 60% of maximum (Fig. 10.22). In thoroughbred horses during heavy exercise, Pa_{CO_2} is actually above normal in spite of a very severe lactacidosis (37, 218). The reason for this hypoventilation might relate to a limitation on $\dot{V}_A$ imposed by the entrainment of breathing frequency and limb movement (114). Absence of a correlation between plasma H^+ and hyperventilation in ponies does not by itself indicate that H^+ has no influence on the hyperventilation. Indeed, it has been shown that ponies hyperventilate when lactic acid is infused intravenously at rest and during mild and moderate exercise (135). Absence of a correlation simply suggests that stimuli other than plasma $[H^+]$ are of importance to the hyperventilation.

The concept of stimulation of $\dot{V}_E$ by metabolic acidosis via the carotid chemoreceptors is supported

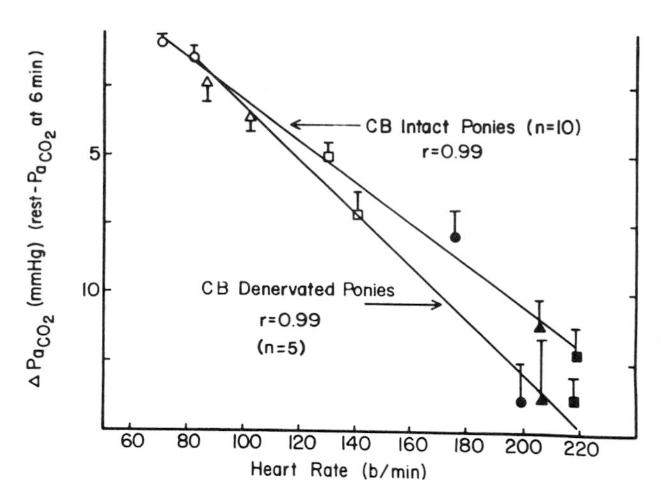

FIG. 10.22. The change in Pa_{CO_2} (ΔPa_{CO_2}) between rest and six levels of steady-state treadmill exercise in carotid body intact and denervated ponies plotted against heart rate used as an index of work intensity. Note the inverse linear relationship between work intensity and ΔPa_{CO_2}, and that the exercise hypocapnia is accentuated by CBD. [Reprinted with permission from Pan et al. (373).]

by a study in humans in whom carotid chemoreceptor activity was blunted by halothane (269) and by a second study in carotid denervated dogs (24). In both of these studies, the $\dot{V}_E$ response to exogenous metabolic acidosis was reduced after attenuation of carotid chemoreceptor activity. However, studies in dogs (241), rabbits (347), goats (450), and ponies (135) have shown that carotid body denervation (CBD) does not attenuate the hyperpnea induced by intravenous acid infusion. Moreover, during acid infusion there are rapid changes in cerebral extracellular fluid $[H^+]$ (464). Presumably, this acidosis increases stimulation at the intracranial chemoreceptor to mediate the hyperventilation during exogenous lactacidosis. These data show that the carotid chemoreceptors are not required for the hyperventilation in response to exogenous lactacidosis; therefore, they do not support the postulate that the hyperventilation during heavy exercise is due to increased H^+ stimulus at the carotid chemoreceptors.

Ponies are the only species without airway disease known to have been studied during maximal exercise before and after CBD (153, 373). Even though ponies with their carotid chemoreceptors denervated are mildly hypercapnic at rest, during maximal exercise their Pa_{CO_2} decreases to 1–2 mm Hg below that during maximal exercise before denervation (Fig. 10.22). This 1–2 mm Hg represents a large difference in alveolar ventilation considering the absolute level of Pa_{CO_2} and rate of CO_2 production. The accentuated exercise hyperventilation suggests that the ventilatory stimulus must be greater after denervation. Conceivably, in normal ponies, the hypocapnia at the carotid chemoreceptors outweighs the effect of the metabolic acids, hyperkalemia, and increased catecholamines so that the level of chemoreceptor activity during maximal exercise is reduced. In other words, denervation removes an inhibitory influence on breathing during heavy exercise so that hyperventilation is greater than it is in normal ponies (135).

The inhibitory effect of hypocapnia on breathing at the carotid chemoreceptors has been documented in studies on awake dogs and goats by isolating and separately perfusing these chemoreceptors (108, 441). A reduction in P_{CO_2} of about 10 mm Hg at only the carotid chemoreceptor in the unanesthetized dog immediately reduces V_T and $\dot{V}_E$ by 25–50% (Fig. 10.23). This inhibitory effect on ventilatory output persists (although at a reduced level) throughout 2 min of perfusion despite significant increases in arterial P_{CO_2} (and presumably significant acidification of the medullary chemoreceptors). This inhibitory effect of carotid body hypocapnia on breathing is equivalent to that of hyperoxia applied to the isolated, perfused carotid chemoreceptor (441).

Summary and conclusions of role during heavy exercise. In summary, many data do not support the theory that the hyperventilation during heavy exercise in humans without airway disease is mediated by increased H^+ stimulation of the carotid chemoreceptors. Alternate theories propose that hyperkalemia and/or catecholamines contribute to the hyperventilation are also not supported by data on ponies who had their carotid chemoreceptors denervated. It appears that the marked hypocapnia during heavy exercise results in reduced chemoreceptor activity in spite of the increase in plasma $[H^+]$, $[K^+]$, and catecholamines. It seems then that alternative explanations for the heavy exercise hyperventilation should be considered. One possibility is the mechanism proposed by Asmussen (12) to explain the augmented ventilation during venous occlusion or during curare neuromuscular blockade. His postulate was that as muscles fatigue, central command must increase out of proportion to metabolic rate in order to accomplish the task. Asmussen et al. (18) proposed that muscle afferents were involved in this increased neural output. This hypothesis warrants additional testing.

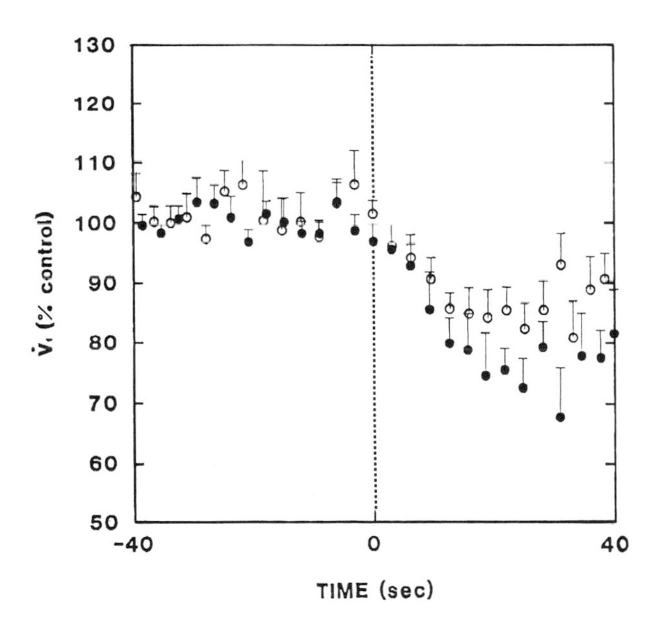

FIG. 10.23. The effect on pulmonary ventilation ($\dot{V}_I$) of reducing P_{CO_2} at the carotid chemoreceptors (unilateral by 7.2 or 13.1 mm Hg in dogs). The perfusion to the carotid chemoreceptors on one side was isolated and P_{CO_2} was reduced (time 0) using an extracorporeal exchange mechanism. Note that carotid chemoreceptor hypocapnia has a rapid and substantial depressant effect on breathing. [Reprinted with permission from Smith et al. (441).]

The Pulmonary Afferents

Basic Structure and Function. There are several different pulmonary receptors (413, 499). The discharge pattern of two of these has a fixed temporal relationship to the breathing cycle. These two are the slowly adapting receptors (SARs) and the rapidly adapting receptors (RARs) found in the extrapulmonary and intrapulmonary airways and innervated by myelinated fibers of the vagus nerve. Both receptors increase discharge rate with inspiration; the SARs sustain a steady discharge rate with a maintained lung inflation, whereas the RARs in the same condition have a rapidly fading activity. The primary function of the SARs is to provide information to the medullary controller regarding lung volume which, in turn, is one of the two determinants of inspiratory duration (a bulbopontine mechanism is the other). Absence of SAR activity (vagotomy) results in a prolonged inspiration and therefore a reduced breathing frequency and increased tidal volume. The importance of these receptors in control of breathing pattern differs between species; its importance is relatively minor in humans. The other major known SAR function is activation of expiratory muscles, which is thought to be a mechanism for keeping a constant end expiratory lung volume with changes in posture. The RARs are also mechanoreceptors whose apparent primary function is mediation of augmented breaths (sighs) that occur spontaneously at irregular intervals. It is thought that during regular breathing, lung compliance decreases gradually and this is sensed by RARs, which initiate the sigh. The function of the sigh is to restore compliance to normal.

Pulmonary and bronchial C-fibers are the other vagal afferents innervating the lungs (86, 413, 499). The bronchial C-fiber receptors are in the tracheobronchial airways and have primarily a chemosensitive function being activated by substances produced, released, and catabolized in the lungs. The pulmonary C-fiber receptors are located between alveolar walls and pulonary capillaries (83). They are more responsive to mechanical events than are the bronchial C-fiber receptors and display activity during conditions such as pulmonary congestion, edema, and microembolism (83, 86). Moreover, some pulmonary C-fibers in spontaneously breathing dogs and cats discharge with an inflationary rhythm (84). Generally, C-fiber afferents are considered to play a protective role in that they initiate reflexes such as a cough, airway constriction, and/or rapid, shallow breathing that reduce and/or eliminate potentially injurious agents.

Role in Hyperpnea of Submaximal Exercise and Hyperventilation of Heavy Exercise

Early studies on potential role of CO_2 receptors. A pulmonary receptor has been hypothesized to mediate the exercise hyperpnea (10, 21, 89, 100, 113, 177). This hypothesis was based on the close correlation between mixed venous P_{CO_2} and pulmonary ventilation during exercise (69, 125). The data of several studies prior to about 1960 indicated that this relationship was not causal (10, 21, 89, 113). For example, Heymans and Heymans (200) found that ventilation did not increase when isolated lungs were perfused with acidotic, hypercapnic, and hypoxemic fluids. Comroe (89) injected NaCN into the right ventricles and found that ventilation did not increase for at least 12 sec, which is sufficient time for the NaCN to reach the carotid chemoreceptors. Comroe concluded that there were no chemoreceptors in the pulmonary circulation. Cropp and Comroe (100) infused blood into the right ventricle with P_{CO_2} increased from 5 to 50 mm Hg. These alterations in mixed venous P_{CO_2} did not increase ventilation of anesthetized dogs and cats and unanesthetized dogs unless there was an increase in Pa_{CO_2} These investigators concluded "that there are no CO_2 receptors in the precapillary pulmonary circulation of importance in the physiological regulation of respiration" (100).

Recent studies supportive of a pulmonary mechanism for exercise hyperpnea. Between 1965 and 1985 there was renewed interest in the concept that pulmonary CO_2 might mediate the exercise hyperpnea. This interest originated in part from the studies summarized earlier that showed that electrically induced exercise in anesthetized mammals evoked a hyperpnea that was not in some studies abolished by spinal cord transection (90, 102, 287, 291). This renewed interest stems also from findings of CO_2-sensitive receptors in the lungs (32, 56, 85, 180, 346, 424). The specific hypothesis was that a mechanism existed in the lungs that was sensitive to the amount of CO_2 delivered. This mechanism reflexly increased ventilation to the same extent proportionately as the increase in CO_2 delivered. Homeostasis of Pa_{CO_2} and Pa_{CO_2} was thereby maintained.

Several investigators have tested the CO_2 flow hypothesis by using an extracorporeal gas exchanger to artificially either decrease (CO_2 scrubbing) or increase (CO_2 loading) venous P_{CO_2}. One of the first studies was by Yamamoto and Edwards (510) who in anesthetized rats intravenously infused CO_2 equal to six times the resting metabolic CO_2 production. They found that ventilation also increased 6-fold to maintain homeostasis of arterial P_{CO_2} and pH. Subsequently, in several additional studies, scrubbing and loading resulted in respective decreases or increases in ventilation to supposedly maintain Pa_{CO_2} homeostasis (286, 296, 380, 381, 454, 488). Several of these studies were in anesthetized animals, but Phillipson et al. studied awake sheep. They found that venous CO_2 loading to increase pulmonary CO_2 excretion up to 350% increased ventilation to the same extent as exercise induced increases in CO_2 excretion (380). They also found in awake sheep that removal of CO_2 from venous blood caused proportionate decreases in ventilation (Fig. 10.24); when CO_2 removal equalled the resting metabolic rate, the sheep stopped breathing (381).

Wasserman et al. (71, 489, 496) have utilized methods other than venous CO_2 loading to test the pulmonary CO_2 flow hypothesis. They have altered CO_2 flow by increasing and decreasing cardiac output, by incremental dynamic exercise, by sinusoidal variation of work rate, and by dietary manipulations. With each method they found proportionate changes in pulmonary CO_2 excretion and ventilation and no measurable changes in Pa_{CO_2}.

Recent studies not supportive of a pulmonary mechanism. Other investigators have found that Pa_{CO_2} changed during scrubbing and loading by an exact amount to account for changes in ventilation (43,

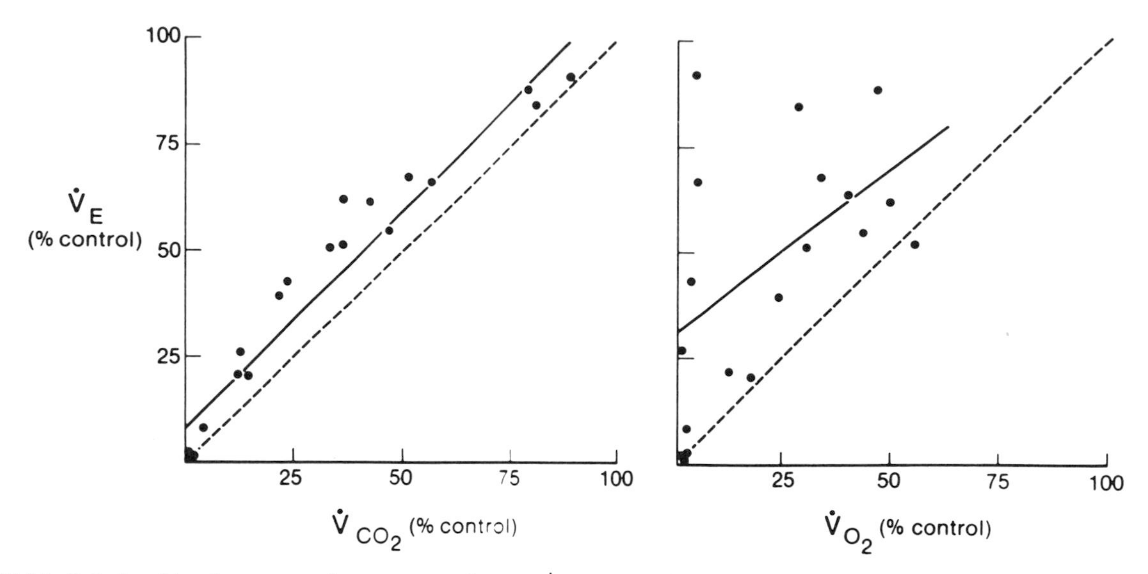

FIG. 10.24. Relationships between pulmonary ventilation ($\dot{V}_E$) and rates of pulmonary CO_2 excretion ($\dot{V}CO_2$) and O_2 uptake ($\dot{V}O_2$) in awake sheep. Changes in $\dot{V}CO_2$ and O_2 were produced by removing CO_2 from and adding O_2 to venous blood through membrane lungs. *Solid lines* are calculated linear regressions; *dashed lines* are lines of identity. [Reprinted with permission from Phillipson, Duffin, and Cooper (381).]

148, 177, 178, 292, 387). To avoid the complications of a potential change in stimulus outside of the lungs, some investigators have surgically isolated the pulmonary and systemic circulation during venous CO_2 loading. In one such study, increasing pulmonary artery P_{CO_2} to 85 mm Hg did increase ventilation (429), but in another, phrenic nerve output was not altered when venous P_{CO_2} was increased to 55 mm Hg (363). Others found that increasing pulmonary blood flow elicited a hyperpnea dependent upon intact vagal nerves (181).

From the above, it appears that breathing can be altered by changing either pulmonary CO_2 or blood flow. However, the data do not provide convincing evidence of a pulmonary receptor and signal with characteristics that would account for the exercise hyperpnea. In other words, the sensitivity of the CO_2 sensor appears to be too low to account for the exercise hyperpnea. Moreover, it has not been shown that a receptor exists that could sense CO_2 flow (CO_2 content × blood flow). In addition, a limitation of these studies is the minimal amount that CO_2 is actually altered (around two to three times normal). In this range of change in $\dot{V}_{CO_2}$, small departures of $\dot{V}_A$ to $\dot{V}_{CO_2}$ matching will cause significant changes in Pa_{CO_2}; thus, in many of these studies the change in breathing could have been mediated by the carotid chemoreceptors (42). In other words, the "noise" of the system is too great for conventional measurement procedures to provide definitive resolution of the question by the methods employed. Furthermore, several of these studies were on anesthetized animals, thus questions always remain regarding the relevance of findings to physiological exercise. Finally, most of the venous CO_2 loading studies were completed in species that are hypocapnic even during mild and moderate exercise. Accordingly, it seems doubtful that the supposed isocapnic hyperpnea during venous CO_2 loading is a suitable model for studying the mechanism of the exercise hyperpnea.

Studies in which lungs were denervated. The hypothesis of pulmonary receptor mediation of the exercise hyperpnea has been directly tested by studying the effect of attenuating or eliminating pulmonary vagal feedback. Humans were studied after lung transplant (28); dogs were studied after anesthetic or cold block of the vagi (5, 382); and dogs and ponies were studied before and after sectioning the hilar branches of the vagus nerves bilaterally (81, 135, 138, 143, 151, 154, 157, 373). In all of these investigations, attenuation of vagal activity decreased breathing frequency and increased tidal volume at rest and during exercise. These findings are predictable from the well-established role of slowly adapting stretch receptors in the control of breathing (413, 499). In addition, in one study cold block of slowly and rapidly adapting stretch receptors during exercise changed the recruitment pattern of respiratory muscles in a manner that increased diaphragm and thoracic expiratory muscle activity (5). However, in virtually all studies in which pulmonary vagal activity was reduced or eliminated, $\dot{V}_E$, $\dot{V}_A$, and Pa_{CO_2} during exercise did not differ from experiments in which the vagus nerves were intact (Figs. 10.25 and 10.26). In six extensive studies on ponies, the hypocapnia during treadmill exercise ranging from submaximal to high levels of intensity did not differ among intact ponies and those with their lungs denervated. The denervated ponies had a markedly attenuated Hering-Breuer inflation reflex that showed no signs of recrudescence; thus, there is little doubt that the lungs were denervated (157). Moreover, when lactic acid was infused intravenously at rest and during mild and moderate exercise in awake ponies, the changes in ventilation and Pa_{CO_2} to this pulmonary and systemic acidosis ($\Delta pH = 0.10$) were not altered by lung denervation (135). Also, in anesthetized cats, infusion of lactic acid into the inferior vena cava while NaOH was infused into the left atrium caused a pulmonary acidosis ($\Delta pH = 0.10$) with a normal arterial pH (363), but failed to increase ventilatory drive.

Summary and conclusions regarding pulmonary mediation of exercise hyperpnea. It seems clear that the activity of slowly adapting stretch receptors does change with changes in CO_2 and it seems clear that small changes near resting levels of metabolic rate can change ventilation through a pulmonary mechanism. However, in the absence of pulmonary innervation, the metabolic demands on ventilation are entirely met. This important point has been dem-

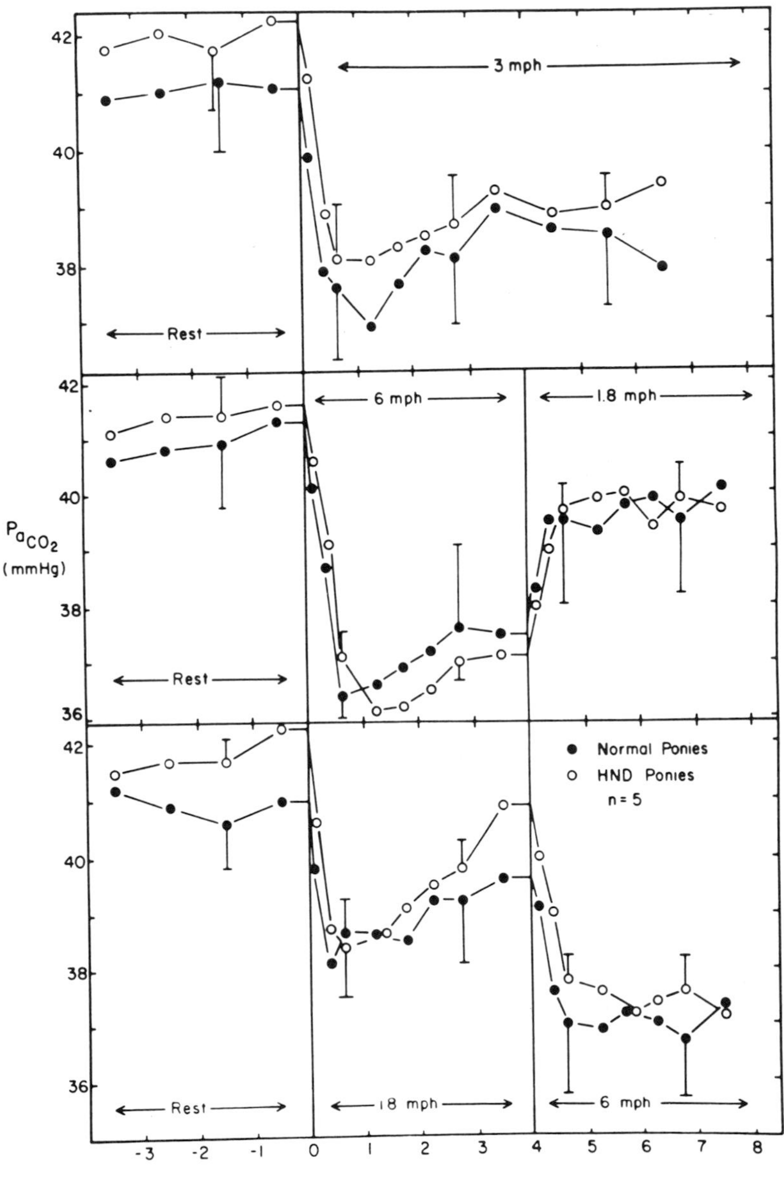

FIG. 10.25. Effect of treadmill exercise on arterial P_{CO_2} (Pa_{CO_2}) in five ponies before (*closed symbols*) and 2–4 weeks after (*open symbols*) hilar nerve denervation (HND). Note that the Pa_{CO_2} responses to all three exercise protocols was not altered by HND. [Reprinted with permission from Flynn et al. (143).]

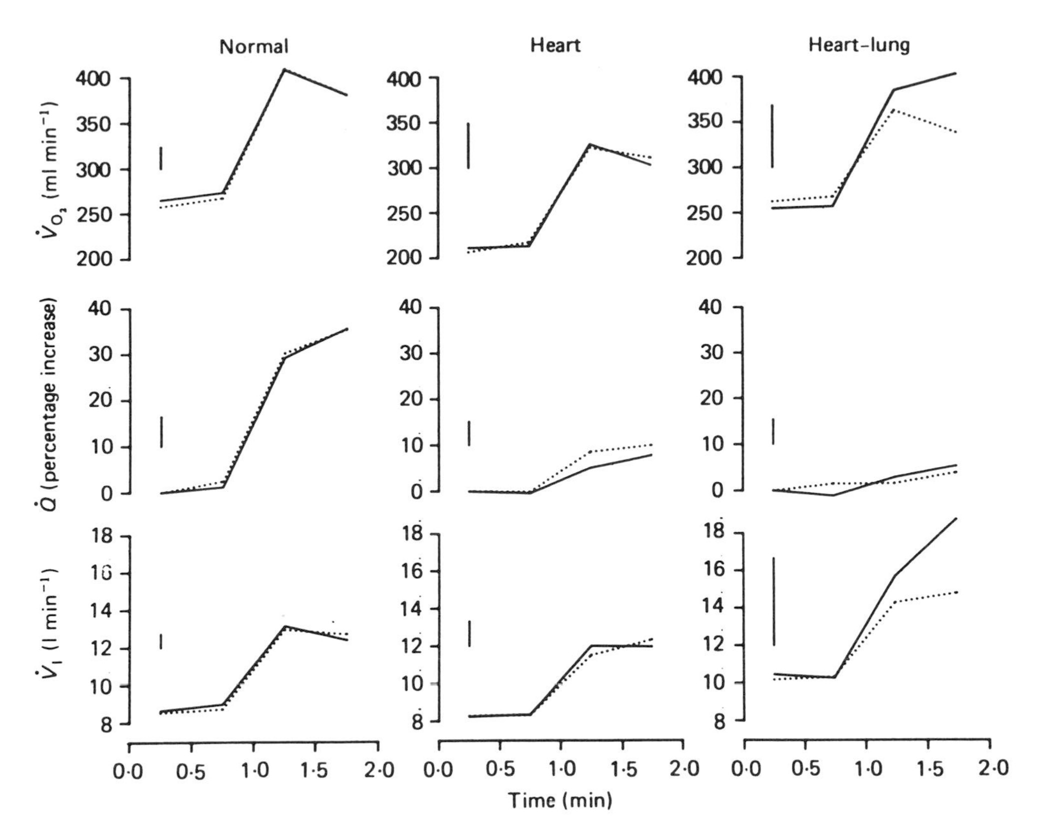

FIG. 10.26. Mean values for two 30 sec periods prior to and following the start of voluntary (*continuous lines*), and electrically (*dotted lines*) induced muscle contractions in the three patient groups (normal, heart transplant, and heart-lung transplant). $\dot{V}_I$, ventilation; $\dot{V}O_2$, oxygen consumption; $\dot{Q}$, cardiac output, expressed as percentage change from the first resting value. The *vertical bars* indicate the Fisher's least-significant difference at the $P<0.05$ level in each case. [Reprinted with permission from Banner et al. (28).]

onstrated during normal dynamic exercise in three species who with intact lung innervation differ greatly in the strength of the pulmonary reflexes. It is therefore concluded that the exercise hyperpnea is not mediated by pulmonary afferents.

Cardiac Afferents

Cardiac mechanoreceptors are activated by changes in atrial and/or ventricular volume or distention, and their primary function is related to autonomic control of cardiac function and arterial blood pressure (9). However, data from several studies suggest that cardiac mechanoreceptors might also influence ventilation. Passive distension of the right ventricle and increases in right ventricular, left ventricular, and pulmonary artery pressure have been shown to increase breathing (237, 272, 273, 299, 469). Conceivably, these receptors mediate the responses observed in anesthetized dogs by Wasserman et al. (489) when they increased cardiac output by intravenous injections of isoproterenol or, in awake humans (63), when they decreased cardiac output by propranolol infusion. In both studies, $\dot{V}_E$ changed directionally as $\dot{Q}_C$ by a precise amount to maintain homeostasis of Pa_{CO_2}. When the cardiac responses to the drugs were blocked, then there were no changes in $\dot{V}_E$. In humans, they also occluded for 2 min venous return from the legs after exercise (225). Upon release of occlusion, $\dot{V}_E$ increased abruptly which was not altered by hyperoxia or CO_2 inhalation, suggesting circulatory mediation. Rowell et al. (402) observed a similar immediate $\dot{V}_E$ increase upon release of venous occlusion, but Dejours et al. (114) observed a delayed hyperpnea that could have been carotid chemoreceptor mediated. As a result of his work, Wasserman et al. (489) proposed a theory known as the "cardiodynamic" mediation of the exercise hyperpnea. Again, it is important to remember that a majority of these data were obtained during stimulation of cardiac afferents by conditions other than normal voluntary exercise.

Several investigators have directly studied the role of cardiac afferents in control of the exercise hyperpnea. In both humans (342) and ponies (370), the temporal pattern of circulatory and ventilatory changes during exercise are not correlated in a manner suggesting interdependence. Three different groups found that the cardiovascular responses to exercise were slower than normal in human heart and heart-lung transplant patients (28, 126, 418). Nevertheless, their ventilatory responses to exercise were normal or even exaggerated (Fig. 10.26). In goats studied before and after complete cardiac denervation (58), just as in the human heart transplant patients, cardiac denervation resulted in a sluggish cardiac response to exercise, but ventilation and Pa_{CO_2} throughout exercise were unaffected. Finally, ventilation did not change directionally with changes in cardiac output (223) during voluntary exercise in animals with artificial hearts.

In summary, it is clear that under specific experimental conditions in anesthetized animals, signals from the heart carried via vagal afferents can stimulate breathing. However, all known direct tests of the cardiodynamic theory using voluntary exercise indicate that cardiac afferents are not critical for the exercise hyperpnea.

Respiratory Muscle Afferents

The diaphragm, the intercostal muscles, and the abdominal expiratory muscles are the primary "pump" muscles of breathing (118, 413, 499). They have primary and secondary muscle spindle endings, Golgi tendon organs, and type III and IV afferents. However, there are relatively few muscle spindle endings in the diaphragm. The function of these afferents is the same as for other skeletal muscles. Muscle spindles mediate a segmental autogenic facilitatory reflex that regulates the muscle contraction to obtain the desired change in length. Tendon organs produce autogenic inhibition on their respective homogenous α-motoneuron. Both of these mechanoreceptors also elicit supraspinal reflexes. The group III and IV afferents are activated by lactate, H^+, and/or K^+. These initiate supraspinal reflexes that in some cases stimulate, whereas at other times they inhibit respiratory drive.

It does not seem reasonable to postulate that respiratory muscle afferents provide a primary drive for the exercise hyperpnea. Indeed, diaphragm deafferentation in ponies slightly increased inspiratory and expiratory times during mild and moderate exercise, but this surgery affected neither ventilation nor Pa_{CO_2} during exercise (151, 154). In addition, sensory denervation of the chest wall in goats by thoracic dorsal rhizotomy did not alter their exercise hyperpnea when the goats were not encumbered with a respiratory mask (335). Nevertheless, even though respiratory muscle afferents do not provide a primary drive to the exercise hyperpnea, these afferents probably do influence the hyperpnea in at least three ways.

Ventilatory Load Compensation. Mild and moderate increases in external inspiratory load at rest elicit reflexes. These reflexes increase inspiratory drive and duration in a manner sufficient to maintain ventilation and blood gas homeostasis (150, 154, 515). However, the same external load during mild and moderate exercise does not increase inspiratory drive; it actually decreases inspiratory drive (154) causing hypoventilation (154, 515). It seems then that at relatively low total (external plus internal) loads, the reflexes facilitate breathing to maintain homeostasis but at high total loads the reflexes inhibit breathing conceivably to prevent fatigue and injury. These reflexes are slightly attenuated after deafferentation of the diaphragm, indicating that diaphragm afferents influence the reflexes (154). Lung denervation also has only a modest affect on these reflexes (154); thus, chest wall and possibly abdominal muscle afferents appear to be the prominent sources of sensory feedback for these reflexes.

Existence of a load-compensating reflex during exercise is also suggested by the effects of reducing flow resistance by ~40% through substitution of helium (He-O_2) for nitrogen in the inspired gas. During mild and moderate exercise, the rate of rise of the integrated EMG from the diaphragm in humans (222) and ponies (151) is reduced by the second or third breath of He-O_2 gas mixture. Presumably, this reduction in inspiratory drive reflects the component of that drive due to reflexes compensating for the internal inspiratory load. However, He-O_2 may affect breathing other than through its effect on airway resistance. For example, in ponies the initial reduction in ventilatory drive with He-O_2 breathing is not sustained; by 2 min of breathing the He-O_2 mixture, drive is at or above control levels. Moreover, the He-O_2 mixture also increases breathing frequency; thus, even though inspiratory drive is reduced, $\dot{V}_E$ during He-O_2 breathing exceeds that measured when breathing room air (151, 222, 348, 372). Neither the initial reduction in inspiratory drive with He-O_2 breathing nor the subsequent return of drive to control levels is altered by deafferenting the diaphragm and the lungs. These changes in breathing are thus not critically dependent on diaphragm and lung receptor mechanisms.

The potential role in the control of breathing of the endogenous ventilatory load has also been studied by reducing load through a pressure assist system (164). Reducing load with this system does not alter breathing at rest or during exercise. Accordingly, it is not clear whether reflex mechanisms exist to compensate for the endogenous ventilatory load. Nevertheless, it seems reasonable to postulate that respiratory muscle afferents influence the exercise hyperpnea in the manner suggested by studies on exogenous load compensatory mechanisms; both facilitatory and inhibitory reflexes exist, with the former dominant to maintain homeostasis until the load becomes potentially injurious and/or fatiguing and at this point inhibition becomes dominant.

Minimization of Work of Breathing. The ventilatory control system has been postulated to function in a manner that minimizes the force generated by the respiratory muscles and thereby minimizes the O_2 cost of breathing (114, 190, 321, 364, 433). Minimization of total elastic and flow-resistive work during exercise is supposedly achieved by appropriate adjustments in: (1) tidal volume and breathing frequency, (2) airway diameter, and (3) recruitment of respiratory muscle.

Tidal volume and breathing frequency responses to exercise. The importance of elastic and flow resistive work in determining tidal volume and breathing frequency is well known (321, 364). Equines provide an example of the influence of high elastance. Their chest wall is relatively stiff so that the elastic work of breathing is high; therefore, it seems appropriate that their exercise hyperpnea is achieved mainly by an increase in breathing frequency (49, 371). Humans have a greater lung and chest wall compliance than equines and, as a consequence, the hyperpnea achieved by increases in tidal volume during mild and moderate exercise is efficient (115, 118). However, as workload and therefore breathing increases, the V_T begins to ventilate the less compliant regions of lung volumes, making it more efficient for increased breathing frequency to contribute more to further increases in ventilation. In ponies and humans, increases in flow resistance work during exercise decreases breathing frequency and increases tidal volume thereby, providing another example of a change to minimize the respiratory work (151, 154, 515).

Airway diameter during exercise. During normal exercise, flow resistive work does not increase appreciably (115). There is a work rate–dependent increase in upper airway volume during exercise that stems from airway dilation (114, 495, 497). In addition, there is a significant bronchodilation initiated by reflexes originating from group III and IV nerve endings in the contracting muscles. Also, the braking (active slowing of expiratory flow) normally evident at rest is eliminated during exercise as a result of both the cessation of diaphragmatic contraction at end inspiration as well as the cessation of laryngeal aperture abduction (134). These changes in airway dimensions permit high flow rates without an increase in flow resistance.

Recruitment of respiratory muscles. The temporal pattern of inspiratory and expiratory flow is actively regulated through appropriate recruitment of inspiratory, expiratory, and airway muscles (114). Theoretically, a rectangular airflow profile is more efficient than a sinusoidal profile. At rest in humans, the profiles tend to be sinusoidal, but during exercise they become more rectangular (512). In some quadrupeds, these profiles are nearly rectangular at rest and during exercise (185, 274). The rectangular profiles are in part due to contraction of the expiratory muscles to reduce end-expiratory lung volume below the passive functional residual capacity (4, 197, 428). Thus, there is an active and passive component to both inspiration and expiration. The reduction in end-expiratory lung volume further enhances efficiency of breathing by lengthening the diaphragm which, in turn, permits generation of increased diaphragmatic muscle tension for the same amount of phrenic nerve activation (115).

The mechanism underlying respiratory work minimization has not been elucidated. It has been postulated and it seems intuitive that afferents from mechanoreceptors in the respiratory muscles and lungs provide crucial information to the medullary controller for efficient breathing (222, 388). Specifically, muscle spindle and tendon organ afferents provide information regarding conditions in the muscles that might underlie the changes in rate, magnitude, and activation pattern of inspiratory, expiratory, and airway muscles to minimize the work of breathing.

Short-Term Modulation. Short-term modulation (STM) refers to a change in the exercise hyperpnea that occurs reversibly within a single exercise trial (23, 334, 335). STM is observed during conditions such as changes in blood and/or brain $[H^+]$ (152, 362), hormonal alterations (270, 379), manipulation of certain neurotransmitters (419), and changes in respiratory dead space (304, 333). At rest, each of these conditions changes ventilation in a manner that usually changes Pa_{CO_2}. During exercise, under these conditions, Pa_{CO_2} is regulated to the same level as at rest. In other words, if a systemic metabolic acidosis causes a hypocapnia of 10 mm Hg at rest, Pa_{CO_2} will also be reduced by 10 mm Hg during exercise. However, to achieve the same decrease in Pa_{CO_2} at rest and during exercise, alveolar ventilation must increase several liters more during exercise. STM refers to the mechanism causing this greater exercise response.

Acute and chronic hypoxia also increase ventilation more during exercise than at rest (116, 117, 156, 336). However, hypoxia differs from the above conditions in that Pa_{CO_2} decreases more during exercise than at rest. This difference indicates that during hypoxia, mechanisms in addition to STM alter the ventilatory response to exercise.

Mitchell et al. (335) originally proposed that STM occurred because thoracic respiratory muscle afferents increased the excitability of respiratory muscle motoneurons. To test this hypothesis, they denervated the chest wall of goats through thoracic dorsal rhizotomy. As already summarized, rhizotomy did not alter the exercise hyperpnea when goats were not wearing a respiratory mask. However, with the mask the goats went into ventilatory failure during exercise even though prior to rhizotomy the goats easily tolerated the masks. The dead space added by the mask worsened the failure after rhizotomy. These data indicate an important contribution of respiratory muscle afferents to the augmented ventilation needed to maintain Pa_{CO_2} at an altered level during exercise. Subsequently, Bach et al. (23) found that the augmented ventilation in response to added dead space during exercise was eliminated when a serotonin receptor antagonist was infused intravenously or administered only to the midcervical spinal cord or below (Fig. 10.27). They concluded that STM results from spinal respiratory motoneuron excitability changes secondary to activation of brainstem serotonergic neurons, and that respiratory muscle afferents contribute to this altered excitability.

The concept of short-term modulation contributing to the exercise hyperpnea under certain circumstances is novel; its mechanism and its importance requires additional studies. Among other reasons, the concept is of importance because it represents a nontraditional approach to the study of the exercise hyperpnea.

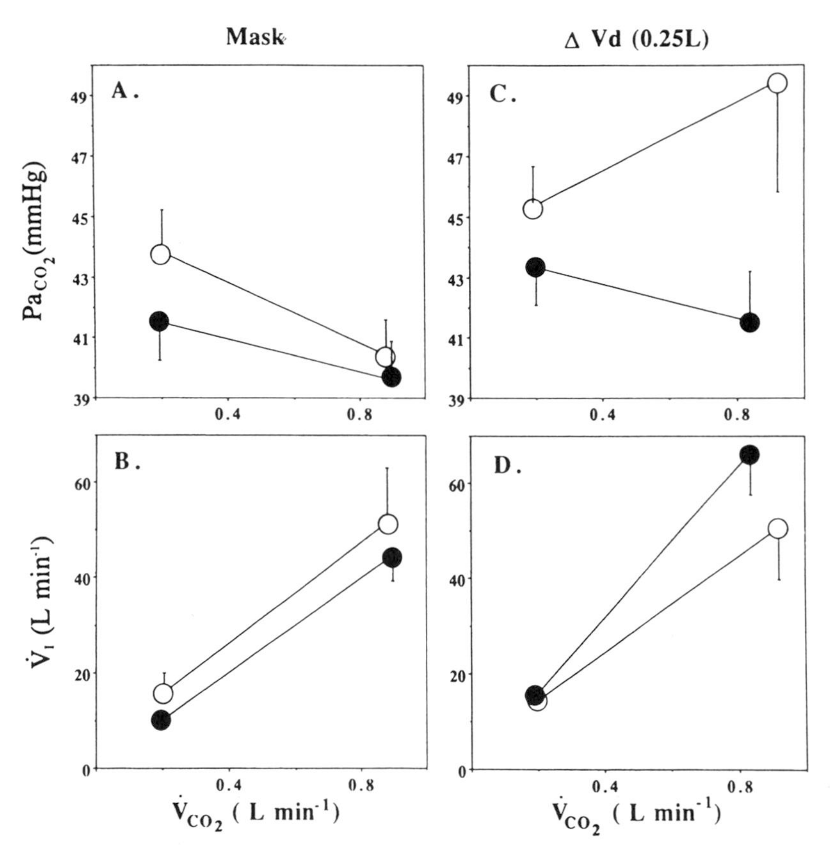

FIG. 10.27. Pulmonary ventilation ($\dot{V}_I$) and Pa_{CO_2} of goats at rest and during one level of mild treadmill exercise. The left panel was obtained with the goats wearing a conventional mask for obtaining $\dot{V}_I$ and the right panel was obtained with addition of 250 ml external dead space ($\dot{V}_D$). *Closed symbols* are prior to drug treatment, while *open symbols* are after methysergide administration, which is an antagonist of serotonin. Note that methyserside attenuated V_I response to increased V_D resulting in exercise hypercapnia. [Reprinted with permission from Buch, Lutcavage, and Mitchell (23).]

Mediation of the Exercise Hyperpnea by Multiple Mechanisms

In contrast to the claim of several physiologists that a single mechanism mediates the exercise hyperpnea, a few physiologists have entertained the concept that multiple mechanisms contribute. Among the latter is Dejours (113) who several decades ago advanced the neurohumoral theory of the exercise hyperpnea. Dejours and others observed that at the onset of submaximal exercise, $\dot{V}_E$ reached about 50% of its steady-state value within a few seconds. He reasoned this response was too rapid to be mediated by a muscle metabolite transported by the blood to a receptor outside of the muscle. Therefore, he felt this increase was *neurally* mediated (either by spinal afferents or central command). The remaining increase in ventilation to the steady state occurred slowly over about 1.5 min. He felt this temporal pattern was inconsistent with neural events but was consistent with a gradual increase in some unidentified muscle metabolite acting outside of the muscle. This second phase of the hyperpnea was termed humoral. Conceivably, slight increases in plasma [K^+], Pa_{CO_2}, catecholamines, pulmonary P_{O_2}, and core temperature might add to provide sufficient stimulation to account for this humoral phase. Alternately, this phase could be mediated by short-term potentiation, which is a neural phenomenon described in Chapter 1. In any event, the concept that more than one mechanism normally contributes to the hyperpnea has never been solidly supported nor has it been convincingly shown to be invalid.

Another version of multiple mechanisms for mediation of the exercise hyperpnea was proposed by Yamamoto (511) who stated that there are "many sufficient mechanisms, each of which in a given isolated circumstance, explains the whole phenomenon. When they act simultaneously, they mask each other." This theory of "redundancy" attempts to reconcile the widely differing theories, many of which claim to be capable of explaining the entire exercise hyperpnea.

Redundancy in a control system could originate from at least three different mechanisms (186). *One* mechanism is occlusion that prevents of summation of two different excitatory influences on a neuron. Theoretically, humoral and peripheral neurogenic afferents (both proportional to metabolic rate) could excite the same medullary neurons. In the absence of summation, activation of medullary neurons and thus the exercise hyperpnea will be the same irrespective of whether both or only one of the afferents are functional. A *second* hypothetical mechanism could involve presynaptic inhibition, which might occur when one excitatory input to a medullary neuron blocks another excitatory input before both synapse at the same medullary neuron. In theory, both humoral and peripheral neurogenic afferents could synapse on the same medullary neurons, but additionally one presynaptically inhibits the other. A *third* potential mechanism of redundancy is through chemoreceptor feedback. Theoretically, neurogenic and/or humoral afferents could normally provide the primary drive for the exercise hyperpnea. In the absence of a primary drive, the normal relationship between ventilation and metabolic rate would be disrupted, causing arterial hypercapnia and hypoxemia that could increase activation of carotid chemoreceptors. Thereby, chemoreceptor mechanisms could contribute to the exercise hyperpnea through error feedback.

One of the two known attempts to test Yamamoto's theory was by Waldrop et al. (480). They found in anesthetized cats that the summed $\dot{V}_E$ response to activation of central command (129) and to peripheral neurogenic feedback when given separately, exceeded the $\dot{V}_E$ response when the two mechanisms were activated simultaneously. Additional data suggested that the central command mechanism normally predominates. These data are consistent with redundancy by occlusion as defined above.

The other study on the possibility of redundant mechanisms was by Pan et al. (374). In awake ponies, they determined whether changes in breathing and Pa_{CO_2} in response to exercise after three lesions (carotid body denervation, hilar nerve denervation, and partial spinal lesion) were predictable from the individual effects of each lesion. They had previously found that at the onset of exercise, carotid body denervation accentuates the exercise hypocapnia; hilar nerve denervation does not alter the normal hypocapnic response; and partial spinal lesion attenuates the exercise hypocapnia. They predicted, therefore, that if redundancy existed among these mechanisms, the exercise hypocapnia would be less than normal after all three lesions and conceivably breathing may not increase enough to prevent hypercapnia. They found though that the exercise hyperpnea and hypocapnia were greater after all three lesions than with any single lesion. The accentuated hyperpnea and hypocapnia were due to a markedly increased V_T during exercise. These data do not provide support for redundancy because the effects of multiple lesions were opposite to those expected. In other words, after lesion of three potential pathways the exercise hyperpnea was accentuated rather than attenuated; if these pathways were redundant, lesioning all three would have attenuated the hyperpnea.

It is presently unclear whether there are redundant pathways for mediation of the exercise hyperpnea. The findings of Waldrop and co-workers support the concept, whereas those of Pan et al. do not. A potentially important difference between these studies is the former tested whether central command was redundant with other mechanisms, whereas the latter study tested potential redundancy among peripheral afferents. Conceivably, then, central command is redundant with peripheral mechanisms. This idea seems reasonable given the redundancy that exists in other aspects of ventilatory control and given the vital nature of the exercise hyperpnea to survival.

SUMMARY AND CONCLUSIONS

Peripheral Afferent Contribution to Circulatory Responses to Exercise

Peripheral afferent mechanisms play an important role in causing at least part of the cardiovascular responses to exercise. In particular, the evidence is strong that a reflex arising from exercising limb muscles (i.e., the exercise pressor reflex) constricts the vascular tree. This constriction may be especially useful not only in increasing the perfusion pressure of exercising muscle but also in countering the severe metabolic vasodilation known to occur in skeletal muscles during exercise. Indeed, if there were no opposing mechanisms, the vasodilator capacity of large muscle groups, such as those used in running, would be sufficient to exhaust the capacity of the heart to provide blood.

The role of the exercise pressor reflex in causing the cardiac responses to exercise is difficult to assess. Central command appears to play an important role in withdrawing vagal tone to the heart during exercise. Nevertheless, evidence has been presented that the exercise pressor reflex can also increase heart rate. The increase is caused definitely by sympathetic excitation, and probably by vagal and withdrawal also.

Whether metabolic or mechanical stimuli evoke the exercise pressor reflex is an important but unresolved issue. At this point, the evidence strongly suggests that a metabolic factor plays an important role in evoking the reflex. However, there is also reasonable evidence that a mechanical factor may be important. Clearly, the concept of a mechanical factor causing part of the exercise pressor reflex is new, and this may well be the reason that there is less evidence for it than there is for a metabolic factor. The value of a mechanical factor may be that it provides the CNS rapid feedback about the demands placed upon the exercising muscles. Two demands requiring mechanoreceptor feedback may be the mass of muscle recruited and the force of contraction.

The nature of the metabolic factor that causes the exercise pressor reflex is unknown, but it appears in some way to be linked with a lack of oxygen delivery to the working muscles. The concept that the metabolic factor evoking the exercise pressor reflex is the same factor that causes vasodilation in the exercising muscles is attractive. Unfortunately, at this point in time, there is no evidence for or against this concept. The evidence that the contraction-induced stimulation of group III and IV muscle afferents evokes the cardiovascular components of the exercise pressor reflex arc is overwhelming. Experiments that employ unphysiological methods to contract hindlimb skeletal muscles have revealed that for the most part group III afferents signal information about mechanical events occurring in the muscle, whereas group IV afferents signal information about metabolic events. Recently, group III afferents have been shown to be stimulated by a true form of dynamic exercise (i.e., treadmill walking); the pattern of response displayed by these thinly myelinated afferents suggested that they were functioning as mechanoreceptors. Finally, preliminary evidence has been consistent with the speculation that group III and IV muscle afferents release in the dorsal horn glutamate as a neurotransmitter and substance P as a neuromodulator. Moreover, the essential circuitry of the reflex arc includes the ventrolateral medulla.

Peripheral Afferent Contribution to Ventilatory Responses to Exercise

There is still no convincing evidence that any of the proposed peripheral afferent mechanisms is the primary mediator of the exercise hyperpnea. The potential role of several of these has been directly studied during normal voluntary exercise. The data indicate that carotid chemoreceptor, pulmonary, cardiac, and respiratory muscle afferents do not provide a primary stimulus for the hyperpnea. Nevertheless, most of these afferent systems influence the hyperpnea. The carotid chemoreceptors "fine tune" alveolar ventilation to metabolic rate, thereby minimizing disturbances in alveolar and arterial P_{O_2} and P_{CO_2}. Pulmonary afferents are important to termination of inspiration and, thereby, the pattern of breathing. Respiratory muscle afferents also affect the pattern of breathing and provide information regarding the mechanical status of the breathing apparatus, which is needed for efficient breathing (minimization of the

O_2 cost of breathing). None of these functions is unique to exercise, but the importance of each probably increases as the metabolic demands of exercise increase and precise adjustments are needed to minimize disruptions in arterial blood gases.

The role of limb afferents in the exercise hyperpnea is less clear. There seems little doubt that limb afferents can influence breathing. Moreover, there is evidence that limb afferents contribute to the hyperpnea during normal voluntary exercise. The simple fact remains that it is impossible to eliminate limb afferents and still be able to perform voluntary exercise. Several imaginative techniques have been used to attenuate or eliminate limb afferents (partial spinal lesions, epidural block, electrically induced contractions in paraplegics), but in each case uncertainty exists regarding the extent of limb afferent attenuation and/or whether muscle contractions are really normal under these conditions. Consequently, the data from these experiments is inconclusive regarding the role of these afferents. Nevertheless, it is conceivable that limb afferents influence the hyperpnea in a supplementary manner and/or their contribution might be redundant with central command. In other words, these afferents may provide information to the medullary controller about conditions in the limbs that enable central mechanisms to function optimally. The importance of these afferents might increase as conditions in the muscles increasingly deviate from rest (e.g., as during heavy exercise, reduced blood flow, altered thermal conditions). Also, the importance might increase in the absence or attenuation of central primary mechanisms. In other words, if there are redundant mechanisms in hierarchial order, then it would seem that limb afferents would be second in line or the primary backup to central command. These hypotheses require additional testing.

The mechanism of the hyperventilation in humans during heavy exercise is also unclear. The traditional explanation of increased H^+ stimulation at carotid chemoreceptors does not seem to satisfactorily account for the hyperventilation. There is good evidence both for and against the postulate that the hyperventilation is mediated in part by increased plasma K^+ and catecholamine concentration acting at the carotid chemoreceptors. This hypothesis requires additional testing. Moreover, hypotheses unrelated to carotid chemoreceptors require testing. For example, Asmussen hypothesized increased central command secondary to increased muscle afferents to account for the increased exercise hyperpnea during neuromuscular blockade and venous occlusion. It is conceivable that with fatigue and ischemia in muscles during heavy exercise, central command and therefore breathing increase proportionately more than metabolic rate resulting in hyperventilation.

Finally, imaginative and nontraditional approaches to studying the exercise hyperpnea must be encouraged. Certainly the concepts of memory, learning, and long-term modulation have only recently appeared in the literature on this topic. These and other yet unformulated concepts need to be tested using conventional whole-animal and relatively newer cellular and molecular approaches.

REFERENCES

1. Abrahams, V. C., B. Lynn, and F. J. R. Richmond. Organization and sensory properties of small myelinated fibres in the dorsal cervical rami of the cat. *J. Physiol. (Lond.)* 347: 177–187, 1984.
2. Adams, L., H. Frankel, J. Garlick, A. Guz, K. Murphy, and S. J. G. Semple. The role of spinal cord transmission in the ventilatory response to exercise in man. *J. Physiol. (Lond.)* 355: 85–97, 1984.
3. Adams, L., J. Garlick, A. Guz, K. Murphy, and S. J. G. Semple. Is the voluntary control of exercise in man necessary for the ventilatory response? *J. Physiol. (Lond.)* 355: 71–83, 1984.
4. Answorth, D. M., C. A. Smith, S. W. Eicker, K. S. Henderson, and J. A. Dempsey. The effects of chemical versus locomotory stimuli on respiratory muscle activity in the awake dog. *Respir. Physiol.* 78: 163–176, 1989.
5. Ainsworth, D. M., C. A. Smith, B. D. Johnson, S. W. Eicker, K. S. Henderson, and J. A. Dempsey. Vagal modulation of respiratory muscle activity in awake dogs during exercise and hypercapnia. *J. Appl. Physiol.* 72: 1362–1367, 1992.
6. Alam, M., and F. H. Smirk. Observation in man upon a blood pressure raising reflex arising from the voluntary muscles. *J. Physiol. (Lond.)* 89: 372–383, 1937.
7. Alam, M., and F. H. Smirk. Observations in man on a pulse-accelerating reflex from the voluntary muscles of the legs. *J. Physiol. (Lond.)* 3: 247–252, 1938.
8. Andres, K. H., M. Von During, and R. F. Schmidt. Sensory innervation of the Achilles tendon by group III and IV afferent fibers. *Anat. Histol. Embryol.* 172: 145–156, 1985.
9. Armour, J. A., R. D. Wurster, and W. C. Randall. Cardiac reflexes. In: *Neural Regulation of the Heart*, edited by W. C. Randall. New York: Oxford University Press, 1977, p. 157–186.
10. Armstrong, B. W., H. H. Hurt, R. W. Blide, and J. M. Workman. The humoral regulation of breathing. *Science* 133: 1897–1906, 1961.
11. Art, T., D. Desmecht, H. Amory, and P. Lekeux. Synchronization of locomotion and respiration in trotting ponies. *J. Vet. Med. A.* 37: 95–103, 1990.
12. Asmussen, E. Exercise and the regulation of ventilation. In: *Physiology of Muscular Exercise*, New York: American Heart Association, 1967, p. 132–145.
13. Asmussen, E. Ventilation at transition from rest to exercise. *Acta Physiol. Scand.* 89: 68–78, 1973.
14. Asmussen, E., E. H. Christensen, and M. Nielsen. Humoral or nervous control of respiration during muscular work? *Acta Physiol. Scand.* 6: 160–167, 1943.

15. Asmussen, E., and M. Nielsen. Studies on the regulation of respiration in heavy work. *Acta Physiol. Scand.* 12: 171–188, 1946.
16. Asmussen, E., and M. Nielsen. Ventilatory responses to CO_2 during work at normal and at low oxygen tensions. *Acta Physiol. Scand.* 39: 27–35, 1957.
17. Asmussen, E., and M. Nielsen. Pulmonary ventilation and effect of oxygen breathing in heavy exercise. *Acta Physiol. Scand.* 43: 365–378, 1958.
18. Asmussen, E., and M. Nielsen. Experiments on nervous factors controlling respiration and circulation during exercise employing blocking of the blood flow. *Acta Physiol. Scand.* 60: 103–111, 1964.
19. Asmussen, E., M. Nielsen, and G. Welth-Pedersen. Cortical or reflex control of respiration during muscular work? *Acta Physiol. Scand.* 6: 168–175, 1943.
20. Aung-Din, R., J. H. Mitchell, and J. C. Longhurst. Reflex α-adrenergic coronary vasoconstriction during hindlimb static exercise in dogs. *Circ. Res.* 48: 502–509, 1981.
21. Aviado, D. M., T. H. Li, W. Kalow, C. F. Schmidt, G. L. Turnbull, G. W. Peskin, M. E. Hess, and A. J. Weiss. Respiratory and circulatory reflexes from the perfused heart and pulmonary circulation of the dog. *Am. J. Physiol.* 165: 261–277, 1951.
22. Azerad, J., C. C. Hunt, Y. Laporte, B. Pollin, and D. Thiesson. Afferent fibres in cat ventral roots: electrophysiological and histological evidence. *J. Physiol. (Lond.)* 379: 229–243, 1986.
23. Bach, K. B., M. E. Lutcavage, and G. S. Mitchell. Serotonin is necessary for short-term modulation of the exercise ventilatory response. *Respir. Physiol.* 91: 57–70, 1993.
24. Bainton, C. R. Canine ventilation after acid-base infusion, exercise, and carotid body denervation. *J. Appl. Physiol.* 44: 28–35, 1978.
25. Band, D. M., I. R. Cameron, and S. J. G. Semple. Oscillations in arterial pH with breathing in the cat. *J. Appl. Physiol.* 26: 261–267, 1969.
26. Band, D. M., R. A. F. Linton, R. Kent, and F. L. Kurer. The effect of peripheral chemodenervation on the ventilatory response to potassium. *Respir. Physiol.* 60: 217–225, 1985.
27. Band, D. M., P. Willshaw, and C. B. Wolff. The speed of response of the carotid body chemoreceptor. In: *Morphology and Mechanisms of Chemoreceptors*, edited by A. S. Paintal. New Delhi, India: Navchetan Press, Ltd., 1976, p. 197–207.
28. Banner, N., A. Guz, R. Heaton, J. A. Innes, K. Murphy, and M. Yacoub. Ventilatory and circulatory responses at the onset of exercise in man following heart or heart-lung transplantation. *J. Physiol. (Lond.)* 399: 437–449, 1988.
29. Bannister, R. G., and D. J. C. Cunningham. The effects on the respiration and performance during exercise of the addition of oxygen to the inspired air. *J. Physiol. (Lond.)* 125: 118–137, 1954.
30. Barman, J. M., M. F. Moreira, and F. Consolazio. The effective stimulus for increased pulmonary ventilation during muscular exertion. *J. Clin. Invest.* 22: 53–56, 1943.
31. Barr, P. O., M. Beckman, H. Bjurstedt, J. Brismar, C. M. Hessler, and G. Matell. Time course of blood gas changes provoked by light and moderate exercise in man. *Acta Physiol. Scand.* 60: 1–17, 1964.
32. Bartoli, A., B. A. Cross, A. Guz, A. K. Jain, M. I. M. Nobel, and D. W. Trenchard. The effect of carbon dioxide in the airways and alveoli on ventilation. A vagal reflex studies in the dog. *J. Physiol. (Lond.)* 240: 91–109, 1974.
33. Bauer, R. M., G. A. Iwamoto, and T. G. Waldrop. Ventrolateral medullary neurons modulate the pressor reflex to muscular contraction. *Am. J. Physiol.* 257 (*Regulatory Integrative Comp. Physiol.* 26): R1154–R1161, 1989.
34. Bauer, R. M., G. A. Iwamoto, and T. G. Waldrop. Discharge patterns of ventrolateral medullary neurons during muscular contraction. *Am. J. Physiol.* 259 (*Regulatory Integrative Comp. Physiol.* 28): R606–R611, 1990.
35. Bauer, R. M., P. C. Nolan, E. M. Horn, and T. G. Waldrop. An excitatory amino acid synapse in the thoracic spinal cord is involved in the pressor response to muscular contraction. *Brain Res. Bull.* 32: 673–679, 1993.
36. Bauer, R. M., T. G. Waldrop, G. A. Iwamoto, and M. A. Holzwarth. Properties of ventrolateral medullary neurons that respond to muscular contraction. *Brain Res. Bull.* 28: 167–178, 1992.
37. Bayly, W. M., B. D. Grant, R. G. Breeze, and J. W. Kramer. The effects of maximal exercise on acid-base balance and arterial blood gas tensions in thoroughbred horses. In: *Equine Exercise Physiology*, edited by D. H. Snow, S. G. Persson, and R. J. Rose. Cambridge: Granta Editions, 1983, p. 400–404.
38. Bayly, W. M., D. R. Hodgson, D. A. Schulz, J. A. Dempsey, and P. D. Gollnick. Exercise induced hypercapnia in the horse. *J. Appl. Physiol.* 67: 1958–1966, 1989.
39. Bazil, M. K., and F. J. Gordon. Spinal NMDA receptors mediate pressor responses evoked from the rostral ventrolateral medulla. *Am. J. Physiol.* 260 (*Heart Circ. Physiol.* 29): H265–H274, 1991.
40. Bechbache, R. R., and J. Duffin. The entrainment of breathing frequency by exercise rhythm. *J. Physiol. (Lond.)* 272: 553–561, 1977.
41. Bennett, F. M. A role for neural pathways in exercise hyperpnea. *J. Appl. Physiol.* 56: 1559–1564, 1984.
42. Bennett, F. M., and W. E. Fordyce. Gain of the ventilatory exercise stimulus: definition and meaning. *J. Appl. Physiol.* 65: 2011–2017, 1988.
43. Bennett, F. M., R. D. Tallman, and F. S. Grodins. Role of $\dot{V}CO_2$ in control of breathing of awake exercising dogs. *J. Appl. Physiol.* 56: 1335–1337, 1984.
44. Bennett, J. A., C. Kidd, A. B. Latif, and P. N. McWilliam. A horseradish peroxidase study of vagal motoneurons with axons in cardiac and pulmonary branches of the cat and dog. *Q. J. Exp. Physiol.* 66: 145–154, 1981.
45. Bessou, P., P. DeJours, and Y. Lapote. Effets ventilatoires réflexes de la stimulation de fibres afférentes de grand diamètre, d'origine musculaire, chez le chat. *C. R. Soc. Biol. (Paris)* 153: 477–481, 1959.
46. Bessou, P., and Y. Laporte. Activation des fibres afférentes amyélinisées de petit calibre, d'origine musculaire (fibre du groupe III). *C. R. Soc. Biol. (Paris)* 152: 1587–1590, 1958.
47. Biscoe, T. J., and M. J. Purves. Factors affecting the cat carotid chemoreceptor and cervical sympathetic activity with special reference to passive hind-limb movements. *J. Physiol. (Lond.)* 190: 425–441, 1967.
48. Bisgard, G. E., and H. V. Forster. Ventilatory responses to acute and chronic hypoxia. In: *Handbook of Physiology, Adaptation to the Environment*, edited by D. B. Dills. Washington, DC: Am. Physiol. Soc., 1995.
49. Bisgard, G. E., H. V. Forster, B. Byrnes, K. Stanek, J. Klein, and M. Manohar. Cerebrospinal fluid acid-base balance during muscular exercise. *J. Appl. Physiol.* 45: 94–101, 1978.
50. Bisgard, G. E., H. V. Forster, J. Messina, and R. G. Sarazin. Role of the carotid body in hyperpnea of moderate exercise in goats. *J. Appl. Physiol.* 52: 1216–1222, 1986.

51. Black, A. M. S., N. W. Goodman, B. S. Nail, P. S. Rao, and R. W. Torrance. The significance of the timing of chemoreceptor impulses for their effect upon respiration. *Acta Neurobiol. Exp.* 33: 139–147, 1973.
52. Black, A. M. S. and R. W. Torrance. Respiratory oscillations in chemoreceptor discharge in control of breathing. *Respir. Physiol.* 13: 221–237, 1971.
53. Bonde-Petersen, F., L. B. Rowell, R. G. Murray, G. G. Blomqvist, R. White, E. Karlsson, W. Campbell, and J. H. Mitchell. Role of cardiac output in the pressor responses to graded muscle ischemia in man. *J. Appl. Physiol.* 45(4): 574–580, 1978.
54. Bonham, A. C., and I. Jeske. Cardiorespiratory effects of DL-homocysteic acid in caudal ventrolateral medulla. *Am. J. Physiol.* 256 (*Heart Circ. Physiol.* 25): H688–H696, 1989.
55. Boyd, I. A., and M. R. Davy. *Composition of Peripheral Nerves*. Edinbugh: Livingstone, 1968.
56. Bradley, G. W., M. I. M. Noble, and D. Trenchard. The direct effect on pulmonary stretch receptor discharge produced by changing lung carbon dioxide concentration in dogs on cardiopulmonary bypass and its action on breathing. *J. Physiol. (Lond.)* 261: 359–373, 1976.
57. Bramble, D. B., and D. R. Carrier. Running and breathing in mammals. *Science* 219: 251–256, 1983.
58. Brice, A. G., H. V. Forster, L. G. Pan, D. R. Brown, A. L. Forster, and T. F. Lowry. Effect of cardiac denervation on cardiorespiration responses to exercise in goats. *J. Appl. Physiol.* 70: 1113–1120, 1991.
59. Brice, A. G., H. V. Forster, L. G. Pan, A. Funahashi, M. D. Hoffman, T. F. Lowry, and C. L. Murphy. Is the hyperpnea of muscle contractions critically dependent on spinal afferents? *J. Appl. Physiol.* 64: 223–226, 1988.
60. Brice, A. G., H. V. Forster, L. G. Pan, A. Funahashi, T. F. Lowry, C. L. Murphy, and M. D. Hoffman. Ventilatory and Pa_{CO_2} response to voluntary and electrically-induced leg exercise. *J. Appl. Physiol.* 64: 218–225, 1988.
61. Brown, D. L., and P. G. Guyenet. Cardiovascular neurons of the brainstem with projections to the spinal cord. *Am. J. Physiol.* 247 (*Regulatory Integrative Comp. Physiol.* 16): R1009–R1016, 1984.
62. Brown, D. R., H. V. Forster, L. G. Pan, A. G. Brice, C. L. Murphy, T. F. Lowry, S. M. Gutting, A. Funahashi, M. D. Hoffman, and S. Powers. Ventilatory response of spinal-cord lesioned subjects to electrically induced exercise. *J. Appl. Physiol.* 68: 2312–2321, 1990.
63. Brown, H. V., K. Wasserman, and B. J. Whipp. Effect of beta-adrenergic blockade during exercise on ventilation and gas exchange. *J. Appl. Physiol.* 41: 886–892, 1976.
64. Brunner, M. J., M. S. Sussman, A. S. Greene, C. H. Kullman, and A. A. Shoukas. Carotid sinus baroreflex control of respiration. *Circ. Res.* 51: 624–636, 1982.
65. Burger, R. E., J. A. Estavillo, P. Kumar, P. L. G. Nye, and D. J. Patterson. Effects of potassium, oxygen, and carbon dioxide on the steady state discharge of cat carotid body chemoreceptors. *J. Physiol. (Lond.)* 401: 519–531, 1988.
66. Cameron, A. A., J. D. Leah, and P. J. Snow. The coexistence of neuropeptides in feline sensory neurons. *Neuroscience* 81: 969–979, 1988.
67. Carcassi, A. M., A. Concu, M. Decandia, M. Onnis, G. P. Orani, and M. B. Piras. Respiratory responses to stimulation of large fibers afferent from muscle receptors in cats. *Pflugers Arch.* 399: 309–314, 1983.
68. Carcassi, A. M., A. Concu, M. Decandia, M. Onnis, G. P. Orani, and M. B. Piras. Effects of long-lasting stimulation of extensor muscle nerves on pulmonary ventilation in cats. *Pflugers Arch.* 400: 409–412, 1984.
69. Casaburi, R., J. Daly, J. E. Hansen, and R. M. Effros. Abrupt changes in mixed venous blood gas composition after the onset of exercise. *J. Appl. Physiol.* 67: 1106–1112, 1989.
70. Casaburi, R., R. W. Stremel, B. J. Whipp, W. L. Beaver, and K. Wasserman. Alteration by hyperoxis of ventilatory dynamics during sinusoidal work. *J. Appl. Physiol.* 48: 1083–1091, 1980.
71. Casaburi, R., B. J. Whipp, S. N. Koyal, and K. Wasserman. Coupling of ventilation to CO_2 production during constant load ergometry with sinusoidally varying pedal rate. *J. Appl. Physiol.* 44: 97–103, 1978.
72. Ciriello, J., and F. R. Calaresu. Lateral reticular nucleus: A site of somatic and cardiovascular integration in the cat. *Am. J. Physiol.* 233 (*Regulatory Integrative Comp. Physiol.* 4): R100–R109, 1977.
73. Ciriello, J., M. M. Caverson, and D. H. Park. Immunohistochemical identification of noradrenaline and adrenaline synthesizing neurons in the cat ventrolateral medulla. *J. Comp. Neurol.* 253: 216–230, 1986.
74. Ciriello, J., M. M. Caverson, and C. Polosa. Function of the ventrolateral medulla in the control of circulation. *Brain Res. Bull.* 11: 359–391, 1986.
75. Clark, J. M., R. D. Sinclair, and J. B. Lenox. Chemical and nonchemical components of ventilation during hypercapnic exercixe in man. *J. Appl. Physiol.* 48: 1065–1076, 1980.
76. Cleland, C. L., and W. Z. Rymer. Functional properties of spinal interneurons activated by muscular free nerve endings and their potential contributions to the clasp-knife reflex. *J. Neurophysiol.* 69: 1181–1191, 1993.
77. Clement, D. L. Neurogenic influences on blood pressure and vascular tone from peripheral receptors during muscular contraction. *Cardiology* 61: 65–68, 1976.
78. Clement, D. L., and J. L. Plannier. Cardiac output distribution during induced static muscular contractions in the dog. *Eur. J. Appl. Physiol.* 45: 199–207, 1980.
79. Clement, D. L., C. L. Pelletier, and J. T. Shepherd. Role of muscular contraction in the reflex vascular responses to stimulation of muscle afferents in the dog. *Circ. Res.* 33: 386–392, 1973.
80. Clifford, P. S., J. T. Litzow, and R. L. Coon. Arterial hypocapnia during exercise in beagle dogs. *J. Appl. Physiol.* 61: 599–602, 1986.
81. Clifford, P. S., J. T. Litzow, J. H. Von Colditz, and R. L. Coon. Effect of chronic pulmonary denervation on ventilatory resonse to exercise. *J. Appl. Physiol.* 61: 603–610, 1986.
82. Coggeshall, R. E., and H. Ito. Sensory fibres in ventral roots L7 and S1 in the cat. *J. Physiol. (Lond.)* 267: 215–235, 1977.
83. Coleridge, H. M., and J. C. G. Coleridge. Impulse activity in afferent vagal C-fibres with endings in the intrapulmonary airways of dogs. *Respir. Physiol.* 29: 125–142, 1977.
84. Coleridge, H. M., and J. C. G. Coleridge. Afferent vagal C-fibers in the dog lung: their discharge during spontaneous breathing, and their stimulation by alloxan and pulmonary congestion. In: *Krough Centenary Symposium on Respiratory Adaptations, Capillary Exchange and Reflex Mechanisms*, edited by A. S. Paintal and P. Gill-Kumar. Delhi: Vallabhbhai Patel Chest Institute, 1977, p. 396–406.
85. Coleridge, H. M., J. C. G. Coleridge, and R. B. Banzett. Effect of CO_2 on afferent vagal endings in the canine lung. *Respir. Physiol.* 34: 135–151, 1978.

86. Coleridge, J. C. G., and H. M. Coleridge. Afferent vagal C fibre innervation of the lungs and airways and its functional significance. *Rev. Physiol. Biochem. Pharmacol.* 99: 2–110, 1984.
87. Coleridge, J. C. G., H. M. Coleridge, A. M. Roberts, M. P. Kaufman, and D. G. Baker. Tracheal contraction and relaxation initiated by lung and somatic afferents in dogs. *J. Appl. Physiol.* 52: 984–990, 1982.
88. Coles, D. R., F. Duff, W. H. T. Shepherd, and R. F. Whelan. The effect on respiration of infusions of adrenaline and noradrenaline into the carotid and vertebral arteries in man. *Br. J. Pharmacol.* 11: 346–350, 1956.
89. Comroe, J. H. The location and function of the chemoreceptors in the aorta. *Am. J. Physiol.* 127: 176–191, 1939.
90. Comroe, J. H., and C. F. Schmidt. Reflexes from the limbs as a factor in the hyperpnea of muscular exercise. *Am. J. Physiol.* 138: 536–547, 1943.
91. Connelly, J. C., L. W. McCallister, and M. P. Kaufman. Stimulation of the caudal ventrolateral medulla decreases total lung resistance in dogs. *J. Appl. Physiol.* 63: 912–917, 1987.
92. Conway, J., D. J. Paterson, E. S. Petersen, and P. A. Robbins. Changes in arterial potassium and ventilation in response to exercise in humans. *J. Physiol. (Lond.)* 374: 26P, 1986.
93. Coote, J. H., and W. N. Dodds. The baroreceptor reflex and the cardiovascular changes associated with sustained muscular contraction in the cat. *Pflugers Arch.* 363: 167–173, 1976.
94. Coote, J. H., S. M. Hilton, and J. F. Perez-Gonzalez. The reflex nature of the pressor response to muscular exercise. *J. Physiol. (Lond.)* 215: 789–804, 1971.
95. Coote, J. H., and J. F. Pérez-González. The response of some sympathetic neurones to volleys in various afferent nerves. *J. Physiol. (Lond.)* 208: 261–278, 1970.
96. Costa, F., and I. Biaggioni. Role of adenosine in the sympathetic activation produced by isometric exercise in humans. *J. Clin. Invest.* 93: 1654–1660, 1994.
97. Craig, A. D., and S. Mense. The distribution of afferent fibers from the gastrocnemius-soleus muscle in the dorsal horn of the cat as revealed by the transport of horseradish peroxidase. *Neurosci. Lett.* 41: 233–238, 1983.
98. Crayton, S. C., R. Aung-Din, D. E. Fixler, and J. H. Mitchell. Distribution of cardiac output during induced isometric exercise in dogs. *Am. J. Physiol.* 236: (*Heart Circ. Physiol.* 7): H218–H224, 1979.
99. Crayton, S. C., J. H. Mitchell, and F. C. Payne, III. Reflex cardiovascular response during the injection of capsaicin into skeletal muscle. *Am. J. Physiol.* 240 (*Heart Circ. Physiol.* 11): H315–H319, 1981.
100. Cropp, G. J. A., and J. H. Comroe, Jr. Role of mixed venous CO_2 in respiratory control. *J. Appl. Physiol.* 16: 1029–1033, 1961.
101. Cross, B. A., A. Davey, A. Guz, P. G. Katona, M. Maclean, K. Murphy, S. J. G. Semple, and R. Stidwell. The role of spinal cord transmission in the ventilatory response to electrically induced exercise in the anesthetized dog. *J. Physiol. (Lond.)* 329: 37–55, 1982.
102. Cross, B. A., A. Davey, A. Guz, P. G. Katona, M. Maclean, K. Murphy, S. J. G. Semple, and R. Stidwell. The pH oscillations in arterial blood during exercise: a potential signal for the ventilatory response in the dog. *J. Physiol. (Lond.)* 329: 57–73, 1982.
103. Cunningham, D. J. C., E. N. Hey, and B. B. Lloyd. The effect of intravenous infusion of noradenaline on the respiratory response to carbon dioxide. *Q. J. Exp. Physiol.* 43: 394–399, 1958.
104. Cunningham, D. J. C., B. B. Lloyd, and J. M. Patrick. The relation between ventilation and end-tidal P_{CO_2} in man during moderate exercise with and without CO_2 inhalation. *J. Physiol. (Lond.)* 169: 104–106, 1963.
105. Cunningham, D. J. C., D. Spurr, and B. B. Lloyd. The drive to ventilation from arterial chemoreceptors in hypoxic exercise. In: *Arterial Chemoreceptors*, edited by R. W. Torrance. Oxford: Blackwell, 1968, p. 301–323.
106. Curtis, D. R., and G. A. R. Johnston. The chemical excitation of spinal neurones by certain acidic amino acids. *J. Physiol. (Lond.)* 150: 656–682, 1960.
107. Dahlstrom, A., and K. Fuxe. Evidence for the existence of monamine neurons in the central nervous II. Experimentally-induced changes in interneuronal amine levels of bulbospinal neurone systems. *Acta Physiol. Scand.* 64: 247, 1964.
108. Daristotle, L., A. D. Berssenbrugge, M. J. Engwall, and G. E. Bisgard. The effects of carotid body hypocapnia on ventilation in goats. *Respir. Physiol.* 79: 123–136, 1990.
109. Davies, C. T. M., and D. W. Starkie. The pressor response to voluntary and electrically evoked isometric contractions in man. *Eur. J. Appl. Physiol.* 53: 359–363, 1985.
110. Davy, K. P., W. G. Herbert, and J. H. Williams. Effect of indomethacin on the pressor responses to sustained handgrip contraction in humans. *J. Appl. Physiol.* 75: 273–278, 1993.
111. Debiasi, S., and A. Rustioni. Glutamate and substance P co-exist in primary afferent terminals in the superficial laminae of the spinal cord. *Proc. Natl. Acad. Sci. U. S. A.* 83: 7820–7824, 1988.
112. Dejours, P. Control of respiration on muscular exercise. In: *Handbook of Physiology, Respiration*, edited by W. O. Fenn and H. Rahn. Washington, DC: Am. Physiol. Soc., 1974, p. 631–648.
113. Dejours, P., J. C. Mithoefer, and A. Teillac. Essai de nise en evidence de chemorecepteurs veineux de ventilation. *J. Physiol. (Paris)* 47: 160–163, 1955.
114. Dempsey, J. A., H. V. Forster, and D. M. Ainsworth. Regulation of hyperpnea, hyperventilation and respiratory muscle recruitment during exercise. In: *Regulation of Breathing*, edited by J. A. Dempsey and A. Pack. New York: Marcel Dekker, Inc., 1994, p. 1065–1134.
115. Dempsey, J. A., H. V. Forster, M. L. Birnbaum, W. G. Reddan, J. Thoden, R. F. Grover, and J. Rankin. Control of exercise hyperpnea under varying durations of exposure to moderate hypoxia. *Respir. Physiol.* 16: 213–231, 1973.
116. Dempsey, J. A., N. Gledhill, W. G. Reddan, H. V. Forster, P. G. Hanson, and A. D. Claremont. Pulmonary adaptation to exercise: effect of exercise type, duration, chronic hypoxia and physical training. In: *The Marathon: Physiological, Medical, Epidemiological, and Psychological Studies*, edited by P. Milvy. New York: Academy of Science, 1977, p. 243–261.
117. Dempsey, J. A., and J. Rankin. Physiologic adaptations of gas transport systems to muscular work in health and disease. *Am. J. Phys. Med.* 46: 582–647, 1967.
118. De Troyer, A. Respiratory muscles. In: *The Lung: Scientific Foundations*, edited by R. G. Crystal and J. B. West. New York: Raven Press, 1991, p. 869–884.
119. Dittmar, C. Ein neuer Beweis für die Reizbarkeit der centripetalen Fasern des Rückenmarks. *Ber. K. Sächs. Ges. Wiss., Math. Phys. KI.* 22: 18–48, 1870.
120. Donaldson, G. C., and C. G. Newstead. In man at rest undergoing haemodialysis reduction in arterial potassium

does not influence minute ventilation. *J. Physiol. (Lond.)* 407: 29P, 1988 (Abstract).

121. Douglas, C. G., and J. S. Haldane. The regulation of normal breathing. *J. Physiol. (Lond.)* 38: 420–440, 1909.
122. Duffin, J., R. R. Bechbache, R. C. Gorda, and S. A. Chung. The ventilatory response to carbon dioxide in hyperoxic exercise. *Respir. Physiol.* 40: 93–105, 1980.
123. Duggan, A. W., P. J. Hope, C. W. Lang, and C. A. Williams. Sustained isometric contraction of skeletal muscle results in release of immunoreactive neurokinins in the spinal cord of the anaesthetized cat. *Neurosci. Lett.* 122: 191–194, 1991.
124. Dutia, M. B., and W. R. Ferrell. The effect of suxamethonium on the response to stretch of Golgi tendon organs in the cat. *J. Physiol. (Lond.)* 306: 511–518, 1980.
125. Edwards, R. H. T., D. M. Denison, G. Jones, C. T. M. Davies, and E. J. M. Campbell. Changes in mixed venous gas tensions at start of exercise in man. *J. Appl. Physiol.* 32: 165–169, 1972.
126. Ehrman, J., S. Keteyian, F. Fedel, K. Rhoads, T. B. Levine, and R. Shepard. Cardiovascular responses of heart transplant recipients to graded exercise testing. *J. Appl. Physiol.* 73: 260–264, 1992.
127. Eiken, O., and H. Bjurstedt. Dynamic exercise in man as influenced by experimental restriction of blood flow in the working muscles. *Acta Physiol. Scand.* 131: 339–346, 1987.
128. Eisele, J. H., B. C. Ritchie, and J. W. Severinghaus. Effect of stellate ganglion blockade on the hyperpnea of exercise. *J. Appl. Physiol.* 22: 966–969, 1967.
129. Eldridge, F. L. Central integration of mechanisms in exercise hyperpnea. *Med. Sci. Sports Exerc.* 26: 319–327, 1994.
130. Eldridge, F. L., P. Gill-Kumar, D. E. Millhorn, and T. G. Waldrop. Spinal inhibition of phrenic motoneurons by stimulation of afferents from peripheral muscles. *J. Physiol. (Lond.)* 311: 67–79, 1981.
131. Eldridge, F. L., D. E. Millhorn, J. P. Kiley, and T. G. Waldrop. Stimulation by central command of locomotion, respiration and circulation during exercise. *Respir. Physiol.* 59: 313–337, 1985.
132. Ellaway, P. H., P. R. Murphy, and A. Tripathi. Closely coupled excitation of gamma-motoneurons by group III muscle afferents with low mechanical threshold in a cat. *J. Physiol. (Lond.)* 331: 481–498, 1982.
133. Ellenberger, H. H., J. L. Feldman, and H. G. Goshgarian. Ventral respiratory group projections to phrenic motoneurons: electron microscopic evidence for monosynaptic connections. *J. Comp. Neurol.* 302: 707–714, 1990.
134. England, S. J., and D. Bartlett. Changes in respiratory movements of the human vocal chords during hyperpnea. *J. Appl. Physiol.* 52: 780–785, 1982.
135. Erickson, B. K., H. V. Forster, L. G. Pan, T. F. Lowry, D. R. Brown, M. A. Forster, and A. L. Forster. Ventilatory compensation for lactacidosis in ponies: role of carotid chemoreceptors and lung afferents. *J. Appl. Physiol.* 70: 2619–2626, 1991.
136. Ettinger, S., K. Gray, S. Whisler, and L. Sinoway. Dichloroacetate reduces sympathetic nerve responses to static exercise. *Am. J. Physiol.* 261 (*Heart Circ. Physiol.* 30): H1653–H1658, 1991.
137. Euler, U. S., and S. Hellner. Excretion of noradrenaline and adrenaline in muscular work. *Acta Physiol. Scand.* 26: 193–191, 1952.
138. Favier, R., G. Kepenekian, D. Desplanches, and R. Flandrois. Effects of chronic lung denervation on breathing pattern and respiratory gas exchange during hypoxia, hypercapnia and exercise. *Respir. Physiol.* 47: 107–119, 1982.
139. Feigl, E. O. Parasympathetic control of coronary blood flow in dogs. *Circ. Res.* 25: 509–519, 1969.
140. Fernandez, A., H. Galbo, M. Kjaer, J. H. Mitchell, N. H. Secher, and S. N. Thomas. Cardiovascular and ventilatory responses to dynamic exercise during epidural anesthesia in man. *J. Appl. Physiol.* 420: 281–293, 1990.
141. Fisher, M. L., and D. O. Nutter. Cardiovascular reflex adjustments to static muscular contraction in the canine hindlimb. *Am. J. Physiol.* 226: 648–655, 1974.
142. Flandrois, R., J. F. Lacour, and J. P. Eclache. Control of respiration in exercising dog: interaction of chemical and physical humoral stimuli. *Respir. Physiol.* 21: 169–181, 1974.
143. Flynn, C., H. V. Forster, L. G. Pan, and G. E. Bisgard. Role of hilar nerve afferents in hyperpnea of exercise. *J. Appl. Physiol.* 59: 798–806, 1985.
144. Folgering, H., J. Ponte, and T. Sadig. Adrenergic mechanisms and chemoreception in the carotid body of the cat and rabbit. *J. Physiol. (Lond.)* 325: 1–21, 1982.
145. Fontana, G. A., T. Pantaleo, F. Bongianni, F. Gresci, F. Lavorini, C. Tostiguerra, and P. Panuccio. Prostaglandin synthesis blockade by ketoprofen attenuates the respiratory and cardiovascular responses to static handgrip. *J. Appl. Physiol.* 78: 449–457, 1995.
146. Ford, T. W., J. A. Bennett, C. Kidd, and P. N. McWilliam. Neurones in the dorsal motor vagal nucleus of the cat with non-myelinated axons projecting to the heart and lungs. *Exp. Physiol.* 75: 459–473, 1990.
147. Ford, T. W., and P. N. McWilliam. The effects of electrical stimulation of myelinated and non-myelinated vagal fibres on heart rate in the rabbit. *J. Physiol. (Lond.)* 380: 341–347, 1986.
148. Fordyce, W. E., and F. S. Grodins. Ventilatory response to intravenous and airway CO_2 administration in anesthetized dogs. *J. Appl. Physiol.* 48: 337–346, 1980.
149. Foreman, R. D., R. F. Schmidt, and W. D. Willis. Effects of mechanical and chemical stimulation of fine muscle afferents upon primate spinothalamic tract cells. *J. Physiol. (Lond.)* 286: 215–231, 1979.
150. Forster, H. V., M. B. Dunning, T. F. Lowry, B. K. Erickson, M. A. Forster, L. G. Pan, A. G. Brice, and R. M. Effros. Effect of asthma and ventilatory loading on Pa_{CO_2} during exercise in humans. *J. Appl. Physiol.* 75: 1385–1394, 1993.
151. Forster, H. V., B. K. Erickson, T. F. Lowry, L. G. Pan, M. J. Korducki, and A. L. Forster. Effect of helium induced ventilatory unloading on breathing and diaphragm EMG in awake ponies. *J. Appl. Physiol.* 77: 452–462, 1994.
152. Forster, H. V., and K. Klausen. The effect of chronic metabolic acidoses and alkalosis on ventilation during exercise and hypoxia. *Respir. Physiol.* 17: 336–346, 1973.
153. Forster, H. V., T. F. Lowry, C. L. Murphy, and L. G. Pan. Role of elevated plasma $[K^+]$ and carotid chemoreceptors in hyperpnea of exercise in awake ponies. *J. Physiol. (Lond.)* 417: 112P, 1990.
154. Forster, H. V., T. F. Lowry, L. G. Pan, B. K. Erickson, M. J. Korducki, and M. A. Forster. Diaphragm and lung afferents contribute to inspiratory load compensation in awake ponies. *J. Appl. Physiol.* 76: 1330–1339, 1994.
155. Forster, H. V., L. G. Pan, G. E. Bisgard, C. Flynn, S. M. Dorsey, and M. S. Britton. Independence of exercise hypocapnia and limb movement frequency in ponies. *J. Appl. Physiol.* 57: 1885–1893 1984.

156. Forster, H. V., L. G. Pan, G. E. Bisgard, R. P. Kaminski, S. C. Dorsey, and M. A. Busch. The hyperpnea of exercise at various P_{IO_2} in normal and carotid body denervated ponies. *J. Appl. Physiol.* 54: 1387–1393, 1983.
157. Forster, H. V., L. G. Pan, C. Flynn, and G. E. Bisgard. Attenuated Hering-Breuer inflation reflex 4 years after pulmonary vagal denervation in ponies. *J. Appl. Physiol.* 69: 2163–2167, 1990.
158. Forster, H. V., L. G. Pan, and A. Funahashi. Temporal pattern of Pa_{CO_2} during exercise in humans. *J. Appl. Physiol.* 60: 653–660, 1986.
159. Freund, P. R., S. F. Hobbs, and L. B. Rowell. Cardiovascular responses to muscle ischemia in man—dependency on muscle mass. *J. Appl. Physiol.* 45: 762–767, 1978.
160. Freund, P. R., L. B. Rowell, T. M. Murphy, S. F. Hobbs, and S. H. Butler. Blockade of pressor response to muscle ischemia by sensory nerve block in man. *Am. J. Physiol.* 236: (*Heart Circ. Physiol.* 7): H433–H439, 1979.
161. Friedman, D. B., J. Brennum, F. Sztuk, O. B. Hansen, P. S. Clifford, F. W. Bach, L. Arendt-Nielsen, J. H. Mitchell, and N. H. Secher. The effect of epidural anaesthesia with 1% lidocaine on the pressor response to dynamic exercise in man. *J. Physiol. (Lond.)* 470: 681–691, 1993.
162. Gaffney, E. R. Thal, W. F. Taylor, B. C. Bastian, J. A. Weigelt, J. M. Atkins, and G. G. Blomqvist. Hemodynamic effects of medical anti-shock trousers (MAST Garment). *J. Trauma* 21: 931–937, 1981.
163. Galbo, H., M. Kjaer, and N. J. Secher. Cardiovascular, ventilatory and catecholamine responses to maximal dynamic exercise in partially curarized man. *J. Physiol. (Lond.)* 389: 557–568, 1987.
164. Gallagher, C. G., and M. Younes. Effect of pressure assist on ventilation and respiratory mechanics in heavy exercise. *J. Appl. Physiol.* 66: 1824–1837, 1989.
165. Gandevia, S. C., and S. F. Hobbs. Cardiovascular responses to static exercise in man: central and reflex contributions. *J. Physiol. (Lond.)* 430: 105–117, 1990.
166. Gandevia, S. C., K. Killian, D. K. McKenzie, M. Crawford, G. M. Allen, R. B. Gorman, and J. P. Hales. Respiratory sensations, cardiovascular control, kinaesthesia and transcranial stimulation during paralysis in humans. *J. Physiol. (Lond.)* 470: 85–107, 1993.
167. Geis, G. S., and R. D. Wurster. Cardiac responses during stimulation of the dorsal motor nucleus and nucleus ambiguus in the cat. *Circ. Res.* 46: 606–611, 1980.
168. Gerber, G., R. Cerne, and M. Randic. Participation of excitatory amino acid receptors in the slow excitatory synaptic transmission in rat spinal dorsal horn. *Brain Res.* 561: 236–251, 1991.
169. Go, V. L. W., and T. L. Yaksh. Release of substance P from the cat spinal cord. *J. Physiol. (Lond.)* 391: 141–167, 1987.
170. Goodman, N. W., B. S. Nail, and R. W. Torrance. Oscillations in the discharge of single carotid chemoreceptor fibres of the cat. *Respir. Physiol.* 20: 251–266, 1974.
171. Gordon, F. J., and L. M. McCann. Pressor responses evoked by microinjection of L-glutamate into the caudal ventrolateral medulla of the rat. *Brain Res.* 457: 251–281, 1988.
172. Gordon, G. The mechanism of the vasomotor reflexes produced by stimulating mammalian sensory nerves. *J. Physiol. (Lond.)* 102: 95–107, 1943.
173. Graham, L. T., R. P. Shank, R. Werman, and M. H. Aprison. Distribution of some synaptic transmitter suspects in cat spinal cord. *J. Neurochem.* 14: 465–472, 1967.
174. Graham, R., Y. Jammes, S. Delpierre, C. Grimaud, and C. Roussos. The effects of ischemia, lactic acid and hypertonic sodium chloride on phrenic afferent discharge during spontaneous diaphragmatic contraction. *Neurosci. Lett.* 67: 257–262, 1986.
175. Granit, R., S. Skoglund, and S. Thesleff. Activation of muscle spindles by succinylcholine and decamethonium. *Acta Physiol. Scand.* 28: 134–151, 1953.
176. Grant, B., and S. J. G. Semple. Mechanisms whereby oscillations in arterial carbon dioxide tension might affect pulmonary ventilation. In: *Morphology and Mechanisms of Chemoreceptors*, edited by A. S. Paintal. New Delhi, India: Navchetan Press, Ltd. 1976.
177. Grant, B. J. B., R. P. Stidweill, B. A. Cross, and S. J. G. Semple. Ventilatory response to inhaled and infused CO_2: relationship to the oscillating signal. *Respir. Physiol.* 44: 365–380, 1981.
178. Greco, E. D., W. E. Fordyce, F. Gonzalez, P. Reischl, and F. S. Grodins. Respiratory responses to intravenous and intrapulmonary CO_2 in awake dogs. *J. Appl. Physiol.* 45: 109–114, 1978.
179. Green, H. J., R. L. Hughson, G. W. Orr, and D. A. Ranney. Anaerobic threshold, blood lactate and muscle metabolites in progressive exercise. *J. Appl. Physiol.* 54: 1032–1038, 1983.
180. Green, J. F., E. R. Schertel, H. M. Coleridge, and J. C. G. Coleridge. Effect of pulmonary arterial P_{CO_2} on slowly adapting pulmonary stretch receptors. *J. Appl. Physiol.* 60: 2048–2055, 1986.
181. Green, J. F., and M. I. Sheldon. Ventilatory changes associated with changes in pulmonary blood flow in dogs. *J. Appl. Physiol.* 54: 997–1102, 1983.
182. Gregory, J. E., P. Kenins, and U. Proske. Can lacate-evoked cardiovascular response be used to identify muscle ergoreceptors? *Brain Res.* 404: 375–378, 1987.
183. Griffiths, T. L., L. C. Henson, D. Huntsman, K. Wasserman, and B. J. Whipp. The influence of inspired O_2 partial pressure on ventilatory and gas exchange kinetics during exercise. *J. Physiol. (Lond.)* 306: 34P, 1980 (Abstract).
184. Grunstein, M. M., J. P. Derenre, and J. Milic-Emile. Control of depth and frequency of breathing during baroreceptor stimulation in cats. *J. Appl. Physiol.* 39: 395–404, 1975.
185. Gutting, S. M., H. V. Forster, T. F. Lowry, A. G. Brice, and L. G. Pan. Respiratory muscle recruitment in awake ponies during exercise and CO_2 inhalation. *Respir. Physiol.* 86: 315–332, 1991.
186. Guyton, A. C. Organization of the nervous system, basic functions of synapsis and transmitter substances. In: *Textbook of Medical Physiology*. Philadelphia: W. B. Saunders Company, 1991, p. 447–494.
187. Hagberg, J. M., J. M., E. F. Coyle, J. E. Carrol, J. M. Miller, W. H. Martin, and M. H. Brooke. Exercise hyperventilation in patients with McArdles disease. *J. Appl. Physiol.* 52: 991–994, 1982.
188. Hagenhauser, G. J. T., J. R. Sutton, and N. L. Jones. Effect of glycogen depletion on the ventilatory response to exercise. *J. Appl. Physiol.* 54: 470–474, 1983.
189. Haggendal, J., L. H. Harley, and B. Saltin. Arterial noradrenaline concentration during exercise in relation to the relative work loads. *Scand. J. Clin. Lab. Invest.* 26: 337–342, 1970.
190. Hamalainen, R. P., and A. A. Viljanen. Modelling the respiratory air-flow pattern by optimizing criteria. *Biol. Cybern.* 29: 143–149, 1978.

191. Hanson, P., A. Claremont, J. Dempsey, and W. Reddan. Determinants and consequences of ventilatory responses to competitive endurance running. *J. Appl. Physiol.* 52: 615–623, 1982.
192. Harrison, T. R., W. G. Harrison, J. A. Calhoun, and J. P. Marsh. Congestive heart failure. The mechanisms of dyspnea on exertion. *Arch. Intern. Med.* 50: 690–720, 1932.
193. Haselton, J. R., P. A. Padrid, and M. P. Kaufman. Activation of neurons in the rostral ventrolateral medulla increases bronchomotor tone in dogs. *J. Appl. Physiol.* 71: 210–216, 1991.
194. Haxhiu, M. A., E. Van Lunteren, J. Mitra, N. S. Cherniack, and K. P. Strohl. Comparison of the responses of the diaphragm and upper airway muscles to central stimulation of the sciatic nerve. *Respir. Physiol.* 58: 65–76, 1984.
195. Hayward, L., U. Wesselmann, and W. Z. Rymer. Effects of muscle fatigue on mechanically sensitive afferents of slow conduction velocity in the cat triceps surae. *J. Neurophysiol.* 65: 360–370, 1991.
196. Helke, C. J., J. J. Neil, V. J. Massari, and A. D. Loewy. Substance P Neurons project from the ventral medulla to the intermediolateral cell column and ventral horn in the rat. *Brain Res.* 243: 147–152, 1982.
197. Henke, K. G., M. Sharratt, D. Pegelow, and J. A. Dempsey. Regulation of end-expiratory lung volume during exercise. *J. Appl. Physiol.* 64: 135–146, 1988.
198. Henneman, E., G. Somjen, and D. O. Carpenter. Functional significance of cell size in spinal motoneurons. *J. Neurophysiol.* 28: 560–580, 1965.
199. Henry, J. L. Effects of substance P on functionally identified units in cat spinal cord. *Brain Res.* 114: 439–451, 1976.
200. Heymans, J. F., and C. Heymans. Sur les modifications directes et sur la regulation reflexes de l'activite du centre respiratoire de la tete isolie du chien. *Arch. Int. Pharmacodyn. Ther.* 33: 273–372, 1927.
201. Hill, J. M., and M. P. Kaufman. Attenuation of reflex pressor and ventilatory responses to static muscular contraction by intrathecal opioids. *J. Appl. Physiol.* 68: 2466–2472, 1990.
202. Hill, J. M., and M. P. Kaufman. Attenuating effects of intrathecal clonidine on the exercise pressor reflex. *J. Appl. Physiol.* 70: 516–522, 1991.
203. Hill, J. M., and M. P. Kaufman. Intrathecal serotonin attenuates the pressor response to static contraction. *Brain Res.* 550: 157–160, 1991.
204. Hill, J. M., J. G. Pickar, and M. P. Kaufman. Attenuation of reflex pressor and ventilatory responses to static contraction by an NK-1 receptor antagonist. *J. Appl. Physiol.* 73: 1389–1395, 1992.
205. Hill, J. M., J. G. Pickar, and M. P. Kaufman. Blockade of non-NMDA receptors attenuates reflex pressor response to static contraction. *Am. J. Physiol.* 266 (*Heart Circ. Physiol.* 35): H1769–H1776, 1994.
206. Hill, J. M., J. G. Pickar, M. Parrish, and M. P. Kaufman. Effects of hypoxia on the discharge on group III and IV muscle afferents in cats. *J. Appl. Physiol.* 73: 2524–2529, 1992.
207. Hník, P., O. Hudlická, J. Kucera, and R. Payne. Activation of muscle afferents by nonproprioceptive stimuli. *Am. J. Physiol.* 217: 1451–1458, 1969.
208. Hodgson, H. J. F., and P. B. C. Matthews. The ineffectiveness of excitation of the primary endings of the muscle spindle by vibration as a respiratory stimulate in the decerebrate cat. *J. Physiol. (Lond.)* 194: 555–563, 1968.
209. Hoffer, J. A., G. E. Loeb, W. B. Marks, M. J. O'Donovan, C. A. Pratt, and N. Sugano. Cat hind limb motoneurons during locomotion. I. Destination, axonal conduction velocity, and recruitment threshold. *J. Neurophysiol.* 57: 510–529, 1987.
210. Hoffer, J. A., M. J. O'Donovan, C. A. Pratt, and G. E. Loeb. Discharge patterns of hindlimb motoneurons during normal cat locomotion. *Science* 213: 466–468, 1981.
211. Hoffer, J. A., N. Sugano, G. E. Loeb, W. B. Marks, M. J. O'Donovan, and C. A. Pratt. Cat hind limb motoneurons during locomotion. II. Normal activity patterns. *J. Neurophysiol.* 57: 530–553, 1987.
212. Hoheisel, U., and S. Mense. Response behaviour of cat dorsal horn neurons receiving input from skeletal muscle and other deep somatic tissues. *J. Physiol. (Lond.)* 426: 265–280, 1990.
213. Hökfelt, T., J. O. Kellerth, G. Nilsson, and B. Pernow. Experimental immunohistochemical studies on the localization and distribution of substance P in cat primary sensory neurons. *Brain Res.* 100: 235–252, 1975.
214. Hollander, A. P., and L. N. Bouman. Cardiac acceleration in man elicited by a muscle-heart reflex. *J. Appl. Physiol.* 38: 272–278, 1975.
215. Honda, Y., S. Myojo, S. Hasegawa, T. Hawegawa, and J. W. Severinghaus. Decreased exercise hyperpnea in patients with bilateral carotid chemoreceptor resection. *J. Appl. Physiol.* 46: 908–912, 1979.
216. Hopkins, D. A., and J. A. Armour. Medullary cells of origin of physiologically identified cardiac nerves in the dog. *Brain Res. Bull.* 8: 359–365, 1982.
217. Hornbein, T. F., S. C. Sorensen, and C. R. Parks. Role of muscle spindles in lower extremities in breathing during bicycle exercise. *J. Appl. Physiol.* 27: 476–479, 1969.
218. Hornicke, J., R. Meixner, and U. Pollmann. Respiration in exercising horses. In: *Equine Exercise Physiology*, edited by D. H. Snow, S. G. Persson, and R. J. Rose. Cambridge: Grants Editions, 1982, p. 7–16.
219. Hughes, E. F., S. C. Turner, and G. A. Brooks. Effect of glycogen depletion and pedaling speed on "anaerobic threshold." *J. Appl. Physiol.* 52: 1598–1607, 1982.
220. Hultman, E., and H. Sjoholm. Blood pressure and heart rate response to voluntary and non-voluntary static exercise in man. *Acta Physiol. Scand.* 115: 499–501, 1982.
221. Hunt, C. C. Relation of function to diameter in afferent fibers of muscle nerves. *J. Gen. Physiol.* 38: 117–131, 1954.
222. Hussain, S. N. A., R. L. Pardy, and J. A. Dempsey. Mechanical impedance as determinant of inspiratory neural drive during exercise in humans. *J. Appl. Physiol.* 59: 365–375, 1985.
223. Huszczuk, A., B. J. Whipp, T. D. Adams, A. G. Fisher, R. O. Crapo, C. G. Elliot, K. Wasserman, and D. B. Olsen. Ventilatory control during exercise in calves with artificial hearts. *J. Appl. Physiol.* 68: 2604–2611, 1990.
224. Iggo, A. Non-myelinated afferent fibers from mammalian skeletal muscle. *J. Physiol. (Lond.)* 155: 52–53P, 1961.
225. Innes, J. A., I. Solarte, A.Huszeyk, E. Yah, B. J. Whipp, and K. Wasserman. Respiration during recovery from exercise: effects of trapping and release of femoral blood flow. *J. Appl. Physiol.* 67: 2608–2613, 1989.
226. Iwamoto, G. A., and B. R. Botterman. Peripheral factors influencing expression of pressor reflex evoked by muscular contraction. *J. Appl. Physiol.* 58: 1676–1682, 1985.
227. Iwamoto, G. A., B. R. Botterman, and T. G. Waldrop. The exercise pressor reflex: evidence for an afferent pressor pathway outside the dorsolateral sulcus region. *Brain Res.* 292: 160–164, 1984.

228. Iwamoto, G. A., R. D. Brtva, and T. G. Waldrop. Cardiorespiratory responses to chemical stimulation of the caudalmost ventrolateral medulla in the cat. *Neurosci. Lett.* 129: 86–90, 1991.
229. Iwamoto, G. A., and M. P. Kaufman. Caudal ventrolateral medullary cells responsive to static muscular contraction. *J. Appl. Physiol.* 62: 149–157, 1987.
230. Iwamoto, G. A., M. P. Kaufman, B. R. Botterman, and J. H. Mitchell. Effects of lateral reticular nucleus lesions on the exercise pressor reflex in cats. *Circ. Res.* 51: 400–403, 1982.
231. Iwamoto, G. A., J. H. Mitchell, M. Mizuno, and N. H. Secher. Cardiovascular responses at the onset of exercise with partial neuromuscular blockade in cat and man. *J. Physiol. (Lond.)* 3842: 39–47, 1987.
232. Iwamoto, G. A., J. H. Mitchell, M. Sadeq, and G. P. Kozlowski. Localization of tyrosine hydroxylase and phenylethanolamine N-methyltransferase immunoreactive cells in the medulla of the dog. *Neurosci. Lett.* 107: 12–18, 1989.
233. Iwamoto, G. A., J. G. Parnaveles, M. P. Kaufman, B. R. Botterman, and J. H. Mitchell. Activation of caudal brainstem cell groups during the exercise pressor reflex as elucidated by 2-[^{14}C] deoxyglucose. *Brain Res.* 304: 178–182, 1984.
234. Iwamoto, G. A., T. G. Waldrop, M. P. Kaufman, B. R. Botterman, K. J. Rybicki, and J. H. Mitchell. Pressor reflex evoked by muscular contraction: contributions by neuraxis levels. *J. Appl. Physiol.* 59: 459–467, 1985.
235. Johansson, B. Circulatory responses to stimulation of somatic afferents. *Acta Physiol. Scand.* 57: 1–91, 1962.
236. Johnson, J. L., and M. H. Aprison. The distribution of glutamic acid, a transmitter candidate, and other amino acids in the dorsal sensory neuron of the cat. *Brain Res.* 24: 285–292, 1970.
237. Jones, P. W., A. Huszczuk, and K. Wasserman. Cardiac output as a controller of ventilation through changes in right ventricular load. *J. Appl. Physiol.* 53: 218–224, 1982.
238. Jordan, D., M. E. M. Khalid, N. Schneiderman, and K. M. Spyer. The location and properties of preganglionic vagal cardiomotor neurones in the rabbit. *Pflugers Arch.* 395: 244–250, 1982.
239. Joyner, M. J. Does the pressor response to ischemic exercise improve blood flow to contracting muscles in humans? *J. Appl. Physiol.* 71: 1496–1501, 1991.
240. Joyner, M. J., and W. Wieling. Increased muscle perfusion reduces muscle sympathetic nerve activity during handgripping. *J. Appl. Physiol.* 75: 2450–2455, 1993.
241. Kaehny, W. D., and J. T. Jackson. Respiratory response to HCL acidosis in dogs after carotid body denervation. *J. Appl. Physiol.* 46: 1138–1142, 1979.
242. Kagawa, J., and H. D. Kerr. Effects of brief graded exercise on specific airway conductance in normal subjects. *J. Appl. Physiol.* 28: 138–144, 1970.
243. Kagerberg, G. S., and A. Bjorklund. Topographic principles in the spinal projections of serotonergic and non-serotonergic brainstem neurons in the rat. *Neuroscience* 15: 445–480, 1985.
244. Kai-Kai, M. M., B. H. Anderton, and P. Keen. A quantitative analysis of the interrelationships between subpopulations of rat sensory neurons containing arginine vasopressin or oxytocin and those containing substance P, fluoride-resistant acid phosphatase or neurofilament protein. *Neuroscience* 18: 475–486, 1986.
245. Kalia, M., J. M. Senapati, B. Parida, and A. Panda. Reflex increase in ventilation by muscle receptors with nonmedullated fibers (C-fibers). *J. Appl. Physiol.* 32: 189–193, 1972.
246. Kangrga, I., and M. Randic. Tachykinins and calcitonin gene-related peptide enhance release of endogenous glutamate and aspartate from the rat spinal dorsal horn slice. *J. Neurosci.* 10: 2026–2038, 1990.
247. Kannan, H., H. Yamashita, K. Koizumi, and C. M. Brooks. Neuronal activity of the cat supraoptic nucleus is influenced by muscle small-diameter afferent (groups III and IV) receptors. *Proc. Natl. Acad. Sci. U. S. A.* 85: 5744–5748, 1988.
248. Kao, F. F. An experimental study of the pathway involved in exercise hyperpnea employing cross-circulation technique. In: *The Regulation of Human Respiration*, edited by D. J. C. Cunningham and B. B. Lloyd. Oxford: Blackwell, 1963, p. 461–502.
249. Kao, F. F., S. Lahiri, C. Wang, and S. S. Mei. Ventilation and cardiac output in exercise: interaction of chemical and work stimuli. *Circ. Res.* 20: 179–191, 1967.
250. Kao, F. F., and L. H. Ray. Respiratory and circulatory responses of anesthetized dogs to induced muscular work. *Am. J. Physiol.* 179: 249–254, 1954.
251. Kao, F. F., and L. H. Ray. Regulation of cardiac output in anesthetized dogs during induced muscular work. *Am. J. Physiol.* 179: 255–260, 1954.
252. Karlsson, J. A., M. J. B. Finney, C. G. A. Persson, and C. Post. Substance P antagonists and the role of tachykinins in non-cholinergic bronchoconstriction. *Life Sci.* 35: 2681–2691, 1984.
253. Kaufman, M. P., G. A. Iwamoto, J. C. Longhurst, and J. H. Mitchell. Effects of capsaicin and bradykinin on afferent fibers with endings in skeletal muscle. *Circ. Res.* 50: 133–139, 1982.
254. Kaufman, M. P., G. P. Kozlowski, and K. J. Rybicki. Attenuation of the reflex pressor response to muscular contraction by a substance P antagonist. *Brain Res.* 333: 182–184, 1985.
255. Kaufman, M. P., J. C. Longhurst, K. J. Rybicki, J. H. Wallach, and J. H. Mitchell. Effects of static muscular contraction on impulse activity of groups III and IV afferents in cats. *J. Appl. Physiol.* 55: 105–112, 1983.
256. Kaufman, M. P., G. A. Ordway, J. C. Longhurst, and J. H. Mitchell. Reflex relaxation of tracheal smooth muscle by thin fiber muscle afferents in dogs. *Am. J. Physiol.* 243 (*Regulatory Integrative Comp. Physiol.* 12): R383–R388, 1982.
257. Kaufman, M. P., and K. J. Rybicki. Muscular contraction reflexly relaxes tracheal smooth muscle in dogs. *Respir. Physiol.* 56: 61–72, 1984.
258. Kaufman, M. P., and K. J. Rybicki. Discharge properties of group III and IV muscle afferents: their responses to mechanical and metabolic stimuli. *Circ. Res.* 61: 160–165, 1987.
259. Kaufman, M. P., K. J. Rybicki, G. P. Kozlowski, and G. A. Iwamoto. Immunoneutralization of substance P attenuates the reflex pressor response to muscular contraction. *Brain Res.* 377: 199–203, 1986.
260. Kaufman, M. P., K. J. Rybicki, and J. H. Mitchell. Hindlimb muscular contraction reflexly decreases total pulmonary resistance. *J. Appl. Physiol.* 59: 1521–1526, 1985.
261. Kaufman, M. P., K. J. Rybicki, T. G. Waldrop, and J. H. Mitchell. Effect on arterial pressure of rhythmically contracting the hindlimb of cats. *J. Appl. Physiol.* 56: 1265–1271, 1984.
262. Kaufman, M. P., K. J. Rybicki, T. G. Waldrop, and G. A. Ordway. Effect of ischemia on responses of group III and

IV afferents to contraction. *J. Appl. Physiol.* 57: 644–650, 1984.
263. Kaufman, M. P., K. J. Rybicki, T. G. Waldrop, G. A. Ordway, and J. H. Mitchell. Effects of static and rhythmic twitch contractions on the discharge of group III and IV muscle afferents. *Cardiovasc. Res.* 18: 663–668, 1984.
264. Kelly, M. A., G. R. Owens, and A. P. Fishman. Hypercapnic ventilation during exercise: effects of exercise methods and inhalation techniques. *Respir. Physiol.* 50: 75–85, 1982.
265. Kiely, J. M., and F. J. Gordon. Non-NMDA receptors in the rostral ventrolateral medulla mediate somatosympathetic pressor responses. *J. Auton. Nerv. Syst.* 43: 231–240, 1993.
266. Kjaer, M., N. H. Secher, F. W. Bach, H. Galbo, D. R. Reeves, Jr., and J. H. Mitchell. Hormonal, metabolic, and cardiovascular responses to static exercise in humans: influence of epidural anesthesia. *Am. J. Physiol.* 261 (*Endocrinol. Metab.* 24): E214–E220, 1991.
267. Klein, C. M., R. E. Coggeshall, S. M. Carlton, K. N. Westlund, and L. S. Sorkin. Changes in calcitonin gene-related peptide immunoreactivity in the rat dorsal horn following electrical stimulation of the sciatic nerve. *Neurosci. Lett.* 115: 149–154, 1990.
268. Kniffki, K., S. Mense, and R. F. Schmidt. Responses of group IV afferent units from skeletal muscle to stretch, contraction and chemical stimuli. *Exp. Brain Res.* 31: 511–522, 1978.
269. Knill, R. L., and J. L. Clement. Ventilatory responses to acute metabolic acidemia in humans awake, sedated, and anesthetized with halothane. *Anesthesiology* 62: 733–745, 1985.
270. Knuttgen, J. G., and K. Emersen. Physiological response to pregnancy at rest and during exercise. *J. Appl. Physiol.* 36: 546–553, 1974.
271. Koizumi, K., J. Ushiyama, and C. M. Brooks. Muscle afferents and activity of respiratory neurons. *Am. J. Physiol.* 200: 679–684, 1961.
272. Kostreva, D. R., F. A. Hopp, E. J. Zuperku, F. O. Ingler, F. L. Coon, and J. P. Kampine. Respiratory inhibition with sympathetic afferent stimulation in the canine and primate. *J. Appl. Physiol.* 44: 718–724, 1978.
273. Kostreva, D. R., F. A. Hopp, E. J. Zuperku, and J. P. Kampine. Apnea, tachypnea, and hypotension elicited by cardiac vagal afferents. *J. Appl. Physiol.* 47: 312–318, 1979.
274. Koterba, A. M., P. C. Kosch, J. Beech, and T. Whitlock. Breathing strategy of the adult horse (*Equus caballus*) at rest. *J. Appl. Physiol.* 64: 337–346, 1988.
275. Kozelka, J. W., G. W. Christy, and R. D. Wurster. Somatoautonomic reflexes in anesthetised and unanesthetised dogs. *J. Auton. Nerv. Syst.* 5: 63–70, 1982.
276. Kozelka, J. W., G. W. Christy, and R. D. Wurster. Ascending pathways mediating somatoautonomic reflexes in exercising dogs. *J. Appl. Physiol.* 62: 1186–1191, 1987.
277. Kozelka, J. W., and R. D. Wurster. Ascending spinal pathways for somato-autonomic reflexes in the anesthetized dogs. *J. Appl. Physiol.* 58: 1832–1839, 1985.
278. Krasney, J. A., M. G. Levitzky, and R. C. Koehler. Sinoaortic contribution to the adjustment of systemic resistance in exercising dogs. *J. Appl. Physiol.* 36: 679–685, 1974.
279. Kretz, R. Local cobalt injection: a method to discriminate presynaptic axonal from postsynaptic neuronal activity. *J. Neurosci. Methods* 11: 129–135, 1984.
280. Krogh, A., and J. Lindhard. The regulation of respiration and circulation during the initial stages of muscular work. *J. Physiol. (Lond.)* 47: 112–136, 1913.
281. Kumada, M., K. Nogami, and K. Sagawa. Modulation of carotid sinus baroreceptor reflex by sciatic nerve stimulation. *Am. J. Physiol.* 228: 1535–1541, 1975.
282. Kumazawa, T., and E. Tadaki. Two different inhibitory effects on respiration by thin-fiber muscular afferents in cats. *Brain Res.* 272: 364–367, 1983.
283. Kumazawa, T. N., and K. Mizumura. Thin-fibre receptors responding to mechanical, chemical and thermal stimulation in the skeletal muscle of the dog. *J. Physiol. (Lond.)* 273: 179–194, 1977.
284. Kunze, D. L. Reflex discharge patterns of cardiac vagal efferent fibres. *J. Physiol. (Lond.)* 222: 1–15, 1972.
285. Lahiri, S. Physiologic responses: peripheral chemoreflexes. In: *The Lung: Scientific Foundations*, edited by R. G. Crystal, J. B. West, et al. New York: Raven Press, 1991, p. 1333–1340.
286. Lamb, T. W. Ventilatory responses to intravenous and inspired carbon dioxide in anesthetized cats. *Respir. Physiol.* 2: 99–104, 1966.
287. Lamb, T. W. Ventilatory responses to hind limb exercise in anesthetized cats and dogs. *Respir. Physiol.* 6: 88–104, 1968.
288. Laporte, Y., P. Bessou, and S. Bouissett. Action réflexe des différents types de fibres afférents d'origine musculaire sur la pression sanguine. *Arch. Ital. Biol.* 98: 206–221, 1960.
289. Lassen, A., J. H. Mitchell, D. R. Reeves, Jr., H. B. Rogers, and N. H. Secher. Cardiovascular responses to brief static contractions in man with topical nervous blockade. *J. Physiol. (Lond.)* 409: 333–341, 1989.
290. Leonard, B., J. H. Mitchell, M. Mizuno, N. Rube, B. Saltin, and N. H. Secher. Partial neuromuscular blockade and cardiovascular resonses to static exercise in man. *J. Physiol. (Lond.)* 359: 365–379, 1985.
291. Levine, S. Ventilatory response to muscular exercise: observations regarding a humoral pathway. *J. Appl. Physiol.* 47: 126–137, 1979.
292. Lewis, S. M. Awake baboon's ventilatory response to venous and inhaled CO_2 loading. *J. Appl. Physiol.* 39: 417–422, 1975.
293. Light, A. R., and E. R. Perl. Spinal termination of functionally identified primary afferent neurons with slowly conducting myelinated fibers. *J. Comp. Neurol.* 186: 133–150, 1979.
294. Linton, R. A. F., and D. M. Band. The effect of potassium on carotid chemoreceptor activity and ventilation in the cat. *Respir. Physiol.* 59: 65–70, 1985.
295. Linton, R. A. F., M. Lim, C. B. Wolff, P. Wilmshurst, and D. M. Band. Arterial potassium measured continuously during exercise in man. *Clin. Sci.* 67: 427–431, 1984.
296. Linton, R. A. F., R. Miller, and R. Cameron. Ventilatory response to CO_2 inhalation and intravenous infusion of hypercapnic blood. *Respir. Physiol.* 26: 383–394, 1976.
297. Liu, C. T., R. A. Huggins, and H. E. Hoff. Mechanisms of intra-arterial K^+-induced cardiovascular and respiratory responses. *Am. J. Physiol.* 217: 969–973, 1969.
298. Liu, G., J. L. Feldman, and J. C. Smith. Excitatory amino acid-mediated transmission of inspiratory drive to phrenic motoneurons. *J. Neurophysiol.* 64: 423–436, 1990.
299. Lloyd, T. C. Effect on breathing of acute pressure rise in pulmonary artery and right ventricle. *J. Appl. Physiol.* 57: 110–116, 1984.
300. Longhurst, J. C. Static contraction of hind limb muscles in cats reflexly relaxes tracheal smooth muscle. *J. Appl. Physiol.* 57: 380–387, 1984.
301. Maqbool, A., T. F. C. Batten, and P. N. McWilliam. Ultrastructural relationships between GABAergic terminals

and cardiac vagal preganglionic motoneurons and vagal afferents in the cat: a combined HRP tracing and immunogold labelling study. *Eur. J. Neurosci.* 3: 501–513, 1991.
302. Marchettini, P. Muscle pain, animal and human experimental and clinical studies. *Muscle Nerve* 16: 1033–1039, 1993.
303. Mark, A. L., R. G. Victor, C. Nerhed, and B. G. Wallin. Microneurographic studies of the mechanisms of sympathetic nerve responses to static exercise in humans. *Circ. Res.* 57: 461–469, 1985.
304. Martin, P. A., and G. S. Mitchell. Long-term modulation of the exercise ventilatory response in goats. *J. Physiol. (Lond.)* 470: 601–617, 1993.
305. Matsukawa, K., P. T. Wall, L. B. Wilson, and J. H. Mitchell. Reflex responses of renal nerve activity during isometric muscle contraction in cats. *Am. J. Physiol.* 259 (*Heart Circ. Physiol.* 28): H1380–H1388, 1990.
306. Matsukawa, K., P. T. Wall, L. B. Wilson, and J. H. Mitchell. Reflex stimulation of cardiac sympathetic nerve activity during static muscle contraction in cats. *Am. J. Physiol.* 267 (*Heart Circ. Physiol.* 36): H821–H827, 1994.
307. McAllen, R. M., and K. M. Spyer. The location of cardiac vagal preganglionic motoneurons projecting in the medulla of the cat. *J. Physiol. (Lond.)* 258: 187–204, 1976.
308. McAllen, R. M., and K. M. Spyer. Two types of vagal preganglionic motoneurons projecting to the heart and lungs. *J. Physiol. (Lond.)* 292: 353–364, 1978.
309. McClain, J., C. Hardy, B. Enders, M. Smith, and L. Sinoway. Limb congestion and sympathoexcitation during exercise. *J. Clin. Invest.* 92: 2353–2359, 1993.
310. McClain, J., J. C. Hardy, and L. I. Sinoway. Forearm compression during exercise increases sympathetic nerve traffic. *J. Appl. Physiol.* 77: 2612–2617, 1994.
311. McCloskey, D. I., and J. H. Mitchell. Reflex cardiovascular and respiratory responses originating in exercising muscle. *J. Physiol. (Lond.)* 224: 173–186, 1972.
312. McCloskey, D. I., and K. A. Streatfeild. Muscular reflex stimuli to the cardiovascular system during isometric contractions of muscle groups of different mass. *J. Physiol. (Lond.)* 250: 431–441, 1975.
313. McCoy, K. W., D. M. Rotto, K. J. Rybicki, and M. P. Kaufman. Attenuation of the reflex pressor response to muscular contraction by an antagonist to somatostatin. *Circ. Res.* 62: 18–24, 1988.
314. McCoy, M., and M. Hargreaves. Potassium and ventilation during incremental exercise in trained and untrained men. *J. Appl. Physiol.* 73: 1287–1290, 1992.
315. McCrimmon, D. R., J. C. Smith, and J. L. Feldman. Involvement of excitatory amino acids in neurotransmission of inspiratory drive to spinal respiratory motoneurons. *J. Neurosci.* 9: 1910–1921, 1989.
316. McMahon, S. E., and P. N. McWilliam. Changes in R-R interval at the start of muscle contraction in the decerebrate cat. *J. Physiol. (Lond.)* 447: 549–562, 1992.
317. McMahon, S. E., P. N. McWilliam, and J. C. Kaye. Hindlimb contraction inhibits evoked activity in baroreceptor-sensitive neurones in the nucleus tractus solitarius (NTS) of the anaesthetized cat. *J. Physiol. (Lond.)* 467: 18P, 1993 (Abstract).
318. McMurray, R. G., and S. W. Ahlborn. Respiratory responses to running and walking at the same metabolic rate. *Respir. Physiol.* 47: 257–265, 1982.
319. McWilliam, P. N., and T. Yang. Inhibition of cardiac vagal component of baroreflex by group III and IV afferents. *Am. J. Physiol.* 260 (*Heart Circ. Physiol.* 29): H730–H734, 1991.
320. McWilliam, P. N., T. Yang, and L. X. Chien. Changes in the baroreceptor reflex by muscle contraction in the decerebrate cat. *J. Physiol. (Lond.)* 436: 549–558, 1991.
321. Mead, J. Control of respiratory frequency. *J. Appl. Physiol.* 49: 528–532, 1980.
322. Melcher, A., and D. E. Donald. Maintained ability of carotid baroreflex to regulate arterial pressure during exercise. *Am. J. Physiol.* 241 (*Heart Circ. Physiol.* 10): H838–H849, 1981.
323. Mense, S. Nervous outflow from skeletal muscle following chemical noxious stimulation. *J. Physiol. (Lond.)* 267: 75–88, 1977.
324. Mense, S. Sensitization of group IV muscle receptors to bradykinin by 5-hydroxytryptamine and prostaglandin E-2. *Brain Res.* 225: 95–105, 1981.
325. Mense, S., and A. D. I. Craig. Spinal and supraspinal terminations of primary afferent fibers from the gastrocnemius-soleus muscle in the cat. *Neuroscience* 26: 1023–1035, 1988.
326. Mense, S., and H. Meyer. Different types of slowly conducting afferent units in cat skeletal muscle and tendon. *J. Physiol. (Lond.)* 363: 403–417, 1985.
327. Mense, S., and H. Meyer. Bradykinin-induced modulation of the response behaviour of different types of feline group III and IV muscle receptors. *J. Physiol. (Lond.)* 398: 49–63, 1988.
328. Mense, S., and N. R. Prabhakar. Spinal termination of nociceptive afferent fibres from deep tissues in the cat. *Neurosci. Lett.* 66: 169–174, 1986.
329. Mense, S., and R. F. Schmidt. Activation of group IV afferent units from muscle by algesic agents. *Brain Res.* 72: 305–310, 1974.
330. Mense, S., and M. Stahnke. Responses in muscle afferent fibers of slow conduction velocity to contractions and ischemia in the cat. *J. Physiol. (Lond.)* 342: 383–397, 1983.
331. Millan, M. J., M. H. Millan, A. Czlonkowski, and A. Herz. Vasopressin and oxytocin in the rat spinal cord: Distribution and origins in comparison to metenkephalin, dynorphin, and related opioids and their irresponsiveness to stimuli modulating neurohypophyseal secretion. *Neuroscience* 13: 179–187, 1984.
332. Miller, K. E., and V. S. Seybold. Comparison of met-enkephalin, dynorphin A- and neurotensin-immunoreactive neurons in the cat and rat spinal cords. I. Lumbar cord. *J. Comp. Neurol.* 255: 293–304, 1984.
333. Mitchell, G. S. Ventilatory control during exercise with increased respiratory dead space in goats. *J. Appl. Physiol.* 69: 718–727, 1990.
334. Mitchell, G. S., K. B. Bach, P. A. Martin, and K. T. Foley. Modulation and plasticity of the exercise ventilatory response. In: *Respiration in Health and Disease*, edited by P. Scheid. Stuttgart: Gustav Fischer Verlag, 1993, p. 269–277.
335. Mitchell, G. S., M. A. Douse, and K. T. Foley. Receptor interactions in modulating ventilatory activity. *Am. J. Physiol.* 259 (*Regulatory Integrative Comp. Physiol.* 28): R911–R920, 1990.
336. Mitchell, G. S., C. A. Smith, and J. A. Dempsey. Changes in the V_I:V_{CO_2} relationship during exercise: role of carotid body. *J. Appl. Physiol.* 57: 1894–1900, 1984.
337. Mitchell, J. H., D. S. Mierzwiak, K. Wildenthal, W. D. J. Willis, and A. M. Smith. Effect on left ventricular performance of stimulation of an afferent nerve from muscle. *Circ. Res.* 22: 507–516, 1968.
338. Mitchell, J. H., W. C. Reardon, and D. I. McCloskey. Reflex effects on circulation and respiration from contracting

skeletal muscle. *Am. J. Physiol.* 233 (*Heart Circ. Physiol.* 2): H374–H378, 1977.

339. Mitchell, J. H., D. R. Reeves, H. B. Rogers, and N. H. Secher. Epidural anesthesia and cardiovascular responses to static exercise in man. *J. Physiol. (Lond.)* 417: 13–24, 1989.
340. Miyamura, J., T. Yamishina, and Y. Honda. Ventilatory response to CO_2 rebreathing at rest and during exercise in untrained subjects and athletes. *Jpn. J. Physiol.* 26: 245–254, 1976.
341. Moore, R. M., R. E. Moore, and A. O. Singleton, Jr. Experiments on the chemical stimulation of pain-endings associated with small blood-vessels. *Am. J. Physiol.* 107: 594–602, 1934.
342. Morikawn, T., Y. Ono, K. Sasaki, Y. Sakokibara, Y. Tonaka, R. Maruzama, Y. Nishibayashi, and Y. Honda. Afferent and cardiodynamic drives in the early phase of exercise hyperpnea in humans. *J. Appl. Physiol.* 67: 2006–2013, 1989.
343. Morrison, S. F., and D. J. Reis. Reticulospinal vasomotor neurons in the RVL mediate the somatosympathetic reflex. *Am. J. Physiol.* 256 (*Regulatory Integrative Comp. Physiol.* 25): R1084–R1097, 1989.
344. Murase, K., and M. Randic. Actions of substance P on rat spinal dorsal horn neurones. *J. Physiol. (Lond.)* 346: 203–217, 1984.
345. Murphy, K., R. P. Stidwell, B. A. Cross, K. D. Leaver, E. Anastassiades, M. Phillips, A. Guz, and S. J. G. Semple. Is hypercapnia necessary for the ventilatory response to exercise in man. *Clin. Sci.* 73: 617–625, 1987.
346. Mustafa, M. E. K. Y., and M. J. Purves. The effect of CO_2 upon discharge from slowly adapting receptors in the lungs of rabbits. *Respir. Physiol.* 16: 197–212, 1972.
347. Nattie, E. E. Ventilation during acute HCL infusion in intact and chemodenervated conscious rabbits. *Respir. Physiol.* 54: 97–107, 1983.
348. Nattie, E. E., and S. M. Tenney. The ventilatory response to resistance unloading during muscular exercise. *Respir. Physiol.* 10: 249–262, 1970.
349. Nery, L. E., K. Wasserman, J. D. Andrews, D. J. Huntsman, J. E. Hansen, and B. J. Whipp. Ventilatory and gas exchange kinetics during exercise in chronic airway obstruction. *J. Appl. Physiol.* 53: 1594–1602, 1982.
350. Nielson, M., and E. Asmussen. Humoral and nervous control of breathing in exercise. In: *The Regulation of Human Respiration*, edited by D. J. C. Cunningham and B. B. Lloyd. Philadelphia, PA: F. A. Davis Company, 1963, p. 504–513.
351. Nòbrega, A. C. L., and C. G. S. Araùjo. Heart rate transient at the onset of active and passive dynamic exercise. *Med. Sci. Sports Exerc.* 25: 37–41, 1993.
352. Nosaka, S., N. Nakase, and K. Murata. Somatosensory and hypothalamic inhibitions of baroreflex vagal bradycardia in rats. *Eur. J. Pharmacol.* 413: 656–666, 1989.
353. Nosaka, S., K. Yasunaga, and M. Kawano. Vagus cardioinhibitory fibers in rats. *Pflugers Arch.* 379: 281–285, 1979.
354. Nosaka, S., K. Yasunaga, and S. Tamai. Vagal cardiac preganglionic neurons: distribution, cell types, and reflex discharges. *Am. J. Physiol.* 243 (*Regulatory Integrative Comp. Physiol.* 12): R92–R98, 1982.
355. Nye, P. C. G. Identification of peripheral chemoreceptor stimuli. *Med. Sci. Sports Exerc.* 26: 311–318, 1994.
356. O'Brien, C., C. J. Woolf, M. Fitzgerald, R. M. Lindsay, and C. Molander. Differences in the chemical expression of rat primary afferent neurons which innervate skin, muscle or joint. *Neuroscience* 32: 493–502, 1989.
357. Ohki, M., M. Hasegawa, N. Kurita, and I. Wantanbe. Effects of exercise on nasal resistance and nasal blood flow. *Acta Otolaryngol.* 104: 328–333, 1987.
358. Ohtake, P. J., and D. B. Jennings. Ventilation is stimulated by small reduction in arterial pressure in the awake dog. *J. Appl. Physiol.* 73: 1549–1557, 1992.
359. Oldenburg, F. A., D. O. McCormack, J. L. C. Morse, and N. L. Jones. A comparison of exercise responses in stair-climbing and cycling. *J. Appl. Physiol.* 46: 510–516, 1979.
360. O'Leary, D. S. Autonomic mechanisms of muscle metaboreflex control of heart rate. *J. Appl. Physiol.* 74: 1748–1754, 1993.
361. Orani, G. P., and M. Decandia. Group I afferent fibers: effects on cardiorespiratory system. *J. Appl. Physiol.* 68: 932–937, 1990.
362. Oren, A., B. J. Whipp, and K. Wasserman. Effect of acid-base status on the kinetics of the ventilatory response to moderate exercise. *J. Appl. Physiol.* 52: 1013–1017, 1982.
363. Orr, J. A., M. R. Fedde, H. Shams, H. Roskenbleck, and P. Scheid. Absence of CO_2 sensitive venous chemoreceptors in the cat. *Respir. Physiol.* 73: 211–224, 1988.
364. Otis, A. B., W. O. Fenn, and H. Rahn. Mechanics of breathing in man. *J. Appl. Physiol.* 2: 592–607, 1950.
365. Overton, J. M., and R. W. Stremel. Hindlimb muscle contraction elicits depressor responses in anesthetized rats. *Physiologist* 35: 238, 1992.
366. Padrid, P. A., J. R. Haselton, and M. P. Kaufman. Ischemia potentiates the reflex bronchodilation evoked by static muscular contraction in dogs. *Respir. Physiol.* 81: 51–62, 1990.
367. Padrid, P. A., J. R. Haselton, and M. P. Kaufman. Role of caudal ventrolateral medulla in reflex and central control of airway caliber. *J. Appl. Physiol.* 71: 2274–2282, 1991.
368. Paintal, A. S. Functional analysis of group III afferent fibres of mammalian muscles. *J. Physiol. (Lond.)* 152: 250–270, 1960.
369. Pan, H.-L., C. L. Stebbins, and J. C. Longhurst. Bradykinin contributes to the exercise pressor reflex: mechanism of action. *J. Appl. Physiol.* 75: 2061–2068, 1993.
370. Pan, L. G., H. V. Forster, G. E. Bisgard, S. M. Dorsey, and M. A. Busch. Cardiodynamic variables and ventilation during treadmill exercise in ponies. *J. Appl. Physiol.* 57: 753–759, 1984.
371. Pan, L. G., H. V. Forster, G. E. Bisgard, R. P. Kaminski, S. M. Dorsey, and M. A. Busch. Hyperventilation in ponies at the onset of and during steady-state exercise. *J. Appl. Physiol.* 54: 1394–1402, 1983.
372. Pan, L. G., H. V. Forster, G. E. Bisgard, T. F. Lowry, and C. L. Murphy. Role of carotid chemoreceptors and pulmonary vagal afferents during helium oxygen breathing in ponies. *J. Appl. Physiol.* 62: 1020–1027, 1987.
373. Pan, L. G., H. V. Forster, G. E. Bisgard, C. L. Murphy, and T. F. Lowry. Independence of exercise hyperpnea and acidosis during high intensity exercise in ponies. *J. Appl. Physiol.* 60: 1016–1024, 1986.
374. Pan, L. G., H. V. Forster, A. G. Brice, T. F. Lowry, C. L. Murphy, and R. D. Wurster. Effect of multiple denervations on the exercise hyperpnea in awake ponies. *J. Appl. Physiol.* 79: 302–311, 1995.
375. Pan, L. G., H. V. Forster, R. D. Wurster, C. L. Murphy, A. G. Brice, and T. F. Lowry. Effect of partial spinal cord ablation on exercise hyperpnea in ponies. *J. Appl. Physiol.* 69: 1821–1827, 1990.
376. Paterson, D. J. Potassium and ventilation in exercise. *J. Appl. Physiol.* 72: 811–820, 1992.

377. Paterson, D. J., J. S. Friedland, D. O. Oliver, and P. A. Robbins. The ventilatory response to lowering potassium with dextrose and insulin in subjects with hyperkalemia. *Respir. Physiol.* 76: 393–398, 1989.
378. Perez-Gonzalez, J. F. Factors determining the blood pressure responses to isometric exercise. *Circ. Res.* 48: I-76–I-86, 1981.
379. Pernoll, M. L., J. Metcalfe, P. A. Kovach, R. Wachtel, and M. Dunham. Ventilation during rest and exercise in pregnancy and postpartum. *Respir. Physiol.* 25: 295–310, 1975.
380. Phillipson, E. A., G. Bowes, E. R. Townsend, J. Duffin, and J. D. Cooper. Role of metabolic CO_2 production in ventilatory response to steady-state exercise. *J. Clin. Invest.* 68: 768–774, 1981.
381. Phillipson, E. A., J. Duffin, and J. D. Cooper. Critical dependence of respiratory rhythmicity on metabolic CO_2 load. *J. Appl. Physiol.* 50: 45–54, 1981.
382. Phillipson, E. A., R. F. Hickey, C. R. Bainton, and J. A. Nadel. Effect of vagal blockade on regulation of breathing in conscious dogs. *J. Appl. Physiol.* 29: 475–479, 1970.
383. Pickar, J. G., J. M. Hill, and M. P. Kaufman. Stimulation of vagal afferents inhibits locomotion in mesencephalic cats. *J. Appl. Physiol.* 74: 103–110, 1993.
384. Pickar, J. G., J. M. Hill, and M. P. Kaufman. Dynamic exercise stimulates group III muscle afferents. *J. Neurophysiol.* 71: 753–760, 1994.
385. Pitetti, K. H., G. A. Iwamoto, J. H. Mitchell, and G. A. Ordway. Stimulating somatic afferent fibers alters coronary arterial resistance. *Am. J. Physiol.* 256 (*Regulatory Integrative Comp. Physiol.* 25): R1331–R1339, 1989.
386. Pomeranz, B., P. D. Wall, and W. V. Weber. Cord cells responding to fine myelinated afferents from viscera, muscle, and skin. *J. Physiol. (Lond.)* 199: 511–532, 1968.
387. Ponte, J., and M. J. Purves. Carbon dioxide and venous return and their interaction as stimuli to ventilation in the cat. *J. Physiol. (Lond.)* 274: 445–475, 1978.
388. Poon, C.-S. Ventilatory control in hypercapnia and exercise: optimization hypothesis. *J. Appl. Physiol.* 62: 2447–2459, 1987.
389. Pryor, S. L., S. F. Lewis, R. G. Haller, L. A. Bertocci, and R. G. Victor. Impairment of sympathetic activation during static exercise in patients with muscle phosphorylase deficiency (McArdle's disease). *J. Clin. Invest.* 85: 1444–1449, 1990.
390. Quest, J. A., and G. L. Gebber. Modulation of baroreceptor reflex by somatic afferent nerve stimulation. *Am. J. Physiol. (Lond.)* 222: 1251–1259, 1972.
391. Radhakrishnan, V., and J. L. Henry. Excitatory amino acid receptor mediation of sensory inputs to functionally identified dorsal horn neurons in cat spinal cord. *Neuroscience* 55: 531–544, 1993.
392. Randic, M., and V. Miletic. Effects of substance P in cat spinal dorsal horn neurones activated by noxious stimuli. *Brain Res.* 128: 164–169, 1977.
393. Richard, C. A., T. G. Waldrop, R. M. Bauer, J. H. Mitchell, and R. W. Stremel. The nucleus reticularis gigantocellularis modulates the cardiopulmonary responses to central and peripheral drives related to exercise. *Brain Res.* 482: 49–56, 1989.
394. Risling, M., C.-J. Dalsgaard, A. Cukierman, and A. C. Cuello. Electron microscopic and immunohistochemical evidence that unmyelinated ventral root axons make u-turns or enter the spinal pia mater. *J. Comp. Neurol.* 225: 53–63, 1984.
395. Roberts, A. M., M. P. Kaufman, D. G. Baker, J. K. Brown, H. M. Coleridge, and J. C. G. Coleridge. Reflex tracheal contraction induced by stimulation of bronchial C-fibers in dogs. *J. Appl. Physiol.* 51: 485–493, 1981.
396. Roberts, P. J. The release of amino acids with proposed neurotransmitter function from the cuneate and gracile nuclei of the rat in vivo. *Brain Res.* 67: 419–428, 1974.
397. Ross, C. A., D. A. Ruggiero, D. H. Park, and D. J. Reis. Rostral ventrolateral medulla: selective projection in the thoracic autonomic cell column from the region containing C1 autonomic neurons. *J. Comp. Neurol.* 228: 168–185, 1984.
398. Rotto, D. M., J. M. Hill, H. D. Schultz, and M. P. Kaufman. Cyclooxygenase blockade attenuates the responses of group IV muscle afferents to static contraction. *Am. J. Physiol.* 259 (*Heart Circ. Physiol.* 28): H745–H750, 1990.
399. Rotto, D. M., and M. P. Kaufman. Effects of metabolic products of muscular contraction on the discharge of group III and IV afferents. *J. Appl. Physiol.* 64: 2306–2313, 1988.
400. Rotto, D. M., H. D. Schultz, J. C. Longhurst, and M. P. Kaufman. Sensitization of group III muscle afferents to static contraction by products of arachidonic acid metabolism. *J. Appl. Physiol.* 68: 861–867, 1990.
401. Rotto, D. M., C. L. Stebbins, and M. P. Kaufman. Reflex cardiovascular and ventilatory responses to increasing H^+ activity in cat hindlimb muscle. *J. Appl. Physiol.* 67: 256–263, 1989.
402. Rowell, L. B., L. Hermansen, and J. R. Blackmon. Human cardiovascular and respiratory responses to graded muscle ischemia. *J. Appl. Physiol.* 41: 693–701, 1976.
403. Rowell, L. B., M. V. Savage, J. Chambers, and J. R. Blackmon. Cardiovascular responses to graded reductions in leg perfusion in exercising humans. *Am. J. Physiol.* 261 (*Heart Circ. Physiol.* 30): H1545–H1553, 1991.
404. Rowell, L. B., and D. D. Sheriff. Are muscle "chemoreflexes" functionally important? *News Physiol. Sci.* 3: 240–253, 1988.
405. Ruggiero, D. A., P. Gatti, R. A. Gillis, W. P. Norman, M. Anwar, D. J. Reis, and D. H. Park. Adrenaline synthesizing neurons in the medulla of the cat. *J. Comp. Neurol.* 252: 532–542, 1986.
406. Russell, J. A. Noradrenergic inhibitory innervation of canine airways. *J. Appl. Physiol.* 48: 16–22, 1980.
407. Rybicki, K. J., and M. P. Kaufman. Stimulation of group III and IV muscle afferents reflexly decreases total pulmonary resistance in dogs. *Respir. Physiol.* 59: 185–195, 1985.
408. Rybicki, K. J., M. P. Kaufman, J. L. Kenyon, and J. H. Mitchell. Arterial pressure responses to increasing interstitial potassium in hindlimb muscle of dogs. *Am. J. Physiol.* 247 (*Regulatory Integrative Comp. Physiol.* 16): R717–R721, 1984.
409. Rybicki, K. J., T. G. Waldrop, and M. P. Kaufman. Increasing gracilis interstitial potassium concentrations stimulates group III and IV afferents. *J. Appl. Physiol.* 58: 936–941, 1985.
410. Sacks, R. D., and R. R. Roy. Architecture of the hindlimb muscles of cats: functional significance. *J. Morphol.* 173: 185–195, 1982.
411. Saito, M., M. Naito, and T. Mano. Different responses in skin and muscle sympathetic nerve activity to static muscle contraction. *J. Appl. Physiol.* 69: 2085–2090, 1990.
412. Sakurai, M., W. Hiba, T. Chonan, Y. Kikuchi, and T. Takishima. Responses of upper airway muscles to gastrocnemius muscle contraction in dogs. *Respir. Physiol.* 84: 311–321, 1991.

413. Sant'Ambrogio, G., and F. B. Sant'Ambrogio. Reflexes from the airway, lung, chest, wall, and limbs. In: *The Lung: Scientific Foundation*, edited by R. G. Crystal, J. B. West, et al. New York: Raven Press, 1991, p. 1383–1395.
414. Sato, A., Y. Sato, and R. F. Schmidt. Heart rate changes reflecting modifications of efferent cardiac sympathetic outflow by cutaneous and muscle afferent volleys. *J. Auton. Nerv. Syst.* 4: 231–241, 1981.
415. Sato, A., Y. Sato, and R. F. Schmidt. Changes in heart rate and blood pressure upon injection of algesic agents into skeletal muscle. *Pflugers Arch.* 393: 31–36, 1982.
416. Sato, A., and R. F. Schmidt. Spinal and supraspinal components of the reflex discharges into lumbar and thoracic white rami. *J. Physiol. (Lond.)* 212: 839–850, 1971.
417. Saunders, K. B. Oscillations of arterial CO_2 tension in a respiratory model: some implications for the control of breathing in exercise. *J. Theor. Biol.* 84: 163–179, 1980.
418. Savin, W. M., W. L. Haskell, J. S. Schroeder, and E. B. Stinson. Cardio-respiratory responses of cardiac transplant patients to graded, symptom-limited exercise. *Circulation* 45: 1183–1194, 1980.
419. Schaefer, S. L., and G. S. Mitchell. Ventilatory control during exercise with peripheral chemoreceptor stimulation: hypoxia versus domperidome. *J. Appl. Physiol.* 67: 2438–2446, 1989.
420. Scherrer, U., S. L. Pryor, L. A. Bertocci, and R. G. Victor. Arterial baroreflex buffering of sympathetic activation during exercise-induced elevations in arterial pressure. *J. Clin. Invest.* 86: 1855–1861, 1990.
421. Schmidt, R. F., and E. Weller. Reflex activity in the cervical and lumbar sympathetic trunk induced by unmyelinated somatic afferents. *Brain Res.* 24: 207–218, 1970.
422. Schneider, S. P., and E. R. Perl. Selective excitation of neurons in the mammalian spinal dorsal horn by asparate and glutamate in vitro: correlation with location and excitatory input. *Brain Res.* 360: 339–343, 1985.
423. Schneider, S. P., and E. R. Perl. Comparison of primary afferent and glutamate excitation of neurons in the mammalian spinal dorsal horn. *J. Neurosci.* 8: 2062–2073, 1988.
424. Schoener, E. P., and H. M. Frankel. Effect of hyperthermia and Pa_{CO_2} on the slowly adapting pulmonary stretch receptor. *Am. J. Physiol.* 222: 62–72, 1972.
425. Schwarcz, R., T. Hökfelt, K. Fuxe, G. Jonsson, M. Goldstein, and L. Terenius. Ibotenic acid induced neuronal degeneration: a morphological and neurochemical study. *Exp. Brain Res.* 37: 199–216, 1979.
426. Seals, D. R. Sympathetic neural discharge and vascular resistance during exercise in humans. *J. Appl. Physiol.* 66: 2472–2478, 1989.
427. Senapati, J. M. Effect of stimulation of muscle afferents on ventilation of dogs. *J. Appl. Physiol.* 21: 242–246, 1966.
428. Sharratt, M. T., K. G. Henke, D. F. Pegelow, E. Aaron, and J. Dempsey. Exercise-induced changes in functional residual capacity. *Respir. Physiol.* 70: 313–326, 1988.
429. Sheldon, J. I., and J. F. Green. Evidence for pulmonary CO_2 chemosensitivity: effects on ventilation. *J. Appl. Physiol.* 52: 1192–1197, 1982.
430. Sheriff, D. D., D. S. O'Leary, A. M. Scher, and L. B. Rowell. Baroreflex attenuates pressor response to graded muscle ischemia in exercising dogs. *Am. J. Physiol.* 258 (*Heart Circ. Physiol.* 27): H305–H310, 1990.
431. Sheriff, D. D., C. R. Wyss, L. B. Rowell, and A. M. Scher. Does inadequate oxygen delivery trigger pressor response to muscle hypoperfusion during exercise? *Am. J. Physiol.* 253 (*Heart Circ. Physiol.* 22): H1199–H1207, 1987.
432. Shin, H. K., J. Kim, S. C. Nam, K. S. Paik, and J. M. Chung. Spinal entry route for ventral root afferent fibers in the cat. *Exp. Neurol.* 94: 714–725, 1986.
433. Silverman, L., G. Lee, T. Plotkin, L. A. Sawyers, and A. R. Yancy. Airflow measurements on human subjects with and without respiratory resistance at several work rates. *Arch. Indust. Hygiene* 3: 461–478, 1951.
434. Simone, D. A., P. Marchettini, G. Caputi, and J. L. Ochoa. Identification of muscle afferents subserving sensation of deep pain in humans. *J. Neurophysiol.* 72: 883–889, 1994.
435. Sinoway, L., S. Prophet, I. Gorman, T. J. Mosher, J. Shenberger, M. Dolecki, R. Briggs, and R. Zelis. Muscle acidosis during static exercise is associated with calf vasoconstriction. *J. Appl. Physiol.* 66: 429–436, 1989.
436. Sinoway, L. I., J. M. Hill, J. G. Pickar, and M. P. Kaufman. Effects of contraction and lactic acid on the discharge of group III muscle afferents in cats. *J. Neurophysiol.* 69: 1053–1059, 1993.
437. Sinoway, L. I., R. F. Rea, T. J. Mosher, M. B. Smith, and A. L. Mark. Hydrogen ion concentration is not the sole determinant of muscle metaboreceptor responses in humans. *J. Clin. Invest.* 89: 1875–1884, 1992.
438. Sinoway, L. I., M. B. Smith, B. Enders, U. Leuenberger, T. Dzwonczyk, K. Gray, S. Whisier, and R. L. Moore. Role of diprotonated phosphate in evoking muscle reflex responses in cats and humans. *Am. J. Physiol.* 267 (*Heart Circ. Physiol.* 36): H770–H778, 1994.
439. Sinoway, L. I., K. J. Wroblewski, S. A. Prophet, S. M. Ettinger, K. S. Gray, S. K. Whisler, G. Miller, and R. L. Moore. Glycogen depletion-induced lactate reductions attenuate reflex responses in exercising humans. *Am. J. Physiol.* 263 (*Heart Circ. Physiol.* 32): H1499–H1505, 1992.
440. Skoglund, C. R. Vasomotor reflexes from muscle. *Acta Physiol. Scand.* 50: 311–327, 1960.
441. Smith, C. A., K. W. Saupe, K. S. Henderson, and J. A. Dempsey. Ventilatory effects of specific carotid body hypocapnia in dogs during wakefulness and sleep. *J. Appl. Physiol.* 79: 689–699, 1995.
442. Smullin, D. H., S. R. Skilling, and A. A. Larson. Interactions between substance P, calcitonin gene-related peptide, taurine and excitatory amino acids in the spinal cord. *Pain* 42: 93–101, 1990.
443. Solomon, I. C., A. M. Motekaitis, M. K. C. Wong, and M. P. Kaufman. NMDA receptors in the caudal ventrolateral medulla mediate the reflex airway dilation arising from the hindlimb. *J. Appl. Physiol.* 77: 1697–1704, 1994.
444. Somjen, G. G. The missing error signal—regulation beyond negative feedback. *News Physiol. Sci.* 7: 184–185, 1992.
445. Stebbins, C. L., B. Brown, D. Levin, and J. C. Longhurst. Reflex effect of skeletal muscle mechanoreceptor stimulation on the cardiovascular system. *J. Appl. Physiol.* 65: 1539–1547, 1988.
446. Stebbins, C. L., O. A. Carretero, T. Mindroiu, and J. C. Longhurst. Bradykinin release from contracting skeletal muscle of the cat. *J. Appl. Physiol.* 69: 1225–1230, 1990.
447. Stebbins, C. L., and J. C. Longhurst. Bradykinin-induced chemoreflexes from skeletal muscle: implications for the exercise reflex. *J. Appl. Physiol.* 59: 56–63, 1985.
448. Stebbins, C. L., and J. C. Longhurst. Potentiation of the exercise pressor reflex by muscle ischemia. *J. Appl. Physiol.* 66: 1046–1053, 1989.
449. Stebbins, C. L., A. Ortiz Acevedo, and J. M. Hill. Spinal vasopressin modulates the reflex cardiovascular response to static contraction. *J. Appl. Physiol.* 72: 731–738, 1992.

450. Steinbrook, R. A., S. Javaheri, R. A. Gabel, J. C. Donovan, D. E. Leith, and V. Fencl. Regulation of chemodenervated goats in acute metabolic acidosis. *Respir. Physiol.* 56: 51–60, 1984.
451. Stornetta, R., S. F. Morrison, D. A. Ruggiero, and D. J. Reis. Neurons of the rostral ventrolateral medulla mediate somatic pressor reflex. *Am. J. Physiol.* 256 (*Regulatory Integrative Comp. Physiol.* 25): R448–R462, 1989.
452. Strange, S., N. H. Secher, J. A. Pawelczyk, J. Karpakka, N. J. Christensen, J. H. Mitchell, and B. Saltin. Neural control of cardiovascular responses and of ventilation during dynamic exercise in man. *J. Physiol. (Lond.)* 470: 693–704, 1993.
453. Streatfeild, K. A., N. S. Davidson, and D. I. McCloskey. Muscular reflex and baroreflex influences on heart rate during isometric contractions. *Cardiovasc. Res.* 11: 87–93, 1977.
454. Stremel, R. W., B. J. Whipp, R. Casaburi, D. J. Huntsman, and K. Wasserman. Hypopnea consequent to reduced pulmonary blood flow in the dog. *J. Appl. Physiol.* 46: 1171–1177, 1979.
455. Strohl, K. P., M. P. Norcia, A. D. Wolin, M. A. Haxhiu, E. Vanlunteren, and E. C. Deal, Jr. Nasal and tracheal responses to chemical and somatic afferent stimulation in anesthetized cats. *J. Appl. Physiol.* 65: 870–877, 1988.
456. Swett, J., and C. J. Woolf. The somatotopic organization of primary afferent terminals in the superficial laminae of the dorsal horn of the rat spinal cord. *J. Comp. Neurol.* 231: 66–77, 1985.
457. Takahashi, E., K. Tejima, and K.-I. Yamakoshi. Entrainment of respiratory rhythm to respiratory oscillations of arterial P_{CO_2} in vagotomized dogs. *J. Appl. Physiol.* 73: 1052–1057, 1992.
458. Tallarida, G., F. Baldoni, G. Peruzzi, F. Brindisi, G. Raimondi, and M. Sangiorgi. Cardiovascular and respiratory chemoreflexes from the hindlimb sensory receptors evoked by intra-arterial injection of bradykinin and other chemical agents in the rabbit. *J. Pharmacol. Exp. Ther.* 208: 319–329, 1979.
459. Tallarida, G., F. Baldoni, G. Peruzzi, G. Raimondi, P. Di Nardo, M. Massaro, G. Visigalli, G. Franconi, and M. Sangiorgi. Cardiorespiratory reflexes from muscles during dynamic and static exercise in the dog. *J. Appl. Physiol.* 58: 844–852, 1985.
460. Tallarida, G., F. Baldoni, G. Peruzzi, G. Raimondi, M. Massaro, A. Abate, and M. Sangiorgi. Different patterns of respiratory responses to chemical stimulation of muscle receptors in the rabbit. *J. Pharmacol. Exp. Ther.* 223: 552–559, 1982.
461. Tallarida, G., F. Baldoni, G. Peruzzi, G. Raimondi, M. Massaro, A. Abate, and M. Sangiorgi. Different patterns of respiratory reflexes originating in exercising muscle. *J. Appl. Physiol.* 55: 84–91, 1983.
462. Tallarida, G., F. Baldoni, G. Peruzzi, G. Raimondi, M. Massaro, and M. Sangiorgi. Cardiovascular and respiratory reflexes from muscles during dynamic and static exercise. *J. Appl. Physiol.* 50: 784–791, 1981.
463. Teppema, L. J. P. W., J. A. Barts, and J. A. M. Evers. The effect of the phase relationship between the arterial blood gas oscillations and central neural respiratory activity on phrenic motoneuronone output in cats. *Respir. Physiol.* 61: 301–316, 1985.
464. Teppema, L. J. P., W. J. A. Barts, H. T. Folgering, and J. A. M. Evers. Effects of respiratory and (isocapnic) metabolic arterial acid-base disturbances on medullary extracellular fluid pH and ventilation in cats. *Respir. Physiol.* 53: 379–395, 1983.
465. Thames, M. D., and F. M. Abboud. Interaction of somatic and cardiopulmonary receptors in control of renal circulation. *Am. J. Physiol.* 237 (*Heart Circ. Physiol.* 6): H560–H565, 1979.
466. Thimm, F., and K. Baum. Response of chemosensitive nerve fibers of group III and IV to metabolic changes in rat muscles. *Pflugers Arch.* 410: 143–152, 1987.
467. Thimm, F., M. Carvalho, M. Babka, and E. M. Zu Verl. Reflex increases in heart rate induced by perfusing the hind leg of the rat with solutions containing lactic acid. *Pflugers Arch.* 400: 286–293, 1984.
468. Tibes, U. Reflex inputs to the cardiovascular and respiratory centers from dynamically working canine muscles: Some evidence for involvement of group III or IV nerve fibers. *Circ. Res.* 41: 332–341, 1977.
469. Uchida, Y. Tachypnea after stimulation of afferent cardiac sympathetic nerve fibers. *Am. J. Physiol.* 230: 1003–1007, 1976.
470. Victor, R. G., L. A. Bertocci, S. L. Pryor, and R. L. Nunnally. Sympathetic nerve discharge is coupled to muscle cell pH during exercise in humans. *J. Clin. Invest.* 82: 1301–1305, 1988.
471. Victor, R. G., S. L. Pryor, N. H. Secher, and J. H. Mitchell. Effects of partial neuromuscular blockade on sympathetic nerve responses to static exercise in humans. *Circ. Res.* 65: 468–476, 1989.
472. Victor, R. G., D. M. Rotto, S. L. Pryor, and M. P. Kaufman. Stimulation of renal sympathetic activity by static contraction: evidence for mechanoreceptor-induced reflexes from skeletal muscle. *Circ. Res.* 64: 592–599, 1989.
473. Victor, R. G., and D. R. Seals. Reflex stimulation of sympathetic outflow during rhythmic exercise in humans. *Am. J. Physiol.* 257 (*Heart Circ. Physiol.* 26): H2017–H2024, 1989.
474. Victor, R. G., D. R. Seals, and A. L. Mark. Differential control of heart rate and sympathetic nerve activity during dynamic exercise. *J. Clin. Invest.* 79: 508–516, 1987.
475. Vissing, J., L. B. Wilson, J. H. Mitchell, and R. G. Victor. Static muscle contraction reflexly increases adrenal sympathetic nerve activity in rats. *Am. J. Physiol.* 261 (*Regulatory Integrative Comp. Physiol.* 30): R1307–R1312, 1991.
476. Vissing, S. F., U. Scherrer, and R. G. Victor. Stimulation of skin sympathetic nerve discharge by central command. *Circ. Res.* 69: 228–238, 1991.
477. Von During, M., and K. H. Andres. Topography and ultrastructure of group III and IV nerve terminals of cat's gastrocnemius-soleus muscle. In: *The Primary Afferent Neuron: A Survey of Recent Morpho-functional Aspects*, edited by W. Zenker and W. L. Neuhuber. New York: Plenum Press, 1990, p. 35–41.
478. Waldrop, T. G., M. C. Henderson, G. A. Iwamoto, and J. H. Mitchell. Regional blood flow responses to stimulation of the subthalamic locomotor region. *Respir. Physiol.* 64: 93–102, 1986.
479. Waldrop, T. G., and J. H. Mitchell. Effects of barodenervation on cardiovascular response to static muscular contraction. *Am. J. Physiol.* 249 (*Heart Circ. Physiol.* 18): H710–H714, 1985.
480. Waldrop, T. G., D. C. Mullins, and M. C. Henderson. Effects of hypothalamic lesions on the cardiorespiratory responses to muscular contraction. *Respir. Physiol.* 66: 215–224, 1986.

481. Waldrop, T. G., K. J. Rybicki, and M. P. Kaufman. Chemical activation of group I and II muscle afferents has no cardiorespiratory effects. *J. Appl. Physiol.* 56: 1223–1228, 1984.
482. Waldrop, T. G., and R. W. Stremel. Muscular contraction stimulates posterior hypothalamic neurons. *Am. J. Physiol.* 256 (*Regulatory Integrative Comp. Physiol.* 25): R348–R356, 1989.
483. Walgenbach, S. C., and D. E. Donald. Inhibition by carotid baroreflex of exercise-induced increases in arterial pressure. *Circ. Res.* 52: 253–262, 1983.
484. Ward, S. A., and B. J. Whipp. Phase-coupling of arterial blood-gas oscillations and ventilatory dynamics during exercise in humans. *FASEB J.* 7: 3664, 1993.
485. Warner, M. M., and G. S. Mitchell. Ventilatory responses to hyperkalemia and exercise in normoxic and hypoxic goats. *Respir. Physiol.* 82: 239–250, 1990.
486. Warren, J. B., S. J. Jennings, and T. J. H. Clark. Effect of adrenergic and vagal blockade on the normal human airway response to exercise. *Clin. Sci.* 66: 79–85, 1984.
487. Wasserman, K., B. J. Whipp, R. Casaburi, M. Golden, and W. L. Beaver. Ventilatory control during exercise in man. *Bull. Eur. Physiopathol. Respir.* 15: 27–47, 1979.
488. Wasserman, K., B. J. Whipp, R. Casaburi, D. J. Huntsman, J. Castagna, and R. Lugliani. Regulation of arterial PCO_2 during intravenous CO_2 loading. *J. Appl. Physiol.* 38: 651–656, 1975.
489. Wasserman, K., B. J. Whipp, and J. Castagna. Cardiohydynamic hyperpnea: hyperpnea secondary to cardiac output increase. *J. Appl. Physiol.* 36: 457–464, 1974.
490. Wasserman, K., B. J. Whipp, S. N. Koyal, and M. G. Cleary. Effect of carotid body resection on ventilatory and acid-base control during exercise. *J. Appl. Physiol.* 39: 354–358, 1975.
491. Webb-Peploe, M. M., D. Brender, and J. T. Shepherd. Vascular responses to stimulation of receptors in muscle by capsaicin. *Am. J. Physiol.* 222: 189–195, 1972.
492. Weil, J. V., E. Byrne-Quinn, I. E. Sodal, J. S. Kline, R. E. McCullough, and G. F. Filley. Augmentation of chemosensitivity during mild exercise in normal man. *J. Appl. Physiol.* 33: 813–819, 1972.
493. Weissman, M. L., B. J. Whipp, D. J. Huntsman, and K. Wasserman. Role of neural afferents from working limbs in exercise hyperpnea. *J. Appl. Physiol.* 49: 239–248, 1980.
494. Wetzel, M. C., and D. G. Stuart. Ensemble characteristics of cat locomotion and its neural control. *Prog. Neurobiol.* 7: 1–98, 1976.
495. Wheatley, J. R., T. C. Amis, and L. A. Engel. Oro-nasal partitioning of ventilation during exercise in man. *J. Appl. Physiol.* 71: 546–551, 1991.
496. Whipp, B. J. Control of exercise hyperpnea. In: *Regulation of Breathing Part II*, edited by T. F. Hornbein. New York: Marcel Dekker, Inc., 1981, p. 1069–1140.
497. Widdicombe, J. B., and J. A. Nadel. Airway volume, airway resistance, and work and force of breathing: theory. *J. Appl. Physiol.* 18: 863–868, 1963.
498. Widdicombe, J. G. Action potentials in parasympathetic and sympathetic efferent fibres to trachea and lungs of dogs and cats. *J. Physiol. (Lond.)* 186: 56–88, 1966.
499. Widdicombe, J. G. Nervous receptors in the respiratory tract and lungs. In: *Regulation of Breathing, Lung Biology in Health and Disease*, edited by T. F. Hornbein. New York: Marcel Dekker, Inc., 1981, p. 429–473.
500. Wiesenfeld-Hallin, Z., T. Hökfelt, J. M. Lundberg, W. G. Forssmann, M. Reinecke, F. A. Tschopp, and J. A. Fischer. Immunoreactive calcitonin gene-related peptide and substance P coexist in sensory neurons to the spinal cord and interact in spinal behavioral responses of the rat. *Neurosci. Lett.* 52: 199–204, 1984.
501. Wildenthal, K., D. S. Mierzwiak, N. S. Skinner, Jr., and J. H. Mitchell. Potassium-induced cardiovascular and ventilatory reflexes from the dog hindlimb. *Am. J. Physiol.* 215: 542–548, 1968.
502. Willette, R. N., S. Punnen, A. J. Krieger, and H. N. Sapru. Interdependence of rostral and caudal ventrolateral medullary areas in the control of blood pressure. *Brain Res.* 231: 169–174, 1984.
503. Williams, C. A., J. R. Roberts, and D. B. Freels. Changes in blood pressure during isometric contractions to fatigue in the cat after brain stem lesions: effects of clonidine. *Cardiovasc. Res.* 24: 821–833, 1990.
504. Williamson, J. W., J. H. Mitchell, H. L. Olesen, P. B. Raven, and N. H. Secher. Reflex increase in blood pressure induced by leg compression in man. *J. Physiol. (Lond.)* 475: 351–357, 1994.
505. Williamson, J. W., P. B. Raven, B. H. Foresman, and B. J. Whipp. Evidence for an intramuscular ventilatory stimulus during dynamic exercise in man. *Respir. Physiol.* 94: 121–135, 1993.
506. Wilson, L. B., I. E. Fuchs, K. Matsukawa, J. H. Mitchell, and P. T. Wall. Substance P release in the spinal cord during the exercise pressor reflex in anaesthetized cats. *J. Physiol. (Lond.)* 460: 79–90, 1993.
507. Wilson, L. B., P. T. Wall, K. Matsukawa, and J. H. Mitchell. The effect of spinal microinjections of an antagonist to substance P or somatostatin on the exercise pressor reflex. *Circ. Res.* 70: 213–222, 1992.
508. Woolf, C. J., and P. D. Wall. Chronic peripheral nerve section diminishes the primary afferent A-fibre mediated inhibition of rat dorsal horn neurons. *Brain Res.* 242: 77–85, 1982.
509. Wyss, C. R., J. L. Ardell, A. M. Scher, and L. B. Rowell. Cardiovascular responses to graded reductions in hindlimb perfusion in exercising dogs. *Am. J. Physiol.* 245 (*Heart Circ. Physiol.* 14): H481–H486, 1983.
510. Yamamoto, I. H., and M. W. Edwards. Homeostasis of CO_2 during intravenous infusion of CO_2. *J. Appl. Physiol.* 15: 807–818, 1960.
511. Yamamoto, W. S. Looking at the regulation of ventilation as a signalling process. In: *Muscular Exercise and the Lung*, edited by J. A. Dempsey and C. E. Reed. Madison, WI: University of Wisconsin, 1977, p. 137–149.
512. Yamashiro, S. M., and F. S. Grodins. Optimal regulation of respiratory airflow. *J. Appl. Physiol.* 30: 597–602, 1971.
513. Yoshimura, M., and T. Jessell. Amino acid-mediated EPSPs at primary afferent synapses with substantia gelatinosa neurones in the rat spinal cord. *J. Physiol. (Lond.)* 430: 315–335, 1990.
514. Young, I. H., and A. J. Woolcock. Changes in arterial blood gas tension during unsteady-state exercise. *J. Appl. Physiol.* 44: 93–96, 1978.
515. Zechman, F., F. G. Hull, and W. E. Hull. Effects of graded resistance to tracheal air flow in man. *J. Appl. Physiol.* 10: 356–362, 1967.
516. Zhan, W.-Z., H. H. Ellenberger, and J. L. Feldman. Monoaminergic and GABAergic terminations in phrenic nucleus of rat identified by immunohistochemical labeling. *Neuroscience* 31: 105–113, 1989.
517. Zuntz, N., and J. Geppert. Ueber die natur der normalen atemreize und den ort ihrer wirkung. *Arch. Gen. Physiol.* 38: 337–338, 1886.

11. Airway, lung, and respiratory muscle function during exercise

JEROME A. DEMPSEY | *Department of Preventive Medicine, University of Wisconsin-Madison, Madison, Wisconsin*

LEWIS ADAMS | *Department of Medicine, Charing Cross and Westminster Medical School, London, United Kingdom*

DOROTHY M. AINSWORTH | *Department of Clinical Science, College of Veterinary Medicine, Cornell University, Ithaca, New York*

RALPH F. FREGOSI | *Department of Physiology, University of Arizona Health Sciences Center, Tucson, Arizona*

CHARLES G. GALLAGHER | *Division of Respiratory Medicine, Royal University Hospital, University of Saskatchewan, Saskatoon, Saskatchewan, Canada*

ABE GUZ | *Department of Medicine, Charing Cross and Westminster Medical School, London, United Kingdom*

BRUCE D. JOHNSON | *Division of Cardiovascular Diseases, Mayo Clinic and Foundation, Rochester, Minnesota*

SCOTT K. POWERS | *Departments of Exercise Science and Physiology, University of Florida, Gainesville, Florida*

CHAPTER CONTENTS

AS THE FIRST LINE OF DEFENSE for oxygen (O_2) transport and the major regulator of acid–base status via carbon dioxide (CO_2) elimination, alveolar ventilation must be provided in large quantities and in a mechanically efficient manner during exercise. These tasks are critically dependent upon both the structural capacities and mechanical properties of the airways, lung, and chest wall and the precision with which their functions are regulated by nervous control mechanisms. This chapter concentrates on these mechanical features of the exercise hyperpnea, thereby complimenting the central and peripheral reflex neural regulatory mechanisms of hyperpnea covered in detail in Chapters 1 and 2 (see also Chapters 9 and 10). We have updated and expanded previous treatments of traditional topics such as effects of exercise on static and dynamic mechanics (430) and mechanisms of exertional dyspnea. The neuromechanical regulation of breathing pattern during the production of the exercise hyperpnea has been given special emphasis. A new topic covered here is the regulation of the upper, extrathoracic airway during exercise, a problem that has received much attention in recent years driven by its clinical relevance to such problems as sleep apnea. A major emphasis of the chapter is on respiratory muscles during exercise—their recruitment, regulation, and energetics; their fatigability and trainability; and their neuromechanical linkage to locomotion. Over the past two decades much has been learned about the fundamental properties of respiratory muscles and their mechanical actions, but only recently have these principles and techniques been applied to questions covering the function and regulation of respiratory muscles during exercise.

There are several limitations to the scope of our treatment of the topic of exercise and respiratory mechanics. First, we do not attempt to detail the fundamentals of the dynamic and static mechanical properties of the respiratory system but rather refer the reader to the classic, elegant treatments of these topics by Mead, Fenn, Rahn, Otis, Agostini, and colleagues contained in the original *American Physiological Society Handbook of Respiration* (128). Second, space limitations have restricted our descriptions and discussions of regulatory mechanisms primarily to healthy young adult humans exercising at sea level (i.e., the "reference standard" for most human exercise studies). Certainly some departures from this practice were made when necessary, as with such topics as locomotor-respiratory coupling *or* measurements of respiratory muscle blood flow *or* physical training effects on respiratory muscle enzymatic capacity. For these purposes, extensive use is made of findings in exercising quadrupeds. Similarly, only limited reference is made to the effects of normal aging *or* environmental insults *or* specific disease states, especially in the treatment of mechanical limitations to ventilation and performance during exercise. Finally, we note the multiple contributors to this chapter and ask the reader to please overlook some unavoidable inconsistencies in style of presentation which we hope are outweighed by the comprehensiveness and depth of the coverage.

REGULATION OF THE UPPER AIRWAY DURING EXERCISE

Anatomy and Physiology of the Upper Airway

The upper airway is composed of the nose, mouth, pharynx, and larynx. The dimensions of these structures can be altered by tonic and respiratory-related activity of intrinsic and extrinsic striated muscles, and also by changes in the vascular capacitance of the mucosal lining, which is partly under central sympathetic control. The features of upper airway anatomy that are relevant to this discussion will be briefly reviewed. Several detailed reviews have been published recently (41, 300, 335, 336; see also Chapter 10).

The Nose. The nose is a major site of respiratory airflow resistance, accounting for 50% of the total pulmonary resistance at rest (129; see below). The principal site of nasal airway resistance occurs at the "nasal valve," which is considered to extend from the posterior end of the vestibule to the anterior end of the inferior turbinates (336). The nasal valve in humans has a cross-sectional area of about 30 mm^2, which is the smallest cross-sectional area in the entire upper airway. As pointed out by Proctor (336), the nasal valve narrows but never closes completely under physiological conditions. Beyond the nasal valve the cross-sectional area widens considerably, to about 260 mm^2 when both the left and right sides of the nose are considered, and then narrows again to 200 mm^2 at the nasopharynx.

Sympathetic vasoconstriction of the richly vascularized nasal mucosa can reduce mucosal thickness and widen the area of the nasal valve (91, 97, 115, 173, 294, 300, 342). The mucosal lining also plays an important role in warming and moistening the inspired air and in the filtering of foreign particles. These "air conditioning" functions are facilitated by the turbinates, which extend out of each lateral wall of the nasal cavity and increase the mucosal surface area.

The diameter of the nasal valve may also be altered to some extent by a group of striated muscles that cover the external nares, and are collectively referred to as the "alae nasi" muscles (Fig. 11.1*A*). The most relevant muscles regarding breathing are the dilator naris muscles, which flare and stabilize the external nares, and increase the diameter of the vestibule. Although the degree to which contraction of these muscles can prevent collapse or change the diameter of the nasal valve is not entirely clear, four observations suggest that activation of the nasal dilator muscles may be important during exercise. First, Strohl (385) has shown that voluntary activation of the nasal dilators can reduce airflow resistance by 30%. Second, when the nasal walls are mechanically "splinted" by inserting hollow, rigid tubes into the vestibule, peak nasal flow increased from 3.5 to 4.3 liters/s (319). Third, the diameter of the nasal valve can decrease and even collapse during forceful inspiration, when the downstream pressure exceeds about −12 cm H_2O (319, 335). Fourth, electromyographic (EMG) activity of the nasal dilator muscles rises as a function of the rate of nasal airflow during exercise (92, 93, 427; see below). Although the "nasal constrictor" muscles can narrow the nasal vestibule when activated, their role during spontaneous breathing in humans is uncertain. All muscles of the external nares are innervated by the facial motor nerve.

The Pharynx. The pharynx extends from the internal nares to the level of the cricoid cartilage of the larynx, and is lined with various skeletal muscles and mucous membrane (Fig. 11.1*a* and *c*). It is subdivided into three main parts: the nasopharynx, which extends from the posterior part of the nasal septum to the lower border of the soft palate; the oropharynx, which lies posterior to the oral cavity and extends from the soft palate to the hyoid bone; and the hypopharynx, which extends from the lower border of the soft palate to the laryngeal opening (Fig. 11.1*a*). Both the oropharynx and hypopharynx serve as conduits for the digestive system as well as the respiratory system, which further complicates the study of respiratory-related upper airway functions.

The diameter of the pharynx is altered principally by muscles that control the position of the soft palate, hyoid, and tongue. Positioning of the soft palate is accomplished by the activity of various palatal muscles (Fig. 11.1*b*). For example, the pharyngeal constrictors and the levator veli palatini muscle bring the soft palate in contact with the posterior pharyngeal wall at a level caudal to the internal

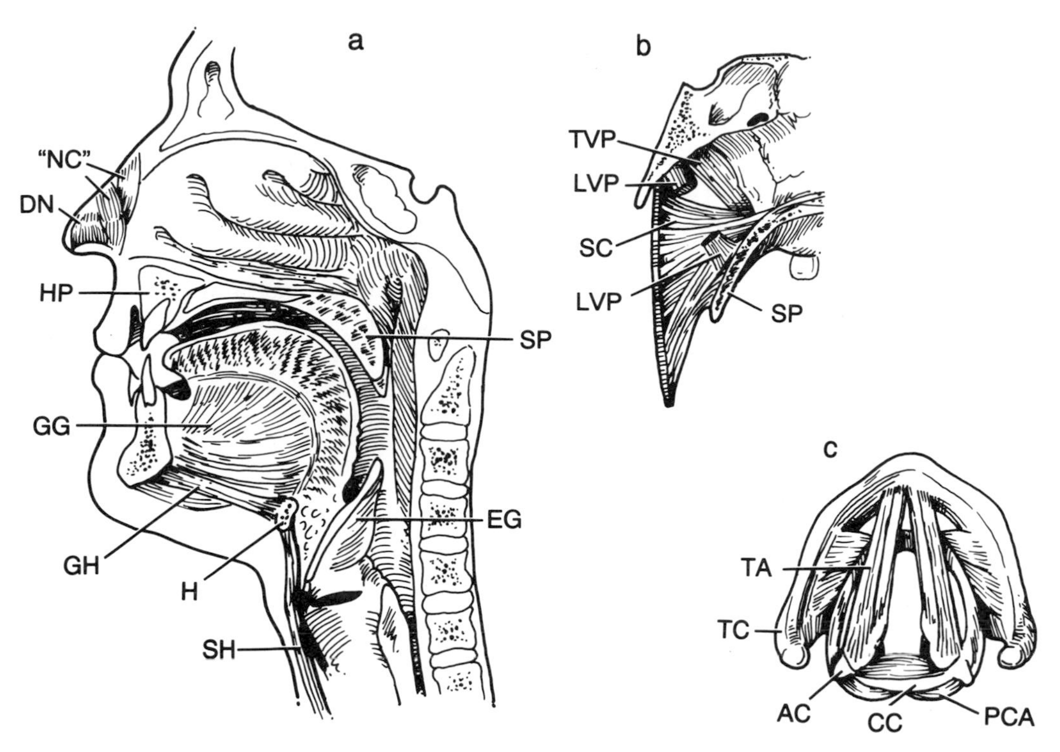

FIG. 11.1. *a*, Sagittal section of the human head and neck, showing the upper airways and some of the associated musculature. NC, nasal constrictor muscles; DN, dilator naris muscle; HP, hard palate; GG, genioglossus muscle; GH, geniohyoid muscle; H, hyoid bone; SH, sternohyoid muscle; SP, soft palate; EG, epiglottis. *b*, Section through the posterior pharynx showing some of the musculature acting on the soft palate and pharyngeal wall. TVP, tensor veli palatini muscle; LVP, levator veli palatini muscle; SC, superior pharyngeal constrictor muscles; SP, soft palate. *c*, Superior view of the larynx, showing the major laryngeal adductor and abductor muscles. TA, thyroarytenoid muscle; PCA, posterior cricoarytenoid muscle; TC, AC, and CC, thyroid, arytenoid and cricoid cartilages, respectively. See test for explanation of anatomy and muscular actions. [Parts *b* and *c* adapted from Bartlett (41) and Warwick and Williams (418), respectively].

nares, thereby stopping nasal airflow. The tensor veli palatini muscle also helps to maintain patency of the pharyngeal airway by stiffening the soft palate. This muscle is active in inspiration, and may be involved in preventing passive relapse of the soft palate onto the posterior pharyngeal wall, which could close the nasal airway (41). It is clear that the position of the soft palate plays a major role in dictating whether or not airflow is nasal, oral, or a combination of nasal and oral flows (i.e., oronasal). This statement is supported by the findings of Rodenstein and Stanescu (346), who used imaging techniques to show that the soft palate closed the oropharyngeal airway during nose breathing, closed the nasopharyngeal airway during mouth breathing, and was positioned midway between the tongue and posterior pharyngeal wall during oronasal breathing. However, in spite of the importance of the soft palate in determining oronasal flow partitioning, there have been no studies on palatal position or muscular activities during exercise.

Other pharyngeal muscles act to move the hyoid bone and tongue in a ventrocaudal direction, thereby widening the pharynx and the oral cavity (Fig. 11.1*a*). For example, the geniohyoid muscle draws the tongue and hyoid bone forward, the genioglossus muscle depresses the tongue and thrusts it forward, and the hyoglossus depresses the tongue and draws its lateral surfaces downward. The genioglossus muscle is thought to be the prime mover of the tongue, especially with regard to its respiratory-related functions (359). It is also important to emphasize that whenever the lips are separated the mouth becomes part of the oropharyngeal airway, so that tongue position has a large impact on "oral airway" diameter. When the lips are slightly parted, as at the onset of oronasal breathing, the oral pathway for flow is a narrow orifice between the tongue and soft palate [Fig. 11.1*a*; (336)]. However, this pathway can widen substantially by parting the lips widely and depressing and protruding the tongue. The pharyngeal and palatal muscles are innervated by motor nerves of the pharyngeal plexus. The geniohyoid muscle is innervated by a small branch of the first cervical spinal nerve that joins the hypoglossal nerve before entering the muscle. The genioglossus and hyoglossus muscles are innervated by the hypoglossal nerve.

The Larynx. The cartilaginous larynx connects the pharynx with the trachea, thereby separating the "upper" and "lower" airways. An important feature of laryngeal anatomy in terms of breathing is that the mucous membrane lining forms two pairs of bilateral folds: the ventricular folds (false vocal cords) and the vocal folds (true vocal folds). It is obvious that the valve-like control of the laryngeal opening has an enormous impact on pulmonary resistance; for example, complete apposition of the ventricular folds closes the glottis and resistance becomes infinite.

The extent of the apposition of the folds is controlled by the coordination of a number of extrinsic and intrinsic muscles. The most relevant external laryngeal muscle in regard to respiratory control is the sternohyoid muscle, which depresses the hyoid bone and dilates the pharynx (Fig. 11.1*a*); it is innervated by branches of the first three cervical nerves. There are three internal laryngeal muscles that have important respiratory-related functions. These are the posterior cricoarytenoid muscle (PCA), the thyroarytenoid (TA) muscle, and the cricothyroid (CT) muscle (Fig. 11.1*c*). The PCA is active during inspiration and serves to widen the opening between the vocal cords (i.e., the rima glottidis); the PCA is the only laryngeal muscle that functions in glottic opening. The thyroarytenoid muscle acts to keep the vocal folds in the midline, and therefore can decrease glottic aperture. Recent studies in decerebrate cats have demonstrated phasic, expiratory activity in the motor nerve that innervates this muscle (353, 354), and have shown that its activity is modulated by chemoreceptor stimulation (354). The cricothyroid muscle tenses and elongates the vocal cords, but its respiratory-related mechanical actions are complex and poorly understood. The cricothyroid is active primarily during inspiration, and its activity increases with hypercapnia and hypoxia (428). The PCA and TA muscles are innervated by separate branches of the recurrent laryngeal nerve, and the CT by the superior laryngeal nerve.

Contractile Properties and Endurance of Upper Airway Muscles

Limited data from both human and animal studies suggest that the upper airway muscles have relatively rapid contraction times and reasonably good endurance (356, 407–409). For example, contraction time of the geniohyoid muscle exceeds that of the diaphragm in the neonatal piglet, but the muscles have similar endurance performance, as assessed by a standard fatigue test (408). A recent study on human upper airway muscle contractile properties (141) shows that the nasal dilator muscles have a faster contraction time than human biceps brachii and diaphragm muscles, but the endurance performance of this upper airway muscle has not been examined. However, Scardella et al. (360) showed that the genioglossus muscle was more fatigable than the muscles of the inspiratory pump in healthy human subjects. This was established by measuring the rate of decline in force of the genioglossus muscle during repetitive, voluntary protrusions of the tongue performed at 80% of the maximal voluntary contraction force. This value was compared to the decline in inspiratory mouth pressure under similar conditions; both muscles were activated intensely before the test by having the subjects breathe against an inspiratory resistive load. The authors suggested that the faster rate of fatigue in the genioglossus muscle is consistent with its high proportion of fast-glycolytic motor units (181).

Changes in Upper Airway Flow Resistance During Exercise

Nasal Resistance. Nasal resistance is variable between subjects, is nonlinear, and also varies between nostrils in a cyclic manner (115). In addition, nasal air flow is partially turbulent even at rest, owing to the complex geometry of the nasal passages (65, 66, 336). The measurement of nasal airflow resistance requires estimation of the pressure drop across the nasopharynx, a technique known as "rhinomanometry." Although various methods have been used to assess nasopharyngeal pressure, the most common is posterior rhinomanometry, which involves the insertion of a catheter into the nasopharyngeal region via the nose or mouth. Nasopharyngeal pressure is measured together with nasal or oronasal airflow and resistance is calculated. Resistance is generally calculated at an arbitrarily chosen flow rate, but this is controversial because upper airway resistance is remarkably flow dependent (see Olson et al. (299) for an excellent review of methodology and of the problems encountered in measuring upper airway flow resistance). The flow dependence of nasal resistance is apparent in the upper part of Figure 11.2. The figure shows the pressure–flow relationship as measured by posterior rhinomanometry when a subject voluntarily hyperventilated before (*control*) and 1 min after incremental cycle ergometer exercise (*exercise*). This figure clearly shows that the curves are nonlinear, and that the reported value for "nasal airflow resistance" will vary widely de-

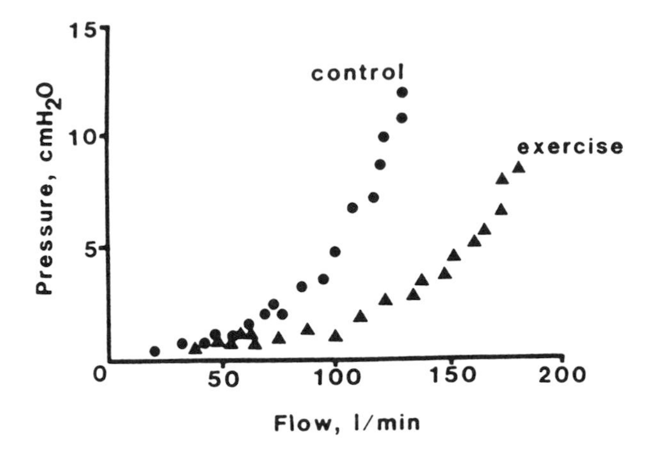

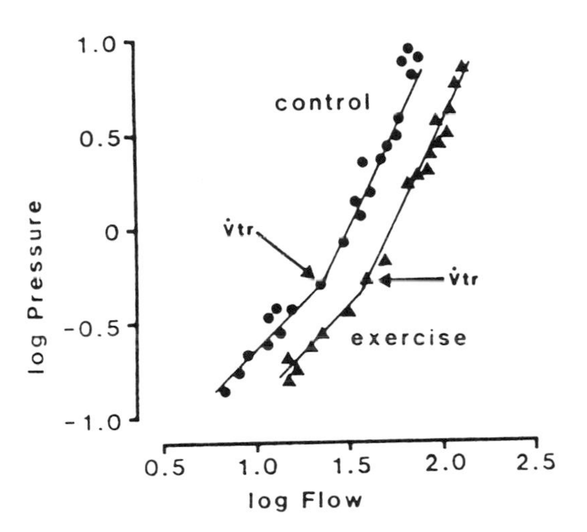

FIG. 11.2. *Top*, Nasal airway pressure–flow relationships obtained during voluntary hyperpnea in a healthy subject. The tests were performed before (control) and after (exercise) exhausting cycle ergometer exercise. Note that the curves are nonlinear, showing the marked flow dependence of upper airway resistance. Also note that prior exercise shifts the pressure–flow curve to the right, indicating that exercise hyperpnea decreases resistance. *Bottom*, Log transformation of the data shown in the top panel, demonstrating the technique for determining the flow rate at the transition (V̇tr) from laminar to turbulent flow. See text for detailed explanation of figure. [From Olson et al. (299).]

pending on the specific pressure–flow point that is arbitrarily chosen. The figure also shows that prior exercise shifts the curve well to the right at flow rates above 50 liters/min, indicating that exercise decreases nasal airflow resistance (see below).

It is clear that reported values for upper airway flow resistance have to be interpreted very carefully, and that useful comparisons cannot be made unless the flow rates are carefully matched and the pressure drop is measured in the same anatomical location. In an effort to understand better the flow conditions in the upper airway during hyperpnea, Richerson and Seebohm (342) and Olson and Strohl (300) have performed log-transformations of the pressure flow data, as shown in the bottom panel of Figure 11.2. It is clear that the log-transformed data are nicely described by the two lines drawn on the figure, which represent slopes of 1.0 and 2.0. Fitting the data to slopes of 1.0 and 2.0 is based on Rohrer's equation that describes the relationship between pressure (P) and flow (V) in nonuniform, rigid tubes:

$$P = k_1V + k_2V^2 \tag{1}$$

where k_1 and k_2 are constants. The equation can be log-transformed so that:

$$\log P = \log k_1 + \log V \tag{2}$$

which represents conditions of (predominately) laminar flow, and

$$\log P = \log k_2 + 2 \log V \tag{3}$$

which represents conditions of (predominately) turbulent flow. Given this analysis, the pressure and flow values that correspond to the intersection of the lines with slopes of 1.0 and 2.0 should represent the *approximate* values of pressure and flow that would be found at the transition from laminar to turbulent flow conditions. The flow rate at this transition point, which Olson et al. (299, 300) have termed "transitional flow" (V̇tr), can be reported and easily compared from one study to the next.

One caveat regarding nasal resistance and its changes with exercise is that almost all of the measurements have been made *following* exercise, when both flow and driving pressure are changing considerably. Nevertheless, the results obtained from many investigations show a consistent postexercise reduction in nasal airflow resistance (89, 91, 97, 294, 300, 342, 394). The mechanism responsible for this appears to be a sympathetically mediated vasoconstriction of the mucosal vasculature. This hypothesis is supported by observations showing that stellate ganglion blockade abolished the decrease in airway resistance that followed exercise (342), and that phenylephrine decreased airway resistance to values that were not different than those found following exercise (300). Further evidence in support of this idea is found in the observation that nasal blood flow and nasal resistance decline with a similar time course after exercise (294). Moreover, Forsyth and colleagues (135) measured changes in nasal resistance *during* exercise and found an intensity-dependent reduction in young healthy subjects that were allowed to select their breathing route spontaneously. Thus, most evidence suggests that nasal resistance falls during exercise.

Although it is generally assumed that this is due to mucosal vasoconstriction, a recent study shows that nasal resistance will rise if the mouth fails to open. Connel and Fregosi (92) measured nasal airway resistance in subjects that were not allowed to open their mouths, and found an intensity-dependent increase in airway resistance and a rise in end-tidal P_{CO_2}. Thus, with nose-only breathing during exercise, subjects hypoventilated when exercising at work rates that allowed maintenance of isocapnia during oronasal breathing. These data demonstrate that the decrease in resistance that results from mucosal vasoconstriction (e.g., 342) cannot overcome the increase in resistance associated with nose breathing even in light to moderately intense exercise.

Oral Resistance. There are only two reports of changes in oral resistance in response to exercise, and in both cases the measurements were made following exercise. The available data suggest that oral resistance is about fourfold lower than nasal resistance at rest, and ninefold lower following exercise (425). In addition, the percentage fall in oral resistance with exercise (77%) was greater than the percentage fall in nasal resistance (48%) (425). It has also been shown that breathing through a mouthpiece decreased oral resistance by 80% (90), suggesting that the extent of mouth opening and caudal depression of the tongue play a major role in determining oral resistance. Cole et al. (90) also found a decrease in oral resistance with exercise in subjects that were not wearing a mouthpiece, suggesting that the oropharynx was dilated. It is possible that the oropharyngeal dilation is the result of active control of the soft palate and tongue, but information on the muscular control of the pharyngeal dilators during exercise is lacking.

Laryngeal Resistance. Although direct measurements of laryngeal resistance either following or during exercise are not available, England and Bartlett (120, 121) made visual estimates of the changes in glottic caliber with a fiberoptic bronchoscope during exercise and hypercapnia. They found that the glottis normally narrowed during expiration and widened on inspiration. When hyperpnea was evoked by either exercise or hypercapnia the glottis widened, and the extent of expiratory narrowing diminished. Moreover, the extent of glottic narrowing was positively correlated with the duration of expiration; shorter expiratory periods, which occur with hypercapnia and especially exercise, were associated with correspondingly less glottic narrowing. The authors suggested that expiratory glottic narrowing in eupnea served to impede expiratory flow, acting as a "brake" that prevents the lungs from passively emptying below the relaxed end-expiratory level. This expiratory braking is then reduced in hyperpnea when the need to increase expiratory flow is increased, and expiratory duration is shortened. These same authors also reported a negative correlation between glottic size and pulmonary flow resistance, suggesting that the widening of the glottis in hyperpnea is associated with reductions in laryngeal resistance (120, 121).

The mechanisms that have been proposed to explain the hyperpnea-induced changes in glottic dimensions are controversial. One idea suggests that the extrinsic laryngeal muscles, which stabilize the larynx during inspiration as the lungs and trachea move caudally, make a major contribution to the widening of the glottis during inspiration; the positive swing in intrathoracic pressure on expiration is associated with the return of the laryngeal folds to their unstressed position (130, 406). The other idea suggests that changes in glottic aperture result primarily from increased activity of the intrinsic laryngeal muscles, with the PCA causing glottic abduction on inspiration, and the thyroarytenoid muscle leading to expiratory adduction (120, 121). However, it is likely that both mechanisms play an important role during exercise, when the intrathoracic pressure swings and caudal reflections of the larynx are large, and drive to the upper airway muscles is also increased. Van De Graaff (406) showed that upper airway flow resistance fell by 50% during maximal stimulation of both phrenic nerves in the anesthetized dog, even though all of the upper airway musculature had been surgically removed. It appears that glottic caliber and laryngeal resistance are actively controlled by both upper airway and respiratory pumping muscles during exercise. It is possible that caudal traction causes pharyngeal and laryngeal dilation, and activation of muscles in these regions serves to stabilize the airway, thereby preventing collapse and perhaps causing further dilation as well. The relative contributions of both mechanisms across a wide range of exercise intensities and durations needs to be established.

Upper Airway Muscle Activities during Exercise

In recent years, substantial progress has been made in our understanding of the respiratory-related discharge of the upper airway muscles in reduced preparations, including their reflex responses to stimulation of central and peripheral chemoreceptors (180, 353, 354, 383), pulmonary stretch receptors (353), and receptors in the upper airway (270, 271, 281, 365, 382, 403, 404, 411). Studies in resting human subjects have demonstrated phasic, respiratory-related activity during eupnea and chemically driven hyperpnea in the nasal dilator muscles (73, 92, 93, 141, 259, 338, 384, 385, 424, 432), the tensor muscles of the soft palate (42, 172, 429), the genioglossus and geniohyoid muscles (191, 295, 301, 302, 359), the posterior cricoarytenoid muscle (68, 230), and the cricothyroid muscle (68, 126, 231, 428). In sharp contrast to these advances in our knowledge of upper airway muscle control in resting subjects, there are few data on the behavior of the upper airway musculature during exercise hyperpnea. Indeed, with one exception, the only unpublished studies that we could find concern the nasal dilator muscles of the alae nasi. There is one published study of the changes in genioglossal EMG activity during exercise (424), but useful data were obtained in only two subjects, only a single intensity of exercise was examined, and the change in activity from rest to exercise was not reported. We are unaware of any studies of laryngeal, pharyngeal, or palatal muscle activities during exercise in humans or in lower mammals.

Although the available data on nasal dilator muscle activities during exercise are by no means complete, some consistent findings have emerged. First, the nasal dilator muscles contract rhythmically in phase with inspiration, and the activity rises monotonically as a function of the rate of nasal airflow (92, 93, 141, 424, 427). These observations are consistent with findings in resting humans and anesthetized animals that show that the shape of the moving time averaged EMG of upper airway muscles closely parallels the pattern of inspiratory airflow (93, 230, 244, 302, 424). Figure 11.3 depicts the changes in nasal and total inspired pulmonary ventilation, the mean inspiratory flow rate (V_T/T_I) and the EMG activities of the nasal dilator muscles in human subjects performing progressive-intensity exercise on a cycle ergometer. In these experiments, the subjects were allowed to select freely their route of breathing and were wearing a mask that covered the nose, but the mouth was unimpeded. Note that nasal dilator muscle EMG activities closely followed the rates of nasal airflow. Thus, both the nasal flow rate and the EMG activities plateaued at 60% of peak power even though total pulmonary ventilation (and therefore central respiratory drive) continued to increase as a function of the exercise intensity. It is clear from this and from other studies using different experimental designs (92, 141, 424, 427) that the drive to the upper airway muscles is highly correlated with the nasal airflow rate.

In spite of the high correlation between the rate of upper airway flow and the drive to the upper airway muscles, three observations suggest that flow may not be the primary factor that determines drive to the upper airway musculature. First, the sudden and surreptitious reduction of nasal airway resistance during exercise (by substituting He-O_2 for air) is associated with a *decrease* in drive to the nasal dilator muscles even though nasal airflow is *increasing* under these conditions (92). Second, in a more recent study the EMG of the nasal dilator muscles was measured during CO_2 rebreathing and during exercise in the same subjects; the subjects breathed through the nose alone in both experiments. When comparisons were made at a constant level of total pulmonary ventilation (and therefore flow through the nose), it was found that exercise resulted in considerably higher EMG activities than hypercapnia (J. Sullivan and R. Fregosi, unpublished observations). Third, the EMG burst of the nasal dilator muscles precedes the onset of inspiratory flow (92, 282, 384, 426, 427), suggesting that central, feedforward mechanisms play an important role in adjusting the drive to the upper airway musculature (see below). These latter data suggest that the determinant of the neural drive to the nasal dilator muscles during exercise is not a simple function of the rate of flow through the nose. It is possible that changes in nasal resistance, intraluminal pressure, or a feedforward mechanism play a role in determining drive to the upper airway muscles during exercise.

An important, yet-unanswered question is whether or not activation of the upper airway muscles can modulate upper airway resistance during exercise. It is obvious that if flow through the upper airways increased without an increase in upper airway dimensions, the flow profile would be largely turbulent and resistance would increase. However, as discussed above, there is ample evidence suggesting that vasoconstriction of the nasal mucosa has a major impact on the overall reduction in upper airway flow resistance, but the contribution of the upper airway musculature to the decline in resistance has not been established. Nevertheless, studies in resting human subjects have shown that voluntary activation of the nasal dilator muscles can decrease upper airway resistance (384), and that a decrease in the tone of the tongue or palatal muscles can lead to large increases in airway resistance, and even airway obstruction (197, 198, 359). In addition, the finding that nasal dilator EMG activity and nasal resistance both decreased within the first breath when the inspirate was changed from air to He-O_2

in exercising subjects indicates that the upper airway muscles respond rapidly to changes in upper airway resistance (92). These observations suggest that the upper airway muscles are likely to play a role in controlling upper airway patency during exercise. Future studies need to establish if and to what extent the activation of various upper airway muscles can modulate resistance in different regions of the upper airway.

Oronasal Distribution of Respiratory Airflow

Oronasal flow partitioning refers to the measurement of the fraction of air passing via the nasal and oral respiratory passages at any point in time. In most studies of the exercise hyperpnea the oronasal distribution is not considered, and total pulmonary ventilation is measured by instrumenting the subjects with nose clips and a large mouthpiece. Although this method is simple, it obviously disrupts the normal pattern of airflow through the respiratory system. The simultaneous and independent measurement of airflow through the nose and mouth is technically difficult, but several investigators have made such measurements using small nasal masks to measure nasal flow, leaving the mouth uninstrumented; total pulmonary ventilation is then measured with a head-out body plethysmograph (e.g., 135), or with inductive plethysmography [Fig. 11.3; (93)]. Oral ventilation is then obtained by subtracting nasal ventilation from the total. Another technique uses one face mask that is partitioned into nasal and oral compartments (426). Such techniques have been used to show that 70%–80% of normal subjects breathe primarily through the nose at rest (115, 135, 259, 292, 293, 319, 335, 426) even though nasal resistance is much greater than oral resistance under these conditions. However, keep in mind that with all of these methods, the masks and associated flow measuring devices add dead space to the airway, which may alter oronasal flow partitioning.

These and other methods have also been used to measure the airflow rate associated with the switch from a primarily nasal to an oronasal breathing pattern during exercise (the "switch point"). The estimates are quite variable, ranging from 22 to 44 liters/min (292, 426). The relative distribution of nasal and oral ventilatory rates during exercise also vary widely. For example, Wheatley et al. (426) reported that nasal ventilation accounted for essentially all of the ventilation at rest, and from 26%–64% of the total ventilation at the start of oronasal breathing during exercise. And Fregosi and Lansing

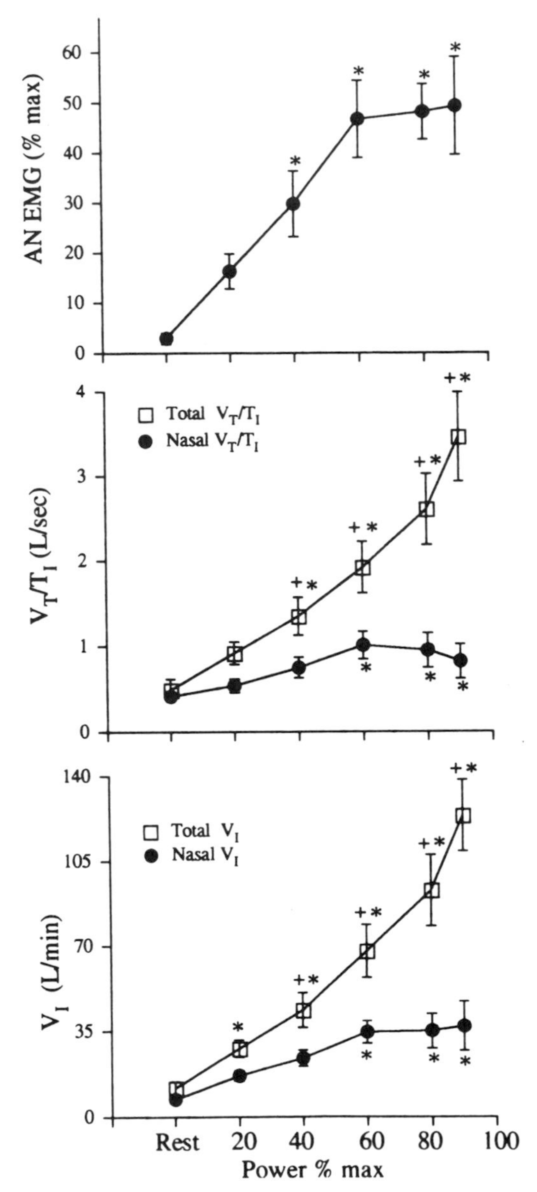

FIG. 11.3. Influence of exercise intensity on the integrated EMG activity of the nasal dilator muscles (AN EMG), mean inspiratory flow (V_T/T_I) and inspired pulmonary ventilation (V_I). Values for both nasal and total V_T/T_I and V_I are given, as indicated on the *insets*. Note that the plateau in both of these variables at exercise intensities exceeding 60% of the peak power coincides with the plateau in the AN EMG. * Significantly different than resting control value ($P < 0.05$); + significantly different than nasal V_I ($P < 0.05$). (From R. F. Fregosi and R. L. Lansing, unpublished observations.)

(unpublished observations) showed that nasal ventilation ranged from 44%–100% of the total at rest, and from 15%–61% of the total during bicycle exercise at 90% of the peak power in seven subjects. The factors underlying the wide range in estimates of the switch point and in oronasal flow distribution are unclear. Although methodological differences probably explain some of the variability, it is noteworthy that all authors who have made such measurements report marked intersubject variability. This is not surprising if one considers that the switch point ranges from zero (mouth breathers) to infinity (nose breathers that never open their mouths).

What Regulates Oronasal Flow Distribution during Exercise? As mentioned above, subjects that fail to open their mouth during exercise bouts that require ventilatory rates in excess of approximately 30–40 liters/min hypoventilate. This observation suggests that maintenance of an appropriate level of alveolar ventilation during exercise requires that oral and nasal flow rates are adjusted in a manner that minimizes upper airway resistance. The fraction of the pulmonary ventilation that enters the nose or mouth is dependent upon the relative resistances of these two pathways, and on the configuration of the face, mouth, and soft palate. The purpose of this section is to review the mechanisms that may govern the drive to the upper airway musculature, and therefore the configuration of the upper airway during exercise.

Two main hypotheses have been advanced to explain the control of oronasal flow partitioning during exercise: an increase in nasal airway resistance, and a feedforward mechanism that somehow adjusts the flow-partitioning mechanisms of the entire pharynx (424). Evidence for a role of airway resistance in determining the switch point is provided by observations showing that the rate of nasal ventilation measured at the transition from (predominantly) laminar to (predominantly) turbulent airflow in the nose ($\dot{V}tr$ in Fig. 11.2) corresponds nicely with the maximal nasal ventilation rate achieved during progressive intensity exercise (300; R. F. Fregosi and R. L. Lansing, unpublished observations). This is illustrated by comparing the $\dot{V}tr$ of roughly 30–35 liters/min shown in Figure 11.2 with peak nasal airflow rates shown in Figure 11.3. This latter observation suggests that the onset of flow turbulence during exercise may initiate mouth opening so that overall pulmonary resistance does not increase. However, where the change in nasal resistance is sensed has not been established, nor have the mechanisms that lead to mouth opening during exercise (see above).

There are receptors in the nasal lumen that monitor increases in the rate of nasal airflow (99, 403), negative pressure in the nasal lumen (270, 404, 411), flow-induced changes in temperature of the mucosal surfaces (403), or the introduction of noxious chemicals into the nasal airway (365). The strongest and most reproducible responses appear to be elicited by negative intraluminal pressure (282, 404, 411). Moreover, these responses appear to depend on the state of central nervous system (CNS) arousal, as they are attenuated during slow-wave sleep (392, 429). If the activity of these receptors is indeed state dependent, they may be good candidates for adjusting drive to the upper airway musculature during exercise, when the state of CNS arousal is high and changes in intraluminal pressure are elevated. However, recent evidence suggests that these local mechanisms are overridden during exercise. For example, neither lidocaine anesthesia of the nasal mucosa (424, J. Sullivan and R. Fregosi, unpublished observations) nor mechanical prevention of collapse of the external nares with nasal "splints" (171) influences the drive to the nasal dilator muscles during exercise significantly. Changes in nasal mucosal temperature have also been considered but do not appear to be involved, in that the inhalation of hot (>40°C), saturated air failed to alter drive to the nasal dilator muscles during exercise, at least in the single workload that was examined (424). Although these observations cast doubt on the ability of nasal receptors to sense changes in upper airway resistance during exercise, it is possible that receptors in pharyngeal, laryngeal, or intrapulmonary structures provide the necessary afferent input to the upper airway motoneuron pools.

Feedforward mechanisms are more difficult to conceptualize, although Wheatley et al. (424) have proposed a model whereby the upper airway muscles (including the muscles that regulate the position of the soft palate) are driven by a feedforward motor program that somehow coordinates the drive to the respiratory pumping muscles and the upper airway muscles. The attractiveness of this hypothesis is obvious, in that increased activity of the diaphragm results in the development of negative pressure in the respiratory system, which if unopposed, could lead to collapse or displacement of the upper airway.

The primary evidence for feedforward control of the upper airway muscles during exercise is provided by the longstanding observation that the discharge onset of upper airway muscles precedes the onset of inspiratory airflow (92, 230, 301, 302, 338, 384, 424, 427), and also the motor output to the diaphragm (180, 383). This "negative onset time" becomes even more negative during exercise (92, 424, 427), which serves to stiffen the upper airway before collapsing pressure is generated by contraction of the diaphragm. Recent experiments by Wheatley and colleagues (424) have shown that the sudden switch from nasal to oral breathing during expiration in exercising subjects leads to a less negative onset time and a reduction in drive to the nasal dilator muscles (Fig. 11.4*A*). When this same maneuver was re-

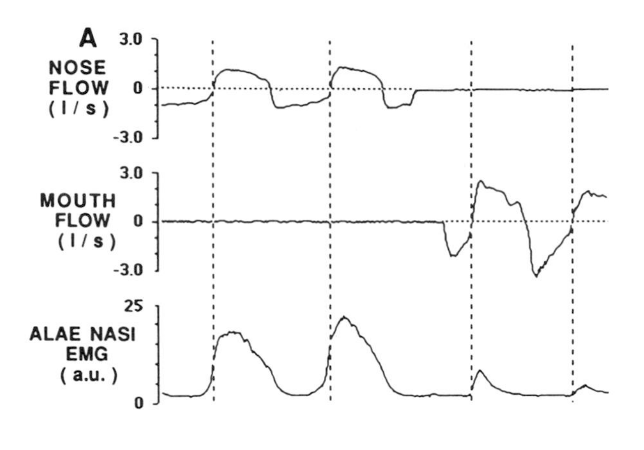

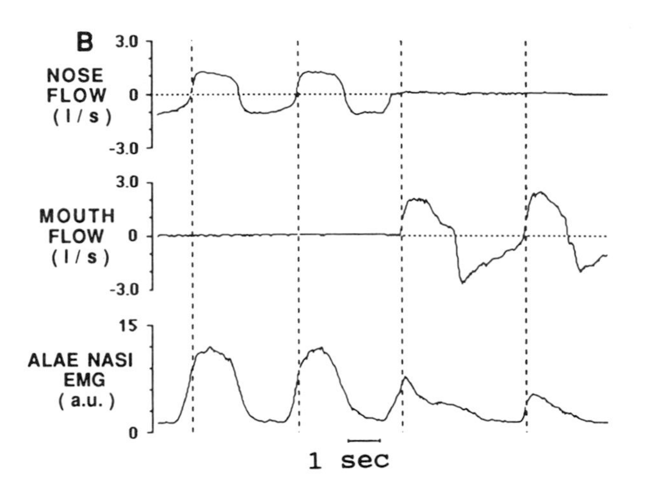

FIG. 11.4. Recordings showing changes in flow through the nose and mouth, and integrated EMG activity of the nasal dilator muscles ("alae nasi") when a representative subject voluntarily changes the breathing route from nasal to oral during cycling exercise. Note that during nose breathing EMG activity is much higher, and the onset of the EMG burst precedes the onset of flow (*vertical dashed lines*). Also note that when the flow route changes from nasal to oral in midexpiration (*A*), the EMG amplitude is diminished but EMG onset no longer precedes the onset of flow. In contrast, when flow route changes at the end of expiration (*B*), EMG amplitude is diminished but onset time does not change. Thus, when the upper airway was configured for oral flow well before the next inspiration (*A*), the nervous system no longer had to activate the alae nasi musculature early and intensely in order to protect the nasal airway from collapse. In contrast, when the switch from nasal to oral flow was made at the very end of expiration (*B*), the system was still configured for a nasal breath, and the EMG burst preceded the onset of flow. However, the system soon sensed the absence of nasal flow and made appropriate adjustments during the breath, resulting in a reduced EMG amplitude. Taken together, these data suggest that *(1)* the configuration of the entire upper airway, presumably determined by a feedforward mechanism, is more important than local reflex mechanisms in determining the onset of upper airway muscle activities, and *(2)* local reflex mechanisms can alter burst amplitude during a breath (see text) [From Wheatley, Amis, and Engel (424).]

peated at the very end of expiration (Fig. 11.4*B*), the onset of the burst was not altered, but its amplitude was still diminished; this was interpreted as evidence for feedforward control of nasal dilator muscle activities during exercise. We interpret these data to indicate that an undefined feedforward mechanism adjusts the timing of the nasal dilator muscle burst relative to nasal airflow, but that reflex mechanisms have a major impact on the amplitude of the burst. This interpretation suggests that the timing and amplitude of nasal dilator muscle activities are independently controlled during exercise. It is clear that more studies are needed to adequately test this and other models of upper airway muscle control during exercise.

EFFECTS OF EXERCISE ON PASSIVE RESPIRATORY MECHANICS

Elastic Properties

A number of studies have reported a fall in dynamic lung compliance during moderate or heavy exercise (153, 207, 387, 444). Dynamic compliance also falls during voluntary hyperventilation at rest (153). However, dynamic compliance is influenced by operating lung volume and respiratory rate, both of which change markedly with exercise. Therefore, the altered dynamic compliance is not necessarily due to a change in lung elastic recoil. Younes and Kivinen (444) found that lung elastic recoil at measured total lung capacity was the same at maximal exercise as at rest. There was a small but significant reduction in recoil pressure during light exercise but at no other work rate during incremental exercise. Therefore, current evidence indicates that elastic recoil at high lung volumes shows little, if any, change during heavy incremental exercise in normal humans. There are few data concerning the effects of exercise on static recoil at low lung volumes and there are technical difficulties in making such measurements.

Total Lung Capacity

Total lung capacity measured by nitrogen washout or body plethysmography has been found to remain unchanged during exercise in humans (30, 387, 444). Radiographic assessment of lung volume also indicates that total lung capacity is unchanged immediately after maximal incremental exercise (144). Total lung capacity was also unchanged when measured immediately after a marathon race (268). The lack of change in total lung capacity is not surprising because it is determined by inspiratory muscle strength and lung and chest wall recoil at high lung volumes, none of which usually change significantly with exercise. The effects of exercise on inspiratory muscle strength are discussed elsewhere in this chapter.

Expiratory Flow Rates, Vital Capacity, and Residual Volume

A number of studies found that pulmonary resistance during exercise was unchanged from that at rest (161, 387). However airway resistance varies with air flow rate and would be expected to increase with the increased $\dot{V}_E$ and flow rates of exercise. When specific airway conductance was measured during a panting maneuver, there was evidence of airway dilatation with exercise (214). More recently, Warren et al. (417) compared a measure of pulmonary resistance during exercise to that during panting with a similar breathing pattern at rest. They found a progressive bronchodilatation during exercise. The improvement in the expiratory flow–volume curve immediately after exercise in many normal humans (201, 207) indicates that this bronchodilatation persists for a short time after exercise.

Bronchodilatation during exercise in normal humans appears to be due to removal of resting vagal tone (417). Based on animal experiments (217), it is likely that removal of vagal bronchoconstrictor tone is a reflex response to stimulation of chemosensitive limb muscle afferents during exercise (also see Chapter 10). Bronchodilatation during exercise is probable at least partly due to tracheal dilatation (351) as well as laryngeal dilatation. Regulation of upper airway caliber was discussed in detail previously in this chapter (see earlier under REGULATION OF THE UPPER AIRWAY DURING EXERCISE).

Whereas there is a good evidence of exercise-induced bronchodilatation, several investigators have reported a fall in vital capacity after heavy exercise, and this is usually associated with a fall in maximum expiratory flow rates, especially at low lung volumes (90, 268, 297). The fall in vital capacity is accompanied by an increase in residual volume so that total lung capacity is unchanged (268). These changes in vital capacity and expiratory flow rates appear to be associated mainly with heavy endurance exercise. However, they have also been reported with maximal incremental exercise and appear more related to exercise intensity than to duration itself (297). These changes persist for some time after exercise (299). Forced expiration volumine in 1 s (FEV_1) was still significantly reduced the morning after an endurance triathalon in one study (186). There is also evidence that closing capacity may increase after intense exercise (282).

The combination of increased residual volume, reduced expiratory flow rates, and increased closing capacity suggests that these changes are probably related to airway/parenchymal abnormalities. Possible mechanisms underlying these changes include interstitial pulmonary edema, or airway/parenchymal damage related to the high ventilatory demands of exercise. The possibility that exercise may be associated with mild pulmonary edema is discussed elsewhere in this *Handbook* (see Chapter 13).

BREATHING PATTERN DURING EXERCISE

The term "breathing pattern" is used here first to refer to the changes in "mechanical" breathing pattern during exercise; that is, the changes in tidal volume, end-inspiratory and end-expiratory lung volumes, inspiratory and expiratory flow rates, and respiratory timing. It is also used to denote the changes in pattern of respiratory muscle contraction that cause these mechanical changes.

Mechanical Breathing Pattern

The increase in $\dot{V}_E$ during progressive exercise is due to increases in both tidal volume (V_T) and respiratory frequency (f_b) (Fig. 11.5). At low levels of exercise, increases in V_T and f_b both contribute to the increasing $\dot{V}_E$ [Fig. 11.5; (143, 185)]. At high levels of exercise, further increases in $\dot{V}_E$ are almost completely due to increasing f_b while V_T remains constant or shows little change (84, 143). This has been referred to as the tachypneic breathing pattern of heavy exercise. In some subjects, further increases in $\dot{V}_E$ at high levels of $\dot{V}_E$ are accomplished by increasing f_b while V_T progressively decreases (145, 201). Tidal volume usually stops increasing when it reaches approximately 50%–60% of vital capacity, although there is significant intersubject variation in this ratio (56, 145, 182). Normal young subjects typically show a three- to fivefold increase in V_T from rest to maximal exercise. Respiratory frequency often shows a one- to threefold increase, but the increase in f_b may be greater than this in fit subjects because of their higher $\dot{V}_E$ at maximal exercise (Fig. 11.5).

The increase in V_T during exercise is due to both a decrease in end-expiratory lung volume (EELV) and an increase in end-inspiratory lung volume (EILV). End-expiratory lung volume falls with even minor increases in $\dot{V}_E$ above resting levels (182, 444), and the fall in EELV precedes the increase in

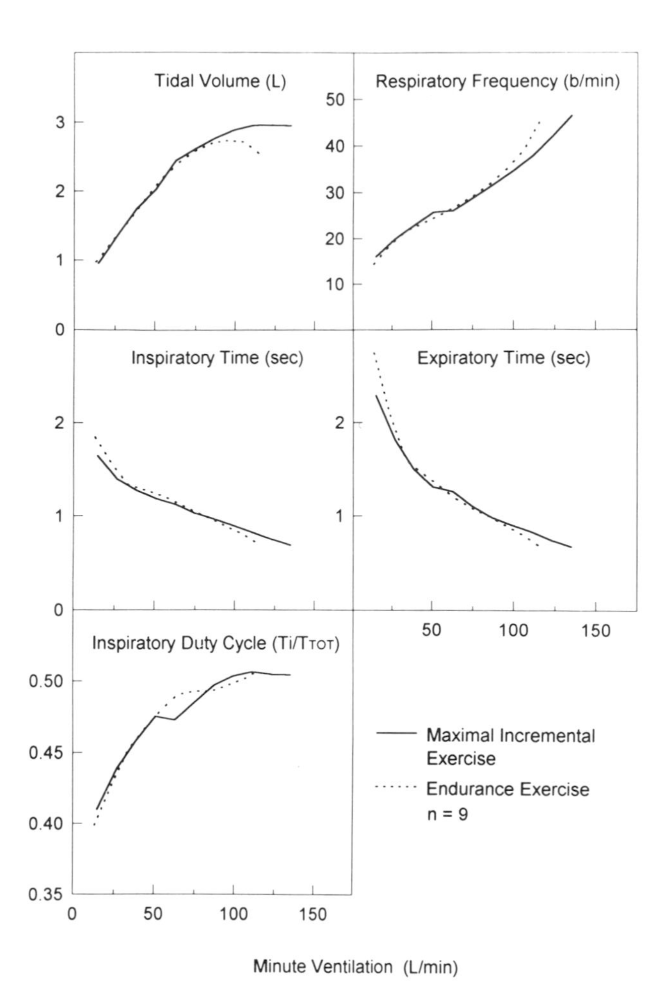

FIG. 11.5. Comparison of breathing pattern in normal humans during maximal incremental exercise and endurance exercise. The initial increase in minute ventilation is due to increases in both tidal volume and respiratory frequency. However, tidal volume stops increasing at high levels of ventilation and further increases in ventilation are due to increasing respiratory frequency alone. Tidal volume is less and respiratory frequency greater during endurance exercise at high levels of ventilation [Data obtained from Syabbalo et al. (395).] See text for details.

EILV with loadless pedaling (30). Most studies of normal humans indicate that, after this initial fall in EELV during mild exercise, EELV stabilizes at a new level (75, 146, 193, 207, 444), and further increases in VT are due to increases in EILV alone (Fig. 11.6). This new EELV is usually approximately 0.4–0.7 liter below resting EELV, although values outside this range may be observed in individual subjects.

Whereas EELV falls early in exercise and remains at this level during moderate exercise, it may increase toward or above resting EELV at higher work rates (Fig. 11.6). This rise in EELV is a consequence of expiratory flow limitation (205, 207, 316). This rise in EELV is beneficial, as it allows higher expiratory flow rates to be generated. However, it increases the load on the inspiratory muscles by increasing the pressure that they have to generate and by decreasing their pressure-generating capacity through the length–tension effect.

The increase in f_b during progressive exercise in humans is due to a fall in both inspiratory (TI) and expiratory (TE) times (Fig. 11.5). There is a greater fractional decrease in TE than in TI so that the inspiratory duty cycle (TI/TTOT) increases from approximately 0.4 at rest to as high as 0.50–0.55 at maximal exercise [Fig. 11.5; (84, 276, 395)]. A similar increase in TI/TTOT also occurs in exercising dogs (11). Because fractional shortening of TE exceeds that of TI, the increase in mean expiratory flow rate (VT/TE) from rest to maximal exercise exceeds the increase in mean inspiratory flow rate (VT/TI). The inspiratory flow profile at rest is usually quasi sinusoidal, with peak inspiratory flow rates seen near midinspiration (Fig. 11.7). In contrast, peak expiratory flow rate during quiet breathing at rest usually occurs during early expiration and expiratory flow rate gradually declines during expiration. As $\dot{V}E$ increases during exercise, the inspiratory and expiratory flow profiles both become more rectangular or square-wave–like [Fig. 11.7; (232)].

Methods of Assessment of Respiratory Muscle Contraction

Minute ventilation and mechanical breathing pattern result from the pattern of respiratory muscle contraction acting on the mechanical properties of the respiratory system. The relation between respiratory muscle output and mechanical breathing pattern is reviewed in detail elsewhere (441). This section will briefly review methods of assessing the pattern of respiratory muscle contraction in exercising humans.

First, the dynamic pressure generated by the diaphragm can be measured directly as follows:

$$Pdi = Pab - Ppl \qquad (4)$$

where Pdi, Pab, and Ppl are transdiaphragmatic, abdominal, and pleural pressures, respectively. Pab and Ppl are measured by catheters in the stomach and esophagus, respectively. At this time, the diaphragm is the only respiratory muscle where the pressure resulting from its contraction can be measured directly.

Second, the net dynamic pressure resulting from the contraction of all the respiratory muscles (Pmus) can be measured or estimated. This method treats the respiratory system as if it is a simple viscoelastic structure with essentially only one or two components, and it involves calculating the net active pres-

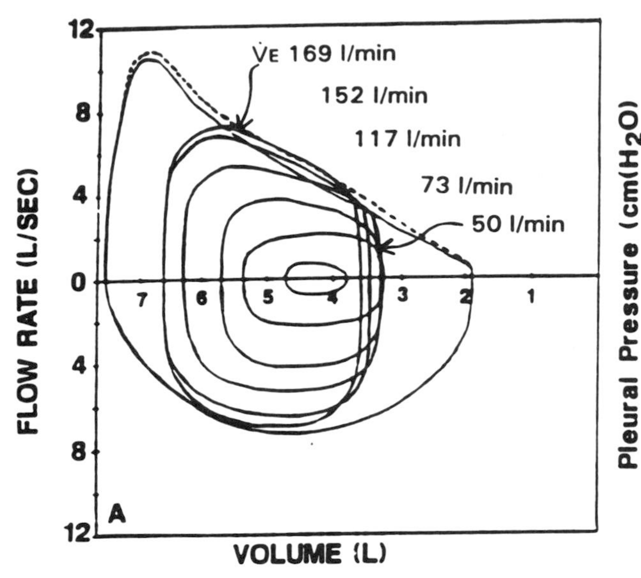

FIG. 11.6. Young adult average tidal flow–volume and pressure–volume loops and minute ventilation ($\dot{V}_E$) for eight athletes during rest and progressive exercise, which averaged 42%, 61%, 83%, 95%, and 100% of maximal oxygen uptake. Tidal flow–volume curves are shown plotted within preexercise (*solid line*) and postexercise (*dashed line*) maximum flow–volume curves. Tidal pressure–volume curves are shown also with constraints for effective pressure generation on expiration (Pmaxe) and the capacity for pressure generation on inspiration (Pcapi). Widths of Pmaxe and Pcapi at a given lung volume indicate 95% confidence intervals. The loops at a minute ventilation of 117 liter $\cdot$ min^{-1} represent the typical response to maximum short-term exercise in an untrained young adult subject (maximum $\dot{V}O_2$ 40–50 ml $\cdot$ kg^{-1} $\cdot$ min^{-1}). The $\dot{V}_E$ of 169 liters/min was the average response to maximum exercise in the trained subject (maximum $\dot{V}O_2$ = 70–80 ml $\cdot$ kg^{-1} $\cdot$ min^{-1}) [From Johnson, Saupe and Dempsey (207).]

sure across the respiratory system. This active pressure is composed of:

$$Pmus = Pel + Pres + Pin \qquad (5)$$

where *P*el, *P*res, and *P*in are the pressures used to overcome the elastic, resistive, and inertial properties of the respiratory system (lungs and chest wall), respectively. Inspiratory *P*mus is arbitrarily assigned a positive value, and expiratory *P*mus is negative. The inertial pressure losses are usually very small, so that equation 5 can be simplified to:

$$Pmus = Pel + Pres \qquad (6)$$

Rearranging equation 6 yields:

$$Pres = Pmus - Pel \qquad (7)$$

In other words, inspiratory flow will begin or continue (i.e., *P*res is positive) only when *P*mus exceeds the recoil pressure of the respiratory system. Expiratory flow will begin or continue only when *P*mus is less than the recoil pressure of the respiratory system.

*P*mus is calculated from the pressures used to overcome chest wall elastance (*P*w,el) and resistance (*P*w,res) and pleural pressure (444):

$$Pmus = Pw,el + Pw,res - Ppl \qquad (8)$$

This method of calculating *P*mus is based on the analysis of Mead and Agostoni (279). The methods used to calculated *P*mus are described in detail elsewhere (146, 227, 444). Figure 11.7 shows average *P*mus from three subjects studied at rest and during light and moderately heavy exercise.

Third, pleural pressure (*P*pl) itself has frequently been used as an index of net respiratory muscle pressure (*P*mus). Measurement of *P*pl is easier than measurement of *P*mus because *P*w,el and *P*w,res are ignored (see equation 8). However, this is also the major disadvantage of using *P*pl alone as an index of respiratory muscle output. While *P*w,el and *P*w,res are difficult to measure, they make up a significant fraction of *P*mus. For example, a young subject with a normal chest wall elastance of 5 cm H_2O/liter and a V_T of 2.8 liters at maximal exercise will have a *P*w,el at end-inspiration 14 cm H_2O greater than that at end-expiration. Therefore, examining *P*pl alone would underestimate the change in *P*mus from end-expiration to end-inspiration by this amount.

Each of these three measures of respiratory muscle pressure (*P*di, *P*mus, and *P*pl) may be expressed as a fraction of the subject's capacity (*P*cap) to generate that pressure. *P*cap varies with muscle length and velocity of shortening, which change with lung vol-

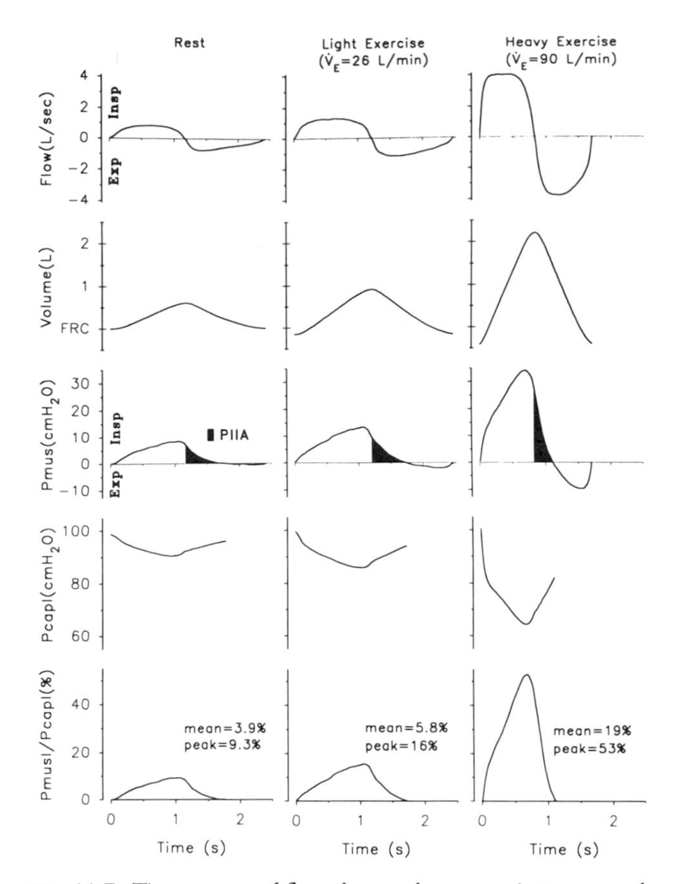

FIG. 11.7. Time course of flow; lung volume; respiratory muscle pressure (Pmus); dynamic capacity of inspiratory muscles to generate pressure (Pcapi); and ratio of inspiratory Pmus to Pcapi before exercise, during light exercise, and during moderately heavy exercise. Data are the average from three subjects during cycle exercise. PIIA is postinspiratory muscle activity. Numbers in the bottom row are mean and peak PmusI/PcapI. See text for details. (From B. Krishnan, T. Zintel, and C. G. Gallagher, unpublished data.)

ume and respiratory flow, respectively. Thus inspiratory *P*mus (*P*musI) at any time during the breathing cycle may be expressed as a fraction of *P*mus during a maximal inspiratory maneuver (i.e., *P*cap) at the same lung volume and flow rate, as shown in Figure 11.7. Clearly *P*mus I/*P*cap varies throughout the breathing cycle (Fig. 11.7). *P*mus I/*P*cap averaged over the respiratory cycle is then the tension time index of the inspiratory muscles (49). Similarly *P*pl and *P*di during exercise have been expressed as a fraction of *P*cap in a number of studies (205, 207, 242).

The activity of different groups of respiratory muscles can be assessed indirectly by relating changes in rib cage and abdominal movements to simultaneous changes in *P*pl and *P*ab. This provides data about the relative mechanical activities of the diaphragm, the intercostal/accessory inspiratory muscles, the abdominal expiratory muscles, and the intercostal/accessory expiratory muscles. These methods are reviewed elsewhere (165). Electromyography and measurement of length changes in the various respiratory muscles during exercise provide more direct information on patterns of muscle recruitment. However, very few data are available in humans and quadrupeds (9, 10, 14).

Pattern of Respiratory Muscle Contraction

End-expiratory lung volume during quiet breathing at rest [functional residual capacity (FRC)] is the relaxation volume of the respiratory system in normal humans. From a respiratory muscle point of view, resting breathing is primarily an inspiratory activity in humans (Fig. 11.7). Inspiratory flow begins as soon as inspiratory muscles generate an inflationary pressure (i.e., *P*mus becomes positive). *P*mus rises in a ramp-like pattern and then declines slowly. Peak *P*mus occurs when there is still inspiratory flow (i.e., peak *P*mus exceeds respiratory recoil pressure at that "lung" volume). Therefore, expiration does not begin until *P*mus has fallen below its peak value (equation 7). *P*mus remains positive for the initial part of expiration, thus slowing the fall in lung volume during expiration (Fig. 11.7). This persistence of inspiratory (positive) *P*mus during expiration is termed postinspiratory activity (PIIA). There is little or no expiratory *P*mus at rest in humans. In contrast, resting EELV is dynamically determined in quadrupeds; it differs from relaxation volume of the respiratory system.

As $\dot{V}_E$ increases during exercise, both rate of rise and peak inspiratory *P*mus increase (Fig. 11.7). The shape of the rising phase of *P*mus changes so that the rate of rise of *P*mus is maximal early in inspiration. As shown in Fig. 11.7, PIIA persists but, at least at high levels of $\dot{V}_E$, for a smaller fraction of T_E. In exercising dogs, the duration of PIIA of the crural diaphragm remained unchanged despite the reduction in T_E with exercise (10). Therefore, the PIIA/T_E ratio increased with exercise. Expiratory muscle activity begins at very low levels of exercise and increases further as $\dot{V}_E$ rises (165, 182, 227). Recent studies using intramuscular wire electrodes also confirm abdominal muscle recruitment during mild exercise in humans (106). The fall in EELV with exercise itself implies expiratory muscle recruitment. Generating expiratory *P*mus, bronchodilatation during exercise, and reducing PIIA cause expiratory flow rates to increase. Expiratory *P*mus is also used to decrease EELV below FRC, which is beneficial in allowing large increases in V_T while breathing on the relatively linear part of the respiratory pressure–volume curve. This spares the inspiratory muscles, as a much greater increase in inspiratory *P*mus would be needed if the same V_T had to be obtained completely above FRC. The fall in EELV is also beneficial, as it allows the diaphragm and other inspiratory muscles to operate on the more efficient part of their length–tension curves.

It should not be assumed that the pattern of change in inspiratory or expiratory *P*mus during exercise necessarily reflects the activity of a particular muscle group. While there are relatively few data at this time, there is accumulating evidence of heterogeneity in the responses of respiratory muscles to exercise. A number of studies provide evidence that the relative contribution of the inspiratory/intercostal muscles to inspiration increases and that of the diaphragm decreases as $\dot{V}_E$ rises during exercise (70, 165, 246). Johnson et al. (207) found that mean *P*di remained constant as $\dot{V}_E$ and mean *P*pl continued to increase during heavy prolonged exercise. It was recently shown that while inspiratory and expiratory *P*mus both increase during light and moderate exercise, the increasing $\dot{V}_E$ of heavy endurance exercise is accompanied by a relatively greater increase in expiratory than in inspiratory *P*mus (226).

Inspiratory flow rate is limited primarily by the ability to generate inspiratory muscle pressure (*P*musI); inspiratory flow at a given lung volume continues to increase as *P*musI increases progressively to maximum. In contrast, expiratory flow rate is limited by airway mechanics, not the ability to generate expiratory muscle pressure (*P*musE). Maximal expiratory flow rate at a given lung volume is reached when *P*musE is only a small fraction of its capacity. The lowest *P*musE that causes maximal expiratory flow at a given lung volume will be termed maximal effective pressure (*P*eff). Further increases in *P*musE greater than Peff cause no further increase in expiratory flow rates. It is clear that humans can generate *P*musE significantly greater than *P*eff; for example, during voluntary hyperventilation at rest (223). Normal subjects generate the required *P*musE during exercise, but usually no more; that is, *P*musE rarely exceeds *P*eff [see Fig. 11.6); (207, 223, 298)]. *P*eff is not exceeded when ventilation is further stimulated by CO_2 inhalation or hypoxia (207). The fact that excessive and ineffective pressures are not generated during exercise, when they could be, probably depends on feedback from airway receptors. This is supported by the observation that changes in gas density (thus changing airway resistance) alter abdominal muscle recruitment within two breaths (182).

As discussed above (see Fig. 11.7), the dynamic pressure generated by inspiratory muscles may be expressed as a fraction of the subject's ability to generate pressure (*P*cap) at the lung volume and flow rate adopted during exercise. This has been performed for inspiratory muscles as a whole (227, 444), as shown in Figure 11.7. This analysis may also be performed using *P*pl as an index of *P*mus (207, 242). *P*di may also be examined in this way (203). These studies show that peak dynamic pressure generated by the inspiratory muscles may exceed 80% of *P*cap at maximal exercise in fit humans (203, 207, 227). For less fit subjects, peak *P*musI/*P*cap is frequently greater than 50% (Fig. 11.7). Mean *P*musI/*P*cap is more important than peak *P*musI/*P*cap where respiratory muscle energetics are concerned. Mean *P*musI/*P*cap is the tension time index of inspiratory muscles and is a major determinant of the energy cost of breathing and of susceptibility to fatigue (see later under Oxygen Cost of Hyperpnea). The subjects whose data are shown in Figure 11.7 had a mean *P*musI/*P*cap of 19% during moderately heavy exercise and, based on the analysis of Bellemare and Grassino (49), this is potentially fatiguing. Values significantly higher than this are seen in more fit subjects. Inspiratory muscle fatigue is reviewed elsewhere in this chapter.

Influence of Sensory Feedback on Breathing Pattern

Studies of exercising dogs and ponies show that vagal feedback from the lungs is important in regulation of breathing pattern. Pulmonary denervation or vagal cooling increased V_T and decreased f_b during exercise (14, 86, 133). The fall in f was due to an increase in T_I with generally no significant change in T_E. This altered breathing pattern is presumably due to loss of lung volume feedback from stretch receptors (Hering-Breuer inflation reflex), but loss of feedback from other receptors may also have had a role. Whereas vagal afferent input influences breathing pattern, it appears to have no significant effect on regulation of $\dot{V}_E$ during exercise (14, 86, 133). Ainsworth et al. (14) recently examined the effects of vagal afferent input on regulation of respiratory muscle output in exercising dogs. Vagal cooling increased the EMG activity of the diaphragm, parasternal (inspiratory rib cage), and triangular sterni (expiratory rib cage) muscles, indicating that vagal feedback normally inhibits these muscles. However, abdominal expiratory muscle activity did not change despite the increase in V_T with vagal cooling, suggesting that vagal feedback usually stimulates abdominal muscle activity (14).

While it has traditionally been believed that the Hering-Breuer reflex is very weak in humans (431), recent evidence indicates that vagal volume feedback influences breathing pattern in resting humans, at least under anesthesia (321). However, there are major logistical problems in assessing the role of vagal afferent input in exercising humans. Sciurba et al. (363) examined breathing pattern during exercise in patients after heart-lung transplantation. They were compared to patients who had received heart transplantation only and therefore would be expected to have intact pulmonary innervation. Routine pulmonary function tests were generally normal or near normal in both patient groups. Inspiratory and expiratory muscle strengths were similarly reduced in both patient groups. The rate of rise in f_b with increasing $\dot{V}_E$ was less and the initial rate of rise in V_T was greater in the heart-lung transplant patients. However, these differences were much less at maximal exercise; the ratio of V_T to vital capacity (VC) at maximal exercise was similar in the two groups and similar to that of normal humans and patients with cardiorespiratory disease who have not had denervation (142, 160). Therefore, this study suggests that vagal afferent input may influence exercise breathing pattern in humans, at least at low levels of $\dot{V}_E$. This is also supported by the finding of Winning et al. (436) that topical airway anesthesia caused breathing pattern to become deeper and slower during incremental exercise in humans.

Heavy exercise in humans increases hydrogen ion concentration, serum potassium, and serum norepinephrine, each of which stimulates the carotid bodies. Syabbalo et al. (396) used hyperoxia to examine the importance of peripheral chemoreceptor feedback in regulation of exercise breathing pattern in humans. As expected, hyperoxia caused a fall in ventilation for a given work rate. However, breathing pattern at matched $\dot{V}_E$ was unaffected by hyperoxia, suggesting that peripheral chemoreceptor input does not influence breathing pattern in exercising humans during room air breathing. However, hypoxic hyperventilation (causing hypocapnia) increases PIIA and inhibits expiratory muscle activity, thus increasing EELV in dogs (377, 378). Hypoxia may have similar affects in exercising humans, as evidenced by the rise (or lack of fall) in EELV in patients who became hypoxemic during exercise but did not have expiratory flow limitation (267).

Addition of external dead space has been shown to cause a deeper slower breathing pattern at high levels of $\dot{V}_E$ during exercise (277). This response is absent, or much less, when ventilation is stimulated by CO_2 inhalation alone (143). It has therefore been suggested that alteration in the P_{CO_2} temporal profile may be responsible for the altered breathing pattern (277). Alteration in the P_{CO_2} temporal profile might be sensed by carotid body or pulmonary/airway chemoreceptors. However, the change in breathing pattern with added dead space also occurs in the presence of carotid body suppression by hyperoxia (396). Therefore, carotid afferent input is not required for the altered breathing pattern with added dead space. The mechanisms underlying the response to dead space loading are unclear.

Influence of Respiratory Mechanics on Breathing Pattern

The choice of breathing patterns that a subject may use at a given level of $\dot{V}_E$ is ultimately limited by the mechanical properties of the respiratory system. At low levels of $\dot{V}_E$, V_T could, at least in theory, equal vital capacity. As $\dot{V}_E$ and therefore, mean inspiratory and expiratory flow rates increase, the maximum possible V_T falls (201, 277). This is because breathing with a sufficiently high V_T must include lung volumes associated with lower maximal inspiratory and expiratory flow rates than does breathing with a small V_T (277). Is the breathing pattern adopted during exercise limited by respiratory mechanics? Because the V_T plateau during incremental exercise rises significantly with dead space loading (277), it is clear that the tachypneic pattern during incremental exercise is not limited by mechanics. However the changes in EELV during heavy exercise are limited by respiratory mechanics in some subjects. Expiratory flow limitation causes EELV to rise (Fig. 11.6).

Influence of Duration of Exercise on Breathing Pattern

$\dot{V}_E$, V_T, and f usually remain constant after about 4 min of exercise at low work rates in humans. However, $\dot{V}_E$ and f continue to increase with increasing exercise during heavy endurance exercise (103, 395, 419). Is this tachypneic breathing pattern unique to endurance exercise? Syabbalo et al. (395) compared breathing pattern during endurance and maximal incremental exercise on a cycle ergometer in the same subjects. There was no significant difference in V_T, f_b, T_I, or T_E at low and moderate levels of $\dot{V}_E$ (Fig. 11.5). However, V_T was less and f_b greater during endurance exercise at high levels of $\dot{V}_E$ (Fig. 11.5). The mechanisms underlying this tachypneic breathing pattern, which occurs near the end of endurance exercise, are unknown. As reviewed elsewhere (103, 395), the major possibilities include inspiratory muscle fatigue, pulmonary edema, and/or altered respiratory mechanics.

Influence of Mode of Exercise on Breathing Pattern

Is breathing pattern during exercise influenced by exercise (including mode of exercise) itself or is breathing pattern during exercise simply the "usual" pattern adopted by the respiratory control system whenever ventilatory demand is increased? It was once believed that the V_T-f_b response to exercise was the same as that when ventilation was stimulated by other means such as hypercapnia or metabolic acidosis (185). However, while there are major similarities in breathing pattern between different forms of ventilatory stimulation, it is also clear that there are significant quantitative differences (308). The pattern of increase in V_T and f_b at low work rates in humans (Fig. 11.5) is qualitatively similar to that when $\dot{V}_E$ is increased by hypercapnia or other methods of ventilatory stimulation (182, 185). However, exercise is associated with greater abdominal muscle recruitment during expiration and accordingly a greater fall in EELV than at the same $\dot{V}_E$ during hypercapnia in both humans and dogs (10, 182). The abdominal muscles function as "accessory locomotor muscles." Grillner et al. (164) suggested that the increased abdominal muscle recruitment during exercise may be partly related to the locomotor function of these muscles.

Breathing pattern during exercise may also vary with the type of exercise. For example, V_T is less and f_b greater during arm-cranking than during cycling (253). It is unclear whether the more tachypneic breathing pattern during arm exercise is because of the smaller muscle mass (resulting in greater sympathetic activation, metabolic acidosis, etc., at a given work rate), entrainment, or the competing respiratory/locomotor roles of arm muscles. However, it is clear that breathing pattern is influenced by the type of exercise even when exercising muscle mass is similar. At matched $\dot{V}_E$, treadmill running causes greater abdominal muscle activation and a greater fall in EELV than occur with walking or cycling (182). The idea that this increased abdominal muscle recruitment is related to the mode of exercise itself is supported by the observation of Henke et al. that this precedes any increase in $\dot{V}_E$ (182).

As reviewed elsewhere in this chapter (see later under LOCOMOTOR-RESPIRATION INTERDEPENDENCE), there is considerable evidence of coupling between respiratory and locomotor rhythms in many species. Possible mechanisms underlying coupling are discussed elsewhere in this chapter. Does coupling influence breathing pattern during exercise? This issue has been addressed in a number of studies where limb movement frequency was changed without significant changes in metabolic rate. Bayly et al. (44) observed changes in f_b with changes in running speed at matched $\dot{V}CO_2$ in horses. Similarly, Loring et al. (252) observed significant increases in f_b related to increased limb movement frequency in humans during treadmill exercise. Minute ventilation was not measured in this study and it is conceivable that the increase in f_b was related to an increase in $\dot{V}_E$. However, this is very unlikely because of the magnitude of the changes in f_b and because estimated metabolic rate remained constant as limb frequency increased. Loring et al. also found that limb frequency influenced f_b on occasions when there was no evidence of entrainment, and this merits further study. Prabhu et al. (333) examined this issue during cycle ergometry in humans. They found no change in V_T, f_b, or respiratory timing at matched $\dot{V}_E$ as pedaling frequency was varied from 40–80 rpm in the same subjects. This was also found in several subjects who had clear evidence of respiratory-locomotor coupling; these subjects varied the coupling ratio without changing f_b as pedaling frequency changed. Therefore, the extent to which limb movement frequency influences breathing pattern clearly varies with the mode of exercise. Possible mechanisms underlying this phenomenon are discussed elsewhere in this chapter.

It has frequently been suggested that physical training causes breathing pattern to become slower and deeper (20, 371). As recently demonstrated by McParland et al. (276), there is little experimental support for this idea.

Breathing Pattern during Recovery from Exercise

Younes and colleagues (443, 444) observed rapid shallow breathing during recovery from maximal exercise in most, but not all, humans. For a given level of $\dot{V}_E$, V_T was less and f_b greater during recovery than during exercise. This phenomenon is limited to very high exercise levels and was only observed when $\dot{V}O_2$ at end exercise exceeded 92% of maximal $\dot{V}O_2$. Caillaud et al. (71) noted greater tachypnea during the recovery period in trained than in untrained subjects. Younes et al. (443) suggested that this tachypnea during recovery may be due to pulmonary edema or inspiratory muscle fatigue developing near maximal exercise. The former possibility is supported indirectly by the observation that rapid shallow breathing during recovery from exercise also occurs, though at much lower work rates, in patients with cardiac failure (145). Exercise-induced diaphragmatic fatigue has been clearly demonstrated in humans and this is reviewed elsewhere in this chapter. Diaphragmatic fatigue appears unlikely to cause the rapid shallow breathing during recovery from exercise because this rapid shallow breathing is unaffected by unloading inspiratory muscles during exercise (146).

Physiological Implications of Exercise Breathing Pattern

The increase in respiratory muscle recruitment during exercise requires increased energy supply to the respiratory muscles (see later under RESPIRATORY MUSCLE PERFUSION AND ENERGETICS). This in turn requires increased blood flow to and increased oxygen extraction by the respiratory muscles. The increased respiratory (especially inspiratory) muscle recruitment is also a major contributor to the sensation of breathlessness that is experienced during exercise. Therefore, increased energy cost of breathing and breathlessness are two of the "costs" of the hyperpneic response to exercise. Does the pattern of breathing adopted during exercise allow these costs to be met in an efficient way? Classic studies by Otis et al. (306) and Mead (278) examined the influence of breathing pattern on work of breathing and mean respiratory muscle pressure. These studies suggested that the respiratory frequency adopted at rest is least costly in terms of respiratory energetics; significant increases or decreases in f_b from this "optimal" level should increase the energy cost of breathing. More recent studies have used more elaborate mathematical models to examine this question (98). Yamashiro and colleagues (438) concluded that the changes in f_b, EILV, and EELV adopted by humans during exercise serve to minimize the work of breathing. The quasi-rectangular flow pattern adopted during exercise (Fig. 11.7) is also efficient in reducing the energy cost of breathing (232).

Apart from overall respiratory muscle energetics, differences in recruitment pattern between different respiratory muscles may have obvious advantages. The significant expiratory muscle recruitment during exercise lessens the pressure that inspiratory muscles have to generate, as well as improving their pressure-generating capacity through the length–tension effect. The increased recruitment of rib cage inspiratory muscles during exercise helps to reduce the work the diaphragm has to perform, thus possibly delaying or preventing the onset of diaphragmatic fatigue. The inspiratory duty cycle of 0.5 adopted during exercise (see Fig. 11.5) may also be optimal in improving diaphragmatic blood flow (189).

The pattern of breathing during exercise also influences the sensation of dyspnea. The intensity of dyspnea appears to be related more to peak, rather than mean, inspiratory pressure (220). Breathing over the linear part of the respiratory pressure–volume curve causes peak inspiratory pressure to be less than if higher lung volumes were used. However, the "need" to maintain EILV in the linear part of the pressure–volume curve appears to be overridden in fit elderly people, who frequently have an EILV that is 95% of total lung capacity (205, 206). There is evidence that respiratory sensation is impaired in the elderly and it is possible that this may be why the elderly tolerate a higher EILV than do younger subjects. The factors that regulate breathlessness during exercise are reviewed elsewhere in this chapter (see later under *An Urge to Breathe*).

The increased tidal volume during exercise is clearly useful in reducing relative dead space ventilation (V_D/V_T). V_T increases further in response to dead space loading, and it has been suggested that this response is directed toward optimizing gas exchange (277). The pattern of respiratory muscle contraction adopted during exercise can also influence cardiac function.

Changes in intrathoracic pressure and lung volume may influence cardiac preload and afterload. Changes in abdominal pressure may also influence venous return. While the effects of changing intrathoracic and abdominal pressures have been investigated extensively at rest (see 317 for a detailed review), there are relatively few data during exercise (152).

Therefore, there are reasons to suggest that the pattern of breathing adopted during exercise might, at least partly, be directed toward optimizing respiratory muscle energetics, respiratory sensation, gas exchange, or cardiac function. There are insufficient data at this time to clearly indicate which (if any) of these is assigned the highest priority by the respiratory control system. We suggest that optimizing respiratory muscle energetics or respiratory sensation is usually most important in humans during heavy exercise. The relative priority of these "costs" may change when the need to optimize gas exchange or cardiac function increases; the increase in V_T with dead space loading is consistent with this idea (277).

IMPORTANCE OF RESPIRATORY LOAD IN REGULATION OF EXERCISE HYPERPNEA

$\dot{V}_E$ and mechanical breathing pattern are the end result of the interaction between the pattern of respiratory muscle contraction and the mechanical properties of the respiratory system. As discussed earlier (see earlier under EFFECTS OF EXERCISE ON PASSIVE RESPIRATORY MECHANICS), passive respiratory mechanics change little with exercise. Therefore, it is the changes in intensity and pattern of respiratory muscle contraction that cause the changes in $\dot{V}_E$ and mechanical breathing pattern during exercise.

How do normal respiratory mechanics influence respiratory muscle output and $\dot{V}_E$ during exercise? This issue has been addressed with two different methods of "unloading" the respiratory system during exercise. One method substitutes helium for nitrogen, and this reduces turbulent airflow and thus decreases airway resistance during exercise. A second method applies a positive-pressure assist, proportional to inspiratory flow rate and/or inspired volume, during inspiration (146, 227, 266, 323, 442). This method essentially applies a "negative resistance" (or elastance) in series with the normal inspiratory resistance. Some of these studies also provided pressure assist during expiration; that is, mouth pressure during expiration was negative in proportion to expiratory flow rate (146, 227).

Helium-Oxygen Unloading

Hussain et al. (193) found a significant fall in average rate of rise of the diaphragm EMG when He-O_2 was substituted for room air during exercise in humans. This fall occurred within the first breath following administration of He-O_2. Similarly, Forster et al. (134) found a significant fall in average rate of rise and duration of the diaphragm EMG signal within three breaths of breathing He-O_2 in exercise in ponies. This rapid fall in diaphragm EMG is presumably a reflex response to activation of respiratory mechanoreceptors, consequent on changing from room air to He-O_2 breathing.

The initial fall in diaphragm activation due to breathing He-O_2 is proportionally less than the change in respiratory load, resulting in an increase in $\dot{V}_E$ with He-O_2 breathing. This hyperventilation is most marked at high levels of $\dot{V}_E$ (64, 104, 193), though it has also been observed at relatively low levels of $\dot{V}_E$ (414). Forster et al. (134) found that diaphragm EMG activity increased gradually after the initial fall in response to He-O_2 substitution. Thereafter, in the steady state of He-O_2 breathing, diaphragm EMG activity was unchanged from the initial room air period. The mechanisms underlying this gradual increase in diaphragm EMG activity are unclear. It should also be noted that the rise in $\dot{V}_E$ due to He-O_2 inhalation in the study of Forster et al. was usually not accompanied by a fall in arterial P_{CO_2}. Therefore, metabolic rate or dead space ventilation must have changed, and factors other than helium itself might contribute to the late increase in diaphragm activation with He-O_2 in ponies. In contrast, He-O_2 breathing during heavy exercise in humans raises $\dot{V}_E$ and lowers arterial P_{CO_2} (104, 141).

Unloading with Pressure Assist

When the second method, pressure assist, was used during exercise in humans, this caused a marked fall in respiratory muscle pressure during exercise (146, 227). This fall in respiratory muscle pressure was such that $\dot{V}_E$ remained constant or showed only minor changes compared to exercise without pressure assist. Krishnan et al. (227) recently examined the effects of pressure assist during endurance exercise to exhaustion. Pressure assist resulted in significant falls in inspiratory and expiratory muscle pressure, with no significant change in $\dot{V}_E$ during exercise; $\dot{V}_E$ (mean $\pm$ SEM) at end exercise was 137 $\pm$ 15 with pressure assist compared to 133 $\pm$ 15 liters/min in control exercise. There was also no significant change in EILV or EELV with unloading.

Conclusion

So what can we conclude about the role of the normal respiratory load in regulation of exercise hyperpnea? Studies using He-O_2 and pressure assist both show that reduction in the normal load reduces respiratory muscle output. Based on data from He-O_2 experiments, this reduction is immediate and presumably involves reflex mechanisms. The reduction in respiratory muscle output with pressure assist is proportional to the change in respiratory load so that $\dot{V}_E$ remains essentially unchanged. The fall in muscle output with He-O_2 breathing is usually less than the fall in load, so that $\dot{V}_E$ increases. Why is there this discrepancy? Pressure-assist and He-O_2 breathing both reduce the pressure that respiratory muscles have to generate for a given $\dot{V}_E$, but the extent of muscle unloading is much greater with pressure assist. He-O_2 reduces airway resistance and changes the distribution of resistance among different parts of the airways, while pressure assist does not do this; if anything, pressure assist may cause a small increase in pulmonary resistance (146, 227). It is possible that the hyperventilation related to He-O_2 is related directly to its effects on airway mechanics; it might be related to the increase in the maximum flow–volume curve due to helium breathing. The lack of significant change in $\dot{V}_E$ with pressure assist during heavy exercise suggests that the work that the respiratory muscles have to perform during exercise does not constrain $\dot{V}_E$ during exercise.

LOCOMOTOR-RESPIRATION INTERDEPENDENCE

During exercise, limb movements and breathing efforts do not remain as independent and isolated events but, rather, the outcome of one activity ultimately influences that of the other. The nature of these locomotor-respiratory interactions can be considered from two basic perspectives: *(1)* the biomechanical effects of tightly linking locomotion with respiration and *(2)* the impact of locomotion per se on respiratory muscle activities, independent of locomotory:respiratory coupling. These two concepts are examined in the following sections.

Entrainment—the Most Obvious Locomotor-Respiratory Interaction

Entrainment or synchronization between limb movements and breathing patterns is commonly observed in exercising humans and quadrupeds (25, 62). In humans, entrainment occurs during running, cycling, and rowing (46, 225, 312, 397) and, although the exact "stimulus" for entrainment remains obscure, several factors are associated with its occurrence. Within a given exercise modality, *experienced* runners, cyclists, or rowers entrain more readily than nonexperienced participants (60, 225, 258). However, entrainment in naive subjects can be promoted through *auditory cues* using metronomes (46, 440). For a particular activity, such as cycling, some subjects will entrain more frequently as the *work intensity* increases (72, 200, 397), but physical fitness alone apparently has no influence on the degree of coordination between breathing and exercise rhythms (151). Finally, the *type of rhythmic exercise* also influences the degree of entrainment. At comparable work intensities, breathing-exercise coordination is higher during running than cycling (46, 54), perhaps because running is a more natural movement form for a bipedal mammal (311).

Cursorial mammals—dogs and horses—also exhibit locomotory:respiratory coupling, although the degree of entrainment here appears to be primarily a function of the *gait* (27, 62, 188) and the *duration* of exercise (24). One-to-one coupling of stride frequency and breathing frequency is found consistently in *cantering* or *galloping* horses—a linkage that remains even if 6% CO_2 challenge is superimposed upon the exercise bout (155)—whereas entrainment is inconsistent in walking or trotting horses (24, 188, 233). Likewise, in exercising dogs, entrainment also can be an inconsistent finding, perhaps due to the variable nature of the canine breathing pattern. (Dogs frequently "pant" or breathe at frequencies > 1.5 Hz during exercise as a means of thermoregulation.) Bramble and colleagues reported 1:1 and 2:1 ratios between breathing and stride frequency in galloping or trotting dogs (62, 63), while Ainsworth et al. did not find strict locomotory:respiratory coupling in dogs walking or trotting on the treadmill while breathing at frequencies either less than 1 Hz (11) or between 2–5 Hz (12).

How Does Entrainment Effect Ventilation?

A biomechanical approach has classically been advanced to explain the generation of airflow during exercise and is appealing from a systems energetic consideration. Because both exercise and respiration rely on cyclical movements impacting upon the thoracic complex, to circumvent any mechanical constraints developing as a result of limb motion, breathing must be made to fit the locomotory cycle (62). Three exercise-associated forces have been postulated to generate airflow in humans and quadrupeds during locomotion. These include *(1)* forces resulting from accelerations and decelerations of the trunk that produce *to-and-fro movements of the liver* ("the visceral piston") that effect diaphragmatic movement; *(2)* concussive forces resulting from *limb impact* which, when transmitted to the thoracic cavity, produce pressure or volume changes; and *(3)* compressive forces developing within the abdominal cavity during *lumbrosacral flexion and extension*, which ultimately produce pressure and volume changes within the thoracic cavity (61, 445). The biomechanical importance of these three forces on the breathing cycle has been developed more extensively for quadrupedal locomotion.

In the *cantering* horse, inhalation begins when the horse first becomes airborne, as the trunk is accelerated forward, causing rearward displacement of the liver and abdominal contents. This action, along with forelimb extension and upward movement of the head, enlarges the rib cage, decreases intrathoracic pressure, and promotes inspiratory flow. Then, as the hindlimbs are extended caudally due to lumbrosacral extension, the abdominal volume increases and the abdominal pressure decreases, aiding diaphragmatic descent. Expiration begins as the concussive forces of forelimb impact are transmitted to the thorax, externally loading and compressing the rib cage. Deceleration of the trunk, due to limb impact, causes cranial development of the "visceral piston" and this, along with abdominal compression due to lumbosacral flexion, further assists with expiratory flow. The emphasis in this model is the generation of airflow due to forces developing secondary to limb or head movement, which by virtue of their muscular attachments to the thoracic complex effect intrathoracic pressure and volume changes. However, although the biomechanical model fits well with the observed locomotory movements and respiratory airflow patterns in galloping horses (27), little conclusive evidence exists to support the relative contributions of these biomechanical forces during exercise. Indeed, Young et al. (445) recently challenged the effectiveness of the "visceral piston." Based upon models of visceral accelerations and decelerations, they estimated visceral displacements to be 230 degrees out of phase with ventilation and concluded that lumbosacral flexions and extensions, rather than visceral piston displacements, exerted a more significant biomechanical effect on ventilation. Furthermore, Frevert and colleagues (140) also have contested the importance of limb impact on respiratory airflow. They studied galloping horses that *occasionally* departed from the usual 1:1 locomotory:respiratory ratios during exercise. During these intervals (when locomotory:respiratory ratios ≠ 1), they ensemble averaged the flow signals using the limb frequency as a trigger. In doing so, flows associated with breathing averaged to zero, allowing them to calculate flows associated with stride. Stride-related volume excursions averaged 10%–20% of the tidal volume, suggesting that only a small part of respiratory airflow resulted from this biomechanical force.

Although biomechanical forces may contribute to the generation of airflow during exercise, one must still acknowledge the *active* contribution of respiratory muscles to breathing, either in the presence or

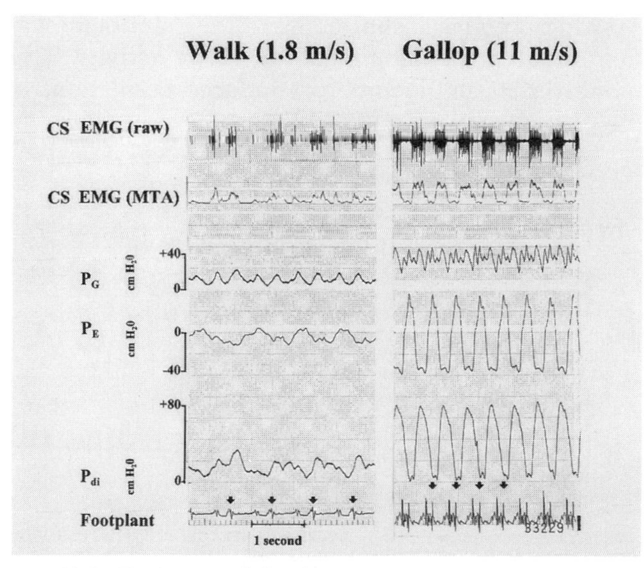

FIG. 11.8. Equine costal diaphragmatic EMG (raw and moving time-averaged); gastric, esophageal, and transdiaphragmatic pressure (PG, PE, and Pdi); and accelerometer tracing indicating left forelimb impact (*arrows*) during walking and during galloping (11 ms). Note that the foot plant activity does not occur during a consistent phase of the respiratory cycle when the horse is walking, whereas phase-linking is apparent during the gallop. (From Ainsworth et al. (9).]

absence of entrainment. Indeed, recent data from Ainsworth et al. (9) have clearly demonstrated that the major inspiratory muscle of the horse—the diaphragm—is electrically active during exercise and that this EMG activity is associated with the development of a concurrent mechanical effect—transdiaphragmatic pressure generation. As shown in Figure 11.8, phasic diaphragmatic electrical activity is apparent in this horse walking on the treadmill (1.8 m/s) when breathing and stride frequency are not tightly linked. During the gallop—when the horse is entrained—a further increase in the phasic electrical activity as well as in the peak inspiratory transdiaphragmatic pressure is apparent. In fact, the exercise-induced increases in diaphragmatic EMG are always positively correlated with increments in transdiaphragmatic pressure, suggesting that the ventilatory demands are met by active recruitment of the diaphragm, even if locomotion and respiration are linked.

Is there Stronger Evidence to Support a Significant Biomechanical Effect of Locomotion on Respiration in Dogs?

Bramble and Jenkins (63) used cineradiographic techniques to assess diaphragmatic and truncal excursions in dogs trotting on a treadmill and breathing at high frequencies (panting). By tracking the craniocaudad and dorsoventrad movements of the diaphragm (relative to a radiodense marker on the tenth thoracic vertebra), they determined that when the diaphragm was "relaxed," craniocaudad and dorsoventrad diaphragmatic displacements were related 1:1 to locomotory-induced truncal accelerations/decelerations. Furthermore, during these periods of "*diaphragmatic relaxation*," inspiratory and expiratory flow also tracked locomotory-induced diaphragmatic displacements 1:1. However, during certain breathing cycles, Bramble and Jenkins noted that *cranial* displacements of the diaphragm became smaller and the rate of diaphragmatic displacement was unrelated to the breathing frequency. As a consequence, airflow rates *exceeded* diaphragmatic contraction rates—ratios varied from 3:1 to 10:1—but airflow rates still remained linked 2:1 with stride frequency. Thus, they concluded that the main function of the diaphragmatic "contractions" was to periodically "reset" the oscillating diaphragm so that displacements induced by locomotion were again initiated from a more caudal diaphragmatic position.

In this biomechanical model, Bramble and Jenkins ascribed a major role to the visceral piston in generating airflow in trotting dogs. In fact, they likened the to-and-fro movement of the liver against the diaphragm, in combination with the alternating compressive forces generated by limb impact, to a system of three individual pistons. Not only did these three forces contribute to respiratory airflow but, because of their asynchronous activity, asymmetric ventilation of the apical and diaphragmatic lung lobes occurred. They argued that, while *craniocaudad* diaphragmatic displacements periodically were unlinked with respiratory flow, *dorsoventral* diaphragmatic displacements (secondary to visceral piston activity) remained synchronized with respiratory airflow. Because this dorsoventrad force impacted predominantly on the diaphragmatic lung lobes, volume changes occurred within these lobar segments. However, when the two sides of the thorax were alternately loaded and unloaded, compression or expansion of the underlying apical lung lobes produced asynchronous emptying and filling.

Additional data supporting the importance of limb impact on airflow generation in exercising dogs has recently become evident. Ainsworth and colleagues (12) found that when dogs walk or trot on the treadmill, they exhibit two basic types of breathing patterns—type A and type B. Type A is a pure high-frequency breathing pattern in which esophageal pressure oscillations occur at frequencies ranging from 2–5 Hz. This pattern is *similar* to the breathing pattern described by Bramble and Jenkins (63) and is demonstrated in the *left panel* of Figure 11.9. However, this is *not* the breathing pattern for which a discernible effect of foot impact on esophageal pressure generation (and hence airflow) could be detected. Rather, it is the second type of breathing pattern, type B, which appears to contain locomotory-associated esophageal pressure fluctuations. Specifically, the type B pattern is characterized by a slower inherent breathing rate (<1 Hz) upon which are superimposed high-frequency oscillations in the esophageal pressure, ranging from 3–6 Hz. As shown in the *right panel* of Figure 11.9, the high-frequency esophageal pressure oscillations occurring during inspiration are associated with electrical activation of the diaphragm and probably represent a "panting" pattern superimposed upon the slower inspiratory time. Note, however, that the high-frequency esophageal pressure fluctuations occurring during expiration are not associated with diaphragmatic EMG but are associated with footplant activity.

Although footplant-associated forces are capable of producing ventilation, other aspects of the biomechanical model of Bramble and Jenkins remain questionable: These investigators used cineradiographic data to *infer* the physiological status—relaxed or contracted—of the diaphragm, and in the absence of direct EMG measurements, such assumptions may be misleading or inaccurate. Indeed, recent EMG and sonomicrometry data from exercising dogs (12) challenge the thesis of *passive* diaphragmatic oscillations and airflow production. Specifically, these investigators found that transpulmonary pressure changes (and hence fluctuations in respiratory airflow) in exercising dogs were directly correlated 1:1 with phasic electrical activation and shortening of costal and crural diaphragm (Fig. 11.10). In addition, phasic shortening of the diaphragm was not apparent in the *absence* of EMG activity. This implied that any locomotory-induced oscillations of

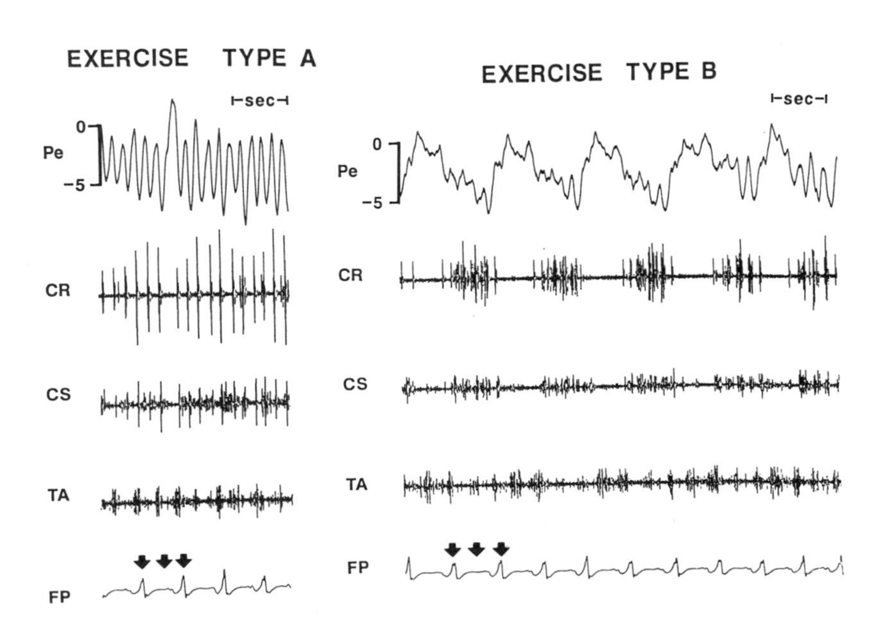

FIG. 11.9. Canine breathing patterns are highly variable, as shown in this figure for one dog trotting on the treadmill while unencumbered by a breathing mask. The two types of patterns—**high-frequency** type A (*left panel*), a pure high frequency oscillation in the esophageal pressure; and **mixed-frequency** type B (*right panel*), a slower inherent breathing pattern with superimposed high-frequency oscillations in the esophageal pressure—are apparent. Esophageal pressure (Pe), crural (CR), costal (CS), transverse abdominal (TA) EMG, and foot plant left hindlimb (FP) are shown. In type A and type B, decrements in esophageal pressure (and airflow) are always associated with electrical activation of the costal and crural diaphragm. In type B, oscillations in the esophageal pressure during expiration occur at intervals related to foot plant and hence TA activation. (From Ainsworth et al. (12).]

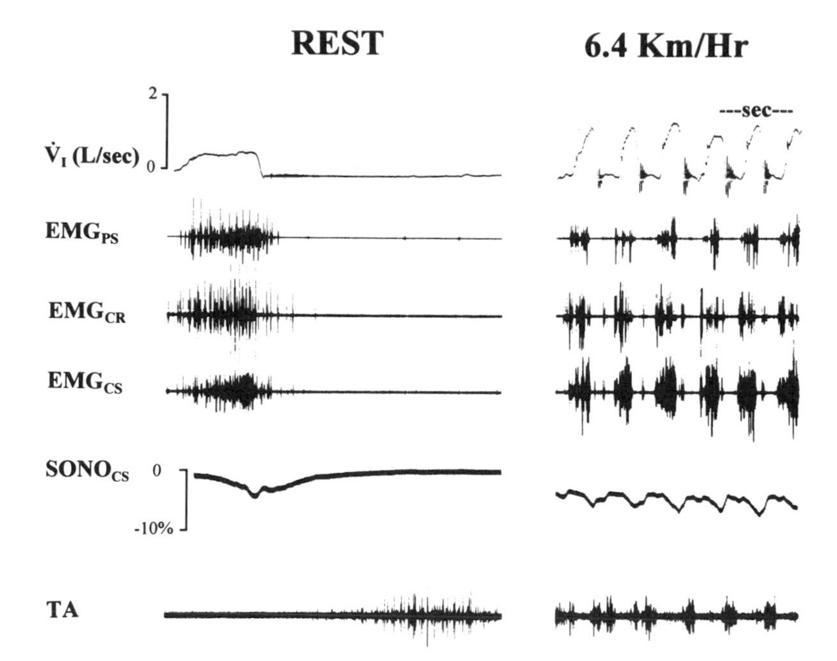

FIG. 11.10. Inspiratory flow (VI); electrical activity of the parasternal (PS, rib cage inspiratory), crural (CR), and costal (CS) diaphragm, and transverse abdominal (TA) muscles and sonomicrometry tracing of the costal diaphragm (SONO CS) in one dog at rest and during trotting. Note that either at rest or during exercise, phasic electrical activity of both inspiratory and expiratory muscles is evident and that phasic shortening of the costal diaphragm (downward displacement of SONO tracing) occurs only during electrical activation. This breathing pattern is representative of high-frequency breathing with f_b = 115 breaths · min^{-1} [From Ainsworth et al. (12).]

the diaphragm due to the visceral piston were either ineffective or occurred at frequencies equal to that of diaphragmatic contraction (3–5 Hz). However, because breathing and stride frequencies were not tightly coupled in these dogs, entrainment of diaphragmatic movement with hepatic excursions seemed unlikely. Thus these investigators provide direct evidence demonstrating that airflow is associated with electrical activation of the diaphragmatic, rib cage inspiratory, and abdominal expiratory muscles in panting dogs during exercise. The only place for passive mechanical effects seems to be during expiration, when the high-frequency oscillations were superimposed upon the slower breathing pattern.

Are Biomechanical Effects Important in Entrainment in Humans?

The actual contribution of the three locomotory-associated forces—visceral piston movement, foot impact, and lumbosacral flexion and extension—on human respiratory patterns has also been difficult to quantify. Furthermore, some physiologists doubt that the visceral piston even produces a significant impact on the diaphragm and chest wall mechanics based upon its vector orientation produced during running (400). Nonetheless, in an attempt to assess its contribution to respiration, MacDonald and colleagues (254) studied the breathing patterns in subjects propelling wheelchairs via arm-thrust movements. They reasoned that, in the absence of bipedal locomotion, impact loading of the lower body would be eliminated, negating any contribution of the visceral piston to breathing. Based upon the low entrainment rates between limb movement and breathing frequency found in their subjects (40%), they concluded that visceral movement was indeed necessary for the development of entrainment. Likewise, Paterson and colleagues (312) studied entrainment in subjects performing arm or leg ergometry exercises and found that entrainment developed only during 25% of the total exercise period. They concluded that the intermittent nature of entrainment during these types of exercises, compared to the higher incidence reported during treadmill running and unrestrained running, could be due to a greater involvement of active muscles and to a piston-like action of the visceral mass enforcing a rhythmicity on the respiratory system.

Banzett and colleagues (40) examined the relative importance of foot impact on breathing in humans walking and running on a treadmill. They hypothesized that upward acceleration of the spine associated with footfall would produce two separate effects—expiratory displacements of the rib cage and inspiratory displacements of the diaphragm and abdomen—as the abdominal mass moved downward relative to the spine. The net effect of these two actions would be reflected in the flow pattern observed at the mouth. To identify the cyclic contributions of locomotion to flow, they used footfall as a trigger to ensemble average the flow signal. So, during periods when breathing and stepping were not synchronized, the ensemble average contained only those flow events associated with the step cycle. They determined that step-related volume changes averaged a mere 1%–2% of the tidal volume excursions and concluded that this biomechanical force produced too small an effect to contribute appreciably to pulmonary ventilation.

Finally, the impact of abdominal compressive forces, secondary to lumbosacral flexion and extension, on breathing patterns also has been examined in studies of elite rowers. Because the cramped body position assumed by the rower at the start of the rowing stroke would presumably impair diaphragmatic excursions (96), one would predict that this biomechanical constraint would affect the pattern of breathing opted by the rowers. Steinacker and colleagues (381) studied oarsmen performing incremental rowing ergometry and found that as work intensity increased, rowers switched from a 1:1 to a 2:1 breath/stroke ratio. They concluded that this transition was due to pulmonary mechanical constraints. As the demand for tidal volume increased with increasing work intensity, breathing efforts encroached upon the flat portion of the pulmonary compliance curve. Hence, a greater portion of the negative intrapleural pressure change was used to overcome pulmonary elastic work. However, although the transition from a 1:1 to a 2:1 ratio circumvented the mechanical limitation of lung distention during inspiration, the respiratory system was now confronted with a different mechanical constraint, that of expiratory flow limitation. Interestingly, given that such mechanical limitations developed, one would have predicted that the onset of inspiration relative to the stroke cycle would have been tightly regulated. This was specifically examined by Mahler et al. (258), who studied the breathing pattern of elite oarswomen. They found that, whereas the rowers consistently entrained breathing and stroke frequencies 1:1 or 2:1, considerable variability in the *onset* of inspiration during the rowing cycle occurred. Some rowers initiated inspiration prior to the "catch" or start of the cycle, some inspired at the point of the catch, and others inspired at the finish of the stroke cycle. Thus, despite the development of a significant biomechanical limitation, optimization of the onset of either inspiration or expiration was not apparent.

Are there Any Benefits to Locomotory:Respiratory Coupling? If respiratory and locomotory muscles could share a common task then, theoretically, the efficiency of respiratory muscles might increase, possibly improving gas exchange and deterring the development of diaphragmatic fatigue (203). Unfortunately, few studies (to date) have specifically addressed these questions. However, Garlando and co-workers (151) examined the relationship between the degree of entrainment (spontaneous or acoustically triggered breathing) and oxygen uptake in cyclists working at moderate loads—50% of their work capacity—while pedaling at 70 cycles/min. Subjects were studied four times and minute ventilation and end-expiratory P_{CO_2} did not vary significantly between runs. They found as the degree of entrainment increased between exercise bouts, $\dot{V}_{O_2}$ decreased approximately 40 ml/min or 2%–3% of the total $\dot{V}_{O_2}$ [Fig. 11.3; (151)]. Based upon the work of Aaron et al. (2), in which the oxygen cost of breathing during moderate exercise is 3%–5% of the total $\dot{V}_{O_2}$ (see Fig. 11.12), the observed reduction reported by Garlando et al. may have represented a 50% decrease in the total oxygen cost of breathing. Although the mechanism underlying such reductions in $\dot{V}_{O_2}$ could not be determined in their study, they proposed that synchronization enabled one to combine the ventilatory and postural functions of the respiratory muscles with a substantial reduction in energy cost.

The impact of entrainment on gas exchange has also been of interest to equine exercise physiologists, especially in lieu of the finding that horses lack an adequate hyperventilatory response during intense exercise (44). Evans and colleagues (125) examined the effect of entrainment on alveolar ventilation in standardbred horses taught to gallop or to pace at 13 m/sec—maximum oxygen consumption. During the gallop, stride and breathing frequencies were linked 1:1, but during the pace, entrainment ratios of 1:3 were observed. Despite the differences in breathing strategies (during the pace the frequency was slower), at comparable metabolic loads, the degree of arterial hypercapnia was the same in both groups. Thus, entrainment did not appear to affect the development or severity of alveolar hypoventilation in this species.

Finally, the potential development of asynchronous ventilation in exercising dogs as a sequela to entrainment has been addressed earlier. One potential benefit of the interlobar exchange may be a more thorough mixing of airway gases, which would improve gas exchange efficiency and minimize dead space ventilation (63).

Locomotory:Respiratory Interactions, Independent of Entrainment

By now it is apparent that while biomechanical forces developing during entrainment may contribute to the generation of airflow, breathing still remains a neurally mediated event. Indeed, ample evidence exists from studies of chronically instrumented quadrupeds demonstrating that *(1)* both inspiratory and expiratory muscles are electrically active during eupnea, *(2)* that this electrical activity is associated with phasic muscle shortening, and *(3)* that phasic EMG activity of both inspiratory and expiratory muscles increases significantly during the hyperpnea of exercise (9, 11–13, 169). However, because coactivation of respiratory and locomotory muscles during exercise occurs, subtle locomotory:respiratory interactions, *independent* of strict entrainment, may develop. For example, locomotion may influence the efficiency of respiratory (diaphragmatic) activity or conversely, respiratory muscles may modulate locomotory functions.

Optimization of Respiratory Muscle Length–Tension Relationships. During exercise in both humans and quadrupeds, tonic and phasic recruitment of abdominal expiratory muscles improves inspiratory muscle function. Specifically, in the absence of glottal narrowing or increases in postinspiration inspiratory activity of the diaphragm, increases in phasic expiratory muscle activity augment mean expiratory airflow and contribute to decrements in end-expiratory lung volume (11, 366). Furthermore, increases in tonic abdominal muscle activity, as evidenced by shifts in either the mean gastric pressure (Fig. 11.11) or in the baseline of the moving time-averaged EMG signal (11, 182) influence inspiratory muscle activity in at least two ways. First, by "stiffening" the abdominal wall and making the abdominal cavity less compliant, the abdominal fulcrum against which diaphragmatic contraction occurs is improved. Second, tonic abdominal muscle activity contributes to significant decreases in end-expiratory lung volume, the net effect of which is an improvement in the length–tension relationships of the inspiratory muscles. (Recall that for a given neural input, a greater degree of tension or pressure is generated when the muscle is lengthened). Finally, an additional benefit of augmented tonic abdominal muscle activity relates not to a respiratory function but rather to a locomotory effect. By increasing the intra-abdominal pressure, the abdominal cavity more efficiently supports the upper part of the body, unloads the spine, and act as a "shock absorber" during exercise (164). The net effect is to lessen the concussive forces transmitted to the vertebral column and cranium. Furthermore, this increase in tonic ab-

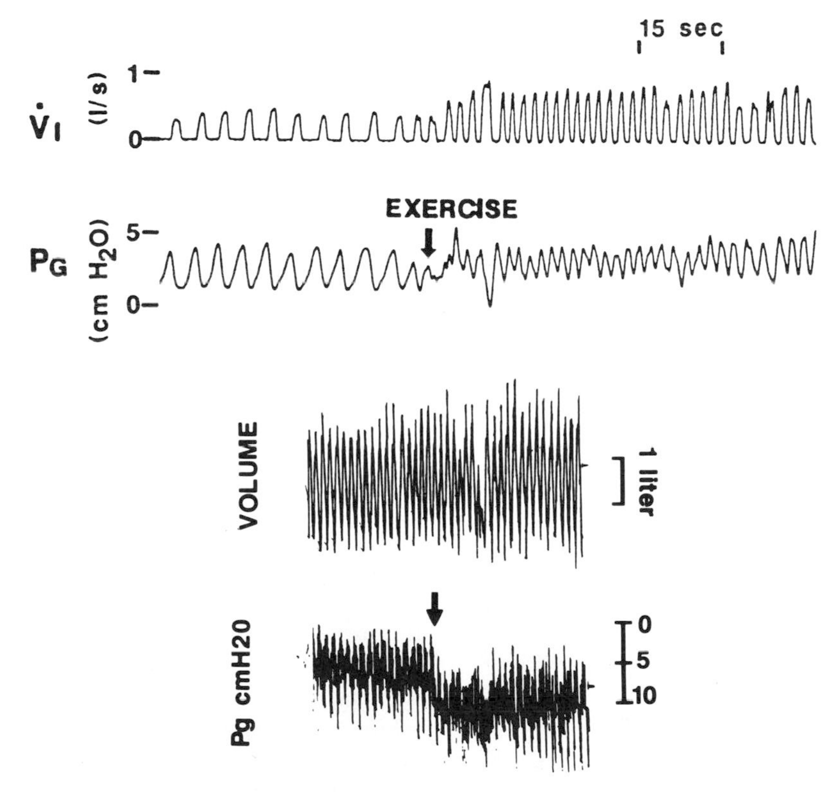

FIG. 11.11. Inspiratory flow (VI) or tidal volume and gastric pressure (PG) traces from a human (*left panel*) and a dog (*right panel*). In the dog, note that at the onset of exercise, mean gastric pressure increases due to tonic increases in abdominal muscle activity. (From Ainsworth et al. (11).] In the human, gastric pressure increases during the transition from the walk to the jog. (From Henke et al. (182).] (Please note, in the dog an increased gastric pressure moves upward in the figure; whereas in the human the PG scales are reversed and increased PG moves down.)

dominal muscle activity and intra-abdominal pressure serves to reduce the magnitude of visceral displacements (164).

Impact of Respiratory Muscle Activities on Locomotory Functions. During quadrupedal exercise, abdominal expiratory muscles may also modulate locomotory effects. Normally, during quiet breathing in awake quadrupeds, the transverse abdominal muscle is phasically active during expiration, as evidenced from both EMG and sonomicrometry studies in awake quadrupeds (169, 243, 377). In exercising dogs, breathing at either slow or fast frequencies, the transverse abdominal muscle exhibits a bursting pattern coincident with footplant (Fig. 11.9), although its expiratory role is still preserved as evidenced from the accentuated EMG occurring during expiration (11, 12). Based upon its anatomical attachments, it is unlikely that the transverse abdominal muscle protracts the hindlimbs. Instead, locomotory-associated activity may serve to limit or counteract truncal rotation, preventing deformations of the chest and abdomen and preserving the configurations of the respiratory muscles so that optimal tension may develop with each breath during exercise.

Conclusion

During exercise, a number of different locomotory: respiratory interactions develop that may ultimately impact upon the efficiency of either activity. If entrainment develops, then the biomechanical forces derived from visceral piston activity, foot impact, and lumbosacral flexion might produce intrathoracic volume changes and contribute to airflow generation. The effect of each of these biomechanical forces on ventilation has been examined in both quadrupeds and humans, and its impact appears to be variable. Nevertheless, these forces are not the sole determinants of airflow, as ample evidence exists from chronically instrumented animals demonstrating the active contribution of the diaphragm (and other respiratory muscles) to breathing. Furthermore, because of coactivation of respiratory and locomotory muscles during exercise, subtle interactions develop that ultimately influence diaphragmatic operating lengths (via alterations in tonic abdominal activity) or modulate the extent of truncal rotation induced by locomotion.

RESPIRATORY MUSCLE PERFUSION AND ENERGETICS

Energy expenditure required by the respiratory muscles during exercise is dependent upon exercise-induced changes in several types of mechanical work by the respiratory muscles (see earlier under Methods of Assessment of Respiratory Muscle Contraction). First, elastic work is expended for lung expansion during inspiration and to overcome elastic work done on the chest wall during expiration. This elastic component will be further affected by any reductions in dynamic compliance or changes in muscle length (i.e., EELV) during exercise. Second, resistive work will increase nonlinearly as increasing flow rate becomes fully turbulent and expiratory work will rise disproportionally at very heavy work rates as airways undergo dynamic compression and expiratory flow limitation occurs to varying degrees. The increased velocity of muscle shortening at any given developed tension will also increase respiratory muscle $\dot{V}O_2$ (273). Third, in heavy exercise it is likely (although not as yet fully described) that extra work will be performed by the inspiratory and expiratory muscles during deformation of the rib cage and abdominal walls (156). Finally, the increased blood flow required for hyperpnea may also require an additional increase in energy expenditure in the form of cardiac work (19).

Oxygen Cost of Hyperpnea

Measuring the O_2 or energy cost of exercise hyperpnea in humans or animals is complex. In experimental animals, respiratory muscle blood flow during exercise is measurable (see below), and since muscle $\dot{V}O_2$ and $\dot{Q}$ usually change together, a good estimate of O_2 requirement can be derived from blood flow measurements (see below). For example, Manohar's microsphere measurements of blood flow to the diaphragm and to all inspiratory and expiratory muscles of the rib cage and abdominal wall showed that "respiratory" muscle $\dot{Q}$ increased up to 15% of total cardiac output at peak exercise in the pony (263). Unfortunately, respiratory muscles are also recruited to a significant extent both tonically and phasically for locomotor and postural purposes during exercise (see earlier under Are there Any Benefits to Locomotory:Respiratory Coupling?); thus, this approach will clearly overestimate the oxygen cost of the hyperpnea alone. In humans, an indirect approach is to measure the change in total body $\dot{V}O_2$ while changing ventilation and ventilatory work by voluntary hyperpnea and/or added CO_2 or added resistances. Not surprisingly, these approaches have produced a wide range of values as representing the oxygen cost of hyperpnea (see review in 2). A recent approach had resting subjects voluntarily duplicate the esophageal and transdiaphragmatic pressures, breathing pattern, end-expiratory lung volume, and $\dot{V}E$ they utilized during moderate and maximum intensity exercise (2). The estimates obtained for the oxygen cost of hyperpnea over a wide range of $\dot{V}E$ were reproducible and consistent with other published values obtained at comparable levels of ventilatory work (19). The values obtained with this approach (i.e., with the subject at rest) represent an estimate of the oxygen cost of the primarily phasic ventilatory work and work expended in chest wall stabilization by the respiratory muscles during exercise but do not include the energy expended for locomotor-related actions of these muscles.

Figure 11.12 shows the oxygen cost per liter of ventilation and the $\dot{V}O_2$ for hyperpnea as a percentage of total body $\dot{V}O_2$ at increasing minute ventilations during moderate, heavy, and maximum exercise. Note that the oxygen cost per liter of $\dot{V}E$ remained fairly constant from 60 to ~110 liters/min, averaging 1.5–2.0 ml $O_2 \cdot liter^{-1} \cdot min^{-1}$ of $\dot{V}E$, but then rose sharply to exceed 3.0 ml $O_2 \cdot liter^{-1} \cdot min^{-1}$ of $\dot{V}E$ as $\dot{V}E$ rose an additional 30–40 liters/min at higher exercise intensities. So with incremental exercise, as $\dot{V}E$ rose and the oxygen cost per liter of $\dot{V}E$ increased with progressive hyperventilation, the oxygen cost of breathing comprised a greater and greater share of the rise in total body $\dot{V}O_2$. This proportion reached 35%–45% of the *increase* in $\dot{V}O_{2TOT}$ that accompanied the transition from very heavy to maximum exercise (i.e., at a time when the slope of the $\dot{V}O_{2TOT}$:work rate relationship is falling while $\dot{V}CO_2$ and $\dot{V}E$ are rising sharply). Thus, unlike some earlier predictions (305, 369), the increase in the O_2 cost of breathing with increasing exercise intensity was never sufficient to require all (or even greater than one-half) of the increase in total body $\dot{V}O_2$. It was estimated that the O_2 cost per liter of $\dot{V}E$ would have to be three to four times greater than the measured values or that $\dot{V}E$ exceed 225 liters/min in order for this critical value of "useful" ventilation to be reached during exercise.

The total oxygen cost of hyperpnea averaged 3%–5% of $\dot{V}O_{2TOT}$ in moderate exercise and about 8%–10% at $\dot{V}O_{2max}$, but the variability was large (see Fig. 11.12*b*), with some subjects in the range of 13%–16% of $\dot{V}O_{2max}$. These higher values occurred in subjects with greater than average $\dot{V}O_{2max}$ who experienced significant expiratory flow limitation, very high levels of inspiratory and expiratory work of breathing, and probably substantial additional work on a distorted chest wall. It was reasoned that these peak values of 15% of total $\dot{V}O_2$ for the oxygen cost of exercise hyperpnea at peak exercise probably represent the upper limit for humans achievable at $\dot{V}O_{2max}$, because peak perfusion of limb locomotor muscle has been consistently estimated to be about 80%–85% of cardiac output (see Chapter 17) and at least some portion of the remaining total available perfusate must be devoted to nonventilatory functions. Of course these estimates presume that the

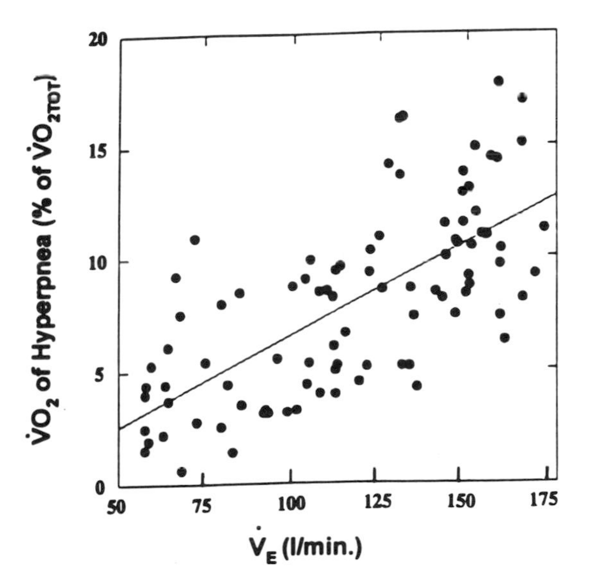

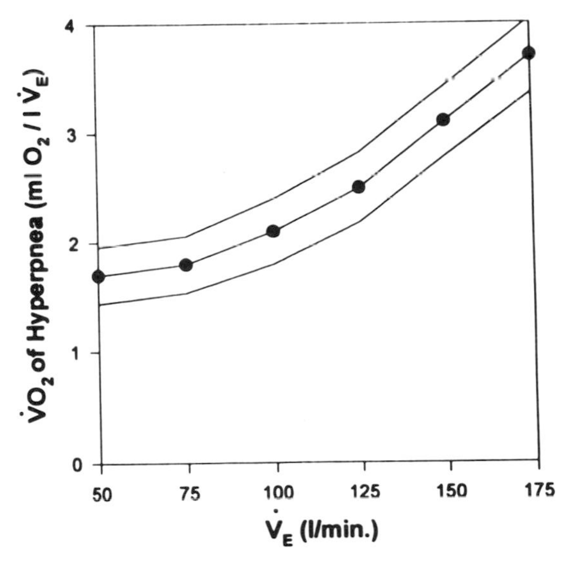

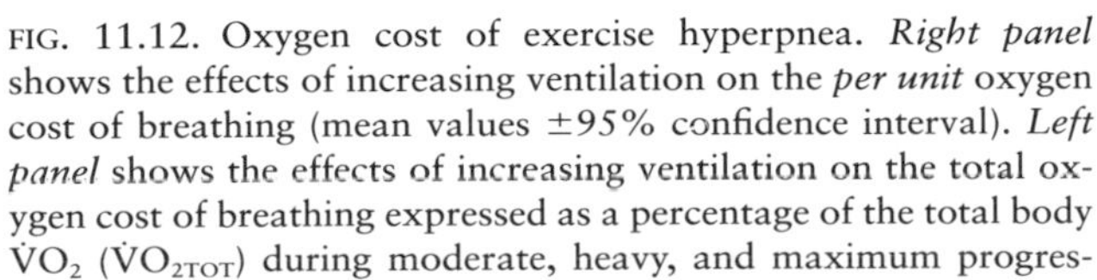

FIG. 11.12. Oxygen cost of exercise hyperpnea. *Right panel* shows the effects of increasing ventilation on the *per unit* oxygen cost of breathing (mean values ±95% confidence interval). *Left panel* shows the effects of increasing ventilation on the total oxygen cost of breathing expressed as a percentage of the total body $\dot{V}O_2$ ($\dot{V}O_{2TOT}$) during moderate, heavy, and maximum progressive exercise. [Individual subject values (N = 9).] Values for the O_2 cost of breathing were obtained in resting subjects from the measured increases in $\dot{V}O_2$ that accompanied steady-state mimicking of the pressure–volume loop, $\int P_{di}$, $\int P_g$, f_b, V_T, and EELV obtained during various exercise intensities. [From Aaron et al. (1, 2).]

working limb locomotor muscles *will* receive their maximum possible $\dot{Q}$ on demand at maximum exercise, but this seems unlikely if hard-working respiratory muscles are competing effectively for their blood flow requirement to support their high energy demand (see below).

Respiratory Muscle Blood Flow

Manohar's comprehensive studies in the exercising pony used phrenic venous cannulation and radionucleotide-labeled microspheres to provide the only model in which respiratory muscle $\dot{Q}$ and $\dot{V}O_2$ have been quantified during exercise (261–265) (see Table 11.1). At $\dot{V}O_{2max}$ in the pony ($\dot{V}O_{2max}$ ~ 120–130 ml · kg^{-1} · min^{-1} and Pa_{CO_2} 25–30 mm Hg), diaphragm $\dot{V}O_2$ (as estimated via the Fick principle) increased from 0.4 ml · 100 g^{-1} · min^{-1} at rest to 45 ml · min^{-1} · 100 g^{-1} because of 20- to 30-fold increases in blood flow and greater than 80% O_2 extraction by the diaphragm. Intercostal muscles also received blood flow at rates many times greater than rest, but their peak blood flow was less than one-half that of the diaphragm. Furthermore, attempts to further lower diaphragm vascular resistance and to increase blood flow at maximum exercise either by infusion of a vasodilator drug or by raising ventilatory work (via airway resistive loading) showed that the diaphragm may have been maximally vasodilated. The myocardium, on the other hand, did show a significant vasodilator reserve at peak exercise. Furthermore, the highest values for diaphragm blood flow were equal to or even slightly greater than blood flow per 100 g to the primary locomotor muscles of the limbs (e.g., gluteus medius and biceps femoris) at peak exercise (see Table 11.1). Thus, the diaphragm may be an exception to the generalization that some degree of sympathetically mediated vasoconstriction occurs during moderate and heavy exercise in active limb muscles (see Chapter 17). Apparently, this ongoing vasoconstriction is deemed necessary for maintaining perfusion pressure. Also, the diaphragm is capable of achieving and maintaining greater than 80% O_2 extraction despite the very high flow rates achieved when maximally dilated during heavy exercise at maximum cardiac output. Perhaps the maximal available capillary blood volume in the diaphragm is sufficiently large to maintain adequately long red cell transit times in order to ensure maximum O_2 offloading and extraction.

How well do respiratory muscles "compete" with locomotor muscles for blood flow during exercise, especially under conditions as described above where respiratory muscle work is increased dramatically during heavy and peak exercise loads at a time when the heart's capacity for increasing cardiac output is limited? This question has not been tested directly, although studies in humans have determined

TABLE 11.1. *Exercise Effects on Respiratory and Locomotor Muscle Perfusion and Oxygen Uptake in the Pony*

Muscle	Rest	Moderate Exercise	Maximum Exercise*
Diaphragm†	10–12	82	265–325
Blood flow			
Arterial-to-phrenic venous O_2 content Δ	3.5	15	17
(% O_2 extraction)	(25%)	(75%)	(80%)
$\dot{V}O_2$	0.4	11	45
External intercostal	8–10	—	150
Blood flow			
Transversus abdominis	30	—	125
Blood flow			
Internal oblique	25	—	250
Blood flow			
Gluteus medius	8–10	—	225–265
Blood flow			
Biceps femoris	8–10	—	240
Blood flow			

*Maximum cardiac output = 600–730 ml · kg^{-1} · min^{-1} (or ~ 5 × rest). The range of maximum cardiac outputs and muscle blood flows reflects the state of training of the animal in different studies (263–265).

†Blood flow and $\dot{V}O_2$ in ml · 100 g^{-1} · min^{-1}; O_2 content in ml · 100 ml^{-1}.

the effects of adding a large muscle mass (arm work) to ongoing exercise with the legs, which are already working at heavy or peak intensities (224, 364; see also Chapter 17). Adding this extra arm work resulted in vasoconstriction and reduced blood flow to the legs; so that increased flow was made available to the working arms in the face of a "fixed" peak cardiac output. Will increased respiratory muscle work at peak exercise also elicit vasoconstriction in working limb muscle and a redistribution of blood flow to the chest wall? Theoretically, this would depend in part upon the relative strength of local and autonomically controlled reflexes in the different muscle vascular beds (see Chapter 17) and probably also the magnitude of the increased respiratory muscle work. Given the diaphragm's excellent capability for autoregulation of flow in the face of changing perfusion pressure and especially the apparently maximum vasodilation achieved in heavy exercise in the pony (see above), we would predict that the respiratory muscles, if placed under sufficient load during heavy exercise, would indeed receive their "share" of blood flow at the expense of limb locomotor muscles under conditions where total cardiac output was at or near capacity. Clearly, we need direct studies to quantify the effects on locomotor muscle blood flow of increasing and reducing the work of breathing normally experienced during exercise of varying intensity and duration.

The pony has also provided extensive data on arterial-to-phrenic venous metabolite differences during prolonged heavy exercise that demonstrate the extraordinary aerobic capacity of the diaphragm and its suitability for meeting and sustaining high metabolic requirements. Over 30 min at high-intensity exercise, the pony showed progressive hyperventilation with very high breathing frequencies and yet maintained blood flow and high O_2 extraction rates of the diaphragm throughout (265). Arterial blood lactate and NH_3 concentrations rose throughout exercise, but no net production of either metabolite by the diaphragm occurred as indicated by the absence of arterial-to-phrenic venous concentration differences (264). Similar findings were obtained across the diaphragm of the awake sheep that was subjected to high resistive loads for prolonged periods (45). These data are consistent with the notion that the working diaphragm, much like cardiac muscle, might take up and utilize lactate as a substrate during prolonged exercise. This was also suggested by the high levels of tissue diaphragmatic lactate found in the absence of substantial glycogen depletion in the rat diaphragm following exhaustive exercise (139; also see later under Fiber Type Recruitment).

EXERCISE-INDUCED RESPIRATORY MUSCLE FATIGUE

Respiratory System Design

The respiratory muscle system and particularly its primary inspiratory muscle, the diaphragm, is highly resistant to fatigue during exercise. Its oxidative capacity is extremely high and fiber cross-sectional area per capillary number (i.e., an index of diffusion distance; see later under Metabolic Properties) is low relative to most locomotor muscles (285, 329).

The diaphragm is made up of motor units that vary considerably in their metabolic properties and their resistance to fatigue (373, 374). During spontaneous breathing, phrenic motoneurons in the cat were recruited in an order related to increasing axonal conduction velocity (110, 111). There is a relationship between axonal conduction velocity and phrenic motoneuron membrane input resistance; therefore, the size principle, as defined by Henneman and Mendell (183), likely predicts the order of diaphragm motor unit recruitment during exercise (421). The slow-twitch fatigue-resistant motor units (composed of type I fibers) are typically recruited first for most ventilatory behaviors, followed by the fast-twitch fatigue-resistant motor units (type IIa fibers) and the fast-twitch fatigable motor units (type IIb) (373, 374). Thus, the natural recruitment order of the diaphragm optimizes its fatigue resistance.

In addition to the metabolic capacity and recruitment order of the diaphragm, the respiratory system has accessory muscles to breathing (i.e., external intercostal, scalene, sternocleidomastoid muscles) that may be recruited to assist the diaphragm in pressure generation during exercise (184, 348). Studies have also suggested a rotation among the inspiratory muscles during conditions of fatigue or impending fatigue (348), whereas at a finer level of control, rotation among motor units within a muscle has been suggested while maintaining force generation and potentially allowing periods of intermittent recovery (122, 318).

As outlined in earlier sections of this chapter (see earlier under Oxygen Cost of Hyperpnea), heavy exercise may place substantial demands on the respiratory muscles to produce and sustain high levels of ventilatory work. The next section deals with the question of whether the elegant design of the respiratory muscles is appropriate to meet these demands.

ASSESSMENT OF DIAPHRAGM FATIGUE IN ANIMAL MODELS

Several techniques have been used to study respiratory muscle fatigue in animal models. For example, diaphragmatic muscle bundles have been excised and bathed in oxygenated physiological solutions to study contractile and fatigue properties. Peripheral failure has been distinguished from neuromuscular transmission failure through intermittent nerve and direct muscle electrical stimulation (229). These techniques have added a great deal of insight into the influence of various factors (e.g., myosin isoforms, oxygen-derived free radicals, hydrogen ion concentration) on diaphragmatic fatigue, but fail to mimic the in vivo condition where blood flow is intact and a natural recruitment order occurs (204, 209, 210, 228, 307, 339, 374). To our knowledge no studies have applied in vitro stimulation of excised muscle bundles to the state of exercise, likely due to the difficulties of tissue removal and preparation and time constraints imposed in dissection. The technique of bilateral phrenic nerve stimulation (BPNS) however, could be applied to the exercising animal, but has not yet been attempted. Thus, we are left with more indirect assessments that imply recruitment or use of metabolic substrates, such as glycogen depletion.

Glycogen Depletion

An association between muscle glycogen levels and muscle performance has been demonstrated; therefore, it is appropriate to presume that if significant glycogen depletion occurs, muscle performance may be affected (53, 215, 358). To date, the results in the diaphragm have been quite variable. Fregosi and Dempsey (139) demonstrated approximately 25%–30% glycogen depletion in the diaphragm of rats who were exercised at various intensities and durations, the most intense being for 38 min at 88% of $\dot{V}O_{2max}$. They also observed increased lactate concentrations in the diaphragm in the presence of only minimal glycogen depletion, presumably due to active uptake of lactate by the diaphragm as a fuel source. Ianuzzo et al. (196), Moore and Gollnick (287), Green et al. (162), and Gorski et al. (158) demonstrated greater but also variable (39%–90%) reductions in diaphragm muscle glycogen content after prolonged running to exhaustion at different work intensities (50% to >100% $\dot{V}O_{2max}$) or after 5 h of swimming. Despite the variability in these studies, as stated previously, it appears significant amounts of glycogen typically remain in the respiratory muscles, and in almost all studies its depletion is substantially less than that observed in locomotor muscles with similar fiber type. It is difficult to determine what these findings mean in terms of diaphragmatic fatigue (131).

Fiber Type Recruitment

Interestingly, in the study by Green et al. (162) glycogen depletion was observed in all fiber types of the diaphragm, implying that even the fast fatigable fibers were recruited. Investigators have argued that the fast fatigable motor units typically composed of type IIb muscle fibers are rarely active during most ventilatory behaviors and are only reserved for expulsive type behaviors such as coughing and sneezing (375). The glycogen depletion data, however, remain controversial because release of catecholamines (e.g., epinephrine) during exercise will deplete glycogen even from nonexercised muscle (275). These effects may especially be true in those studies in which rats were forced to run on a treadmill with the increased stress of an electric grid or forced to swim for survival. Thus, basing estimates of muscle fiber or motor unit recruitment on glycogen depletion may be in error. On the other hand, the increase in succinate dehydrogenase activity (SDH) in all fiber types of the diaphragm in response to training supports the view that all fiber types are recruited during exercise, even the highly fatigable fibers (159). Furthermore, assessments of motor unit recruitment in skeletal muscle are often based on observations of only a select number of motor units and are technically difficult to perform. Thus, the influence on motor unit recruitment of enhanced muscle shortening and increased velocity of shortening, as occurs in the diaphragm during exercise, remains unresolved. There have been reports of a reversal of the proposed normal recruitment order in the intercostal muscles of humans during volitional tasks (420). If true for the majority of motor units, this could greatly increase the susceptibility of the respiratory muscles to fatigue. It remains to be determined if the highly fatigable motor units of the diaphragm are ever truly recruited during heavy whole-body exercise.

DEFINITION OF FATIGUE

Task Failure vs. Objective Assessment of Fatigue

Classically, skeletal muscle fatigue has been defined by Edwards (117) as "a failure to maintain the required or expected force." This definition has often been applied to respiratory muscle studies in which human subjects are required to maintain a target pleural or transdiaphragmatic pressure or a given force by volitional means until they cannot continue (called "task failure"). This approach should be distinguished from those that objectively assess peripheral muscle fatigue by the use of direct stimulation of muscle or nerve. "Task failure" could occur without peripheral muscle fatigue if "motivation" were a factor in the loss of force generation. Similarly, peripheral muscle fatigue could occur prior to or in the absence of "task failure" if the amount of fatigue is not sufficient to reduce maximal force generation to the target force. The original definition of Edwards (117) was recently extended to include a reduction in force that recovers with rest in order to distinguish muscle fatigue from muscle weakness (291a).

Contractile Changes with Fatigue

Other changes occur in skeletal muscle function during fatigue along with the fall in force (343). A slowing of the maximal speed of shortening as well as a prolongation of contraction time (116) have been observed. Maneuvers that require high velocities of muscle shortening may cause a preferential decline in maximal shortening velocity relative to the decline in maximal tetanic force production of the muscle (17, 18, 100, 116). Others have observed a slowing of the rate of relaxation as well as reduced ability of the muscle to shorten under load in conjunction with the loss of muscle force development (124, 343). Thus, fatigue in this context should be considered as any alteration in the normal performance of the muscle that is relieved by rest (117, 118, 122, 291a).

PREDICTING RESPIRATORY MUSCLE FATIGUE DURING EXERCISE

Is there evidence that the ventilatory demands of whole-body exercise on the respiratory muscles is sufficient to cause fatigue? Early studies by Roussos et al. (348, 350) suggested that diaphragmatic fatigue will occur when transdiaphragmatic pressures exceed 40% of maximum, while fatigue of the inspiratory muscles will occur when pleural pressures exceed 50%–70% of maximum. Classical studies by Bellemare and Grassino (49) found a critical time tension index for the diaphragm (TTdi = 0.15) during inspiratory resistive loading using a controlled "square-wave" breathing pattern to "task failure." This index was based on the transdiaphragmatic pressures produced as a percentage of maximum multiplied by the duty cycle. If this critical index was exceeded, the time to "task failure" decreased as a function of the TTdi. Rarely in normal humans during exercise does the peak transdiaphragmatic or pleural pressures exceed 20%–30% of the maximal static pressures, nor does the TTdi ever approach 0.15 (33, 70, 203). Based on these criteria, neither diaphragmatic or inspiratory muscle fatigue would be expected to occur with exercise. This is in contrast to studies which suggest that sustainable ventilation during voluntary hyperpnea above 60% of the maximal breathing capacity can only be maintained for a finite period of time (401). Although variable, 75%–80% of the 12 or 15 s maximum voluntary ventilation (MVV) can be sustained (to "task failure") only over a range of 4–20 min (34, 59, 401). Clearly, heavy exercise often results in ventilatory demands that approach or exceed 70% of the MVV and this would imply that respiratory muscle fatigue may occur.

Application of Resting Tests to Respiratory Muscle Function During Exercise

Exercise hyperpnea results in high flow rates and relatively high velocities of muscle shortening relative to the studies using resistive breathing to define fatigue thresholds for the respiratory muscles. These differences probably cause important differences in fatigability. For example, during voluntary efforts against resistive loads, the oxygen cost of breathing ($\dot{V}O_{2RM}$) was shown to be the best predictor of task failure by the respiratory muscles (274). However, when similar increments in $\dot{V}O_{2RM}$ (300–600 ml/min) were produced by high levels of unloaded hyperpnea (3), the time to task failure was markedly longer (>5×) than would be predicted from the resistive load studies. In addition, at rest with voluntary inspiratory efforts against loads, the recruitment order of the respiratory muscles and/or motor units within specific muscles may differ from the exercise state. Furthermore, blood flow competition between active muscular beds (i.e., respiratory muscles vs. locomotor muscles) most likely occurs in whole-body exercise (see earlier under Respiratory Muscle Blood Flow), but does not exist when hyperpnea is produced at rest. Thus it is difficult to apply these predictors of respiratory muscle fatigue to the state of exercise hyperpnea.

ASSESSMENT OF RESPIRATORY MUSCLE FATIGUE IN HUMANS

Volitional Tests

Techniques applied to humans to determine whether respiratory muscles fatigue with whole-body exercise include volitional tests that measure alterations in pulmonary function; MVV; and maximal mouth, pleural, or transdiaphragmatic pressure development (*P*di) (70, 88, 192, 251). Other studies have relied on "task failure" as an index of fatigue and had subjects mimic at rest the ventilation or the pressures produced during exercise for given time periods (2, 3, 370).

Volitional Tests Applied to Exercise

Shephard (370) observed that the MVV performed after 20 min of exercise at a work load of 80% of $\dot{V}O_{2max}$ was significantly less than that after 5 min of exercise, implying that respiratory muscle fatigue may occur. Warren (416) noted a 17% fall in the 12 s MVV in ultramarathon runners, but only after 24 h of running. Further evidence for respiratory muscle fatigue during exercise was presented by Mahler and Loke (257) and Loke (251), who demonstrated a decrease in vital capacity as well as decreases in maximum inspiratory and expiratory pressure development after a marathon. In contrast, several other studies have not demonstrated alterations in volitional measurements of ventilatory performance after exercise (20, 291). Thus, the results of the volitional tests have been inconclusive due to these conflicting results and because the test conditions themselves are difficult to control and may not be sufficiently objective or independent of whole-body fatigue.

Nonvolitional Tests

Spectral Changes of the EMG. Shifts in the frequency spectrum of the integrated EMG activity of the diaphragm with fatigue may be related to alterations in neuromuscular transmission and sarcolemmal excitability. A shift in the power spectral content of diaphragm EMG toward lower frequencies appears to precede or accompany fatigue (50, 168, 289). However, the validity of using the shift in the EMG spectral frequency as an index of fatigue (70, 168, 309) has been challenged (374). Whole-muscle EMG reflects the summation of individual motor unit action potentials. The EMG signal must depend in part on which motor units are activated, their frequency of activation, and the timing of their activation relative to other units. Thus, changes in the EMG signal coincident with fatigue could result from changes in individual motor unit action potentials, number of activated muscle units, motor unit discharge rates, or synchrony between the discharges of different units. Changes in the EMG signal during exercise may be independent of fatigue. An additional serious problem with the use of the EMG spectral frequency approach to quantifying fatigue is the inability of current techniques to obtain accurate, artifact-free diaphragmatic EMG measurements in exercising humans.

Bilateral Phrenic Nerve Stimulation (BPNS)

More recently, the technique of BPNS has been applied in humans for the assessment of diaphragm function. The technique of BPNS allows objective assessment of diaphragm function without influence of motivation, whole-body fatigue, or other central factors. The technique involves supramaximal stimulation of the phrenic nerves (usually transcutaneously or through needle or wire electrodes) bilaterally behind the sternocleidomastoid muscles in the neck (28, 29, 47, 190). Typically, twitches with short pulses (100–150 μs duration) are used. However, a few studies have applied short-duration tetanic stimulations either bilaterally or unilaterally (34, 203). The reliability of the technique is dependent on several key elements, including supramaximal phrenic nerve stimulation, quasi-isometric conditions, muscle length, and abdominal compliance. Studies using this technique must carefully control for each of these potential sources of error. Even with careful control of these variables, the diaphragm will likely shorten an indeterminate amount during phrenic stimulation. Use of the BPNS technique following resistive breathing to the point of task failure demonstrated that the human diaphragm can indeed be fatigued (34, 47, 150).

CHARACTERISTICS OF DIAPHRAGM FATIGUE

High- vs. Low-Frequency Fatigue

Based on initial studies using BPNS, investigators subdivided diaphragm fatigue into high-frequency and low-frequency fatigue (28, 289). High-frequency fatigue was characterized by an inability to maintain a given *P*di at high rates of phrenic nerve stimulation (typically 50–100 Hz), whereas low-frequency fatigue was characterized by failure to maintain adequate pressures at low stimulus frequencies (1–20 Hz). Several investigators demonstrated that loaded and unloaded hyperpnea at rest can elicit both low- and high-frequency fatigue in conscious humans (28, 34, 289). They also suggested that the high-frequency fatigue recovers quickly, after 10–20 min, whereas the low-frequency component may require hours. Based on the type of fatigue (low vs. high), as well as changes occurring in the compound muscle action potential (M-wave) in response to a supramaximal twitch or twitches combined with maximal volitional maneuvers, different sites of fatigue can be determined and have generally been separated into three categories: central fatigue, failure of neuromuscular transmission, or pheripheral mechanism of fatigue (55).

Sites and Mechanisms of Respiratory Muscle Fatigue

Major potential sites of fatigue have been summarized by Bigland-Ritchie (55). Central fatigue was described as a reduced excitatory input to higher motor centers and/or excitatory drive to lower motoneurons. Failure of neuromuscular transmission could result from decreased motor nerve excitability, altered synaptic transmission, and/or reduced sarcolemma excitability. Peripheral fatigue could originate from altered excitation contraction coupling or contractile mechanisms, from alterations in metabolic energy supply, and/or from accumulation of metabolites (22, 122, 131, 132, 344, 380). Considerable controversy exists regarding the role of these sites in the etiology of muscle fatigue, in particular the relative importance of central factors and failure of neuromuscular transmission vs. peripheral mechanisms (47, 150).

Central Fatigue in Humans

Investigators have attempted to asses central fatigue of the diaphragm following resistive breathing by using the "twitch occlusion" method (47, 150). This method is based on the finding that most subjects can maximally contract the diaphragm through combined inspiratory and expulsive maneuvers against an occluded airway. BPNS is applied transcutaneously in combination with the volitional maneuver, and if additional force output by the diaphragm is obtained, a component of central fatigue is implied (i.e., failure to activate the total motoneuronal pool by volitional efforts). The technique is critically dependent upon motivational influences and is technically difficult for the subject to perform. Evidence of "central fatigue" obtained in this way cannot be equated with "reflex inhibition" of motor output to the diaphragm, which might occur as a consequence of afferent feedback from a fatiguing, contracting muscle (199, 347). Thus, the relevance of this technique to the physiological condition of exercise hyperpnea where motor unit recruitment is based on precise neurohumoral regulation rather than voluntary effort and motivation remains questionable.

Neurotransmission Fatigue

Neuromuscular transmission fatigue has typically been inferred by a reduction in the mass action potential (M-wave) with electrical stimulation of the motor nerves. Several studies have demonstrated a fall in the M-wave as a result of maximal voluntary contractions sustained for various periods of time in different muscles (48, 114, 122). The time course of recovery appears to be very fast, often less than 1–2 min (48). At present no such reports of a reduced M-wave amplitude of the diaphragm in response to electrical stimulation after exercise have been reported; however, shifts in the EMG power spectrum possibly implying changes in muscle excitability have been observed during heavy exercise (70). Most studies examining diaphragm fatigue using BPNS after exercise have not been able to stimulate the nerves within the first few minutes after exercise, possibly missing this type of fatigue.

BILATERAL PHRENIC NERVE STIMULATION APPLIED TO EXERCISE

Short-Term Exercise

Only recently has the technique of BPNS been applied to exercise (31, 33, 203, 247, 256). Levine and Henson (247) performed BPNS before and after short-term maximal progressive exercise to exhaustion lasting 12–15 min and found no changes in the supramaximal twitch. They subsequently added an inspiratory resistance (38 cm H_2O liter^{-1} · s^{-1}) and repeated the phrenic nerve stimulation before and after a progressive exercise test. By adding the resistance, approximately half of the subjects demonstrated a significant decline in the supramaximal twitch with no change in M-wave amplitude. This initial study demonstrated several important findings dealing with diaphragm fatigue. First, acute short-term exercise does not cause diaphragm fatigue in healthy humans with average levels of fitness. Second, spontaneously breathing humans will drive themselves to the point of diaphragm fatigue during exercise while breathing against an inspiratory resistance; that is, the degree of dyspnea did not cause subjects to stop prior to respiratory muscle fatigue developing. Third, the fatigue was primarily peripheral in origin, since M-wave amplitude did not change. Finally, those who demonstrated the greatest fall in twitch *P*di were the subjects who developed the most diaphragmatic pressure over time (an index of diaphragmatic force output).

Endurance Exercise

Bilateral phrenic nerve stimulation was subsequently applied to endurance exercise to exhaustion at a fixed work rate (203, 256). Subjects with a range of fitness levels exercised to exhaustion at workloads that elicited 80%–95% of $\dot{V}O_{2max}$. A significant reduction in the twitch *P*di, measured at FRC was found, averaging between 15% and 26%. A few subjects demonstrated reductions as high as 40%–50% in BPNS *P*di. Similar exercise effects were obtained when BPNS was carried out at lung volumes above and below FRC and at 10 and 20 Hz stimulation frequencies (203). Johnson et al. (203) tested relatively fit subjects who were able to maintain 85% and 95% of $\dot{V}O_{2max}$ for 30 and 14 min, respectively, while Mador et al. (256) tested relatively unfit subjects who were only able to maintain 80% of $\dot{V}O_{2max}$ for 8 min. A similar average reduction in the twitch *P*di was observed between studies at the lower exercise loads despite the marked difference in exercise duration, while subjects exercising at the higher exercise load averaged a 60% greater reduction in the twitch *P*di. It was interesting that diaphragm fatigue was observed in the subjects studied by Mador (256) despite the fact that the $\dot{V}E$ near the end of exercise averaged only 50% of the 12 s MVV. An example of BPNS at 1 and 10 Hz before and after exercise at 95% of $\dot{V}O_{2max}$ is shown in Figure 11.13 (203). M-wave amplitude was constant; however, significant declines were noted in both esophageal (*Pe*) and gastric (*Pg*) pressures causing the decline in *P*di. Stimulated *P*di values generally recovered by 70 min following exercise. No changes were observed in time to peak tension of the *P*di waveform, M-wave area, or amplitude. Significant correlations with the amount of fatigue observed following exercise were found between the relative intensity (expressed as a percentage of maximum) that subjects reached near the end of the endurance test, as well as with the relative increase in an index of diaphragmatic force output (the time integral for the *P*di waveform multiplied by breathing frequency) (203). In particular, subjects who truly were working above 85% of $\dot{V}O_{2max}$ near end exercise tended to demonstrate the most consistent and significant diaphragmatic fatigue.

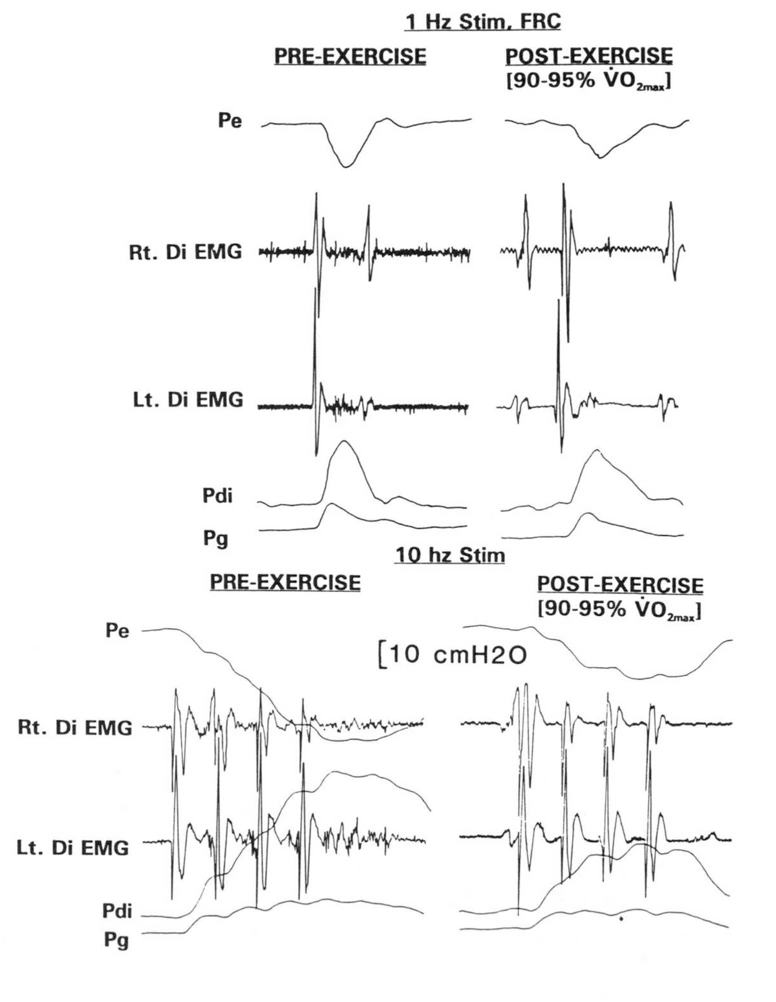

FIG. 11.13. Example of bilateral phrenic nerve stimulation (BPNS) performed before and after exercise at 1 and 10 Hz. Both esophageal (Pe) and gastric (Pg) pressure fell following exercise, causing the reduction in the Pdi waveform amplitude. At 1 Hz stimulation, a prolongation in relaxation rate of the Pdi waveform was also observed. No changes were observed in the amplitude of the M-waves from either the left or right hemidiaphragm. [From Johnson et al. (203).]

Accordingly, these studies were the first to demonstrate objectively that the diaphragm muscle is susceptible to exercise-induced low-frequency fatigue, especially when exercise intensity progressed beyond 85% of $\dot{V}O_{2max}$ and was of the endurance type.

Factors Contributing to the Decline in Twitch Pdi *Following Exercise*

Each of the preceding studies demonstrated a relationship between an index of diaphragmatic "pressure production" over time and the degree of fatigue observed following exercise, indicating that diaphragmatic force output was a likely factor contributing to the fatigue. The fact that exercise intensity was also highly correlated to the degree of fatigue suggested that perhaps mechanisms precipitated by —or dependent upon—whole-body heavy endurance exercise [e.g., blood flow competition, per se, might contribute significantly to diaphragmatic fatigue (412)].

Role of Diaphragmatic Force Output in Fatigue

Babcock et al. (33) investigated the role of diaphragmatic force output as the cause of exercise-induced diaphragmatic fatigue. Subjects mimicked at rest the essential mechanical components of breathing during exercise (i.e., VT, f_b, EELV), as well as the diaphragmatic pressure production ($\int Pdi \cdot f_b$) for a similar time period that subjects achieved during exercise at 95% of $\dot{V}O_{2max}$. Subjects at rest also voluntarily produced and sustained diaphragmatic force outputs that were 150%–200% of those found during whole-body endurance exercise. Figure 11.14 shows the amount of observed diaphragm fatigue vs. the diaphragmatic force output achieved during voluntary hyperpnea at rest (*hatched area*) (33) and during exercise (*symbols*) (33, 203, 256). A threshold for significant diaphragmatic fatigue in the resting subject was observed when the diaphragmatic force output was increased to approximately four to five times the resting values. This fatigue "threshold" also approximated a TTdi of less than 0.15 or a peak *P*di of greater than 70% of dynamic $Pcap_{di}$. During whole-body exercise, only a small fraction of the subjects clearly exceeded these critical thresholds for the development of diaphragmatic fatigue during exercise. Thus, diaphragm force output during exercise cannot by itself account for the majority of the fatigue observed in most subjects.

At least two types of additional factors might determine exercise-induced diaphragmatic fatigue.

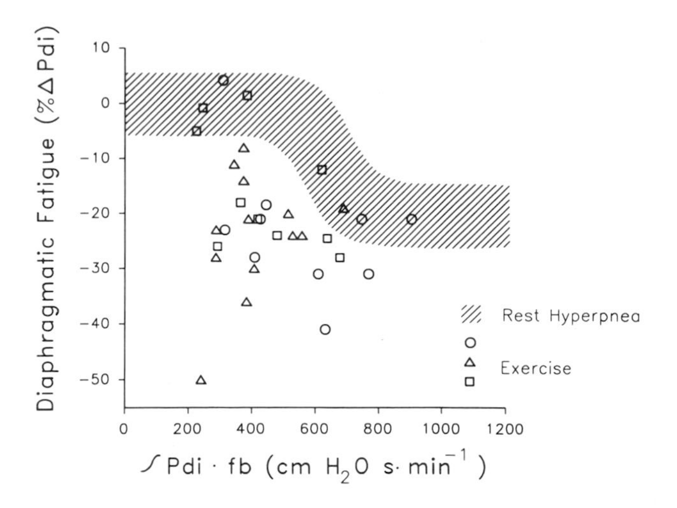

FIG. 11.14. Comparison of diaphragmatic fatigue produced by exercise vs. that produced by mimicking various levels of diaphragmatic force at rest. Plotted is the diaphragmatic force index (time integral for *P*di multiplied times breathing frequency) achieved during exercise in the studies by Johnson et al. (203) (*circles*), Babcock et al. (33) (*triangles*), and Mador et al. (256) (*squares*) vs. the percentage fall in *P*di amplitude with supramaximal stimulation. This is shown relative to the force produced during resting hyperpnea vs. the fall in the *P*di waveform amplitude after this voluntary maneuver. Note that after performing the resting hyperpnea for the same time period as achieved during exercise (95% $\dot{V}O_{2max}$), significant fatigue does not occur until a time integral of 600 cm H_2O s · min^{-1}, whereas during exercise significant fatigue occurs at much lower levels of diaphragmatic work.

First, during intense endurance exercise the levels of circulating metabolic by-products increase and a number of these substances (i.e., lactate, H^+, K^+, P_i and oxygen-derived free radicals) have been implicated in the fatigue process (131, 202, 339, 344, 372). In the rat, following heavy endurance exercise to exhaustion, lactate content in the blood and the diaphragm tissue was shown to increase substantially (139). Since only minimal reductions occurred in the glycogen concentration of the rat diaphragm, it was presumed that the elevated tissue lactate levels were due primarily to lactate uptake from the blood rather than lactate production by the diaphragm. Similarly, during leg exercise in humans, lactate uptake by forearm muscle occurs and does so in proportion to the intensity of the forearm contraction as demonstrated by increased arterial-to-venous lactate differences across the muscle (74, 248). Perhaps, then, the diaphragm fatigue observed following whole-body endurance exercise may be due to the accumulation of lactate and [H^+] by the diaphragm. If this proposed acidification of the diaphragm does play a role in its fatigue, it is also probable that the amount of diaphragm work incurred during whole-body exercise must also play an important interactive role. Babcock et al. (33) also observed that the "rested" first dorsal interosseous muscle of the hand showed no fatigue in response to supramaximal ulnar nerve stimulation following the same intensity and duration of whole-body endurance exercise that causes significant diaphragm fatigue. This would imply that the exercise-induced increase in lactate and/or H^+ or other circulating metabolites do not cause fatigue in a nonexercised muscle.

Second, a significant difference in the competition for blood flow distribution may also explain the greater diaphragmatic fatigue incurred following the whole-body exercise than for similar amounts of diaphragmatic force produced at rest. At rest, voluntary hyperpnea comparable to the levels experienced during exercise would be accompanied by blood flow to the diaphragm that was adequate to meet metabolic demands. On the other hand, in whole-body exercise, the diaphragm must now compete with existing locomotor muscles for the increase in blood flow. Thus, one might expect a reduced diaphragmatic flow for a given amount of ventilatory work during exercise as compared to the voluntary hyperpnea trials conducted at rest. Accordingly, the relatively lower blood flow during exercise would mean an inadequate oxygen transport in relation to the metabolic demand placed on the diaphragm, and this imbalance would contribute to the observed greater diaphragmatic fatigue induced by exercise than by the hyperpnea alone. This conjecture remains untested and highly speculative. Definitive answers on the cause of exercise-induced diaphragmatic fatigue must await information on blood flow distribution during exercise (see earlier under Respiratory Muscle Blood Flow).

CONSEQUENCES OF EXERCISE-INDUCED DIAPHRAGMATIC FATIGUE

Fatigue vs. Task Failure

The evidence summarized in the foregoing demonstrates that the diaphragm, like other skeletal muscles, is susceptible to fatigue during exhaustive endurance exercise—but what is the significance of this fatigue? As explained earlier (see Predicting Respiratory Muscle Fatigue during Exercise), we cannot assume that the observed reductions in *P*di of 20%–30% or even 40%–50% in a few extreme cases are synonymous with "task failure" by the diaphragm. To the contrary, diaphragm fatigue can occur in the *absence* of task failure. When Babcock et al. (33) had resting subjects sustain levels of force output by the diaphragm that averaged 80% greater than those obtained during exercise, significant "fatigue" of the diaphragm occurred in the majority of cases (as evaluated with BPNS), but "task failure" was rarely evident (one of seven trials), as shown by the subject's ability to maintain voluntarily these high levels of diaphragmatic force output. Furthermore, since the time integral of esophageal pressure ($\int Pe$) and minute ventilation continued to rise throughout long-term exercise and adequate CO_2 elimination was maintained throughout, it is also likely that the inspiratory muscles as a whole did not undergo "task failure." Breathing frequency does rise over time during sustained heavy exercise; some might attribute this to respiratory muscle "fatigue" (see below). However, it is only in very rare, extreme circumstances such as competitive endurance running in a very hot, humid environment that tachypnea becomes severe enough to actually affect the adequacy of alveolar ventilation or CO_2 elimination and to reduce the efficiency of the ventilatory response (177). In other words, the ventilatory response to heavy endurance exercise is adequate with respect to gas exchange requirements. Finally, those experiments discussed earlier (see earlier under Unloading with Pressure Assist) in which the inspiratory muscles were partially unloaded during prolonged exercise, reported no effect on $\dot{V}_E$ or exercise performance time. If this partial "assist" to the inspiratory muscles also alleviated some of the exercise-induced diaphragmatic fatigue (which seem likely), then these data would also support the notion that diaphragm fatigue is without significant consequence to ventilatory response or exercise performance.

Respiratory muscle fatigue may, if sufficient in magnitude, be of physiologic significance to the regulation of ventilation. The voluntary performance of fatiguing ventilatory efforts to the point of task failure in resting subjects was shown to cause subsequent alterations in breathing pattern at rest and exercise (255) and even led to reductions in exercise performance (269). However, studies of similar design have not shown these significant after-effects of fatiguing respiratory efforts (113, 291). Perhaps one explanation for these discrepant effects might be differences in the magnitude of the respiratory muscle fatigue or the rate of recovery from fatigue incurred by the volitional maneuvers. For example, the average reduction in stimulated *P*di following exercise is, with few exceptions, only about one-half that usually incurred by voluntary efforts against added resistive loads to the point of task failure (439) (see below). These extreme levels of diaphragmatic fatigue might occur in some highly trained athletes during very high intensities of endurance exercise. If so, they might explain the enhancing effect on ventilation, exercise performance, and relief of dyspnea observed with He-O_2 breathing under these conditions (1). However, He-O_2 may also have effects other than relieving respiratory muscle fatigue (see earlier under Unloading with Pressure Assist). In summary, we conclude that it must be extremely rare, if at all, that exercise-induced respiratory muscle fatigue to the point of "task failure" is incurred during whole-body exercise (see below).

Does Training of Respiratory Muscles Affect Exercise Performance?

Several studies in recent years have examined the effects of specific respiratory muscle endurance training on the performance of both the respiratory muscles and exercise performance itself. These types of studies speak to the question of whether the aerobic capacity of the respiratory muscles, which in turn should have a bearing on their fatigability, will affect performance. All studies are in agreement in finding an increased respiratory muscle endurance, as assessed by voluntary hyperpnea to the point of "task failure" (see later under Respiratory Sensation during Exertion), in both endurance athletes and nonathletes (57, 58, 127, 288). Most studies also report that heavy endurance exercise performance or maximum $\dot{V}O_2$ were unaffected by respiratory muscle training (127, 176, 288). The two studies of Boutellier et al. (57, 58) are exceptions in that endurance performance at about 75%–80% of $\dot{V}O_{2max}$ was increased by 38% in nonathletes and 50% in athletes; and these changes were accompanied by substantial but highly variable reductions in the ventilatory response to exercise. The discrepancies among studies may reflect differences in exercise intensities and durations used for testing and the markedly different experimental designs among the various studies. These studies also do not include carefully matched control groups in their experimental design; this is important, especially in these longitudinal studies, which use volitional end-points in their testing procedures. Thus, interpretation of these respiratory muscle training data to mean that exercise-induced respiratory muscle fatigue may or may not be an important determinant of exercise performance must await more definitive study.

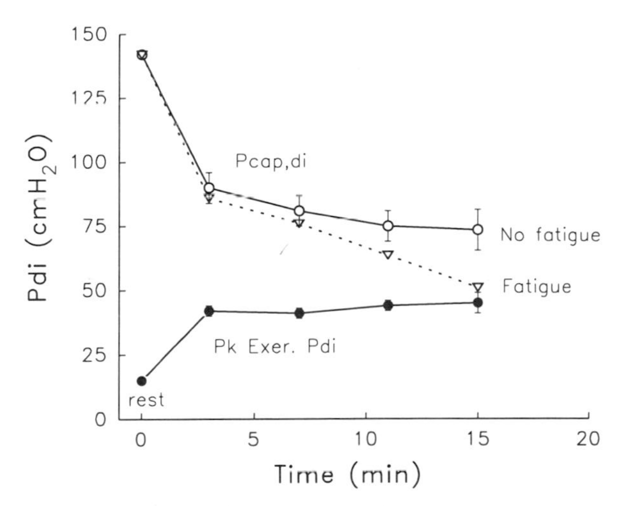

FIG. 11.15. Influence of fatigue on the dynamic capacity for pressure generation by the diaphragm. Note during heavy exercise (95% of $\dot{V}O_{2max}$) that the peak diaphragmatic pressure produced during exercise (*closed circles*) approaches 70% of the dynamic capacity for producing transdiaphragmatic pressures (*open circles*). When a 20%–25% reduction in the maximal force-generating capacity of the diaphragm is considered, peak Pdi produced during exercise approaches 90%–95% of this capacity (*open circles*).

Altered Respiratory Muscle Recruitment with Fatigue

Although exercise-induced respiratory muscle fatigue may have little impact on the ventilatory response to exercise or exercise performance, fatigue specific to the diaphragm may be sufficient to alter the normal recruitment of the respiratory muscles. As noted previously, the pressures produced by the diaphragm during exercise approach 50%–70% of the dynamic capacity for pressure generation (203). However, when a 20%–25% reduction in force-generating capacity is considered as shown in Figure 11.15, peak pressures produced by the diaphragm during exercise do approach 75%–95% of this capacity. In studies of endurance exercise (33, 203, 256), the peak pressure generated by the diaphragm and the pressure time integral rose steeply early in exercise but then plateaued or even fell slightly as exercise continued despite a continued rise in minute ventilation and pleural pressure. Thus, it is possible that, during heavy whole-body exercise, accumulation of metabolites in the diaphragm may cause a reduction of diaphragm force production during exercise via reflex inhibition (i.e., central fatigue). Little change in overall breathing pattern or performance may occur due to the ability of other inspiratory muscles to maintain an adequate pleural pressure sufficient to maintain the appropriate alveolar ventilation. Furthermore, the inhibition of diaphragm force output may prevent the recruitment of fatigable motor units (see earlier under DEFINITION OF FATIGUE), thereby protecting the primary inspiratory muscle from undergoing extreme fatigue to the point of "task failure."

PHYSICAL TRAINING EFFECTS ON RESPIRATORY MUSCLES

Studies examining the effects of training on the muscles of the chest wall are relatively few compared to the numerous reports of the effects of training on locomotor muscles. However, several recent investigations have examined alterations in human respiratory muscle performance as well as the cellular changes that occur in animal ventilatory muscles in response to "whole-body" endurance exercise training. These studies include evaluations of the effects of specific ventilatory muscle training (i.e., voluntary hyperpnea or inspiratory resistive loading) on human respiratory muscle strength and endurance. In this section, we review the effects of both whole-body endurance training and specific ventilatory muscle training on human and animal respiratory muscles. We begin with a brief overview of human respiratory muscle fiber morphology.

Respiratory Muscle Morphology and Contractile Properties

By definition, any skeletal muscle that changes the dimensions of the chest wall is a respiratory muscle. There are many muscles located between the waist and head that can move the chest wall; however, only the diaphragm, parasternal intercostals, internal and external intercostals, scalenes, and sternocleidomastoids have been morphologically examined in humans.

Shortening Velocity and Fiber Type. Although skeletal muscle phenotype can be categorized in several ways, histochemical staining for myofibrillar adenosine triphosphatase (ATPase) activity has been the dominant procedure employed to characterize human respiratory muscles. The Brooke and Kaiser (67) myosin ATPase-based scheme of fiber classification can be used to separate skeletal muscle fibers into three major categories: *(1)* type I; *(2)* type IIa; and *(3)* type IIb (see 320 for review). The physiological significance of various muscle fiber types is the differences between fibers in oxidative capacity and maximal shortening velocity (V_{max}). In general, when compared to types IIa and IIb, human type I fibers have the highest oxidative capacity and slowest V_{max} (87, 175, 229, 340). Type IIb fibers have the highest V_{max} and the lowest capacity (87, 175, 229, 340). Finally, the oxidative capacity and V_{max} of type IIa fibers are often between type I and type IIb fibers (87, 175, 229, 340).

Although most mammalian skeletal muscles contain a mixture of all three fiber types, the ratio of type I to type II fibers in a muscle is commonly linked with the muscle's activity pattern (21). For example, in untrained subjects, tonically active postural muscles generally possess a greater ratio of type I to type II fibers when compared to phasically active (nonpostural) locomotor muscles. In general, most human respiratory muscle fibers contain a high percentage of type I and type IIa fibers and relatively few type IIb fibers. For example, the sum of type I and type IIa fibers in the costal diaphragm, internal intercostals, and parasternal intercostals ranges between 77% and 99% of the total fiber pool (285). This observation is consistent with the notion that human respiratory muscles contain fibers with a relatively high oxidative capacity.

Capillary Density: Fiber Cross-Sectional Area/Capillary Ratio. The number of capillaries surrounding each muscle fiber is surprisingly similar across most human skeletal muscles (285). However, a factor in untrained humans that distinguishes key respiratory muscles from less active locomotor muscles is the fiber cross-sectional area (CSA)/capillary ratio (Fig. 11.16). This ratio is significantly lower in the costal diaphragm compared to the vastus lateralis. The physiological significance of this observation is that this ratio provides an index of diffusion distance between capillaries and muscle fibers (285, 286); that is, the lower the ratio, the shorter the diffusion distance. Although there is not always a tight coupling between capillary supply and oxidative capacity across species, in humans, the ratio is closely linked to the oxidative potential of muscle fibers and to the endurance capacity of the muscle (358).

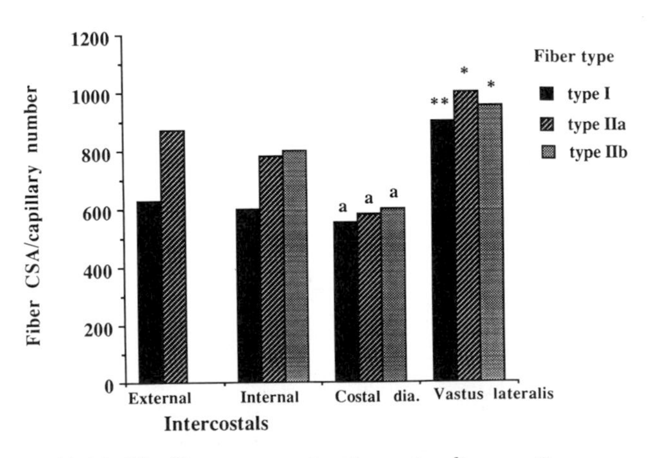

FIG. 11.16. The fiber cross-sectional area (μm^2) to capillary number in three human respiratory muscles compared to a mixed fiber locomotor muscle. [Data are from Mizuno (285).] a, different ($P < 0.05$) from all other muscle; **, different ($P < 0.05$) from internal and external intercostals; *, different ($P < 0.05$) from internal intercostals.

Bioenergetic Enzyme Activities. Published reports of quantitative biochemical analysis of glycolytic and mitochondrial enzyme activities in human respiratory muscles are few. Furthermore, most of the biochemical data available on human respiratory muscles are measurements from patients admitted for surgery or from individuals who were physically inactive during hospitalization (286). Although some studies have examined respiratory muscles obtained from healthy subjects following accidental death, respiratory muscle enzyme activity measurements from postmortem studies are difficult to interpret because of the long and varying time periods between death and tissue removal. Therefore, it is difficult to compare oxidative and glycolytic enzyme activities between human respiratory and locomotor muscles. In contrast, numerous animal studies have demonstrated that the activity of oxidative (i.e., Krebs cycle) enzymes in healthy sedentary rats is 35%–65% greater in the costal diaphragm compared to mixed fiber locomotor muscles (i.e., plantaris) (167, 324, 325). Such large differences in oxidative capacity between the diaphragm and locomotor muscles of untrained animals are not surprising, given the metabolic plasticity of skeletal muscles in response to regular contractile activity. For example, a relatively sedentary (caged) rat has little opportunity to exercise the plantaris muscle; however, the diaphragm is chronically active, as the resting breathing rate is reported to be 70–100 breaths/min (95).

Whole-Body Training: Effects on Rodent Respiratory Muscles

Investigators studying the effects of training on respiratory muscles have used either whole-body endurance exercise training or specific respiratory muscle training as a means of providing a training stimulus. We begin our discussion by considering the effects of whole-body endurance exercise on rodent respiratory muscles.

Metabolic Properties. Most of the literature on this topic has focused on the rat diaphragm. When examining how the diaphragm adapts to exercise training, the crural and costal diaphragm regions must be treated as separate muscles because these two areas appear to have different ventilatory responsibilities (108, 109) and vary in metabolic characteristics (331, 391). Although once controversial, it is now clear that endurance training results in small (i.e., 20%–30%) but significant increases in costal diaphragmatic mitochondrial enzyme activity (e.g., citrate synthase, succinate dehydrogenase) and antioxidant enzyme activity (i.e., superoxide dismutase and glutathione peroxidase) in rodents (159, 167, 195, 286, 325, 327, 328, 329, 330). Surprisingly, the magnitude of these adaptations is relatively independent of the exercise duration and intensity [Fig. 11.17; (325)]. The explanation for this observation is unclear. However, one possible explanation is that the costal diaphragm reaches a plateau in motor unit recruitment prior to meeting the ventilatory requirements during heavy or prolonged exercise; therefore, any further increase in ventilation can only be achieved by recruitment of additional inspiratory muscles. Indirect evidence suggests that both the crural diaphragm and parasternal intercostals may be involved in this process (325). For example, endurance exercise of short duration (e.g., 30 min/day) or low intensity does not significantly increase the oxidative capacity of the crural diaphragm and parasternal intercostal muscles. In contrast, long-duration exercise training (e.g., ≥60 min/day) at high work rates significantly improves the oxidative capacity in both the crural diaphragm and parasternal intercostal muscles [Fig. 11.18; (325)]. These data indicate that these muscles are recruited to assist the diaphragm in meeting the ventilatory requirements during medium- to high-intensity endurance exercise.

Fiber Cross-sectional Area. Endurance training appears to decrease the CSA of costal diaphragmatic fibers with no change in the capillary/fiber ratio (163, 326, 327, 398). Furthermore, a reduction in fiber CSAs may be responsible for a portion of the training-induced increase in relative SDH activity in the costal diaphragm (326, 327). For example, if the total SDH activity in the cell remains unchanged, a reduction in fiber CSAs can result in increased relative SDH activity. Powers et al. (327) found that the mean increase in relative SDH activity in diaphragmatic type I and IIa fibers in trained animals was approximately 16% and 18%, respectively. However, training reduced type I and IIa fiber CSAs by approximately 10% and 15%, respectively. Therefore, the increase in total SDH activity in both type I and IIa fibers accounted for only a portion of the training-induced increase in SDH activity. In short, these findings demonstrate that the training-induced increase in the relative oxidative capacity of the diaphragm is due to both an increase in the quantity of oxidative enzymes and a decrease in fiber CSA.

The regulatory mechanism responsible for the training-induction reduction in diaphragmatic fiber CSA is unclear. Furthermore, the logic in this type of adaptive strategy is subject to debate. It appears that both type I and IIa fibers improve their relative oxidative function, in part, by selective fiber atrophy,

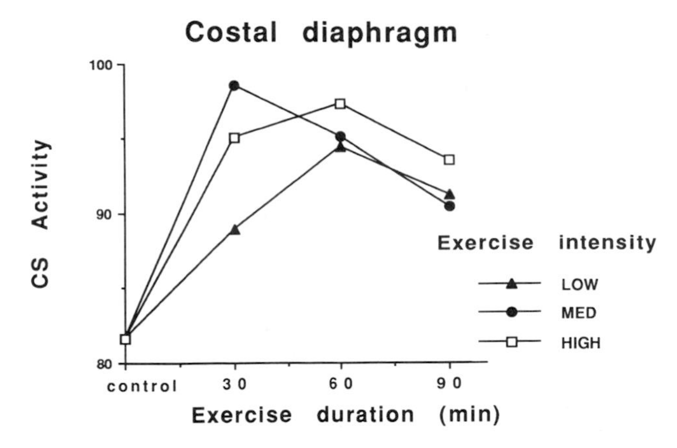

FIG. 11.17. Influence of exercise intensity and duration on the increase in citrate synthase (CS) activity in the costal diaphragm of rats following a 10-week endurance running training program. Nine groups of animals trained at each of three exercise intensities (low = ~55% Vo_{2max}; medium = ~65% Vo_{2max}; high = ~Vo_{2max} 75%) and each of three exercise durations (30, 60, and 90 min · day^{-1}). [Data are from Powers et al. (325).]

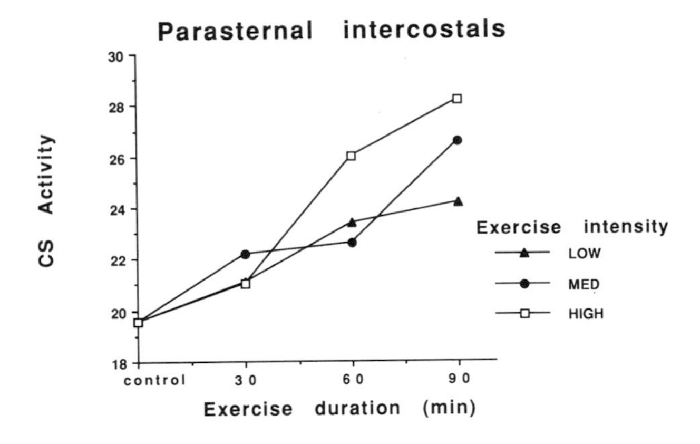

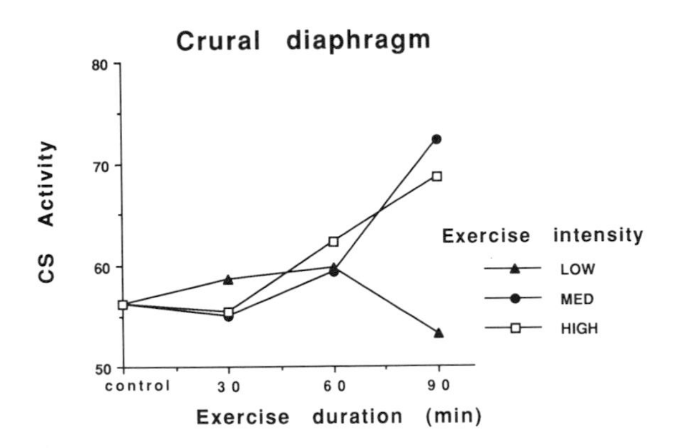

FIG. 11.18. Influence of exercise intensity and duration on the increase in citrate synthase (CS) activity in the crural diaphragm and parasternal intercostal muscles of rats following a 10-week endurance running training program. Nine groups of animals trained at each of three exercise intensities (low = ~55% Vo_{2max}; medium = ~65% Vo_{2max}; high = ~Vo_{2max} 75%) and each of three exercise durations (30, 60, 90 min · day^{-1}). [Data are from Powers et al. (325).]

which may reduce their force-producing ability. The functional importance of a reduction in fiber CSA may be related to a reduced distance for diffusion of gases, metabolites, and/or substrates. Thus, muscle fiber size, oxidative capacity, and fatigue resistance may be interrelated (376).

Endurance training appears to have little effect on costal diaphragm glycolytic enzymes. Two possible exceptions are hexokinase and lactate dehydrogenase (LDH). Endurance training results in small but significant increases in hexokinase activity (+20%) within the costal diaphragm (195). Furthermore, total LDH activity in the diaphragm tends to decrease with endurance training (330). It is unclear if endurance training results in a significant shift in diaphragmatic LDH isoforms.

Diaphragmatic Fiber Types. Does whole-body endurance training alter fiber types in the diaphragm? Investigations using ATPase histochemistry to examine diaphragmatic fiber type do not report exercise training–induced shifts in fiber type (326, 327). However, recent studies have demonstrated that both low-intensity endurance running (389) and low- to moderate-intensity swimming (390) result in small but significant changes in the myosin heavy chain (MHC) composition of the costal diaphragm without altering the MHC pool within the crural diaphragm. Specifically, these investigations reported a reduction in the percentage of costal diaphragmatic type IIb MHC and increases in MHC type IId and type IIa. The physiological significance of these changes is unclear.

Training and Metabolic Properties in Accessory Respiratory Muscles. Endurance training also stimulates increases in the oxidative and antioxidant capacity of other key rodent inspiratory muscles such as the parasternal and external intercostals (163, 325). Furthermore, endurance training results in small (~10%) increases in the oxidative capacity of abdominal (expiratory) muscles (167, 405).

Training and Diaphragmatic Contractile Properties. To date, only one study has examined the effects of whole-body exercise training on the contractile performance of the diaphragm. Metzger and Fitts (281) studied the effects of 6 weeks of interval training (i.e., treadmill running) on the in vitro contractile properties of the rat costal and crural diaphragm. These data demonstrated that this type of exercise training did not alter diaphragmatic maximal force production or the maximal speed of shortening (V_{max}). Furthermore, training did not alter diaphragmatic endurance as defined by an isometric "fatigue test." These findings are predictable, given that the training protocol did not alter diaphragm fiber type or increase the oxidative capacity of the muscle. However, it seems possible that a more aggressive exercise training protocol (i.e., longer duration), resulting in a fast-to-slow shift in myosin isoforms, could alter diaphragmatic V_{max}. This is a testable hypothesis using in vitro techniques and should be addressed in future studies.

Future Experiments. There is a need for additional animal experiments to evaluate the effects of rigorous and prolonged exercise training on diaphragmatic endurance. Whereas in vitro techniques are adequate for measurement of rodent diaphragmatic force production and maximal shortening velocity, questions remain about the validity of this method in assessing diaphragmatic endurance. A general criticism of the in vitro method of measuring diaphragmatic endurance is that the vascular supply to the muscle is removed. This could result in problems of oxygen delivery and removal of metabolites in fibers located in deep regions of the muscle. For example, in this preparation, oxygen is supplied to the diaphragm via dissolved oxygen within the aqueous medium surrounding the muscle. Whether or not adequate oxygen reaches all diaphragmatic fibers during an intense contractile activity in this type of preparation is unknown; hence, this potential gas exchange limitation makes interpretation of in vitro experiments difficult. Future experiments examining the effects of whole-body exercise training on rodent diaphragmatic endurance should consider in situ or in vivo techniques to assess diaphragmatic performance.

In summary, endurance training results in small but significant increases in both mitochondrial and antioxidant enzyme activities of rodent respiratory muscles. A key question remains: Does the improvement in respiratory oxidative capacity and antioxidant enzyme activity enhance respiratory muscle performance? In theory, an increase in mitochondrial volume should increase fat utilization, reduce the rate of muscle glycogen degradation, and decrease lactate formation (157, 187). Furthermore, any training-induced up-regulation of superoxide dismutase and glutathione peroxidase activity in respiratory muscles would improve the tissue's ability to eliminate superoxide radicals and hydroperoxides. Hence, respiratory muscles would be more effective in reducing the oxidative stress caused by an exercise-induced increase in mitochondrial respiration. When considered in total, these changes may delay fatigue during periods of high-intensity contractile activity (187, 339).

Whole-Body Exercise: Effects on Human Respiratory Muscle Performance

Studies examining the effects of whole-body exercise on human respiratory muscle strength and endurance have involved healthy subjects as well as patients with obstructive airway disease. Unfortunately, a meta-analysis of these studies is difficult because of the complication of comparing studies that have used different exercise modalities, varied training regimens, and different tests of ventilatory muscle function. Nonetheless, the literature suggests that whole-body endurance exercise training results in improved ventilatory muscle performance as evidenced by increases in the maximal sustainable ventilation and maximal voluntary ventilation (83, 296). Furthermore, studies comparing ventilatory performance of highly trained subjects with that of untrained subjects reveal that endurance training improves the ability of respiratory muscles to maintain a high-power output (88), but the evidence is indirect. That is, previous studies have evaluated the changes in respiratory "task performance" and have not directly measured alterations in respiratory muscle work capacity (e.g., measurement of transdiaphragmatic pressure). Clearly, additional work is needed to objectively evaluate the effects of whole-body training on respiratory muscle performance.

Specific Respiratory Muscle Training

In addition to the whole-body exercise training, several investigators have also examined the effects of specific respiratory muscle training on ventilatory muscle performance. Most specific respiratory muscle training studies have used two general modes of ventilatory muscle training: *(1)* voluntary isocapnic hyperpnea, and *(2)* inspiratory resistive loading.

Voluntary Isocapnic Hyperpnea. Voluntary isocapnic hyperpnea training is accomplished by having subjects maintain high target levels of ventilation for varying periods up to 20 min (245, 288, 296). Subjects generally train three to five times per week and the training effect is evaluated by monitoring the maximal isocapnic ventilation that can be maintained for an established time period (e.g., 15 min). Both healthy subjects and patients with airway disease appear to show improvement in respiratory muscle endurance with this type of training (51, 52, 127, 245, 288, 296).

Inspiratory Resistive Loading. During inspiratory resistive loading training, loads are applied to inspiratory muscles three to five times per week for a duration of 5–15 min. The training effect is evaluated as the increase in time that a fixed resistive load can be tolerated or the increase in the maximal resistance that can be sustained over a specified amount of time. Although this type of training may improve respiratory muscle endurance (15, 82), these findings should be interpreted with caution (52, 310). With the exception of the work of Clanton et al. (82), the studies of inspiratory resistance cited above have controlled neither lung volume nor the breathing strategy during pre- and post-training evaluation of respiratory muscle endurance. This is significant because adoption of a breathing pattern using slow inspirations during inspiratory loading is better tolerated by subjects; the reason is that slow inspirations lower inspiratory (mouth) pressures, slow the rate of development of respiratory muscle fatigue, and reduce the sensation of effort in breathing (52). Indeed, during inspiratory resistance experiments on naive subjects, Belman et al. (52) have shown that changing the normal (freely chosen) breathing pattern to a pattern of long slow breaths immediately improved respiratory muscle endurance. Clearly, subsequent studies employing resistive breathing as a method of respiratory muscle training should monitor and control both the lung volume and breathing pattern during the pre- and post-training evaluations (310). Again, future human studies should also provide objective measurements of changes in respiratory muscle performance following respiratory muscle training programs.

RESPIRATORY SENSATION DURING EXERTION

Common experience tells us that the increase in ventilation that accompanies exercise changes our perception of respiratory-related sensations. Early on in exercise, we become aware that we are breathing more, and as exercise progresses, we can continue to assess the rise in ventilation. At some point during increasingly intense exercise, most individuals will report an uncomfortable sensation commonly referred to as "shortness of breath" or "breathlessness," which grows in intensity as the exercise continues. This sensation assumes great significance in many disease states, when even mild exertion can lead to debilitating levels of breathlessness or dyspnea; the symptom of dyspnea related to disease has recently been reviewed (388). Although some authors have argued that dyspnea associated with pathological states should be regarded as distinct from the breathlessness reported by healthy subjects on exertion (even though patients themselves use the same terms), there is no good evidence as to whether the sensory experiences are different. For the purposes of this review, the terms will be used interchangeably.

Mechanisms of Respiratory Sensations during Exercise

In view of the potentially complex nature of respiratory sensation during exercise, we will examine separately the neurophysiological basis of its main components before considering how different types of neural information might interact; the reader is referred to several reviews on this topic (7, 78, 147, 220, 362, 368). Figure 11.19 shows a possible schema for the neurophysiological substrate of respiratory sensations (considered below) in terms of the peripheral and central nervous structures known to be associated with respiratory control.

Methods of Assessing Respiratory Sensations

Psychophysical techniques developed for the study of perception of sensory phenomena (for review, see 382) have permitted us to systematically investigate perceived sensations associated with breathing during exercise. If the magnitude of a stimulus giving rise to a sensation can be measured (e.g., the volume of a breath or the value of an external inspiratory resistance), then it is possible to establish the absolute sensitivity of sensory discrimination (by assessing "just noticeable" differences), as well as the quantitative relationship between the stimulus and sensation intensities (by assessing the relative ratio changes in their magnitudes). Such studies have provided valuable insights into the physiological basis of sensations of respiratory mechanical events (for review, see 446). However, for other respiratory sensations experienced during exercise, the specific stimuli are not known (e.g., the sensation of an urge to breathe) or are not easily measurable (e.g., sensations related to a conscious awareness of the efferent activity to respiratory muscles). In these cases, sensory scaling techniques in which the subject is asked to assess the intensity of their sensation relative to fixed notional criteria have been employed. Two such approaches that have been widely used in studies on respiratory sensation are the Borg Category Scale and the Visual Analogue Scale. Both scales have been shown to be valid for the assessment of respiratory sensations and are generally comparable with one another (4, 69, 290, 379, 434).

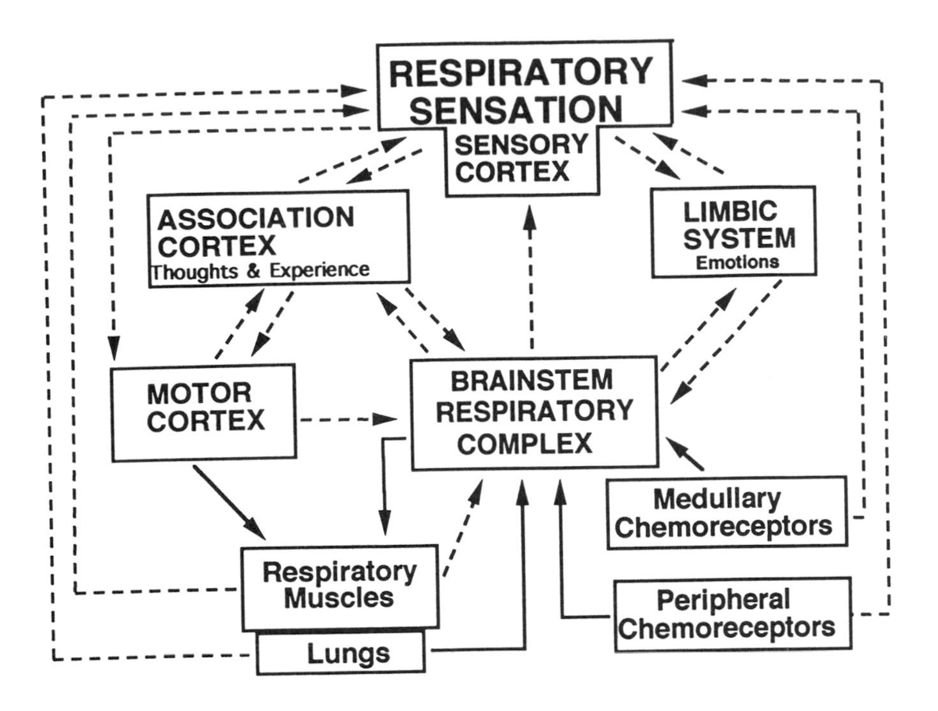

FIG. 11.19. A schematic representation of known (*solid lines*) and putative (*broken lines*) neural pathways showing possible interactions between areas of respiratory control and respiratory-related sensations during respiratory stimulation (e.g., exercise). The figure is intended to provide an "anatomical" basis to which the reader can refer, with respect to some of the research findings and ideas discussed in this review.

Respiratory Movements

Spontaneous respiratory movements require a centrally generated efferent command to respiratory muscles and are associated with afferent feedback from receptors within the lungs (pulmonary receptors), the respiratory muscles (muscle spindles and Golgi tendon organs), the rib cage (joint receptors), and the upper airways (airflow and temperature receptors). Banzett et al. (37) have demonstrated that patients with spinal lesions above the level of efferent and afferent connections to the main respiratory muscle (i.e., C_1–C_2) are able to perceive ventilator-delivered changes in tidal volume with the same acuity as normal subjects. By exclusion, these results suggest that vagal afferent information from pulmonary receptors (likely to be slowly adapting stretch receptors in view of their known sensitivity to lung expansion) can be perceived as volume displacement in the absence of efferent activity to respiratory muscles or afferent feedback from respiratory muscles or rib cage receptors; however, there is no direct evidence on this point. On the other hand, evidence from experiments in normal subjects indicates that volume perception may depend on both the level of central command (148, 337) and afferent feedback from the chest wall (386, 437). The upper airway seems unlikely to be an important source of afferent information for judging volume changes (112, 137).

An Urge to Breathe

During progressive exercise in normal subjects, the level of ventilation at which a sensation of an uncomfortable need to breathe is first reported varies widely (5, 351) but is generally well above that at which there is the first awareness that breathing has increased (216, 423). Ventilatory stimulation with hypercapnia or hypoxia induces sensations of an urge to breathe, although it is not clear to what extent these are qualitatively similar to the experience during exercise (4). Certainly, the sensations associated with exercise are judged by most people to be qualitatively different from those accompanying breathholding or ventilatory stimulation, when increases in breathing are constrained (38). The interaction between ventilatory stimulation and respiratory movements does indeed appear to be crucial in the genesis of an uncomfortable urge to breathe (see below) and may be relevant in patients with respiratory mechanical limitation who experience severe dyspnea at low levels of exertion.

In considering the neurophysiological basis of the urge to breathe during exercise, a key observation is that isocapnic *voluntary* hyperventilation to a level associated with substantial discomfort during exercise or hypercapnia causes little or no discomfort even in patients with severe mechanical limitation (8, 138). Moreover, in normal exercising subjects the urge to breathe is substantially reduced if ventilation is sustained with isocapnic voluntary breathing at a lower level of exercise (239). Thus, this sensation appears to depend not simply on the fact that breathing has increased but that the increase has resulted from automatic rather than volitional ventilatory stimulation. In this respect, the urge to breathe during exercise is analogous to that experienced during hypoxia or hypercapnia (5) but occurs in the absence of any appreciable change in blood gas levels. A common feature would appear to be that activation of respiratory-related neurons in the brainstem (assuming exercise hyperpnea is mediated via this pathway), in addition to stimulating respiratory muscles, also gives rise to neural information that is perceived by higher central nervous structures as an unpleasant sensation referred to the lungs/chest. A neurophysiological correlate for such a pathway has recently been shown by Chen et al. (76, 77), who have demonstrated in decorticate cats the existence of pathways ascending from the brainstem that are activated in response to respiratory chemostimulation. They demonstrated mesencephalic and thalamic neurons that develop rhythmic activity related to breathing and graded in magnitude according to the level of medullary neural respiratory drive. However, whether this activity is relaying respiratory-related information to the sensorium and whether it would be present during exercise is not known. Anatomical connections from medulla to diencephalon certainly lend support to this physiological evidence (43).

We have recent direct evidence from conscious, normal humans in support of the thesis that the urge-to-breathe sensation derives from reflex stimulation of respiratory-related CNS structures. This evidence comes from experiments in which voluntary breathing was prevented by complete neuromuscular blockade in conscious humans. When their mechanical ventilation was fixed, small amounts of CO_2 added to the ventilator induced an urge to breathe in the presumed absence of any change in proprioceptive feedback from the lungs, respiratory muscle, or rib cage receptors (38, 149). The data from one of these studies (38) are presented in Figure 11.20. In addition, studies in patients following heart-lung transplantation (35) or with lung disease following inhalation of anesthetic aerosol (435) do not support any important role for pulmonary receptors in the genesis of exercise-induced breathlessness; similarly the ability of patients with C1–C2 spinal cord lesions (39) and respiratory muscle paralysis (304) to feel an urge to breathe during mild hypercapnia is not consistent with an important role for chest wall/respiratory muscle afferent receptors in giving rise to this sensation.

The extent to which the perception of an urge to breathe during exercise in normal subjects derives directly from activation of pontomedullary structures is uncertain. An early study in children with congenital hypoventilation during sleep (Ondine's curse—presumed to be associated with dysfunction of the automatic respiratory controller in the brainstem) reported marked hypoventilation during exercise in the absence of any appreciable respiratory discomfort (194). However, studies in children with this condition indicate a more normal ventilatory response to exercise (313, 367), even though there is complete absence of response to chemostimulation with hypoxia and hypercapnia and associated respiratory sensations at rest. Whether these individuals experience an urge to breathe during exercise is unclear (367). Anecdotal evidence in patients with medullary disease affecting automatic respiratory control (acquired Ondine's curse) seems to indicate little respiratory discomfort during exercise despite a normal ventilatory response (7).

As mentioned above, hypoxia and hypercapnia, like exercise, induce an uncomfortable sensation of a need to breathe associated with ventilatory stimulation. Early studies suggested that for a given degree of ventilatory stimulation in normal subjects, hypercapnia and hypoxia induced at rest a greater urge to breathe than did exercise (4, 379) suggesting that chemosensitivity per se was *dyspnogenic*. However, a further study, better controlled for the distracting influence of exercise, has indicated that the urge to breathe associated with exercise alone is not different from that reported for the same degree of ventilatory stimulation induced by steady-state hypercapnia or isocapnic hypoxia coupled with a lower level of exercise (237). Similar findings were reported by Ward and Whipp (413) with respect to hypercapnia during exercise; however, these authors found that hypoxia during exercise induced a greater respiratory discomfort than the same ventilation resulting from exercise alone. In addition, transient hypoxia during exercise does appear to induce rapid changes in sensation that precede the slower ventilatory changes (81). These observations leave open the possibility that hypoxia during exercise is associated with a degree of discomfort disproportionate to its effect on ventilation at least in the nonsteady state. Similarly, there is clear evidence that hyperoxia during exercise alleviates respiratory discomfort both in normal subjects (36, 81) and in patients with respiratory disease (238, 393), although it is not clear if this effect is disproportionately greater than the accompanying fall in ventilation.

In assessing the onset of an urge to breathe during progressive exercise in normal subjects, a num-

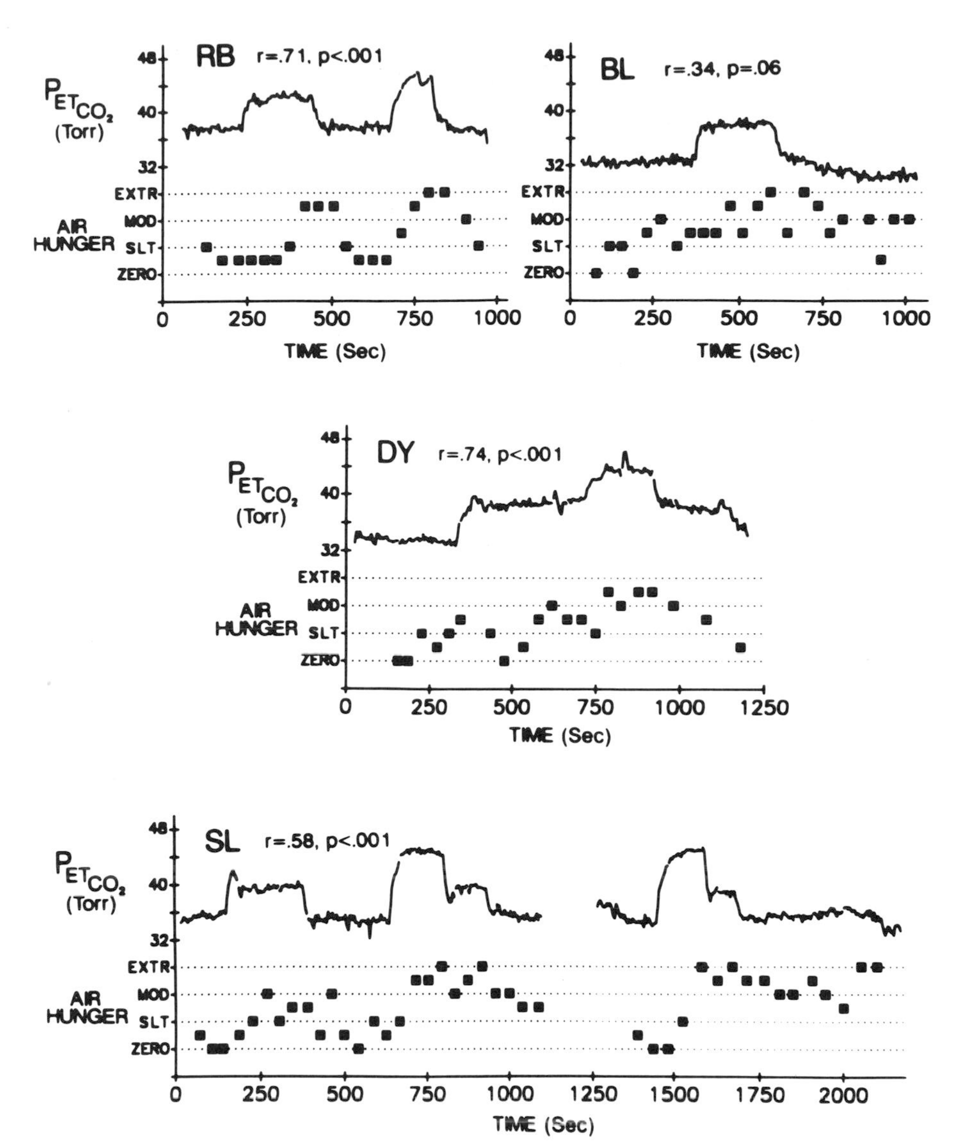

FIG. 11.20. Time course of end-tidal P_{CO_2} (PET_{CO_2}) and subjective ratings of air hunger (urge to breathe) in four subjects (RB, BL, DY, and SL) during complete neuromuscular paralysis. Subjects underwent fixed mechanical ventilation and made ratings (via a tourniqueted arm) as inspired CO_2 concentration was surreptitiously increased; ratings were made using a seven-point scale ranging from zero through slight (SLT) and moderate (MOD) to extreme (EXTR) with intermediate rating options. Nonparametric correlation coefficients (*r*) were calculated between ratings and the level of PET_{CO_2} two min earlier (to allow for "equilibration" of medullary P_{CO_2}. [From Banzett et al. (38).]

ber of investigators have been struck by an apparent association between this and the onset of lactic acidosis (81). Moreover, for a given degree of exercise-induced ventilation, the intensity of respiratory discomfort seems to be inversely correlated with physical fitness (5), which may reflect individual differences in the level of exercise at which anaerobiosis becomes established. However, a recent study in normal subjects has failed to show any difference in the urge to breathe during exercise in the presence of experimentally induced normocapnic metabolic acidosis compared with ordinary higher intensity exercise inducing the same level of ventilation (235). Thus, a specific role for acidosis in the genesis of respiratory discomfort during exercise remains speculative.

Table 11.2 summarizes a series of studies by our group (discussed above) in which we assessed the effect of a second ventilatory stimulus during exercise on intensity of the urge to breathe. Our main interpretation was that the intensity of the urge to breathe reflects the degree of "reflex" respiratory stimulation irrespective of the nature of the specific stimulus.

TABLE 11.2. *Average Results from Three Studies in Normal Subjects in which Exercise was Paired with a Second Ventilatory Stimulus to Achieve the Same Levels of Ventilation as with Exercise Alone**

Experimental Condition	Number of Subjects	Workload (watts)	PET_{CO_2} (mm Hg)	Sa_{O_2} (%)	Urge to Breathe at 50 liter · min^{-1} (%VAS)
Exercise alone[†]	18	150	44	96	38
Exercise + hypercapnia[†]	18	110	54	96	37
Exercise + hypoxia[†]	18	105	45	89	36
Exercise alone[‡]	6	110	40	96	31
Exercise + acidosis[‡]	6	85	41	96	29
Exercise alone[§]	9	130	39	96	29
Exercise + volition[§]	9	85	38	96	9

*The mean intensity of the sensation of an urge to breathe (breathlessness) at a mean ventilation of 50 liter·min^{-1} was assessed using a Visual Analogue Scale (VAS). Mean levels of workload, end-tidal PCO_2 (PET_{CO_2}), and ear oximetry estimates of arterial oxygen saturation (Sa_{O_2}) at which measurements were made are shown.

[†]Results taken from Lane et al. (237).

[‡]Results taken from Lane and Adams (235).

[§]Results taken from Lane et al. (238).

A Sense of Respiratory Effort

It has been suggested that humans can perceive the intensity of the motor command to respiratory muscles as a sense of respiratory effort and that this may be related to the dyspnea sensation (147). Studies employing experimentally induced respiratory muscle fatigue (148) and increases in lung volume (221) suggests that under these conditions subjects are able to distinguish changes in the sense of motor command from changes in inspiratory muscle force (inspiratory pressure) created by the addition of respiratory loads. Moreover, imposition of inspiratory loads during exercise in normal subjects (119) has led to the suggestion that the sensation of breathlessness may be related to the perception of respiratory effort. This view has been supported by exercise studies in patients with cardiorespiratory disease (241). However, under these conditions it is unclear to what extent a "sense of effort" is a feature of automatic respiratory motor output from the brainstem as opposed to increased efferent activity from the motor cortex (16). Certainly, if asked, normal subjects are able to perceive an increase in the "work" or "effort" associated with increased breathing during exercise, but this sensation appears to be quite distinct from the "urge to breathe" sensation (101, 236).

Notwithstanding the importance of efferent neural activity in the perception of respiratory sensations, there is considerable evidence that afferent feedback from receptors in respiratory muscles (tendon organs and muscle spindles) and rib cage (joint receptors) is integral to the perception of respiratory muscle tension or pressure, the magnitude of volume or ventilation (see above), and the magnitude of added respiratory loads (for review, see 446). However, the exact neural mechanisms by which such afferent information interacts with efferent output to respiratory muscles leading to perception of respiratory mechanical events during exercise remains to be defined.

Respiratory Sensation as a Respiratory Controller during Exercise

Over the years, a view has arisen that in achieving a required level of alveolar ventilation (e.g., in response to exercise), a pattern of breathing is adopted that minimizes respiratory work or respiratory muscle force (278, 438), although no specific "work receptors" have been proposed. However, under conditions of increased mechanical constraint in normal subjects (loaded breathing) and in patients with respiratory disease, the spontaneously adopted pattern of breathing was not necessarily appropriate for the minimizing tension or work of breathing (213, 219), and it has been suggested that the "sense of effort" was being minimized. In this way, the level of tidal volume and respiratory frequency adopted during exercise would depend not only on the tension being developed by the respiratory muscles but also on their length and velocity of shortening (212).

More recently, Poon (322) has proposed an optimization model that could account for the level and pattern of ventilation adopted during exercise. In this way, breathing would be regulated to minimize both blood gas changes (monitored by chemoreceptors) and increases in respiratory mechanical work (monitored either consciously or subconsciously as "respiratory mechanical discomfort"). Cherniack and co-workers (78, 79) have further modified this idea and suggested (80, 179) that breathing during ventilatory stimulation (including exercise) might be determined by a behavioral need to minimize perceived sensations of respiratory discomfort. Chonan et al. (80) demonstrated that for a given level of hypercapnia induced in normal subjects, volitional increases or decreases in ventilation away from the spontaneous level cause additional respiratory discomfort. Moreover, Harty and Adams (179) have recently demonstrated that in exercising normal subjects, increases in the sensation of breathlessness are associated with very modest degrees of volitional ventilatory suppression. Current evidence indicates that in normal subjects the act of breathing per se can ameliorate sensations of respiratory discomfort even in the absence of changes in blood gases (136, 260, 341). This effect has also been observed in patients with C1–C2 spinal cord lesions (260) and in patients following heart-lung transplantation (179a), suggesting that neither afferent information from the chest wall/respiratory muscles nor from pulmonary receptors is obligatory for this "mechanically related" relief of respiratory discomfort. In the context of respiratory sensation as a respiratory controller during exercise, recent studies have used positron emission tomography (PET) to image cerebral function during and following exercise. They show evidence of control of respiratory muscles for the motor cortex at a time when subjects perceive an exercise-related urge to breathe (6). Whether this association between respiratory sensation and higher center control of breathing represents a causal relationship, perhaps operating by associative learning, remains speculative.

Respiratory Sensation as a Limiting Factor during Exercise

Whereas it is generally accepted that dyspnea is a major symptom limiting exercise performance during cardiorespiratory and other diseases (388), work by Killian et al. (222) has shown that patients with respiratory disease identify both leg fatigue and dyspnea as important in limiting their performance during incremental exercise on a bicycle ergometer. More surprisingly, the same study revealed that at maximal exercise capacity, healthy subjects rated leg fatigue as very severe and dyspnea as severe to very severe, with many subjects identifying dyspnea as a more important or as important a symptom as leg fatigue in limiting exercise. More recently, the same group (174) has shown that during extreme exertion for short durations, although normal subjects rated leg fatigue as the major limiting symptom, dyspnea levels were also rated highly. Such high work intensities in normal subjects will be associated with marked changes in both respiratory mechanics and humoral changes in the blood, and hence the respiratory sensations reported as dyspnea are likely to reflect a complex combination of sensations of "urge," "effort," and other sensory continuae (see above). It is also possible that during heavy or sustained exercise, ratings of respiratory sensations may be "masked" by the general discomfort associated with other exercise-related symptoms such as leg pain, fatigue, and increased body temperature. In this respect it is significant that a number of workers have reported increases in breathlessness with continued exercise in the absence of changes in ventilation or respiratory mechanics (303).

Conclusions

Considerable progress has been made in terms of our understanding of the neurophysiological basis of respiratory sensations on exertion, although much still remains to be learned. Inevitably, studies in humans are necessary for progress in this area, and while this presents limitations it also provides exciting opportunities. In addition to the need for more studies during exercise with careful assessment of associated respiratory sensations, it is likely that new techniques that permit functional imaging of the brain as well as the continued study of patients with well-defined neurological lesions (both in the brainstem and cerebrum) will shed further light on this difficult problem.

SUMMARY—PULMONARY SYSTEM LIMITATIONS AND THEIR EFFECTS ON EXERCISE PERFORMANCE

There are a number of ways in which pulmonary function might be limited during exercise of short and long duration, and they could act independently or in concert with other influences to limit exercise performance. These possibilities are briefly outlined in the following list.

1. Alveolar end-capillary O_2 disequilibrium may occur in heavy exercise, causing arterial hypoxemia and thereby limiting maximal systemic O_2 transport, the capability for maximizing the arterial-to-venous O_2 content difference across the working muscle, and therefore $\dot{V}O_{2max}$ (see Chapter 12, this volume).
2. When mechanical limits of the airways and lung parenchyma to flow rate and volume are

reached, alveolar ventilation is unable (or "unwilling") to increase further with increasing work rate, alveolar P_{O_2} falls or is unable to rise normally and O_2 transport and CO_2 elimination are diminished.

3. The dynamic capacity of the respiratory muscles for the generation of pleural pressure may be insufficient to meet or sustain ventilatory requirements.

4. Respiratory muscles fatigue to such an extent that they are incapable of generating and/or maintaining sufficient tension to ensure adequate tidal volume and alveolar ventilation to meet metabolic requirements or may induce a highly tachypneic breathing pattern, thereby reducing alveolar ventilation.

5. The work and metabolic cost of breathing incurred by the primary respiratory and stabilizing muscles of the chest wall plus their demand for perfusion to meet this O_2 cost may "steal" blood flow from locomotor muscles, thereby, limiting their work output.

6. The sum of sensory inputs from all chemoreceptors and mechanoreceptors to the higher CNS gives rise to sufficiently severe dyspneic sensations so as to bring about symptom-limited exercise performance.

7. There also may be interactive effects of pulmonary function limitations with other determinants of oxygen transport and performance. For example: *(1)* the effects of high intrathoracic negative pressures or intra-abdominal positive pressures on venous return and stroke volumes (see Chapter 15, this volume); *(2)* conversely, the effects of a limited cardiac output on perfusion of the respiratory muscles; and *(3)* the synergistic effects on motivation to continue exercise from the combined sensations of exertional dyspnea with locomotor muscle fatigue (218).

Given these possibilities, we now use the findings and principles discussed throughout this chapter to determine the answer to the following question: If any of these limitations are in fact achieved, under what circumstances this might happen and what consequences would be there for $\dot{V}_{O_{2max}}$ or exercise performance?

Absence of Pulmonary System Limitations in the Normally Fit

In the prototype human subject we have used throughout this chapter (i.e., the young, healthy, untrained adult working at sea level) it is safe to conclude that the lung and chest wall—with a few notable exceptions (see below)—operate highly efficiently and well within their relative capacities at all exercise intensities up to maximum and for long durations of exercise at high intensity. Thus, up to an average $\dot{V}_{O_{2max}}$ approximating 50–55 ml · min^{-1} · kg^{-1} or within about 30%–40% greater than the normal mean, the following evidence supports this conclusion:

1. Significant exercise-induced arterial hypoxemia does not occur, as even though $\dot{V}_A$:$\dot{Q}$ distribution is less than perfect and the alveolar-to-arterial P_{O_2} difference widens to about 25 mm Hg, sufficient alveolar hyperventilation occurs at maximal exercise (Pa_{CO_2} <35 mm Hg), so the arterial P_{O_2} remains within 10 mm Hg of resting levels and Sa_{O_2} >93%.

2. Expiratory or inspiratory flow limitation is minimal at maximal exercise, end-expiratory lung volume remains well below resting values, and V_T operates principally along the steepest (most efficient) portion of the pressure/volume relationship (see Fig. 11.6). Ventilation at maximum exercise increases further when additional CO_2 stimulation (85) or dead space breathing are superimposed (396). Thus, there is clearly significant ventilatory reserve at maximal exercise in healthy untrained adults.

3. The generation of pleural pressure by inspiratory muscles during tidal breathing at maximum exercise is less than 50%–60% of dynamic capacity.

4. The oxygen cost of breathing per liter ventilation only begins to rise appreciably at the levels of ventilatory work obtained at $\dot{V}_{O_{2max}}$ and the total O_2 cost of hyperpnea is less than 10% of $\dot{V}_{O_{2max}}$ (see Fig. 11.12).

5. The work done by the respiratory muscles is not, by itself, fatiguing at maximal V_{O_2} or during long-term exercise of moderate intensity (see Fig. 11.14). In very heavy endurance exercise to exhaustion, the diaphragm does show "significant" fatigue that recovers slowly following exercise.

6. Given the negative effects of partial unloading of the respiratory muscles (see earlier under Unloading with Pressure Assist), it is unlikely that either the mechanical work or O_2 cost of breathing or dyspneic sensations or probably even the degree of respiratory muscle fatigue experienced during maximum exercise or long-term endurance exercise affects either the ventilatory response or exercise performance.

Thus, under these conditions of heavy exercise in the standard reference subject, it is clear that while O_2 transport remains the critical limiting factor to $\dot{V}_{O_{2max}}$, maximum cardiovascular transport capacity to working muscle and specifically maximum stroke volume are probably the dominant limiting factor to $\dot{V}_{O_{2max}}$ (see Chapter 17). Furthermore, with heavy endurance exercise the negative data obtained with unloading (see earlier under Unloading with Pressure

Assist) would support the conclusion that the fatigue of locomotor muscles must proceed during endurance exercise at a faster rate than that of the respiratory muscles.

CONTRASTING ADAPTABILITIES: DEMAND VS. CAPACITY

Structural capacities of each link in the gas transport chain from alveolar gas to locomotor muscle mitochondria differ markedly relative to the maximum demands imposed by exercise. As summarized in the preceding discussion, the lung, airways, and respiratory muscles are clearly overbuilt in the untrained human healthy subject; however, these pulmonary system structures would appear to be the least malleable in response to changing fitness levels and in this respect contrast sharply with the marked changes that occur in the metabolic capacity of the locomotor muscles and in the functional capacity of the cardiovascular system (102, 105). Accordingly, as either the capacity to transport or consume O_2 ($\dot{V}O_{2max}$) or endurance exercise performance increase greater than the normal reference standard (by means of physical training and/or genetic endowment), it is likely that the primary determinants of exercise limitation will change. Over the past two decades these relationships between demand and capacity in several of the organ systems involved in gas transport have been analyzed both within and among a variety of a mammalian species. We consider both gas exchange and respiratory mechanics in our present analysis but refer the reader to Chapters 12 and 13 in this *Handbook* for a detailed analysis of alveolar-to-arterial (A-a) O_2 exchange during exercise.

Alveolar Capillary Diffusion Surface of the Lung

This index of pulmonary diffusion capacity does not—with very few exceptions (see below)—adapt to match increasing levels of fitness or $\dot{V}O_{2max}$. This has been documented by the similarities found in functional measurements of diffusion capacity in sedentary vs. athletic humans who differ by as much as twofold in $\dot{V}O_{2max}$ (102). Most strikingly, in athletic vs. sedentary animals who are similar in body mass but vary by as much as threefold in $\dot{V}O_{2max}$, morphologic dimensions of the lung's diffusion surface are only slightly higher in the athletic species (399, 422). Accordingly, in very heavy exercise (i.e., at >80% $\dot{V}O_{2max}$), excessive widening of the A-a DO_2 (to 45 mm Hg) and arterial hypoxemia (80%–92% SaO_2) occur with a significant prevalence in highly trained athletes ($\dot{V}O_{2max}$ 65–85 ml/kg) and in most thoroughbred horses studied ($\dot{V}O_{2max}$ 140–170 ml · kg^{-1} · min^{-1}) (44, 104, 107, 123, 178, 332). In turn, when this exercise-induced hypoxemia is prevented via the use of mild hyperoxia in inspired gas, $\dot{V}O_{2max}$ increases significantly and roughly in proportion to the magnitude of the original hypoxemia [i.e., about 5%–15% in humans (332) and 10%–25% in the thoroughbred horse (211) (P. D. Wagner et al., personal communication). So the lung's capabilities for O_2 exchange are limited because of the limited plasticity in its diffusion surface. This adaptive failure will present a significant limitation to $\dot{V}O_{2max}$. This emphasie that (in humans) the maximum metabolic demand must be at least 70%–80% greater than normal[1] before the diffusion reserve is exhausted. Even under these extreme conditions exercise-induced hypoxemia does not occur in all highly fit human subjects (107).

Ventilatory Limitations/Constraints

These issues of demand vs. capacity also apply to ventilatory limitation during exercise. Maximum ventilatory requirement must rise commensurate with any rise in maximal metabolic rate (see Fig. 11.21). The upper limits to maximum exercise breathing frequency, tidal volume, and ventilation are determined structurally by the lung's resistive and elastic properties and the force-velocity characteristics of the inspiratory muscles (see earlier under BREATHING PATTERN DURING EXERCISE). Among subjects of widely varying $\dot{V}O_{2max}$, the dynamic capacity for pressure generation by the inspiratory muscles and the area of the maximum flow–volume envelope are—with some notable exceptions (23)—quite similar (83, 207, 250). So as $\dot{V}O_{2max}$ (and $\dot{V}CO_{2max}$) increase, are the normal mechanical reserves sufficient to accommodate the accompanying increase in maximum ventilatory requirement? As shown in Figure

[1]It is important to emphasize that it is not just the magnitude of the $\dot{V}O_{2max}$ (demand) that determines whether exercise-induced hypoxemia occurs. Morphologic capacity of the lung is also important in assessing this balance. For example, species such as the dog, pony, and rat have maximal metabolic rates that exceed those in the most elite humans by 50%–80% and yet do not experience exercise-induced arterial hypoxemia (44, 103, 139). Most impressive in this regard is a recent report in the pronged-horn antelope who has a maximal $\dot{V}O_2$ that is >400 ml · kg^{-1} · min^{-1} or five to six times that of a nonathletic animal (goat) of similar body mass (249). The antelope also has a lung diffusion surface that is also six times that of the nonathletic animal and equal to the magnitude of the adaptive increases in muscle mitochondrial volume and cardiac output (249). Thus, this species presents as a unique example among highly fit athletic species of lung morphology scaling in proportion to maximum metabolic requirements. Among human endurance-trained athletes, the highly trained swimmer might also be exceptional in showing pulmonary diffusion capacities and lung volumes that exceed those in their sedentary contemporaries (23, 83).

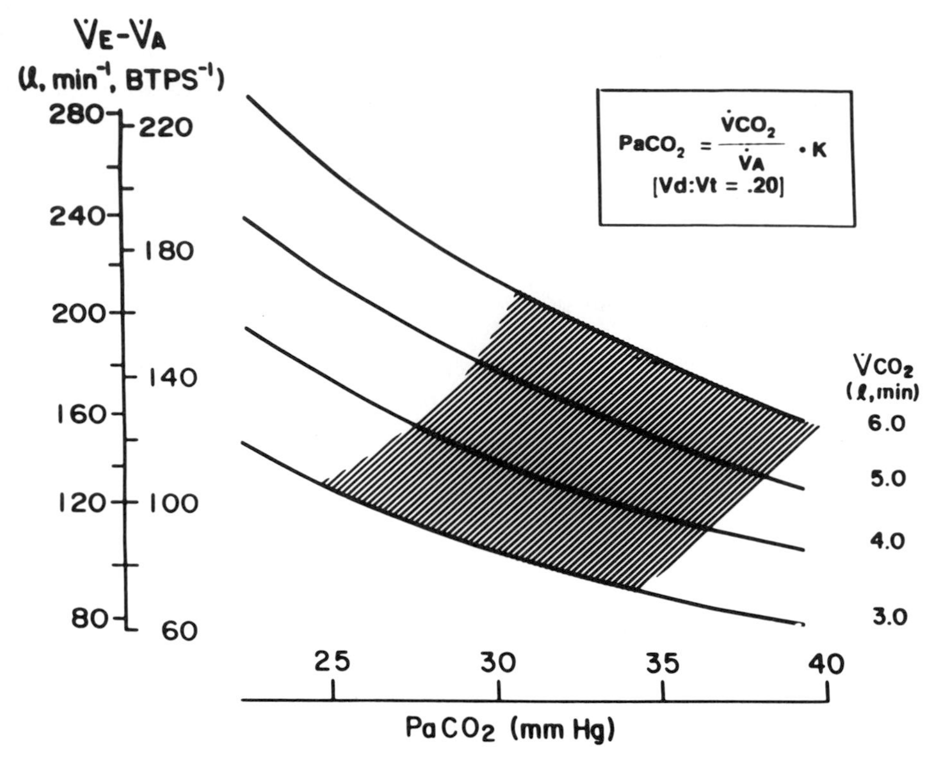

FIG. 11.21. Relationship of alveolar ventilation ($\dot{V}_A$) to arterial P_{CO_2} (Pa_{CO_2}) at various levels of maximum exercise ($\dot{V}_{CO_2}$) according to the alveolar air equation. Values shown for total minute ventilation ($\dot{V}_E$) assume a V_D/V_T of 0.20 at maximum exercise. Note that to achieve a given level of hyperventilation at maximum exercise (e.g., a Pa_{CO_2} = 30 mm Hg), the ventilatory requirements are markedly different for the sedentary subject ($\dot{V}_{CO_2}$ = 3 liter · min^{-1}, $\dot{V}_E \approx$ 120 liter · min^{-1}) vs. that achieved in the highly fit ($\dot{V}_{CO_2}$ = 6 liter · min^{-1}; $\dot{V}_E$ > 190 liter · min^{-1}). The *shaded areas* show the wide range of alveolar hyperventilation achieved at maximum exercise among healthy subjects across the fitness continuum with substantial overlap but a tendency for less hyperventilation at the higher maximum $\dot{V}_{CO_2}$ in the highly fit.

11.6, highly fit humans do achieve substantial expiratory flow limitation (i.e., 40%–50% of V_T) at maximal exercise even when maximal $\dot{V}_{O_2}$ and $\dot{V}_E$ are only 20%–30% greater than the untrained reference subject. Furthermore, in the endurance athlete whose $\dot{V}_{O_{2max}}$ is greater than 70 ml · kg^{-1} · min^{-1} and $\dot{V}_E$ is greater than 160 liters/min, truly mechanical limits to $\dot{V}_E$ may often appear to be reached. V_T is 70%–90% flow limited on expiration and expiratory pressures reach critical "effective" levels; peak inspiratory flow rate and inspiratory pressures are near maximal dynamic capacity; EELV has risen to or near resting levels; and finally, end-EILV is greater than 85% of total lung capacity (TLC) (166, 207).

Is $\dot{V}_E$ truly mechanically limited or "constrained" under these extreme conditions? On the one hand, $\dot{V}_E$ at $\dot{V}_{O_{2max}}$ has not reached the conventional criterion of maximal mechanical ventilation (i.e., the 12–15 s maximal voluntary ventilation). However, this measure may not be an appropriate estimate of the highest available ventilation for exercise because it is commonly carried out at high lung volumes and excessive expiratory pressures and frequencies and is not sustainable for more than a few seconds (208). Further support of the occurrence of significant mechanical limitation to $\dot{V}_E$ at these high exercise levels includes the failure of $\dot{V}_{E_{max}}$ to increase further with added substantial amounts of CO_2 or hypoxemia (207) as opposed to the immediate and sustained increase in $\dot{V}_E$ obtained with He-O_2 in these highly fit subjects (104) and in equine athletes [see below (123)]. This effect of He-O_2 on increasing ventilation exceeded the effects of added chemoreceptor stimuli in the same subjects (104), thereby suggesting that He-O_2 was probably exerting its effect by increasing the maximum envelope of the flow–volume loop, thereby increasing mechanical reserve and permitting increased frequency and tidal volume. Furthermore, the slope of the ventilatory response to added CO_2 has been shown to remain unchanged over a wide range of submaximal exercise loads, but this response slope begins to show a systematic reduction in heavy submaximal work loads as $\dot{V}_E$ enters the range of 120–140 liters/min (85) and at flow rates where significant expiratory flow limitation usually begins to appear (see Fig. 11.6). Perhaps then the constraint of ventilatory drive, by reflex inhibition responding to the increased mechanical load, might begin to exert a significant inhibitory influence on both $\dot{V}_E$ and breathing pattern. This might begin to occur at high levels of exercise intensity that are significantly below these extreme cases where ventilation is completely nonresponsive to added stimuli (see below).

The regulation of the hyperventilatory response to heavy exercise and the differences in the magnitude of this response among subjects remains—much like the hyperpnea of more moderate exercise—very poorly understood. A fundamental question here is whether inhibitory mechanical feedback secondary to increasing flow limitation *or* increasing muscle work *or* respiratory muscle fatigue ever play an important role in regulating ventilation as work rates increase during heavy and very heavy exercise. Gradually declining CO_2 response slopes in heavy exercise might suggest this to be the case (see above); but this implied so-called feedback neural reflex inhibition of ventilation has never been documented during heavy exercise. Alternatively, feedforward mechanisms such as multiple chemoreceptor stimuli and/or rising central command (414 see also Chapter 9) are extremely strong and may be so dominant that ventilation will continue to respond until exercise is simply terminated (at $\dot{V}O_{2max}$) or "complete" mechanical limitation of ventilation is reached (see above) or both occur simultaneously (207).

The study of some highly trained humans during very heavy exercise revealed ventilatory responses that support all of these views of ventilatory control (207). We now present three examples to illustrate the diversity of relationships between ventilatory response and mechanical reserve. First, most of these highly fit subjects show substantial flow limitation, high elastic loads, and very high inspiratory muscle pressure generation at maximal exercise; this coincides with subnormal levels of alveolar hyperventilation. Second, a few subjects show progressive and clearly adequate hyperventilation even in the face of marked increases in flow limitation, elastic loads, and near maximum dynamic pressure generation by the inspiratory muscles. Third, others show inadequate hyperventilation (with resulting hypoxemia) but with only minimal levels of mechanical limitation to flow. As discussed earlier, interventions such as resistive loading, mechanical unloading of the respiratory muscles, expanding the maximal flow–volume envelope, or added chemoreceptor stimuli give some clues as to the role of mechanical constraint on ventilation but remain unsatisfying because of: *(1)* the heterogeneity among subjects in their response; *(2)* the inability to quantify changes in neural drive during these interventions; and *(3)* our ignorance of the specific stimuli that (normally) mediate the neural drive to hyperventilation in heavy exercise (see Chapter 10). Accordingly, because of the added complexities of potential mechanical limitations imposed by the lung and/or chest wall, the regulation of breathing during heavy and maximal exercise may be viewed as equally, if not more, complex and mysterious than the traditional dilemma of the hyperpnea of (moderate) exercise.

Inadequate Alveolar Ventilation and $\dot{V}O_{2max}$ Limitations

In healthy humans, compensatory hyperventilation and hypocapnia normally accompany the metabolic acidosis and hyperkalemia of heavy exercise (see Fig. 11–21), but the magnitude of this alveolar hyperventilation is highly variable among normal subjects (Pa_{CO_2} ~ 25–40 mm Hg). In those highly fit subjects with exercise-induced arterial hypoxemia as described above, the A-a D_{O_2} is consistently wider than normal, and those with the most significant arterial hypoxemia also tend to hyperventilate the least (Pa_{CO_2} 35–40 mm Hg, P_{AO_2} < 110 mm Hg) (104, 178, 332). A combination of the increased $\dot{V}_E$ reported with He-O_2 (see above) and findings of low ventilatory responses to chemoreceptor stimuli in many of these athletic subjects suggests that both mechanical constraint and low chemoreceptor responsiveness may have contributed to the sluggish hyperventilatory responses to maximal exercise (104, 178, 207, 332).

Unlike any human athlete, the thoroughbred horse retains substantial amounts of CO_2 above resting levels during heavy and maximum exercise (Pa_{CO_2} > 50 mm Hg) (44, 123) despite very high levels of chemoreceptor stimuli in the form of progressive metabolic acidosis and arterial hypoxemia. This alveolar hypoventilation in the equine athlete appears to be attributable at least in part to mechanical limitations, as He-O_2 inhalation in these animals caused significant and sustained increases in V_T, f_b, and $\dot{V}_E$ and lowered Pa_{CO_2} to (preexercise) resting levels (123). Furthermore, CO_2 inhalation superimposed on heavy exercise failed to stimulate ventilation further (234). On the other hand, other findings show that this suppressed "limited" $\dot{V}_E$ and V_T can be increased further and Pa_{CO_2} reduced if hypoxia is superimposed (315), or even if the heavy exercise bout is continued for a few more minutes during which circulating lactate and H^+ are rising markedly (44). Unfortunately, just as described above for the human, in this equine athlete we are also unable to specify the factors responsible for the hyperventilatory response, or its absence, in heavy exercise.

Reduced levels of hyperventilation during severe exercise will contribute to the limitation of $\dot{V}O_{2max}$ in the highly trained when, in the face of excessively widened A-a DO_2, alveolar PO_2 will not be increased sufficiently to prevent arterial O_2 saturation from falling below a critical level (104, 332).[2] An additional factor attributable to chest wall mechanics that might contribute to limitation of exercise performance would be an excessive O_2 cost of breathing ($\dot{V}O_{2RM}$) secondary to the high ventilatory work at peak exercise (see Fig. 11.12). As discussed earlier (see earlier under Respiratory Muscle Blood Flow), this possibility seems likely, especially under conditions when $\dot{V}O_{2RM}$ is in the range of 15% of $\dot{V}O_{2TOT}$; however, we are lacking direct evidence that the respiratory muscle metabolic requirements are sufficient to actually result in a reduced blood flow to locomotor muscles at a time when cardiac output is maximum.

Adding resistive loads also will reduce $\dot{V}E_{max}$ and $\dot{V}O_{2max}$, and the effect varies markedly among subjects. Lindstedt et al. (250) showed recently that if graded inspiratory resistances are added progressively during maximal exercise, reductions in maximal $\dot{V}E$ and $\dot{V}O_{2max}$ occurred with much smaller increases in external resistance (and reductions in maximal inspiratory flow rate) in the highly fit vs. the unfit subject. These data support the concept, as illustrated in Figure 11.6, of a much smaller (and sometimes nonexistent) mechanical reserve for ventilatory response at $\dot{V}O_{2max}$ in the highly fit.

Endurance Exercise Performance

The issues of demand vs. capacity have not been examined extensively in terms of a role for ventilation and ventilatory mechanics in the limitation of endurance exercise performance. An important determinant of respiratory muscle fatigue and the ability to sustain ventilation during prolonged exercise is the aerobic capacity of the respiratory muscles. As reviewed previously (see earlier under Capillary Density), heavy exercise training in animals and humans will result in a significant adaptation in endurance capacity of the respiratory muscles and the aerobic enzymatic capacity of the diaphragm. This adaptation has apparent significance to the endurance athlete who, like his untrained contemporary, still experiences significant diaphragm fatigue during heavy endurance exercise carried out to exhaustion at similar relative intensities and durations in both trained and untrained. However, the magnitude of the athlete's diaphragm fatigue and the time course of its recovery following exercise is similar to that in the untrained even though the athlete is sustaining a substantially higher $\dot{V}CO_2$, $\dot{V}E$, and diaphragmatic work throughout the exercise (32). These findings suggest that the increased aerobic capacity of the highly fit subject's diaphragm has adapted appropriately to the increased demand for sustained ventilation and diaphragmatic power output because of enhanced exercise capacity.

The endurance-trained athlete maintains very high levels of ventilation throughout prolonged heavy exercise. While the absolute levels of $\dot{V}E$ exceed those in the less fit at any given heavy exercise intensity (and therefore increased absolute $\dot{V}O_2$ and $\dot{V}CO_2$), the athlete generally hyperventilates less than his less fit contemporary. Nevertheless, the level of alveolar ventilation is sufficient during prolonged submaximal exercise to prevent exercise-induced hypoxemia, except in very rare cases (103, 203).

The magnitude of the ventilatory response in the highly trained, coupled with their normal maximal flow–volume envelope means that expiratory flow limitation is significant and progressive and increases progressively throughout prolonged heavy exercise. As a consequence, the work and the oxygen cost of this progressive hyperventilation is quite high, and ratings of dyspnea often match those for sensations of locomotor muscle fatigue. Under these extreme conditions (>90% maximal $\dot{V}O_2$ in the highly fit), He-O_2 breathing has been shown to prolong endurance time and even significantly reduce $\dot{V}O_2$ (1), suggesting that perhaps some manifestation of high levels of sustained ventilatory work may actually have a bearing on endurance exercise capacity in the very fit individual. This enhanced effect on performance of reducing respiratory muscle work may result from a significant increase in the blood flow to locomotor muscles that in the normally "loaded" air breathing state was required by the respiratory muscles. As explained earlier (see earlier under Respiratory Muscle Blood Flow), this important question of blood flow distribution during heavy exercise among competing vascular beds of the limbs and chest wall needs direct study.

[2]Theoretically any significant reduction in SaO_2 should reduce arterial O_2 content (to less than what it would be if SaO_2 had been maintained at 96%–98%) and thereby limit the maximum a-vO_2 difference and the $\dot{V}O_{2max}$. The sensitivity of $\dot{V}O_{2max}$ to different levels of exercise-induced arterial O_2 desaturation was tested by preventing any reduction in SaO_2 (332). Systematic measurable effects on $\dot{V}O_{2max}$ were observed when SaO_2 was reduced to <93%.

SPECIAL CIRCUMSTANCES FAVORING PULMONARY LIMITATIONS TO EXERCISE PERFORMANCE IN HEALTH

Hypoxia of High Altitudes

In the hypoxia of high altitudes, limitations to pulmonary gas exchange, ventilation, and respiratory muscle function are more readily achieved, especially in the highly trained, and in turn become a more serious threat to exercise limitation than at sea level. Rhinehold Messner's recollections as he approached the summit of Mount Everest in 1978 (without the aid of supplementary oxygen) expresses the overwhelming dominance of pulmonary system limitations during exercise under conditions where Pa_{O_2} approaches 25 mm Hg and $\dot{V}_{O_{2max}}$ is reduced to less than one-third its sea-level value (280):

> After very few steps, we huddle over our axes, mouth agape, struggling for sufficient breath . . . as we get higher it becomes such a strenuous business that we scarcely have strength to go on. In my stage of spiritual abstraction, I no longer belong to myself and to my eyesight. I am nothing more than a single, narrow gasping lung, floating over the mists and the summits.

An increased propensity for *diffusion limitation and therefore exercise-induced hypoxemia* are among the best documented effects of high altitude. No beneficial adaptations in any of the major determinants of alveolar–capillary diffusion occur that would serve to counteract the reduced rate of alveolar–capillary equilibrium in hypoxia (see Chapter 12, this volume) with short-term hypoxic exposure. The highly trained with their elevated maximal $\dot{V}_{O_2}$ and their marginal diffusion reserve (see above) are especially susceptible to severe exercise-induced hypoxemia in hypoxic environments, even at only moderately high altitudes (1200–1500 m, P_{IO_2} 125–135 mm Hg) (104). In addition to diffusion limitation, many highly trained subjects working at very heavy submaximal exercise loads or at $V_{O_{2max}}$ *can* not (because of mechanical limits) and/or *will* not (because of reflex inhibition) increase their alveolar ventilation in response to added hypoxic chemostimulation (207). This enhanced susceptibility to exercise-induced hypoxemia probably explains the greater reductions in maximal $\dot{V}_{O_2}$ in hypoxic environments obtained in highly trained vs. untrained subjects (240).

The maximum flow–volume envelope is also unchanged in hypoxia, thus the pronounced tachypneic hyperventilatory response to exercise in hypoxia, especially following acclimatization, will cause *greater expiratory flow limitation and increased ventilatory work* for any given exercise work rate (31, 402). In hypobaric hypoxia, the reduced gas density will alleviate some of the flow-resistive work of breathing (especially at altitudes > 4000 m); however, this effect is outweighed by the magnitude of the hyperventilatory response. Thus, the respiratory muscles are subjected to increased workloads, reduced O_2 transport, and increased circulating catecholamines during exercise in hypoxia. Accordingly, in rats subjected to heavy endurance exercise in hypoxia, glycogen depletion and lactacidosis were markedly accentuated in the diaphragm (139). In the healthy human, the magnitude of exercise-induced diaphragmatic fatigue following endurance exercise to exhaustion, as assessed by the BPNS technique (see earlier under Phrenic Nerve Stimulation), was found to be similar in hypoxia and normoxia; but this fatigue occurred in a much briefer exercise time and was significantly slower to recover following endurance exercise in hypoxia (31). Dyspneic sensations are also especially pronounced in both heavy short-term and long-term exercise in hypoxia. Thus, while the hyperventilatory response to exercise in hypoxia is certainly a key protector of O_2 transport and probably an important determinant of successful acclimatization to high altitudes (361), it also is accomplished at very high cost and may contribute significantly to limitations of exercise performance, especially in endurance exercise. Exactly how important this increased ventilatory work is to the limitation of endurance exercise performance in hypoxic environments has not been evaluated.

Aging Effects on Pulmonary Limitations

The normal aging process both decreases the capacity of maximum ventilatory response and increases its oxygen cost because of the age-dependent reduction in lung elastic recoil and the increasing stiffness of the chest wall (94, 204). These changes are manifested in reduced vital capacity and expiratory flow rates and in hyperinflation at rest and have been shown to occur in healthy, nonsmoking adults, with the most marked changes occurring in the 55- to 75-year-old age range (415). Cross-sectional comparisons of high and normal fit subjects show less expiratory flow limitation in the high fit (in higher FEV, and MEF_{50} (170, 204, 206). However, these differences among subjects might only reflect a preselection bias, because longitudinal studies show these aging effects to occur to the same extent in both the physically active and in sedentary subjects (272). Thus, with healthy aging the maximum envelope of the flow–volume loop is reduced, and even in moderate exercise significant expiratory flow limitation begins to occur. Ventilatory work is increased throughout exercise, EELV returns to and sometimes even above resting levels, and end-inspiratory lung volume often exceeds 90% of TLC during heavy or maximum exercise (205, 206). In many highly active older subjects with increased $\dot{V}O_{2max}$ and therefore increased maximum ventilatory requirement relative to their sedentary contemporaries, complete ventilatory limitation is often achieved at or near $\dot{V}O_{2max}$, just as in younger subjects (see Fig. 11.6). However, in the older athlete this ventilatory limitation occurs at a much lower $\dot{V}E$ (i.e., in the 110–130 liters/min range of $\dot{V}E$ in the aged and at >150 liters/min in the young).

Diffusion capacity is also reduced with aging (94), and in heavy exercise in the highly fit, significant arterial hypoxemia (<93% SaO_2) has been observed in some older subjects, secondary to a widened A-a O_2 difference and because of limited hyperventilation (204, 334). However, unlike the exercise-induced hypoxemia in younger athletes, in the older subjects this occurred at a much lower maximal $\dot{V}O_2$ in the 40–55 $ml \cdot kg^{-1} \cdot min^{-1}$ range. We emphasize that the prevalence of this exercise-induced hypoxemia in the fit elderly is not nearly as extensive as in the young athlete, suggesting that for the most part the normal aging effects on the healthy lung and chest wall must parallel fairly closely those in the cardiovascular/metabolic determinants of $\dot{V}O_{2max}$. In other words—recognizing many notable exceptions and the need for further longitudinal study of larger populations—reductions in maximum demand (i.e., $\dot{V}O_{2max}$), with healthy aging most often parallel those in functional capacities of the lung and chest wall.

We are grateful to several persons who provided valuable review and constructive criticism of this chapter, including Mark Babcock, Robert Banzett, Richard Coast, Jeff Coombes, Louise Fletcher, Craig Harms, Robert Herb, David Leith, Murli Manohar, and Steven McClaran. Editor Loring Rowell also provided invaluable feedback on all phases of the chapter. We also thank Basel Taha for his help in computer coordination of the chapter.

Granting agencies who funded much of the original research in this chapter include: NHLBI (HL41790, R.F.F.; HL15469 J.A.D.); Canadian Medical Research Council (C.G.G.); American Lung Association-Florida Affiliate (S.K.P.); Harry M. Zweig Memorial Fund for Equine Research, Horsemen's Benevolent Protection Association, Cornell Unrestricted Alumni Fund (D.M.A.); and the Welcome Trust Programme Grant (A.G., A.L.).

We are especially grateful to Ms. Gundula Birong for her excellent preparation of the manuscript. J.A.D. wishes to acknowledge the extra special team efforts of the "Gang of Eight."

REFERENCES

1. Aaron, E. A., K. G. Henke, D. F. Pegelow, and J. A. Dempsey. Effects of mechanical unloading of the respiratory system on exercise and respiratory muscle endurance. *Med. Sci. Sports Exerc.* 17: 290, 1985.
2. Aaron, E. A., B. D. Johnson, C. K. Seow, and J. A. Dempsey. Oxygen cost of exercise hyperpnea: measurement. *J. Appl. Physiol.* 72: 1810–1817, 1992.
3. Aaron, E.A., K. C. Seow, B. D. Johnson, and J. A. Dempsey. Oxygen cost of exercise hyperpnea: implications for performance. *J. Appl. Physiol.* 72: 1818–1825, 1992.
4. Adams, L., N. Chronos, R. Lane, and A. Guz. The measurement of breathlessness induced in normal subjects: validity of two scaling techniques. *Clin. Sci.* 69: 7–16, 1985.
5. Adams, L., N. Chronos, R. Lane, and A. Guz. The measurement of breathlessness induced in normal subjects: individual differences. *Clin. Sci.* 70: 131–140, 1986.
6. Adams, L., G. Fink, B. Wuyam, K. Murphy, J. Watson, J. A. Innes, I. Kobayashi, D. R. Corfield, R. S. J. Frackowiak, T. Jones, and A. Guz. Use of positron emission tomography to study motor cortical control of breathing during and following exercise in man. *Proceedings of the Sixth International Symposium on Modelling and Control of Ventilation*, London, 1995 (in press).
7. Adams, L., and A. Guz. Dyspnea on exertion. In: *Exercise: Pulmonary Physiology and Pathophysiology*, edited by B. J. Whipp and K. Wasserman. New York: Marcel Dekker. Inc., 1991, p. 449–494.
8. Adams, L., R. Lane, S. A. Shea, A. Cockcroft, and A. Guz. Breathlessness during different forms of ventilatory stimulation: a study of mechanisms in normal subjects and respiratory patients. *Clin. Sci.* 69: 663–672, 1985.
9. Ainsworth, D. M., S. W. Eicker, N. G. Ducharme, and R. P. Hackett. Exercise-induced activation of the equine diaphragm. *Proc. Vet. Resp. Symp.* 13: A19, 1994.
10. Ainsworth, D. M., C. A. Smith, S. W. Eicker, K. S. Henderson, and J. A. Dempsey. The effects of chemical versus locomotory stimuli on respiratory muscle activity in the awake dog. *Respir. Physiol.* 78: 163–176, 1989.
11. Ainsworth, D. M., C. A. Smith, S. W. Eicker, K. S. Henderson, and J. A. Dempsey. The effects of locomotion on respiratory muscle activity in the awake dog. *Respir. Physiol.* 78: 145–162, 1989.
12. Ainsworth, D. M., C. A. Smith, K. S. Henderson, and J. A. Dempsey. High frequency breathing in exercising dogs requires respiratory muscle activity. *Proceedings of the Sixth International Symposium on Modelling and Control of Ventilation*, London, 1995 (in press).
13. Ainsworth, D. M., C. A. Smith, B. D. Johnson, S. W. Eicker, K. S. Henderson, and J. A. Dempsey. Vagal contributions to respiratory muscle activity during eupnea in the awake dog. *J. Appl. Physiol.* 72: 1355–1361, 1992.
14. Ainsworth, D. M., C. A. Smith, B. D. Johnson, S. W. Eicker, K. S. Henderson, and J. A. Dempsey. Vagal modulation of respiratory muscle activity in awake dogs during exercise and hypercapnia. *J. Appl. Physiol.* 72: 1362–1367, 1992.
15. Aldrich, T., and J. Karpel. Inspiratory muscle resistive training in respiratory failure. *Am. Rev. Respir. Dis.* 131: 461–462, 1985.
16. Altose, M. D., N. S. Cherniack, and A. P. Fishman. Respiratory sensations and dyspnea. *J. Appl. Physiol.* 58: 1051–1054, 1985.
17. Ameredes, B. T., W. F. Brechue, G. M. Andrew, and W. N. Stainsby. Force-velocity shifts with repetitive isometric and isotonic contractions of canine gastrocnemius in situ. *J. Appl. Physiol.* 73: 2105–2111, 1992.
18. Ameredes, B. T., B. D. Johnson, and G. C. Sieck. Depression of diaphragm maximal velocity of unloaded short-

ening after repetitive isovelocity contractions. *Am. J. Respir. Crit. Care Med.* 149: A797, 1994.
19. Anholm, J. D., R. L. Johnson, and M. Ramanthon. Changes in cardiac output during sustained maximal ventilation in humans. *J. Appl. Physiol.* 63: 181–187, 1987.
20. Anholm, J. D., J. Stray-Gundersen, M. Ramanathan, and R. L. Johnson, Jr. Sustained maximal ventilation after endurance exercise in athletes. *J. Appl. Physiol.* 67: 1759–1763, 1989.
21. Ariano, M., R. Armstrong, and V. Edgerton. Hindlimb muscle fiber populations of five mammals. *J. Histochem. Cytochem.* 21: 51–55, 1973.
22. Armstrong, R. B. Mechanisms of exercise-induced delayed onset muscular soreness: a brief review. *Med. Sci. Sports Exerc.* 16: 529–538, 1984.
23. Armour, J., R. M. Donnelly, and P. T. Bye, The large lungs of elite swimmers: an increased alveolar number. *Eur. Resp. J.* 6: 237–247, 1993.
24. Art, T., D. Desmecht, H. Amory, and P. Lekeux. Synchronization of locomotion and respiration in trotting ponies. *J. Exp. Biol.* 155: 245–259, 1991.
25. Asmussen, E. Muscular exercise. In: *Handbook of Physiology, Respiration*, edited by W. O. Fenn and H. Rahn. Washington, DC: Am. Physiol. Soc., 1964, p. 939–978.
26. Astrand, P. O., and K. Rodhal. Physical training. In: *Textbook of Work Physiology*, New York: McGraw-Hill, 1985, p. 412–485.
27. Attenburrow, D. P. Time relationship between the respiratory cycle and limb cycle in the horse. *Equine Vet. J.* 14: 69–72, 1982.
28. Aubier, M., G. Farkas, A. D. Troyer, R. Mozes, and C. Roussos. Detection of diaphragmatic fatigue in man by phrenic stimulation. *J. Appl. Physiol. Respir. Environ. Exerc. Physiol.* 50: 538–544, 1981.
29. Aubier, M., D. Murciano, Y. Lecocguic, N. Vires, and R. Pariente. Bilateral phrenic stimulation: a simple technique to assess diaphragmatic fatigue in humans. *J. Appl. Physiol.* 58: 58–64, 1985.
30. Babb, T. G., and J. R. Rodarte. Lung volumes during low-intensity steady-state cycling. *J. Appl. Physiol.* 70: 934–937, 1991.
31. Babcock, M. A., B. D. Johnson, D. F. Pegelow, O. E. Suman, D. Griffin, and J. A. Dempsey. Hypoxic effects on exercise-induced diaphragmatic fatigue in normal healthy humans. *J. Appl. Physiol.* 78: 82–92, 1995.
32. Babcock, M. A., D. F. Pegelow, and J. A. Dempsey. Aerobic fitness effects on exercise-induced diaphragmatic fatigue. *Am. J. Respir. Crit. Care Med.* 149: A799, 1994.
33. Babcock, M. A., D. F. Pegelow, S. R. McClaran, O. E. Suman, and J. A. Dempsey. Contribution of diaphragmatic force output to exercise-induced diaphragm fatigue. *J. Appl. Physiol.* 78: 1710–1719, 1995.
34. Bai, T. R., B. J. Rabinovitch, and R. L. Pardy. Near maximal voluntary hyperpnoea and ventilatory muscle function. *J. Appl. Physiol.* 57: 1742–1748, 1984.
35. Banner, N. R., M. H. Lloyd, R. D. Hamilton, J. A. Innes, A. Guz, and M. H. Yacoub. Cardiopulmonary response to dynamic exercise after heart and combined heart-lung transplantation. *Br. Heart J.* 61: 215–223, 1989.
36. Bannister, R. G., and D. J. C. Cunningham. The effects on the respiration and performance during exercise of adding oxygen to the inspired air. *J. Physiol. (Lond.)* 125: 118–137, 1954.
37. Banzett, R. B., R. W. Lansing, and R. Brown. High level quadriplegics perceive lung volume change. *J. Appl. Physiol.* 62: 567–573, 1987.
38. Banzett, R. B., R. W. Lansing, R. Brown, G. P. Topulos, D. Yager, S. M. Steele, B. Londono, S. H. Loring, M. B. Reid, L. Adams, and C. S. Nations. "Air hunger" from increased PCO2 persists after complete neuromuscular block in humans. *Respir. Physiol.* 81: 1–17, 1990.
39. Banzett, R. B., R. W. Lansing, M. B. Reid, L. Adams, and R. Brown. "Air hunger" arising from increased PCO2 in mechanically ventilated quadriplegics. *Respir. Physiol* 76: 53–68, 1989.
40. Banzett, R. B., J. Mead, M. B. Reid, and G. P. Topulos. Locomotion in men has no appreciable mechanical effect on breathing. *J. Appl. Physiol.* 72: 1922–1926, 1991.
41. Bartlett, D. J. Upper airway motor systems. In: *Handbook of Physiology, The Respiratory System, Control of Breathing*, edited by N. S. Cherniack and J. G. Widdicombe. Bethesda, MD: Am. Physiol. Soc., 1986, p. 223–245.
42. Basmajian, J. V., and C. R. Dutta. Electromyography of the pharyngeal constrictors and levator palati in man. *Anat. Rec.* 139: 561–563, 1961.
43. Bayev, K. V., V. K. Beresovskii, T. G. Kebkalo, and L. A. Savoskina. Afferent and efferent connections of brainstem locomotor regions: study by means of horseradish-peroxidase transport technique. *Neuroscience* 26: 871–891, 1988.
44. Bayly, W. M., D. R. Hodgson, D. A. Schulz, J. A. Dempsey, and P. D. Gollnick. Exercise-induced hypercapnia in the horse. *J. Appl. Physiol.* 67: 1958–1966, 1989.
45. Bazzy, A. R., L. M. Pang, S. R. Akabas, and G. G. Haddad. O_2 metabolism of the sheep diaphragm during flow resistive loaded breathing. *J. Appl. Physiol.* 66: 2305–2311, 1989.
46. Bechbache, R. R., and J. Duffin. The entrainment of breathing frequency by exercise rhythm. *J. Physiol. (Lond.)* 272: 553–561, 1977.
47. Bellemare, F., and B. Bigland-Ritchie. Central components of diaphragmatic fatigue assessed by phrenic nerve stimulation. *J. Appl. Physiol.* 62: 1307–1316, 1987.
48. Bellemare, F., and N. Garzaniti. Failure of neuromuscular propagation during human maximal voluntary contraction. *J. Appl. Physiol.* 64: 1084–1093, 1988.
49. Bellemare, F., and A. Grassino. Effect of pressure and timing of contraction on human diaphragm fatigue. *J. Appl Physiol. Respir. Environ. Exerc. Physiol.* 53: 1190–1195, 1982.
50. Bellemare, F., and A. Grassino. Evaluation of human diaphragm fatigue. *J. Appl. Physiol.* 53: 1196–1206, 1982.
51. Belman, M., and G. Gaesser. Ventilatory muscle training in the elderly. *J. Appl. Physiol.* 64: 899–905, 1988.
52. Belman, M., S. Thomas, and M. Lewis. Resistive breathing training in patients with chronic obstructive pulmonary disease. *Chest* 90: 663–670, 1986.
53. Bergstrom, J., L. Hermansen, E. Hultman, and B. Saltin. Diet, muscle glycogen and physical performance. *Acta Physiol. Scand.* 71: 140–150, 1967.
54. Bernasconi, P., and J. Kohl. Analysis of co-ordination between breathing and exercise rhythms in man. *J. Physiol. (Lond.)* 471: 693–706, 1993.
55. Bigland-Ritchie, B. Muscle fatigue and the influence of changing neural drive. *Clin. Chest Med.* 5: 21–34, 1984.
56. Blackie, S. P., M. S. Fairbarn, N. G. McElvaney, P. G. Wilcox, N. J. Morrison, and R. L. Pardy. Normal values and ranges for ventilation and breathing pattern at maximal exercise. *Chest* 100: 136–142, 1991.
57. Boutellier, U., R. Buchel, A. Kundert, and C. Spengler. The respiratory system as an exercise limiting factor in normal

trained subjects. *Eur. J. Appl. Physiol.* 65: 347–353, 1992.
58. Boutellier, U., and P. Piwko. The respiratory system as an exercise limiting factor in normal sedentary subjects. *Eur. J. Appl. Physiol.* 64: 145–152, 1992.
59. Bradley, M. E., and D. E. Leith. Ventilatory muscle training and the oxygen cost of sustained hyperpnea. *J. Appl. Physiol.* 45: 885–892, 1978.
60. Bramble, D. M. Respiratory patterns and control during unrestrained human running. In: *Modelling and Control of Breathing*, edited by B. J. Whipp and D. M. Wiberg. New York: Elsevier Biomedical, 1983, p. 213–220.
61. Bramble, D. M. Axial-appendicular dynamics and the integration of breathing and gait in mammals. *Am. Zool.* 29: 171–186, 1989.
62. Bramble, D. M., and D. R. Carrier. Running and breathing in mammals. *Science* 219: 251–256, 1983.
63. Bramble, D. M., and F. A. Jenkins. Mammalian locomotor-respiratory integration: implication for diaphragmatic and pulmonary design. *Science* 262: 235–240, 1993.
64. Brice, A. G., and H. G. Welch. Metabolic and cardiorespiratory responses to He-O_2 breathing during exercise. *J. Appl. Physiol.* 54: 387–392, 1983.
65. Bridger, G. P., and D. F. Proctor. Maximum nasal inspiratory flow and nasal resistance. *Ann. Otol.* 79: 481–488, 1970.
66. Brody, A. W., R. R. Stoughton, T. L. Connoly, J. J. Shehan, J. J. Navin, and E. E. Kobald. Experimental value of the Reynolds critical flow in the human airway. *J. Lab. Clin. Med.* 67: 43–57, 1966.
67. Brooke, M., and K. Kaiser. Three myosin adenosine triphosphatase systems: the nature of their pH lability and sulfhydryl dependence. *J. Histochem. Cytochem.* 18: 670–672, 1970.
68. Buchtal, F., and A. K. Faaborg. Electromyography of laryngeal and respiratory muscles. *Ann. Otol. Rhinol. Laryngol.* 73: 118–123, 1964.
69. Burdon, J. G. W., E. F. Juniper, K. J. Killian, F. E. Hargreave, and E. J. M. Campbell. The perception of breathlessness in asthma. *Am. Rev. Respir. Dis.* 126: 825–828, 1982.
70. Bye, P. T. P., S. A. Esau, K. R. Walley, P. T. Macklem, and R. L. Pardy. Ventilatory muscles during exercise in air and oxygen in normal men. *J. Appl. Physiol. Respir. Environ. Exerc. Physiol.* 56: 464–471, 1984.
71. Caillaud, C., F. Anselme, J. Mercier, and C. Prefaut. Pulmonary gas exchange and breathing pattern during and after exercise in highly trained athletes. *Eur. J. Appl. Physiol.* 67: 431–437, 1993.
72. Caretti, D. M., P. C. Szlyk, and I. V. Sils. Effects of exercise modality on patterns of ventilation and respiratory timing. *Respir. Physiol.* 90: 201–211, 1992.
73. Carlo, W. A., R. J. Martin, E. F. Abboud, E. N. Bruce, and K. P. Strohl. Effects of sleep state and hypercapnia on alae nasi and diaphragm EMG in preterm infants. *J. Appl. Physiol.* 54: 1590–1596, 1983.
74. Catchside, P. G., and G. C. Scroop. Lactate kinetics in resting and exercising forearms during moderate-intensity supine leg exercise. *J. Appl. Physiol.* 74: 435–443, 1993.
75. Cha, E. J., D. Sedlock, and S. M. Yamashiro. Changes in lung volume and breathing pattern during exercise and CO_2 inhalation in humans. *J. Appl. Physiol.* 62: 1544–1550, 1987.
76. Chen, Z., F. L. Eldridge, and P. G. Wagner. Respiratory-associated rhythmic firing of midbrain neurones in cats: relation to level of respiratory drive. *J. Physiol. (Lond.)* 437: 305–325, 1991.
77. Chen, Z., F. L. Eldridge, and P. G. Wagner. Respiratory-associated thalamic activity is related to level of respiratory drive. *Respir. Physiol.* 90: 99–113, 1992.
78. Cherniack, N. S., and M. D. Altose. Mechanisms of dyspnea. *Clin. Chest Med.* 8: 207–214, 1987.
79. Cherniack, N. S., Y. Oku, G. M. Saidel, E. N. Bruce, and M. D. Altose. Optimization of breathing through perceptual mechanisms. In: *Control of Breathing and Dyspnea*, edited by T. T. Takishima and N. S. Cherniack. Oxford: Pergamon Press, 1991, p. 337–345.
80. Chonan, T., M. B. Mulholland, M. D. Altose, and N. S. Cherniack. Effects of changes in level and pattern of breathing on the sensation of dyspnea. *J. Appl. Physiol.* 69: 1290–1295, 1990.
81. Chronos, N., L. Adams, and A. Guz. Effect of hyperoxia and hypoxia on exercise-induced breathlessness in normal subjects. *Clin. Sci.* 74: 531–537, 1988.
82. Clanton, T., G. Dixon, and J. Drake. Inspiratory muscle conditioning using a threshold loading device. *Chest* 87: 62–66, 1985.
83. Clanton, T. L., G. F. Dixon, J. Drake, and J. E. Gadek. Effects of swim training on lung volumes and inspiratory muscle conditioning. *J. Appl. Physiol.* 62: 39–46, 1987.
84. Clark, J. M., F. C. Hagerman, and R. Gelfand. Breathing patterns during submaximal and maximal exercise in elite oarsmen. *J. Appl. Physiol.* 55: 440–446, 1983.
85. Clark, J. M., R. E. Sinclair, and J. B. Lennox. Chemical and non-chemical components of ventilation during hypercapnic exercise in man. *J. Appl. Physiol.* 48: 1065–1076, 1980.
86. Clifford, P. S., J. T. Litzow, J. H. von Colditz, and R. L. Coon. Effect of chronic pulmonary denervation on ventilatory responses to exercise. *J. Appl. Physiol.* 61: 603–610, 1986.
87. Close, R. Dynamic properties of mammalian muscles. *Physiol. Rev.* 52: 129–197, 1972.
88. Coast, J. R., P. S. Clifford, T. W. Henrich, J. Stray-Gunderson, and R. L. Johnson. Maximal inspiratory pressure following maximal exercise in trained and untrained subjects. *Med. Sci. Sports Exerc.* 22: 811–815, 1990.
89. Cole, P. Nasal airflow resistance. In: *Respiratory Function of the Upper Airway*, edited by O. P. Mathew and G. S. Ambrogio. New York: Marcel Dekker, Inc., 1988, p. 391–414.
90. Cole, P., R. Forsyth, and J. S. Haight. Respiratory resistance of the oral airway. *Am. Rev. Respir. Dis.* 22: 363–365, 1982.
91. Cole, P., R. Forsyth, and J. S. Haight. Effects of cold air and exercise on nasal patency. *Ann. Otol. Rhinol. Laryngol.* 92: 196–198, 1983.
92. Connel, D., and R. F. Fregosi. Influence of nasal airflow and resistance on nasal dilator muscle activities during exercise. *J. Appl. Physiol.* 74: 2529–2536, 1993.
93. Connel, D., R. Lansing, and R. F. Fregosi. Influence of exercise intensity and nasal flow resistance on activities of human nasal dilator muscles. *FASEB J.* 5: A1476, 1991.
94. Crapo, R. O. The aging lung. In: *Pulmonary Disease in the Elderly Patient*, edited by D. A. Mahler. New York: Marcel Dekker, Inc., 1993, p. 1–25.
95. Crossfilt, M., and J. Widdicombe. Physical characteristics of the chest and lungs and the work of breathing in different mammalian species. *J. Physiol. (Lond.)* 158: 1–14, 1961.

96. Cunningham, D. A., P. B. Goade, and J. B. Critz. Cardiorespiratory response to exercise on a rowing and bicycle ergometer. *Med. Sci. Sports* 7: 37–43, 1975.
97. Dallimore, N. S., and R. Eccles. Changes in human nasal resistance associated with exercise, hyperventilation and rebreathing. *Acta Otolaryngol.* 84: 416–421, 1977.
98. Daubenspeck, J. A. Mechanical factors in breathing pattern regulation in humans. *Ann. Biomed. Eng.* 9: 409–424, 1981.
99. Davies, A. M., and R. Eccles. The effects of nasal airflow on the electromyographic activity of nasal muscles in the anaesthetized cat. *J. Physiol. (Lond.)* 358: 102P, 1984.
100. Dehann, A., M. A. N. Lodder, and A. J. Sergeant. Age related effects of fatigue and recovery from fatigue in rat medial gastrocnemius muscle. *Q. J. Exp. Physiol.* 74: 715–726, 1989.
101. Demediuk, B. H., H. Manning, J. Lilly, V. Fencl, S. E. Weinberger, J. W. Weiss, and R. M. Schwartzstein. Dissociation between dyspnea and respiratory effort. *Am. Rev. Respir. Dis.* 146: 1222–1225, 1992.
102. Dempsey, J. A. Is the lung built for exercise? *Med. Sci. Sports Med.* 18: 143–155, 1986.
103. Dempsey, J. A., E. Aaron, and B. J. Martin. Pulmonary function and prolonged exercise. In: *Perspectives in Exercise. Science and Sports Medicine*, edited by D. R. Lamb and R. Murray. Indianapolis: Benchman Press, 1988, p. 75–124.
104. Dempsey, J. A., P. G. Hanson, and K. S. Henderson. Exercise-induced arterial hypoxaemia in healthy human subjects at sea level. *J. Physiol. (Lond.)* 355: 161–175, 1984.
105. Dempsey, J. A., and B. D. Johnson. Demand vs capacity in the healthy pulmonary system. *Schweiz. Z. Sportmed. Jahrgang* 40: 55–64, 1992.
106. Dempsey, J. A., B. D. Johnson, and K. W. Saupe. Adaptations and limitations in the pulmonary system during exercise. *Chest* 97: 81S–87S, 1990.
107. Dempsey, J. A., S. Powers, and N. Gledhill. Cardiovascular and pulmonary adaptations to physical activity: discussion. In: *Exercise, Fitness and Health*, edited by C. Bouchard, et al. Champaign, IL: Human Kinetics, 1994, p. 205–216.
108. DeTroyer, A., M. Sampson, S. Sigrist, and P. Macklem. The diaphragm: two muscles. *Science* 213: 237–238, 1981.
109. DeTroyer, A., M. Sampson, S. Sigrist, and P. Macklem. Action of the costal and crural parts of the diaphragm during breathing. *J. Appl. Physiol.* 53: 30–39, 1982.
110. Dick, T. E., F. J. Kong, and A. J. Berger. Correlation of recruitment order with axonal conduction velocity for supraspinally driven motor units. *J. Neurophysiol.* 57: 245–259, 1987.
111. Dick, T. E., F. J. Kong, and A. J. Berger. Recruitment order of diaphragmatic motor units obeys Hennemans's size principle. In: *Respiratory Muscles and Their Neuromotor Control*, edited by G. C. Sieck, S. G. Gandevia, and W. E. Cameron. New York: Alan R. Liss, 1987, p. 249–261.
112. DiMarco, A. F., D. A. Wolfson, S. B. Gottfried, and M. D. Altose. Sensation of inspired volume in normal subjects and quadriplegic patients. *J. Appl. Physiol.* 53: 1481–1486, 1982.
113. Dodd, S. L., S. K. Powers, D. Thompson, G. Landry, and J. Lawler. Exercise performance following intense short-term ventilatory work. *Int. J. Sports Med.* 10: 48–52, 1989.
114. Duchateau, J., and K. Hainaut. Electrical and mechanical failures during sustained and intermittent contractions in humans. *J. Appl. Physiol.* 58: 942–947, 1985.
115. Eccles, R. The central rhythm of the nasal cycle. *Acta Otolaryngol.* 86: 464–468, 1978.
116. Edman, K. A. P., and A. R. Mattiazzi. Effects of fatigue and altered pH on isometric force and velocity of shortening at zero load in frog muscle fibers. *J. Muscle Res. Cell Motil.* 2: 321–334, 1981.
117. Edwards, R. H. T. Human muscle function and fatigue. *Human Muscle Fatigue: Physiological Mechanisms*, edited by R. Porter and J. Whelan. London: Pitman, 1981, p. 1–18.
118. Edwards, R. H. T. Biochemical basis of fatigue in exercise performance: catastrophic theory of muscular fatigue. In: *Biochemistry of Exercise*, edited by H. Knuttgen, J. Vogel, and J. Poortmans. Champaign, IL: Human Kinetics, 1983, p. 3–28.
119. El-Manshawi, A., K. J. Killian, E. Summers, and N. L. Jones. Breathlessness during exercise with and without resistive loading. *J. Appl. Physiol.* 61: 896–905, 1986.
120. England, S. J., and D. Bartlett, Jr. Changes in respiratory movements of the human vocal cords during hyperpnea. *J. Appl. Physiol.* 52: 780–785, 1982.
121. England, S. J., D. Bartlett, Jr., and S. L. Knuth. Comparison of human vocal cord movements during isocapnic hypoxia and hypercapnia. *J. Appl. Physiol.* 53: 81–86, 1982.
122. Enoka, R. M., and D. G. Stuart. Neurobiology of muscle fatigue. *J. Appl. Physiol.* 72: 1631–1648, 1992.
123. Erickson, B. K., J. Seavon, K. Kubo, A. Hiraga, M. Kai, Y. Yamaya, and P. D. Wagner. Mechanisms of reduction in alveolar-arterial PO_2 difference by helium breathing in the exercising horse. *J. Appl. Physiol.* 76: 2794–2801, 1994.
124. Esau, S. A., P. T. Bye, and R. L. Pardy. Changes in rate of relaxation of sniffs with diaphragmatic fatigue in humans. *J. Appl. Physiol.* 55: 731–735, 1983.
125. Evans, D. L., E. B. Silverman, D. R. Hodgson, M. D. Eaton, and R. J. Rose. Gait and respiration in standardbred horses when pacing and galloping. *Res. Vet. Sci.* 37: 233–239, 1994.
126. Faaborg-Andersen, K. L. Electromyographic investigation of intrinsic laryngeal muscles in humans. *Acta Physiol. Scand.* 41: 1–149, 1957.
127. Fairbarn, M. S., K. C. Coutts, R. L. Pardy, and D. C. McKenzie. Improved respiratory muscle endurance of highly trained cyclists and the effects on maximal exercise performance. *Int. J. Sports Med.* 12: 66–70, 1991.
128. Fenn, W. O., and H. Rahn. *Handbook of Physiology. Respiration.* Washington, DC: Am. Physiol. Soc., 1964.
129. Ferris, B. G., J. Mead, and L. H. Opie. Partitioning of respiratory flow resistance in man. *J. Appl. Physiol.* 19: 653–658, 1964.
130. Fink, B. R. *The Human Larynx.* New York: Raven Press, 1975.
131. Fitts, R. H. Cellular mechanisms of muscle fatigue. *Physiol. Rev.* 74: 49–94, 1994.
132. Fitzgerald, R. S., M. X. Hauer, G. G. Bierkamper, and H. Raff. Responses of in vitro rat diaphragm to changes in acid base environment. *J. Appl. Physiol.* 57: 1202–1210, 1984.
133. Flynn, C., H. V. Forster, L. G. Pan, and G. E. Bisgard. Role of hilar nerve afferents in hyperpnea of exercise. *J. Appl. Physiol.* 59: 798–806, 1985.

134. Forster, H. V., B. K. Erickson, T. F. Lowry, L. G. Pan, M. J. Korducki, and A. L. Forster. Effect of helium-induced ventilatory unloading on breathing and diaphragm EMG in awake ponies. *J. Appl. Physiol.* 77: 452–462, 1994.
135. Forsyth, R. D., P. Cole, and R. J. Shephard. Exercise and nasal patency. *J. Appl. Physiol.* 55: 860–865, 1983.
136. Fowler, W. S. Breaking point of breath-holding. *J. Appl. Physiol.* 6: 539–545, 1954.
137. Fox, J., H. Kreisman, A. Colacone, and N. Wolkove. Respiratory volume perception through the nose and mouth determined noninvasively. *J. Appl. Physiol.* 61: 436–439, 1986.
138. Freedman, S., R. Lane, and A. Guz. Breathlessness and respiratory mechanics during reflex or voluntary hyperventilation in patients with chronic airflow limitation. *Clin. Sci.* 73: 311–318, 1987.
139. Fregosi, R. F., and J. A. Dempsey. Effects of exercise in normoxia and acute hypoxia on respiratory muscle metabolites. *J. Appl. Physiol.* 60: 1274–1283, 1986.
140. Frevert, C. S., C. S. Nations, H. J. Seeherman, S. H. Loring, and R. B. Banzett. Airflow associated with stride in the horse. *Physiologist* 33: A83, 1990.
141. Fuller, D., J. Sullivan, E. Essif, K. Personius, and R. F. Fregosi. Measurement of the EMG-force relationship during voluntary and exercise-induced contractions in a human upper airway muscle. *J. Appl. Physiol.* 79: 270–278, 1995.
142. Gallagher, C. G. Exercise and chronic obstructive pulmonary disease. *Med. Clin. North Am.* 74: 619–641, 1990.
143. Gallagher, C. G., E. Brown, and M. Younes. Breathing pattern during maximal exercise and during submaximal exercise with hypercapnia. *J. Appl. Physiol.* 63: 238–244, 1987.
144. Gallagher, C. G., W. Huda, M. Rigby, D. Greenberg, and M. Younes. Lack of radiographic evidence of interstitial pulmonary edema after maximal exercise in normal subjects. *Am. Rev. Respir. Dis.* 137: 474–476, 1988.
145. Gallagher, C. G., and M. Younes. Breathing pattern during and after maximal exercise in patients with chronic obstructive disease, interstitial lung disease, and cardiac disease, and in normal subjects. *Am. Rev. Respir. Dis.* 133: 581–586, 1986.
146. Gallagher, C. G., and M. Younes. Effect of pressure assist on ventilation and respiratory mechanics in heavy exercise. *J. Appl. Physiol.* 66: 1824–1837, 1989.
147. Gandevia, S. C. Neural mechanisms underlying the sensation of breathlessness: kinesthetic parallels between respiratory and limb muscles. *Aust. N. Z. J. Med.* 18: 83–91, 1988.
148. Gandevia, S. L., K. J. Killian, and E. J. M. Campbell. The effect of respiratory muscle fatigue on respiratory sensations. *Clin. Sci.* 60: 463–466, 1981.
149. Gandevia, S. C., K. J. Killian, D. K. Mckenzie, M. Crawford, G. M. Allen, R. B. Gorman, and J. P. Hales. Respiratory sensation, cardiovascular control, kinaesthesia and transcranial stimulation during complete paralysis in humans. *J. Physiol. (Lond.)* 470: 85–108, 1993.
150. Gandevia, S. C., and D. K. McKenzie. Activation of the human diaphragm during maximal static efforts. *J. Physiol. (Lond.)* 367: 45–56, 1985.
151. Garlando, F., J. Kohl, E. A. Koller, and P. Pietsch. Effect of coupling the breathing and cycling rhythms on oxygen uptake during bicycle ergometry. *Eur. J. Appl. Physiol.* 54: 497–501, 1985.
152. Giesbrecht, G. G., F. Ali, and M. Younes. Short-term effect of tidal pleural pressure swings on pulmonary blood flow during rest and exercise. *J. Appl. Physiol.* 71: 465–473, 1991.
153. Gilbert, R., and J. J. Auchincloss. Mechanics of breathing in normal subjects during brief, severe exercise. *J. Lab. Clin. Med.* 73: 439–450, 1969.
154. Gillespie, D. J., and R. E. Hyatt. Respiratory mechanics in the unanesthetized dog. *J. Appl. Physiol.* 36: 98–102, 1974.
155. Gillespie, J. R., G. L. Landgren, and D. E. Leith. 1: 2 ratio of breathing to stride frequencies in a galloping horse breathing 6% CO_2. *Equine Exerc. Physiol.* 3: 66–70, 1991.
156. Goldman, M., G. Grimby, and J. Mead. Mechanical work of breathing derived from rib cage and abdominal V-P partitioning. *J. Appl. Physiol.* 41: 752–764, 1976.
157. Gollnick, P., M. Riedy, J. Quintinskie, and L. Bertocci. Difference in metabolic potential of skeletal muscle fibres and their significance for metabolic control. *J. Exp. Biol.* 115: 191–199, 1985.
158. Gorski, J., Z. Namiot, and J. Giedrojc. Effect of exercise on metabolism of glycogen and triglycerides in the respiratory muscles. *Pflugers Arch.* 377: 251–254, 1978.
159. Gosselin, L. E., M. Betlach, A. C. Vailas, and D. P. Thomas. Training induced alterations in young and senescent rat diaphragm muscle. *J. Appl. Physiol.* 72: 1506–1511, 1992.
160. Gowda, K., T. Zintel, C. McParland, R. Orchard, and C. G. Gallagher. Diagnostic value of maximal exercise tidal volume. *Chest* 98: 1351–1354, 1990.
161. Granath, A., E. Horie, and H. Linderholm. Compliance and resistance of the lungs in the sitting and supine positions at rest and during work. *Scand. J. Clin. Lab. Invest.* 11: 226–234, 1959.
162. Green, H. J., M. E. Ball-Burnett, M. A. Morrissey, J. Kile, and G. C. Abraham. Glycogen utilization in rat respiratory muscles during intense running. *Can. J. Physiol. Pharmacol.* 66: 917–923, 1988.
163. Green, H., M. Plyley, D. Smith, and J. Kile. Extreme endurance training and fiber type adaptation in rat diaphragm. *J. Appl. Physiol.* 66: 1914–1920, 1986.
164. Grillner, S., J. Nilsson, and A. Thorstensson. Intra-abdominal pressure changes during natural movements in man. *Acta. Physiol. Scand.* 103: 275–283, 1978.
165. Grimby, G., M. Goldman, and J. Mead. Respiratory muscle action inferred from rib cage and abdominal V-P partitioning. *J. Appl. Physiol.* 41: 739–751, 1976.
166. Grimby, G., B. Saltin, and L. Wilhemson. Pulmonary flow volume and pressure volume relationship during submaximal and maximal exercise in young well-trained men. *Bull. Physiopathol. Respir.* 7: 57–168, 1971.
167. Grinton, S., S. Powers, J. Lawler, D. Criswell, S. Dodd, and W. Edwards. Endurance training-induced increases in expiratory muscle oxidative capacity. *Med. Sci. Sports Exerc.* 24: 551–555, 1992.
168. Gross, D., A. Grassino, W. R. D. Ross, and P. T. Macklem. Electromyogram pattern of diaphragmatic fatigue. *J. Appl. Physiol. Respir. Environ. Exerc. Physiol.* 46: 1–7, 1979.
169. Gutting, S. M., H. V. Forster, T. F. Lowry, A. G. Brice, and L. G. Pan. Respiratory muscle recruitment in awake ponies during exercise and CO_2 inhalation. *Respir. Physiol.* 86: 315–332, 1991.

170. Hagberg, J. M., J. E. Yerg, and D. R. Seals. Pulmonary function in young and older athletes and untrained men. *Appl. Physiol.* 65: 101–105, 1988.
171. Haight, J., and P. Cole. Site and function of the nasal valve. *Laryngoscope* 93: 49–55, 1983.
172. Hairston, L. E., and E. K. Sauerland. Electromyography of the human palate: discharge patterns of the levator and tensor veli palatini. *Electromyogr. Clin. Neurophysiol.* 21: 287–297, 1981.
173. Hamilton, L. H. Nasal airway resistance: its measurement and regulation. *Physiologist* 22: 43–49, 1979.
174. Hamilton, A., G. Obminski, E. Summers, M. L. Jones, and K. J. Killian. Endurance capacity and symptom limitation during extreme exertion. *Am. J. Respir. Crit. Care Med.* 149: A776, 1994.
175. Hamm, T., P. Nemeth, L. Solanki, D. Gordon, R. Reinking, and D. Stuart. Association between biochemical and physiological properties in single motor units. *Muscle Nerve* 11: 245–254, 1988.
176. Hanel, B., and N. Secher. Maximal oxygen uptake and work capacity after inspiratory muscle training: a controlled study. *J. Sports Sci.* 9: 43–52, 1991.
177. Hanson, P. A., A. Claremont, J. A. Dempsey, and W. G. Reddan. Determinants and consequences of ventilatory responses to competitive endurance running. *J. Appl. Physiol.* 52: 615–623, 1982.
178. Harms, C. A., and J. M. Stager. How peripheral chemosensitivity and inadequate hyperventilation contribute to exercise-induced hypoxemia. *J. Appl. Physiol.* 79: 575–580, 1995.
179. Harty, H. R., and L. Adams. Dose dependency of perceived breathlessness on hypoventilation during exercise in normal subjects. *J. Appl. Physiol.* 77: 2666–2674, 1994.
179a. Harty, H. R., C. J. Mummery, L. Adams, R. B. Banzatt, I. G. Wright, N. R. Banner, M. H. Yacoub, and A. Guz. Ventilatory release of the urge to breathe sensation in humans: are pulmonary receptors important? *J. Physiol. (Lond.)* 490: 805–815, 1996.
180. Haxhiu, M. A., E. van Lunteren, J. Mitra, and N. S. Cherniack. Responses to chemical stimulation of upper airway muscles and diaphragm in awake cats. *J. Appl. Physiol.* 56: 397–403, 1984.
181. Hellstrand, E. Morphological and histochemical properties of tongue muscles in cats. *Acta Physiol. Scand.* 110: 187–198, 1980.
182. Henke, K. G., M. Sharratt, D. Pegelow, and J. A. Dempsey. Regulation of end-expiratory lung volume during exercise. *J. Appl. Physiol.* 64: 135–146, 1988.
183. Henneman, E., and L. M. Mendell. Functional organization of motoneuron pool and its inputs. In: *Handbook of Physiology, The Nervous System, Motor Control*, edited by V. B. Brooks. Bethesda, MD: Am. Physiol. Soc., 1981, p. 423–507.
184. Hershenson, M. B., Y. Kikuchi, and S. H. Loring. Relative strengths of the chest wall muscles. *J. Appl. Physiol.* 65: 852–862, 1988.
185. Hey, E. N., B. B. Lloyd, D. Cunningham, M. Jukes, and D. Bolton. Effects of various respiratory stimuli on the depth and frequency of breathing in man. *Respir. Physiol.* 1: 193–205, 1966.
186. Hill, N. S., C. Jacoby, and H. W. Farber. Effect of an endurance triathalon on pulmonary function. *Med. Sci. Sports Exerc.* 23: 1260–1264, 1991.
187. Holloszy, J., and E. Coyle. Adaptations of skeletal muscle to endurance exercise and their metabolic consequences. *J. Appl. Physiol.* 56: 831–838, 1984.
188. Hornicke, H., R. Meixner, and U. Pollman. Respiration in exercising horses. In: *Equine Exercise Physiology*, edited by D. H. Snow, S. G. M. Persson, and R. J. Rose. Cambridge: Granta Editions, 1983, p. 7–16.
189. Hu, A., F. H. Comtois, and A. E. Grassino. Optimal diaphragmatic blood perfusion. *J. Appl. Physiol.* 72: 149–157, 1992.
190. Hubmayr, R. D., W. J. Litchy, P. C. Gay, and S. B. Nelson. Transdiaphragmatic twitch pressure: effects of lung volume and chest wall shape. *Am. Rev. Respir. Dis.* 139: 647–652, 1989.
191. Hudgel, D. W., K. R. Chapman, C. Faulks, and C. Hendricks. Changes in inspiratory muscle electrical activity and upper airway resistance during periodic breathing induced by hypoxia during sleep. *Am. Rev. Respir. Dis.* 135: 899–906, 1987.
192. Hussain, S. N. A., and R. L. Pardy. Inspiratory muscle function with restrictive chest wall loading during exercise in normal humans. *J. Appl. Physiol.* 58: 2027–2032, 1985.
193. Hussain, S. N. A., R. L. Pardy, and J. A. Dempsey. Mechanical impedance as determinant of inspiratory neural drive during exercise in humans. *J. Appl. Physiol.* 59: 365–375, 1985.
194. Hyland, R. H., N. L. Jones, A. C. P. Powles, S. C. M. Lenkie, R. G. Vanderlinden, and S. W. Epstein. Primary alveolar hypoventilation treated with nocturnal electrophrenic respiration. *Am. Rev. Respir. Dis.* 117: 165–172, 1978.
195. Ianuzzo, C. D., E. Noble, N. Hamilton, and B. Dabrowski. Effects of streptozotocin diabetes, insulin treatment, and training on the diaphragm. *J. Appl. Physiol.* 52: 1471–1475, 1982.
196. Ianuzzo, C. D., M. J. Spalding, and H. Williams. Exercise-induced glycogen utilization by the respiratory muscles. *J. Appl. Physiol.* 62: 1405–1409, 1987.
197. Issa, F. G., P. Edwards, E. Szeto, D. Lauff, and C. Sullivan. Genioglossus and breathing responses to airway occlusion: effect of sleep and route of occlusion. *J. Appl. Physiol.* 64: 543–549, 1988.
198. Issa, F. G., and C. E. Sullivan. Upper airway closing pressures in obstructive sleep apnea. *J. Appl. Physiol.* 57: 520–527, 1984.
199. Jammes, Y., B. Buchler, S. Delpierre, A. Rasidakis, C. Grimaud, and C. Roussos. Phrenic afferents and their role in inspiratory control. *J. Appl. Physiol.* 60: 854–860, 1986.
200. Jasinskas, C. L., B. A. Wilson, and J. Hoare. Entrainment of breathing rate to movement frequency during work at two intensities. *Respir. Physiol.* 42: 199–209, 1980.
201. Jensen, J. I., S. Lyager, and O. F. Pedersen. The relationship between maximal ventilation, breathing pattern and mechanical limitation of ventilation. *J. Physiol. (Lond.)* 309: 521–532, 1980.
202. Johnson, B. D., M. L. Austrup, and G. C. Sieck. Diaphragm contractile properties in transgenic mice overexpressing CuZn-superoxide dismutase. *Am. J. Respir. Crit. Care Med.* 149: A322, 1994.
203. Johnson, B. D., M. A. Babcock, O. E. Suman, J. A. Dempsey. Exercise-induced diaphragmatic fatigue in healthy humans. *J. Physiol. (Lond.)* 460: 385–405, 1993.
204. Johnson, B. D., M. S. Badr, and J. A. Dempsey. Impact of the aging pulmonary system on the response to exercise. *Clin. Chest Med.* 15: 229–246, 1994.

205. Johnson, B. D., W. G. Reddan, D. F. Pegelow, K. C. Seow, and J. A. Dempsey. Flow limitation and regulation of function residual capacity during exercise in a physically active aging population. *Am. Rev. Respir. Dis.* 143: 960–967, 1991.
206. Johnson, B. D., W. G. Reddan, K. G. Seow, and J. A. Dempsey. Mechanical constraints on exercise hyperpnea in a fit aging population. *Am. Rev. Respir. Dis.* 143: 968–977, 1991.
207. Johnson, B. D., K. W. Saupe, and J. A. Dempsey. Mechanical constraints on exercise hyperpnea in endurance athletes. *J. Appl. Physiol.* 73: 874–886, 1992.
208. Johnson, B. D., P. D. Scanlon, and K. C. Beck. Regulation of ventilatory capacity during exercise in asthmatics. *J. Appl. Physiol.* (in press).
209. Johnson, B. D., and G. C. Sieck. Activation-induced reduction of SDH activity in diaphragm muscle fibers. *J. Appl. Physiol.* 75: 2689–2695, 1993.
210. Johnson, B. D., and G. C. Sieck. Differential susceptibility of diaphragm muscle fibers to neuromuscular transmission failure. *J. Appl. Physiol.* 75: 341–348, 1993.
211. Jones James H. Circulatory function during exercise: Integration of convection and diffusion. *Adv. Vet. Sci. Comp. Med.* 38A: 217–251, 1994.
212. Jones, N. L. Determinants of breathing patterns. In: *Exercise: Pulmonary Physiology and Pathophysiology*, edited by B. J. Whipp and K. Wasserman. New York: Marcel Dekker, Inc., 1991, p. 99–119.
213. Jones, N. L., K. J. Killian, and D. G. Stubbing. The thorax during exercise. In: *The Thorax*, edited by C. Roussos and P. Macklem. New York: Marcel Dekker, Inc., 1985, p. 627–661.
214. Kagawa, J., and H. D. Kerr. Effects of brief graded exercise on specific airway conductance in normal subjects. *J. Appl. Physiol.* 28: 138–144, 1970.
215. Karlsson, J., and B. Saltin. Diet, muscle glycogen and endurance performance. *J. Appl. Physiol.* 31: 203–206, 1971.
216. Katz-Salamon, M., C. Von Euler, and O. Franzen. Perception of mechanical factors in breathing. In: *Physical Work and Effort*, edited by G. Borg. Oxford: Pergamon Press, 1976, p. 101–113.
217. Kaufman, M. P., K. J. Rybicki, and J. H. Mitchell. Hindlimb muscular contraction reflexly decreases total pulmonary resistance in dogs. *J. Appl. Physiol.* 59: 1521–1526, 1985.
218. Killian, K. J. Limitation of exercise by dyspnea. *Can. J. Sport Sci.* 12: 53S–60S, 1987.
219. Killian, K. J., D. D. Bucens, and E. J. M. Campbell. Effect of breathing patterns on the perceived magnitude of added loads to breathing. *J. Appl. Physiol.* 52: 578–584, 1982.
220. Killian, K. J., and E. J. Campbell. Mechanisms of dyspnea. In: *Dyspnea*, edited by D. A. Mahler. New York: Futura Publishing Co., 1990, p. 55–73.
221. Killian, K. J., S. C. Gandevia, E. Summers, and E. J. M. Campbell. Effect of increased lung volume on perception of breathlessness, effort and tension. *J. Appl. Physiol.* 57: 686–691, 1984.
222. Killian, K. J., P. Leblanc, D. H. Martin, E. Summers, N. L. Jones, and E. J. M. Campbell. Exercise capacity and ventilatory, circulatory, and symptom limitation in patients with chronic airflow limitation. *Am. Rev. Respir. Dis.* 146: 935–940, 1992.
223. Klas, J. V., and J. A. Dempsey. Voluntary vs reflex regulation of maximal exercise flow: volume loop. *Am. Rev. Respir. Dis.* 139: 150–156, 1989.
224. Klausen, K., N. H. Secher, J. P. Clausen, O. Hartling, and J. Trap-Jensen. Central and regional circulatory adaptations to one-leg training. *J. Appl. Physiol. Respir. Environ. Exerc. Physiol.* 52: 976–983, 1982.
225. Kohl, J., E. A. Koller, and M. Jager. Relation between pedalling and breathing rhythm. *Eur. J. Appl. Physiol.* 47: 223–237, 1981.
226. Krishnan, B., T. Zintel, C. McParland, and C. G. Gallagher. The evolution of respiratory motor output in constant load heavy exercise. *FASEB J.* 5: A1480, 1991.
227. Krishnan, B., T. Zintel, C. McParland, and C. G. Gallagher. Lack of importance of respiratory muscle load in ventilatory regulation during heavy exercise. *J. Physiol. (Lond.)* 1995 (in press).
228. Kuei, J. H., R. Shadmehr, and G. C. Sieck. Relative contribution of neurotransmission failure to diaphragm fatigue. *J. Appl. Physiol.* 68: 174–180, 1990.
229. Kugelberg, E. Histochemical composition, contraction speed, and fatigability of rat soleus motor units. *J. Neurol. Sci.* 20: 177–198, 1973.
230. Kuna, S. T., R. A. Day, G. Insalaco, and R. D. D. Villeponteaux. Posterior cricoarytenoid activity in normal adults during involuntary and voluntary hyperventilation. *J. Appl. Physiol.* 70: 1377–1385, 1991.
231. Kurtz, D., J. Krieger, and J. C. Stierle. EMG activity of cricothyroid and chin muscles during wakefulness and sleeping in the sleep apnea syndrome. *Electroencephalogr. Clin. Neurophysiol.* 45: 777–784, 1978.
232. Lafortuna, C. L., A. E. Minetti, and P. Mognoni. Inspiratory flow pattern in humans. *J. Appl. Physiol. Respir. Environ. Exerc. Physiol.* 57: 1111–1119, 1984.
233. Lafortuna, C. L., and F. Saibene. Mechanics of breathing in horses at rest and during exercise. *J. Exp. Biol.* 155: 245–259, 1991.
234. Landgren, G. L., J. R. Gillespie, and D. E. Leith. No ventilatory response in thoroughbreds galloping at 14 $m \cdot s^{-1}$. In: *Equine Exercise Physiology*, edited by S. G. Persoon, A. Lindholm, and L. B. Jeffcott. Davis, CA: ICEEP, 1991, p. 59–65.
235. Lane, R., and L. Adams. Metabolic acidosis and breathlessness during exercise and hypercapnia in man. *J. Physiol. (Lond.)* 461: 47–61, 1993.
236. Lane, R., L. Adams, and A. Guz. Is low-level respiratory resistive loading during exercise perceived as breathlessness? *Clin. Sci.* 73: 627–634, 1987.
237. Lane, R., L. Adams, and A. Guz. The effects of hypoxia and hypercapnia on perceived breathlessness during exercise in humans. *J. Physiol. (Lond.)* 428: 579–593, 1990.
238. Lane, R., A. Cockcroft, L. Adams, and A. Guz. Arterial oxygen saturation and breathlessness in patients with chronic obstructive airways disease. *Clin. Sci.* 72: 693–698, 1987.
239. Lane, R., A. Cockcroft, and A. Guz. Voluntary isocapnic hyperventilation and breathlessness during exercise in normal subjects. *Clin. Sci.* 73: 519–523, 1987.
240. Lawler, J., S. K. Powers, and D. Thompson. Linear relationships between $\dot{V}O_{2max}$ and $\dot{V}O_{2max}$ decrement during exposure to acute hypoxia. *J. Appl. Physiol.* 64: 1486–1492, 1988.
241. Leblanc, P., D. M. Bowie, E. Summers, N. L. Jones, and K. J. Killian. Breathlessness and exercise in patients with

cardiorespiratory disease. *Am. Rev. Respir. Dis.* 133: 21–25, 1986.

242. Leblanc, P., E. Summers, M. D. Inman, N. L. Jones, E. Campbell, and K. J. Killian. Inspiratory muscles during exercise: a problem of supply and demand. *J. Appl. Physiol.* 64: 2482–2489, 1988.
243. Leevers, A. M., and J. D. Road. Abdominal muscle activation by expiratory threshold loading in awake dogs. *Respir. Physiol.* 93: 289–303, 1993.
244. Leiter, J. C., S. L. Knuth, and D. B. Bartlett, Jr. Dependence of pharyngeal resistance on genioglossal EMG activity, nasal resistance and flow. *J. Appl. Physiol.* 73: 584–590, 1992.
245. Leith, D., and M. Bradley. Ventilatory muscle strength and endurance training. *J. Appl. Physiol.* 41: 508–516, 1976.
246. Levine, S., M. Gillen, P. Weiser, G. Feiss, M. Goldman, and D. Henson. Inspiratory pressure generation: comparison of subjects with COPD and age-matched normals. *J. Appl. Physiol.* 65: 888–899, 1988.
247. Levine, S., and D. Henson. Low-frequency diaphragmatic fatigue in spontaneously breathing humans. *J. Appl. Physiol.* 64: 672–680, 1988.
248. Lindinger, M. I., G. J. F. Heigenhauser, R. S. McKelvie, and N. L. Jones. Role of nonworking muscle on blood metabolites and ions with intense intermittent exercise. *Am. J. Physiol.* 258 (*Regulatory Integrative Comp. Physiol.* 27): R148–R149, 1990.
249. Lindstedt, S. L., J. F. Hokanson, D. J. Wells, S. D. Swain, H. Hoppeler, and V. Navarra. Running energetics in the prong horn antelope. *Nature* 353: 748–750, 1991.
250. Lindstedt, S. L., R. G. Thomas, and D. E. Leith. Does peak inspiratory flow contribute to setting $\dot{V}O_{2max}$? *Respir. Physiol.* 95: 109–118, 1994.
251. Loke, J. D. M., and J. A. Virgulto. Respiratory muscle fatigue after marathon running. *J. Appl. Physiol.* 52: 821–824, 1982.
252. Loring, S. H., J. Mead, and T. B. Waggener. Determinants of breathing frequency during walking. *Respir. Physiol.* 82: 177–188, 1990.
253. Louhevaara, V., A. Sovijarvi, J. Ilmarinen, and P. Teraslinna. Differences in cardiorespiratory responses during and after arm crank and cycle exercise. *Acta Physiol. Scand.* 138: 133–143, 1990.
254. MacDonald, M. E., R. L. Kirby, S. T. Nugent, and D. A. MacLeod. Locomotor-respiratory coupling during wheelchair propulsion. *J. Appl. Physiol.* 72: 1375–1379, 1992.
255. Mador, M. J., and F. A. Acevedo. Effect of respiratory muscle fatigue on breathing pattern during incremental exercise. *Am. Rev. Respir. Dis.* 143: 462–468, 1991.
256. Mador, M. J., U. J. Magalang, A. Rodis, and T. J. Kufel. Diaphragmatic fatigue after exercise in healthy human subjects. *Am. Rev. Respir. Dis.* 148: 1571–1575, 1993.
257. Mahler, D. A., and J. Loke. Lung function after marathon running at warm and cold ambient temperatures. *Am. Rev. Respir. Dis.* 124: 154–157, 1981.
258. Mahler, D. A., C. R. Shuhart, E. Brew, and T. A. Stukel. Ventilatory responses and entrainment of breathing during rowing. *Med. Sci. Sports Exerc.* 23: 186–192, 1991.
259. Mann, D. G., C. S. Sasaki, H. Fukuda, M. Suzuki, and J. R. Hernandez. Dilator naris muscle. *Ann. Otol.* 86: 362–370, 1977.
260. Manning, H. L., S. A. Shea, R. M. Schwartzstein, R. W. Lansing, R. Brown, and R. B. Banzett. Reduced tidal volume increases "air hunger" at fixed PCO2 in ventilated quadriplegics. *Respir. Physiol.* 90: 19–30, 1992.
261. Manohar, M. Blood flow to the respiratory and limb muscles and to abdominal organs during maximal exertion in ponies. *J. Physiol. (Lond.)* 377: 25–35, 1986.
262. Manohar, M. Vasodilator reserve in respiratory muscles during maximal exertion in ponies. *J. Appl. Physiol.* 60: 1571–1577, 1986.
263. Manohar, M. Costal vs. crural diaphragmatic blood flow during submaximal and near-maximal exercise in ponies. *J. Appl. Physiol.* 65: 1514–1519, 1988.
264. Manohar, M., and A. S. Hassan. The diaphragm does not produce ammonia or lactate during high density short-term exercise. *Am. J. Physiol.* 259 (*Heart Circ. Physiol.* 28): H1185–H1189, 1990.
265. Manohar, M., and A. S. Hassan. Diaphragmatic energetics during prolonged exhaustive exercise. *Am. Rev. Respir. Dis.* 144: 415–418, 1991.
266. Marciniuk, D., D. McKim, R. Sanii, and M. Younes. Role of central respiratory muscle fatigue in endurance exercise in normal subjects. *J. Appl. Physiol.* 76: 236–241, 1994.
267. Marciniuk, D. D., G. Sridhar, R. E. Clemens, T. A. Zintel, and C. G. Gallagher. Lung volumes and expiratory flow limitation during exercise in interstitial lung disease. *J. Appl. Physiol.* 77: 963–973, 1994.
268. Maron, M. B., L. H. Hamilton, and M. G. Maksud. Alterations in pulmonary function consequent to competitive marathon running. *Med. Sci. Sports Exerc.* 11: 244–249, 1979.
269. Martin, B., M. Heintzelman, and H. Chen. Exercise performance after ventilatory work. *J. Appl. Physiol.* 52: 1581–1585, 1982.
270. Mathew, O. P., Y. K. Abu-Osba, and B. T. Thach. Influence of upper airway pressure changes on genioglossus muscle respiratory activity. *J. Appl. Physiol.* 52: 438–444, 1982.
271. McBride, B., and W. A. Whitelaw. A physiological stimulus to upper airway receptors in humans. *J. Appl. Physiol.* 51: 1189–1197, 1981.
272. McClaran, S. R., M. Babcock, D. Pegelow, W. Reddan, and J. Dempsey. Longitudinal effects of aging on lung function at rest and exercise in the healthy active fit elderly adult. *J. Appl. Physiol.* 78: 1957–1968, 1995.
273. McCool, F. D., D. R. McCann, D. E. Leith, and F. G. Hoppin, Jr. Pressure-flow effects on endurance of inspiratory muscles. *J. Appl. Physiol.* 60: 299–303, 1986.
274. McCool, F. D., G. T. Tzelepis, D. E. Leith, and F. G. Hoppin, Jr. Oxygen cost of breathing during fatiguing inspiratory resistive loads. *J. Appl. Physiol.* 66: 2045–2055, 1989.
275. McDermott, J. C., G. C. Elder, and A. Bonen. Adrenal hormones enhance glycogenolysis in nonexercising muscle during exercise. *J. Appl. Physiol.* 63: 1275–1283, 1987.
276. McParland, C., B. Krishnan, J. Lobo, and C. G. Gallagher. Effect of physical training on breathing pattern during progressive exercise. *Respir. Physiol.* 90: 311–323, 1992.
277. McParland, C., J. Mink, and C. G. Gallagher. Respiratory adaptations to dead space loading during maximal incremental exercise. *J. Appl. Physiol.* 70: 55–62, 1991.
278. Mead, J. Control of respiratory frequency. *J. Appl. Physiol.* 15: 325–336, 1960.
279. Mead, J., and E. Agostoni. Dynamics of breathing. In: *Handbook of Physiology, Respiration*, edited by W. O. Fenn and H. Rahn. Washington, DC: Am. Physiol. Soc., 1964, p. 411–427.
280. Messner, T. *Everest: Expedition to the Ultimate.* London: Kaye and Ward, 1979.

281. Metzger, J., and R. Fitts. Contractile and biochemical properties of diaphragm: effects of exercise and fatigue. *J. Appl. Physiol.* 60: 1752–1758, 1986.
282. Mezzanotte, W. S., D. J. Tangel, and D. P. White. Mechanisms of control of alae nasi muscle activity. *J. Appl. Physiol.* 72: 925–933, 1992.
283. Miles, D. S., A. D. Enoch, and S. C. Grevey. Interpretation of changes in DLCO and pulmonary function after running five miles. *Respir. Physiol.* 66: 135–145, 1986.
284. Mitchinson, A. G., and J. M. Yoffey. Respiratory displacement of the larynx, hyoid bone and tongue. *J. Anat.* 81: 118–121, 1947.
285. Mizuno, M. Human respiratory muscles: fibre morphology and capillary supply. *Eur. Respir. J.* 4: 587–601, 1991.
286. Mizuno, M., and N. H. Secher. Histochemical characteristics of human expiratory and inspiratory intercostal muscles. *J. Appl. Physiol.* 67: 592–598, 1989.
287. Moore, R. L., and P. D. Gollnick. Response of ventilatory muscles of the rat to endurance training. *Pflugers Arch.* 392: 268–271, 1982.
288. Morgan, D., W. Kohrt, B. Bates, and J. Skinner. Effects of respiratory muscle endurance training on ventilatory and endurance performance of moderately trained cyclists. *Int. J. Sports Med.* 8: 88–93, 1987.
289. Moxham, J., R. H. T. Edwards, M. Aubier, A. Detroyer, G. Farkas, P. T. Macklem, and C. Roussos. Changes in EMG power spectrum (high to low) with force fatigue in humans. *J. Appl. Physiol.* 53: 1094–1099, 1982.
290. Muza, S. R., M. T. Silverman, G. C. Gilmore, H. K. Hellerstein, and S. G. Kelsen. Comparison of scales used to quantitate the sense of effort to breathe in patients with chronic obstructive pulmonary disease. *Am. Rev. Respir. Dis.* 141: 909–913, 1990.
291a. National Heart, Lung and Blood Institute. Workshop Summary. Respiratory Muscle Fatigue: Report of the Respiratory Muscle Fatigue Workshop Group. *Am. Rev. Respir. Dis.* 142: 474–480, 1990.
291b. Nava, S., E. Zanotti, C. Rampulla, and A. Rossi. Respiratory muscle fatigue does not limit exercise performance during moderate endurance run. *J. Sports Med. Phys. Fitness* 32: 39–44, 1992.
292. Niinimaa, V., P. Cole, S. Mintz, and R. J. Shephard. The switching point from nasal to oro-nasal breathing. *Respir. Physiol.* 42: 61–71, 1980.
293. Niinimaa, V., P. Cole, S. Mintz, and R. J. Shephard. Oronasal distribution of respiratory airflow. *Respir. Physiol.* 43: 69–75, 1981.
294. Ohki, M., M. Hasegawa, N. Kurita, and I. Watanabe. Effects of exercise on nasal resistance and nasal blood flow. *Acta Otolaryngol.* 104: 328–333, 1987.
295. Okabe, S., T. Chonan, W. Hida, M. Satoh, Y. Kikuchi, and T. Takishima. Role of chemical drive in recruiting upper airway and inspiratory intercostal muscles in patients with obstructive sleep apnea. *Am. Rev. Respir. Dis.* 147: 190–195, 1993.
296. O'Kroy, J., and J. Coast. Effects of flow and resistive training on respiratory muscle strength and endurance. *Respiration* 60: 279–283, 1993.
297. O'Kroy, J., R. A. Loy, and J. R. Coast. Pulmonary function changes following exercise. *Med. Sci. Sports Exerc.* 24: 1359–1364, 1992.
298. Olafsson, S., and R. E. Hyatt. Ventilatory mechanics and expiratory flow limitation during exercise in normal subjects. *J. Clin. Invest.* 48: 564–573, 1969.
299. Olson, L. G., J. M. Fouke, P. L. Hoekje, and K. P. Strohl. A biomechanical view of upper airway function. In: *Regulation of Breathing*, edited by O. P. M. Ambrogio. New York: Marcel Dekker, 1988, p. 359–389.
300. Olson, L. G., and K. P. Strohl. The response of the nasal airway to exercise. *Am. Rev. Respir. Dis.* 135: 356–359, 1987.
301. Onal, E., M. Lopata, and T. D. O'Connor. Diaphragmatic and genioglossal electromyogram responses to CO_2 rebreathing in humans. *J. Appl. Physiol.* 50: 1052–1055, 1981.
302. Onal, E., M. Lopata, and T. D. O'Connor. Diaphragmatic and genioglossal electromyogram responses to isocapnic hypoxia in humans. *Am. Rev. Respir. Dis.* 124: 215–217, 1981.
303. O'Neill, P. A., R. D. Stark, S. C. Allen, and T. B. Stretton. The relationship between breathlessness and ventilation during steady state exercise. *Clin. Respir. Physiol.* 22: 247–250, 1986.
304. Opie, L. H., A. C. Smith, and J. M. K. Spalding. Conscious appreciation of the effects produced by independent changes of ventilation volume and end-tidal PCO_2 in paralysed patients. *J. Physiol. (Lond.)* 149: 494–499, 1959.
305. Otis, A. B. The work of breathing. In: *Handbook of Physiology, Respiration*, edited by W. O. Fenn and H. Rahn. Washington, DC: Am. Physiol. Soc., 1964, p. 463–476.
306. Otis, A. B., W. A. Fenn, and H. Rahn. Mechanics of breathing in man. *J. Appl. Physiol.* 2: 592–607, 1950.
307. Pagala, M. K. D., T. Namba, and D. Grob. Failure of neuromuscular transmission and contractility during muscle fatigue. *Muscle Nerve* 7: 454–464, 1984.
308. Painter, R., and D. Cunningham. Analyses of human respiratory flow patterns. *Respir. Physiol.* 87: 293–307, 1992.
309. Pardy, R. L., and P. T. P. Bye. Diaphragmatic fatigue in normoxia and hyperoxia. *J. Appl. Physiol.* 58: 738–742, 1985.
310. Pardy, R., W. D. Reid, and M. Belman. Respiratory muscle training. In: *Clinics in Chest Medicine: Respiratory Muscles: Function in Health and Disease*, edited by M. Belman. Philadelphia: W. B. Saunders Company, 1988, p. 287–296.
311. Paterson, D. J., G. A. Wood, R. N. Marshall, A. R. Morton, and A. Harrison. Entrainment of respiratory frequency to exercise rhythm during hypoxia. *J. Appl. Physiol.* 62: 1767–1771, 1987.
312. Paterson, D. J., G. A. Wood, A. R. Morton, and J. D. Henstridge. The entrainment of ventilation frequency to exercise rhythm. *Eur. J. Appl. Physiol. Occup. Physiol.* 55: 530–537, 1986.
313. Paton, J. Y., S. Swaminathan, C. W. Sargent, A. Hawksworth, and T. G. Keens. Ventilatory response to exercise in children with congenital central hypoventilation syndrome. *Am. Rev. Respir. Dis.* 147: 1185–1191, 1993.
314. Pearce, D. H., and H. J. Milhorn. Dynamic and steady-state respiratory responses to bicycle exercise. *J. Appl. Physiol.* 41: 959–967, 1977.
315. Pelletier, N., and D. E. Leith. Ventilation and CO_2 exchange in exercising horses: effect of inspired O_2 fraction. *J. Appl. Physiol.* 78: 654–662, 1995.
316. Pelligrino, R., V. Brussasco, J. R. Rodarte, and T. G. Babb. Expiratory flow limitation and regulation of end-expiratory lung volume during exercise. *J. Appl. Physiol.* 74: 2552–2558, 1993.

317. Permutt, S., and R. A. Wise. Mechanical interaction of respiration and circulation. In: *Handbook of Physiology, The Respiratory System, Mechanics of Breathing*, edited by P. T. Macklem and J. Mead. Bethesda, MD: Am. Physiol. Soc., 1986, p. 647–656.
318. Person, R. S. Rhythmic activity of a group of human motoneurons during voluntary contraction of a muscle. *Electroencephalogr. Clin. Neurophysiol.* 36: 585–595, 1974.
319. Pertuze, J., A. Watson, and N. B. Pride. Maximum airflow through the nose. *J. Appl. Physiol.* 70: 1369–1376, 1991.
320. Pette, D., and R. Staron. Cellular and molecular diversities of mammalian skeletal muscle fibers. *Rev. Physiol. Biochem. Pharmacol.* 116: 2–76, 1990.
321. Polacheck, J., R. Strong, J. Arens, C. Davies, I. Metcalf, and M. Younes. Phasic vagal influence on inspiratory motor output in anesthesized human subjects. *J. Appl. Physiol. Respir. Environ. Exerc. Physiol.* 49: 609–619, 1980.
322. Poon, C. S. Ventilatory control in hypercapnia and exercise: optimization hypothesis. *J. Appl. Physiol.* 62: 2447–2459, 1987.
323. Poon, C. S., S. A. Ward, and B. J. Whipp. Influence of inspiratory assistance on ventilatory control during moderate exercise. *J. Appl. Physiol.* 62: 551–560, 1987.
324. Powers, S., D. Criswell, J. Lawler, L. Ji, D. Martin, R. Herb, and G. Dudley. Influence of exercise and fiber type on antioxidant enzyme activity in rat skeletal muscle. *Am. J. Physiol.* 266 (*Regulatory Integrative Comp. Physiol.* 35): R375–R380, 1994.
325. Powers, S., D. Criswell, J. Lawler, D. Martin, L. Ji, R. Herb, and G. Dudley. Regional training-induced alterations in diaphragmatic oxidative and antioxidant enzymes. *Respir. Physiol.* 95: 227–237, 1994.
326. Powers, S., D. Criswell, F. K. Lieu, S. Dodd, and H. Silverman. Diaphragmatic fiber type specific adaptation. *Respir. Physiol.* 89: 195–207, 1992.
327. Powers, S. K., D. Criswell, F. Lieu, S. Dodd, and H. Silverman. Exercise-induced cellular alterations in the diaphragm. *Am. J. Physiol.* 263 (*Regulatory Integrative Comp. Physiol.* 32): R1093–R1096, 1992.
328. Powers, S., S. Grinton, J. Lawler, D. Criswell, and S. Dodd. High intensity exercise training-induced metabolic alterations in respiratory muscles. *Respir. Physiol.* 89: 169–177, 1992.
329. Powers, S., J. Lawler, D. Criswell, S. Dodd, S. Grinton, G. Bagby, and H. Silverman. Endurance training-induced cellular adaptations in respiratory muscles. *J. Appl. Physiol.* 68: 2114–2118, 1990.
330. Powers, S., J. Lawler, D. Criswell, K. L. Fu, and D. Martin. Aging and respiratory muscle metabolic plasticity: effects of endurance training. *J. Appl. Physiol.* 72: 1068–1073, 1992.
331. Powers, S., J. Lawler, D. Criswell, H. Silverman, V. F. H. S. Grinton, and D. Harkins. Regional metabolic differences in the rat diaphragm. *J. Appl. Physiol.* 69: 648–650, 1990.
332. Powers, S. K., J. Lawler, J. A. Dempsey, S. Dodd, and G. Landry. Effects of incomplete pulmonary gas exchange on VO2 max. *J. Appl. Physiol.* 66: 2491–2495, 1989.
333. Prabhu, B., T. Zintel, D. Marciniuk, R. Clemens, and C. G. Gallagher. Lack of effect of pedalling frequency on breathing pattern during bicycle ergometry. *Am. Rev. Respir. Dis.* 145: A582, 1992.
334. Préfaut, C., F. Anselme, C. Caillaud, and J. Massé-Biron. Exercise-induced hypoxemia in older athletes. *J. Appl. Physiol.* 76: 120–126, 1994.
335. Proctor, D. F. The upper respiratory tract. In: *Pulmonary Diseases and Disorders*, edited by A. P. Fishman. New York: McGraw-Hill, 1979, p. 3–17.
336. Proctor, D. F. Form and function of the upper airways and larynx. In: *Handbook of Physiology, The Respiratory System, Mechanics of Breathing*, edited by P. T. Macklem and J. Mead. Bethesda, MD: Am. Physiol. Soc., 1986, p. 63–73.
337. Redline, S., S. B. Gottfried, and M. D. Altose. Effect of changes in inspiratory muscle strength on the sensation of respiratory force. *J. Appl. Physiol.* 70: 240–245, 1991.
338. Redline, S., and K. P. Strohl. Influence of upper airway sensory receptors on respiratory muscle activation in humans. *J. Appl. Physiol.* 63: 368–374, 1987.
339. Reid, M. B., K. E. Haack, K. M. Franchek, P. A. Valberg, L. Kobzik, and M. S. West. Reactive oxygen in skeletal muscle. I. Intracellular oxidant kinetics and fatigue in vitro. *J. Appl. Physiol.* 73: 1797–1804, 1992.
340. Reiser, P., R. Moss, G. Giulian, and M. Greaser. Shortening velocity in single fibers from adult rabbit soleus muscle is correlated with myosin heavy chain composition. *J. Biol. Chem.* 260: 9077–9080, 1985.
341. Remmers, J. E., J. G. Brooks, and S. M. Tenney. Effect of controlled ventilation on the tolerable limit of hypercapnia. *Respir. Physiol.* 4: 78–90, 1968.
342. Richerson, H. B., and P. M. Seebohm. Nasal airway response to exercise. *J. Allergy* 41: 269–284, 1968.
343. Road, J., R. Vahi, P. Del Rio, and A. Grassino. In vivo contractile properties of fatigued diaphragm. *J. Appl. Physiol.* 63: 471–478, 1987.
344. Roberts, D., and D. J. Smith. Biochemical aspects of peripheral muscle fatigue, a review. *Sports Med.* 7: 125–138, 1989.
345. Robertson, E., and J. Kjeldgaard. Improvement in ventilatory muscle function with running. *J. Appl. Physiol.* 52: 1400–1406, 1982.
346. Rodenstein, D. O., and D. C. Stanescu. Soft palate and oronasal breathing in humans. *J. Appl. Physiol.* 57: 651–657, 1984.
347. Roussos, C. Ventilatory muscle fatigue governs breathing frequency. *Bull. Eur. Physiopathol. Respir.* 20: 445–451, 1984.
348. Roussos, C. Respiratory muscle fatigue and ventilatory failure. *Chest* 97: 89S–96S, 1990.
349. Roussos, C., M. Fixley, D. Gross, and P. T. Macklem. Fatigue of inspiratory muscles and their synergistic behaviour. *J. Appl. Physiol.* 46: 897–904, 1979.
350. Roussos, C. S., and P. T. Macklem. Diaphragmatic fatigue in man. *J. Appl. Physiol.* 43: 189–197, 1977.
351. Rubinstein, I., N. Zamel, A. S. Rebuck, V. Hoffstein, A. D. D'Urzo, and A. S. Slutsky. Dichotomous airway response to exercise in asthmatic patients. *Am. Rev. Respir. Dis.* 138: 1164–1168, 1988.
352. Saibene, F., P. Mognoni, C. L. Lafortuna, and R. Mostardi. Oro-nasal breathing during exercise. *Pflugers Arch.* 378: 65–69, 1978.
353. St John, W. M., and D. Zhou, Differing control of neural activities during various portions of expiration in the cat. *J. Physiol. (Lond.)* 418: 189–204, 1989.
354. St John, W. M., D. Zhou, and R. F. Fregosi. Expiratory neural activities in gasping. *J. Appl. Physiol.* 66: 223–231, 1989.
355. Salman, D. S., D. F. Proctor, D. L. Swift, and S. A. Evering. Nasal resistance: description of a method and effect of temperature and humidity changes. *Ann. Otol.* 80: 736–743, 1971.

356. Salomone, R. J., and E. van Lunteren. Effects of hypoxia and hypercapnia on geniohyoid contractility and endurance. *J. Appl. Physiol.* 71: 709–715, 1991.
357. Saltin, B., and J. Karlsson. Muscle glycogen utilization during work of different intensities. In: *Advances in Experimental Medicine and Biology. Muscle Metabolism During Exercise*, edited by B. Pernow and B. Saltin. New York: Plenum Press, 1971, p. 289–299.
358. Saltin, B., and L. Rowell. Functional adaptations to physical activity and inactivity. *Federation Proc.* 39: 1506–1513, 1980.
359. Sauerland, E. K., and R. M. Harper. The human tongue during sleep: electromyographic activity of the genioglossus muscle. *Exp. Neurol.* 51: 160–170, 1976.
360. Scardella, A. T., N. Krawciw, J. T. Petrozzino, M. A. Co, T. V. Santiago, and N. H. Edelman. Strength and endurance characteristics of the normal human genioglossus. *Am. Rev. Respir. Dis.* 148: 179–184, 1993.
361. Schoene, R. B., S. Lahiri, P. H. Hackett, R. M. Peters, Jr., J. S. Milledge, C. J. Pizzo, F. H. Sarnquist, S. J. Boyer, D. J. Graber, K. H. Maret, and J. B. West. Relationship of hypoxic ventilatory response to exercise performance on Mount Everest. *J. Appl. Physiol.* 56: 1478–1483, 1984.
362. Schwartzstein, R. M., H. L. Manning, J. W. Weiss, and S. E. Weinberger. Dyspnea: a sensory experience. *Lung* 168: 185–199, 1990.
363. Sciurba, F. C., G. R. Owens, M. H. Sanders, P. G. Bartley, R. L. Hadesty, I. L. Paradis, and J. P. Costantino. Evidence of an altered pattern of breathing during exercise in recipients of heart-lung transplants. *N. Engl. J. Med.* 319: 1186–1192, 1988.
364. Secher, N. H., J. P. Clausen, K. Klausen, I. Noer, and J. Trap-Jensen. Central and regional circulatory effects of adding arm exercise to leg exercise. *Acta Physiol. Scand.* 100: 288–297, 1977.
365. Sekizawa, S., and H. Tsubone. Nasal receptors responding to noxious chemical irritants. *Respir. Physiol.* 96: 37–48, 1994.
366. Sharratt, M. T., K. G. Henke, E. A. Aaron, D. F. Pegelow, and J. A. Dempsey. Exercise-induced changes in functional residual capacity. *Respir. Physiol.* 70: 313–326, 1987.
367. Shea, S. A., L. P. Andres, D. C. Shannon, and R. B. Banzett. Ventilatory response to exercise in humans lacking ventilatory chemosensitivity. *J. Physiol. (Lond.)* 468: 623–640, 1993.
368. Shea, S. A., R. B. Banzett, and R. W. Lansing. Respiratory sensations and their role in the control of breathing. In: *Regulation of Breathing*, edited by J. A. Dempsey and A. I. Pack. New York: Marcel Dekker, Inc., 1994, p. 923–957.
369. Shephard, R. J. The oxygen cost of breathing during vigorous exercise. *Q. J. Exp. Physiol.* 51: 336–350, 1966.
370. Shephard, R. J. The maximum sustained voluntary ventilation in exercise. *Clin. Sci.* 32: 167–176, 1967.
371. Shephard, R. J. Effects of training upon respiratory function. *Med. Sport* 33: 9–17, 1980.
372. Shindoh, C., A. DiMarco, A. Thomas, P. Manubay, and G. Supinski. Effect of N-acetylcysteine on diaphragm fatigue. *J. Appl. Physiol.* 68: 2107–2113, 1990.
373. Sieck, G. C. Diaphragm muscle: structural and functional organization. *Clin. Chest Med.* 9: 195–210, 1988.
374. Sieck, G. C., and M. Fournier. Changes in diaphragm motor unit EMG during fatigue. *J. Appl. Physiol.* 68: 1917–1926, 1990.
375. Sieck, G. C., and M. Fournier. Diaphragm motor unit recruitment during ventilatory and nonventilatory behaviors. *J. Appl. Physiol.* 66: 2539–2545, 1989.
376. Sieck, G. C., M. Lewis, and C. Blanco. Effects of undernutrition on diaphragm fiber size, SDH activity and fatigue resistance. *J. Appl. Physiol.* 66: 2196–2205, 1989.
377. Smith, C. A., D. M. Ainsworth, K. S. Henderson, and J. A. Dempsey. Differential responses of expiratory muscle to chemical stimuli in awake dogs. *J. Appl. Physiol.* 66: 384–391, 1989.
378. Smith, C. A., D. M. Ainsworth, K. S. Henderson, and J. A. Dempsey. Differential timing of respiratory muscles in response to chemical stimuli in awake dogs. *J. Appl. Physiol.* 66: 392–399, 1989.
379. Stark, R. D., S. A. Gambles, and J. A. Lewis. Methods to assess breathlessness in healthy subjects: a critical evaluation and application to analyze the acute effects of diazepam and promethazine on breathlessness induced by exercise or by exposure to raised levels of carbon dioxide. *Clin. Sci.* 61: 429–439, 1981.
380. Stauber, W. T. Eccentric action of muscles: physiology, injury, and adaptation. In: *Exercise and Sport Sciences Reviews*, edited by K. B. Pandolf. Baltimore, MD: Williams & Wilkins, 1989, p. 157–185.
381. Steinacker, J. M., M. Both, and B. J. Whipp. Pulmonary mechanics and entrainment of respiration and stroke rate during rowing. *Int. J. Sports Med.* 14: S15–S19, 1993.
382. Stevens, S. S. Sensation and measurement. In: *Psychophysics. Introduction to its Perceptual, Neural and Social Prospects*, edited by G. Stevens. New York: John Wiley & Sons, 1975, p. 37–62.
383. Strohl, K. P. Respiratory activation of the facial nerve and alar muscles in anaesthetized dogs. *J. Physiol. (Lond.)* 363: 351–362, 1985.
384. Strohl, K. P., J. Hensley, M. Hallett, N. A. Saunders, and R. H. Ingram. Activation of upper airway muscles before onset of inspiration in normal humans. *J. Appl. Physiol.* 49: 638–642, 1980.
385. Strohl, K. P., C. F. O'Cain, and A. S. Slutsky. Alae nasi activation and nasal resistance in healthy subjects. *J. Appl. Physiol.* 52: 1432–1437, 1982.
386. Stubbing, D. G., K. J. Killian, and E. J. M. Campbell. The quantification of respiratory sensations by normal subjects. *Respir. Physiol.* 44: 251–260, 1981.
387. Stubbing, D. G., L. D. Pengelly, J. Morse, and N. L. Jones. Pulmonary mechanics during exercise in normal males. *J. Appl. Physiol.* 49: 506–510, 1980.
388. Stulbarg, M. S., and L. Adams. Manifestations of respiratory disease: dyspnea. In: *Textbook of Respiratory Medicine, Vol. 1, Part 2*, edited by J. F. Murray and J. A. Nadel. Philadelphia: W. B. Saunders Company, 1994, p. 511–528.
389. Sugiura, T., A. Morimoto, and N. Murakami. Effects of endurance training on myosin heavy-chain isoforms and enzyme activity in the rat diaphragm. *Pflugers Arch.* 421: 77–81, 1992.
390. Sugiura, T., A. Morimoto, Y. Sakata, T. Watanabe, and N. Murakami. Myosin heavy chain isoform changes in rat diaphragm are induced by endurance training. *Jpn. J. Physiol.* 40: 759–763, 1990.
391. Sugiura, T., S. Morita, A. Morimoto, and N. Murakami. Regional differences in myosin heavy chain isoforms and enzyme activities of the rat diaphragm. *J. Appl. Physiol.* 73: 506–509, 1992.

392. Suratt, P. M., R. McTier, and S. C. Wilhoit. Alae nasi electromyographic activity and timing in obstructive sleep apnea. *J. Appl. Physiol.* 58: 1252–1256, 1985.
393. Swinburn, C. R., J. M. Wakefield, and P. W. Jones. Relationship between ventilation and breathlessness during exercise in chronic obstructive airways disease is not altered by prevention of hypoxemia. *Clin. Sci.* 67: 515–519, 1984.
394. Syabbalo, N. C., A. Bundgaard, and J. G. Widdicombe. Effects of exercise on nasal airflow resistance in healthy subjects and in patients with asthma and rhinitis. *Bull. Eur. Physiopathol. Respir.* 21: 507–513, 1985.
395. Syabbalo, N. C., B. Krishnan, T. Zintel, and C. G. Gallagher. Differential ventilatory control during constant work rate and incremental exercise. *Respir. Physiol.* 97: 175–187, 1994.
396. Syabbalo, N., T. Zintel, R. Watts, and C. G. Gallagher. Carotid chemoreceptors and respiratory adaptations to dead space loading during incremental exercise. *J. Appl. Physiol.* 75: 1378–1384, 1993.
397. Szal, S. E., and R. B. Schoene. Ventilatory response to rowing and cycling in elite oarswomen. *J. Appl. Physiol.* 67: 264–269, 1989.
398. Tamaki, N. Effect of endurance training on muscle fiber composition and capillary supply in rat diaphragm. *Eur. J. Appl. Physiol.* 56: 127–131, 1987.
399. Taylor, C. R., R. H. Karns, E. W. Weibe, and H. Hoppeler. Adaptive variation in the mammalian respiratory system in relation to energetic demand. *Respir. Physiol.* 69: 1–28, 1987.
400. Tenney, S. M., and J. C. Leiter. The control of breathing: an uninhibited survey from the perspective of comparative physiology. In: *Regulation of Breathing*, edited by J. A. Dempsey and A. I. Pack. New York: Marcel Dekker, Inc., 1994, p. 3–39.
401. Tenney, S. M., and R. E. Reese. The ability to sustain great breathing efforts. *Respir. Physiol.* 5: 187–201, 1968.
402. Thoden, J. S., J. A. Dempsey, W. G. Reddan, M. L. Birnbaum, H. V. Forster, R. F. Grover, and J. Rankin. Ventilatory work during steady-state response to exercise. *Federation Proc.* 28: 1316–1321, 1969.
403. Tsubone, H. Nasal flow receptors of the rat. *Respir. Physiol.* 75: 51–64, 1989.
404. Tsubone, H. Nasal "pressure" receptors. *Jpn. J. Vet. Sci.* 52: 225–232, 1990.
405. Uribe, J., C. Stump, C. Tipton, and R. Fregosi. Influence of exercise training on the oxidative capacity of rat abdominal muscles. *Respir. Physiol.* 88: 171–180, 1992.
406. Van de Graaff, W. B. Thoracic influence on upper airway patency. *J. Appl. Physiol.* 65: 2124–2131, 1988.
407. Van Lunteren, E., and P. Manubay. Contractile properties of feline genioglossus, sternohyoid and sternothyroid muscles. *J. Appl. Physiol.* 72: 1010–1015, 1992.
408. Van Lunteren, E., and R. J. Martin. Pharyngeal dilator muscle contractile and endurance properties in neonatal piglets. *Respir. Physiol.* 92: 65–75, 1993.
409. Van Lunteren, E., R. J. Salomone, P. Munaby, G. S. Supinski, and T. E. Dick. Contractile and endurance properties of geniohyoid and diaphragm muscles. *J. Appl. Physiol.* 69: 1992–1997, 1992.
410. Van Lunteren E., and K. P. Strohl. The muscles of the upper airway. In: *Clinics of Chest Medicine*, edited by J. Widdicombe. Philadelphia: W. B. Saunders Company, 1986, p. 171–188.
411. Van Lunteren E., W. B. Van de Graaff, D. M. Parker, J. Mitra, M. A. Haxhiu, K. P. Strohl, and N. S. Cherniack. Nasal and laryngeal reflex responses to negative upper airway pressure. *J. Appl. Physiol.* 56: 746–752, 1984.
412. Ward, M. E., S. A. Magder, and S. N. Hussain. Oxygen delivery-independent effect of blood flow on diaphragm fatigue. *Am. Rev. Respir. Dis.* 145: 1058–1063, 1992.
413. Ward, S. A., and B. J. Whipp. Effects of peripheral and central chemoreceptor activation on the isopneic rating of breathing in exercise in humans. *J. Physiol. (Lond.)* 411: 27–43, 1989.
414. Ward, S. A., B. J. Whipp, and C. S. Poon. Density-dependent airflow and ventilatory control during exercise. *Respir. Physiol.* 49: 267–277, 1982.
415. Ware, J. H., D. W. Dockery, T. A. Louis, X. Xu, B. K. Ferris, and F. E. Speizer. Longitudinal cross-sectional estimates of pulmonary function decline in never-stroking adults. *Am. J. Epidemiol.* 132: 685–700, 1990.
416. Warren, G. L., K. J. Cureton, and P. B. Sparling. Does lung function limit performance in a 24-hour ultramarathon? *Respir. Physiol.* 78: 253–264, 1989.
417. Warren, J. B., S. J. Jennings, and T. J. H. Clark. Effect of adrenergic and vagal blockade on the normal human airway response to exercise. *Clin. Sci.* 66: 79–85, 1984.
418. Warwick, R., and P. L. Williams. *Gray's Anatomy*. Philadelphia: W. B. Saunders Company, 1973, p. 1245–1248.
419. Wasserman, K., B. J. Whipp, and R. Casaburi. Respiratory control during exercise. In: *Handbook of Physiology, The Respiratory System, Mechanics of Breathing*, edited by P. T. Macklem and J. Mead. Bethesda, MD: Am. Physiol. Soc., 1986, p. 595–620.
420. Watson, T. W. J., and W. A. Whitelaw. Voluntary hyperventilation changes recruitment order of parasternal intercostal motor units. *J. Appl. Physiol.* 62: 187–193, 1987.
421. Webber, C. L., and K. Pleschka. Structural and functional characteristics of individual phrenic motoneurons. *Pflugers Arch.* 364: 113–121, 1976.
422. Weibel, E. R., L. B. Marques, M. Constantinopol, F. Doffey, P. Gehr, and C. R. Taylor. The pulmonary gas exchanger. *Respir. Physiol.* 69: 81–100, 1987.
423. West, D. W., C. G. Ellis, and E. J. M. Campbell. Ability of man to detect increases in his breathing. *J. Appl. Physiol.* 39: 372–376, 1975.
424. Wheatley, J. R., T. C. Amis, and L. A. Engel. Influence of airflow temperature and pressure on alae nasi electrical activity. *J. Appl. Physiol.* 71: 2283–2291, 1991.
425. Wheatley, J. R., T. C. Amis, and L. A. Engel. Nasal and oral airway pressure-flow relationships. *J. Appl. Physiol.* 71: 2317–2324, 1991.
426. Wheatley, J. R., T. C. Amis, and L. A. Engel. Oronasal partitioning of ventilation during exercise. *J. Appl. Physiol.* 71: 546–551, 1991.
427. Wheatley, J. R., T. C. Amis, and L. A. Engel. Relationship between alae nasi activation and breathing route during exercise in humans. *J. Appl. Physiol.* 71: 118–124, 1991.
428. Wheatley, J. R., A. Brancatisano, and L. A. Engel. Cricothyroid muscle responses to increased chemical drive in awake normal humans. *J. Appl. Physiol.* 70: 2233–2241, 1991.
429. Wheatley, J. R., D. J. Tangel, W. S. Mezzanotte, and D. P. White. Influence of sleep on response to negative airway pressure of tensor palatini muscle and retropalatal airway. *J. Appl. Physiol.* 75: 2117–2124, 1993.
430. Whipp, B. J., and R. L. Pardy. Breathing during exercise. In: *Handbook of Physiology, The Respiratory System, Mechanics of Breathing*, edited by P. T. Macklem and J.

Mead. Bethesda, MD: Am. Physiol. Soc., 1986, p. 605–630.

431. Widdicombe, J. G. Respiratory reflexes in man and other mammalian species. *Clin. Sci.* 21: 163–170, 1961.
432. Wilhoit, S. C., and P. M. Suratt. Effect of nasal obstruction on upper airway muscle activation in normal subjects. *Chest* 92: 1053–1055, 1987.
433. Wilson, D. G., and H. G. Welch. Effects of varying concentrations of N_2/O_2 and He/O_2 on exercise tolerance in man. *Med. Sci. Sports Exerc.* 12: 380–384, 1980.
434. Wilson, R. C., and P. W. Jones. A comparison of the visual analogue scale and modified Borg scale for the measurement of dyspnoea during exercise. *Clin. Sci.* 76: 277–282, 1989.
435. Winning, A. J., R. D. Hamilton, and A. Guz. Ventilation and breathlessness on maximal exercise in patients with interstitial lung disease after local anaesthetic aerosol inhalation. *Clin. Sci.* 74: 275–281, 1988.
436. Winning, A. J., R. D. Hamilton, S. A. Shea, C. Knott, and A. Guz. The effect of airway anaesthesia on the control of breathing and the sensation of breathlessness in man. *Clin. Sci.* 68: 215–225, 1985.
437. Wolkove, N., M. D. Altose, S. G. Kelsen, P. G. Kondapalli, and N. S. Cherniack. Perception of changes in breathing in normal human subjects. *J. Appl. Physiol.* 50: 78–83, 1981.
438. Yamashiro, S. M., and F. S. Grodins. Respiratory cycle optimization in exercise. *J. Appl. Physiol.* 62: 337–345, 1973.
439. Yan, S., I. Lichros, S. Zakynthinos, and P. T. Macklem. Effect of diaphragmatic fatigue on control of respiratory muscles and ventilation during CO_2 rebreathing. *J. Appl. Physiol.* 75(3): 1364–1370, 1993.
440. Yonge, R. P., and E. S. Petersen. Entrainment of breathing in rhythmic exercise. In: *Modelling and Control of Breathing*, edited by B. J. Whipp and D. M. Wilberg. New York: Elsevier Biomedical, 1983, p. 197–204.
441. Younes, M. Determinants of thoracic excursions. In: *Exercise—Pulmonary Physiology and Pathophysiology*, edited by B. J. Whipp and K. Wasserman. New York: Marcel Dekker, Inc., 1991, p. 1–66.
442. Younes, M., D. Bilan, D. Jung, and H. Kroker. An apparatus for altering the mechanical load of the respiratory system. *J. Appl. Physiol.* 62: 2491–2499, 1987.
443. Younes, M., and J. Burks. Breathing pattern during and after exercise of different intensities. *J. Appl. Physiol.* 59: 898–908, 1985.
444. Younes, M., and G. Kivinen. Respiratory mechanics and breathing pattern during and following maximal exercise. *J. Appl. Physiol.* 57: 1773–1782, 1984.
445. Young, I. S., R. M. Alexander, A. J. Woakes, P. J. Butler, and L. Anderson. The synchronization of ventilation and locomotion in horses (*Equus caballus*). *J. Exp. Biol.* 166: 19–31, 1992.
446. Zechman, F. W., and R. L. Wiley. Afferent inputs to breathing: Respiratory sensation. In: *Handbook of Physiology, The Respiratory System, Control of Breathing*, edited by N. S. Cherniack and J. G. Widdicombe. Bethesda, MD: Am. Physiol. Soc., 1986, p. 449–474.

12. Determinants of gas exchange and acid–base balance during exercise

ROBERT L. JOHNSON, JR. | *Departments of Internal Medicine and Pulmonary Research, University of Texas Southwestern Medical Center, Dallas, Texas*

GEORGE J. F. HEIGENHAUSER | *Department of Medicine, McMaster University Health Sciences Center, Hamilton, Ontario, Canada*

CONNIE C. W. HSIA | *Department of Internal Medicine, University of Texas Southwestern Medical Center, Dallas, Texas*

NORMAN L. JONES | *Department of Medicine, McMaster University Health Sciences Center, Hamilton, Ontario, Canada*

PETER D. WAGNER | *Department of Medicine, University of California-San Diego, La Jolla, California*

CHAPTER CONTENTS

ENERGY TRANSDUCTION DURING EXERCISE requires high levels of oxygen (O_2) and carbon dioxide (CO_2) transport and generates large acid loads from CO_2 and lactate production; at the same time intracellular hydrogen ion concentrations, $[H^+]$, must be controlled within a narrow range required for optimal neural function and muscle metabolic and contractile functions. How these requirements for gas exchange and acid–base regulation are met is the concern of this chapter, which is organized in the following way.

The first section, STRUCTURAL AND FUNCTIONAL DETERMINANTS OF GAS EXCHANGE, concerns mechanisms of distributive and diffusive gas transport in lungs and tissues and mechanisms by which the allosteric properties of hemoglobin at peak exercise help to maximize the arteriovenous (A-V) O_2 content difference, minimize the A-V P_{CO_2} difference, and reduce the rise of $[H^+]$ in muscle.

The second section, METHODS OF ASSESSMENT, discusses methods used to define and assess individual steps in gas transport; that is, rates of gas mixing in the lung, distribution of ventilation with respect to perfusion, and lung and tissue diffusing capacities. Conceptually, the individual steps can only be completely understood within the context of the methods used for measurement.

The third section, PULMONARY GAS EXCHANGE DURING EXERCISE, discusses how each step in the transport chain adapts or fails to adapt to exercise and how adaptation is modified by acute and chronic exposure to high altitude.

The fourth section, ACID–BASE REGULATION DURING EXERCISE, discusses acid–base regulation during exercise, using a physicochemical approach. Normally the kidneys are required to excrete only about 50 mEq of fixed acid per day, but during heavy exercise about 140 mEq of carbonic and lactic acid are produced each minute. Yet, $[H^+]$ in muscle must be maintained within a narrow range during this high rate of acid production in order to maintain contractile function of skeletal muscle.

The fifth section, COMPARATIVE ASPECTS OF GAS EXCHANGE, discusses aspects of gas exchange during exercise in dogs and horses that have helped to clarify important issues concerning gas exchange during exercise in humans.

STRUCTURAL AND FUNCTIONAL DETERMINANTS OF GAS EXCHANGE

The Nature of O_2 and CO_2 Binding and Chemical Equilibria in Blood

Hemoglobin, an Allosteric Carrier of O_2 and CO_2. Hemoglobin behaves almost as if it were a mobile allosteric enzyme carrying out its transport functions for both O_2 and CO_2; this will be a recurring theme in explaining feedback control of gas transport. In fact, hemoglobin has provided the basic model for understanding how allosteric enzymes work in controlling a metabolic pathway. Such enzymes are usually oligomers (i.e., have multiple subunits each of which bind the primary ligand). The primary ligand for hemoglobin is oxygen. Binding at one primary site tends to change the configuration of the oligomer (called an allosteric transition) to make the remaining binding sites more accessible; these are called homotropic effects and result in what is called "cooperativity" between binding sites. Other secondary ligands or "effectors" can either inhibit or enhance binding at the primary site by enhancing or inhibiting the allosteric transition; these are called heterotropic effects and $[H^+]$, CO_2, and 2,3-diphosphoglycerate (2-3-DPG) are effector molecules that bind to and act upon hemoglobin. The homotropic effects of oxygen binding to hemoglobin are responsible for the sigmoidal shape of the oxyhemoglobin dissociation curve and for the Haldane effect on the CO_2 dissociation curve in whole blood; the heterotropic effects of CO_2, $[H^+]$ and 2,3-DPG are responsible for the Bohr effect on the oxyhemoglobin dissociation curve.

Shape of the Oxymyoglobin and Oxyhemoglobin Dissociation Curves. Hemoglobin is a tetramer (four subunits) with a molecular weight of 64,458 (112). Theoretically, it should bind 1.39 ml of oxygen per gram of hemoglobin; however, because of inactive hemoglobin in vivo (212), physiologic O_2 binding capacity lies in the range of 1.34–1.36 ml of O_2 per gram of hemoglobin as originally defined by Hüfner in 1894 (129, 172). Hüfner assumed one iron binding site per hemoglobin molecule to yield the following reversible reaction:

$$Hb + O_2 \rightleftharpoons HbO_2$$

Based on the law of mass action, he predicted a hyperbolic relationship between O_2 binding and O_2 tension. Myoglobin, with only one oxygen binding site per molecule, exhibits such a relationship [Fig. 12.1; (243)]:

$$S = \frac{K[O_2]}{1 + K[O_2]} = \frac{\left(\frac{P}{P_{50}}\right)}{1 + \left(\frac{P}{P_{50}}\right)} \quad (1)$$

where S is the fractional saturation of myoglobin; $[O_2]$ is concentration of physically dissolved oxygen in mM/liter; K is an association constant; P is oxygen tension in mm Hg; and P_{50} is the oxygen tension at 50% saturation. However, contrary to Hüfner's prediction, Bohr, Hasselbalch, and Krogh (22) experimentally found a sigmoidal relationship between O_2 saturation and tension (Fig. 12.1). Based on the latter findings, A. V. Hill (109) assumed that hemoglobin must be an aggregate with more than one binding site and hypothesized the following reaction: $Hb_n + nO_2 \leftrightarrow Hb_n(O_2)_n$, where n is the number of binding sites per hemoglobin aggregate. Hill then predicted the following relationship, also based on the law of mass action, between the number of binding sites, n, and the oxyhemoglobin dissociation curve:

$$S = \frac{K[O_2]^n}{1 + K[O_2]^n} = \frac{\left(\frac{P}{P_{50}}\right)^n}{1 + \left(\frac{P}{P_{50}}\right)^n} \quad (2)$$

where K is a constant and P_{50} = the oxygen tension at 50% saturation. Equation 2 can be logarithmically transformed as follows:

$$\log\left(\frac{S}{1 - S}\right) = n \cdot \log(P) - n \cdot \log P_{50} \quad (3)$$

By plotting $\log [S/(1 - S)]$ with respect to log(P) the experimental slope of the relationship should yield an estimate of the number of binding sites, n. But when experimentally measured, n was not an integer and was not constant over the entire relationship (Fig. 12.2). At low oxygen saturations n was near 1 but rose to a maximum of 2.7 in the midregion of the O_2 tension–saturation relationship and then approached 1 again at high O_2 tensions; n is unaffected by either changes in temperature, pH, P_{CO_2}, or

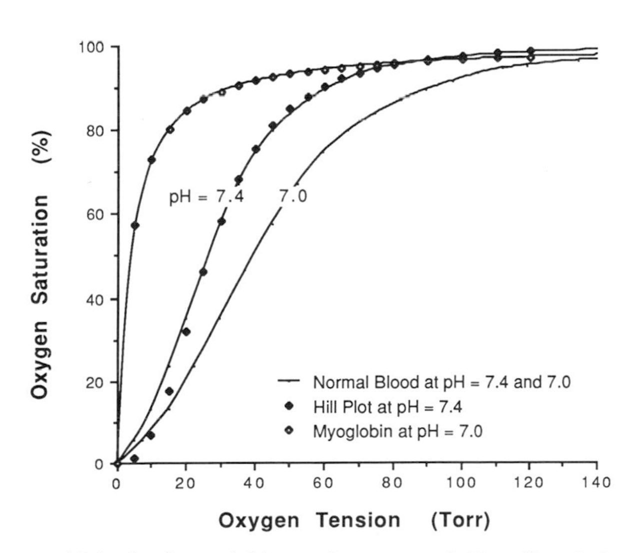

FIG. 12.1. Oxyhemoglobin and oxymyoglobin dissociation curves at different levels of pH. The oxyhemoglobin dissociation curve at pH 7.4 is compared to that calculated from the Hill equation at the same P_{50}.

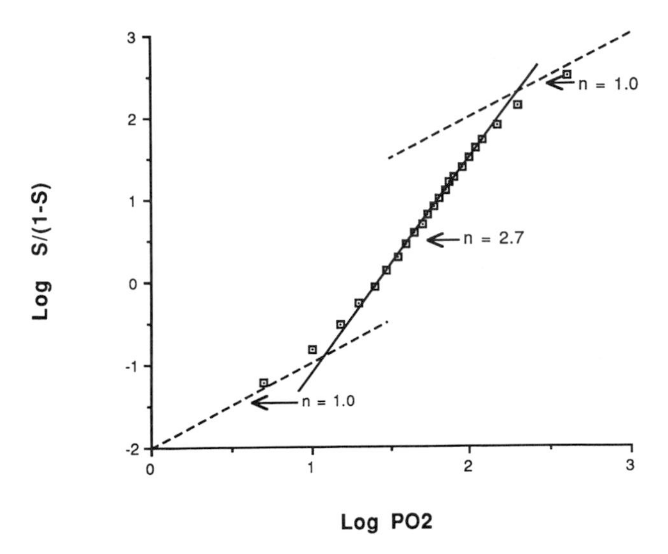

FIG. 12.2. Hill plot for human whole blood to determine the value of n as defined in equation 3. At low oxygen saturations, the slope of the relationship approaches 1 as predicted for a second-order reaction as the first heme binding site becomes filled. The steepest slope yields an n of 2.7. At very high oxygen saturations, the slope again approaches 1 as the last binding site is being filled.

changes in the concentration of 2,3-DPG. Hill was correct that hemoglobin is an aggregate, and Hill's equation is still used as a convenient approximation to the oxyhemoglobin dissociation curve (Fig. 12.1), but n does not reflect the number of binding sites. Rather n reflects what is termed "cooperative interaction" between the four O_2 binding sites on hemoglobin (284); the higher the value of n, the greater the cooperativity and the sharper the bend in the O_2-hemoglobin dissociation curve. In the absence of oxygen, the four protein subunits of hemoglobin tend to be bound together tightly by electrostatic bonds or salt bridges. This has been called the T (tense) or less reactive molecular configuration (176, 191). When oxygen initially binds to reduced hemoglobin, data plotted in the form of equation 3 approach a straight line with $n = 1$ as predicted by Hüfner for a monomer. Oxygen binding, however, imposes a stress on the bonds between subunits, weakens adjacent salt bridges, and causes a change in configuration of the tetramer. This configuration has been called the R (relaxed) form, in which the globin subunits change shape in such a way that makes the remaining binding sites more accessible to oxygen (176, 191). This cooperativity between subunits during oxygen binding causes the sigmoidal shape of the oxyhemoglobin dissociation curve (Fig. 12.2).

Secondary ligands for an allosteric enzyme (effector molecules) can inhibit, enhance, or eliminate cooperativity, thereby altering affinity of the enzyme for the primary ligand. In this way small effector molecules can exert control over the rate of metabolic pathway, and this will also be shown to be true for effector molecules acting on hemoglobin. Effectors usually do not change shape of the binding curve between an enzyme and its ligand but rather alter position of the curve as reflected by the K_m (i.e., the ligand concentration at which 50% of the binding sites on the enzyme are occupied); for hemoglobin, P_{50} is equivalent to K_m (i.e., the oxygen tension at which 50% of the oxygen binding sites are occupied). The effector molecules acting on hemoglobin are CO_2, $[H^+]$, and 2,3-DPG. The effect of CO_2 on hemoglobin reported by Bohr and his colleagues in 1904 (22) is recognized now to be a consequence of the fact that high levels of P_{CO_2} and $[H^+]$ stabilize the T configuration of hemoglobin and inhibit oxygen binding; hence, increases in P_{CO_2} and $[H^+]$ increase the P_{50} of hemoglobin (Bohr effect). Increases in concentration of 2,3-DPG and in temperature also raise the P_{50} (Table 12.1). The P_{50} provides a reference point for describing how the oxyhemoglobin dissociation curve changes position in response to changes in P_{CO_2}, pH, 2,3-DPG, or temperature; if P_{50} is altered by a factor k, the P_{O_2} at all other saturations are changed by the same factor and the entire oxyhemoglobin dissociation curve can be reconstructed from just one number. Quantitative effects of pH, P_{CO_2}, 2,3-DPG, and temperature on the P_{50} are given in Table 12.1.

In subsequent sections we will show how differences in shape and reactivity of the O_2 dissociation curves of myoglobin and hemoglobin constitute important attributes of these two molecules, which facilitate oxygen transport at heavy exercise. We will show that hemoglobin, through allosteric transitions, tends to optimize O_2 and CO_2 transport in the lungs and tissues through shifts in P_{50} induced by changes in pH, P_{CO_2}, temperature, and by oxygen itself. These influences on hemoglobin are further modulated through chemical and neural feedback induced by changes in P_{O_2}, P_{CO_2}, pH, and temperature to the respiratory center to cause appropriate changes in ventilation. Each of these mechanisms will be discussed in more detail later relative to their importance in optimizing oxygen transport during exercise; first we must discuss some aspects of the CO_2 dissociation curve and some concepts related to gas diffusion and chemical reaction rates.

Shape of the CO_2 Dissociation Curve. Carbon dioxide transport in blood is in many ways more complex and difficult to describe rigorously than oxygen transport because more interacting chemical reactions and equilibria are involved in determining the

TABLE 12.1. *Effects of Temperature, pH, P_{CO_2}, Base Excess, and 2,3-DPG on P_{50}*

	Relationship	Reference
Hemoglobin	Normal P_{50} = 26.5 mmHg at pH 7.4, 37°C	
Temperature (°C)	$\Delta\log P_{50} = 0.024\ \Delta t$	Severinghaus (227)
pH (pH Units) & P_{CO_2} mm Hg	$\Delta\log P_{50} = -0.40\ \Delta ph + 0.06\ \Delta\log P_{CO_2}$	Severinghaus (227)
pH (pH units) & B E (mEq/liter)	$\Delta\log P_{50} = -0.48\ \Delta ph + 0.0013$ Be	Severinghaus (227)
DPG (molar ratio to hemoglobin)	P_{50} = 10.36 DPG + 17.63 at pH 7.4	Bellingham et al. (15)
pH & BE (DPG molar ratio = 0.89)	$\Delta\log P_{50} = -0.52\ \Delta pH + 0.0022$ BE	Wranne et al. (283)
pH & BE (DPG molar ratio = 0.15)	$\Delta\log P_{50} = -0.67\ \Delta pH + 0.0052$ BE	Wranne et al. (283)
Myoglobin	Normal P_{50} = 3.7 mm Hg at pH 7.0, 37°C	
Temperature (°C)	$\Delta\log P_{50} = 0.048\ \Delta t$	Theorell (243)
pH (pH units)	$\Delta\log P_{50} = -0.10\ \Delta pH$	Theorell (243)

final distribution of CO_2 in its different forms between the plasma and red cell milieu. Carbon dioxide is carried as physically dissolved CO_2, H_2CO_3, HCO_3^-, CO_3^{2-}, and bound to hemoglobin as carbamate (R-$NHCO_2^-$). The physical chemical determinants of how these various forms of CO_2 are distributed between plasma and red cells will be described in more detail in a later section on acid–base balance. The most important consideration in this section is the shape and interaction of the CO_2 and oxyhemoglobin dissociation curves. Changes of blood CO_2 tension and $[H^+]$ alter the position of the oxyhemoglobin dissociation curve (i.e., the P_{50}); this is the Bohr effect. The reciprocal of the Bohr effect is the Haldane effect, in which changes in oxyhemoglobin saturation alter the position of the CO_2 dissociation curve. The Haldane effect was not recognized until 10 years after Bohr, Hasselbalch, and Krogh made their observations of the related Bohr effect (35). Both are mediated through the same changes in configuration of the hemoglobin molecule. A low oxyhemoglobin saturation increases the affinity of hemoglobin for hydrogen ions, which in turn increases the formation of bicarbonate and enhances CO_2 binding as carbamate (R-$NHCO_2^-$) on each terminal α-amino group of the four subunits of hemoglobin; the net result is that lowering oxygen saturation of blood raises the carrying capacity of blood for CO_2 and vice versa. The effect can be illustrated with the following equation of electrical neutrality, which must be satisfied in whole blood (237):

Whole blood strong ion difference
= total negative charges on ionized forms of CO_2
+ total negative charges on proteins

or

$$[SID^+]_b = [[R\text{-}NHCO_2^-]_b + [HCO_3^-]_b + 2[CO_3^{2-}]] + [[Hb^-]_b + [P^-]_b] \quad (4)$$

where $[R\text{-}NHCO_2^-]_b$ and $[HCO_3^-]_b$ and $[CO_3^{2-}]_b$ are the concentrations of carbamate, bicarbonate and carbonate respectively in milliequivalents per liter of whole blood; $[SID^+]_b$ is the strong ion difference; that is, the difference between the concentration of strong cations (Na^+ and K^+) and anions (Cl^-, and lactate$^-$), in milliequivalents per liter of whole blood; $[Hb^-]_b$ and $[P^-]_b$ are the net negative charges on hemoglobin and on serum proteins in milliequivalents per liter of whole blood. $[H^+]$ and $[OH^-]$ concentrations are neglected here because their concentrations remain extremely low within the physiologic range owing to buffering by $[Hb^-]_b + [P^-]_b$. The strong ion difference, $[SID^+]_b$, remains constant unless strong cations or anions are added or removed by an outside source; hence, the total negative charges on the right hand side of equation 4 also are fixed and any change in milliequivalents per liter of negative charge on one component must be balanced by a corresponding change in the opposite direction of another component to satisfy equation 4. The net negative charge on the hemoglobin molecule, $[Hb^-]_b$, controls interactions between the CO_2 and oxyhemoglobin dissociation curves. Increasing oxygen saturation of hemoglobin raises its net negative charge by lowering its pK, causing a release of protons; this causes reciprocal decreases in $[R\text{-}NHCO_2^-]_b$, $[HCO_3^-]_b$, and $[CO_3^{2-}]_b$ and an increase in uncharged physically dissolved CO_2 without changing whole blood CO_2 content (i.e., causing an increase in P_{CO_2} at a fixed CO_2 content). The net result is shown in Figure 12.3. Changing the oxygen saturation of blood shifts the position of the CO_2 dissociation curve; this is the Haldane effect. The *arrows* in Figure 12.3 indicate that, at any given CO_2 content, oxygenation of hemoglobin raises the P_{CO_2} of blood as the blood passes through the lung and deoxygenation lowers the P_{CO_2} in blood as the blood passes through tissues, both caused by the Haldane effect. The important physiological result of this biochemical change is a reduction in the ar-

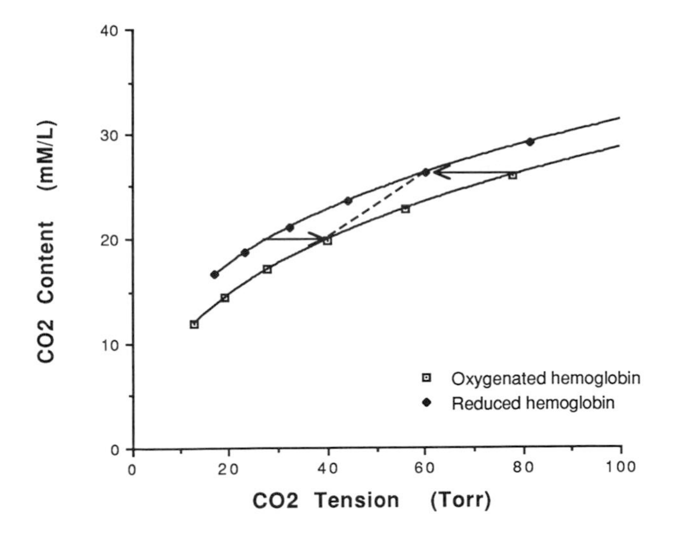

FIG. 12.3. The CO_2 dissociation curve for reduced and oxygenated blood. CO_2 is primarily carried in the plasma as bicarbonate, but must be rapidly hydrated in the red cell by the enzyme, carbonic anhydrase, to form bicarbonate and then transported into the plasma in exchange for chloride. Part of the CO_2 is bound to hemoglobin and carried as carbamate without requiring hydration or dehydration during transport. The change in shape of the hemogobin molecule as it releases oxygen in tissues enhances both the formation of bicarbonate and carbamate inside the red cell, so that more CO_2 is carried at any given CO_2 tension (Haldane shift). The *horizontal arrows* indicate the shift in P_{CO_2} that occurs at a given CO_2 content when oxyhemogobin saturation falls in tissues (*upper arrow*) or rises in the lung (*lower arrow*). The *dashed line* would be the effective CO_2 dissociation curve. At maximal oxygen uptake, the Haldane shift minimizes the arteriovenous P_{CO_2} and $[H^+]$ differences required for a given CO_2 output.

teriovenous P_{CO_2} and $[H^+]$ differences required for a given arteriovenous CO_2 content difference (i.e., it makes the CO_2 dissociation curve steeper as shown by the *dashed line* in Figure 12.3). Thus, for a given CO_2 production in exercising muscle, it allows the muscle to operate at a lower P_{CO_2} and $[H^+]$. It also makes it easier for an increase in ventilation to lower the P_{CO_2} and $[H^+]$ in exercising muscle, thereby protecting contractile function (see equations 6 and 8, below). Here is another indication of how the allosteric properties of hemoglobin exert control over a major metabolic pathway.

Alveolar Gas Composition at Equilibrium with End-Capillary Blood

The subject whose data at maximal exercise will be used to illustrate the calculations applied in the next few sections was a young college athlete; demographic characteristics and measurements at peak exercise are listed in Table 12.2.

Alveolar Ventilation and Gas Tensions. Mean alveolar gas composition weighted for alveolar ventilation (not alveolar volume) are given by the following relationship; physiologic dead space ventilation ($\dot{V}_D$ and alveolar ventilation ($\dot{V}_A$) are defined functionally as follows:

$$\dot{V}_D/\dot{V}_E = \frac{F_{A_{CO_2}} - F_{E_{CO_2}}}{F_{A_{CO_2}} - F_{I_{CO_2}}} \text{ and} \qquad (5)$$

$$\dot{V}_A/\dot{V}_E = 1 - \dot{V}_D/\dot{V}_E$$

Equation 5 is referred to as the Bohr dead space equation, where $F_{A_{CO_2}}$, $F_{E_{CO_2}}$, and $F_{I_{CO_2}}$ are fractional concentrations of alveolar, end-expired and inspired CO_2 measured dry (20), and $\dot{V}_E$ is expired ventilation.

In the 1940s and 1950s, Rahn and Fenn (202) and Riley et al (158, 208) developed a body of theory to explain pulmonary gas exchange based on mass conservation principles. Development of these equations is clearly summarized by Otis (182). A key concept was that in a homogeneous lung, the alveolar gas P_{O_2} and P_{CO_2} must be closely related. Briefly, alveolar gas tensions are determined by inspired gas concentrations, O_2 uptake, ($\dot{V}_{O_2}$), CO_2 output ($\dot{V}_{CO_2}$), and respiratory quotient $R = \dot{V}_{CO_2}/\dot{V}_{O_2}$ in accord with the following relationships:

$$P_{A_{CO_2}} = (\dot{V}_{CO_2}/\dot{V}_A) \cdot C_f \qquad (6)$$

$$P_{A_{O_2}} = (P_B - P_{H_2O})F_{I_{O_2}} - P_{A_{CO_2}} \cdot \left[F_{I_{O_2}} + \frac{1 - F_{I_{O_2}}}{R}\right] \qquad (7)$$

where $\dot{V}_{CO_2}$ is always given at 0°C, 760 mm Hg, dry (STPD); $\dot{V}_A$ is under body conditions of temperature, ambient pressure, and saturated with water vapor (BTPS); $P_{A_{O_2}}$, $P_{A_{CO_2}}$, and $P_{I_{CO_2}}$ are alveolar O_2, alveolar CO_2, and inspired CO_2 tensions, respectively, under BTPS conditions; $F_{I_{O_2}}$ is the fractional inspired O_2 concentration in dry air; C_f is a conversion factor $[(273 + t) \cdot 760/273]$ translating fractional concentration (BTPS) to mm Hg; t is body temperature in degrees Celsius, 273°C is 0° kelvin and 760 is 1 atmosphere pressure in mm Hg; P_B is ambient barometric pressure and P_{H_2O} is water vapor tension at body temperature (t). P_{H_2O} is 47 mm Hg at normal resting body temperature but will increase during prolonged exercise and can be estimated from body temperature in degrees Celsius using the following relationship, accurate to within 1% between 37° and 42°C:

$$P_{H_2O} = 5.556e^{0.058t}$$

TABLE 12.2. *Demographics and Measurements at Maximal O_2 Uptake*

Measurements	Units	Data
Age	Years	19
Height	cm	180
Weight	kg	70
Maximal O_2 uptake	(ml/min)/kg	62.6
Body temperature	°C	39°
Respiratory exchange ratio (R)		1.05
Expired ventilation ($\dot{V}E$)	liters/min (BTPS)	152
Alveolar ventilation ($\dot{V}A$)	liters/min (BTPS)	111
Cardiac output ($\dot{Q}$)	liters/min	27.3
Memb. diffusing capacity for CO (DM_{CO})	(ml/min)/mm Hg	80
Pulm. capillary blood volume (Vc)	ml	257
Blood O_2 capacity at exercise (O_2 Cap)	ml/dl	20.28
Mixed venous O_2 content ($C\bar{v}_{O_2}$)	ml/dl	3.13
Mixed venous CO_2 content ($C\bar{v}_{CO_2}$)	mM/l	23.4
Mixed venous saturation ($S\bar{v}_{O_2}$)	%	15.2
Femoral venous O_2 tension (Pv_{O_2})	mm Hg	15.0
Femoral venous CO_2 tension (Pv_{CO_2})	mm Hg	66.0
Arterial O_2 content (Cc'_{O_2})	ml/dl	19.13
Arterial O_2 saturation (S)	%	93.3
Arterial CO_2 tension (Pa_{CO_2})	mm Hg	36
Alveolar O_2 tension (Ideal PA_{O_2})	mm Hg	112
Arterial O_2 tension (Pa_{O_2})	mm Hg	84
Arterial pH (pHa)	pH units	7.32
Base excess (BE)	mEq/liter	−7.0

From the data in Table 12.2, at 39°C P_{H_2O} = 53.4 mm Hg, and C_f = 868.6. Arterial CO_2 tension (Pa_{CO_2}) was 36 mm Hg; assuming that $PA_{CO_2} = Pa_{CO_2}$, equation 6 was solved for $\dot{V}A$ = 111 liters/min and equation 7 was solved to give PA_{O_2} = 112 mm Hg.

Ratio of Alveolar Ventilation to Perfusion ($\dot{V}A/\dot{Q}c$). Equations 6 and 7 can be combined with the Fick equations for CO_2 and O_2, respectively, to provide a description of how the ratio of ventilation to perfusion ($\dot{V}A/\dot{Q}c$) affects alveolar capillary gas exchange in a region of lung. The Fick equation for CO_2 is:

$$\dot{V}CO_2 = 0.0222\,\dot{Q}_C(C\bar{v}_{CO_2} - Cc'_{CO_2}) \quad (8)$$

where $\dot{Q}_C$ is pulmonary blood flow in liters per minute; $C\bar{v}_{CO_2}$ and Cc'_{CO_2} are mixed venous CO_2 contents and 0.0222 is liters of CO_2 gas (STPD) per mM CO_2. The Fick equation for O_2 is:

$$\dot{V}O_2 = \dot{Q}_C(Cc'_{O_2} - C\bar{v}_{O_2}) \quad (9)$$

where Cc'_{O_2} and $C\bar{v}_{O_2}$ are end-capillary and mixed venous O_2 content, respectively, in milliliters of O_2 per milliliter of blood. Combining equations 6 and 8 for CO_2:

$$Cc'_{CO_2} = C\bar{v}_{CO_2} - \left[\frac{\dot{V}A/\dot{Q}_C}{19.33}\right] PA_{CO_2} \quad (10)$$

Combining equations 7 and 9 for O_2:

$$Cc'_{O_2} = C\bar{v}_{O_2} + \left(\frac{(PI_{O_2} - PA_{CO_2} \cdot FI_{O_2}) \cdot \dot{V}A/\dot{Q}_C}{C_f \cdot FI_{O_2}}\right) - \left[\frac{\dot{V}A/\dot{Q}_C}{C_f \cdot FI_{N_2}}\right] PA_{O_2} \quad (11)$$

where C_f is the same conversion factor defined in equation 6 and FI_{N_2} is the nitrogen fraction.

These are mass conservation equations that indicate that any change in CO_2 and O_2 content in blood between entrance into and exit from the lung in a given time must be matched by a corresponding change in the opposite direction of CO_2 and O_2 content in alveolar gas leaving the lung in the same interval. The equations yield linear relationships between end-capillary blood CO_2 content (Cc'_{CO_2}) and alveolar CO_2 tension (PA_{CO_2}) and between end-capillary oxygen content (Cc'_{O_2}) and alveolar O_2 tension (PA_{O_2}), shown in Figure 12.4 and calculated from the data in Table 12.2; slopes of the relationships (the bracketed terms of equations 10 and 11) are determined by the ventilation–perfusion ratios ($\dot{V}A/\dot{Q}c$). Equilibrium for CO_2 and O_2 between end-capillary blood and alveolar air is indicated by the intersections between equations 10 and 11 with the respective CO_2 and O_2 dissociation curve. The CO_2 dissociation curve is constructed for an oxygen

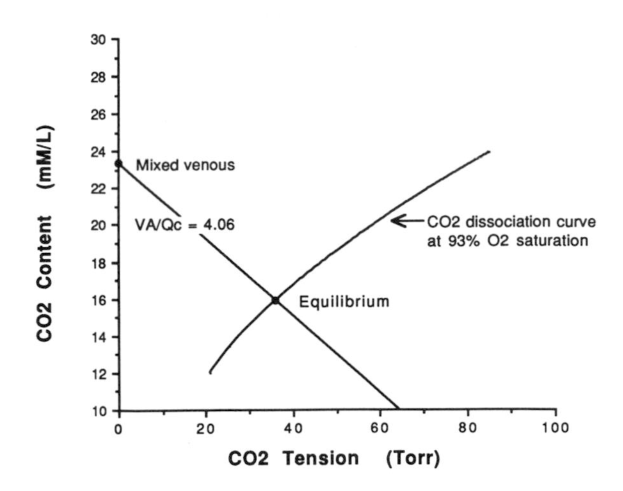

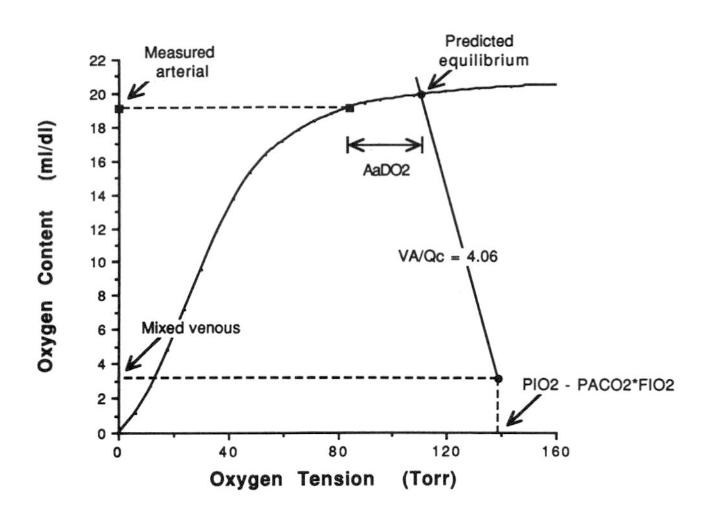

FIG. 12.4. Estimating O_2 and CO_2 equilibrium in the lung or in a region of lung if mixed venous blood gases, the $\dot{V}A/\dot{Q}c$ ratio and the dissociation curves for oxygen and oxyhemoglobin are known. Results are derived from data collected at maximal oxygen uptake in a young high school athlete. The *straight diagonal lines* were calculated from equations 5 and 6, which were solved simultaneously for a respiratory exchange ratio of 1.05 and $\dot{V}A/\dot{Q}c$ ratio of 4.06. Equilibrium is indicated by the intersection between the *straight diagonal lines* with the corresponding dissociation curve.

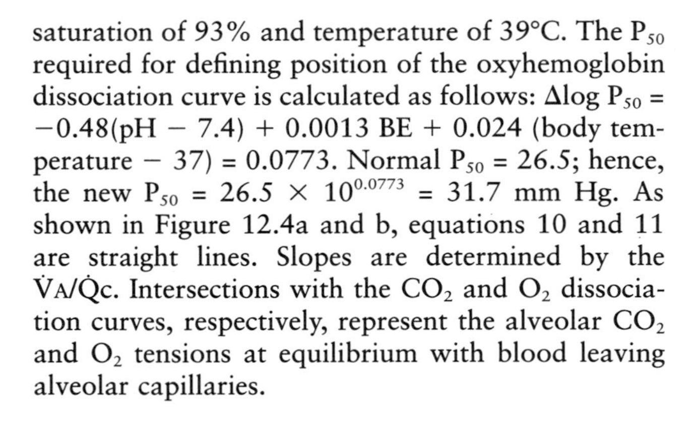

saturation of 93% and temperature of 39°C. The P_{50} required for defining position of the oxyhemoglobin dissociation curve is calculated as follows: $\Delta \log P_{50} = -0.48(\text{pH} - 7.4) + 0.0013\ \text{BE} + 0.024$ (body temperature $- 37) = 0.0773$. Normal $P_{50} = 26.5$; hence, the new $P_{50} = 26.5 \times 10^{0.0773} = 31.7$ mm Hg. As shown in Figure 12.4a and b, equations 10 and 11 are straight lines. Slopes are determined by the $\dot{V}A/\dot{Q}c$. Intersections with the CO_2 and O_2 dissociation curves, respectively, represent the alveolar CO_2 and O_2 tensions at equilibrium with blood leaving alveolar capillaries.

Alveolar–Arterial Oxygen Tension Difference. The difference between alveolar and arterial oxygen tension (AaP_{O_2}) is an index of the efficiency of blood gas exchange. Arterial oxygen tension (Pa_{O_2}) is easily measured and unambiguous, but alveolar oxygen tension can have different values depending on the method of estimation. End-tidal oxygen tension is a mean weighted for regional alveolar ventilation. "Ideal" alveolar oxygen tension as defined by Riley and Cournand (208) is approximated by substituting arterial for alveolar CO_2 tension in both equations 6 and 7; the resulting PA_{O_2} is approximately weighted for regional blood flow, since the CO_2 dissociation curve of blood is almost linear over a limited range; the latter technique will yield smaller AaP_{O_2} values than those estimated using end-tidal PA_{O_2}. From Table 12.2, the AaP_{O_2} was 28 mm Hg at maximal oxygen uptake, much greater than that normally existing in young healthy subjects at rest.

Diffusive Gas Transport

Background and Physical Principles. Rates of diffusion for a gas are defined by the Fick equation:

$$\frac{dV}{dt} = Ad\frac{\partial C}{\partial x} \tag{12}$$

where dV/dt is the volume transferred per unit time in the x direction; $\partial C/\partial x$ is the concentration gradient in centimeters along the x direction normal to the area (A) in square centimeters through which the exchange is occurring; d is the diffusion coefficient of the gas in square centimeters per second. The Fick equation in this form leads to inconveniences in describing diffusive exchange between a gas and liquid phase or between different liquid phases. At a gas–liquid interface, the concentrations of gases in the two phases at equilibrium may be quite different, yet no net exchange occurs by diffusion as would be suggested by equation 12; this results from the fact that differences in solubility between phases will partition the concentrations at equilibrium differently. Net diffusive exchange occurs only when the partial pressures of the gases in the different phases are different. Thus, in describing diffusive transfer between two different phases, differential solubilities must be taken into account; in order to address this problem, Krogh modified the Fick equation:

$$\frac{dV}{dt} = A\left[\frac{60 \cdot \alpha d}{760}\right]\frac{\partial P}{\partial x} \tag{13}$$

where α is the Bunsen solubility coefficient at body temperature in milliliters gas per milliter of blood per atmosphere of pressure (i.e., atm^{-1}); $\partial P/\partial x$ is the partial pressure gradient of the gas in mm Hg per centimeter in the x direction; 60 is s/min and 760 is mm Hg/atm; $[60 \cdot \alpha d/760]$ is known as the Krogh diffusion constant. Incorporation of solubility (α) in the Krogh constant has led to some confusion in interpreting data involving respiratory gases as explained below.

Rates of diffusion are dependent upon the velocities of random motion of molecules. Since average kinetic energies of different molecules at a given temperature (i.e., $Mv^2/2$ where M is molecular weight and v is velocity) are the same, heavier molecules move slower and have correspondingly lower diffusion coefficients; diffusion coefficients are directly proportional to mean velocity and inversely proportional to the square root of molecular weight (Graham's law). Based on Graham's law, $D_{CO_2} = 0.85\ D_{O_2}$. However, because of the greater solubility of CO_2 ($\alpha_{CO_2} = 24 \cdot \alpha_{O_2}$), the Krogh diffusion constant for CO_2 is 20 times that for oxygen. Even though CO_2 diffuses slower for a given concentration gradient than does O_2, CO_2 diffuses 20 time faster than O_2 for a given partial pressure gradient because the higher solubility of CO_2 generates a concentration difference for CO_2 that is 24 times that for O_2. Table 12.3 lists some important constants required to describe diffusive exchange for different respiratory gases.

Based on the Krogh diffusion constants for plasma in Table 12.1, the relative diffusivities of CO, NO, and CO_2 to that of O_2 in the pulmonary membrane are approximately 0.88, 2.0, and 19, respectively.

Krogh Diffusing Capacity of the Alveolar Capillary Membrane. Based on the above considerations, diffusing capacity of the alveolar capillary membrane (D_M) is defined as follows:

$$D_M = \left[\frac{60 \cdot \alpha d}{760}\right] \cdot \left[\frac{\text{membrane area}}{\text{mean barrier thickness}}\right]$$

$$= D_K \cdot \left[\frac{\text{membrane area}}{\text{mean barrier thickness}}\right]$$

This is the morphometric or structural definition of diffusing capacity. The membrane area is alveolar surface area. Mean barrier thickness is the mean harmonic diffusion path across the alveolar capillary membrane to the surface of the red cell. The mean length of the molecular diffusion path across the alveolar-capillary-plasma barrier will vary with spacing between red cells and also with red cell shapes (65, 261). The physiological definition of lung diffusing capacity for oxygen (DL_{O_2}) would be the oxygen uptake divided by the difference between alveolar oxygen tension (PA_{O_2}) and mean oxygen tension in red cells ($P\bar{c}_{O_2}$) passing through lung capillaries; that is:

$$DL_{O_2} = \frac{\dot{V}O_2}{PA_{O_2} - P\bar{c}_{O_2}} \qquad (14)$$

This estimate includes components of resistance due to both diffusion and chemical reaction velocities as described in the next section.

Binding Affinities and Reaction Kinetics. The importance of binding affinities of different respiratory gases to hemoglobin as determinants of diffusive transport was recognized before the turn of the century by Haldane, Bohr, and August and Marie Krogh (21, 89, 154). At this time it was not possible to measure oxygen diffusing capacity of the lung; arterial blood oxygen tension could not be measured,

TABLE 12.3. *Constants Determining Rates of Diffusion of Respiratory Gases*

	Diffusion Coefficient (d), $cm_2 \cdot sp^{-1}$ at 37°C			Bunsen Solubility Coef., (α) atm^{-1} at 37°C			Krogh Diffusion Constant (DK), $cm_2 \cdot min^{-1} \cdot$ mm Hg		
Gas	Air*	Tissue†	Plasma†	Air*	Tissue‡	Plasma§	Air	Tissue	Plasma
CO	0.237	$2.46 \cdot 10^{-2}$	$1.99 \cdot 10^{-5}$	0.882	$1.79 \cdot 10^{-2}$	$1.84 \cdot 10^{-2}$	$1.65 \cdot 10^{-2}$	$3.48 \cdot 10^{-8}$	$2.97 \cdot 10^{-8}$
NO	0.237	$2.46 \cdot 10^{-2}$	$1.99 \cdot 10^{-5}$	0.882		$4.39 \cdot 10^{-2}$	$1.65 \cdot 10^{-2}$		$6.90 \cdot 10^{-8}$
O_2	0.257	$2.30 \cdot 10^{-2}$	$1.86 \cdot 10^{-5}$	0.882	$2.13 \cdot 10^{-2}$	$2.14 \cdot 10^{-2}$	$1.79 \cdot 10^{-2}$	$3.87 \cdot 10^{-8}$	$3.38 \cdot 10^{-8}$
CO_2	0.181	$1.96 \cdot 10^{-2}$	$1.59 \cdot 10^{-5}$	0.883		$51.4 \cdot 10^{-2}$	$1.26 \cdot 10^{-2}$		$64.5 \cdot 10^{-8}$

*Diffusion coefficients were measured for all gases except NO, which is assumed to be the same as CO based on Graham's law (281, 282); †Measurements were made for O_2 in human plasma, others being calculated based on Graham's law (84, 288); ‡Data from Powers (197). CO and NO measurements are in water (5, 279), O_2 and CO_2 measurements in plasma (36, 226). Both the diffusion coefficient (d) and the Krogh diffusion constant (DK) increase with temperature; temperature coefficients for d and DK are approximately 2% and 1% per degree Celsius, respectively. Solubility decreases with temperature. Bunsen solubility coefficients for oxygen and CO_2 in plasma at different temperatures can be estimated within ± 1% error between 33° and 43°C as follows:

$\alpha O_2 = 0.041796 - 0.000889 \cdot t + 0.00000913 \cdot t^2$

$\alpha CO_2 = 0.884 - 0.01t$

where t is temperature in degrees Celsius.

much less mean capillary oxygen tension, which was necessary to measure DM_{O_2} using equation 14. However, it was recognized that the binding affinity of hemoglobin for CO was more than 200 times that for O_2. Quantitatively, this can be expressed as follows:

$$\frac{S_{CO}}{S_{O_2}} = \frac{215 \cdot P_{CO}}{P_{O_2}} \quad (15)$$

where S_{CO} and S_{O_2} are carboxy- and oxyhemoglobin saturations, respectively, and P_{CO} and P_{O_2} are CO and O_2 tensions, respectively. Normally, the CO saturation of blood is less than 1%. If CO and O_2 saturations are 1% and 97% at a P_{O_2} of 100 mm Hg, CO tension would be (100/97)/215 = 0.005 mm Hg. Even at CO and O_2 saturations of 10% and 90%, respectively, at a P_{O_2} of 100 mm Hg, CO tension would be only about 0.05 mm Hg. Thus, it was recognized that if CO uptake could be measured for brief intervals at alveolar CO tensions of 1–2 mm Hg, CO diffusing capacity could be estimated, based on the following equation:

$$DL_{CO} = \frac{\dot{V}_{CO}}{PA_{CO}} \quad (16)$$

where CO back-pressure from carboxyhemoglobin is neglected. Thus, DL_{CO} could be measured from CO uptake and alveolar CO tension without requiring any blood samples. Then DL_{CO} was used to provide an estimate of DL_{O_2}, based on the ratio of the Krogh diffusion constant for the two gases, as follows:

$$DL_{O_2} = DL_{CO} \cdot \left[\frac{\alpha_{O_2} \cdot d_{O_2}}{\alpha_{CO} \cdot d_{CO}}\right] = DL_{CO} \cdot \frac{DK_{O_2}}{DK_{CO}} \quad (17)$$

The bracketed term, assuming the solubilities in a watery membrane, was 1.23; so that conventionally it was assumed that $DL_{O_2} = 1.23 \cdot DL_{CO}$. Early investigators assumed that the velocity of CO and O_2 reactions with hemoglobin in the red cell were instantaneous.

The potential importance of reaction kinetics as determinants of rates of gas exchange across the alveolar capillary membrane was recognized much later by Hartridge and Roughton in the 1920s (93–95). Hartridge and Roughton measured the first rapid reaction velocities between O_2 and hemoglobin and between CO and hemoglobin in the early 1920s. Meldrum and Roughton (171) in 1933 isolated carbonic anhydrase from the red cell and demonstrated that without this enzyme, equilibrium of CO_2 tension between capillary blood and alveolar air and between capillary blood and peripheral tissues would be far from complete, even at rest. Application of this knowledge that reaction kinetics could offer a significant resistance to alveolar capillary gas transfer for reactive gases such as O_2, CO_2, CO, and NO was not applied physiologically or clinically until the 1940s and 1950s. Then it became apparent that measurements of DL_{O_2} and DL_{CO} might not accurately reflect true membrane diffusing capacity (DM) for these gases.

Relative binding affinities and reaction velocities of three primary ligands for hemoglobin are shown in Table 12.4. Both CO and NO, because of their high binding affinities for hemoglobin, can be used for measuring diffusion capacity of the lung based on equation 16. However, because of the marked differences in reaction velocities between CO and NO with hemoglobin, measurements of DL_{CO} and DL_{NO} provide uniquely different and complementary information about the pulmonary capillary bed that will become evident later (see later under Diffusing Capacity of the Lung).

Relative Importance of Diffusion and Reaction Kinetics in Gas Exchange. Roughton and Forster (213) were able to formulate the interrelationship between diffusion and reaction kinetics with the following simple equation:

Total resistance = membrane resistance + red cell resistance

or

$$\frac{1}{DL} = \frac{1}{DM} + \frac{1}{\theta Vc} \quad (18)$$

TABLE 12.4. *Binding Affinities and Reaction Velocities of Respiratory Gases with Hemoglobin*

Gas	Binding Affinity Relative to O_2	Reaction Velocity Relative to O_2
O_2	1	1
CO*	215	0.2
NO†	250,000	39

*Estimated for human blood at 37°C (4, 77).
†Estimated indirectly from measurements relative to CO sheep hemoglobin at 3° and 20°C (32, 78).

DL is diffusing capacity of the lung in milliliters per minute per mm Hg, and its reciprocal represents total resistance offered by the sum of diffusion barriers and reaction kinetics to gas exchange; DM is membrane diffusing capacity, incorporating diffusive resistances offered by both alveolar capillary membrane and plasma barriers, in milliliters per minute per mm Hg; θ is a complex term representing both diffusion and reaction kinetics within red cells contained in a milliliter of blood with a normal hematocrit and O_2 capacity. Values of θ were determined by in vitro measurements of reaction kinetics and expressed in milliliters per minute per mm Hg per milliliter of whole blood for both carbon monoxide (θCO) and oxygen (θO_2); Vc is the pulmonary capillary blood volume in milliliters; the reciprocal of θVc is the resistance offered by all of the pulmonary capillary red cells participating in gas exchange. One of the problems in utilizing equation 18 has been obtaining reproducible and accurate measurements of θ (Table 12.5); nevertheless, the equation has been a valuable tool for understanding gas exchange.

The magnitude of θCO was measured by Roughton et al. in vitro at different oxygen tensions yielding an approximately linear relationship between 1/θCO and PO_2 (214):

$$\frac{1}{\theta\mathrm{CO}} = (0.73 + 0.0058\ \mathrm{PO_2}) \cdot \frac{14.9}{[\mathrm{Hb}]} \qquad (19)$$

where θCO is in milliliters per minute per ml of blood at a normal O_2 capacity of 20 ml/dl (Hb = 14.9 g/dl); θCO varies directly with the blood hematocrit or hemoglobin (Hb). Since 1/θCO increases as oxygen tension increases based on equation 19, DL_{CO} will decreases as alveolar oxygen tension increases. From measurements of DL_{CO} at more than one alveolar oxygen tension (PA_{O_2}), a linear relationship is obtained between 1/DL_{CO} and PA_{O_2} from which physiologic estimates of DM_{CO} and Vc can be made based on equation 18.

There have been theoretical concerns over θCO. Data were collected under conditions requiring much higher CO tensions than those used for measuring DL_{CO}. The data were constrained to fit theoretical relationships between 1/θCO and PO_2 for a given ratio of permeability of the red cell membrane to red cell interior (λ). Based on these theoretical relationships, λ was estimated from kinetic data at different oxygen tensions and ranged between 0.86 at a PO_2 of 570 mm Hg, and 2.5 at an O_2 tension of 100 mm Hg; since λ is more reliably estimated at lower oxygen tensions, equation 19, based on an assumption that $\lambda = 2.5$, is most often used. There has always been concern that λ was an artifact caused by unstirred layers around the red cells that would behave as a membrane resistance to diffusion. Figure 12.5 shows relationships between 1/θCO and PO_2 estimated for assumed values of λ between 1.5 and ∞; these estimates are compared with the unconstrained data of Roughton et al. (214) and more recent data of Reeves and Park (187, 207). Measurements of Reeves and Park were made with a thin-film tech-

TABLE 12.5. *Kinetics of Respiratory Gas Uptake by Human Red Cells*

Gas $\frac{1}{\theta}$ (min · mm Hg) at 37°C	ΔE, kcal/M*	References
CO		
0.73 + 0.0058 · PO_2		Roughton & Forster (213)
1.08 + 0.00647 · PO_2	21.4	Holland (117)
0.0156 + 0.0080 · PO_2		Reeves & Park (208)
1.20 + 0.0041 · PO_2		Forster (71)
O_2		
0.357		Staub et al. (239)
0.333 (corrected for unstirred layer)		Holland et al. (116, 118)
0.263		Yamaguchi et al. (286)
Variable but < Yamaguchi et al.		Heidelberger & Reeves (98)
CO_2†		
0.192 (based on the hydration of CO_2)		Constantine et al. (42)
0.544 (based on chloride exchange)		Wagner & West (258)

*ΔE = Activation energy for CO displacement of oxygen from hemoglobin and can be used to correct the slope of the relationship between 1/θ and PO_2 from that measured at 37°C to any existing body temperature using the Arrhenius equation:

$$\mathrm{Ln}\frac{\text{slope 2}}{\text{slope 1}} = -\frac{\Delta E}{R}\left(\frac{1}{T_1} - \frac{1}{T_2}\right)$$

where ΔE is in kcal/mole and R is 1.987×10^{-3} kcal/mole degree.

†based on a half-time of 0.024 s for CO_2 hydration in the red cell or on a half-time of 0.15 s for the $[HCO_3^-]-Cl^-$ exchange between red cells and plasma.

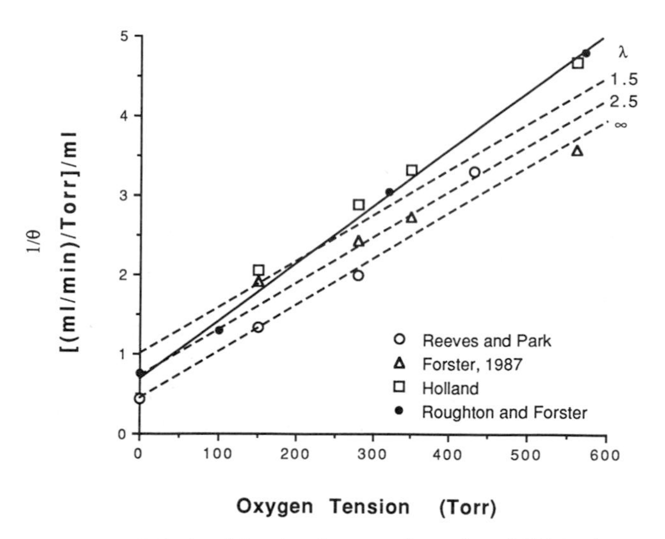

FIG. 12.5. Relationships for the rate of uptake of CO by human red cells in suspension ($1/\theta_{CO}$) to oxygen tension measured in vitro in two different laboratories. *Closed circles* represent measurements reported by Roughton, Forster, and Cander in 1957 using a steady-state turbulent flow-mixing technique (214) at CO tensions of about 90 mm Hg. *Open circles* represent measurements by a thin film technique at CO tensions of about 2 mm Hg (i.e., a value similar to the alveolar CO tension during physiological measurements of $D_{L_{CO}}$). The kinetic data of Roughton et al. for CO uptake were corrected to a low CO tension: (P_{CO}/P_{O_2}) < 0.03. The measurements of Roughton and Forster also were constrained to a theoretical equation developed by Nicholson and Roughton to define the interaction between CO diffusion and reaction kinetics describing the CO displacement of O_2 from oxyhemoglobin (180). The equation employs a ratio of diffusive permeability of the red cell membrane to that of the red cell interior (λ). *Dashed lines* are the constrained relationships reported by Roughton and Forster for different assumed value of λ between 1.5 and ∞. Average λ fit to the kinetic data was 1.5. Data of Park and Reeves, which are measured by a technique that minimizes error from unstirred layers, fall within the original constrained relationships of Roughton and Forster and yield similar estimates of D_M and V_C from $D_{L_{CO}}$ measured at different O_2 tensions (187, 207).

nique that minimizes unstirred layers and employs CO tensions of only 2 mm Hg, similar to those used in actual measurements of $D_{L_{CO}}$; their data are unconstrained by theory but fall within the same range as the original estimates of Roughton and Forster, reducing the uncertainty in application of θ_{CO} to either physiological or morphometric data. On the other hand, uncertainty is greater for measurements of θ_{O_2} than for θ_{CO} because the reaction velocities for O_2 with hemoglobin and rates of uptake by red cells are much faster (98, 239, 286); hence, errors caused by unstirred layers become exaggerated. Unstirred layers have been estimated to slow O_2 uptake by red cells by a factor of about 2 (116). In addition, θ_{O_2} declines as the fraction of unoccupied heme binding sites decreases above an O_2 saturation of about 80% (239). Based on the latter assumption and applying it to Yamaguchi's estimate of θ_{O_2} (Table 12.5), $\theta_{O_2} = 19 \cdot (1 - S_{O_2})$ above a fractional O_2 saturation of 0.8.

Equation 18 has been applied to alveolar capillary exchange of CO, NO, O_2, and CO_2 and allows a means of translating and comparing resistances relative to uptake and release between any two gases. Some important physical constants for these gases are listed in Tables 12.3, 12.4, and 12.5.

Structural Determinants. The largest structural unit of gas exchange is the pulmonary acinus, which consists of respiratory airways beginning with the transitional bronchiole, a series of dichotomously branching respiratory bronchioles and alveolar ducts ending in alveolar sacs. The number of alveolar units arising from each airway generation increases progressively. Within each acinus, molecular diffusion becomes increasingly important as the mechanism of gas transport along intra-acinar airways and alveolar spaces as well as across the alveolar-capillary-plasma barrier. Pulmonary acini in the human lung number some 30,000, and the acinar airways are fully developed at birth. The number of alveoli is about 20 to 50 million at birth (53, 57, 155) and continues to increase during childhood to about 300 million (264), associated with an increase in alveolar surface area from about 2.8 m^2 at birth to between 40 and 120 m^2 at adulthood (57, 244, 264). Fully developed acinar volume follows a log-normal distribution and averages from as low as 30 mm^3 (24, 199) in early estimates to about 187 mm^3 (88, 92) in later estimates, depending on the level of lung inflation. The number of generations of intra-acinar airway branching ranges between 6 (199) and 12 (88, 92, 188, 224). Estimates of mean longitudinal acinar path length also varies from 4 mm (224) to 8.25 mm (88), possibly related to the level of lung inflation. The structural components determining the overall resistance to alveolar gas diffusion can be conceptualized in a simple electrical analog model of series resistances:

$$\frac{1}{D_L} = \frac{1}{D_G} + \frac{1}{D_M} + \frac{1}{D_E} \quad (20)$$

where D_L is the overall rate of uptake (diffusing capacity) of a given marker gas across the acini; D_G is the rate of diffusion of the gas through the alveolar air space from the acinar airways to the tissue membrane; D_M is the rate of uptake of the gas across the tissue membrane and plasma barrier; D_E is the combined rate of uptake across the erythrocyte membrane and subsequent reaction with hemoglobin.

Structural basis of gas phase diffusion resistance ($1/D_G$). Transport of respired gases in airways occurs by a combination of convection and diffusion. The relative importance of these mechanisms depends on whether transport is occurring in larger conductive airways (generations 0–16) or in smaller alveolated air passages of the acinus; that is, respiratory bronchioles (generations 17–19) and alveolar ducts (generations 20–23), which lie in the last 0.7 cm of the peripheral airways. Total cross-sectional area progressively increases from generation 3 toward the lung periphery and increases very rapidly within the acinus (50). At a given rate of inspiration, convective flux (flow/unit area) is inversely proportional to total airway cross-sectional area; therefore, convective flux will progressively decrease as the interface of inspired air moves peripherally even though total flow (flux × cross-sectional area) remains fixed. In contrast, diffusive flux of an inspired component gas is independent of total airway cross-sectional area; therefore, diffusive flux will progressively increase with respect to the concentration gradient as the convective interface moves peripherally while total diffusive transport (flux × cross-sectional area) will progressively increase. A peripheral location in small airways will be reached where the rate of diffusive transport exceeds the rate of convective transport. Paiva showed that as the convective interface moves during inspiration, it reaches a point in the small acinar airways where it moves so slowly that it almost stabilizes at a fixed level (183); depth of this interface penetration increases as the rate and depth of inspiration increase. Mixing between inspired and alveolar gases beyond this relatively stationary convective front is achieved almost entirely by diffusion.

Incomplete diffusion equilibrium within acinar airways can cause *stratified inhomogeneity* in the distribution of ventilation (51, 184, 221) and theoretically could impose a significant gas phase diffusion limitation to gas transport at rest or exercise. The existence and importance of stratified inhomogeneity has been a continuing source of experimental and theoretical study over the past 50 years and remains incompletely resolved. Rauwerda (205) in 1946 argued on theoretical grounds that diffusive transport in the acinus was so rapid that the upward slope of the alveolar plateau must be caused by uneven ventilation distribution between acinar units rather than by stratified inhomogeneity within units. The issue was raised again by Cumming et al. (50) in 1966 with both theoretical and experimental arguments that intra-acinar equilibration was not complete at the end of inspiration and that stratified inhomogeneity exists even in the normal lung. The most sophisticated theoretical arguments supporting stratified inhomogeneity have been advanced by Paiva and Scherer based on morphometric models of conducting and acinar airways (183, 222).

Scheid, Hlastala, and Piiper (113, 220) have modeled stratified inhomogeneity as gas phase resistance to diffusive transport of inert gases in the acinus ($1/D_G$) where D_G is diffusing capacity of the gas phase; their objective was to determine the potential effect of stratified inhomogeneity on measurements of ventilation–perfusion inhomogeneity by the multiple inert gas elimination technique. The magnitude of intra-acinar P_{O_2} drop has been estimated to be about 5 mm Hg in the rat lung (113, 247). In a similar approach, we can utilize an electrical analog (Fig. 12.6) to model the gas phase diffusing capacity

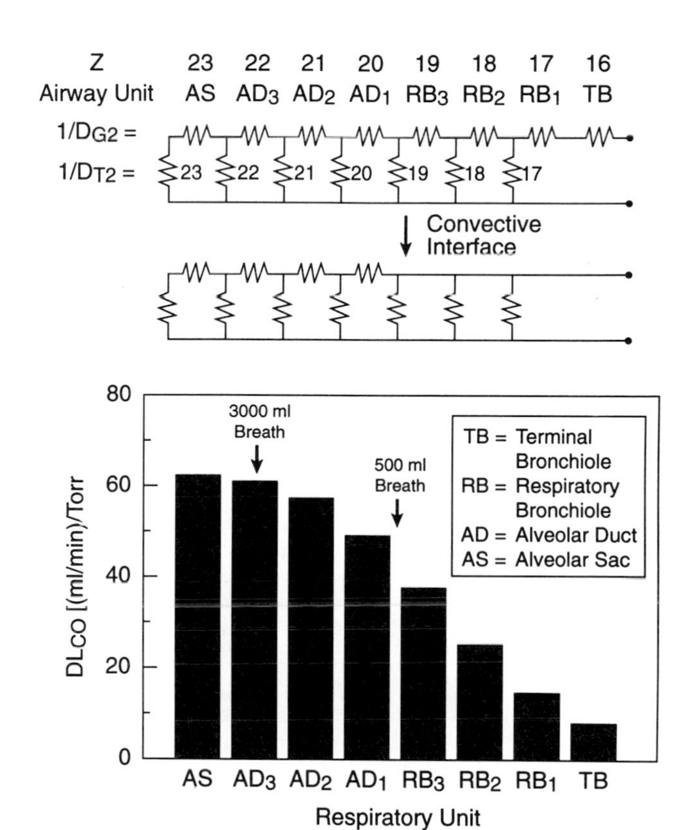

FIG. 12.6. Predicted effects of increasing the depth of inspiration on DL_{CO} based on an electrical analog of resistances to gas phase and tissue diffusion in the lung acinus. Resistors oriented from right to left across the page represent gas phase resistance to CO diffusion in respired air. There is a resistor for each airway generation from the terminal bronchiole (TB) at the mouth of the acinus to the alveolar sac (AS) at the end. Resistors perpendicular to these represent tissue resistance to diffusive CO uptake in capillaries of alveoli arising from each airway generation. Approximate changes in depth of penetration of the convective interface at different inspired volumes are shown. DL_{CO} increases with depth of convective penetration owing to the progressive decrease in gas phase resistance. Calculations are based on airway length and total cross-sectional area in each generation and the fraction of total alveoli arising from each generation as reported by Weibel (191).

for CO (DG_z in milliliters per min per mm Hg) across each airway generation z in the human acinus as:

$$DG_z = \frac{60 \cdot DCO}{760} \cdot \left[\frac{S_z}{l_z}\right] \quad (22)$$

where DCO = the diffusion coefficient for CO in alveolar air in square centimeters per second (281); S_z = total cross-sectional area of the airways in generation z and l_z is the length of airways in generation z. The diffusing capacity of the alveolar tissue phase (DT_z) in each generation z is estimated as:

$$DT_z = VA + f_z \cdot \left[\frac{DT}{VA}\right] \quad (23)$$

where f_z = fraction of total alveoli arising from airways of generation z, VA is total alveolar volume, and [DT/VA] is diffusing capacity of the tissue phase per milliliter alveolar volume. Total resistance to diffusion across the lung (gas phase and alveolar tissue phase) at generation z ($1/DL_z$) is the sum of resistance in the gas and tissue phases; that is:

$$\left(\frac{1}{DL_z}\right) = \left(\frac{1}{DG_z} + \frac{1}{DT_z}\right) \quad (24)$$

Total lung diffusing capacity can then be approximately using Weibel's morphometric description of the dimensions of the human acinus (264).

In the circuit diagram of Figure 12.6*A*, each generation beyond the terminal bronchiole (TB) incorporates a resistor representing gas phase and a resistor representing the alveolar tissue phase. As the depth of inspiration increases, the proximal gas phase resistors are shunted out as shown in the lower panel of Figure 12.6*A*. This model can be used to illustrate how changing depth of penetration of the gas phase interface into the acinus might affect CO diffusing capacity (DL_{CO}) at rest and during exercise (Figure 12.6*B*). DL_{CO} should increase as depth of convective penetration into the acinus increases (50) both at rest and during exercise. At present, the importance of gas phase resistance to oxygen transport at rest or heavy exercise is unclear in health or disease.

Structural basis of pulmonary membrane resistance (1/DM). By assuming that 1/DG is negligible, Weibel utilized equation 20 to develop a model for estimating pulmonary diffusing capacity DL (28, 69, 75, 230, 265–267, 273) based on stereological principles (49) and quantitative estimates of structural dimensions in the lung instilled with fixatives. In this "morphometric model" of gas exchange, the lungs are fixed in vivo by the instillation of glutaraldehyde into the trachea under a constant hydrostatic pressure while the heart is still beating, in order to preserve the normal configuration of the pulmonary capillary bed. The fixation pressure generally employed (25 cm H_2O) results in a postmortem lung volume somewhere between functional residual capacity (FRC) and total lung capacity (TLC). The fixed lungs are removed and subsequently sectioned serially. Representative samples are taken using various unbiased systematic random schemes for microscopic examination at different levels of magnification (268). From selected samples, volume of capillary blood is estimated by point counting. DM is estimated from mean alveolar and capillary surface area (Sa and Sc, respectively) and the harmonic mean thickness of the tissue-plasma barrier (τ_{hb}) measured from random linear intercepts overlaid on representative electron micrographs sampled from the fixed lung. For CO or O_2:

$$DM = \alpha \cdot D \cdot \frac{Sa + Sc}{2 \cdot \tau_{hb}} \quad (25)$$

where α is the Bunsen solubility coefficient and D is the diffusion coefficient for CO (84, 197) or O_2 (271) in tissue and plasma taken from the literature. In the original conceptualization of the model, the tissue and plasma components of membrane resistance were assumed to constitute separate resistances (1/Dt and 1/Dp, respectively) arranged in series; that is:

$$\frac{1}{DM} = \frac{1}{Dt} + \frac{1}{Dp} \quad (26)$$

This early conceptualization created some insoluble mathematical difficulties; therefore, in a recent modification (123, 269) the tissue and plasma components were combined and treated as a single membrane barrier resistance. The modification results in approximately 30%–40% reduction in DM and 10%–20% reduction in DL compared with the original model.

SURFACE AREA OF ALVEOLAR MEMBRANE. The functionally effective membrane surface area for diffusive gas exchange depends on the matching between alveolar surface area and capillary surface area; the former is usually greater than the latter in various species (76, 123, 271); hence, an average of the two generally is used in estimating structural membrane diffusing capacity (DM) by equation 25. Alveolar surface may be expanded by unfolding and/or stretching related to lung inflation (9). Gil et al. (79) showed in rats that alveolar surface area is significantly higher in fluid-inflated lungs, where surface tension has been eliminated, than in air-inflated lungs. Estimated alveolar surface area also increases as lung volume increases, both in indirect studies during life (41) and in postmortem fixed human lungs studied by morphometry (76, 244), presumably because of the unraveling of previously atelectactic folds. The physiologic increase in DL_{CO} associated with lung inflation is variable but generally small, generally less than 20% of overall physiological increase in DL_{CO} from rest to exercise (31, 124, 175). How much of this increase is due to true membrane unfolding (reduction in 1/DM), and how much is due to deeper acinar penetration of the larger inspired gas volume (reduction in 1/DG) has yet to be clarified.

SURFACE AREA OF CAPILLARY MEMBRANE. Capillary surface may be expanded by opening of capillaries and/or distention related to greater microvascular perfusion or pressure, although its mechanisms and regional regulation are still topics of debate. It is important to recognize the two-phase nature of blood; each phase, plasma and erythrocyte, supports independent functions that can be recruited separately. Anatomical capillary recruitment may occur via augmentation of either plasma or red cell flow; both will increase perfused surface area, but only the augmentation of red cell flow contributes toward gas exchange (132). Wagner and colleagues used in vivo videomicroscopy of subpleural lung capillaries in dogs to show that capillary segments perfused with red cells increase as perfusion pressure increases (259, 260); recruitment of red cell perfusion is associated with an increase in DL_{CO} (30) and does not reach a plateau up to pressures of about 40 mm Hg (260). This is consistent with data in normal foxhounds in whom DL_{CO} does not reach a plateau up to maximal O_2 uptake at which pulmonary artery pressure reaches about 45 mm Hg (124, 126). Thus, capillary reserves for diffusion are vast and not completely exhausted in normal animals or man even at maximal exercise; recruitment of capillary reserves involves close interaction between functional and structural variables, which will be discussed in more detail later under Comparison of Structural and Physiologic Diffusing Capacity.

HARMONIC MEAN BARRIER THICKNESS. Harmonic mean thickness of the tissue-plasma barrier (τ_{hb}) is the average of the reciprocal local barrier thicknesses estimated from random linear intercept lengths that cross from the epithelium to the erythrocyte membrane on representative electron micrographs (86, 270):

$$\frac{1}{\tau_{hb}} = \text{magnification} \cdot \left(\frac{\sum_{i=1}^{m} \frac{n_i}{l_i}}{\sum_{i=1}^{m} n_i} \right) \tag{27}$$

where n is the number of linear intercepts of length l. Formerly, the right hand side of equation 27 was multiplied by a stereologic correction factor. This factor was to correct for the variable angles of intersection of the random test lines with a perpendicular drawn to the epithelial surface, and it essentially translated random path lengths between the alveolar and red cell surfaces into the shortest average distance between points of intersection with the red cell to the epithelial surface. The appropriateness of this construct has been called into question as will be discussed below.

Structural basis of erythrocyte resistance (1/DE). The resistance to gas uptake within 1 ml of blood (1/DE) consists of the combined resistances offered by the red cell membrane and the reaction rate with hemoglobin ($1/\theta$) and by the total volume of capillary blood (1/Vc):

$$\frac{1}{DE} = \frac{1}{\theta \cdot Vc} \tag{28}$$

The estimation of θ is discussed elsewhere in this chapter. Stereologically, Vc may be estimated by simple point counting on representative micrographs from fixed lung specimens. As capillaries are recruited during exercise, capillary blood volume progressively increases, a response that attenuates the decline of erythrocyte transit time through the pulmonary capillary bed and helps ensure full oxygenation of end-capillary blood. Full structural capacity of the pulmonary capillary bed is unknown; comparisons between morphometric estimates and physiologic estimates at exercise have so far been confounded by interpretative difficulties due to differences in experimental conditions.

Potential errors in morphometric estimation of diffusive transport. Both the physiologic (213) and morphometric (265) descriptions of diffusive gas exchange employ a lumped parameter model to describe a distributed process; this assumption can be a source of systematic errors. To illustrate this error, a finite element method (FEM) technique (12) has been utilized to describe the distribution of CO flux into a hypothetical alveolar capillary containing one or more red cells exposed to a low alveolar CO concentration (Fig. 12.7). The finite element method is an engineering modeling technique, used to study relationships between structure and function in engineering. Examples include mechanical stress distribution in a body when placed under force loads, distribution of temperature gradients and associated heat flux due to energy transfer in an engine, or distribution of concentration gradients and flux in diffusive transport of a substance in a chemical plant. The two-

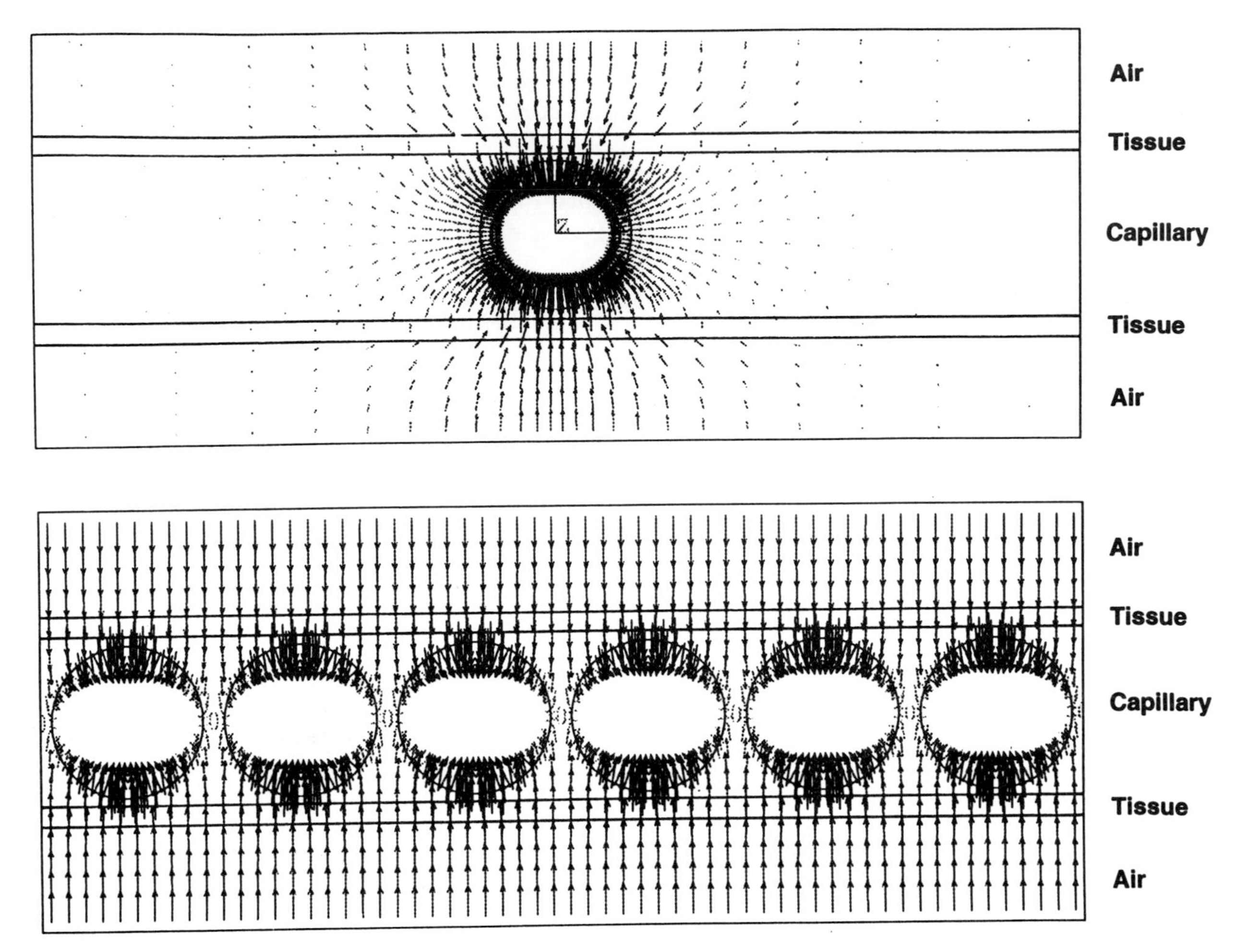

FIG. 12.7. Vector diagrams demonstrate the fluxes of CO from alveolar air into red cells, which act as infinite sinks. Results are shown at two levels of capillary hematocrit. Magnitude and direction of the flux are represented by the size and orientation of the *arrows*, respectively. *A*, one cell per 50 μm capillary (hematocrit = 12%). *B*, 6 cells per 50 μm capillary (hematocrit = 66%). [Reproduced with permission from Hsia et al. (121).]

dimensional or three-dimensional space that is being modeled by the FEM technique is subdivided ito small contiguous finite elements; then well-established physical principles are utilized to describe spatial distribution of the modeled parameters among and between the multiple elements; a computer is utilized to solve a system of simultaneous equations equivalent to the number of finite spatial elements employed. The larger the number of finite elements, the closer to reality the model appraoches. Figure 12.7 illustrates the application of an FEM model to describe the diffusive uptake of CO in a hypothetical capillary. These diagrams indicate that the distribution of flux across the capillary is not uniformly distributed and that average trajectories of CO molecules from alveolar air to red cells are not linear as assumed in the morphometric description. Hence the application of the factor of 3/2 in equation 27 of the morphometric model to calculate DM_{CO} or DM_{O_2} may be inappropriate and causes an underestimate of mean linear path lengths and an overestimate of membrane diffusing capacity. Furthermore, as pointed out by Federspiel (65), each red cell utilizes only a limited part of the red cell membrane for oxygen exchange; hence, effective diffusing capacity is a function of hematocrit.

Rate of Equilibration between Alveolar Air and Capillary Blood

Oxygen. Oxygen diffusing capacity of the lung (DL_{O_2}) for the data in Table 12.2 can be estimated from equation 18, assuming that DM_{O_2} = 1.15 × DM_{CO} (1.15 × 80 = 92) and that θO_2 = 3.9 (ml/min)/mm Hg per ml of blood (286); this yields a DL_{O_2} of 84 (ml/min)/mm Hg. In Table 12.2 mean transit time through lung capillaries is (257/27,300) × 60 = 0.56 s and the ratio of $DL_{O_2}/\dot{Q}c$ = 84/27.3 = 3.08. Eliminating the oxygen subscripts for simplicity, the rate at which oxygen tension in an element of capillary blood approaches equilibrium with the alveolar air as it passes through a lung capillary obeys the following relationship:

$$(O_2Cap) \cdot \frac{\partial S}{\partial t} = \frac{D_L}{V_C} (P_A - P_C) \qquad (29)$$

where $\partial S/\partial t$ = the rate of increase of oxygen saturation; D_L is O_2 diffusing capacity as defined by equation 18 in milliliters per minute per mm Hg, and D_L/V_C is the oxygen diffusing capacity per milliliter of capillary blood; P_A and P_C are alveolar and capillary intraerythrocyte O_2 tensions in mm Hg, respectively. According to Staub (239), θO_2 remains approximately constant from 0%–80% saturation but at higher saturations falls in proportion to the number of unoccupied O_2 binding sites remaining. This will cause $D_{L_{O_2}}$ to fall by about 10% between 80% and 93% O_2 saturation; we have neglected this change in $D_{L_{O_2}}$ in our calculations. Rearranging equation 29 and integrating both sides we obtain the following:

$$\Delta t = \frac{(O_2Cap)V_c}{D_L} \int_{S\bar{v}}^{Sc'} \frac{\partial S}{(P_A - P_C)} \qquad (30)$$

where Δt is the transit time required to reach an end-capillary oxygen saturation of Sc' from a starting mixed venous saturation, $S\bar{v}$, when exposed to an alveolar oxygen tension, P_A. From equation 30 we can construct the time required to reach any given oxygen saturation as blood passes through lung capillaries if $D_{L_{O_2}}$, $P_{A_{O_2}}$, and the position and shape of the oxyhemoglobin dissociation curve are known. A good approximation to this time course can be obtained using the Hill equation as an approximation of the oxyhemoglobin dissociation curve to define intraerythrocyte O_2 tension (Pc) in terms of intraerythrocyte O_2 saturation (Sc) as follows:

$$P_{C_{O_2}} = P_{50} \left(\frac{Sc}{1 - Sc}\right)^{0.37} \qquad (31)$$

Such an approximation using equations 30 and 31 is shown in Figure 12.8*A* for the data in Table 12.2. Calculations were made assuming a normal P_{50} of 26.5 mm Hg as well as the actual P_{50} of 31.7 mm Hg. Raising the P_{50} reduces the rate at which blood becomes oxygenated as it passes through the lung. This can be deduced by examining equations 30 and 31. Substituting the right hand side of equation 31 for $P_{C_{O_2}}$ in equation 30, one can see when P_{50} increases as in response to acidosis or to a rise in body temperature during exercise, $P_{C_{O_2}}$ correspondingly increases at any given oxygen saturation and thereby

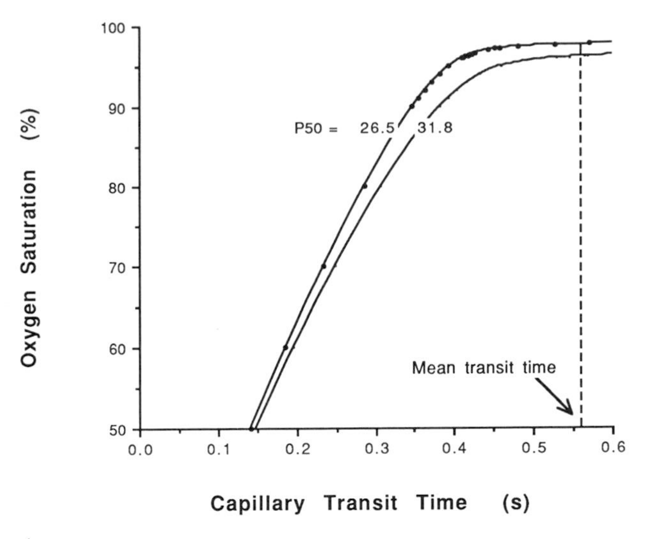

A

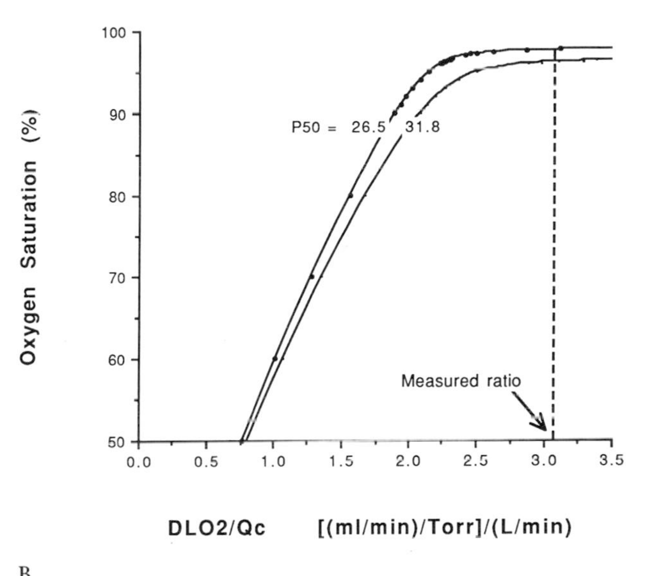

B

FIG. 12.8. Rates at which oxygen equilibrates with oxyhemoglobin during blood transit through lung capillaries were calculated from the data in Table 12.2 at maximal exercise. *A*, Constructed based on equations 29 and 30, showing the rate of increase in oxygen saturation at an alveolar oxygen tension of 112 mm Hg and at an estimated in vivo P_{50} of 31.8 mm Hg. Mean transit time was 0.565 s, insufficient for complete equilibrium; oxygen tension in blood leaving the lung was estimated at approximately 104 mm Hg. *B*, The same data plotted in a different way based on equations 30 and 31, yielding the same information but illustrating the fact that at a given alveolar oxygen tension and P_{50} arterial oxygen saturation will begin to fall sharply as the ratio of $D_{L_{O_2}}/\dot{Q}c$ falls below a critical level. Calculations in both graphs were repeated at a normal resting P_{50} of 26.5 mm Hg to illustrate the more rapid approach to equilibrium at a lower P_{50} owing to the higher average oxygen tension difference between alveolar air and capillary blood during red cell transit when P_{50} is lower.

lowers the pressure gradient driving oxygen into blood; this reduces the denominator of the integral and makes Δt larger (i.e., makes the rise in oxygen saturation slower during capillary transit). Reducing the P_{50} has the opposite effect. In summary, a rise in P_{50} will slow the rate of oxygenation of blood as it passes through the lung exposed to a given alveolar oxygen tension; a fall in P_{50} will speed up the oxygenation of blood as it passes through the lung.

Equation 30 can be rearranged in another way to provide additional insight concerning determinants of the rate of oxygenation of blood during its transit through the lung. Since $Vc/\Delta t$ = pulmonary capillary blood flow ($\dot{Q}c$), equation 30 can be rearranged to give:

$$\frac{D_L}{\dot{Q}c} = (O_2Cap) \int_{S\bar{v}}^{Sc'} \frac{\partial Sc}{(P_A - Pc)} \tag{32}$$

Equation 32 indicates that, at a given alveolar oxygen tension, mixed venous oxygen saturation and P_{50}, the oxygen saturation of the blood leaving capillaries in a region of lung is determined by the ratio of $D_L/\dot{Q}c$ just as the equilibrium saturation of blood leaving a lung region is determined by $\dot{V}_A/\dot{Q}c$. The relationship between the $D_L/\dot{Q}c$ ratio and end-capillary blood oxygen saturation derived from equations 31 and 32 for the data in Table 12.2 at maximal oxygen uptake is shown in Figure 12.8*B*. In Figure 12.8*A* and *B* the intersection of the *vertical dashed line* with the *plotted curve* indicates the predicted oxygen saturation of blood leaving the lung. In Figure 12.8*A*, the *dashed line* is placed at the mean capillary transit time of 0.56 s; in Figure 12.8*B*, the *dashed line* is placed at the measured ratio of $D_L/\dot{Q}c$ = 3.08. Both methods yield equivalent end-capillary oxygen saturations. It will also be shown in a subsequent section that uneven red cell transit times through lung capillaries in an otherwise homogeneous lung can cause the same impairment of gas exchange as regional differences in the $D_L/\dot{Q}c$ ratio.

The concept of $D/\beta\dot{Q}$. The ratio of $D_L/\beta\dot{Q}c$ was introduced by Piiper and Scheid as a convenient means of comparing diffusive gas exchange in different species (194): β is the average slope of the O_2 or CO_2 dissociation curve between mixed venous and end-capillary blood in the lung; $D_L/\dot{Q}c$ is the ratio of diffusing capacity to pulmonary capillary blood flow for O_2 or CO_2. Applying equation 29, where we assume that the O_2 dissociation curve is linear with a slope, $\beta = O_2Cap\ \partial S/\partial P$, expressed in milliliters of O_2 per milliliter of blood per mm Hg, equation 34 by substitution then becomes:

$$\beta \frac{\partial P}{\partial t} = -\frac{D_L}{Vc}(P_A - Pc)$$

Collecting terms and integrating

$$Ln\frac{(P_A - Pc')}{(P_A - P\bar{v})} = -\frac{D_L}{\beta Vc}\Delta t$$

where Δt = transit time in minutes

but
$$\frac{Vc}{\Delta t} = \dot{Q}c$$

hence
$$Ln\frac{(P_A - Pc')}{(P_A - P\bar{v})} = -D_L/\beta\dot{Q}c$$

Taking the exponential of both sides:

$$\frac{(P_A - Pc')}{(P_A - P\bar{v})} = e^{-D_L/\beta\dot{Q}c} \tag{33}$$

Equation 33 is an approximation for describing diffusive exchange of O_2 or CO_2 in the lung. It is only accurate under conditions where the dissociation curves approach linearity (e.g., under hypoxic conditions for oxygen exchange); however, even under conditions where the dissociation curve is curvilinear, the equation can often be used as an aid in conceptualizing how changes in O_2 capacity, P_{50}, or the region of the O_2 dissociation curve being utilized affect gas exchange (see later under Diffusion Limitation). In the next section equation 33 will be used to estimate the rate of CO_2 exchange in the lung assuming an approximately linear CO_2 dissociation curve.

Carbon dioxide. Rough approximations can be made to the rate of CO_2 equilibrium in lung capillaries, but the chemical reaction kinetics are much more complex than for oxygen. During exercise, CO_2 diffuses from muscle through plasma into erythrocytes, where part reacts directly with hemoglobin to form carbamate and the remainder is hydrated to carbonic acid (H_2CO_3) by the enzyme carbonic anhydrase with a time constant of about 0.045 s (42); bicarbonate (HCO_3^-) is formed almost instantaneously by dissociation of the H_2CO_3. Although the CO_2 is transported principally as HCO_3^- in plasma, there is no carbonic anhydrase in plasma, and hydration of CO_2 in the absence of carbonic anhydrase is slow; hence most of the HCO_3^- is formed in the erythrocytes and returned to plasma in exchange for Cl^- by a carrier-mediated process. This HCO_3^-–Cl^- exchange has a time constant estimated to be between 0.1 and 0.22 s (34, 103, 144). During these events, allosteric changes in hemoglobin enhance the rate of bicarbonate and carbamate formation with a time constant of 0.1–0.12 s (47, 143). The reverse sequence of events occurs in the lung to that during loading of CO_2 from muscle to blood. The time constants for CO_2 reactions in lung and tissues are relatively slow with respect to the time spent by blood in lung capillaries at heavy exercise (~0.5 s); as a consequence, the $HCO_3^- - Cl^-$ exchange may still be incomplete by the time blood leaves lung capillaries. If the $HCO_3^- - Cl^-$ exchange is still incomplete by the time blood leaves the lung capillaries, postcapillary exchange will continue to occur until equilibrium is reached at a higher Pa_{CO_2}. In Figure 12.9 the assumption has been made that $HCO_3^- - Cl^-$ exchange is imposing the primary rate limitation to CO_2 uptake and release from blood with a half-time of 0.15 s. θCO_2 can be estimated from the half-time (∂t) as follows:

$$\theta CO_2 = \frac{0.693 \cdot 0.0224 \cdot 60 \cdot m}{\partial t} \qquad (34)$$

where 0.693 = Ln(0.5), 0.0224 = ml CO_2 gas (STPD)/(mM CO_2/ml blood), 60 = s/min, m = slope of the CO_2 dissociation curve over the limited range of interest in units of (mM/liter)/mm Hg, ∂t = half-time in s. From the data in Table 12.2, $\theta CO_2 = 1.84$ ml $\cdot$ min^{-1} $\cdot$ mm Hg^{-1} per ml blood based on the units defined for equation 33. Based on equation 18 and assuming $DM_{CO_2} = 19 \cdot DM_{O_2}$, DL_{CO_2} at maximal oxygen uptake should be 372 ml $\cdot$ min^{-1} $\cdot$ mm Hg^{-1}, approximately 4.4 times that of the DL_{O_2}. Assuming an approximately linear CO_2 dissociation curve, equation 33 has been used to estimate the alveolar-arterial CO_2 tension difference that can be explained by the estimated DL for CO_2.

Based on the data in Table 12.2, if $Pc'_{CO_2} = 36$ mm Hg, $P\bar{v}_{CO_2} = 61$ mm Hg, $\beta = 0.296$ (mM/liter)/mm Hg and transit time is 0.565 s, PA_{CO_2} can be estimated from equation 34 to be 32.3 mm Hg, yielding an alveolar arterial CO_2 tension difference of 3.7 mm Hg after postcapillary adjustments of CO_2 tension caused by continued $HCO_3^- - Cl^-$ exchange. Postcapillary adjustment of CO_2 tension would classically be interpreted as caused by alveolar dead space rather than as diffusion–reaction rate disequilibrium. The calculations from the data in Table 12.2 indicate that the relatively slow $HCO_3^- - Cl^-$ exchange could cause a significant postcapillary CO_2 tension difference even in normal subjects at heavy exercise. However, more recent data suggest that carbonic anhydrase exists on the luminal surface of the pulmonary capillaries; endothelial carbonic anhydrase would provide a parallel pathway for direct conversion of plasma HCO_3^- to CO_2, bypassing the red cell and thereby significantly reducing but not completely eliminating this predicted postcapillary rise in Pa_{CO_2} (44, 61, 145). Even so, CO_2 exchange across the alveolar capillary membrane is slower than would be suggested by the 19-fold greater diffusivity of CO_2 in the alveolar capillary membrane relative to that for O_2. The magnitude of postcapillary adjustments of Pa_{CO_2} remains experimentally unclear at this point.

Nonuniformity of Regional Gas Exchange

Regional Differences in $\dot{V}A/\dot{Q}c$ Ratios. The measured arterial blood oxygen tension from Table 12.2 was less than that predicted at equilibrium in a single-compartment lung (Fig. 12.4); hence, there was an alveolar-arterial oxygen tension gradient of 28 mm Hg, indicating some kind of inefficiency in gas exchange during heavy exercise. One possibility would be that there are multiple lung compartments with different ratios of ventilation to perfusion ($\dot{V}A/\dot{Q}c$). A two-compartment example using data from Table 12.2 is illustrated in Figure 12.10, in which one compartment receives 6 liters/min of the $\dot{Q}c$ and 6 liters/min of the $\dot{V}A$; the other compartment receives 21.3 liters/min of $\dot{Q}c$ and 104.8 liters/min of the alveolar ventilation. Thus, in the region with the $\dot{V}A/\dot{Q}c$ ratio of 1.0, equilibrium is achieved with Cc'_{O_2} of 15.7 ml/dl and Cc'_{CO_2} of 20.1 mM/liter with a Pa_{CO_2} of 59 mm Hg. In the compartment with the larger $\dot{V}A/\dot{Q}c$ ratio of 4.92, equilibrium is achieved with a Cc'_{O_2} of 20.05 ml/dl and a Cc'_{CO_2} of 16.1 ml/dl with a Pa_{CO_2} of 32 mm Hg. When mixed in a ratio of 6:21.3, the mixture has a Cc'_{CO_2} of 16 mM/liter, a Pa_{CO_2} of 36 mm Hg, a Cc'_{O_2} of 19.13 ml/dl, and Pa_{O_2} of 84 mm Hg. A single two-compartment solution is all that can be defined for these data. A method for obtaining a more accurate estimate of the distribution of $\dot{V}A/\dot{Q}c$ with respect to both ventilation and perfusion in a multicompartment lung can be obtained by the multiple inert gas elimination technique (MIGET), discussed later under Ventilation/Perfusion ($\dot{V}A/\dot{Q}$) Relationships.

Regional Differences in $DL/\dot{Q}c$ Ratios. About 25% of the 28 mm Hg AaP_{O_2} for the subject described in Table 12.2 can be explained by diffusion disequilibrium alone at maximal oxygen uptake if the lung is entirely homogeneous. However, all of the measured AaP_{O_2} can be explained by diffusion disequilibrium in an otherwise homogeneous lung (i.e., uniform alveolar oxygen tension and uniform $\dot{V}A/\dot{Q}c$ ratios) if we assume two compartments with unequal red cell transit times or alternatively two compartments with different $DL/\dot{Q}c$ ratios. Figure 12.11*A* and *B* are local magnifications of Figure 12.8*A* and *B* to demonstrate these possibilities. Given the qualifying assumptions (uniform alveolar oxygen tension and uniform $\dot{V}A/\dot{Q}c$ ratios), Figure 12.11*A* and *B* represent different ways of graphing the same solution. Two compartments with different capillary red cell transit times are equivalent to two compartments of unequal DL/Q̇c exposed to the same alveolar oxygen tension. In Figure 12.11*A* the AaP_{O_2} can be explained by 50% of the red cells with a transit time of 0.38 s and 50% with a transit time of 0.76 s; in Figure 12.11*B* the same thing is represented by 50% of the pulmonary blood flow distributed through 66.7% of the DL_{O_2} (i.e., DL/Q̇c = 4.1) and the remaining 50% through 33.3% of the DL_{O_2} [i.e., DL/Q̇c = 2.05]. Fifty percent of the Q̇c (13.65 liters/min) passing through 33.3% of the pulmonary capillary bed (Vc = 85.6 ml) yields a transit time of approximately 0.38 s, and the remainder going through 66.7% of the capillary bed (Vc = 171.4) yields a transit time of approximately 0.76 s where alveolar oxygen tension is uniformly distributed throughout; this implies that uneven transit times exist in each alveolus. Figure 12.11*A* and *B* represent one of an infinite number of possible solutions for this kind of two-compartment model that can explain the measured AaP_{O_2}. Differences in DL/Q̇c also could be partitioned in different regions of the lung as well as in each alveolus, although this complicates the calculations and yields a different set of solutions, since different alveolar oxygen tensions will occur in the two regions if V̇A/Q̇c ratios are assumed to be uniform; this results from the fact that oxygen uptake would be less and alveolar oxygen tension correspondingly higher in the region with the low DL/Q̇c ratio.

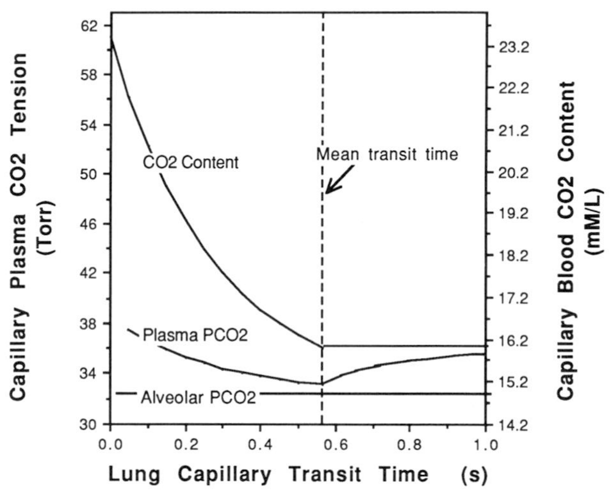

FIG. 12.9. Rates of alveolar capillary CO_2 equilibrium were calculated for data in Table 12.2 at maximal O_2 uptake assuming that the rate-limiting process is the HCO_3–Cl^- shift between red cells and plasma during CO_2 elimination in the lung. This shift has a half-time for completion of about 0.15 s. Others have made similar calculations based on more sophisticated approaches involving a more comprehensive analysis of the different chemical reactions involved in CO_2 transport, but similar conclusions are reached (18, 110). Theoretically, these slow exchanges would be incomplete during short capillary transit times, and after red cells leave lung capillaries HCO_3 would continue to enter the cells and liberate CO_2 gas; hence, postcapillary CO_2 tension will rise. The final difference between alveolar and arterial CO_2 tension was estimated to be 3.7 mm Hg. Endothelial carbonic anhydrase in the lung will reduce this alveolar-arterial CO_2 tension gradient but not completely eliminate it (133).

Optimizing Transport between Lung and Muscle

Importance of Myoglobin in Red Muscle. Myoglobin provides important feedback control for maintaining a high rate of oxygen transport within muscle fibers at heavy exercise, even at very low intracellular oxygen tension gradients; this is a consequence of facilitation of oxygen diffusion by myoglobin. Scholander was the first to demonstrate facilitated oxygen transport by a respiratory pigment; he showed that diffusion of oxygen through a hemoglobin solution was faster than through water and clearly described the mechanism involved (223) as follows. Oxygen is relatively insoluble in water; hence, for a given oxygen tension difference there is a low concentration difference for driving diffusive transport, but hemoglobin concentrates oxygen on heme binding sites and thereby facilitates oxygen diffusion by carrying oxygen molecules piggyback; thus, oxyhemoglobin molecules diffuse along their own concentration gradient. More important, however, with respect to exercise, is the fact that myoglobin within muscle fibers provides a similar facilitation of oxygen diffusion to mitochondria. Wyman developed a general formulation of the facilitated diffusion mechanism (285), which was used in a slightly modified form by Wittenberg (280) to provide a steady-state description of flux across a hypothetical sheet of muscle:

Oxymyoglobin diffusion
+ free O_2 diffusion = total O_2 flux

or

$$D_p n C_p \frac{\Delta S}{\Delta x} + D_c \frac{\Delta C}{\Delta x} = \text{flux} \qquad (35)$$

where D_p = diffusion coefficient of the protein molecules in millimoles per centimeter per second, C_p is the concentration of the protein in millimoles per milliliter, n = number of binding sites on the protein, S = saturation of binding sites, and x = distance; D_c = the diffusion coefficient of the facilitated molecule in millimoles per centimeter per second, C = concentration of the facilitated molecule in millimoles per milliliter, and flux is in millimoles per square centimeter per second. The equation is a statement that

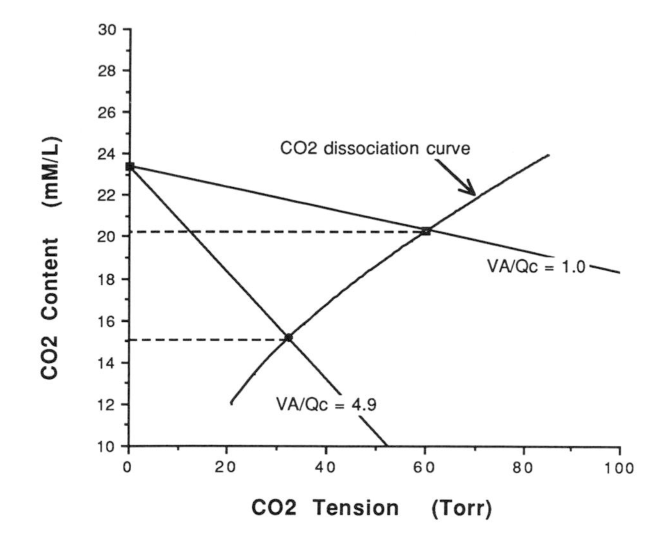

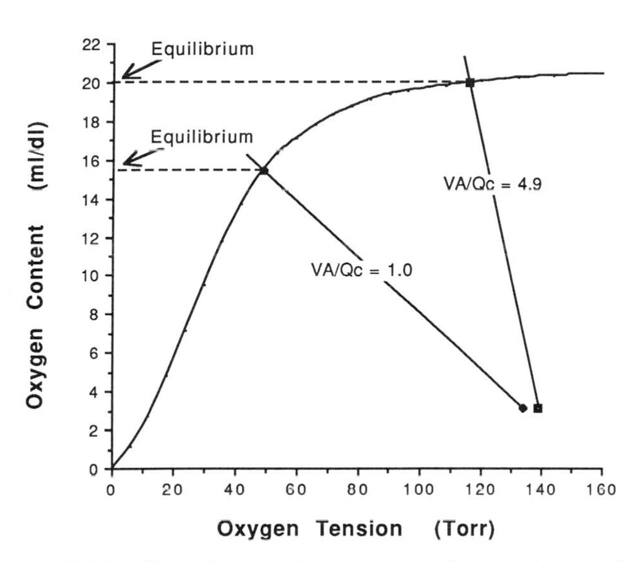

FIG. 12.10. Effect of unequal distribution of ventilation–perfusion ($\dot{V}A/\dot{Q}c$) ratios on efficiency of gas exchange. The same principals employed to estimate O_2 and CO_2 equilibrium in a homogeneous lung (Fig. 12.4) can be applied to individual regions of lung if regional $\dot{V}A/\dot{Q}c$ ratios, mixed venous gas contents, inspired gas concentrations, and the dissociation curves for oxyhemoglobin and CO_2 are known. The two-compartment model illustrated above for CO_2 and O_2 can explain the measured $AaPo_2$ at maximal oxygen uptake, but it is not the only explanation. For example, Figure 12.11 will illustrate another possible explanation based on either uneven red cell transit times through lung capillaries or uneven distribution of $DL_{O_2}/\dot{Q}c$ ratios in the lung.

oxygen transport in muscle involves parallel diffusion of two molecules, oxymyoglobin and free oxygen. For myoglobin, $n = 1$. For dealing with facilitated oxygen diffusion across a sheet of muscle it is helpful to translate equation 35 into terms of partial pressure differences as in Krogh's modification of the Fick equation (equation 13). The translation is easily done. The term nC_p becomes O_2 capacity provided by the myoglobin in muscle (in units of O_2 per milliliter of muscle); if we make the simplifying assumption that the oxymyoglobin dissociation curve is linear over the O_2 saturation of interest, then the term $(O_2Cap)\Delta S/\Delta P$ represents the effective solubility of oxygen bound to myoglobin (in milliliters of O_2 per milliliter of muscle per mm Hg); for free oxygen dissolved in the muscle water $\Delta C = (\alpha/760) \cdot \Delta P$ where ΔP is in mm Hg and α is the Bunsen solubility coefficient of oxygen in muscle in atmospheres and 760

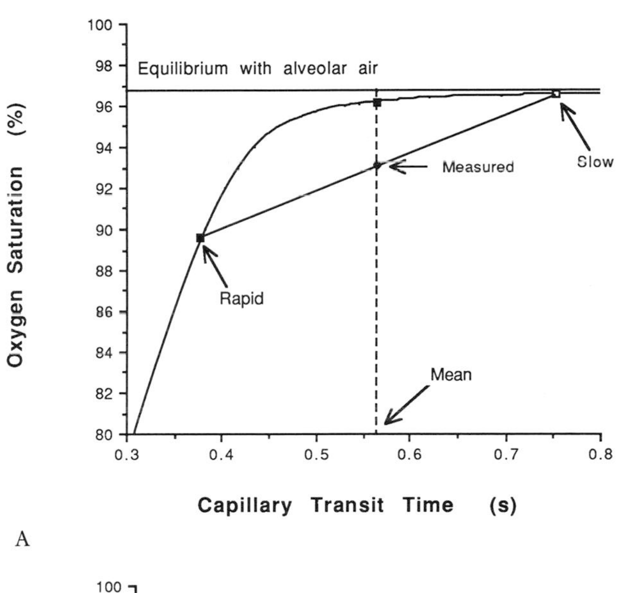

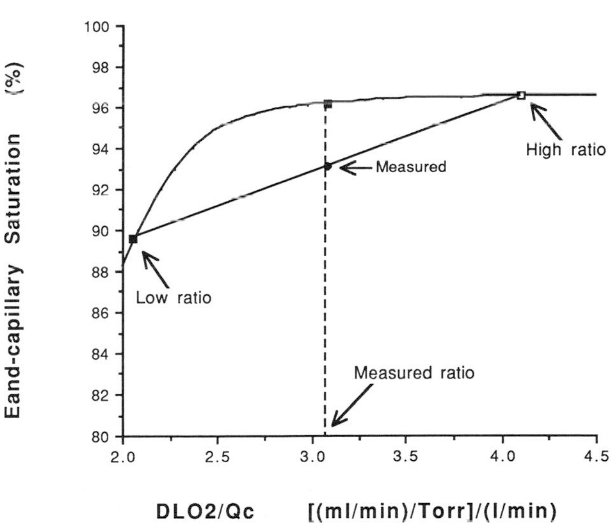

FIG. 12.11. Effect of uneven red cell transit times through lung capillaries or uneven ratios of $DL_{O_2}/\dot{Q}c$ on the alvelar–arterial oxygen tension difference ($AaPo_2$) based on the data from Table 12.2. Panels a and b illustrate graphically how unequal red cell transit times or unequal ratios of $DL_{O_2}/\dot{Q}c$ can explain the measured 28 mm Hg $AaPo_2$. There are an infinite number of these two-compartment solutions that are equally plausible.

is mm Hg per atmosphere. Making these substitutions in equation 35:

Oxymyoglobin diffusion

+ free O_2 diffusion = total O_2 flux

or

$$\text{DMb}\frac{(O_2\text{Cap})\Delta S}{\Delta P}\cdot\frac{\Delta P}{\Delta x} + \text{D}O_2\frac{\alpha}{760}\cdot\frac{\Delta P}{\Delta x} = \text{flux} \quad (36)$$

where the diffusion coefficients DMb and DO_2 are now expressed in units of square centimeters per second and flux is in milliliters of O_2 per second per square centimeter. If we let ΔP represent the difference in oxygen tension (P) from the surface of the muscle to that at the site of removal (P_r), then based upon the Hill equation for myoglobin,

$$\backslash F\ \frac{\Delta S}{\Delta P} = \frac{P_{50}}{(P + P_{50})(P_r + P_{50})}$$

Furthermore, diffusivity of free dissolved oxygen is 20 times that of oxymyoglobin (i.e., $DO_2 = 20 \cdot$ DMb). Making these further substitutions in equation 36:

$$\text{D}O_2\left(\frac{1}{20}\left[\frac{(O_2\text{Cap})P_{50}}{(P + P_{50})(P_r + P_{50})}\right] + \left[\frac{\alpha}{760}\right]\right)\frac{\Delta P}{\Delta x} = \text{flux} \quad (37)$$

The bracketed terms represent effective solubilities of bound and free oxygen in muscle; $\Delta P/\Delta x$ is the pressure difference across the muscle sheet; the factor 1/20 reflects the ratio of the diffusivities of myoglobin and free oxygen (i.e., DMb/DO_2). If myoglobin concentration in muscle is 5×10^{-4} mM/ml, then oxygen capacity of muscle myoglobin would be $22.4 \times 5 \times 10^{-4} = 0.0112$ ml/ml; if PO_2 at the surface of the muscle were 20 mm Hg and at the site of removal 1 mm Hg, effective solubility of oxygen bound to myoglobin becomes about 13.3 times that of free oxygen, but since diffusivity of the oxymyoglobin is only 1/20 that of free oxygen, the oxygen bound to myoglobin will diffuse at a rate that is 66% of that for free oxygen. By this mechanism myoglobin enhances oxygen diffusion by a factor of 1.66. As the oxygen tension at the surface of the muscle falls, the ratio of the effective solubility of bound to free oxygen progressively increases. At a PO_2 of 3.5 mm Hg at the muscle surface, diffusive transport by oxymyoglobin now becomes 2.23 times that by free oxygen; hence, oxygen diffusion is increased by a factor of 3.23. At 2 mm Hg, diffusive O_2 transport is enhanced by 3.8-fold. If the site of oxygen removal is the mitochondria, one can see that as oxygen utilization increases during exercise and PO_2 at the surface of muscle fibers decreases there is a compensatory increase in oxygen diffusivity owing to facilitated transport by myoglobin. Oxygen transport can be sustained at relatively shallow oxygen tension gradients from the surface of the fiber to sites of mitochondrial utilization (119). Thus, myoglobin maintains a low oxygen tension at the surface of muscle fibers; at the same time the sigmoidal shape of the oxyhemoglobin dissociation curve maintains a high driving pressure for diffusion of oxygen between capillary red cells and the muscle surface. The principal resistance to oxygen extraction is located within the capillary and surrounding interstitium between the capillary and muscle surface; resistance within muscle fibers is minimized by myoglobin. Physiologically, *effective* muscle diffusing capacity, Dt_{O_2}, the reciprocal of resistance, has been estimated at maximal oxygen uptake in vascularly isolated perfused canine muscle during electrical stimulation from measurements of $\dot{V}O_2$, $\dot{Q}c$, and arterial and venous PO_2 using a reverse Bohr integral (equation 32) as follows (115):

$$\frac{\text{Dt}}{\dot{Q}c} = (O_2\text{Cap})\int_{Sa}^{S\bar{v}}\frac{\partial Sc}{-Pc} \quad (38)$$

If muscle capillary blood flow ($\dot{Q}c$), the O_2 carrying capacity of blood (O_2Cap), the input oxygen saturation (Sa), and the output oxygen saturation (Sv) are known, Dt_{O_2} can be calculated. This relationship will be used in the next section to define the optimal P_{50} for oxygen transport.

Effect of Position of the Oxyhemoglobin Dissociation Curve (P_{50}). An allosteric enzyme provides feedback control for a metabolic pathway through changes in K_m for the substrate (i.e., the concentration of the primary ligand at which 50% of the binding sites are filled) induced by small effector molecules. The same is true for hemoglobin; for hemoglobin K_m is referred to as P_{50} and the primary effectors are H^+, CO_2, 2,3-DPG, and blood temperature. The importance of the P_{50} can be rapidly grasped from Figure 12.12. By shifting the P_{50} up or down, the partition of the pressure gradient available for loading oxygen in the lung and unloading it in the tissues can be varied (Fig. 12.12*A*). The optimal position of the oxyhemoglobin dissociation curve (i.e., level of the P_{50}) is one that partitions the pressure gradient appropriate to the relative resistance to diffusive trans-

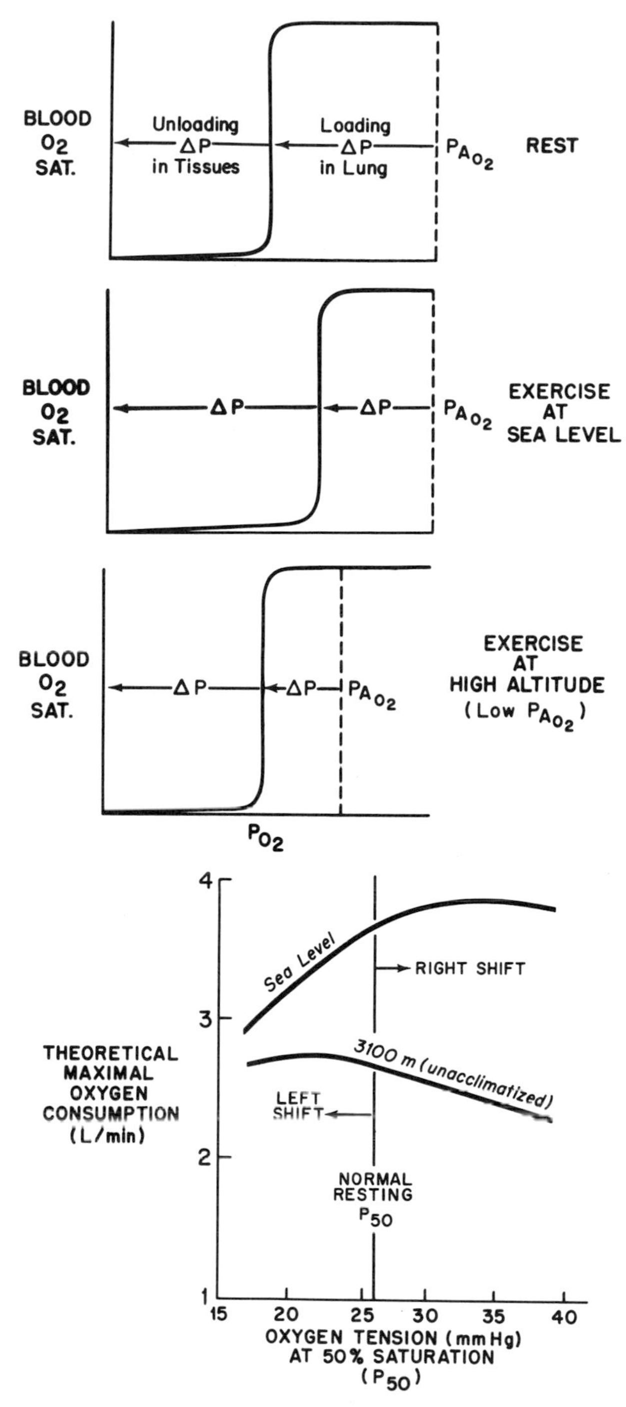

FIG. 12.12. An illustration of how the position of the oxyhemoglobin dissociation curve (P_{50}) affects oxygen loading of blood in the lung and unloading in the tissues. *A*, Position of the oxyhemoglobin dissociation curve has the potential to match optimally the diffusive resistance in the lung and tissues with the pressure gradient available for oxygen loading and unloading respectively, as illustrated by this exaggeration ofthe sigmoidal shape of the dissociation curve. *B*, Optimal P_{50} will vary with altitude because of differences in alveolar O_2 tension. Oxygen transport at sea level will be enhanced at a low pH (high P_{50}) because of the relatively high muscle resistance to diffusive O_2 uptake. Oxygen transport at high altitude will be enhanced at a more alkaline pH (lower P_{50}) which enhances oxygen loading in the lung at the low alveolar oxygen tension.

port in the lung and in muscle during exercise so as to maximize the mass transport of O_2; that is:

$$\frac{P_{A_{O_2}}}{P_{50}} = \frac{D_{T_{O_2}}}{D_{L_{O_2}}}$$

Feedback control to provide optimal positioning of the oxyhemoglobin dissociation curve during exercise is provided in part by the effector molecules and in part by ventilatory control mechanisms. For example, during exercise, if oxygen delivery to exercising muscle is insufficient, lactic acid is released; the resulting acidosis increases the P_{50}, which in turn enhances the rate of oxygen diffusion to muscle mitochondria. The acidosis also stimulates peripheral chemoreceptors to increase ventilation and raise alveolar oxygen tension to partially offset the reduced pressure gradient for loading oxygen in the lung. If the primary resistance to diffusive transport is in the lung, the resulting fall in arterial P_{O_2} will stimulate the carotid body to increase ventilation; this both raises alveolar oxygen tension and reduces $P_{A_{CO_2}}$ and H^+, shifting the P_{50} down, which enhances the pressure gradient for loading oxygen more rapidly in the lung. Thus, a finely tuned feedback control mechanism exists to optimize oxygen transport during exercise based on interplay among *(1)* lactic acid release from muscle; *(2)* ventilatory control of Pa_{O_2}, H^+, and Pa_{CO_2} through chemoreceptor feedback; and *(3)* chemical control of hemoglobin P_{50} through changes in $[H^+]$, P_{CO_2}, and 2,3-DPG.

Optimization of the ratio of alveolar oxygen tension to P_{50}, $P_{A_{O_2}}/P_{50}$, is an important mechanism for achieving maximal oxygen utilization at a given cardiac output. The optimum ratio of $P_{A_{O_2}}/P_{50}$ at maximal exercise is determined by the ratio of effective diffusing capacity of the lung to effective diffusing capacity of muscle, $D_{L_{O_2}}/D_{t_{O_2}}$, as implied in Figure 12.12*A*. Incorporating the Hill approximation to the oxyhemoglobin dissociation curve and dividing equation 32 by equation 38, the following relationship becomes apparent (O_2 subscripts are eliminated to reduce complexity):

$$\frac{D_L}{D_t} = \frac{\displaystyle\int_{S\bar{v}}^{Sa} \frac{\partial Sc}{(P_A/P_{50}) - [Sc/(1 - Sc)]^{0.37}}}{\displaystyle\int_{Sa}^{S\bar{v}} \frac{\partial Sc}{[Sc/(1 - Sc)]^{0.37}}} \quad (39)$$

For any given ratio of diffusing capacity of lung (D_L) to that of muscle (D_t), iterative solutions of equation 29 show that there is an optimum ratio of P_A/P_{50} that provides a maximum A-V O_2 content difference; that is, the difference between the limits of the two integrals, $Sc' - S\bar{v}$. A P_A/P_{50} that is higher than optimum entered into equation 39 yields a solution in which arterial O_2 saturation (Sc′) is high but muscle oxygen extraction, (Sc′ − S$\bar{v}$)/Sc′, is too low for optimization. A P_A/P_{50} that is less than optimum entered into equation 39 yields a solution in which oxygen extraction is high but arterial oxygen saturation, Sc′, is too low for optimization. These points will be illustrated later with actual data from horses and dogs at maximal exercise. Equation 39 also emphasizes the two levels of important feedback control that operate through the ratio of P_A/P_{50}; there is feedback control of ventilation, which determines the alveolar oxygen tension (Pa_{O_2}), and feedback control through the allosteric properties of hemoglobin, which determines the P_{50}.

Maximizing the A-V O_2 saturation difference at peak exercise by optimizing the ratio of $P_{A_{O_2}}/P_{50}$ also minimizes the A-V P_{CO_2} difference required for a given CO_2 output by virtue of the Haldane effect (Fig. 12.3); the latter will keep the $[H^+]$ in exercising muscle at a minimum, thereby preserving contractile function. Thus, optimizing oxygen transport by shifts in the P_{50} will automatically optimize CO_2 transport by the reciprocal actions of the Bohr and Haldane effects.

METHODS OF ASSESSMENT

Rates of Inert Gas Mixing in the Lung

As discussed earlier under Diffusive Gas Transport, gas mixing in the respiratory zone of the lung involves convective as well as diffusive mechanisms, and the complexity of the gas phase transport process raises questions about adequacy of mixing, not only at rest but also during exercise. In fact, one could argue that mixing is challenged more during exercise than at rest. To assess the adequacy of gas mixing, methods have been devised to separate diffusive and convective mechanisms.

The obvious tactic for examining the diffusive component of gas mixing is to compare mixing of two (or more) gases with different molecular weights. Kinetic theory accords all gas molecules at any given temperature the same kinetic energy:

$$(E) = \frac{1}{2} M\dot{V}^2$$

where M is molecular mass and $\dot{V}$ is the velocity of random thermally induced molecular movement (i.e., diffusion). Consequently, rates of diffusion should be inversely proportional to $\sqrt{M}$. While mixtures of several different gases may complicate this simple law, molecular weight is still the dominant factor in a given anatomical structure. A further major determinant of overall gas transport in the lung is the physical solubility of the gas. Thus, *poorly soluble* gases that are inhaled can be used to study diffusive components in the airways independently of complicating influences caused by exchange of molecules between alveolar gas and capillary blood. *Soluble* gases, while reflecting gas phase mixing similarly as for insoluble gases, are additionally affected by capillary exchange. Thus, proper choice of test gases can elucidate different components of the gas exchange process.

Such gases can be presented to the lungs either in the inspired gas, forcing net gas uptake into the blood, or in the venous blood perfusing the lungs, forcing gas elimination from the blood to alveolar gas and then to the environment. The former requires simply the inhalation of the desired gas mixture; the latter method requires initially dissolving the gases to be used in saline or dextrose and a peripheral venous infusion of the mixture. The advantage of the inhaled approach is its simplicity and also the naturally high gas concentrations that can be achieved, enabling high signal-to-noise ratios and therefore the use of rapidly responding analyzers to capture events in short time periods. The disadvantage is that steady-state gas exchange cannot be achieved. The intravenous infusion technique suffers from lower signal-to-noise ratio but does enable steady-state exchange to be studied simultaneously.

Several such approaches have been applied, although relatively few during exercise. While the initial question is always, Is there evidence of incomplete gas mixing on the basis of insufficient time for diffusive process?, a second and more practical question becomes, If so, what is its quantitative importance for a gas like O_2? Does such a mixing defect significantly affect arterial oxygenation?

Inhaled Techniques

Single breath. A convenient gas pair used to evaluate gas mixing is He and SF_6. Their molecular weight ratio of 146/4 predicts a roughly sixfold difference in gas phase diffusion coefficient. Their advantage is their extremely low blood solubility (partition coefficient of 0.01 or less, implying that at equilibrium, 99% of the molecules will remain in the gas phase). Inhalation of a single bolus of a mixture of He and SF_6, followed by mass spectrometric measurement of the concentration on succeeding expirations, has been a classic method (185). Impaired diffusive mixing would be evident from a separation of the alveolar plateaus based on molecular weight, providing an index of how deeply each gas penetrated into the lung acinus.

Multiple breath washout. A more complex approach based on similar general principles has been evolved by Engel, Crawford, and Paiva using the conventional multibreath N_2 washout (48). Here, the slope of the alveolar plateau is measured on each breath after replacing inspired air with pure O_2. This method gives information on the interaction between diffusive and convective processes in gas mixing, but details of the technique are beyond the scope of this chapter.

Infusion Techniques

Two inert gases with similar solubilities but different molecular weights. Simultaneous intravenous infusion of solutions of two dissolved gases of different molecular weights was first used by Adaro and Farhi (1). Acetylene (MW = 26) and a fluorocarbon (MW = 85.5) of similar solubility give a 1.8-fold difference in rates of diffusion that can be exploited to determine steady-state consequences of incomplete diffusive mixing. Another gas pair that has been employed is He and SF_6 (221). The physiological limitation of these methods is in the fact that blood solubilities are not identical between such gas pairs. How to adjust for such solubility differences requires quantitative knowledge of the ventilation/perfusion distribution within the lung—these data are not generally available. Small differences in solubility can considerably affect interpretation of apparent effects of differences in molecular weight.

Multiple inert gases with widely different solubilities and molecular weights. To overcome the above limitations, a "cocktail" of several inert gases of different solubilities *and* molecular weights can be infused. While seemingly more complex than the two-gas pair, the advantage is that the effects of different solubilities are accounted for, leaving molecular weight differences detectable if present. More specifically, the differential elimination of the various gases in the cocktail is used to calculate a *convectively based* $\dot{V}_A\backslash\dot{Q}$ distribution (of blood flow and ventilation). In so doing, a computer algorithm fits the measured elimination data to a simple convective model of compartmental $\dot{V}_A$, $\dot{Q}$, and thus $\dot{V}_A\backslash\dot{Q}$ ratio. The bottom line is that if this mathematical fit is adequate (i.e., within the range expected from experimental error), additional influences due to molecular weight differences cannot be recognizably present. On the other hand, significant molecular weight–based perturbations due to impaired diffusive mixing will produce a poor mathematical fit to the inert gas data. Such poor fits are distinguished from simple measurement error because the former will be nonrandom; higher molecular weight gases will yield a poorer fit because they are less efficiently eliminated than those of lower molecular weight, owing to the lower gas phase diffusivity of the higher molecular weight gases (126, 209).

Ventilation/Perfusion ($\dot{V}_A/\dot{Q}$) Relationships

It is generally accepted that while diffusive processes play a role in gas mixing and exchange, particularly during exercise and at altitude (see below), the phenomenon of convective $\dot{V}_A/\dot{Q}$ inequality can also be important in interfering with O_2 uptake (and CO_2 output) in the lung. $\dot{V}_A/\dot{Q}$ inequality is defined as the occurrence within the lung of regions whose *ratio* of ventilation ($\dot{V}_A$) to blood flow ($\dot{Q}$) vary from one another. If all alveoli had the same *ratio* of $\dot{V}_A$ to $\dot{Q}$ this ratio would equal the ratio of total lung alveolar ventilation to cardiac output; there would be no $\dot{V}_A/\dot{Q}$ inequality and the most commonly used parameter of $\dot{V}_A/\dot{Q}$ inequality, the alveolar-arterial P_{O_2} difference, would be zero, assuming no diffusion-limited exchange.

The assessment of inequality is not easy. The traditional approaches have been to use measurements of gas exchange to infer $\dot{V}_A/\dot{Q}$ inequality, but the preceding section should make one aware that $\dot{V}_A/\dot{Q}$ inequality, which is based on convective distribution of $\dot{V}_A$ and $\dot{Q}$ to the alveoli, is not the only factor influencing gas exchange: incomplete diffusive mixing, discussed above, as well as other phenomena such as intrapulmonary and postpulmonary shunts will, if present, interfere with O_2 exchange. Thus, to be useful in identifying $\dot{V}_A/\dot{Q}$ inequality, it becomes necessary to have tools that can dissect apart these various contributing factors, or to develop other methods that are not subject to these uncertainties. This has been a daunting problem, and while relatively good approaches have been developed, not all problems have yet been solved as will be indicated.

Use of Radioactive Tracer Techniques to Assess $\dot{V}_A/\dot{Q}$ Inequality. In clinical medicine, patients suspected of pulmonary embolism are routinely examined by radioactive scanning methods that produce independent topographical maps of blood flow and of ventilation. Radioactive xenon or krypton can be inhaled and then exhaled over several breaths and the regional radioactivity disappearance curve recorded by a gamma camera. This yields a regional map of ventilation rates (that can be referenced to regional gas volume). In the same patient, corresponding tracer techniques can be used to mark the regional distribution of blood flow. Broad patterns of $\dot{V}A/\dot{Q}$ distribution can be directly measured in this way both at rest and moderate exercise; however, the limited spatial resolution of this approach does not reveal all of the $\dot{V}A/\dot{Q}$ inequality actually present, since mismatch is evidently occurring at anatomical levels too small to be identified by the gamma camera.

The Alveolar–Arterial PO_2 Difference. Based on the concept of "ideal" alveolar gas, alveolar oxygen tension (PA_{O_2}) can be calculated by substituting the measured arterial CO_2 tension (Pa_{CO_2}) for the alveolar CO_2 tension in equation 7. Subtracting the measured arterial PO_2 (Pa_{O_2}) from this calculated value of "ideal" PA_{O_2}, the classical parameter, AaP_{O_2} (the alveolar-arterial PO_2 difference). In a perfectly homogeneous lung with an infinite diffusing capacity, alveolar and arterial PO_2 are the same and AaP_{O_2} = 0; regional inequalities of $\dot{V}A/\dot{Q}$ causes AaP_{O_2} to increase. As $\dot{V}A/\dot{Q}$ inequality progressively gets worse, Pa_{O_2} falls but Pa_{CO_2} rises only little if at all (assuming adequate ventilatory compensation), and the AaP_{O_2} therefore will correspondingly increase. However, *any* cause of inadequate gas exchange such as *(1)* incomplete diffusive gas mixing in lung acini, *(2)* diffusion limitation of O_2 transfer across the blood-gas barrier, and *(3)* intrapulmonary and *(4)* extrapulmonary right to left shunt will also produce an increase in AaP_{O_2}.

Consequently, the AaP_{O_2} is a general index of inadequate gas exchange and *not* solely reflective of any one physiological limitation. Its strength is its availability and ease of application, its weakness is its lack of specificity.

To improve the resolution in detecting increases in AaP_{O_2} due to $\dot{V}A/\dot{Q}$ mismatch and those due to diffusion limitation, Lilienthal, Riley, and co-workers 50 years ago showed that if $\dot{V}A/\dot{Q}$ inequality or shunt is responsible, alveolar hypoxia will dramatically reduce the AaP_{O_2} (158). Conversely, if the AaP_{O_2} is caused by diffusion limitation, it will become accentuated by alveolar hypoxia. The effects of alveolar hypoxia are even more pronounced during exercise, where the reduced red cell transmit time in the lung capillaries (i.e., low $DL/\dot{Q}c$) accentuates any such diffusion limitation. Thus, measurements of the AaP_{O_2} (during exercise) made breathing both air and hypoxic gas (FI_{O_2} 0.12–0.15 is typical) give additional insight into causes of gas exchange inefficiency. This approach does have its limitations, however, because both $\dot{V}A/\dot{Q}$ mismatch and diffusion limitation are usually present during heavy exercise and many combinations of the two could be present and compatible with a given set of findings. Another potential source of error is that $\dot{V}A/\dot{Q}$ mismatch often changes when different gas mixtures are breathed.

The Multiple Inert Gas Elimination Technique (MIGET) to Assess $\dot{V}A/\dot{Q}$ Mismatch. Because of the above problems, approaches were developed some years ago to directly measure the distribution of $\dot{V}A/\dot{Q}$ ratios. The most well-developed of these has become known as the MIGET and uses a simple principle: quantitative exchange of any inert gas (in the steady state) is a unique function of the solubility of the gas (in blood) and the $\dot{V}A/\dot{Q}$ ratio of lung region that is exchanging the gas. This function is given by the following equation:

$$PA = Pc' = P\bar{v} \cdot \left(\frac{\lambda}{\lambda + \dot{V}A/\dot{Q}}\right)$$

where PA = alveolar gas tension, Pc' = end-capillary gas tension, $P\bar{v}$ is pulmonary artery (mixed venous) gas tension, λ is the partition coefficient (blood solubility), and $\dot{V}A/\dot{Q}$ is the $\dot{V}A/\dot{Q}$ ratio of a small homogeneous lung region. This equation assumes *no* diffusion limitation for the inert gas (i.e., $PA = Pc'$) and is derived from simple steady-state mass conservation considerations (141).

Because λ is easily measured in vitro, in vivo measurements of PA (or Pc') and $P\bar{v}$ provide the data necessary to calculate the $\dot{V}A/\dot{Q}$ ratio of the homogeneous lung region from the above equation.

However, one can measure only mixed expired, mixed venous, and mixed arterial inert gas levels—not levels for each small homogeneous unit. We then must add up the contributions (using the above equation for each unit) of all lung units, weighting the contribution of each unit by its fractional blood flow:

$$P_{\overline{ARTERIAL}} = P\bar{v} \cdot \sum \dot{Q} \left(\frac{\lambda}{\lambda + \dot{V}A/\dot{Q}}\right)$$

$$P_{\overline{EXPIRED}} = P\bar{v} \cdot \sum \dot{V}A \left(\frac{\lambda}{\lambda + \dot{V}A/\dot{Q}}\right)$$

From measurement of $P_{\overline{ARTERIAL}}$, $P_{\overline{EXPIRED}}$, $P\bar{v}$, and λ and appropriate computer-assisted mathematical analysis, it is possible to calculate over the $\dot{V}A/\dot{Q}$ range present in the lung, the quantitative values of $\dot{V}A$ and $\dot{Q}$ that have to be present to account for the measured mean arterial and expired concentrations. The more gases we use (with different values of λ), the more information will be obtained. Ideally, we need as many different gases as there are different $\dot{V}A/\dot{Q}$ regions, but it has been repeatedly shown that a satisfactory analysis is routinely possible using only six gases of well-chosen λ (solubility values: low, medium, and high) (63, 73, 204). Successful application of MIGET also demands high experimental accuracy. Thus, gas concentrations (measured by gas chromatography) must have no more than ±5% coefficient of variation (CV), and the data will be that much more precise if this can be further reduced. Most laboratories can achieve a ±3% CV with good techniques.

MIGET thus directly determines the extent and pattern of $\dot{V}A/\dot{Q}$ mismatch. It does so even if there is alveolar-capillary diffusion limitation for O_2 causing an AaP_{O_2}, because the inert gases used are invulnerable to diffusion limitation in any lungs that are still able to sustain enough O_2 uptake for survival (70). MIGET also separates $\dot{V}A/\dot{Q}$ inequality from right to left *intrapulmonary* shunting, which it quantifies directly along with the $\dot{V}A/\dot{Q}$ distribution. MIGET will not detect *postpulmonary* right-to-left shunting, however (i.e., bronchial or thebesian venous admixture).

Because MIGET is insensitive to alveolar-capillary diffusion limitation that could affect O_2, it provides an intrinsically simple way to quantify O_2 diffusion limitation: the MIGET-determined $\dot{V}A/\dot{Q}$ distribution, based only on inert gas data, can be used to compute an expected value for AaP_{O_2}, using standard computer algorithms (275). If the AaP_{O_2} so predicted agrees with the actual value of AaP_{O_2} measured simultaneously but independently of MIGET, there can be no diffusion limitation for O_2 across the blood-gas barrier (or postpulmonary shunt). If, on the other hand, the measured AaP_{O_2} exceeds the value predicted from the MIGET data, either diffusion limitation or a postpulmonary shunt must be present. Application of this technique to estimate DL_{O_2} is discussed in the next section (see later under Extension of the MIGET Technique to Measure DL_{O_2}).

Finally, as mentioned earlier, the MIGET can also be used to assess completeness of gas phase diffusive mixing by looking for a poor fit between the measured inert gas data and the $\dot{V}A/\dot{Q}$ distribution that comes closest to matching these data.

MIGET measurements can be carried out at rest and during exercise at any desired FI_{O_2}. A necessary condition is a steady state of gas exchange (just as for using the AaP_{O_2}). Since exercise, especially of high intensity, cannot be endured for long periods, it becomes important to address this issue to avoid misinterpreting data. This can be approached experimentally by making two or more entire MIGET measurements in rapid time sequence. This is feasible because, while the inert gases used are being continuously infused into a peripheral vein, to make a measurement requires only the withdrawal of about 7 ml of arterial (± mixed venous) blood and 20 ml of mixed expired gas, all over a 10–20 s period. With all subsequent analysis performed off-line, such multiple measurements are feasible and become very useful to establish a steady state. A steady state would be inferred if the multiple measurements all gave the same $\dot{V}A/\dot{Q}$ distribution rather than revealing some progressive trend. At a theoretical level, the approach to steady-state gas exchange after a step change in inert gas infusion, ventilation, or cardiac output is explained by a single exponential function describing classic compartmental kinetics:

$$P_{(t)} = P_{(o)}e^{-kt}$$

where $P_{(o)}$ is inert gas tension prior to the step change, $P_{(t)}$ is subsequent tension at time t, and k is the rate constant equal to the conductance (of the lung) for the inert gas divided by the storage capacitance (of the lung) for the inert gas. Conductance (C) occurs by ventilation and perfusion so that

$$C = \dot{V}A + \lambda\dot{Q}$$

while capacitance (CAP) reflects storage in gas and tissue spaces:

$$CAP = VOL + \lambda Vt$$

Here VOL = lung gas volume and Vt is lung tissue volume. Thus,

$$k = \frac{\dot{V}A + \lambda\dot{Q}}{VOL + \lambda Vt}$$

For an insoluble gas (small λ), k approximates $\dot{V}A/VOL$ (k_{INSOL}). For a soluble gas (large λ), k approximates $\dot{Q}/Vt$ (k_{SOL}). At rest, $\dot{V}A \approx \dot{Q} \approx 6$ liters/min; VOL = FRC ≈ 4 liters; and Vt approximates 0.6 liters.

$$k_{INSOL} = 6/4 = 1.5 \text{ min}^{-1}$$

$$k_{SOL} = 6/0.6 = 10 \text{ min}^{-1}$$

Thus, for 99% equilibration (experimentally indistinguishable from a steady state), an insoluble gas requires only 3 min ([Ln 100] ÷ 1.5) and a soluble gas only 30 s ([Ln 100] ÷ 10).

During exercise, VOL and VT can be taken to be unchanged for the purposes of these calculations, but $\dot{V}A$ can exceed 100 liters/min while $\dot{V}T$ commonly reaches 25 liters/min.

$$\therefore k_{INSOL} = 100/4 = 25 \text{ min}^{-1}$$

and

$$k_{SOL} = 25/0.6 = 42 \text{ min}^{-1}$$

with 99% time to steady state thus being 11 s for the insoluble gas and 7 s for the soluble gas. Generally, even heavy exercise lasts 3–4 min, so that for

MIGET purposes, the lungs are in an adequate steady state for appropriate data interpretation.

Diffusing Capacity of the Lung

Carbon Monoxide Diffusing Capacity (DL_{CO}) and the Controversy over O_2 Secretion. The carbon monoxide method for measuring diffusing capacity arose in response to a controversy over whether oxygen uptake in the lung could be entirely explained by simple diffusion or whether active oxygen secretion must occur. Although there was no method for collecting arterial blood or directly measuring blood oxygen tension at the turn of this century, Haldane and Smith in 1896 reported an ingenious method for indirect estimation of arterial oxygen tension (Pa_{O_2}) from venous blood (89). A subject breathed a small inspired CO tension (PI_{CO}), about 0.3 mm Hg, until CO uptake stopped and venous blood was fully equilibrated with the inspired CO tension (i.e., $Sa_{CO} = Sv_{CO}$). Use was made of the fact that hemoglobin has a binding affinity for CO that is over 200 times that for O_2 (equation 15). After equilibrium, arterial blood would be fully saturated with about 35% CO and 65% O_2 (i.e., $Sa_{O_2} = 1 - Sv_{CO}$ where saturation is expressed as a fraction). Since at equilibrium $Pa_{CO} = PI_{CO}$, Pa_{O_2} could be calculated directly from venous CO–hemoglobin saturation using equation 15. They unexpectedly found that arterial O_2 tension exceeded alveolar O_2 tension. They concluded that O_2 must be actively secreted into blood. Based on the original data of Haldane and Smith, Bohr made the first measurements of CO diffusing capacity (DL_{CO}) (21). Bohr recognized that, because of the high affinity of hemoglobin for CO, CO back-pressure would be negligibly small during the early part of equilibration in the subjects that Haldane and Smith studied and that it should be possible to estimate DL_{CO} from the rate of CO uptake ($\dot{V}_{CO}$) divided by the alveolar CO tension (equation 16). Thus, Bohr estimated resting DL_{CO} from the careful measurements of Haldane and Smith. Then, using Graham's law (equation 17) and assuming a watery alveolar capillary membrane, he translated his estimates into terms of DL_{O_2} (i.e., $DL_{O_2} = 1.23 \cdot DL_{CO}$). Using his famous Bohr integral (equations 30, 32, and 39), he estimated the DL_{O_2} required to sustain a maximal oxygen uptake of 2552 ml/min by diffusive transport alone would be about 38 ml $\cdot$ min^{-1} $\cdot$ mm Hg^{-1}; the DL_{O_2} estimated from the resting CO measurements of Haldane and Smith was 16.1 ml $\cdot$ min^{-1} $\cdot$ mm Hg^{-1}. Thus, Bohr interpreted his calculations as indicating simple diffusion alone was inadequate to support exercise O_2 uptake, consistent with Haldane's oxygen secretion theory. Bohr's conclusions were in error because he failed to consider that DL_{CO} might increase with exercise. A year later, 1910, Marie and August Krogh reported that DL_{CO} measured by a breath-holding method increased from rest to exercise to a level that was adequate to explain oxygen uptake by simple diffusion. It was Marie Krogh's arguments and expanded measurements of DL_{CO} at rest and exercise, in her doctoral thesis published in 1914, that signaled the beginning of the end of the oxygen secretion hypothesis. Accurate estimates of alveolar-arterial oxygen tension differences were necessary for its final demise.

Lilienthal-Riley Method for Measuring O_2 Diffusing Capacity (DL_{O_2}). Reliable estimates of arterial oxygen tension were also required to lay the groundwork for a more direct method for estimating oxygen diffusing capacity. A method was introduced in the mid-1940s by Lilienthal, Riley, and associates (158) for estimating the relative importance of uneven $\dot{V}A/\dot{Q}c$ ratios and a low ratio of diffusing capacity to blood flow ($DL/\dot{Q}c$) as sources of a measured AaP_{O_2} difference at rest or exercise. The method is based on the fact that the portion of the AaP_{O_2} attributable to diffusion limitation is accentuated and that portion due to regions of unequal $\dot{V}A/\dot{Q}c$ ratios is reduced by breathing a low inspired oxygen tension. By making repeated measurements of blood gas exchange for O_2 and CO_2 at rest and exercise, breathing two or more different inspired oxygen concentrations, these investigators partitioned the measured AaP_{O_2} between a component caused by $\dot{V}A/\dot{Q}c$ nonuniformity and another caused by alveolar capillary diffusion limitation. From these data they calculated an end-capillary oxygen saturation (Sc'_{O_2}); using an assumed or measured mixed venous oxygen saturation ($S\bar{v}_{O_2}$), they employed equation 32 (with the famous Bohr integral) to estimate DL_{O_2}. Previous to these estimates, DL_{O_2} could only be indirectly estimated from DL_{CO}. Since the method requires measurements of the AaP_{O_2} at different inspired oxygen concentrations at rest and exercise, there is an implicit assumption that changing inspired oxygen tension does not alter the distribution of blood flow, ventilation, or diffusing capacity. The latter assumption has been shown to be unreliable and hence a potential source of significant error (90, 255); nevertheless, the method has been of conceptual importance and has provided estimates of DL_{O_2} at heavy exercise that are within a reasonable range.

Extension of the MIGET Technique to Measure DL_{O_2}. The Lilienthal-Riley method for measuring DL_{O_2} has been conceptually expanded in the past 20 years to employ measurements of blood gas exchange of CO_2

and O_2 simultaneously with the MIGET (255, 256); this combination of techniques can define patterns of multicompartment $\dot{V}A/\dot{Q}c$ distributions in the lung as well as estimates of that component of the AaP_{O_2} attributable to diffusion disequilibrium. Thus, knowing the distribution of $\dot{V}A/\dot{Q}c$ ratios in a multicompartment lung with respect to blood flow and alveolar ventilation in each compartment and knowing inspired and mixed venous gas concentrations, it is possible to estimate the equilibrium blood gas and alveolar concentrations that should exist in each compartment (Fig. 12.4). Mixed alveolar and arterial blood gas tensions can also be calculated from the fractional contributions made by each compartment to expired alveolar air and arterial blood. This yields a predicted AaP_{O_2} from the inert gas measurements to compare with those estimated by direct blood gas measurements. If the directly measured AaP_{O_2} is larger than that predicted from MIGET, incomplete diffusion equilibrium is suggested. Hammond and Hempleman, assuming a uniform $DL/\dot{Q}c$ among compartments, estimated how low $DL/\dot{Q}c$ would have to be in order to explain the measured AaP_{O_2} discrepancy between measurement and prediction by MIGET (91, 104); knowing total cardiac output DL_{O_2} can be estimated. A separate estimate can be made based on similar principles assuming the same $DL/\dot{V}A$ among the compartments. These methods yield more reliable and reproducible results during measurements at exercise and at low inspired oxygen tensions, which accentuate diffusion limitations.

Current Methods for DL_{CO} Three basic methods now exist: *(1)* steady state, *(2)* breath-holding, and *(3)* rebreathing, all modifications of the original methods of Bohr and of August and Marie Krogh.

Steady state. The steady-state method, a modification of the original Bohr technique, was introduced by Filley in 1954 (67) and modified by Bates in 1955 (11). It involves having a subject inspire a gas mixture containing a small concentration of CO (~ 0.1%) during normal breathing at rest or exercise by an open-circuit technique until a steady state of CO uptake ($\dot{V}CO$) is achieved; DL_{CO} is estimated with equation 16. Advantages of the steady-state method are that it can be applied during normal breathing and can easily be used for exercise measurements. Disadvantages are that it is susceptible to variability caused by uneven distribution of ventilation even in normal subjects. There is a high variability in resting measurements; exercise measurements are much more stable.

Single breath. In the original Krogh breath-holding method, the subject exhaled fully to residual volume (RV) and then rapidly inspired air containing 0.3% or 0.4% CO from a spirometer to TLC; this was followed by rapid exhalation to midway between TLC and FRC, where an initial end-tidal gas sample was collected to measure the alveolar CO fraction (FA_1); the breath was then held 10–15 s (Δt) followed by a rapid exhalation to obtain a second sample (FA_2). DL_{CO} was estimated by the following equation:

$$DL_{CO} = \frac{60 \cdot VA\ (STPD)}{(PB - PH_2O)} \cdot \frac{LnFA_1/FA_2}{\Delta t} \qquad (40)$$

where VA is the volume of the lung at breath-holding, estimated as (RV + inspired volume − the volume of the first exhalation) and converted to standard conditions (STPD). One objection to this method was that it required two expired samples that might not represent the same region of lung. Forster and associates (181) modified the original Krogh breath-holding method in an important and innovative way by adding insoluble, inert He to the inspired mixture. DL_{CO} could be estimated from one alveolar sample collected at the end of breath-holding. The initial CO concentration could be calculated from the helium dilution. Otherwise the technique was the same. The subject exhales to RV followed by rapid inspiration of a gas mixture containing 0.3% CO (FI_{CO}) and 10% He (FI_{He}) in air or oxygen to a measured lung volume; the breath is held a measured time interval (Δt) and then rapidly exhaled to measure end-tidal alveolar fractional concentrations of He and CO, FA_{He} and FA_{CO}, respectively. The initial alveolar CO fraction (FA_{CO_0}) is estimated from the helium dilution, $FA_{CO_0} = FI_{CO} \cdot (FA_{He}/FI_{He})$. DL_{CO} is estimated from the following modification of equation 40 (subscripts for CO are eliminated for simplicity):

$$DL_{CO} = \frac{60 \cdot VA\ (STPD)}{(PB - PH_2O)} \cdot \frac{LnFA_o/FA}{\Delta t} \qquad (41)$$

The original Ogilvie-Forster technique (181) measured Δt from the start of inspiration to end of alveolar gas collection; the Jones-Meade method includes 0.7 of the inspiratory time and half of the sampling time (136) and provides a more reproducible measurement.

There are two modifications of the single-breath method that may have special applications.

THREE-EQUATION METHOD. This is a refinement of the single-breath technique that takes into account the fact that CO disappears differently during the inspiratory and expiratory components of the single breath than during the period of breath-holding (82, 166). Inspiration, breath-holding, and expiration each require a separate equation to describe CO disappearance. There is no closed solution to these equations; DL must be determined by an iterative method assuming that DL remains constant throughout all maneuvers.

SLOW-EXHALATION METHOD. This is a method that takes advantage of the fact that disappearance of CO after inspiration of a small CO concentration can be continuously followed during a subsequent slow exhalation (163, 179). The equation utilized is the same as the slow-exhalation equation in the previous section. Estimates of DL can be made over arbitrarily small segments of $\Delta \dot{V}E$ and Δt throughout exhalation if gas concentrations and expired volumes are continuously followed. This method has the advantage that cardiac output can also be measured simultaneously with DL_{CO} at rest and light exercise if acetylene is excluded in the gas mixture (128).

REBREATHING. The rebreathing technique was originally introduced by Lewis in the 1950s (157) and modified later by Sackner to include acetylene for measuring pulmonary blood flow and tissue volume (216). The current technique involves having a subject rebreathe a gas mixture from an anesthesia bag containing 0.3%–0.4% CO; 0.4%–0.6% acetylene; and an inert and relatively insoluble tracer gas such as He, Ne, or CH_4 in a balance of oxygen and nitrogen. The mixture is rebreathed from the bag for 6–15 s. Volume of gas mixture in the bag is set to whatever tidal volume is desired and the subject is instructed to empty the bag with each inspiration. Gas concentrations at the mouth are followed continuously with a rapid gas analyzer. The inert insoluble gas (e.g., He) is rapidly diluted during rebreathing and exponentially approaches a constant alveolar concentration (FA_{He}); from dilution of the inert insoluble gas ($FA_{He}\infty/FI_{He}$) the volume of the lung and rebreathing system (Vs) is calculated:

$$Vs\ (STPD) = VB \frac{FI_{He}}{FA_{He}\infty} \cdot \frac{PB}{760} \cdot \frac{273}{(273 + t)}$$

where t is room temperature in degrees Celsius, PB is barometric pressure in mm Hg, and gas fractions are measured dry. Diffusing capacity and pulmonary blood flow ($\dot{Q}c$) are estimated from the negative slopes, (m)CO and (m)C_2H_2, respectively, of the time decay in minutes of the natural logarithms of end-tidal FA_{CO} and $FA_{C_2H_2}$ with respect to FA_{He} during rebreathing.

$$DL_{CO} = \frac{Vs}{(PB - PH_2O)} \cdot (m)CO$$

$$\dot{Q}c = (Vs + \alpha_t V_t) \cdot \frac{760}{\alpha_b(PB - PH_2O)} \cdot (m)C_2H_2$$

where α_t and α_b are Bunsen solubility coefficients of acetylene in tissue and blood, respectively, at body temperature; V_t is fine septal tissue volume in the lung. V_t is estimated from the initial dilution of acetylene in fine septal tissues; this dilution is estimated from the depression of the intercept of the relationship between $LnFA_{C_2H_2}/FA_{He}$ and time of rebreathing obtained by extrapolation to time = 0. Tissue dilution = the ratio (R) of $FA_{C_2H_2}/FA_{He}$ measured from the intercept to that predicted from the inspired gas mixture, $FI_{C_2H_2}/FI_{He}$:

$$V_t = \frac{Vs}{\alpha_t \cdot R} \cdot (1 - R)$$

Acetylene measurements of cardiac output have been validated against both dye dilution (244) and standard Fick measurements (124) at rest and heavy exercise.

The rebreathing technique has the advantages of being applicable to heavy exercise, requiring little cooperation from the subject, allowing simultaneous measurements of cardiac output, and minimizing effects of uneven distribution of ventilation with respect to blood flow and diffusing capacity by continual mixing of the gases in the lung. It has the disadvantages of being more expensive and complex.

Roughton-Forster Technique for Separating DL_{CO} into its Component Parts. By making measurements of DL_{CO} at more than one oxygen tension, it is possible to utilize the Roughton-Forster equation (equation 18) to solve for the membrane diffusing capacity (DM_{CO}) and the pulmonary capillary volume (Vc); the goal is then to use equation 18 to translate measurements of DM_{CO} and Vc into terms of oxygen diffusing capacity (DL_{O_2}). This is exactly what August and Marie Krogh were trying to accomplish in 1910 and 1914 as a means of examining the oxygen secretion hypothesis of Haldane. One problem with application of the Roughton-Forster technique has been the uncertainty about θ, the specific rate of uptake of CO by red cells at different oxygen tensions. As can be seen in Table 12.5 the slopes and intercepts of the relationship between $1/\theta$ and PO_2 extend over a seemingly wide range obtained in different laboratories, often using different methods. On the other hand, when the combined data are plotted together within the physiologic range at which measurements are made, the results yield a reasonably close relationship, with a correlation coefficient of 0.91 and a slope and intercept close to that originally reported by Roughton, Forster, and Cander.

Recently, the nitric oxide and CO methods have been used simultaneously as a means of eliminating the requirement of measuring DL_{CO} at more than one oxygen tension to measure DM_{CO} and Vc. Since θNO is exceedingly high, the $1/\theta Vc$ term in equation 18 becomes negligibly small for NO uptake; hence DL_{NO} is taken to be equivalent to DM_{NO}. Based on Graham's law, then $DM_{CO} = 0.418 \times DL_{NO}$. From simultaneous measurements of DL_{CO} and DL_{NO}, Vc can be estimated as follows:

$$Vc = \frac{1}{\theta NO} \cdot \frac{0.418 DL_{NO} DL_{CO}}{DL_{CO} - 0.418 DL_{NO}}$$

Using this technique yields values of DM_{CO} and Vc that are not significantly different from those estimated by the original Roughton-Forster method.

We have used the standard Roughton-Forster equation listed in Table 12.5 for comparisons of DL_{CO}, DL_{O_2}, and DL_{NO} in the next section.

Nitric Oxide Method. Nitric oxide is also a primary ligand of hemoglobin that combines with the heme binding sites more rapidly than does O_2 and binds more tightly than does CO (Table 12.3). With these attributes, NO should also be an ideal gas for measuring diffusing capacity of the lung, and its use has been pioneered by three groups (23, 85, 173). Measurements can be made with a mass spectrometer or with a chemiluminescence analyzer using identical computational algorithms as are used for carbon monoxide; the breath-holding or rebreathing methods can be employed (85, 173). Since the reaction kinetics between NO and hemoglobin is so rapid, red cell resistance to NO uptake ($1/\theta NO$) in the context of the Roughton-Forster equation (equation 18) is considered negligible; the principal resistance to NO uptake in the lung should be the alveolar capillary membrane.

Comparisons of DL_{CO}, DL_{O_2}, and DL_{NO} at Rest and Exercise. Results using the rebreathing technique in 22 normal subjects are summarized in Figure 12.13; 4 males and 18 females ranging in age from 17 to 54. Included are six Olympic bicyclists on the 1968 Swedish team. Measurements were made at rest, at an intermediate workload and at maximal oxygen uptake. DL_{CO}, DM_{CO}, and Vc all increased from rest to maximal exercise.

The data in Figure 12.13 have been translated into terms of DL_{O_2} and DL_{NO} using the Roughton-Forster equation. The assumptions are based on data from Tables 12.3, 12.4, and 12.5 that $\theta O_2 = 3.9\ min^{-1} \cdot mm\ Hg^{-1}$, $\theta NO = \infty$, $DM_{O_2} = 1.15 \times DM_{CO}$, and that $DM_{NO} = 2.39 \times DM_{CO}$. DL_{O_2} by the different methods are compared with respect to simultaneous measurements of both pulmonary blood flow and oxygen uptake where this is possible (Fig. 12.14). Measurements of DL_{NO} are only available at rest, and neither oxygen uptakes or cardiac outputs are recorded. In order to make the comparisons in Figure 12.14C, a normal cardiac index was assumed.

Important information is available from these comparisons:

1. All of the techniques give similar results, suggesting that all measure approximately the same thing.
2. Diffusing capacity increases with exercise; if it didn't, as originally pointed out by Bohr, diffusion limitation should be apparent at relatively low levels of exercise.
3. No clear plateau in the relationship between DL and $\dot{Q}c$ exists, which is surprising because it seems obvious that an upper limit should exist; the sources of continued recruitment are unclear.
4. The relationship between DL and $\dot{V}O_2$ for the same data does suggest an upper limit; however, this may simply be a consequence of the alinear relationship between oxygen uptake and cardiac output that is apparent early in exercise.

PULMONARY GAS EXCHANGE DURING EXERCISE

This section will complement and integrate with the preceding ones dealing with basic and methodological approaches. First, changes in arterial blood gases in response to exercise are described. Subsequently, based on the methods described earlier, physiological interpretation of these data is presented. Finally, speculation on the structural and physiological basis of normal blood gas responses is offered.

Changes in Arterial PCO_2 and PO_2 at Incremental Workloads

In general, exercise-induced changes from values at rest have to be interpreted with care because resting data commonly reflect hyperventilation. Consequently, resting arterial PO_2 is unusually high and PCO_2 low. For a young normal subject aged 20–40, a truly resting arterial blood sample would reveal a PO_2 of 95–100 mm Hg and a PCO_2 of 35–40 mm Hg. Typical values for such subjects anticipating exercise are PO_2 = 100–120 mm Hg and PCO_2 = 25–35 mm Hg, depending on the degree of hyperventilation. Because of reduced arterial PCO_2, tissue CO_2 stores are washed out and transiently, respiratory exchange ratio (R) normally about 0.80–0.85 at rest, increases to 1 or greater. An alveolar-arterial PO_2 difference ($AaPO_2$) calculation assuming a nor-

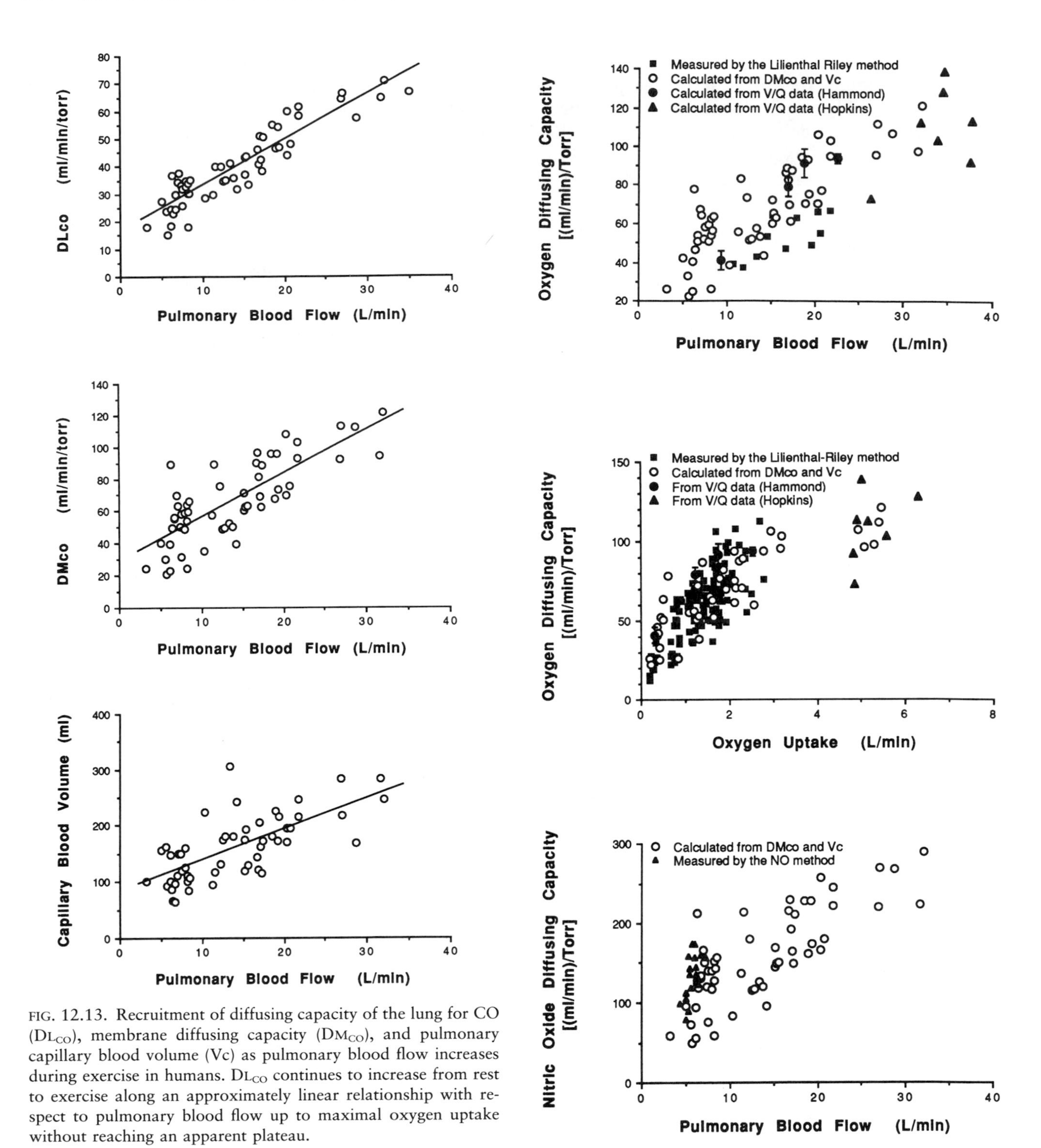

FIG. 12.13. Recruitment of diffusing capacity of the lung for CO (DL_{CO}), membrane diffusing capacity (DM_{CO}), and pulmonary capillary blood volume (Vc) as pulmonary blood flow increases during exercise in humans. DL_{CO} continues to increase from rest to exercise along an approximately linear relationship with respect to pulmonary blood flow up to maximal oxygen uptake without reaching an apparent plateau.

FIG. 12.14. Comparison of DL_{O_2} and DL_{NO} at rest and exercise calculated from the data in Figure 12.13 with measurements of DL_{O_2} by the Lilienthal-Riley technique (40, 158, 228, 229, 248) and by application of MIGET (91, 120) and with measurements of DL_{NO} by a breath-holding method (23, 164). Comparisons are made with respect to blood flow where measurements of cardiac output are available (Panel 1) and with respect to oxygen uptake (Panel b). Neither oxygen uptake nor cardiac output were available for measurements of DL_{NO}, which were all obtained at rest; hence, a cardiac index of 3.0 was assumed for each measurement of DL_{NO}.

mal value of R of 0.8 would yield an artificially small AaP_{O_2}.

As soon as even light exercise begins, arterial P_{O_2} and P_{CO_2} almost always "settle down" and are not systematically different from truly resting values (P_{O_2} 95–100, P_{CO_2} 35–40 mm Hg). As exercise intensity is increased to moderate levels short of pro-

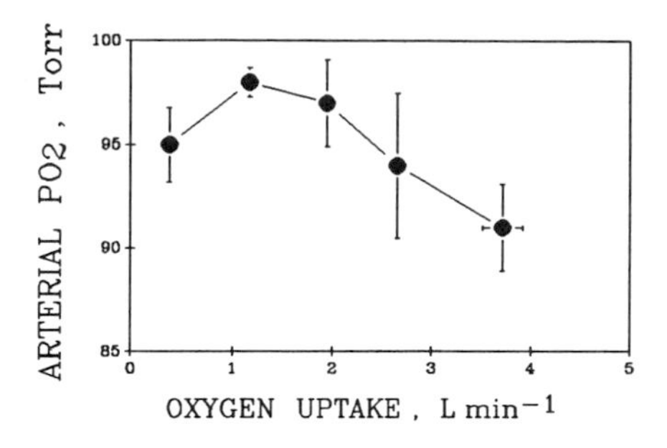

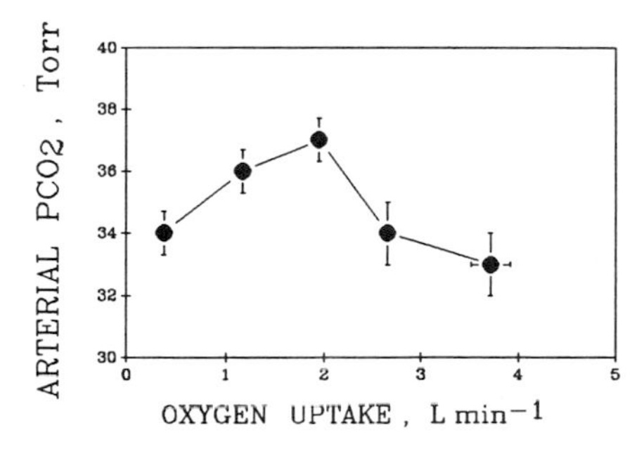

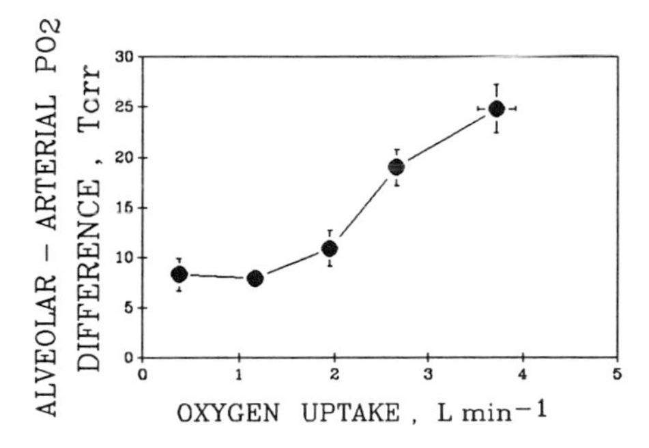

FIG. 12.15. Arterial PO_2, arterial PCO_2, and alveolar–arterial PO_2 difference as a function of exercise intensity (oxygen uptake). At heavy levels of exercise, both arterial PO_2 and PCO_2 fall, and as a result the alveolar–arterial PO_2 difference increases markedly (253).

ducing lactic acidosis, there is little further change in values, although arterial PO_2 may decline slightly. Because of this and a small increase in R, the $AaPO_2$ increases (261).

As the lactic threshold is reached and passed, ventilatory stimulation increases out of proportion to metabolic demand and arterial PCO_2 generally falls to 30–35 mm Hg. Arterial PO_2, on the other hand, does not usually rise as the alveolar gas equation would predict from this change in PCO_2. Rather, PO_2 remains relatively constant or even falls, perhaps to 90–95 mm Hg. This, together with further increases in R to above 1.0, keep the $AaPO_2$ steadily growing as exercise intensity is increased. At such values of PO_2, there is virtually no desaturation of hemoglobin because of the flat O_2 dissociation curve in this region. This is despite the rightward shift of the O_2 dissociation curve produced by the combination of acidosis and increased blood temperature.

In some endurance athletes, at high work intensities, arterial PO_2 falls more substantially to levels in the 60–70 mm Hg range and arterial saturation to less than 90% (55, 213). Figure 12.15 shows the typical progression of PO_2, PCO_2, and $AaPO_2$ with increasing exercise intensity (253).

Physiological Basis of Arterial Blood Gas Changes

The classic framework of the four causes of hypoxemia is a good way to examine the effects of exercise on gas exchange. They are *(1)* hypoventilation, *(2)* right-to-left shunting, *(3)* diffusion limitation, and *(4)* ventilation/perfusion ($\dot{V}A/\dot{Q}$) inequity. In the context of exercise, hypoventilation is a term that expresses a relative insufficiency of ventilation for the metabolic load (i.e., O_2 or CO_2), even as the absolute level of ventilation clearly exceeds resting values. In normal subjects, most workers define such hypoventilation on the basis of arterial PCO_2 being elevated (and conversely, hyperventilation is said to occur when arterial PCO_2 is below normal). This is convenient and eliminates the need for measuring both ventilation and O_2/CO_2 (to more directly assess the presence of hypoventilation). Use of arterial PCO_2 further eliminates the need for knowing fractional airway dead space, which is necessary to compute *alveolar* ventilation from *minute* ventilation.

Note that just as at rest, the $AaPO_2$ will be unaffected by steady-state hyper- or hypoventilation: while hypoventilation causes PO_2 to fall, the corresponding rise in PCO_2 will automatically compensate this fall, resulting in no change in $AaPO_2$.

Since the hallmarks of exercise-induced gas exchange, at least up to moderate exercise levels, are little or no hypoxemia, with a progressive rise in $AaPO_2$ and essentially constant PCO_2, hypoventilation as defined is not able to account for any changes in PO_2/PCO_2 with exercise. However, in elite athletes at or near their peak O_2 levels, some increase in arterial PCO_2 occurs, due probably to insufficient ventilation in relation to extremely high levels of CO_2 output. The corresponding fall in PO_2 (as predicted from the alveolar gas equation) is explained similarly (55). However, any increase in $AaPO_2$ reflects shunt, $\dot{V}A/\dot{Q}$ inequality, or diffusion limitation, alone or in combination.

Intrapulmonary shunt is essentially nonexistent according to many studies using the MIGET (81, 90, 253) as the technique for measuring gas exchange.

Postpulmonary shunt, not directly measurable with any accuracy in intact man, is generally considered to amount to no more than 1% of the cardiac output. This would have no effect on arterial P_{CO_2}, but would cause P_{O_2} to fall by 3–7 mm Hg and AaP_{O_2} to rise by the same amount. While its presence is difficult to determine, the repeated observation that from rest through modest exercise levels (i.e., to two-thirds to three-fourths of peak O_2) the arterial P_{O_2} measured directly is not different from that predicted from simultaneously obtained MIGET data suggests negligible contributions of postpulmonary shunt to arterial P_{O_2}. This conclusion is based on the fact that MIGET does not detect postpulmonary shunts, so that if such were significant, measured arterial P_{O_2} would be less than that predicted by MIGET. This is underscored by the additional observation that due to high O_2 extraction during exercise, postpulmonary shunted blood should have a very low P_{O_2}, making its effect on arterial P_{O_2} that much greater.

Since shunt and hypoventilation are not present, the two reasons for the exercise-induced AaP_{O_2} are therefore $\dot{V}_A/\dot{Q}$ mismatch and diffusion limitation, the only remaining possible factors. A number of studies have documented the development of increased levels of $\dot{V}_A/\dot{Q}$ mismatch in perhaps 50% of normal subjects during exercise. Contrasted to clinically important $\dot{V}_A/\dot{Q}$ mismatch seen in patients with pulmonary diseases, this worsening of $\dot{V}_A/\dot{Q}$ relationships is minimal and accounts for maybe 5–10 mm Hg increase in AaP_{O_2} from rest to $\dot{V}_{O_{2max}}$. Why $\dot{V}_A/\dot{Q}$ inequality worsens is not known; this will be discussed below.

Diffusion limitation of O_2 transport between alveolar gas and capillary blood becomes a contributing factor to the increased AaP_{O_2} of exercise, but only at $\dot{V}_{O_2}$ greater than about 3 liters/min. This is shown by the agreement between measured arterial P_{O_2} and the MIGET-predicted value below such levels of $\dot{V}_{O_2}$ and the progressive disparity between the two at higher exercise levels (MIGET predicted arterial P_{O_2} > measured P_{O_2}), as shown in Figure 12.16. As argued by Piiper and Scheid (193), such diffusion limitation occurs when the *ratio* of the O_2 diffusive conductance of the blood-gas barrier to the blood perfusive conductance of O_2 falls to a value low enough to measurably prevent O_2 equilibration in the available contact time in the lung capillaries. Thus, while diffusive conductance is known to rise progressively with exercise, blood flow rises relatively even more (127). Since blood flow is the major determinant of the blood O_2 perfusive conductance, the above-mentioned conductance ratio falls and evident diffusion limitation ensues.

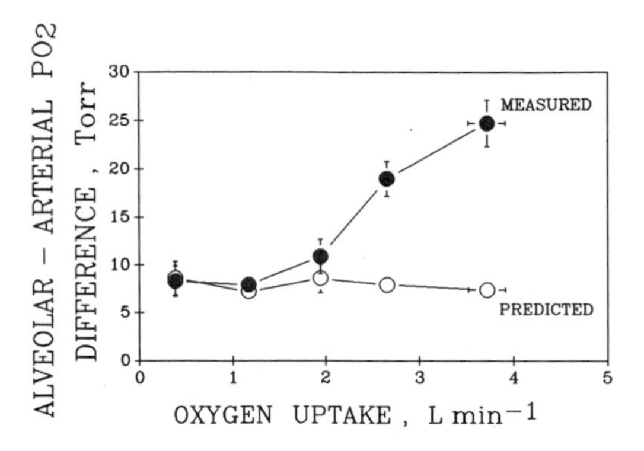

FIG. 12.16. Measured and predicted alveolar–arterial P_{O_2} differences from the same data as in Figure 12.15. The predicted value represents the effects of ventilation–perfusion inequality, while the measured value also includes the effects of diffusion limitation. Up to 2 liter/min $\dot{V}_{O_2}$ ventilation–perfusion inequality accounts for virtually all of the alveolar–arterial P_{O_2} difference. At higher exercise intensities, the contribution of ventilation–perfusion mismatching does not change, while diffusion limitation becomes increasingly important.

Is there evidence of diffusion-limited gas-phase mixing in normal subjects during exercise? The methods described for studying this phenomenon have revealed very minor degrees of impaired exchange of high-molecular-weight gases compared to otherwise similar gases of lower molecular weight, but estimates of the effect of this phenomenon on AaP_{O_2} are on the order of only 1–2 mm Hg. Given that AaP_{O_2} increases from 0–10 mm Hg to 20–40 mm Hg from rest to $\dot{V}_{O_{2max}}$, impaired gas mixing plays essentially no role in the exchange problems of exercise. MIGET data have never revealed molecular weight-determined inert gas exchange, consistent with the above conclusion. Pneumonectomized foxhounds may indeed show such gas-phase mixing impairment based on MIGET data, but even here it is a small (≈ 5%) contributor to the overall AaP_{O_2}.

In summary, the most important contributors to the progressive and considerable increase in AaP_{O_2} with exercise are incomplete alveolar-capillary equilibration due to a fall in $D_L/\dot{Q}$ with exercise coupled with $\dot{V}_A/\dot{Q}$ mismatch. While not contributing to the AaP_{O_2}, insufficient ventilation can additionally depress arterial P_{O_2}, but usually only in truly elite athletes. On the other hand, shunts play a minor and mostly undetectable role. Whether these conclusions apply to older normal subjects during exercise has not been studied. Since such subjects probably have more $\dot{V}_A/\dot{Q}$ mismatch (at rest) than younger subjects, the possibility exists that exercise has a greater deleterious effect on arterial P_{O_2} in older subjects, and this remains to be refuted.

Physiological Basis of $\dot{V}_A/\dot{Q}$ Mismatch and Diffusion Limitation

$\dot{V}_A/\dot{Q}$ Mismatch. The reason for the modest increase in $\dot{V}_A/\dot{Q}$ inequality remains somewhat speculative. First, only about 50% of subjects demonstrate this response (218); those that do, appear to have higher cardiac output values and more lactic acidosis than those who do not (218). The actual $\dot{V}_A/\dot{Q}$ distribution simply becomes a little broader; alternate patterns, such as development of separate regions of very low $\dot{V}_A/\dot{Q}$ ratio, are rarely if ever observed in normal subjects. The changes produced by exercise are greater in acute hypoxia (e.g., $F_{I_{O_2}} = 0.12$) than in normoxia, despite not reaching as high a $\dot{V}_{O_{2max}}$ under hypoxic conditions (253), and are rapidly reversed by exercising in hyperoxia. The effects of hypoxia are similar whether produced by hypobaric or normobaric gas mixtures of reduced $P_{I_{O_2}}$ (90). Over a matrix of conditions involving different altitudes, exercise rates, and $F_{I_{O_2}}$ values, the degree of $\dot{V}_A/\dot{Q}$ mismatch bears a unique relationship to mean pulmonary arterial pressure. However, an equally unique relationship to total ventilation is seen, and cause and effect cannot be established. The increase in $\dot{V}_A/\dot{Q}$ mismatch lasts for some 15–20 min following the cessation of exercise, sometime after overall ventilation and cardiac output have returned to close to resting values. Finally, when measured, spirometric indices of airways obstruction such as FEV_1 and FEV_{25-75} are not impaired immediately after exercise.

The possible pathophysiological causes of increased $\dot{V}_A/\dot{Q}$ mismatch on exercise are likely to come from these lists:

1. Airway-related events
   a. Ventilatory inhomogeneity from transient peribronchial fluid accumulation (causing airway obstruction) due to the high transcapillary fluid flux (39).
   b. Ventilatory inhomogeneity from transient interstitial alveolar wall edema (causing regional loss of tissue compliance).
   c. Accentuated small anatomical asymmetries (amongst airways) that are unimportant at low resting flow rates but which create inequality during high air flow rates during exercise.
   d. Similarly minor degrees of accumulated peripheral airway secretion, stimulated by the inflammatory effects of high gas flow rates on airway epithelia.
   e. Frank (if mild) bronchoconstriction from irritant effects of effects of high airway gas flow rates.
2. Blood flow–related events
   a. Transient interstitial edema causing perivascular fluid accumulation and thus vascular obstruction in different regions.
   b. Mechanical effects of alveolar wall fluid accumulation reducing adjacent capillary blood flow.
   c. Altered distribution of vasomotor tone due to the high flow and pressures of exercise, perhaps overcoming the normal regulatory process of adjusting tone and hence local blood flow to more uniformly match local ventilation via the hypoxic vasoconstrictor mechanism.

How can the previously mentioned observations help us to exclude any of the above possibilities? There is clearly no frank bronchoconstriction, 1e. Potential factors 1a, 1b, 2a, and 2b all center on mild, transient interstitial pulmonary edema. There is only circumstantial evidence for this, since no techniques available today have yet shown directly the development of small degrees of edema in man. We recently found that exercise did produce perivascular cuffing in the pig (219), but its importance in causing $\dot{V}_A/\dot{Q}$ mismatch in that animal has not been determined. The close relationship of $\dot{V}_A/\dot{Q}$ mismatch to pulmonary artery pressure and its accentuation by hypoxia fits with edema as a cause, and the relatively long resolution time beyond that required for ventilation and cardiac output to subside, also argues for a structural lesion such as edema (and against causes directly related to high air or blood flows and pressures such as increased effect of small anatomical asymmetries). However, clearance of peripheral airway secretions could also require 15–20 min.

In Chapter 13, the argument is made that in the face of exercise, the balance of forces determining fluid movement out of the capillaries should not lead to edema on the basis of available data. Yet at the same time, animal models unequivocally show greatly increased lung lymph flow rates during exercise (39). Postexercise measures of lung volumes and diffusing capacity following prolonged high-intensity exercise such as running a marathon (64, 165, 174) have also pointed to the possibility of mild edema. Consequently, the cause of exercise-induced $\dot{V}_A/\dot{Q}$ mismatch is presently unclear, with transient edema as the favored but unproved hypothesis. Whatever the cause turns out to be, the important issue is not the clinical effect of this $\dot{V}_A/\dot{Q}$ mismatch on pulmonary gas exchange (a minor effect on overall O_2 transport). The important question is, What is the basis of this $\dot{V}_A/\dot{Q}$ inequality telling us about the limit to lung function in exercise? The answer could have implications for understanding pulmonary responses to disease.

If this $\dot{V}A/\dot{Q}$ inequality is the product of edema, perhaps this is the same basic phenomenon as seen in a small number of otherwise normal subjects who, when exercising vigorously at even modest altitudes, develop life-threatening degrees of clinical pulmonary edema known as high-altitude pulmonary edema (HAPE). Recent work by West and colleagues (274) has shown that physical breakdown of the alveolar capillaries can be seen under physiological conditions such as exercise, due to the naturally developing high pulmonary vascular pressures. Clearly, this would have the potential for causing edema and consequently $\dot{V}A/\dot{Q}$ inequality. However, if this is so, there remains an enigma—the horse develops very high pulmonary arterial and left atrial pressures during exercise, yet little increase in $\dot{V}A/\dot{Q}$ inequality is seen. If all is indeed based on pulmonary hemodynamics, this paradox requires that the horse has an extremely strong capillary structure capable of withstanding transmural pressures that may reach 70 mm Hg or more.

Diffusion Limitation. The development of diffusion limitation is much less problematic to explain. When evident, it becomes greater with increasing work rate. It is rarely seen (at sea level) below an O_2 level of about 3 liters/min, but as the subject is made more and more hypoxic, diffusion limitation is seen at lighter and lighter exercise loads, but again increasing in prominence with exercise intensity. This all makes perfect sense when one realizes that whether diffusion equilibration is complete or not depends simply on the ratio of the diffusional conductance (DL) of the blood-gas barrier for oxygen to the perfusional conductance ($\beta\dot{Q}c$) of the pulmonary vasculature for oxygen (194). Here, β is the slope of the O_2 dissociation curve, while $\dot{Q}c$ is blood flow. If for the purposes of simplified discussion the O_2 dissociation curve is taken to be linear, it was shown earlier under *The Concept of D/βQ̇* that:

$$\frac{PA - Pc'}{PA - P\bar{v}} = e^{-DL/\beta\dot{Q}c} \qquad (33)$$

where PA, $P\bar{v}$, and Pc′ are alveolar, mixed venous, and end-capillary PO_2 values, respectively.

As exercise intensity increases, DL increases as more capillary surface and volume become available via recruitment and distention; however, β also increases because mixed venous PO_2 falls dramatically and $\dot{Q}c$ increases as well [Fig. 12.17; (252)]. As a result, $DL/\beta\dot{Q}c$ falls, and when this reaches a low enough value, alveolar and end-capillary PO_2 values will not equilibrate, given the time available.

In acute hypoxia, $\dot{Q}c$ is even higher at a given submaximal exercise load than in normoxia, while β is also higher than in normoxia (Fig. 12.18). Thus, the ratio $DL/\beta\dot{Q}c$ falls even more in hypoxia, increasing the degree of diffusion limitation.

Lack of differences in DL between subjects who develop $\dot{V}A/\dot{Q}$ mismatch compared to those who do not (218) suggests that the explanation given above is sufficient: whatever causes $\dot{V}A/\dot{Q}$ mismatch on exercise is not deleteriously affecting DL and thus is not further contributing to diffusion limitation.

There is, however, one rather odd observation made recently (196): after 48 h of residence at 3800 m where PI_{O_2} is 90 mm Hg and arterial O_2 saturation is 85%–90% at rest, DL appears to be lower at a given $\dot{V}O_2$ during exercise than at the same PI_{O_2} at sea level, without significant worsening of $\dot{V}A/\dot{Q}$ relationships. This mysterious phenomenon requires independent confirmation and explanation.

It appears in conclusion that the development of diffusion limitation during exercise is explained by the $DL/\beta\dot{Q}$ concept, and in particular by β and $\dot{Q}c$ increasing rather than by DL falling. Conversely, DL increases with exercise, but not by as much as $\beta\dot{Q}c$. This is consistent with observations in elite athletes who are typified by greater arterial hypoxemia during exercise as well as a higher cardiac output than their less elite counterparts. The equine athlete is an even better example: not only is maximum cardiac output roughly twice as high (per kilogram) as in man, the phenomenon of splenic contraction increases [Hb] to 20–22 g/dl at peak O_2. Thus, both β and $\dot{Q}c$ are significantly greater in the horse, and while DL is also greater, the $DL/\beta\dot{Q}$ ratio accounts for the high degree of diffusion limitation exhibited by the horse at peak $\dot{V}O_2$ (254). Following splenectomy, the exercise-induced increases in both [Hb] (reflected by reduced β) and $\dot{Q}$ are attenuated therefore diffusion limitation is much less in evidence (252).

If blood flow is a prominent component of pulmonary diffusion limitation, it is so because of its effect on capillary transit time. It is important to recognize that not all red cells enjoy the same transit time; rather, there is a distribution of such times about a mean (72). Even if the mean of this distribution is calculated to be sufficient to allow complete diffusion equilibration (139), those cells with a longer than mean transit time obviously can gain no additional O_2 and thus cannot compensate for those red cells whose transit time, less than the mean, is too short for complete equilibration.

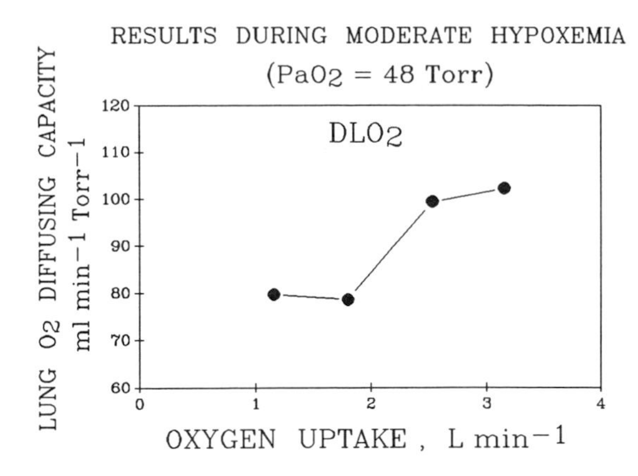

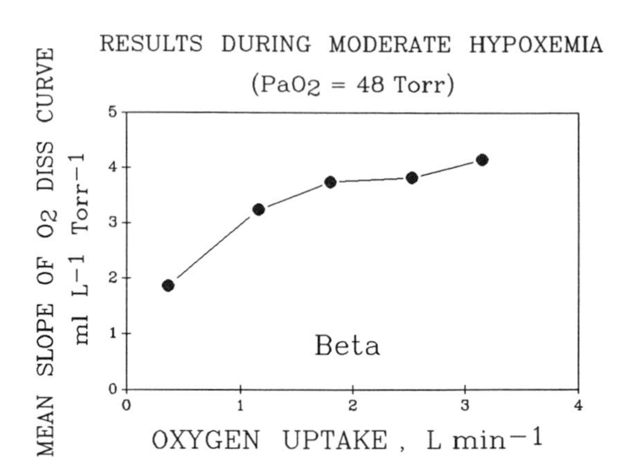

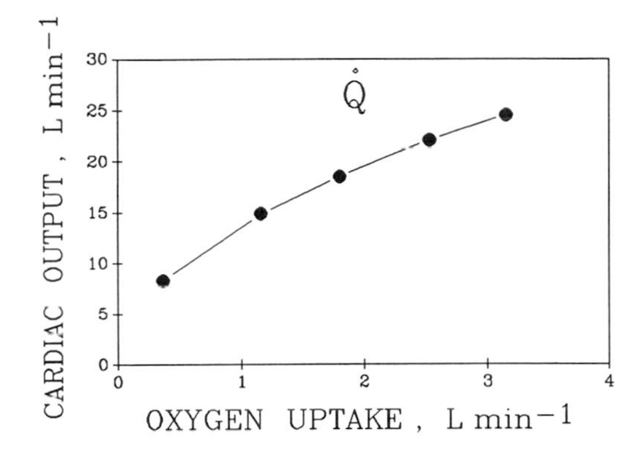

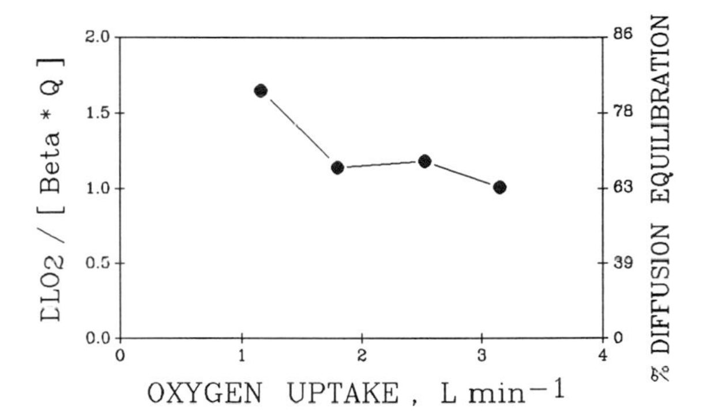

FIG. 12.17. At simulated altitude of 10,000 feet (barometric pressure = 523 mm Hg), considerable diffusion limitation of oxygen uptake occurs during exercise, which permits calculation of the oxygen diffusing capacity. $D_{L_{O_2}}$ increases essentially linearly with increasing exercise. As explained in the text, the importance of diffusion limitation depends upon the ratio $D_L/\beta\dot{Q}$ falling from 1.6 (light exercise) to 1 (heavy exercise) under these conditions, resulting in incomplete diffusive equilibration as shown in the *bottom right panel*. Thus during moderate and heavy exercise at this altitude, diffusion equilibration proceeds but only to two-thirds completion (253).

Effects of Chronic Hypoxia on Pulmonary Gas Exchange in Exercise. Effects of acute hypoxia/ascent to altitude were integrated into the immediately preceding section in the context of both $\dot{V}_A/\dot{Q}$ inequality and diffusion limitation. Such effects are of course limited to modest degrees of hypoxia equivalent to exposure to about 15,000 ft (4500 m) altitude. The descriptions above of both increased diffusion limitation and greater $\dot{V}_A/\dot{Q}$ mismatch than in normoxia, at a given $\dot{V}_{O_2}$, imply that the AaP_{O_2} is greater in acute hypoxia than at normal sea level P_{O_2} [Fig. 12.19; (252)]. Does this persist during acclimatization? In fact it does not persist; the AaP_{O_2}–$\dot{V}_{O_2}$ relationship after as little as 2 weeks reverts to the initial sea level relationship. This may be explained partly by the corresponding reduction in the cardiac output–$\dot{V}_{O_2}$ relationship and partly to the rise in alveolar oxygen tension that occurs during initial acclimatization at high altitude (14, 217); this will tend to reduce $\beta\dot{Q}$ and increase the $D_L/\beta\dot{Q}$ ratio, thereby permitting a greater degree of diffusion equilibration and reducing AaP_{O_2}. With time, this is further complicated by a rise in hematocrit and hemoglobin concentration, which will increase β but may simultaneously increase D_L by more efficient use of capillary surface area through closer red cell spacing (65) (see also earlier under Krogh Diffusing Capacity of the Alveolar Capillary Membrane). Importance of the latter mechanism is still uncertain.

Data from altitudes above 15,000 ft are rare. From Operation Everest II, results showed an inconsistent effect of extreme (simulated) altitude on pulmonary gas exchange (257). Thus, at the equivalent of 20,000 ft there were clinically significant, major perturbations of $\dot{V}_A/\dot{Q}$ mismatch and exercise-induced diffusion limitation. When restudied several days later at 25,000 ft, the same subjects displayed much less gas exchange abnormality. This paradox may well be due to the fact that just before the subjects reached 20,000 ft, the rate of ascent was much

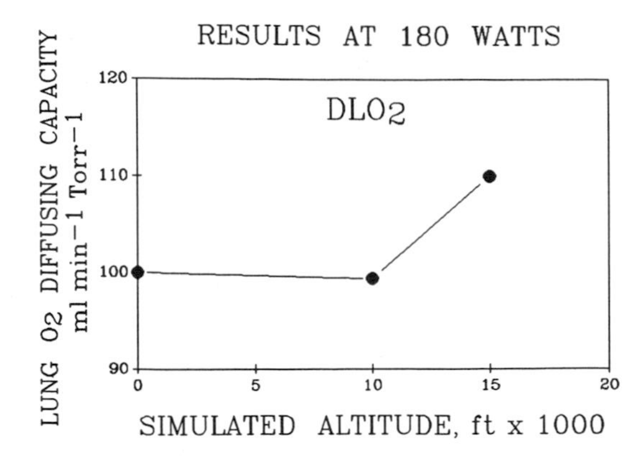

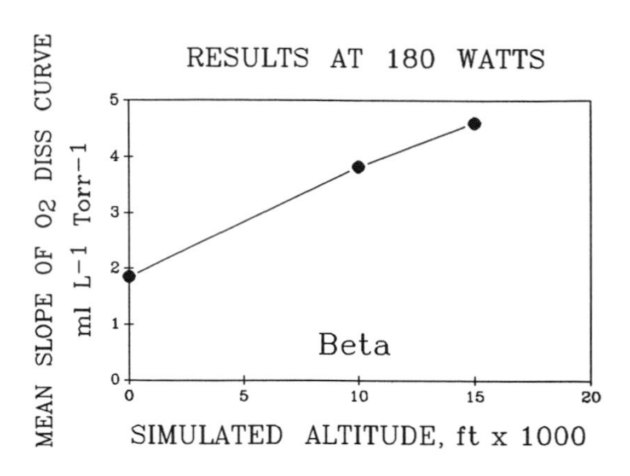

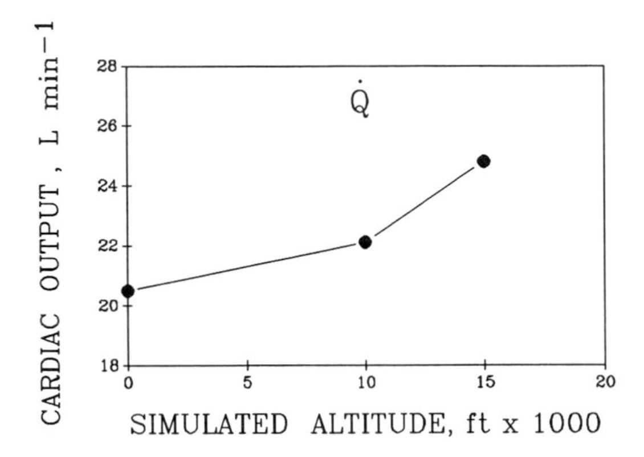

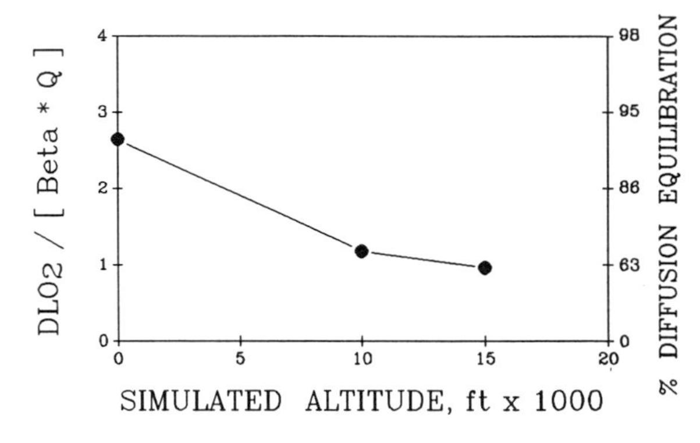

FIG. 12.18. Effects of altitude (simulated in a hypobaric chamber) on diffusional limitation of oxygen at a constant level of exercise (180 W). DL_{O_2} increases at altitude, at this submaximal level, presumably as a consequence of increasing blood flow causing a combination of distention and recruitment. The effective slope of the oxyhemoglobin dissociation curve (β) increases with increasing altitude as arterial and venous P_{O_2} fall, and the result of these changes is that the ratio $DL_{O_2}/\beta\dot{Q}$ progressively falls with altitude.

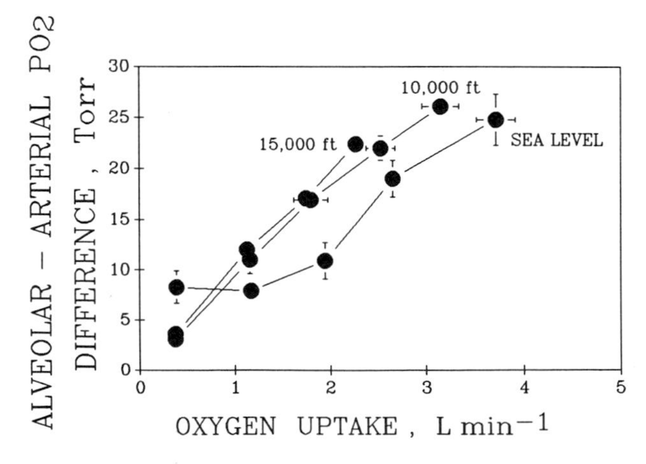

FIG. 12.19. Alveolar–arterial P_{O_2} difference during exercise as a function of altitude. During submaximal exercise the alveolar–arterial P_{O_2} difference is significantly higher at altitude than at sea level. This is the result of greater diffusion limitation (252).

faster than when approaching 25,000 ft, where a more conservative ascent profile was adopted. Thus, just as with more conventional HAPE seen at much lower altitudes in the field, the rate of ascent is hypothesized to be more injurious than the altitude per se in terms of pulmonary gas exchange. In Operation Everest II, at 20,000 ft, the gas exchange disturbances were, remarkably, quantitatively similar to what is seen in critically ill patients on ventilators in the intensive care unit and were associated in one subject with clinically obvious pulmonary edema (Fig. 12.20).

ACID–BASE REGULATION DURING EXERCISE: A PHYSICOCHEMICAL APPROACH

Exercise of increasing intensity is initially accompanied by little change in acid–base status, but when 50% of aerobic power is exceeded, an acidosis develops, characterized by a fall in arterial pH, an in-

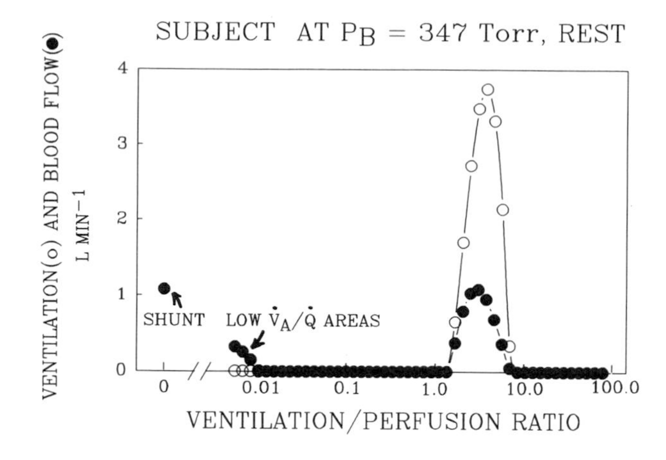

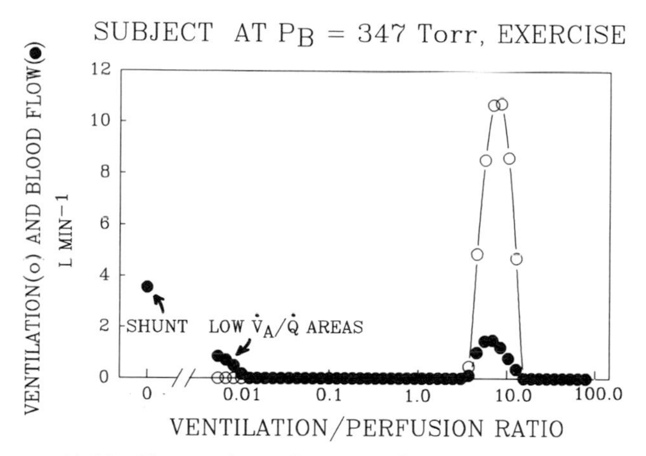

FIG. 12.20. Abnormal ventilation–perfusion ratio distributions caused by HAPE in one subject at a simulated altitude of 20,000 ft. At rest, there was a 15% shunt and an additional 10% of the cardiac output perfusing abnormally low $\dot{V}A/\dot{Q}$ areas. On exercise, the shunt increased to 29%, with 17% of the cardiac output perfusing areas of low $\dot{V}A/\dot{Q}$ ratio.

crease in lactate concentration, and a fall in CO_2 pressure, indicating hyperventilation. Most studies of $[H^+]$ homeostasis in exercise have been based on these changes in arterial blood and interpreted in terms of lactic acid production and the control of ventilation. However, when viewed from a broader viewpoint in which the maintenance of muscle function becomes preeminent, there is a need to consider changes occurring within muscle. It then becomes apparent that arterial blood provides a poor reflection of changes occurring in other fluid compartments, that many systems and processes are involved, and that the ventilatory response during exercise is contributing not only toward homeostasis in arterial blood but also in exercising muscle.

It is now clear that large increases in intramuscular $[H^+]$ occur during muscle contraction and may profoundly influence the capacity to exercise. As early as 1927, measurements of pH in homogenates of cat muscle by Furasawa and Kerridge showed that intramuscular pH at rest was 7.04 ($[H^+]$ 100 nEq/liter), falling to 6.26 ($[H^+]$ 550 nEq/liter) when electrical stimulation could not elicit further force production (178). It was almost 50 years before this approach was applied to samples of human muscle obtained by needle biopsy (106). More recently, intramuscular pH has been derived noninvasively by ^{31}P nuclear magnetic resonance (NMR) (29, 201). There is virtual agreement that intramuscular pH is around 7.0 at rest and 6.3–6.5 at fatigue in maximal exercise. Furthermore, studies employing experimental manipulations of acid–base state have shown profound effects on metabolism and performance in exercise. Thus, an appreciation of the mechanisms contributing to acid–base homeostasis is essential for an understanding of the factors limiting exercise. On the one hand, experimental increases in muscle $[H^+]$ and P_{CO_2} are associated with a variety of effects known to contribute to muscle fatigue, and on the other, many situations in which exercise cannot be maintained are accompanied by marked ionic and acid–base changes. Recent research has employed innovative methods and concepts that have clarified both the changes and their effects.

Basic Concepts of Acid–Base Physiology

Physical chemists of the last century classified ions as acids and bases, depending on whether they were able to combine with hydrogen ions or hydroxyl ions, respectively, due to their electrical charge. The law of mass action put forward by Guldberg and Waage in 1867 became fundamental for understanding ionic equilibria and was used by L. J. Henderson in 1909 (105) to define the hydrogen ion concentration for any weak acid, HA, dissociating to H^+ and A^-:

$$[H^+] = K_A \cdot [HA]/[A^-]$$

where K_A is the equilibrium constant expressing the degree of dissociation, in terms of the $[H^+]$ at which HA is half dissociated (105). Henderson explored the regulation of $[H^+]$ in blood plasma, recognizing that the important contributing systems were the plasma proteins acting as weak acids, and carbonic acid. He derived the following equation, since then known as Henderson's equation:

$$[H^+] = K \cdot [CO_2]/[HCO_3^-]$$

Hasselbalch (96) used the convention introduced by Sørensen in 1909 (233), in which the $[H^+]$ was expressed by pH, where p is the negative power of 10, and rearranged this equation to obtain

$$pH = pK + \log[HCO_3^-]/[CO_2]$$

or expressed in terms of P_{CO_2}

$$pH = 6.1 + \log[HCO_3^-]/0.0301\ P_{CO_2}$$

The Henderson-Hasselbalch equation has continued to provide the basic description of relationships between pH and P_{CO_2} in plasma, and from which plasma $[HCO_3^-]$ can be calculated. Since arterial plasma P_{CO_2} is determined by the ratio of CO_2 output to alveolar ventilation, as expressed by $Pa_{CO_2} = 863(\dot{V}CO_2/\dot{V}A)$, Pa_{CO_2} is generally used to indicate the respiratory component of an acid–base disturbance and changes in $[HCO_3^-]$ to quantify the nonrespiratory, or "metabolic," component. This led to the Henderson equation being used to describe the physiological control of $[H^+]$. For example, Pitts (195) emphasized that "Regulation of the concentrations of the components of this one buffer pair fixes the hydrogen ion concentration and thereby determines the ratios of all the other buffer pairs."

However, it was recognized at an early stage that the independent effects of P_{CO_2} on $[HCO_3^-]$ expose a basic flaw in any approach to acid–base balance based solely on the P_{CO_2}–$[HCO_3^-]$ system in plasma. Changes in $[HCO_3^-]$ could not be used quantitatively to indicate "metabolic" changes without taking into account the independent effects of P_{CO_2} on $[HCO_3^-]$. Several approaches were used to overcome this problem, culminating in the graphical approach of Siggaard-Andersen (231), which was based on titration studies of plasma and whole blood with CO_2 in order to calculate a standard plasma $[HCO_3^-]$ at a whole blood P_{CO_2} of 40 mm Hg and a given hemoglobin concentration. These advances led to the concept of "base excess," the excess $[HCO_3^-]$ in plasma for which respiratory changes had been allowed for. Although solidly based for unseparated plasma, having been established by in vitro titrations, the approach was not in agreement with plasma changes in studies where the "titrations" were carried out in vivo; for example, by having animals breathe gas with a high P_{CO_2}. Schwartz and Relman (225), on the basis of such studies, criticized the concept of base excess, beginning what Bunker (26) termed "The Great Transatlantic Acid–Base Debate," which centered on the validity of in vitro relationships applied to in vivo situations. The debate was resolved from a mathematical, if not conceptual, point of view when it was recognized that by using in vitro data based on whole blood having a hemoglobin concentration of 5 g/dl, the approximate hemoglobin concentration in total extracellular fluid, an accurate reflection of in vivo behavior was obtained (8).

The "classic" approach to interpretation of acid–base changes in exercise, in which the focus is lactic acid production by muscle, has spawned a number of concepts which, although they are conceptually simple and have proved useful, are flawed when taken too literally. Foremost among these is the concept of lactic acid buffering by bicarbonate in muscle and blood. Conceptually, this is described in the linked reactions

$$LaH + HCO_3^- \rightleftharpoons La^- + H_2CO_3$$
$$H_2CO_3 \rightleftharpoons CO_2 + H_2O$$

Mathematically, this suggests that lactate production is associated with an equimolar reduction in bicarbonate and increase in CO_2 production. The fact that increases in arterial whole blood lactate concentration usually correlate reasonably well with reductions in plasma $[HCO_3^-]$ and increases in CO_2 output (38, 262) suggests that the system behaves *as if* these reactions took place (262). However, the concept breaks down when it is applied to other fluid compartments, as described in more detail below; furthermore, whilst plasma may be considered as a single fluid compartment, whole blood consists of two compartments—erythrocytes and plasma—between which ionic exchanges occur. Also, the interpretation is based on the concept that $[H^+]$ actually react with HCO_3^-, with control of $[H^+]$ being exerted through changes in P_{CO_2} and $[HCO_3^-]$, and it ignores other ionic and fluid changes. The flaws in the approach are mainly due to the confusion of dependent with independent variables, and are readily identified by returning to the physical chemistry and applying simple systems analysis to $[H^+]$ changes. Such a physicochemical approach allows a quantitative assessment of the various independent contributing mechanisms and systems, and provides a sounder basis for the analysis of acid–base disturbances. Furthermore, the factors that influence $[H^+]$ in muscle as well as other body compartments have been clarified. No longer can measurements in arterial plasma alone be used to infer the adequacy of, or contributors to, acid–base homeostasis.

Physicochemical Approach to Factors Influencing [H⁺]

The physicochemical properties of physiological aqueous solutions can be completely described by the equilibration between three "systems"—*strong ions, weak acids*, and CO_2. These systems interact within the constraints imposed by the three physical laws of mass action, electrical neutrality, and conservation of mass. The law of mass action implies that reactions may be characterized in terms of the reactants and products, with equilibrium state being defined by the equilibrium constants. Electrical neutrality implies that the activities of positively and negatively charged ions are equal in physiological solutions. Conservation of mass implies that the interconversion of substances, larger into smaller and vice versa, does not lead to a net loss or gain in the total mass of the constituent molecules.

In the present context, a system is defined as a number of linked molecules, whose concentrations may be predicted in terms of its constituent independent variables and the associated constants or parameters. An *independent variable* is defined as one whose concentration cannot be changed within the system, and is unaffected by changes that take place in the other systems. For example, the concentrations of strong ions in a solution will not be affected by any changes in CO_2 (another system) or in $[H^+]$ (a dependent variable within the strong ion system). A *dependent variable* is one whose concentration changes whenever the independent variable changes within its system and, as it may appear in several systems, its concentration is a function of the interaction between systems. For example, for a solution in a beaker we can only change the concentration of sodium or chloride by adding these ions from the outside; the concentration of hydrogen ions will then be changed but also will be changed by adding buffers or bubbling CO_2 through the solution. If we can describe the behavior of the systems involved in H^+ homeostasis in terms of the independent variables and acting within the constraints imposed by the physicochemical laws, constants, and parameters, we may calculate all the dependent variables at equilibrium. Furthermore, we may use the mathematical relationships to predict what the effect of any change in an independent variable will be on the dependent variables that appear in all the interacting systems within a fluid compartment.

Although this concept was understood more than 50 years ago, its mathematical expression was so complex as to be practically impossible. The late Peter Stewart (240–242) pointed out that computers can readily provide a surprisingly simple quantitative solution for the equations that express the equilibration between systems. Probably of greater importance than the purely technical solution of equations, Stewart's approach emphasized the distinction between variables capable of acting independently and those whose concentrations are dependent on equilibration between all the systems. He identified the *independent variables* as the net charge difference between strong ions [the *strong ion difference*, (SID)], the total concentration of weak electrolyte ($[A_{tot}]$), and the partial pressure of CO_2 (P_{CO_2}). Dependent variables include $[H^+]$, $[HCO_3^-]$ and $[A^-]$, the dissociated portion of the weak electrolyte. Changes in water content due to osmotic or other factors influence $[H^+]$ by changing the independent variables either in absolute terms or relative to one another. These systems can be best understood from the viewpoint of the law of mass action acting in physiological solutions. The constraint of electrical neutrality required of biological solutions may be graphically presented in the form of histograms in which two columns of equal height contain the concentrations of the negatively charged anions side by side with the positively charged cations (Fig. 12.21). This teaching aid was popularized by J. L. Gamble (74), and has ever since been known as a "Gamblegram."

In presenting the approach mathematically, an assumption is made that equilibrium is achieved in the reactions. In this chapter we will not address the rates of reactions in any detail, even though during exercise large changes in many variables may occur with great rapidity. In vitro, the only system at risk of not reaching equilibrium is CO_2 (146), but physiologically equilibration may involve ion exchange via active transport, simple or mediated diffusion between fluid compartments, and changes in water content brought about by osmotic or hydrostatic forces; all these processes have finite rates that mitigate against complete equilibration during exercise.

The Law of Mass Action; "Strong" and "Weak" Electrolytes. The law of mass action states that the rate of a reaction proceeding between reactants is proportional to their respective concentrations. In the reaction expressed by the equation

$$A + B \rightleftharpoons C + D$$

the rate of reaction in the forward and reverse directions is proportional to the product of the reactants [A][B] and products [C][D], respectively. If the constants that govern the rates of the respective forward and reverse reactions are denoted k_1 and k_2, at equilibrium

$$k_1[A][B] = k_2[C][D]$$

or

$$k_1/k_2 = K = [C][D]/[A][B]$$

where K is the equilibrium constant. Considering an acid, HX, in aqueous solution, "dissociation"—or release of protons—is represented by

$$HX \rightleftharpoons H^+ + X^-$$

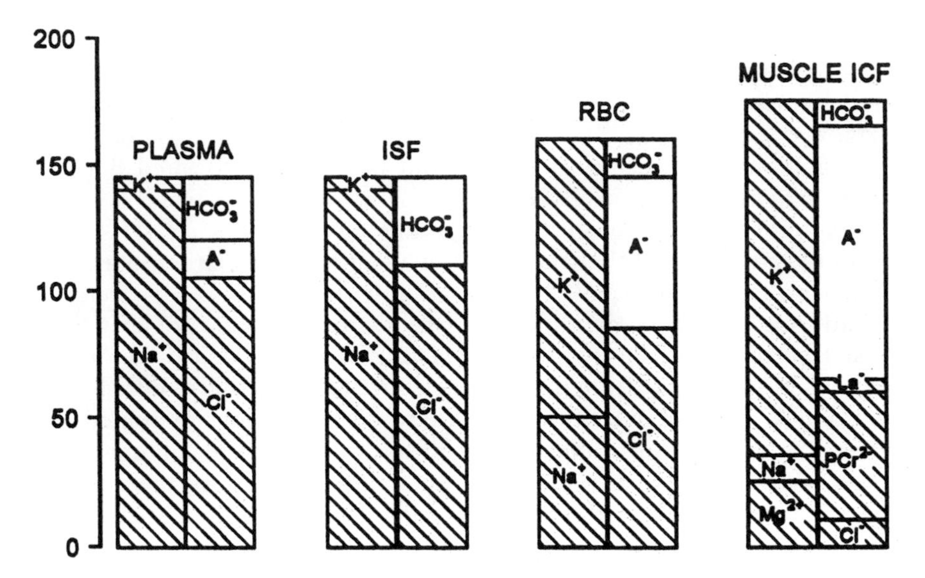

FIG. 12.21. Gamblegrams to show the systems contributing to H^+ ion concentration in different compartments. Independent variables are [SID], A_{tot}, and P_{CO_2}. The two bars of the histogram represent net negative and positive changes, and are of equal height to indicate the constraint of electrical neutrality, and in which [SID] equals the sum of the dependent variables $[A^-]$ and $[HCO_3^-]$.

and at equilibrium

$$k_1/k_2 = K_x = [H^+][X^-]/[HX]$$

The weaker the strength of the bond between X^- and H^+, the larger will be the dissociation constant K_x. The greater the magnitude of K_x, the further the reaction will proceed to the right and the higher will be the relative concentration of H^+ to HX. Thus, $[H^+]$ can be expressed in terms of the other variables as follows:

$$[H^+] = K_x[HX]/[X^-] \quad (42)$$

Using the pH notation, equation 3 becomes

$$pH = pK_x + \log([X^-]/[HX]) \quad (43)$$

where pH = $-\log [H^+]$ and $pK_x = -\log K_x$. When HX is half-dissociated, $[X^-] = [HX]$ and pH = pK; thus, the pK of an acid or base is the pH at which it is half dissociated.

Strong acids may be defined as acids having a high K (low pK). Similarly, strong bases will have low K values, or high pK. Strong acids are defined as those that are fully dissociated in physiological solutions. Weak acids are those that are only partially dissociated. The extent of the dissociation may be expressed in terms of the ratio of the dissociated to undissociated forms. The term $[A_{tot}]$ is used to denote the total available anionic charge of the weak acids, consisting of dissociated ($[A^-]$) and undissociated ([HA]) portions. For most weak organic electrolytes $[A_{tot}]$ represents the net concentration of available negative charges usually due to free carboxyl (COO^-) groups exceeding the free amino (NH_2^+) groups.

Equation 43 may be expressed graphically as in Figure 12.22, in which the ratio of $[A^-]$ to [AH] has been plotted in relation to pH for three weak electrolytes having pK values of 5, 7, and 9. If we consider the pH range 6–8 to be of physiological relevance during exercise, it can be seen from Figure 12.22 that the electrolyte with a pK of 5 is virtually

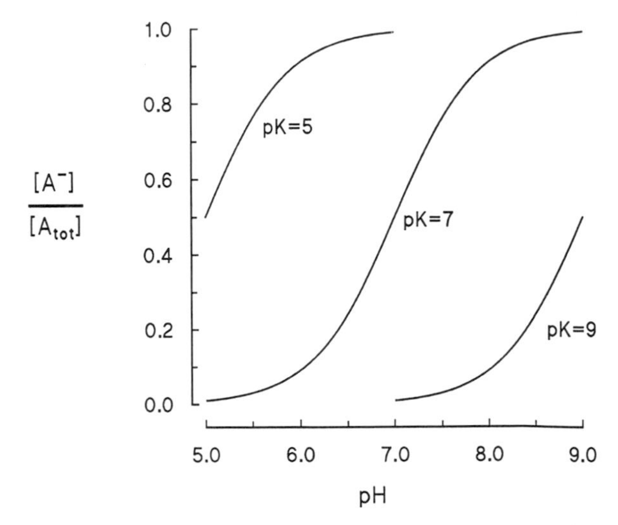

FIG. 12.22. The proportion of dissociated (A^-) to undissociated (HA) forms of three weak electrolytes having pK values of 5, 7, and 9. In the physiological range of pH (6.4–7.6), the first is fully dissociated and the third is undissociated.

fully dissociated and that with a pK of 9 is virtually undissociated. Thus, when considering ionic concentrations in body tissue fluids we may arbitrarily classify electrolytes having a pK between 5 and 9 as "weak" and those outside this range as strong acids (pK < 5) or strong bases (pK > 9).

Strong *inorganic* acids and bases are completely dissociated at the pH in body fluids; they have a dissociation constant (K_A) that is far removed from that of water, and usually have a pK (log 1/K) of less than 3 or greater than 10. These include the salts, acids, and bases of Na^+, K^+, Cl^-, and SO_4^{2-}. Strong *organic* acids such as lactic acid and creatine phosphate are not as fully dissociated as the strong inorganic electrolytes, but from their pK values of 3.9 and 4.5, respectively, they act as strong ions in body fluids, and can be viewed as being completely dissociated to anion and H^+. Strong bases, such as NH_3, are completely dissociated to the cation and OH^-. Other organic acids, such as organic and inorganic phosphates, having pKs closer to 7 and being only partially dissociated at body pH, are classed as weak electrolytes. Weak electrolytes exist to a measurable extent in both their dissociated and undissociated forms and are often viewed as buffers, because any tendency to change $[H^+]$ is resisted through an increase or decrease in the proportion of the total that is in the dissociated form ($A^-/[A_{tot}]$). Uncharged molecules, such as Cr^0, do not influence ionic state directly, although they may generate changes in water content osmotically.

Water. Dissociation of H_2O to protons and hydroxyl ions is described by the following reaction:

$$H_2O \leftrightarrow OH^- + H^+$$

Applying the law of mass action we obtain

$$K_w = [H^+][OH^-]/[H_2O] \qquad (44)$$

In this equation, $[H_2O]$ in pure water is 55 mol/liter and as $[H^+]$ and $[OH^-]$ are 10^{-7} Eq/liter or less, $[H_2O]$ may be taken as constant; by multiplying with K_w we obtain the apparent dissociation constant for water, K'_w:

$$K_w \cdot [H_2O] = K'_w = [H^+][OH^-]$$

At 25°C,

$$K'_w = [H^+][OH^-] = 10^{-14} \text{ Eq/liter}$$

Thus, $[H^+]$ is 1×10^{-7} Eq/liter; the negative logarithm, or pH, is 7.0 and this is usually considered the pH of neutrality. However, as temperature increases, the strength of bonds holding the two protons to oxygen becomes weaker, K'_w becomes greater, and both $[H^+]$ and $[OH^-]$ increase (206). Consequently, pH will fall, yet electrical neutrality is maintained and $[H^+] = [OH^-]$. At 37°C in pure water, $K'_w = 2.4 \cdot 10^{-14}$ Eq/liter. However, in addition to temperature, ionic strengths and concentrations of different substances also influence K'_w so that in body fluids at 37° $K'_w = 4.4 \cdot 10^{-14}$ Eq/liter. Hence, at 37° in body fluids,

$$[H^+] = (4.4 \cdot 10^{-14})/[OH^-] \text{ Eq/liter} \qquad (45)$$

As a consequence, at 37°C in body fluids, neutral $[H^+]$ will be $2.1 \cdot 10^{-7}$ Eq/liter (a pH of 6.8). The temperature dependence of the apparent equilibrium constant for water, as for all other equilibrium constants, has to be kept in mind in considering changes during exercise, in which relatively large increases in muscle and core temperature may occur (60).

Systems Contributing to [H⁺] Regulation

Strong Electrolytes. The concentration of strong inorganic ions in the various body fluid compartments is controlled by numerous, integrated physiological control systems that regulate exchange of ions between the plasma, extracellular, and intracellular fluid. The normal arterial plasma Na^+, Cl^-, and K^+ concentrations in plasma are 142 mEq/liter, 104 mEq/liter, and 4 mEq/liter, respectively. These concentrations may be achieved in vitro by combining 100 mEq NaCl, 4 mEq KCl, and 42 mEq NaOH in 1 liter of water. We know intuitively that the concentration of strong ions in water may be predicted from knowledge of how many equivalents of each species were added and the volume of water; in this example we have added 42 mEq of OH^-. However, it is not readily apparent what the resulting $[H^+]$ or $[OH^-]$ will be because the added hydroxyl ions will react with the protons and drive the equilibrium reaction for water back to the left according to the law of mass action. Thus, we can state that $[H^+]$ and $[OH^-]$ are not a function of how many protons are put into or taken away from a given compartment. Instead, the respective concentrations are functions of the equilibrium reactions in which they take part. The $[H^+]$ must be calculated from these equilibrium reactions, observing the constraint of electrical neutrality.

The constraint of electrical neutrality means that in a solution of KCl and NaCl, the following two equations have to be fulfilled:

$$K'_w = [H^+][OH^-] \text{ (mass action)}$$

and

$$[Na^+] + [K^+] + [H^+] - [Cl^-] - [OH^-] = 0 \text{ (neutrality)}$$

Since

$$[OH^-] = K'_w/[H^+],$$

$$[Na^+] + [K^+] + [H^+] - [Cl^-] - K'_w/[H^+] = 0 \quad (46)$$

This expression can be simplified by combining the concentrations of strong cations and strong anions into a single term; that is, in this solution [SID] = $[Na^+] + [K^+] - [Cl^-]$. Because [SID] influences the system but can only be altered by ionic changes imposed from outside the system, it obeys the operating criteria for an *independent variable.*

Equation 46 may be simplified to

$$[SID] + [H^+] - K'_w/[H^+] = 0$$

and clearing fractions

$$[H^+]^2 + [SID][H^+] - K'_w = 0$$

Inspection of this equation shows that $[H^+]$ is a function of both [SID] and the equilibrium constant for water, and $[H^+]$ fulfills the criteria for a *dependent variable.* Although a change in [SID] will inevitably be accompanied by changes in $[H^+]$, changes in $[H^+]$ due to the action of some other system—for example, by equilibrating the solution with CO_2—can have no effect on [SID].

In addition to Na^+, Cl^-, and K^+, strong organic ions such as lactate and ketones may influence extracellular [SID], and in muscle, intracellular lactate, creatine phosphate, ammonium, calcium, magnesium, and sulphate also act as strong ions.

Weak Acids. As discussed above, weak electrolytes are those that exist in a partially dissociated and partially undissociated form in the physiological range of $[H^+]$. They act as buffers by changing the proportion of their total available electronic charges ($[A_{tot}]$), which is present in a dissociated form ($[A^-]$). Often, buffers are considered to reduce $[H^+]$, but it needs to be remembered that they are acids and, if added to a solution, will tend to increase $[H^+]$. Their ability to act as buffers to minimize changes in $[H^+]$ depends on how close their pK is to the pH, and on their total concentration. Also, as they are large charged molecules they exchange very poorly between fluid compartments.

In plasma the only group of weak acids that exists in appreciable concentration is the amino acids in plasma proteins; other weak acids such as phosphates are normally in very low concentration in plasma and thus exert a negligible effect. The ionic equivalents and dissociation characteristics of the amino acids in plasma proteins have been obtained by titration studies, which have shown that they behave as if their pK was uniform at 6.63, or a K_A of $3 \cdot 10^{-7}$. The extent to which A_{tot} is dissociated into A^- is a function of the factors that control $[H^+]$, and is thus a variable that is *dependent* on the equilibrium between all the systems involved. Thus, two additional equations are needed to describe $[H^+]$. The first is the dissociation reaction for weak acids:

$$[H^+] \cdot [A^-] = (3 \cdot 10^{-7}) \cdot [HA] \text{ Eq/liter} \quad (47)$$

In addition to their K_A, the effectiveness of buffers in any site is dependent on their total concentration ($[A_{tot}]$). Although the proportion of weak acid that is dissociated, or ionized, may vary, the sum remains constant (conservation of mass):

$$[HA] + [A^-] = [A_{tot}] \quad (48)$$

In this system $[A_{tot}]$ is the *independent variable*; [HA], $[H^+]$, and $[A^-]$ are *dependent variables.* For plasma, $[A_{tot}]$ may be calculated (mEq/liter) by multiplying the plasma protein concentration (g/dl) by 0.24 (211).

In considering acid–base control in a wide range of vertebrates with widely variable body temperature, Rahn, Reeves, and colleagues (203, 206) identified that the control systems did not act to maintain $[H^+]$ activity constant, but rather maintained a constant protein ionization state (A^-/HA). The change in $[H^+]$ with changing temperature suggested the peptide histidine imadozole groups where extremely important in this control, having a pK value of 7.05 at 20°C and 6.76 at 37°C. Hochachka and Somero (114) have pointed out that imadozole groups occupy key positions in enzyme binding sites, strengthening the arguments that maintenance of their ionization state under varying conditions of temperature and (H^+).

In considering changes in $[H^+]$ intracellularly, such as in muscle, the situation is more complex due to the greater total concentration and number of weak organic acids; as discussed below, during exercise and metabolic interconversions between different organic phosphates are extensive, adding another order of complexity. Titration studies in animal muscle have been used to characterize the "effective" or "apparent" $[A_{tot}]$ and K_A (159), but in our present state of understanding these values are influenced by numerous factors, which may not be entirely predictable.

Carbon Dioxide. The concentration of carbon dioxide in any fluid compartment represents the balance between its entry into the compartment from metabolism and diffusion, and its removal by blood flow and alveolar ventilation.

The reaction involved in CO_2 removal and the variables taking part in the CO_2 system are summarized as follows:

$$CO_2 + H_2O \rightleftharpoons H_2CO_3 \rightleftharpoons HCO_3^- + H^+$$

Approaching these reactions from the left, carbon dioxide dissolves in water to form carbonic acid, catalyzed by carbonic anhydrase, and spontaneously dissociates to HCO_3^- and H^+. The resulting increase in $[H^+]$ will then retard further dissociation and eventually equilibrium will be reached among the physically dissolved CO_2, $[H^+]$, and $[HCO_3^-]$ according to the following equation:

$$[H^+] = K_{a'}\ [CO_2]/[HCO_3^-]$$

where $K_{a'}$ is an apparent dissociation constant incorporating the dissociation constants for H_2CO_3 to CO_2 and H_2O and for dissociation of H_2CO_3 to H^+ and HCO_3^-. The amount of dissolved CO_2 may be derived from the P_{CO_2} and the solubility constant of CO_2 ($3.01 \cdot 10^{-5}$ Eq · liter^{-1} · mm Hg^{-1} (139); the equation may then be rewritten as:

$$[H^+] = K_{a'} \cdot 3.01 \cdot 10^{-5}\ P_{CO_2}/[HCO^-3]\ \text{Eq/liter}$$

$K_{a'}$, which is $7.94 \cdot 10^{-7}$, may be combined with the solubility coefficient to yield

$$[H^+] = K_c \cdot P_{CO_2}/[HCO_3^-]\ \text{Eq/liter} \qquad (50)$$

where $K_c = (7.94 \cdot 10^{-7}) \cdot (3.01 \cdot 10^{-5})$ Eq/liter $= 2.4 \cdot 10^{-11}$ Eq/liter and for $[H^+]$ expressed in nEq/liter

$$[H^+] = 24 \cdot P_{CO_2}/[HCO_3^-]\ \text{nEq/liter}$$

(Henderson's equation)

Since arterial P_{CO_2} is controlled outside the system by alveolar ventilation, it is the *independent variable* in this equation, with $[H^+]$ and $[HCO_3^-]$ both being *dependent variables.*

In logarithmic form, equation 50 becomes the Henderson-Hasselbalch equation:

$$pH = 6.1 + \log([HCO_3^-]\ /\ 0.0301\ P_{CO_2})$$

The total CO_2 content ($[CO_{2tot}]$ is the molar concentration of dissolved CO_2 gas plus $[H_2CO_3^-]$:

$$[CO_{2tot}] = [HCO_3^-] + (0.0301\ P_{CO_2})$$

In considering changes in the CO_2 system in muscle during exercise, $[CO_{2tot}]$ increases in relation to metabolic rate and the clearance of CO_2 by muscle blood flow, and becomes the *independent variable*, with P_{CO_2} and $[HCO_3^-]$ then becoming dependent on changes occuring in [SID] and $[A_{tot}]$, as discussed below.

The hydration of CO_2 proceeds slowly in the absence of carbonic anhydrase (CA), having an estimated half-time of 5–8 s (142), but CA increases the velocity by four orders. The assumption of equilibration in a fluid compartment containing CA is thus valid; however, the tissue distribution of CA is not uniform, and because CA is absent in plasma, the movement of CO_2 and ions will slow the physiological equilibration of the CO_2 system. During exercise, when large changes occur in CO_2 and ions in plasma it seem likely that CO_2 is never in full equilibrium.

Bicarbonate spontaneously dissociates to carbonate (CO_3^{2-}), and another proton:

$$HCO_3^- \rightleftharpoons H^+ + CO_3^{2-}$$

The dissociation constant for this reaction (K_3) is $6 \cdot 10^{-11}$; hence,

$$[H^+] = K_3\ [HCO_3^-]/[CO_3^{2-}]\ \text{Eq/liter} \qquad (51)$$

or

$$[H^+] = (6 \cdot 10^{-11})\ [HCO_3^-]/[CO_3^{2-}]\ \text{Eq/liter}$$

Although frequently $[CO_3^{2-}]$ tends to be ignored because its concentration is so small compared to $[HCO_3^-]$, it is in fact several orders of magnitude more concentrated than $[H^+]$. The reactions show that $[CO_3^{2-}]$ increases as $[H^+]$ falls, with important physiological implications when it interacts with Ca^{2+}.

Interaction between Systems

Regulation of $[H^+]$ may be described by simultaneous solution of the following six equations describing water dissociation (equation 42), and the three reactive systems—carbon dioxide (equations 50 and 51), weak acids (equations 47 and 48), and strong electrolytes (equation 46):

equation 42:

$K'_w = [H^+] \cdot [OH^-]$

($K'_w = 4.4 \cdot 10^{-14}$)

equation 50:

$K_c \cdot P_{CO_2} = [H^+]/[HCO_3^-]$

($K_c = 2.4 \cdot 10^{-11}$)

equation 51:

$K_3 \cdot [HCO_3^-] = [H^+]/[CO_3^{2-}]$

($K_3 = 6.0 \cdot 10^{-11}$)

equation 47:

$K_A \cdot [HA] = [H^+] \cdot [A^-]$

[K_A defined by compartment composition (Table 12.6)]

equation 48:

$[HA] + [A^-] = [A_{tot}]$

equation 46:

$$[SID] + [H^+] - [HCO_3^-] - [CO_3^{2-}] - [A^-] - K'_w[H^+] = 0$$

Each of the independent variables, [SID], $[A_{tot}]$, and PCO_2, appears only once in this series of equations, whereas the dependent variables ($[H^+]$, $[HCO_3^-]$, $[CO_3^{2-}]$, $[OH^-]$ and $[A^-]$ appear more than once, since each is dependent on equilibrium among all the systems. A fourth-order polynomial expression may be derived (see Appendix) that can be solved for $[H^+]$, given any combination of the three independent variables (241):

$$A[H^+]^4 + B[H^+]^3 + C[H^+]^2 + D[H^+] + E = 0 \quad (52)$$

where $A = 1$, $B = K_A + [SID]$, $C = (K_A[SID] - [A_{tot}]) - (K_c \cdot PCO_2 + K'_w)$, $D = [K_A (K_c \cdot PCO_2 + K'_w) + (K_3 \cdot K_c \cdot PCO_2)]$, $E = K_A \cdot K_3 \cdot K_c \cdot PCO_2$.

This equation may be used to calculate the effects of changes in the independent variables either singly or in combination. Table 12.6 lists the approximate values for K_A and pK_A of important weak acids at 37°C.

Determinants of [H⁺] in Different Body Compartments

Systems involved in acid-base status exert differing effects in different fluid compartments, due to differences in the relative magnitude of the three independent variables (Fig. 12.21). The distribution of $[H^+]$ in different tissues is determined solely by the distribution of the independent variables contributing to acid-base regulation, identified above.

In Muscle. Intracellular [SID] is large, dominated by high $[K^+]$, low $[Cl^-]$, and creatine phosphate (CrP^{2-}) acting as a strong acid (159). During exercise, decreases in intramuscular [SID] tend to increase $[H^+]$ and are mainly due to decreases in $[K^+]$ and increases in $[La^-]$; a decrease in CrP^{2-} (a strong acid) increases [SID), which tends to counterbalance a rise in $[La^-]$ and attenuates potential increases in $[H^+]$.

TABLE 12.6. *Approximate* K_A *and* pK_A *for Important Weak Acids**

	K_A	pK_A
Plasma proteins	3.0×10^{-7}	6.52
Hemoglobin (oxy)	2.5×10^{-7}	6.60
hemoglobin (red)	6.31×10^{-8}	7.20
Inorganic phosphate (Pi)	1.58×10^{-7}	6.78
Hexose phosphate	7.76×10^{-7}	6.11
ATP	1.75×10^{-7}	6.50
ADP	1.78×10^{-7}	6.30

*Equation 47.

The high protein and phosphate concentrations in muscle contribute to a high weak acid concentration $[A_{tot}]$ that is ten times that in plasma; the high $[A_{tot}]$ provides important buffers so that decreases in $[A^-]$ minimize the effects of decreases in [SID]. PCO_2 in tissues is higher than in arterial blood at rest, and $[HCO_3^-]$ is less than half the plasma level. During exercise, CO_2 production increases at a faster rate than its removal by blood flow, and total CO_2 content ($[CO_{2tot}]$) increases and acts as an independent variable; since [SID] tends to fall and $[H^+]$ rises, the result is a large increase in PCO_2 in muscle, aiding its diffusion into venous blood. Until recently, carbonic anhydrase was thought not to be present in muscle, and it was argued that during exercise this was an advantage, by slowing the formation of HCO_3^-, which would not move as rapidly out of muscle as CO_2. However, as HCO_3^- is a dependent variable, its formation probably only occurs at low intensities of exercise when only small changes in [SID] occur. Also, during the last 15 years, at least three isozymes of CA have been demonstrated in muscle (83). Finally, in heavy exercise there are increases in intracellular water, due to osmotic and hydrostatic forces, that tend to reduce the concentration of ions and the other variables.

In Interstitial Fluid. The weak acid system plays virtually no part in fluids that are ultrafiltrates of plasma (e.g., lymph, cerebrospinal fluid), because of the low concentration of protein ($[A_{tot}]$ is effectively zero), and $[H^+]$ is only influenced by changes in [SID], with exchange of strong ions between the intracellular fluid and plasma, and PCO_2, in equilibrium with the PCO_2 in these two adjacent compartments. As [SID] and PCO_2 are close to the values in plasma, the $[A^-]$ is zero, $[HCO_3^-]$ is equal to [SID] and only slightly less than the sum of $[HCO_3^-]$ and $[A^-]$ in plasma (Fig. 12.21).

In Plasma. The balance between the systems is towards [SID], but large variations in $PaCO_2$ may effect large and rapid changes in arterial $[H^+]$. Increases in $[H^+]$ during exercise are usually related to reductions in [SID] associated with increases in $[La^-]$ but modulated by changes in inorganic strong ions, mainly Cl^-. Shifts in water between plasma and cells will also modify the concentrations of strong ions and A_{tot}. However, the buffering effect of $[A_{tot}]$ is limited, because the ratio of $[A^-]$ to $[A_{tot}]$ is about 1/10 in the physiological pH range.

In Erythrocytes. All three systems have similar weighting because [SID] is high, $[A_{tot}]$ is also high due to hemoglobin, and PCO_2 is in equilibrium with the P_{CO_2} of the surrounding plasma. The changes in $[H^+]$ are further affected by the K_A of hemoglobin, which is influenced by its state of oxygenation, being 2.5×10^{-7} in the oxygenated state but only 6.3×10^{-8} when deoxygenated. This has a large effect on $[A^-]$, and consequently $[HCO_3^-]$; for example, if we keep [SID] (60 mEq/liter), $[A_{tot}]$ (60 mEq/liter), and P_{CO_2} (40 mm Hg) constant, and change only K_A from $2.5 \cdot 10^{-7}$ to 6.3×10^{-8}, $[A^-]$ falls from 47 mEq/liter to 36 mEq/liter, and $[HCO_3^-]$ increases from 13 mEq/liter to 24 mEq/liter. Combined with the high activity of CA in erythrocytes aiding the rate of formation of HCO_3^-, this leads to a very large and rapid increase in erythrocyte $[HCO_3^-]$ as blood flows through exercising muscle, losing its O_2 and gaining CO_2. In the lung there is an equally large and rapid reduction in erythrocyte $[HCO_3^-]$. Of course, this simple statement ignores the transient increases in P_{CO_2} that occur during this process, which serve to aid diffusion of CO_2 from the erythrocyte. Also ignored are the effects of movements in strong ions, mainly Cl^-, which will change the relationships between $[A^-]$ and $[HCO_3^-]$.

These differences between fluid compartments emphasize the importance of fluid and ion shifts between them, in the acid–base perturbations occurring in exercise.

Contributors to [H⁺] in Muscle at Rest and Exercise

At Rest. (See Fig. 12.23, *upper right hand panel*). The dominant strong cation is K^+, with Na^+, Mg^{2+} and Ca^{2+} being in much lower concentration; the main strong anion is creatine phosphate (CrP^{2-}); Cl^-, La^-, and Py^- are in relatively low concentration in resting muscle, resulting in a large [SID] of about 110 mEq/liter. Proteins and phosphates act as buffers in an effective concentration ($[A_{tot}]$) of approximately 140 mEq/liter. P_{CO_2} is higher than in arterial blood at around 50 mm Hg. The interactions between these independent variables result in $[H^+]$ being about 100 nEq/liter (pH 7.0), and $[HCO_3^-]$ of about 10 mEq/liter in resting muscle.

During Maximal Exercise. (See Fig. 12.23, *lower right hand panel*). A number of changes occur that are more or less closely related to the intensity of exercise. These include an increase in water content, exchange of strong ions between intracellular and extracellular water, changes in the concentration of metabolites acting as strong or weak ions, and increases in CO_2 production by aerobic metabolism of glycogen/glucose and fats.

Water. Changes in water content exert their main effect through changes in the concentrations of other variables that influence [SID] and $[A_{tot}]$. Such changes are secondary to hydrostatic and osmotic changes associated with exercise, with increases in intramuscular water and reductions in plasma volume; thus, the effects are in opposite directions in the intracellular and extracellular compartments. The increases that occur in muscle water are closely related to increases in glycolytic flux; the production of lactate ions, and to a lesser extent glycolytic intermediates such as glucose-6-phosphate, from the much larger glycogen molecule increase osmolality; breakdown of CrP^{2-} will also contribute to this effect. The shift of water into muscle is related to the intensity of muscle contraction and in heavy "sprint" exercise may be as much as 14% (160, 162), when it is associated with reductions in plasma water of similar extent. Generally, these changes tend to minimize increases in muscle $[H^+]$. Increases

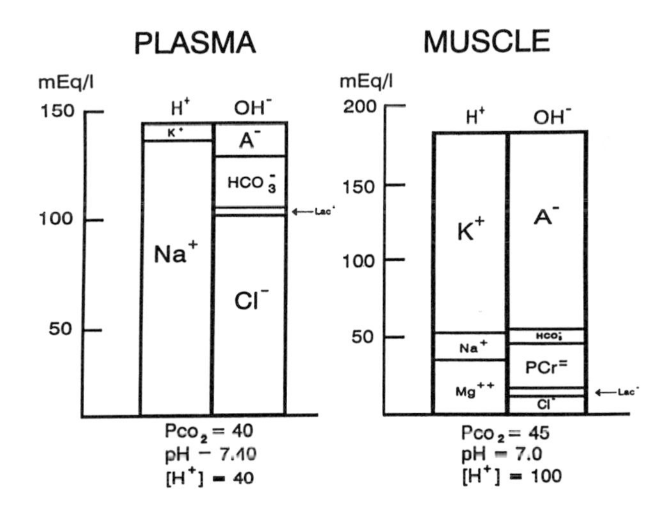

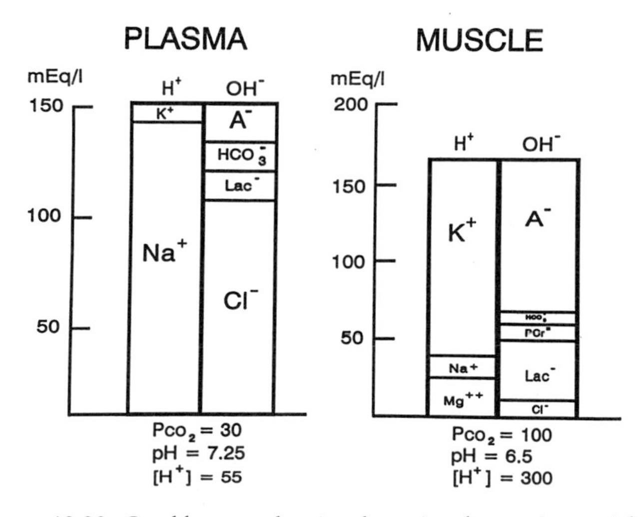

FIG. 12.23. Gamblegrams showing the major changes in arterial plasma and muscle ionic status from rest (*upper panels*) to maximum exercise (*lower panels*).

in intramuscular temperature during exercise (60) will tend to increase K'_w, but this effect is small.

Ion exchanges and [SID]. The concentration of strong inorganic ions is influenced by changes in water content by exchange with extracellular water. Increases in plasma [K^+] are proportional to the relative exercise intensity (168), and are related to reductions in muscle [K^+] that occur when the efflux of K^+ exceeds its reuptake into muscle by Na^+/K^+ ATPase pumps (37, 170), and is also partly secondary to changes in water content. Efflux of K^+ is related mainly to the outward rectifying current during repolarization of the membrane potential. Although the efflux of K^+ may be due to increased conductance of ATP or Ca^{2+}-sensitive K^+ channels, or to increases in K^+ permeability due to osmotic factors, these effects have yet to be established (37). During light and moderate exercise (up to 80% capacity) there is little change in any of the strong inorganic ions, but in very heavy exercise (159) the reduction in muscle [K^+] may amount to as much as 50 mEq/liter. Although ion exchange mechanisms between muscle and extracellular fluid have also been described for both Na^+ and Cl^-, there are only small increases in their concentrations, and the relevance of these mechanisms in humans during exercise is not clear (167).

Effect of metabolite concentrations on [SID] and [A_{tot}]. The interrelationships between metabolic reactions and acid-base state in muscle are complicated by the fact that protons are produced or absorbed in many reactions, and conversely H^+ ions may influence the activity of several rate limiting enzymes. Although many reactions involved in energy metabolism are stoichiometrically associated with the generation or absorption of protons, the actual changes in [H^+] are the result of many complex relationships that are most easily understood in terms of the physicochemical interactions outlined above. Thus, although examining classic biochemical relationships may suggest proton production, the actual change in [H^+] may be quite different because what matters is the change in the concentrations of the strong and weak ions that act as substrates or products in the reactions. These effects are quantified by considering the pK of these acids and bases. In this way, the biochemical processes associated with exercise may influence [SID], [A_{tot}], and K_a.

Calcium release from the sarcoplasmic membrane initiates muscle contraction, serving to couple the electrical, mechanical, and biochemical events and hydrolysis of ATP required to maintain cross-bridge cycling:

$$ATP^{4-} + H_2O \rightleftharpoons ADP^{3-} + Pi^{2-} + H^+$$

The effect of this reaction on H^+ production is very small because ATP is constantly being regenerated, changes in the total concentration of the reactants are small, and they are all weak acids, as expressed in their pK values: 6.79 for ATP^{4-}, 6.75 for ADP^{3-}, and 6.78 for Pi^{2-}. Only small falls in ATP^{4-} have been observed even at high exercise, or about 25%, with negligible effect on [A_{tot}] and K_A (234).

The most rapid restoration of ATP is accomplished through the creatine kinase reaction and the adenine nucleotide cycle. The creatine kinase reaction enables ATP to be regenerated in the absence of glycolysis and also acts to shuttle energy equivalents between the cytosol and the mitochondria (17):

$$PCr^{2-} + ADP^{3-} + H^+ \rightleftharpoons Cr^0 + ATP^{4-}$$

The forward reaction is associated with a large reduction in the concentration of PCr^{2-}, a strong acid (pK = 4.5) compared to its product creatine, which is uncharged, and thus has no effect on [H^+]. Thus, this reaction increases [SID] and exerts a strong alkalinizing effect as shown by studies employing ^{31}P NMR (54). As ATP concentration is effectively maintained, the net balance of the last two reactions is expressed by:

$$PCr^{2-} \rightleftharpoons Cr^0 + Pi^{2-}$$

Increases in inorganic phosphate concentration from the breakdown of PCr^{2-} may reach 20–30 mM/kg (100) in heavy exercise, thereby increasing [A_{tot}], and changing the net K_A. Increasing intramuscular [H^+] is associated with an increase in the ratio of the diprotonated to monoprotonated form of phosphate according to the reaction

$$HPO_4^{2-} + H^+ \rightleftharpoons H_2PO_4^-$$

As the pK of this reaction is 6.78, the fraction of total phosphate as the diprotonated form ($H_2PO_4^-$) increases from 0.4 at pH 7.0 to 0.8 at pH 6.4.

During heavy exercise, ATP breakdown is associated with increases in ADP and AMP, which act to increase adenine nucleotide degradation to IMP with concomitant production of ammonia; increases in plasma NH_3 concentration approximately parallel increases in [La^-], but they are an order of magnitude lower (130) and thus do not have an impact on [SID], in spite of the high pK of ammonium dissociation (pK = 9.3).

The flux-generating step for muscle glycogenolysis is the glycogen phosphorylase (GP) reaction, and the main nonequilibrium enzyme in the pathway is phosphofructokinase (PFK). For glucose oxidation, the flux-generating step is hepatic glucose release, with glucose uptake across the sarcolemma acting as an additional rate-limiting step. Once in the muscle, oxidation of glucose is controlled by similar factors controlling glycolysis, with the addition of the hexokinase reaction. Many of the intermediate reactions involve protons, but unless substantial changes in the concentration of reactants occur, the effect on $[H^+]$ is small. The major source for changes in $[H^+]$ caused by glycolysis is lactate formation. The formation of lactate from pyruvate is catalyzed by lactate dehydrogenase, an equilibrium enzyme:

$$Py^- + NADH + H^+ \rightleftharpoons La^- + NAD^+$$

The reaction suggests that protons will be absorbed during the formation of La^-, but the mass action equation indicates that changes in $[La^-]$ will always be at least tenfold greater than changes in $[Py^-]$, and the resulting decreases in [SID] will actually increase $[H^+]$. Although the "anaerobic" or lactate threshold concept implicates formation of La^- in conditions of oxygen lack when the $[NADH]/[NAD^+]$ ratio increases, with the reaction maintaining $[NAD^+]$, most studies have not been able to demonstrate this change. While this topic remains a matter of current debate (276), lactate formation may be more appropriately considered in terms of an imbalance between pyruvate production by glycolysis, and its oxidation in the pyruvate dehydrogenase reaction and subsequently in the citric acid cycle. As lactic acid is a strong acid (p*K*-3.9), and large increases in $[La^-]$ occur in heavy exercise, there is a very large effect on intramuscular $[H^+]$ through a reduction in [SID] (Fig. 12.23, *lower right hand panel*).

The citric acid cycle links electron transport to ATP production; the first step in this link is the oxidation of NADH. Although the flux through the cycle is substrate dependent, it is mainly regulated by the ratios of mitochondrial ADP/ATP and NAD^+/NADH. Aerobic regeneration of ATP through oxidation of glycogen and glucose appears to absorb protons:

$$C_6H_{12}O_6^0 + 36ADP^{4-} + 36Pi^{2-} + 36H^+ + 6O_2 \rightleftharpoons 36ATP^{4-} + 6CO_2 + 6H_2O$$

However, as the change in ion concentrations is small and p*K*s of the reactants are all 6.5–6.9, the main independent acid–base variable in this reaction is the production of CO_2, with an increase in muscle $[CO_{2tot}]$ and rise in P_{CO_2}.

Lipolysis of triglycerides into free fatty acids (FFA), both in muscle and in adipose tissue, does not contribute to the acidosis of exercise. Because FFA are carried in plasma bound to albumin, it is possible that a small reduction in $[A_{tot}]$ might result, but it seems unlikely that this effect could ever exceed 2 mM/liter (97). The oxidation of FFA in muscle mitochondria does not appear to affect muscle $[H^+]$, but for a given metabolic energy production, much less CO_2 is produced when fat is burned as a fuel than glycogen. This may be appreciated from the stoichiometry of the reactions; for glycolysis, as seen in the above reaction, 1 mole of CO_2 is produced in regenerating 6 moles of ATP. For a representative FFA (palmitate):

$$C_{16}H_{32}O_2^0 + 129ADP^{4-} + 129Pi^{2-} + 23O_2 \leftrightarrow 129ATP^{4-} + 16H_2O + 16CO_2$$

shows that 1 mole of CO_2 is produced for 8 moles of ATP, indicating a substantially more efficient energy source, from the acid–base point of view. Increases in P_{CO_2} in muscle are associated with increases in $[H^+]$; as discussed more fully below, although in most situations diffusion of CO_2 is very rapid, in heavy exercise not all the CO_2 produced can be removed instantly, and P_{CO_2} may rise to well above 100 mm Hg. In addition to its effects on $[H^+]$, theoretically CO_2 may influence the flux through some metabolic pathways that involve decarboxylation.

Muscle buffer capacity. When viewed in conventional terms, "buffer capacity" refers to the factors that minimize a change in $[H^+]$ for a given influx of H^+ ions. As lactic acid is the main source of H^+ ions, the relationship between increases in $[La^-]$ and reductions in pH in muscle has been used as an index of muscle buffering. Although this concept appears straightforward, it becomes potentially misleading in physicochemical terms because of the many factors that influence $[H^+]$; in different forms of exercise variable but potentially large changes occur in [SID], $[A_{tot}]$, K_A, and P_{CO_2}. Also, the concept creates confusion through vague usage of the term "buffer," which has been inconsistently and variably used to include [SID], $[A_{tot}]$ and $[HCO_3^-]$. Finally, differences between buffering characteristics have been interpreted in terms of differing transmembrane fluxes of H^+, OH^-, or HCO_3^-; however, it is clear that movement of these dependent variables will have no effect on pH unless they are accompanied by movement of ions, water, or CO_2 that will influence the independent variables defined above.

The changes in muscle pH occurring as a result of titrations in vitro or changes in lactic acid and other metabolites in vivo have been extensively studied (130). Some authors have isolated one important factor such as increases in lactate concentration, and examined the accompanying changes in $[H^+]$ as an index of buffering capacity. Others have titrated muscle samples with HCl and NaOH (156), or CO_2

(102); such studies have shown differences in buffer capacity between different muscles that appear mainly to be due to variation in muscle ionic composition related to muscle fiber types. For example, in rat hindlimb muscles, type 2 glycolytic fibers have higher glycogen concentrations and glycolytic rates, but also the largest [SID], due to their higher [K^+] (159). Thus, a given increase in [La^-] will be accompanied by a smaller increase in [H^+] than in the type 1 fibers having a smaller [SID]. Studies in humans suggest that differences in ionic composition between fiber types are less important in human muscle (232). Studies comparing in vitro with in vivo data have shown differences between the two (101) that are presumably related to ionic shifts between fluid compartments. During exercise, changes in water content and ion shifts will influence [SID], and changes in [A_{tot}] and, less importantly, K_A may accompany changes in the concentration of organic and inorganic phosphates. The effects of the weak acid buffer systems may be expressed in the extent of falls in [A^-], which may amount to 50 mEq/liter or more, acting to counter the reduction in [SID]. It is clear that intracellular buffering of protons generated by metabolic processes and ion shifts is handled by these weak acids, and that HCO_3^- plays virtually no part in intracellular buffering, since it is capable of only small reductions in its concentration.

The parameter that defines the power of buffers (A_{tot}) in muscle is K_A. Many organic compounds contribute to an effective K_A, and as large changes occur in their relative proportions during exercise, it might be expected that large changes occur in exercise compared to rest. However, titration studies of rat skeletal muscle samples at rest and after maximal exercise are consistent with only small changes in K_A, from 1.64×10^{-7} at rest to 1.97×10^{-7} at maximum exercise (159).

Carbon dioxide. Carbon dioxide production by muscle increases with increases in power and oxygen consumption, and in relation to the balance between glycogen and fat for fuel; the balance between these two fuels depends on exercise intensity and duration. Carbon dioxide is also generated in other reactions in which aerobic metabolism has not gone to completion. For example, the production of acetyl CoA from pyruvate is associated with CO_2 production; in heavy exercise, acetate production may exceed the rate at which it can enter into the TCA cycle and both acetyl carnitine and CO_2 accumulate (200).

The total content of CO_2 in muscle increases during exercise in relation to the balance between its production by metabolism and its removal by muscle blood flow; the proportion of [CO_{2tot}] existing as dissolved CO_2 (reflected in P_{CO_2}) or as HCO_3^-, is determined by the other independent variables [SID]and [A_{tot}]. Although P_{CO_2} cannot be directly measured within muscle, during leg exercise there is an increase in femoral venous P_{CO_2}, to over 100 mm Hg in maximal effort (149), indicating an intramuscular P_{CO_2} of at least this high in very heavy work. This will tend to markedly increase muscle [H^+], and also to aid rapid diffusion of CO_2 into venous blood draining muscle. Muscle [HCO_3^-] at rest is much lower than in extracellular fluid, 8–12 mM/liter, due mainly to the high [SID] and [A_{tot}] in muscle, and during exercise there is a fall to even lower levels, due to reductions in [SID]. It has often been held that a major source of CO_2 in muscle is due to the "buffering" of acid by bicarbonate. However, the modulation of increases in [H^+] secondary to lactate increases is mainly related to changes in [SID], including reductions in [PCr^{2-}], and the ratio of [A^-] to [A_{tot}]. In muscle [HCO_3^-] is in low concentration and the evolution of CO_2 requires a relatively much larger increase in [H^+] than in plasma. Increases in pulmonary CO_2 output associated with increases in plasma [La^-] are not simply due to a reaction between lactic acid and HCO_3^- but are the result of more complex changes in [SID] and P_{CO_2} in both venous and arterial blood (see below).

Muscle [H^+]. The main changes outlined above—increase in water content, reduction in PCr^{2-}, increase in inorganic and organic Pi^{2-}, reduction in [K^+], increase in P_{CO_2}—all occur during exercise, although we lack data regarding the extent of all these changes in relation to exercise intensity, in order to quantify the relative contributions of different factors as muscle increases power output from rest to maximum. *Upper* and *lower right hand panels* of Figure 12.23 present a comparison between rest and maximal exercise. Although effects of a fall in [SID] and increased P_{CO_2} are countered by the intramuscular buffer systems, intramuscular [H^+] may still reach 400 nEq/liter (pH 6.4) in heavy exercise (149). The relative roles of different factors contributing to this increase in [H^+] have been estimated by Heigenhauser et al. (168) from studies in exercising humans; immediately after 30 s of maximal cycling exercise, up to 30% may be due to increases in P_{CO_2}, 40% or more may be due to reductions in [SID], and 30% may be due to changes in [A_{tot}] and K_A. These relative contributors change rapidly during recovery from this form of exercise, mainly due to the rapidity with which CO_2 leaves muscle.

Effects on muscle of acid–base changes in exercise. Theoretically, many of the ionic changes occurring in exercise could affect muscle function and metabolism, and several have been proposed as contributing to fatigue. Increases in intramuscular [H^+]

may result in inhibition of excitation-contraction coupling (19), reduction in cross-bridge cycling with decrease in ATP turnover (43), and inhibition of rate-limiting enzymes controlling glycolytic flux (246). Changes in $[H^+]$ will also influence the dissociation, and thus the ratio of A^- to AH, of potentially critical amino acids such as histidine (203) in enzymes. Hochachka and Somero (114) have argued that as histidine is located in a key regulatory position in many enzyme systems, the change in ionization will profoundly influence enzyme activity. Whilst increases in $[H^+]$ are generally felt to inhibit enzyme activity, this conclusion is based on studies of a relatively small number of reactions studied in vitro. Kinases, such as phosphofructokinase, show inhibition, whereas phosphatases and dehydrogenases may show enhanced activity with increased $[H^+]$. The situation is made more complex by the fact that most rate-limiting enzymes exist in inactive and active forms, with the interconversion being catalyzed by a kinase and phosphatase. For example, glycogen phosphorylase is converted to an active form by a kinase, whereas for pyruvate dehydrogenase the conversion is catalyzed by a phosphatase; thus, an increase in muscle $[H^+]$ may inhibit phosphorylase but activate pyruvate dehydrogenase. It is interesting that these two effects will act to reduce muscle lactate and H^+ accumulation.

Finally, the metabolic effects of CO_2 are generally ignored. Carbon dioxide is produced in rate-limiting reactions involving dehydrogenases with conversion of NADH to NAD^+; pyruvate dehydrogenase is the flux-controlling step for entry of pyruvate into the citric acid cycle, and isocitrate dehydrogenase and α-ketoglutarate dehydrogenase are regulatory enzymes within the cycle. Dalziell and Londesborough (52) built on an initial observation of Krebs and Roughton (153) and showed that CO_2 influenced the rate of these reactions, suggesting that CO_2 buildup in muscle may reduce the flux through oxidative phosphorylation. These studies employed carbonic anhydrase inhibitors to show that the enzyme effects were mediated by CO_2 rather than HCO_3^-. Several physiological studies have suggested that increases in perfusate P_{CO_2} impair muscle function (235). However, this question is far from settled, as CO_2 affects a number of mechanisms in different ways; changes in perfusate CO_2 influence ion fluxes between the muscle cell and plasma (161), and twitch tension is increased when CO_2 is increased in the perfusate, whether by increasing P_{CO_2} or $[HCO_3^-]$ (186).

Changes in Extracellular Fluid in Exercise

In addition to the reactions in muscle associated with increased energy turnover, the ionic status in muscle will be influenced by the changes occurring in blood as it traverses the exercising muscle, involving changes in both venous and arterial blood.

Venous Plasma and Erythrocytes

Water. Increases in intramuscular water content, due to osmotic and hydrostatic factors, are associated with reductions in plasma volume that are approximately linear with exercise intensity and reach 10%–15% in heavy exercise. There is an associated hemoconcentration and increase in the concentration of ions (160). There are no changes in erythrocyte volume, suggesting that the effects of water shifts between muscle and blood are confined to plasma (168).

Strong ions. Increases in plasma strong ion concentrations are partly due to plasma volume reductions, explaining increases in $[Na^+]$; increases in $[K^+]$ and $[La^-]$ are relatively greater, indicating significant efflux of both ions (Fig. 12.24). Reductions in plasma $[Cl^-]$ are related to movement of Cl^- into muscle and erythrocytes. The result of these ion changes is that [SID] increases between the arterial and venous sides of the muscle in spite of an increase in $[La^-]$, and leads to the apparently paradoxical increase in $[HCO_3^-]$ associated with an increase in $[La^-]$ [Fig. 12.24; (149)]. This adaptation is crucial for CO_2 removal from muscle, as the total CO_2 in venous blood is critically dependent on plasma [SID] and P_{CO_2}.

Venous erythrocytes show an increase in $[La^-]$ that is half that of plasma. There is also an increase in $[K^+]$ of as much as 10–15 mEq/liter, which teleologically minimizes the increase in plasma $[K^+]$ and offsets the increase in $[Cl^-]$ (168), thus helping to maintain erythrocyte $[HCO_3^-]$.

Weak acids. Increases in plasma protein concentration, secondary to water shifts, increase $[A_{tot}]$ to a small extent and are related to exercise intensity. In erythrocytes, reductions in oxygen saturation with increasing exercise are associated with increases in reduced Hb with an accompanying fall in K_A. For a given reduction in [SID], this effect leads to lower $[A^-]$, tending to limit increases in erythrocyte $[H^+]$, and increase $[HCO_3^-]$.

Carbon dioxide pressure. Carbon dioxide pressure in venous plasma is mainly a function of the balance between muscle CO_2 production and blood flow. In short-term maximal exercise, P_{CO_2} increases to above 100 mm Hg; there is an increase at the onset of submaximal exercise, but in steady-state exercise the increase above rest values is much less, to an extent that is partly related to decreases in arterial P_{CO_2} (162).

$[H^+]$ and $[HCO_3^-]$ in venous blood. Hydrogen ion

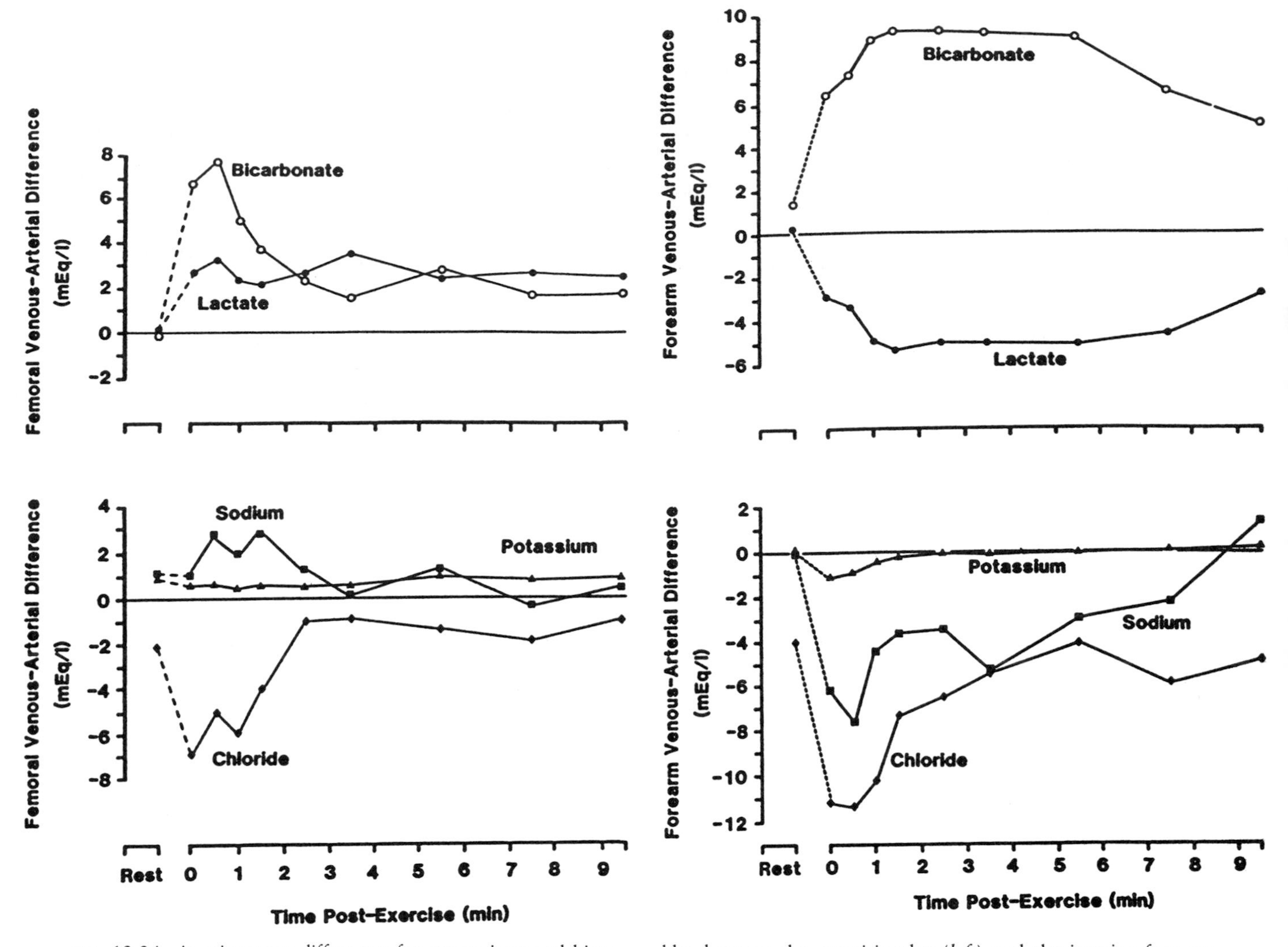

FIG. 12.24. Arteriovenous differences for strong ions and bicarbonate following 30 s maximal exercise, contrasting changes in blood across the exercising leg (*left*) and the inactive forearm (*right*). [From Kowalchuk et al. (148, 149), with permission.]

concentration in venous plasma and erythrocytes increase linearly with increases in exercise intensity, with erythrocyte $[H^+]$ being maintained approximately 20 nEq/liter above that in plasma; increases in $[H^+]$ to over 100 nEq/liter are observed in arterial plasma obtained in maximal exercise (106). In spite of an increase in plasma $[La^-]$, venous plasma $[HCO_3^-]$ increases (149), due to increases in [SID] and increases in P_{CO_2}.

Arterial Blood. Changes in arterial blood parallel the venous changes, but there are important differences related to the ventilatory adaptations to exercise, the effects of nonexercising tissues on ionic changes, and differences in HbO_2 saturation.

Water. Reductions in arterial plasma volume are similar in extent to those in venous blood, tending to increase $[A_{tot}]$ to a similar extent (160, 162).

Strong ions. There are small increases in $[Na^+]$ and $[Cl^-]$ that are quantitatively accounted for by reductions in plasma volume. Increases in plasma $[La^-]$ and $[K^+]$ are less than found in venous blood draining active muscle, due mainly to the uptake of La^- by inactive tissue (see below). Erythrocyte $[La^-]$ is half the plasma value, with no other important changes (168).

Weak acids. Increases in plasma $[A_{tot}]$ secondary to reductions in plasma volume contribute to increases in $[A^-]$.

Carbon dioxide. Pulmonary ventilation increases during exercise in relation to CO_2 output, the relationship being linear at low and moderate work but alinear at heavy intensities. The peripheral and central factors contributing to increases in ventilation remain one of the more controversial unsolved problems in physiology (68), and are beyond the scope of this chapter. However, it is of interest that studies of ventilation in resting animals have shown a closer relationship to cerebrospinal fluid (CSF) [SID] changes than to $[H^+]$ (177). Furthermore, recently Anderson and Jennings have shown that changes in arterial plasma osmolality may influence the control of breathing (6). Arterial P_{CO_2}, as expected from the alveolar ventilation equation, is unchanged from rest (35–45 mm Hg) at the lower work intensities and falls to 30–35 mm Hg at higher levels. In addition, because the CO_2 dissociation curve is steeper at low P_{CO_2}, a fall in arterial P_{CO_2} helps to increase the venoarterial CO_2 content difference and reduce muscle tissue P_{CO_2}.

Control of arterial $[H^+]$. Although $[H^+]$ is up to 10 nEq/liter less in arterial than venous plasma at low and moderate workloads, at higher levels they are virtually identical. The explanation for this is a greater fall in [SID] in arterial plasma, related to a higher $[Cl^-]$, coupled with a lower P_{CO_2} (Fig. 12.24). The higher $[Cl^-]$ is due to exchange across the erythrocyte membrane, through the band 3 protein ion carrier (146).

Lactate Oxidation and the Role of Inactive Muscle

Lactate produced by active muscle may be oxidized or resynthesized into stored glycogen (see also Chapter 14). As La^- leaving exercising muscle is distributed through the extracellular fluid, there is a large potential role for less active muscle to take up La^- and oxidize it (33, 148). In addition to acting as an aerobic fuel source, La^- oxidation acts to reduce the systemic acidosis that accompanies increases in extracellular $[La^-]$. Increased $[H^+]$ in extracellular fluid increases uptake by muscle having a low $[La^-]$. Movement of La^- across cell membranes is enhanced in both directions according to any change in $[H^+]$; thus, uptake of La^- will occur into inactive muscle if the $[H^+]$ of arterial plasma is increased.

The initial rapid uptake of La^- by inactive muscle acts as a sink for La^-, aiding in limiting its accumulation in plasma; further reduction in plasma $[La^-]$ depends on its oxidation. Evidence from measurement of arteriovenous $[La^-]$ differences across inactive muscle (148) and studies of radiolabeled La^- (238) indicate extensive La^- uptake and oxidation. Hermansen and Stensvold (107) showed that the rate at which plasma $[La^-]$ fell following heavy exercise was increased by moderate exercise. It is evident that this process can occur even in heavy exercise that is continued for a long period (134, 238) or carried out intermittently (234). Studies in the perfused rat hindlimb (235) showed that acidemic perfusion increased the oxidation of La^-, and implied that a number of ions may be involved in the regulation of La^- transfer across the cell membrane and its oxidation in the mitochondria.

Lactate oxidation provides an adaptation to reduce the severity of exercise-induced acidosis; the simplistic stoichiometry of the reaction suggests that bicarbonate will be reformed as follows:

$$La^- + 3O_2 \rightleftharpoons 2CO_2 + HCO_3^- + 3H_2O$$

However, the situation is not this simple, and as in every other acid–base situation, all the variables need to be taken into account. What appears to happen is that La^- is taken up by muscle, and thus tends to decrease [SID] and increase $[H^+]$ within the muscle, and increase [SID] in plasma. As $[HCO_3^-]$ in muscle is low, and muscle behaves as a closed system for CO_2, the result is an increase in P_{CO_2} and diffusion of CO_2 out of muscle and into venous blood. P_{CO_2} in venous blood leaving inactive muscle that has taken up La^- is markedly increased, often to over 75 mm Hg (148), and consequently $[HCO_3^-]$ and total CO_2 output from inactive muscle increase. Another possibility is as follows: uptake of lactate leads to an increase in pyruvate and its conversion to acetyl CoA with the generation of CO_2; as the energy turnover and thus citric acid cycle activity in inactive muscle are low, storage of acetyl groups may occur as acetyl carnitine, without any increase in O_2 consumption. Thus, in the unsteady state of heavy exercise or in the early recovery period, an improvement in lactic acidosis is bought at the expense of a tissue "respiratory" acidosis.

During exercise, the main fate of La^- is uptake and oxidation (7), both processes being increased by acidosis (80). La^- also takes part in gluconeogenesis in liver—the Cori cycle—which occurs mainly in low-intensity exercise (2), and may be inhibited in very heavy exercise. Gluconeogenesis in previously exercised muscle is important in recovery, and is activated rapidly (108). The reaction requires input of energy:

$$2La^- + 4ATP^{4-} + 2GTP^{4-} + 6H_2O \rightleftharpoons Glu^0 + 4ADP^{3-} + 2GDP^{3-} + 6Pi^{2-} + 4H^+$$

and the stoichiometry indicates the potential for $[H^+]$ changes, mainly related to reductions in $[La^-]$ and increases in $[Pi^{2-}]$, but to our knowledge no data exist regarding the extent of these potential changes.

Integration of Mechanisms in Acid–Base Balance and CO_2 Excretion

Exercise imposes a considerable challenge to homeostasis in the exercising muscle, which is countered by an integrated series of physicochemical and physiological mechanisms tending to minimize increases in intracellular [H^+] and remove CO_2. Locally within muscle these include changes tending to increase [SID], including breakdown of PCr^{2-} and ion exchanges to maintain [K^+], and reductions in A_{tot} and increases in K_a. Uptake of La^- and Cl^- by erythrocytes and inactive muscle tend to increase [SID] in plasma. However, the integration between physiological mechanisms is particularly important for the removal of CO_2 from muscle, involving increases in blood flow and ventilation and allosteric changes in hemoglobin molecule as pointed out earlier under Effect of Position of the Oxyhemoglobin Dissociation Curve (P_{50}).

The topic of CO_2 removal during exercise has never received the same attention as O_2 delivery; however, the two processes are inextricably linked and cooperative in nature. Aspects of CO_2 output during exercise are often explained in terms that, at best, are tautological. For example, it has long been appreciated that the time constant of CO_2 output at the onset of exercise is about twice as long as that for O_2 intake; this is usually "explained" as being due to the larger CO_2 stores or a lag in ventilation. A clearer understanding of the factors influencing CO_2 excretion may be obtained by taking a physicochemical approach to changes that occur during exercise in the muscle and venous circulation on the one hand, and the lungs and arterial circulation on the other. This separation is helpful, because in the former the CO_2 "system" is partly "closed," and in the latter it is "open." The implications are that when closed, the system's independent variable is mainly the total content of CO_2 ([CO_{2tot}]) in tissue or blood, and when open it is the P_{CO_2} in the alveoli and arterial blood.

The excretion of CO_2 involves movement between fluid compartments and carriage within them. As early as 1920, Jacobs (131) demonstrated that transfer of CO_2 across biological membranes occurred by diffusion of CO_2 down a pressure gradient, and did not occur as HCO_3^-, presumably because of its extremely poor solubility in the lipids of cell membranes. Carriage of CO_2, on the other hand, is mainly in the form of HCO_3^- because CO_2 is not highly soluble. In the discussion that follows, equilibration between all forms of CO_2 is assumed to be complete, and thus quantitatively described by the equations above. However, the rate of interconversion of CO_2 between all its forms is dependent on carbonic anhydrase, present in muscle, on capillary walls, and in erythrocytes but absent in plasma. The slow hydration of CO_2 in plasma may mean that during heavy exercise the assumption of full equilibration is not justified (111, 146); this may mean that P_{CO_2} measured in plasma by electrodes may underestimate the actual P_{CO_2} during exercise. Studies of carbonic anhydrase inhibitors during exercise in the horse (210) and humans (150, 151), have demonstrated marked effects, which interestingly are accompanied by metabolic effects, including a reduction in lactate accumulation.

In Muscle. The CO_2 system is influenced (*1*) by metabolic rate; (*2*) by changes in [SID], influencing P_{CO_2} and thus the pressure head for diffusion; (*3*) by changes in blood [SID], influencing the whole blood CO_2 dissociation curve; and (*4*) by muscle blood flow. At the onset of exercise, muscle blood flow increases rapidly, but more slowly than the muscle's oxygen demands; however, in exercise of moderate or low intensity, any deficit is made up by an increase in oxygen extraction. The arteriovenous O_2 content difference can increase instantly at least threefold to make up for any delay; the venoarterial CO_2 difference cannot increase with the same rapidity. We assume CO_2 production increases at least as fast as O_2 consumption, increasing the muscle CO_2 content ([CO_{2tot}]) and P_{CO_2}. For a given change in [CO_{2tot}], the change in P_{CO_2} depends on changes in [SID]; as shown in Figure 12.25, if [SID] increases there may be little increase in P_{CO_2}, but if there is a fall in [SID], very large increases in P_{CO_2} will occur, to establish a large gradient of P_{CO_2} between muscle and perfusing plasma. Although increases in [SID] are less common than decreases, they may occur at

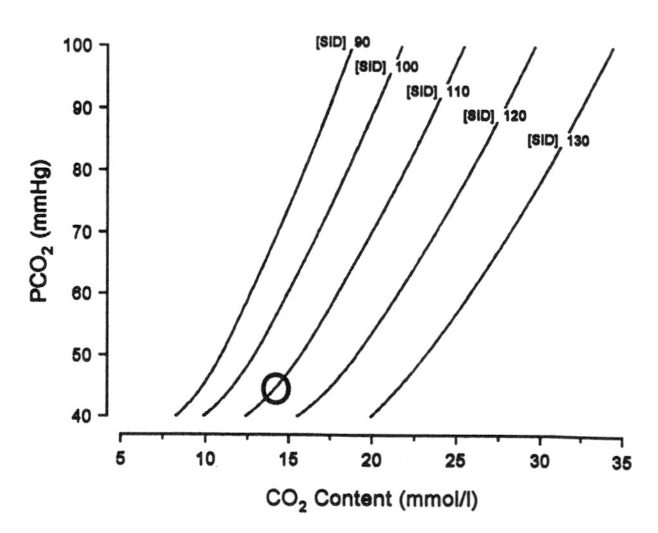

FIG. 12.25. Effects of increases in muscle CO_2 content, due to metabolism in exercise, on intracellular P_{CO_2}; resting values indicated by *circle*. Note that if [SID] is unchanged or increases, CO_2 may accumulate without a large change in P_{CO_2}, but a fall in [SID] will lead to large accompanying increases in P_{CO_2}.

the initiation of heavy exercise, when the fall in $[PCr^{2-}]$ may exceed the increase in $[La^-]$ (135).

In Venous Blood. The venous CO_2 content increases to an extent dictated mainly by the P_{CO_2} and the plasma [SID], but initially the increase in P_{CO_2} is insufficient to generate the required venoarterial content difference (Fig. 12.26) for muscle blood flow to completely remove the metabolically generated CO_2. Thus there is a delay in CO_2 washout, an accumulation of CO_2, and a further increase in P_{CO_2} in muscle, until the blood flow and venoarterial difference have increased sufficiently to carry all the CO_2 produced. In addition to an increase in venous P_{CO_2}, which probably equilibrates fully with muscle P_{CO_2}, increases in venous CO_2 content and thus the venoarterial content difference are mainly dependent on increases in venous plasma [SID] (Fig. 12.26); these are achieved through reductions in plasma $[Cl^-]$ and increases in $[Na^+]$, but hindered by any increases in $[La^-]$, as blood passes through muscle. The situation is made more complex by the different rates at which some of the ionic shifts take place, between muscle and plasma and the erythrocyte; movement of Cl^- and La^- exchange are both carrier-mediated and relatively slow processes (25, 137, 138).

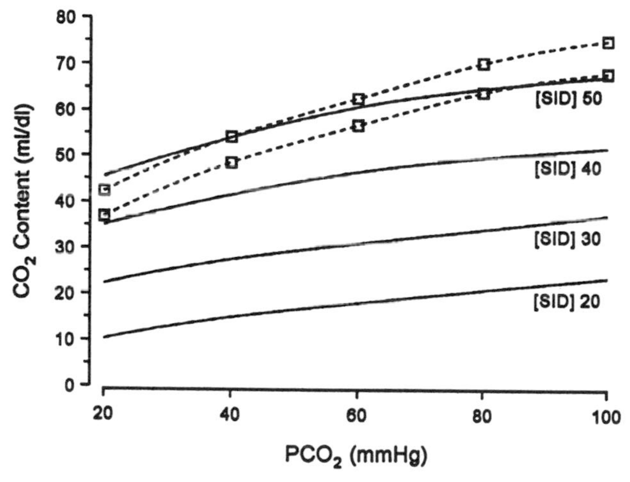

FIG. 12.26. The CO_2 "dissociation curve" for whole blood, with isopleths of plasma [SID], constructed for blood having a hemoglobin content of 14 g/dl and O_2 saturation of 97%. The points plot the classical whole blood curve of content vs. P_{CO_2} (87) for fully oxygenated blood (*lower curve*), and only 25% saturated (*upper curve*). Note that the increase in content shown by the classical relationships due to increases in P_{CO_2} and desaturation are in part due to increases in plasma [SID]. Also, note that a sufficient venoarterial difference in CO_2 content during exercise cannot be achieved through an increase in P_{CO_2} alone; an increase in [SID] is also required by virtue of the HCO_3^-–Cl^- shift to avoid a very large increase in $P_{V_{CO_2 1}}$ or decrease in Pa_{CO_2}.

The position of the whole blood CO_2 dissociation curve (Figs. 12.3 and 12.26) is shifted upwards by falls in O_2 saturation, with a greater CO_2 content at any given P_{CO_2} in unsaturated blood. This effect is mainly accounted for by the uptake of H^+ by hemoglobin, resulting in a greater chloride shift from plasma into the erythrocyte and a larger [SID] and pH in plasma. Thus, the potential increase in erythrocyte CO_2 content due to reduction in O_2 saturation per se is offset by a reduction in erythrocyte [SID] due to increases in $[Cl^-]$ and $[La^-]$ in the red cell; because of this, CO_2 content is only 0.2–0.7 ml/dl higher in blood 25% saturated than at 100% saturation, for a given plasma [SID] [Fig. 12.26 (87)]. Thus, the reduction in K_A due to deoxygenated hemoglobin may be equally as important in buffering increases in $[H^+]$ accompanying increases in erythrocyte $[Cl^-]$ as in increasing erythrocyte $[HCO_3^-]$ and $[CO_{2tot}]$. The movement of Cl^- across the erythrocyte membrane mainly takes place via the band 3 carrier protein and is a process that is sufficiently slow for it to be a limiting factor for CO_2 equilibration during heavy exercise.

CO_2 Dissociation Curve. The content of CO_2 in whole blood ($C_{CO_{2wb}}$), may be calculated by modifications of the equation of Visser (251) as a function of plasma pH, P_{CO_2}, hemoglobin, and arterial O_2 saturation, as validated by Douglas et al. (56):

$$C_{CO_{2wb}} = C_{CO_{2pl}} \{1 - [(0.0289\mathrm{Hb})/(3.352 - 0.456\mathrm{S}_{O_2}) \cdot (8.142 - \mathrm{pH})]\}$$

In this equation, plasma CO_2 content ($C_{CO_{2pl}}$) is calculated from a modification of the Henderson-Hasselbalch equation:

$$C_{CO_{2pl}} = 2.226 \cdot s \cdot P_{CO_2} \cdot (1 + 10^{\mathrm{pH}-\mathrm{p}K'})$$

where s is the solubility constant for CO_2. As changes in plasma $[A_{tot}]$ are small and due to hemoconcentration, the relationship between whole blood $[CO_{2tot}]$ and P_{CO_2} may be calculated in terms of plasma [SID] at different values of Sa_{O_2} (Fig. 12.26). The equation is empirical, and in addition to dissolved CO_2 and bicarbonate includes CO_2 carried as carbamate, in combination with hemoglobin. Carbamate formation is expressed in the reaction:

$$CO_2 + \mathrm{R\text{-}NH_2} \leftrightarrow \mathrm{R\text{-}NHCOO^-} + H^+$$

where R is a protein such as hemoglobin; the pK of the reaction is well above 7.5, indicating that the undissociated carbamic acid may be ignored in body fluids. Carbamate concentration is a function of [Hb], O_2 saturation, and pH (87), all factors that are used in the equation as parameters.

It can be seen that there may be several reasons why the venoarterial CO_2 content difference may be insufficient for complete CO_2 removal from exercising muscle, even where the blood flow and arteriovenous O_2 difference are adequate for O_2 delivery.

Pulmonary Ventilation. Ventilation increases during exercise in close relation to the flow of CO_2 to the lung (277, 278) but, clearly, additional factors play a role, particularly in heavy exercise, when a relative increase in ventilation has the effect of reducing P_{CO_2}. Increased P_{CO_2} fluctuation in arterial plasma (3, 287), increases in plasma $[K^+]$ (189), and increased efferent neural stimuli from muscle mechano- and chemoreceptors (62) have been implicated (see Chapter 10), in addition to the changes in plasma [SID] and osmolality noted above. While this relative alveolar hyperventilation is usually seen as homeostatic with respect to arterial plasma $[H^+]$, it may equally be considered as an important adaptation to aid removal of CO_2 from muscle. Because of the shape of the whole blood CO_2 dissociation curve (Fig. 12.26), a lower CO_2 content in arterial blood helps to increase the venoarterial content difference, so that in a "steady state" of heavy exercise CO_2 removal matches the metabolic demands. However, in very heavy exercise such a steady state may never be achieved, and muscle P_{CO_2} progressively increases to contribute to a marked fall in muscle pH and fatigue.

The Physicochemical Approach: Advantages and Drawbacks

In this chapter we have detailed an approach that allows a quantitative description of the factors influencing $[H^+]$ in both intracellular and extracellular fluids. We would emphasize that the approach has its roots in the classic physical chemistry of the 1920s to 1940s (105, 225), and thus cannot be considered new. What is new, and a departure from the conventional approach, is the conceptual distinction between dependent and independent variables, and in which $[HCO_3^-]$ and $[H^+]$ are clearly dependent on the interaction between several acid–base systems. This may seem a truism, and some examples may help to make the distinction explicit. In conventional discussions of acid–base changes, reactions are often considered to "provide" or "release" protons and thereby influence $[H^+]$ directly; the oxygenation of hemoglobin and lactate production are two examples. However, protons can never be provided or released without another ionic change, and even if they could be the effects cannot be predicted. Thus, in these two examples the important changes are an increase in $[K^+]$ and [SID], respectively; the potential effects of the changes on $[H^+]$ can be calculated, whereas the addition of H^+ ions is meaningless and incalculable.

A major advantage of the approach is that it frees us from the concepts developed as part of the conventional approach in which acid–base changes are described in terms of the CO_2 system. In this approach, changes in P_{CO_2} are used to characterize the respiratory contributions, and changes in $[HCO_3^-]$ at a given P_{CO_2} (40 mm Hg) are classed as metabolic and quantified in terms of "base excess" and "base deficit." Such an approach only makes sense when applied to arterial plasma and leaves us without much insight into the relative contributions of different variables. The approach also frees us from the notion that $[H^+]$ is "controlled" by the balance between P_{CO_2} and $[HCO_3^-]$. An example of the contrast between approaches related to exercise is the concept of bicarbonate buffering of lactic acid as depicted in the reaction:

$$LaH + HCO_3^- \rightleftharpoons La^- + CO_2 + H_2O$$

This scheme suggests that $[HCO_3^-]$ falls equally to the increase in $[La^-]$ and a stoichiometrically equal excess CO_2 evolution occurs; it ignores the contribution of other variables, and only "works" when applied to arterial plasma. In the past, changes in the relationships between $[La^-]$ and $[HCO_3^-]$ or $[H^+]$ have been used to infer changes in buffer capacity or as evidence that La^- and H^+ ions were leaving muscle at different rates (16, 169). Later work has clarified these controversies by showing that they were accounted for by differences in [SID] in muscle or plasma (99), and by the different behavior of acid–base variables in different fluid compartments. The reason that the concept works approximately in arterial plasma is that lactate is the only strong ion to change much, and it dominates [SID].

Once the systems and the related dependent and independent components have been defined, the variables influencing changes in $[H^+]$ are clarified. When applied to physiology, some long-held concepts are shown in a different light. For example, once $[HCO_3^-]$ is accepted as being dependent on the interaction between several systems it is difficult to accept that $[H^+]$ is "controlled" by changes in $[HCO_3^-]$, or that movement of H^+ or HCO_3^- ions are of any relevance to acid–base regulation by themselves. Furthermore, the present approach has the other distinct advantage of linking acid–base changes to other physiological functions that are influenced by ion concentration changes, such as membrane potentials, cell volume, and other aspects of fluid and electrolyte regulation.

The approach remains a source of controversy, at least in part because of confusion between the concepts involved and the mathematics used to quantify the contributions of independent variables. Conceptually, the approach may call into question some long-held mechanisms that influence ionic state in different fluid compartments (e.g., Na^+/H^+ and Cl^-/HCO_3^- exchanges). However, the approach cannot identify the mechanisms by which changes are brought about, but can quantify the effects; in these two examples it is able to quantify the effects on $[H^+]$ and $[HCO_3^-]$ in a given compartment resulting from changes in $[Na^+]$ and $[Cl^-]$.

The mathematical implications are also controversial. Although $[H^+]$ may be calculated using the approach, obviously this is not a primary objective, for $[H^+]$ may be measured. There is good concordance between measured and calculated $[H^+]$ in plasma, but accuracy is dependent on the accuracy with which the independent variables are measured; for example, at low levels of [SID] a small error has a large effect on calculated $[H^+]$ (152). A more valid criticism relates to the confidence that may be placed in the equation parameters. The most critical of these are $[A_{tot}]$ and K_A. In plasma these values were linked to plasma protein content and the results of classic titration studies (250). These established "effective" $[A_{tot}]$ and K_A; more recently it has been pointed out that these values for plasma represent the combined effects of many amino acids with widely varying K_A, and new mathematical expressions have been derived (66, 192). Such studies are of great theoretical importance, but in the practical application of the approach have not shown significant advantages (152). In the case of exercising muscle the problem is far more complex, because $[A_{tot}]$ and K_A change; titration studies have established "effective" values for them (159), but much more work is required to place them on a similar footing to plasma. Added to these problems are difficulties in measurement of ion concentrations and P_{CO_2} in muscle. Other criticisms that do not appear to be practically important include the fact that ion concentrations are measured, but $[H^+]$ is influenced by ionic activities that may be altered by changes in osmolality and by the unknown combination of free fatty acids to ionic binding sites on plasma albumin (249). The resolution of such problems awaits innovations in plasma and tissue ion measurements.

In summary, the application of a physicochemical approach to the regulation of acid–base status in muscle and extracellular fluid in exercise is in its infancy, but it has already clarified many observations and led to a rethinking of classical concepts. Furthermore, it has opened the door to understanding the close links between fluid and electrolyte control and the physiological and biochemical events occurring during exercise in muscle, the circulation, and respiration.

COMPARATIVE ASPECTS OF GAS EXCHANGE

Comparative physiology has two important objectives: *(1)* to understand important interrelationships among the many different species and their environments (ecology), and *(2)* to clarify basic functional mechanisms (anatomical, physiological, or biochemical) by taking advantage of the multiple ways that different species have modified and deployed similar mechanisms to adapt to a wide range of environmental stress and physiological requirements. Two animals that are of particular interest in understanding mechanisms of adaptation to exercise are the dog and the horse, two particularly athletic species. Both achieve maximal levels of O_2 and CO_2 exchange that are twice those in human Olympic athletes.

Comparison of Structural and Physiologic Estimates of Diffusing Capacity

Comparisons of $D_{L_{CO}}$, $D_{M_{CO}}$, and Vc estimated by physiological and morphometric methods have yielded conflicting results that remain to be clarified (45, 46, 122, 272). These comparisons between techniques are best accomplished in animal studies in which comparisons by physiological and morphometric techniques can be accomplished on the same animals. However, when compared to resting physiological measurements, morphometric estimates of $D_{L_{CO}}$ are about twice that of physiological estimates and the $D_{M_{CO}}$ about ten times that of physiological estimates in the same animal (45, 46). This gross discrepancy largely results from a failure to account for the normal physiological reserves of diffusing capacity that may be recruited from rest to exercise. It is thought that the completely unfolded membrane surface utilized by the morphometric method reflects the maximal structural capacity for diffusion, a capacity not approached physiologically except perhaps at peak exercise. Indeed, when compared to physiological measurement at peak exercise in the same animals, morphometric and physiologic estimates of $D_{L_{CO}}$ are found to be in good agreement [Fig. 12.27; (122)]. There are also significant correlations between morphometric and physiological estimates of $D_{M_{CO}}$ and Vc, however, $D_{M_{CO}}$ is still higer (by a factor of two) by the morphometric than by the physiological method, while Vc is lower (by a factor of one-half) by the morphometric than by the

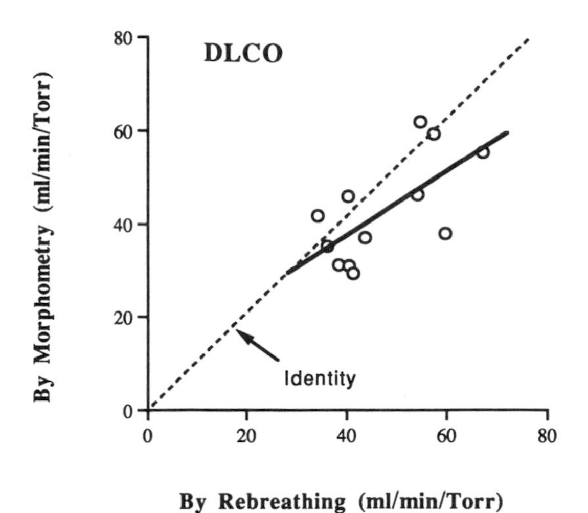

FIG. 12.27. Comparison of DL_{CO} estimates by physiologic (rebreathing) method in dogs during heavy exercise with that in the same animals by morphometric methods at postmortem. The physiological estimate of DL_{CO} at peak exercise is actually sightly greater than estimated by morphometry at postmortem. This result is misleading, however, because the membrane diffusing capacity by morphometry is twice the physiological estimate and the pulmonary capillary blood volume by morphometry is half that estimated physiologically at peak exercise. These differences remain unresolved.

physiologic method (C. C. W. Hsia and E. R. Weibel, unpublished findings). The remaining differences may be attributable to differences in both experimental conditions as well as model assumptions as discussed below.

Discrepancy Due to Experimental Conditions. A number of methodological issues arise that make direct comparisons between these two techniques difficult. As mentioned above, morphometric estimates are obtained from lungs fixed at a resting cardiac output and a lung volume intermediate between FRC and TLC (i.e., conditions not consistent with the exercise state). On the other hand, the elimination of surface tensions and the consequent complete unfolding of available alveolar membrane simulates the recruitment of diffusion surface during heavy exercise. Tissue shrinkage and deformation during fixation and processing may distort the true in vivo structural dimensions. Artificial capillary hemoconcentration as a result of the fixation process leads to a consistent overestimation of capillary hematocrit by morphometry (27). It is inherently difficult to account for dynamic inhomogeneities on fixed specimens (e.g., distribution of erythrocytes with respect to plasma flow and its possible interaction with capillary membrane). Federspiel (65), in a theoretical model, first demonstrated that erythrocyte spacing is an important determinant of effective membrane diffusing capacity for O_2 (DM_{O_2}). Wang et al. (59, 26) also showed in theoretical formulations that distorted erythrocyte shapes assumed under high-flow conditions may affect the oxygen transport characteristics of the blood. Such dynamic variables necessarily influence any physiologic measurements, but they cannot be incorporated into the present morphometric analysis.

Discrepancy Due to Model Assumptions. Systematic discrepancies between the two methods may also arise from oversimplifying assumptions or from conceptual errors in their respective models. To explore these possible conceptual errors, an independent "gold standard" is needed with which the two methods can be compared. In this regard we have applied the finite element method (FEM) (12) by using principles of heat exchange to analyze CO diffusion in a longitudinal cross section through a single hypothetical pulmonary capillary segment of defined dimensions containing an arbitrary number of equally spaced spherical red blood cells (RBCs) [see Figure 12.7; (261)]. If anatomical dimensions of a lung capillary, spacing of intracapillary RBCs, θCO per RBC, and diffusion and solubility coefficients for CO in tissue and plasma are known, the FEM can predict the distribution of CO tension as well as the CO flux into capillary red cells. By integrating these fluxes over the entire capillary and over each RBC, the total CO uptake (DL_{CO}) and effective membrane diffusing capacity (DM_{CO}) of the capillary can be estimated. DL_{CO} of the capillary model estimated at two different O_2 tensions by FEM are then introduced into the classical Roughton-Forster model (211) to determine if the anatomically defined DM_{CO} and Vc (or the number of RBCs) could be accurately recovered. Similarly, the same hypothetical capillary segment can be subjected to standard morphometric analysis to obtain estimates of DM_{CO} and Vc.

Preliminary results with this approach by one of the authors have suggested that application of the lumped parameter model developed by Roughton and Forster to a distributed process may be a source of systematic errors in both the physiologic and morphometric interpretations of DL_{CO} and DL_{O_2}. The magnitude of these potential errors needs further study; however, the results suggest that application of the stereologic construct of correcting the morphometrically estimated harmonic mean barrier thickness by a factor of two-thirds, is inappropriate; this will cause a 50% overestimate of DM by morphometry.

Recruitment of Diffusing Capacity during Exercise

There has been controversy over whether diffusing capacity of the lung reaches an upper limit at submaximal workloads. Early results with the Lilienthal-Riley method suggested such a limit for DL_{O_2} at low workloads (40). Observations by intravital microscopy (198) and by morphometry (10, 147) also have suggested that maximum recruitment of the pulmonary capillary bed occurs when pulmonary blood flow is increased only slightly above resting levels. However, as illustrated in Fig. 12.17 and 12.18, observations in human subjects fail to demonstrate an upper limit of DL_{CO} up to maximal oxygen uptake. An upper limit of DL_{CO} could not be found in dogs from rest up to maximal oxygen uptake; an upper limit for recruitment of pulmonary capillary surface markers related to metabolic function [i.e., norepinephrine receptors (58) and angiotensin-converting enzyme (59)] also could not be demonstrated in dogs. After pneumonectomy, all of the cardiac output at rest and exercise must be directed through the remaining lung; yet in foxhounds after pneumonectomy an upper limit of DL_{CO} could not be demonstrated, even at levels of pulmonary blood flow through the remaining lung equivalent to a cardiac output of 35 liters/min through both lungs in a normal foxhound (Fig. 12.28*A*). These data suggest a very extensive capillary reserve in the lung of normal mammals that continues to be recruited up to the heaviest sustainable workloads. Continued recruitment of this reserve does not, however, ensure that at heavy workloads diffusion will not impose a significant resistance to diffusive gas transport. As shown in Figure 12.28*B*, even though DL_{CO} continues to rise as pulmonary blood flow ($\dot{Q}c$) rises, $DL/\dot{Q}c$ falls to a point that diffusion imposes a significant resistance to gas exchange at heavy workloads. Sources of recruitment remain unclear. If, on the other hand, this recruitment did not occur, impairment of diffusive transport for oxygen would become evident at relatively low levels of exercise.

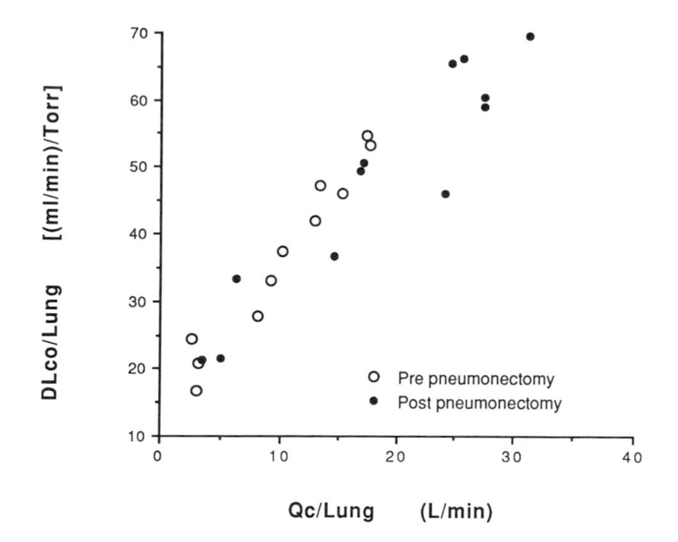

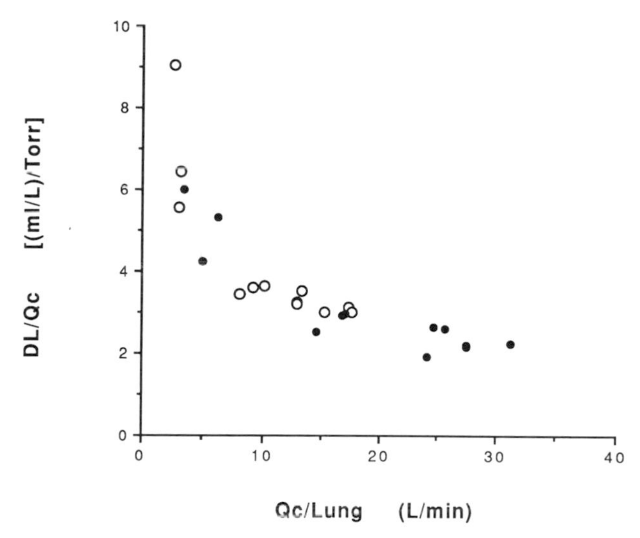

FIG. 12.28. *A*, Comparison of DL_{CO} with respect to pulmonary blood flow before and after left pneumonectomy in foxhounds. Data are normalized with respect to the normal lung and show that DL_{CO} continues to rise after pneumonectomy as blood flow is increased to a level equivalent to 35 liters/min through two normal lungs without reaching a plateau. *B*, Comparison for the relationship between $DL_{CO}/\dot{Q}c$ with respect to pulmonary blood flow from rest to peak exercise for the same data as that in *A*. The data show that in spite of continued recruitment after pneumonectomy, $DL/\dot{Q}c$ falls to a lower level after pneumonectomy than before so that diffusion became a significant source of exercise limitation.

Importance of Blood Volume and Hematocrit

Acute short-term exercise insufficient to cause significant overall body fluid loss is accompanied in man by a minor increase in hemoglobin concentration of perhaps 0.5 g/dl. This is a roughly 3% change, and appears due to a volume shift of plasma out of the vascular compartment based on higher mean vascular pressures seen during exercise. In man, there is evidence of splenic contraction during exercise, but this has little or no impact on circulating blood volume or [Hb].

However, in the dog and horse (the two most well-studied examples), the spleen undergoes massive contraction under sympathetic control. The circulation is thus augmented greatly, both in terms of circulating blood volume and systemic [Hb]. Both augmented volume and [Hb] would be expected to enhance overall performance but would not necessarily be of benefit to all steps in the O_2 transport pathway.

As regards pulmonary gas exchange, the concept of $D/\beta\dot{Q}$ should be reviewed (see earlier under Rate of Equilibration between Alveolar Air and Capillary Blood). Recall that D is pulmonary diffusing capacity; β is the slope of the O_2 dissociation curve, proportional to [Hb]; and $\dot{Q}$ is cardiac output. $D/\beta\dot{Q}$, the ratio of diffusive to perfusive conductance in the lung, determines whether diffusive equilibration of O_2 between alveolar gas and capillary blood will be complete.

Splenic contraction in the average 500-kg horse increases the [Hb] from about 14–22 g/dl and blood volume by about 12 liters. Splenectomy, of course, prevents both of these adjustments. When horses are compared before and after splenectomy, there is a dramatic change in pulmonary gas exchange. Instead of desaturation of 75%–80% (arterial O_2 saturation at $\dot{V}O_{2max}$), saturation is preserved in the mid to low 90s (at rest, 95%–97% saturation is the rule). Without using the MIGET to sort through the possible reasons for this remarkable improvement in arterial oxygenation, some speculation is warranted:

1. Splenectomy, in reducing $\dot{V}O_{2max}$, reduces the ventilatory requirements at peak exercise. The horse, however, does not reduce maximal ventilation, probably because of greater metabolic acidosis from earlier lactate production following splenectomy. Consequently, arterial PCO_2 is reduced some 10 mm Hg, while arterial PO_2 is correspondingly higher.
2. Maximal cardiac output is some 20% lower after splenectomy, thereby tending to prolong average capillary transit time. This is the consequence of a lower total blood volume (30 liters vs. 40 liters, roughly) and consequently lower cardiac filling pressures. We do not know to what degree this is offset by a reduced pulmonary capillary blood volume.
3. The failure of [Hb] to rise after splenectomy correspondingly causes β (as defined above) to remain low.
4. There may be a reduction in D if it is dependent on [Hb] as is the case in man.

The last three changes make projection of the overall $D\beta\dot{Q}$ ratio speculative, but on balance, the reductions in β and $\dot{Q}$ probably exceed that of D, increasing the $D/\beta\dot{Q}$ ratio and thus favoring diffusion equilibration. If blood doping in man acts similarly, both the volume and [Hb] augmentation may have multiple, interactive, and partially offsetting effects despite the net overall improvement in maximum $\dot{V}O_2$.

Another aspect of changes in hematocrit on gas exchange may be derived from dog studies. Figure 12.29*A* shows the increase in hematocrit in normal foxhounds from rest to heavy exercise; this represents about a 40% increase in hematocrit in the foxhound compared to only about a 3% increase in humans. Figure 12.29*B* shows the increase in DL_{CO} with respect to cardiac output in the foxhound compared with the human from rest to peak exercise normalized for body weight. There is a significantly steeper slope of recruitment of DL_{CO} in the foxhound than in the human. Normalizing the data for body

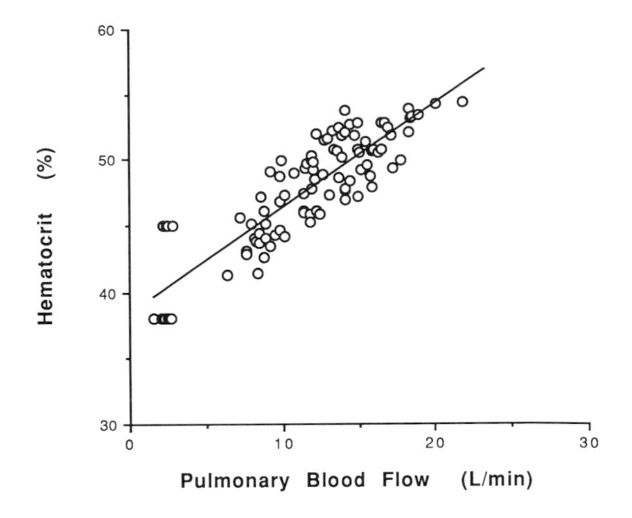

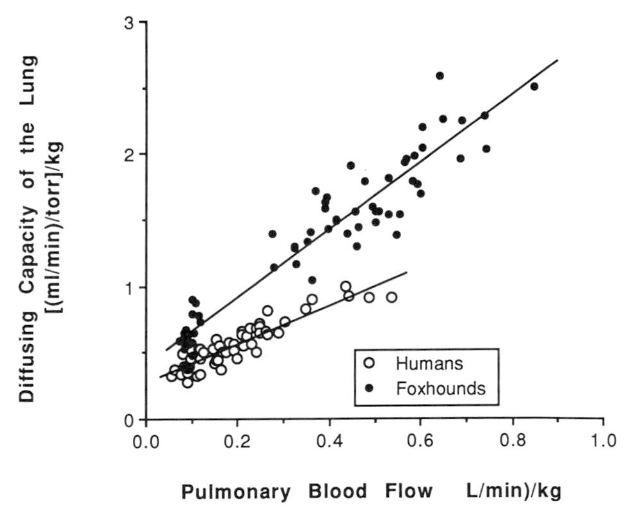

FIG. 12.29. *A*, Change in hematocrit in normal foxhounds from rest to peak exercise. There is an approximately 40% increase in hematocrit in foxhounds owing to injection of red cells into the circulation by splenic contraction. In humans the increase of hematocrit is only about 3% under similar conditions, primarily due to a fall in plasma valume. *B*, Comparison of the recruitment of DL_{CO} in foxhounds with that in humans as pulmonary blood flow increases during exercise. Recruitment of diffusing capacity is significantly steeper in foxhounds than in humans, very likely a result of the large expansion of circulating blood volume in the foxhound from exercise-induced splenic contraction.

weight does not alter the slope of these relationships, since both DL_{CO} and $\dot{Q}c$ are normalized by the same factor; slopes are significantly different in absolute as well as relative terms. The foxhound's lung is one-half to two-thirds that of the human in size; yet the foxhound is able to recruit DL_{CO} much more effectively during exercise than the human, and DL_{CO} in the dog approaches in absolute terms the DL_{CO} in human Olympic athletes. How is this accomplished? There are two potential mechanisms: *(1)* the pulmonary capillary bed in the dog is structurally different (e.g., more compliant to changes in pressure in the dog than in the human); and *(2)* splenic contraction augments both blood volume and hematocrit in the dog, which enhances capillary and surface area recruitment for gas exchange during exercise. The latter mechanism is unavailable in the human, in whom the small increase in hematocrit actually reflects a decrease in plasma volume rather than splenic contraction. Both the horse and the dog blood dope themselves during exercise by a direct transfusion of red cells into the circulation that seems to occur in direct proportion to the intensity of the exercise. This augmentation of volume and hematocrit in the horse and in the dog may enhance not only convective transport due to the increase in O_2 carrying capacity of the blood but also by increasing diffusive transport in the lung and perhaps in muscle. The latter mechanisms, if true, may be extremely important in human adaptive responses to high altitude, where an increase in oxygen carrying capacity of the blood if unaccompanied by enhancement in diffusive transport in lung and muscle would be relatively ineffective in raising exercise capacity at high altitude, where exercise is predominantly limited by diffusion in the lungs and in the muscle rather than by cardiac output.

Optimization of O_2 Transport—The Role of Hemoglobin P_{50}

Time-honored arguments state that while a right-shifted (high P_{50}) oxyhemoglobin dissociation curve favors peripheral unloading of O_2 in the muscle, a left-shifted (low P_{50}) curve favors loading of oxygen in the pulmonary capillaries (see equation 39). Therefore, both pulmonary and tissue oxygen exchange must be somewhat compromised for overall optimization of O_2 transport. The horse and the foxhound both present good examples for asking the question of whether the O_2 hemoglobin dissociation curve is optimally positioned for maximizing O_2 transport at peak exercise. This is because both are athletic species that exhibit prominent O_2 desaturation during peak exercise (13, 126, 190) due to acidosis and hypercapnia (Bohr effects), hyperthermia, and diffusion limitation (Table 12.7). Thus, O_2 sat-

TABLE 12.7. *O_2 and CO_2 Transport Data on Horses and Foxhounds at $\dot{V}O_{2max}$*

		Horse	Foxhound	
		Normal	Normal	Right Pnx*
Weight	kg		25.4	23.7
DL_{O_2}	ml · min^{-1} mm Hg^{-1}	1075	66.5	46.2
Dt_{O_2}	ml · min^{-1} · mm Hg^{-1}	1700	79.0	62.5
O_2 uptake	liters · min^{-1}	65.6	3.57	2.77
CO_2 output	liters · min^{-1}	79.0	3.76	3.03
Temperature	°C	41.9	41.5	41.2
PA_{O_2}	mm Hg	101	106	113
Hemoglobin	g/dl	20.3	19.4	20.5
Pa_{O_2}	mm Hg	73	84.7	86.1
Pa_{CO_2}	mm Hg	52.5	46.0	40.3
pHa		7.16	7.25	7.26
Sa_{O_2}	%	81.6	86.2	86.4
Arterial O_2 content	ml/dl	23.22	23.03	24.2
$P\bar{v}_{O_2}$	mm Hg	15.3	23.0	23.5
$P\bar{v}_{CO_2}$	mm Hg	112	82.8	78.5
pHv			7.13	7.14
$S\bar{v}_{O_2}$	%	8.1	13.3	16.0
Venous O_2 content	ml/dl	2.32	3.12	4.17
Arterial lactate	mM/l	8.6	4.2	4.1
Standard P_{50}	mm Hg	25.0	29.0	29.0
In vivo arterial P_{50}	mmHg	41.5	43.1	41.6

*Foxhounds that had undergone right pneumonectomy 9 months earlier.

uration is commonly in the range of only 80%–85%, and one could easily imagine that this deficit cannot be made up by the better peripheral unloading afforded by the rightward shift produced by the above factors.

Calculations can be performed to elucidate this question and to test the effectiveness of feedback control provided by the allosteric properties of hemoglobin using data. Knowing at $\dot{V}O_{2max}$ and O_2 diffusing capacity of both lungs and muscle, together with alveolar PO_2 and PCO_2 (under ventilatory control), cardiac output, and standard blood-based variables (Hb, temperature, acid–base status), it is possible to compute muscle and venous PO_2, saturation, and O_2 content (and thus expected $\dot{V}O_{2max}$) as a function of P_{50}. In these calculations, the in vivo P_{50} has been translated back to the standard P_{50} at pH 7.4, $PaCO_2$ 40 mm Hg and zero base excess. The *upper two panels* of Figure 12.30 show the conflicting effects of P_{50} on arterial O_2 saturation (and thus on arterial O_2 delivery) and on peripheral O_2 extraction. As a result, in the horse, $\dot{V}O_{2max}$ peaks at a P_{50} in the low 20 mm Hg range (Fig. 12.30, *lower panel*). As can be seen, actual $\dot{V}O_{2max}$ is only minimally less than optimum, occurring at a standard P_{50} of 25 mm Hg. Similar effects occur for the dog, despite differences between the two species in actual standard P_{50} and the peak at which $\dot{V}O_{2max}$ is expected to occur.

Thus, despite significant arterial desaturation, the large increase of in vivo P_{50} happens to have been at the optimal vale for overall O_2 transport in both species at the measured alveolar oxygen tension. From the parabolic shapes of these predicted relationships between $\dot{V}O_{2max}$ and P_{50} it is possible to see how important and effective feedback control provided by the allosteric properties of hemoglobin is in optimizing oxygen transport. As pointed out in an earlier section, an optimal P_{50} not only achieves a maximal O_2 saturation difference at peak exercise but also minimizes the A-V PCO_2 and $[H^+]$ difference required for a given maximal CO_2 output through the Haldane effect. Thus, in effect both O_2 and CO_2 transport are optimized.

CONCLUSION

Gas exchange should not be considered as a separate component of exercise but rather should be considered as one of multiple linked components in a metabolic pathway that includes glycolysis, the tricarboxylic acid cycle, and the electron transport chain. All components and mechanisms of control in this pathway are inextricably linked. This linkage provides the necessary control for rapid minute-to-minute or second-to-second changes in metabolic rate and oxygen supply, which in man may increase by 20-fold from rest to maximal exercise and in some athletic animals such as the horse and dog by 40-fold. Supply is maintained by rapid changes in cardiac output and ventilation. However, we also emphasize the molecular control exerted by the allosteric properties of hemoglobin in maintaining optimal matching of resistances imposed on rates of gas exchange in the lung and muscle; the importance

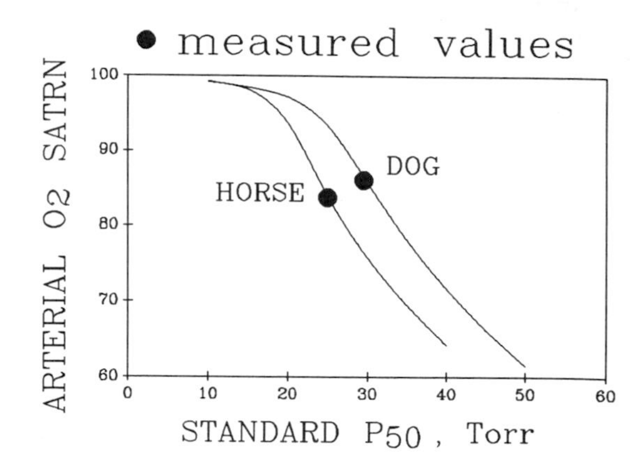

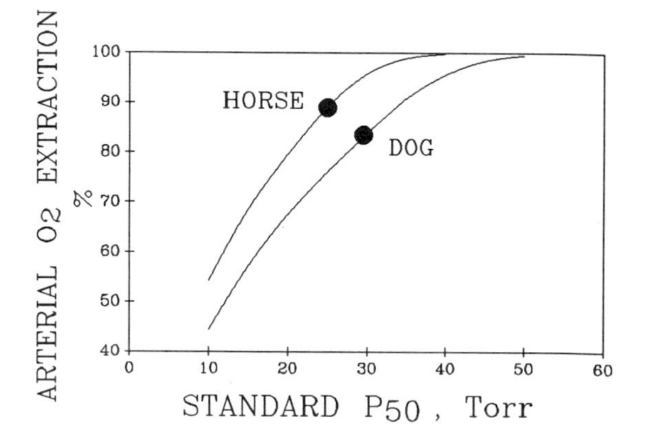

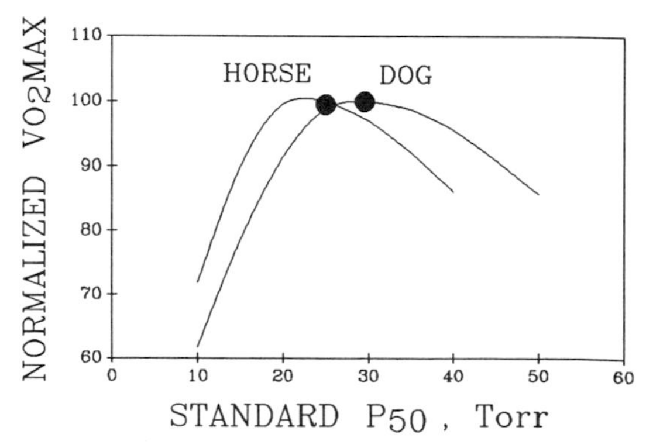

FIG. 12.30. Effect of P_{50} in optimizng maximal oxygen uptake. The principles illustrated with equation 39 were applied to available data on horses and foxhounds at maximal oxygen uptake.

of this mechanism is illustrated in Figure 12.30. Thus, hemoglobin provides a mechanism to maximize A-V O_2 and CO_2 content differences at any given levels of ventilation and cardiac output at maximal exercise, while minimizing A-V P_{CO_2} differences and pH changes in muscle. Control of O_2 and CO_2 transport are absolutely essential to the integrity of the metabolic pathways in muscle not only in supplying sufficient oxygen but also in eliminating CO_2 and to prevent intramuscular $[H^+]$ from rising to levels that would inhibit enzymatic and contractile function.

REFERENCES

1. Adaro, F., and L. E. Fahri. Effects of intralobular gas diffustion on alveolar gas exchange. *Federation Proc.* 30: 437, 1971 (Abstract).
2. Ahlborg, G., P. Felig, L. Hagenfeldt, R. Hendler, and J. Wahren. Substrate turnover during prolonged exercise in man. Splanchnic and leg metabolism of glucose, free fatty acids, and amino acids. *J. Clin. Invest.* 53: 1080–1090, 1974.
3. Allen, C. J., and N. L. Jones. Rate of change in alveolar carbon dioxide and the control of ventilation during exercise. *J. Physiol. (Lond.)* 355: 1–9, 1984.
4. Allen, T. A., and W. S. Root. Partition of carbon monoxide and oxygen between air and whole blood of rats, dogs and men as affected by plasma pH. *J. Appl. Physiol.* 10: 186–190, 1957.
5. Altman, P. L., and D. S. Dittman. *Respiration and Circulation, 2nd Ed. Biological Handbooks*, edited by P. L. Altman and D. S. Dittmer. Bethesda, MD: Federation of American Societies for Experimental Biology, 1971, p. 930.
6. Anderson, J. W., and D. B. Jennings. Osmolality, NaCl dietary intake, and regulation of ventilation by CO_2. *Am. J. Physiol.* 255 (*Regulatory Integrative Comp. Physiol.* 24): R105–R112, 1988.
7. Åstrand, P.-O., F. Hultman, A. Juhlin-Dannfelt, and G. Reynolds. Disposal of lactate during and after strenuous exercise in humans. *J. Appl. Physiol.* 61: 338–343, 1986.
8. Astrup, P., and J. W. Severinghaus. *History of Acid-Base Physiology*. Stockholm: Munksgaard, 1986.
9. Bachofen, H., S. Schürch, M. Urbinelli, and E. R. Weibel. Relations among alveolar surface tension, surface area, volume, and recoil pressure. *J. Appl. Physiol.* 62: 1878–1887, 1987.
10. Bachofen, H., D. Wangensteen, and E. R. Weibel. Surfaces and volumes of alveolar tissue under zone II and zone III conditions. *J. Appl. Physiol. Respir. Environ. Exerc. Physiol.* 53: 879–885, 1982.
11. Bates, D. V., N. G. Boucot, and A. E. Dormer. The pulmonary diffusing capacity in normal subjects. *J. Physiol. (Lond.)* 129: 237–252, 1955.
12. Bathe, K. *Finite Element Procedures in Engineering Analysis*. Englewood Cliffs, NJ: Prentice-Hall, 1932.
13. Bayly, W. M., B. D. Grant, R. G. Breeze, and J. W. Kramer. The effects of maximal exercise on acid-base balance and arterial blood gas tension in thoroughbred horses. In: *Equine Exercise Physiology*, edited by D. H. Snow, S. G. B. Persson, and R. J. Rose. Cambridge, UK: Granta, 1983, p. 400–407.
14. Bebout, D. E., D. Story, J. Roca, M. C. Hogan, D. C. Poole, C. R. Gonzalez, O. Ueno, P. Haab, and P. D. Wagner. Effects of altitude acclimatization on pulmonary gas exchange during exercise. *J. Appl. Physiol.* 67: 2286–2295, 1989.
15. Bellingham, A. J., J. C. Detter, and C. Lenfant. Mechanisms of hemoglobin oxygen affinity in acidosis and alkalosis. *J. Clin. Invest.* 50: 700–706, 1971.
16. Benadé, A. J. S., and N. Heisler. Comparison of efflux rates of hydrogen and lactate ions from isolated muscles *in vitro*. *Respir. Physiol.* 32: 369–380, 1978.
17. Bessman, S. P., and F. Savabi. The role of the phosphocreatine energy shuttle in exercise and muscular hypertrophy. In: *Biochemistry of Exercise VII*, edited by A. W. Taylor, P. D. Gollnick, H. J. Green, C. D. Ianuzzo, E. G. Noble, G. Métivier, and J. R. Sutton. Champaign, IL: Human Kinetics Press, 1990, p. 167–178.
18. Bidani, A., E. D. Crandall, and R. E. Forster. Analysis of post capillary pH changes in blood in vivo after gas exchange. *J. Appl. Physiol.* 44: 770–781, 1978.
19. Blanchard, E. M., B. Pan, and R. J. Solero. The effect of acidic pH on the ATPase activity and tronin CA^{2+} binding of rabbit skeletal myofilaments. *J. Biol. Chem.* 259: 3181–3186, 1984.
20. Bohr, C. Ueber die Lungenatmung. *Scand. Arch. Physiol.* 2: 236–268, 1891.
21. Bohr, C. Uber die spesifische Tatigkeit der Lungen bei der respiratorischen Gasaufnahme und ihr Verhalten zu der durch die alveolarwand stattfinden Gasdiffusion. *Scand. Arch. Physiol.* 22: 221–280, 1909.
22. Bohr, C., K. A. Hasselbach, and A. Krogh. Uber inen in biologischen Beziehung wichtigen Einfluss, den die Kohlensaurespannung de Blutes auf dessen Saurstoffbindung ubt. *Scand. Arch. Physiol.* 16: 401–412, 1904.
23. Borland, C. D. R., and T. Higgenbottam. A simultaneous single breath measurement of pulmonary diffusing capacity with nitric oxide and carbon monoxide. *Eur. Respir. J.* 2: 56–63, 1989.
24. Boyden, E. A. The structure of the pulmonary acinus in a child of six years and eight months. *Am. J. Anat.* 132: 275–300, 1971.
25. Brooks, G. A. The lactate shuttle during exercise and recovery. *Med. Sci. Sports Exerc.* 18: 355–364, 1986.
26. Bunker, J. P. The great trans-Atlantic acid-base debate. *Anesthesia* 26: 591–594, 1965.
27. Bur, S., H. Bachofen, P. Gehr, and E. R. Weibel. Lung fixation by airway instillation: effects on capillary hematocrit. *Exp. Lung Res.* 9: 57–66, 1985.
28. Burri, P. H., and E. R. Weibel. Morphometric estimation of pulmonary diffusion capacity. II. Effect of P_{O_2} on the growing lung, adaption of the growing rat lung to hypoxia and hyperoxia. *Respir. Physiol.* 11: 247–264, 1971.
29. Burt, C. T., J. Koutcher, J. T. Roberts, R. E. London, and B. Chance. Magnetic resonance spectroscopy of the musculoskeletal system. *Radiol. Clin. North Am.* 24: 321–331, 1986.
30. Capen, R. L., L. P. Latham, and W. W. Wagner, Jr. Diffusing capacity of the lung during hypoxia: role of capillary recruitment. *J. Appl. Physiol. Respir. Environ. Exerc. Physiol.* 50: 165–171, 1981.
31. Carlin, J. I., C. C. W. Hsia, S. S. Cassidy, M. Ramanathan, P. S. Clifford, and R. L. Johnson, Jr. Recruitment of lung diffusing capacity with exercise before and after pneumonectomy in dogs. *J. Appl. Physiol.* 70: 135–142, 1991.

32. Cassoly, R., and Q. H. Gibson. Conformation, cooperativity and ligand binding in human hemoglobin. *J. Mol. Biol.* 91: 301–313, 1975.
33. Chin, E. R., M. I. Lindinger, and G. J. F. Heigenhauser. Lactate metabolism in inactive skeletal muscle during lactacidosis. *Am. J. Physiol.* 261 (*Regulatory Integrative Comp. Physiol.* 30): R93–R105, 1991.
34. Chow, E. I., E. D. Crandall, and R. E. Forster. Kinetics of bicarbonate-chloride exchange across the human red cell membrane. *J. Gen. Physiol.* 68: 633–652, 1976.
35. Christianson, J., C. G. Douglas, J. S. Haldane, and J. B. S. Haldane. The absorption and dissociation of carbon dioxide from human blood. *J. Physiol. (Lond.)* 48: 244–271, 1914.
36. Christoforides, C., L. H. Laasberg, and J. Hedley-Whyte. Effect of temperature on solubility of O_2 in human plasma. *J. Appl. Physiol.* 26: 56–60, 1969.
37. Clausen, T. Significance of the Na^+-K^+ pump regulation in skeletal muscle. *News Physiol. Sci.* 5: 148–151, 1990.
38. Clode, M., and E. J. M. Campbell. The relationship between gas exchange and changes in blood lactate changes during exercise. *Clin. Sci.* 37: 263–272, 1969.
39. Coates, G., H. O'Brodovich, A. L. Jeffries, and G. W. Gray. Effects of exercise on lymph flow in sheep and goats during normoxia and hypoxia. *J. Clin. Invest.* 74: 133–141, 1984.
40. Cohn, J. E., B. W. Carroll, B. W. Armstrong, R. H. Shephard, and R. L. Riley. Maximal diffusing capacity in the lung in normal male subjects of different ages. *J. Appl. Physiol.* 6: 588–597, 1954.
41. Colebatch, H. J. H., and C. K. Y., Ng. Estimating alveolar surface area during life. *Respir. Physiol.* 88: 163–170, 1992.
42. Constantine, H. P., M. R. Craw, and R. E. Forster. Rate of reaction of carbon dioxide with human red blood cells. *Am. J. Physiol.* 208: 801–811, 1965.
43. Cooke, R., K. Franks, G. B. Luciani, and E. Pate. The inhibition of rabbit skeletal muscle contraction by hydrogen ions and phosphate. *J. Physiol. (Lond.)* 395: 77–97, 1988.
44. Crandall, E. D., and J. E. Obrasky. Direct evidence for participation of rat lung carbonic anhydrase in CO_2 reactions. *J. Clin. Invest.* 62: 618–622, 1978.
45. Crapo, J. D., and R. O. Crapo. Comparison of total lung diffusion capacity and the membrane component of diffusion capacity as determined by physiologic and morphometric techniques. *Respir. Physiol.* 51: 183–194, 1983.
46. Crapo, J. D., R. O. Crapo, R. L. Jensen, R. R. Mercer, and E. R. Weibel. Evaluation of lung diffusing capacity by physiological and morphometric techniques [published erratum appears in *J. Appl. Physiol.* 65:following 2800, 1988.]. *J. Appl. Physiol.* 64: 2083–2091, 1988.
47. Craw, M. R., H. P. Constantine, J. A. Morello, and R. E. Forster. Rate of the Bohr shift in human red cell suspensions. *J. Appl. Physiol.* 18: 317–374, 1963.
48. Crawford, A. B. H., M. Makowska, M. Paiva, and L. A. Engel. Convection and diffusion-dependent ventilation maldistribution in normal subjects. *J. Appl. Physiol.* 49: 838–846, 1985.
49. Cruz-Orive, L. M., and E. R. Weibel. Recent stereological methods for cell biology: brief surgery. *Am. J. Physiol.* 258 (*Lung Cell. Mol. Physiol.* 2): L148–L156, 1990.
50. Cumming, G., J. Crank, K. Horsefield, and I. Parker. Gaseous diffusion in the airways of the human lung. *Respir. Physiol.* 1: 58–54, 1966.
51. Cumming, G., K. Horsfireld, J. G. Jones, and D. C. F. Muir. The influence of gaseous diffusion on the alveolar plateau at different lung volumes. *Respir. Physiol.* 2: 386–398, 1967.
52. Dalziel, K., and J. C. Londesborough. The mechanisms of reductive carboxylation reactions. Carbon dioxide or bicarbonate as substrate of nicotinamide-adenine dinucleotide phosphate-linked isocitrate dehydrogenase and malic enzyme. *Biochem. J.* 110: 223–230, 1968.
53. Davies, G., and L. Reid. Growth of the alveoli and pulmonary arteries in childhood. *Thorax* 25: 669–681, 1970.
54. Dawson, M. J., D. G. Gadian, and D. R. Wilkie. Muscular fatigue investigated by phosphorus nuclear magnetic resonance. *Nature* 274: 861–865, 1978.
55. Dempsey, J. A., P. G. Hanson, and K. S. Henderson. Exercise induced arterial hypoxemia in healthy human subjects at sea level. *J. Physiol. (Lond.)* 355: 161–175, 1984.
56. Douglas, A. R., N. L. Jones, and J. W. Reed. Calculation of whole blood CO_2 content. *J. Appl. Physiol.* 65: 473–477, 1988.
57. Dunnill, M. S. Postnatal growth of the lung. *Thorax* 17: 329–333, 1962.
58. Dupuis, J., C. A. Goresky, C. Junear, A. Calderone, J. L. Rouleau, C. P. Rose, and S. Goresky. Use of norepinephrine uptake to measure lung capillary recruitment with exercise. *J. Appl. Physiol.* 68: 700–713, 1990.
59. Dupuis, J., C. A. Goresky, J. W. Ryan, J. L. Rouleau, and G. G. Bach. Pulmonary angiotensin-converting enzyme substrate hydrolysis during exercise. *J. Appl. Physiol.* 75: 1868–1886, 1992.
60. Edwards, R. H. T. Human muscle function and fatigue. *Ciba Found. Symp.* 82: 1–18, 1981.
61. Effros, R. M., L. Shapiro, and P. Silverman. Carbonic anhydrase activity of rabbit lungs. *J. Appl. Physiol.* 49: 589–600, 1980.
62. Eldridge, F. L. Central integration of mechanisms in exercise dyspnea. *Med. Sci. Sports Exerc.* 26: 319–327, 1994.
63. Evans, J. W., and P. D. Wagner. Limits on $\dot{V}_A/\dot{Q}$ distribution from analysis of experimental inert gas elimination. *J. Appl. Physiol.* 42: 889–898, 1977.
64. Farrell, P. A., M. B. Maron, L. H. Hamilton, M. G. Maksud, and C. Foster. Time course of lung volume changes during prolonged treadmill exercise. *Med. Sci. Sports Exerc.* 15: 319–324, 1983.
65. Federspiel, W. J. Pulmonary diffusing capacity: implications of two-phase blood flow in capillaries. *Respir. Physiol.* 77: 119–134, 1989.
66. Figge, J., T. Mydosh, and V. Fencl. Serum proteins and acid-base equilibria: a follow-up. *J. Lab. Clin. Med.* 120: 713–719, 1992.
67. Filley, G. F., D. J. Mac Intosh, and G. W. Wright. Carbon monoxide uptake and pulmonary diffusing capacity in normal subjects at rest and during exercise. *J. Clin. Invest.* 33: 530–539, 1954.
68. Filley, G. F., G. D. Swanson, and N. B. Kindig. Chemical breathing controls: slow, intermediate and fast. *Clin. Chest Med.* 1: 13–32, 1980.
69. Forrest, J. B., and E. R. Weibel. Morphometric estimation of pulmonary diffusion capacity. VII. The normal guinea pig lung. *Respir. Physiol.* 24: 191–202, 1975.
70. Forster, R. E. Exchange of gases between alveolar air and pulmonary capillary blood: pulmonary diffusing capacity. *Physiol. Rev.* 37: 391–452, 1957.
71. Forster, R E. Diffusion of gases across the alveolar capillary membrane. In: *Handbook of Physiology*, *The Respiratory System, Gas Exchange*, edited by L. E. Fahri and S. M. Tenney. Washington, DC: Am. Physiol. Soc., 1987, p. 71–88.

72. Fung, Y. C. B., and S. S. Sobin. Pulmonary alveolar blood flow. In: *Bioengineering Aspects of the Lung*, edited by J. B. West. New York and Basel: Marcel Dekker, Inc., 1977, p. 267–359.
73. Gale, G. E., J. R. Torre-Bueno, R. E. Moon, H. A. Saltzman, and P. D. Wagner. Ventilation/perfusion inequality in normal humans during exercise at sea level and simulated altitude. *J. Appl. Physiol.* 58: 978–988, 1985.
74. Gamble, J. L. *Chemical Anatomy, Physiology and Pathology of Extracellular Fluid.* Cambridge, MA: Harvard University Press, 1949.
75. Geelhaar, A., and E. R. Weibel. Morphometric estimation of pulmonary diffusion capacity. 3. The effect of increased oxygen consumption in Japanese waltzing mice. *Respir. Physiol.* 11: 354–366, 1971.
76. Gehr, P., M. Bachofen, and E. R. Weibel. The normal human lung: ultrastructure and morphometric estimation of diffusion capacity. *Respir. Physiol.* 32: 121–140, 1978.
77. Gibson, Q. H., F. Kreuzer, E. Medu, and F. J. W. Roughton. The kinetics of human hemoglobin in solution and in the red cell at 37°C. *J. Physiol. (Lond.)* 129: 65–89, 1955.
78. Gibson, Q. H., and F. J. W. Roughton. The reactions of sheep hemoglobin with nitric oxide. *J. Physiol. (Lond.)* 128: 69P, 1955.
79. Gil, J., H. Bachofen, P. Gehr, and E. R. Weibel. Alveolar volume-surface area relation in air- and saline-filled lungs fixed by vascular perfusion. *J. Appl. Physiol. Respir. Environ. Exerc. Physiol.* 47: 990–1001, 1979.
80. Gladden, L. B. Lactate uptake by skeletal muscle. In: *Exercise and Sports Sciences Reviews*, edited by K. B. Pandolf. Baltimore: Williams & Wilkins, 1989, p. 115–116.
81. Gledhill, N., A. B. Froese, and J. A. Dempsey. Ventilation to perfusion distribution during exercise in health. In: *Muscular Exercise and the Lung*, edited by J. A. Dempsey and C. E. Reed. Madison, WI: University of Wisconsin Press, 1977, p. 325–344.
82. Graham, B. L., J. T. Mink, and D. J. Cotton. Improved accuracy and precision of single-breath CO diffusing capacity measurements. *J. Appl. Physiol. Respir. Environ. Exerc. Physiol.* 51: 1306–1313, 1981.
83. Gros, G., and S. J. Dodgson. Velocity of CO_2 exchange in muscle and liver. *Ann. Rev. Physiol.* 50: 669–694, 1988.
84. Grote, J. Die Sauerstoffeddiffusionscostanten im lungengewebe and wasser und ihre temperaturebhangikeit. *Pflugers Arch. Ges. Physiol.* 295: 245–254, 1967.
85. Guenard, H., N. Varene, and P. Vaida. Determination of lung capillary blood volume and membrane diffusing capacity in patients in man by the measurements of NO and CO transfer. *Respir. Physiol.* 70: 113–120, 1987.
86. Gundersen, H. J. G., T. B. Jensen, and R. Østerby. Distribution of membrane thickness determined by lineal analysis. *J. Microsc.* 113: 27–43, 1978.
87. Gutierrez, G., and J. J. Ronco. Tissue gas exchange. In: *Pulmonary and Critical Care Medicine*, edited by R. C. Bone. St Louis: Mosby, 1994, p. 1–18.
88. Haefeli, B. B., and E. R. Weibel. Morphometry of the human pulmonary acinus. *Anat. Rec.* 220: 401–414, 1988.
89. Haldane, J., and J. L. Smith. The oxygen tension of arterial blood. *J. Physiol. (Lond.)* 20: 497–518, 1896.
90. Hammond, M. D., G. E. Gale, K. S. Kapitan, A. Ries, and P. D. Wagner. Pulmonary gas exchange in humans during normobaric hypoxic exercise. *J. Appl. Physiol.* 61: 1749–1757, 1986.
91. Hammond, M. D., and S. C. Hempleman. Oxygen diffusing capacity estimates derived from measured VA/Q distributions in man. *Respir. Physiol.* 69: 129–147, 1987.
92. Hansen, J. E., and E. P. Ampaya. Human air space shapes, sizes, areas and volumes. *J. Appl. Physiol.* 38: 990–995, 1975.
93. Hartridge, H., and F. J. W. Roughton. A method for measuring the velocity of very rapid reactions. *Proc. R. Soc. Lond. A* 104: 376–394, 1923.
94. Hartridge, H., and F. J. W. Roughton. The velocity with which carbon monoxide displaces oxygen from combination with hemoglobin. Part I. *Proc. R. Soc. Lond., B* 94: 336–367, 1923.
95. Hartridge, H., and F. J. W. Roughton. The velocity with which oxygen combines with reduced hemoglobin. Part III. *Proc. R. Soc. Lond. A* 107: 654–683, 1925.
96. Hasselbalch, K. Neutralitatsregulation und reizbarkeit des atemzentrums in ihren Wirkungen auf die koklensauresspannung des Blutes. *Bioochem. Z.* 46: 403–439, 1912.
97. Havel, R. J., B. Pernow, and N. L. Jones. Uptake and release of fatty acids and other metabolites in legs of exercising men. *J. Appl. Physiol.* 23: 90–99, 1967.
98. Heidelberger, E., and R. B. Reeves. O2 transfer kinetics in a whole blood unicellular thin layer. *J. Appl. Physiol.* 68: 1854–1890, 1990.
99. Heigenhauser, G. J. F., N. L. Jones, J. M. Kowalchuk, and M. I. Lindinger. The role of the physicochemical systems in plasma in acid-base control in exercise. In: *Biochemistry of Exercise VII*, edited by A. W. Taylor, P. D. Gollnick, H. J. Green, C. D. Ianuzzo, E. G. Noble, G. Metivier, and J. R. Sutton. Champaign, IL: Human Kinetics, 1990, p. 359–374.
100. Heigenhauser, G. J. F., and M. I. Lindinger. The total ionic status of muscle during intense exercise. In: *Oxygen Transfer from Atmosphere to Tissues*, edited by N. C. Gonzales and M. R. Fedde. New York: Plenum Press, 1988, p. 237–242.
101. Heisler, N., and J. Piiper. The buffer value of rat diaphragm muscle tissue determined by P_{CO_2} equilibration of homogenates. *Respir. Physiol.* 12: 169–178, 1971.
102. Heisler, N., and J. Piiper. Determination of intracellular buffering properties in rat diaphragm muscle. *Am. J. Physiol.* 222: 747–753, 1972.
103. Hemingway, A., C. J., Hemingway, and F. J. W. Roughton. The rate of chloride shift of respiration studied with a rapid filtration method. *Respir. Physiol.* 10: 1–9, 1970.
104. Hempleman, S. C., and A. T. Gray. Estimating steady-state $D_{L_{O2}}$ with nonlinear dissociation curves and VA/Q inequality. *Respir. Physiol.* 732: 279–288, 1988.
105. Henderson, L. J. *Blood: A Study in General Physiology.* New Haven, CT: Yale University Press, 1928.
106. Hermansen, L., and J.-B. Osnes. Blood and muscle pH after maximal exercise in man. *J. Appl. Physiol.* 32: 304–308, 1972.
107. Hermansen, L., and Stensvold. Production and removal of lactate during exercise in man. *Acta Physiol. Scand.* 86: 191–201, 1972.
108. Hermansen, L., and O. Vaage. Lactate disappearance and glycogen synthesis in human muscle after maximal exercise. *Am. J. Physiol.* 233 (*Endocrinol. Metab. Gastrointest. Physiol.* 2): E422–E429, 1977.
109. Hill, A. V. The possible effects of the aggregation of the hemoglobin molecules of hemoglobin on the dissociation curve. *J. Physiol. (Lond.)* 40: iv–vii, 1910.
110. Hill, E. P., G. G. Power, and R. D. Gilbert. Mathematical simulation of pulmonary O2 and CO2 exchange. *Am. J. Physiol.* 224: 904–917, 1973.

111. Hill, E. P., G. G. Power, and R. D. Gilbert. Rate of pH changes in blood plasma in vitro and in vivo. *J. Appl. Physiol.* 42: 928–934, 1977.
112. Hill, R. J. W., G. Konigsberg, G. Guidotti, and L. C. Craig. The structure of human hemoglobin I. The separation of the α- and β- chains and their amino acid composition. *J. Biol. Chem.* 237: 1549–1554, 1962.
113. Hlastala, M. P., P. Scheid, and J. Piiper. Interpretation of inert gas retention and excretion in the presence of stratified inhomogeneity. *Respir. Physiol.* 46: 247–259, 1981.
114. Hochachka, P. W., and G. N. Somero. *Biochemical Adaptation.* Princeton, NJ: Princeton University Press, 1984.
115. Hogan, M. C., D. E. Bebout, A. T. Gray, P. D. Wagner, J. B., West, and P. E. Haab. Muscle maximal O2 uptake at constant O2 delivery with and without CO in the blood. *J. Appl. Physiol.* 69: 830–836, 1990.
116. Holland, R. A., H. Shibata, P. Scheid, and J. Piiper. Kinetics of O2 uptake and release by red cells in stopped-flow apparatus: effects of unstirred layer. *Respir. Physiol.* 59: 71–91, 1985.
117. Holland, R. A. B. Rate at which CO replaces O_2 from O_2Hb in red cells of different species. *Respir. Physiol.* 7: 43–63, 1969.
118. Holland, R. A. B., W. Van Hezewijk, and J. Zubzanda. Velocity of oxygen uptake by partly saturated adult and fetal human red cells. *Respir. Physiol.* 29: 303–314, 1977.
119. Honig, C. L., T. E. J. Gayeski, W. J. Federspiel, A. Clark, Jr., and P. Clark. Gradients from hemoglobin to cytochrome: new concepts, new complexities. *Adv. Exp. Med. Biol.* 169: 23–38, 1984.
120. Hopkins, S. R., A. S. Belzberg, B. R. Wiggs, and D. C. McKenzie. Pulmonary transit time and diffusion limitation during heavy exercise in athletes. *Respir. Physiol.* 1995 (in press).
121. Hsia, C. C. W., C. J. C. Chuong, and R. L. Johnson, Jr. Critique of the conceptual basis of diffusing capacity estimates: a finite element analysis. *J. Appl. Physiol.* 1995 (in press).
122. Hsia, C. C. W., F. Fryder-Doffey, V. Stalder-Navarro, J. Johnson, R. C. Reynods, and E. R. Weibel. Structural changes underlying compensatory increase of diffusing capacity after left pneumonectomy in adult dogs. *J. Clin. Invest.* 92: 758–764, 1993.
123. Hsia, C. C. W., L. F. Herazo, F. Frydor-Doffey, and E. R. Weibel. Compensatory lung growth occurs in dogs after right pneumonectomy. *J. Clin. Invest.* 94: 758–764, 1994.
124. Hsia, C. C. W., L. F. Herazo, M. Ramanathan, and R. L. Johnson, Jr. Cardiopulmonary adaptations to pneumonectomy in dogs. IV. Total diffusing capacity, membrane diffusing capacity and capillary blood volume. *J. Appl. Physiol.* 77: 998–1005, 1994.
125. Hsia, C. C. W., L. F. Herazo, M. Ramanathan, and R. L. Johnson, Jr. Cadiac output during exercise measured by acetylene rebreathing, thermodilution and Fick techniques. *J Appl. Physiol.* 78: 1612–1616, 1995.
126. Hsia, C. C. W., L. F. Herazo, M. Ramanathan, R. L. Johnson, Jr., and P. D. Wagner. Cardiopulmonary adaptations to pneumonectomy in dogs. II. Ventilation-perfuson relationships and microvascular recruitment. *J. Appl. Physiol* 74: 1299–1309, 1993.
127. Hsia, C. C. W., M. Ramanathan, and A. S. Estrera. Recruitment of diffusing capacity with exercise in patients after pneumonectomy. *Am. Rev. Respir. Dis.* 145: 811–816, 1992.
128. Huang, Y. T., M. J. Helms, and N. R. MacIntyre. Normal values for single exhalation diffusing capacity and pulmonary capillary blood flow in sitting, supine positions and during mild exercise. *Chest* 105: 501–508, 1994.
129. Hufner, G. Neue Versuche zu Bestimmung der Saurstoffecapacitat des Blutfarbstoffes. *Arch. Physiol. (Leipzig)*: 130–176, 1894.
130. Hultman, E., and K. Sahlin. Acid-base balance during exercise. *Exerc. Sport Sci. Rev.* 8: 41–127, 1980.
131. Jacobs, M. H. The production of intracellular acidity by neutral and alkaline solutions containing carbon dioxide. *Am. J. Physiol.* 53: 457–463, 1920.
132. Johnson, R. L., Jr., and C. C. W. Hsia. Functional recruitment of pulmonary capillaries. *J. Appl. Physiol.* 76: 1405–1407, 1994.
133. Johnson, R. L., Jr., and M. Ramanathan. Buffer equilibria in the lungs. In: *the Kidney, Physiology and Pathophysiology*, edited by D. W. Seldin and G. Giebisch. New York: Raven Press, 1985, p. 193–218.
134. Jones, N. L., G. J. F. Heigenhauser, A. Kuksis, C. G. Matsos, J. R. Sutton, and C. J. Toews. Fat metabolism in heavy exercise. *Clin. Sci.* 59: 469–478, 1980.
135. Jones, N. L., N. McCartney, T. Graham, L. L. Spriet, J. M. Kowalchuk, G. J. F. Heigenhauser, and J. R. Sutton. Muscle performance and metabolism in maximal isokinetic cycling at slow and fast speeds. *J. Appl. Physiol.* 59: 132–136, 1985.
136. Jones, R. S., and F. A. Meade. A theoretical and experimental analysis of anomalies in the estimation of pulmonary diffusing capacity by the single breath method. *Q. J. Exp. Physiol.* 46: 131–143, 1961.
137. Juel, C. Potassium and sodium shifts during in vitro isometric muscle contraction, and the time course of the ion-gradient recovery. *Pflugers Arch.* 406: 458–463, 1986.
138. Juel, C. Intracellular pH recovery and lactate efflux in mouse soleus muscles stimulated *in vitro*: the involvement of sodium/proton exchange and a lactate carrier. *Acta Physiol. Scand.* 132: 363–371, 1988.
139. Karas, R. H., C. R. Taylor, J. H. Jones, S. L. Lindstedt, R. B. Reeves, and E. R. Weibel. Adaptive variation in the mammalian respiratory system in relation to energetic demand: VII. Flow of oxygen across the pulmonary gas exchanger. *Respir. Physiol.* 69: 101–115, 1987.
140. Kelman, G. R. Digital computer procedure for the conversion of PCO_2 into blood content. *Respir. Physiol.* 3: 111–115, 1967.
141. Kety, S. The theory and applications of the exchange of inert gas at the lungs and tissues. *Pharmacol. Rev.* 3: 1–41, 1951.
142. Klocke, R. A. Mechanism and kinetics of the Haldane effect in human erythrocytes. *J. Appl. Physiol.* 35: 673–681, 1973.
143. Klocke, R. A. Mechanism and kinetics of the Haldane effect on human erythrocytes. *J. Appl. Physiol.* 35: 678–681, 1973.
144. Klocke, R. A. Rate of bicarbonate-chloride exchange in human red cells at 37°C. *J. Appl. Physiol.* 40: 707–714, 1976.
145. Klocke, R. A. Catalysis of CO2 reactions by lung carbonic anhydrase. *J. Appl. Physiol.* 44: 882–888, 1978.
146. Klocke, R. A. Velocity of CO_2 exchange in blood. *Ann. Rev. Physiol.* 50: 625–637, 1988.
147. Konig, M. F., J. M. Lucocq, and E. R. Weibel. Demonstration of pulmonary vascular perfusion by electron and light microscopy. *J. Appl. Physiol.* 75: 1877–1883, 1993.
148. Kowalchuk, J. M., G. J. F. Heigenhauser, M. I. Lindinger, G. Obminski, J. R. Sutton, and N. L. Jones. Role of lungs

and inactive muscle in acid-base control after maximal exercise. *J. Appl. Physiol.* 65: 2090–2096, 1988.
149. Kowalchuk, J. M., G. J. F. Heigenhauser, M. I. Lindinger, J. R. Sutton, and N. L. Jones. Factors influencing hydrogen ion concentration in muscle after intense exercise. *J. Appl. Physiol.* 65: 2080–2089, 1988.
150. Kowalchuk, J. M., G. J. F. Heigenhauser, J. R. Sutton, and N. L. Jones. Effect of chronic acetazolamide administration on gas exchange and acid-base control after maximal exercise. *J. Appl Physiol.* 76: 1211–1219, 1994.
151. Kowalchuk, J. M., G. J. F. Heigenhauser, J. R. Sutton, and N. L. Jones. Effect of acetazolamide on gas exchange and acid-base control after maximal exercise. *J. Appl. Physiol.* 72: 278–287, 1992.
152. Kowalchuk, J. M., and B.W. Scheuermann. Acid-base regulation: a comparison of quantitative methods. *Can. J. Physiol. Pharmacol.* 72: 818–826, 1994.
153. Krebs, H. A., and F. J. W. Roughton. Carbonic anhydrase as a tool in studying the mechanisms of reactions involving H_2CO_3, CO_2 or HCO^{3-} *Biochem. J.* 43: 550–555, 1948.
154. Krogh, A., and M. Krogh. On the rate of diffusion of carbonic oxide into the lungs of man. *Scand. Arch. Physiol.* 23: 236–247, 1909.
155. Langston, C., K. Kida, M. Reed, and W. M. Thurlbeck. Human lung growth in late gestation and in the neonate. *Am. Rev. Respir. Dis.* 129: 607–613, 1984
156. Larsen, L. A., and J. M. Burnell. Muscle buffer values. *Am. J. Physiol.* 234 (*Renal Fluid Electrolyte Physiol.* 3): F432–F436, 1978.
157. Lewis, B. M., T. Lin, F. E. Noe, and E. J. Hayford-Welsing. the measurement of pulmonary diffusing capacity for carbon monoxide by a rebreathing method. *J. Clin. Invest.* 38: 2073–2086, 1959.
158. Lilienthal, J. L., Jr., R. L. Riley, D. D. Proemmel, and R. E. Franke. An experimental analysis in man of the pressure gradient from alveolar air to arterial blood during rest and exercise at sea level and at high altitude. *Am. J. Physiol.* 147: 199–216, 1946.
159. Lindinger, M. I., and G. J. F. Heigenhauser. Acid-base systems in skeletal muscle and their response to exercise. In: *Biochemistry of Exercise VII*, edited by P. D. Gollnick, A. W. Taylor, H. J. Green, C. D. Ianuzzo, E. G. Noble, G. Metivier, and J. R. Sutton. Champaign, IL: Human Kinetics, 1990, p. 341–357.
160. Lindinger, M. I., G. J. F. Heigenhauser, R. S. McKelvie, and N. L. Jones. Blood ion regulation during repeated maximal exercise and recovery in humans. *Am. J. Physiol.* 262 (*Regulatory Integrative Comp. Physiol.* 31): R126–R136, 1992.
161. Lindinger, M. I., G. J. F. Heigenhauser, and L. L. Spriet. Effects of alkalosis on muscle ions at rest and with intense exercise. *Can. J. Physiol. Pharmacol.* 68: 820–829, 1990.
162. Lindinger, M. I., L. L. Spriet, E. Hultman, T. Putman, R. S. McKelvie, L. C. Lands, N. L. Jones, and G. J. F. Heigenhauser. Plasma volume and ion regulation during exercise after low- and high-carbohydrate diets. *Am. J. Physiol.* 266 (*Regulatory Integrative Comp. Physiol.* 35): R1896–R1906, 1994.
163. MacIntyre, N. R., and J. A. Nadel. Regional diffusing capacity in normal lungs during a slow exhalation. *J. Appl. Physiol. Respir. Environ. Exerc. Physiol.* 52: 1487–1492, 1983.
164. Manier, G., J. Moinard, P. Techoueryres, N. Varene, and H. Guenard. Pulmonary diffusion limitation after prolonged strenuous exercise. *Respir. Physiol.* 83: 143–154, 1991.
165. Maron, M. B., and L. H. Hamilton, and M. G. Maksud. Alterations in pulmonary function consequent to competitive marathon running. *Med. Sci. Sports Exerc.* 11: 244–249, 1979.
166. Martonen, T. B., and A. F. Wilson. Theoretical basis of single breath gas absorption tests. *J. Math. Biol.* 14: 203–220, 1982.
167. McKelvie, R. S., N. L. Jones, and G. J. F. Heigenhauser. Factors contributing to increased muscle fatigue with β-blockers. *Can. J. Physiol. Pharmacol.*, 69: 254–261, 1991.
168. McKelvie, R. S., M. I. Lindinger, G. J. F. Heigenhauser, and N. L. Jones. Contribution of erythrocytes to the control of the electrolyte changes of exercise. *Can. J. Physiol. Pharmacol.* 69: 984–993, 1996.
169. Medbø, J. I., and O. M. Sejersted. Acid-base and electrolyte balance after exhausting exercise in endurance-trained and sprint-trained subjects. *Acta Physiol. Scand.* 125: 97–109, 1985.
170. Medbø, J. I., and O. M. Sejersted. Plasma potassium changes with high intensity exercise. *J. Physiol. (Lond.)* 421: 105–122, 1990.
171. Meldrum, N. U., and F. J. W. Roughton. Carbonic anhydrase. Its preparation and properties. *J. Physiol. (Lond.)* 80: 113–142, 1933.
172. Merlot-Benichou, C., M. Sinet, M. C. Blayo, and C. Gaudebout. Oxygen-combining capacity in dog. In vitro and in vivo determination. *Respir. Physiol.* 21: 87–99, 1974.
173. Meyer, M., K. Schuster, H. Schulz, M. Mohr, and J. Piiper. Pulmonary diffusing capacities for nitric oxide and carbon monoxide determined by rebreathing in dogs. *J. Appl. Physiol.* 68: 2344–2357, 1990.
174. Miles, D. S., and R. J. Durbin. Alterations in pulmonary function consequent to a 5-mile run. *J. Sports Med.* 25: 90–97, 1985.
175. Miller, J. M., and R. L. Johnson, Jr. Effect of lung inflation on pulmonary diffusing capacity at rest and exercise. *J. Clin. Invest.* 45: 493–500, 1966.
176. Monod, J., J. Wyman, and J. Changeux. One the nature of allosteric transitions: a plausible model. *J. Mol. Biol.* 12: 88–118, 1965.
177. Nattie, E. E., and Y. N. Cai. CSF and plasma ions and blood gases during organic metabolic acidosis in conscious rabbits. *J. Appl. Physiol.* 57: 68–76, 1984.
178. Needham, D. *Machina Carnis. The Biochemistry of Muscular Contraction in its Historical Development.* New York: Cambridge University Press, 1976.
179. Newth, C. J. L., D. J. Cotton, and J. A. Nadel. Pulmonary diffusing capacity measured at multiple intervals during a slow exhalation in man. *J. Appl. Physiol. Respir. Environ. Exerc. Physiol.* 43: 617–625, 1977.
180. Nicholson, P., and F. J. W. Roughton. A theoretical study of the influence of diffusion and chemical reaction velocity on the rate of exchange of carbon monoxide and oxygen between the red blood corpuscle and the surrounding fluid. *Proc. R. Soc. Lond. B* 138: 241–264, 1951.
181. Ogilvie, C. M., R. E. Forster, W. S. Blakemore, and J. W. Morton. A standardized breath holding technique for the clinical measurement of the diffusing capacity of the lung for carbon monoxide. *J. Clin. Invest.* 36: 1–17, 1957.
182. Otis, A. B. Quantitative relationships in steady-state gas exchange. In: *Handbook of Physiology, Respiration*, edited by W. O. Fenn and H. Rahn, Washington, DC: Am. Physiol. Soc., 1964, p. 681–698.
183. Paiva, M. Gas transport in the lung. *J. Appl. Physiol.* 35: 401–410, 1973.

184. Paiva, M. Gas mixing and distribution in the human lung. In: *Lung Biology in Health and Disease*, edited by L. A. Engel and M. Paiva. New York: Marcel Dekker, Inc., 1985, p. 221–285.
185. Paiva, M., S. Verbank, and A. van Muylem. Diffusion-dependent contribution to the slope of the alveolar plateau. *Respir. Physiol.* 72: 257–270, 1988.
186. Pannier, J. L., J. Weyne, and I. Leusen. Effects of PCO_2, bicarbonate and lactate on the isometric contractions of isolated soleus muscle of the rat. *Pflugers Arch.* 320: 120–132, 1970.
187. Park, H. K., and R. Reeves. Thin film measurements of Q(CO) in human red cells at zero, partial and full oxygen saturation. *FASEB J.* 4: 901, 1990.
188. Parker, H., K. Horsefield, and G. Cumming. Morphology of distal airways in the human lung. *J. Appl. Physiol.* 31: 386–391, 1971.
189. Patterson, D. J. Potassium and ventilation in exercise. *J. Appl. Physiol.* 72: 811–820, 1992.
190. Persson, S. G. B., P. Kallings, and C. Ingvast-Larsson. Relationsips between arterial oxygen tension and cardiopulmonary function during submaximal exercise in the horse. In: *Equine Exercise Physiology 2*, edited by J. R. Gillespie, N. E. Robinson, and C. A. Davis. Davis, CA: ICEEP Publications, 1987, p. 161–171.
191. Perutz, M. F. Stereochemistry of cooperative effects in hemoglobin. *Nature* 228: 726–739, 1970.
192. Pieschl, R. L., P. W. Toll, D. E. Leith, L. J. Peterson, and M. R. Fedde. Acid-base changes in the running greyhound: contributing variables. *J. Appl. Physiol.* 73: 2297–2304, 1992.
193. Piiper, J., and P. Scheid. Model for capillary-alveolar equilibration with special refernce to O2 uptake in hypoxia. *Respir. Physiol.* 46: 193–208, 1981.
194. Piiper, J., and P. Scheid. Models for a comparative functional analysis of gas exchange organs in vertebrates. *J. Appl. Physiol. Respir. Environ. Exerc. Physiol.* 53: 1321–1329, 1982.
195. Pitts. R. F. The role of ammonia production and excretion in regulation of acid-base balance. *N. Engl. J. Med.* 284: 32–38, 1971.
196. Podolsky, A., R. S. Eldridge, R. S. Richardson, D. R. Knight, E. C. Johnson, S. R. Hopkins, B. Michimata, B. Grassi, S. S. Feiner, S. S. Kurdak, J. M. Uribe, D. C. Poole, P. E. Bickler, J. W. Severinghause, and P. D. Wagner. Relationship between susceptibility to high altitude pulmonary edema and to exercise induced ventilation/perfusion mismatch. *Am. J. Respir. Crit. Care Med.* 149: A818, 1994.
197. Powers, G. P. Solubility of O2 and CO in blood and pulmonary and placental tissue. *J. Appl. Physiol.* 24: 468–474, 1968.
198. Presson, R. G., C. C. Hanger, P. S. Godbey, J. A. Graham, T. C. Lloyd, Jr., and W. W. Wagner, Jr. Effect of increasing flow on distribution of pulmonary transit times. *J. Appl. Physiol.* 76: 1701–1711, 1994.
199. Pump, K. K. Morphology of the acinus of the human lung. *Dis. Chest* 56: 126–134, 1969.
200. Putman, C. T., L. L. Spriet, E. Hultman, M. I. Lindinger, L. C. Lands, R. S. McKelvie, G. Cederblad, N. L. Jones, and G. J. F. Heigenhauser. Pyruvate dehydrogenase activity and acetyl group accumulation during exercise after different diets. *Am. J. Physiol.* 265 (*Endocrinol. Metab.* 28): E752–E760, 1993.
201. Radda, G. K. The use of NMR spectroscopy for the understanding of disease. *Science* 233: 640–645, 1986.
202. Rahn, H., and W. O. Fenn. *A Graphical Analysis of Respiratory Gas Exchange: The O2–CO2 Diagram.* Washington, DC: Am. Physiol. Soc., 1955.
203. Rahn, H., R. B. Reeves, and B. J. Howell. Hydrogen ion regulation, temperature and evolution. *Am. Rev. Respir. Dis.* 112: 165–172, 1975.
204. Ratner, E. R., and P. D. Wagner. Resolution of the multiple inert gas method for estimating VA/Q distributions. *Respir. Physiol.* 49: 293–313, 1982.
205. Rauwerda, P. E. *Unequal Ventilation of Different Parts of the Lung and Determination of Cardiac Output* (thesis). University of Groningen, 1946.
206. Reeves, R. B. An imidazole alphastat hypothesis for vertebrate acid-base regulation: tissue carbon dioxide content and body temperature in bullfrogs. *Respir. Physiol.* 14: 219–236, 1972.
207. Reeves, R. B., and H. K. Park. CO uptake kinetics of red cells and CO diffusing capacity. *Respir. Physiol.* 88: 1–21, 1992.
208. Riley, R. L., and A. Cournand. "Ideal" alveolar air and analysis of ventilation-perfusion relationships in the lungs. *J. Appl. Physiol.* 1: 825–847, 1949.
209. Robertson, H. T., J. Whitehead, and M. P. Hlastala. Diffusion-related differences in elimination of inert gases from the lung. *J. Appl. Physiol.* 61: 1162–1172, 1986.
210. Rose, R. J., D. R. Hodgson, T. B. Kelso, L. J. McCutcheon, W. M. Bayly, and P. D. Gollnick. Effects of acetazolamide on metabolic and respiratory responses to exercise at maximal O_2 uptake. *J. Appl. Physiol.* 68: 617–626, 1990.
211. Rossing, T. H., N. Maffeo, and V. Fencl. Acid-base effects of altering plasma protein concentration in human blood in vitro. *J. Appl. Physiol.* 61: 2260–2265, 1986.
212. Roughton, F. J. W., R. C. Darling, and W. S. Root. Factors affecting the determination of oxygen capacity, content and pressure in human arterial blood. *Am. J. Physiol.* 147: 708–720, 1944.
213. Roughton, F. J. W., and R. E. Forster. Relative importance of diffusion and chemical reaction rates in determining the rate of exchange of gases in the human lung, with special reference to true diffusing capacity of the pulmonary membrane and volume of bood in lung capillaries. *J. Appl. Physiol.* 11: 290–302, 1957.
214. Roughton, F. J. W., R. E. Forster, and L. Cander. Rate at which carbon monoxide replaces oxygen from combination with human hemoglobin in solution and in the red cell. *J. Appl. Physiol.* 11: 269–276, 1957.
215. Rowell, L. B., H. L. Taylor, Y. Wang, and W. S. Carlson. Saturation of arterial blood with oxygen during maximal exercise. *J. Appl. Physiol.* 19: 284–286, 1964.
216. Sackner, M. A., D. Greenletch, M. Heiman, S. Epstein, and N. Atkins. Diffusing capacity, membrane diffusing capacity, capillary blood volume, pulmonary tissue volume and cardiac output by a rebreathing technique. *Am. Rev. Respir. Dis.* 111: 157–165, 1975.
217. Saltin, B., R.F. Grover, C. G. Blomqvist, H. Hartley, and R. L. Johnson, Jr. Maximal oxygen uptake and cardiac output after 2 weeks at 4,300 m. *J. Appl. Physiol.* 25: 400–409, 1968.
218. Schaffartzik, W., D. C. Poole, T. Derion, K. Tsukimoto, M. C. Hogan, J. P. Arcos, D. E. Bebout, and P. D. Wagner. V_A/Q distribution during heavy exercise and recovery in humans: implications for pulmonary edema. *J. Appl. Physiol.* 72: 1657–1667, 1992.
219. Schaffartzik, W. J., J. Arcos, K. Tsukimoto, O. Mathieu-Costello, and P. D. Wagner. Pulmonary interstitial edema

in the pig after heavy exercise. *J. Appl. Physiol.* 74: 2586–2594, 1993.

220. Scheid, P., M. P. Hlastala, and J. Piiper. Inert gas elimination from lungs with stratified in homogeneity: theory. *Respir. Physiol.* 44: 299–309, 1981.
221. Scherer, P. W., S. Gobran, S. J. Aukburg, J. E. Baumgardner, R. Bartkowski, and G. R. Neufeld. Numerical and experimental study of steady-state CO2 and the inert gas washout. *J. Appl. Physiol.* 64: 1022–1029, 1988.
222. Scherer, P. W., L. H. Schendalman, and N. M. Greene. Simultaneous diffusion and convection in single breath lung washout. *Bull. Math. Biophys.* 34: 393–412, 1972.
223. Scholander, P. F. Oxygen transport through hemoglobin solutions. *Science* 131: 585–590, 1960.
224. Schreider, J. P., and O. G. Raabe. Structure of the human respiratory acinus. *Am. J. Nat.* 162: 221–232, 1981.
225. Schwartz, W. B., and A. S. Relman. A critique of the parameters used in the evaluation of acid-base disorders. "Whole-blood buffer base" and "standard bicarbonate" compared with blood pH and plasma bicarbonate concentration. *N. Engl. J. Med.* 268: 1382–1388, 1963.
226. Sendroy, J., Jr., R. T. Dillon, and D. D. Van Slyke. Studies of gas and electrolyte equilibria in blood. XIX. The solubility and physical state of uncombined oxygen in blood. *J. Biol. Chem.* 105: 597–632, 1934.
227. Severinghaus, J. W. Blood gas calculator. *J. Appl. Physiol.* 21: 1108–1116, 1966.
228. Shepard, R. H., E. Varnauskas, H. B. Martin, J. E. Cotes, and R. L. Riley. Relationship between cardiac output and apparent diffusing capacity of the lung in normal men during treadmill exercise. *J. Appl. Physiol.* 13: 205–210, 1958.
229. Siebens, A. A., N. R. Frank, D. C. Kent, M. M. Newman, R. A. Rauf, and B. L. Vestal. Measurements of the pulmonary diffusing capacity for oxygen during exercise. *Am. Rev. Respir. Dis.* 80: 806–824, 1959.
230. Siegwart, B., P. Gehr, J. Gil, and E. R. Weibel. Morphometric estimation of pulmonary diffusion capacity. IV. The normal dog lung. *Respir. Physiol.* 13: 141–159, 1971.
231. Siggaard-Andersen, O. Blood acid-base alignment nomogram. *Scand. J. Clin. Lab. Invest.* 15: 211–217, 1963.
232. Sjøgaard, G. Electrolytes in slow and fast muscle fibers of humans at rest and with dynamic exercise. *Am. J. Physiol.* 245 (*Regulatory Integrative Comp. Physiol.* 14): R25–R31, 1933.
233. Sørensen, S. P. L. Enzyme studien II. Uber die Messung und die bedeutung der Wasserstoffionen Koncentration bei enzymatischen Prozessen. *Biochem. Z.* 21: 131–304, 1909.
234. Spriet, L. L., M. I. Lindinger, R. S. McKelvie, G. J. F. Heigenhauser, and N. L. Jones Muscle glycogenolysis and H^+ concentration during maximal intermittent cycling. *J. Appl. Physiol.* 66: 8–13, 1989.
235. Spriet, L. L., C. G. Matsos, S. J. Peters, G. J. F. Heigenhauser, and N. L. Jones. Effects of acidosis on rat muscle metabolism and performance during heavy exercise. *Am. J. Physiol.* 248 (*Cell Physiol.* 17): C337–C347, 1985.
236. Spriet, L. L., K. Söderlund, M. Bergstöm, and E. Hultman. Skeletal muscle glycogenolysis, glycolysis, and pH during electrical stimulation in men. *J. Appl. Physiol.* 62: 616–621, 1987.
237. Stadie, W. C., and H. O'brien. The carbamate equilibrium II. The equilibrium between oxyhemoglobin and reduced hemoglobin. *J. Biol. Chem.* 117: 439–470, 1937.
238. Stanley, W. C., E. W. Gertz, J. A Wisnecki, R. A. Neese, D. L. Morris, and G. A. Brooks. Lactate extraction during net lactate release in legs of humans during exercise. *J Appl. Physiol.* 60: 1116–1120, 1986.
239. Staub, N. C., J. M. Bishop, and R. E. Forster. Velocity of O2 uptake by human red cells. *J. Appl. Physiol.* 17: 511–516, 1961.
240. Stewart, P. A. Independent and dependent variables of acid-base control. *Respir. Physiol.* 33: 9–26, 1978.
241. Stewart, P. A. *How to Understand Acid-Base. A Quantitative Acid-Base Primer for Biology and Medicine.* New York: Elsevier/North Holland, 1981.
242. Stewart, P. A. Modern quantitative acid-base chemistry. *Can. J. Physiol. Pharmacol.* 61: 1444–1461, 1983.
243. Theorell, H. Krisallinesches Myoglobin V. Mitteilung: Die Sauerstoffbindungskurve des Myoglobin. *Biochem. Z.* 268: 73–82, 1934.
244. Thurlbeck, W. M. The internal structure of nonemphysematous lungs. *Am. Rev Respir. Dis.* 95: 765–773, 1967.
245. Triebwasser, J. H., R. L. Johnson, Jr., R. P. Burpo, J. C. Campbell, W. C. Reardon, and C. G. Blomqvist. Noninvasive determination of cardiac output by a modified acetylene rebreathing procedure utilizing mass spectrometer measurements. *Aviat. Space Environ. Med.* 48: 203–209, 1977.
246. Trivedi, B., and W. H. Danforth. Effects of pH on the kinetics of frog muscle phosphofructokinase. *J. Biol. Chem.* 241: 4110–4112, 1966.
247. Truog, W. E., M. P. Hlastala, T. A. Standaert, H. P. McKenna, and W. A. Hodson. Oxygen-induced alteration of ventilation-perfusion relationship in rats. *J. Appl. Physiol. Respir. Environ. Exerc. Physiol.* 47: 1112–1117, 1979.
248. Turino, G. M., E. H. Bergofsky, R. M. Goldring, and A. P. Fishman. Effect of exercise on pulmonary diffusing capacity. *J. Appl. Physiol.* 18: 447–456, 1963.
249. van Leeuwen, A. M. Net cation equivalency ("base binding power") of the plasma proteins. A study of ion-protein interaction in human plasma by means of in vivo ultrafiltration and equilibrium dialysis. *Acta Med. Scand.* 176 (suppl. 422): 3–212, 176, 1964.
250. van Slyke, D. D., A. B. Hastings, A. Hiller, and J. Sendroy. Studies of gas and electrolyte equilibria in blood. XIV. Amounts of alkali bound by serum albumin and globulin. *J. Biol. Chem.* 79: 769–780, 1928.
251. Visser, B. F. Pulmonary diffusion of CO_2. *Phys. Med. Biol.* 5: 155–166, 1960.
252. Wagner, P. D., B. K. Erikson, K. Kubo, A. Hiraga, M. Kai, Y. Yamaya, R. S. Richardson, and J. Seaman. Maximum O2 transport and utilization before and after splenectomy. In: *Equine Exercise Physiology 4*: Proceedings of the Fourth International Conference on Equine Exercise Physiology, Korralbyn, Queensland, Australia: *Equine Vet. J.* 1994.
253. Wagner, P. D., G. E. Gale, R. E. Moon, J. R. Torre-Bueno, B. W. Stolp, and H. A. Saltzman. Pulmonary gas exchange in humans exercising at sea level and simulated altitude. *J. Appl. Physiol.* 61: 260–270, 1986.
254. Wagner, P. D., J. R. Gillespie, G. L. Landgren, M. R. Feede, B. W. Jones, R. M. DeBowes, R. L. Pieschl, and H. H. Erickson. Mechanism of exercise-induced hypoxemia in horses. *J. Appl. Physiol.* 66: 1227–1233, 1989.
255. Wagner, P. D., R. B. Laravuso, R. R. Uhl, and J. B. West Continuous distributions of ventilation-perfusion ratios in normal subjects breathing air and 100% CO_2. *J. Clin. Invest.* 54: 54–68, 1974.
256. Wagner, P. D., H. A. Saltzman, and J. B. West. Measurements of continuous distributions of ventilation-perfusion ratios: theory. *J. Appl. Physiol.* 36: 588–599, 1974.

257. Wagner, P. D., J. R. Sutton, J. T. Reeves, A. Bymerman, B. M. Groves, and M. K. Malconian Operation Everest II: pulmonary gas exchange during a simulated ascent of Mt. Everest. *J. Appl. Physiol.* 63: 2348–2359, 1987.
258. Wagner, P. D., and J. B. West. Effects of diffusion impairment on O2 and CO2 time courses in pulmonary capillaries. *J. Appl. Physiol.* 33: 62–71, 1972.
259. Wagner, W. W., Jr., and L. P. Latham. Pulmonary capillary recruitment during airway hypoxia in the dog. *J. Appl. Physiol.* 39: 900–905, 1975.
260. Wagner, W. W., L. P. Latham, and R. L. Capen. Capillary recruitment during airway hypoxia: role of pulmonary artery pressure. *J. Appl. Physiol.* 47: 383–387, 1979.
261. Wang, C.-W., and A. S. Popel. Effect of red bood cell shape on oxygen transport in capillaries. *Math. Biosci.* 116: 89–110, 1992.
262. Wasserman, K. The anaerobic threshold measurement to evaluate exercise performance. *Am. Rev. Respir. Dis.* 129: S35–S40, 1984.
263. Wasserman, K. W., and B. J. Whipp. Exercise physiology in health and disease. *Am. Rev. Respir. Dis.* 112: 219–249, 1975.
264. Wiebel, E. R. *Morphometry of the Human Lung.* New York: Academic Press, Inc., 1963.
265. Weibel, E. R. Morphometric estimation of pulmonary diffusion capacity. I. Model and method. *Respir. Physiol.* 11: 54–75, 1970.
266. Weibel, E. R. Morphometric estimation of pulmonary diffusion capacity. V. Comparative morphometry of alveolar lungs. *Respir Physiol.* 14: 26–43, 1972.
267. Weibel, E. R. A simpified morphometric method for estimating diffusing capacity in normal and emphysematous human lungs. *Am Rev. Respir Dis.* 107: 579–588, 1973.
268. Weibel, E. R. Morphometric and stereological methods in respiratory physiology, including fixation techniques. Techniques in the life sciences. *Respir. Physiol.* P401: 1–35, 1984.
269. Weibel, E. R., W. J. Federspiel, F. Frydor-Doffey, C. C. W. Hsia, M. Konig, V. Stalder-Navarro, and R. Vock. Morphometric model for pulmonary diffusing capacity I. Membrane diffusing capacity. *Respir. Physiol.* 93: 125–149, 1993.
270. Weibel, E. R., and B. W. Knight. A morphometric study on the thickness of the pulmonary air-blood barrier. *J. Cell Biol.* 21: 367–384, 1964.
271. Weibel, E. R., L. B. Marques, M. Constantinopol, F. Doffey, P. Gehr, and C. R. Taylor. Adaptive variation in the mammalian respiratory system in relation to energetic demand: VI. The pulmonary gas exchanger. *Respir. Physiol.* 69: 81–100, 1987.
272. Weibel, E. R., C. R. Tayor, J. J. O'Neil, D. E. Leith, P. Gehr, H. Hoppeler, V. Langman, and R. V. Baudinette. Maximal oxygen consumption and pulmonary diffusing capacity: a direct comparison of physiologic and morphometric measurements in canids. *Respir. Physiol.* 54: 173–188, 1983.
273. Weibel, E. R., P. Untersee, J. Gil, and M. Zulauf. Morphometric estimation of pulmonary diffusion capacity. VI. Effect of varying positive pressure inflation of air spaces *Respir. Physiol.* 18: 285–308, 1973.
274. West, J. B., K. Tsukimoto, O. Matthieu-Costello, and R. Predilleto. Stress failure in pulmonary capillaries. *J. Appl. Physiol.* 70: 1731–1742, 1991.
275. West, J. B., and P. D. Wagner. Pulmonary gas exchange. In: *Bioengineering Aspects of the Lung,* edited by J. B. West. New York and Basel: Marcel Dekker, Inc., 1980.
276. Whipp, B. J. The bioenergetic and gas exchange basis of exercise testing. *Clin. Chest Med.* 15: 173–192, 1994.
277. Whipp, B. J., J. A. Davis, and K.Wasserman. Ventilatory control of the "isocapnic buffering" region in rapidly-incremental exercise. *Respir. Physiol.* 76: 357–368, 1989.
278. Whipp, B. J., and S. A. Ward. Coupling of ventilation to pulmonary gas exchange during exercise. In: *Exercise. Pulmonary Physiology and Pathophysiology,* edited by B. J. Whipp and K. Wasserman. New York: Marcel Dekker, Inc. 1991, p. 271–307.
279. Wilhelm, E., R. Balting, and J. Wilcock. Low pressure solubility of liquid gases in water. *Chem. Rev.* 77: 219–262, 1977.
280. Wittenberg, J. B. Myogobin-facilitated oxygen diffusion: role of myoglobin in oxygen entry into muscles. *Physiol. Rev.* 50: 559–636, 1970.
281. Worth, H., W. Nusse, and J. Piiper Determination of binary diffusion coefficients of various gas species used in respiratory physiology. *Respir. Physiol.* 32: 15–26, 1978.
282. Worth, H., and J. Piiper. Diffusion of helium, carbon monoxide and sulfur hexafluoride in gas mixtures similar to alveolar gas. *Respir. Physiol.* 32: 155–166, 1978.
283. Wranne, B., R. D. Woodson, and J. C. Detter. Bohr effect: interaction between H^+, CO2, and 2,3 DPG in fresh and stored blood. *J. Appl. Physiol.* 32: 749–754, 1972.
284. Wyman, J., Jr. Heme proteins. *Adv. Protein Chem.* 4: 407–531, 1948.
285. Wyman, J. Facilitated diffusion and the possible role of myoglobin as a transport mechanism. *J. Biol. Chem.* 241: 115–121, 1966.
286. Yamaguchi, K., P. D. Nguyen, P. Scheid, and J. Piiper. Kinetics of O2 uptake and release by human erythrocytes studied by a stopped-flow technique. *J. Appl. Physiol.* 58: 1215–1224, 1985.
287. Yamamoto, W. S., and M. W. Edwards, Jr. Homeostatis of carbon dioxide during intravenous infusion of carbon dioxide. *J. Appl. Physiol.* 15: 807–818, 1960.
288. Yoshida, F., and N. Oshima. Diffusivity of oxygen in blood serum. *J. Appl. Physiol.* 21: 915–919, 1966.

13. Pulmonary hemodynamics and fluid exchange in the lungs during exercise

JOHN T. REEVES | *Departments of Medicine and Pediatrics, Developmental Lung Biology Laboratory, University of Colorado Health Sciences Center, Denver, Colorado*

AUBREY E. TAYLOR | *Department of Physiology, University of South Alabama School of Medicine, Mobile, Alabama*

CHAPTER CONTENTS

IN HUMANS, MUSCULAR EXERCISE can increase oxygen (O_2) uptake and carbon dioxide (CO_2) output some 20-fold above resting values. The question is, How does the lung circulation provide for such a massive increase in gas transport? Oxygen, being ~1/30 as soluble as CO_2, poses the more difficult transport problem. Evolution has apparently solved the O_2 transport problem by developing an extensive and thin alveolar-capillary membrane across which O_2 can diffuse. Possibly as a result of these requirements for O_2 transfer, vascular pressures in oxygenating circuits of mammals are low, being about one-fifth of those in the systemic circulation. As a result of this low transmural pressure, the walls of the arteries and veins are thinner than those in the systemic circulation. In essence, the lung microcirculation is delicately enclosed by the alveoli in such a fashion that O_2 transport into the blood actually begins in the arteries before the blood reaches the extensive capillaries. In addition, since the lung circulation is in series with the systemic circulation, these delicate lung vessels receive the entire cardiac output and are greatly influenced by the left ventricular filling pressures.

In this chapter we will examine the extent to which lung vascular function is dominated by changes in the systemic circulation. In particular, it is important to consider left ventricular filling pressure, which increases during exertion and both distends and recruits these thin-walled blood vessels. Vascular distension at a given transmural pressure, which is determined by vascular compliance, lowers vascular resistance. It is essential that capillary surface area and volume be increased in exercise to allow red cells a transit time through the lung that is sufficiently long for them to take on their full complement of O_2. This permits the transport of large quantities of O_2 in a setting of high flow, as required for exercise. In addition, the pulmonary vessels must not leak large amounts of fluid into the alveoli, since that would severely limit the O_2 and CO_2 exchange in the lungs. Although recent reviews are available (67, 86, 85, 84), this chapter will present these issues in more detail than previously, and will integrate current data into our understanding of how the lung circulation copes with the huge blood flow increases occurring in exercise.

PRESSURES AND FLOWS IN THE HUMAN LUNG CIRCULATION

Historical Notes

From earliest days of physiological study, investigators of the lung circulation have shown remarkable agreement in that the lung circulation is a low pressure system. Even Harvey (27) commented that "... the right [ventricle] neither reaches to the apex of the heart, nor is it of such strength, being three times thinner in its walls. ... The right has only to drive the blood through the lungs, whilst the left has to propel it through the whole body." The low pressure in the right, compared to the left, ventricle was demonstrated by Chaveau and Marey (9), who measured simultaneous pressures in the two ventricles. Studies by Lichtheim in 1876, Tigerstedt in 1903 (as quoted in 17), and von Euler and Liljestrand in 1947 (17) all showed that occlusion of blood flow to one lung, which probably doubled flow to the other lung, did not increase pressure significantly, suggesting a remarkable capacity of the lung's circulation to decrease its resistance with increased flow. Cournand, who received the Nobel Prize for cardiac catheterization commented on the "capacity and flexibility of the small vessels in the lungs" and that under "physiologic conditions a clear cut demonstration of vaso-motor activity ... is still lacking" (12).

The first exercise measurements were performed nearly simultaneously in three different laboratories (17, 31, 70), and all of them confirmed the capacity of the normal lung vascular bed to accept increased flow. Von Euler and Liljestrand (17), using electrical stimulation of muscles to simulate exercise in the anesthetized cat, reported only a small increase in pulmonary arterial pressure. They thought it likely that there was a large increase in blood flow. The first reports of exercise per se were in supine (31) and upright (70) man. The two studies agreed that "the normal pulmonary vascular bed can accommodate a large increase in the rate of pulmonary blood flow with little or no increase in pressure" (31) and that there was "a large drop in pulmonary vascular resistance" (70).

But how was the lung circulation controlled, and in particular, how could a large increase in flow occur without an increased pressure gradient? In 1938 Barcroft (3) predicted that during exercise there was "the opening up of vascular areas, either by increasing the calibre of vessels already open, or opening up those hitherto shut." Because the vessels are thin walled, small pressure increases could "open up vascular areas." The first measurements relating to left atrial pressure made during exercise were done in humans by Dexter et al. in 1951 (15), showing an increased pressure in six of the seven persons studied. In the 1960s, Scandinavian investigators found evidence of elevated left atrial pressure during heavy exercise (7, 34), particularly in the elderly (22). These findings suggested a rise in left ventricular diastolic pressure occurring with exercise, the finding of which was confirmed years later (60, 89).

Early investigators provided clues as to the mechanisms associated with the increased left ventricular diastolic pressure occurring during exercise. Starling showed that increased ventricular work is accompanied by an increased ventricular filling pressure (79). In 1898, Barnard (5) found that the pericardium could withstand more strain than the myocardium, and he hypothesized that the pericardium "limits passive dilation of the heart." He also speculated that during exercise the heart would be "supported by its pericardium." Kuno (45) reported in 1915 that, "When the pericardium is intact, the heart, in order to perform a certain amount of work, requires a higher venous pressure than when the pericardium is opened." These early studies provided clues that the left ventricle, including perhaps the pericardium, had a potentially important influence on the outflow pressures of the lung circulation.

Henderson and Prince (29) developed the concept that filling pressure of the left ventricle might regulate the volume of blood in the lungs, and stated that the "left heart acts somewhat like a dam of moderate height across the outlet of a reservoir." At the same time, Marie Krogh (44) reported that during exercise, "due to changes in circulation rate," the lung increased its capacity to allow O_2 to diffuse into the blood, a finding that was finally confirmed 30 and 40 years later (48, 71). Johnson et al. (39) showed that the exercise-induced increase in diffusing capacity was accompanied by an increased pulmonary capillary blood volume. Also, in 1956 Rahn et al. (65) developed the concept that the pulmonary blood flow at rest was unevenly distributed, with gravity, "favoring (greater flow in) the dependent portions of the lung."

Thus, for some decades knowledge has been available that (*1*) the lung's vasculature is distensible, (*2*) the vessels are relatively passive, (*3*) the vessels are affected by left heart pressures, (*4*) left atrial pressures rise in exercising humans, (*5*) increased ventricular work and restriction of ventricular filling by the pericardium would increase pulmonary venous filling pressure, and (*6*) increased pulmonary venous pressures increase pulmonary capillary volume and probably distribute more evenly the blood flow through the lungs. Therefore, published clues have long been available concerning mechanisms by which the lung circulation can provide for O_2 transport during exercise. The present chapter will integrate and evaluate the currently available information, and will assess more precisely the mechanisms regulating exercise pulmonary hemodynamics and fluid flux changes.

Human Data

With the advent of cardiac catheterization, hemodynamic measurements have been made in both men and women, during upright and supine cycle exercise. For our analyses we used published data (69, 67, 81, 89) and other data provided by R. E. Moon and P. D. Wagner (personal communication). Comparisons of measurements in upright and supine positions provide more insight into the mechanisms associated with the role of the pulmonary circulation in exercise that can be obtained by the examination of either position alone. Regarding individual data, 67 supine subjects had resting measurements and 47 of them had two or more exercises at different intensities, giving a total of 185 measurements of the pulmonary circulation during rest and exercise. A total of 85 measurements were also made in 16 upright subjects sitting at rest and during several bicycle exercises of increasing intensity. Measurements in animals are also evaluated in order to provide additional insight into the circulatory changes occurring within the lung during exercise.

Arterial, Intrathoracic, and Left Heart Pressures

Systemic Arterial and Wedge Pressure. Changing systemic arterial pressure, via its effects on left ventricular emptying, could influence pulmonary hemodynamics by altering pulmonary blood flow and left atrial pressure. As discussed in detail elsewhere (see Chapter 17), mean systemic arterial pressure increases with increasing exercise effort (Fig. 13.1*A*). In addition, left atrial and ventricle diastolic pressures also increase. Assuming "wedge" pressure reflects left atrial pressure, it is not surprising that an exercise-related increase in arterial pressure is accompanied by an increase in pulmonary wedge pressure (Fig. 13.1*B*). However, it is important to consider measurement of intrathoracic pressures, the relation of atrial to ventricular filling pressures, and the reliability of the "wedge" pressure as a measure of left ventricular filling pressure.

Intrathoracic Pressure Changes during Exercise. Because the heart and lungs reside in the thorax, pressures within the cardiac chambers and lung vessels are influenced by respiratory changes in intrathoracic pressure. For example, with inspiration, intrathoracic and intracardiac pressures fall, and with expiration, they rise. Exercise, which increases the respiratory effort, increases the negative and positive pressure swings with inspiration and expiration, respectively, an extreme example of which is the exercising horse [Fig. 13.2; (16)]. Conventionally, intracardiac pressures are measured with respect to the atmosphere, rather than to intrathoracic pressure, even though the latter would more closely approximate instantaneous transmural pressures (Fig. 13.2). Fortunately, however, when the lungs are normal, intrathoracic pressure averaged over several respi-

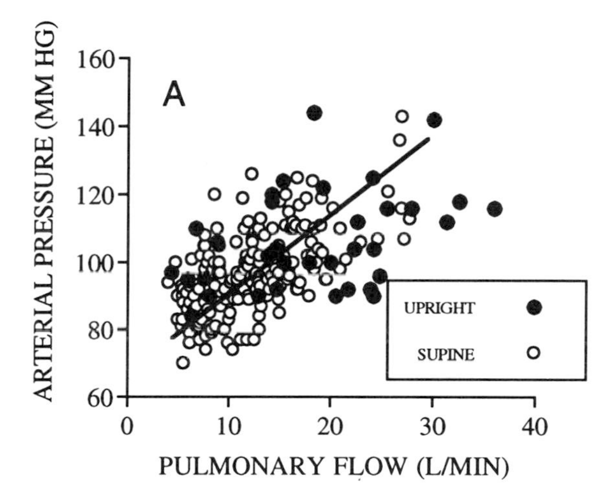

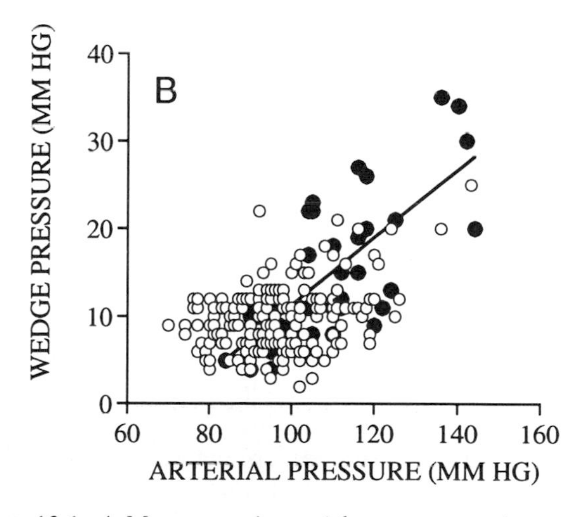

FIG. 13.1. *A*, Mean systemic arterial pressure vs. pulmonary flow during upright and supine cycle exercise for repeated measurements in 8 upright and 67 supine subjects. For all subjects pressure increased ($r = 0.62$) with increasing flow. *B*, Wedge pressure increased ($r = 0.62$) with increasing mean systemic arterial pressure during upright and supine cycle exercise for the same measurements as in *A*.

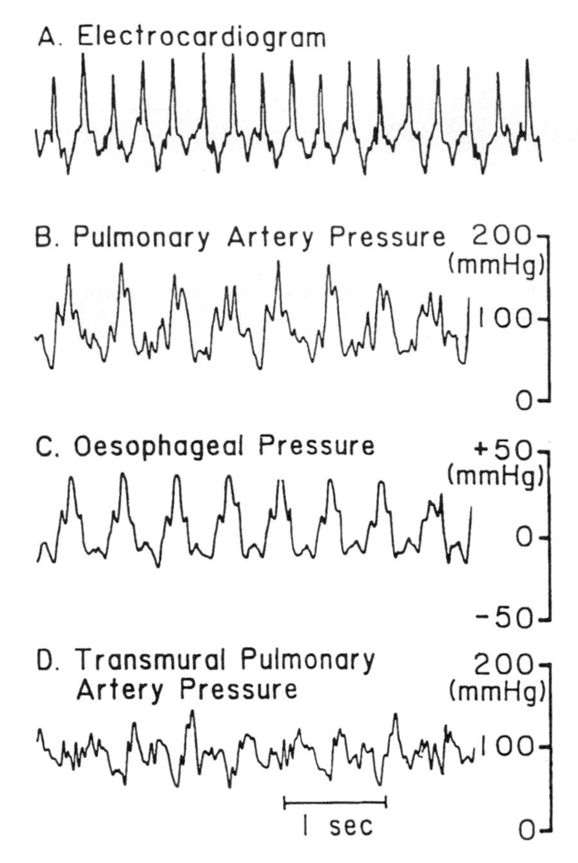

FIG. 13.2. Tracings from an exercising horse showing the large intrathoracic respiratory (esophageal) pressure. However, the mean pulmonary arterial pressure averaged over several respiratory cycles is approximately the same no matter whether the reference pressure is the atmosphere (*B*) or the esophageal pressure (*D*). [From Erickson et al. (16), permission.]

ratory cycles is near zero and is little changed from the resting value. Thus, ignoring the intrathoracic respiratory pressure swings introduces little error into the normal mean intravascular cardiopulmonary pressure changes with exercise. Furthermore, when left atrial pressure is subtracted from pulmonary arterial pressure to obtain the atrioventricular pressure gradient, the intrathoracic pressure component is eliminated mathematically.

Atrial Pressures and Ventricular Filling. Exercise increases venous return to both ventricles and therefore increases right and left ventricular filling volumes, filling pressures and, via the Starling mechanism, stroke volume. The ventricular end-diastolic pressures reflect the brief elevation of ventricular pressure from atrial contraction and approximate true ventricular filling pressure. With exercise, the rising end-diastolic pressures in the two ventricles (69) are strongly correlated (r = 0.93), but the right ventricular pressure rises less than does that in the left ventricle (68).

As mentioned above, the exercise-related increase in left ventricular filling pressure has important implications for the lung circulation. Because left ventricular pressures are not often measured during exercise, we must use another means to evaluate left ventricular filling pressure, namely some estimate of mean left atrial pressure. Because the mean left atrial pressure is the average throughout the cardiac cycle, it will be less than the left ventricular end-diastolic pressure (LVEDP). However, both pressures are important because the former defines downstream pressure for the lung circulation, and the latter defines ventricular filling.

"Wedge" and Left Ventricular End-Diastolic Pressures. Mean left atrial pressure in man is usually estimated indirectly when a balloon-tipped flotation catheter is "wedged" by inflating the balloon, which occludes a lobar branch of the pulmonary artery. The flow in the branch is stopped, and the pressure measured distal to the occlusion (the wedge pressure) is that in the first downstream channel (a lobar vein or left atrium) in which flow is occurring. (Conceivably, when a small catheter is wedged into a small pulmonary artery, the downstream pressure will be that in a small pulmonary vein.) The question is, How well does pressure measured distal to a wedged balloon relate to LVEDP? Measurements are available at rest and during cycle exercise in ten normal men studied in both the supine and sitting positions [Table 13.1; (89)]. Gravity pools blood in the lower extremity in subjects sitting at rest, causing both ventricular filling pressures and the cardiac output to be lower than in supine subjects. As shown above during exercise, systemic arterial systolic, diastolic, and mean pressures increased. LVEDP and wedge pressures also rose, independent of body position. The comparison of 36 simultaneous wedge pressures and LVEDP measurements showed a high degree of correlation (Fig. 13.3), confirming that the wedge pressure reliably tracks left ventricular filling pressure during exercise.

Wedge and Pulmonary Arterial Pressures

Rise in Wedge Pressure with Exercise. Figure 13.4*A* shows the increase in wedge pressure with increasing exercise intensity. Wedge pressure increases along with pulmonary blood flow no matter whether the subjects are sitting (*left panel*) or are supine (*right panel*). The increase seems real because (*1*) it is a consistent finding, (*2*) it correlates with the rise in LVEDP (Fig. 13.3) above, and (*3*) it is accompanied by a rise in pulmonary arterial pressure (Fig. 13.4*B*).

TABLE 13.1. *Rest and Exercise Measurements in Ten Healthy Men during Right and Left Heart Catheterization*

State	HR	Pressures, mm Hg						Flow, liters·min^{-1}·m^{-2}
		A_s	A_d	A_m	LV_{EDP}	P_W	P_{PA}	CI
Rest supine	73	130	76	96	8	6	13	3.5
Exercise supine	128	178	84	119	16	13	24	7.7
Rest sitting	84	132	82	99	4	4	13	2.8
Exercise sitting	146	184	89	121	11	8	22	7.3

HR, heart rate; A_s, peripheral systemic arterial systolic pressure; A_d, peripheral systemic arterial diastolic pressure; A_m, peripheral systemic arterial mean pressure; LVEDP, left ventricular end-diastolic pressure; P_w, pulmonary arterial wedge; P_{PA}, mean pulmonary arterial pressure; CI, cardiac index. From Parker, Digiorgi, and West (60).

The linear relationship between wedge pressure and flow, however, was variable between individuals. At one end of the spectrum of responses is subject # 6 [*left panel* Fig. 13.4*A*; (24, 69)] who increased his wedge pressure by 27 mm Hg to 35 mm Hg upon going from rest to an exercise that increased his lung blood flow to 35 liters/min, and his O_2 uptake to 90% of his maximal value. When the exercise was repeated while breathing 100% O_2, the flow and wedge pressure were similar to values obtained during air breathing, suggesting that hypoxemia did not contribute to this large increase in wedge pressure. Furthermore, wedge pressures above 20 mm Hg were observed in this subject at lower exercise intensities that could be sustained for many minutes during a long-distance run.

At the low end of the spectrum (Fig. 13.4*A*, *left*) is subject # 9, whose wedge pressure rose only 2 mm Hg from rest to 84% of maximal capacity (24, 69).

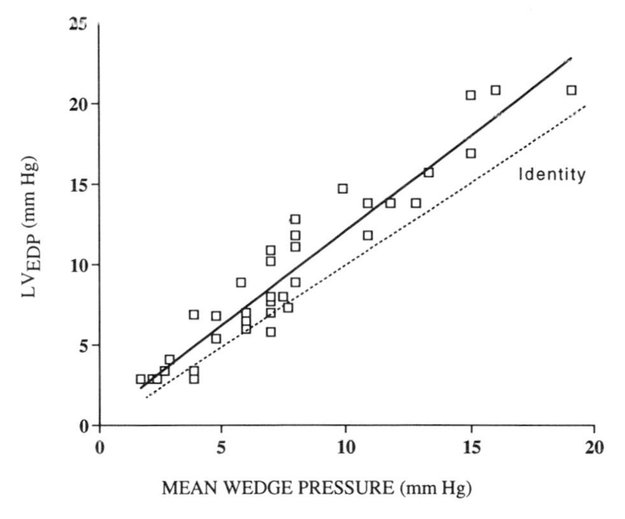

FIG. 13.3. Relation of left ventricular end-diastolic pressure (LV_{EDP}), y, to simultaneously measured wedge pressure, x, at rest and during exercise, supine and upright in ten healthy men. The two variables were closely related (y = 1.18x + 0.3; $r > 0.9$, $P < 0.001$). Identity is shown as a *broken line*. [Redrawn from Thadani and Parker (89).]

Presumably, this subject performs heavy exercise with little or no increase in wedge pressure. Maximum O_2 uptake was only slightly greater in the former than in the latter subject (49.9 vs. 43.5 ml·kg^{-1}·min^{-1}). As discussed below, the intersubject variability in wedge pressure increase indicates that subject # 6, more than subject # 9, will have a greater tendency to increase filtration of water out of the microcirculation into the lung interstitium during exercise, since capillary pressure must be higher in the former.

Relation of Pulmonary Arterial to Wedge Pressure. Pulmonary arterial mean pressure also increases with blood flow during cycling exercise (Fig. 13.4*B*), and the magnitude of the pressure rise depends largely on wedge pressure. For example (Fig. 13.4*B*, *left*), in subject # 6, the mean pulmonary arterial pressure rose by 26 mm Hg from rest to maximal exercise, which was similar to the rise in the wedge pressure. But for subject # 9, the rise in pulmonary arterial pressure of only 5 mm Hg compares with the rise of 2 mm Hg in the wedge pressure. For subjects in either the sitting or supine position, the pulmonary arterial pressure is highly correlated with the wedge pressure (Fig. 13.5). Analysis suggests that the variation in wedge pressures accounts for approximately 80% of the variation in the pulmonary arterial pressure. This dependence of the normal pulmonary arterial pressure on pressure distal to the capillaries during exercise (i.e., the left atrium) occurs for the lung, but not the systemic, circulation. In the systemic circulation, where the arteriolar pressure is much higher than in the lung, venous pressure must rise to very high levels before pressure rises in the aorta.

Causes of the Exercise-Related Rise in Wedge Pressure

The Starling mechanism. The correlation shown above (Fig. 13.1*B*) between wedge and systemic arterial pressures is consistent with the operation of the Starling mechanism (79), where increased ven-

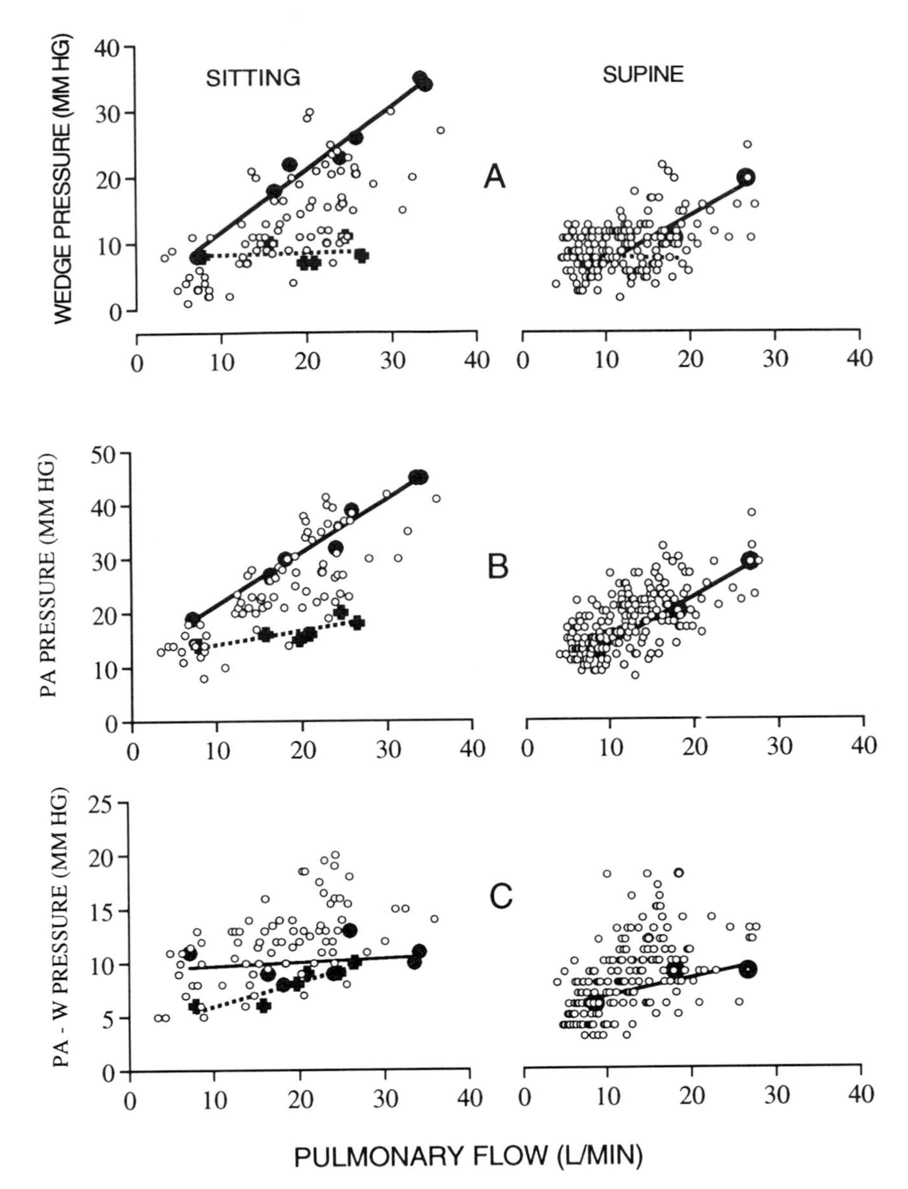

FIG. 13.4. Pulmonary wedge (*A*), mean pulmonary arterial (*B*), and pulmonary arterial minus wedge (*C*), pressures at rest and during cycle exercise vs. pulmonary blood flow in sitting (*left panels*) and supine subjects (*right panels*). Averaged slopes for the individual subjects were, sitting and supine, 0.8 and 0.3 for *A*, 1.0 and 1.0 for *B*, and 0.5 and 0.4 for *C*. Serial measurements (sitting) in subject # 6 (*filled circles* and *unbroken line*) and in subject # 9 (*crosses* and *broken line*) as taken from published reports (24, and the reviews 67, 69) are indicated. Serial measurements in one supine subject is also indicated.

tricular filling pressure and volume allows increased myocardial work. Thus, one expects that a rise in filling pressure would increase diastolic ventricular volume, and such is the case when subjects go from rest to mild exercise. The evidence comes from simultaneous measurements of volume (by radionuclide methods) combined with pressures from the left ventricle (81). Thus, mild exercise increased wedge pressure, left ventricular end-diastolic volume, and stroke volume (Fig. 13.6). These changes are consistent with the Starling mechanism, where an increase in filling pressure and volume increases stroke volume (35) (see Chapter 15). With heavier exercise, however, the pattern of response changes.

Dissociation of ventricular end-diastolic volume from filling pressure. For progressively heavier exercises, the wedge pressure continues to rise but the end-diastolic ventricular volume does not continue to increase (Fig. 13.6). Because stroke volume relates to diastolic volume, it too becomes independent of wedge pressure (Figs. 13.6 and 13.7). The key point for the present chapter is that heavy exercise dissociates end-diastolic volume from wedge pressure. If so, we can only conclude that the resistance to filling

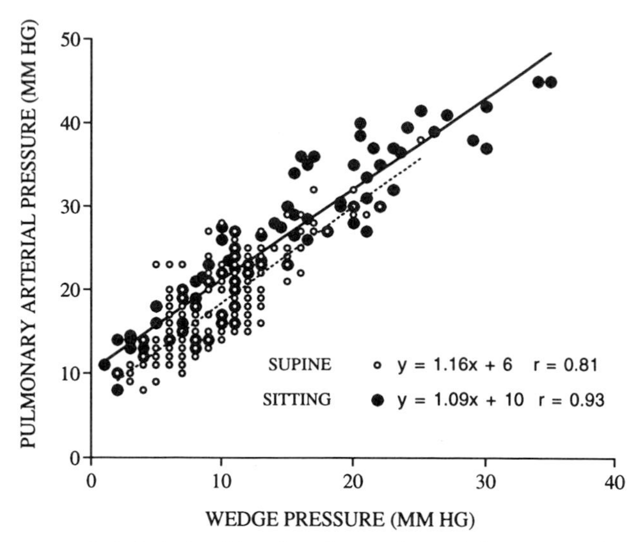

FIG. 13.5. Relationship of resting and exercising mean pulmonary arterial (x) to wedge (y) pressure for upright and supine normal men and women.

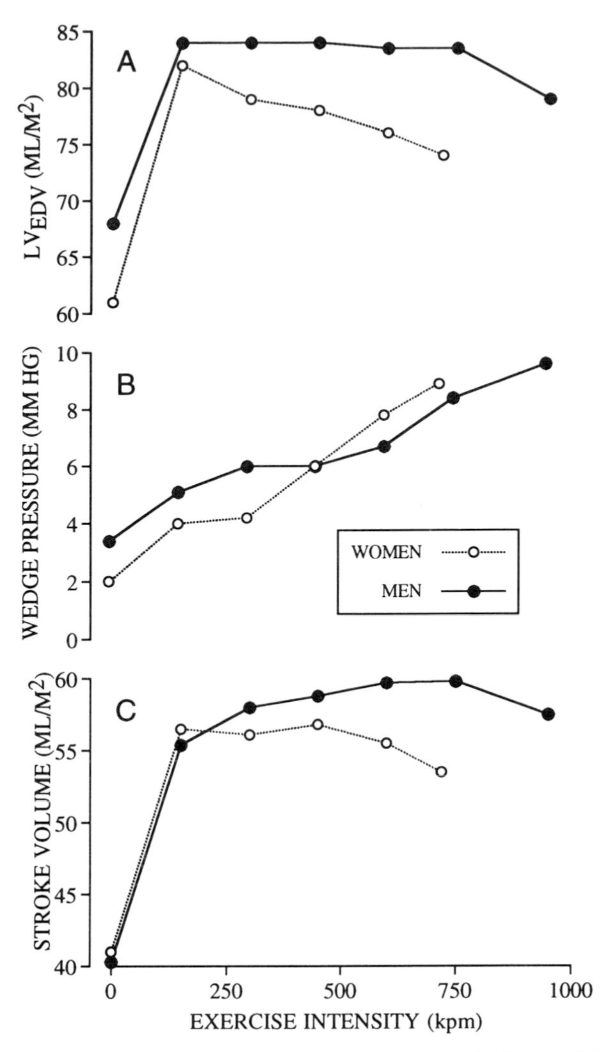

FIG. 13.6. Simultaneous average measurements during upright cycle exercise for men and women of left ventricular end-diastolic volume index (LV_{EDV}) (*A*), wedge pressure (*B*), and stroke volume index (*C*). [Redrawn from Sullivan, Cobb, and Higgenbotham (81).]

of the left ventricle is small for mild exercise but increases with increasing effort.

Pericardial limitation of ventricular filling. Because the normal pericardium has a high elastance and snugly encloses its contents, even small increases of heart volume cause the pericardium to rapidly approach the limits of its compliance (63) (see Chapter 15). When a subject goes from rest to mild exercise, end-diastolic volume in the left ventricle increases approximately 35 ml (81), and one would assume that the volume in the right ventricle increases the same amount. If an increase in combined ventricular volume of approximately 70 ml results in pericardial stretch, then further increments in LUEDP would only slightly increase end-diastolic or stroke volume.

Pericardial limitation of ventricular filling has been proposed as the mechanism that produces very high wedge pressures when humans inspire against a closed glottis [Müller maneuver (63)]. Pericardial limitation of both ventricles accounts for the high filling pressures observed in dogs when saline is infused to increase intravascular volume [Fig. 13.8*A*; (19)]; and it may facilitate the equalization of stroke volumes between the two sides of the heart (19). Following pericardial removal in pigs, the ventricle dilates over several days and becomes more compliant (Fig. 13.8*B*). Then, when the pigs exercise, maximal stroke volume and cardiac output increase (26), as discussed in Chapter 15. When present, then, the pericardium limits ventricular filling during the Müller maneuver, plasma volume expansion, and exercise. It is likely that the pericardium participates in the elevation of wedge pressure during heavy exercise in normal humans.

Do sympathetics change ventricular diastolic compliance? While augmented sympathetic activity during exercise increases cardiac contractility (35, 74), it has not been reported to increase ventricular tone during diastole. Furthermore, the human data suggest that ventricular compliance may even increase during exercise because some subjects increase their stroke volumes without increasing filling pressures (Fig. 13.7). Thus, it seems unlikely that sympathetic tone which increases systolic function would impair diastolic filling.

Limitations of diastolic filling time. Another possible mechanism that may contribute to the rise in wedge pressure during heavy exercise is the tachycardia

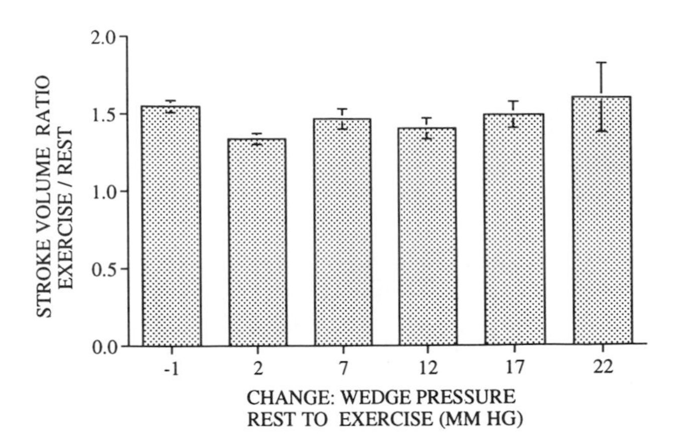

FIG. 13.7. Measurements of stroke volume as related to wedge pressure showing the change from rest to exercise within 16 seated subjects. Although there tended to be a small increase in wedge pressure stroke volume with increasing wedge, the relationship was not significant.

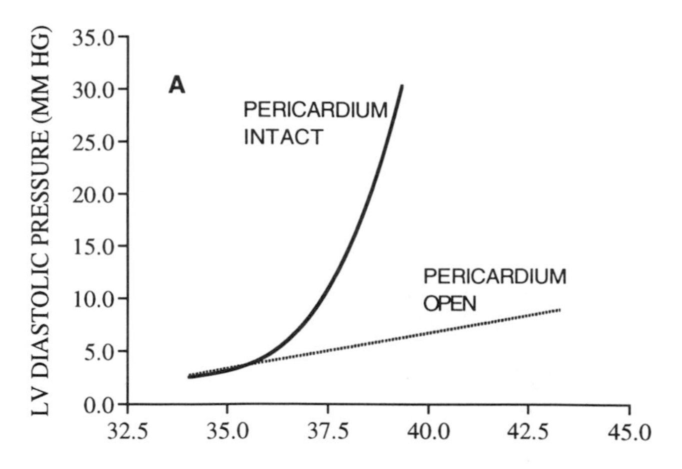

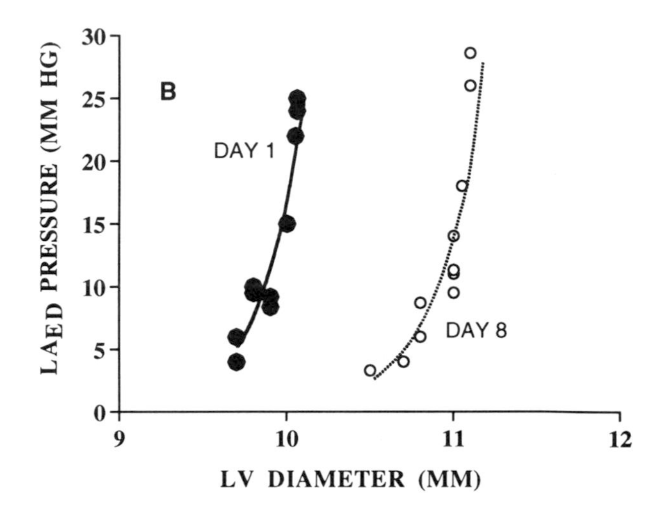

FIG. 13.8. *A*, Pressure–diameter relationship for the dog with an intact (*unbroken line*) and an open (*broken line*) pericardium. [Redrawn from Glantz et al. (19).] *B*, Left atrial end-diastolic pressure vs. a measure of left ventricular diameter with changes in intrathoracic volume in an unanesthetized resting pig showing progressive left ventricular dilation from 1 day to 8 days after pericardiectomy. [Redrawn from Hammond et al. (26).]

that limits diastolic filling time and results in the creation of a diastolic pressure gradient between the left atrium and left ventricle. Such pressure gradients are known to occur in early diastole, but they are less well defined at end-diastole. Exercise echocardiograms show that at heart rates of approximately 100 bpm, the mitral valve remains open throughout diastole; that is, it no longer closes in middiastole as seen with slower resting heart rates (92). At exercise rates of 200 bpm similar diastolic flow occurs across the valve in approximately half the time, suggesting the presence of a pressure gradient across the mitral valve. A large mitral valve gradient is expected in early diastole but does not apparently occur in man at end-diastole, as already seen in Figure 13.3.

Summary of Wedge Pressure Changes with Exercise. The above analysis implies that the rise in wedge pressure with exercise has several components in exercising humans. For very mild exercise, the Starling mechanisms operates to increase stroke volume via increased ventricular filling pressure and volume. With heavier exercise, atrial pressure rises but no longer serves to increase ventricular filling, probably because the pericardium limits left ventricular volume. There may also be an early diastolic pressure gradient across the mitral valve during heavy exercise. It is important that future work establish whether these or other mechanisms are responsible for the rise in the wedge pressure that occurs during exercise, because wedge pressure is the primary determinant of the increased pulmonary arterial pressure during exercise in normal humans.

Arteriovenous Pressure Gradient (Driving Pressure)

Individual Variability as Flow Increases. Since 80% of the interindividual variation in exercise pulmonary arterial pressure is accounted for by the wedge pressure, the remaining 20% variation appears to be related to vascular resistance in the lung. The classical demonstration of resistance is the pressure–flow relationship, as shown Figure 13.4C. Although the arteriovenous pressure gradient (driving pressure) clearly increases with increasing flow, the driving pressure for a given flow is variable among both supine and upright subjects. For most subjects (see examples Fig. 13.4C, *left*), a straight line describes the increased driving pressure with increasing flow, suggesting the variability is largely between, rather than within, individuals.

Furthermore, for a given individual, the slope of this pressure–flow line can be used to approximate the subject's total pulmonary resistance. The greater the slope, the greater the resistance to flow during exercise. We were able to compute exercise-related slopes from 16 upright and 47 supine subjects. Because the distribution of slopes (or calculated resistances, see below) did not appear to depend on body position, we combined both populations to obtain the distribution of exercise-related resistances in the 63 healthy young persons (Fig. 13.9). The slopes ranged from 0 to 2 units, which supported the concept that substantial interindividual variation occurred in pulmonary arterial pressure with increasing blood flow. Also, therefore, the calculated pulmonary vascular resistances in response to exercise also varies among individuals in response to exercise.

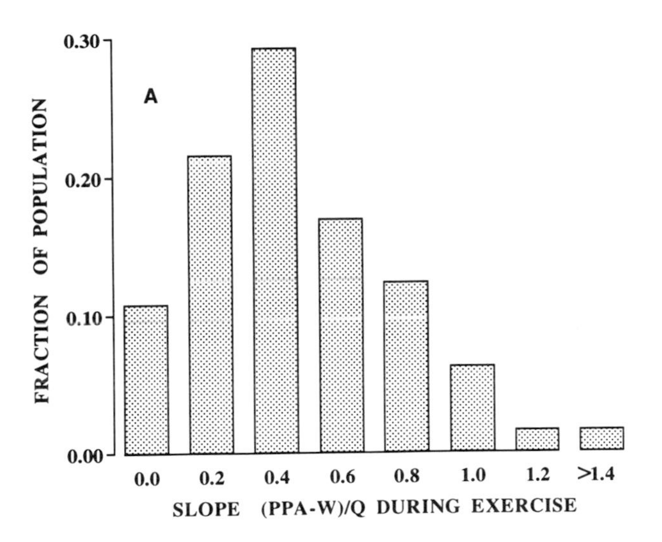

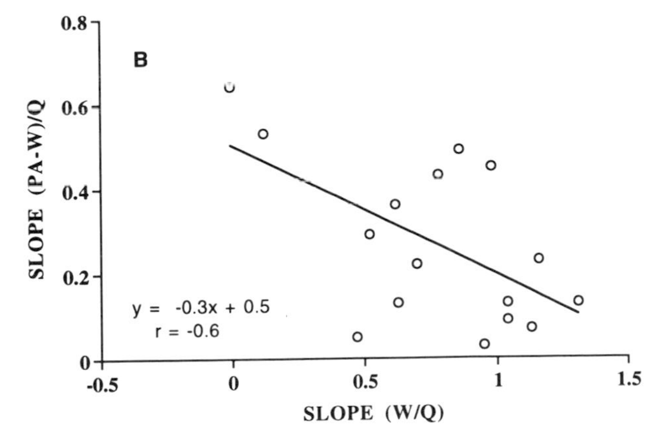

FIG. 13.9. *A*, Distribution in humans of the relationship of pulmonary artery minus wedge pressure to pulmonary blood flow during cycle exercise. A regression line was calculated for each of the 63 persons, and the distribution of the slopes is represented here. For the 47 supine persons, the regression included the resting measurement. *B*, Exercise slopes, (PA-W)/Q as related to (W/Q) for the 16 subjects performing upright exercise. The statistically significant relationship ($P < 0.05$) suggests that those persons having large wedge pressure increments during exercise have smaller increments in the pulmonary pressure gradient from artery to vein.

Pulmonary Vasodilation with Exercise; Effect of Body Position. Despite the interindividual variation, Figure 13.9 shows that more than 95% of this population can increase blood flow 1 liter/min with only 1 mm Hg (or less) increase in driving pressure, compatible with the occurrence of pulmonary vasodilation during exercise. Furthermore, for a given flow, the similar driving pressures for supine vs. upright exercising subjects (Fig. 13.10*A*) suggested that body position had little influence on the pressure–flow relationship. Extrapolation of the exercise measurements in Figure 13.10*A* to zero O_2 uptake (or zero flow) yields a small positive intercept (7–9 mm Hg) on the pressure axis. Because the extrapolated

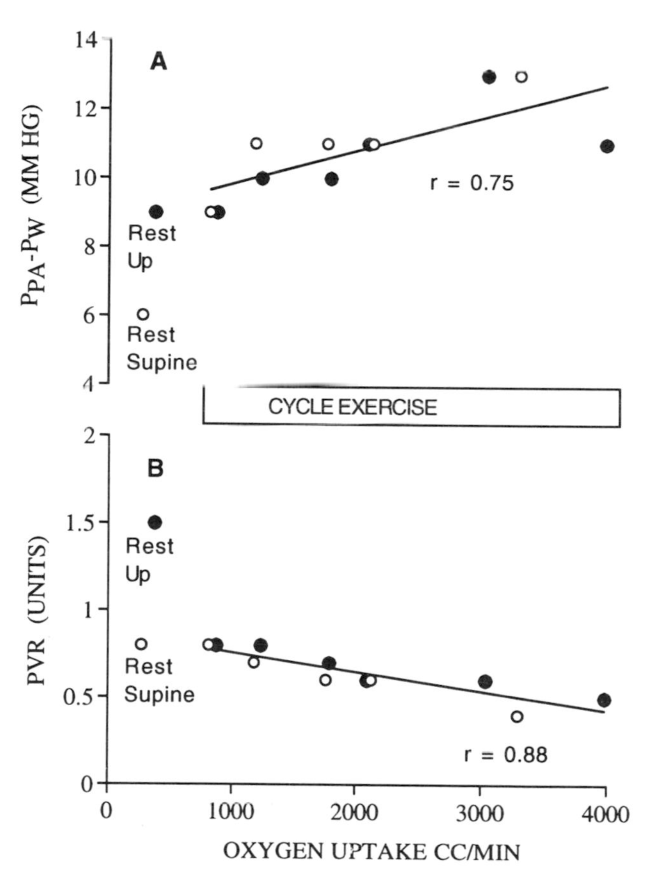

FIG. 13.10. Pulmonary arterial minus wedge pressure (*A*) and (*B*) pulmonary vascular resistance (PVR) as related to oxygen uptake in upright (*filled circles*) compared to supine (*open circles*) subjects at rest and during cycle exercise as indicated. [Data are the mean values taken from the review in Reeves, Dempsey, and Grover (67).]

pressure–flow relationship had a positive pressure intercept (rather than passing through the origin), calculated resistance fell, where the magnitude of the decrease was about 50% from light to heavy exercise (Fig. 13.10*B*). Thus, the analysis indicated that pulmonary vasodilation occurred during exercise and was independent of body position. The relatively high resting resistance in the sitting subjects was probably related to their lower wedge pressures (Table 13.1).

Is there Chemical Mediation of the Vasodilation with Exercise? The exercise-related increase in flow velocity, particularly during systole, increases endothelial shear stress, which could possibly cause the endothelial release of vasodilating substances such as prostacyclin and nitric oxide (NO). Although data are not available in man, studies in chronically instrumented animals suggest that endogenously produced vasodilators (prostacyclin and NO) do not cause the reduction in vascular resistance seen during exercise. Cyclooxygenase inhibition with meclofenamate in dogs (49) and sheep (57) raised the resting pulmonary vascular resistance. However, during exercise the resistance fell by the same amount as in the untreated animals, so that the pulmonary vasodilation could not be attributed to vasodilator prostaglandins. Also in sheep, inhibition of NO synthase with *N*-nitro-L-arginine raised resting pulmonary vascular resistance but did not inhibit the decreased resistance associated with exercise (40). Therefore, prostacyclin and/or NO can contribute to the low resting pulmonary vascular tone, but neither appears responsible for the vasodilation occurring with exercise.

Mechanical Factors Mediating Vasodilation. If powerful endogenous vasodilators such as prostacyclin and NO do not cause the pulmonary vasodilation during exercise, one wonders if regulation of these thin-walled, compliant vessels may be mediated by purely mechanical factors. Increasing transmural pressure in exercise could both recruit lung vessels (opening those previously closed or not flowing) and distend open vessels. In supine subjects, we can assume that the lung venous pressure exceeds alveolar pressure (zone 3), and the blood vessels are essentially fully recruited. Indeed, in these subjects, resting resistance lies near the extrapolated exercise line (Fig. 13.10*B*). However, in upright subjects, the onset of mild exercise causes a large fall in resistance, which could reflect vascular recruitment and/or distention. It is interesting to predict changes in pressure and flow in humans during exercise by mathematical models of vascular distention derived from studies in dog lungs, where segmental resistance and compliances have been carefully analyzed.

Lung vascular distention. Indicator dilution studies in whole dog lobes suggest that pulmonary vascular volumes and compliances are distributed approximately 27:53:20 in arteries, capillaries, and veins (14), with about 50% of total volume or compliance being in the capillaries. Of particular interest is that the total lung vascular compliance was about 8 ml/mm Hg in a 30 kg dog. Thus, only small increases in vascular pressure can cause measurable distention of the lung vasculature, consistent with a relatively compliant vascular system.

Injection of liquids with varying viscosities (13) has supported the concept that a bimodal site of vascular resistance occurs in the lung (Fig. 13.11). Thus, the capillary compartment with its relatively low resistance per unit volume is bounded upstream and downstream by arterial and venous compartments with higher resistances per volume contained, where the major resistance is the arterial site.

In the dog lung, the distensibility of lung arteries, ~100–1000 μm diameter, studied in vitro was surprisingly constant for a wide range of arterial diameters (2), showing approximately a 2% increase in diameter per mm Hg pressure rise. Recently, a model that relates pressure–flow curves and vascular distensibility has been developed for the dog lung assuming that all vessels are in zone 3 conditions (50). Dawson applied this model to the human data shown above in order to estimate the distensibility of resistance vessels, designated alpha (α) for the human lung vasculature. The model states:

$$Pa = \frac{[(1 + \alpha^* Pv)^5 + 5^*\alpha^* R_0{}^* Q]^{1/5} - 1}{\alpha}$$

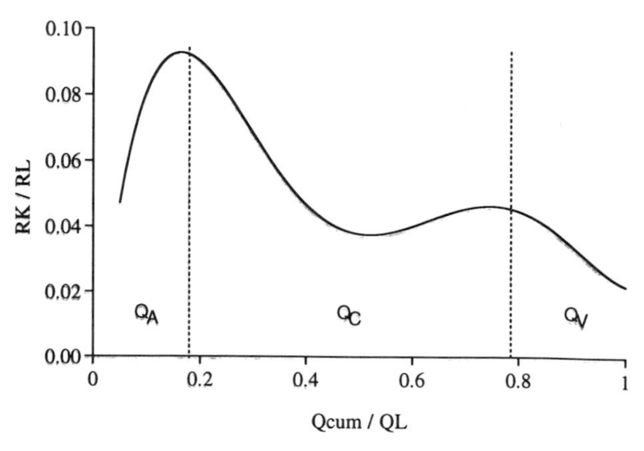

FIG. 13.11. The relation of segmental (RK) to total (RL) lung resistance as related to cumulative volume longitudinaly along the lung vasculature. *Vertical lines* mark the average end of the arterial volume (Q_A) and capillary volume (Q_C). [Adapted from Dawson et al. (14).]

where Pa is mean pulmonary artery pressure, Pv is mean pulmonary venous (wedge) pressure, α is distensibility of the resistance vessels, and R_0 is the hemodynamic resistance of the undistended vessels. The calculations indicate that with an $\alpha = 1.35\%/$ mm Hg and for an R_0 of 1.54 mm Hg · $\text{min}^{-1}\cdot\text{liter}^{-1}$, the model fits the actual measurements for both simple and upright exercising humans (Fig. 13.12). Both upright and supine data sets can be explained by the effects of posture on the relationship between wedge pressure and cardiac output. Given that the model provides a reasonable fit to the data, and that the distention of the resistance vessels is the only mechanisms in the model for changing pulmonary vascular resistance with increasing flow, mechanical distention of the lung vessels is a possible explanation of the resistance changes occurring with exercise. However, because overall exercise resistance is quite low, and because little of that resistance is located in the capillaries (13, 14), the model does not exclude a role for capillary recruitment (see below).

The small pulmonary arteries of dogs have a compliance of approximately 1%/mm Hg (32). For arterioles and venules (diameters 0.2–2 mm), compliances in the dog were 1.7% and 1.2%/mm Hg, respectively, and published human data suggest compliances of 2% and 1.4%. Thus, arterioles are slightly more distensible than veins. The distensibility coefficient of 1.35% found in the present analysis is consistent with that measured directly in human vessels in vitro. This quantitative consistency tends to support the concept that distensibility provides the major mechanism for the decrease in pulmonary vascular resistance during exercise in humans.

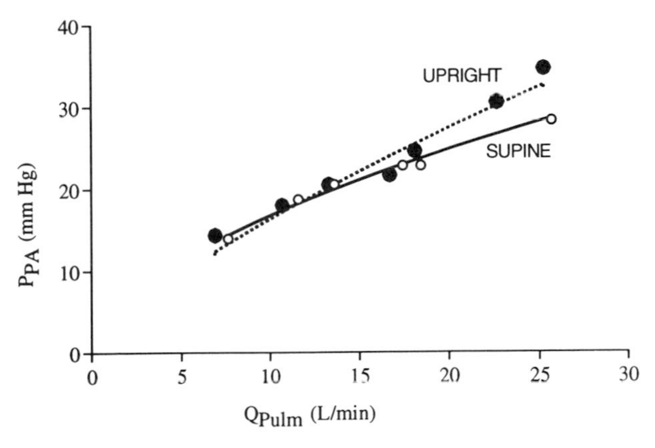

FIG. 13.12. Relation of mean pulmonary arterial pressure to pulmonary blood flow for supine (*unfilled circles*) and upright (*filled circles*) subjects at rest and during exercise. For supine and upright posture respectively, the *unbroken* and *broken lines* represent a good fit to the data points assuming the coefficient of distensibility (α) is 1.35%/mm Hg pressure rise, and the resistance to flow at zero pressure (R_0) is 1.54 mm Hg·$\text{min}^{-1}\cdot\text{liter}^{-1}$. The equation as derived by Linehan et al. (50) is shown in the text.

If so, one would expect that persons with large increases in wedge pressure during exercise would dilate their lung vessels (4) and show less increase in driving pressure with increasing flow. That such occurs is suggested by Figure 13.4*C*, *left*. The subject with a large increase in wedge pressure with increasing exercise intensity showed no increase in driving pressure (a nearly zero slope) as flow increased. However, the subject with little increase in wedge pressure did shown an increased slope. The issue is whether the large distribution of slopes relating driving pressure to flow, as shown in Figure 13.9*A*, is dependent on the magnitude of the increase in wedge pressure with increasing flow. An analysis of the 16 upright subjects showed that such was the case (Fig. 13.9*B*), indicating that an increase in the downstream pressure during exercise contributed to the decrease in resistance to blood flow through the lung.

Vascular recruitment. The above analysis assumes that the lung vasculature is in zone 3 condition. However, when man is upright and at rest the lung apices may be in zone 2, since the alveolar pressure approximates or exceeds the capillary pressure. The larger pulmonary pressure gradient for flow (artery-wedge pressure) in resting upright, as compared to supine, subjects and the larger calculated resting resistance upright than supine (Fig. 13.10) suggests that all lung capillaries are not perfused in the upright position. If so, the more basal portions of the lungs should have a large percentage of the capillaries open, and fewer of the capillaries are perfused in the apices. With even mild exercise, however, the supine and upright hemodynamic data become similar, suggesting that only mild exertion is necessary to open all or nearly all pulmonary vessels, including capillaries. Consistent with this concept is an in vitro study suggesting that with small increments of microvascular pressure, nearly all capillaries contain red cells, and with further pressure increments, only capillary distention results (20).

Carbon monoxide measurements. Can we use measurements of diffusing capacity to determine whether recruitment is complete in exercising man? Consider upright exercise: after all, most exertion, except that occurring during swimming or procreation, is performed upright. If our analysis is correct, with even mild exercise the entire lung circulation becomes perfused, probably because a particularly powerful mechanism for opening the microcirculation is an increase in venous pressure (4, 94). Thus, diffusing capacity should reflect the greater microcirculatory volume.

The diffusion from lung alveoli to capillary blood of carbon monoxide (carbon monoxide diffusion capacity or DL_{CO}) depends upon the surface area of the blood gas barrier, its thickness, and the capillary blood volume (see Chapter 12). Indeed, carbon monoxide diffusion capacity increases progressively with increasing exercise intensity (39) and pulmonary blood flow (Fig. 13.13). That is, the DL_{CO} does not become asymptotic to some limiting value as exercise capacity is approached. The implication is that the volume of red cells in the pulmonary microcirculation has also not reached its limit, which could be attributed to progressively increasing recruitment. However, the progressive increase in DL_{CO} can also be due to capillary dilation and increased capillary hematocrit, both of which contribute to the increased capillary blood volume (see Chapter 12). The carbon monoxide method cannot distinguish between recruitment and distension occurring during exercise. Thus, the precise roles of capillary recruitment vs. distensibility in exercise is unresolved and awaits the development of future methodology.

Erythrocyte transit times through capillaries. Capillary volume has important implications for red cell transit time through the lung microcirculation. Recent direct visualization of fluorescent dye flowing from arteriole to venule on the surface of the dog lung lobe provides additional insight into the question of capillary recruitment and transit time of blood through the capillaries (64). When flow through the lobe was doubled, which occurs in mild exercise, the number of perfused capillaries increased (i.e., more capillaries were recruited). Simultaneously, the mean transit times became shorter, and the relative dispersion (SD of the transit times/mean transit time) became smaller and the minimum transit time shortened from approximately 1.2 s to 0.9 s. Thus, both capillary perfusion and the distributions of capillary transit times became more homogenous. However, when flow was again doubled, further recruitment and a further decrease in relative dispersion was not observed, although mean minimum transit time shortened further (Fig. 13.14). These findings in the dog lobes support the hemodynamic analysis that full recruitment of capillaries occurs with modest increments of flow. Higher flows are accompanied by higher capillary pressures and, because of their compliance, increased capillary volumes. The increase in volume maximizes transit time of red cells through the lung as flows increase. Extrapolation of these data suggests that a minimum transit time of about 0.25 s would occur at a pulmonary flow of about 20 liters/min (i.e., near the limit of maximal flow for the exercising dog) (64).

Summary of mechanical factors. The "purpose" of increasing blood flow during exercise is to increase O_2 transport, which implies that O_2 uptake from alveolus to lung capillary blood increases. The system design apparently calls for several sequential strategies to occur, depending on the amount of O_2 to be transported. On initiating mild exertion, the upright subject recruits fully, or nearly so, the entire pulmonary microcirculation. As exercise intensity and flow increase, microcirculatory pressures rise dilat-

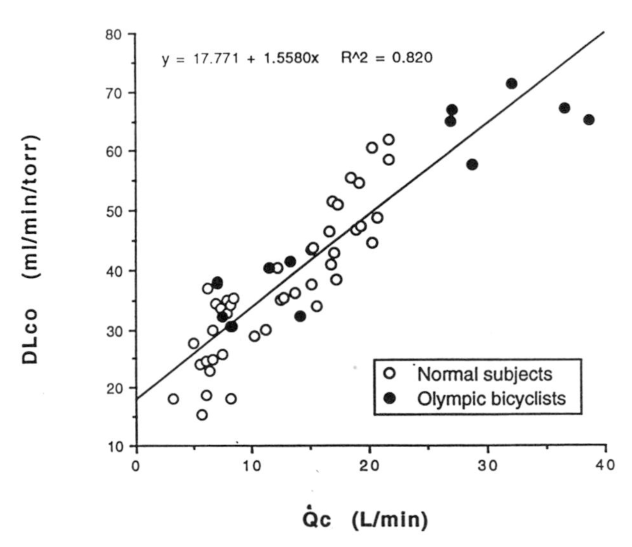

FIG. 13.13. Carbon monoxide pulmonary diffusion values at rest and during cycle exercise. (Unpublished Data provided by C. C. W. Hsia and R. L. Johnson.)

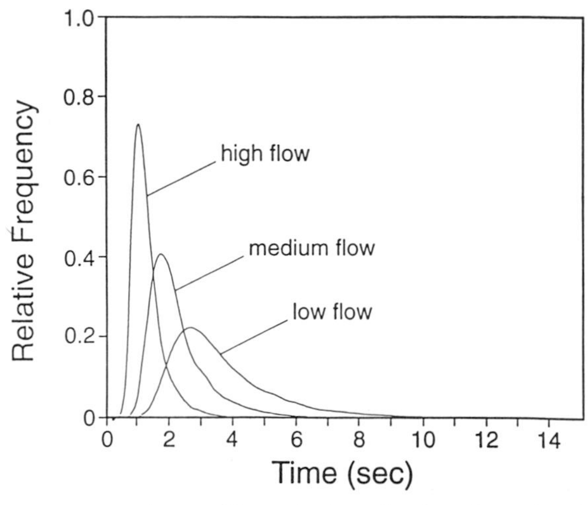

FIG. 13.14. Distribution of transit times for flow through a dog lung lobe when the flow was 400 ml/min (low), 800 ml/min (medium), and 1600 ml/min (high). The values of flow are approximately equivalent to cardiac outputs of 1.6, 3.2, and 6.4 liters/min, respectively, in the intact dog. [From Presson et al. (64), with permission.]

ing the vasculature, reducing the resistance to flow, and increasing microcirculatory (particularly capillary) volume. The increase in volume serves to increase the diffusing surface and to maximize transit time of red cells through the lung, both factors serving to preserve arterial oxygenation in high-flow states. Because of the distensibility of the lung vessels, the important thread that runs through all of the pulmonary hemodynamic changes in normal exercising man is the extent to which there is an increase in left ventricular filling pressure and mean left atrial pressure.

Exercise and Compliance in Large Pulmonary Arteries

The main pulmonary artery and its branches are under control of the sympathetics (37) which, when activated, increase the stiffness of the large pulmonary arteries without increasing peripheral pulmonary vascular resistance. In dogs, central nervous system (CNS) stimulation simulates many of the responses of exercise (82) and stiffens the large pulmonary arteries. Measurements in exercising man indicate that the large conduit arteries, in both the pulmonary and systemic circulation, stiffen as the peripheral resistance falls. The stiffening of large pulmonary arteries serves to match the output impedance of the right ventricle to the input impedance of the pulmonary circulation. However, the stiffening of these conduit arteries during exercise increases the pulse wave velocity in the large arteries and the systolic–diastolic pulse pressure, which increases pulsatile flow in the microcirculation and the shear stress on its endothelium.

A novel investigation on the role of the sympathoadrenal system during exercise has been conducted in the exercising sheep (40, 41). β-Adrenergic (β) blockade by the administration of propranolol was found to increase resting pulmonary vascular resistance and to blunt the exercise-related fall in resistance. α-Adrenergic (α) blockade by phentolamine tended to enhance the fall in resistance, and with administration of both α- and β-blockade, hemodynamics were not different from those without drug treatment. These findings suggested that in exercise an increased neurogenic tone occurs in the pulmonary arteries, but this increased vasoconstrictor tone is opposed by β-induced vasodilation.

The question that remains is, Which blood vessels respond to the sympathoadrenal stimuli, particularly those affected by the α-adrenergic system? The α-neural supply is predominantly to large pulmonary arteries, but the pattern of innervation differs substantially among species (37), and larger pulmonary veins are also innervated (28). When α-mediated vasoconstriction is unopposed during exercise (*1*) increased arterial tone could "spill over" to smaller conduit arteries and raise prearteriolar resistance, (*2*) venous tone could increase sufficiently to raise venous resistance, and (*3*) a sufficient neural supply is present in the arterioles to raise the arteriolar resistance. While these issues are currently unresolved, the most efficient matching of right ventricular to pulmonary arterial impedance would be to dilate the arterioles, yet also to stiffen the large pulmonary arteries.

HEMODYNAMICS DURING EXERCISE IN ANIMALS

Sheep

The sheep is becoming an important animal in which to study exercise, since (*1*) it can be trained to run on a treadmill, (*2*) it is large enough for hemodynamic measurements, and (*3*) lung fluid flux can be measured during exercise. Therefore, one can compare hemodynamic measurements in sheep to those in man. It is important to recall that this comparison not only crosses species, but it also involves a quadruped that has had a pulmonary flow probe placed during a recent thoracotomy and the pericardium has often been removed. Furthermore, a pressure gradient from a small wedged catheter to the left atrium is present in sheep (58), a gradient not present in man and which suggests a greater venous resistance in the pulmonary circulation of sheep than in man. Removal of the pericardium prior to making the measurements in sheep may account for some of the hemodynamic differences between sheep and man (J. H. Newman, personal communication). In the absence of a pericardium, when the sheep triples its pulmonary blood flow, pulmonary arterial pressure rises, but left atrial pressure does not (Fig. 13.15*A* and *B*), and the pressure gradient from pulmonary artery to left atrium is rather great (Fig. 13.15*C*). Preliminary data suggest that when the sheep's pericardium is left intact, left atrial pressure rises as expected during exercise (J. H. Newman, personal communication).

Data obtained in exercising sheep provide measurements that are not possible to obtain in man (58). For example, instantaneous and continuous measurements of variables from the onset of exercise (Fig. 13.16*A* and *B*) indicate that within a minute of beginning exercise, pulmonary blood flow and arterial pressure rise. During this initial minute

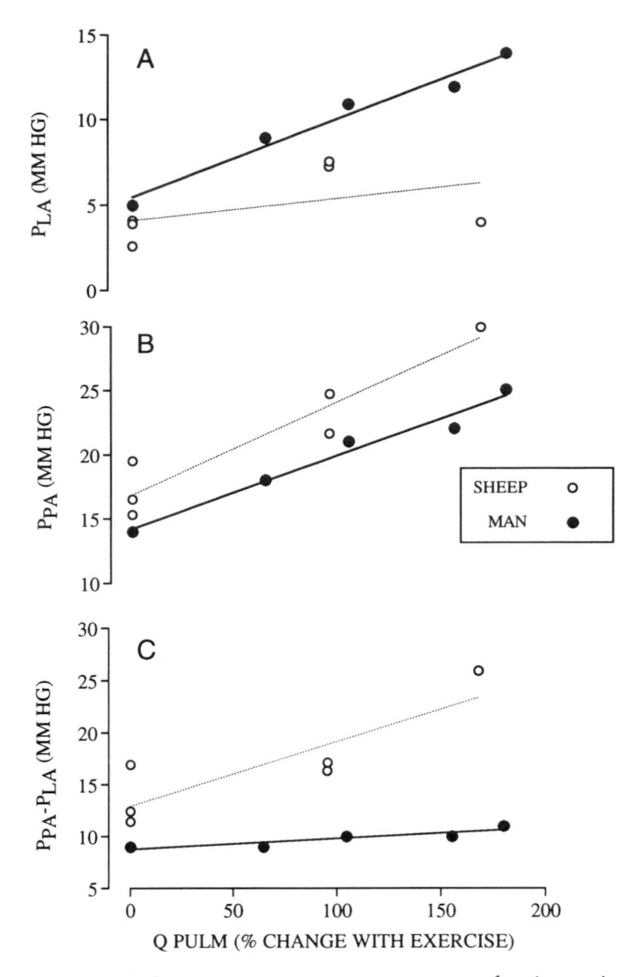

FIG. 13.15. Pulmonary pressure measurements for increasing pulmonary flow (Q PULM, expressed as percentage change from rest to exercise) in sheep (*unfilled circles* and *broken line*) and upright man (*filled circles* and *unbroken line*). From above downward are shown (*A*) left atrial (sheep) or wedge pressure (man), (*B*) mean pulmonary arterial pressure, and (*C*) pulmonary arterial minus left atrial pressure. [Human measurements are from Reeves et al. (40), and sheep measurements are redrawn from Newman et al. (58) and Kane et al. (41).]

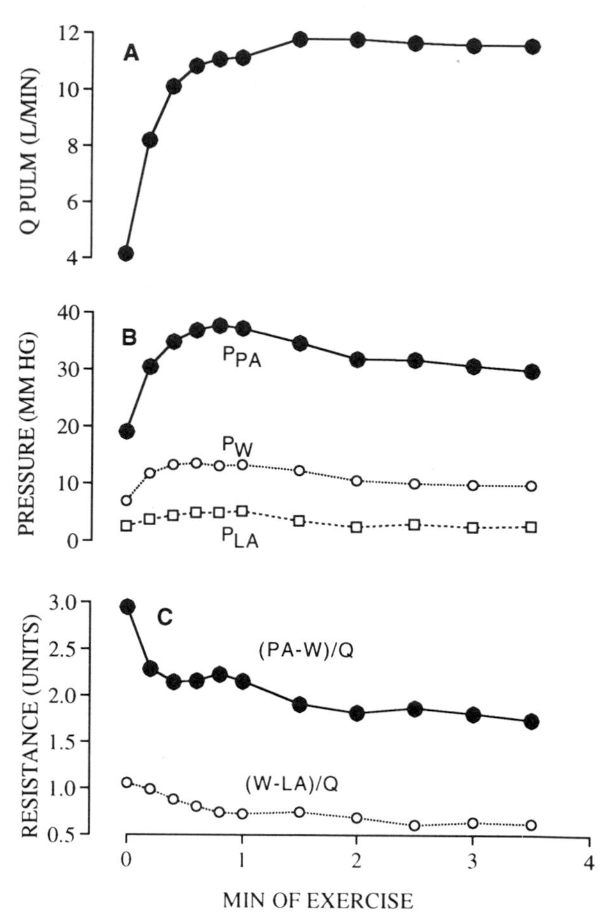

FIG. 13.16. Measurements at rest (time 0) and during 3.5 min of treadmill exercise at a 10% grade and 4 mph in six young adult sheep. *A*, Pulmonary blood flow (Q PULM) using a main pulmonary arterial flow probe. *B*, Mean pressures from the pulmonary artery (P_{PA}) wedge (P_W), and left atrium (P_{LA}). C, Resistances (pressure gradient/flow) from pulmonary artery to wedge and from wedge to left atrium. [Redrawn from Newman et al. (58).]

of exercise, the flow rises more than pressure, indicating an initial fall in pulmonary vascular resistance (Fig. 13.16*C*). The peak pressure is not sustained and flow continues to rise after pressure has peaked. By 2 min flow reaches a plateau, which is sustained. Calculated pulmonary vascular resistance continues to fall. The fall in calculated resistance has a rapid phase followed by a slower phase. The rise in microvascular pressure is greater than that in left atrial pressure, suggesting the presence of venous resistance. These pressure and flow transients indicate that complex changes are occurring within the lung vasculature very rapidly during exercise in sheep.

Dogs

Clues relative to how recruitment and distension participate in the falling resistance in lungs have been obtained from the flow distributions measured in exercising dogs. The dog, like the sheep, is a quadruped with its heart lying on the sternum at the "bottom" of the lung. The lung has a vertical distance from the most dependent (ventral) to the most dorsal part of approximately 16 cm (Fig. 13.17*A*). Unlike the human lung with its large base and small apex, dog lungs have small ventral volumes but large dorsal volumes. Preliminary studies (W. W. Wagner, unpublished observations) using horizontal dog lung slices 1 cm thick (Fig. 13.17*B*) confirm that lung volume increases with vertical distance from ventral to dorsal areas. Because most of the lung volume is well above the heart, the question arises as to the relative

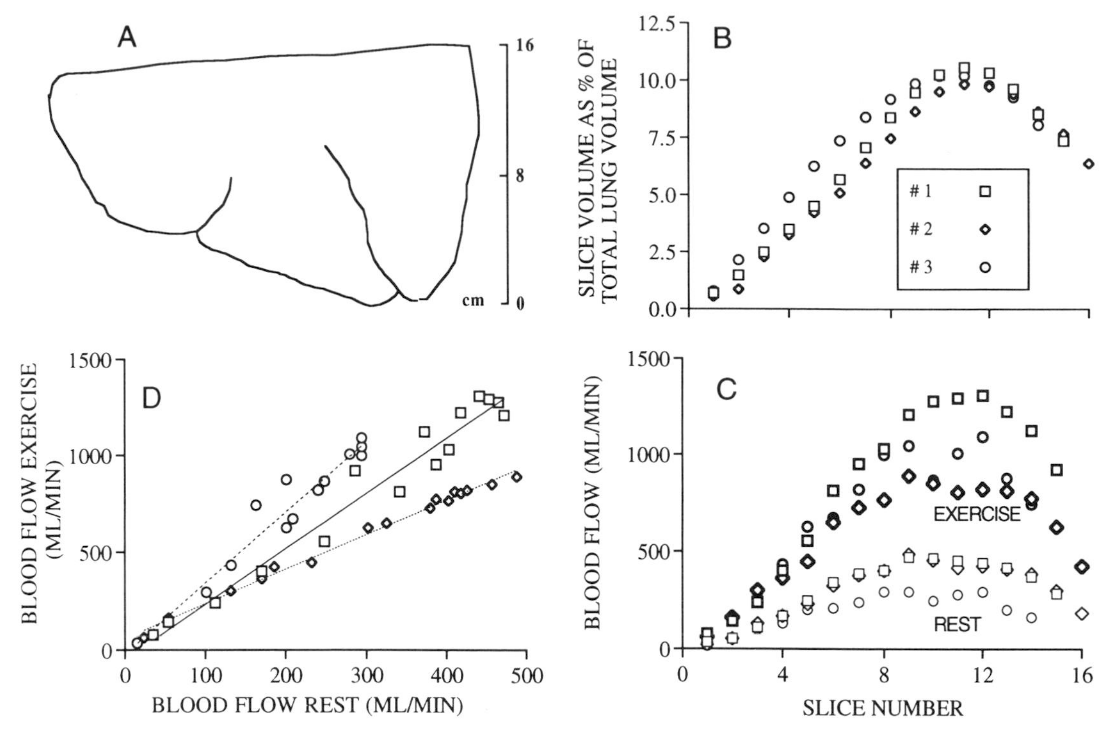

FIG. 13.17. Measurements in dogs. *A*, Drawing showing a 16 cm vertical distance, ventral to dorsal, for a lung in an adult, standing, facing leftward. *B*, Volume distribution in lung slices, 1 cm thick, from ventral (#1) to dorsal surface (#16) for each of three dogs. Note that most of the lung volume is dorsal. (The inflated lung was air dried prior to being sliced.) *C*, Estimated blood flow distribution for each lung slice in *B*. Note that for both rest and exercise, the distribution of blood flow resembles distribution of lung volume. (Flow determination was by microspheres injected intravenously in the living dog at rest and during one steady state exercise bout.) *D*, Ratio, for each lung slice, of exercise to resting blood flow. Note that for all slices in each dog, exercise flow was proportional to resting flow, where the constant of proportionality (slope) was the ratio of exercise to resting cardiac output for each dog. (Data, unpublished, were provided by W. W. Wagner.)

roles of vascular recruitment vs. distention with exercise in the dog lung compared to humans. Microsphere studies have indicated that at rest, both ventral and dorsal areas are perfused, with most flow going to the large dorsal lung volume (Fig. 13.17C). With steady-state exercise, flow increases in all lung areas, and for each dog, the exercise flows in all lung slices are proportional to the resting flows (Fig. 13.17*D*). Because the increase in flow in the upper lung zones was nearly proportional to the increase in the lower zones, a disproportionately large recruitment in the upper zones seems unlikely. Such findings suggest that dorsal recruitment of new arterial vessels with exercise is relatively unimportant in the dog, and raises the possibility that the fall in resistance with exercise is primarily arterial distention.

Horses

Pulmonary hemodynamics in the exercising horse deserve special consideration, given the lung's large ventral to dorsal vertical distance (>60 cm) and the horse's capacity to increase O_2 uptake nearly 40-fold and pulmonary arterial pressure fourfold in heavy exercise (16, 33, 46, 52, 62, 90, 93; and W. W. Wagner, personal communication). Possibly related to their large size, horses have high pulmonary arterial pressures (Fig. 13.18), and the values are higher than those for man both at rest and during exercise, even when the flow is adjusted per kilogram of body weight (46). The exercise measurements of vascular pressures within the chest are noisy in the horse, being complicated by the very large intrathoracic (esophageal) pressure swings (from about −15 to +35 mm Hg) from inspiration to expiration (16, A. K. Shima et al., personal communication).

Despite the horse's large size and high pulmonary pressures and flows, its pulmonary hemodynamic response to exercise is similar to that of man in that pulmonary arterial and wedge pressure rise progressively with increasing flow (Fig. 13.18). When the two pressures have been measured together, pulmonary arterial pressure correlates very strongly (r = 0.98) with wedge, suggesting that the variation in wedge pressure accounts largely for the variation in

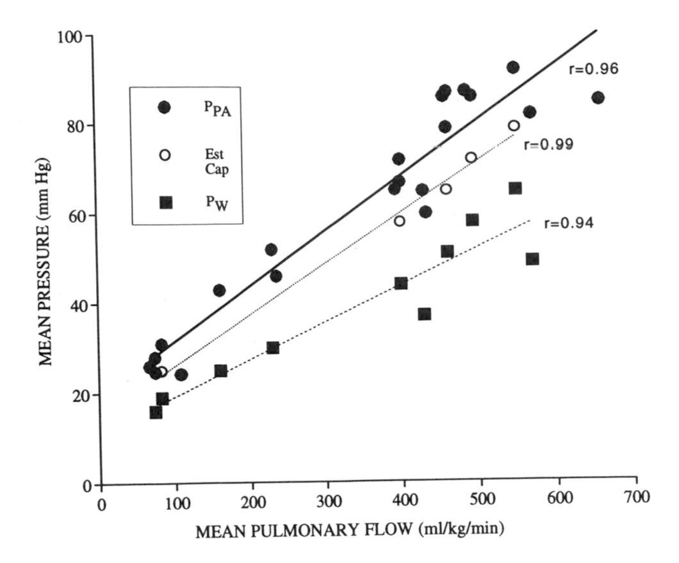

FIG. 13.18. Pressure–flow relationships for the horse at rest and during exercise showing the mean pulmonary arterial pressure (P_{PA}), estimated capillary pressure (Est Cap), and wedge pressure (P_W). Shown are composite mean and individual values from references 16, 33, 46, 52, 62, 90, 93 and W. W. Wagner, personal communication. Where flow data were not available, they were estimated from heart rate.

pulmonary arterial pressure, as in man. However, the pressure gradient from pulmonary artery to wedge is greater in the horse than in man, dog, or sheep. The possibility that much of this pressure gradient is in the pulmonary veins is suggested by the estimated pulmonary capillary pressure measurements (52), which are closer to the pulmonary arterial pressures than to the wedge pressure (Fig. 13.18).

If so, the capillary pressures in the horse during heavy exercise are very close to pressures in the pulmonary artery, which implies that capillary pressures greater than 70 mm Hg are possible. Such levels are capable of rupturing capillaries and inducing pulmonary hemorrhage (52, 95), but one wonders what protects the horse from high pressure–induced pulmonary edema during this process.

LUNG FLUID EXCHANGE

From the previous sections it is obvious that cardiac output and left atrial pressure (P_{wedge}) increase during exercise in humans and animals. Therefore, pulmonary microvessel pressures must increase, which should drive fluid out of the pulmonary circulation into lung tissue. Usually only small amounts of fluid enter the lung interstitial tissues with moderate elevations in capillary pressure; however, when capillary pressures are large, intra-alveolar edema develops (21, 25, 58, 56, 76). The following sections will describe transmicrovascular fluid exchange in general and specifically in the lung. These introductory sections will be followed by sections that evaluate lung fluid exchange in exercising animals and humans.

General Concepts

Figure 13.19 shows an idealized pulmonary microvessel lined by a continuous layer of endothelial cells and surrounded by a basement membrane and an interstitial compartment containing interstitial fluid and an interstitial matrix. An initial lymphatic that drains the interstitial space is also shown. The term "capillary" has been used classically to describe a generalized area of the microcirculation where fluid is exchanged between plasma and interstitium (85, 88). But since small arteries and venules, as well as anatomical alveolar capillaries, can exchange fluid and solutes with the interstitium, we have chosen to use the term "microcirculation" to describe that portion of the pulmonary circulation where fluid and solute exchanges with the interstitium (76).

In each microvessel some average hydrostatic pressure (P_{MV}) is present that tends to drive fluid out of the circulation into the interstitium. This hydro-

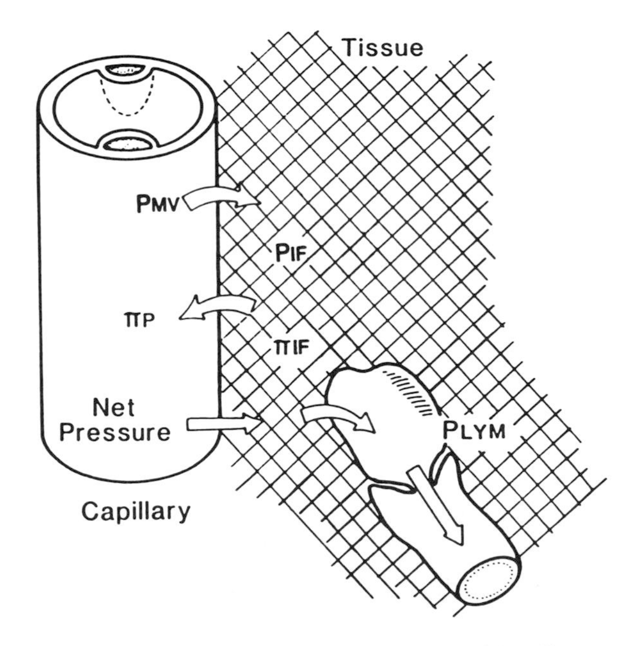

FIG. 13.19. Schematic representation of the Starling forces operating between pulmonary capillaries and the interstitium. Note that the alveolar surface tension is exactly opposed by the subatmospheric interstitial fluid pressure (−5) and the lymphatic filling pressure (P_{IF} − P_{LYM}) [−5−(−6)] is positive, which promotes the filling of lymphatic vessels. (Redrawn from Guyton, *Textbook of Medical Physiology*, 7th edition, Saunders, 1986.)

static pressure is opposed by the hydrostatic pressure existing in interstitial fluid (P_{IF}). The difference between these two hydrostatic forces (ΔP_{MV}) has been defined as the *capillary (or microvascular) filtration pressure* (51, 55, 57, 61):

$$\text{Microvascular filtration pressure} = \Delta P_{MV} = P_{MV} - P_{IF} \quad (1)$$

Plasma contains many small solutes, which exchange easily with the interstitium in most organs, since they exert no lasting effective osmotic pressure across the microvascular wall. The plasma, however, contains large proteins that cannot easily cross the capillary wall to enter the interstitial fluid. Consequently, they exert an important force governing transvascular fluid exchange, the osmotic pressure of plasma, and interstitial fluid. The osmotic pressure exerted by the plasma proteins is defined as the protein osmotic (or oncotic) pressure (78). Since all tissue fluids with the exception of the brain interstitium contain plasma proteins, the protein osmotic gradient acting across the microvascular barrier ($\Delta\pi_{MV}$) is equal to the difference between the protein osmotic pressure of plasma (π_P) and the protein osmotic pressure of the interstitial fluid (π_{IF}). This protein osmotic pressure gradient $\Delta\pi_{MV}$ is defined as the *capillary (or microvascular) absorptive force*, since it acts in a direction opposite to the microvascular filtration pressure; that is:

$$\text{Microvascular absorptive pressure} = \Delta\pi_{MV} = \pi_P - \pi_{IF} \quad (2)$$

Equation 3 below is the basic equation that defines the forces responsible for transmicrovascular fluid exchange. The forces contained in this equation, P_{MV}, P_{IF}, π_P and π_{IF} are defined as Starling forces to honor E. H. Starling, the great English physiologist, who first postulated the mechanisms responsible for regulating transmicrovascular fluid exchange (78); that is:

$$\Delta P_{MV} = \Delta\pi_{MV},$$

or

$$P_{MV} - P_{IF} = \pi_P - \pi_{IF} \quad (3)$$

This equation states that when P_{MV} increased, P_{IF} and $\pi_P - \pi_{IF}$ increase to oppose the change in microvascular pressure. Equation 3 is the mathematical statement of the Starling-Landis law of the capillary and simply states that within physiological limits, microvascular filtration is *self-regulating* because the protein osmotic and interstitial fluid pressure changes in a direction to oppose changes in the microvascular pressure. Normally, these phenomena regulate interstitial volume within narrow limits over a wide range of microvascular pressures.

The actual system is, of course, not this simple, since we now know that increasing microvascular pressure increases lymph flow (i.e., the Starling forces are not in a perfect balance). A small amount of fluid always leaks out of the circulation into the tissues to form lymph, and a more complex equation is required to explain the actual solvent flux occurring between plasma and the interstitial spaces (54, 57, 61).

$$J_{MV} = K_{FC}[\Delta P_C - \sigma_d \Delta\pi_{MV}] = J_L \quad (4)$$

In equation 4, J_{MV} represents the net microvascular filtration and is equal to lymph flow (J_L) when the tissues are neither shrinking nor swelling. Note that equation 4 contains two constants: K_{FC}, which is the microvascular filtration coefficient, and σ_d, the osmotic reflection coefficient of all plasma proteins. K_{FC} is a function of the number and size of pores available (surface area) for fluid exchange in the microvascular walls. The osmotic reflection coefficient of plasma proteins is a function of the selectivity of the microvascular membrane to plasma proteins. σ_d equals 1 if proteins cannot leave the plasma and equals 0 if the microvascular wall is freely permeable to the protein; that is, if $\sigma_d = 1$, the calculated or measured protein osmotic pressure is totally exerted across the microvascular barrier. There are several different proteins in plasma—albumin (4.5 g/dl, 29 cm H_2O), γ-globulin (2.5 g/dl, 8 cm H_2O), fibrinogen (0.3 g/dl, 0.3 cm H_2O)—that provide a total plasma protein concentration and protein osmotic pressure of 7.3 $g \cdot dl^{-1}$ and 37.3 cm H_2O, respectively. The osmotic pressure generated by the plasma proteins is a nonlinear cubic function of protein concentration. Also, one-third of the protein osmotic pressure in plasma is caused by the negative charge on the molecules holding sodium ions in the plasma.

The actual protein osmotic pressure represents the sum of all protein osmotic gradients multiplied by their respective reflection coefficients, but for the purpose of our discussion, we will simply use the *total plasma protein osmotic pressure* and assume σ_d is near 1. The reader should realize that this represents a lumped average protein osmotic gradient and reflection coefficient for all proteins contained in plasma and interstitial fluid.

Not only do fluid and small molecules exchange easily between plasma and the interstitial fluid, but even the largest plasma proteins enter the interstitium in most organs, albeit slowly. This is a complex biophysical phenomenon and the net protein flux occurring across the microcirculation (J_S) is described by the following solute flux equation developed by Granger and Taylor (23, 87):

$$J_S = (1 - \sigma_d)\, J_{MV} C_P + \frac{x}{e^x - 1} PS\Delta C \qquad (5)$$

C_P in equation 5 is the plasma concentration of the protein, PS is the permeability-surface area product for the protein–membrane system, ΔC is the difference in the concentration of the proteins in plasma (C_P) minus their interstitial fluid protein concentration (C_{IF}) and x is a coefficient that is equal to:

$$x = \frac{(1 - \sigma_d) J_{MV}}{PS} \qquad (6)$$

Equation 6 explains the nonlinear nature of transcapillary protein flux because x increases as a function of J_{MV}.

Assuming that the first term in equation 5 is the convective flux and the second term is diffusive flux, then the protein flux equation (equation 5) reduces to $C_{IF}/C_P = 1 - \sigma_d$ when transmicrovascular filtration is large (13). This requires that the diffusional term approaches zero at high filtration rates. In fact, this behavior of protein flux has been used to measure σ_d in many organs by increasing microvessel pressure to levels that maximally dilute C_{IF}.

For a complete analysis of the protein flux equation as it relates to the microcirculation, the reader should consult Reed et al. (66), Taylor and Parker (88), Taylor and Granger (87), and Taylor (85). The major factors to remember about transmicrovascular protein flux are: (*1*) when J_{MV} increases, C_{IF} decreases because the protein concentration in the microvascular filtrate is lower than the interstitial concentration; (*2*) the convective component of protein flux into the interstitium increases as the transvascular filtration increases; and (*3*) at low rates of transmicrovascular filtration, the convective flux of protein is small and proteins move out of the circulation by diffusion into the tissues down their concentration gradients (66).

Table 13.2 shows the Starling forces: microvascular pressure (P_{MV}), tissue fluid pressure (P_{IF}), and plasma (π_P) and tissue (π_{IF}) protein osmotic pressures and lymph flow for several organs (86). Note that the normal imbalance in the Starling forces $[(P_{MV} - P_{IF}) - (\pi_P - \pi_{IF})]$ is positive and small in most organs. These data indicate that only small amounts of transmicrovascular fluid filtration occurs for normal microvascular pressures. Only in the brain, the absorbing small intestine, and renal peritubular capillaries are the sum of Starling forces negative (i.e., the microvessels in these organs are removing fluid from the interstitium). Also, π_{IF} varies among different organs relative to their microvascular protein permeability and lymph flows. Interestingly, P_{IF} can be subatmospheric or positive depending on the hydration state of the tissues (i.e., less hydrated tissues have smaller interstitial fluid pressures and, in fact, some are actually subatmospheric).

Factors that Oppose Edema Formation

Table 13.3 shows the change in each Starling force and lymph flow when P_{MV} was increased by about 20 mm Hg (28 cm H_2O) in several different organs as compared to the total change in each force (86). Although increasing microvascular pressure by this amount causes almost no interstitial edema, edema does accompany further increases in microvascular pressure. Note that π_{IF} decreased, causing ($\pi_P - \pi_{IF}$) to increase in all tissues except the liver. Both P_{IF} and lymph flow increase to oppose edema formation, but P_{IF} increases only slightly in the colon. These alter-

TABLE 13.2. *Starling Forces in Selected Animal Tissues*[*,†]

Tissue	P_{MV}	P_{IF}	π_p	π_{IF}	LF	ΔP
Lung	7	−5	23	12	0.10	+1
Subcutaneous	13	−5	21	4	0.015	+1
Skeletal muscle	9	−3	20	8	0.005	0
Brain	11	7	14	0	—	−10
Intestine (normal)	16	2	23	10	0.08	+1
Intestine (absorbing)	16	3	23	5	0.10	−5
Liver	7	6	22	20	0.10	−1
Cardiac muscle	23	15	21	13	0.12	0
Glomerular	50	15[‡]	28	0[‡]	2.0	+7
Renal peritubular	25	7	32	7	2.0	−7

*Modified from Taylor, A. E. Molecular fluid and solute exchange. In: *Encyclopedia of Human Biology*, New York: Academic Press, 1991, p. 35, with permission. P_{MV}, P_{IF}, π_p, π_{IF}, and LF denote capillary and tissue hydrostatic pressure, plasma and tissue protein osmotic pressure, and lymph flows, respectively. ΔP is the sum of the forces $[(P_{MV}\text{-}P_{IF}) - (\pi_p\text{-}\pi_{IF})]$ and represents filtration when negative. A sum of zero indicates no filtration or absorption.
‡This represents tubular protein osmotic pressures rather than renal interstitial pressure.

TABLE 13.3. *Safety Factors in Various Animal Tissues*[*,†]

Tissue	Percentage of Total Safety Factor		
	$(\Delta_p\text{-}\Delta_{IF})$	Lymph flow	P_{IF}
Lung	50	17	33
Hindpaw	14	24	62
Small intestine	45	20	35
Colon	52	4	44
Liver	0	42	58
Heart	7	12	81

*Modified from Taylor, A. E. Molecular fluid and solute exchange. *In: Encyclopedia of Human Biology*. New York: Academic press, 1991, P. 35, with permission. †$(\pi_p\text{-}\pi_{IF})$ is the absorptive force and P_{IF} is the tissue fluid pressure. The values are shown as percentage of the total safety factor measured when capillary pressure was increased 20 mm Hg above control values.

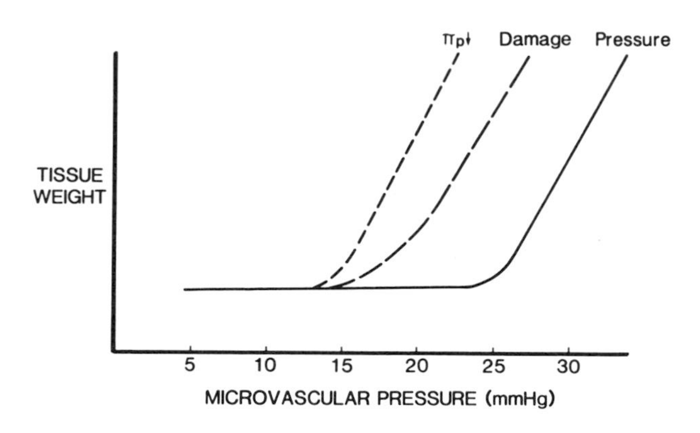

FIG. 13.20. Effect of capillary pressure on lung edema when only capillary pressure is increased (pressure), plasma proteins are decreased ($\pi_P\downarrow$), and endothelial damage (damage). [Redrawn from Newman et al. (56).]

ations in Starling forces greatly limit the formation of interstitial edema until filtration increases to levels at which these forces and lymph flow can no longer change. These changes in forces and lymph flows have been defined as "edema safety factors" (83, 88). These forces can change to oppose transvascular filtration pressures of approximately 25–30 mm Hg in all tissues before excessive edema develops. However, in liver, heart, and hind paw, the protein osmotic pressure gradients cannot change to any significant degree, and interstitial fluid pressure and lymph flow increase to provide the major edema safety factors in these organs. Although the Starling forces in all organs change to oppose increases in microvascular pressures, the contributions of each Starling force relative to the overall edema safety factor varies considerably between organs.

Edema Safety Factors in Lung

Figure 13.20 shows the effect of increasing microvascular pressure on edema formation in lungs. Note that microvascular pressure must increase to 25–30 mm Hg in normal lungs before edema develops (*solid line*) (25). As can be seen from Table 13.2, this ability to oppose edema formation in lungs occurs because: (*1*) $(\pi_P - \pi_T)$ decreased by almost 10 mm Hg, (*2*) P_{IF} increases by 5 mm Hg, and (*3*) lymph flow increases sufficiently to provide a safety factor of about 5 mm Hg (76, 83, 86).

The *small dashed line* in Figure 13.20 shows the effects of decreasing plasma protein concentration to one-half the normal value on edema formation. Note that edema now occurs at lower microvascular pressures, since the microvascular absorptive force $(\Delta\pi_{MV})$ cannot change to the same magnitude that develops when plasma protein concentration is normal (25).

Damage to the microvascular wall affects edema formation because proteins leak across the microvascular walls and increase π_{IF}. Subsequently, the protein osmotic pressure gradient cannot increase to buffer the increased microvascular filtration. This ability of $\Delta\pi_{MV}$ to increase declines because interstitial protein concentration does not decrease with increased transvascular filtration, and also σ_d decreases. These changes decrease the microvascular absorption force to very low values because the effect is not additive but multiplicative, since both σ_d and $(\pi_p - \pi_{IF})$ decrease (86, 88).

However, when the microvascular membrane has been damaged, intra-alveolar edema does not develop until capillary pressure is higher than that produced by only decreasing plasma osmotic pressure as shown by the *dashed lines* in Figure 13.20. This ability to withstand increased filtration pressures when the microvascular wall is more permeable to plasma protein occurs because damaged microvessels may release substance(s), such as nitric oxide and prostaglandins, that could increase the effectiveness of the lymphatics to remove interstitial fluid. Although interstitial edema does develop at lower microvascular pressures, intra-alveolar edema does not develop until pressures increase to higher levels, in contrast to that observed by only decreasing plasma protein osmotic pressure. This occurs because lymph flow can remove a larger amount of transvascular filtration when the endothelial barrier is damaged (90). The reason that damaged endothelial barriers increase the effectiveness of the lymphatic system to remove transvascular filtration is not known, but it must be caused by increasing tissue motion, increasing pumping effectiveness of the lymphatic systems, and/or increasing lymphatic filling to promote greater lymph flows.

Lung Microvascular Fluid Exchange

The discussion presented in the previous section relates to generalized fluid balance across the microcirculation and only applies to events measured in the normal animal tissues. Each organ system contains a unique anatomy and distribution of microvascular pressures, interstitial protein concentrations, and lymph flows that are determined by the normal structural–functional properties of a particular organ. Table 13.2 shows the Starling forces change in an absorbing small intestine as compared to a nonabsorbing intestine. Note that because the transported fluid contains no protein, the interstitial protein concentration decreases causing ($\pi_P - \pi_{IF}$) to increase, and the microcirculation actually reverts from a filtering to an absorbing state in order to remove the transported fluid.

The lung's alveolar epithelial membrane can also transport alveolar fluid into the interstitium, which decreases π_{IF}, promoting the reabsorption of transported fluid by microvessels because ($\pi_P - \pi_{IF}$) favors absorption, Also, the lymphatics will remove a portion of the edema fluid from the airways. Obviously, during most forms of exercise, no net fluid is being removed from the alveoli, unless of course intra-alveolar edema has developed.

Obviously, the Starling forces and lymph flow must change to oppose the increased P_{MV} occurring in human lungs, since cardiac output increases three to four times above normal values and left atrial pressure increases during strenuous exercise! It is theoretically possible that alveolar transport could increase to maintain relatively "dry" alveoli during exercise because the ameloride-sensitive sodium channels are activated when intra-alveolar edema occurs with lung injury. Then, greater amounts of alveolar fluid can be pumped back into the lung's interstitium (42) and drained by a more active lymphatic system.

Fluid Drainage Patterns in Lung Tissue

Since the lung tissues are both above and below heart level, the microvascular hydrostatic pressures will be higher at the bottom than at the top of the lung (76, 88). This implies that microvascular filtration is higher at the bottom than at the top of the lung because P_{MV} is higher. However, this need not be the case, since the change that occurs in microvascular pressure (1 cm H_2O change in P_{MV} per centimeter distance above and below the heart level) is apparently opposed by tissue fluid pressures changing by about 0.75 cm H_2O/cm lung height, being more subatmospheric at the top of the lung (53). In addition, the tissue protein osmotic pressure changes by approximately 0.25 cm H_2O/cm change in lung height, being higher at the top of the lung (55). It is possible that an almost identical Starling force balance can exist at both the top and bottom of the lungs resulting in no greater tendency for fluid to filter at the bottom than at the top of the lung.

However, some investigators believe that a greater tendency for edema formation is present in the dependent areas of the lung because of the higher microvessel pressures. If so, the lymphatic transport at the bottom of the lung may also be more efficient in removing microvascular filtration.

To add to the complexity associated with the different transvascular forces at the top and bottom of the lung, one must also realize that hydrostatic pressure decreases between the arterial inflow vessels and the venous outflow portions of the microcirculation throughout the lung. The term "capillary" has often been used to describe filtration occurring across general microvascular beds, but it is well known that small pulmonary blood vessels exchange fluid with the interstitium in the prealveolar vessels (arterioles), alveolar vessels (capillaries), and postalveolar vessels (venules). The partition of filtration in these various microvessels is approximately 25% in both arterial and venous extra-alveolar vessels and 50% in the alveolar vessels (54). This means that fluid exchanges at many sites within the pulmonary circulation and varies not only in a horizontal direction, but in a vertical direction as well. The amount of filtration occurring in each area of the pulmonary microcirculation to form lymph and expand the interstitial spaces depends on the Starling force imbalance present at each tissue site. Yet, we must measure lymph flow or lung weight to estimate transvascular filtration rate, both of which are lumped parameters now used to describe transvascular filtration.

Obviously, this arrangement of microvascular pressure, tissue fluid pressure, protein osmotic pressure, and possibly lymph flows causes a heterogeneous force balance to be present in each horizontal slice of the lung from the top to the bottom. A simple analysis of interstitial and intra-alveolar edema development cannot incorporate all the possible force distributions, since the data are not available for resting animals and certainly not for exercising animals. It should be clear to the reader by now that a simple force balance analysis is an oversimplification of the real fluid exchange system in the lung, but a simple analysis is quite useful in explaining the physiological changes occurring in the microcirculation during different perturbations such as exercise.

When fluid does filter out of the lung's microcirculation, and especially in the alveolar capillaries, it initially fills small lymphatic capillaries that are not in the alveoli per se, but are located in perialveolar interstitial tissue spaces. Lymphatics then carry the fluid into larger interstitial spaces, from which it moves rapidly into the spaces surrounding the larger arterioles, veins, and airways, and forms perivascular and peribronchial fluid cuffs. The potential spaces around vessels and airways serve as important sumps that drain fluid from the alveolar regions and therefore protect gas exchange (77). Only after intra-alveolar edema is present does fluid leak across the visceral pleura and enter the pleural space (1). However, the extensive pleural lymphatic system could remove substantial amounts of the transcapillary filtrate (53). Until the alveoli actually fill with fluid, the lung is able to maintain blood oxygenation remarkably well.

Effects of Intra-alveolar Edema on Gas Exchange

Figure 13.21 shows the effects of intra-alveolar edema on arterial oxygen tension ($Pa_{O}{}^2$) in an animal study. Plasma volume was expanded by saline infusions and $Pa_{O}{}^2$ (left ordinate) and extravascular lung water (right ordinate) were measured. Note that an increase in lung water of 25%–50% (which occurs before the alveoli flood) caused little change in $Pa_{O}{}^2$, probably because the edema was sequestered in perivascular spaces away from gas exchanging

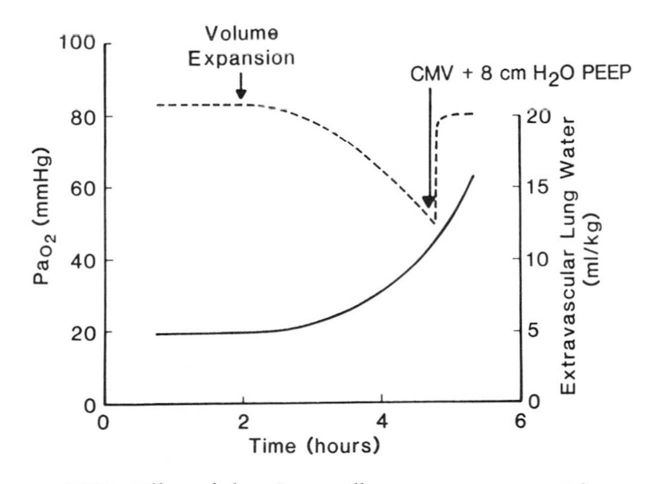

FIG. 13.21. Effect of elevating capillary pressure on arterial oxygen tension (Pa_{O_2} *dashed line*) and extravascular lung water (*solid line*). At the *left arrow*, capillary pressure was increased by volume expansion. Mechanical ventilation (CMV) at 8 cm PEEP was applied at the *right arrow*. Note the dramatic improvement of (Pa_{O_2} when mechanical ventilation (CMV) with PEEP was applied. (Modified from Noble, W. H.: Pulmonary oedema: a review. *Can. Anesth. Soc. J.* 27: 286–302, 1981.)

surfaces. However, after intra-alveolar edema occurred, $Pa_{O}{}^2$ began to decrease. During moderate exercise in humans, P_{PA}, P_{wedge}, and cardiac output do increase, which should increase transvascular fluid filtration. As discussed in the following sections, the extent to which lung water accumulates during exercise depends on the degree of capillary pressure change and the ability of edema-preventing mechanisms to buffer the increased microvascular pressures.

However, we also know that carbon monoxide diffusion capacity may increase in exercise (21; see also Chapter 12), P_{PA} increases, and pulmonary lymph flow and the protein osmotic gradient acting across the microcirculatory barrier increase (10, 11, 40, 56–59, 76). Some of these factors tend to oppose edema formation, while others accelerate the process. In order to develop the status of lung fluid balance during exercise in humans, we will first evaluate data obtained in awake animals to describe their lung fluid exchange status during exercise and extrapolate these findings to explain why intra-alveolar edema does not develop in lungs of exercising humans where more exact measures of Starling forces and transvascular filtration have not been made.

FLUID EXCHANGE IN EXERCISING ANIMAL MODELS

We will consider the data in Table 13.4 obtained by Newman et al. (58) in awake sheep that were exercised at 4 mph on a 10% grade. Rest and exercise measurements included mean pulmonary arterial pressure (P_{PA}), mean left atrial pressure (P_{LA}), cardiac output, and lymph flow. Also, a small arterial catheter was wedged, which we will assume closely approximates microvascular pressure (P_{MV}), since the actual microvessel pressure was not measured. We assume that the pulmonary circulation can be described by a single premicrovascular resistance (r_A) where the pressure gradient (ΔP_{PA}) is from P_{PA} to P_{MV}, and a single postmicrovascular resistance (r_V) where the pressure gradient (ΔP_V) is from P_{MV} to P_{LA}.

Before exercise (Table 13.4, *Control*), P_{PA} was 20 cm H_2O, P_{MV} 8 cm H_2O, and P_{LA} 3 cm H_2O when cardiac output was 4 liters (Table 13.4, *Control*). Precapillary resistance was 12/4 or 3 cm $H_2O \cdot liter^{-1} \cdot min^{-1}$, postcapillary resistance was 5/4, or 1.2 cm $H_2O \cdot liter^{-1} \cdot min^{-1}$, and total pulmonary vascular resistance was 4.2 cm $H_2O \cdot liter^{-1} \cdot min^{-1}$. Note, that when P_{MV} is 8 cm H_2O, $\Delta\pi_P$ is approximately (37–26) = 11 cm H_2O. If P_{IF} is −4, then the imbalance in Starling forces would be [8 − (−4) − 11] = 12 − 11 = only 1 cm H_2O. This calculation

TABLE 13.4. *Microvascular Pressure Changes with Exercise in Sheep**

	cm H_20					cm $H_2O \cdot liter^{-1} \cdot min^{-1}$				
	P_{PA}	ΔP_A	P_{MV}	ΔP_V	P_{LA}	Q, liter/min	r_A	r_V	r_A/r_V	r_T
Control*	20	12	8	(5)	3	4	3.0	1.2	2.5	4.2
Maximum†	37	23	14	(8)	6	11	2.1	0.7	3.0	2.8
New Steady-State‡	30	19	11	(7)	4	12	1.6	0.6	2.7	2.2

P_{PA}, mean pulmonary arterial pressure; ΔP_A, pressure gradient occurring between P_{PA} and the microvascular pressure [(P_{MV}) assumed equal to the small catheter measurement]; ΔP_V, pressure gradient between the P_{MV} and the left atrial pressure (P_{LA}); Q, pulmonary blood flow; r_A, r_u, and r_T refer to precapillary, postcapillary and total pulmonary vascular resistance, respectively. *Measurements in sheep at rest (Control), and after 1 min (Maximum) and 4 min (New Steady State) of treadmill exercise at 4 mph and a 10% grade. From Newman et al. (58).

indicates that the imbalance in transcapillary forces is normally very low in sheep lungs as shown in Table 13.2 (85).

At 1 min of exercise (Table 13.4, *Maximum*), P_{PA} increased to 37 cm H_2O, P_{LA} to 6.2 cm H_2O, and P_{MV} increased from 8 cm H_2O to 14 cm H_2O. The increased flow caused such a small change in P_{MV} because r_V decreased dramatically to 0.7. After 4 min of exercise (Table 13.4, *New steady state*), estimated P_{MV} had decreased from 14 cm H_2O to 11 cm H_2O, which was only 3 cm H_2O above control levels! The low P_{MV} reflected a further reduction in total vascular resistance to 2.3 cm $H_2O \cdot liter^{-1} \cdot min^{-1}$, which in turn was associated with a decrease in P_{PA} to 30 cm H_2O. $\Delta\pi_{MV}$ increased to 37 − 23) = 14 cm H_2O. If P_{IF} did not change, then the imbalance in forces would be $[11 - (-4) - 14] = 1$ cm H_2O, which is not different than the filtration pressure calculated for control conditions.

This small increase in microvascular pressure would not produce much interstitial edema and certainly no intra-alveolar edema (see Fig. 13.20). (The removal of the pericardium in sheep and the relatively low exercise intensity may account for the small increase in left atrial pressure, relative to that measured in man.) The lymph-to-plasma ratios decreased from 0.62 to 0.52, indicating that transvascular fluid filtration increased and lymph flow increased from 0.08 ml/min to 0.26 ml/min. When lymph flow increases, and the lymph-to-plasma protein concentration ratio decreases, then a greater transvascular filtration has occurred. Thus, π_{IF} decreased, while ($\pi_P - \pi_{IF}$) and lymph flow increased.

If tissue pressure increased to higher positive values, then the imbalance in forces would actually be subatmospheric, which is impossible with transmicrovascular filtration occurring to form lymph. Since the microcirculation was filtering, then the interstitial fluid pressure must have become more subatmospheric to provide the necessary force to generate the larger transmicrovascular filtration occurring in exercise.

The protein osmotic safety factor and lymph flow obviously changed to prevent intra-alveolar fluid accumulation during exercise, but the most important factor that changed to accommodate this increased microvascular filtration was an increased lymph flow. But what caused lymph flow to increase to this high level if microvascular pressure only changed by 3 cm H_2O?

A portion of the lymph flow increase may be related to the greater surface area for filtration (recruitment or distensibility) occurring during exercise (see Chapter 12). This was the conclusion reached in a set of studies conducted in sheep exercised at less strenuous levels (10, 11, 59). Johnson et al. have also shown that diffusion capacity increased twofold with moderate exercise (39; see also Chapter 12).

Although we do not know the magnitude of the interstitial pressure changes in exercise, it is well known that interstitial fluid pressure surrounding the perivascular spaces becomes more subatmospheric with higher lung volumes (54). If tissue fluid pressure becomes more subatmospheric during exercise, then the imbalance in forces could easily be $[11 - (-8)] - 14 = 19 - 14 = 5$ cm H_2O or greater, which produces a large increase in transmicrovascular filtration pressure. If this occurs without excessive interstitial edema, then an increased filtration pressure caused by a more subatmospheric tissue fluid pressure would explain the large pulmonary lymph flows seen in exercising sheep.

Obviously, there should be no interstitial fluid volume accumulation in the lungs of moderately exercising animals, since any tendency for excessive filtration to occur is easily accommodated by the increased lymph flow and the changes in Starling forces (P_{IF} and $\pi_{MV} - \pi_{IF}$).

More insight into the mechanisms responsible for the higher lymph flow in exercise can also be obtained from Figure 13.22, which is reproduced from the study of Newman et al. (58). This figure shows lymph flow and prevailing microvascular pressure (P_{MV}) occurring during exercise in the sheep model

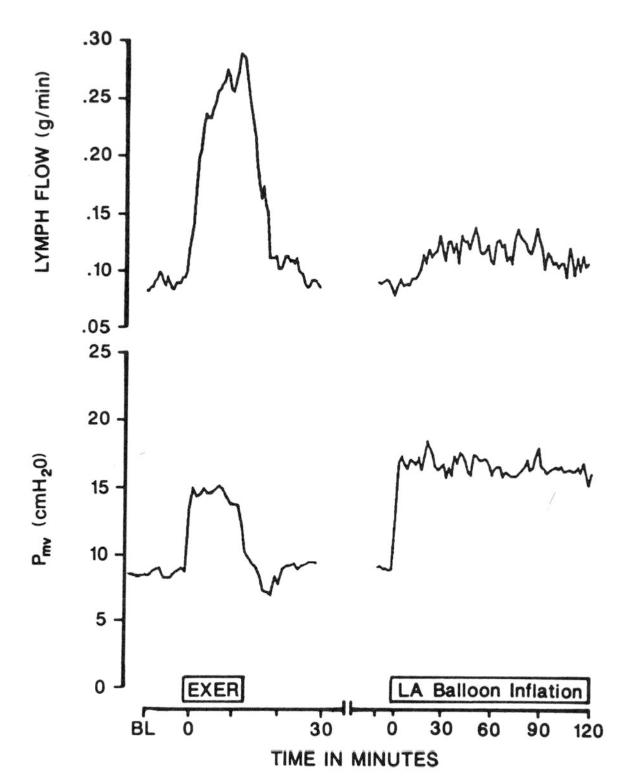

FIG. 13.22. Microvascular pressure and lymph flow as a function of time during either exercise or passive left atrial hypertension from four sheep under conditions shown in Figure 13.22. Estimated microvascular pressure was approximately 15 cm H_2O during exercise and 17 cm H_2O during left atrial hypertension. [Reproduced with permission of A. Holmgren (33).]

(*left*) as compared to only increasing left atrial pressure to a similar microvascular pressure level (*right*). If the increased lymph flow observed in exercise was only a function of an increased P_{MV}, then the lymph flow should have increased to the same extent for both cases; however, the lymph flow increased much more rapidly and to a much higher level with exercise than with comparable increases in left atrial pressure.

Lung motion provides an effective pumping action on the lung's lymphatic system. Since the lung lymphatics have valves, then greater lung interstitial pressure would empty them, and when the lungs recoil during inspiration, the lymphatics would refill. Therefore, the increased lung lymph flow seen in exercising sheep is likely due to effective lymphatic pumping action of increased ventilation. In fact, pumps are used in many animal experimental preparations that increase lymph flow by a massaging action. Koizumi et al. have shown that the effects of hyperpnea and increased microvascular pressures are additive in increasing lymph flow during exercise (43). Also, breathing against a higher outflow resistance or increasing lung volume would also cause P_{IF} to become more subatmospheric (as discussed above) and provide the transvascular force to increase the transmicrovascular filtration (51). In addition, some substance(s) may be released during exercise that would cause the intrinsic pumping ability of the lung's lymphatic system to become more effective, such as seen when microvessels are damaged by different pathological conditions. In fact, the data from exercising sheep studies indicate (41) that NO is released during exercise. This vasodilator has been shown to increase both lymphatic rate and strength of contraction in some lymphatic studies (96).

Unfortunately, the published data do not allow us to define clearly the mechanism(s) responsible for the rapid and large increase in lung lymph flow that occurs during exercise in contrast to the much smaller increase caused by simply increasing microvascular pressure. However, we can approximate the effect of several factors. Increased surface area (see Chapter 12) and lung motion (43) can each double lymph flow, and increased microvascular pressure can add another 50% (58). These changes would only provide a change in lymph flow of 2.5 time normal. Yet in exercise, lymph flow increases rapidly to at least five times control! Therefore, other mechanisms such as decreased P_{IF} and/or an increased effectiveness of the lymphatic "pump" must be responsible for the additional increased lymph flow seen in lungs of exercising sheep; however, the heterogeneity of lung tissue filtration can certainly mask the interpretation of the actual mechanism(s) responsible for producing this remarkable and important increase in lymph flow. Future studies should be done to evaluate this important physiological mechanism that prevents alveolar edema from forming in humans during exercise.

LUNG FLUID EXCHANGE IN EXERCISING HUMANS

Increases in Microvascular Pressures

We have evaluated lymph flow and Starling force changes in the lungs of exercising animals, and the data for exercising humans also indicate that little edema, if any, occurs in the lungs. Thus, mechanisms similar to those of other animals are likely operating to oppose edema formation in exercising humans. At the onset of exercise, P_{LA} increased in humans as cardiac output increases. For example, Figure 13.23*B* shows P_{wedge} for eight exercising humans. At an exercise intensity of only 50 W, P_{wedge} increased from 6 mm Hg to about 14 mm Hg, but vascular resistance (R_T; Fig. 13.23*C*) decreased by almost 50%.

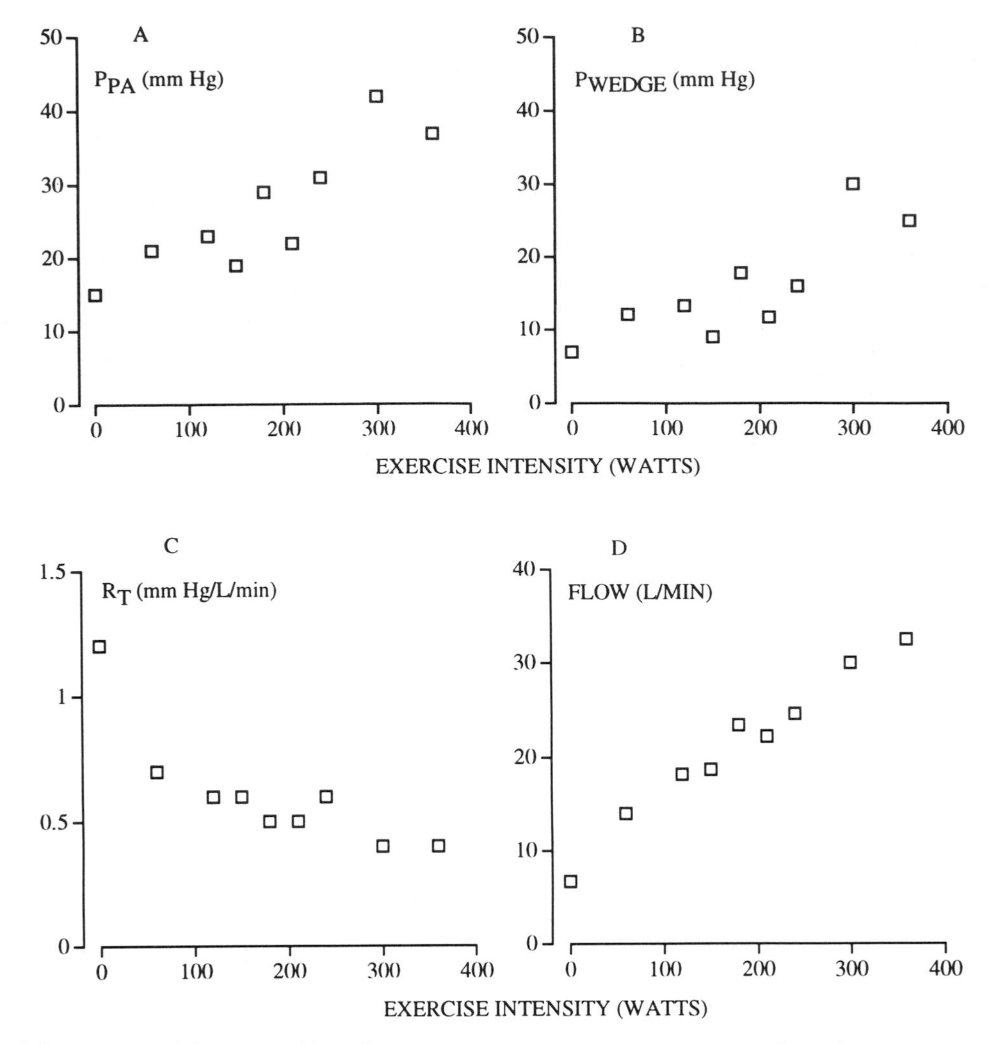

FIG. 13.23. *A*, Pulmonary arterial pressure; *B*, wedge pressure; *C*, vascular resistance; and *D*, cardiac output as a function of exercise intensity in upright cycling men at sea level (24, 69) and from the Operation Everest II data base.

Cardiac output also increased from 6 to 15 liters/min (Fig. 13.23*C*), while P_{PA} increased from 15 to about 20 mm Hg (Fig. 13.23*A*). At the highest workloads, cardiac output was greater than 30 liters/min, P_{wedge} was about 25 mm Hg, and P_{PA} was about 40 mm Hg (67). Barman and Taylor (4) have shown that when P_{LA} was increased to only 15 mm Hg in dogs that their pulmonary microvascular pressure became almost equal to P_{LA}. P_{LA} and P_{MV} were equalized because venous resistance greatly decreased so that the pressure gradient responsible for producing the blood flow remained almost constant and even decreased slightly as P_{LA} increased to higher levels.

The large initial decrease in total pulmonary vascular resistance upon exercise in humans most likely is due to a decreased postmicrovascular resistance that serves as an important edema safety factor, since P_{MV} remains low and not much higher than P_{wedge} (i.e., r_V is almost zero). This low pulmonary venous resistance at the onset of exercise is found in the data from both sheep and humans and justifies to some extent the extrapolation of the animal data to humans.

If we assume that the venous and arterial resistances are similar in exercising humans and sheep (58), then the estimated microvascular pressure in humans during heavy exercise would be:

$$\begin{aligned} P_{MV} &= P_{LA} + [r_V/r_A + r_V]\ (P_{PA} - P_{LA}) \\ &= 25 + r_V/r_A + r_V\ (40 - 25) \\ &= 25 + 0.6/2.2\ (15) \\ &= 25 + 4 = 29 \text{ mm Hg} \end{aligned}$$

Since pulmonary edema does not develop until microvascular pressure exceeds 25–30 mm Hg, then intra-alveolar edema would not likely develop in these exercising subjects, but interstitial edema could be present. Since hyperpnea is also present in exercising humans, the lung motion would increase lymph flow as described for sheep in Newman's study and the lymphatic drainage would become more efficient. Obviously, little or no edema occurred in these exercising individuals. Such data are difficult to obtain from exercising humans, but morphological data from exercising pigs is shown in Figure 13.24. Note only slight perivascular cuffing occurs and intra-alveolar edema was absent. It is hoped that measures of microvascular pressures can be made in exercising humans, but there is little doubt that r_V decreases and lymph flow increases in exercising humans. Exercise results in a more efficient clearance of interstitial fluid, a decreased pulmonary venous resistance that minimizes microvascular pressure, and an increased $\Delta\pi_{MV}$.

Microvascular Stress Failure in Exercise

West has described a condition of "stress failure" involving damage that occurs in lung microvessels (95) when either microvascular pressures are increased to levels above 40–50 mm Hg (72) or when airway distending pressures are increased above 40–45 mm Hg (30, 61). When lungs that have been subjected to high airway pressures are evaluated microscopically, uniform fractures appear in both the endothelial and epithelial barriers (91). Although vascular and alveolar pressure of these magnitudes are not present in exercising humans, it has been thought that high microvessel pressures can be attained in horses during a strenuous race (59). Often, horses during a race produce a bloody, fulminating pulmonary edema, and it is likely that their pulmonary vascular pressures are greatly affected as their back legs move back and forth causing alternating stretch and compression of lung tissue. Shina et al. (personal communication) have recently measured pulmonary capillary pressures in exercising horses by analyzing pulmonary arterial wedge pressure transients. They found that the average pulmonary arterial and wedge pressures increased from 30 mm Hg to 60 mm Hg and 19 mm Hg to 31 mm Hg during exercise in horses, respectively, causing the microvascular pressure to increase to 20–34 mm Hg. Although the pulmonary arterial pressure transients increased from 30 mm Hg in diastole to over 90 mm Hg in systole and the pressure recordings were very noisy, these authors concluded that microvascular pressure increases of this magnitude could produce interstitial edema but were too small to produce "stress failure." However, if the horse suffers

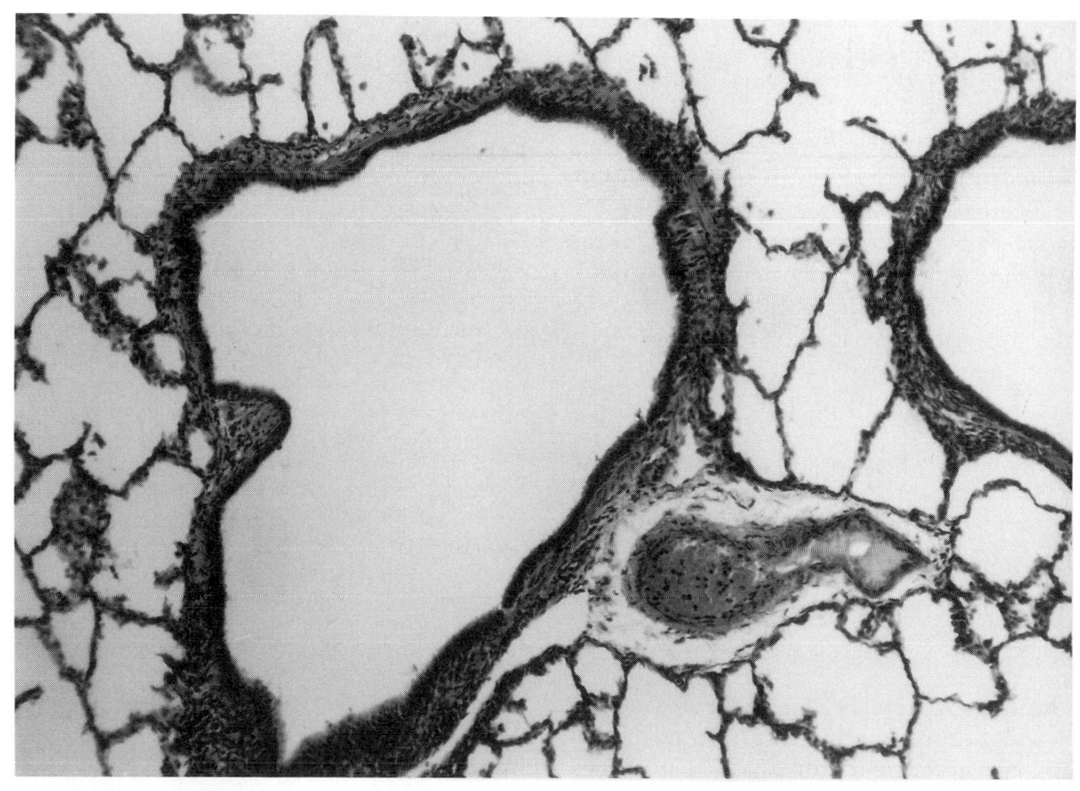

FIG. 13.24. Histological slide provided by P. D. Wagner from pig lungs after exercise (print shows 850 × 600 μm area). Only slight perivascular cuffing was present and no intra-alveolar edema.

some degree of alveolar hypoxia because of edema formation or vascular damage occurring in the arterial segments of the circulation, then pressures upstream from the associated vasoconstriction could produce stress failure and microvascular damage in some lung areas. In fact, this phenomenon has been postulated as an explanation of high-altitude pulmonary edema, since patients with this condition have high protein concentrations in the alveolar fluid, indicating that their microvascular walls have been damaged (36).

CONCLUSIONS

An understanding of the pressure–flow relationships in the human lung circulation during exercise depends upon at least three major concepts.

1. The most significant effect of exercise on the lung circulation is the increase in the wedge (left atrial) pressure, which is progressive with exercise intensity and accounts for ~80% of the increase in pulmonary arterial pressure. This marked effect of downstream pressure on upstream pressure is unique for the lung circulation, as the systemic arterial pressure during exercise is largely independent of right atrial pressure. It is the marked interindividual variation in the wedge pressure with exercise that accounts largely for the variability of pulmonary arterial pressure among individuals.
2. The remaining 20% of the variation in pulmonary arterial pressure with exercise reflects interindividual variability in driving pressures as flows increase. Because of the high total vascular compliance in the normal lung microcirculation, the increased left atrial pressure and that resulting from the increased flow act to distend the small vessels, accounting largely for the dramatic fall in pulmonary vascular resistance during exercise. Microcirculatory recruitment, in this view, is limited primarily to the transition from rest to mild exercise in the upright posture.
3. Microcirculatory distention increases the surface area for diffusion and slows passage of the red cell through the lung, which facilitates O_2 transfer. Possible disadvantages of such dilation are an increased pulsatile flow in the capillaries, and an elevated capillary pressure, which would increase filtration of fluid into the interstitium.

Nevertheless, it is extremely doubtful that exercise at sea level will produce pulmonary edema to any significant extent in normal humans. Edema does not occur because lymph flow and the protein osmotic pressure gradient ($\pi_{MV} - \pi_{IF}$) increase to oppose edema formation. The effects of hyperpnea appear to promote microvascular filtration and to increase lymph flow as well. An increase in P_{LA} in humans causes the postmicrovascular resistance to decrease to low levels, and for upright subjects it causes the vascular resistance to decrease by 50% during even moderate exercise. In addition, the low postmicrovascular resistance minimizes the rise in P_{MV}. The passive distention of pulmonary veins is probably the mechanism for the fall in venous resistance in exercising humans. In the exercising sheep, P_{LA} only moderately increased but resistance fell significantly, the mechanisms for which are not entirely clear. The possibilities that increased flow and vascular distention contribute to vasodilation of exercise still require further research.

It seems to us that these are the main findings that physiologists must use to frame their future work in this area. Clearly, further lung circulation research is needed to confirm or refute the concepts presented in this chapter and to place them in the proper perspective relative to the control of pulmonary vascular resistance and lung microvessel fluid exchange in exercising humans and animals.

The authors wish to thank Chris Dawson, Larry Horwitz, Robert Johnson, John Newman, Sol Permutt, and Wiltz Wagner for their considerable help in the preparation of this manuscript. This work was supported by National Institutes of Health grants HL46481 and HL22549.

REFERENCES

1. Allen, S., J. Gabel, and R. Drake. Left atrial hypertension causes pleural effusion in unanethetized sheep. *Am. J. Physiol.* 257 (*Heart Circ. Physiol.* 26): H690–H692, 1989.
2. Al-Tinawi, A., J. A. Madden, C. A. Dawson, J. H. Linehan, D. H. Harder, and D. A. Rickaby. Distensibility of small arteries in the dog lung. *J. Appl. Physiol.* 71: 1714–1722, 1991.
3. Barcroft, J. *Features in the Architecture of Physiological Function.* London: Cambridge University Press, 1938.
4. Barman, S. A., and A. E. Taylor. Effect of pulmonary venous pressure elevation on vascular resistance and compliance. *Am. J. Physiol.* 258 (*Heart Circ. Physiol.* 27): H1164–H1170, 1990.
5. Barnard, H. L. The functions of the pericardium. *J. Physiol. (Lond.)* 22: 43–48, 1898.
6. Bartle, S. H., H. J. Hermann, J. W. Cavo, R. A. Moore, and J. M. Costenbader. Effect of the pericardium on left ventricular volume and function in acute hypervolemia. *Cardiovasc. Res.* 2: 284–289, 1968.
7. Bevegard, S. The effects of cardioacceleration by methylscopalamine nitrate on the circulation at rest and during exercise in supine position with special reference to stroke volume. *Acta Physiol. Scand.* 57: 61–80, 1963.
8. Brower, R., and S. Permutt. Exercise and the pulmonary circulation in exercise. In: *Lung Biology in Health and Disease,*

edited by B. J. Whipp and K. Wasserman. New York: Marcel Dekker, Inc., 1991, p. 201–221.

9. Chaveau, A., and J. Marey. Détermination graphique des rapports du choc avec les mouvements des oreilles et des ventricles: experience fait à l'aide d'un appareil enregisteur (sphygmographe). *C. R. Acad. Sci.* 111 622, 1861.
10. Coates, G., H. O'Brodovich, and G. Goeree. Hindlimb and lung lymph flows during prolonged exercise. *J. Appl. Physiol.* 75: 633–638, 1993.
11. Coates, G., H. O'Brodovich, A. L. Jefferies, and G. W. Gray. Effects of exercise on lung lymph flow in sheep and goats during normoxia and hypoxia. *J. Clin. Invest.* 74: 133–141, 1984.
12. Cournand, A. Recent observations on the dynamics of the pulmonary circulation. *Bull. N. Y. Acad. Sci.* 23: 27–50, 1947.
13. Dawson, C. A., T. A. Bronikowski, J. H. Linehan, and D. A. Rickaby. Distribution of vascular pressure and resistance in the lung. *J. Appl. Physiol.* 64: 274–284, 1988.
14. Dawson, C. A., D. A. Rickaby, J. H. Linehan, and T. A. Bronikowski. Distributions of vascular volume and compliance in the lung. *J. Appl. Physiol.* 64: 266–273, 1988.
15. Dexter, L., J. L. Whittenberger, F. W. Haynes, W. T. Goodale, R. Gorlin, and C. G. Sawyer. Effect of exercise on circulatory dynamics of normal individuals. *J. Appl. Physiol.* 3: 439–453, 1951.
16. Erickson, B. K., H. H. Erickson, and J. R. Coffman. Pulmonary, aortic and oesophageal pressure changes during high intensity treadmill exercise in the horse: a possible relation to exercise-induced hemorrhage. *Equine Vet. J.* 9: 47–52, 1990.
17. Euler, U. S. von, and G. Liljestrand. Observations on the pulmonary arterial blood pressure in the cat. *Acta Physiol. Scand.* 12: 301–320, 1947.
18. Fishman, A. P., H. W. Fritts, Jr., and A. Cournand. Effects of acute hypoxia and exercise on the pulmonary circulation. *Circulation* 22: 204–215, 1960.
19. Glantz, S. A., G. A. Misbach, W. Y. Moores, D. G. Mathey, J. Levken, D. F. Stowe, W. W. Parmley, and J. V. Tyberg. The pericardium substantially affects the left ventricular diastolic pressure-volume relationship in the dog. *Circ. Res.* 42: 433–441, 1978.
20. Glazier, J. B., J. M. B. Hughes, J. E. Maloney, and J. B. West. Measurements of capillary dimensions and blood volume in rapidly frozen capillaries. *J. Appl. Physiol.* 26: 65–76, 1969.
21. Goresky, C. A., J. W. Warnica, J. H. Burgess, and B. E. Nadeau. Effect of exercise on dilution estimates of extravascular lung water and on carbon monoxide diffusing capacity in normal lung. *Circ. Res.* 37: 379–389, 1975.
22. Granath, A., and T. Strandell. Relationships between cardiac output, stroke volume and intracardiac pressures at rest and during exercise in supine position and some anthropomorphic data in healthy old men. *Acta Med. Scand.* 176: 447–466, 1964.
23. Granger, D. N., and A. E. Taylor. Permeability of intestinal capillaries to endogenous macromolecules. *Am. J. Physiol.* 238 (*Heart Circ. Physiol.* 7): H455–H464, 1980.
24. Groves, B. M., J. T. Reeves, J. R. Sutton, P. D. Wagner, A. Cymerman, M. K. Malconian, P. B. Rock, P. M. Young, and C. S. Houston. Operation Everest II: elevated high altitude pulmonary resistance unresponsive to oxygen. *J. Appl. Physiol.* 63: 521–530, 1987.
25. Guyton, A. C., and A. E. Lindsey. Effects of elevated left atrial pressures and decreased plasma protein in the development of pulmonary edema. *Circ. Res.* 7: 649–655, 1959.
26. Hammond, H. K., F. C. White, V. Bhargava, and R. Shabetai. Heart size and maximal cardiac output are limited by the pericardium. *Am. J. Physiol.* 263 (*Heart Circ. Physiol.* 32): H1675–H1681, 1992.
27. Harvey, W. On the motion of the heart and blood in animals. In: *Harvey and the Circulation of the Blood*, edited by A. Bowie. London: George Bell & Sons, 1889.
28. Hebb, C. Motor innervation of the pulmonary blood vessels of mammals. In: *Pulmonary Circulation and Interstitial Space*, edited by A. P. Fishman and H. H. Hecht. Chicago: University of Chicago Press, 1969.
29. Henderson, Y., and A. L. Prince. The relative systolic discharges of the right and left ventricles and their bearing on pulmonary congestion and depletion. *Heart* 5: 217–226, 1913–1914.
30. Hernandez, L. A., K. J. Peevy, A. A. Moise, and J. C. Parker. Chest wall restriction limits high airway pressure-induced lung injury in young rabbits. *J. Appl. Physiol.* 66: 2364–2368, 1989.
31. Hickam, J. B., and W. H. Cargill. Effect of exercise on cardiac output and pulmonary arterial pressure in normal persons and in patients with cardiovascular disease and pulmonary emphysema. *J. Clin. Invest.* 27: 10–23, 1948.
32. Hillier, S. C., P. S. Godbey, C. C. Hanger, J. A. Graham, R. G. Presson, O. Okada, J. H. Linehan, C. A. Dawson, and W. W. Wagner. Direct measurement of pulmonary microvascular distensibility. *J. Appl. Physiol.* 75: 2106–2111, 1993.
33. Holmgren, A. Circulatory changes during muscular work in man. *Scand. J. Clin. Lab. Invest.* 8(Suppl. 24): 1–97, 1956.
34. Holmgren, A., B. Jonsson, and T. Sjostrand. Circulatory data in normal subjects at rest and during exercise in recumbent position, with special reference to the stroke volume at different working intensities. *Acta Physiol. Scand.* 49: 343–363, 1960.
35. Horwitz, L. D., J. M. Atkins, and S. L. Leshin. Role of the Frank-Starling mechanism in exercise. *Circ. Res.* 31: 868–875, 1972.
36. Hultgren, H. N. High altitude pulmonary edema. In: *Biomedicine Problems of High Terrestrial Altitude*, edited by A. H. Hegnauer. New York: Springer-Verlag, 1969, p. 131–141.
37. Hyman, A. L., H. L. Lippton, C. W. Dempsey, C. J. Fontana, D. E. Richardson, R. W. Rieck, and P. J. Kadowitz. Autonomic control of the pulmonary circulation. In: *Pulmonary Vascular Physiology and Pathophysiology*, edited by E. K. Weir and J. T. Reeves, 38: 291–324, vol. 38 *Lung Biology in Health and Disease*, exec. ed. C Lenfant, New York: Marcel Dekker, Inc., 1989.
38. Ingram, R. H., J. P. Szidon, R. Skalak, and A. P. Fishman. Effects of sympathetic nerve stimulation on the pulmonary arterial tree of the isolated lobe perfused in situ. *Circ. Res.* 22: 801, 1968.
39. Johnson, R. L., W. S. Spicer, J. M. Bishop, and R. E. Forster. Pulmonary capillary blood volume, flow, and diffusing capacity during exercise. *J. Appl. Physiol.* 15: 893–902, 1960.
40. Kane, D. W., T. Tesauro, T. Koizumi, R. Gupta, and J. H. Newman. Exercise induced vasoconstriction during combined blockade of nitric oxide (NO) synthase and beta adrenergic receptors. *J. Clin. Invest.* 93: 677–683, 1994.
41. Kane, D. W., T. Tesauro, and J. H. Newman. Adrenergic modulation of the pulmonary circulation during strenuous exercise in the sheep. *Am. Rev. Respir. Dis.* 147: 1233–1238, 1993.
42. Khimenko, P. L., J. W. Barnard, T. M. Moore, P. S. Wilson, S. T. Ballard, and A. E. Taylor. Vascular permeability and epithelial transport effects on lungs edema formation in is-

chemia and reperfusion. *J. Appl. Physiol.* 77: 1116–1121, 1994.
43. Koizumi, T., D. Johnston, L. Bjertnaes, M. Banerjee, and J. H. Newman. Clearance of filtrate during passive pulmonary capillary hypertension versus exercise: role of hyperpnea *Am. J. Resp. Crit. Care Med.* 149: A820, 1994.
44. Krogh, M. The diffusion of gases through the lungs of man. *J. Physiol. (Lond.)* 49: 271–300, 1914–1915.
45. Kuno, Y. The significance of the pericardium. *J. Physiol. (Lond.)* 50: 1–36, 1915–1916.
46. Landgren, G. L. Ventilation, gas transport, and responses to CO2 breathing in horses at rest and during heavy exercise. Ph.D. Thesis, Manhattan, KS: Kansas State University, 1989.
47. Lekeux, P., and T. Art. The respiratory system: anatomy, physiology, and adaptations to exercise and training. In: *The Athletic Horse*, edited by D. R. Hodgson and R. J. Rose. Philadelphia, W. B. Saunders Company, 1994, p. 79–127.
48. Lillienthal, J. L., R. L. Riley, D. D. Proemel, and R. E. Franke. An experimental analysis in man of the oxygen pressure gradient from the alveolar air to arterial blood during rest and exercise at sea level and at altitude. *Am. J. Physiol.* 147: 199–216, 1946.
49. Lindenfeld, J., J. T. Reeves, and L. D. Horwitz. Low exercise pulmonary resistance is not dependent on vasodilator prostaglandins. *J. Appl. Physiol.* 55: 558–561, 1983.
50. Linehan, J. H., S. T. Haworth, L. D. Nelin, G. S. Krenz, and C. A. Dawson. A simple distensible model for interpreting pulmonary vascular pressure-flow curves. *J. Appl. Physiol.* 73: 987–994, 1992.
51. Loyd, J. E., K. B. Nolop, R. E. Parker, R. J. Roselli, and K. L. Brigham. Effects of increased respiratory resistance loading on lung fluid balance in awake sheep. *J. Appl. Physiol.* 60: 198–203, 1986.
52. Manohar, M., E. Hutchens, and E. Coney. Frusemide attenuates the exercise-induced rise in pulmonary capillary blood pressure in horses. *Equine Vet. J.* 26: 51–54, 1994.
53. Miserocchi, A., and D. Negrini. Pleural dynamics as regulators of pleural fluid dynamics. *News Physiol. Sci.* 6: 153–158, 1991.
54. Mitzner, W., and J. C. Rubotham. Distribution of interstitial compliance and filtration coefficients in canine lung. *Lymphology* 12: 140–148, 1979.
55. Molstad, L. S., and A. E. Taylor. Effects of hydrostatic height on pulmonary lymph protein circulation. *Microvasc. Res.* 11: 124, 1976.
56. Newman, J. H., B. J. Butka, R. E. Parker, and R. J. Roselli. Effect of progressive exercise on lung fluid balance in sheep. *J. Appl. Physiol.* 64: 2125–2131, 1988.
57. Newman, J. H., B. J. Butka, and K. L. Brigham. Thromboxane A_2 and prostacyclin do not modulate pulmonary hemodynamics during exercise in sheep. *J. Appl. Physiol.* 61: 1706–1711, 1986.
58. Newman, J. H., C. P. Cochran, R. J. Roselli, R. E. Parker, and L. S. King. Pressure and flow changes in the pulmonary circulation in exercising sheep: evidence for elevated microvascular pressure. *Am. Rev. Respir. Dis.* 147: 921–926, 1993.
59. O'Brodovich, H. M., and G. Coates. Effect of isoproterenol or exercise on pulmonary lymph flow and hemodynamics. *J. Appl. Physiol.* 60: 38–44, 1986.
60. Parker, J. O., S. Digiorgi, and R. O. West. A hemodynamic study of acute coronary insufficiency precipitated by exercise. *Am. J. Cardiol.* 17: 470–483, 1966.
61. Parker, J. C., M. I. Townsley, B. Rippe, A. E. Taylor, and J. Thigpen. Increased microvascular permeability in dog lungs due to high peak airway pressures. *J. Appl. Physiol.* 57: 1809–1816, 1984.
62. Pelletier, N., and D. E. Leith. Cardiac output but not high pulmonary artery pressure varies with FIO_2 in exercising horses. *Respir. Physiol.* 91: 83–97, 1993.
63. Permutt, S., R. A. Wise, and J. T. Sylvester. Interaction between the circulatory and ventilatory pumps. In: *The Thorax, Part B*, Vol. 29, edited by C. Roussos and P. T. Macklem. *Lung Biology in Health and Disease*, exec. ed. C. Lenfant. New York: Marcel Dekker, Inc., 1985.
64. Presson, R. G., C. C. Hanger, P. S. Godbey, J. A. Graham, T. C. Lloyd, and W. W. Wagner. The effect of increasing flow on the distribution of pulmonary capillary transit times. *J. Appl. Physiol.* 76: 1701–1711, 1994.
65. Rahn, H., P. Sadoul, L. E. Fahri, and J. Shapiro. Distribution of ventilation and perfusion in the lobes of the dog's lung in the supine and erect position. *J. Appl. Physiol.* 8: 417–426, 1956.
66. Reed, R. K., M. I. Townsley, R. J. Korthuis, and A. E. Taylor. Analysis of lymphatic protein flux data vs unique PS products and s_{AS} at low lymph flux. *Am. J. Physiol.* 261 (*Heart Circ. Physiol.* 30): H728–H740, 1991.
67. Reeves, J. T., J. A. Dempsey, and R. F. Grover. Pulmonary circulation during exercise. In: *Pulmonary Vascular Physiology and Pathophysiology*, edited by E. K. Weir and J. T. Reeves, Vol. 38 of *Lung Biology in Health and Disease*, C. Lenfant, exec. ed. New York: Marcel Dekker, Inc., 1988, p. 107–133.
68. Reeves, J. T., B. M. Groves, A. Cymerman, J. R. Sutton, P. D. Wagner, D. Turkevich, and C. S. Houston. Operation Everest II: cardiac filling pressures during cycle exercise at sea level. *Respir. Physiol.* 80: 147–154, 1990.
69. Reeves, J. T., B. M. Groves, J. R. Sutton, P. D. Wagner, A. Cymerman, M. K. Malconian, P. B. Rock, P. M. Young, and C. S. Houston. Operation Everest II: preservation of cardiac function at extreme altitude. *J. Appl. Physiol.* 63: 531–539, 1987.
70. Riley, R. L., A. Himmelstein, H. L. Motley, H. M. Weiner, and A. Cournand. Studies of the pulmonary circulation at rest and during exercise in normal individuals and in patients with chronic pulmonary disease. *Am. J. Physiol.* 152: 372–380, 1948.
71. Riley, R. L., R. H. Shepard, J. E. Cohn, D. G. Carroll, and B. W. Armstrong. Maximal diffusion capacity of the lungs. *J. Appl. Physiol.* 6: 573–587, 1954.
72. Rippe, B., M. Townsley, J. Thigpen, J. Parker, et al. Effects of vascular pressure on the pulmonary microvasculature in isolated dog lungs. *J. Appl. Physiol.* 57: 233–239, 1984.
73. Rushmer, R. F. Constancy of the stroke volume in ventricular responses to exertion. *Am. J. Physiol.* 196: 745–750, 1959.
74. Rushmer, R. F., Q. A. Smith, and E. P. Lasher. Neural mechanisms of cardiac control during exertion. *Physiol. Rev.* 40: 27–34, 1960.
75. Slonim, N. B., A. Ravin, O. J. Balchum, and S. H. Dressler. The effect of mild exercise in the supine position on the pulmonary arterial pressure of five normal human subjects. *J. Clin. Invest.* 33: 1022–1030, 1954.
76. Staub, N. C. Pulmonary edema. *Physiol. Rev.* 54: 687–811, 1974.
77. Staub, N. C., H. Nagam, and M. C. Pearce. Pulmonary edema in dogs, especially the sequence of fluid accumulation in lung. *J. Appl. Physiol.* 22: 227–240, 1967.
78. Starling, E. H. On the absorption of fluid from the convective tissue spaces. *J. Physiol. (Lond.)* 19: 312–326, 1898.
79. Starling, E. H. *The Linacre Lecture on the Law of the Heart given at Cambridge, 1915*. London: Longmans, 1918.

80. Stokes, D. L., N. R. MacIntyre, and J. A. Nadel. Nonlinear increase in diffusing capacity during exercise by seated and supine subjects. *J. Appl. Physiol.* 51: 858–863, 1981.
81. Sullivan, M. J., F. R. Cobb, and M. B. Higgenbotham. Stroke volume increases by similar mechanisms during upright exercise in normal men and women. *Am. J. Cardiol.* 67: 1405–1412, 1991.
82. Szidon, J. P., and J. F. Flint. Significance of sympathetic innervation of pulmonary vessels in response to acute hypoxia. *J. Appl. Physiol.* 43: 65–71, 1977.
83. Taylor, A. E. Capillary fluid filtration Starling forces and lymph flow. *Circ. Res.* 49: 557–575, 1981.
84. Taylor, A. E. The lymphatic edema safety factors: the role of edema dependent lymphatic factors (EDLF). *Lymphatic* 23: 111–123, 1990.
85. Taylor, A. E. Molecular fluid and solute exchange. In: *Encyclopedia of Human Biology*. New York: Academic Press, 1991, p. 35.
86. Taylor, A. E., J. W. Barnard, S. A. Barman, and W. K. Adkins. *Fluid Balance in the Lung*, edited by R. G. Crystal, J. B. West, et al. New York: Raven Press, 1991, p. 1142–1167.
87. Taylor, A. E., and D. N. Granger. Exchange of micromolecules across the microcirculation. In: *Handbook of Physiology, The Cardiovascular System, Microcirculation*, edited by E. M. Renkin, and C. C. Michael. Bethesda, MD: Am. Physiol. Soc., 1984, p. 467–520.
88. Taylor, A. E., and J. C. Parker. Pulmonary interstitial spaces and lymphatics. In: *Handbook of Physiology. The Respiratory System, Circulation and Nonrespiratory Functions*, edited by A. P. Fishman and A. B. Fisher. Bethesda, MD: Am. Physiol. Soc., 1985, p. 167–230.
89. Thadani, U., and J. O. Parker. Hemodynamics at rest and during supine and sitting bicycle exercise in normal subjects. *Am. J. Cardiol.* 41: 52–59, 1978.
90. Thomas, D. P., G. F. Fregin, N. H. Gerber, and N. B. Ailes. Effects of training on cardiorespiratory function in the horse. *Am. J. Physiol.* 245 (*Regulatory Integrative Comp. Physiol.* 14): R160–R165, 1983.
91. Tsukimoto, K., O. Mathieu-Costello, R. Prediletto, A. R. Elliot, and J. B. West. Ultrastructural appearances of pulmonary capillaries at high transmural pressures. *J. Appl. Physiol.* 71: 573–582, 1991.
92. Turkevich, D., A. Micco, and J. T. Reeves. Noninvasive measurement of the decrease in left ventricular filling time during maximal exercise in normal subjects. *Am. J. Cardiol.* 62: 650–652, 1988.
93. Wagner, P. D., J. R. Gillespie, G. L. Landgren, M. R. Fedde, B. W. Jones, R. M. DeBowes, R. L. Pieschl, and H. H. Erickson. Measurement of exercise-induced hypoxemia in horses. *J. Appl. Physiol.* 66: 1227–1233, 1989.
94. Wagner, W. W., and L. P. Latham. Pulmonary capillary recruitment during airway hypoxia in the dog. *J. Appl. Physiol.* 39: 900–905, 1975.
95. West, J. B., O. Mathieu-Costello, J. H. Jones, E. K. Birks, R. B. Logemann, J. R. Pascoe, and W. S. Tyler. Stress failure of pulmonary capillaries in racehorses with exercise-induced pulmonary hemorrhage. *J. Appl. Physiol.* 75: 1097–1109, 1993.
96. Yokoyama, S., and T. Ohhashi. Effects of acetylcholine on spontaneous contractions in isolated bovine mesenteric lymphatics. *Am. J. Physiol.* 264 (*Heart Circ. Physiol.* 33): H1460–H1464, 1993.

14. Lactate transport and exchange during exercise

L. BRUCE GLADDEN | *Department of Health & Human Performance, Auburn University, Auburn, Alabama*

CHAPTER CONTENTS

LACTIC ACID HAS A dissociation constant, pK, of ~3.7 (73). Therefore, at normal muscle and blood pH values ranging from 6.4–7.4 or greater, more than 99% of the lactic acid that is present in body fluids is dissociated into the lactate anion and a hydrogen ion. Accordingly, lactic acid is commonly referred to simply as "lactate." Lactate is perhaps the most thoroughly studied exercise metabolite, and numerous roles have been assigned to it, many incorrectly. At one time or another, lactate has been considered the immediate energy donor for muscle contraction (88), a primary factor in muscle soreness (8), the central cause of oxygen (O_2) debt (64), and a causative agent in muscle fatigue (59). These views have changed dramatically.

Perhaps most often studied is the response to progressive, incremental exercise. In this case, blood lactate concentration ([La]) rises gradually at first and then more rapidly as the exercise becomes more intense. Primary issues in the study of data of this type have been identification and interpretation of the lactate threshold, frequently known as the anaerobic threshold (200).

WHY DOES [La] INCREASE DURING EXERCISE?

Muscle Hypoxia: The Traditional Hypothesis

Why do muscle and blood lactate concentrations increase with increasing exercise intensity? This question has received greatest attention in the context of the lactate threshold (LT) during progressive incremental exercise. Operationally, the LT has been defined as the exercise intensity at which blood [La] begins to increase abruptly and progressively (43, 74), or as the exercise intensity at which some fixed blood lactate concentration such as 2 mM (43) or 2.5 mM (4) is achieved. Wasserman and colleagues

(198–200) have argued that this threshold is caused by an imbalance between O_2 supply and O_2 requirement in the exercising muscles; that is, by muscle hypoxia. This explanation emphasizes an increased rate of lactate production by exercising muscles and places minimal emphasis on the role of lactate removal mechanisms. In the terminology recommended by Connett et al. (40), the Wasserman hypothesis (198–200) suggests dysoxia, O_2-limited cytochrome turnover, and therefore O_2-limited oxidative phosphorylation.

Wasserman's anaerobic threshold hypothesis is straightforward. As exercise intensity increases and more motor units are recruited, the O_2 requirement of the contracting muscles increases. At some submaximal exercise intensity that varies among subjects, the O_2 requirement exceeds the O_2 supply to the exercising muscles at the cellular level. As a result, the rate of adenosine triphosphate (ATP) generation from oxidative mechanisms becomes insufficient, and anaerobic glycolysis is increased to supply ATP at the required rate (66, 198–200). Table 14.1 summarizes the anaerobic threshold explanation for the increasing muscle and blood lactate concentrations during exercise. For simplicity, this scheme is referred to as the "traditional" hypothesis.

Evidence Against Muscle Hypoxia

Are there sites of inadequate O_2 supply within submaximally exercising muscle? This is the central question in the debate over the validity of the traditional hypothesis. A great deal of circumstantial evidence supports the notion that lactate production during exercise is the result of O_2-limitation. Wasserman (198) and Katz and Sahlin (120) have summarized numerous studies showing that perturbations that decrease O_2 delivery to muscle (such as decreasing $P_{I_{O_2}}$, isovolemic anemia, and breathing carbon monoxide) also elevate muscle and blood [La] (e.g., 119, 130, 171, 195, 214). Conversely, under conditions of increased O_2 delivery to muscle (such as increased $P_{I_{O_2}}$), [La] in muscle and blood is decreased (e.g., 95, 130, 204).

TABLE 14.1. *"Traditional" Hypothesis for the Lactate (Anaerobic) Threshold*

1. Muscle hypoxia occurs at ~50%–70% of $\dot{V}O_{2max}$
2. Insufficient O_2 ⇒ Inhibition of the electron transport chain ⇒ inadequate aerobic ATP generation and ↑ mitochondrial [NADH]
3. Mitochondrial NADH build-up inhibits NADH shuttles ⇒ ↑ cytosolic [NADH] and ↓ cytosolic [NAD]
4. ↑ Mitochondrial [NADH]/[NAD] inhibits TCA cycle ⇒ ↓ pyruvate use ⇒ ↑ mitochondrial [pyruvate] ⇒ ↑ cytosolic [pyruvate]
5. Pyruvate becomes H^+ acceptor in cytosol ⇒ ↑ lactic acid production
6. Inadequate aerobic ATP generation ⇒ ↓ [ATP], ↓ [PC] and ↑ [ADP], ↑ [Pi], ↑ [AMP] → increased glycolytic rate and more lactic acid production
7. ↑ Lactic acid production ⇒ ↑ muscle and blood [La]

Two main pieces of evidence appear to refute the idea that muscle and blood lactate concentrations increase during submaximal exercise because of muscle dysoxia (120, 184). Jöbsis and Stainsby (106) first argued against the idea in 1968. Stainsby and Welch (186) had earlier observed that lactate output from stimulated dog gastrocnemius muscle in situ was transient, beginning at the onset of contractions and reaching a peak in 5–20 min. Jöbsis and Stainsby (106) reasoned that if the lactate output was caused by O_2-limited oxidative phosphorylation, then there should be an accompanying reduction of members of the respiratory chain, including the NADH/NAD$^+$ pair. Upon stimulation of the gastrocnemius at rates previously shown to elicit peak twitch $\dot{V}O_2$ and high rates of net lactate output, the signal from their surface fluorometric technique indicated oxidation of NADH/NAD$^+$ in comparison to the resting condition (140). Based on these results, Jöbsis and Stainsby (106) concluded that muscle lactate production and output were not caused by O_2-limitation at the level of the respiratory chain.

Connett and colleagues (36–38) took an even more direct approach to question the role of O_2-limitation in muscle lactate production. They (36–38) used myoglobin cryomicrospectroscopy to obtain the distribution of PO_2 in subcellular volumes of dog gracilis muscles that were frozen at rest and during twitch contractions. Lactate concentration was also measured in the population of cells used for spectroscopy. In order to interpret the observed distribution of PO_2 values at the mitochondrial level, one must know the critical PO_2 (PO_{2crit}) for $\dot{V}O_2$ and oxidative ATP synthesis. PO_{2crit} is the partial pressure of O_2, below which maximal cytochrome aa_3 turnover (maximal mitochondrial respiratory rate) is reduced. In isolated mitochondria, PO_{2crit} has been estimated to be between 0.1 and 0.5 mm Hg (32). The relationship between respiratory rate and PO_2 in isolated mitochondria is illustrated in Figure 14.1. Connett and co-workers (37) have argued that PO_{2crit} is also about 0.5 mm Hg in vivo. At stimulation frequencies of 1/s and 4/s, Connett et al. (37) found no loci with PO_2 less than 2 mm Hg in dog gracilis muscles either at steady state or during the transition from rest to contractions. These contraction rates elicited 10% and 70% of peak twitch $\dot{V}O_2$ for these muscles. Muscle [La] rose from 1 mmol/kg wet muscle to ~2 mmol/kg at 1/s and to 6 mmol/kg at 4/s. From these data, they (37) concluded that [La] in-

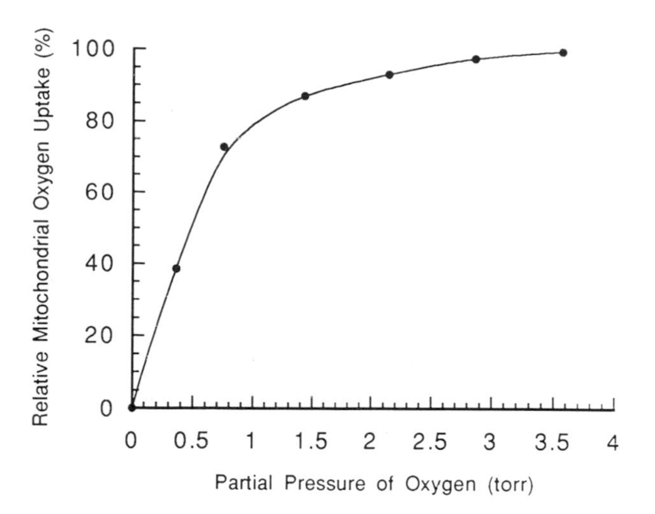

FIG. 14.1. Relationship between oxygen consumption and partial pressure of oxygen in mitochondria isolated from rat heart. Note that oxygen consumption is maximal down to very low partial pressures. Other techniques have shown that mitochondrial oxygen consumption is independent of oxygen partial pressure down to ~0.5 mm Hg. See text for details. [Redrawn with permission from Rumsey, W. L., C. Schlosser, E. M. Nuutinen, M. Robiolio, and D. F. Wilson. Cellular energetics and the oxygen dependence of respiration in cardiac myocytes isolated from adult rat. *J. Biol. Chem.* 265: 15392–15399, 1990 (172).]

creases in fully aerobic, exercising muscle; therefore, the lactate accumulation must be caused by factors other than a simple O_2-limited mitochondrial ATP synthesis rate.

Multiple Factors

Biochemical Regulation. Investigators who accept the arguments against O_2-limited lactate production have generally relied on a multifactorial explanation instead. First, from the perspective of biochemical regulation, cellular lactic acid production depends on the balance of competition for pyruvate and NADH between lactate dehydrogenase (LDH) on the one hand, and alanine transaminase, the NADH shuttles, and the mitochondrial pyruvate transporter (86) on the other hand (66). LDH is well suited to compete favorably for pyruvate and NADH because it catalyzes a near-equilibrium reaction (151) and is located in the cytosol, where it should have easy access to its substrates. As work rate increases, the glycolytic rate is increased due to activation of key regulatory enzymes in the pathway, primarily the nonequilibrium enzymes phosphorylase and phosphofructokinase (PFK). A complete presentation of the controlling factors of glycolytic rate is provided by Connett and Sahlin (see Chapter 19).

Sympathoadrenal Activity. Another key component of the multifactorial explanation is the progressive elevation of sympathoadrenal activity that occurs with increasing exercise intensity. The resulting increase in circulating epinephrine concentration may stimulate glycolysis via phosphorylase activation (15, 24, 54, 87, 151), and conceivably by way of PFK activation as well (121). Some investigators find a correlation between blood [La] and plasma epinephrine concentration during progressive incremental exercise (137, 158), even to the extent of a catecholamine threshold that is coincident with the LT (137). Furthermore, the sympathetic nervous system plays a major role in redistributing blood flow from inactive tissues to active skeletal muscle (24, 107). As a result, blood flow to potential lactate removal sites such as the liver, kidney, and inactive muscle may be reduced as exercise intensity increases (24, 34, 170, 189). This can cause less gluconeogenesis from lactate, less lactate oxidation, and less total lactate removal, leading in turn to an increase in blood [La].

Motor Unit Recruitment. Type S motor units are recruited at low exercise intensities; then, as exercise intensity increases, there is a progressive recruitment of type FR motor units and finally type FF units (6, 24, 27). The tendency for lactate production by muscle fibers increases in the same order as the recruitment pattern (i.e., S < FR < FF). This trend has been correlated with the relative proportion of muscle (M) -type LDH as compared to the heart (H) -type LDH in the different muscle fiber types (24, 118, 151). It has been suggested that a preponderance of the M-type LDH predisposes muscle fibers to lactate production (118). However, a cause-and-effect relationship is difficult to justify, since LDH catalyzes a near-equilibrium reaction (151). In any event, muscle fibers of type FR and FF motor units are recruited to a greater extent as exercise intensity increases, and these same fibers are more likely to produce lactate. Therefore, another possible cause of increased muscle and blood lactate concentrations during progressive exercise is the added recruitment of type FR and FF motor units. Moritani et al. (145) have recently identified a threshold for neuromuscular fatigue during progressive cycling exercise. This threshold is based on rising electromyographic (EMG) activity originating from progressive recruitment of additional motor units and/or increased firing frequency of already recruited motor units. The threshold for neuromuscular fatigue is consistent with a role for motor unit recruitment in the LT.

Lactate Appearance vs. Disappearance. The multifactorial explanation for increased [La] during exercise proposes that several processes act in combination to stimulate lactate production and to inhibit lactate removal. As exercise intensity increases, both lactate appearance and disappearance increase. At low exercise intensities, the rate of lactate appearance only slightly exceeds the rate of disappearance. However, as the work rate becomes more intense, the rate of lactate appearance outstrips the rate of disappearance, leading to elevations of [La] in active muscles and blood at first, and later on in inactive muscles and other tissues as well. Radioactive tracer studies provide the foundational data for this scheme (19, 20, 22, 24, 184). Figure 14.2 illustrates the relationship between lactate appearance and disappearance with increasing work rate, and also shows the resultant response of blood [La]. Table 14.2 summarizes the multifactorial explanation for elevations in muscle and blood lactate concentrations during progressive exercise.

TABLE 14.2. *Multifactorial Explanation for the Lactate (Anaerobic) Threshold*

1. Lactic acid production depends on a competition for pyruvate and NADH between LDH vs. the NADH shuttles and the mitochondrial pyruvate transporter
2. Phosphorylase is activated by increased work rate probably due to calcium; this increases the glycolytic rate
3. With increased exercise intensity; [ATP] ↓, [ADP] ↑, [AMP] ↑, [Pi] ↑, and [ammonia] ↑ ⇒ PFK activation and increases lactic acid production
4. Sympathoadrenal activity increases with work rate—epinephrine activates phosphorylase and thereby stimulates glycolysis
5. Sympathoadrenal activity also causes vasoconstriction and decreased blood flow to liver, kidney, and inactive muscle ⇒ less lactate oxidation and removal
6. Fast-twitch fiber recruitment increases lactic acid production
7. Lactic acid production exceeds removal ⇒ ↑ muscle and blood [La]

Criticism of Evidence Against O_2-limitation

Important criticisms have been directed against the two major pieces of evidence against O_2-limitation: surface NADH/NAD^+ fluorometry (106) and myoglobin cryomicrospectroscopy (36–38). First, those who use laser fluorometry have reported NADH/NAD^+ reduction rather than oxidation during tetanic contractions of isolated rat slow-twitch and fast-twitch muscles (55) and during static contractions at 50% and 100% of maximal voluntary knee extension force in humans (84). Also, the surface fluorometry technique is unable to distinguish between NADH and NADPH (2, 120, 194), or to distinguish between oxidation/reduction changes within the mitochondria vs. the cytosol (120, 129, 152). Movement artifacts were possible during the contractions (56, 120, 205) as was damage to the microcirculation of the muscle during surgery and exposure to the fluorometer (56, 120). The signal acquisition of the surface fluorometry technique was limited to a small surface area and a shallow depth below the surface thus preventing the detection of possible changes within larger volumes of the muscle (2, 56, 120). Finally, it has been argued that Jöbsis and Stainsby (106) should have compared the NADH/NAD^+ reduction between a lower work rate associated with only slight lactate output (or even uptake) and a higher work rate at which lactate output was significantly greater, rather than making an exercise to rest comparison (56, 101).

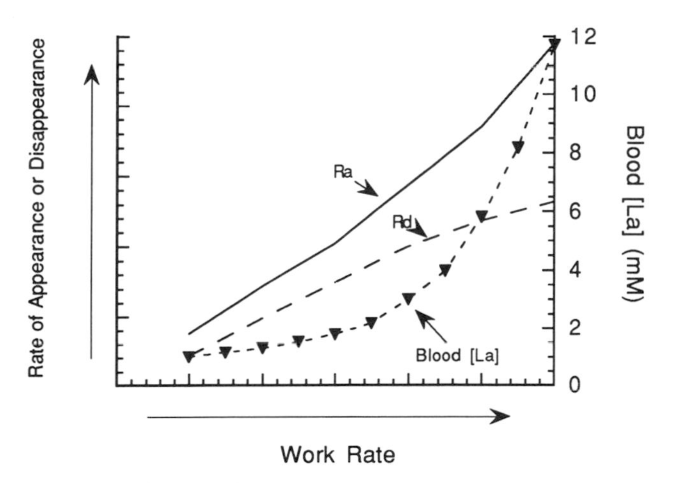

FIG. 14.2. Schematic illustration of relationship between lactate rate of appearance, lactate rate of disappearance, and resulting blood [La] during progressive, incremental exercise. [Redrawn with permission from Brooks, G. A. Anaerobic threshold: review of the concept and directions for future research. *Med. Sci. Sports Exerc.* 17: 22–31, 1985 (18).]

With regard to the myoglobin cryomicrospectroscopy method, Jones et al. (109, 123) have questioned the ability of this technique to achieve the accuracy required to determine O_2 dependence of mitochondrial function. Kennedy and Jones (123) state that the analysis of Honig et al. (100) "does not provide corrections for possible vapor layers, does not consider capture of O_2 concentration gradients, and does not consider heterogeneous freezing patterns due to heterogeneous ultrastructure." They (123) also argue that the measurement of myoglobin oxygenation in frozen muscle may have insufficient resolution and accuracy to detect O_2 gradients with the required precision. Possible complicating factors include internal reflectance of ice crystals, possible heterogeneity of crystal structure in cellular structures, possible refractive and reflective effects due to surface irregularities, and nonuniform light scatter at the microscopic level (123). These concerns have been echoed by other investigators (56, 121).

Clearly, a major point of contention remains. Are there intracellular locales within submaximally exercising muscles at which mitochondrial respiration ($\dot{V}O_2$ and oxidative phosphorylation) is limited by inadequate O_2? Whereas O_2-limitation is a matter of intense debate, there is universal agreement that the intramuscular O_2 level does decrease with increasing exercise intensity. For example, Doll et al. (50) and Knight et al. (125) reported that femoral venous PO_2 (and, therefore, presumably exercising leg muscle PO_2) declined with progressive increases in work rate during cycle ergometer exercise. Similar results were reported by Andersen and Saltin (5) for knee extensor contractions of one limb in humans. Bylund-Fellenius and colleagues (28, 29, 99) introduced an O_2 probe through a cannula into the gastrocnemius muscle of human subjects to estimate intramuscular PO_2 during leg exercise performed on a foot ergometer. Intramuscular PO_2 decreased in proportion to the work rate performed. Connett et al. (39) have also reported a decrease in median PO_2 as determined via the myoglobin cryomicrospectroscopy method with increasing metabolic rate in the contracting dog gracilis muscle. Furthermore, there is almost universal agreement that lactate production and accumulation are reduced during hyperoxia (130, 198, 203). Prime examples of this response are reported by Hogan et al. (95) and Graham et al. (78) for humans during cycle ergometer exercise, by Hogan and Welch (97) for contracting canine skeletal muscle, and by Idström et al. (104) for contracting rat skeletal muscle.

Near-Equilibrium Steady State: A Unifying Hypothesis?

There are both supporting arguments and condemning refutations for the two opposing views concerning the causes of lactate production during progressive exercise. Can these opposing points of view (O_2-limitation vs. multifactorial, non–O_2-limitation) be reconciled? The salient facets of the two views may be less contradictory in the context of the "near-equilibrium steady-state hypothesis" (57, 126, 144, 210) for the control of mitochondrial oxidative phosphorylation. The following outline paraphrases the description of Wilson (210). The near equilibrium hypothesis has two parts: *(1)* the first two sites of oxidative phosphorylation are near equilibrium under physiological conditions, and *(2)* the third site of phosphorylation is irreversible and therefore is the rate-determining step in the overall process. The first two sites of oxidative phosphorylation that are postulated to be near equilibrium in this hypothesis are summarized in the following overall reaction:

$$NADH_i + 2c^{3+} + 2ADP_e + 2Pi_e \leftrightarrow NAD_i^+ + 2c^{2+} + 2ATP_e + H^+ \quad (1)$$

where c^{3+} and c^{2+} are the oxidized and reduced forms of mitochondrial cytochrome c and the subscripts i and e represent the intramitochondrial and extramitochondrial pools of reactants, respectively. The cytochrome c oxidase [cytochrome aa_3; (126)] reaction is the irreversible, rate-determining step:

$$2c^{2+} + 1/2O_2 + ADP_e + Pi_e + 2H^+ \Rightarrow 2c^{3+} + H_2O + ATP_e \quad (2)$$

The rate of the cytochrome c oxidase reaction (and therefore of oxidative phosphorylation and mitochondrial O_2 consumption) is a function of the concentrations of O_2 and of reduced cytochrome c, both of which are substrates for the reaction (57, 126, 210). Since reduced cytochrome c (c^{2+}) is a product of the near equilibrium reactions summarized in equation 1, it is, in turn, a function of the intramitochondrial $[NAD_i^+]/[NADH_i]$ redox couple and of the cytosolic phosphorylation potential, $[ATP]/[ADP] \cdot [Pi]$. Accordingly, *under acute conditions*, mitochondrial oxidative phosphorylation rate and O_2 consumption are hypothesized to depend on three interrelated factors (57, 126, 210):

1. Intramitochondrial $[NAD_i^+]/[NADH_i]$, which depends on substrate availability and the status of intermediary metabolism.
2. Cytosolic $[ATP]/[ADP] \cdot [Pi]$, which is determined by the rate of cellular ATP demand.
3. The available concentration of molecular O_2.

With saturating levels of O_2, an increase in work rate by muscles is powered by an increased rate of ATP breakdown which in turn results in some decrease in [ATP] and larger increases in [ADP] and [Pi] (through PC hydrolysis). The result is a decrease in the cytosolic $[ATP]/[ADP] \cdot [Pi]$ which activates mitochondrial oxidative phosphorylation to match the rate of ATP utilization, at the price of a lower cellular energy state (210). Depending on the magnitude of changes in $[ATP]/[ADP] \cdot [Pi]$ and the exact balance between the various energetic pathways, there may also be changes in $[NAD_i^+]/[NADH_i]$ that will play a role in the increase in oxidative phosphorylation as well as regulation of other energy pathways (57).

As noted earlier, intramuscular O_2 tension does decrease as work rate increases; in the framework of the near-equilibrium steady-state hypothesis, this will be a regulating factor of oxidative phosphorylation. As the Po_2 declines, the mitochondrial oxidative phosphorylation rate and O_2 consumption can be maintained only through a decrease in either the cytosolic [ATP]/[ADP] · [Pi], the intramitochondrial $[NAD_i^+]/[NADH_i]$, or a combination of both factors (57, 126, 210–212). These adjustments to declining Po_2 will also be reflected in a more reduced redox state of cytochrome c to drive the nonequilibrium reaction in equation 2 (57, 126, 210–212). Figures 14.3 and 14.4 provide schematic examples of the required responses of cytosolic [ATP]/[ADP] · [Pi] and intramitochondrial $[NAD_i^+]/[NADH_i]$ in order to maintain maximal oxidative phosphorylation with declining Po_2; these figures are redrawn from the mathematical models of Wilson et al. (212). Figure 14.3 shows the effect of cytosolic [ATP]/[ADP] · [Pi] at constant intramitochondrial $[NAD_i^+]/[NADH_i]$ on the O_2 dependence of mitochondrial oxygen consumption, while Figure 14.4 shows the effect of intramitochondrial $[NAD_i^+]/[NADH_i]$ at constant [ATP]/[ADP] · [Pi].

It is impossible to separate the regulatory roles of O_2, cytosolic [ATP]/[ADP] · [Pi], and intramitochondrial $[NAD_i^+]/[NADH_i]$ from each other in the near-equilibrium steady-state hypothesis. However, the central link among increasing work rate, declining Po_2, and increasing lactate production is the cytosolic [ATP]/[ADP] · [Pi]. For example, as work rate increases, the rate of ATP utilization increases. There

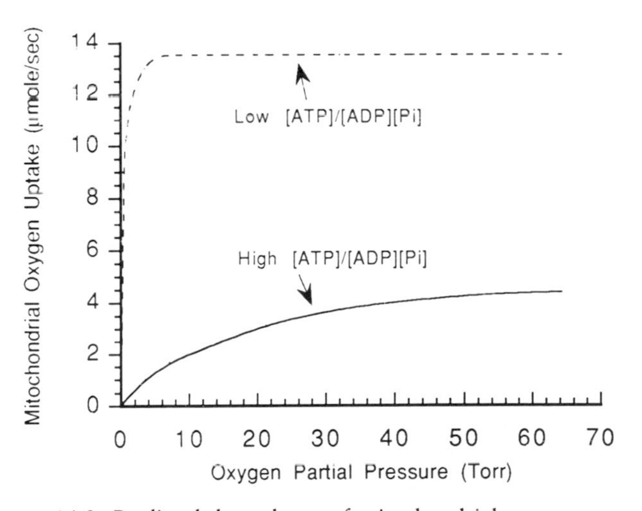

FIG. 14.3. Predicted dependence of mitochondrial oxygen consumption on partial pressure of oxygen at high- and low-energy states with constant $[NAD^+]/[NADH]$ of 1.0. Note that oxygen independence is preserved to low partial pressures when energy state is low. [Based on mathematical models of, and redrawn with permission from, Wilson, D. F., C. S. Owen, and M. Erecinska. Quantitative dependence of mitochondrial oxidative phosphorylation on oxygen concentration: a mathematical model. *Arch. Biochem. Biophys.* 195: 494–504, 1979 (212).]

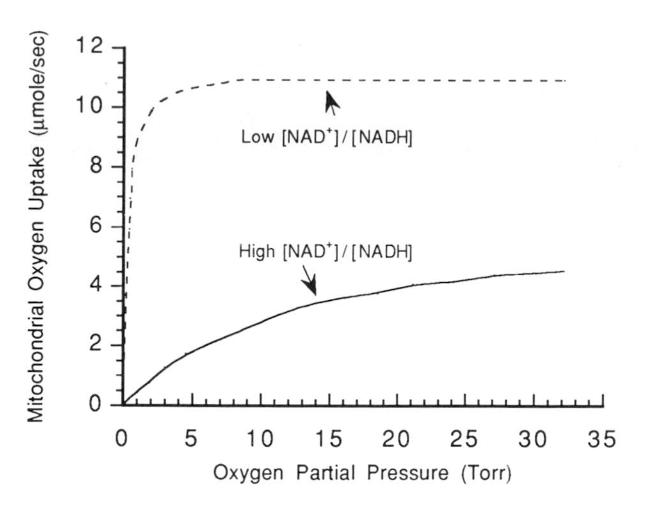

FIG. 14.4. Predicted dependence of mitochondrial oxygen consumption on partial pressure of oxygen at high and low $[NAD^+]/[NADH]$ with constant [ATP]/[ADP][Pi] of 500 · M^{-1}. Note that oxygen independence is preserved to low partial pressures when $[NAD^+]/[NADH]$ is low. [Based on mathematical models of, and redrawn with permission from, Wilson, D. F., C. S. Owen, and M. Erecinska. Quantitative dependence of mitochondrial oxidative phosphorylation on oxygen concentration: a mathematical model. *Arch. Biochem. Biophys.* 195: 494–504, 1979 (212).]

will be a transient imbalance between ATP utilization and ATP synthesis that will lead to a decrease in the cytosolic [ATP]/[ADP] · [Pi], which in turn will stimulate oxidative phosphorylation to match the required rate of ATP breakdown. If intramuscular Po_2 declines at the same time as work rate increases (and the evidence suggests that it does), there is an additional contribution to the imbalance between ATP utilization and ATP synthesis. This will require a greater decrease in the cytosolic [ATP]/[ADP] · [Pi] to stimulate oxidative phosphorylation than would have been necessary if Po_2 had not gone down. The link between declining Po_2 and increasing lactate production is the fact that the individual changes in [ATP], [ADP], and [Pi] that constitute the decrease in cytosolic [ATP]/[ADP] · [Pi] are all powerful stimuli for increased glycolytic activity and, therefore, increased lactate production (120, 121, 181, 190).

Therefore, the near-equilibrium steady-state hypothesis does suggest a role for O_2 in the elevated muscle and blood concentrations that occur during progressive exercise. However, this role does not exclude the causative effects of many of the agents supported by the multifactorial explanation of increasing lactate concentration. There is also a subtle but major difference between the role allocated to O_2 by the near-equilibrium steady-state hypothesis and the role espoused by the O_2-limitation explanation for increasing lactate concentration. The O_2-limitation explanation argues that oxidative phosphorylation is limited by inadequate O_2. However, the extrapolation from the near-equilibrium steady-state hypothesis does not argue for sustained O_2-limited oxidative phosphorylation. In this explanation, any imbalances between ATP utilization and synthesis are transient and are immediately corrected by changes in the near-equilibrium stimuli of oxidative phosphorylation. Note that this entire discussion has addressed the role and adequacy of O_2 at submaximal work rates, and does not extend to the question of O_2-limitation at maximal O_2 uptake.

Clearly, there are other hypotheses concerning the regulation of oxidative phosphorylation, and they have their merits (57, 126, 144, 210). However, considerable evidence supports the notion that the regulatory factors for oxidative phosphorylation change when the oxygen level is changed (7, 94, 96). For example, Hogan et al. (94) studied the canine gastrocnemius in situ during alterations of tissue oxygenation. Tissue oxygenation was altered by reducing O_2 delivery via decreasing Pa_{O_2}. $\dot{V}_{O_2}$ and metabolites were measured in contracting muscles at three different levels of oxygen delivery. The important finding was that greater changes in proposed regulators of mitochondrial oxidative phosphorylation ([PC], [ADP], and [ATP]/[ADP] · [Pi]) were required to achieve a given $\dot{V}_{O_2}$ as Pa_{O_2} was decreased (see Fig. 14.5). Concomitant muscle lactate output and accumulation were greater, with the greater changes in proposed regulators at the lower Pa_{O_2} values. These results (94) and others like them (7, 96) from Hogan's group are consistent with a link between mitochondrial regulation and stimulation of glycolysis.

Numerous investigators (55, 84, 119–121, 173, 174) have reported an increased reduction of the $NADH/NAD^+$ pair during exercise that is of greater than moderate intensity. These results have sometimes been used to argue that oxidative phosphorylation is O_2-limited and that this limitation in turn causes an increase in muscle and blood lactate concentrations (120, 121). However, progressive reduction of $NADH/NAD^+$ more likely represents a regulatory response to maintain oxidative phosphorylation at the required rate (174). This interpretation is consistent with the near-equilibrium steady-state hypothesis and suggests that reduction of $NADH/NAD^+$ does not provide any direct evaluation of O_2-limitation of oxidative phosphorylation. Duhaylongsod et al. (56) have recently used near-infrared spectroscopy to evaluate the redox state of cytochrome aa_3 in contracting canine gracilis muscle as contraction intensity and the corresponding metabolic rate were increased progressively. They (56) reported that the concentration of oxidized mitochondrial cytochrome aa_3 decreased in a near-linear fashion as metabolic rate increased from rest to $\dot{V}_{O_{2max}}$. Lactate efflux from the muscles increased progressively with metabolic rate. Again, these responses suggest a link between mitochondrial regulation and stimulation of glycolysis as proposed in the near-equilibrium steady-state hypothesis (190). *At submaximal work rates*, these findings do not necessarily imply that oxidative phosphorylation and $\dot{V}_{O_2}$ are O_2-limited.

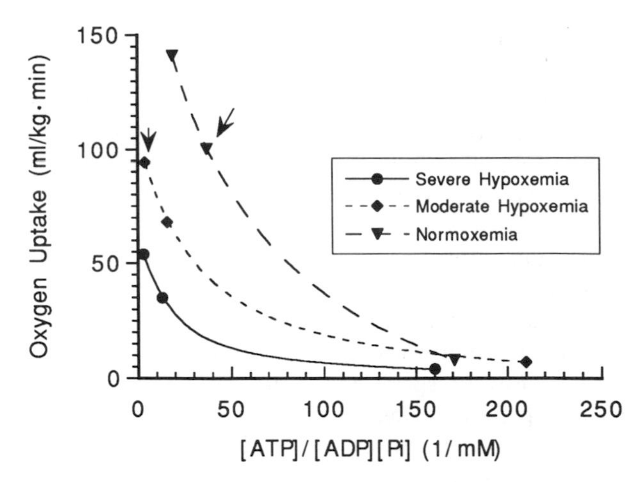

FIG. 14.5. Relationship between energy state and oxygen uptake in dog gastrocnemius muscle in situ at rest and two stimulation rates for normoxemia, moderate hypoxemia, and severe hypoxemia. The important point is that a greater decrease in energy state is required in order to stimulate a given oxygen uptake when the oxygen delivery is low. Note especially the two points indicated by *arrows*. The oxygen uptake is approximately the same, but a much lower energy state is required with moderate hypoxemia in comparison to normoxemia. [Redrawn with permission from Hogan, M. C., P. G. Arthur, D. E. Bebout, P. W. Hochachka, and P. D. Wagner. Role of O_2 in regulating tissue respiration in dog muscle working in situ. *J. Appl. Physiol.* 73: 728–736, 1992 (94).]

Summary

The cause of the LT during progressive exercise remains a subject of debate. The first major hypothesis holds that muscle and blood lactate concentrations increase with exercise intensity because of O_2-limited mitochondrial respiration (i.e., muscle hypoxia). The major competing hypothesis argues that muscle oxygenation is adequate for optimal mitochondrial function, and that lactate production is increased due to the effects of several interacting factors. These factors include biochemical regulation, sympathoadrenal activity, motor unit recruitment, and the balance between lactate production and removal. There is no definitive answer to the question of whether there are mitochondria within submaximally exercising muscles in which respiration is limited by inadequate O_2. However, there is general agreement that PO_2 in contracting muscles does decline as exercise intensity increases.

The near-equilibrium steady-state hypothesis for the control of mitochondrial oxidative phosphorylation may provide an explanation that reconciles the opposing points of view concerning O_2 availability and elevated [La] during exercise. In the near-equilibrium steady-state hypothesis, a lower PO_2 requires a lower phosphorylation potential ([ATP]/[ADP] · [Pi]) in order to stimulate a given rate of oxidative phosphorylation by mitochondria. Therefore, as exercise intensity increases and muscle PO_2 declines, cellular phosphorylation potential must decrease in order to stimulate ATP synthesis by mitochondrial oxidative phosphorylation. An obligatory consequence of the decreasing phosphorylation potential is progressive stimulation of key enzymes that regulate glycolytic rate. The end result is increased lactate production and elevations of muscle and blood [La]. The near-equilibrium steady-state hypothesis retains a regulatory role for muscle PO_2 but does not exclude an important role for the numerous factors identified in the multifactorial explanation of exercise lactate concentrations.

THE LACTATE SHUTTLE

In the past, lactate was viewed as a dead-end waste product that could move rapidly across muscle membranes by simple diffusion. These out-dated notions of lactate transport and metabolism contrast sharply with the modern concept of lactate exchange within living organisms. Current understanding of the metabolic role of lactate is embodied in the "lactate shuttle hypothesis" developed by Brooks (19, 20, 22, 184). Briefly, the lactate shuttle hypothesis holds that lactate formation and the subsequent distribution of lactate throughout the body is a major mechanism whereby the coordination of intermediary metabolism in different tissues, and cells within those tissues, can be accomplished. This shuttle probably functions during all metabolic conditions—resting postabsorptive and postprandial conditions as well as sustained, submaximal exercise. Furthermore, the shuttle and its different components are probably important in clinical lactic acidosis, which is most often due to circulatory insufficiency (35).

Within the shuttle concept, lactate is a useful metabolic intermediate because it can be exchanged rapidly among tissue compartments. Once formed in muscle cells that may have high glycogenolytic and glycolytic rates, lactate can be transported to other sites where it may serve as an energy source and a gluconeogenic precursor. Lactate oxidation can occur in nearby oxidative muscle cells, or at other sites such as the heart, or other oxidative skeletal muscles that might be either at rest or engaged in light to moderate exercise. At the same time, lactate can be taken up in the liver and used for glucose production or liver glycogen storage. As pointed out by Stainsby and Brooks (184):

> Lactate can be exchanged between muscle and blood, between blood and muscle, between active and inactive muscles, between inactive and active muscles, between active and active muscles, between blood and heart, between active muscle and liver, between liver and other tissues such as exercising muscle, between skin and blood, between intestine and portal blood, between portal blood and liver, and along pH and concentration gradients within muscle tissue.

Function of the lactate shuttle during postprandial conditions is an important component of the glucose paradox whereby most glucose from dietary carbohydrate bypasses the liver and is converted to lactate by skeletal muscle (21, 149). Subsequently, much of this glucose-derived lactate is taken up by the liver and converted to glycogen.

Stainsby and Brooks (184) have suggested that there may also be an intracellular lactate shuttle. Net lactate production occurs in the cytosol, while net lactate consumption should occur adjacent to mitochondria. This creates a source (cytosolic glycolysis) and a sink (mitochondria) for intracellular lactate flux. The much higher concentration of lactate in comparison to either pyruvate or NADH, particularly during exercise, would contribute to the functioning of an intracellular lactate shuttle. In such a shuttle, lactate diffusion from cytosolic sites to mitochondria might represent an important enhancement in the rate of delivery of pyruvate and reducing equivalents to the mitochondria. Figure 14.6 provides a schematic representation of such a shuttle. Tissue-to-tissue and cell-to-cell aspects of the lactate shuttle have been nicely illustrated previously (21).

The importance of lactate as a major component of intermediary metabolism is underscored by the fact that during moderate-intensity exercise, blood lactate flux may exceed glucose flux (22). During altitude exposure, blood lactate flux exceeds glucose flux even at rest (22). With the advent of the lactate shuttle hypothesis, a major shift has occurred in the role that has been hypothesized for skeletal muscle in lactate metabolism. Previously, skeletal muscle was believed to be predominantly a producer of lactate; however, skeletal muscle is now viewed as not

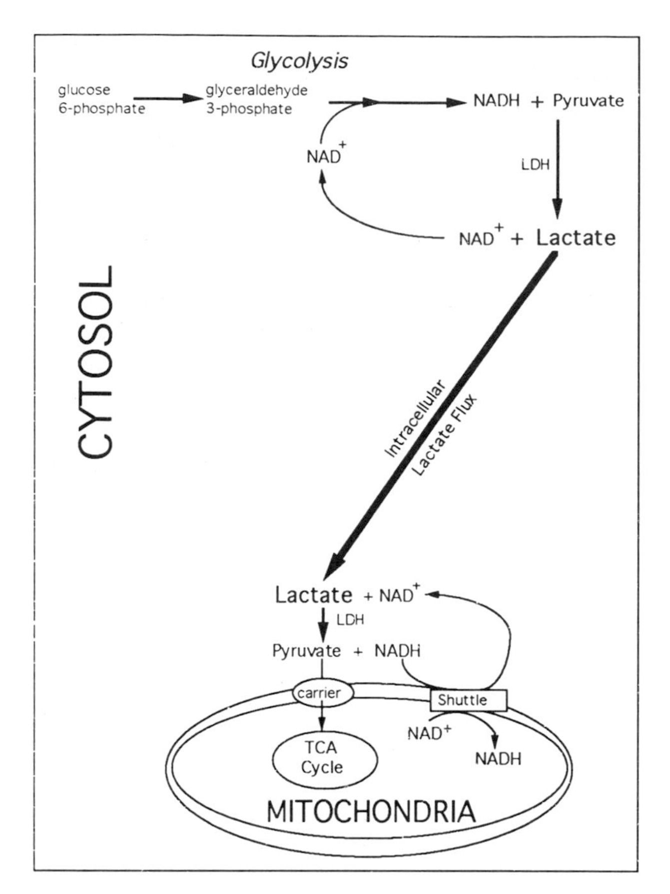

FIG. 14.6. Illustration of a hypothetical intracellular lactate shuttle. Lactate produced in the cytosol might diffuse to mitochondria where the [La] is lower because of lactate consumption. At the mitochondria, the LDH reaction would operate to produce pyruvate and NADH from lactate and NAD^+. Due to the higher concentration of lactate in comparison to pyruvate and NADH, such a shuttle might enhance the delivery of pyruvate and reducing equivalents to the mitochondria, particularly during exercise.

only the most important source of lactate, but also as the most likely primary consumer of lactate as well (166).

At rest, muscles slowly release lactate into the blood on a net basis, although at times they may show a small net uptake. During exercise, particularly short-term high-intensity exercise, muscles produce lactate rapidly, while lactate clearance is slowed. This results in an increased intramuscular [La] and an increased net output of lactate from the muscles into the blood. Later, during recovery from short-term exercise, or even during continued, prolonged exercise; there is net lactate uptake ($\dot{L}$) from the blood by resting muscles or by other muscles that are doing mild to moderate exercise. During prolonged exercise of low to moderate intensity, the muscles that originally showed net lactate output at the onset of the exercise may actually reverse to net $\dot{L}$. This shuttling of lactate between adjacent muscles and between muscles and blood (and among other tissues as noted earlier) raises important questions concerning how and at what rates lactic acid is able to cross the muscle membrane. Functioning of the lactate shuttle is difficult to envision in the absence of a well-developed carrier system for lactate.

CARRIER-MEDIATED LACTATE TRANSPORT

In the past, investigators merely assumed that lactate moves rapidly across muscle membranes by simple diffusion. More recent studies have provided strong evidence of a carrier-mediated transport system for lactate in skeletal muscle. For example, Juel (111) observed lactate efflux from mouse soleus muscles in vitro during 30 min of recovery from contractions induced by short trains of electrical stimulation. Lactate efflux from the muscles was inhibited to varying degrees by α-cyano-4-hydroxycinnamate (CIN), *p*-chloromercuribenzenesulphonic acid (*p*CMBS), and phloretin, all known blockers of lactate carriers in other tissues. However, the anion-exchange inhibitors, 4-acetamido-4′-isothiocyanostilbene (SITS), 4,4′-diisothiocyano-2,2′-stilbenedisulfonic acid (DIDS), and tetrathionate did not inhibit lactate efflux. Overall, Juel's results (111) indicated the existence of a lactate transporter in skeletal muscle that accounted for more than half of the lactate output during recovery from contractions in his model. In a subsequent study, Juel and Wibrand (117) followed lactate transport into isolated mouse soleus muscles in vitro with a ^{14}C-lactate tracer. CIN and *p*CMBS inhibited tracer uptake by 80%, suggesting that the major part of the transport involves a carrier. The remaining 20% of the lactate uptake was noninhibitable, nonsaturable, and reduced at high pH; it was attributed to diffusion of undissociated lactic acid.

Lactate Transport in Sarcolemmal Vesicles

Study of membrane transport of lactate has now been extended to the level of sarcolemmal vesicles, beginning with Roth and Brooks (166–168), who were the first to perform such experiments on skeletal muscle. In all of their experiments, Roth and Brooks (167, 168) studied lactate influx into sarcolemmal vesicles from rat mixed skeletal muscle under zero *trans* conditions; that is, isotopic lactate with varied unlabeled lactate concentrations was always present outside the vesicles while there was initially neither labeled nor unlabeled lactate inside the vesicles. When the initial rates of influx were plotted as a function of the extravesicular [La], L(+)-lactate influx displayed saturation kinetics in the typical hyperbolic form as shown in Figure 14.7. Overall, they (167, 168) reported evidence of a membrane-bound carrier that is stereospecific for the L(+) isomer, with V_{max} = 139.4 nmol · mg^{-1} · min^{-1}, and apparent K_m = 40.1 mM.

DIDS inhibited lactate transport by 13%, suggesting a minor role for lactate exchange with either Cl^- or HCO_3^-. CIN and *p*CMBS inhibited lactate transport by ~70% and 83%, respectively. Ten mM pyruvate inhibited the influx of 1 mM radioisotopic L(+)-lactate by 71% as compared to an inhibition of 82% by 10 mM unlabeled L(+)-lactate; this indicates that the carrier is a monocarboxylate carrier rather than a lactate-only carrier. This carrier was also pH gradient-sensitive (168); lactate transport into the vesicles was stimulated by an inwardly directed hydrogen ion gradient. This gradient increased carrier-mediated transport but also appeared to increase passive diffusion via undissociated lactic acid. The increased lactate influx into vesicles was not affected by the absolute pH level, but rather by the pH gradient between the external medium and the intravesicular space. Obviously, a carrier that is predominant in the transmembrane transport of lactate could be extremely important in regulating net fluxes of lactate, thereby influencing metabolism and intracellular pH regulation as well.

Juel and colleagues (113, 115) obtained sarcolemmal vesicles by collagenase treatment of rat skeletal muscle. These vesicles were referred to as giant sarcolemmal vesicles because their median diameter (~6 μm) was three or more times greater than that of vesicles obtained by standard methods (<1 μm) such as those used by Roth and Brooks (167, 168). Also, Juel (113) studied lactate *efflux* from the vesicles under zero *trans* conditions with isotopic lactate and varied unlabeled lactate concentrations inside the vesicles and neither labeled nor unlabeled lactate in the efflux medium. Nevertheless, the lactate efflux results of Juel's experiments on the giant sarcolemmal vesicles were similar in most respects to the influx experiments of Roth and Brooks (167, 168) on the smaller, classical vesicles. A notable difference, however, was that the giant vesicles had a lower K_m (20.9 mM vs. 40.1 mM); and the V_{max} was estimated by Juel to be approximately ten times greater than that reported by Roth and Brooks (167, 168) for the smaller vesicles. From these results, Juel (113) argued that the giant sarcolemmal vesicles are more representative of intact muscles. This is an extremely interesting and important possibility, but Juel's assertions require considerably more verification than has been provided to date. Direct comparisons between the results of Juel et al. (113, 115) and of Roth and Brooks (167, 168) are somewhat difficult because Juel et al. (113, 115) studied lactate efflux from vesicles and expressed the results in relation to vesicle surface area, whereas Roth and Brooks (167, 168) studied lactate influx into vesicles and expressed the results in relation to vesicular protein content.

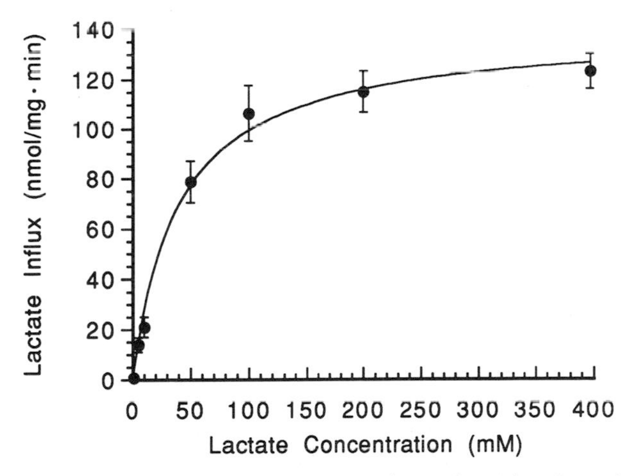

FIG. 14.7. L(+)-lactate influx into sarcolemmal vesicles. Curve is best fit to Michaelis-Menten hyperbolic function. V_{max} = 139.4 nmol · mg^{-1} · min^{-1}; K_m = 40.1 mM. [Redrawn with permission from Roth, D. A., and G. A. Brooks. Lactate transport is mediated by a membrane-bound carrier in rat skeletal muscle sarcolemmal vesicles. *Arch. Biochem. Biophys.* 279: 377–385, 1990 (167).]

Recently, McDermott and Bonen (140) have also studied lactate influx into classical, small vesicles isolated from rat hindlimb muscles with no lactate initially inside the vesicles. Again, their results were in general agreement with the previous results of Roth and Brooks (167, 168). However, McDermott and Bonen (140) found a K_m for lactate influx of ~12.5 mM that is not only much lower than the value of ~40 mM reported by Roth and Brooks (167, 168), but is also about half the K_m of ~21 mM reported by Juel (113) for giant sarcolemmal vesicles. V_{max} in the study of McDermott and Bonen (140) was about three times higher than the V_{max} found by Roth and Brooks (167, 168), but still lower than the value reported by Juel (113) in giant vesicles. McDermott and Bonen (140) speculated that the quantitative differences between their results and those of Roth and Brooks (167, 168) might be due to the use of male rats (McDermott and Bonen) rather than female rats, or to differences in the preparation of sarcolemmal vesicles. Roth and Brooks (167, 168) used the sarcolemmal isolation procedures described by Grimditch et al. (83), whereas McDermott and Bonen (140) used the techniques of Klip et al. (124). The important point is that all of the investigators agree that there is a sarcolemmal lactate transporter that could function in the lactate shuttle. This transporter has a higher affinity for lactate than other monocarboxylates including pyruvate, and is apparently bidirectional and symmetrical (26).

It appears that lactate transport across the membrane of sarcolemmal vesicles occurs by three pathways: *(1)* mainly via a monocarboxylate carrier, which accounts for ~70%–90% of lactate transport across the physiological range of lactate concentrations; *(2)* a minor, probably negligible amount by way of an inorganic anion exchanger (lactate anion exchange for either Cl^- or HCO_3^-); and *(3)* diffusion of undissociated lactic acid, a pathway that makes greater contributions at higher lactate concentrations (140, 142, 167–169). Overall, this pattern for muscle membrane transport is analogous to the three pathways of monocarboxylate transport in red blood cells (RBCs) (161). This is not to say that lactate transport is identical in both muscle and RBCs; it is not. Poole and Halestrap (161) have suggested that there is a family of lactate transporters with differing characteristics that are distributed throughout various tissues (161).

Juel (113) also studied *trans* acceleration and equilibrium exchange in giant sarcolemmal vesicles. In these experiments, the vesicles were loaded with isotopic tracer lactate and a high unlabeled [La] (50 mM). The initial [La] outside the vesicles in the efflux medium was varied from 0 mM (zero *trans* conditions) to 50 mM (equilibrium exchange conditions). The rate of lactate efflux was increased in a hyperbolic manner by the higher lactate concentrations in the extravesicular medium until a maximal rate was reached under equilibrium exchange conditions (intravesicular [La] = efflux medium [La]). However, the K_m was not greatly affected. *Trans* acceleration also occurs in small vesicles (26). Results of this type have been used to develop a model for the skeletal muscle monocarboxylate carrier (113, 116, 161); the model is believed to be generally similar to that previously proposed for RBCs (161).

As illustrated in Figure 14.8, it is postulated that the carrier first binds H^+ and then lactate, after which a conformational change translocates the lactate across the membrane. [It is believed that the intermediate form of the carrier with only H^+ bound is either immobile or else translocates only very slowly (113, 116).] The substrates are then released in the reverse order of loading, lactate first and then H^+. Next, the unloaded carrier undergoes a conformational change to return to the other side of the membrane and continue the transport process. Translocation of the unloaded carrier is believed to be the rate-limiting process for transport. According to this model, *trans* acceleration occurs because the

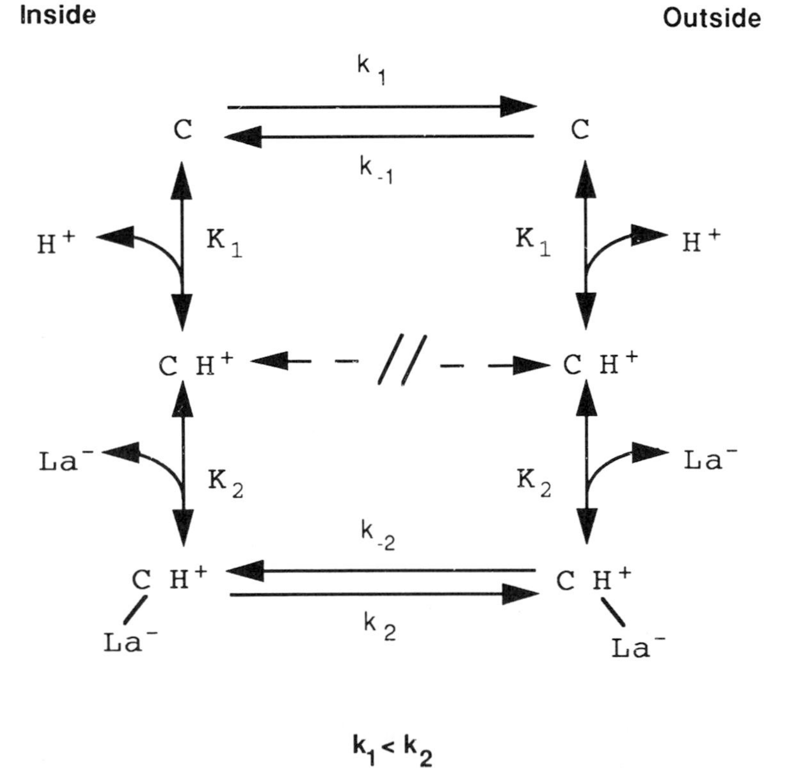

FIG. 14.8. Schematic of proposed model for the monocarboxylate carrier of lactate transport in red blood cells (161). Lactate transport in sarcolemmal vesicles has been proposed to be qualitatively similar (113, 161). The various K's represent binding rates while the k's represent translocation rates. It is postulated that the carrier first binds H^+ and then lactate. The carrier with only H^+ bound is believed to be either immobile or else translocates only very slowly. See text for additional details. [Redrawn with permission from Poole, R. C., and A. P. Halestrap. Transport of lactate and other monocarboxylates across mammalian plasma membranes. *Am. J. Physiol.* 264 (*Cell Physiol.* 33): C761–C782, 1993 (161).]

presence of lactate on both sides of the membrane decreases the probability that a carrier will undergo conformation and translocation in the unloaded state. The closer the *trans* acceleration conditions come to equilibrium conditions, the more likely it becomes that the carrier is in the loaded state and, therefore, the faster its reorientation from one side of the membrane to the other. Accordingly, Juel (113, 116) has reported V_{max} for equilibrium exchange conditions to be ~2.3 times greater than V_{max} measured during efflux under zero *trans* conditions.

The giant sarcolemmal vesicle technique has been extended to the study of lactate transport in human skeletal muscle by Juel et al. (112, 116). Needle biopsy samples of human skeletal muscle were treated with a collagenase solution to cause vesicle formation. The results were generally similar to those previously obtained by Juel et al. (113, 115) on rat giant sarcolemmal vesicles and, for the first time, provided strong, direct evidence of a lactate carrier in human skeletal muscle.

Lactate Transport in Isolated Cells

Beaudry et al. (11) reported that lactate uptake into L6 myoblasts was due to simple diffusion. The initial rate of lactate uptake was linearly related to [La] in the incubation medium, and CIN had no effect on the uptake rate. The L6 myoblasts are undifferentiated muscle cells of an established cell line obtained from rat muscles. Subsequent experiments by Beaudry's group (1) revealed that a carrier was involved in lactate uptake by L6 myotubes, which are formed by cellular fusion of myoblasts in a later stage of development. Lactate uptake by the myotubes displayed saturation kinetics and was inhibited by CIN. Thus, it seems that the lactate carrier only appears after terminal differentiation.

Nagesser et al. (147) have recently measured lactate efflux from fatigued fast-twitch muscle fibers of the toad *Xenopus laevis*. Single fibers were isolated from the iliofibularis muscle and fatigued by intermittent tetanic stimulation at 20°C in both phosphate and bicarbonate buffer solutions at two different pH levels, 7.2 and 7.8. Lactate efflux was measured and found to be constant during 10 min of stimulation. In some experiments, lactate efflux was measured in the presence of 5 mM CIN. Based on a comparison of lactate efflux between the different buffer solutions, with and without CIN, the data suggested that *(1)* combined diffusion of lactic acid and the lactate anion accounted for ~20%, *(2)* lactate anion for bicarbonate ion exchange accounted for ~61%, and *(3)* lactate-proton cotransport (monocarboxylate carrier) accounted for ~19% of the total lactate efflux. The surprising result is the predominant role of inorganic anion exchange and the relatively small contribution of the monocarboxylate carrier. Whether this reflects a species difference between amphibians and mammals is unknown.

Reconstitution of the Lactate Carrier

Recently, Wibrand and Juel (209) were the first investigators to reconstitute the lactate carrier from rat skeletal muscle sarcolemma in a functionally active form. The characteristics of lactate transport in reconstituted phospholipid vesicles were similar to those observed in native giant sarcolemmal vesicles. Allen and Brooks (3) have also reconstituted the sarcolemmal lactate transporter from rat skeletal muscle. SDS-polyacrylamide gel electrophoresis in the same study (3) provided evidence that the lactate transporter is a polypeptide of about 34 kd in rat skeletal muscle. McCullagh and Bonen (139) found that labeled lactate was bound to membrane protein(s) in the 30–40 kd molecular mass range. The skeletal muscle lactate transporter is probably slightly smaller than the RBC lactate transporter [35–50 kd (160, 161)].

Garcia et al. (65) have recently reported the cloning of a cDNA encoding a monocarboxylate transporter that resembled the erythrocyte monocarboxylate transporter with regard to properties such as proton symport, *trans* acceleration, and sensitivity to CIN. They (65) referred to the transporter derived from wild-type Chinese hamster ovary cells as *MCT1*. Garcia et al. (65) used a rabbit polyclonal antibody to *MCT1* to detect the largest amounts of the transporter in hamster RBCs, cecum, heart, eye, lung, epididymis, and testis; intermediate levels in brain and kidney; and low levels in gastrocnemius and liver. The muscle fibers richest in *MCT1* appears to be those that were also rich in mitochondria. The apparent molecular mass of *MCT1* on SDS-polyacrylamide gels was 43 kd, which is in the range of the RBC transporter. *MCT1* seems unlikely to be the predominant transporter in skeletal muscle, although this low K_m carrier could be important in lactate transport under resting conditions with low [La].

Lactate Transport In Situ

Studies of lactate transport in sarcolemmal vesicles are extremely important because they allow investigators to focus on the properties of sarcolemmal transfer alone. Sarcolemmal vesicles offer the advantage of alleviating confounding problems of metabolism, capillary diffusional resistance and flow, interstitial concentration variabilities, and uncontrolled intracellular solute compositions (166, 167). As discussed above, sarcolemmal vesicles also provide the material for isolation, purification, and eventually, sequencing of the lactate transporter protein. However, sarcolemmal membrane preparations separate the lactate transport processes from the metabolic processes that they serve, and thereby remove regulatory interaction between transport and metabolism (142). Some questions regarding lactate transport require models other than sarcolemmal vesicles. For example, there is presently no way to estimate the physiological lactate transport capacity from the vesicle studies because the lactate carrier has not been specifically isolated and there is no high-affinity ligand that will bind to the lactate transporter and allow measurement of the density of muscle lactate carriers in the membrane of intact muscles. Furthermore, experiments with sarcolemmal vesicles do not provide any way to directly evaluate the possible effects of physiological factors such as blood flow, muscle contractions, and changes in hormonal concentrations on the lactate transport process. In order to investigate membrane transport into vascularly perfused skeletal muscle in situ, the paired-tracer dilution method has been used.

The paired-tracer dilution technique involves arterial injection of an extracellular reference tracer (e.g., D-[^{3}H]mannitol or L-[^{3}H]glucose) and the transportable substance; in this case, L-[^{14}C]lactate (103, 218). The method relies on differential movement of the transportable substance into the tissue relative to the extracellular tracer, as calculated from the fractional recoveries of the tracers in the venous effluent samples taken immediately after arterial injection of the tracers. The paired-tracer dilution method was first employed in the study of lactate transport in skeletal muscle by Watt et al. (202). They (202) concluded that the transport of lactate across the sarcolemma of the rat hindlimb occurs by two major pathways. One pathway was nonsaturable and accounted for 70% of lactate movement at normal lactate concentrations and 90% of transport at 50 mM. The other pathway appeared to be saturable and was inhibited to varying degrees by 25 mM pyruvate, 5 mM CIN, and 0.2 mM *p*CMBS. V_{max} and K_m for the artificially perfused rat hindlimb were reported to be 0.84 mmol · kg^{-1} · min^{-1} and 21 mM, respectively (202).

Despite the widespread use of the paired-tracer dilution method since its introduction in the early 1980s, there are a number of concerns with regard to the underlying assumptions of the technique for measurement of rapid influx into tissue and across parenchymal cell membranes. Criticisms and potential limitations of the method have been discussed in some detail previously (71). Careful critique of the method suggests that it is a qualitative indicator of rapid tracer lactate influx into the entire muscle tissue rather than a quantitative measure of influx across the sarcolemmal membrane. Recently, Gladden et al. (71) used the paired-tracer dilution method to make qualitative assessments of rapid tracer lactate influx into perfused dog gastrocnemii in situ. The results of these experiments were generally supportive of previous studies of muscle membrane lactate transport in more isolated systems and provided additional evidence of a physiological role for the lactate carrier in skeletal muscle.

These paired-tracer experiments (71) support the notion that lactate influx into canine skeletal muscle is a function of both a linear (possibly diffusive) component and a Michaelis-Menten (carrier-mediated) component. However, due to the qualitative nature of the paired-tracer method, reliable quantitative measures of membrane transport of lactate are unavailable. Multiple tracer methods and models such as those developed by Bassingthwaighte's group (e.g., 10, 128) offer great promise for providing quantitative answers to many of the questions that have been raised about lactate transport. Unlike the paired-tracer methods (103, 218), the multiple tracer methods employ realistic, and necessarily more complex, models of capillary–tissue exchange. Wolfe's group (33) has also presented a new model to quantify regional pyruvate and lactate transmembrane transport, shunting, exchange, production, and oxidation in vivo. The model relies on systemic infusion of pyruvate or lactate stable isotopic carbon tracers, and the measurement of pyruvate and lactate enrichment at several vascular sites and in tissues.

Summary

It is now firmly established that a significant, perhaps major, portion of lactate transfer across the sarcolemma is by way of cotransport with a proton on a monocarboxylate carrier. The carrier is bidirectional and probably symmetrical as well. There may be different isoforms of the carrier in different tissues or even within the same tissue, but this has not been established. Diffusion (primarily undissociated lactic acid) is also important and makes a greater contribution to transmembrane flux as the [La] increases and the monocarboxylate carrier approaches saturation. While the qualitative pattern of lactate transport across the sarcolemma is generally accepted, the quantitative aspects are unknown. For example, the reported values for V_{max} and K_m of the lactate carrier vary considerably. The carrier protein has not yet been identified, and the study of the molecular biology of lactate transport is in its infancy.

Clearly, characterization and understanding of the skeletal muscle membrane transport process for lactate is important. The presence of efficient lactate transport systems in different tissues throughout the body is essential for functioning of the lactate shuttle. However, it should be recognized that these transport processes may not be rate-limiting, and that they may not be primary regulators of lactate metabolism. Concentration gradients for lactate that are routinely observed between different tissue compartments and between tissue and blood may reflect the end result of rapid membrane transport of lactate to achieve an equilibrium that is dependent on the transmembrane [H^+] gradient (67, 164).

Lactate entry into and disposal by muscles in vivo or in situ quite obviously involves other processes in addition to muscle membrane transport. When lactate is presented to muscle in the blood stream, the uptake of that lactate (or at least a portion of it) is a complex event. As a minimum, lactate passes from the plasma through capillary pores into the interstitium, is transported across the sarcolemmal membrane, and at least a portion is metabolized. The process is further complicated by the presence of RBCs, which have three parallel pathways of lactate transport across their membrane (see below), and by the likelihood that some lactate is taken up by endothelial cells, with a portion being transported through the endothelial cells into the interstitium. Matters are further complicated by the fact that both [La] and [H^+] vary in different body compartments (e.g., intracellular vs. interstitial); this leads to variable *trans* acceleration effects and variable [H^+] gradient effects (see below) on lactate transport. Obviously, the reverse pathway for lactate efflux from muscle cells into the blood stream is equally complex.

MUSCLE AS A CONSUMER OF LACTATE: REGULATING FACTORS

Muscle lactate metabolism is affected by numerous factors. Many of the possible regulators of lactate production have been addressed earlier in this review. In addition, there have been several previous reviews that have discussed the causation of lactate production and the effect of factors such as exercise intensity, hypoxia, and aerobic training (19, 22, 40, 75, 98, 120, 121, 184, 198, 199, 203). Less attention has been given to the factors that may regulate lactate uptake and consumption by muscle. A partial list of the most important factors studied to date includes [La], metabolic rate, blood flow, [H^+], fiber type, and exercise training.

Lactate Concentration

Since the decline in blood [La] following exercise has usually been described by an exponential equation, it was proposed early on that the rate of removal of lactate from the body is directly proportional to the concentration of lactate (150). This point of view is supported by numerous studies in which the absolute rate of decline in blood [La] after exercise slows as the [La] itself decreases (e.g., 49). Radioactive tracer studies in dogs (105) and rats (62) have suggested that lactate uptake increases as the blood [La] increases. Pagliassotti and Donovan (154) examined the issue more directly by artificially perfusing three different skeletal muscle preparations (glycolytic, gracilis muscle; oxidative, soleus muscle; mixed, gastrocnemius, plantaris, and soleus) in anesthetized rabbits. Net lactate output reversed to net $\dot{L}$ in all three preparations as the perfusate [La] was increased, and net $\dot{L}$ increased with each further elevation of perfusate [La]. The relationship between net $\dot{L}$ and perfusate [La] was curvilinear, suggesting that the uptake would eventually approach a saturation limit.

Gladden et al. (68–70, 73, 159) have shown that net $\dot{L}$ by canine gastrocnemius muscle in situ increases in proportion to arterial blood [La]. In one of these studies (70), lactate/lactic acid solution was infused into arterial blood supplying the gastrocnemius at five different rates. These infusion rates ranged from zero, which allowed baseline plasma [La] of ~3 mM, to rates yielding plasma arterial inflow [La] of ~30 mM. The 30 min infusions provided plasma lactate concentrations that were within the physiological range for greyhounds following sprint exercise (48). Figure 14.9 illustrates that increasing plasma [La] increased net $\dot{L}$, with a tendency for net $\dot{L}$ to approach a plateau at the higher plasma lactate concentrations (~20–30 mM). These results raised another important and unanswered question: Is net $\dot{L}$ limited by the muscle's ability to metabolize lactate or is the limit imposed by the plasma membrane-bound lactate transport system?

Richter et al. (163) measured lactate exchange across human quadriceps muscle during different exercise conditions. The quadriceps released lactate during rest and contractions. However, when arm

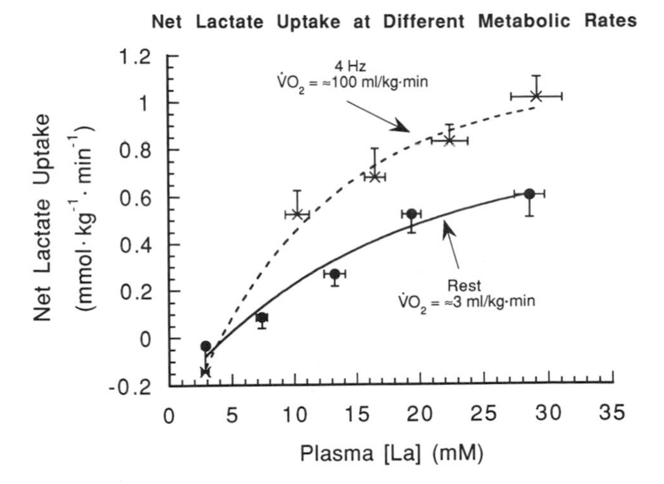

FIG. 14.9. Net lactate uptake by canine gastrocnemius in situ at rest and during contractions (twitches at 4 Hz) at a high metabolic rate with increasing plasma [La]. Two points are important: *(1)* with increasing [La], net lactate uptake approaches a plateau; and *(2)* net lactate uptake is higher with the higher metabolic rate of contractions. [Redrawn with permission from Gladden, L. B., R. E. Crawford, and M. J. Webster. Effect of lactate concentration and metabolic rate on net lactate uptake by canine skeletal muscle. *Am. J. Physiol.* 266 (*Regulatory Integrative Comp. Physiol.* 35): R1095–R1101, 1994 (70).]

exercise was added to the leg exercise, arterial [La] increased and the quadriceps reversed from net lactate output to net $\dot{L}$. Radioactive tracer studies in exercising humans also support an important role for [La] in determining net $\dot{L}$. When lactate metabolism was determined during progressive supine cycle ergometer exercise, extraction of continuously infused tracer lactate by the legs during rest and light exercise was linearly related to arterial blood [La] (188). Similarly, net $\dot{L}$ by the nonexercising arms was linearly related to arterial [La] throughout the progressive exercise. In a subsequent study of lactate appearance during exercise at altitude, Brooks et al. (25) observed that total lactate extraction (both labeled and unlabeled lactate) was a linear function of arterial [La]. Thus, both tracer and nontracer measurements indicate that net $\dot{L}$ by muscle is dependent on the [La] of the perfusing medium.

As discussed in some detail above, studies of sarcolemmal vesicles show that membrane transport of lactate is related to the transmembrane [La] gradient in a manner that is well described by a linear function (most likely simple diffusion) plus a Michaelis-Menten function (most likely the lactate carrier). Qualitative evaluations of lactate influx into skeletal muscle in situ via the paired-tracer dilution method support the conclusions of the sarcolemmal vesicle studies.

Metabolic Rate

Metabolic Rate: Effects on Lactate Metabolism. Resting skeletal muscle can take up significant amounts of lactate during periods of elevated blood [La] (67, 73, 154). What is the effect of an increase in metabolic rate on net $\dot{L}$? Typically, an elevated metabolic rate is associated with a faster glycolytic rate and concomitant lactate production. However, if the metabolic rate is elevated without a large increment in glycolysis, then net lactate utilization might be increased as a result of a faster rate of pyruvate and NADH oxidation. These requirements are likely met during steady-state submaximal exercise. Net lactate utilization may also be increased during more intense exercise after the contracting muscles have gone through the initial transient period (first 10–15 min) of rapid lactate release (23, 67).

The notion that net muscle $\dot{L}$ is stimulated by an increase in muscle metabolic rate is supported by numerous studies (e.g., 49) showing that the rate of blood [La] decline during recovery from intense exercise is enhanced by mild to moderate exercise during the recovery period. The increased rate of lactate decline during recovery with exercise may be a consequence of increased utilization of lactate as a fuel by the contracting muscles (67). Several groups have used isotopically labeled lactate to study lactate metabolism during exercise in intact rats (51), dogs (105), and men (136, 187), and across exercising muscle groups in rats (176), dogs (42, 79), and men (25, 188). The conclusions from these lactate tracer studies are as follows: *(1)* Oxidation is a major route of lactate disposal during both rest (40%–50% of lactate produced) and exercise (55%–87% of lactate produced during light exercise); *(2)* the rate of lactate production increases during exercise, but so does the rate of lactate removal; and *(3)* lactate removal occurs to a large extent in exercising muscles, most likely by way of oxidation. Lactate oxidation is linearly related to metabolic rate ($\dot{V}O_2$).

Gladden et al. (68, 70) have directly addressed the role of metabolic rate in net $\dot{L}$ by the canine gastrocnemius in situ. Lactate/lactic acid was infused to elevate arterial plasma [La] while maintaining normal acid–base status. As illustrated in Figure 14.9, net $\dot{L}$ was greater during 4 Hz twitch contractions (high metabolic rate) in comparison to rest (low metabolic rate) across a wide range of elevated lactate concentrations. These results support the idea that skeletal muscle is not simply a producer of lactate and that muscle can be a significant consumer of lactate even during contractions at a high metabolic rate. Since the net $\dot{L}$ measurements were done under steady-state conditions, this also supports the idea that the increased uptake represents an increased utilization of the lactate.

Metabolic Rate: Effects on Lactate Transport. Before the muscle can metabolize lactate from an external source, the lactate must cross the sarcolemmal membrane. Since muscle lactate utilization appears to be enhanced by an increased metabolic rate, it might be expected that increases in metabolic rate will also stimulate membrane transport of lactate. In one study, McDermott and Bonen (142) electrically stimulated the hindlimb muscles of anesthetized rats, and then muscle strips from the soleus muscle were incubated and used to determine rapid lactate influx. Thirty minutes of contractions did not increase the rate of lactate uptake by the muscle strips even though 2-deoxy-D-glucose uptake was stimulated by 47%. Subsequently, Bonen and McCullagh (14) extracted intact soleus and extensor digitorum longus muscles from mice that had been made to run on a treadmill. These muscles were then incubated and rapid lactate uptake was measured in vitro. Lactate uptake by the previously exercised muscles was increased by ~9%–28% above the uptake rate for nonexercised muscles. Watt et al. (201) investigated the effect of contractions on rapid lactate influx as determined via the paired-tracer dilution method in the perfused rat hindlimb. Electrical stimulation of the hindlimb muscles at perfusate [La] of 1 mM doubled the hindlimb $\dot{V}O_2$ and increased net lactate output by more than tenfold; however, rapid tracer lactate influx was unchanged, suggesting that there was no increase in lactate transport. Overall, it appears that any enhancement of lactate transport by exercise is minimal, especially when compared to the increases that are typically reported for muscle glucose uptake (~62%–400%) in response to exercise (76, 148, 178). This also supports a predominant role for lactate metabolism rather than lactate transport in the determination of rate of lactate exchange.

Blood Flow

In the case of net $\dot{L}$, it could be argued that if all other factors remain constant, an increased blood flow should increase lactate and proton delivery to the muscle, thereby maintaining more favorable extracellular to intracellular lactate and proton gradients, thus promoting $\dot{L}$. Influx of lactate for net $\dot{L}$ involves at least two processes in series (69): *(1)* influx of lactate from the blood into the interstitial space, and *(2)* the influx of lactate from the interstitial space into the muscle cell. Because most of the net $\dot{L}$ will involve either undissociated lactic acid or coupled lactate and proton movement (113, 140, 166, 168, 202), maintenance of both a high $[H^+]$ and [La] in the interstitial fluid could be important. In this context, an adequate blood flow with appropriate distribution might be expected to promote net $\dot{L}$ by ensuring that an adequate supply of both hydrogen and lactate ions is delivered to the interstitial space.

Gladden et al. (69) investigated the possible effect of blood flow on net $\dot{L}$ in the dog gastrocnemius in situ. In all trials, metabolic rate and blood [La] were controlled while blood flow was varied. Lactate/lactic acid was infused to establish a blood [La] of ~12 mM while maintaining normal acid–base status. In one series, the gastrocnemius was stimulated to contract with twitches at 1 Hz while blood flow was adjusted by a pump to either *(1)* the spontaneous level for 1 Hz contractions, or *(2)* a level that was ~65% greater than the spontaneous level. The increase in blood flow had no effect on net $\dot{L}$. In a second series, four different perfusion pressures were presented to each gastrocnemius as it contracted at 1 Hz; the different perfusion pressures caused a twofold variation in blood flow to the gastrocnemius. In this series, net $\dot{L}$ was greater only at the highest perfusion pressure and blood flow. Altogether, these experiments suggested that blood flow probably has little effect on net $\dot{L}$ over a fairly wide low-to-middle range of normal flow rates for the gastrocnemius. The possibility remains that blood flow may have an independent effect on net $\dot{L}$ at the upper extreme of the normal blood flow range during contractions of the dog gastrocnemius.

Possible effects of flow on the transport process for lactate influx into muscle tissue are difficult to evaluate. Watt et al. (201) attempted to assess the effects of perfusate flow on rapid tracer lactate influx into isolated, resting rat hindlimb. Rapid tracer lactate influx as measured by the paired-tracer dilution method was dependent on perfusate flow at rates less than $0.5\ ml \cdot g^{-1} \cdot min^{-1}$. The apparent dependence of rapid tracer lactate influx on flow at the lower perfusate flow rates could be due to the rapid movement of lactate across skeletal muscle membranes. At lower flows, rapid tracer lactate influx might be followed by rapid efflux of some of the tracer during the course of the measurement. This would have the effect of lowering the measured influx rate, so the observed dependency of lactate influx may not be a real occurrence but rather a reflection of back-flux of tracer. Limitations of the paired-tracer method prevent definitive conclusions.

Hydrogen Ion Concentration

There has been extensive study of the possible effects of $[H^+]$ on lactate production both directly by inhibition of key glycolytic enzymes (see 59, 131, 181) and indirectly by inhibition of the contractile process (see 59, 131). However, less attention has been given to possible effects of [H^+] on lactate utilization, which would most likely be related to intramuscular (intracellular) [H^+]. It is a reasonable assumption that *if* increased intracellular [H^+] inhibits lactate production in the presence of an adequate exogenous [La], then lactate utilization will be enhanced. In this context, Graham et al. (77) reported that acidosis, induced by hypercapnia, resulted in net $\dot{L}$ by dog gastrocnemii in situ after 20 min of contractions at 3 Hz. Under normal acid–base conditions, the gastrocnemii were still releasing lactate after 20 min of contraction at 3 Hz. Bonen et al. (16) have also reported that glycogen synthesis from lactate in mouse fast-twitch (EDL) and slow-twitch (soleus) muscles in vitro was stimulated by decreases in external pH over the physiological range. Glycogen formation from lactate (10 mM) was increased by 49% in the soleus and by 39% in the EDL at external pH of 6.5 as compared to pH 7.4. Whether this enhancement of glyconeogenesis was due to a reduced intracellular pH that inhibited PFK activity thus promoting reversal of glycolysis or was due to a greater transmembrane [H^+] gradient that increased membrane transport of lactate is unclear. Further study of the interaction between intracellular [H^+] and lactate utilization is needed.

Several studies (14, 113, 116, 140, 142, 168) have addressed the relationship between [H^+] and membrane transport of lactate. The most thorough study of [H^+] and membrane lactate transport is that of Roth and Brooks (168), in which both intra- and extravesicular [H^+] were manipulated in experiments with sarcolemmal vesicles. When the extravesicular [H^+] was greater than intravesicular [H^+], the initial rate of lactate influx into the vesicles was always enhanced in parallel with the increased [H^+] gradient from outside to inside. At an extravesicular pH of 5.6 with intravesicular pH at 7.4, lactate influx was about ten times faster at 1 mM [La] and greater than five times faster at 10 mM extravesicular [La]. Similar results were obtained when intravesicular [H^+] was varied. Any increase in the [H^+] gradient across the vesicular membrane stimulated flux across the membrane in the direction of high [H^+] to low [H^+]. Lactate flux was markedly inhibited when the direction of the [H^+] gradient was counter to the [La] gradient. Lactate transport inhibitors were less effective with greater transmembrane [H^+] gradients in the study of Roth and Brooks (168). For example, at intravesicular pH 7.4, ~85% of lactate influx could be blocked at extravesicular pH 7.4, but only ~63%–83% at extravesicular pH 5.9. This suggests that the lactate carrier may account for less of the total lactate transport at higher [H^+] gradients while undissociated lactic acid (HLa) diffusion accounts for more. At a [La] of 1 mM, ~30 times as much HLa is present at pH 5.9 as at pH 7.4 (168).

Unlike the case for [H^+] manipulations on only one side of the membrane, simultaneous changes of [H^+] on both sides of the vesicular membrane with no [H^+] gradient results in similar rates of lactate transport, suggesting that absolute [H^+] is much less important than the [H^+] gradient (168). Juel (113) has argued that H^+ may be stimulatory to transport if lactate is present, but inhibitory in the absence of lactate. He (113) postulated that the H^+ might bind to the lactate carrier first, and then if lactate is not bound, the protonated carrier might not be able to reorient itself. If this is the case, then simultaneous changes of [H^+] on both sides of the membrane might counteract each other when lactate is present on only one side. In other words, additional H^+ on the side with lactate would stimulate lactate binding to the carrier and transport to the other side. However, additional H^+ on the side without lactate would inhibit carrier reorientation because of the increased likelihood of H^+ binding without lactate binding.

In experiments with giant sarcolemmal vesicles, Juel et al. (113, 116) have also found that efflux of lactate from vesicles with intravesicular pH of 7.4 was reduced when the extravesicular pH was decreased below 7.4, whereas lactate efflux was increased at extravesicular pH values above 7.4. Again, lactate transport is stimulated in the direction of the [H^+] gradient. In equilibrium exchange experiments, equal increases in [H^+] on both sides of the vesicular membrane stimulated lactate flux (113, 116). This was attributed mainly to an increase in simple diffusion of undissociated HLa because of the greater concentration of HLa at higher [H^+].

Bonen and colleagues (14, 140, 142) have reported effects of [H^+] on lactate uptake by sarcolemmal vesicles, small strips of rat soleus muscle, and small intact mouse EDL and soleus muscles. Although their (14, 140, 142) findings were generally similar to those of Roth and Brooks (168) and Juel et al. (113, 116), they suggest in contrast that the stimulation of lactate influx by an increased inwardly directed [H^+] gradient is not entirely due to the concomitant increase in [HLa] on the low pH, external side. Bonen et al. (140, 142) manipulated external [HLa] in two ways: *(1)* constant external pH of 7.4 with different external lactate concentrations from 0.5–25 mM, and *(2)* constant external [La] with different external pH values from 6.0–8.0.

Subsequently, lactate uptake into both sarcolemmal vesicles and muscle strips was plotted as a function of external [HLa] for the two different manipulations. For a given increase in external [HLa], lactate influx was stimulated more when the ionic [La^-] was greater. This supports the notion that H^+ ions in the presence of lactate promote the loading of lactate onto the carrier and thus enhance the rate of lactate transport.

The physiological significance of the results reported from sarcolemmal vesicles and muscle strips in vitro is supported by experiments on the perfused rat hindlimb in situ (202). Watt et al. (202) used the paired-tracer method and found that rapid tracer lactate influx was increased by 30% at 1 mM [La] and by 12% at 50 mM [La] when the perfusate pH was decreased from 7.4 to 6.8. When perfusate pH was increased from 7.4 to 7.7, rapid tracer lactate influx was decreased by ~20% at both 1 mM and 50 mM [La].

Note that changes in [H^+] in vivo can have opposing effects (146). For example, blood acidosis may stimulate lactate uptake by muscles that have a [La] lower than blood, but at the same time inhibit lactate output from those muscles which have a [La] higher than blood. Another important point is that whereas the effects of respiratory and nonrespiratory acid–base changes appear to be generally similar (138, 182, 183), there may be some potentially confounding differences. It has been suggested that changes in extracellular [H^+] due to variations in P_{CO_2} are more effective than nonrespiratory extracellular [H^+] changes in altering intracellular [H^+] (196). This could occur because of a greater cell membrane permeability to CO_2 than to nonrespiratory acids. If this is the case, then nonrespiratory [H^+] changes should generate a greater transmembrane [H^+] difference and therefore have a greater effect on membrane transport of lactate. On the other hand, respiratory [H^+] changes should cause a greater change in intracellular [H^+], but a smaller change in transmembrane [H^+] difference. This might translate into a greater effect on lactate production and thereby utilization, and a lesser effect on membrane transport of lactate (67).

Muscle Fiber Type

Net Lactate Uptake and Disposal. Lactate uptake and disposal appears to vary greatly among the different fiber types. Baldwin et al. (9) investigated the capacity of muscle homogenates from different fiber types to oxidize lactate at 2–10 mM [La]. Lactate oxidation was greatest in homogenates from fast, oxidative glycolytic muscles, intermediate in the homogenates from oxidative muscles, and lowest in the homogenates from glycolytic muscles. The lactate oxidation was highly correlated with the total LDH H-isozyme activity. Soon afterwards, McLane and Holloszy (143) measured lactate incorporation into glycogen in rat hindlimb muscles during perfusion with medium containing 12 mM lactate as the only substrate. There was minimal incorporation of lactate into glycogen in the soleus muscle, which consists predominantly of slow-twitch red muscle fibers. In contrast, lactate was rapidly incorporated into glycogen in both fast-twitch white and fast-twitch red muscle fibers. These findings were confirmed in experiments by Shiota, Golden, and Katz (176), in which rat hindlimb muscles were perfused with medium containing 10 mM lactate as the only substrate.

Pagliassotti and Donovan (153–155) performed elegant experiments on lactate uptake and metabolism in resting muscles of three different fiber types in anesthetized rabbits. The three preparations were the glycolytic gracilis muscle (99.1% type IIb fibers); the oxidative soleus muscle (97.5% type I fibers); and a mixed preparation comprised of gastrocnemius, plantaris, and soleus together (25% type I, 31% type IIa, and 44% type IIb fibers). Oxidative muscle preparations first began to take up lactate at ~2.5 mM [La], whereas net $\dot{L}$ was first observed at 4 mM in glycolytic and mixed muscle preparations. The rate of net $\dot{L}$ was greatest in the mixed muscles, intermediate in the oxidative muscles, and lowest in the glycolytic muscles. Oxidation was the primary fate of the lactate taken up by the oxidative and mixed preparations, whereas glyconeogenesis was the major fate of lactate removal in the glycolytic preparation. At 8 mM [La], apparent oxidation accounted for 51%, 39%, and 28% of total net lactate removal by the oxidative, mixed, and glycolytic preparations, respectively (154). Lactate incorporation into glycogen at 8 mM [La] accounted for 2%, 26%, and 48% of the total net $\dot{L}$ by the oxidative, mixed, and glycolytic preparations, respectively (155). The work of Bonen et al. (16) on both mouse fast- and slow-twitch muscle in vitro supports the findings of Pagliassotti and Donovan (153–155). Bonen et al. (16) found that glycogen synthesis from lactate (5–20 mM [La] in incubation medium) was three- to fourfold greater in the fast-twitch EDL than in the slow-twitch soleus. These studies clearly show that both the rate of muscle lactate uptake and the route of disposal for lactate depends on the fiber-type composition of the muscle.

Lactate Transport. Two studies (14, 115) have investigated lactate transport in different muscle fiber types. First, Juel et al. (115) found that giant sarcolemmal vesicles from "red" rat muscle fibers had a 50% greater equilibrium exchange rate for carrier-mediated lactate transport capacity than did the vesicles from "white" muscles. Additionally, the rate constant for lactate efflux from giant vesicles derived from rabbit soleus (97.5% type I fibers) was 39% faster than the rate constant for efflux from vesicles derived from the gracilis (99.1% type IIb fibers). In a second study of lactate transport and fiber type, Bonen and McCullagh (14) investigated rapid lactate uptake into isolated EDL (fast-twitch) and soleus (slow-twitch) muscles from mice. Lactate uptake was significantly faster in the soleus muscles across a range of external lactate concentrations from ~5–50 mM; at 30 mM [La], uptake by the soleus was ~40% faster than that by the EDL.

The finding that lactate transport is faster in oxidative muscle fibers than in glycolytic fibers runs counter to the notion that glycolytic muscle fibers are prone to high lactate production rates during contractions/exercise and that they should be equipped for rapid transport of lactate out to the extracellular environment. However, oxidative fibers do produce lactate and they are usually active for longer periods of time than are glycolytic fibers. A greater ability to transport lactate (and H^+ ions at the same time) out of oxidative fibers might partially explain the greater resistance to fatigue in oxidative fibers (115). Furthermore, peak lactate production by oxidative muscle fibers may be greater than is usually appreciated. For example, peak lactate output by contracting, oxidative canine gastrocnemius muscle in situ is similar to peak lactate output by contracting, glycolytic feline gastrocnemius muscle in situ (185). Finally, the faster lactate transport rates in oxidative fibers may reflect the role of lactate as an energy substrate for those fibers, whereas the slower lactate transport rates in glycolytic fibers may coincide with greater retention of lactate during recovery from intense exercise. The retained lactate in glycolytic fibers following exercise is then more likely to be resynthesized into glycogen (154, 155).

Exercise Training

Lactate Metabolism. Blood and muscle lactate concentrations are lower at the same absolute and relative work rates following endurance training (98). This has most often been attributed to a lower lactate production by skeletal muscle as the result of increased muscle mitochondrial density, a concomitant increase in oxidative capacity, a decrease in muscle LDH activity, a decrease in the percentage of the M-type isozyme of LDH, and increased reliance on fat oxidation as a source of energy (98); see Part III of this *Handbook*.

Endurance training may also cause an increase in lactate utilization by muscles. Donovan and Brooks (51) studied the effects of endurance training on lactate metabolism in rats by radioactive lactate tracer techniques. They (51) found that the metabolic clearance rate of lactate was 107% greater in trained animals than in sedentary animals during hard exercise. Presumably, a large proportion of the metabolic clearance of lactate occurred in skeletal muscle. Studies of lactate infusion into resting rats have also shown that lactate clearance is faster following endurance training (52, 53). With increasing rates of lactate infusion, blood [La] rose in a curvilinear fashion, reaching greater than 11 mM in sedentary rats as compared to ~5.5 mM in endurance-trained rats. This training response was due to a more rapid rise in net lactate removal with increases in blood [La]. Further analysis of the net lactate removal rates as a function of blood [La] revealed that the K_m was dramatically lowered after training to a value that was one-third that of the sedentary animals (4 vs. 12 mM). Although this improved clearance of lactate with endurance training can be attributed to changes in the ability of a number of different organs to handle lactate (e.g., liver, heart), it is quite likely that changes in lactate removal capacity of skeletal muscle constitute a major component of the overall response (141).

In the first longitudinal investigation of the effects of endurance training on lactate appearance and clearance in humans, MacRae et al. (132) applied radioisotope dilution measurements during progressive exercise before and after a 9 week endurance training program. As expected, there was a slower rise in blood [La] with increasing work rate after the training period. The tracer technique revealed that the lower blood [La] response was due to a reduced rate of lactate appearance at the lower work rates and an increased metabolic clearance rate of lactate at the higher work rates. This study generally agrees with previous studies on animals and supports the view that endurance training not only reduces muscle lactate production, but also increases muscle lactate utilization.

Lactate Transport. Enhancement of lactate clearance by training could be due to an increased facility for lactate utilization as reviewed above and/or an increased ability to transport lactate into and out of muscles. Improved membrane transport of lactate would promote lactate efflux from muscles that are producing lactate, and aid influx into less active muscles for oxidation and/or glyconeogenesis (141).

Roth and Brooks (169) examined zero-*trans* lactate influx into sarcolemmal vesicles from mixed rat hindlimb skeletal muscles in control animals, endurance-trained animals, and sprint-trained animals. Neither endurance training nor sprint training affected K_m or V_{max} for the transport process. In other words, lactate transport rate and capacity were unaltered by training.

In contrast, Pilegaard et al. (157) found that equilibrium exchange lactate efflux rate (30 mM [La]) from giant sarcolemmal vesicles from rat hindlimb muscles was significantly faster (+58%) after moderate-intensity (~90% $\dot{V}O_{2max}$) treadmill training. Similarly, high-intensity (~112% $\dot{V}O_{2max}$) treadmill training resulted in an increase in the equilibrium exchange lactate efflux rate at 10, 30 (+76%), and 60 mM [La]. These results suggest that training may lower the K_m and increase the V_{max} for carrier-mediated lactate transport in the sarcolemmal membrane. A lower K_m implies that the transport protein has a higher affinity for lactate after training, while a higher V_{max} implies greater membrane density of the transport protein and/or an increased turnover rate through the membrane for the individual transport proteins. Another possibility is that the muscle fiber-type composition might have shifted to a greater percentage of oxidative fibers. Since the oxidative fibers have been shown to have a faster lactate transport rate, this could explain the faster rates of lactate flux after training.

McDermott and Bonen (141) investigated the effects of endurance treadmill training (~78% of $\dot{V}O_{2max}$) on lactate influx into classical, small sarcolemmal vesicles under zero-*trans* conditions at 1 and 50 mM [La]. The initial lactate influx rate at 1 mM [La] was increased by 59% as the result of training. However, there was no difference in lactate influx between vesicles from control animals and trained animals at 50 mM [La]. The interpretation of these data was that endurance training reduced the K_m, implying a higher affinity of the carrier for lactate, and that the training had no effect on the maximal lactate transport capacity (V_{max}), implying no increase in transport protein density in the membrane and no increase in the turnover speed (141). McDermott and Bonen (141) also offered a more complex explanation for the reduction in K_m. If the muscle membrane contains a family of lactate carriers, each with a different affinity for lactate, then endurance training could have caused a shift in the protein isoform composition such that there was a greater percentage of isoforms with high lactate affinity in the trained muscles (141).

The only investigation of the effect of training on lactate transport in humans is the cross-sectional study of Pilegaard et al. (156). Muscle biopsies were obtained from the vastus lateralis of three groups of subjects (untrained, trained, and athletes) and treated with collagenase solution to generate giant sarcolemmal vesicles. The mean efflux rate with 30 mM intravesicular [La] under zero-*trans* conditions was significantly higher from the vesicles of the athletes as compared to vesicles from the untrained and trained groups. However, no subject with $\dot{V}O_{2max}$ less than 68 ml · kg^{-1} · min^{-1} had a greater than average lactate transport capability. When the athletic group was further subdivided, the results suggested that two factors were required to improve lactate transport ability: *(1)* a high volume (frequency and duration) of training combined with *(2)* regular high-intensity training. The highest vesicular lactate transport rates were found in two 4 km bicyclists, one of whom was a bronze medalist at the 1992 Olympic Games.

To summarize, investigations of the effects of training on membrane transport of lactate have been contradictory. Training has been reported to *(1)* have no effect on membrane lactate transport ability (169), *(2)* increase the V_{max} and decrease the K_m for membrane transport of lactate (157), *(3)* decrease the K_m, but have no effect on the V_{max} for transport (141), and *(4)* cause an increase in lactate transport rate in human athletes when the training volume and intensity are extremely high (156). Some of the apparent discrepancies may arise from differences in experimental procedures such as the gender of animals studied, training programs, and methods of lactate transport measurement.

Possible benefits of an improved membrane transport ability for lactate could be realized in several ways. Faster lactate transport rates could accelerate the efflux of lactate and protons from rapidly glycolyzing muscle fibers to neighboring fibers that are less active and/or more oxidative. Lactate and protons could also be moved more quickly across the sarcolemma into the interstitial fluid and into the blood. The faster lactate transport would also hasten uptake of lactate into less active and/or more oxidative fibers, both in the active muscles and at sites distant to the sites of work output. However, before these ideas can be accepted, the role of membrane lactate transport in the regulation of lactate dynamics must be determined. At this time, it appears that the metabolic effects of an increased mitochondrial density have the major impact on lactate kinetics after endurance training. It is likely that the sarcolemma provides only minimal resistance to the overall lactate exchange between cells (169), although this concept has been challenged (33).

Summary

In the lactate shuttle hypothesis, intermediary metabolism is coordinated among different tissues and cells by the conversion of glucose and glycogen to lactate and the subsequent exchange of lactate between and among those tissues and cells. This shuttle may be especially active during dynamic exercise. Because of its large mass and metabolic capacity, skeletal muscle is perhaps the major component of the lactate shuttle, not only in terms of lactate production but also in terms of net $\dot{L}$ and utilization. In this context, the major determinants of net $\dot{L}$ by muscle appear to be the [La] gradient from blood to muscle, the metabolic rate, the hydrogen ion concentration, muscle fiber type, and the training state. Most of these factors affect not only the rate of metabolic utilization of lactate by muscle, but also the rate of sarcolemmal lactate transport.

BLOOD TRANSPORT OF LACTATE

The blood is a key component in the lactate shuttle because it distributes lactate to all tissues. The transport of lactate across the RBC membrane proceeds by three distinct pathways: *(1)* nonionic diffusion of the undissociated acid; *(2)* an inorganic anion exchange system, often referred to as the band 3 system; and *(3)* a monocarboxylate-specific carrier mechanism (47). Lactate transport into the RBCs has been recently reviewed in detail by Poole and Halestrap (161). Since metabolism in the RBCs is anaerobic and forms lactate, an efficient system of lactate efflux is essential (85). However, the small amount of lactate produced by the RBCs can probably be handled by nonionic diffusion and the band 3 system, and does not necessarily require the monocarboxylate carrier (45). On the other hand, intense exercise causes an intramuscular accumulation of lactate and hydrogen ions that can inhibit muscular function. Lactate and hydrogen ions move out of muscles into the interstitial fluid via the transport pathways discussed earlier. From the interstitial fluid, lactate and hydrogen ions gain access to the blood through endothelial clefts and probably across endothelial cells as well. Although lactate can be taken up and utilized as a fuel by endothelial cells (127), the extent to which lactate and H^+ ions move from interstitial fluid to blood or vice versa by way of a transendothelial cell route is unknown.

Within whole blood, lactate can be found in both RBCs and plasma. During intense exercise, a system designed to cotransport lactate and hydrogen ions from the plasma into the RBCs could aid in establishing a gradient between the plasma and interstitial fluid, and enhancing the available space for efflux of lactate and H^+ ions from the exercising muscles (45, 166). Additionally, a coupled cotransport system for monocarboxylates and hydrogen ions may be advantageous with regard to RBC buffering capacity and acid–base homeostasis. Once in the blood, lactate and H^+ ions are transported away from the exercising muscles to sites of lactate removal such as the liver, heart, inactive muscle, and mild to moderately active muscle. Whole blood [La] before, during, and after exercise depends on the balance between net entry of lactate into the blood primarily from active skeletal muscles and the redistribution to and removal from the blood by various sites of net lactate uptake.

Lactate Distribution between Plasma and RBCs

At rest, the distribution of lactate between the plasma and intraerythrocyte compartments is unequal, with approximately one-third of the total whole blood lactate being found within the RBCs and two-thirds within the plasma (61, 72, 108, 114, 179). As an example, at a resting whole blood water [La] of 0.8 mM, RBC water [La] might be 0.5 mM, while the plasma water [La] is 1.0 mM. The gradients between plasma and RBCs for lactate and other ions appear to be largely due to a Donnan equilibrium (17, 60, 63, 108). In such a system, ions that can move across the cell membrane are distributed in relation to nonpenetrating ions on either side of the membrane. In the case of the RBCs, hemoglobin is the major nonpenetrating constituent, and it has a net negative charge. Accordingly, negative ions such as chloride, bicarbonate, and lactate, which can traverse the membrane, will be in higher concentrations in the plasma than in RBCs, whereas positive ions such as H^+ will be at higher concentrations in the RBCs than in the plasma (17, 60, 63, 108). For example, the RBC/plasma [La] ratio is mirrored by the plasma/RBC [H^+] ratio (17, 60, 63).

As lactate is released into the blood from contracting muscles during exercise, the lactate first enters the plasma phase and then moves into the RBCs, primarily via the monocarboxylate transport system. If lactate enters the plasma at a rate that can be handled by the membrane transport pathways of the RBC membrane, then both plasma and RBC lactate concentrations will rise proportionally. Consequently, the [La] gradient from plasma to RBCs will increase, but the ratio of RBCs to plasma [La] will not change from the value at rest. However, if lactate were to enter the plasma at a rate exceeding the ability of the RBCs to take up lactate and equilibrate with the plasma, then the result would be a disproportionate increase in plasma [La] relative to RBCs [La] and therefore a decline in the RBC/plasma [La] ratio. Both Smith et al. (180) and Foxdal et al. (61) found that the [La] gradient from plasma to RBCs increased with exercise intensity during progressive incremental exercise. However, the RBC/plasma [La] ratio (~0.60) was unchanged from rest through the highest exercise intensity. These results were not affected by the duration of the work rate increment (1, 4, and 5 min) (61, 180).

In another study, Smith et al. (179) followed plasma and RBC lactate concentrations during 30 min of steady-state cycle ergometer exercise at two different work rates, 40% of $\dot{V}O_{2peak}$ (<LT) and 70% $\dot{V}O_{2peak}$ (>LT). During >LT exercise, plasma [La] rose above 6 mM. There was a sizeable [La] gradient (~3.5 mM) from plasma to RBCs during most of the >LT trial. In the <LT exercise, plasma [La] increased only slightly above rest (2.4 mM) and the [La] gradient from plasma to RBCs averaged 0.8 mM. Despite drastically different plasma-to-RBC [La] gradients in the >LT and <LT exercises, the ratio of RBCs to plasma [La] was the same for both (0.58) and not significantly different from rest. These results suggest that an equilibration between plasma and RBCs was reached with respect to [La].

The greatest demand on blood lactate transport occurs during and immediately after intense exercise of short duration in which whole blood [La] commonly reaches 11–20 mM (75). These large increases in [La] are the result of rapid lactate production by contracting muscles and a concomitant rapid entry of lactate and protons into the blood. Juel et al. (114) examined this situation in a study of lactate distribution in the blood following exhaustive dynamic exercise with the knee extensors of one leg. During and immediately following the exhaustive exercise, a large [La] gradient developed between plasma and RBCs in both arterial blood (Δ[La] = ~7 mM) and femoral venous blood (Δ[La] = ~13 mM). Plasma [La] was not in equilibrium with the RBCs [La], as evidenced by a decrease in the RBC/plasma [La] ratio from ~0.5 at rest to ~0.2 in femoral venous blood and ~0.3 in arterial blood at exhaustion. The ratio returned towards the normal resting value during resting recovery. Similar results were reported by Gladden et al. (72) in a preliminary report in which subjects performed 1 min of maximal cycling. Immediately after the exercise, the RBC/plasma [La] ratio had declined to ~0.3 from ~0.6 at rest.

Together, these studies of lactate transport in blood suggest that under most exercise conditions, RBCs can take up lactate at a rate that is proportional to its rate of entry into the plasma. As a result, RBC [La] reaches an equilibrium with plasma [La] and causes an RBC/plasma [La] ratio that is similar to the resting value even when there is a large [La] gradient from plasma to RBCs. Under most conditions, the plasma will contain ~70% and the RBCs ~30% of the increased [La] in the blood occurring between rest and peak exercise. The exception to [La] equilibration between plasma and RBCs occurs immediately following intense "all-out" exercise, when lactate entry into the plasma occurs at a proportionally faster rate than uptake of lactate into the RBCs. Overall, equilibration of plasma and RBC lactate concentrations must depend on several factors including the rate of lactate release from the contracting muscles, the rate of RBC membrane transport of lactate, the hematocrit of blood perfusing the active muscles, and the blood flow rate to the active muscles.

These conclusions must be tempered by two practical experimental issues. First, immediately upon collection of blood samples, exchange of lactate between plasma and RBCs must be minimized. The half-time for equilibration of RBC lactate with plasma lactate has been reported to be between 50 s (114) and 2 min (108) at 37°C. Lactate exchange can be stopped by immediate, rapid centrifugation (114) or rapid cooling to near 0°C followed by centrifugation (72, 179). Second, the site of blood collection has important implications. In most of the studies cited above, blood was sampled from a forearm vein during leg exercise. During the return of blood from the legs to the central circulation and eventually to a forearm vein, lactate can be taken up from the plasma into the RBCs, allowing partial if not complete equilibration of lactate across the RBC membrane during the circulation time. Clearly, disequilibrium is more likely to be found if blood is sampled from a vein that drains the muscles producing lactate.

Comparative Aspects of Lactate Transport in RBCs

As noted above, the transport of lactate across the RBC membrane proceeds by three parallel pathways. The significance of these pathways with regard to lactate transport varies among species (46, 161). The monocarboxylate-specific carrier is the predominant pathway in the RBCs of some mammals (humans, rabbits, and rats), while the band 3 system is the preferred pathway for lactate transport in the RBCs of other mammals (e.g., ox) (46). Skelton et al. (177) compared lactate influx into RBCs of "athletic" animals versus "nonathletic" animals. The animals were categorized on the basis of known differences in oxidative capability. Dogs and horses were chosen as aerobic athletes, since they demonstrate a $\dot{V}O_{2max}$ that is two to three times higher than that of their "same size" nonathletic counterparts, goats and cattle (41, 110, 193). As illustrated in Figure 14.10, the RBCs of the athletic species (horses and dogs) had a significantly enhanced lactate influx rate in comparison to the RBCs of the nonathletic species (cattle and goats) at lactate concentrations from 1.6–41 mM extracellular [La]. These differences in lactate influx were correlated with the predominant pathway of transport. The monocarboxylate carrier was the primary pathway in RBCs of the athletic species (~90% of total lactate influx), whereas the band 3 system was the primary pathway in RBCs of nonathletic species (56%–83% of total lactate influx at various lactate concentrations). The band 3 pathway appears to be a slow system of lactate exchange, whereas the monocarboxylate pathway provides rapid movement of lactate across the erythrocyte membrane (46). Prevalence of the monocarboxylate system as the major pathway of lactate transport in the RBCs of athletic species may give them a faster lactate influx.

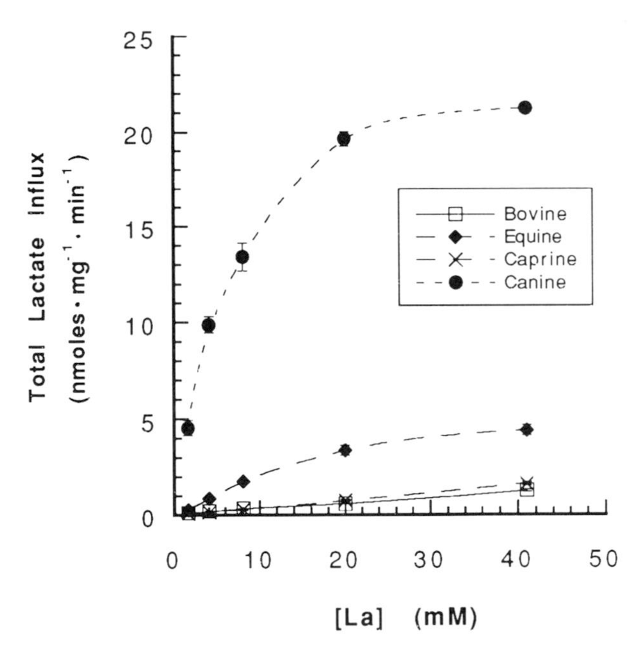

FIG. 14.10. Total lactate influx via all three parallel pathways of lactate transport in the RBCs of "athletic" (equine and canine) and "nonathletic" (bovine and caprine) species. Lactate influx was much more rapid in the RBCs of the "athletic" species. [Redrawn with permission from Skelton, M. S., D. E. Kremer, E. W. Smith, and L. B. Gladden. Lactate influx into red blood cells of "athletic" and "nonathletic" species. *Am. J. Physiol.* 268 (*Regulatory Integrative Comp. Physiol.* 37): R1121–R1128, 1995 (177).]

What is the physiological relevance of the differences in RBC lactate influx observed by Skelton et al. (177)? Possibly, athletic animals with high capacity for oxidative metabolism are more likely to engage in "exercise" at a high metabolic rate. The use of the monocarboxylate-specific carrier mechanism as the primary pathway of lactate transport may be advantageous during exercise conditions that result in an increased production of lactic acid. Transport of the resulting lactate and hydrogen ions away from the exercising muscle and into the blood by the rapid, cotransport design of the monocarboxylate pathway may reduce the potential for muscle acidosis and eventual fatigue (177). On the other hand, the band 3 system of lactate transport involves the entry of a lactate anion into the erythrocyte by a nonspecific anion transporter analogous to the carrier-mediated action for chloride, sulfate, phosphate, and bicarbonate anions (44, 85). Reliance on this system as the primary pathway for lactate transport might be a disadvantage during intense exercise, since it is a slower transporter and would not remove the fatigue-causing hydrogen ions as rapidly (59, 177). The lactate shuttle may be more highly developed or function differently in aerobic animals than in glycolytic animals.

ALTITUDE

Muscle and blood lactate concentrations represent the combined effects of several regulating factors including intracellular PO_2, biochemical agents that affect enzyme activity, sympathoadrenal activity, and rate of lactate appearance vs. disappearance. Each of these regulators may be influenced by exposure to high altitude. Accordingly, altitude represents a natural environment that has differing effects on various components of the lactate shuttle and warrants special consideration. A surprising result of these complex interactions is the lactate paradox phenomenon.

The Lactate Paradox

Acute exposure to high altitude or hypoxia results in higher blood lactate concentrations at any given work rate; but at exhaustion, the maximal blood [La] is the same as at sea level under normoxic conditions. However, with acclimatization to high altitude, the blood [La] at a given work rate is lower than during acute exposure, and approaches the concentration observed at sea level (13, 23, 81, 82, 133,

135, 162, 206, 207, 217) (see Fig. 14.11 for an example of this response). In fact, the higher the altitude of acclimatization, the lower the blood lactate concentrations observed after acclimatization (133). Furthermore, when acclimatized individuals exercise to exhaustion, the maximal blood [La] is lower than that observed at sea level or upon acute exposure to high altitude (82, 122, 206, 207). Again, the higher the altitude of acclimatization, the lower the maximal blood [La] observed [see Fig. 14.12; (122, 206, 207)]. One might expect that with continued hypoxia during the period of acclimatization, individuals might continue to rely heavily on glycolytic metabolism to supply energy for work performance; hence the paradox that blood lactate concentrations are actually lower than during initial exposure to the hypoxia of high altitude (89).

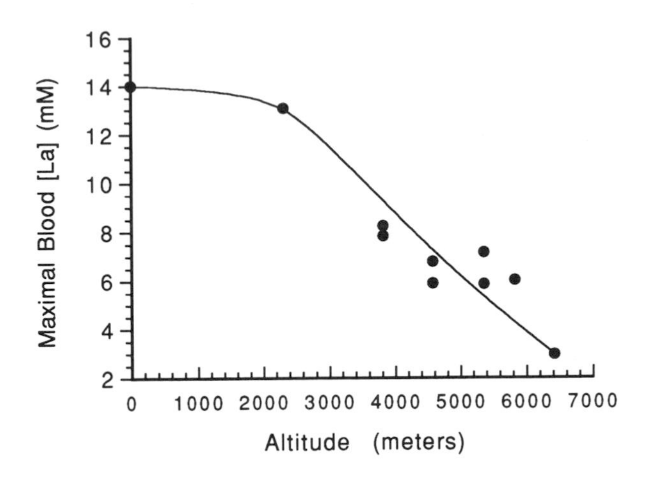

FIG. 14.12. Maximal blood [La] following exhaustive exercise in high-altitude natives and acclimatized sea level natives (data combined). Note that maximal blood [La] declines as altitude increases. [Data are from Cerretelli et al. (31) and West et al. (208) and are redrawn with permission from West, J. B. Acid-base status and blood lactate at extreme altitude. In: *Hypoxia, Metabolic Acidosis, and the Circulation*, edited by A. I. Arieff. New York: Oxford University Press, 1992, p. 33–44 (207).]

Explanations for the Lactate Paradox

What is (are) the underlying mechanism(s) for the lactate paradox? A number of hypotheses have been offered to explain the phenomenon, including: *(1)* sequestration of lactate inside muscle cells, *(2)* improvement of O_2 supply to muscle during acclimatization, *(3)* muscle glycogen depletion during acclimatization, *(4)* inability to fully activate skeletal muscles, *(5)* low blood bicarbonate concentration, *(6)* enzymatic adaptations, *(7)* increased efficiency of performing external work, *(8)* improved coupling efficiency of metabolic signals to oxidative phosphorylation, and *(9)* changes in plasma epinephrine concentration during acclimatization. These postulates are discussed in the following sections.

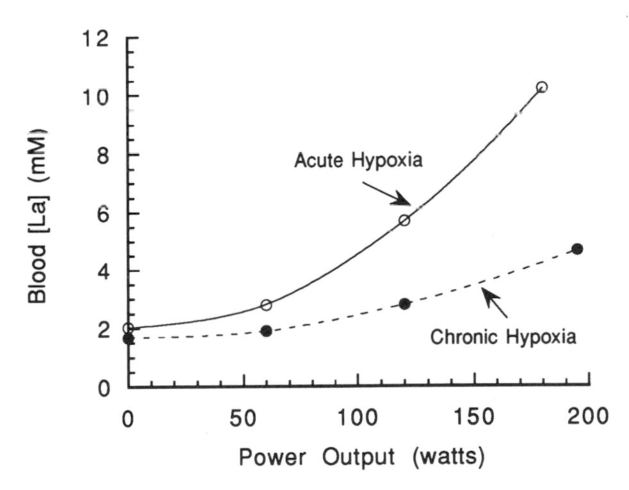

FIG. 14.11. Blood [La] responses to exercise at high altitude in unacclimatized (acute hypoxia) and acclimatized subjects (chronic hypoxia) exposed to altitudes (429 mm Hg, unacclimatized; 347 mm Hg, acclimatized) resulting in the same arterial O_2 pressure in both groups (33–35 mm Hg). [Based on data from Wagner et al. (197) and Sutton et al. (192) and redrawn with permission from Reeves, J. T., E. E. Wolfel, H. J. Green, R. S. Mazzeo, A. J. Young, J. R. Sutton, and G. A. Brooks. Oxygen transport during exercise at altitude and the lactate paradox: lessons from Operation Everest II and Pikes Peak. *Exerc. Sport Sci. Rev.* 20: 275–296, 1992 (162).]

Sequestration of Lactate Inside Muscle Cells. The reduced blood [La] with altitude acclimatization is not due to sequestration of lactate inside muscle cells. In an investigation in which subjects were acclimated to progressive hypobaria over a 40-day period, Green et al. (82, 162) observed a marked reduction in maximal muscle [La] at the point of exhaustion during progressive exercise at 282 mm Hg in comparison to sea level conditions. Subsequently, Green and colleagues (81) measured muscle [La] after the same absolute submaximal work intensity at sea level, upon acute exposure to 4300 m altitude, and after 3 weeks of acclimatization to 4300 m. Muscle [La] was significantly elevated during acute altitude exposure but declined to the sea level concentration with acclimatization. Bender et al. (13) have also shown that net lactate release by exercising muscles during progressive exercise is decreased by acclimatization to 4300 m. During submaximal exercise, Brooks et al. (25) observed that net lactate output by contracting muscles after 5 min of activity was greatest at acute altitude exposure, intermediate after altitude acclimatization, and lowest at sea level. Apparently, the lower blood and muscle lactate concentrations and the decreased net lactate release from contracting muscles following acclimatization reflect a decreased lactate production. Stable isotope tracer kinetics have also been used by Brooks et al. (23, 25) to reveal that the rate of lactate appearance during submaximal exercise is increased upon acute exposure to altitude, but then declines towards the sea level rate with acclimatization. In addition there was evidence that changes in muscle lactate production and release were only partially responsible for the observed changes in muscle and blood lactate concentrations (25). It could be argued that the lower blood and muscle lactate concentrations after acclimatization are due to a faster than normal rate of lactate removal relative to production; but this is not the case. Brooks et al. (23, 25) have shown that lactate disappearance mimicks the response of lactate appearance at sea level, upon acute altitude exposure, and after 3 weeks of acclimatization to altitude.

Improved Oxygen Supply to Muscle during Acclimatization. Upon exposure to altitude or hypobaria and the attendant decrease in $P_{I_{O_2}}$, there is a significant decline in arterial O_2 concentration (12, 13, 162, 213). One might expect that the decreased arterial O_2 concentration would reduce O_2 delivery to muscle, decrease muscle P_{O_2}, increase muscle lactate production, and increase muscle and blood lactate concentrations in comparison to sea level. With acclimatization, ventilatory adaptations occur and hemoglobin concentration rises (12, 13, 162, 213). As a result, arterial O_2 concentration is increased after acclimatization, leading to the expectation that O_2 delivery to muscle would be improved and that muscle and blood lactate concentrations would be lower than during acute altitude exposure. However, muscle O_2 delivery is unchanged by acclimatization because blood flow to exercising muscle is decreased, thus offsetting the increased arterial O_2 concentration (12, 13, 162, 213). Therefore, it does not appear that improved O_2 delivery is responsible for the acclimatization-induced reduction of [La] during exercise.

Perhaps the best evidence against improved O_2 delivery as an explanation for the lactate paradox is provided by the studies of Bender et al. (13). Their experiments were designed to permit measurements during hypoxia before and after acclimatization, and also during normoxia before and after acclimatization. Accordingly, the subjects were studied during exercise at sea level and during acute simulation of 4300 m in a hypobaric chamber, and then again after acclimatizing for 18 days at 4300 m while breathing the ambient air and while breathing 35% O_2. In all experiments, net lactate release by one exercising leg was measured during steady-state cycle ergometer exercise. Net lactate release at a given $\dot{V}_{O_2}$ was lower during hypoxia after acclimatization than during acute altitude exposure. This is the expected lactate paradox response. Net lactate release at a given $\dot{V}_{O_2}$ was also lower (in comparison to sea level before acclimatization) when the hypoxia was corrected by O_2 breathing. In other words, altitude acclimatization lowered net lactate release regardless of the O_2 supply (i.e., either normoxia or hypoxia). Apparently, acclimatization depresses muscle lactate production independently of any potential improvement in O_2 delivery to the muscles.

Muscle Glycogen Depletion during Acclimatization. It has been suggested that the lower lactate production and lower lactate concentrations observed after acclimatization might be caused by a progressive depletion of muscle glycogen during the period of acclimatization (191, 206). Depletion might result from the low carbohydrate/hypocaloric diet that is often consumed by altitude sojourners (191). However, this explanation for the lactate paradox has now been disproven by several studies that have consistently reported muscle glycogen concentrations that are not significantly reduced by acclimatization (81, 82, 215). Therefore, the lower muscle lactate production following acclimatization is not caused by an inadequate glycogen concentration.

Inability to Fully Activate Skeletal Muscles. As noted above, one aspect of the lactate paradox is the fact that maximal muscle and blood lactate concentrations following exhaustive exercise are lower than the values observed at sea level or upon acute exposure to high altitude. Some have proposed that this might stem from incomplete neuromuscular activation in chronic hypobaric hypoxia (82, 122, 133). In this case the central nervous system could become the limiting factor to muscle contraction and, thereby, lactate production (122). Green et al. (82) proposed that incomplete activation of the contractile apparatus might represent a beneficial adaptive response that would protect against potentially harmful effects of metabolic acidosis under the adverse conditions of extreme hypoxia and its concomitant decreased buffering capability. In addition to, or instead of, reduced activation of the motoneuron pool, there could also be an insufficient release of calcium by the sarcoplasmic reticulum or a reduced sensitivity to the calcium stimulus because of alterations in regulatory and contractile proteins (82).

There appears to have been no direct experimental evaluation of contractile activation during the acclimatization process. Whereas incomplete muscle activation might explain lower maximal lactate concentrations following exhaustive exercise, it is an unlikely explanation for the submaximal [La] response following acclimatization. Since the muscle and blood lactate concentrations during submaximal exercise following acclimatization are similar to the lactate concentrations observed at sea level at the same work rates, it appears that muscle activation is similar under the two submaximal conditions. Furthermore, this hypothesis cannot explain the lactate paradox at moderate altitudes where there is little change in cerebral oxygenation (133). Additional evidence against inadequate muscle activation is the fact that the lactate paradox did not deacclimate in Andean natives during 6 weeks of residence at sea level (92, 133).

Low Blood Bicarbonate Concentration. After altitude acclimatization, buffer capacity is reduced because of lower tissue and blood bicarbonate concentrations. Many investigators (31, 122, 206, 208) have proposed that this reduced buffer capacity might explain the lower maximal lactate concentrations observed after exhaustive exercise following altitude acclimatization. With the reduced buffer capacity, a given accumulation of lactic acid would result in a greater than normal decrease in muscle and blood pH values. Indeed, Cerretelli (30) found a greater decrease in blood pH for a given increase in blood [La] in acclimatized lowlanders and Sherpas (high-altitude natives of the Himalayan mountains) in comparison to sea level natives. The greater decrease in pH could in turn inhibit regulatory enzymes in the glycolytic pathway to reduce lactate production.

The bicarbonate hypothesis has now been directly tested. Kayser et al. (122) studied six men who performed supramaximal exercise to exhaustion at sea level and again after 1 month of acclimatization at 5050 m. Under both sea level and altitude conditions, the subjects were tested without (control) and with oral sodium bicarbonate loading (0.3 g/kg body weight). Maximal blood [La] at sea level increased from 12.9 mM in the control condition to 16.6 mM after bicarbonate loading. After altitude acclimatization, maximal blood [La] was reduced to 6.9 mM. Bicarbonate loading at altitude normalized blood bicarbonate concentration and base excess such that the subjects were returned to the normal buffer line, although they remained in a condition of respiratory alkalosis. However, the increase in maximal blood [La] from 6.9 to 8 mM was not significant. These experiments provide strong evidence against the hypothesis that the decreased buffer capacity accompanying high-altitude acclimatization is the cause of the decrease in maximal [La].

Enzymatic Adaptations. Hochachka et al. (90, 93) have proposed that the low lactate concentrations observed during exercise in high-altitude natives is at least partially explained by two enzymatic adaptations: *(1)* a high pyruvate kinase (PK) activity relative to LDH activity, and *(2)* a high malate dehydrogenase (MDH) activity relative to LDH activity. In this hypothesis, the relatively high PK and MDH would promote glycolytic pyruvate and NADH formation with most of the NADH being oxidized within mitochondria. At the same time, the relatively low LDH would limit lactate formation in comparison to the ongoing glycolytic rate. Hochachka et al. (93) compared the PK/LDH (1.4) and MDH/LDH (1.9–3.9) ratios of muscle from Sherpas and Quechuas (high-altitude Indian natives of the Andes mountains), both representing populations of lifelong high-altitude natives, to the same ratios from muscles of other vertebrates. The ratios for the high-altitude natives were generally much greater.

However, in a subsequent study of muscle fibers from three Quechuas, Rosser and Hochachka (165) did not find a greater MDH/LDH ratio in comparison to three lowlanders. In fact, MDH activity was ~20% less and LDH activity ~28% more in the type 1 fibers of the Quechuas. The findings of Green et al. (80) are also counter to the hypothesis of Hochachka et al. (93). Green et al. (80) reported no change in the PK/LDH ratio in eight healthy sea level natives exposed to progressive hypobaric acclimatization. The PK/LDH ratio ranged from 1.5 to 1.6 over the 40-day transition from sea level to 282 mm Hg. Overall, studies of muscle enzyme adaptations during altitude acclimatization have produced inconsistent findings. Young et al. (216) found no changes in the enzyme activities of either the glycolytic pathway or tricarboxylic acid cycle (TCA) during four weeks of altitude acclimatization in sea level natives. However, Saltin et al. (175) observed reductions in TCA cycle enzymes and fatty acid oxidation enzymes, with no change in the enzymes of other metabolic pathways in lowlanders acclimatizing to altitude over 6–44 weeks. Howald et al. (102) studied seven participants in a Swiss expedition to Mount Everest during a period of 6 weeks and reported that the enzyme activities of terminal substrate oxidation (TCA cycle, fatty acid oxidation, ketone body utilization, respiratory chain) decreased, while the enzyme activities of glycolysis increased. The MDH/LDH ratio was 2.7 at the end of the acclimatization period as compared to 3.3 before. Overall, it appears that enzymatic adaptations cannot explain the lactate paradox.

Improved Mechanical Efficiency. In sea level natives acclimatizing to high altitude, there is no change in the efficiency with which external work is performed. This is evidenced by a constant $\dot{V}O_2$ for a given work rate at sea level and throughout the period of acclimatization (13, 81, 213). However, Hochachka et al. (92) argue that Quechuas are more efficient in performing external work than are sea level natives. The reported efficiencies reflect substantially lower energy input for a given work output in the high-altitude natives. Obviously, a higher efficiency would contribute to less lactate production and lower lactate concentrations at any given work rate.

The mechanism for a higher efficiency in the Quechuas is unknown. However, Hochachka et al. (92) noted that plots of power output vs. net metabolic power input (gross metabolic power input minus resting metabolic rate) did not extrapolate to the origin, implying that there is an amount of energy expenditure required during exercise that is not converted to mechanical work. This "lost" energy is less in Quechuas than in sea level natives. They (92) speculated that lower energy "loss" in the high-altitude natives may be related to more efficient Ca^{2+} cycling and/or a down-regulation of muscle sensitivity to thyroid hormones (92). [For further details, see Hochachka et al. (92).]

In contrast to the report of Hochachka et al. (92) concerning Quechuas, Favier et al. (58) found no difference in net work efficiency between another group of Andean natives (mostly Mestizo of predominantly Amerindian ancestry) and lowland natives acclimatized to high altitude. Favier et al. (58) attributed the findings of Hochachka et al. (92) to a relative anemia in their (92) Quechuan subjects ([Hb] = 15.7 g/dl) in comparison to normal values for high altitude natives ([Hb] = ~18–20 g/dl).

Improved Coupling Efficiency of Metabolic Signals to Oxidative Phosphorylation. The phosphorylation potential is an important stimulus for the activation of oxidative phosphorylation during exercise. Individual components of the phosphorylation potential ([ATP], [ADP], and [Pi]) are also important in stimulating glycolysis and thereby lactate production. If oxidative phosphorylation were more closely coupled to the phosphorylation potential and other regulators, then smaller changes in phosphorylation potential and related factors would be required to engender the necessary $\dot{V}O_2$ for a particular work rate. In turn, the smaller changes in [ATP], [ADP], [Pi], [PC], and [AMP] would offer less stimulation of glycolysis and less lactate production. This scenario has been proposed as a possible explanation for the lactate paradox (81, 133).

During calf muscle exercise, ^{31}P nuclear magnetic spectroscopy measures showed a reduced perturbation of all variables related to the phosphorylation potential in Quechuas as compared to sedentary sea level natives at equivalent work rates (133). It appears that oxidative phosphorylation is more tightly coupled to changes in its regulators, thus allowing less stimulation of lactate production. Matheson et al. (133) attributed their results to the higher mechanical efficiency discussed above. With a higher mechanical efficiency, a lower oxidative phosphorylation rate is required at any given work rate. The lower phosphorylation rate in turn requires less perturbation of the phosphorylation potential for stimulation of electron transport chain activity, and concomitantly less stimulation of lactate formation.

Green et al. (81) have also suggested that tighter metabolic control is responsible for the reduction in glycolysis between acute altitude exposure and acclimatization in sea level natives. After acclimatization, free [ADP] was lower and the [ATP]/free [ADP] ratio was increased in comparison to acute altitude exposure. However, unlike the case for the Quechuas, there was no improvement in mechanical efficiency during the acclimatization period. Therefore, the mechanism for the improved coupling efficiency during altitude acclimatization of sea level natives is unknown. In summary, metabolic coupling is tighter after acclimatization. A higher mechanical efficiency may explain the tighter coupling in altitude natives, but the origin of tighter coupling in acclimatized sea level natives is unknown.

Changes in Epinephrine Concentration. Epinephrine may stimulate glycolysis via phosphorylase activation and perhaps PFK stimulation as well. The correlation between blood [La] and epinephrine concentration during exercise is high. In this context, blood [La] (134, 162) and rate of blood lactate appearance (23, 162) are both correlated with changes in plasma epinephrine concentration during acute and chronic high-altitude exposure. The epinephrine concentration is in turn related to arterial oxygen saturation across the conditions of sea level, acute altitude exposure, and chronic altitude exposure (acclimatization) (134).

Young et al. (217) and Mazzeo et al. (135) have performed more direct tests of the involvement of β-adrenergic stimulation in the acute and chronic [La] response of newcomers to altitude. In the study of Young et al. (217), sea level residents were studied during 30 min of steady-state exercise at sea level, and after 3, 8, and 20 days of residence at 4300 m. The work rate required the same percentage of $\dot{V}O_{2max}$ (80%) during each test session, and half of the subjects ingested the β-adrenergic blocker, propranolol, while half ingested a placebo from 3 days prior to ascent through day 15 at altitude. The study of Mazzeo et al. (135) was quite similar, with the main difference being that subjects exercised for 45 min at the same absolute work rate (~50% of sea level $\dot{V}O_{2max}$) at sea level, 4 h after reaching 4300 m, and after 3 weeks of high-altitude residence. Both of these studies (135, 217) reached essentially the same conclusions, which are perhaps best illustrated by the results of Mazzeo et al. (135) as shown in Figure 14.13. First, β-adrenergic blockade reduced the blood [La] upon acute altitude exposure by ~50%; this along with the fact that epinephrine concentration was elevated upon acute exposure with both placebo and β-blockade suggests that the initial increase in [La] is largely due to β-adrenergic stimulation. However, the major finding is that β-blockade does not prevent the decline in blood [La] for a particular work rate during acclimatization to altitude. The results show that both the subjects on placebo and the β-blocked subjects experienced lower lactate concentrations with acclimatization. It appears that an increase in circulating epinephrine during exercise upon arrival at altitude followed by a progressive decline in epinephrine with acclimatization explains part but not all of the decreased [La] response that occurs with acclimatization.

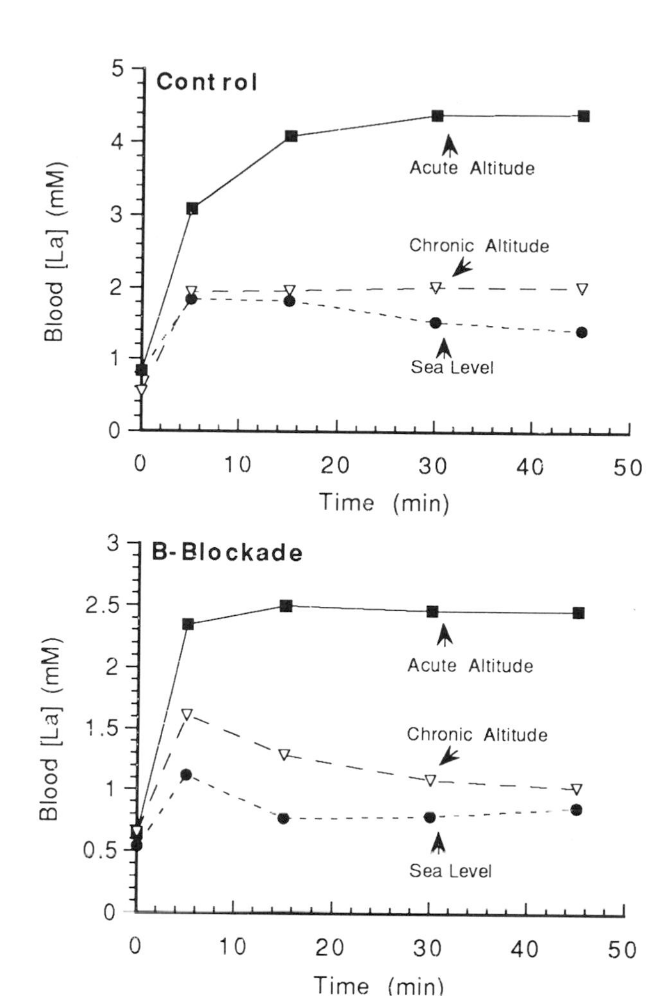

FIG. 14.13. Arterial blood [La] values at rest and during 45 min of submaximal exercise in control and β-blocked subjects at sea level, acute, and chronic altitude exposure at 4300 m. Note that β-blockade caused a reduction in [La] under all conditions including acute exposure. Also, note that acclimatization (chronic altitude) resulted in a decrease in [La] in both control and β-blockade groups. [Redrawn with permission from Mazzeo, R. S., G. A. Brooks, G. E. Butterfield, A. Cymerman, A. C. Roberts, M. Selland, E. E. Wolfel, and J. T. Reeves. β-Adrenergic blockade does not prevent the lactate response to exercise after acclimatization to high altitude. *J. Appl. Physiol.* 76: 610–615, 1994 (135).]

Summary

The evidence reviewed above eliminates some of the proposed hypotheses for the lactate paradox. The discredited hypotheses include: sequestration of lactate inside muscle cells, improved oxygen delivery to muscle by blood during acclimatization, muscle glycogen depletion during acclimatization, low blood bicarbonate concentration, and enzymatic adaptations. While incomplete muscle activation has not been directly evaluated during acclimatization, this also appears to be an unlikely explanation of the lactate paradox. Improved mechanical efficiency may contribute to the lactate paradox in high-altitude natives, but this concept is controversial. Improved mechanical efficiency is not a factor in the lactate paradox observed in sea level natives undergoing acclimatization.

There is an improved coupling efficiency of metabolic signals to oxidative phosphorylation in both high-altitude natives and acclimatized lowlanders. The improved coupling efficiency in high-altitude natives may result from an improved mechanical efficiency that in turn is postulated to derive from more efficient Ca^{2+} cycling and/or a down-regulation of muscle sensitivity to thyroid hormones. The underlying cause of the improved coupling efficiency in acclimatized sea level natives is unknown. A lessening of the epinephrine response to exercise at altitude explains part of the lactate paradox observed in acclimatizing sea level natives, but the catecholamine responses of high-altitude natives to exercise has apparently not been studied. The mechanisms for lower lactate concentrations in high-altitude natives and acclimatized sea level natives are likely to be different in some respects. In acclimatized sea level natives, the lactate paradox disappears in about 2 to 3 weeks upon return to sea level (92, 122). However, there was no evidence of deacclimation of the lactate paradox in Quechuas during 6 weeks at sea level, suggesting that the underlying mechanism(s) may be developmentally or genetically fixed (92). On the other hand, it has been argued that the responses of the Quechuas (92, 122) were unique to a relative anemia in these subjects in comparison to typical high-altitude natives (58).

At the beginning of this chapter, evidence for and against muscle hypoxia as the cause of increased muscle and blood lactate concentrations during exercise under normoxic conditions was reviewed. It should be emphasized that the role of muscle oxygenation as a major factor in the increased lactate concentrations upon acute altitude exposure and the subsequent decline in lactate concentrations with acclimatization has also been questioned (162). Brooks and colleagues (25) used stable isotopes to study lactate metabolism during exercise at sea level, on acute exposure to 4300 m, and after 3 weeks of acclimatization to 4300 m. Their results revealed that active skeletal muscle is not the sole source of blood lactate during exercise at either sea level or high altitude. In fact, during a 45 min period of steady-state exercise, active muscle was a site of both lactate production and utilization, not just net release. Accordingly, future studies of the lactate paradox should not focus entirely on active skeletal muscle, but should instead examine all aspects of the lactate shuttle.

I am grateful to Dr. Dave Pascoe for his assistance in preparation of the manuscript. This work was supported in part by National Institutes of Health grant 1R01AR40342.

REFERENCES

1. Abida, K. El, A. Duvallet, L. Thieulart, M. Rieu, and M. Beaudry. Lactate transport during differentiation of skeletal muscle cells: evidence for a specific carrier in L6 myotubes. *Acta Physiol. Scand.* 144: 469–471, 1992.
2. Akerboom, T. P. M., R. Van Der Meer, and J. M. Tager. Techniques for the investigation of intracellular compartmentation. In: *Techniques in the Life Sciences. Biochemistry. Techniques in Metabolic Research*, edited by H. L. Kornberg, J. C. Metcalfe, and D. H. Northcote. Amsterdam: Elsevier, 1979, p. 1–33.
3. Allen, P. J., and G. A. Brooks. Partial purification and reconstitution of the sarcolemmal L-lactate carrier from rat skeletal muscle. *Biochem. J.* 303: 207–212, 1994.
4. Allen, W. K., D. R. Seals, B. F. Hurley, A. A. Ehsani, and J. M. Hagberg. Lactate threshold and distance-running performance in young and older endurance athletes. *J. Appl. Physiol.* 58: 1281–1284, 1985.
5. Andersen, P., and B. Saltin. Maximal perfusion of skeletal muscle in man. *J. Physiol. (Lond.)* 366: 233–249, 1985.
6. Armstrong, R. B. Muscle fiber recruitment patterns and their metabolic correlates. In: *Exercise, Nutrition, and Energy Metabolism*, edited by E. S. Horton and R. L. Terjung. New York: Macmillan Publishing Company, 1988, p. 9–26.
7. Arthur, P. G., M. C. Hogan, D. E. Bebout, P. D. Wagner, and P. W. Hochachka. Modeling the effects of hypoxia on ATP turnover in exercising muscle. *J. Appl. Physiol.* 73: 737–742, 1992.
8. Asmussen, E. Observations on experimental muscular soreness. *Acta Rheum. Scand.* 2: 109–116, 1956.
9. Baldwin, K. M., A. M. Hooker, and R. E. Herrick. Lactate oxidative capacity in different types of muscle. *Biochem. Biophys. Res. Commun.* 83: 151–157, 1978.
10. Bassingthwaighte, J. B., I. S. J. Chan, and C. Y. Wang. Computationally efficient algorithms for convection-permeation diffusion models for blood-tissue exchange. *Ann. Biomed. Eng.* 20: 687–725, 1992.
11. Beaudry, M., A. Duvallet, L. Thieulart, K. El Abida, and M. Rieu. Lactate transport in skeletal muscle cells: uptake in L6 myoblasts. *Acta Physiol. Scand.* 141: 379–381, 1991.
12. Bender, P. R., B. M. Groves, R. E. McCullough, R. G. McCullough, S.-Y. Huang, A. J. Hamilton, P. D. Wagner, A. Cymerman, and J. T. Reeves. Oxygen transport to exercising leg in chronic hypoxia. *J. Appl. Physiol.* 65: 2592–2597, 1988.
13. Bender, P. R., B. M. Groves, R. E. McCullough, R. G. McCullough, L. Trad, A. J. Young, A. Cymerman, and J. T. Reeves. Decreased exercise muscle lactate release after high altitude acclimatization. *J. Appl. Physiol.* 67: 1456–1462, 1989.
14. Bonen, A., and K. J. A. McCullagh. Effects of exercise on lactate transport into mouse skeletal muscles. *Can. J. Appl. Physiol.* 19: 275–285, 1994.
15. Bonen, A., J. C. McDermott, and C. A. Hutber. Carbohydrate metabolism in skeletal muscle: an update of current concepts. *Int. J. Sports Med.* 10: 385–401, 1989.
16. Bonen, A., J. C. McDermott, and M. H. Tan. Glycogenesis and glyconeogenesis in skeletal muscle: effects of pH and hormones. *Am. J. Physiol.* 258 (*Endocrinol. Metab.* 21): E693–E700, 1990.
17. Bromberg, P. A., J. Theodore, E. D. Robin, and W. N. Jensen. Anion and hydrogen ion distribution in human blood. *J. Lab. Clin. Med.* 66: 464–475, 1965.
18. Brooks, G. A. Anaerobic threshold: review of the concept and directions for future research. *Med. Sci. Sports Exerc.* 17: 22–31, 1985.
19. Brooks, G. A. The lactate shuttle during exercise and recovery. *Med. Sci. Sports Exerc.* 18: 360–368, 1986.
20. Brooks, G. A. Lactate production under fully aerobic conditions: the lactate shuttle during rest and exercise. *Federation Proc.* 45: 2924–2929, 1986.
21. Brooks, G. A. Blood lactic acid: sports "bad boy" turns good. *Gatorade Sports Science Exchange*, No. 2, April, 1988.
22. Brooks, G. A. Current concepts in lactate exchange. *Med. Sci. Sports Exerc.* 23: 895–906, 1991.
23. Brooks, G. A., G. E. Butterfield, R. R. Wolfe, B. M. Groves, R. S. Mazzeo, J. R. Sutton, E. E. Wolfel, and J. T. Reeves. Decreased reliance on lactate during exercise after acclimatization to 4,300 m. *J. Appl. Physiol.* 71: 333–341, 1991.

24. Brooks, G. A., and T. D. Fahey. *Exercise Physiology: Human Bioenergetics and Its Applications.* New York: John Wiley & Sons, 1984, p. 84–89, 208–213.
25. Brooks, G. A., E. E. Wolfel, B. M. Groves, P. R. Bender, G. E. Butterfield, A. Cymerman, R. S. Mazzeo, J. R. Sutton, R. R. Wolfe, and J. T. Reeves. Muscle accounts for glucose disposal but not blood lactate appearance during exercise after acclimatization to 4,300 m. *J. Appl. Physiol.* 72: 2435–2445, 1992.
26. Brown, M. A., and G. A. Brooks. *Trans*-stimulation of lactate transport from rat sarcolemmal membrane vesicles. *Arch. Biochem. Biophys.* 313: 22–28, 1994.
27. Burke, R. E. Motor units: anatomy, physiology, and functional organization. In: *Handbook of Physiology, The Nervous System, Motor Control*, edited by V. B. Brooks. Bethesda, MD: Am. Physiol. Soc., 1981, p. 345–422.
28. Bylund-Fellenius, A.-C., J.-P. Idström, and S. Holm. Muscle respiration during exercise. *Am. Rev. Respir. Dis.* 129(Suppl.): S10–S12, 1984.
29. Bylund-Fellenius, A.-C., P. M. Walker, A. Elander, S. Holm, J. Holm, and T. Scherstén. Energy metabolism in relation to oxygen partial pressure in human skeletal muscle during exercise. *Biochem. J.* 200: 247–255, 1981.
30. Cerretelli, P. Gas exchange at high altitude. In: *Pulmonary Gas Exchange*, edited by J. B. West. New York: Academic Press, 1980, p. 97–147.
31. Cerretelli, P., A. Veicsteinas, and C. Marconi. Anaerobic metabolism at high altitude: the lactacid mechanism. In: *High Altitude Physiology and Medicine*, edited by W. Brendel and R. A. Zink. New York: Springer-Verlag, 1982, p. 94–102.
32. Chance, B., and B. Quistorff. Study of tissue oxygen gradients by single and multiple indicators. *Adv. Exp. Med. Biol.* 94: 331–338, 1978.
33. Chinkes, D. L., X.-J. Zhang, J. A. Romijn, Y. Sakurai, and R. R. Wolfe. Measurement of pyruvate and lactate kinetics across the hindlimb and gut of anesthetized dogs. *Am. J. Physiol.* 267 (*Endocrinol. Metab.* 30): E174–E182, 1994.
34. Clausen, J. P. Effect of physical training on cardiovascular adjustments to exercise and thermal stress. *Physiol. Rev.* 57: 779–815, 1977.
35. Cohen, R. D. Clinical implications of the pathophysiology of lactic acidosis: the role of defects in lactate disposal. In: *Hypoxia, Metabolic Acidosis, and the Circulation*, edited by A. I. Arieff. New York: Oxford University Press, 1992, p. 85–98.
36. Connett, R. J., T. E. J. Gayeski, and C. R. Honig. Lactate production in a pure red muscle in absence of anoxia: mechanisms and significance. *Adv. Exp. Med. Biol.* 159: 327–335, 1983.
37. Connett, R. J., T. E. J. Gayeski, and C. R. Honig. Lactate accumulation in fully aerobic, working, dog gracilis muscle. *Am. J. Physiol.* 246 (*Heart Circ. Physiol.* 15): H120–H128, 1984.
38. Connett, R. J., T. E. J. Gayeski, and C. R. Honig. Energy sources in fully aerobic rest-work transitions: a new role for glycolysis. *Am. J. Physiol.* 248 (*Heart Circ. Physiol.* 17): H922–H929, 1985.
39. Connett, R. J., T. E. J. Gayeski, and C. R. Honig. Lactate efflux is unrelated to intracellular P_{O_2} in a working red muscle in situ. *J. Appl. Physiol.* 61: 402–408, 1986.
40. Connett, R. J., C. R. Honig, T. E. J. Gayeski, and G. A. Brooks. Defining hypoxia: a systems view of V_{O_2}, glycolysis, energetics, and intracellular P_{O_2}. *J. Appl. Physiol.* 68: 833–842, 1990.
41. Constantinopol, M., J. H. Jones, E. R. Weibel, C. R. Taylor, A. Lindholm, and R. H. Karas. Oxygen transport during exercise in large mammals: II. Oxygen uptake by the pulmonary gas exchanger. *J. Appl. Physiol.* 67: 871–878, 1989.
42. Corsi, A., M. Zatti, M. Midrio, and A. L. Granata. In situ oxidation of lactate by skeletal muscle during intermittent exercise. *FEBS Lett.* 11: 65–68, 1970.
43. Davis, J. A., V. J. Caiozzo, N. Lamarra, J. F. Ellis, R. Vandagriff, C. A. Prietto, and W. C. McMaster. Does the gas exchange anaerobic threshold occur at a fixed blood lactate concentration of 2 or 4 mM? *Int. J. Sports Med.* 4: 89–93, 1983.
44. Deuticke, B. The transmembrane exchange of chloride with hydroxyl and other anions in mammalian red blood cells. In: *Oxygen Affinity of Hemoglobin and Red Cell Acid Base Status*, edited by M. Rorth and P. Astrup. New York: Academic Press, 1972, p. 307–319.
45. Deuticke, B. Monocarboxylate transport in erythrocytes. *J. Membr. Biol.* 70: 89–103, 1982.
46. Deuticke, B. Monocarboxylate transport in red blood cells: kinetics and chemical modification. *Methods Enzymol.* 173: 300–329, 1989.
47. Deuticke, B., E. Beyer, and B. Forst. Discrimination of three parallel pathways of lactate transport in the human erythrocyte membrane by inhibitors and kinetic properties. *Biochim. Biophys. Acta* 684: 96–110, 1982.
48. Dobson, G. P., W. S. Parkhouse, J.-M. Weber, E. Stuttard, J. Harman, D. H. Snow, and P. W. Hochachka. Metabolic changes in skeletal muscle and blood of greyhounds during 800-m track sprint. *Am. J. Physiol.* 255 (*Regulatory Integrative Comp. Physiol.* 24): R513–R519, 1988.
49. Dodd, S., S. K. Powers, T. Callender, and E. Brooks. Blood lactate disappearance at various intensities of recovery exercise. *J. Appl. Physiol.* 57: 1462–1465, 1984.
50. Doll, E., J. Keul, and C. Maiwald. Oxygen tension and acid-base equilibria in venous blood of working muscle. *Am. J. Physiol.* 215: 23–29, 1968.
51. Donovan, C. M., and G. A. Brooks. Endurance training affects lactate clearance, not lactate production. *Am. J. Physiol.* 244 (*Endocrinol. Metab.* 7): E83–E92, 1983.
52. Donovan, C. M., and M. J. Pagliassotti. Endurance training enhances lactate clearance during hyperlactatemia. *Am. J. Physiol.* 257 (*Endocrinol. Metab.* 20): E782–E789, 1989.
53. Donovan, C. M., and M. J. Pagliassotti. Enhanced efficiency of lactate removal after endurance training. *J. Appl. Physiol.* 68: 1053–1058, 1990.
54. Drummond, G. I., J. P. Harwood, and C. A. Powell. Studies on the activation of phosphorylase in skeletal muscle by contraction and by epinephrine. *J. Biol. Chem.* 244: 4235–4240, 1969.
55. Duboc, D., M. Muffat-Joly, G. Renault, M. Degeorges, M. Toussaint, and J. R. Pocidalo. In situ NADH laser fluorimetry of rat fast and slow twitch muscles during tetanus. *J. Appl. Physiol.* 64: 2692–2695, 1988.
56. Duhaylongsod, F. G., J. A. Griebel, D. S. Bacon, W. G. Wolfe, and C. A. Piantadosi. Effects of muscle contraction on cytochrome a,a_3 redox state. *J. Appl. Physiol.* 75: 790–797, 1993.
57. Erecińska, M., and D. F. Wilson. Regulation of cellular energy metabolism. *J. Memb. Biol.* 70: 1–14, 1982.
58. Favier, R., H. Spielvogel, D. Desplanches, G. Ferretti, B. Kayser, and H. Hoppeler. Maximal exercise performance in chronic hypoxia and acute normoxia in high-altitude natives. *J. Appl. Physiol.* 78: 1868–1874, 1995.

59. Fitts, R. H. Cellular mechanisms of muscle fatigue. *Physiol. Rev.* 74: 49–94, 1994.
60. Fitzsimons, E. J., and J. Sendroy, Jr. Distribution of electrolytes in human blood. *J. Biol. Chem.* 236: 1595–1601, 1961.
61. Foxdal, P., B. Sjödin, H. Rudstam, C. Östman, B. Östman, and G. C. Hedenstierna. Lactate concentration differences in plasma, whole blood, capillary finger blood and erythrocytes during submaximal graded exercise in humans. *Eur. J. Appl. Physiol.* 61: 218–222, 1990.
62. Freminet, A., E. Bursaux, and C. F. Poyart. Effect of elevated lactataemia in the rates of lactate turnover and oxidation in rats. *Pflugers Arch.* 346: 75–86, 1974.
63. Funder, J., and J. O. Wieth. Chloride and hydrogen ion distribution between human red cells and plasma. *Acta Physiol. Scand.* 68: 234–245, 1966.
64. Gaesser, G. A., and G. A. Brooks. Metabolic bases of excess post exercise oxygen consumption: a review. *Med. Sci. Sports Exerc.* 16: 29–43, 1984.
65. Garcia, C. K., J. L. Goldstein, R. K. Pathak, R. G. W. Anderson, and M. S. Brown. Molecular characterization of a membrane transporter for lactate, pyruvate, and other monocarboxylates: implications for the Cori cycle. *Cell* 76: 865–873, 1994.
66. Gladden, L. B. Current "anaerobic threshold" controversies. *Physiologist* 27: 312–318, 1984.
67. Gladden, L. B. Lactate uptake by skeletal muscle. *Exerc. Sport Sci. Rev.* 17: 115–155, 1989.
68. Gladden, L. B. Net lactate uptake during progressive steady-level contractions in canine skeletal muscle. *J. Appl. Physiol.* 71: 514–520, 1991.
69. Gladden, L. B., R. E. Crawford, and M. J. Webster. Effect of blood flow on net lactate uptake during steady-level contractions in canine skeletal muscle. *J. Appl. Physiol.* 72: 1826–1830, 1992.
70. Gladden, L. B., R. E. Crawford, and M. J. Webster. Effect of lactate concentration and metabolic rate on net lactate uptake by canine skeletal muscle. *Am. J. Physiol.* 266 (*Regulatory Integrative Comp. Physiol.* 35): R1095–R1101, 1994.
71. Gladden, L. B., R. E. Crawford, M. J. Webster, and P. W. Watt. Rapid tracer lactate influx into canine skeletal muscle. *J. Appl. Physiol.* 78: 205–211, 1995.
72. Gladden, L. B., E. W. Smith, and M. S. Skelton. Lactate distribution in blood during passive and active recovery after intense exercise. *Med. Sci. Sports Exerc.* 26 (Suppl.): S35, 1994.
73. Gladden, L. B., and J. W. Yates. Lactic acid infusion in dogs: effects of varying infusate pH. *J. Appl. Physiol.* 54: 1254–1260, 1983.
74. Gladden, L. B., J. W. Yates, R. W. Stremel, and B. A. Stamford. Gas exchange and lactate anaerobic thresholds: inter- and intraevaluator agreement. *J. Appl. Physiol.* 58: 2082–2089, 1985.
75. Gollnick, P. D., W. M. Bayly, and D. R. Hodgson. Exercise intensity, training, diet, and lactate concentration in muscle and blood. *Med. Sci. Sports Exerc.* 18: 334–340, 1986.
76. Goodyear, L. J., M. F. Hirshman, P. A. King, E. D. Horton, C. M. Thompson, and E. S. Horton. Skeletal muscle plasma membrane glucose transport and glucose transporters after exercise. *J. Appl. Physiol.* 68: 193–198, 1990.
77. Graham, T. E., J. K. Barclay, and B. A. Wilson. Skeletal muscle lactate release and glycolytic intermediates during hypercapnia. *J. Appl. Physiol.* 60: 568–575, 1986.
78. Graham, T. E., P. K. Pedersen, and B. Saltin. Muscle and blood ammonia and lactate responses to prolonged exercise with hyperoxia. *J. Appl. Physiol.* 63: 1457–1462, 1987.
79. Granata, A. L., M. Midrio, and A. Corsi. Lactate oxidation by skeletal muscle during sustained contraction in vivo. *Pflugers Arch.* 366: 247–250, 1976.
80. Green, H. J., J. R. Sutton, A. Cymerman, P. M. Young, and C. S. Houston. Operation Everest II: adaptations in human skeletal muscle. *J. Appl. Physiol.* 66: 2454–2461, 1989.
81. Green, H. J., J. R. Sutton, E. E. Wolfel, J. T. Reeves, G. E. Butterfield, and G. A. Brooks. Altitude acclimatization and energy metabolic adaptations in skeletal muscle during exercise. *J. Appl. Physiol.* 73: 2701–2708, 1992.
82. Green, H. J., J. Sutton, P. Young, A. Cymerman, and C. S. Houston. Operation Everest II: muscle energetics during maximal exhaustive exercise. *J. Appl. Physiol.* 66: 142–150, 1989.
83. Grimditch, G. K., R. J. Barnard, S. A. Kaplan, and E. Sternlicht. Insulin binding and glucose transport in rat skeletal muscle sarcolemmal vesicles. *Am. J. Physiol.* 249: 398–408, 1985.
84. Guezennec, C. Y., F. Lienhard, F. Louisy, G. Renault, M. H. Tusseau, and P. Portero. In situ NADH laser fluorimetry during muscle contraction in humans. *Eur. J. Appl. Physiol.* 63: 36–42, 1991.
85. Halestrap, A. P. Transport of pyruvate and lactate into human erythrocytes. *Biochem. J.* 156: 193–207, 1976.
86. Halestrap, A. P., R. D. Scott, and A. P. Thomas. Mitochondrial pyruvate transport and its hormonal regulation. *Int. J. Biochem.* 11: 97–105, 1980.
87. Hargreaves, M., and E. A. Richter. Regulation of skeletal muscle glycogenolysis during exercise. *Can. J. Sport Sci.* 13: 197–203, 1988.
88. Hill, A. V. The energy degraded in the recovery processes of stimulated muscles. *J. Physiol. (Lond.)* 46: 28–80, 1913.
89. Hochachka, P. W. The lactate paradox: analysis of underlying mechanisms. *Ann. Sport Med.* 4: 184–188, 1988.
90. Hochachka, P. W. Muscle enzymatic composition and metabolic regulation in high altitude adapted natives. *Int. J. Sports Med.* 13 (Suppl. 1): S89–S91, 1992.
91. Hochachka, P. W., and G. O. Matheson. Regulating ATP turnover rates over broad dynamic work ranges in skeletal muscles. *J. Appl. Physiol.* 73: 1697–1703, 1992.
92. Hochachka, P. W., C. Stanley, G. O. Matheson, D. C. McKenzie, P. S. Allen, and W. S. Parkhouse. Metabolic and work efficiencies during exercise in Andean natives. *J. Appl. Physiol.* 70: 1720–1730, 1991.
93. Hochachka, P. W., C. Stanley, D. C. McKenzie, A. Villena, and C. Monge. Enzyme mechanisms for pyruvate-to-lactate flux attenuation: a study of Sherpas, Quechuas, and hummingbirds. *Int. J. Sports Med.* 13 (Suppl. 1): S119–S122, 1992.
94. Hogan, M. C., P. G. Arthur, D. E. Bebout, P. W. Hochachka, and P. D. Wagner. Role of O_2 in regulating tissue respiration in dog muscle working in situ. *J. Appl. Physiol.* 73: 728–736, 1992.
95. Hogan, M. C., R. H. Cox, and H. G. Welch. Lactate accumulation during incremental exercise with varied inspired oxygen fractions. *J. Appl. Physiol.* 55: 1134–1140, 1983.
96. Hogan, M. C., S. Nioka, W. F. Brechue, and B. Chance. A ^{31}P-NMR study of tissue respiration in working dog muscle during reduced O_2 delivery conditions. *J. Appl. Physiol.* 73: 1662–1670, 1992.
97. Hogan, M. C., and H. G. Welch. Effect of altered arterial O_2 tensions on muscle metabolism in dog skeletal muscle

during fatiguing work. *Am. J. Physiol.* 251 (*Cell Physiol.* 20): C216–C222, 1986.

98. Holloszy, J. O., and E. F. Coyle. Adaptations of skeletal muscle to endurance exercise and their consequences. *J. Appl. Physiol.* 56: 831–838, 1984.
99. Holm, S., and A.-C. Bylund-Fellenius. Continuous monitoring of oxygen tension in human gastrocnemius muscle during exercise. *Clin. Physiol.* 1: 541–552, 1981.
100. Honig, C. R., T. E. J. Gayeski, W. Federspiel, A. Clark, and P. Clark. Muscle O_2 gradients from hemoglobin to cytochrome: new concepts, new complexities. *Adv. Exp. Med. Biol.* 169: 23–38, 1984.
101. Horstman, D. H., M. Gleser, and J. Delehunt. Effects of altering O_2 delivery on $\dot{V}O_2$ of isolated, working muscle. *Am. J. Physiol.* 230: 327–334, 1976.
102. Howald, H., D. Petté, J.-A. Simoneau, A. Uber, H. Hoppeler, and P. Cerretelli, III. Effects of chronic hypoxia on muscle enzyme activities. *Int. J. Sports Med.* 11 (Suppl. 1): S10–S14, 1990.
103. Hundal, H. S., M. J. Rennie, and P. W. Watt. Characteristics of L-glutamine transport in perfused rat skeletal muscle. *J. Physiol. (Lond.)* 393: 283–305, 1987.
104. Idström, J.-P., V. H. Subramanian, B. Chance, T. Scherstén, and A.-C. Bylund-Fellenius. Oxygen dependence of energy metabolism in contracting and recovering rat skeletal muscle. *Am. J. Physiol.* 248 (*Heart Circ. Physiol.* 17): H40–H48, 1985.
105. Issekutz, B., Jr., W. A. S. Shaw, and A. C. Issekutz. Lactate metabolism in resting and exercising dogs. *J. Appl. Physiol.* 40: 312–319, 1976.
106. Jöbsis, F. F., and W. N. Stainsby. Oxidation of NADH during contractions of circulated mammalian skeletal muscle. *Respir. Physiol.* 4: 292–300, 1968.
107. Johnson, J. M. Circulation to skeletal muscle. In: *Textbook of Physiology, Vol. 2*, edited by H. D. Patton, A. F. Fuchs, B. Hille, A. M. Scher, and R. Steiner. Philadelphia: W. B. Saunders Company, 1989, p. 887–897.
108. Johnson, R. E., H. T. Edwards, D. B. Dill, and J. W. Wilson. Blood as a physicochemical system: the distribution of lactate. *J. Biol. Chem.* 157: 461–473, 1945.
109. Jones, D. P. Intracellular diffusion gradients of O_2 and ATP. *Am. J. Physiol.* 250 (*Cell Physiol.* 19): C663–C675, 1986.
110. Jones, J. H., K. E. Longworth, A. Lindholm, K. E. Conley, R. H. Karas, S. R. Kayar, and C. R. Taylor. Oxygen transport during exercise in large mammals: I. Adaptive variation in oxygen demand. *J. Appl. Physiol.* 67: 862–870, 1989.
111. Juel, C. Intracellular pH recovery and lactate efflux in mouse soleus muscles stimulated *in vitro*: the involvement of sodium/proton exchange and a lactate carrier. *Acta Physiol. Scand.* 132: 363–371, 1988.
112. Juel, C. Human muscle lactate transport can be studied in sarcolemmal giant vesicles made from needle-biopsies. *Acta Physiol. Scand.* 142: 133–134, 1991.
113. Juel, C. Muscle lactate transport studied in sarcolemmal giant vesicles. *Biochim. Biophys. Acta* 1065: 15–20, 1991.
114. Juel, C., J. Bangsbo, T. Graham, and B. Saltin. Lactate and potassium fluxes from human skeletal muscle during and after intense, dynamic, knee extensor exercise. *Acta Physiol. Scand.* 140: 147–159, 1990.
115. Juel, C., A. Honig, and H. Pilegaard. Muscle lactate transport studied in sarcolemmal giant vesicles: dependence on fibre type and age. *Acta Physiol. Scand.* 143: 361–365, 1991.
116. Juel, C., S. Kristiansen, H. Pilegaard, J. Wojtaszewski, and E. A. Richter. Kinetics of lactate transport in sarcolemmal giant vesicles obtained from human skeletal muscle. *J. Appl. Physiol.* 76: 1031–1036, 1994.
117. Juel, C., and F. Wibrand. Lactate transport in isolated mouse muscles studied with a tracer technique—kinetics, stereospecificity, pH dependency and maximal capacity. *Acta Physiol. Scand.* 137: 33–39, 1989.
118. Kaplan, N. O., and J. Everse. Regulatory characteristics of lactate dehydrogenases. *Adv. Enzyme Regul.* 10: 323–336, 1972.
119. Katz, A., and K. Sahlin. Effect of decreased oxygen availability on NADH and lactate content in human skeletal muscle during exercise. *Acta Physiol. Scand.* 131: 119–128, 1987.
120. Katz, A., and K. Sahlin. Regulation of lactic acid production during exercise. *J. Appl. Physiol.* 65: 509–518, 1988.
121. Katz, A., and K. Sahlin. Role of oxygen in regulation of glycolysis and lactate production in human skeletal muscle. *Exerc. Sport Sci. Rev.* 18: 1–28, 1990.
122. Kayser, B., G. Ferretti, B. Grassi, T. Binzoni, and P. Cerretelli. Maximal lactic capacity at altitude: effect of bicarbonate loading. *J. Appl. Physiol.* 75: 1070–1074, 1993.
123. Kennedy, F. G., and D. P. Jones. Oxygen dependence of mitochondrial function in isolated rat cardiac myocytes. *Am. J. Physiol.* 250 (*Cell Physiol.* 19): C374–C383, 1986.
124. Klip, A., T. Ramlal, D. A. Young, and J. O. Holloszy. Insulin-induced translocation of glucose transporters in rat hindlimb muscles. *FEBS Lett.* 224: 230, 1987.
125. Knight, D. R., W. Schaffartzik, D. C. Poole, M. C. Hogan, D. E. Bebout, and P. D. Wagner. Effects of hyperoxia on maximal leg O_2 supply and utilization in men. *J. Appl. Physiol.* 75: 2586–2594, 1993.
126. Krisanda, J. M., T. S. Moreland, and M. J. Kushmerick. ATP supply and demand during exercise. In: *Exercise, Nutrition, and Energy Metabolism*, edited by E. S. Horton and R. L. Terjung. New York: Macmillan Publishing Company, 1988, p. 27–44.
127. Krützfeldt, A., R. Spahr, S. Mertens, B. Siegmund, and H. M. Piper. Metabolism of exogenous substrates by coronary endothelial cells in culture. *J. Mol. Cell. Cardiol.* 22: 1393–1404, 1990.
128. Kuikka, J., M. Levin, and J. B. Bassingthwaighte. Multiple tracer dilution estimates of D- and 2-deoxy-D-glucose uptake by the heart. *Am. J. Physiol.* 250 (*Heart Circ. Physiol.* 19): H29–H42, 1986.
129. Kushmerick, M. J. Energetics of muscle contraction. In: *Handbook of Physiology, Skeletal Muscle*, edited by L. D. Peachey. Bethesda, MD: Am. Physiol. Soc., 1983, p. 189–236.
130. Linnarsson, D., J. Karlsson, N. Fagraeus, and B. Saltin. Muscle metabolites and oxygen deficit with exercise in hypoxia and hyperoxia. *J. Appl. Physiol.* 36: 399–402, 1974.
131. MacLaren, D. P. M., H. Gibson, M. Parry-Billings, and R. H. T. Edwards. A review of metabolic and physiological factors in fatigue. *Exerc. Sport Sci. Rev.* 17: 29–66, 1989.
132. MacRae, H. S.-H., S. C. Dennis, A. N. Bosch, and T. D. Noakes. Effects of training on lactate production and removal during progressive exercise in humans. *J. Appl. Physiol.* 72: 1649–1656, 1992.
133. Matheson, G. O., P. S. Allen, D. C. Ellinger, C. C. Hanstock, D. Gheorghiu, D. C. McKenzie, C. Stanley, W. S. Parkhouse, and P. W. Hochachka. Skeletal muscle metabolism and work capacity: a ^{31}P-NMR study of Andean natives and lowlanders. *J. Appl. Physiol.* 70: 1963–1976, 1991.
134. Mazzeo, R. S., P. R. Bender, G. A. Brooks, G. E. Butterfield, B. M. Groves, J. R. Sutton, E. E. Wolfel, and J. T. Reeves.

Arterial catecholamine responses during exercise with acute and chronic high-altitude exposure. *Am. J. Physiol.* 261 (*Endocrinol. Metab.* 24): E419–E424, 1991.
135. Mazzeo, R. S., G. A. Brooks, G. E. Butterfield, A. Cymerman, A. C. Roberts, M. Selland, E. E. Wolfel, and J. T. Reeves. β-Adrenergic blockade does not prevent the lactate response to exercise after acclimatization to high altitude. *J. Appl. Physiol.* 76: 610–615, 1994.
136. Mazzeo, R. S., G. A. Brooks, D. A. Schoeller, and T. F. Budinger. Disposal of blood [1-^{13}C]lactate in humans during rest and exercise. *J. Appl. Physiol.* 60: 232–241, 1986.
137. Mazzeo, R. S., and P. Marshall. Influence of plasma catecholamines on the lactate threshold during graded exercise. *J. Appl. Physiol.* 67: 1319–1322, 1989.
138. McCartney, N., G. J. F. Heigenhauser, and N. L. Jones. Effects of pH on maximal power output and fatigue during short-term dynamic exercise. *J. Appl. Physiol.* 55: 225–229, 1983.
139. McCullagh, K. J. A., and A. Bonen. L(+)-Lactate binding to a protein in rat skeletal muscle plasma membranes. *Can. J. Appl. Physiol.* 20: 112–124, 1995.
140. McDermott, J. C., and A. Bonen. Lactate transport by skeletal muscle sarcolemmal vesicles. *Mol. Cell. Biochem.* 122: 113–121, 1993.
141. McDermott, J. C., and A. Bonen. Endurance training increases skeletal muscle lactate transport. *Acta Physiol. Scand.* 147: 323–327, 1993.
142. McDermott, J. C., and A. Bonen. Lactate transport in rat sarcolemmal vesicles and intact skeletal muscle, and after muscle contraction. *Acta Physiol. Scand.* 151: 17–28, 1994.
143. McLane, J. A., and J. O. Holloszy. Glycogen synthesis from lactate in the three types of skeletal muscle. *J. Biol. Chem.* 254: 6548–6553, 1979.
144. Meyer, R. A., and J. M. Foley. Testing models of respiratory control in skeletal muscle. *Med. Sci. Sports Exerc.* 26: 52–57, 1994.
145. Moritani, T., T. Takaishi, and T. Matsumoto. Determination of maximal power output at neuromuscular fatigue threshold. *J. Appl. Physiol.* 74: 1729–1734, 1993.
146. Morrow, J. A., R. D. Fell, and L. B. Gladden. Respiratory alkalosis: no effect on blood lactate decline or performance. *Eur. J. Appl. Physiol.* 58: 175–181, 1988.
147. Nagesser, A. S., W. J. van der Laarse, and G. Elzinga. Lactate efflux from fatigued fast-twitch muscle fibres of *Xenopus laevis* under various extracellular conditions. *J. Physiol. (Lond.)* 481: 139–147, 1994.
148. Nesher, R., I. E. Karl, and D. M. Kipnis. Dissociation of effects of insulin and contraction on glucose transport in rat epitrochlearis muscle. *Am. J. Physiol.* 249 (*Cell Physiol.* 18): C226–C232, 1985.
149. Newgard, C. B., L. J. Hirsch, D. W. Foster, and J. D. McGarry. Studies on the mechanism by which exogenous glucose is converted into liver glycogen in the rat. A direct or an indirect pathway? *J. Biol. Chem.* 258: 8046–8052, 1983.
150. Newman, E. V., D. B. Dill, H. T. Edwards, and F. A. Webster. The rate of lactic acid removal in exercise. *Am. J. Physiol.* 118: 457–462, 1937.
151. Newsholme, E. A., and A. R. Leech. *Biochemistry for the Medical Sciences.* New York: John Wiley & Sons, 1983, p. 204–207.
152. Paddle, B. M. A cytoplasmic component of pyridine nucleotide fluorescence in rat diaphragm: evidence from comparisons with flavoprotein fluorescence. *Pflugers Arch.* 404: 326–331, 1985.
153. Pagliassotti, M. J., and C. M. Donovan. Influence of cell heterogeneity on skeletal muscle lactate kinetics. *Am. J. Physiol.* 258 (*Endocrinol. Metab.* 21): E625–E634, 1990.
154. Pagliassotti, M. J., and C. M. Donovan. Role of cell type in net lactate removal by skeletal muscle. *Am. J. Physiol.* 258 (*Endocrinol. Metab.* 21): E635–E642, 1990.
155. Pagliassotti, M. J., and C. M. Donovan. Glycogenesis from lactate in rabbit skeletal muscle fiber types. *Am. J. Physiol.* 258 (*Regulatory Integrative Comp. Physiol.* 27): R903–R911, 1990.
156. Pilegaard, H., J. Bangsbo, E. A. Richter, and C. Juel. Lactate transport studied in sarcolemmal giant vesicles from human muscle biopsies: relation to training status. *J. Appl. Physiol.* 77: 1858–1862, 1994.
157. Pilegaard, H., C. Juel, and F. Wibrand. Lactate transport studied in sarcolemmal giant vesicles from rats: effect of training. *Am. J. Physiol.* 264 (*Endocrinol. Metab.* 27): E156–E160, 1993.
158. Podolin, D. A., P. A. Munger, and R. S. Mazzeo. Plasma catecholamines and lactate response during graded exercise with varied glycogen conditions. *J. Appl. Physiol.* 71: 1427–1433, 1991.
159. Poole, D. C., L. B. Gladden, S. Kurdak, and M. C. Hogan. L-(+)-Lactate infusion into working dog gastrocnemius: no evidence lactate per se mediates $\dot{V}O_2$ slow component. *J. Appl. Physiol.* 76: 787–792, 1994.
160. Poole, R. C., and A. P. Halestrap. Identification and partial purification of the erythrocyte L-lactate transporter. *Biochem. J.* 283: 855–862, 1992.
161. Poole, R. C., and A. P. Halestrap. Transport of lactate and other monocarboxylates across mammalian plasma membranes. *Am. J. Physiol.* 264 (*Cell Physiol.* 33): C761–C782, 1993.
162. Reeves, J. T., E. E. Wolfel, H. J. Green, R. S. Mazzeo, A. J. Young, J. R. Sutton, and G. A. Brooks. Oxygen transport during exercise at altitude and the lactate paradox: lessons from Operation Everest II and Pikes Peak. *Exerc. Sport Sci. Rev.* 20: 275–296, 1992.
163. Richter, E. A., B. Kiens, B. Saltin, N. J. Christensen, and G. Savard. Skeletal muscle glucose uptake during dynamic exercise in humans: role of muscle mass. *Am. J. Physiol.* 254 (*Endocrinol. Metab.* 17): E555–E561, 1988.
164. Roos, A. Intracellular pH and distribution of weak acids across cell membranes. A study of D- and L-lactate and of DMO in rat diaphragm. *J. Physiol. (Lond.)* 249: 1–25, 1975.
165. Rosser, B. W. C., and P. W. Hochachka. Metabolic capacity of muscle fibers from high-altitude natives. *Eur. J. Appl. Physiol.* 67: 513–517, 1993.
166. Roth, D. A. The sarcolemmal lactate transporter: transmembrane determinants of lactate flux. *Med. Sci. Sports Exerc.* 23: 925–934, 1991.
167. Roth, D. A., and G. A. Brooks. Lactate transport is mediated by a membrane-bound carrier in rat skeletal muscle sarcolemmal vesicles. *Arch. Biochem. Biophys.* 279: 377–385, 1990.
168. Roth, D. A., and G. A. Brooks. Lactate and pyruvate transport is dominated by a pH gradient-sensitive carrier in rat skeletal muscle sarcolemmal vesicles. *Arch. Biochem. Biophys.* 279: 386–394, 1990.
169. Roth, D. A., and G. A. Brooks. Training does not affect zero-*trans* lactate transport across mixed rat skeletal muscle sarcolemmal vesicles. *J. Appl. Physiol.* 75: 1559–1565, 1993.
170. Rowell, L. B. Human cardiovascular adjustments to exercise and thermal stress. *Physiol. Rev.* 54: 75–159, 1972.

171. Rowell, L. B., J. R. Blackmon, M. A. Kenny, and P. Escourrou. Splanchnic vasomotor and metabolic adjustments to hypoxia and exercise in humans. *Am. J. Physiol.* 247 (*Heart Circ. Physiol.* 16): H251–H258, 1984.
172. Rumsey, W. L., C. Schlosser, E. M. Nuutinen, M. Robiolio, and D. F. Wilson. Cellular energetics and the oxygen dependence of respiration in cardiac myocytes isolated from adult rat. *J. Biol. Chem.* 265: 15392–15399, 1990.
173. Sahlin, K. NADH in human skeletal muscle during short-term intense exercise. *Pflugers Arch.* 403: 193–196, 1985.
174. Sahlin, K., A. Katz, and J. Henriksson. Redox state and lactate accumulation in human skeletal muscle during dynamic exercise. *Biochem. J.* 245: 551–556, 1987.
175. Saltin, B., E. Nygaard, and B. Rasmussen. Skeletal muscle adaptation in man following prolonged exposure to high altitude. *Acta Physiol. Scand.* 109: 31A, 1980.
176. Shiota, M., S. Golden, and J. Katz. Lactate metabolism in the perfused rat hindlimb. *Biochem. J.* 222: 281–292, 1984.
177. Skelton, M. S., D. E. Kremer, E. W. Smith, and L. B. Gladden. Lactate influx into red blood cells of athletic and nonathletic species. *Am. J. Physiol.* 268 (*Regulatory Integrative Comp. Physiol.* 37): R1121–R1128, 1995.
178. Slentz, C. A., E. A. Gulve, K. J. Rodnick, E. J. Henriksen, J. H. Youn, and J. O. Holloszy. Glucose transporters and maximal transport are increased in endurance-trained rat soleus. *J. Appl. Physiol.* 73: 486–492, 1992.
179. Smith, E. W., M. S. Skelton, and L. B. Gladden. Plasma to red blood cell lactate distribution in high and low intensity steady-state exercise. *Med. Sci. Sports Exerc.* 26 (Suppl.): S35, 1994.
180. Smith, E. W., M. S. Skelton, D. E. Kremer, and L. B. Gladden. Effect of increment duration on blood lactate distribution during graded exercise. *FASEB J.* 9: A359, 1995.
181. Spriet, L. L. Phosphofructokinase activity and acidosis during short-term tetanic contractions. *Can. J. Physiol. Pharmacol.* 69: 298–304, 1991.
182. Spriet, L. L., M. I. Lindinger, G. J. F. Heigenhauser, and N. L. Jones. Effects of alkalosis on skeletal muscle metabolism and performance during exercise. *Am. J. Physiol.* 252 (*Regulatory Integrative Comp. Physiol.* 21): R833–R839, 1986.
183. Spriet, L. L., C. G. Matsos, S. J. Peters, G. J. F. Heigenhauser, and N. L. Jones. Effects of acidosis on rat muscle metabolism and performance during heavy exercise. *Am. J. Physiol.* 248 (*Cell Physiol.* 17): C337–C347, 1985.
184. Stainsby, W. N., and G. A. Brooks. Control of lactic acid metabolism in contracting muscles and during exercise. *Exerc. Sport Sci. Rev.* 18: 29–63, 1990.
185. Stainsby, W. N., and P. D. Eitzman. Lactic acid output of cat gastrocnemius-plantaris during repetitive twitch contractions. *Med. Sci. Sports Exerc.* 18: 668–673, 1986.
186. Stainsby, W. N., and H. G. Welch. Lactate metabolism of contracting dog skeletal muscle *in situ*. *Am. J. Physiol.* 211: 177–183, 1966.
187. Stanley, W. C., E. W. Gertz, J. A. Wisneski, D. L. Morris, R. A. Neese, and G. A. Brooks. Systemic lactate kinetics during graded exercise in man. *Am. J. Physiol.* 249 (*Endocrinol. Metab.* 12): E595–E602, 1985.
188. Stanley, W. C., E. W. Gertz, J. A. Wisneski, R. A. Neese, D. L. Morris, and G. A. Brooks. Lactate extraction during net lactate release by the exercising legs of man. *J. Appl. Physiol.* 60: 1116–1120, 1986.
189. Stone, H. L., and I. Y. S. Liang. Cardiovascular response and control during exercise. *Am. Rev. Respir. Dis.* 129 (Suppl.): S13–S16, 1984.
190. Sussman, I., M. Erecinska, and D. F. Wilson. Regulation of cellular energy metabolism: the Crabtree effect. *Biochim. Biophys. Acta* 591: 209–223, 1980.
191. Sutton, J. R., N. L. Jones, and L. G. C. E. Pugh. Exercise at altitude. *Annu. Rev. Physiol.* 45: 427–437, 1983.
192. Sutton, J. R., J. T. Reeves, P. D. Wagner, B. M. Groves, A. Cymerman, M. K. Malconian, P. B. Rock, P. M. Young, S. D. Walter, and C. S. Houston. Operation Everest II: oxygen transport during exercise at extreme simulated altitude. *J. Appl. Physiol.* 64: 1309–1321, 1988.
193. Taylor, C. R., R. H. Karas, E. R. Weibel, and H. Hoppeler. Adaptive variation in the mammalian respiratory system in relation to energetic demand: II. Reaching the limits to oxygen flow. *Respir. Physiol.* 69: 7–26, 1987.
194. Unkefer, C. J., R. M. Blazer, and R. E. London. In vivo determination of the pyridine nucleotide reduction charge by carbon-13 nuclear magnetic resonance spectroscopy. *Science* 222: 62–85, 1983.
195. Vogel, J. A., and M. A. Gleser. Effect of carbon monoxide on oxygen transport during exercise. *J. Appl. Physiol.* 32: 234–239, 1972.
196. Waddell, W. J., and R. G. Bates. Intracellular pH. *Physiol. Rev.* 49: 285–329, 1969.
197. Wagner, P. D., G. E. Gale, R. E. Moon, J. R. Torre-Bueno, B. W. Stolp, and H. H. Saltzman. Pulmonary gas exchange in humans exercising at sea level and simulated altitude. *J. Appl. Physiol.* 61: 260–270, 1986.
198. Wasserman, K. The anaerobic threshold measurement to evaluate exercise performance. *Am. Rev. Respir. Dis.* 129 (Suppl.): S35–S40, 1984.
199. Wasserman, K. Anaerobiosis, lactate, and gas exchange during exercise: the issues. *Federation Proc.* 45: 2904–2909, 1986.
200. Wasserman, K., B. J. Whipp, S. N. Koyal, and W. L. Beaver. Anaerobic threshold and respiratory gas exchange during exercise. *J. Appl. Physiol.* 35: 236–243, 1973.
201. Watt, P. W., L. B. Gladden, H. S. Hundal, and R. E. Crawford. Effects of flow and contraction on lactate transport in the perfused rat hindlimb. *Am. J. Physiol.* 267 (*Endocrinol. Metab.* 30): E7–E13, 1994.
202. Watt, P. W., P. A. MacLennan, H. S. Hundal, C. M. Kuret, and M. J. Rennie. L(+)-Lactate transport in perfused rat skeletal muscle: kinetic characteristics and sensitivity to pH and transport inhibitors. *Biochim. Biophys. Acta* 944: 213–222, 1988.
203. Welch, H. G. Hyperoxia and human performance: a brief review. *Med. Sci. Sports Exerc.* 14: 253–262, 1982.
204. Welch, H. G., F. Bonde-Petersen, T. Graham, K. Clausen, and N. Secher. Effects of hyperoxia on leg blood flow and metabolism during exercise. *J. Appl. Physiol.* 44: 385–390, 1977.
205. Wendt, I. R., and J. B. Chapman. Fluorometric studies of recovery metabolism of rat fast- and slow-twitch muscles. *Am. J. Physiol.* 230: 1644–1649, 1976.
206. West, J. B. Lactate during exercise at extreme altitude. *Federation Proc.* 45: 2953–2957, 1986.
207. West, J. B. Acid-base status and blood lactate at extreme altitude. In: *Hypoxia, Metabolic Acidosis, and the Circulation*, edited by A. I. Arieff. New York: Oxford University Press, 1992, p. 33–44.
208. West, J. B., S. J. Boyer, D. J. Graber, P. H. Hackett, K. H. Maret, J. S. Milledge, R. M. Peters, Jr., C. J. Pizzo, M. Samaja, F. H. Sarnquist, R. B. Schoene, and R. M. Winslow. Maximal exercise at extreme altitudes on Mount Everest. *J. Appl. Physiol.* 55: 688–698, 1983.

209. Wibrand, F., and C. Juel. Reconstitution of the lactate carrier from rat skeletal-muscle sarcolemma. *Biochem. J.* 299: 533–537, 1994.
210. Wilson, D. F. Factors affecting the rate and energetics of mitochondrial oxidative phosphorylation. *Med. Sci. Sports Exerc.* 26: 37–43, 1994.
211. Wilson, D. F., M. Erecińska, C. Drown, and I. A. Silver. The oxygen dependence of cellular energy metabolism. *Arch. Biochem. Biophys.* 195: 485–493, 1979.
212. Wilson, D. F., C. S. Owen, and M. Erecinska. Quantitative dependence of mitochondrial oxidative phosphorylation on oxygen concentration: a mathematical model. *Arch. Biochem. Biophys.* 195: 494–504, 1979.
213. Wolfel, E. E., B. M. Groves, G. A. Brooks, G. E. Butterfield, R. S. Mazzeo, L. G. Moore, J. R. Sutton, P. R. Bender, T. E. Dahms, R. E. McCullough, R. G. McCullough, S.-Y. Huang, S.-F. Sun, R. F. Grover, H. N. Hultgren, and J. T. Reeves. Oxygen transport during steady-state submaximal exercise in chronic hypoxia. *J. Appl. Physiol.* 70: 1129–1136, 1991.
214. Woodson, R. D., R. E. Wills, and C. Lenfant. Effect of acute and established anemia on transport at rest, submaximal and maximal work. *J. Appl. Physiol.* 44: 36–43, 1978.
215. Young, A. J., W. J. Evans, A. Cymerman, K. B. Pandolf, J. J. Knapik, and J. T. Maher. Sparing effect of chronic high-altitude exposure on muscle glycogen utilization. *J. Appl. Physiol.* 52: 857–862, 1982.
216. Young, A. J., W. J. Evans, E. C. Fisher, R. L. Sharp, D. L. Costill, and J. T. Maher. Skeletal muscle metabolism of sea-level natives following short-term high-altitude residence. *Eur. J. Appl. Physiol.* 52: 463–466, 1984.
217. Young, A. J., P. M. Young, R. E. McCullough, L. G. Moore, A. Cymerman, and J. T. Reeves. Effect of beta-adrenergic blockade on plasma lactate concentration during exercise at high altitude. *Eur. J. Appl. Physiol.* 63: 315–322, 1991.
218. Yudilevich, D. L., and G. E. Mann. Unidirectional uptake of substrates at the blood side of secretory epithelia: stomach, salivary gland, pancreas. *Federation Proc.* 41: 3045–3053, 1982.

15. Cardiac output during exercise: contributions of the cardiac, circulatory, and respiratory systems

JOSEPH S. JANICKI | *Department of Physiology and Pharmacology, Auburn University, Auburn, Alabama*

DON D. SHERIFF | *Division of Cardiovascular Research, St. Elizabeth's Medical Center, Boston, Massachusetts*

JAMES L. ROBOTHAM | *Department of Anesthesiology and Critical Care Medicine, Johns Hopkins University, Baltimore, Maryland*

ROBERT A. WISE | *Department of Medicine, Johns Hopkins University, Baltimore, Maryland*

CHAPTER CONTENTS

THE CARDIAC, RESPIRATORY, AND PERIPHERAL CIRCULATORY SYSTEMS all contribute in an integrated fashion to ensure that, for a wide range of physical activity, cardiac output is matched to the metabolic requirements of the body. To this end, cardiac output is capable of a seven- to eightfold increase from its normal resting value of 5 liters/min (66). This is accomplished by increases in stroke volume and heart rate where stroke volume increments are the direct result of *(1)* elevations in venous return, which lead to increases in ventricular diastolic volume; *(2)* enhanced myocardial contractility; and *(3)* adjustments in systemic vascular impedance during systole.

In addition to the gradient between aortic and central venous pressures generated by the heart, adjustments in the peripheral circulatory system together with the combined actions of the skeletal muscle, abdominal, and respiratory pumps are essential to provide sufficient venous return to the heart during increased physical activity. The relationship among the circulatory and respiratory systems and the heart is schematically depicted in Figure 15.1. Here venous filling of the right heart is conceptualized as being proportional to the height of a blood-filled reservoir with respect to the right atrium; as the height of the venous reservoir above the level of the right atrium is increased, so is the filling of the right heart. Alterations in the pressure within the thorax also affect this height. For example, a decrease in intrathoracic pressure results in a similar decrease in right atrial pressure, when measured with respect to atmospheric pressure. This effectively raises the height or pressure gradient between the extrathoracic venous reservoir and the right heart. Likewise, the systemic circulation external to the thorax is depicted as a reservoir whose distance above the left ventricle (LV) represents the pressure head during systole that the left ventricle must generate and maintain in order to eject a portion of its volume. The relative height of this reservoir is affected by adjustments to the resistances of the peripheral circulatory beds and variations in intrathoracic pressure. Other factors within the thorax that influence cardiac output include the filling pressure gradient between the pulmonary circulation and the left heart (i.e., height of pulmonary reservoir relative to left heart in Fig. 15.1), the degree to which the pericardium and lungs resist cardiac distention, and cardiac chamber interdependence.

The purpose of this chapter is to consider in depth how each of these systems contributes to the cardiac output response during exercise. Accordingly, it is divided into three major sections, the first focused on the heart, the second on the peripheral circulation and its coupling to the heart, and the third on the respiratory system. The integration of these systems and their neurohumoral control are covered in more detail in Chapter 17.

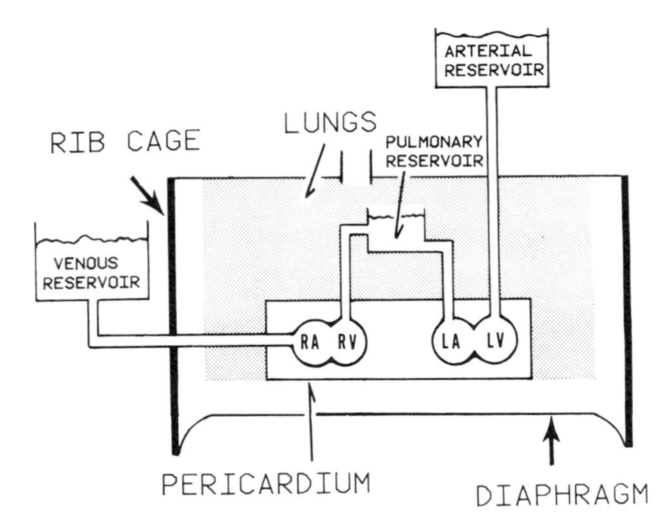

FIG. 15.1. Schematic representation of the relationship between the heart and the respiratory and circulatory systems. The systemic arterial and venous circulations and the pulmonary circulation are conceptualized as extra- and intrathoracic reservoirs, respectively. The heart is depicted as two pumps coupled in series. R, right; L, left; A, atrium; V, ventricle. (Reprinted with permission from Janicki, J. S., S. G. Shroff, and K. T. Weber. Influence of extracardiac forces on the cardiopulmonary unit. In: *Ventricular/Vascular Coupling*, edited by F. C. P. Yin. New York: Springer-Verlag, 1986, p. 262–287.)

INTRINSIC PROPERTIES OF THE HEART

Cardiac output is a function of heart rate and the following determinants of stroke volume: filling volume of the left ventricle (preload), force or stress which the ventricle must generate and sustain in order to eject blood into the aorta (afterload), and myocardial contractility. Indirect determinants are therefore considered to be those factors, external to the left ventricle (Fig. 15.1), that affect the amount of venous return to the heart or filling of the left ventricle (i.e., preload), and/or the vascular impedance of the systemic circulation (i.e., afterload). In this section, the role of the direct determinants and two of the indirect determinants, the pericardium and cardiac chamber interdependence, on the cardiac output response to exercise in normal, young and elderly, males and females, and in conditioned athletes is considered. The other indirect determinants are covered later under COUPLING OF THE HEART AND PERIPHERAL CIRCULATION and RESPIRATORY SYSTEM. Also in this section, the myocardial structural remodeling that occurs with conditioning and aging that may affect these determinants is examined.

Heart Rate (Exercise Response)

With either isotonic or isometric exercise, heart rate (HR) increases initially by parasympathetic inhibition and, subsequently, by sympathetic stimulation. The importance of neural control of heart rate is clearly demonstrated in heart failure patients after orthotopic heart transplantation (Fig. 15.2). As a result of total cardiac denervation, resting heart rate is elevated to a value that is close to the inherent rate of the sinoatrial node (130, 285) and, with the onset of exercise, the increase in heart rate, being dependent primarily on the level of circulating catecholamines (208), is delayed and markedly blunted (65, 281, 343). The relationship between HR and oxygen uptake (i.e., a measure of exercise intensity) is linear, with the slope being dependent on the mass of muscle involved (22). That is, when dynamic exercise is performed with progressively smaller groups of muscle, the slope was found to increase (22). At any given level of exercise, there is a tendency for HR to be faster in young subjects (i.e., <35 years of age) than in older subjects, particularly near peak exercise (286, 287, 342), as the maximal achievable HR decreases with age by approximately 0.75 bpm/year (109). For any level of submaximal oxygen uptake, HR is greater in females than in age-matched males, because of a lower hemoglobin in females (10). However, when the level of work is expressed as a percentage of maximal oxygen uptake, there is

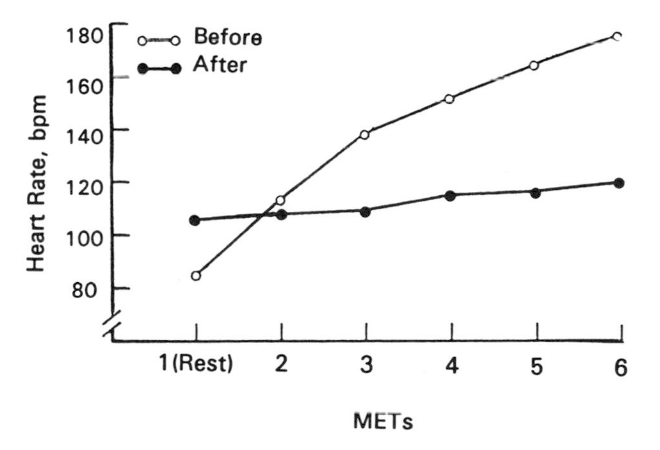

FIG. 15.2. Heart rate responses to graded exercise before and after orthotopic cardiac transplantation. As a result of cardiac denervation, the resting heart rate is elevated and the response to exercise, being dependent primarily on the level of circulating catecholamines, is delayed and blunted. (Reprinted with permission from Squires, R. W. Exercise training after cardiac transplantation. Med. Sci. Sports. Exerc. 23: 686–694, 1991.

no gender difference in the heart rate–work rate relation (10, 243, 342).

The heart rate responses to static and dynamic handgrip or two-knee extension exercise performed to local muscular fatigue are similar despite differences in oxygen uptake (151). Studies concerning the effect of age on the HR response to static exercise have consistently shown it to be greater in young individuals than in the elderly (138, 199, 215, 235). Regardless of age and gender, dynamic exercise training leads, via central reflex and peripheral adaptations (47; see also Chapter 17), to a decrease in heart rate at rest and at any given submaximal level of work (23, 254); maximum HR, however, is either unaffected or slightly decreased. This training-induced bradycardia is apparent after as little as 2 (53) to 10 (243) weeks of endurance conditioning. Thus, one beneficial consequence of conditioning is a broadening of the range of heart rates available during exercise. Unfortunately, such a conditioning effect is quickly lost within a few weeks of inactivity (166, 302).

Stroke Volume (Exercise Response)

Cardiac output in a normal nontrained individual performing maximal upright treadmill exercise increases approximately fourfold (Fig. 15.3). The relative contribution of heart rate and stroke volume (SV) to this rise in cardiac output is dependent on whether the exercise is being performed in the upright or supine position. Resting SV is always greater in the supine position compared to that in the upright position because of the increase in central blood volume and ventricular diastolic volume that occurs in the supine position. In going from the sitting to the supine position, the resting SV typically increases to a value that is approximately 20% less than maximum SV (305). In the upright position, exercise tachycardia is responsible for 63% of the increase in cardiac output and the remainder is due to an elevation in SV, with most of the one- to two-fold increase in SV occurring during the transition from rest to the moderate work levels. At levels of exercise greater than 60%–70% of maximum oxygen consumption (e.g., >20 ml · min^{-1} · kg^{-1} in Fig. 15.3), SV has been reported to decrease (3, 108, 254, 279, 287), to plateau (48, 75, 87, 254), or to continually increase (10, 75, 87, 140, 244, 279).

Effects of Training. The type of SV response at higher levels of work appears to be related to the degree of fitness. For example, in young sedentary individuals, SV at higher intensities of exercise has been noted to decline, whereas following training it was found

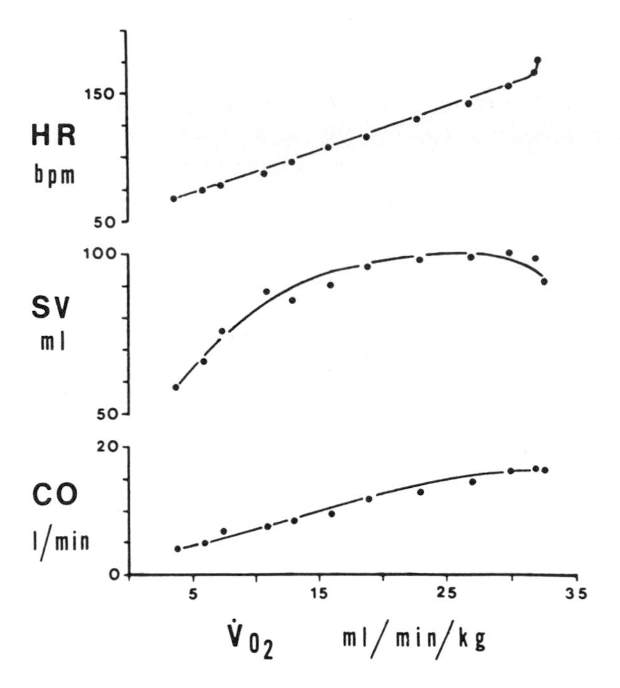

FIG. 15.3. Heart rate (HR), stroke volume (SV), and cardiac output (CO) responses to incremental treadmill exercise obtained in a normal, untrained individual. Increased heart rate is responsibile for 63% of the augmented cardiac output. Larger stroke volumes account for the remainder, primarily from rest to moderate levels of work. Oxygen uptake ($\dot{V}O_2$) indicates the level of work. (Reprinted with permission from Weber, K. T. Gas transport and the cardiopulmonary unit. In: *Cardiopulmonary Exercise Testing: Physiologic Principles and Clinical Application*, edited by K. T. Weber and J. S. Janicki. Philadelphia: W. B. Saunders Company, 1986, p. 15–33.)

to remain constant (279). In endurance-trained young (87) and elderly (75, 254) athletes, SV was found to increase continually as oxygen uptake approached a maximum.

Dynamic or endurance training. In general, dynamic or endurance training is associated with an increase in SV at any given level of isotonic exercise intensity (3, 23, 75, 136, 243, 244, 254, 278). At rest, the difference is usually not sufficiently large to reach the level of statistical significance. However, at mild to moderate levels of exercise, SV index (i.e., SV divided by body surface area) in young (20–40 years old) and elderly (60–68 years old) highly trained endurance athletes are 8–24 ml/m^2 (3, 27, 87, 136, 244) and 6–15 ml/m^2 (75, 254), respectively, greater than that in age-matched healthy untrained individuals. Stroke volume during dynamic exercise is also augmented as a result of short-term training for 3 months in young adults (279) and 9–12 months in elderly males (278). Interestingly, 9–12 months of conditioning did not elicit similar improvements in elderly females (280). Also, regardless of the period of training, the SV conditioning effect is lost within 4 weeks of becoming inactive (166).

Power training. In contrast to dynamic exercise, SV at rest in individuals who are involved in sports requiring predominantly static exercise and power training is similar to that in untrained individuals (155). Regardless of training status and type of training, SV remains invariant during moderate [i.e., 20%–40% of maximum voluntary contraction (MVC)] static exercise (136, 155, 274) and tends to decline as the level of isometric work approaches 80% of the MVC (136).

Effects of Aging. In a group of active males and females who were carefully screened for occult coronary artery disease, SV at rest has been found to increase slightly over the age range of 30–80 years (235). In addition, this trend was more pronounced during exercise, indicating an age-related reliance on SV for the maintenance of cardiac output during exercise. The fact that no age relation was seen for SV index in a group of men aged 20–50 years (107) indicates that this age-related compensation in the SV response to exercise becomes apparent in individuals older than 50 years.

Determinants of Stroke Volume

Afterload

Definition. Afterload describes the mechanical load opposing ventricular ejection. In the context of coupling of the arterial system to the left ventricle, afterload is best described by the hydraulic input impedance spectrum of the arterial circulation (171, 191, 200). Input impedance is derived from aortic pressure and flow measurements and is a complex quantity consisting of frequency-dependent modulus and phase components. Accordingly, one has to examine not only the impedance modulus at each frequency but also its phase in order to determine whether impedance is changing. Because of this and also because impedance units (i.e., dyne-s/cm^5 or dyne-s/cm^3) are not the units of stress (dyne/cm^2), impedance is not typically used by exercise or cardiac physiologists. Instead, afterload is taken to be the pressure, force, or stress (i.e., force per unit area of muscle) that the ventricle must generate to overcome the load imposed by the circulatory system. This practice has its origins in the classic papillary muscle preparation in which the stimulated muscle, with known cross-sectional area, had to lift a weight (276). Subsequently, this concept has been extended to the left ventricle where, with certain assumptions regarding chamber geometry and transmural distribution of the generated force or stress, myocardial stress becomes a function of ventricular pressure and volume (328). Thus, since chamber size and pressure are changing throughout the ejection period, myocardial stress is a time dependent variable, which typically peaks shortly after ejection begins and then continually declines for the remainder of ejection.

During exercise, both systolic pressure and ventricular filling volume are elevated, thus requiring a greater developed force or stress within the myocardium (i.e., ventricular afterload is increased). When one is concerned with muscle mechanics or the mechanical determinants of myocardial oxygen consumption during exercise, a knowledge of myocardial stress is essential. However, when considering the heart as a pump and the influence of afterload on SV, the dominant afterload factor is blood pressure. This is demonstrated in Figure 15.4, where it can be seen that when left ventricular end-diastolic pressure (LVEDP), contractility, and heart rate are experimentally held constant, SV is an inverse linear function of the level of pressure the ventricle must produce and maintain in order to eject a portion of its volume into the aorta (331). Such a linear relation is obtained regardless of the level of ventricular filling or contractility (Fig. 15.4). The net effect of increasing filling volume is to shift this relation to the right so that, for any given level of ejection pressure, a greater SV is realized. The x-axis intercept of this relation represents the maximal pressure that the ventricle can generate for the given set of experimental conditions (i.e., preload, contractility, and heart rate) and is referred to as the peak isovolumetric pressure. The relationship between end-diastolic volume (EDV) and its associated peak isovolumetric pressure is used to describe contractility (see below).

Blood pressure response to dynamic exercise. As shown in Figure 15.5, brachial arterial cuff systolic, diastolic, and mean blood pressure all increase, albeit at different rates, with the level of upright bicycle exercise. It should be noted that, because of amplification of the arterial pulse as it travels peripherally, brachial systolic and diastolic pressures do not always reflect the corresponding pressures in the ascending aorta. This is particularly true of systolic pressure during exercise. Rowell et al. (241) have shown that radial systolic arterial pressure measured directly at the midforearm level overestimated ascending aortic systolic pressure by as much as 80 mm Hg at maximal upright treadmill exercise. Thus, during exercise, pulse pressure at the peripheral site increased by a factor of 2.6, whereas the increase at the central site was only 1.95. Mean pres-

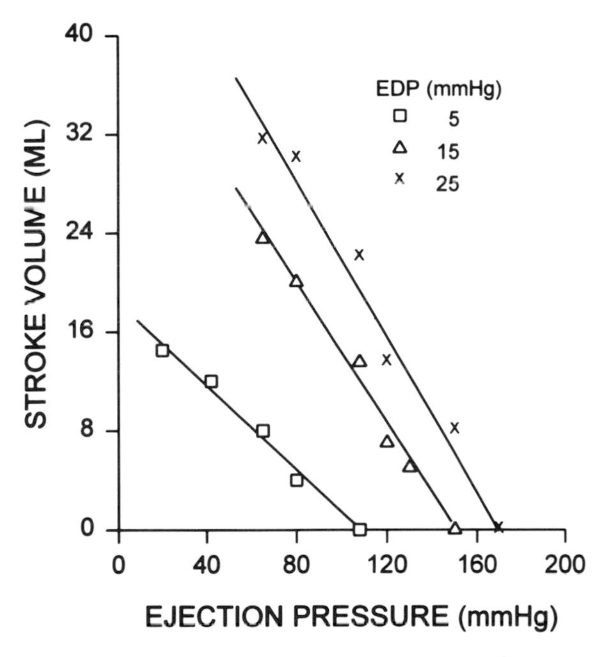

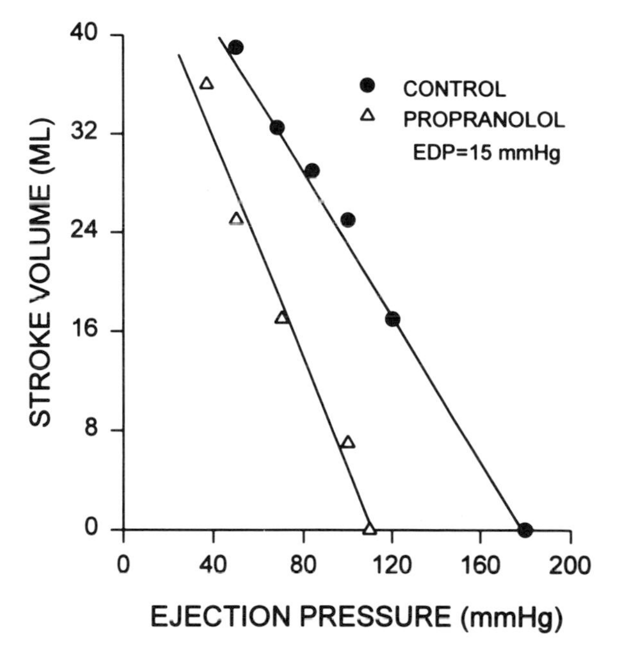

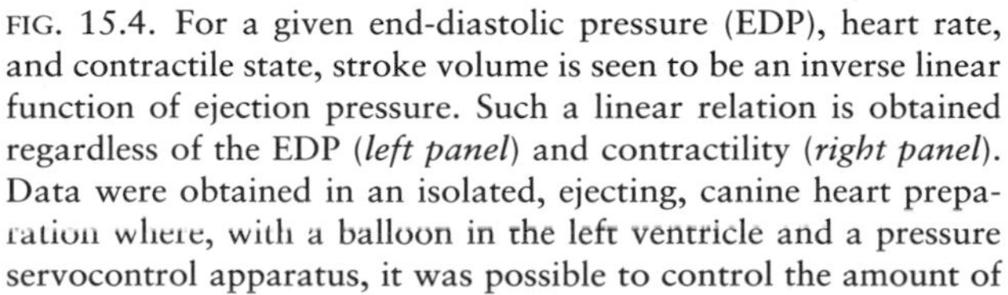
FIG. 15.4. For a given end-diastolic pressure (EDP), heart rate, and contractile state, stroke volume is seen to be an inverse linear function of ejection pressure. Such a linear relation is obtained regardless of the EDP (*left panel*) and contractility (*right panel*). Data were obtained in an isolated, ejecting, canine heart preparation where, with a balloon in the left ventricle and a pressure servocontrol apparatus, it was possible to control the amount of filling volume at the end of diastole and to maintain a constant level of pressure (i.e., ejection pressure) during ejection. (Reprinted with modifications and permission from Weber, K. T., J. S. Janicki, W. C. Hunter, S. Shroff, E. S. Pearlman, and A. P. Fishman. The contractile behavior of the heart and its functional coupling to the circulation. *Prog. Cardiovasc. Dis.* 24: 375–400, 1982.)

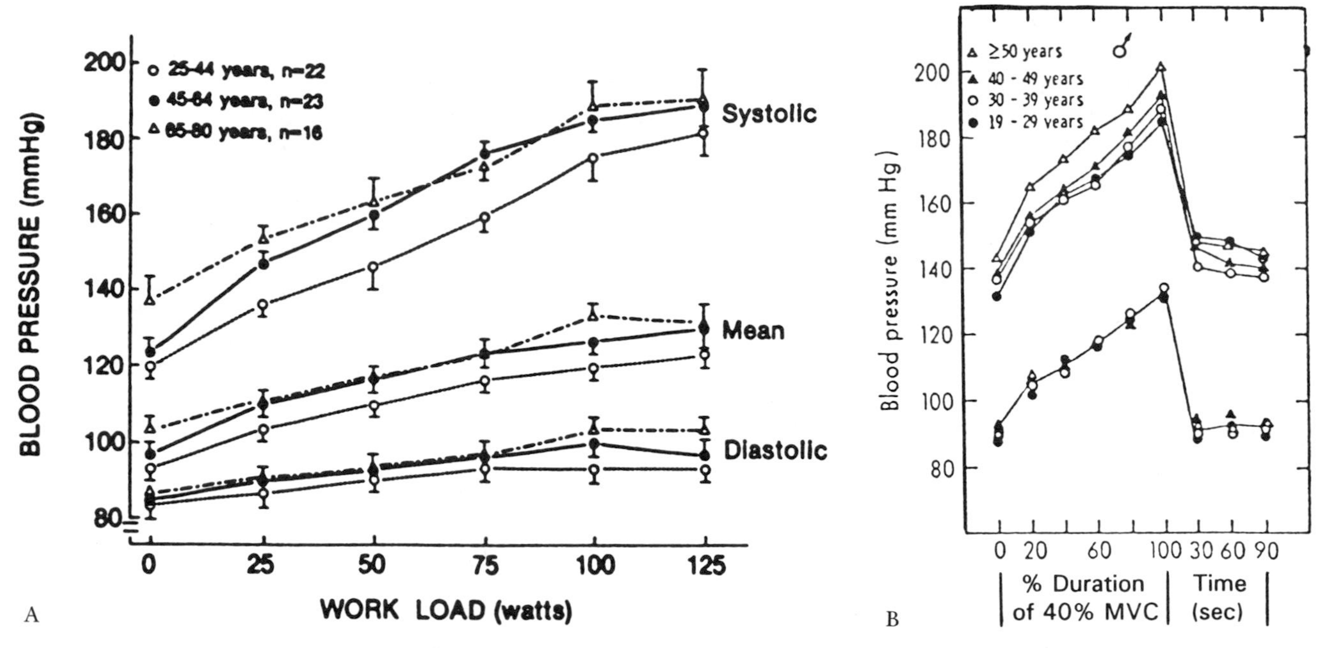

FIG. 15.5. *A*, Brachial artery cuff systolic, mean, and diastolic blood pressure responses to progressive upright bicycle exercise for three age groups. All three pressures continually increase with elevations in work load. For any level of work, there is a tendency for systolic and mean pressures to be lower in the youngest group. (Reprinted with permission from Gerstenblith, G., D. G. Renlund, and E. G. Lakatta. Cardiovascular response to exercise in younger and older men. *Federation Proc.* 46: 1834–1839, 1987.) *B*, Diastolic and systolic blood pressure responses to isometric exercise at 40% of maximal voluntary contraction (MVC) in normal individuals of different ages. These pressures were measured by auscultation of the noncontracting arm. Both pressures increase at the same rate and there is a significant correlation between systolic pressure and age. (Reprinted with permission from Petrofsky, J. S., and A. R. Lind. Aging, isometric strength and endurance, and cardiovascular responses to static effort. *J. Appl. Physiol.* 38: 91–95, 1975).

sures at the central and peripheral sites, however, were found to be nearly identical (241).

The brachial arterial mean and systolic blood pressure responses depicted in Figure 15.5*A* are similar to those reported in other recent studies (2, 3, 27, 72, 108, 254, 278, 306). However, diastolic blood pressure in these studies has been reported to either increase (2, 83, 108, 306), remain unchanged (3, 278), or decrease (72) during progressive exercise.

EFFECTS OF AGING. Also demonstrated in Figure 15.5*A* is the similarity in the pressor response for three age groups. While there was a trend for systolic and mean blood pressures to be lower in the 25- to 44-year-old group, significant correlations between blood pressure and age during exercise have (343) and have not been observed (107, 215, 235). There is, however, a tendency for resting systolic blood pressure to be significantly greater in elderly individuals (9, 215, 235). Blood pressure responses during exercise also appear to be similar in men and women (278, 342). Here, too, one must be mindful of pressure wave amplification effects with age. Studies of wave transmission between the central aorta and brachial artery in humans have indicated a marked decrease in amplification with age (190). Thus, the systolic pressure response to exercise is more representative of central pressure in the 65- to 80-year-old group than the responses in the other two age groups, and it is highly likely that peak systolic central pressure during exercise is greater in the oldest group than in the other two groups.

Blood pressure response to isometric exercise and effects of aging. Brachial artery diastolic and systolic blood pressure responses to isometric exercise are presented in Figure 15.5*B* for four decades of age. In contrast to dynamic exercise, these pressures as well as mean pressure continuously increase during the exercise by approximately the same rate; following termination of the exercise there was a rapid return to baseline levels (215, 320). As seen here and noted by others, there is a significant correlation between systolic blood pressure and age both at rest and during static exercise (215, 294). This was not the case for diastolic pressure. Again, it should be emphasized that, because of pressure amplification, peak systolic blood pressure during exercise in the brachial artery is greater than that in the ascending aorta, particularly in younger individuals (190, 241).

Blood pressure response to isometric and dynamic exercise. The blood pressure responses to static and dynamic exercise (i.e., handgrip or two-knee extension) are similar despite a higher oxygen uptake for the dynamic mode of contraction (151). Also, with both types of exercise, the pressor response appears to be proportional to the mass of muscle actively involved in the performance of the exercise (36, 151, 174, 187, 252, 253, 255). However, this may not be the case when the isometric contraction is brief and of high force as opposed to one that is sustained and of moderate force (338). When the two modes of contraction are combined, the systolic blood pressure response to handgrip is preserved during submaximal (i.e., <50% maximal oxygen uptake) dynamic exercise, but at greater dynamic work the handgrip response is either markedly attenuated or abolished (137). The level to which the sympathetic nervous system is activated is proportional to active muscle size (252, 253) and is thought to play a major role in determining the blood pressure response to combined modes of exercise (137).

Effects of training. When exercise blood pressure levels in trained and untrained individuals are expressed as a function of percentage maximal oxygen uptake and compared, conditioning does not seem to alter the blood pressure response to exercise—static or dynamic—in any consistent fashion or to any measurable degree (3, 155, 254, 260, 278). However, conditioning results in a greater maximal oxygen uptake. Consequently, blood pressure comparisons at absolute levels of submaximal work reveal significant reductions in blood pressure as a result of conditioning (16, 72, 75, 87).

Systemic vascular resistance. By definition of systemic vascular resistance, mean blood pressure equals the product of cardiac output and systemic vascular resistance. As the intensity of physical activity rises, systemic vascular resistance continually decreases because of the vasodilation that occurs in working skeletal muscle (see later under COUPLING OF THE HEART AND PERIPHERAL CIRCULATION). From rest to maximal exercise the drop in resistance is between 50% and 60% of the resting value. These vascular changes accommodate the seven- to eight-fold elevation in cardiac output, with only a slight rise in mean arterial blood pressure.

Influence of afterload on stroke volume. With the above information regarding the blood pressure response to exercise, the issue of how such an exercise-induced increase in pressure might influence SV can be addressed. Recall that when contractility, heart rate, and filling volume were experimentally held constant, SV was shown to be an inverse, linear function of ejection pressure with a representative slope of −0.3 ml/mm Hg (Fig. 15.4). The average pressure during ejection, or ejection pressure (EP), can be approximated from arterial systolic (SBP) and diastolic (DBP) pressures using the formula: EP = DBP + 0.8*[SBP-DBP] (323). For representative central aortic blood pressure values reported by Rowell et al. (241) for rest (112/68 mm Hg) and peak dynamic exercise (154/70 mm Hg), the corresponding EP values are calculated to be 103 and 137 mm Hg. Assuming for man a similar slope between SV and EP as that for the dog (e.g., −0.3 ml/mm Hg; Fig. 15.4), this 34 mm Hg exercise-related elevation in EP would be predicted to bring about a 10 ml reduction in SV if filling volume and contractility were to remain unchanged.

Preload

Left ventricular end-diastolic volume

DEFINITION. As regards the cardiac myocyte, preload is measured by the degree to which it is stretched or by its sarcomere length. In papillary muscle experiments, the muscle fibers are arranged in a parallel fashion and, therefore, muscle length or resting stress is used as an indicator of preload. In the ventricle where muscle fiber orientation varies from epicardium to endocardium, preload is not homogenous. Thus, it is taken to be proportional to either the volume in the ventricle or to the force or stress that exists in the muscle wall prior to contraction. Direct measurement indicates wall force or stress to be proportional to the pressure and volume in the ventricular chamber (105). However, to estimate average wall force or stress from these measurements, assumptions regarding the shape of the ventricle have to be made (170) and, for this reason, volume or some other measure of ventricular size such as diameter are typically used as indicators of ventricular preload when considering the heart as a pump and the influence of preload on SV.

LVEDV RESPONSE TO DYNAMIC EXERCISE. Most of our knowledge of ventricular volume in humans during exercise has come from measurements made with either echocardiography or ventriculography. Both of these techniques, however, require that the upper portion of the torso be motionless. Accordingly, our present knowledge regarding the LV volume response during dynamic exercise in humans has been obtained using cycle ergometry with the subject either supine, seated at an angle, or seated upright. Like stroke volume, LVEDV at rest declines in going from the supine to the upright seated position [e.g., 97 ± 25 to 68 ± 18 ml/m^2 (108)]. Other limitations associated with these techniques are discussed elsewhere (217, 307, 340).

In their 1985 review, Schaible and Scheuer (249) concluded that the effect of exercise on LVEDV was not clear, with different studies reporting an increase, no change, or even a decrease. While most subsequent investigations indicate that LVEDV becomes larger during exercise, reports of no significant change still appear (250, 251, 310). In studies where LVEDV is found to rise with progressive exercise, the response is reported to be either a continual rise (3) or an increase up to work levels of 40%–70% of maximal, after which it becomes invariant (48, 68, 107, 140, 342) or declines (2, 107, 244, 254, 342). The response of LVEDV to exercise appears to be age related (Fig. 15.6). Rodeheffer et al. (235) found LVEDV to either continually increase during progressive exercise in individuals who were between 65 and 80 years of age, initially increase and then plateau at higher levels of work in subjects aged between 45 and 64 years, or initially increase and then decline at higher work levels in younger individuals (25–44 years). This observation was confirmed in approximately half of the above-cited studies (2, 48, 107, 244, 342).

LVEDV RESPONSE TO ISOMETRIC EXERCISE. In contrast to dynamic exercise, light to moderate static exercise is not accompanied by large elevations in LVEDV (155, 207, 294), and with heavy isometric work it typically decreases (136). For handgrip efforts of 30% of the MVC, LV internal diameter was noted to significantly increase by 3% (294) to 12% (207). During leg static exercise greater than 75% MVC, 14%–22% and 30% decreases in chamber volume index (16) and in LVEDV (148), respectively, have been noted. The increase in LVEDV with light to moderate static exercise is probably related to the accompanying increase in arterial blood pressure (see above). The decrease in LVEDV with heavy static exercise involving a large muscle mass is probably related to a throttling of blood flow to the contracting muscles and a Valsalva-induced decrease in systemic venous return to the heart (see later under RESPIRATORY SYSTEM).

EFFECTS OF TRAINING. Endurance or dynamic training is associated with significant LV chamber enlargement and a higher SV. Thus, chronic chamber dilatation is a prominent compensatory adaptation responsible for the maintenance of cardiac output at a reduced heart rate. This remodeling occurs in young and old male (27, 48, 72, 131, 250, 254, 317, 340) and young female (51, 243) endurance athletes, and after endurance training for periods of 4 weeks (53), 10 weeks (243), and 9–12 months (68). One notable exception is the study by Spina and coworkers (280), where LV enlargement was not seen in a group of elderly females after 9–12 months of endurance training.

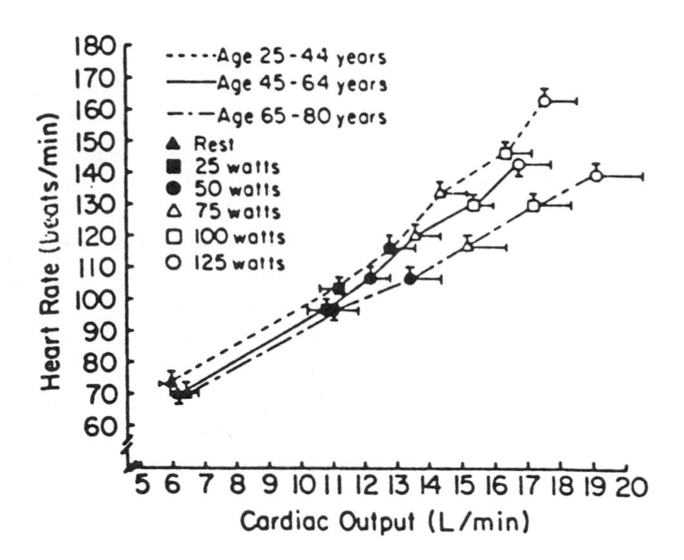

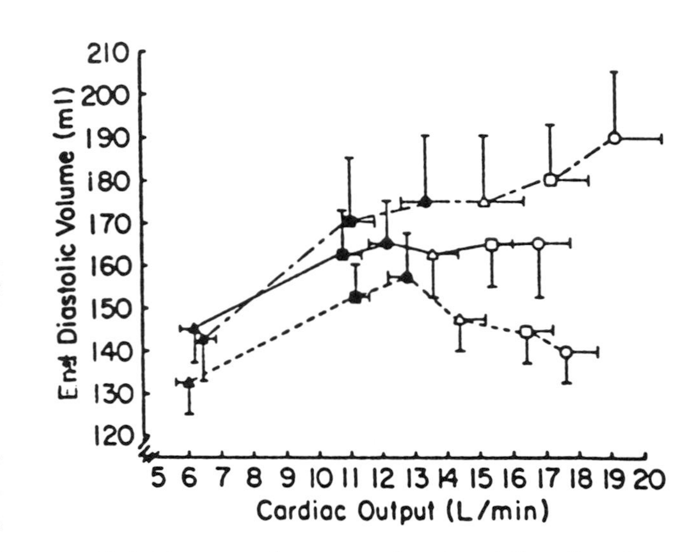

FIG. 15.6. Heart rate (*upper panel*) and end-diastolic volume (*lower panel*) as a function of cardiac output for three age groups of normal individuals performing progressive, upright bicycle exercise. Typically, end-diastolic volume increases and then declines in the 25- to 40-year group, while in the 45- to 64-year group it initially increases and then becomes invariant and in the 65- to 80-year group it continually increases. The heart rate at which the response differences become apparent (i.e., 115 bpm) is similar in the three age groups. (Reprinted with permission from Rodeheffer, R. J., G. Gerstenblith, L. C. Becker, J. L. Fleg, M. L. Weisfeldt, and E. G. Lakatta. Exercise cardiac output is maintained with advancing age in healthy human subjects: cardiac dilatation and increased stroke volume compensate for a diminished heart rate. *Circulation* 69: 203–213, 1984.)

Ventricular size remodeling in power-trained individuals also differs from that seen with endurance training. Basically, no change in LV internal dimensions are seen in resistance-trained individuals when expressed in absolute terms or relative to body surface area (74, 136, 156, 181, 206).

EFFECTS OF AGING. No significant age-related relationship for LVEDV at rest has been found for the age range of 25–80 years (107, 235, 294). As mentioned above, there is a tendency for LVEDV during dynamic exercise to be greater in the elderly (235, 342). This age-related cardiac enlargement was statistically apparent at intermediate levels of exercise intensity. As a result of this enhanced exercise preload, SV increased in a parallel fashion, thereby offsetting the age-related attenuation of the exercise heart rate response.

INFLUENCE OF PRELOAD ON SV. The relation between SV and preload is the well-known Frank-Starling mechanism or "law of the heart," which states that there is a direct proportion between the diastolic volume of the heart and the force of contraction. In the isolated heart preparation with contractility, ejection pressure, and heart rate held constant, SV is directly related to end-diastolic volume. Under these conditions, end-systolic volume remained either unchanged or increased slightly as EDV was increased as shown in Figure 15.7 and the increment in SV was found to be equal to or slightly less than the amount by which EDV was raised (290, 331).

In four recent studies (68, 72, 254, 278) where absolute resting and peak exercise values of LVEDV were determined using supine cycle ergometry, the average rest and peak exercise values were 122 and 139 ml, respectively. From the experimental results shown in Figure 15.7, it can be seen that if afterload and contractility were to remain constant, this 17 ml increase in LVEDV would be expected to result in a similar increase in SV. With upright cycle ergometric exercise, LVEDV at rest was reported (48) to be less (87 ml) than that for the supine position and the exercise-induced increase to be greater (24 ml). In all likelihood, the increase in LVEDV with maximal treadmill exercise would be even larger because of this positional dependence and the fact that a larger muscle mass is involved.

Left ventricular end-diastolic pressure–volume relation. As discussed later under COUPLING OF THE HEART AND PERIPHERAL CIRCULATION, the increase in preload during exercise is primarily the result of adjustments to the peripheral circulatory system that collectively are responsible for an enhanced venous return to the heart. In addition, the diastolic properties of the cardiac chambers will influence the degree to which they are filled. That is, for a given level of ventricular filling or EDP, the filling or EDV is a function of the following: *(1)* myocardial mechanical properties, *(2)* compressive forces external to the ventricle (e.g., those originating from the other cardiac chambers, the pericardium, and the lung), and *(3)* other physiological variables including heart rate and coronary arterial pressure (84, 86, 119, 121). Also, in isolated functioning hearts, variations in arterial pressure with constant coronary perfusion pressure were noted to alter the relation between EDV and EDP (123).

The left ventricular EDP-EDV relation obtained over the range of EDP from 0–25 mm Hg is typically nonlinear, so that chamber stiffness (slope of the relation, ΔEDP/ΔEDV) becomes progressively greater as EDV is increased (Fig. 15.8). Also, a nonparallel shift of this relation to the right or left would indicate an overall decrease or increase, respectively,

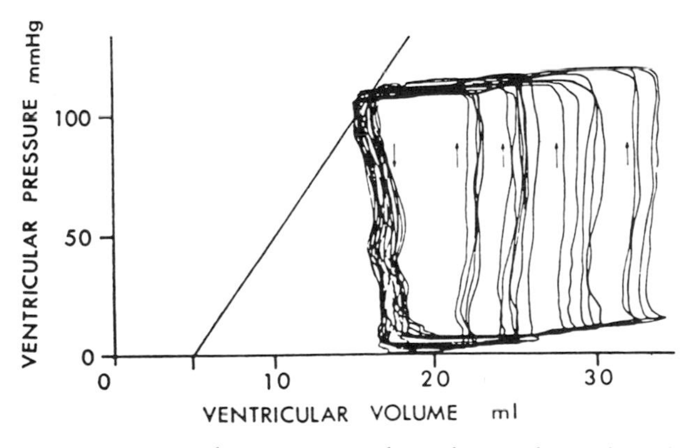

FIG. 15.7. Ventricular pressure–volume loops obtained in the isolated heart preparation at varying end-diastolic volumes. With constant contractility, ejection pressure, and heart rate, end-systolic volume remains invariant and the increase in stroke volume is equal to the amount by which EDV is raised. (Reprinted with permission from Suga, H., K. Sagawa, and A. A. Shoukas. Load independence of the instantaneous pressure-volume ratio of the canine left ventricle and effects of epinephrine and heart rate on the ratio. *Circ. Res.* 32: 314–322, 1973.

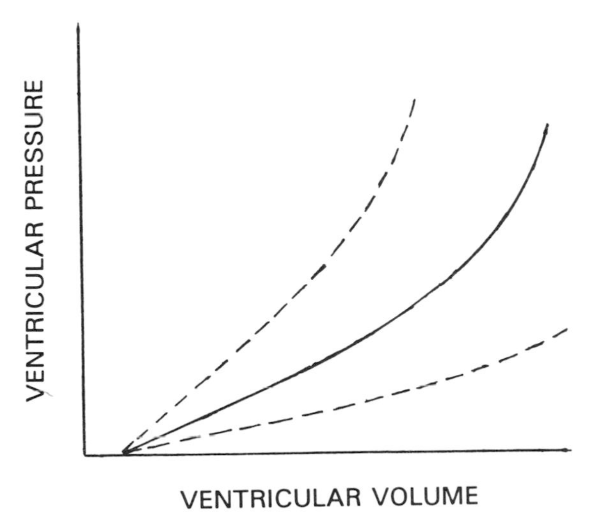

FIG. 15.8. The left ventricular end-diastolic pressure–volume relation over the physiologic range of end-diastolic pressure is typically nonlinear, with the ventricle becoming stiffer as it is dilated. A nonparallel shift to the left or right indicates that ventricular stiffness has increased or decreased, respectively.

in chamber stiffness. For example, at a given EDP, EDV would be less as a result of the EDP-EDV relation shifting to the left.

EFFECTS OF HEART RATE. Increases in heart rate disproportionately shorten the mid-diastolic slow filling portion of the cardiac cycle, allowing less time for filling and possibly complete relaxation. From heart rates between 65 and 70 bpm to heart rates between 150 and 160 bpm, LV filling time (i.e., time between mitral valve opening and closure) decreases by 70% (198). However, experimental results indicate that, in dogs, the EDP-EDV relation is insensitive to a reduced diastolic interval, provided heart rate remains less than 170 bpm (28, 173, 277, 303, 333). Heart rates above this value result in a nonparallel shift of the EDP-EDV curve to the left. This is the result of insufficient time for complete relaxation. This was demonstrated in studies in which rapid pacing greater than 170 bpm was combined with stellate ganglion stimulation to increase the rate of ventricular relaxation. This ensured that relaxation prior to the end of diastole was completed despite the high heart rate. Consequently, EDP decreased to a level identical to that obtained at lower pacing rates (173, 277). Weisfeldt et al. (333) determined that complete relaxation required an additional time period of 3.5 time constants from the time at which maximal negative dP/dt (i.e., the rate of change of LV pressure) occurred. Here, the time constant, which is measured in seconds, represents the time required for the LV pressure at maximal negative dP/dt to decrease by 63.2%. It was only at heart rates greater than 170 bpm that the next contraction occurred before complete relaxation.

It is not known in humans whether elevated heart rates experienced during heavy, dynamic exercise play a significant role in determining ventricular stiffness and hence in limiting ventricular filling and, if so, to what extent. That is, the two- to fourfold rest to peak exercise increase in peak filling rate (18, 27, 46, 251, 310) may counteract or blunt the influence of heart rate on the EDP-EDV relation. Higginbotham and co-workers (108) reported that, in a group of individuals aged 20–50 years, pulmonary capillary wedge pressure (PCWP), a measure of LVEDP, continually increased during progressive upright cycle exercise. However, at high levels of exercise, this increase in PCWP was not accompanied by elevations in EDV or SV. In fact, there was a trend for EDV to decrease near maximal exercise in a majority of the subjects. The authors concluded that this apparent increase in ventricular diastolic stiffness was the result of a disproportionally shortened diastolic portion of the cardiac cycle at the high heart rates (167 ± 16 bpm) encountered during maximal exercise. If this is the case, then it appears to be confined to the age of the individuals examined. As seen in Figure 15.6, LVEDV responses during exercise are age related despite similar heart rate responses. In the young group (25–44 years of age), LVEDV decreased once heart rate exceeded 115 bpm, while in the elderly group (65–80 years) it continually increased up to the maximum heart rate of 140 bpm achieved in this group. As discussed below, pericardial constraint and/or ventricular interdependence could also account for the findings of Higginbotham et al. (108). Also of interest here is the observation that, despite similar heart rates and blood pressures, exercise training abolishes the typical reduction in SV and presumably LVEDV that occurs in young sedentary male and females at work levels between 50% and 100% of maximum oxygen uptake (279). Here, too, training-induced alterations in diastolic properties of the myocardium and/or pericardium may be responsible.

EFFECTS OF CORONARY ARTERIAL PRESSURE. It is well known that the left ventricle becomes stiffer with elevations in coronary arterial pressure via the "erectile" or "garden hose" effect (81, 246). With increments in coronary pressure and intracoronary blood volume, there is a swelling and increased stiffening of the ventricular wall (81, 182). This stiffening shifts the left ventricular EDP-EDV relation to the left (Fig. 15.8). However, a review of experimental results indicates that coronary arterial pressure appears to influence the stiffness of the ventricle only when this pressure is varied over the range of 0–60 mm Hg (1, 81, 246, 304). For coronary perfusion pressures within the range 60–150 mm Hg, where coronary blood flow is expected to be autoregulated (183), the EDP-EDV relation is unaffected (1, 304). However, during exercise, the coronary bed dilates at the same time coronary arterial pressure is increasing. Thus, it is possible that the resulting exercise-induced increase in coronary flow may, via the erectile effect, influence preload.

EFFECTS OF AFTERLOAD. In addition to the erectile effect, exercise-induced increases in arterial pressure appear to influence preload via a different mechanism (85, 123, 177). In an isolated dog heart, LVEDP declined immediately as the level of ejection pressure was increased despite constant contractility, coronary perfusion pressure, and LVEDV (123). The magnitude of change in LVEDP (i.e., 0.2–6.0 mm Hg) depended on the increment in ejection pressure and the volume in the ventricle before the perturbation in pressure. While the mechanism for this decrease in ventricular stiffness as ejection pressure is increased is unknown, it may serve to negate any exercise-induced increases in stiffness related to the erectile effect.

The fact that LVEDP falls following an elevation in ejection pressure indicates that this maneuver shifts the EDP-EDV curve to the right; that is, the left ventricle becomes more distensible (Fig. 15.9). As demonstrated in Figure 15.4, a linear, inverse relation between SV and EP is obtained when EDP and contractility are maintained constant. If, instead, EDV is held constant, then EDP decreases and the SV-EP relation becomes nonlinear and steeper as EP approaches higher values (331). In this nonlinear region, SV is less for any given EP value. Thus, if filling pressure remains constant, the net effect of this afterload-dependent increase in ventricular distensibility would partially counter the afterload-dependent decrease in SV. This effect has been estimated from experimental data to result in a SV increase as high as 3 ml (123). In terms of the example discussed in the subsection on the effects of afterload, the reduction in SV due to the exercise-induced elevation in EP would have been 17% larger in the absence of an afterload-related increase in distensibility.

EFFECTS OF VENTRICULAR INTERDEPENDENCE. The function of one ventricle is inextricably related to that of the other ventricle by the common muscular wall that surrounds the chambers, the interventricular septum, and the pericardium (25, 86, 120). "Ventricular interdependence" is the term that has come to be used to describe the mechanical interaction or interplay between the ventricles. Ventricular interdependence is best demonstrated in the isolated heart where the in-series coupling of the ventricles, the influence of the atria, and the effects of reflexogenic alterations in contractility are removed and ventricular volumes are controlled and directly measurable. Also, the influence of the pericardium on ventricular interdependence can be assessed. Accordingly, with volume held constant in one ventricle, the end-diastolic pressure is noted to rise with that of the other ventricle. An increasing EDP in a ventricle with constant volume indicates a shift of its EDP-EDV relation to the left as illustrated in Figure 15.10. This stiffening of the ventricle is the direct result of a compressive force generated by the septum and free wall of the chamber. For example, an increase in right ventricular (RV) volume shifts the septum towards the left ventricle. Also, the outward movement of the RV free wall stretches the common muscle fibers that surround both ventricles so that the free wall of the LV is pulled inward (see Fig.

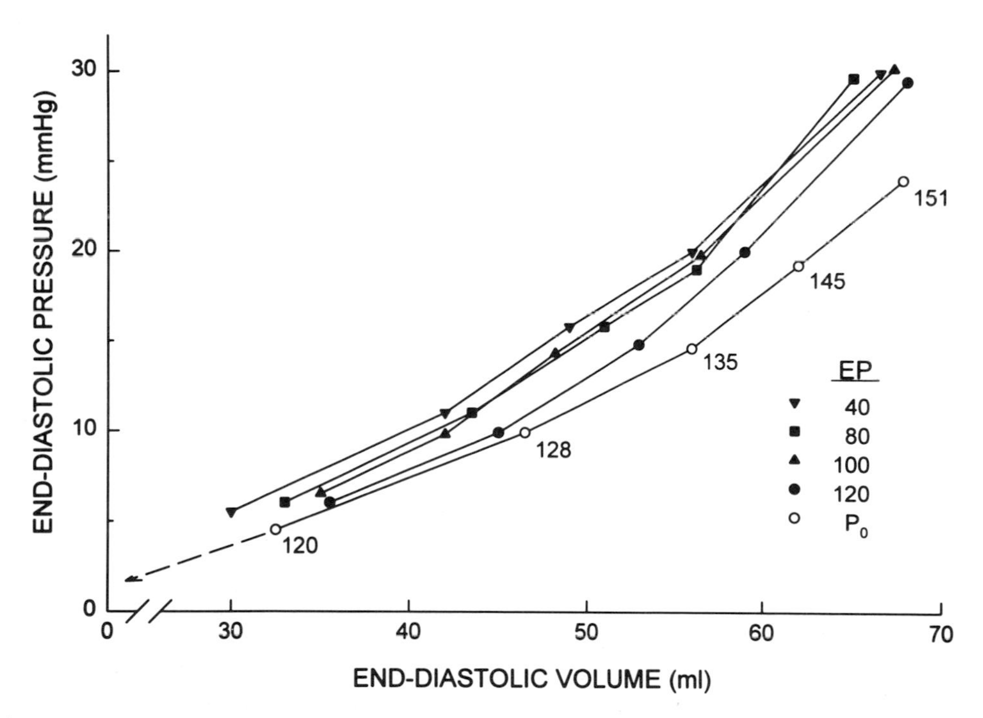

FIG. 15.9. End-diastolic pressure (EDP) –end-diastolic volume (EDV) relations obtained at constant contractility, heart rate, and ejection pressure (EP) or the isovolumetric state (P_0). As EP (mm Hg) is increased, the EDP-EDV relation is shifted downward or to the right, with the lowest curve obtained with the ventricle contracting isovolumetrically. Thus, the ventricle becomes less stiff as ejection pressure is raised. Numbers next to open circle EDP-EDV data points represent corresponding peak isovolumetric pressures (mm Hg). [Reprinted with permission from Janicki, J. S., K. T. Weber, and L. L. Hefner. Ejection pressure and the left ventricular pressure-volume relation. *Am. J. Physiol.* 232 (*Heart Circ. Physiol.* 1): H545–H552, 1977.]

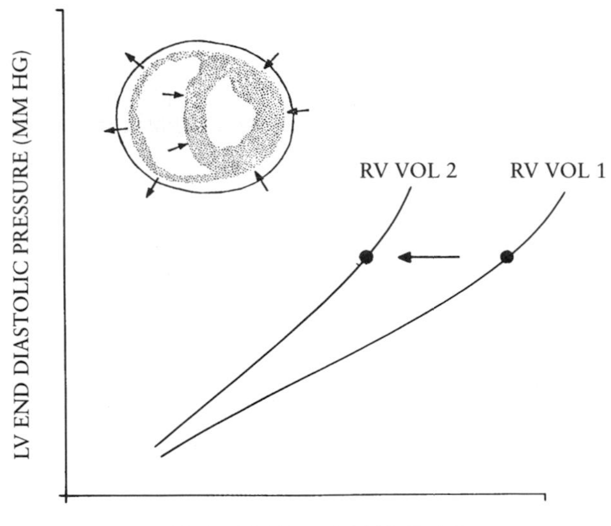

FIG. 15.10. The left ventricular pressure (EDP) –volume (EDV) relation obtained at two different levels of right ventricular (RV) volume (VOL). As a result of ventricular interdependence, the EDP-EDV relation is shifted to the right as RV VOL is increased from RV VOL 1 to RV VOL 2. As depicted in the *inset*, this is the result of the septum being shifted toward the left ventricle and the outward movement of the RV free wall stretching the common muscle fibers and pericardium that surround both ventricles and causing an inward pull of the LV free wall.

15.10, *inset*). At a constant EDV in the left ventricle, pressure will increase as a result of increased right ventricular filling. If instead LV diastolic pressure is maintained constant when the RV is distended, then its volume would decrease.

In nondiseased hearts with normal chamber volumes, ventricular interdependence helps ensure that right and left ventricular cardiac output remain equal over a respiratory cycle. That is, when RV volume increases during inspiration, LV volume and therefore its output are transiently reduced because of ventricular interdependence (110). This reduced LV output over several subsequent cardiac cycles will result in a reduction in RV filling volume and, via interdependence, a restoration of LV volume to its preinspiration value. At the same time LV output is reduced, RV output is increased, which over several cardiac cycles will transiently increase LV filling and output. This respiratory-linked ventricular interdependence is expected to coordinate right and left ventricular function in a similar fashion during exercise despite a markedly elevated ventilation (see later under RESPIRATORY SYSTEM).

The degree of interdependence can be expressed as the ratio of the increase in EDP in one ventricle with fixed EDV to the increase in EDP in the other ventricle undergoing expansion of its volume. This ratio is referred to as the ventricular interaction or cross-talk gain (270). Accordingly, the right-to-left interaction gain is defined as $(LVEDP_b - LVEDP_a)/(RVEDP_b - RVEDP_a)$, where the subscripts, b and a, refer to before and after the increase in RV volume. Right-to-left interaction gain is a direct function of LVEDV and the degree to which the RV is expanded (i.e., $RVEDP_b - RVEDP_a$). In the isolated dog heart, the average gain is approximately 0.26 (122). A slightly higher gain of 0.33 is found in vivo (270). When the pericardium is removed the interaction gain decreases two- to fourfold (67, 122, 265, 269).

Ventricular interdependence also occurs during systole. In the isolated heart contracting isovolumetrically, the peak systolic pressure in the ventricle with fixed volume increases as volume in the other ventricle is augmented (122). The interdependence-related rise in peak pressure in the LV was twice that in the RV. Systolic interdependence, therefore, results in a parallel shift to the left in the peak isovolumetric and end-systolic pressure–volume relations (332). This leftward shift indicates a decrease in the end-systolic volume or a greater SV. Indeed, others (269, 271) have shown that the reduction in LV end-systolic volume secondary to systolic interdependence partially compensates for the decrease in filling volume and output secondary to diastolic interdependence. Systolic interdependence is not influenced by the pericaridum (122).

EFFECTS OF THE PERICARDIUM. The enhancement in interaction gain by the pericardium is a direct consequence of its pressure–volume relationship. That is, as the size of one ventricle is expanded to a point where the pericardium is stretched, the resulting increase in intrapericardial pressure is transmitted to the other ventricle, causing a rise in its EDP and/or a fall in its volume. Accordingly, the ventricles as well as the atria are competing for intrapericardial space, the overall size of which is limited by the constraining properties of the pericardium. When one of the chambers disproportionally increases in size, it effectively limits the intrapericardial space available to the other chambers. Thus, with the pericardium intact, there is also the possibility of atrial-ventricular interdependence (167).

As mentioned earlier, a major functional role of the pericardium is to provide a mechanical constraint to acute variations in heart size (113). This is evidenced by the fact that, when the pericardium is removed, the EDP-EDV relation for both ventricles shifts such that the ventricles are able to accommodate a larger filling volume for the same filling pressure (122). Thus, an exercise-induced acute increase in heart size may result in stretching the pericardium to the point where its elastic properties restrict further cardiac dilation and utilization of the Frank-Starling mechanism. Direct experimental evidence of pericardial constraint during maximal exercise has been reported by Stray-Gundersen et al. (288). Using untrained dogs, they found maximal SV to significantly increase from 65 ± 4 ml to 76 ± 6 ml following the removal of the pericardium. This increase in maximal SV resulted in a 3.5 liters/min or 20% increase in maximal cardiac output and a 7.7 ml O_2 per min/kg or 7% increase in maximal oxygen uptake. More recently, it has been shown in pigs that these increases in SV, cardiac output, and oxygen uptake following pericardiectomy were the result of a 10% increase in LV end-diastolic dimension and an estimated 33% increase in LVEDV (103). Thus, in dogs and pigs, maximal cardiac output is limited by the pericardium, suggesting that the Frank-Starling mechanism is more fully utilized by removal of the pericardium. Also, maximal oxygen delivery is limited by the pericardium, confirming that active skeletal muscle can utilize more oxygen if provided.

The roles of the pericardium and ventricular interdependence in humans have been difficult to assess. However, evidence exists which indicates that, in patients undergoing elective surgery for aortic valve replacement or coronary artery bypass, the nondiseased pericardium contributes substantially to atrial and ventricular intracavitary pressures (24, 313). In addition, Janicki (118) found evidence of pericardial constraint during exercise in 31 of 61 patients with heart failure of varying degree and diverse etiology. The occurrence of pericardial constraint was characterized by SV becoming invariant despite continuing increases in right atrial and pulmonary capillary wedge pressures as the level of treadmill work was further raised (Fig. 15.11). The fact that right atrial and pulmonary capillary wedge pressures continued to increase by equal amounts despite a constant SV (responses R2 and R3 in Fig. 15.11), implies that exercise-induced increments in intracardiac blood volume had increased intrapericardial volume to the steep portion of the pericardial pressure–volume relation. Subsequent increases in intracardiac volume, atrial and/or ventricular, further stretched the pericardium and produced elevations in intrapericardial pressure. The concordant increases in right atrial and pulmonary capillary wedge pressures that occurred after SV had reached a peak were, therefore, reflections of these increases

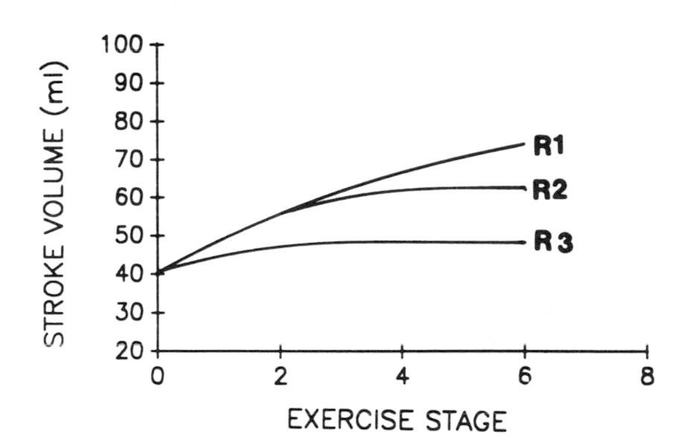

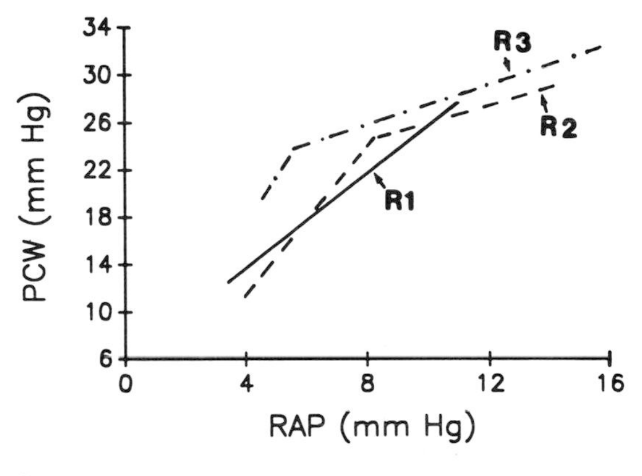

FIG. 15.11. Summary of three exercise hemodynamic responses (R1, R2, and R3) to progressive upright treadmill exercise observed in heart failure patients with similar degrees of impairment. PCW, pulmonary capillary wedge pressure; RAP, right atrial pressure. In responses R2 and R3, the fact that PCW and RAP continue to rise with a slope of 1 despite an invariant stroke volume indicates pericardial constraint to further exercise-induced ventricular expansion. (Reprinted with permission from Janicki, J. S. Influence of the pericardium and ventricular interdependence on left ventricular diastolic and systolic function in patients with heart failure. *Circulation* 81: III-15–III-20, 1990.)

in intrapericardial pressure. In contrast, when pericardial constraint was not apparent during exercise, SV did not become constant and the increments in PCWP were two- to threefold greater than that of right atrial pressure (response R1 in Fig. 15.11). Reeves et al. (223) also found PCWP to be closely coupled to right atrial pressure during upright cycle exercise in normal volunteers and speculated that failure of SV to increase with increasing right atrial and wedge pressures most likely reflected a restriction by the pericardium.

As mentioned earlier, Higginbotham et al. (108) have also reported PCWP to rise continually throughout upright cycle ergometry exercise, and at high levels of exercise this increase was not accompanied by increases in EDV or SV. While the authors reasoned that these results were due to a disproportionally shortened filling period, their findings also support the existence of pericardial constraint at or near maximal work. Further support of pericardial constraint in normal individuals during exercise is obtained from a much earlier report by Robinson et al. (226). In this study, cardiac output and central venous pressure responses to maximal upright exercise were compared before and after a 1- to 2-liter infusion of blood. At rest there was a substantial increase in cardiac output, with only a small rise in central venous pressure following blood volume expansion. During exercise, the increase in central venous pressure with infusion was markedly greater than that obtained before infusion, while maximal cardiac output remained unchanged. Thus, it would appear that the inappropriate rise in central venous pressure was a reflection of an elevation in intrapericardial pressure resulting from the expanded, circulating blood volume.

The fact that clinical evidence for significant pericardial constraint has been obtained under conditions of expanded cardiac volumes has fostered the impression of an inconsequential role for the pericardium at rest and at modest levels of dynamic exercise. However, recent experimental and clinical studies indicate that this may not be the case. Left ventricular mass has been noted to increase 14–21 days after pericardiectomy in pigs (103). Similar findings were noted in patients 6 weeks after coronary artery bypass surgery, which necessitated removal of the pericardium (309). Echocardiographic data obtained 1 day prior and 6 weeks after surgery indicated LV volume and mass had significantly increased from 51 $\pm$ 11 ml/m^2 to 62 $\pm$ 14 ml/m^2 and 109 $\pm$ 23 g/m^2 to 127 $\pm$ 24 g/m^2, respectively. Thus, it would appear that some degree of pericardial constraint may be present at rest so that, after removal of the pericardium, a chronic volume overload develops and leads to ventricular hypertrophy. However, neither study documented the postsurgical level of physical activity of the pigs or humans. It is possible that the LV dilatation and hypertrophy seen at rest resulted from a larger than normal increase in LV volume with moderate levels of activity because of the absence of pericardial constraint. Also, the humans as part of a risk reduction program may have engaged in an aerobic conditioning program.

With chronic distention, the pericardium will accommodate the volume overload by growth (79) that effectively increases its unstressed volume (i.e., the volume at zero distending pressure), shifting the pericardial pressure–volume curve to the right. Thus, it is reasonable to hypothesize that the mechanism for the training-induced increase in LVEDV and SV may, in part, be growth of the pericardium. Stray-Gundersen et al. (288) noted that the degree to which SV was elevated following removal of the pericardium was similar to reported increases in SV following dynamic training (23, 308). It is not known whether an increase in maximal SV would also occur following pericardiectomy in trained dogs.

EFFECTS OF MYOCARDIAL REMODELING. As seen above, the degree to which the ventricle is filled during diastole is dependent on the interaction of multiple physiological factors other than the material properties of the myocardium. Here, alterations to the myocardium that occur as a result of training or aging will be considered along with their potential effect on preload.

Training. LV mass in the athlete is significantly greater than that in age-matched sedentary groups (249). In young male endurance- and power-trained athletes, the average LV mass was 232 g compared to 175 g in the age-matched untrained males (72, 131, 181, 206, 244, 250). Young female athletes also had a significantly greater LV mass (192 g vs. 123 g) than comparable untrained females (51, 243). This cardiac growth is a result of a thickening of the ventricular wall and ventricular enlargement. In trained endurance athletes, septal and posterior lateral wall thicknesses increase on the average of 13% and 19%, respectively (27, 51, 69, 72, 131, 181, 206, 243, 244, 249, 250). There is a similar or slightly greater increase in LV wall thickness as a result of static power training compared to endurance training (74, 136, 181, 206). However, the thickness/chamber radius ratio is greater in the power-trained individual due to the absence of a training-related ventricular dilatation. That is, compensated hypertrophy in power-trained individuals is concentric (i.e., wall thickness increases without chamber enlargement or thickness/chamber radius ratio increases) while that in the endurance athlete is eccentric (i.e., wall thickness increases and chamber volume enlarges without a significant change in the wall thickness/chamber radius ratio). The reason for the use of the term "eccentric" to describe this type of hypertrophy is that the heart becomes "eccentric," or enlarges to the left, with respect to the midline of the chest.

In both young men and women, LV mass (243) and wall thickness (279) increased following 10 weeks of endurance conditioning. This was not the case in a 4-week training study (53). Increases in LV wall thickness were also seen in elderly males (64 ± 3 years) after 9 to 12 months of training (68). However, in a similar study involving elderly females, no change in ventricular wall thickness was observed after 9–12 months of endurance training (280). Interestingly, a training-related increase in SV was also absent in this group of elderly females despite an improved maximal oxygen uptake. Instead, all of the increase in oxygen uptake was accounted for by a greater arteriovenous oxygen content difference. Thus, the adaptive increase in LV wall thickness or muscle mass to endurance training of sufficient duration in older men is similar to that found in young people. The reason why this adaptive mechanism is absent following training in elderly females is unknown.

In the young and old athlete with a significantly greater LV mass than normal and, therefore, a presumably physiological hypertrophy, diastolic function is normal at rest and during exercise (27, 53, 150, 160, 192, 251, 259, 301, 317). In contrast, hypertensive patients with an increase in LV mass less than that seen in the athletes are found to have significant diastolic dysfunction (259). In view of the fact that myocardial collagen concentration is increased in humans with systemic hypertension (204) and that diastolic abnormalities in hypertensive patients are not related to increases in LV mass (258, 296), it is reasonable to assume that this impaired diastolic function is the result of excessive myocardial collagen. That excessive myocardial collagen and not myocyte hypertrophy is responsible for pathologic hypertrophy and the accompanying diastolic dysfunction has been verified in recent studies on experimental animals. Narayan et al. (189) used hydralazine to prevent myocyte hypertrophy, but this did not prevent the abnormal accumulation of collagen in the spontaneously hypertensive rat. They found the excess collagen to produce an abnormal passive myocardial stiffness that was similar to that measured in the untreated spontaneous hypertensive rat with hypertrophy but significantly greater than the stiffness obtained in the genetic control. Finally, Gelpi et al. (82) and Douglas and Tallant (62) found no change in myocardial collagen concentration and LV diastolic chamber compliance in dogs with stable perinephritic hypertension despite significant hypertrophy. Thus, cellular hypertrophy can be thought of as adaptive or physiologic as long as the components of the myocardium remain in proper balance. This would appear to be the case with the myocardial hypertrophy associated with conditioning, since diastolic function remains normal despite a significant increase in myocardial mass.

Aging. The aging human myocardium is characterized by an increase in the proportion of interstitial collagen in contrast to the functional parenchyma (139, 141). The fibrosis is due to scarring, increased interstitial and perivascular collagen, or both. The fibrotic replacement of lost myocardium is usually of vascular origin and is prevalent in the subendocardial zone. The interstitial fibrosis, which does not replace myocytes but instead encircles them, consists of a uniformly distributed, fine network of fibrillar collagen. In the elderly heart, this increased prominence of the interstitium occurs not only in the left ventricle but also in the right ventricle and both atria; and it takes place with little increase in ventricular mass (141, 205). This pattern of interstitial remodeling is similar to that seen with the pressure overload that is secondary to activation of the renin-angiotensin-aldosterone system or to excess mineralocorticoids (326). It suggests that circulating hormones may be an active participant in the aging process of the heart.

With age the heart becomes stiffer, with altered filling parameters. As can be seen in Figure 15.12, diastolic function is significantly altered with decreased early filling and an increased atrial contribution to late filling (116, 149, 251, 294, 317). It is not known whether the fibrosis in the senescent human heart is sufficient to cause this decrease in diastolic function. However, the marked elevations in myocardial collagen seen in the senescent rat have been identified as the cause for its abnormal increased myocardial stiffness (7, 334). Thus, there is experimental evidence to hypothesize a cause-and-effect relation between collagen remodeling of the senescent myocardium and decreased diastolic ventricular function. It remains to be determined whether training with an increase in myocyte mass would correct this abnormal accumulation of interstitial collagen and diastolic dysfunction.

Contractility

Definition. Contractility can be defined as the property of cardiac muscle that determines its ability

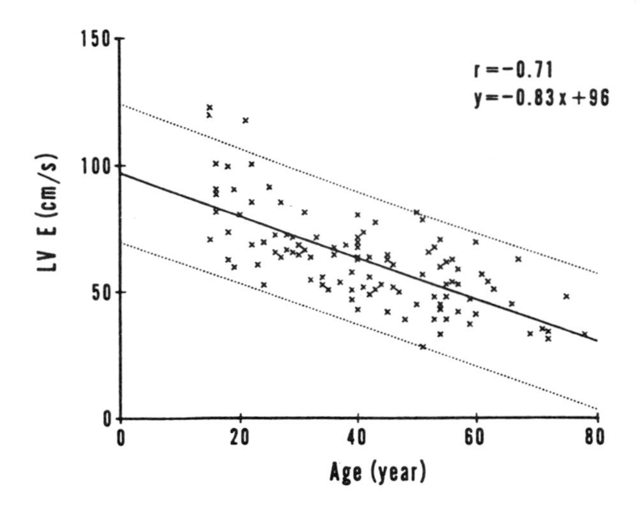

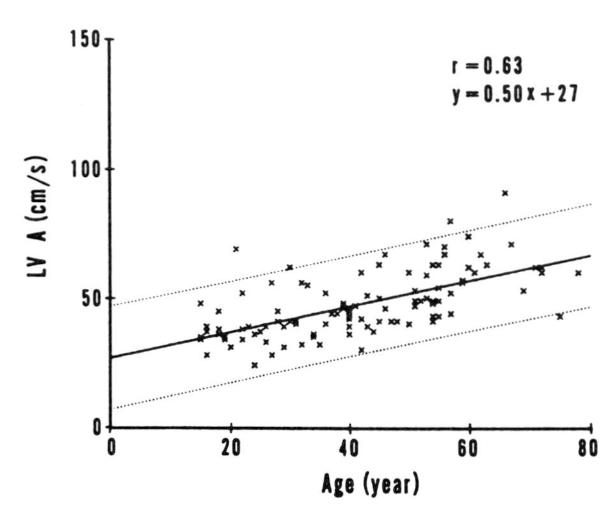

FIG. 15.12. Doppler measured left ventricular (LV) peak early (E) and peak atrial systole (A) filling flow velocity values as a function of age. As a consequence of the ventricle becoming stiffer with age, the magnitude of the E wave decreases and that of the A wave increases. (Reprinted with permission from Iwase, M., K. Nagata, H. Izawa, M. Yokota, S. Kamihara, H. Inagaki, and H. Saito. Age-related changes in left and right ventricular filling velocity profiles and their relationship in normal subjects. (*Am. Heart J.* 126: 419–426, 1993.)

to shorten independent of preload and afterload. Accordingly, it describes in mechanical or functional terms the biochemical characteristics of myocardium, such as its state of β_1-adrenergic receptor responsiveness and sarcolemmal/sarcoplasmic calcium kinetics, and the degree to which the myocardium is being stimulated by neurohumoral influences. Thus, unlike ventricular preload and afterload, which can be directly measured, contractility must be inferred or derived from other measurable variables. Furthermore, the index used to quantify contractility by definition must be independent of preload and afterload. Over the years, many indices for measuring contractility of the ventricle have been proposed and tested, with most being sensitive to some degree to changes in loading conditions. Most of them are based on the time rate of change of the ventricular pressure (e.g., max dP/dt) or aortic flow (e.g., max dQ/dt). Even though they are sensitive to changes in contractile state, none is completely insensitive to changes in preload and afterload (203, 314).

One index, the slope of the linear peak isovolumetric pressure–volume relation (Figs. 15.7 and 15.13), has been shown in the isolated canine heart to be sensitive to pharmacological changes in contractility and independent of preload and afterload; positive and negative inotropic agents result in larger and smaller slope values, respectively (289, 290, 329). Another important aspect of this isovolumetric relation is the close association between it and the end-systolic pressure–volume (ESP-ESV) values from ejecting contractions as demonstrated in Figures 15.7 and 15.13. That is, regression lines fit to peak isovolumetric pressure–volume and ESP-ESV data points are statistically indistinguishable. Thus, this index of contractility can be assessed clinically upon the attainment of three ESP-ESV points. However, in obtaining these points, care must be taken to avoid reflexogenic adjustments of contractility

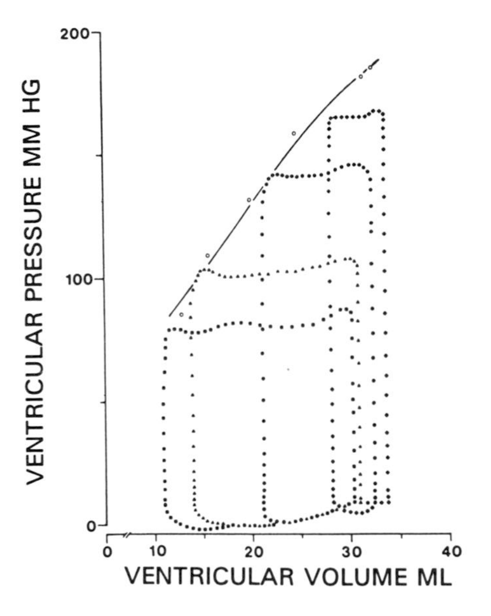

FIG. 15.13. Left ventricular pressure–volume loops obtained at different levels of afterload and the peak isovolumetric pressure–volume relation (*solid line*) obtained in the isolated heart are depicted. As can be seen, the end-systolic pressure–volume points lie on or near the peak isovolumetric pressure–volume curve. The slope of the peak isovolumetric or end-systolic pressure–volume relations is an index of contractility. (Reprinted with permission from Weber, K. T., J. S. Janicki, and L. L. Hefner. Left ventricular force-length relations of isovolumic and ejecting contractions. *Am. J. Physiol.* 231: 337–343, 1976.)

(268). Also, the linearity of the ESP-ESV relation in the intact animal has recently been challenged (39, 134, 193, 315). Nevertheless, this concept is useful for determining the response in contractility during exercise and its contribution to SV.

Following the administration of a positive inotropic agent, the ESP-ESV is shifted to the left with an increased slope. For a constant EDV and ejection pressure, the net effect of this inotropic intervention is a greater SV secondary to a reduced ESV. Thus, with a knowledge of ejection pressure and ESV, it is possible to deduce the contractility response to exercise. As discussed previously, a change in EDV does not affect the volume at end-systole. Also, during exercise there is an increase in ejection pressure which, if contractility remained invariant, would result in a larger ESV and a smaller SV (Figs. 15.4 and 15.13). If, on the other hand, ESV remains constant or decreases with an exercise-induced rise in ejection pressure, then this is clear evidence that contractility has increased.

Contractility during exercise

DYNAMIC EXERCISE. A sampling of the literature reveals that, in individuals below the age of 55 years, ESV significantly decreases from rest to peak exercise in both supine and upright cycle ergometry (2, 18, 72, 108, 244, 249, 251, 310, 342). When a decrease was not seen in this age group, ESV typically remained unchanged (3). Thus, according to the above logic, a decreasing or constant ESV during exercise where ejection pressure is increasing is strong evidence of an enhanced myocardial contractility. Many studies reported ESV normalized to body surface area: end-systolic volume index (ESVI). Typically, ESVI at rest is 30 ml/m^2, and the exercise-induced reduction amounts to 9 ml/m^2 or 30% (18, 108, 310, 342). Assuming the body surface area to be 2.0 m^2 (i.e., height and weight of 180 cm and 81 kg, respectively), the average decline in ESV is 18 ml. This value, together with the average exercise-related increase in LVEDV of 17 ml discussed earlier, would result in an expected 35 ml increase in SV from rest to maximal upright exercise. This is approximately the amount by which SV increased in the example presented in Figure 15.3.

ISOMETRIC EXERCISE. In contrast to dynamic exercise, static efforts appear to result in parallel changes in LVEDV and LVESV. That is, both dimensions have been reported to either increase or decrease depending on whether the effort is less than 50% MVC (155, 207, 294) or greater than 75% MVC (16, 148), respectively. For example, Swinne et al. (294) reported LV end-diastolic and end-systolic dimensions to significantly increase by 1.4 and 2.0 mm, respectively, as a result of a 30% MVC handgrip maneuver; Perez-Gonzales et al. (207) found both dimensions to increase by 2.5 mm with the same effort. In contrast, significant decreases in LVEDV and LVESV were found to occur with larger (i.e., >75% MVC) static efforts involving both legs (16, 148); the decline in LVEDV was approximately twice that of LVESV. With these isometric efforts, ejection pressure rose in proportion to the level of static work. The fact that systolic volume decreased with the larger levels of work indicates that contractility was enhanced and effectively blunted the reduction in SV that would have otherwise occurred secondary to the decrease in preload and increase in afterload (16, 148).

Effects of training. In trained endurance athletes, LV end-systolic size is typically larger both at rest and during exercise than that of age-matched sedentary individuals regardless of age and gender (27, 51, 72, 155, 243, 250, 254, 317). In studies where volumes were reported, the amount of increase in end-systolic size was around 15 ml (51, 72, 243, 254) or approximately one-half the compensatory increase in end-diastolic size common to endurance athletes (see above). Thus, the greater SV in these athletes both at rest and during exercise is the result of an enhanced contractility and LVEDV, where the larger ventricular volume is primarily due to growth of the pericardium.

Similar trends in resting LVESV are experienced as a result of conditioning programs. In men of all ages, and in females less than 55 years, end-systolic size at rest tends to increase but not to the level of statistical significance following dynamic conditioning for periods as short as 4 weeks (53, 68, 243). In elderly females, end-systolic size both at rest and at peak exercise was unchanged after 9–12 months of dynamic training (280). In contrast, elderly men after a similar conditioning program experienced a significant decrease in end-systolic size during exercise compared to essentially no exercise-related change before conditioning (68).

Effects of aging. In elderly men and women (i.e., >60 years), decreases in ESV with dynamic exercise do not occur (68, 140, 254, 278) or become much less than that observed in younger individuals (2). However, contractility does increase during exercise because end-systolic volume remains unchanged despite higher ejection pressures. The relation between end-systolic size and age is less clear. At rest, either no change (235, 294) or a decrease (108, 317) has been observed. Similarly, at peak exercise, either no change (108) or a significant increase (235) has been reported. When significant age-related changes in size were seen, they were small. Thus, those studies that could not demonstrate significant differences may have had a smaller sampling size or age range and/or less sensitive equipment.

COUPLING OF THE HEART AND PERIPHERAL CIRCULATION

This section deals with the mechanical coupling between the heart and the peripheral circulation during dynamic exercise. The term "coupling" refers to a hemodynamic interrelationship between the heart and the peripheral circulation that causes the performance of one to affect the performance of the other. In particular, we draw attention to the importance of the peripheral circulation in determining both cardiac performance and at the same time its own blood flow.

Right atrial pressure and aortic pressure are commonly selected as variables in any analysis of the coupling of the central circulation (heart and pulmonary circulation) to the arteries and veins of the peripheral circulation. Right atrial pressure represents, on the one hand, the back-pressure for venous return and, on the other hand, it is the filling pressure for the right ventricle. Accordingly, right atrial pressure can be viewed as the pressure that influences the rate of blood flow back to the heart (99). Right atrial pressure can also be viewed as the pressure that influences the SV (when aortic pressure is not elevated) and thus the flow of blood out of the heart, or cardiac output. This is the central concept of the Guyton venous return and cardiac function curves (99). Likewise, aortic pressure represents both the back-pressure impeding left ventricular ejection and the pressure head driving blood flow through the peripheral circulation. Thus, the blood flow generated by the heart affects the pressures in the aorta and vena cava, and the pressures in the aorta and vena cava affect the blood flow generated by the heart. The analysis here will center mainly on atrial pressure because it has more profound effects on SV than do normally encountered changes in aortic pressure (106). An early example of the large influence of changes in filling pressure on SV, in contrast to the relatively small influence of changes in aortic pressure, was revealed in the paradoxical rise in cardiac output that accompanied occlusion of the descending throacic aorta (14). As long as the occlusion was made above the origin of the arteries supplying the splanchnic circulation, the blood volume released from that circulation raised right atrial pressure, which in turn increased SV and cardiac output despite the large increase in afterload caused by aortic constriction (14). Cardiac output rose 30% during occlusion of the descending thoracic aorta after reflexes that would oppose the rise were blocked.

Particular attention is given to factors that affect blood volume distribution because atrial pressure (and pressures throughout the central circulation) is strongly influenced by central blood volume (the volume of blood contained in the four cardiac chambers and in the pulmonary vasculature). Many stresses, including exercise, change central blood volume, which in turn can profoundly affect the filling pressure of the ventricles. Inasmuch as even maximal increases in heart rate and contractility cannot offset the negative effects of a large fall in cardiac filling pressure on SV, the successful regulation of cardiac output relies heavily on control that is exerted outside of the heart for maintenance of its filling pressure.

Coupling of Left Ventricle to Arterial System

Sunagawa et al. (292) proposed a scheme for evaluating the coupling of the left ventricle to the arterial system. The analysis was done graphically in the left ventricular pressure–volume plane so that the characteristics of the left ventricle and the arterial system could be described in similar terms. The ventricle was characterized by the end-systolic pressure–volume relation. As discussed in the first section of this chapter, the slope of this relation, called end-systolic elastance, provides a measure of ventricular contractility. The arterial system was characterized by the ratio of end-systolic arterial (or ventricular) pressure to stroke volume, called the effective arterial elastance. Stroke work of the left ventricle was near maximal when the ratio of end-systolic elastance to arterial elastance was near unity. That is, the arterial system and ventricle are effectively coupled to maximize stroke work when the two values of elastance are well matched to each other. The left ventricle and the arterial system are mechanically well matched for energy transfer in conscious, resting dogs (104, 153). Ventricular elastance and arterial elastance both rise during exercise such that the two remain effectively coupled during exercise (104, 153).

Ventricular Filling Pressure

Measures of Cardiac Filling Pressure. Common measures used as indices of ventricular filling pressure include right atrial pressure, CVP (vena caval pressure), and ventricular end-diastolic pressure. In general, compared to end-diastolic pressure, atrial or central venous pressure better reflect the volume of blood made available to the heart by the peripheral circulation. Although end-diastolic pressure is of primary importance in determining end-diastolic volume cardiac fiber length, and thus stroke volume, this pressure can be less than atrial pressure at end-diastole. An atrioventricular pressure gradient may occur at end-diastole during severe exercise because blood flow from the atria to the ventricles (cardiac filling) need not cease before end-diastole (223). Mean values of atrial and central venous pressures are usually reported so that phasic variations are ignored. In contrast, end-diastolic pressure is established at a particular moment in the cardiac cycle. The use of time-averaged pressure ignores the influence of beat-by-beat changes in cardiac filling on beat-by-beat stroke volume. Nevertheless, time-averaged atrial and central venous pressures adequately reflect the importance that net changes in cardiac filling pressure can have on stroke volume. An important limitation of most measures of filling pressure is that they are referenced to atmospheric pressure rather than to intrathoracic pressure. This means that potential changes in transmural pressure due to alterations in intrapericardial pressure or intrathoracic pressure, of which the phasic variation can become pronounced during exercise-induced hyperpnea, are often ignored (these influences are covered later under RESPIRATORY SYSTEM).

Factors Influencing Cardiac Filling Pressure. The pressure within an isolated segment of vessel when there is no blood flow through it is determined by the volume of blood contained within it and also by its capacitance. By extension, the pressure within any defined vascular segment, whether it be an artery, a venule, or a central vein, is also determined by its volume and capacitance even when there is blood flow through it. For example, it is as valid to view arterial pressure as a function of arterial blood volume and arterial capacitance (with or without flow) as it is to view it as a function of cardiac output and peripheral resistance. The key concept is that there must be a virtual, "static" volume of blood within a vascular segment that has flow through it so long as pressure is not changing (311). These concepts are fundamental to understanding why systemic arterial pressure and volume suddenly fall, and central venous pressure and volume suddenly rise, at the onset of dynamic exercise when cardiac output is rising and changes in peripheral resistance have not yet occurred (see below).

A rise or fall in cardiac filling pressure is normally attributable to transfer of blood volume into or out of the central circulation. Since total blood volume is constant over long periods, acute changes in central blood volume must be accompanied by reciprocal changes in peripheral blood volume. A number of events can bring about the reciprocal transfer of blood volume between the central and peripheral vasculatures.

The following four events can alter the distribution of blood volume in exercise.

1. A reduction in blood flow decreases the flow-dependent pressure gradient across veins so that venous transmural pressure falls. The elastic recoil of less distended capacious veins will passively expel a portion of their volume, mainly from venules and small veins. This blood will be transferred back toward the heart along a pressure gradient that is still declining centripetally. This process will continue until flow is reduced to zero and no pressure gradient exists. Opposite changes will accompany a rise in flow. Passive effects of changes in blood flow on blood volume distribution are greatest in organs where blood flow and venous compliance are high (e.g., splanchnic circulation) and least in organs where compliance is low (even in skeletal muscle where blood flow can be extremely high). Organ blood flow can change owing to a change in cardiac output or to a change in vasomotor tone, elicited by sympathetic neural constriction or metabolic vasodilation of arteriolar smooth muscle, for example.
2. Sympathetic constriction within well-innervated portions of the venous system, particularly the capacious splanchnic veins, can actively expel blood volume centrally (31).
3. A fall in arterial pressure reduces arterial blood volume. The passive release of arterial volume and its uptake by the venous system can raise central venous blood volume and pressure.
4. Contraction of skeletal muscle expels muscle venous blood centrally (muscle pump) and can expel abdominal blood volume centrally (abdominal pump). Respiration can also alter the distribution of blood volume (respiratory pump).

Relation Between Cardiac Output and Filling Pressure at Rest

The following two subsections focus on the importance of the mechanical properties of the circulation in determining the relationship between cardiac output and right atrial pressure (i.e., in the absence of reflexes). The potential for reflexes to influence the purely mechanical aspects of this relationship by their action on the heart and peripheral circulation is considered afterward. An understanding of the hydraulic properties of the resting circulation is needed in order to gain an appreciation of the regulatory problems faced by the cardiovascular system in exercise.

Retrograde Analysis of the Relationship between Right Atrial Pressure and Venous Return. Guyton and his co-workers (100) established a pivotal concept that the ability to increase cardiac output in the resting circulation by raising the pumping performance of the heart alone is limited by the capacitive properties of the peripheral circulation. They opened the circulation surgically and bypassed the right ventricle with a mechanical pump so that cardiac output would not be limited by the pumping effectiveness of the right ventricle. Autonomic reflexes were blocked so that the mechanical properties of the circulation could be studied in isolation. The blood returning to the right atrium was led to the bypass pump through thin-walled, collapsible tubing. They lowered this tubing below the level of the right atrium so as to reduce the atrial hydrostatic pressure, the back-pressure for venous return, to negative values (relative to the atmospheric pressure at the level of the right atrium). This would be expected to increase venous return, and thus cardiac output, by raising the pressure gradient that drives the flow of blood back to the right atrium. However, once right atrial pressure was reduced to −1 to −2 mm Hg, the flow of blood back to the heart (venous return) could not be increased further—i.e., no matter how much right atrial pressure was reduced or how much further the pressure gradient from arteries to atrium was increased (100).

The limitation in the ability to raise cardiac output by lowering right atrial pressure in these open-chest dogs was shown to be due to the propensity for the caval veins near the heart to collapse when their luminal pressure falls below atmospheric pressure. Guyton and co-workers (98) also recognized the equally important point that the ability to increase cardiac output by increasing only heart rate and myocardial contractility in the intact circulation would also be limited by this same phenomenon of central venous collapse (98). In closed-chest animals, veins would collapse at the sites where they enter the thoracic cavity (63, 98). Moreover, the heart ordinarily works near this limit in the intact, resting circulation, meaning that cardiac output can only be raised a few percent by increases in cardiac pump performance alone (98). For cardiac output to rise to the extent it does in dynamic exercise, some event(s) in the peripheral circulation must prevent central veins from collapsing when heart rate rises.

In essence, Guyton's (100) experiments provide a "retrograde" analysis of the effects of changes in right atrial pressure on the rate of venous return to the heart. In this analysis, right atrial pressure is viewed as the back-pressure for the return flow of blood from the peripheral circulation. Thus, a lower right atrial pressure produces a larger gradient for venous return, which must equal cardiac output in the steady state.

Anterograde Analysis of the Relationship between Cardiac Output and Right Atrial Pressure. The converse to the approach taken by Guyton et al. (100) is to examine how changes in cardiac output affect right atrial pressure, i.e. rather than examining the effect of right atrial pressure on cardiac output. This was done by bypassing the right ventricle with a pump in a manner similar to that carried out by Guyton et al. (100) (described above) but without inserting a collapsible tube between the right atrium and the mechanical pump. Those who used this preparation found that increases in pump output were accompanied by decreases in right atrial pressure or vice versa (93, 95, 149). Importantly, manipulation of either right atrial pressure, as in the experiment of Guyton (100), or cardiac output with a pump produced similar relationships between cardiac output and right atrial pressure. An example of this relationship is depicted in Figure 15.14*A*, which shows the relationship between cardiac output and cardiac filling pressure when cardiac output is manipulated by changing ventricular pacing rate after autonomic blockade in conscious, resting dogs with a surgically produced atrioventricular block. Data from heart-block patients in whom cardiac output was manipulated at rest by changing ventricular pacing rate show the same negative slope relationship of cardiac output to central venous pressure as shown in Figure 15.14 (see Fig. 15.17).

An anterograde approach to studying the interrelation between left ventricular output and right ventricular filling pressure attributes the negative relationship between these two variables to a flow-dependent distribution of blood volume in the peripheral circulation (99, 149, 311). This should not be confused with the positive relationship between right atrial pressure (independent or "x-axis" variable) and cardiac output, which is a function of the effect of increased ventricular fiber length on ventricular stroke volume (Frank-Starling). In the one case an increase in ventricular filling pressure causes an increase in stroke volume and cardiac output, whereas in the other case an increase in cardiac output causes a decrease in ventricular filling pressure (unless something outside of the heart occurs to prevent this decrease). One key to understanding the cardiovascular adjustments to dynamic exercise is to observe how the system counteracts the negative effect of increased cardiac output on right atrial pressure so that cardiac output and right atrial pressure rise together.

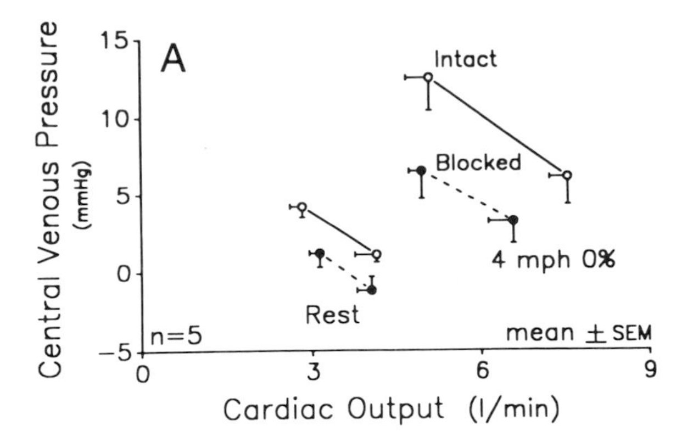

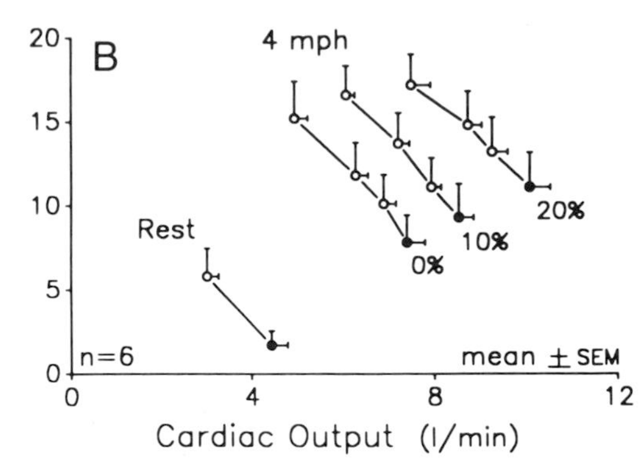

FIG. 15.14. Influence of cardiac output on central venous pressure during rest and treadmill exercise. Cardiac output was changed by changing ventricular pacing rate in conscious dogs with a surgically produced atrioventricular (AV) blockade. *A*, Responses after autonomic blockade with hexamethonium. Autonomic blockade (*dashed lines*) shifts curves downward (presumably owing to loss of peripheral sympathetic tone) with no change in slope compared to control (*solid lines*). Exercise shifts curves upward and rightward to an equal extent with no change in slope despite blockade of autonomic function. *B*, Reflexes intact. *Filled circles* depict normal flow and pressure; these data collected during AV-linked pacing (ventricles stimulated after each atrial depolarization). *Open circles*, Data collected during periods in which pacing rate was reduced below normal AV-linked values. Graded exercise shifts curves upward and rightward with no change in slope. [Reprinted with permission from Sheriff, D. D., X. P. Zhou, A. M. Scher, and L. B. Rowell. Dependence of cardiac filling pressure on cardiac output during rest and dynamic exercise in dogs. *Am. J. Physiol.* 265 (*Heart Circ. Physiol.* 34): H316–H322, 1993.]

The fall in right atrial pressure caused by a rise in cardiac output is attributable to the resistive and capacitive properties of the blood vessels throughout the cardiovascular system. Transmural pressures in the peripheral circulation rise as blood flow increases because the vessels offer resistance to blood flow. Veins also offer resistance to blood flow, and as a consequence a flow-dependent pressure profile also exists along them from venules to the venae cavae. As blood flow increases, so does this pressure gradient across the veins. This venous pressure gradient is increased by *(1)* a rise in pressure in venules and small veins, and *(2)* by the fall in right atrial pressure that accompanies a rise in cardiac output. If one elects to think in terms of "mean circulatory filling pressure" (237), then those pressures that exceed mean circulatory filling pressure will rise when cardiac output rises and those pressures below mean circulatory filling pressure will fall when cardiac output rises. Although the concept of a mean circulatory filling pressure is useful, its practical application is problematic. Mean circulatory filling pressure is a "virtual" pressure in that it does not exist at any anatomically defined location, and its putative location is not the same under all conditions (237). Furthermore, in dynamic exercise the concept of a mean circulatory filling pressure is confounded by the action of the skeletal muscle pump (see below). Nevertheless, inasmuch as mean circulatory filling pressure is about 7 mm Hg (98, 99, 100, 237) and directly measured venular pressures are typically reported to be much higher [e.g., 10–25 mm Hg (224)], a rise in cardiac output must raise the pressure within the capacious postcapillary venules and small veins in most if not all organs. Since the capacity and compliance are both large in venules and small veins, peripheral venous volume expands in proportion to the increments in blood flow and distending pressure.

Conversely, the volume of blood contained in arteries increases only slightly when pressure and flow rise owing to their relative stiffness, which is 30 times greater than that of veins. During the time that blood volume accumulates in the periphery, there is a transient imbalance between left ventricular output and venous return. Left ventricular output transiently exceeds venous return by depleting the volume of blood in pulmonary vessels (pulmonary sump). The balance between left and right ventricular outputs is restored by the effects on stroke volume of the reductions in right atrial pressure, central blood volume, and left atrial pressure. The effect of changing cardiac output at rest, when cardiac output is distributed to the various organs in proportion to their fractions of the total vascular conductance, is shown schematically by *line A* in Figure 15.15. Inasmuch as the splanchnic circulation comprises 25% of total vascular conductance, a large fraction of cardiac output at rest goes to this compliant region. Therefore, the fall in central venous pressure below *line B* in Figure 15.15 that accompanies a rise in cardiac output above its normal resting level can be attributed in part to the rise in splanchnic blood vol-

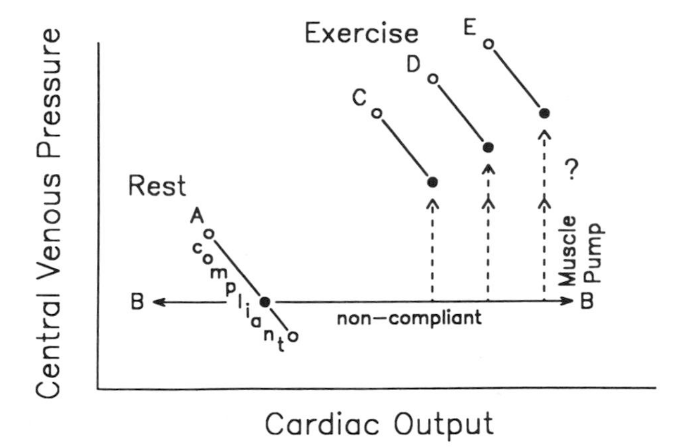

FIG. 15.15. Schematic representation of flow-dependent and flow-independent effects on central venous pressure (CVP). *Line A*, Effect on CVP when changes in blood flow to compliant regions occur as when cardiac output (CO) is changed at rest. *Line B*, Lack of change in CVP when changes in CO are directed to a noncompliant region (e.g., to muscle). *Muscle pump*, Effect on CVP of blood volume mobilized by the muscle pump. Additional increments in CVP related to increments in work rate may be of autonomic origin. *Lines C–E*, Effects on CVP when CO is changed during graded exercise; these changes in CVP are attributed to changes in blood flow to compliant regions. [Reprinted with permission from Sheriff, D. D., X. P. Zhou, A. M. Scher, and L. B. Rowell. Dependence of cardiac filling pressure on cardiac output during rest and dynamic exercise in dogs. *Am. J. Physiol.* 265 (*Heart Circ. Physiol.* 34): H316–H322, 1993.]

ume that accompanies a rise in blood flow through this region.

In summary, the manipulation of right atrial pressure in the retrograde analysis performed by Guyton (100) or of cardiac output in the anterograde analysis promoted by Levy (149) yields consistent results. In a retrograde analysis, a decrease in right atrial pressure is viewed as causing an increase in cardiac output. It does this by increasing the pressure gradient for venous return to the right heart. In an anterograde analysis, an increase in cardiac output is viewed as causing a decrease in right atrial pressure because of the flow-dependent transfer of blood volume away from the central to the peripheral vasculature. Either explanation is valid when viewed within the context of the specific model used for analysis. However, some prefer the anterograde explanation because traditional, retrograde analysis of venous return has blurred the distinction between volume and flow (311). For example, heart failure is often characterized by both a decrease in cardiac output and an increase in venous return—two conditions that are mutually exclusive in the steady state (202). Again, the ability to escape the interdependence among cardiac output, peripheral vascular volume, and ventricular filling pressure is fundamental if a normal increase in cardiac performance is to be achieved during dynamic exercise.

Relative Contributions of Active and Passive Mechanisms. The combined active and passive effects of changing cardiac output on the distribution of blood volume among major organs has been examined indirectly by observing how right atrial pressure changes when cardiac output is raised or lowered by ventricular pacing (263). Sheriff et al. (263) found that central venous pressure rose 3.9 mm Hg when cardiac output was reduced by an amount that reduced arterial pressure by 17 mm Hg. The fall in arterial pressure presumably caused 0.7 ml of blood per kilogram body weight to be transferred from arteries into veins (assuming an arterial compliance of 0.04 ml · mm Hg^{-1} · kg^{-1} body weight). If the fall in arterial pressure could be prevented, thereby causing this volume to remain within the arterial system, central venous pressure would have risen somewhat less; that is, 3.6 vs. 3.9 mm Hg (assuming a venous compliance of 2.5 ml · mm Hg^{-1} · kg^{-1} body weight). This rise in filling pressure is far larger than the rise caused by strong baroreflex activation alone (see below), suggesting that the passive redistribution of blood volume may account for as much as three-quarters of the total rise in central venous pressure that accompanies a reduction in cardiac output. This estimate is substantiated by the lack of effect of autonomic blockade on the slope of the relationship between cardiac output and central venous pressure found by Sheriff et al. (263) and shown in Figure 15.14*A*.

Further support of the predominance of passive effects in causing a change in filling pressure in response to a change in cardiac output is provided by the results of a study by Raymundo et al. (222). They found that arterial baroreceptor denervation had little effect on the changes in central venous pressure that accompanied increments and decrements in cardiac output induced by ventricular pacing in awake dogs with atrioventricular block (222). This finding suggests a small role for active changes in capacitance (venoconstriction) in changing filling pressure in response to changes in cardiac output. Likewise, Rothe and Gaddis (238) found a small (21%) effect of autonomic blockade on the volume of blood expelled into a reservoir at constant venous outflow pressure when cardiac output was reduced in animals on right heart bypass. [Numao and Iriuchijima (195) found a larger (50% vs. 21%) contribution of active changes in capacitance in experiments virtually identical to those of Rothe and Gaddis (238)].

Another way in which to separate out the active and passive effects of changing cardiac output on the distribution of blood volume is to determine the ability of arterial baroreceptor reflexes to raise right atrial pressure in isolation, and then compare this rise to the rise that accompanies a fall in cardiac output. The ability of baroreflexes to raise right atrial pressure in isolation can be accomplished by altering carotid sinus pressure while cardiac output is maintained constant. Tests of the ability of venoconstriction to alter the distribution of blood volume and filling pressure are most meaningful when they are performed on the closed circulation, because the rise in right atrial pressure places a physiological restraint on the volume of blood that can be shifted centrally by venoconstriction. For example, arterial baroreflex activation causes a large volume of blood to be expelled into an external reservoir (opened circulation) when cardiac output and venous outflow pressure (into the reservoir) are held constant (267), because the volume transfer is unopposed by a rise in right atrial pressure. Conversely, less blood volume is mobilized in the closed circulation, because the rise in venous outflow pressure (right atrial pressure) works to retard further mobilization of blood volume (245).

Bennett et al. (17) examined the ability of the carotid sinus baroreceptor reflex to alter right atrial pressure in the closed circulation. They occluded the carotid arteries of awake dogs whose vagus nerves were blocked (to eliminate the buffering action of aortic and cardiopulmonary afferent nerves) while cardiac output was maintained constant. They found that carotid occlusion raised central venous pressure by 0.8 mm Hg and raised arterial pressure by 48 mm Hg. This rise in filling pressure was probably caused by active changes in capacitance (venoconstriction) alone; that is, the change in the distribution of cardiac output between compliant and noncompliant circulations induced by baroreflexes is in the wrong direction to cause central mobilization of blood volume (55, 262). Central venous pressure would have risen by a total of 1.5 mm Hg had the rise in arterial pressure been prevented (same assumptions as above). Thus, when corrected for the different changes in arterial pressure, the rise in central venous pressure caused by carotid occlusion (17) was only 40% as large as the rise that accompanied a reduction in cardiac output in the study by Sheriff et al. (263). This was so despite the far stronger baroreflex activation caused by carotid occlusion than by cardiac output reduction, based on the twofold greater rise in peripheral resistance elicited by carotid occlusion (17, 263). These findings [with one exception (195)] indicate that the rise in right atrial pressure induced by a fall in cardiac output originates primarily from the volume of blood that is passively transferred from peripheral veins to central vasculature rather than from active vasoconstriction and venoconstriction.

Functional Significance. The inverse relationship between cardiac output and cardiac filling pressure benefits circulatory homeostasis by providing a self-regulating feature that helps to maintain a stable level of cardiac output (238). For example, an attempt to raise resting cardiac output is accompanied by a fall in right atrial pressure that reduces stroke volume via the Starling mechanism and provides a self-limiting constraint on the rise in cardiac output. Similarly, a decrease in cardiac output is opposed by a rise in filling pressure and stroke volume until further elevation of end-diastolic volume is restricted mechanically by the stretched pericardium.

On the other hand, the inverse relationship between cardiac output and filling pressure can impede circulatory adjustments. For example, in hyperthermia, the increase in cardiac output needed to increase skin blood flow will eventually be limited by a fall in filling pressure owing to the high compliance of the cutaneous circulation (see Fig. 17.4). Furthermore, the limited ability to raise cardiac output at rest falls far short of the needs for increased cardiac output in dynamic exercise.

At this point there are two pivotal questions: Given the physical interaction among cardiac output, its distribution, and central and peripheral vascular volumes, what adjustments make it possible to raise cardiac output by 400%–700% during dynamic exercise? What is the effect of competing demands for cardiac output during exercise (e.g., demands for greater blood flow to regions other than active muscle)? The preceding discussion of the relationship between cardiac output and right atrial pressure at rest is fundamental to understanding how such a relationship could exist during steady-state exercise, even through cardiac output and central venous pressure normally rise together at exercise onset.

Relation Between Cardiac Output and Right Atrial Pressure in Dynamic Exercise

This subsection puts together the above concepts on the effects of changing regional blood flow and cardiac output at rest and fits them into a scheme that explains the consequences of imposing similar changes in regional blood flow and cardiac output during dynamic exercise. Until recently there was little basis on which to predict the consequences of imposing a change in cardiac output above or below its normal steady-state value during exercise. The question is whether a superimposed rise or fall in cardiac output would have the same effect on right atrial pressure that one sees at rest. Do the muscle pump and the augmented sympathetic vasomotor control so change the physical characteristics of the vascular system that the negative influence of an increase in cardiac output at a given work rate—and a given muscle pumping rate—is no longer evident?

Normal Responses to Exercise. Dynamic exercise is characterized by the great rise in cardiac output, which can exceed 40 liters/min in endurance athletes exercising at their maximal oxygen uptake (66). In contrast to the responses at rest, the rise in cardiac output in dynamic exercise is usually accompanied by increases in cardiac filling pressure measured as central venous pressure, right atrial pressure, and also indirectly as end-diastolic volume (44, 223, 263; see also earlier under INTRINSIC PROPERTIES OF THE HEART and Chapter 17). Filling pressure (and end-diastolic volume) normally rises abruptly at the onset of exercise (Fig. 15.16*A* and Fig. 17.2) and remains elevated thereafter. Right atrial pressure rises in proportion to the severity of exercise in dogs [Fig. 15.14*B*; (44)], but less so in humans (223), and is usually highest when maximal cardiac output is attained in dogs and humans (e.g., Fig. 17.1). Central blood volume rises from rest during exercise in seated (73) and upright humans (242). Thus, the inverse relationship between cardiac output and right atrial pressure seen at rest is reversed by the initiation of dynamic exercise. This subsection deals with those factors that cause this reversal and promote the rise in right atrial pressure that accompanies rising cardiac output in exercise.

Passive and Mechanical Factors Influencing Ventricular Filling Pressure during Exercise

Distribution of blood flow

IMPORTANCE OF REGIONAL COMPLIANCES. A primary reason why right atrial pressure does not fall along with the normally occurring rise in cardiac output in dynamic exercise as it does at rest is that the entire increase in cardiac output during exercise is directed to a noncompliant vascular bed—active muscle. Were a significant fraction of the increase directed to compliant regions, right atrial pressure would decrease (or at least subtract from some of the rise). The specific compliance of *resting* skeletal muscle is about one-eighth that of the circulation as a whole (161, 236). Furthermore, rhythmic muscle contractions reduce muscle vascular compliance by one-half (194), making it $^{1}/_{16}$ of total systemic vascular com-

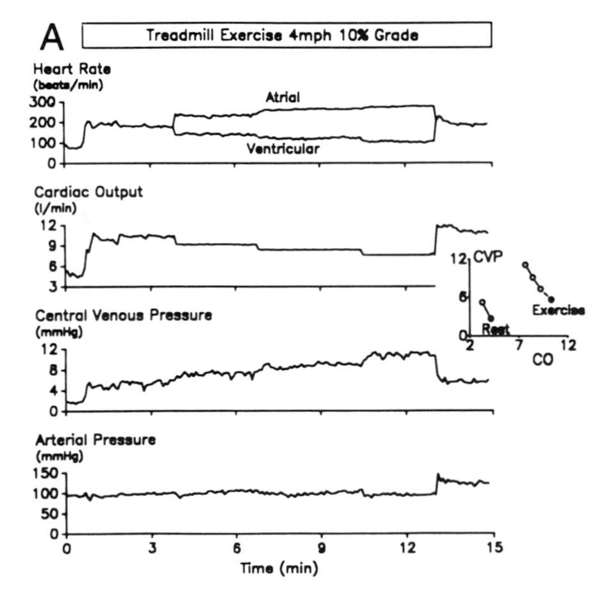

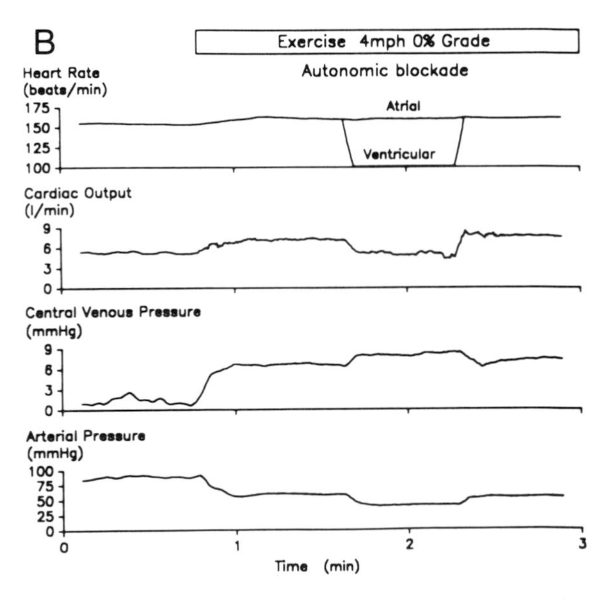

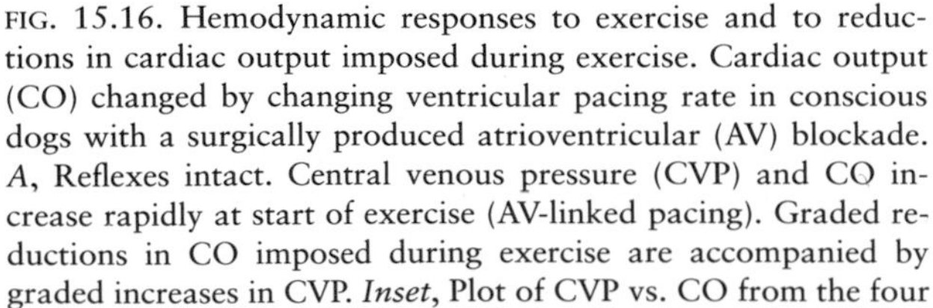

FIG. 15.16. Hemodynamic responses to exercise and to reductions in cardiac output imposed during exercise. Cardiac output (CO) changed by changing ventricular pacing rate in conscious dogs with a surgically produced atrioventricular (AV) blockade. *A*, Reflexes intact. Central venous pressure (CVP) and CO increase rapidly at start of exercise (AV-linked pacing). Graded reductions in CO imposed during exercise are accompanied by graded increases in CVP. *Inset*, Plot of CVP vs. CO from the four steady-state levels of CO during exercise. *B*, Responses after autonomic blockade with hexamethonium. CVP rises rapidly at start of exercise and a reduction in CO imposed during exercise is accompanied by an increase in CVP. [Reprinted with permission from Sheriff, D. D., X. P. Zhou, A. M. Scher, and L. B. Rowell. Dependence of cardiac filling pressure on cardiac output during rest and dynamic exercise in dogs. *Am. J. Physiol.* 265 (*Heart Circ. Physiol.* 34): H316–H322, 1993.]

pliance. The low vascular compliance of muscle ensures that the rise in cardiac output forces little or no blood volume to accumulate within the peripheral vasculature; that is, as long as the entire rise in cardiac output goes to active muscle. When this is the case, the heart receives nearly all of what it pumps out so there is no transient imbalance between left ventricular output and venous return, and thus no change in central blood volume and central venous pressure. This is illustrated schematically by moving rightward along horizontal *line B* in Figure 15.15, which shows the entire rise in cardiac output going to muscle. Again, the contrast in Figure 15.15 is with a descent along *line A* showing that a rise in resting cardiac output lowers central venous pressure when it is distributed to the various organs in proportion to their fractions of the total vascular conductance.

Importantly, the propensity for filling pressure to remain constant when cardiac output rises normally in dynamic exercise does not depend on a net transfer of blood volume out of muscle veins by the muscle pump (see below). For example, filling pressure is well maintained (but not increased) when cardiac output rises in dynamic leg exercise even when the muscle pump is made ineffective by congenital absence of venous valves (*line* C in Fig. 15.17).

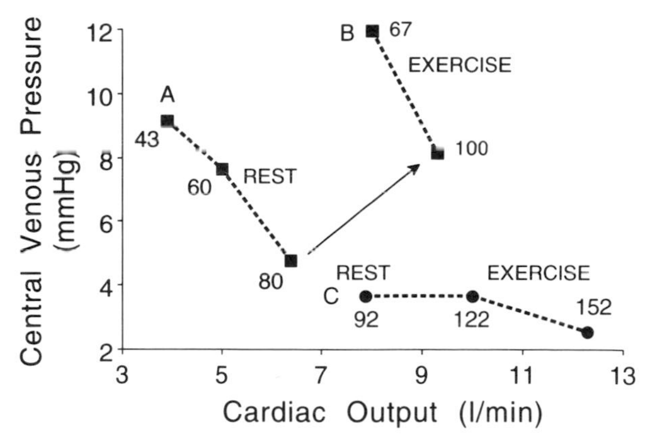

FIG. 15.17. Influence of cardiac output on central venous pressure during rest (*line A*) and bicycle exercise (*line B*). Cardiac output (CO) changed by changing ventricular pacing rate (numerical data labels) in heart-block patients (*dashed lines*). [Data from Bevegard et al. (20).] Central venous pressure (CVP) and CO rise normally from rest to exercise (*arrow*, subjects recumbent). Decreases in CO are accompanied by increases in CVP in rest and exercise. Also shown is response to bicycle exercise in patients with congenital absence of venous valves (*line* C). Lack of change in CVP when CO rises indicates that CVP is maintained without an effective muscle pump when the rise in CO is directed to noncompliant skeletal muscle (data averaged from exercise in supine and sitting postures). [Data from Bevegård and Lodin (21).]

EVIDENCE THAT THE BASIC PATTERN OF BLOOD FLOW DISTRIBUTION IN EXERCISE IS DETERMINED BY NONAUTONOMIC FACTORS. The entire rise in cardiac output in dynamic exercise is directed to active muscle, owing to the action of the muscle pump (see below) and local vasodilator systems residing in muscle (see Chapter 16). This pattern of response can be considered a "passive" adjustment in that it does not depend on the action of the autonomic nervous system. When autonomic responses are blocked in dogs, *calculated* total vascular conductance and muscle vascular conductance rise markedly in dynamic exercise, owing to an exaggerated fall in arterial pressure coupled with normal increments in cardiac output, muscle blood flow, and central venous pressure (261, 263). Likewise, dynamic exercise causes a large fall in arterial pressure in supine humans with impaired sympathetic function despite the normal increments in cardiac output achieved during exercise in this position (19, 164). In both species, blood flow to inactive regions will be passively reduced by the fall in arterial pressure. The passive decreases in blood flow will be diverted to active muscle. Parenthetically, active reductions in blood flow to inactive regions increase the percentage of cardiac output directed to active muscle when autonomic function is intact in humans but not in dogs (see below and Chapter 17). Thus, all of the rise in cardiac output, plus the blood flow diverted from inactive regions, is directed to active muscle during mild dynamic exercise even when global sympathetic function is blocked in dogs and supine humans.

EVIDENCE THAT THE MUSCLE PUMP IS A TRUE (FLOW-GENERATING) PUMP. In tall or upright animals with long hydrostatic columns of blood in veins and arteries of the legs, activation of the muscle pump effectively raises muscle blood flow by increasing muscle perfusion pressure, specifically the arteriovenous pressure difference. It achieves this by reducing the hydrostatic pressure in dependent veins while at the same time arterial pressure remains elevated by 50–100 mm Hg depending on the distance below the heart. Immediately after each contraction of muscle, its veins are empty and venous valves prevent backflow so that muscle venous pressure is close to (or below) zero. Thus, both the hydrostatic and dynamic components of pressure combine on the arterial side to raise driving pressure (76). This may explain why peak muscle blood flow and oxygen consumption during leg exercise are so much higher in upright than in supine cycling (77).

It was tacitly assumed that without the increased hydrostatic pressure on the arterial side of the limb circulation, the muscle pump could not effectively raise muscle blood flow by increasing the arterial-venous pressure difference across the muscle. Laughlin (146) observed that the highest muscle blood flows at a given perfusion pressure were obtained during voluntary rhythmic contractions (running); such high blood flows were unattainable with various modes of electrical stimulation to induce muscle contractions or with pharmacological vasodilation of resting muscle. Laughlin (146) proposed that even without the added hydrostatic pressure on the arterial side, the muscle pump could still be effective in increasing muscle perfusion pressure and muscle blood flow in small animals that lack large hydrostatic forces in their working limbs. This maintained effectiveness would be possible if, during relaxation from a contraction, intramuscular venous pressure falls to subatmospheric values (146). The thinking is that muscle veins are so well tethered to surrounding muscle (12, 157) that they are "pulled-open" by the rapidly relaxing muscle as it rebounds to its relaxed shape and is re-extended to its precontraction length. Because the valves prevent retrograde refilling of muscle veins, negative intravenous pressure is created in the muscles and this draws blood through the microcirculation of the muscle into these veins from the arterial side. In this way the muscle pump could greatly widen the arterial-venous pressure difference without requiring a large hydrostatic component to blood pressure. It should be even more effective in giraffes and humans.

Sheriff et al. (261) provided evidence that dynamic exercise causes a large rapid rise in calculated muscle vascular conductance not explained by hydrostatic influences and too fast to be explained by known neural, metabolic, or myogenic influences on conductance (261). They attributed this sudden rise to a pump-induced rise in "virtual" conductance across the muscle; that is, to a so-called delta conductance caused by the pumping effect of contractions and relaxations on the arterial minus venous pressure difference. The term "virtual conductance" signified that a true ohmic conductance does not exist across a pump that by itself directly increases the blood flow through the organ. In short, they concluded that the initial fall in arterial pressure and increases in blood flow at exercise onset caused calculated "vascular conductance" to rise; this is in contrast to the traditional view that an increase in vascular conductance causes arterial pressure to fall and blood flow to rise.

Support for the postulate that muscle venous pressure falls to negative values after each contraction comes from the finding that drainage of cutaneous veins into deep veins via perforators during muscle relaxation occurred so quickly that there must have been a negative pressure in the deep muscle veins (6). No other significant force is known that could rapidly drive blood flow through the small (high-resistance) perforators connecting superficial and deep veins. Others also propose that active muscle is an active, pumping circulation and not a passive conduit through which blood is driven exclusively from the energy imparted by the left ventricle (312).

Distribution of blood volume. The observation that right atrial pressure often rises suddenly at the onset of exercise signifies that central blood volume rises suddenly as well. The fact that right atrial pressure remains elevated as exercise continues means that the central shift in blood volume is somehow maintained. How is blood volume mobilized and its central distribution maintained?

EFFECT OF MUSCLE PUMP ON MUSCLE BLOOD VOLUME. Muscle contraction raises muscle tissue pressure and compresses muscle veins, causing intramuscular blood volume to be rapidly expelled toward the heart owing to the orientation of its venous valves. This pumping action can be a particularly potent mechanism for the redistribution of blood volume. Stegall (282) found that forceful contractions of calf muscles reduced calf volume (calculated from changes in calf circumference) by 2.3% (23 ml/kg of calf) when subjects were in a 15-degree head-down position, when muscle blood flow and muscle blood volume are reduced somewhat by gravity. In as much as muscle is reported to contain 27–39 ml of blood per kilogram of tissue (45, 59), of which presumably 20–30 ml/kg is contained in veins, this finding indicates that the muscle pump has a high ejection fraction. Conceivably, the muscle pump could mobilize as much as 12 ml/kg body weight given that muscle constitutes 50% of body weight in dogs (186)—probably less (perhaps 40%) in humans—if all muscle contracted simultaneously.

The finding that the muscle pump can expel blood from an elevated limb (282) means that calf veins contain a functionally significant volume of blood despite having a luminal pressure that is possibly less than right atrial pressure. This indicates that limb veins (presumably intramuscular and intermuscular veins) are tethered open by their firm connections to the surrounding tissue (12, 157). The venous blood content of muscle is probably more strongly influenced by the surrounding tissue than by transmural pressure and compliance in the usual sense.

The effect of contraction force on the effectiveness of the muscle pump in expelling blood volume has received little attention. Barendsen and Van den Berg (15) found that contractions generating a force equal to that seen during quiet walking, and contractions generating one-half this force, expelled equal volumes of blood from the calf. This suggests that contraction force is not an important determinant of the effectiveness of the muscle pump in expelling blood volume.

The stride frequencies normally encountered during dynamic exercise prevent extensive refilling of muscle veins between contractions (76, 263). Consider, for example, a human running at 2 strides/s with a heart rate of 2 beats/s and a left ventricular stroke volume of 100 ml. Presumably, about 60% of each stroke volume (i.e., 60% of cardiac output) or 60 ml of blood is distributed to about 15 kg of muscle, or 4 ml/kg of muscle for each stride. In this situation, muscle venous blood content will rise from a nadir of perhaps 2ml/kg, occurring immediately after a contraction ceases, to a peak volume of 6 ml/kg, occurring at the start of the next contraction. Since venous blood volume is probably 2 ml/kg throughout the period of contraction and then rises progressively to 6 ml/kg over the noncontraction phase of a stride, the time-averaged volume would be about 3 ml/kg tissue weight during exercise. If the venous blood content of resting muscle is 23 ml/kg tissue weight, this form of running could produce a net mobilization of 20 ml of blood per kilogram of muscle.

In humans during quiet standing, an estimated 600 ml of blood enters the legs and collects in intramuscular, intermuscular, and cutaneous veins and an additional 250 ml enters into the buttock and pelvic veins (240). Hydrostatic pressures in veins of the legs range from 50–100 mm Hg, depending on the distance below the heart. Importantly, the muscle pump can overcome a pressure of 90–100 mm Hg when such a pressure is generated by partially occluding, with a cuff, the large veins draining muscle (13). Estimates of the ability of muscle pumps to expel the additional blood volume displaced into the leg veins by gravity are conflicting. Stegall (282) found that calf volume (vascular plus tissue) rose by 3% during standing. Contractions reduced calf volume to the same volume whether subjects were upright or in the head-down position. This means that contractions expelled all of the blood added from assuming the upright position (3%) plus the initial blood content (2%) for a total change in volume of 5%. Others have found that contractions reduce calf volume by only 3% when subjects are sitting (15) or are upright (284), indicating that contractions expel only about one-third of the additional blood volume displaced into legs by gravity [assuming that two-thirds of the 3% change is attributable to expulsion of initial (pre-upright) blood volume]. Ludbrook (157) estimated that of the 600 ml of blood that enters the lower limbs on standing, about 220 ml is mobilized centrally during exercise.

Taken together, these factors suggest that the muscle pump could mobilize as much as 20 ml of blood per kilogram of tissue weight or 10 ml/kg of body weight in dogs when they activate a large percentage of their total muscle mass during locomotion (90). This assumes that the muscle pumps in dogs are as effective as those of the human calf, on which most of the above estimates are based. As a function of body weight, less volume is probably mobilized in humans because they have less muscle as a percentage of body weight and probably use a smaller percentage of their total muscle mass during running than do quadrupeds. An estimate of 5 ml/kg body weight seems reasonable, meaning about 400 ml of blood might be mobilized from muscle in a 75 kg human during dynamic exercise.

EFFECT OF BLOOD VOLUME MOBILIZED BY THE MUSCLE PUMP ON RIGHT ATRIAL PRESSURE. Guyton et al. (98) investigated the ability of hindlimb muscle pumps to raise right atrial pressure in anesthesized dogs on right heart bypass with blocked autonomic ganglionic transmission to abolish reflexes. After the bypass pump was stopped, right atrial pressure rose to 3.8 mm Hg ("mean circulatory filling pressure"). Sustained contractions of the lower body musculature elicited by spinal cord stimulation suddenly raised right atrial pressure to 11.3 mm Hg. This sudden rise in pressure was attributed to the muscle pump because reflexes were blocked and any passive effects of changes in blood flow on blood volume distribution were precluded by the stop-flow condition. Inasmuch as neuromuscular blockade of the skeletal muscles prevented the rise, it must have been that their contraction caused the rise in central blood volume and right atrial pressure. Two factors in addition to the hindlimb muscle pumps probably contributed to the large rise in right atrial pressure: *(1)* the timing of the pressure measurement, and *(2)* the abdominal "pump." First, Guyton et al. (98) measured this pressure a few seconds after the contraction began. At that time right atrial pressure was at its maximum because most of the blood volume mobilized from the muscle must have been moved to the cardiopulmonary compartment, owing to the venous valves in the forelimbs and other organs (excluding perhaps the liver, which contains no venous valves). During normal dynamic exercise, the increments in right atrial pressure (back-pressure to venous drainage) will be transmitted to the venules of all organs. As a consequence, blood volume in these organs will eventually rise and diminish the final extent to which right atrial pressure rises, unless some compensatory adjustment prevents it (e.g., vasoconstriction or venoconstriction). Second, sustained, forceful contractions of abdominal muscles probably drove blood volume out of abdominal organs and back to the heart, thereby contributing further to the rise in right atrial pressure; at least the elevated abdominal pressure prevented the muscle pump from redistributing blood volume from muscle to abdominal vessels.

The muscle pump appears to be the major cause of the rise in right atrial pressure that normally accompanies dynamic exercise. If during dynamic exercise the blood volume pumped out of muscle veins is redistributed to the entire circulation (excluding of course the active muscle itself) and the vascular compliance of the recipient regions is 2.2 ml · mm Hg^{-1} · kg^{-1} of body weight (i.e., total vascular compliance less the compliance contributed by muscle), then mobilization of 10 ml/kg body weight in dogs would be expected to raise right atrial pressure by 4.5 mm Hg. This estimate assumes that blood flow to compliant regions is unchanged, as appears to be the case in dogs during mild to moderate exercise (318). This expected rise in right atrial pressure is close to that observed in dogs during mild dynamic exercise (263), suggesting that the muscle pump caused it. Further support for the suggestion that this rise is caused by the muscle pump and not by reflexes is provided in Figure 15.14*A*, which shows that increments in cardiac output and right atrial pressure in response to mild exercise were the same before and after autonomic blockade. In patients with impaired sympathetic function, central venous pressure can rise normally during mild supine leg exercise (legs above heart level) (19). There are, however, sources of blood volume in addition to the volume translocated by the muscle pump even when reflexes are blocked.

In humans and in dogs, exercise causes an exaggerated fall in arterial pressure when autonomic function is impaired. The exaggerated fall in arterial pressure will passively mobilize blood volume out of arteries and into veins. This volume, along with blood displaced out of muscle veins, could contribute to the rise in right atrial pressure. Furthermore, this hypotension must have reduced blood flow to inactive regions as well and as a consequence blood volume could eventually be mobilized from the veins of compliant regions as well as from active muscle. However, this second factor is probably unimportant to the initial rise in right atrial pressure at the onset of exercise [Fig. 15.16*B*); (263)]. This sudden rise was far too fast to be explained by passive mobilization of blood volume from inactive regions inasmuch as the time constant of venous drainage from compliant regions is estimated to be 30 s (41). Therefore, the blood volume suddenly mobilized by the muscle pump could account for most if not all of the immediate rise in filling pressure at the onset of mild dynamic exercise. In short, the facts that the time course of the immediate rise in right atrial pressure matched the time course of muscle pumping (218), and that autonomic blockade did not significantly alter either the time course or the magnitude of this rise, point to the muscle pump as the dominant factor raising central venous pressure at the onset of dynamic exercise. Thus, when exercise began, the increase in the flow of blood propelled back to the heart by the muscle pump exceeded the rapid increase in cardiac output (Fig. 15.16*A*), causing filling pressure to rise. Thereafter, the stable, elevated filling pressure in exercise signifies that muscle pumping and ventricular pumping remain balanced.

EFFECT OF BLOOD FLOW GENERATED BY THE MUSCLE PUMP ON SYSTEMIC HEMODYNAMICS. This subsection deals with the impact on the circulation of the sudden activation of a second pump (muscle) that generates blood flow. Figure 15.18 illustrates the effect of the muscle pump on central circulatory variables at the onset of dynamic exercise in dogs with blocked autonomic reflexes. Beat-by-beat cardiac output was maintained constant by ventricular pacing. The sudden and marked fall in arterial pressure at the onset of exercise occurs too soon and proceeds too rapidly to be caused by metabolic vasodilation within active muscle (Fig. 15.18). Muscle vasodilation in response to rhythmic muscle contractions occurs after a delay of 5–20 s and thereafter proceeds slowly, taking 20–30 s to reach a steady state (89, 165). Metabolic vasodilation likely accounts for the secondary rise in conductance beginning after 10 s of exercise in Figure 15.18. Since blood flow (left ventricular output) and "true" vascular resistance did not change in the first seconds of exercise, neither the fall in arterial pressure nor the rise in central venous pressure can be explained by traditional pressure–flow analysis of systemic hemodynamics. Furthermore, arterial pressure can fall even when cardiac output rises normally at the onset of exercise [Fig. 17.13; (261)]. These responses are better explained by pressure–volume analysis, in which the muscle pump suddenly withdraws blood volume from the arterial system; this causes arterial pressure to fall in proportion to arterial compliance. This blood is withdrawn and pulled through the muscle microcirculation, and is subsequently propelled centrally along with muscle venous blood to cause a rise in central venous pressure in proportion to central venous compliance. Thus, these changes in arterial and central venous pressure, which occur without a change in cardiac output and before relaxation of peripheral resistance vessels can occur, must reflect the mechanical effects of the muscle pump on the pressure–volume char-

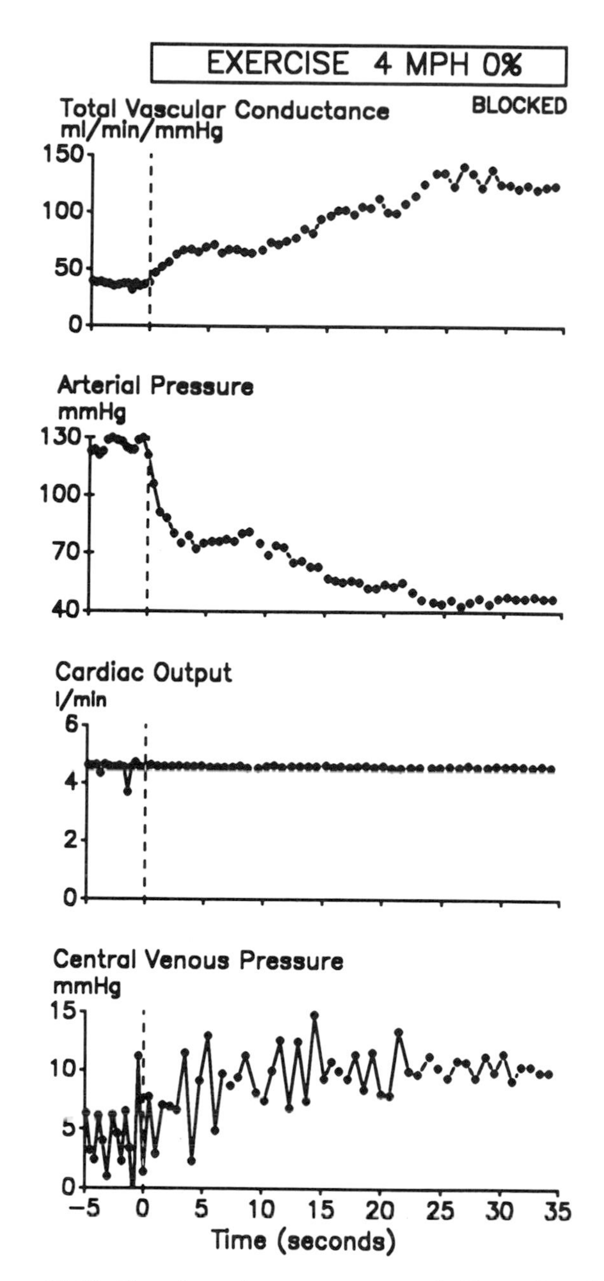

FIG. 15.18. Hemodynamic response to treadmill exercise when cardiac output is held constant at pre-exercise level by ventricular pacing in a dog with a surgically produced atrioventricular block. Data collected while autonomic reflexes were blocked with hexamethonium. See text for interpretation of changes induced by exercise. [Reprinted with permission from Sheriff, D. D., L. B. Rowell, and A. M. Scher. Is rapid rise in vascular conductance at onset of dynamic exercise due to muscle pump? *Am. J. Physiol.* 265 (*Heart Circ. Physiol.* 34): H1227–H1234, 1993.]

acteristics of the circulation. Arterial pressure falls until the rate of flow of blood into the muscle pump chambers (and hence the rate at which blood is pumped back to the heart) equilibrates with the rate of blood flow out of the left ventricle, and central venous pressure rises until the output of the muscle pump equilibrates with the output of the right ventricle. In this example, arterial volume and pressure, and central venous volume and pressure, all stabilize when the rates of the two pumps equilibrate.

CONSEQUENCE OF A DEFECTIVE MUSCLE PUMP. Bevegard and Lodin (21) investigated the impact of defective muscle pumping in humans with congenital absence of venous valves. Central venous pressure not only failed to undergo the rise normally seen in supine exercise but often fell in response to upright cycle exercise. *Line* C in Figure 15.17 shows the lack of effect of exercise on central venous pressure in subjects lacking venous valves. Data were averaged from experiments conducted with subjects in supine and seated postures. Compare *line* C with line B in Figure 15.17, which shows the rise in central venous pressure that accompanied exercise in recumbent heart-block patients (in whom the rate of pacing during exercise was raised from the rate at rest). As pointed out previously, central venous pressure falls little during exercise despite the lack of muscle pumping in patients lacking venous valves, suggesting that most of the rise in cardiac output was directed to muscle. Grimby et al. (94) examined responses to exercise in patients with varicose veins and found that stroke volume was markedly reduced compared to normal subjects; stroke volume could be raised by firmly wrapping the legs with bandages to reduce their venous blood content.

ABDOMINAL AND RESPIRATORY PUMPS. In addition to the skeletal muscle pump, the largest and most effective, there is an abdominal pump that expresses blood volume from abdominal organs and the inferior vena cava and a respiratory pump that aspirates blood from the inferior vena cava when intrathoracic pressure is negative. The respiratory pump also influences the release of blood volume from the liver back to the right atrium. These pumps are discussed later under RESPIRATORY SYSTEM and in Chapter 17.

Summary. Passive (nonautonomic) factors determine the basic pattern of response to exercise of the major hemodynamic variables except for arterial pressure. The muscle pump withdraws blood from its arterial supply and forces it through muscle and then expels this volume along with blood from muscle veins into thoracic vessels to raise central venous pressure. By reducing arterial pressure and raising central venous pressure, the muscle pump decreases the arteriovenous pressure difference across inactive regions and thereby reduces blood flow to these regions. At the same time, the muscle pump appears to increase muscle blood flow by lowering the pressure within intramuscular veins to negative values during each muscular relaxation. In this way the muscle pump ensures a passive redistribution of cardiac output and increases the fraction of total blood flow directed to active muscle. The rise in central venous pressure (along with a much smaller contribution by the fall in arterial pressure; see earlier under INTRINSIC PROPERTIES OF THE HEART) increases stroke volume and cardiac output. For example, Sheriff et al. (263) found that mild dynamic exercise increased cardiac output from 4.0 liters/min to 6.6 liters/min when reflex changes in heart rate and contractility were blocked. Dogs and supine humans are able to successfully carry out mild dynamic exercise relying only on these passive adjustments. Increments in work rate cause further decrements in arterial pressure and, as a consequence, exercise tolerance is presumably limited when cerebral perfusion pressure falls below limits of adequate autoregulation of cerebral blood flow. That is, when reflexes are blocked during exercise, cardiac output and muscle blood flow are above levels that are well tolerated when autonomic function is intact and arterial pressure is normal (261, 263).

Neural Factors Influencing the Response of Filling Pressure to Exercise. This subsection examines the potential role of active regional vasomotor adjustments and how they might contribute to the maintenance of and to the increases in ventricular filling pressure, stroke volume, and cardiac output during exercise.

Quadrupeds. When sympathetic function is intact, arterial pressure is well maintained and tends to rise during dynamic exercise. In dogs, blood flow to inactive regions is little changed (at least in mild to moderate exercise) (186, 318). This has been interpreted to mean that vasoconstriction within inactive regions occurs in direct proportion to the rise in arterial pressure (240). However, this interpretation missed the observation that central venous pressure can rise in parallel with arterial pressure during exercise such that the arteriovenous pressure difference across inactive regions can change little or not at all (263). Accordingly, increments in sympathetic activity directed to inactive regions during exercise may not always be required to maintain constant regional blood flow. Nevertheless, sympathetic vasoconstriction must prevent blood flow to inactive regions from rising whenever arterial pressure increases more than central venous pressure during exercise.

Active muscles vasoconstrict in response to dynamic exercise [see Figs. 17.12 and 17.13; also see Chapter 16; (261, 319)]. This vasoconstriction is of critical importance in controlling arterial pressure in dynamic exercise, but it has no direct effect on right atrial pressure. That is, right atrial pressure would be affected only if muscle vasoconstriction or vasodilation diverted blood flow to or from compliant regions. Figure 17.13 shows the severe hypotension that attends mild exercise in dogs after autonomic blockade, despite the fact that cardiac output was raised by ventricular pacing to the level normally seen at that work rate (261). Inasmuch as inactive regions are not strongly vasoconstricted in normal dogs during mild exercise, these findings suggest that active muscle may be a preferential target of sympathetic vasoconstriction. In a traditional pressure–flow analysis of circulatory hemodynamics, muscle vasoconstriction is viewed as a means of "matching" total vascular conductance to cardiac output so that arterial pressure is well maintained or raised in exercise. An alternative view, based on a pressure–volume analysis, is that muscle vasoconstriction occurs to match the rates of muscle pumping and cardiac pumping, thereby providing a means of regulating the pressure and volume in the arterial "reservoir."

The rise in right atrial pressure in response to mild exercise is little changed by global sympathetic blockade (see above), suggesting only a small role for regional vasoconstriction in raising right atrial pressure in dogs (but not in upright humans—see below). Conversely, selective denervation of the splanchnic circulation combined with adrenal medullectomy in dogs markedly reduced stroke volume and cardiac output during voluntary dynamic exercise of moderate intensity; arterial pressure rose sightly in exercise (from 110 mm Hg to 114 mm Hg) and was unaffected by denervation (8). This result suggests an important role for regional vasoconstriction in raising (or maintaining) right atrial pressure during exercise. The reason why this procedure reduced stroke volume is unknown. For example, this region is only mildly vasoconstricted during exercise in this species, so its denervation would not be expected to greatly alter its flow or volume. Splanchnic vasoconstriction could have prevented splanchnic blood flow and volume from rising passively in those studies where arterial blood pressure rose substantially during exercise in dogs (e.g., 44).

Splanchnic vasoconstriction during severe exercise in dogs (186) could passively reduce splanchnic blood volume and thereby contribute to the further increments in right atrial pressure seen with increasing work rate (44, 263). Splanchnic venoconstriction could contribute as well by actively expelling blood volume from splanchnic veins (31, 33). The spleen is of particular importance in raising circulating blood volume and circulating red blood cell mass in dogs and other quadrupeds. Splenic contraction in dogs can release blood into circulation (~2.5 ml/kg body weight) (266), enough to raise right atrial pressure by 1 mm Hg (assuming a systemic compliance of 2.5 ml · mm Hg^{-1} · kg body weight).

Humans. In humans, blood flow to inactive regions is progressively reduced during dynamic exercise by sympathetic vasoconstriction that occurs in proportion to increases in heart rate above a rate of about 100 bpm (239). Regional vasoconstriction in humans diverts blood flow from inactive regions to active muscle. The reduction in splanchnic blood flow may cause blood volume to be passively released centrally, thereby raising right atrial pressure; at least it will act in conjunction with the abdominal pump to prevent blood expelled from muscle veins from eventually accumulating in abdominal organs. Splanchnic blood volume is reported to fall by approximately 300 ml during mild dynamic exercise (321). Splanchnic venoconstriction and the abdominal pump could expel blood volume as well. The effect of vasoconstriction on splanchnic blood volume is probably more important than its other role of diverting blood flow away from inactive regions to supplement blood flow (and oxygen delivery) to working muscle (240). For example, the increased oxygen delivery attributable to the higher cardiac output that can be achieved owing to the rise in filling pressure caused by central mobilization of splanchnic blood volume may exceed any increase in oxygen delivery provided by the diversion of flow from splanchnic to muscle vasculature. This latter adjustment is most important in cardiac patients unable to raise cardiac output normally in response to exercise.

Patients with severely impaired sympathetic function are unable to exercise in the upright posture because of severe hypotension (19). This is caused by the gravitational displacement of blood volume into dependent cutaneous vasculature and other unconstricted regions. Presumably this is also attributable in part to volume sequestration in the unconstricted splanchnic region prior to the fall in arterial pressure. The exaggerated gravitational displacement of blood volume decreases ventricular filling pressure, leading to a fall in stroke volume, cardiac output, and finally arterial pressure culminating in collapse. Selective denervation of the splanchnic circulation also leads to the same series of events (316), but they occur much more slowly then occurs with more global impairment of sympathetic function, which leads to precipitous hypotension in upright humans during exercise. Presumably, normal function of the muscle, abdominal, and respiratory pumps in these subjects is not sufficient to provide an adequate filling pressure during upright exercise. Regional vasoconstriction is critical to maintenance of both arterial blood pressure and ventricular filling pressure (discussed in more detail in Chapter 17).

Effects of Changes in Cardiac Output Imposed during Dynamic Exercise. The question dealt with here is how an increase or decrease in cardiac output that is superimposed on the normal "steady-state" value for a particular work rate might effect right atrial pressure. Any effect on ventricular filling pressure will depend on how the rise or fall in cardiac output is distributed.

Changes in cardiac output by ventricular pacing. When cardiac output increases in response to dynamic exercise, the entire rise in cardiac output is directed to active muscle. As the severity of exercise increases, the fraction of cardiac output going to muscle in humans increases even further because inactive regions become more and more vasoconstricted. Because skeletal muscle circulation is relatively noncompliant, changes in its blood flow will cause little change in its blood volume. When cardiac output is altered during steady-state exercise (e.g., by ventricular pacing), a substantial fraction of the change should be absorbed by muscle because muscle vascular "conductance" (including its pump function) comprises the major fraction of the total vascular conductance. Accordingly, the effect of a change in cardiac output on right atrial pressure would be far less than if the same change was imposed at rest. This idea is quantitatively expressed in the two-compartment model of Caldini et al. (41).

Caldini and co-workers (41) developed a quantitative two-compartment model of the circulation, based on an earlier model proposed by August Krogh in 1912 (143). In Krogh's model, the amount of blood available to fill the right ventricle was determined by the fraction of cardiac output distributed between compliant and noncompliant vascular circuits (or compartments). In Caldini and colleagues' modification of the Krogh model, the distribution of blood volume, and thus the slope relating cardiac output to right atrial pressure, is a function of the time constants (equal to the product of venous resistance and compliance) governing the rates of venous drainage from each compartment (lumped regional circulations) and the fraction of cardiac output each compartment receives. Compliant circulations (e.g., the splanchnic circulation) have "long" or "slow" time constants and noncompliant circulations (e.g., muscle) have "short" or "fast" time constants. Maximal cardiac output was viewed as a function of *(1)* the fraction of cardiac output directed to beds with "fast" vs. "slow" time constants and *(2)* the values of these time constants. The concept is that blood cannot be forced through the circulation any faster than it drains back to the right heart as governed by the time constants of venous drainage (210). This model provides a reasonable explanation for how cardiac output and its distribution among organs affect blood volume distribution during rest. However, its conceptual usefulness is limited when it is applied to dynamic exercise, because blood does not passively drain from the active skeletal muscles that receive most of the cardiac output in this setting. Rather, the blood is actively propelled back to the heart by a second pump—namely, the active muscles.

Based on the knowledge that the fraction of cardiac output directed to noncompliant muscle rises in proportion to the intensity of exercise (reaching a maximum of approximately 85%), Green and Jackman (92) used the model of Caldini et al. (41) to predict that exercise would decrease the slope of the relationship between cardiac output and right atrial pressure as shown in Figure 15.19. Sheriff et al. (263) tested this prediction by measuring right atrial pressure during rest and graded exercise when cardiac output was changed by altering ventricular pacing rate in dogs. Exercise shifted the relationship between cardiac output and right atrial pressure rightward toward higher cardiac output and upward to higher atrial pressure in proportion to the severity of exercise (Fig. 15.14). Surprisingly, exercise did not alter the slope of this relationship as shown in Figures 15.14 and 15.17. The slope was not significantly altered even when the fraction of cardiac output directed to muscle reached 80% during heavy exercise (263). Why is the slope of the relationship between cardiac output and right atrial pressure not changed by exercise, as predicted by Green and Jackman (92)?

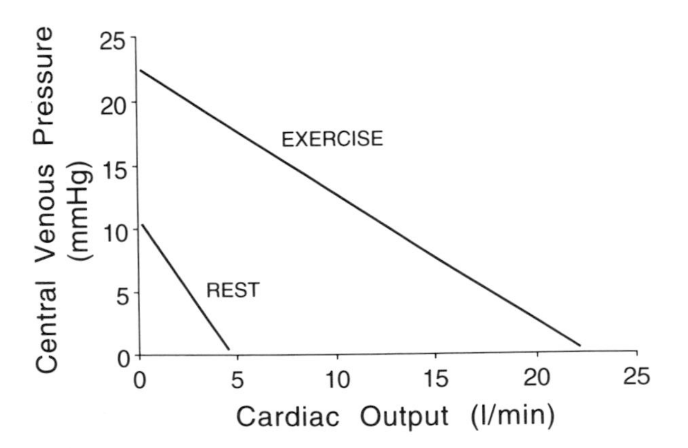

FIG. 15.19. Model prediction of relationship between cardiac output and right atrial pressure during rest and exercise. Exercise is predicted to decrease the slope of the relationship between these two variables. [Adapted from Green and Jackman (92).]

In their prediction of the influence of exercise on the relationship between cardiac output and filling pressure shown in Figure 15.19, Green and Jackman (92) assumed that the fraction of cardiac output directed to muscle was 38% at rest and 95% during exercise. They also assumed that irrespective of whether a change in cardiac output was imposed during rest or exercise, the fraction of cardiac output directed to muscle would remain constant at whatever it had been in either state (e.g., at rest 38% of an increase in cardiac output would go to muscle and in exercise 95% of an increase would go to active muscle). Sheriff and Zhou (262) tested this assumption by estimating the fraction of cardiac output directed to all active muscle from measurements of blood flow to the hindlimbs and cardiac output when cardiac output was altered by ventricular pacing at rest and during graded dynamic exercise. The fraction of cardiac output directed to muscle did not remain constant when cardiac output was manipulated. Rather, this fraction *fell* from 53% to 45% when cardiac output was reduced at rest, and *rose* from 69% to 76% when cardiac output was reduced during mild (4 mph 0% grade) exercise as shown in Figure 15.20*A*. That is, the percentage fall in muscle blood flow exceeded the percentage fall in cardiac output at rest, whereas the opposite response occurred during 4 mph exercise. The potential effect on the relationship between cardiac output and cardiac filling pressure of these directionally opposite changes in the distribution of cardiac output are shown schematically in Figure 15.20*B*. The slope at rest is decreased by the "curve jumping" that occurs when the fraction of cardiac output directed to muscle falls when a reduction in cardiac output is imposed at rest. Conversely, the slope is steepened by the "curve jumping" that occurs when this fraction rises when a reduction in cardiac output is imposed during exercise. The directionally opposite changes in the distribution of cardiac output could equalize the slopes relating cardiac output to right atrial pressure of rest and during exercise as shown in Figure 15.20*B*.

FUNCTIONAL SIGNIFICANCE. The functional significance of an inverse relationship between cardiac output and right atrial pressure in exercise is the same as that at rest. The inverse relationship benefits circulatory homeostatis by providing a passive (hydraulic) self-regulating feature that helps to maintain a stable level of cardiac output (238). This stabilization occurs except when cardiac performance falls at a time when the ventricles are operating at the limit of mechanical restraint on stroke volume imposed by the pericardium (see earlier under INTRINSIC PROPERTIES OF THE HEART). In this case the rise

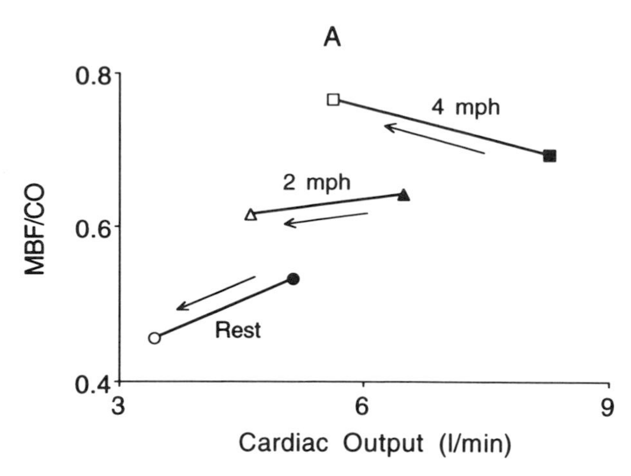

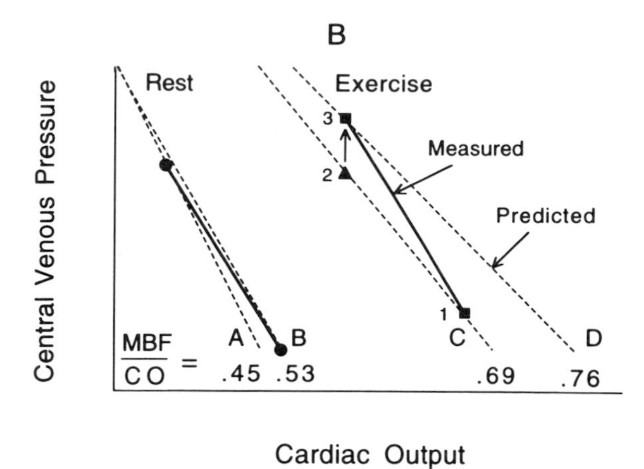

FIG. 15.20. Influence of exercise intensity and of changes in cardiac output (CO) on the estimated fraction of cardiac output directed to active muscle (MBF/CO). Cardiac output was changed by changing ventricular pacing rate at rest and during 0% grade treadmill exercise in conscious dogs with a surgically produced atrioventricular block. *A*, MBF/CO rises with increasing exercise intensity. Direction of change in MBF/CO in response to a reduction in CO (*arrows*) depends on exercise intensity (e.g., MBF/CO falls when CO is reduced at rest but rises when CO is reduced during 4 mph exercise). *B*, Schematic illustration of potential effects of changes in cardiac output distribution on cardiac filling pressure. Changes in CO distribution (MBF/CO) change the slope of the relationship predicted between CO and filling pressure in (*dashed lines A, B, C,* and *D*). "Curve jumping" from *line B* to *line A* when CO is reduced at rest lowers the slope (*circles*), whereas "curve jumping" from *line C* to *line D* when CO is reduced during exercise increases the slope (*squares*). These directionally opposite changes in the distribution of cardiac output tend to equalize the slope of the curves relating CO to filling pressure measured in rest and exercise (*solid lines*). *Arrow* shows effect on filling pressure of diverting flow from a compliant to a noncompliant region when cardiac output does not change. [Adapted with permission from Sheriff, D. D., and X. P. Zhou. Influence of cardiac output distribution on cardiac filling pressure during rest and dynamic exercise in dogs. *Am. J. Physiol.* 267 (*Heart Circ. Physiol.* 36) H2378–2380, 1999.]

in filling pressure that accompanies a fall in cardiac output will no longer increase end-diastolic volume and stroke volume so as to partially counteract the decline in cardiac output. Conversely, this relationship can impede the ability to raise cardiac output when increases in blood flow to compliant regions are required (see below).

The change in the distribution of blood flow induced by changes in cardiac output during dynamic exercise (or during rest) means that curves relating cardiac output to filling pressure cannot be extrapolated to a right atrial pressure that reliably reflects the "mean circulatory filling pressure." Furthermore, the concept of a mean circulatory filling pressure in exercise is confounded by the action of a second (muscle) pump. Even if ventricular function were reduced to zero, the muscle pump would continue to pull blood out of arteries and propel this blood back toward the heart, meaning pressures within the circuit would not be equal as is required by the concept of a mean circulatory filling pressure. Even if blood flow ceased, intramuscular pressure would greatly exceed pressures elsewhere in the circulation, owing to the high tissue pressure (often >200 mm Hg) generated during muscle contraction (256). In effect, exercise divides the skeletal muscle circulation, which becomes a true pressure–flow generating pump, and the remainder of the circulation into two hydraulically separate compartments. Pressure within the skeletal muscle compartment has no physical relationship to (or is mechanically "uncoupled" from) the pressure within the remainder of the circulation. As for the remainder of the circulation, it is passively distended by the volume it contains after blood flow has stopped and pressure between arteries and veins has equilibrated. This equilibrated pressure would represent the mean circulatory filling pressure for this compartment only. Accordingly mean circulatory filling pressure during dynamic exercise lacks a physical meaning and the concept does not apply.

Changes in distribution of cardiac output by competing demands for flow

WHAT ARE COMPETING DEMANDS? This subsection examines how the cardiovascular system adjusts during exercise when additional demands are imposed on the circulation. Additional demands can take the form of added requirements for blood flow to organs other than skeletal muscle. Demands for these other organs either compete for a greater fraction of cardiac output, or cardiac output must rise above its highly predictable value at a given oxygen consumption in order to meet them. Clearly, there is a point at which cardiac output cannot rise further to meet additional demands, and at this point these demands clearly compete. This occurs when cardiac output and oxygen consumption are approaching their maxima. Only an adaptation over weeks will permit cardiac output to rise further and reach a new and higher maximum.

The question to be answered here is, Which demands actually must "compete" for cardiac output because of the passive (hydraulic) regulation that serves as a self-limiting negative feedback and stabilizes cardiac output? Alternatively, why are some demands simply met by raising cardiac output without this self-limiting negative feedback?

HYPERTHERMIA. Exercise in a hot environment places an extra demand on the circulation for more blood flow at any given rate of work. Blood flow to skin, a compliant and capacious vascular bed like the splanchnic region, must be increased in order to increase the transfer of heat to the environment. Figure 17.4 shows that a heat-induced rise in cardiac output at rest reduces central venous pressure along a slope similar to that shown by *line A* in Figure 15.17. Figure 17.4 also shows that a similar relationship between cardiac output and right atrial pressure exists during mild dynamic exercise (i.e., similar to *line B* in Figure 15.17). In short, for the reasons already discussed, the ability to raise cardiac output during exercise to meet the competing demands (here they do compete) for increased skin blood flow is restricted by the limited ability to increase cardiac output. When hyperthermia becomes more severe, this self-limiting effect on cardiac output becomes more pronounced as the total blood flow directed to the skin increases. Eventually, the cardiovascular system cannot raise cardiac output further to meet the added, competing demands for skin blood flow (239).

HYPOXEMIA. A reduction in arterial oxygen tension caused by the reduction in barometric pressure at high altitude is accompanied by an increase in cardiac output during exercise. In acute hypoxemia, cardiac output rises to the same maximal values seen during exercise at sea level conditions, but total oxygen extraction and oxygen consumption are much lower. Data from two studies (283, 322) indicate that the additional rise in cardiac output induced by hypoxemia during submaximal exercise occurs without a fall in right atrial pressure (e.g., along *line B* in Fig. 15.15). Right atrial pressure may even increase. Stenberg et al. (283) observed no significant effect of hypoxemia on stroke volume (consistent with no change in right atrial pressure), on arterial blood pressure, or on maximal cardiac output (again maximal oxygen consumption was reduced). During submaximal levels of exercise, cardiac output was increased by the added demands for increased muscle blood flow—blood flow to other organs, except heart and brain, probably does not increase (239).

Wagner et al. (322) compared central circulatory responses to exercise up to maximal oxygen consumption at sea level and simulated altitudes of 3048 and 4573 m. Stroke volume was unaffected by simulated altitude and even tended to increase at the highest work rate at 4573 m. At sea level, pulmonary wedge pressure rises approximately parallel with right atrial pressure during exercise (223) (see Fig. 17.1). At simulated altitudes, pulmonary wedge pressure rose just as it did at sea level, and the maintained stroke volume suggests that right atrial pressure still rose in parallel with wedge pressure. Therefore, hypoxia appears to represent a case in which demands for increased cardiac output are confined to the perfusion of active muscle, a noncompliant region where an increase in blood flow does not significantly alter right atrial pressure.

ADAPTATION. The adaptation of the heart and circulation to chronic heavy exercise is discussed in the first section of this chapter and in Chapter 17. The primary question raised in Chapter 17 is whether the higher maximum cardiac output is achieved by increased myocardial contractile force, reduced afterload, or increased ventricular preload. The authors of Chapter 17 conclude that most evidence supports a mechanical adaptation in the form of increased pericardial volume in response to repeated exposure to a high preload. Evidence that increased central blood volume and increased right atrial pressure contributed to the rise in maximal stroke volume (which accounts for the rise in cardiac output with no change in maximal heart rate) is lacking. Instead, maximal stroke volume seems to be limited by pericardial constraints. The evidence also points to the entire increase in cardiac output (from its old to new maximum) being distributed to active muscle. The rise in peak muscle blood flow with conditioning is probably due to a progressive withdrawal of tonic vasoconstrictor outflow to working muscle (tonic restraint is required because its capacity to vasodilate and pump blood through itself outstrips cardiac pumping capacity). Therefore, the adaptation to physical conditioning is unopposed by the self-limiting feedback on cardiac output that would attend a rise in blood flow to nonpumping or compliant organs.

RESPIRATORY SYSTEM

A great deal is known about the effect of ventilatory mechanical stresses on the circulation. Most of this comes from studies of normal or loaded breathing in resting individuals, or from the effects of artificial ventilators on the circulation. The way that exercise induces changes in respiratory mechanics, pleural and abdominal pressure, and lung volumes has been studied in both humans and animals. There is, however, little direct information about the way that respiratory stresses during exercise affect the circulation. In this section, we will review what is known about the effects of ventilatory stresses on the circulation, but we must largely speculate about the way that exercise-induced changes in ventilation might modulate the circulation in health and disease.

The mechanical stresses placed on the circulation by respiratory maneuvers can be conveniently categorized as follows: *(1)* changes in pleural pressure, *(2)* changes in lung volume, *(3)* changes in the local constraints of the heart (cardiac fossa and pericardium), *(4)* ventricular interdependence (how one ventricle affects the pressure volume characteristics of the other), and *(5)* changes in abdominal pressure.

In recent years, our understanding of how these stresses affect cardiac output and the distribution of blood volumes and flow within the circulation has increased. Because of the interrelated and complex nature of the circulation, however, the effect of any one of these stresses may not be readily predictable without understanding the behavior of the system as a whole. For example, a rise in pleural pressure may have opposite effects on cardiac output depending upon the pump function of the heart—falling under conditions where pump function is good, and rising under conditions where pump function is very poor. The effect of an elevation in lung volume may have opposite effects on pulmonary venous return—impeding pulmonary venous return when the pulmonary blood volume is low, and transiently augmenting pulmonary venous return when the pulmonary blood volume is high.

In the following subsections, we will discuss how these stresses affect the circulation. Specifically, we will address the way that respiratory stresses affect: *(1)* systemic venous return, *(2)* right ventricular output, *(3)* pulmonary venous return, and *(4)* left ventricular output.

Effects of Exercise on Respiratory Mechanics

The increase in ventilation that accompanies exercise is the result of an increase in both respiratory frequency and tidal volume. At low levels of exercise, the increase in ventilation is largely the consequence of increasing tidal volume. With increasing levels of exercise, the tidal volume reaches a plateau at about 50%–60% of vital capacity and, thereafter, further increases in ventilation are achieved through increases in respiratory frequency (127, 129). Because both tidal volume and inspiratory and expiratory flow rates have effects on pleural pressure, with increasing exercise there is an increase in the swings in pleural pressure; peak inspiratory pleural pressure becomes more negative and peak expiratory pleural pressure becomes more positive. At high levels of exercise, the maximum negative pleural pressure is about −30 cm H_2O (compared to about −8 cm H_2O at rest) and the maximum positive pleural pressure ranges from about 5–30 cm H_2O (compared to −5 cm H_2O at rest) (147, 197).

In young healthy individuals at levels of exercise exceeding 100 W, the end-expiratory lung volume is reduced as a consequence of recruitment of expiratory abdominal muscles (129). The end-inspiratory lung volume increases progressively, and may reach 80%–90% of total lung capacity (TLC) with severe exercise (341). However, in patients with chronic obstructive lung disease (COPD), end-expiratory lung volume rises progressively with exercise (11). This is thought to be a mechanism to enhance expiratory flow rates at the cost of increased inspiratory work of breathing (60, 219). Despite the limitation of expiratory airflow, COPD patients actively expire during exercise, possibly attempting to maintain optimal configuration and length of the diaphragm for subsequent inspiratory efforts. Similarly, elevation of end-expiratory lung volumes and airflow limitation may occur in older trained individuals as a consequence of the age-related loss of lung elastic recoil and the necessity to achieve high levels of expiratory airflow by breathing at high lung volumes (127).

When the arms are used for aerobic exercise, rather than the legs, adjustments are made in the activation of the respiratory muscles. There is less utilization of the inspiratory muscles of the rib cage, which normally maintain the domed configuration of the diaphragm. Thus, arm exercise leads to greater swings in abdominal pressure relative to pleural pressure, possibly altering the dynamics of venous return (43). During heavy resistance exercise, such as weight lifting, maximum loads are accompanied by a Valsalva maneuver of 30–50 mm Hg (159).

Systemic Venous Return

Systemic venous return can be visualized as the passive drainage of blood from the compliant regions of the peripheral circulation back to the right atrium. In the steady state, the heart replenishes the drainage volume in the peripheral compliant regions, while the peripheral circulation controls the distribution of volume among parallel circuits and the pressure–volume characteristics of each of the regions. As developed in the previous section, during exercise, redistribution of blood flow toward skeletal muscle contributes to the increase in systemic venous return by perfusing beds with rapid drainage characteristics (41, 295). Venous return is additionally augmented by the reduction in unstressed volume and decreased venous compliance that accompanies sympathetic stimulation (34, 55).

Effect of Lowering Right Atrial Pressure on Venous Return. During exercise, each inspiration is accompanied by a fall in right atrial pressure, and each expiration is accompanied by an elevation in right atrial pressure, with the mean right atrial pressure falling slightly (126). The effect of a reduction in pressure surrounding the right atrium and an increase in the pressure surrounding the abdominal vessels on blood flow has been considered in some detail. In the eighteenth century, Rev. Stephen Hales made the first measurements of arterial and venous blood pressures and noted respiratory fluctuation in vascular pressures with respiration, which he attributed to blood being expressed from the lungs by the respiratory movements (102). Donders is credited with first suggesting a century ago that the negative pressures in the pleural space could augment the return of blood to the heart (231). Holt, however, used both model systems and animal experiments and concluded that an inspiratory fall in pressure in the right atrium relative to the pressure in the peripheral vessels did not cause an increase in blood flow. He concluded that this was due to the collapse of the vena cava, increasing the inflow resistance to the heart (111, 112). Duomarco and Rimini in 1954 analyzed pressure gradients along the veins and concluded that a lowering of downstream pressure should have no effect on return flow to the heart due to collapse of the veins. They suggested the hydrostatic analogy of a waterfall, which is uninfluenced by changes in pressure at its base (63). Guyton confirmed Holt's findings and validated Duomarco's prediction showing that a reduction of right atrial pressure below −2 mm Hg did not cause any augmentation of venous return, an effect which he also attributed to collapse of the great veins entering the thorax (97). The waterfall concept has been analyzed extensively by Permutt and colleagues with respect to flow of air through the airways and flow of blood through the pulmonary and systemic vessels (209, 212). They pointed out the similarity between the mechanical principles governing both a waterfall and a collapsible tube, where maximal flow is uninfluenced by changes in downstream pressures.

Effect of Spontaneous Respiration on Phasic Venous Return. A number of studies have shown that there is a phasic increase in inferior vena cava (IVC) blood flow during inspiration (4, 29, 52, 64, 96, 176, 180, 257). Review of the tracings and descriptions of the patterns of IVC blood flow from these studies show little uniformity of the pattern of flow. Some studies show the IVC blood flow to peak early in inspiration, while others show that it continues to increase throughout inspiration. In contrast to these studies, there are several studies that have shown decreasing IVC blood flow with inspiration. Wexler and colleagues found that blood flow velocity in the IVC in some subjects increases with inspiration, but falls in others (335). Nakhjavan et al. observed that the inspiratory transmural femoral venous pressure rose in subjects who had inspiratory falls in IVC flow, whereas it fell in the others (188). The fall in IVC blood flow with inspiration was present in 6 of 15 patients with emphysema and hyperinflation of the lungs, but not in normal subjects. The fall in flow was thought to be due to mechanical obstruction of the vena cava by the contracting diaphragm, as originally suggested by Franklin in 1937 (78). Inspiratory collapse of the vena cava at the thoracic inlet was also observed by Jardin et al. in patients with acute asthma, which they ascribed to inspiratory IVC blood flow limitation (124). A similar finding was noted by Doppman et al. using contrast radiography, but their conclusion was that the diaphragm directly obstructed IVC blood flow (61).

Several authors have challenged the notion that the dynamics of blood flow along the IVC can be modeled as a waterfall or Starling resistor. Moreno and colleagues found variability in IVC flow patterns with respiration, usually consisting of a biphasic pattern in which flow initially increases and then falls. If they added saline-filled packs around the liver to prevent direct contact, they found that inspiration was associated with a fall in inspiratory IVC blood flow. They concluded that the major effect of diaphragm contraction was to enhance hepatic venous return through local compression of the liver, while obstructing infrahepatic venous flow (178, 179). Lloyd (154) demonstrated that blood flow in the IVC was increased with diaphragm contraction when the downstream pressure in the thoracic vena cava was high, but that IVC flow was decreased when the downstream venous pressure was low. In the intact animal, however, he found that under normal conditions, there was always an inspiratory augmentation of IVC blood flow. This observation was similar to that made in earlier studies (29, 176). He concluded that "a Starling resistor analog of abdominal veins based solely on abdominal and venous pressures is inappropriate" (154). Focal compression of the liver during diaphragmatic contraction has been subsequently confirmed (54, 297, 299) and demonstrated to be associated with movement of blood from a fast time constant compartment in the liver into the thorax (297, 299). The increase in downstream pressure caused by this rapid increase in IVC flow produces a decrease in the gradient for nonsplanchnic IVC flow (299). Thus, apparent conflicts in the effects of respiration on venous return from the abdominal compartment may in part reflect differential phasic contributions from interdependent hepatic, splanchnic, and nonsplanchnic venous beds. For example, the greater increase in pressure over the liver compared to generalized abdominal pressure with diaphragmatic descent will empty a fast time constant hepatic venous bed, but will reduce flow from both the portal vein and nonsplanchnic IVC. If the inspiration is prolonged or if the mobile blood volume in the liver is small, a gradient for anterograde nonsplanchnic IVC and portal flow could be established. While diaphragmatic contraction clearly can produce increased pressures over the liver, particularly in the crural region (54, 56), the mechanical freedom permitting diaphragmatic descent into the abdomen is also important. Thus, if the airway is obstructed such that, for the same decrease in intrathoracic pressure with diaphragmatic contraction the change in lung volume is minimized and diaphragmatic motion is limited, both the generalized and focal perihepatic increases in abdominal pressure will be less (297). Whether this same phenomenon occurs under exercise conditions in which the diaphragm remains relatively motionless and lung volume increases mainly through rib cage expansion has not been evaluated.

Elevation of lung volume may also affect systemic venous return independent of the effect on pleural pressure. Fessler et al. showed in dogs that lung inflation can directly compress the thoracic vena cava and impair systemic venous return irrespective of the effect on pleural pressure (70, 71). This may explain why persons with moderate COPD who, with exercise develop lung volumes that approach total lung capacity, appear to have circulatory exercise limitation (11). Thus, most investigators studying respiration have found that inspiration causes transient increases in IVC flow with no change or an increase in steady-state flow with the important exceptions noted above.

Effect of Increased Abdominal Pressure on Systemic Venous Return. Investigators studying the effect of pathologic increases in abdominal pressure have found different effects on cardiac output, sometimes increasing it and sometimes decreasing it. Ivankovich et al. found that increases in abdominal pressure with insufflation of gas to 20 mm Hg led to an increase in cardiac output (117). Similarly, Kelman et al. found increases in cardiac output in humans during laparoscopy with increases in abdominal pressure up to 40 mm Hg (135). However, Richardson and Trinkle found no change in cardiac output with increases in abdominal pressure up to 10 mm Hg, and decreases when abdominal pressure was raised above this level (225). Lynch et al. had similar results in newborn piglets (158). Masey et al., studying newborn lambs, also found that increasing abdominal pressure led to a decreased cardiac output (168). Diamant et al. found that the fall in cardiac output with increasing abdominal pressure to 40 mm Hg was exaggerated by hypovolemia and anesthesia, concluding that increases in abdominal pressure must obstruct the inferior vena cava (58). A possible resolution to these disparate findings comes from Kashtan and Green, who measured venous return curves in dogs with increased abdominal pressure (133). They found that in the hypovolemic animal the predominant effect of increasing abdominal pressure is an increase in the calculated resistance to venous return, which would tend to decrease blood flow. In the hypervolemic animal, however, the predominant effect was an increase in mean systemic pressure, which would tend to increase systemic venous return. In summary, an elevation of abdominal pressure can lead to either an increase or a decrease in systemic venous return depending upon the magnitude of the stress and the condition of the circulation.

These apparently conflicting findings have been largely resolved by the work of Takata et al. (300), who showed that the effect of a change in abdominal pressure on systemic venous return depends upon the blood volume of the abdominal compartment, which in turn depends upon the relationship between abdominal pressure and central venous pressure. When the central venous pressure is low relative to abdominal pressure (analogous to West's zone II in the lung), an increase in abdominal pressure reduces systemic venous return by compressing the conducting veins. In contrast, when the central venous pressure is high relative to the abdominal pressure (analogous to West's zone III in the lung), then an increase in abdominal pressure causes an increase in systemic venous return (300, 337). An increase in abdominal pressure, regardless of the abdominal vascular zone condition, will transiently reduce the gradient for flow from the lower extremities (300, 337).

Right Ventricular Output

The RV is a relatively flat, crescent-shaped chamber with a septal wall in common with the LV and a free wall contiguous with LV free-wall fibers. The irregular geometry makes assessment of volume changes in the RV very difficult. It is generally agreed, however, that spontaneous inspiration will increase RV volume due predominantly to an increase in venous return and, to a variable degree, a simultaneous increase in RV afterload as lung volume increases (231, 337, 339) (see later under Effect of Changes in Lung Volume).

In general, the RV is considered as having a free wall anchored to the septum (and possibly to the LV via fiber continuity), with the septum considered as a single muscle mass, dominantly related to the LV, and only indirectly assisting the RV during systole. However, studies suggest that the septum may function mechanically as if it had independent right and left sides (115, 162, 344). It was observed that, under the experimental condition of acutely increasing RV afterload by embolizing the pulmonary vascular bed, a biochemical indicator of metabolic activity was greatly increased in both the RV free wall and the right side of the septum, but not in either the left side of the septum or the LV free wall (115). If metabolic activity is related to mechanical stress (an assumption on which much of cardiac physiology rests), then the right side of the septum must experience a different stress than the left side. Since the same upstream coronary artery supplies the two sides of the septum, this also implies that downstream local signals can differentially regulate the coronary flow to the two sides of the septum. In the presence of an increased pulmonary vascular resistance that increases substantially with exercise, the ability of the septal RV component to contribute to RV pump performance may be critical to maintaining venous return. If acute overdistention of the RV leads to pericardial constraint limiting coronary flow to the RV free wall (125, 201), it would seem likely that the septal contribution becomes proportionately more important. Under exercise conditions in which substantial increases in pulmonary arterial pressure occur, these factors could come into play.

The Role of the Pericardium and Ventricular Interdependence in Ventilatory Modulation of Ventricular Performance. With the inspiratory increase in RV volume, the LV diastolic pressure must also increase for a constant LV volume (228). This will decrease the gradient for pulmonary venous return to the LV and lead to diminished LV inflow. Thus, ventricular interdependence may influence the back-pressure to RV output. Experimental and clinical studies have shown that an elevated PCWP, reflecting an increased left atrial pressure (Pla), can occur with severe RV afterloading and dilation. This results from the RV occupying an increasing proportion of the total intrapericardial space, the septum is shifted leftward, the LV diastolic pressure increases, and hence its volume is decreased (i.e., LV compliance is decreased) (57, 115, 227). In conditions when pulmonary pressure (Ppa) > Pla > alveolar pressure (Palv) (i.e., pulmonary vascular zone III), Pla is the downstream pressure for flow across the pulmonary vasculature, and thus any increase in Pla due to right heart distention could increase the back-pressure to flow. Application of pressure–flow relationship analysis to a vascular bed allows its characterization with respect to a slope of the relationship that defines an incremental resistance, and a zero-flow intercept that defines a static back-pressure that is independent of flow (175). Therefore, not only LV failure or hypervolemia can produce increases in Pla, but also a respiratory-induced change in right heart volume will change LV compliance and, hence, influence flow characteristics across the pulmonary vascular bed. It has not been defined to what degree ventricular interdependence contributes to elevated pulmonary arterial pressures seen in severe exercise under normal conditions, but it would be increasingly likely with underlying obstructive airway or pulmonary vascular disease processes. Under conditions in which exercise occurs in a hypoxic environment with a degree of baseline hypoxic pulmonary vasoconstriction (e.g., at high altitudes), a close correlation between increases in right and left atrial pressure as workload increases (223) might be expected. This also implies that chronic increases in total heart volume with endurance training must include coordinated increases in pericardial size in order to maintain low atrial filling pressures at baseline and during exercise (see earlier under INTRINSIC PROPERTIES OF THE HEART).

Although the influence of the LV, via ventricular interdependence, on RV systolic performance is rarely considered, experimental studies have uniformly demonstrated that, as the LV enlarges, RV systolic pressure increases (25, 122). The mechanism for this is not well understood. At one extreme, the RV free wall can be replaced by a synthetic noncompliant prosthesis and RV performance maintained if pulmonary vascular resistance is normal, presumptively by transfer of mechanical force across the septum (248). Creation of a prosthetic passive septum results in LV systolic bulging into the RV (264). At the other extreme, the ability of the RV to generate a systolic pressure is compromised substantially by cutting the LV free wall (247). These experiments suggest that optimal LV function is required to maintain RV pump performance in conditions with elevations of pulmonary vascular resistance that might occur with exercise. Decrements in RV performance leading to increases in right atrial pressure will decrease the gradient for venous return, which must be overcome by increases in the upstream driving pressure produced during exercise by the "muscle pump" [see earlier under Evidence that the Muscle Pump is a True (Flow-Generating) Pump].

Effect of Changes in Lung Volume. Changes in lung volume, which by definition mean a change in alveolar pressure relative to intrathoracic pressure, have a variable effect on pulmonary vascular resistance. At minimal lung volume (residual volume), the pulmonary vascular resistance is elevated and falls to a minimum as long volume increases toward functional residual capacity (FRC), then increases as lung volume increases toward total lung capacity [Fig. 15.21; (336)]. Thus, from a normal functional residual capacity (FRC), normal tidal volume inspiration produces minimal increases in afterload/impedance (184, 216). However, large tidal volumes or tidal volumes superimposed on an elevated lung volume produced by airway obstruction (e.g., small airways obstruction in asthma) can significantly increase RV afterload. Thus, a markedly elevated lung volume implies an elevated pulmonary vascular resistance.

In addition, an increase in lung volume can mechanically constrain the heart, analogous to some degree to pericardial constraint. Thus, regardless of whether lung volume increases due to a spontaneous inspiration with an associated decrease in pleural pressure, or due to a positive-pressure inspiration with an associated increase in pleural pressure, the lungs can apply a mechanical force to the cardiac surface. This pressure could, at high lung volumes, substantially affect the gradient for venous return (163, 298, 327). Analogous to pericardial mediated ventricular interdependence, lung constraint of cardiac filling has been termed "heart-lung interdependence." As would be intuitively expected, conditions that lead to increases in cardiac size for the same lung volume will also increase heart-lung interdependence. Marked increases in both cardiac and lung volumes, with constant chest wall mechanical properties, will further enhance this interaction. Exercise normally leads to increases in lung volumes at peak inspiration. However with underlying obstructive disease, exercise leads to increases in lung volumes throughout the respiratory cycle (11, 219); this would tend to limit maximum venous return.

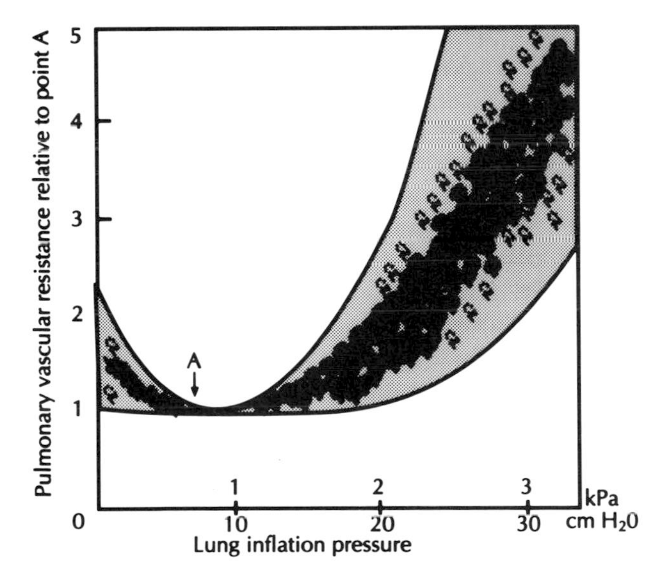

FIG. 15.21. Representation of pooled experimental data on the change in pulmonary vascular resistance with lung inflation in normal lungs. It is evident that pulmonary vascular resistance is minimal at *point A*, which corresponds to functional residual capacity. From that point, with either decreasing or increasing lung inflation, pulmonary vascular resistance increases. (Reprinted with permission from Nunn, J. F. *Applied Respiratory Physiology* London: Butterworth's 1977, p. 259.)

Pulmonary Venous Return

In the steady state, pulmonary venous return is equal to pulmonary arterial (RV) output. Pulmonary arterial and venous vascular volumes will increase as the respective pressure rises, limited only by the upper limits of their distensibility (275). A number of general principles describing the shifts of pulmonary vascular volumes can be derived from studies of changes in lung volume (32, 114, 211). The effect of increasing lung volume has opposite effects on the extra- and intra-alveolar vessels. Extra-alveolar vessels will expand as the lung is inflated, tethered by the surrounding attached pulmonary parenchyma in a process termed "pulmonary vascular interdependence" (275). Inflating the lung enlarges both pulmonary extra-alveolar arteries and veins by creating a negative pressure around the vessel, thus increasing its local transmural pressure (145, 275). Therefore, lung inflation will produce an increased extra-alveolar vascular volume as extra-alveolar arteries and veins expand and take up volume. This would tend to transiently reduce pulmonary venous outflow until a steady state again is reached (32). Conversely, reducing lung volume will diminish extra-alveolar vessel blood volume and tend to produce a transient increase in pulmonary venous outflow. The contribution of changes in lung volume to changes in left heart filling have been investigated in both isolated lungs and in human subjects (32, 101).

However, blood volume in the alveolar vascular bed changes in exactly the opposite direction to the extra-alveolar vessels (32, 211, 275). Enlarging the alveolar gas volume stretches the alveolar capillaries, reducing their capacitance. With a pulmonary valve in place, blood squeezed out of the alveolar bed will move anterograde toward the left heart. Considering the effects of lung inflation of extra-alveolar vessels discussed above and again assuming constant pulmonary artery inflow, the effects of phasic ventilation on pulmonary venous return can be categorized according to the predominant lung zone. In zone III Ppa > Pla > Palv, with high pulmonary vascular pressures expected in vigorous exercise, the extravascular vessels, even during expiration, are near their maximum volume. With lung inflation, the dominant effect is anterograde translocation of the alveolar blood volume displaced by alveolar distention. Whatever volume is not taken up by the extra-alveolar venous bed then exits from the lung. The more congested the alveolar vascular bed and the larger the tidal volume, the greater the volume of blood "ejected" from the lung. In a lung predominantly in zone II (Ppa > Palv > Pla), the alveolar vascular bed is relatively empty during expiration. This zonal state could occur with hypovolemia lowering Pla or with underlying obstructive lung disease and increased respiratory rates during exercise leading to substantial alveolar gas trapping and thus increase in Palv. With a tidal inflation in a zone II lung there is very little blood translocated out of the alveolar bed, while both the pulmonary arterial and venous extra-alveolar vessels will take up volume, dependent on the initial lung volume. Additionally, the inspiratory increase in pulmonary vascular resistance will further reduce flow across the lung. The net result is a diminution in pulmonary venous outflow, depending on the vascular pressures and lung volumes, as opposing events occur in the alveolar and extra-alveolar beds (32). Thus, the mechanical aspects of ventilation during exercise could significantly affect RV performance and venous return.

Extending the above analysis of pulmonary venous return to the intact circulatory systems, two other factors must be considered: *(1)* ventricular interdependence, and *(2)* variable pulmonary arterial inflow. During inspiration, the increase in right heart volume causes, via ventricular interdependence, decreases in LV compliance and, therefore, the downstream pressure for pulmonary venous return is elevated. This will limit increases in LV diastolic filling and hence limit the maximum LV SV as total intrapericardial volume increases and pericardial constraint limits LV filling (see earlier under INTRINSIC PROPERTIES OF THE HEART). Increased pulmonary arterial inflow during inspiration will contribute to increases in both left heart pressures and volumes, and augment LV output (101). The opposite events will occur during expiration. Thus, an increase in systemic venous return will increase RV diastolic volume, tending to reduce pulmonary venous return via pericardial mediated ventricular interdependence, and simultaneously contribute to an increase in pulmonary venous return by augmenting RV output. Limited studies in two human subjects are consistent with studies in dogs, in finding increases in LV SV, cardiac output, or maximum oxygen delivery after pericardiectomy (101, 288).

In summary, pulmonary venous return results from contributions of systemic venous return, RV performance, pulmonary arterial and venous resistances and compliances, lung volume, and ventricular interdependence.

Left Ventricular Output

The prototypical effect of spontaneous respiration on the LV is an inspiratory decrease in LV SV and the associated arterial pressure. Modulation of LV preload during diastole with ventilation may be influenced by ventricular interdependence, pericardial constraint, heart-lung interdependence, and LV contractility. As discussed in the first section of this chapter, modulation of LV systolic performance for a given preload can be altered by changes in afterload and contractility (293). The normal LV is remarkably insensitive to a wide range of acute changes in afterload (38), while the LV end-diastolic volume (preload) is exquisitely sensitive to small changes in pressure. In contrast, the failing LV is insensitive to changes in preload but is sensitive to changes in afterload.

Lowering the intrathoracic pressure around the LV during ventilation is mechanically equivalent to raising the pressure around the extrathoracic vasculature (i.e., an increase in afterload; see Fig. 15.1). The afterload is imposed by the gradient produced between vascular compartments. During expiration, an isolated increase in pleural pressure around the LV effectively decreases the gradient for arterial flow to extrathoracic compartments with constant surrounding pressures. If pleural and abdominal pressures increase equally, as during a Valsalva maneuver, no gradient is produced between the thorax and abdomen, but there is a gradient in surrounding pressures that will enhance blood flow to the head and upper and lower extremities.

The major hypotheses advanced to account for the inspiratory fall in LV SV can be divided into two groups, one ascribing the decrease in LV SV to a diminution in ventricular filling (a diastolic event), the second ascribing the decrease in LV SV to an increase in afterload or a decrease in contractility (systolic events) (229). A primary decrease in LV end-diastolic volume (preload), produces a secondary decrease in the LV end-systolic volume.

While the majority of studies lead to the conclusion that a diminished LV preload is the cause of the inspiratory fall in LV SV, other factors are clearly present. Increases in either the RV volume (ventricular interdependence) or lung volume (heart-lung interdependence) constraining LV filling are commonly believed to contribute to the inspiratory decrease in LV preload (30, 101, 124, 221, 227, 327). Either an increase in afterload and/or a decrease in contractility could explain increases in LV end-systolic and, secondarily, end-diastolic volumes when stroke volume diminishes (37, 42, 132, 291). The cardiac cycle can be divided into a diastolic period (ventricular filling altering preload) and a systolic period (ventricular ejection altered by afterload and contractility). Since respiration affects ventricular performance, it must affect some or all parts of a cardiac cycle. If ventilation influences only diastole, it could increase or decrease ventricular filling. Assuming a constant preload, if ventilation influenced only systole, the resultant stroke volume could increase, decrease, or be unchanged, depending on the relative changes in LV afterload and/or contractility.

Efforts to separate the potential diastolic and systolic influences of respiration on cardiac diastolic and systolic performance required studies in anesthetized dogs using acutely implanted electromagnetic flow probes seated over the mitral valve and on the ascending aorta. Comparison of changes in the integrated mitral and ascending aortic blood flows allows assessment of LV inflow and outflow, independent of any assumptions about LV shape. Clear respiratory variation was evident in both mitral and ascending aortic integrated flows [Fig. 15.22; (232, 233)]. Consistent with a role for ventricular interdependence mediating this relationship, removal of the pericardium markedly attenuated the decrease in mitral flow (232), consistent with the findings by Guz et al. in human subjects (101).

The use of brief periods of ECG-triggered bilateral phrenic nerve stimulation gated to the cardiac cycle allows precise control of intrathoracic pressure within specific periods of a cardiac cycle, with rapid decreases of 15–25 mm Hg in intrathoracic pressure confined to either systole or diastole. This approach permits definition of separate diastolic and systolic events during respiration, since the influence of the RV output in series with the LV is eliminated (213).

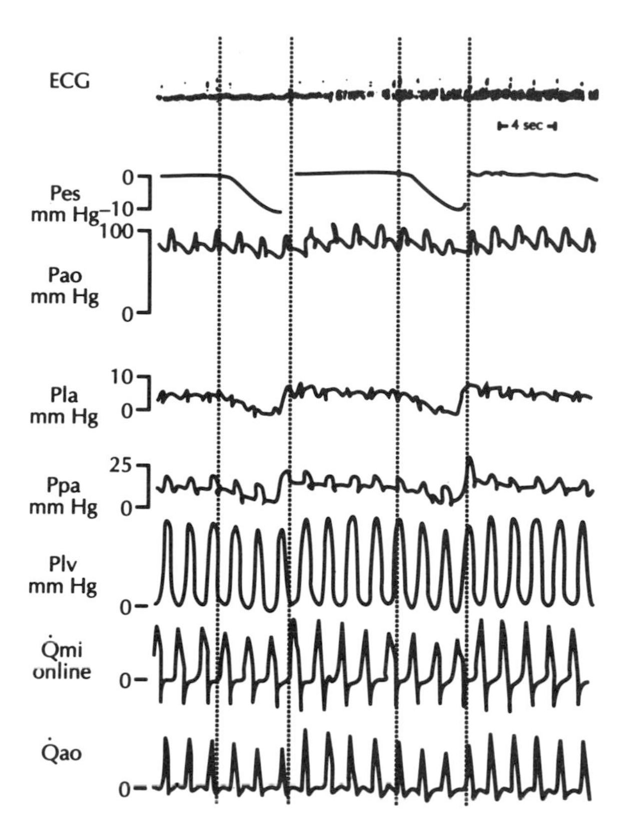

FIG. 15.22. Two consecutive respiratory cycles during partial inspiratory airway obstruction in an anesthetized dog postvagotomy. *Vertical dashed lines* indicate the two periods during which esophageal pressure (Pes) is reduced during inspiration. Both integrated mitral (Q̇mi) and ascending aortic (Q̇ao) flows diminish during inspiration and increase with expiration. There is a large expiratory increase in mitral flow preceding the large increase in aortic flow in both respiratory cycles. Although the rapid increase in esophageal pressure occurs during systole in the second breath, there is little effect on aortic flow. These two respiratory cycles demonstrate the dominance of mitral flow leading aortic flow during partial inspiratory obstruction. Pes, esophageal pressure; Pao, aortic pressure; Pla, left atrial pressure; Ppa, pulmonary artery pressure; Plv, left ventricular pressure. (Reprinted with permission from Robotham, J. L., R. S. Stuart, K. Doherty, M. A. Borkon, and W. Baumgartner. Mitral and aortic flows during spontaneous respiration in dogs. *Anesthesiology* 69: 516–526, 1988.)

Figure 15.23 demonstrates the influence of a phrenic nerve stimulation confined to diastole. When the fall in intrathoracic pressure is confined to diastole, there is a substantial decrease in both the peak mitral flow and the integrated area under the mitral flow tracing, reflecting a decrease in LV filling

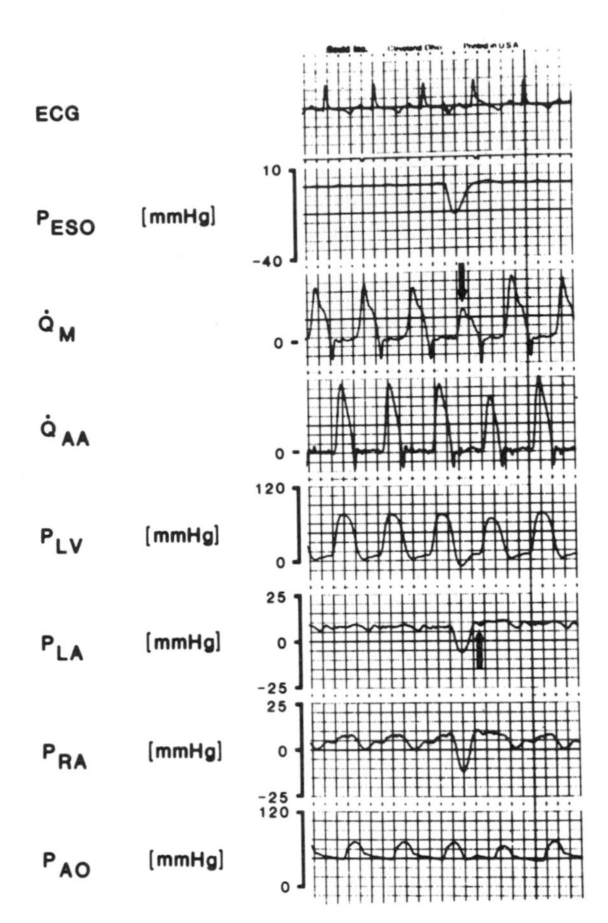

FIG. 15.23. Diastolic phrenic nerve stimulation producing a transient decrease in esophageal pressure (P_{ESO}) confined to diastole in an acutely instrumented anesthetized dog during phrenic nerve stimulation. Steady-state mitral ($\dot{Q}_M$) and ascending aortic ($\dot{Q}_{AA}$) flows are observed prior to the transient fall in intrathoracic pressure. There is an immediate substantial decrease in peak and total mitral flow indicated by a *vertical arrow* pointing down. The subsequent LV stroke volume is similarly reduced at a time when intrathoracic pressure has returned to its baseline value such that there could be no effect on LV ejection. The subsequent mitral flow and LV stroke volume demonstrates compensatory increases. Of critical importance, LV end-diastolic pressure (P_{LV}), left atrial pressure (P_{LA}) (at *upward pointed vertical arrow*), and right atrial pressure (P_{RA}) are all increased relative to atmospheric pressure at end-diastole when esophageal pressure has returned to baseline values. Since LV inflow has diminished, LV end-diastolic volume is reduced and its pressure increased; thus, LV effective compliance must be reduced. The increase in right atrial pressure and pattern of change of mitral flow are consistent with ventricular interdependence being responsible for the reduction in LV preload. P_{AO}, aortic pressure. (Reprinted with permission from Robotham, J. L., and J. Peters. Cardiorespiratory interactions. In: *Adult Respiratory Distress Syndrome*, edited by W. Zapol. New York: Marcel Dekker, Inc., 1991, p. 223–251.)

(213). The subsequent LV SV as defined by the area under the ascending aortic flow for the subsequent systole when esophageal pressure has returned to baseline is reduced, as would be expected from Starling's law with a diminished preload. With esophageal pressure remaining at baseline conditions, the subsequent diastolic and systolic periods demonstrate an increase in both the peak and the integrated mitral and aortic flows consistent with the blood volume dammed up in the pulmonary bed during the transient fall in intrathoracic pressure and then augmenting LV filling. When esophageal pressure had returned to baseline at the end of the diastolic period with phrenic nerve stimulation, both atrial pressures relative to atmosphere were elevated compared to their previous values during apnea, as was the LV end-diastolic pressure. The right atrial pressure, both absolute and transmural (relative to esophageal pressure), is elevated due to its increased volume, while both the absolute and transmural left-sided pressures are increased consistent with a diminished LV end-diastolic volume due to a decreased compliance. With an increase in lung volume occurring during the fall in intrathoracic pressure, either ventricular (25) and/or heart-lung interdependence (325) could account for these findings, both events being compatible with the observed increase in right atrial pressure. The dominant mechanism appears to be ventricular interdependence based on the following observations. First when lung volume is maintained constant, the same basic findings are observed in this experimental preparation (213). Second, in human subjects, the decrease in LV SV observed during a completely obstructed inspiratory effort with no change in lung volume is only slightly less than the decrease in LV SV during an unobstructed inspiration with a similar change in intrathoracic pressure in which lung volume increases (101). Third, changes in LV geometry in chronically instrumented dogs during an increase in lung volume suggest lateral compression of the heart consistent with heart-lung interdependence playing a role in diminishing LV compliance (227). However, the dominant role of ventricular interdependence in reducing LV compliance as the RV volume rapidly increases during the inspiratory fall in intrathoracic pressure seems clear. The increased right heart volume decreases left heart compliance, thus reducing mitral inflow and the subsequent LV SV. Consistent with this, the LV septal–to–free lateral wall dimension decreases during a transient diastolic negative intrathoracic pressure (230).

The influence of a fall in intrathoracic pressure confined to systole is illustrated in Figure 15.24. There is an immediate decrease in the peak and total

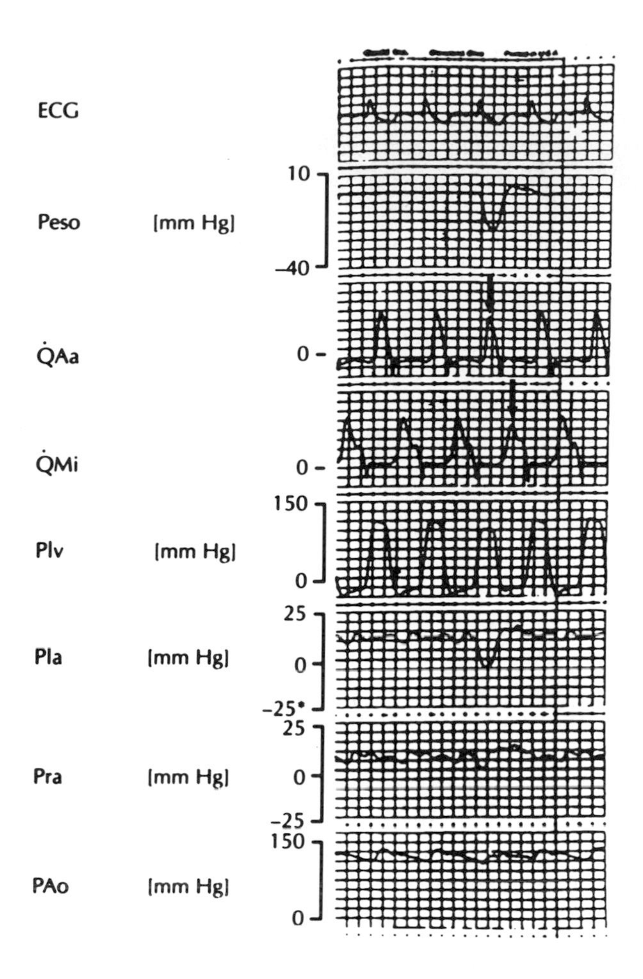

FIG. 15.24. Original recording with negative intrathoracic pressure confined to systole and the airway unobstructed, allowing lung volume to increase during phrenic nerve stimulation. The decrease in esophageal pressure (Peso) begins during isovolumic contraction (i.e., after diastolic mitral flow (Q̇Mi) has stopped) and is associated with a fall in ascending aortic flow (Q̇Aa) and LV stroke volume (integrated (Q̇Aa) indicated by the *downward pointing arrow*. An unchanged LV preload before the systolic negative intrathoracic pressure is indicated by constant (Q̇Mi, end-diastolic left ventricular (Plv) and atrial (Pla) pressures in the immediately preceding beats. In the diastolic period following the systolic fall in intrathoracic pressure, mitral inflow is decreased as indicated by the *downward pointing arrow* consistent with the increased end-systolic volume. Thus, a fall in intrathoracic pressure during systole alone is sufficient to decrease LV stroke volume. P_{AO}, aortic pressure; P_{RA}, right artrial pressure. [Reprinted with permission from Peters, J., C. Fraser, R. S. Stuart, W. Baumgartner, and J. L. Robotham. Negative intrathoracic pressure decreases independently left ventricular filling and emptying. *Am. J. Physiol.* 257 (*Heart Circ. Physiol.* 26): H120–H131, 1989.]

integrated ascending aortic flow. The subsequent mitral flow was decreased, consistent with the presence of an acute increase in the LV end-systolic volume. The fall in LV SV during systolic phrenic nerve stimulation proves that a separate systolic mechanism contributes to the inspiratory fall in LV SV. This means either an acute decrease in contractility or increase in afterload. To address this issue, intrathoracic aortic dimensions were measured to "transduce" the true aortic transmural pressure during systolic phrenic nerve stimulation. The sonomicrometer crystals sutured to the aortic adventitia provide a direct measure of aortic size, and assuming the smooth muscle of the aortic wall does not change its tone during systole, the aortic cross-sectional area must be directly proportional to the local aortic transmural pressure. If a primary decrease in contractility accounts for the fall in LV SV, then with less LV output, the peak systolic aortic volume should decrease. Figure 15.25 illustrates that with a transient fall in intrathoracic pressure confined to systole, the intrathoracic aortic dimensions increase as the LV SV diminishes. This is consistent with an effective increase in afterload imposed where the aorta leaves the intrathoracic compartment (214); that is, the same findings would be expected if an afterload were imposed on the LV with the intrathoracic pressure remaining constant and the pressure surrounding the extrathoracic abdominal aorta, cranial, and upper extremity arterial beds increased. In both cases, LV SV will decrease and intrathoracic aortic volume will increase.

In summary, as negative intrathoracic pressure continues for longer than one cardiac cycle: *(1)* the increased systemic venous return will lead to a gradual increase in LV SV volume despite an increase in LV afterload; *(2)* the increased afterload will tend to preserve the end-diastolic volume by increasing the end-systolic volume; and *(3)* increased, decreased, or zero net change in LV volumes can occur during a fall in intrathoracic pressure. Thus, it is not surprising that conflicting and confusing results exist among studies. The opposite effects are produced by an increase in pleural pressure, effectively reducing LV afterload, increasing LV SV, and decreasing aortic transmural pressure. Steady-state increases in intrathoracic pressure decrease venous return as expected under normal physiologic conditions, but may increase cardiac output in the presence of LV dysfunction (91, 169). The functional status of the heart and peripheral vascular system will define how ventilatory mechanical forces affect the integrated cardiovascular system.

Implications of Ventilatory Stresses during Exercise

The major changes in respiratory mechanics that might be expected to affect cardiovascular function during exercise, compared to the resting state, would

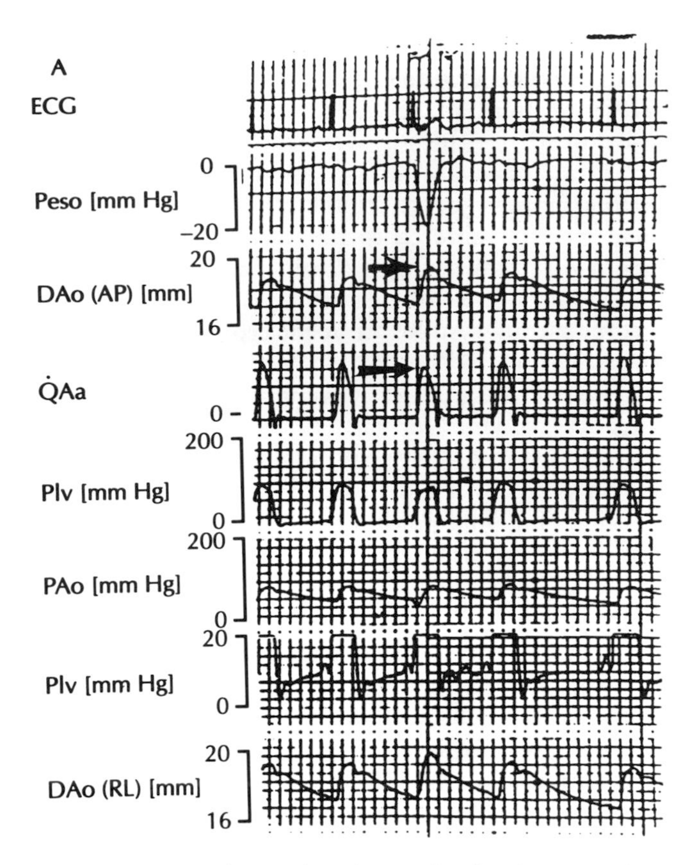

FIG. 15.25. Recording with early systolic phrenic nerve stimulation (PNS) and the airway obstructed to keep lung volume constant in an anesthetized dog. The decrease of esophageal pressure (Peso) causes an increase in the systolic anteroposterior intrathoracic aortic diameter [DAo(AP)], indicated by the *horizontal arrow*, but a fall in left ventricular stroke volume derived from the ascending aortic blood flow ($\dot{Q}$Aa), indicated by the *lower horizontal arrow*. Both systolic left ventricular (Plv) and aortic pressures (PAo) fall relative to atmospheric pressure. Neither the LV end-diastolic pressure (recorded with a fluid-filled catheter) immediately before phrenic nerve stimulation nor the R-R interval change compared with the preceding cardiac cycle. Congruent with the increase in systolic DAo(AP), right-to-left aortic diameter [DAo(RL)] also increases. The decrease in LV stroke volume associated with increased DAo is compatible with an increased LV afterload. The same qualitative changes are observed when lung volume is allowed to increase with the fall in esophageal pressure, such that a decrease of intrathoracic pressure alone, with or without a change in lung volume, is sufficient to explain the fall in ($\dot{Q}$Aa) and LV stroke volume and the increase in DAo. (Reprinted with permission from Peters, J., M. K. Kindred, and J. L. Robotham. Transient analysis of cardiopulmonary interactions. II. Systolic events. *J. Appl. Physiol.* 64: 1518–1526, 1988.)

be increases in respiratory rate, pleural and abdominal pressure swings, and increases in lung volumes and minute ventilation. End-expiratory lung volume (EELV) first decreases, and then returns toward resting functional residual capacity (FRC) as the workload increases. Inspiratory tidal volume increases such that end-inspiratory capacity approaches 80% of total lung capacity. In the presence of obstructive lung disease, EELV does not decrease, but increases above an already elevated baseline FRC such that end-inspiratory lung volume (EILV) approaches 90% of TLC. These changes in lung volumes affect respiratory muscle function, recruitment, and the inspiratory and expiratory pressures generated in the thoracic and abdominal compartments (11, 43, 49, 50, 127–129, 219).

In absolute terms, the peak inspiratory pressure observed in the thoracic and abdominal compartments is approximately −25 mm Hg, or 25%–30% of the maximum negative pressures voluntarily produced during inspiration from a low lung volume, and approximately 10–30 mm Hg during expiration at a high lung volume (40). Abdominal pressure, which rises during inspiration as the diaphragm descends, also exhibits a late expiratory increase in normal subjects with inspiratory resistive loading (220) and in patients with chronic obstructive disease (60) during exercise. Presumptively, an increase in abdominal pressure will affect both diaphragmatic and lower chest wall configuration. The result is that changes in intrathoracic and abdominal pressures are not simply 180 degrees out of phase, but will exhibit phasic relationships that will vary not only with the work rate but also with baseline respiratory state. Thus, the net effect of ventilation on cardiac function will vary as these variables change.

The distribution of time spent in inspiration as a fraction of the total respiratory cycle time (Ti/Ttot) is reported to be quite stable in both humans and animals with increasing work rates, averaging 0.4 for normal subjects and 0.5 for subjects with COPD (49, 126, 128, 220). Thus, although the mean pleural pressure changes very little in absolute terms, the number of respiratory cycles and the amplitude of the variance around the mean increases markedly. Precisely how the phasic changes around a relatively constant mean in ventilation-induced mechanical forces can produce alterations in cardiovascular performance by differentially affecting different portions of the cardiac cycles is intriguing but not well understood. Figures 15.23 and 15.24 demonstrate that these phasic relationships between respiratory cycle–induced changes in intrathoracic pressure and cardiac cycle–induced changes in LV elastance (i.e., systole vs. diastole) may have profoundly different effects on LV volumes. A cyclical force applied that produces only increased oscillation around the same mean should not be expected to alter cardiovascular function. However, if the applied force results in blood volume displacement in one direction only (e.g., the presence of a one-way valve, or marked differences in anterograde vs. retrograde time constants), then the oscillation may act effectively as a unidirectional pump. Studies in running dogs suggest that regional differences in chest wall forces during running will act to improve ventilation to these lung regions, as if there were a regional pump in addition to respiratory muscle activity (5, 26). It seems likely that these regional mechanical forces may contribute to augment both ventilation and perfusion.

Recently, it has been recognized that ventilation-induced changes in abdominal pressure affect venous return to a substantial degree, in some cases to a greater degree than the simultaneous changes in intrathoracic pressure (142). There is little question that mean abdominal pressure increases during exercise, which, depending on the zone condition, will augment or decrease venous return from the infradiaphragmatic compartments. However, regardless of the effect on venous return, an increase in abdominal pressure relative to pleural pressure will effectively increase the afterload on the LV (234). To the extent that abdominal pressure increases relative to the surrounding pressure of the arterial compartments of the upper body, blood flow will be redistributed to the upper body (Fig. 15.26). This can result in increased flow to arms and head despite a net decrease in total cardiac output (i.e., in the extreme, analogous to cross-clamping the aorta at the level of the diaphragm). The implications of ventilation-induced abdominal pressure changes on distribution of arterial blood flow to the legs during running have not been explored to our knowledge, in contrast to the well-recognized increase in venous flow with exercise due to the muscle pump (see earlier under Distribution of Blood Flow). The marked reduction in arterial resistance in the leg or arm muscles with exercise leads to markedly increased flow (35, 172, 324). If increases in abdominal pressure are minimal or similar to increases in intrathoracic pressure, then combined with increased sympathetic outflow reducing flow to the intra-abdominal organs (see Chapter 17), arterial flow to the limbs would be facilitated. Since venous return increases, it would seem reasonable to assume that the exercising "muscle pump" more than compensates for the increased abdominal/thoracic back pressures to venous return.

Compared to the unconditioned subject, in highly conditioned athletes and subjects with baseline right or left ventricular dysfunction, ventilatory stresses would be expected to produce very different effects during exercise-imposed increases in workload. Under normal baseline conditions, the elastance of the pericardium is the dominant factor defining effective atrial compliance (272, 273, 313) and, as such, the downstream pressure for venous return. As discussed in the first section of this chapter, endurance-

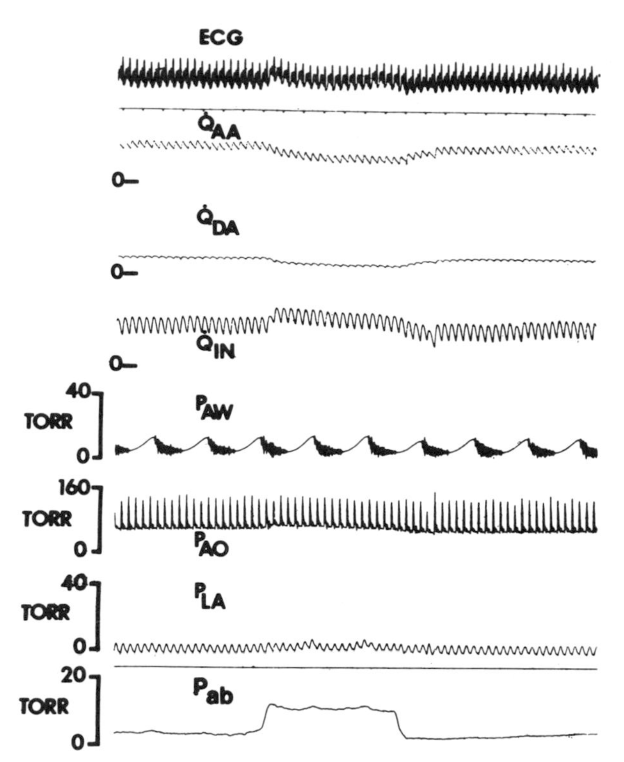

FIG. 15.26. Tracings recorded in one dog during an increase in abdominal pressure (P_{ab}) followed by maintenance of a quasi-steady state and the acute release of abdominal compression. There were no arrhythmias in the ECG. Mean flow in both the ascending aorta ($\dot{Q}_{AA}$) and descending aorta ($\dot{Q}_{DA}$) decreased while flow in the innominate artery ($\dot{Q}_{IN}$) increased. Airway pressure (P_{AW}) measured at the trachea demonstrated a small peak inspiratory increase during abdominal compression. The expiratory airway pressure reflected transmission of 2 cm H_2O of positive end-expiratory pressure. The aortic pressure (P_{AO}) and left atrial pressure (P_{LA}) both increased as P_{ab} increased. (Reprinted with permission from: Robotham, J. L., R. A. Wise, and B. Bromberger-Barnea. Effects of changes in abdominal pressure on left ventricular performance and regional blood flow. Crit. Care Med. 13: 803–809, 1985.)

trained athletes exhibit slow heart rates and develop enlarged hearts without evidence of pathologic wall hypertrophy found with chronic increases in afterload (e.g., hypertension). In contrast, athletes performing brief, highly strenuous exercise (e.g., weight lifters) may exhibit an upper limit of normal left ventricular wall thickness, if not pathologic hypertrophy. It seems reasonable to assume the two different responses reflect differences in the loading conditions, the endurance training requiring maximal venous return/cardiac output over an extended time, the weight lifter a transient ability to respond to a transient acute increase in afterload.

The enlarged heart of the endurance athlete presumably leads to parallel chronic distention and growth of the pericardium, resulting in a downshift of the pericardial pressure–volume relationship (lower pressure for the same or higher volume). Freeman and LeWinter observed that the pericardium adapts to chronic changes in cardiac volumes by reestablishing a pressure–volume relationship (79) that maintains its normal stress–strain relationship and hence a normal back-pressure for venous return. This is clearly true during normal growth and development, since the same absolute right and left atrial pressures exist throughout most of postnatal life despite the increase in cardiac size. The signal transduction pathways that lead to cardiac dilation without muscle hypertrophy and parallel growth in the pericardium during endurance training offer an attractive method to permit maximal venous return by "removing" the pericardial constraint in that range of cardiac volumes, keeping atrial pressures low (see earlier under INTRINSIC PROPERTIES OF THE HEART). It also maintains the inherent safety factor of the pericardium in limiting acute increases in cardiac volumes above the established baseline. For a weight lifter, thickened ventricular walls will limit ventricular interdependence, increase ventricular power, and, combined with the pericardial elastance, limit acute overdistention of the heart. During the brief 3–4 s Valsalva maneuver (forced expiratory effort against a closed glottis) during a lift, there should be a sufficient blood volume in the thorax plus venous return from the abdomen (as no gradient is established between the thorax and abdomen, assuming equal changes in pressure) to maintain LV output and perfusion to the heart and brain. The Valsalva maneuver effectively reduces the afterload (supported by any pericardial elastance) imposed by the massive contraction of the extrathoracic/extra-abdominal musculature that can raise systemic arterial pressures to 350/180 (159). The importance of the pericardium in limiting cardiac overdistention with massive acute pulmonary (88) or systemic hypertension (144), and the Valsalva maneuver reducing the increased load on the LV (80, 152) while simultaneously increasing flow to the limbs and head, has not been adequately evaluated. The reported dizziness of weight lifters immediately after a lift is consistent with emptying of the abdominal venous capacitance beds which, following the Valsalva maneuver, then fill before contributing to venous return. Since more than half of all venous return passes through the abdominal veins (and more during exercise using predominantly the lower limbs), a Valsalva maneuver will decrease venous return depending in large part on the ratio of increase in pleural pressure relative to the increase in abdominal pressure. As described earlier, if both pleural and abdominal pressures were to increase equally with a Valsalva maneuver, there would be no change in the gradient for either venous return between the abdominal and thoracic compartment or change in gradient for arterial flow between the two compartments. However, venous return from the legs to the abdomen would be diminished (300, 337) and arterial inflow to the legs enhanced. Similarly, the venous return from the arms and head would be diminished but arterial inflow enhanced as long as the LV had sufficient venous return to maintain its preload.

The type of exercise and the body position would also be predicted to affect the interactions between respiratory mechanics and the cardiovascular system. For example, the horizontal position will increase blood volume in the thoracic compartment compared to the vertical head-up position at rest. Reflex changes in peripheral vascular resistances and capacitances can, in theory, rapidly readjust these differences to provide adequate venous return to meet the cardiac output demands (see Chapter 17). The contribution of the rib cage and abdominal muscles to maintaining body position or their involvement in voluntary exercise (e.g., accessory neck muscle and upper rib cage muscles during arm exercise) requires that other respiratory muscles (e.g., the diaphragm and abdominal muscles) must make up the difference to maintain appropriate minute ventilation (43, 50). This implies that the distribution and quantity of respiratory-related forces imposed on the circulatory system may vary considerably depending on specific characteristics of the exercise (e.g., swimming, bicycling, running, rowing).

Thus, mechanical ventilatory stresses will interact with cardiovascular events during exercise to modulate both venous return and arterial flow. It is likely that the pericardium may play a major role in this process and that the underlying status of the cardiovascular system will determine both the quantitative and qualitative effects produced.

REFERENCES

1. Abel, R. S., and R. L. Reis. Effects of coronary blood flow and perfusion on left ventricular contractility in dogs. *Circ. Res.* 27: 961–971, 1970.
2. Adams, F. K., Jr., S. M. McAllister, H. El-Ashmawy, S. Atkinson, G. Koch, and D. S. Sheps. Interrelationships between left ventricular volume and output during exercise in healthy subjects. *J. Appl. Physiol.* 73: 2097–2104, 1992.
3. Ahmad, M., and J. P. Dubiel. Left ventricular response to exercise in regular runners and controls. *Clin. Nucl. Med.* 15: 630–635, 1990.
4. Alexander, R. S. Influence of the diaphragm upon portal blood flow and venous return. *Am. J. Physiol.* 167: 738–748, 1951.
5. Alexander, R. M. Breathing while trotting. *Science* 262: 196–197, 1993.

6. Almen, T., and G. Nylander. Serial phlebography of the normal lower leg during muscular contraction and relaxation. *Acta Radiol. (Stockh.)* 57: 264–272, 1962.
7. Anversa, P., E. Puntillo, P. Nikitin, G. Olivetti, J. M. Capasso, and E. H. Sonnenblick. Effects of age on mechanical and structural properties of myocardium of Fischer 344 rats. *Am. J. Physiol.* 256 (*Heart Circ. Physiol.* 25): H1440–H1449, 1989.
8. Askar, E. Effects of bilateral splanchnicectomy on circulation during exercise in dogs. *Acta Physiol. Lat. Am.* 23: 171–177, 1973.
9. Asmussen, E., K. Fruensgaard, and S. Norgaard. A follow-up study of selected physiological functions in former physical education students after forty years. *J. Am. Geriatr. Soc.* 23: 442–450, 1975.
10. Åstrand, P. O., T. E. Cuddy, B. Saltin, and J. Stenberg. Cardiac output during submaximal and maximal work. *J. Am. Physiol.* 19: 268–274, 1964.
11. Babb, T. G., R. Viggiano, B. Hurley, B. Staats, and J. R. Rodarte. Effect of mild-to-moderate airflow limitation on exercise capacity. *J. Appl. Physiol.* 70: 223–230, 1991.
12. Bader, H. The anatomy and physiology of the vascular wall. In: *Handbook of Physiology, Circulation*, edited by W. F. Hamilton and P. Dow. Washington, DC: Am. Physiol. Soc., 1963, p. 865–889.
13. Barcroft, H., and A. C. Dornhorst. Demonstration of the "muscle pump" in the human leg. *J. Physiol. (Lond.)* 108: 39P, 1949.
14. Barcroft, H., and A. Samaan. Explanation of the increase in systemic flow caused by occluding the descending thoracic aorta. *J. Physiol. (Lond.)* 85: 47–61, 1935.
15. Barendsen, G. J., and J. W. van den Berg. Venous capacity, venous refill time and the effectiveness of the calf muscle pump in normal subjects. *Angiology* 35: 163–172, 1984.
16. Ben-Ari, E., R. Gentile, H. Feigenbaum, D. Hess, E. Z. Fisman, A. Pines, Y. Drory, and M. Motro. Left ventricular dynamics during strenuous isometric exercise in marathon runners, weight lifters and healthy sedentary men: comparative echocardiographic study *Cardiology* 82: 75–80, 1993.
17. Bennett, T. D., C. R. Wyss, and A. M. Scher. Changes in vascular capacity in awake dogs in response to carotid sinus occlusion and administration of catecholamines. *Circ. Res.* 55: 440–453, 1984.
18. Bergovec, M., M. Zigman, H. Prpic, S. Mihatov, and D. Vukosavic. Global and regional parameters of left ventricular performance in healthy subjects during rest and exercise assessed by radionuclide ventriculography. *Int. J. Card. Imaging* 9: 39–48, 1993.
19. Bevegård, S., B. Jonsson, and I. Karlof. Circulatory responses to recumbent exercise and head-up tilting in patients with disturbed sympathetic cardiovascular control (postural hypotension). *Acta Med. Scand.* 172: 623–636, 1962.
20. Bevegård, S., B. Jonsson, I. Karlof, H. Lagergren, and E. Sowton. Effect of changes in ventricular rate on cardiac output and central venous pressures at rest and during exercise in patients with artificial pacemakers. *Cardiovasc. Res.* 1: 21–33, 1967.
21. Bevegård, S., and A. Lodin. Postural circulatory changes at rest and during exercise in five patients with congenital absence of valves in the deep veins of the legs. *Acta Med. Scand.* 172: 21–29, 1962.
22. Blomqvist, C. G., S. F. Lewis, W. F. Taylor, and R. M. Graham. Similarity of the hemodynamic responses to static and dynamic exercise of small muscle groups. *Circ. Res.* 48: I87–I92, 1981.
23. Blomqvist, C. G., and B. Saltin. Cardiovascular adaptations to physical training. *Annu. Rev. Physiol.* 45: 169–189, 1983.
24. Boltwood, C. M., A. Skulsky, D. C Drinkwater, S. Lang, D. G. Mulder, and P. M. Shah. Intraoperative measurement of pericardial constraint: role in ventricular diastolic mechanics. *J. Am. Coll. Cardiol.* 8: 1289–1297, 1986.
25. Bove, A. A., and W. P. Santamore. Ventricular interdependence. *Prog. Cardiovasc. Dis.* 23: 365–388, 1981.
26. Bramble, D. M., and F. A. Jenkins, Jr. Mammalian locomotor-respiratory integration: implications for diaphragmatic and pulmonary design. *Science* 262: 235–240, 1993.
27. Brandao, M. U. P., M. Wajngarten, E. Rondon, M. C. P. Giorgi, F. Hironaka, and C. E. Negrao. Left ventricular function during dynamic exercise in untrained and moderately trained subjects. *J. Appl. Physiol.* 75: 1989–1995, 1993.
28. Braunwald, E., R. L. Frye, and J. Ross, Jr. Studies on Starling's law of the heart. Determinants of the relationship between left ventricular end-diastolic pressure and circumference. *Circ. Res.* 34: 498–504, 1960.
29. Brecher, G. A., and C. A. Hubay. Pulmonary blood flow and venous return during spontaneous respiration. *Circ. Res.* 3: 210–214, 1965.
30. Brinker, J. A., J. L. Weiss, D. L. Lappe, J. L. Rabson, W. R. Summer, S. Permutt, and M. L. Weisfeldt. Leftward septal displacement during right ventricular loading in man. *Circulation* 61: 626–633, 1980.
31. Brooksby, G. A., and D. E. Donald. Release of blood from the splanchnic circulation in dogs. *Circ. Res.* 31: 105–118, 1972.
32. Brower, R., R. A. Wise, C. Hassapoyannes, B. Bromberger-Barnea, and S. Permutt. Effect of lung inflation on lung blood volume and pulmonary venous flow. *J. Appl. Physiol.* 58: 954–963, 1985.
33. Brunner, M. J., A. S. Greene, A. E. Frankle, and A. A. Shoukas. Carotid sinus baroreceptor control of splanchnic resistance and capacity. *Am. J. Physiol.* 255 (*Heart Circ. Physiol.* 24): H1305–H1310, 1988.
34. Brunner, M. J., A. A. Shoukas, and C. L. MacAnespie. The effect of the carotid sinus baroreceptor reflex on blood flow and volume redistribution in the total systemic vascular bed of the dog. *Circ. Res.* 48: 74–285, 1981.
35. Bryan, G., A. Ward, and J. M. Rippe. Athletic heart syndrome. *Clin. Sports Med.* 11: 259–272, 1992.
36. Buck, J. A., L. R. Amundsen, and D. H. Nielsen. Systolic blood pressure responses during isometric contractions of large and small muscle groups. *Med. Sci. Sports Exerc.* 12: 145–147, 1980.
37. Buda, A. J., M. R. Pinsky, and N. B. Ingels, Jr. Effect of intrathoracic pressure on left ventricular performance. *N. Engl. J. Med.* 301: 453–459, 1979.
38. Bugge-Asperheim, B., and F. Kiil. Cardiac response to increased aortic pressure. Changes in output and left ventricular pressure pattern at various levels of inotropy. *Scand. J. Clin. Lab. Invest.* 24: 345–360, 1969.
39. Burkhoff, D., S. Sugiura, D. T. Yue, and K. Sagawa. Contractility-dependent curvilinearity of end-systolic pressure-volume relations. *Am. J. Physiol.* 252 (*Heart Circ. Physiol.* 21): H1218–H1227, 1987.
40. Bye, P. T. P., S. A. Esau, K. R. Walley, P. T. Macklem, and R. L. Pardy. Ventilatory muscles during exercise in air and oxygen in normal men. *J. Appl. Physiol. Respir. Environ. Exerc. Physiol.* 56: 464–471, 1984.

41. Caldini, P., S. Permutt, J. A. Waddell, and R. Riley. Effects of epinephrine on pressure, flow, and volume relationships in the systemic circulation of dogs. *Circ. Res.* 34: 606–623, 1974.
42. Cassidy, S. S. Stimulus-response curves of the lung inflation cardio-depressor reflex. *Respir. Physiol.* 57: 259–268, 1984.
43. Celli, B., G. Criner, and J. Rassulo. Ventilatory muscle recruitment during unsupported arm exercise in normal subjects. *J. Appl. Physiol.* 64: 1936–1941, 1988.
44. Cerretelli, P., J. Piiper, F. Mangili, F. Cuttica, and B. Ricci. Circulation in exercising dogs. *J. Appl. Physiol.* 19: 29–32, 1964.
45. Chihara, E., T. Morimoto, K. Shigemi, T. Natsuyama, and S. Hashimoto. Vascular viscoelasticity of perfused rat hindquarters. *Am. J. Physiol.* 260 (*Heart Circ. Physiol.* 29): H1834–H1840, 1991.
46. Clausell, N., E. Ludwig, F. Narro, and J. P. Ribeiro. Response of left ventricular diastolic filling to graded exercise relative to the lactate threshold. *Eur. J. Appl. Physiol.* 67: 222–225, 1993.
47. Crawford, M. H. Physiologic consequences of systematic training. *Cardiol. Clin.* 10: 209–218, 1992.
48. Crawford, M. H., M. A. Petru, and C. Rabinowitz. Effect of isotonic exercise training on left ventricular volume during upright exercise. *Circulation* 72: 1237–1243, 1985.
49. Criner, G. J., and B. R. Celli. Ventilatory muscle recruitment in exercise with O_2 in obstructed patients with mild hypoxemia. *J. Appl. Physiol.* 63: 195–200, 1987.
50. Criner, G. J., and B. R. Celli. Effect of unsupported arm exercise on ventilatory muscle recruitment in patients with severe chronic airflow obstruction. *Am. Rev. Respir. Dis.* 138: 856–861, 1988.
51. Crouse, S. F., J. J. Rohack, and D. J. Jacobsen. Cardiac structure and function in women basketball athletes: seasonal variation and comparisons with nonathletic controls. *Res. Q. Exerc. Sport* 63: 393–401, 1992.
52. Cruz, J. C., P. Cerretelli, and L. E. Farhi. Role of ventilation in maintaining cardiac output under positive pressure breathing. *J. Appl. Physiol.* 22: 900–904, 1967.
53. Dart, A. M., I. T. Meredith, and G. L. Jennings. Effect of 4 weeks endurance training on cardiac left ventricular structure and function. *Clin. Exp. Pharmacol. Physiol.* 19: 777–783, 1992.
54. Decramer, M., A. DeTroyer, A. Kelly, L. Zocchi, and P. T. Macklem. Regional differences in abdominal pressure swings in dogs. *J. Appl. Physiol.* 57: 1682–1687, 1984.
55. Deschamps, A., and S. Magder. Baroreflex control of regional capacitance and blood flow distribution with or without α-adrenergic blockade. *Am. J. Physiol.* 263 (*Heart Circ. Physiol.* 32): H1755–H1763, 1992.
56. DeTroyer, A., M. Sampson, S. Sigrist, and P. T. Macklem. Diaphragm: two muscles. *Science* 213: 237–238, 1981.
57. Dhainaut, J. F., J. Y. Devaux, J. F. Monsallier, F. Brunet, D. Villemant, and M. F. Huyghebaert. Mechanisms of decreased left ventricular preload during continuous positive pressure ventilation in ARDS. *Chest* 90: 74–80, 1986.
58. Diamant, M., J. L. Benumof, and L. J. Saidman. Hemodynamics of increased intra-abdominal pressure: interaction with hypovolemia and halothane anesthesia. *Anesthesiology* 48: 23–27, 1978
59. Diana, J. N., and C. A. Shadur. Effect of arterial and venous pressure on capillary pressure and vascular volume. *Am. J. Physiol.* 225: 637–650, 1973.
60. Dodd, D. S., T. Brancatisano, and L. A. Engel. Chest wall mechanics during exercise in patients with severe chronic air-flow obstruction. *Am. Rev. Respir. Dis.* 129: 33–38, 1984.
61. Doppman, J. R., R. M. Robinson, S. D. Rockoff, J. S. Vasko, R. Shapiro, and A. G. Morrow. Mechanism of obstruction on the infradiaphragmatic portion of the inferior vena cava in the presence of increased intra-abdominal pressure. *Invest. Radiol.* I: 37–53, 1986.
62. Douglas, P. S., and B. Tallant. Hypertrophy, fibrosis, and diastolic dysfunction in early canine experimental hypertension. *J. Am. Coll. Cardiol.* 17: 530–536, 1991.
63. Duomarco, J. L., and R. Rimini. Energy and hydraulic gradient along systemic veins. *Am. J. Physiol.* 178: 215, 1954.
64. Eckstein, R. W., C. J. Wiggers, and G. R. Graham. Phasic changes in inferior cava flow of intravascular origin. *Am. J. Physiol.* 148: 740–744, 1947.
65. Ehrman, J., S. Keteyian, F. Fedel, K. Rhoads, T. B. Levine, and R. Shepard. Cardiovascular responses of heart transplant recipients to graded exercise testing. *J. Appl. Physiol.* 73: 260–264, 1992.
66. Ekblom, B., and L. Hermansen. Cardiac output in athletes. *J. Appl. Physiol.* 25: 619–625, 1968.
67. Elzinga, G., R. Van Grondelle, N. Westerhof, and G. C. Van Den Bos. Ventricular interference. *Am. J. Physiol.* 226: 941–947, 1974.
68. Eshani, A. A., T. Ogawa, T. R. Miller, R. J. Spina, and S. M. Jilka. Exercise training improves left ventricular systolic function in older men. *Circulation* 83: 96–103, 1991.
69. Fagard, R., A. Aubert, J. Staessen, E. V. Eynde, L. Vanhees, and A. Amery. Cardiac structure and function in cyclists and runners: comparative echocardiographic study. *Br. Heart J.* 52: 124–129, 1984.
70. Fessler, H. E., R. G. Brower, E. P. Shapiro, and S. Permutt. Effects of positive end-expiratory pressure and body position on pressure in the thoracic great veins. *Am. Rev. Respir. Dis.* 148: 1657–1664, 1993.
71. Fessler, H. E., R. G. Brower, R. A. Wise, and S. Permutt. Effects of positive end-expiratory pressure on the canine venous return curve. *Am. Rev. Respir. Dis.* 146: 4–10, 1992.
72. Fisman, E. Z., A. G. Frank, E. Ben-Ari, G. Kessler, A. Pines, Y. Drory, and J. J. Kellermann. Altered left ventricular volume and ejection fraction responses to supine dynamic exercise in athletes. *J. Am. Coll. Cardiol.* 15: 582–588, 1990.
73. Flamm, S. D., J. Taki, R. Moore, S. F. Lewis, F. Keech, F. Maltais, M. Ahmad, R. Callahan, S. Dragotakes, N. Alpert, and H. W. Strauss. Redistribution of regional and organ blood volume and effect on cardiac function in relation to upright exercise in healthy human subjects. *Circulation* 81: 1550–1559, 1990.
74. Fleck, S. J. Cardiovascular adaptations to resistance training. *Med. Sci. Sports Exerc.* 20: S146–S151, 1988.
75. Fleg, J. L., S. P. Schulman, F. C. O'Connor, G. Gerstenblith, L. C. Becker, S. Fortney, A. P. Goldberg, and E. G. Lakatta. Cardiovascular responses to exhaustive upright cycle exercise in highly trained older men. *J. Appl. Physiol.* 77: 1500–1506, 1994.
76. Folkow, B., P. Gaskell, and B. A. Waaler. Blood flow through limb muscles during heavy rhythmic exercise. *Acta Physiol. Scand.* 80: 61–72, 1970.
77. Folkow, B., U. Haglund, M. Jodal, and O. Lundgren. Blood flow in the calf muscle of man during heavy rhythmic exercise. *Acta Physiol. Scand.* 81: 157–163, 1971.
78. Franklin, K. J. *Monograph on Veins.* Springfield, IL: Charles C Thomas, 1937, p. 256.

79. Freeman, G. L., and M. M. LeWinter: Pericardial adaptations during chronic dilation in dogs. *Circ. Res.* 54: 294–300, 1984.
80. Fuenmayor, A. J., A. M. Fuenmayor, D. M. Winterdaal, and G. Londono. Cardiovascular responses to Valsalva maneuver in physically trained and untrained normal subjects. *J. Sports Med. Phys. Fitness* 32: 293–298, 1992.
81. Gaasch, W. H., O. H. L. Bing, A. Franklin, D. Rhodes, S. A. Bernard, and R. M. Weintraub. The influence of acute alterations in coronary blood flow on left ventricular diastolic compliance and wall thickness. *Eur. J. Cardiol.* 7 (Suppl): 147–161, 1978.
82. Gelpi, R. J., A. Pasipoularides, A. S. Lader, T. A. Patrick, N. Chase, L. Hittinger, R. P. Shannon, S. P. Bishop, and S. F. Vatner. Changes in diastolic cardiac function in developing and stable perinephritic hypertension in conscious dogs. *Circ. Res.* 68: 555–567, 1991.
83. Gerstenblith, G., D. G. Renlund, and E. G. Lakatta. Cardiovascular response to exercise in younger and older men. *Federation Proc.* 46: 1834–1839, 1987.
84. Gilbert, J. C., and S. A. Glantz. Determinants of left ventricular filling and of the diastolic pressure-volume relation. *Circ. Res.* 64: 827–852, 1989.
85. Gilmore, J. P., H. E. Cingolani, R. R. Taylor, and R. H. McDonald, Jr. Physical factors and cardiac adaptation. *Am. J. Physiol.* 211: 1227–1231, 1966.
86. Glantz, S. A., and W. W. Parmley. Factors which affect the diastolic pressure-volume relation. *Circ. Res.* 42: 171–180, 1978.
87. Gledhill, N., D. Cox, and R. Jamnik. Endurance athletes' stroke volume does not plateau: major advantage is diastolic function. *Med. Sci. Sports Exerc.* 26: 1116–1121, 1994.
88. Goetz, T. E., and M. Manohar. Pressures on the right side of the heart and esophagus (pleura) in ponies during exercise before and after furosemide administration. *Am. J. Vet. Res.* 47: 270–276, 1986.
89. Gorczynski, R. J., B. Klitzman, and B. R. Duling. Interrelations between contracting striated muscle and precapillary microvessels. *Am. J. Physiol.* 235 (*Heart Circ. Physiol.* 4): H494–H504, 1978.
90. Goslow, G. E., Jr., H. J. Seeherman, C. R. Taylor, M. N. McCutchin, and N. C Heglund. Electrical activity and relative length changes of dog limb muscles as a function of speed and gait. *J. Exp. Biol.* 94: 15–42, 1981.
91. Grace, M. P., and D. M. Greenbaum. Cardiac performance in response to PEEP in patients with cardiac dysfunction. *Crit. Care Med.* 10: 358–360, 1982.
92. Green, J. F., and A. P. Jackman. Peripheral limitations to exercise. *Med. Sci. Sports Exer.* 16: 299–305, 1984.
93. Greene, A. S., and A. A. Shoukas. Changes in canine cardiac function and venous return curves by the carotid baroreflex. *Am. J. Physiol.* 251 (*Heart Circ. Physiol.* 20): H288–H296, 1986.
94. Grimby, G., N. J. Nilsson, and H. Sanne. Cardiac output during exercise in patients with varicose veins. *Scand. J. Clin. Lab. Invest.* 16: 21–30, 1964.
95. Grodins, F. S., W. H. Stuart, and R. L. Veenstra. Performance characteristics of the right heart bypass preparation. *Am. J. Physiol.* 198: 552–560, 1960.
96. Guntheroth, W. G., B. C. Morgan, and G. L. Mullins. Effect of respiration on venous return and stroke volume in cardiac tamponade. Mechanism of pulsus paradoxus. *Circ. Res.* 20: 381–390, 1967.
97. Guyton, A. C., and L. H. Adkins. Quantitative aspects of the collapse factor in relation to venous return. *Am. J. Physiol.* 177: 523–527, 1954.
98. Guyton, A. C., B. H. Douglas, J. B. Langston, and T. Q. Richardson. Instantaneous increase in mean circulatory pressure and cardiac output at onset of muscular activity. *Circ. Res.* 11: 431–441, 1962.
99. Guyton, A. C., C. E. Jones, and T. G. Coleman. *Circulatory Physiology: Cardiac Output and its Regulation*, 2nd edition. Philadelphia: W. B. Saunders Company, 1973.
100. Guyton, A. C., A. W. Lindsey, B. Abernathy, and T. Richardson. Venous return at various right atrial pressures and the normal venous return curve. *Am. J. Physiol.* 189: 609–615, 1957.
101. Guz, A., J. A. Innes, and K. Murphy. Respiratory modulation of left ventricular stroke volume in man measured using pulsed Doppler ultrasound. *J. Physiol. (Lond.)* 393: 499–512, 1987.
102. Hales, S. Statistical essays containing haemastatics, or, an account of some hydraulic and hydrostatical experiments made on the blood and blood vessels of animals. In: *Cardiac Classics*, edited by F. A. Willius and T. E. Keys. St. Louis: C. V. Mosby, 1941.
103. Hammond, H. K., F. C. White, V. Bhargava, and R. Shabetai. Heart size and maximal cardiac output are limited by the pericardium. *Am. J. Physiol.* 263 (*Heart Circ. Physiol.* 32): H1675–H1681, 1992.
104. Hayashida, K., K. Sunagawa, M. Noma, M. Sugimachi, H. Ando, and M. Nakamura. Mechanical matching of the left ventricle with the arterial system in exercising dogs. *Circ. Res.* 71: 481–489, 1992.
105. Hefner, L. L., L. T. Sheffield, G. C. Cobbs, and W. Klip. Relation between mural force and pressure in the left ventricle of the dog. *Circ. Res.* 11: 654–663, 1962.
106. Herndon, C. W., and K. Sagawa. Combined effects of aortic and right atrial pressures on aortic flow. *Am. J. Physiol.* 201: 102–108, 1969.
107. Higginbotham, M. B., K. G. Morris, R. S. Williams, R. E. Coleman, and F. R. Cobb. Physiologic basis for the age-related decline in aerobic work capacity. *Am. J. Cardiol.* 57: 1374–1379, 1986.
108. Higginbotham, M. B., K. G. Morris, R. S. Williams, P. A. McHale, R. E. Coleman, and F. R. Cobb. Regulation of stroke volume during submaximal and maximal upright exercise in normal man. *Circ. Res.* 58: 281–291, 1986.
109. Hodgson, J. L., and E. R. Buskirk. Physical fitness and age, with emphasis on cardiovascular function in the elderly. *J. Am. Geriatr. Soc.* 25: 385–392, 1977.
110. Hoffman, J. I. E., A. Guz, A. A. Charlier, and D. E. L. Wilcken. Stroke volume in conscious dogs: effect of respiration, posture and vascular occlusion. *J. Appl. Physiol.* 20: 865–877, 1965.
111. Holt, J. P. The collapse factor in the measurement of venous pressure: the flow of fluid through collapsible tubes. *Am. J. Physiol.* 134: 292–299, 1941.
112. Holt, J. P. The effect of positive and negative intrathoracic pressure on cardiac output and venous pressure in the dog. *Am. J. Physiol.* 135: 594–603, 1942.
113. Holt, J. P. The normal pericardium. *Am. J. Cardiol.* 26: 455–465, 1970.
114. Howell, J. B. L., S. Permutt, D. F. Proctor, and R. L. Riley. Effect of inflation of the lung on different parts of pulmonary vascular bed. *J. Appl. Physiol.* 16: 64–70, 1961.
115. Hurford, W. E., M. Barlai-Kovach, W. Strauss, W. M. Zapol, and E. Lowenstein. Canine biventricular performance during acute progressive pulmonary microembolization: re-

gional myocardial perfusion and fatty acid uptake. *J. Crit. Care* 2: 270–281, 1987.
116. Iwase, M., K. Nagata, H. Izawa, M. Yokota, S. Kamihara, H. Inagaki, and H. Saito. Age-related changes in left and right ventricular filling velocity profiles and their relationship in normal subjects. *Am. Heart J.* 126: 419–426, 1993.
117. Ivankovich, A. D., D. J. Miletich, R. F. Albrecht, H. J. Heyman, and R. F. Bonnet. Cardiovascular effects of intraperitoneal insufflation with carbon dioxide and nitrous oxide in the dog. *Anesthesiology* 42: 281–287, 1975.
118. Janicki, J. S. Influence of the pericardium and ventricular interdependence on left ventricular diastolic and systolic function in patients with heart failure. *Circulation* 81: III-15–III-20, 1990.
119. Janicki, J. S., S. G. Shroff, and K. T. Weber. Influence of extracardiac forces on the cardiopulmonary unit. In: *Ventricular/Vascular Coupling*, edited by F. C. P. Yin. New York: Springer-Verlag, 1986, p. 262–287.
120. Janicki, J. S., S. G. Shroff, and K. T. Weber. Ventricular interdependence. In: *Heart-Lung Interactions in Health and Disease*, edited by S. M. Scharf and S. Cassidy. New York: Marcel Dekker, Inc., 1989, p. 283–307.
121. Janicki, J. S., and K. T. Weber. Factors influencing the diastolic pressure-volume relation. *Federation Proc.* 39: 113–140, 1980a.
122. Janicki, J. S., and K. T. Weber. The pericardium and ventricular interaction, distensibility and function. *Am. J. Physiol.* 238 (*Heart Circ. Physiol.* 7): H494–H503, 1980.
123. Janicki, J. S., K. T. Weber, and L. L. Hefner. Ejection pressure and the left ventricular pressure-volume relation. *Am. J. Physiol.* 232 (*Heart Circ. Physiol.* 1): H545–H552, 1977.
124. Jardin, F., J. C. Farcot, L. Boisante, J. F. Prost, P. Gueret, and J. P. Bourdarias. Mechanism of paradoxic pulse in bronchial asthma. *Circulation* 66: 887–894, 1982.
125. Jarmakani, J. M., P. A. McHale, and J. C. Greenfield, Jr. The effect of cardiac tamponade on coronary haemodynamics in the awake dog. *Cardiovasc. Res.* 9: 112–117, 1975.
126. Jayaweera, A. R., and W. Ehrlich. Changes of phasic pleural pressure in awake dogs during exercise: potential effects on cardiac output. *Ann. Biomed. Eng.* 15: 311–318, 1987.
127. Johnson, B. D., W. G Reddan, D. G. Pegelow, K. C. Seow, and J. A. Dempsey. Flow limitation and regulation of functional residual capacity during exercise in a physically active aging population. *Am. Rev. Respir. Dis.* 143: 960–967, 1991.
128. Johnson, B. D., W. G. Reddan, K. C. Seow, and J. A. Dempsey. Mechanical constraints on exercise hyperpnea in a fit aging population. *Am. Rev. Respir. Dis.* 143: 968–977, 1991.
129. Johnson, B. D., K. W. Saupe, and J. A. Dempsey. Mechanical constraints on exercise hyperpnea in endurance athletes. *J. Appl. Physiol.* 73: 874–886, 1992.
130. Jose, A. D., and D. Collison. The normal range and determinants of the intrinsic heart rate in man. *Cardiovasc. Res.* 4: 160–167, 1970.
131. Kaimal, K. P., B. A. Franklin, T. W. Moir, and H. K. Hellerstein. Cardiac profile of national class walkers. *Chest* 104: 935–938, 1993.
132. Karam, M., R. A. Wise, T. K. Natarajan, S. Permutt, and H. N. Wagner. Mechanism of decreased left ventricular stroke volume during inspiration in man. *Circulation* 69: 866–873, 1984.
133. Kashtan, J., J. F. Green, E. Q. Parsons, and J. W. Holcroft. Hemodynamic effect of increased abdominal pressure. *J. Surg. Res.* 30: 249–255, 1981.
134. Kass, D. A., R. Beyar, E. Lankford, M. Heard, W. L. Maughan, and K. Sagawa. Influence of contractile state on curvilinearity of in situ end-systolic pressure-volume relations. *Circulation* 79: 167–178, 1989.
135. Kelman, G. R., G. H. Swapp, I. Smith, R. J. Benzie, and N. L. M. Gordon. Cardiac output and arterial blood-gas tension during laparoscopy. *Br. J. Anaesth.* 44: 1155–1161, 1972.
136. Keul, J., H. H. Dickhuth, G. Simon, and M. Lehmann. Effect of static and dynamic exercise on heart volume, contractility, and left ventricular dimensions. *Circ. Res.* 48: I162–I170, 1981.
137. Kilbom, A., and J. Persson. Cardiovascular response to combined dynamic and static exercise. *Circ. Res.* 48: I93–I97, 1981.
138. Kino, M., V. Q. Lance, A. Shammatpour, and D. Spodick. Effects of age on response to isometric exercise. *Am. Heart J.* 90: 575–581, 1975.
139. Kitzman, D. W., and W. D. Edwards. Age-related changes in the anatomy of the normal human heart. *J. Gerontol.* 45: M33–M39, 1990.
140. Kitzman, D. W., M. B. Higginbotham, F. R. Cobb, K. H. Sheikh, and M. J. Sullivan. Exercise intolerance in patients with heart failure and preserved left ventricular systolic function: failure of the Frank-Starling mechanism. *J. Am. Coll. Cardiol.* 17: 1065–1072, 1991.
141. Klima, M., T. R. Burns, and A. Chopra. Myocardial fibrosis in the elderly. *Arch. Pathol. Lab. Med.* 114: 938–942, 1990.
142. Krayer, S., M. Decramer, J. Vettermann, E. L. Ritman, and K. Rehder. Volume quantification of chest wall motion in dogs. *J. Appl. Physiol.* 65: 2213–2220, 1988.
143. Krogh, A. Regulation of the supply of blood to the right heart (with a description of a new circulation model). *Scand. Arch. Physiol.* 27: 227–248, 1912.
144. Kuno, Y. The mechanical effect of fluid in the pericardium on the function of the heart. *J. Physiol.* 51: 221–234, 1917.
145. Lai-Fook, S. J., R. E. Hyatt, and J. R. Rodarte. Effect of parenchymal sheer modulus and lung volume on bronchial pressure-diameter behavior. *J. Appl. Physiol.* 44: 859–968, 1978.
146. Laughlin, M. H. Skeletal muscle blood flow capacity: role of muscle pump in exercise hyperemia. *Am. J. Physiol.* 253 (*Heart Circ. Physiol.* 22): H993–H1004, 1987.
147. Leblanc, P., E. Summers, M. D. Inman, N. L. Jones, E. J. M. Campbell, and K. J. Killian. Inspiratory muscles during exercise: a problem of supply and demand. *J. Appl. Physiol.* 64: 2482–2489, 1988.
148. Lentini, A. C., R. S. McKelvie, N. McCarteny, C. W. Tomlinson, and J. D. MacDougall. Left ventricular response in healthy young men during heavy-intensity weight-lifting exercise. *J. Appl. Physiol.* 75: 2703–2710, 1993.
149. Levy, M. N. The cardiac and vascular factors that determine systemic blood flow. *Circ. Res.* 44: 739–746, 1979.
150. Levy, W. C, M. D. Cerqueira, I. B. Abrass, R. S. Schwartz, and J. R Stratton. Endurance exercise training augments diastolic filling at rest and during exercise in healthy young and older men. *Circulation* 88: 116–126, 1993.
151. Lewis, S. F., P. G. Snell, W. F. Taylor, M. Hamra, R. M. Graham, W. A. Pettinger, and C. G. Blomqvist. Role of muscle mass and mode of contraction in circulatory responses to exercise. *J. Appl. Physiol.* 58: 146–151, 1985.

152. Little, W. C., W. K. Barr, and M. H. Crawford. Altered effect of the Valsalva maneuver on left ventricular volume in patients with cardiomyopathy. *Circulation* 71: 227–233, 1985.
153. Little, W. C., and C. P. Cheng. Effect of exercise on left ventricular-arterial coupling assessed in the pressure-volume plane. *Am. J. Physiol.* 264 (*Heart Circ. Physiol.* 33): H1629–H1633, 1993.
154. Lloyd, T. C. Effect of inspiration on inferior vena caval blood flow in dogs. *J. Appl. Physiol.* 55: 1701–1706, 1983.
155. Longhurst, J. C., A. R. Kelly, W. J. Gonyea, and J. H. Mitchell. Cardiovascular responses to static exercise in distance runners and weight lifters. *J. Appl. Physiol.* 49: 676–683, 1980.
156. Longhurst, J. C., A. R. Kelly, W. J. Gonyea, and J. H Mitchell. Echocardiographic left ventricular masses in distance runners and weight lifters. *J. Appl. Physiol.* 48: 154–162, 1980.
157. Ludbrook, J. *Aspects of Venous Function in the Lower Limbs*. Springfield, IL: Charles C Thomas, 1966.
158. Lynch, F. P., O. Tomoshige, J. M. Scully, M. L. Williamson, and D. L. Dudgeon. Cardiovascular effects of increased intra-abdominal pressure in newborn piglets. *J. Pediatr. Surg.* 9: 621–626, 1974.
159. MacDougall, J. D., D. Tuxen, D. G. Sale, J. R. Moroz, and J. R. Sutton. Arterial blood pressure response to heavy resistance exercise. *J. Appl. Physiol.* 58: 785–790, 1985.
160. MacFarlane, N., D. B. Northridge, A. R. Wright, S. Grant, and H. J. Dargie. A comparative study of left ventricular structure and function in elite athletes. *Br. J. Sports Med.* 25: 45–48, 1991.
161. Magder, S. Vascular mechanics of venous drainage in dog hindlimbs. *Am. J. Physiol.* 259 (*Heart Circ. Physiol.* 28): H1789–H1795, 1990.
162. Manohar, M., G. E. Bisgard, V. Bullard, et al. Regional myocardial blood flow and myocardial function during acute right ventricular pressure overload in calves. *Circ. Res.* 44: 531–539, 1979.
163. Marini, J. J., B. H. Culver, and J. Butler. Mechanical effect of lung distention with positive pressure on cardiac function. *Am. Rev. Respir. Dis.* 124: 382–386, 1981.
164. Marshall, R. J., A. Schirger, and J. T. Shepherd. Blood pressure during supine exercise in idiopathic orthostatic hypotension. *Circulation* 14: 76–81, 1961.
165. Marshall, J. M., and H. C. Tandon. Direct observations of muscle arterioles and venules following contraction of skeletal muscle fibres in the rat. *J. Physiol.* 350: 447–459, 1984.
166. Martin, W. H., III, E. F. Coyle, S. A. Bloomfield, and A. A. Ehsani. Effects of physical deconditioning after intense endurance training on left ventricular dimensions and stroke volume. *J. Am. Coll. Cardiol.* 7: 982–989, 1986.
167. Maruyama, Y., K. Ashikawa, S. Isoyama, H. Kanatsuka, E. Ino-Oka, and T. Takishima. Mechanical interactions between four heart chambers with and without the pericardium in canine hearts. *Circ. Res.* 50: 86–100, 1982.
168. Masey, S. A., R. C. Koehler, J. R. Rock, J. M. Pepple, M. C. Rogers, and R. J. Traystman. Effect of abdominal distention on central and regional hemodynamics in neonatal lambs. *Pediatr. Res.* 19: 1244–1249, 1985.
169. Mathru, M., T. L. K. Rao, A. A. El-Etr, and R. Pifarre. Hemodynamic response to changes in ventilatory patterns in patients with normal and poor left ventricular reserve. *Crit. Care Med.* 10: 423–426, 1982.
170. McHale, P. A., and J. C. Greenfield, Jr. Evaluation of several geometric models for estimation of left ventricular circumferential wall stress. *Circ. Res.* 33: 303–312, 1973.
171. Milnor, W. R. Arterial impedance as ventricular afterload. *Circ. Res.* 36: 565–570, 1975.
172. Mitchell, J. H., and G. Blomqvist. Maximal oxygen uptake. *N. Engl. J. Med.* 284: 1018–1022, 1971.
173. Mitchell, J. H., R. J. Linden, and S. J. Sarnoff. Influence of cardiac sympathetic and vagal nerve stimulation on the relation between left ventricular diastolic pressure and myocardial segment length. *Circ. Res.* 8: 1100–1107, 1960.
174. Mitchell, J. H., F. C. Payne, B. Saltin, and B. Schibye. The role of muscle mass in the cardiovascular response to static contractions. *J. Physiol. (Lond.)* 309: 45–54, 1980.
175. Mitzner, W. Resistance of the pulmonary circulation. *Clin. Chest Med.* 4: 127–137, 1983.
176. Mixter, G. Respiratory augmentation of inferior vena caval flow demonstrated by a low resistance phasic flowmeter. *Am. J. Physiol.* 172: 446–456, 1953.
177. Monroe, R. G., C. G. LaFarge, W. J. Gamble, A. Rosenthal, and S. Honda. Left ventricular pressure-volume relations and performance as affected by sudden increases in developed pressure. *Circ. Res.* 22: 333–344, 1968.
178. Moreno, A. H., A. R. Burchell, R. Van der Woude, and J. H. Burke. Respiratory regulation of splanchnic and systemic venous return. *Am. J. Physiol.* 213: 455–465, 1967.
179. Moreno, A. H., A. I. Katz, and L. D. Gold. An integrated approach to the study of the venous system with steps toward a detailed model of the dynamics of venous return to the right heart. *IEEE Trans. Biomed. Eng.* 16: 308–324, 1969.
180. Morgan, B. C., F. L. Abel, G. L. Mullins, and W. G. Guntheroth. Flow patterns in cavae, pulmonary artery, pulmonary vein, and aorta in intact dogs. *Am. J. Physiol.* 210: 903–909, 1966.
181. Morganroth, J., B. J. Maron, W. L. Henry, and S. E. Epstein. Comparative left ventricular dimensions in trained athletes. *Ann. Intern. Med.* 82: 521–524, 1975.
182. Morgenstern, C., U. Holjes, G. Arnold, and W. Lochner. The influence of coronary pressure and coronary flow on intracoronary blood volume and geometry of the left ventricle. *Pflugers Arch.* 340: 101–111, 1973.
183. Mosher, P., J. Ross, Jr., P. A. McFate, and R. F. Shaw. Control of coronary blood flow by an autoregulatory mechanism. *Circ. Res.* 14: 250–259, 1964.
184. Murgo, J. P., and N. Westerhof. Input impedance of the pulmonary arterial system in normal man: effects of respiration and comparison to systemic impedance. *Circ. Res.* 54: 666–673, 1984.
185. Musch, T. I., D. B. Friedman, K. H. Pitetti, G. C. Haidet, J. Stray-Gundersen, J. H. Mitchell, and G. A. Ordway. Regional distribution of blood flow of dogs during graded dynamic exercise. *J. Appl. Physiol.* 63: 2269–2277, 1987.
186. Musch, T. I., G. C. Haidet, G. A. Ordway, J. C. Longhurst, and J. H. Mitchell. Dynamic exercise training in foxhounds I: oxygen consumption and hemodynamic responses. *J. Appl. Physiol.* 59: 183–189, 1985.
187. Nagle, F. J., D. R. Seals, and P. Hanson. Time to fatigue during isometric exercise using different muscle masses. *Int. J. Sports Med.* 9: 313–315, 1988.
188. Nakhjavan, F. K., W. H. Palmer, and M. McGregor. Influence of respiration on venous return in emphysema. *Circulation* 33: 8–16, 1966.
189. Narayan, S., J. S. Janicki, S. G. Shroff, R. Pick, and K. T. Weber. Myocardial collagen and mechanics after prevent-

ing hypertrophy in hypertensive rats. *Am. J. Hypertens.* 2: 675–682, 1989.
190. Nichols, W. W., and M. O'Rourke. Aging, high blood pressure and disease in humans. In: *McDonald's Blood Flow In Arteries,* edited by W. W. Nichols and M. F. O'Rourke. London: Edward Arnold, 1990, p. 398–420.
191. Nichols, W. W., M. F. O'Rourke, A. P. Avolio, T. Yaginuma, J. P. Murgo, C. J. Pepine, and C. R. Conti. Age-related changes in left ventricular/arterial coupling In: *Ventricular/Vascular Coupling,* edited by F. C. P. Yin. New York: Springer-Verlag, 1987, p. 79–114.
192. Nixon, J. V., A. R. Wright, T. R. Porter, V. Roy, and J. A. Arrowood. Effects of exercise on left ventricular diastolic performance in trained athletes. *Am. J. Cardiol.* 68: 945–949, 1991.
193. Noda, T., C. P. Cheng, P. P. de Tombe, and W. C. Little. Curvilinearity of LV end-systolic pressure-volume and dP/dtmax-end-diastolic volume relations. *Am. J. Physiol* 265 (*Heart Circ. Physiol.* 34): H910–H917, 1993.
194. Notarius, C. F., and S. Magder. Changes in the vascular mechanics of skeletal muscle during muscle contractions—an important factor for increased venous return. *FASEB J.* 7: A762, 1993.
195. Numao, Y., and J. Iriuchijima. Effect of cardiac output on circulatory blood volume. *Jpn. J. Physiol.* 27: 145–156, 1977.
196. Nunn, J. F. *Applied Respiratory Physiology.* London: Butterworths, 1977, p. 259.
197. Olafsson, S., and R. E. Hyatt. Ventilatory mechanics and expiratory flow limitation during exercise in normal subjects. *J. Clin. Invest.* 48: 564–573, 1969.
198. Oldershaw, P. J., K. D. Dawkins, D. E. Ward, and D. G. Gibson. Diastolic mechanisms of impaired exercise tolerance in aortic valve disease. *Br. Heart J.* 49: 568–573, 1983.
199. Ordway, G. A., and D. R. Wekstein. Effect of age on cardiovascular responses to static (isometric) exercise. *Proc. Soc. Exp. Biol. Med.* 161: 189–192, 1979.
200. O'Rourke, M. F., A. P. Avolio, and W. W. Nichols. Left ventricular-systemic arterial coupling in disease states. In: *Ventricular/Vascular Coupling*, edited by F. C. P. Yin. New York: Springer-Verlag, 1987, p. 1–19.
201. O'Rourke, R. A., D. P. Fischer, E. E. Escobar, S. Bishop, and E. Rapaport. Effect of acute pericardial tamponade on coronary blood flow. *Am. J. Physiol.* 212: 549–552, 1967.
202. Packer, M. Abnormalities of diastolic function as a potential cause of exercise intolerance in chronic heart failure. *Circulation* 81: III-78–III-86, 1990.
203. Patterson, R. E., B. B. Kent, and E. C. Pierce. A comparison of empirical contractile indices in intact dogs. *Cardiology* 57: 277–294, 1972.
204. Pearlman, E. S., K. T. Weber, J. S. Janicki, C. G. Pietra, and A. P. Fishman. Muscle fiber orientation and connective tissue content in the hypertrophied human heart. *Lab. Invest.* 46: 158–164, 1982.
205. Pearson, A. C., C. V. Gudipati, and A. J. Labovitz. Effects of aging on left ventricular structure and function. *Am. Heart J.* 121: 871–875, 1991.
206. Pelliccia, A., A. Spataro, G. Casell, and B. J. Maron. Absence of left ventricular wall thickening in athletes engaged in intense power training. *Am. J. Cardiol.* 72: 1048–1054, 1993.
207. Perez-Gonzales, J. F., N. B. Schiller, and W. W. Parmley. Direct and noninvasive evaluation of the cardiovascular response to isometric exercise. *Circ. Res.* 48: I138–I148, 1981.
208. Perini, R., C. Orizio, A. Gamba, and A. Veicsteinas. Kinetics of heart rate and catecholamines during exercise in humans. *Eur. J. Appl. Physiol.* 66: 500–506, 1993.
209. Permutt, S., B. Bromberger-Barnea, and H. Bane. Alveolar pressure, pulmonary venous pressure, and the vascular waterfall. *Med. Thorac.* 19: 239–260, 1962.
210. Permutt, S., and P. Caldini. Regulation of cardiac output by the circuit: venous return. In: *Cardiovascular System Dynamics*, edited by J. Baan, A. Noordergraaf, and J. Raines. Cambridge, MA: MIT Press, 1978, p. 465–479.
211. Permutt, S., J. B. L. Howell, D. F. Proctor, and R. L. Riley. Effect of lung inflation on static pressure-volume characteristics of pulmonary vessels. *J. Appl. Physiol.* 16: 64–70, 1961.
212. Permutt, S., and R. L. Riley. Hemodynamics of collapsible vessels with tone: the vascular waterfall. *J. Appl. Physiol.* 18: 924–932, 1963.
213. Peters, J., C. Fraser, R. S. Stuart, W. Baumgartner, and J. L. Robotham. Negative intrathoracic pressure decreases independently left ventricular filling and emptying. *Am. J. Physiol.* 257 (*Heart Circ. Physiol.* 26): H120–H131, 1989.
214. Peters, J., M. K. Kindred, and J. L. Robotham. Transient analysis of cardiopulmonary interactions. II. Systolic events. *J. Appl. Physiol.* 64: 1518–1526, 1988.
215. Petrofsky, J. S., and A. R. Lind. Aging, isometric strength and endurance, and cardiovascular responses to static effort. *J. Appl. Physiol.* 38: 91–95, 1975.
216. Piene, H., and A. Hauge. Influence of moderate vasoconstriction on the wave reflection properties of the pulmonary arterial bed. *Acta Physiol. Scand.* 93: 37–43, 1976.
217. Pochis, W. T., B. D. Collier, A. T. Isitman, R. S. Hellman, D. W. Palmer, A. Z. Krasnow, L. S. Wann, and J. M. Knobel. Diagnostic reliability of radionuclide ventriculography in detecting left ventricular hypertrophy: echocardiographic and ECG correlations. *Clin. Nucl. Med.* 17: 168–170, 1992.
218. Pollack, A. A., and E. H. Wood. Venous pressure in the saphenous vein at the ankle in man during exercise and changes in posture. *J. Appl. Physiol.* 1: 649–662, 1949.
219. Potter, W. A., S. Olafsson, and R. E. Hyatt. Ventilatory mechanics and expiratory flow limitation during exercise in patients with obstructive lung disease. *J. Clin. Invest* 50: 910–919, 1971.
220. Romonatxo, M., J. Mercier, R. Cohendy, and C. Prefaut. Effect of resistive loads on pattern of respiratory muscle recruitment during exercise. *J. Appl. Physiol.* 71: 1941–1948, 1991.
221. Rankin, J. S., C. O. Olsen, C. E.Arentzen, G. S. Tyson, G. Maier, P. K. Smith, J. W. Hammon, Jr., J. W. Davis, P. A. McHale, R. W. Anderson, and D. C. Sabiston, Jr. The effects of airway pressure on cardiac function in intact dogs and man. *Circulation* 66: 108–120, 1982.
222. Raymundo, H., A. M. Scher, D. S. O'Leary, and P. D. Sampson. Cardiovascular control by arterial and cardiopulmonary baroreceptors in awake dogs with atrioventricular block. *Am. J. Physiol.* 257 (*Heart Circ. Physiol.* 26): H2048–H2058, 1989.
223. Reeves, J. T., B. M. Groves, A. Cymerman, J. R. Sutton, P. D. Wagner, D. Turkevich, and C. S. Houston. Operation Everest II: cardiac filling pressures during cycle exercise at sea level. *Respir. Physiol.* 80: 147–154, 1990.
224. Renkin, E. M. Control of microcirculation and blood-tissue exchange. In: *Handbook of Physiology, The Cardiovascular System, Microcirculation*, edited by E. M. Renkin and C. C. Michel. Bethesda, MD: Am. Physiol. Soc., 1984, p. 627–687.

225. Richardson, J. D., and J. K. Trinkle. Hemodynamic and respiratory alterations with increased intra-abdominal pressure. *J. Surg. Res.* 20: 401–404, 1976.
226. Robinson, B. F., S. E. Epstein, R. L. Kahler, and E. Braunwald. Circulatory effects of acute expansion of blood volume: studies during maximal exercise and at rest. *Circ. Res.* 19: 26–32, 1966.
227. Robotham, J. L., F. R. Badke. M. K. Kindred, and M. K. Beaton. Regional left ventricular performance during normal and obstructed spontaneous respiration. *J. Appl. Physiol.* 55: 569–577, 1983.
228. Robotham, J. L., and W. Mitzner. A model of the effects of respiration on left ventricular performance *J. Appl. Physiol.* 46: 411–418, 1979.
229. Robotham, J. L., and J. Peters. Mechanical effects of intrathoracic pressure on ventricular performance. In: *Heart/Lung Interactions*, edited by S. Scharf and S. Cassidy. New York: Marcel Dekker, Inc., 1989, p. 251–283.
230. Robotham, J. L., and J. Peters. Cardiorespiratory interactions. In: *Adult Respiratory Distress Syndrome*, edited by W. Zapol. New York: Marcel Dekker, Inc., 1991, p. 223–251.
231. Robotham, J. L., J. Peters, and M. Takata. Cardiorespiratory interactions. In: *Pulmonary and Critical Care Medicine*, Vol. 2, edited by R C. Bone. St. Louis: Mosby-Year Book, 1993, p. 1–25.
232. Robotham, J. L., R. S. Stuart, M. A. Borkon, K. Doherty, and W. Baumgartner. Effects of changes in left ventricular loading and pleural pressure on mitral flow. *J. Appl. Physiol.* 65: 1662–1675, 1988.
233. Robotham, J. L., R. S. Stuart, K. Doherty, M. A. Borkon, and W. Baumgartner. Mitral and aortic flows during spontaneous respiration in dogs. *Anesthesiology* 69: 516–526, 1988.
234. Robotham, J. L., R. A. Wise, and B. Bromberger-Barnea. Effects of changes in abdominal pressure on left ventricular performance and regional blood flow. *Crit. Care Med.* 13: 803–809, 1985.
235. Rodeheffer, R. J., G. Gerstenblith, L. C. Becker, J. L. Fleg, M. L. Weisfeldt, and E. G. Lakatta. Exercise cardiac output is maintained with advancing age in healthy human subjects: cardiac dilatation and increased stroke volume compensate for a diminished heart rate. *Circulation* 69: 203–213, 1984.
236. Rothe, C. F. Venous system: Physiology of the capacitance vessels. In: *Handbook of Physiology, The Cardiovascular System, Peripheral Circulation and Organ Blood Flow*, edited by J. T. Sheperd and F. M. Abboub. Bethesda, MD: Am. Physiol. Soc., 1983, p. 397–452.
237. Rothe, C. F. Mean circulatory filling pressure: its meaning and measurement. *J. Appl. Physiol.* 74: 499–509, 1993.
238. Rothe, C. F., and M. L. Gaddis. Autoregulation of cardiac output by passive elastic characteristics of the vascular capacitance system. *Circulation* 81: 360–368, 1990.
239. Rowell, L. B. *Human Circulation: Regulation During Physical Stress.* New York: Oxford University Press, 1986.
240. Rowell, L. B. *Human Cardiovascular Control.* New York: Oxford University Press, 1993.
241. Rowell, L. B., G. L. Brengelmann, J. R. Blackmon, R. A. Bruce, and J. A. Murray. Disparities between aortic and peripheral pulse pressures induced by upright exercise and vasomotor changes in man. *Circulation* 37: 954–964, 1968.
242. Rowell, L. B., H. J. Marx, R. A. Bruce, R. D. Conn, and F. Kusumi. Reductions in cardiac output, central blood volume, and stroke volume with thermal stress in normal men during exercise. *J. Clin. Invest.* 45: 1801–1816, 1966.
243. Rubal, B. J., A. R. Al-Muhailani, and J. Rosentswieg. Effects of physical conditioning on the heart size and wall thickness of college women. *Med. Sci. Sports Exerc.* 19: 423–429, 1987.
244. Rubal, B. J., J. M. Moody, S. Damore, S. R. Bunker, and N. M. Diaz. Left ventricular performance of the athletic heart during upright exercise: a heart rate-controlled study. *Med. Sci. Sports Exerc.* 18: 134–140, 1986.
245. Rutlen, D. L., F. G P. Welt, and A. Ilebekk. Passive effect of reduced cardiac function on splanchnic intravascular volume. *Am. J. Physiol.* 262 (*Heart Circ. Physiol.* 31): H1361–H1364, 1992.
246. Salisbury, P. F., C. E. Cross, and P. A. Rieben. Influence of coronary artery pressure upon myocardial elasticity. *Circ. Res.* 8: 794–800, 1960.
247. Santamore, W. P., P. R. Lynch, G. Meier, J. Heckman, and A. A. Bove. Myocardial interaction between the ventricles. *J. Appl. Physiol.* 4: 362–368, 1976.
248. Sawatani, S., G. Mandell, E. Kusaba, W. Schraut, P. Cascade, W. J. Wajszczuk, and A. Kantrowitz. Ventricular performance following ablation and prosthetic replacement of right ventricular myocardium. *Trans. Am. Soc. Artific. Intern. Organs* 20: 629–636, 1974.
249. Schaible, T. F., and J. Scheuer. Cardiac adaptations to chronic exercise. *Prog. Cardiovasc. Dis.* 27: 297–324, 1985.
250. Schairer, J. R., S. Keteyian, J. W. Henry, and P. D. Stein. Left ventricular wall tension and stress during exercise in athletes and sedentary men. *Am. J. Cardiol.* 71: 1095–1098, 1993.
251. Schulman, S. P., E. G. Lakatta, J. L. Lakatta, L. C. Becker, and G. Gerstenblith. Age-related decline in left ventricular filling at rest and exercise. *Am. J. Physiol.* 263 (*Heart Circ. Physiol.* 32): H1932–H1938, 1992.
252. Seals, D. R. Influence of muscle mass on sympathetic neural activity during isometric exercise. *J. Appl. Physiol.* 67: 1801–1806, 1989.
253. Seals, D. R. Influence of active muscle size on sympathetic nerve discharge during isometric contractions in humans. *J. Appl. Physiol.* 75: 1426–1431, 1993.
254. Seals, D. R., J. M. Hagberg, R. J. Spina, M. A. Rogers, K. B. Schechtman, and A. A. Ehsani. Enhanced left ventricular performance in endurance trained older men. *Circulation* 89: 198–205, 1994.
255. Seals, D. R., R. A. Washburn, P. G. Hanson, P. L. Painter, and F. J. Nagle. Increased cardiovascular response to static contraction of large muscle groups. *J. Appl. Physiol.* 54: 434–437, 1983.
256. Sejersted, O. M., A. R. Hargens, K. R. Kardel, P. Blom, O. Jensen, and L. Hermansen. Intramuscular fluid pressure during isometric contraction of human skeletal muscle. *J. Appl. Physiol.* 56: 287–295, 1984.
257. Shabetai, R., N. O. Fowler, J. C. Fenton, and M. Masnakay. Pulsus paradoxus. *J. Clin. Invest.* 44: 1882–1898, 1965.
258. Shahi, M., S. Thom, N. Poulter, P. S. Sever, and R. A. Foale. Regression of hypertensive left ventricular hypertrophy and left ventricular diastolic function. *Lancet* 336: 458–461, 1990.
259. Shapiro, L. M., and W. J. McKenna. Left ventricular hypertrophy: relation of structure to diastolic function in hypertension. *Br. Heart J.* 51: 637–642, 1984.
260. Sheldahl, L. M., T. J. Ebert, B. Cox, and F. E. Tristani. Effect of aerobic training on baroreflex regulation of car-

diac and sympathetic function. *J. Appl. Physiol.* 76: 158–165, 1994.
261. Sheriff, D. D., L. B. Rowell, and A. M. Scher. Is rapid rise in vascular conductance at onset of dynamic exercise due to muscle pump? *Am. J. Physiol.* 265 (*Heart Circ. Physiol.* 34): H1227–H1234, 1993.
262. Sheriff, D. D., and X. P. Zhou. Influence of cardiac output distribution on cardiac filling pressure during test and dynamic exercise in dogs. *Am. J. Physiol.* 267 (*Heart Circ. Physiol.* 36): H2378–H2380, 1994.
263. Sheriff, D. D., X. P. Zhou, A. M. Scher, and L. B. Rowell. Dependence of cardiac filling pressure on cardiac output during rest and dynamic exercise in dogs. *Am. J. Physiol.* 265 (*Heart Circ. Physiol.* 34): H316–H322, 1993.
264. Shimazaki, Y., Y. Kawashima, T. Mori, H. Matsuda, S. Kitamura, and K. Yokota. Ventricular function of single ventricle after ventricular septation. *Circulation* 61: 653–660, 1980.
265. Shirato, K., R. Shabetai, V. Bhargava, D. Franklin, and J. Ross, Jr. Alterations of the left ventricular diastolic pressure-segment length relation produced by the pericardium. *Circulation* 57: 1191–1198, 1978.
266. Shoukas, A. A., C. L. MacAnespie, M. J. Brunner, and L. Watermeier. The importance of the spleen in blood volume shifts of the systemic vascular bed caused by the carotid sinus baroreceptor reflex in the dog. *Circ. Res.* 49: 759–766, 1981.
267. Shoukas, A. A., and K. Sagawa. Control of total systemic vascular capacity by the carotid sinus baroreceptor reflex. *Circ. Res.* 33: 22–33, 1973.
268. Shroff, S. G., K. T. Weber, and J. S. Janicki. End systolic relations: their usefulness and limitations in assessing left ventricular contractile state. *Int. J. Cardiol.* 5: 253–259, 1984.
269. Slinker, B. K., and S. A. Glantz. End-systolic and end-diastolic ventricular interdependence. *Am. J. Physiol.* 251 (*Heart Circ. Physiol.* 20): H1062–H1075, 1986.
270. Slinker, B. K., Y. Goto, and M. M. LeWinter. Direct diastolic ventricular interaction gain measured with sudden hemodynamic transients. *Am. J. Physiol.* 256 (*Heart Circ. Physiol.* 25): H567–H573, 1989.
271. Slinker, B. K., Y. Goto, and M. M. LeWinter. Systolic direct ventricular interaction affects left ventricular contraction and relaxation in the intact dog circulation. *Circ. Res.* 65: 307–315, 1989.
272. Smiseth, O. A., M. A. Frais, I. Kingma, E. R. Smith, and J. V. Tyberg. Assessment of pericardial constraint in dogs. *Circulation* 71: 158–164, 1985.
273. Smiseth, O. A., M. A. Frais, I. Kingma, A. V. M. White, M. L. Knudtson, J. M. Cohen, D. E. Manyari, E. R. Smith, and J. V. Tyberg. Assessment of pericardial constraint: the relation between right ventricular filling pressure and pericardial pressure measured after pericardiocentesis. *J. Am. Coll. Cardiol.* 7: 307–314, 1986.
274. Smith, D. L., J. E. Misner, D. K. Bloomfield, and L. K. Essandoh. Cardiovascular responses to sustained maximal isometric contractions of the finger flexors. *Eur. J. Appl. Physiol.* 67: 48–52, 1993.
275. Smith, J. C., and W. Mitzner. Analysis of pulmonary vascular interdependence in excised dog lobes. *J. Appl. Physiol.* 48: 450–467, 1980.
276. Sonnenblick, E. H. Force-velocity relations in mammalian heart muscle. *Am. J. Physiol.* 202: 931–939, 1962.
277. Sonnenblick, E. H., J. H. Siegel, and S. J. Sarnoff. Ventricular distensibility and pressure-volume curve during sympathetic stimulation. *Am. J. Physiol.* 204: 1–4, 1963.
278. Spina, R. J., T. Ogawa, W. M. Kohrt, W. H. Martin, III, J. O. Holloszy, and A. A. Ehsani. Differences in cardiovascular adaptations to endurance exercise training between older men and women. *J. Appl. Physiol.* 75: 849–855, 1993.
279. Spina, R. J., T. Ogawa, W. H. Martin, III, A. R. Coggan, J. O. Holloszy, and A. A. Ehsani. Exercise training prevents decline in stroke volume during exercise in young healthy subjects. *J. Appl. Physiol.* 72: 2458–2462, 1992.
280. Spina, R. J., T. Ogawa, T. R. Miller, W. M. Kohrt, and A. A. Ehsani. Effect of exercise training on left ventricular performance in older women free of cardiopulmonary disease. *Am. J. Cardiol.* 71: 99–104, 1993.
281. Squires, R. W. Exercise training after cardiac transplantation. *Med. Sci. Sports Exerc.* 23: 686–694, 1991.
282. Stegall, H. F. Muscle pumping in the dependent leg. *Circ. Res.* 19: 180–190, 1966.
283. Stenberg, J., B. Ekblom, and R. Messin. Hemodynamic response to work at simulated altitude, 4,000 m. *J. Appl. Physiol.* 21: 1589–1594, 1966.
284. Stick, C., H. Jaeger, and E. Witzleb. Measurements of volume changes and venous pressure in the human lower leg during walking and running. *J. Appl. Physiol.* 72: 2063–2068, 1992.
285. Stinson, E. B., R. B. Griepp, J. S. Schroeder, E. Dong, and N. E. Shumway. Hemodynamic observations one and two years after cardiac transplantation. *Circulation* 45: 1183–1194, 1972.
286. Strandell, T. Heart rate, arterial lactate concentration and oxygen uptake during exercise in old men compared to young men. *Acta Physiol. Scand.* 60: 197–201, 1964.
287. Stratton, J. R., W. C. Levy, M. D. Cerqueira, R. S. Schwartz, and I. B. Abrass. Cardiovascular responses to exercise: effects of aging and exercise training in healthy men. *Circulation* 89: 1648–1655, 1994.
288. Stray-Gundersen, J., T. I. Musch, G. C. Haidet, D. P. Swain, G. A. Ordway, and J. H. Mitchell. The effect of pericardiectomy on maximal oxygen consumption and maximal cardiac output in untrained dogs. *Circ. Res.* 58: 523–530, 1986.
289. Suga, H., and K. Sagawa. Instantaneous pressure-volume relationships and their ratio in the excised, supported canine left ventricle. *Circ. Res.* 35: 117–126, 1974.
290. Suga, H., K. Sagawa, and A. A. Shoukas. Load independence of the instantaneous pressure-volume ratio of the canine left ventricle and effects of epinephrine and heart rate on the ratio. *Circ. Res* 32: 314–322, 1973.
291. Summer, W. R., S. Permutt, and K. Sagawa. Effects of spontaneous respiration on canine left ventricular function. *Circ. Res.* 45: 719–728, 1979.
292. Sunagawa, K., W. L. Maughan, D. Burkhoff, and K. Sagawa. Left ventricular interaction with arterial load studied in isolated canine ventricle. *Am. J. Physiol.* 245 (*Heart Circ. Physiol.* 14): H773–H780, 1983.
293. Sunagawa, K., W. L. Maughan, and K. Sagawa. Effect of regional ischemia on the left ventricular end-systolic pressure-volume relationship of isolated canine hearts. *Circ. Res.* 52: 170–178, 1983.
294. Swinne, C. J., E. P. Shapiro, S. D. Lima, and J. L. Fleg. Age-associated changes in left ventricular diastolic performance during isometric exercise in normal subjects. *Am. J. Cardiol.* 69: 823–826, 1992.
295. Sylvester, J. T., H. S. Goldberg, and S. Permutt. The role of the vasculature in the regulation of cardiac output. *Clin. Chest Med.* 4: 111–126, 1983.

296. Szlachcic, J., J. F. Tubau, B. O'Kelly, and B. M. Massie. Correlates of diastolic filling abnormalities in hypertension: a Doppler echocardiographic study. *Am. Heart J.* 120: 386–391, 1990.
297. Takata, M., S. Beloucif, M. Shimada, and J. L. Robotham. Superior and inferior vena caval flows during respiration: pathogenesis of Kussmaul's sign. *Am. J. Physiol.* 262 (*Heart Circ. Physiol.* 31): H763–H770, 1992.
298. Takata, M., and J. L. Robotham. Ventricular external constraint by the lung and pericardium during positive end-expiratory pressure. *Am. Rev. Respir. Dis.* 143: 872–875, 1991.
299. Takata, M., and J. L. Robotham. Effects of inspiratory diaphragmatic descent on inferior vena caval venous return. *J. Appl. Physiol.* 72: 597–607, 1992.
300. Takata, M., R. A. Wise, and J. L. Robotham. Effects of abdominal pressure on venous return: Abdominal vascular zone conditions. *J. Appl. Physiol.* 69: 1961–1972, 1990.
301. Takemoto, K. A., L. Bernstein, J. F. Lopez, D. Marshak, S. H. Rahimtoola, and P. A. N. Chandraratna. Abnormalities of diastolic filling of the left ventricle associated with aging are less pronounced in exercise-trained individuals. *Am. Heart J.* 124: 143–148, 1992.
302. Takenaka, K., Y. Suzuki, K. Kawakubo, Y. Haruna, R. Yanagibori, H. Kashihara, T. Igarashi, F. Watanabe, M. Omata, F. Bonde-Petersen, and A. Gunji. Cardiovascular effects of 20 days rest in healthy young subjects. *Acta Physiol. Scand.* 150 (Suppl. 616): 59–63, 1994.
303. Templeton, G. H., R. R. Ecker, and J. H. Mitchell. Left ventricular stiffness during diastole and systole: the influence of changes in volume and inotropic state. *Cardiovasc. Res.* 6: 95–100, 1972.
304. Templeton, G. H., K. Wildenthal, and J. H. Mitchell. Influence of coronary blood flow on left ventricular contractility and stiffness. *Am. J. Physiol.* 223: 1216–1220, 1972.
305. Thadani, U., and J. O. Parker. Hemodynamics at rest and during supine and sitting bicycle exercise in normal subjects. *Am. J. Cardiol.* 41: 52–59, 1978.
306. Thomas, S. G., D. H. Paterson, D. A. Cunningham, D. G. McLellan, and W. J. Kostuk. Cardiac output and left ventricular function in response to exercise in older men. *Can J. Physiol. Pharmacol.* 71: 136–144, 1993.
307. Thorley, P. J., K. L. Sheard, and M. R. Rees. A comparison of methods for estimating left ventricular volumes from radionuclide ventriculography. *Physiol. Meas.* 14: 23–32, 1993.
308. Tipton, C. M., R. A. Carey, W. C. Eastin, and H. H. Erickson. A submaximal test for dogs: evaluation of effects of training, detraining, and cage confinements. *J. Appl. Physiol.* 37: 271–275, 1974.
309. Tischler, M. D., M. Rowan, and M. M. LeWinter. Increased left ventricular mass after thoracotomy and pericardiectomy. A role for relief of pericardial constraint? *Circulation* 87: 1921–1927, 1993.
310. Tomai, F., M. Ciavolella, F. Crea, A. Gaspardone, F. Versaci, C. Giannitti, D. Scali, L. Chiariello, and P. A. Gioffre. Left ventricular volumes during exercise in normal subjects and patients with dilated cardiomyopathy assessed by first-pass radionuclide angiography. *Am. J. Cardiol.* 72: 1167–1171, 1993.
311. Tyberg, J. V. Venous modulation of ventricular preload. *Am. Heart J.* 123: 1098–1104, 1992.
312. Tyberg, J. V., and S. E. Baker. Venous capacitance changes in congestive heart failure and exercise. In: *Veins: Their Functional Role in the Circulation*, edited by S. Hirakawa, C. F. Rothe, A. A. Shoukas, and J. V. Tyberg. Tokyo: Springer-Verlag, 1993.
313. Tyberg, J. V., G. C. Taichman, E. R. Smith, N. W. S. Douglas, O. A. Smiseth, and W. J. Keon. The relationship between pericardial pressure and right atrial pressure: an intraoperative study. *Circulation* 73: 428–432, 1986.
314. Van den Bos, G. C., G. Elzinga, N. Westerhof, and N. I. M. Noble. Problems in the use of indices of myocardial contractility. *Cardiovasc. Res.* 7: 834–848, 1973.
315. Van der Velde, E. T., D. Burkhoff, P. Steendijk, J. Karsdon, K. Sagawa, and J. Baan. Nonlinearity of end-systolic pressure-volume relation of canine left ventricle in vivo. *Circulation* 83: 315–327, 1991.
316. Van Lieshout, J. J. *Cardiovascular Reflexes in Orthostatic Disorders.* Amsterdem: Rodopi, 1989.
317. Vanoverschelde, J. L. J., B. Essamri, R. Vanbutsele, A. M. D'Hondt, J. R. Cosyns, J. M. R. Detry, and J. A. Melin. Contribution of left ventricular diastolic function to exercise capacity in normal subjects. *J. Appl. Physiol.* 74: 2225–2233, 1993.
318. Vatner, S. F. Effects of exercise on distribution of regional blood flows and resistances. In: *The Peripheral Circulations*, edited by R. Zelis. San Francisco: Grune & Stratton, p. 211–233, 1975.
319. Vatner, S. F., D. Franklin, R. L. Van Citters, and E. Braunwald. Effects of carotid sinus nerve stimulation on blood-flow distribution in conscious dogs at rest and during exercise. *Circ. Res.* 27: 495–503, 1970.
320. Vitcenda, M., P. Hanson, J. Folts, and M. Besozzi. Impairment of left ventricular function during maximal isometric dead lifting. *J. Appl. Physiol.* 69: 2062–2066, 1990.
321. Wade, O. L., B. Combes, A. W. Childs, H. O. Wheeler, A. Cournand, and S. E. Bradley. The effects of exercise on the splanchnic blood flow and splanchnic blood volume in normal man. *Clin. Sci.* 15: 457–463, 1956.
322. Wagner, P. D., G. E. Gale, R. E. Moon, J. R. Toore-Bueno, B. W. Stolp, and H. A. Saltzman. Pulmonary gas exchange in humans exercising at sea level and simulated altitude. *J. Appl. Physiol.* 61: 260–270, 1986.
323. Walker, A. A., J. S. Janicki, K. T. Weber, R. O. Russell, and C. E. Rackley. Equations for the calculation of mean ejection pressure. *Cardiovasc. Res.* 7: 567–571, 1973.
324. Wallace, A. G. The heart in athletes. In: *The Heart, Arteries and Veins*, edited by J. W. Hurst. New York: McGraw-Hill, Inc., 1982, p. 1540–1545.
325. Wallis, T., J. L. Robotham, R. Compean, and M. K. Kindred. Mechanical heart-lung interaction with positive end-expiratory pressure. *J. Appl. Physiol.* 54: 1039–1047, 1983.
326. Weber, K. T., C. G. Brilla, and J. S. Janicki. Myocardial fibrosis: functional significance and regulatory factors. *Cardiovasc. Res.* 27: 341–348, 1993.
327. Weber, K. T. Gas transport and the cardiopulmonary unit. In: *Cardiopulmonary Exercise Testing: Physiologic Principles and Clinical Application*, edited by K. T. Weber and J. S. Janicki. Philadelphia: W. B. Saunders Company, 1986, p. 15–33.
328. Weber, K. T., and J. S. Janicki. The heart as a muscle-pump system and the concept of heart failure. *Am. Heart J.* 98: 371–384, 1979.
329. Weber, K. T., J. S. Janicki, and L. L. Hefner. Left ventricular force-length relations of isovolumic and ejecting contractions. *Am. J. Physiol.* 231: 337–343, 1976.
330. Weber, K. T., J. S. Janicki, W. C. Hunter, S. Shroff, E. S. Pearlman, and A. P. Fishman. The contractile behavior of

the heart and its functional coupling to the circulation. *Prog. Cardiovasc. Dis.* 24: 375–400, 1982.

331. Weber, K. T., J. S. Janicki, R. C. Reeves, L. L. Hefner, and T. J. Reeves. Determinants of stroke volume in the isolated canine heart. *J. Appl. Physiol.* 37: 742–747, 1974.
332. Weber, K. T., J. S. Janicki, S. Shroff, and A. P. Fishman. Contractile mechanics and interaction of the right and left ventricles. *Am. J. Cardiol.* 47: 686–695, 1981.
333. Weisfeldt, M. L., J. W. Frederiksen, F. C. P. Yin, and J. L. Weiss. Evidence of incomplete left ventricular relaxation in the dog: prediction from time constant for isovolumic pressure fall. *J. Clin. Invest.* 62: 1296–1302, 1978.
334. Weisfeldt, M. L., W. A. Loeven, and N. W. Schock. Resting and active mechanical properties of trabeculae carnae from aged male rats *Am. J. Physiol.* 220: 1921–1927, 1971.
335. Wexler, L. D., D. H. Bergel, I. T. Gabe, G. S. Makin, and C. J. Mills. Velocity of blood flow in normal human venae cavae. *Circ. Res.* 23: 349–359, 1968.
336. Whittenberger, J. L., M. McGregor, E. Berglund and H. G. Borst. Influence of state of inflation of the lung on pulmonary vascular resistance. *J. Appl. Physiol.* 15: 878–882, 1960.
337. Willeput, R., C. Rondeaux, and A. De Troyer. Breathing affects venous return from legs in humans. *J. Appl. Physiol.* 57: 971–976, 1984.
338. Williams, C. A. Effect of muscle mass on the pressor response in man during isometric contractions. *J. Physiol. (Lond.)* 435: 573–584, 1991.
339. Wise, R. A., J. L. Robotham, and W. R. Summer. Effects of spontaneous ventilation on the circulation. *Lung* 159: 175–186, 1981.
340. Wolfe, L. A., D. A. Cunningham, and D. R. Boughner. Physical conditioning effects on cardiac dimensions: a review of echocardiographic studies. *Can. J. Appl. Spont. Sci.* 11: 66–79, 1986.
341. Younes, M., and G. Kivenen. Respiratory mechanics and breathing pattern during and following maximal exercise. *J. Appl. Physiol. Respir. Environ. Exerc. Physiol.* 57: 1773–1782, 1984.
342. Younis, L. T., J. A. Melin, A. R. Robert, and J. M. R. Detry. Influence of age and sex on left ventricular volumes and ejection fraction during upright exercise in normal subjects. *Eur. Heart J.* 11: 916–924, 1990.
343. Younis, L. T., J. A. Melin, J. C. Schoevaerdts, M. Van Dyck, J. M. Detry, A. Robert, C. Chalant, and M. Goenen. Left ventricular systolic function and diastolic filling at rest and during upright exercise after orthotopic heart transplantation: comparison with young and aged normal subjects. *J. Heart Transplant.* 9: 683–692, 1990.
344. Zwissler, B., R. Schosser, C. Schwickert, P. Spengler, M. Weiss, V. Iber, and K. Messmer. Perfusion of the interventricular septum during ventilation with positive end-expiratory pressure. *Crit. Care Med.* 19: 1414–1424, 1991.

16. Control of blood flow to cardiac and skeletal muscle during exercise

M. HAROLD LAUGHLIN — *Department of Veterinary Biomedical Sciences, University of Missouri, Columbia, Missouri*

RONALD J. KORTHUIS — *Department of Physiology and Biophysics, Louisiana State University Medical Center, Shreveport, Louisiana*

DIRK J. DUNCKER — *Experimental Cardiology, Thoraxcenter, Erasmus University Rotterdam, Rotterdam, The Netherlands*

ROBERT J. BACHE — *Department of Medicine, Cardiovascular Division, University of Minnesota Medical School, Minneapolis, Minnesota*

CHAPTER CONTENTS

TO MAINTAIN EXERCISE FOR MORE THAN A FEW SECONDS, adequate blood flow to skeletal muscle is essential. Providing adequate blood flow to skeletal muscle during high-intensity exercise produces the greatest burden on the cardiovascular system of any stress in normal life. As shown in Figure 16.1, only 5–10 ml of blood is distributed to 100 g of quiescent skeletal muscle. During high-intensity exercise, skeletal muscle blood flow can increase to 150–500 ml $\cdot$ min^{-1} $\cdot$ 100 g^{-1} (307, 310, 448, 449). During exercise at various intensities, blood flow is greater in high oxidative skeletal muscles than in low oxidative skeletal muscles (Fig. 16.1). In large mammals, reported peak skeletal muscle blood flows are in the range of 250–400 ml $\cdot$ min^{-1} $\cdot$ 100 g^{-1} (11, 310, 449, 450), whereas in rodents skeletal muscle blood flows approach 500 ml $\cdot$ min^{-1} $\cdot$ 100 g^{-1} [Fig. 16.1; (307, 310)]. Although coronary blood flow is also increased during exercise, the magnitude of increase during high-intensity exercise is only four- to fivefold because coronary flow is about tenfold greater than skeletal muscle blood flow in resting subjects [Figs. 16.2 and 16.3; (53, 76, 314, 350)]. Relative blood flow in skeletal and cardiac muscle of resting subjects and the effects of increasing intensities of exercise on blood flow to these muscles can be appreciated by comparing Figure 16.1 with Figures 16.2 and 16.3. Resting blood flow in skeletal muscle is much less than coronary blood flow at rest, but during high-intensity exercise blood flow to high oxidative skeletal muscle is similar in magnitude to coronary blood flow.

The increases in blood flow to cardiac and skeletal muscle provided during exercise requires a four- to fivefold increase in cardiac output combined with dramatic increases in vascular conductance in these muscles. Figure 16.4 presents the results of measurements of total cardiac output and cardiac and skeletal muscle blood flow in pigs performing voluntary exercise on a treadmill. These data illustrate the dramatic increase in cardiac output that occurs as exercise intensity increases up to an intensity that produces maximal oxygen consumption ($\dot{V}O_{2max}$) and the increase in the fraction of cardiac output distributed to cardiac and skeletal muscle that occurs as exercise intensity increases. As in the studies illustrated in Figure 16.4, humans at rest distribute only 15%–20% of cardiac output to skeletal muscle, while coronary blood flow represents only 4%–5% of total cardiac output (449). During exercise all of the increased cardiac output is distributed to cardiac and skeletal muscle, and muscle blood flow is further increased because blood flow is diverted from viscera and other nonmuscle tissues (Fig. 16.4). Accordingly, during exercise at $\dot{V}O_{2max}$ 85%–90% of cardiac output is distributed to cardiac and skeletal muscle (449). To summarize, adequate blood flow to cardiac and skeletal muscle during exercise is provided by coordinated increases in: (*1*) cardiac activity and venous return (which increase cardiac output); (*2*) vascular resistance in viscera, skin, and other inactive tissues; and (*3*) vascular conductance in cardiac and skeletal muscle. Decreased conductance in nonmuscle tissue combined with increased conductance in muscle tissue alters the regional distribution of cardiac output. These striking changes in cardiac output and its distribution have captured the interest of scientists in this field for many years (449). Mechanisms that regulate cardiac output and its distribution during exercise are discussed in detail in Chapters 15 and 17. In this chapter we discuss mechanisms believed to be responsible for increasing vascular conductance in cardiac and skeletal muscle during dynamic exercise and we review the current state of understanding of the relative importance of these mechanisms. In addition, we discuss exercise training–induced changes in cardiac and skeletal

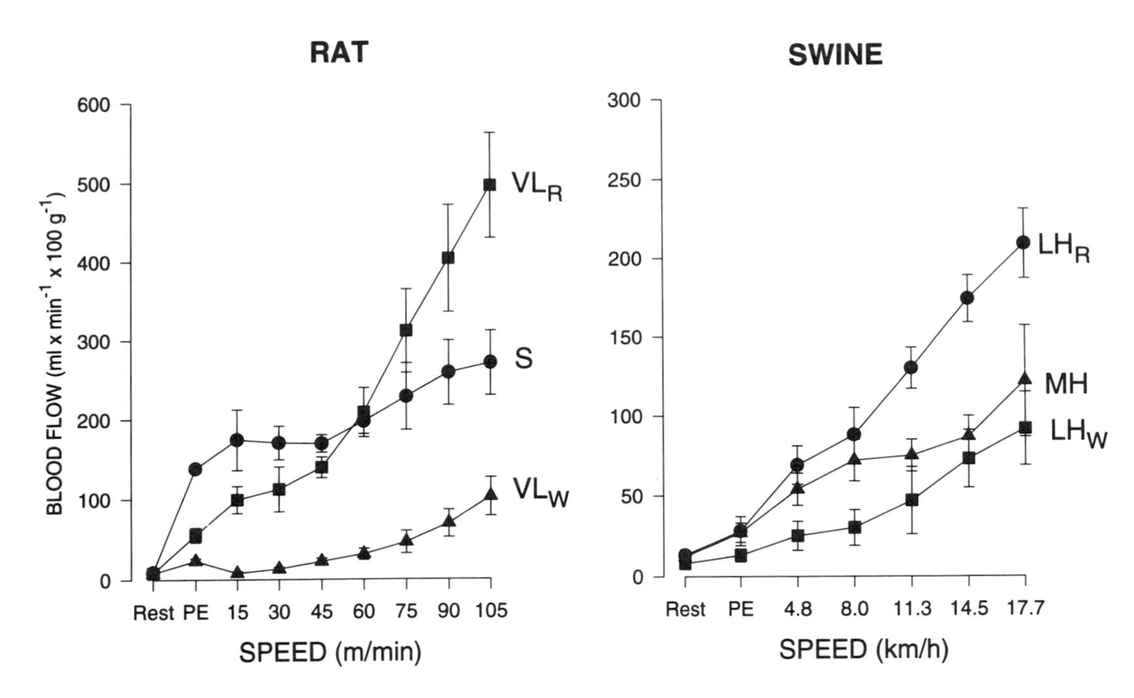

FIG. 16.1. Relationship between blood flow and exercise intensity in skeletal muscles of different fiber-type composition in rats and miniature swine. *A*, Data for the red (VL_R) and white (VL_W) portions of the vastus lateralis muscle and the soleus muscle (S) for rat skeletal muscles are shown on the left. The percentage fiber-type compositions for these muscle are: VL_R = 2% SO (slow-twitch, oxidative), 64% FOG (fast-twitch, oxidative, glycolytic), 34% FG (fast-twitch, glycolytic); VL_W = 0% SO, 1% FOG, 99% FG; S = 77% SO, 23% FOG, 0% FG (311). Rest data are from Laughlin and Armstrong (310) for anesthetized rats. PE = preexercise (i.e. data collected with the animals standing on the treadmill involved in normal activity). PE data and data for rats running on the treadmill at speeds of 15–105 m/min are from Laughlin and Armstrong (311) and Armstrong and Laughlin (25). *B*, Data for the medial head (MH) and the deep (LH_R) and superficial (LH_W) portions of the long head of triceps brachii muscles of miniature swine are presented on the right. The percentage fiber-type compositions for these muscles are: LH_R = 46% SO, 43% FOG, 12% FG; LH_W = 8% SO, 38% FOG, 54% FG; MH = 91% SO, 9% FOG, 0% SO. Rest data are unpublished observations from anesthetized pigs. PE data and data for pigs running on a treadmill at speeds of 4.8–17.7 km/h are from Armstrong et al. $\dot{V}O_{2max}$ was demonstrated at a running speed of 14.5 km/h in these pigs (20).

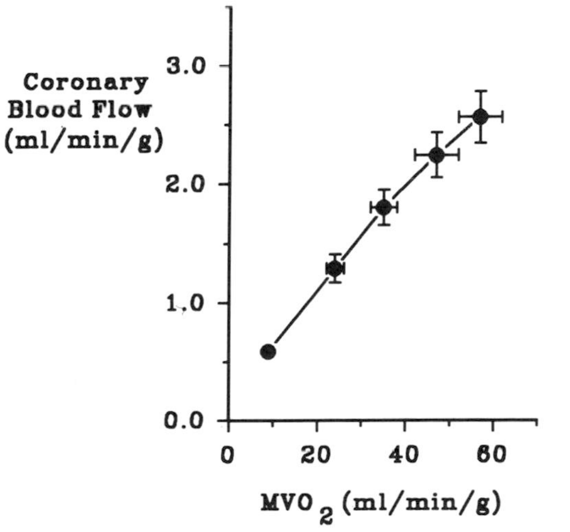

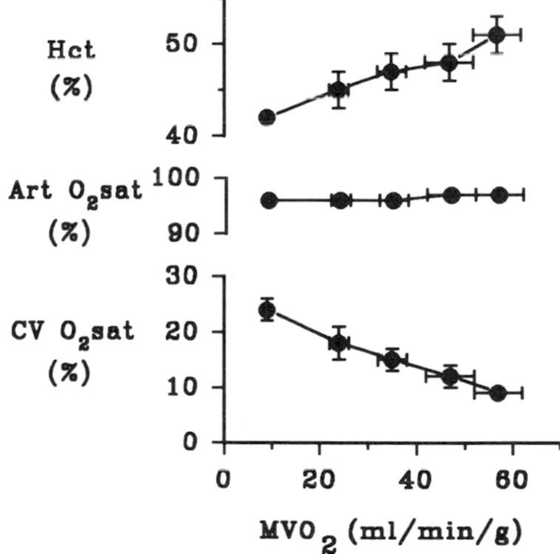

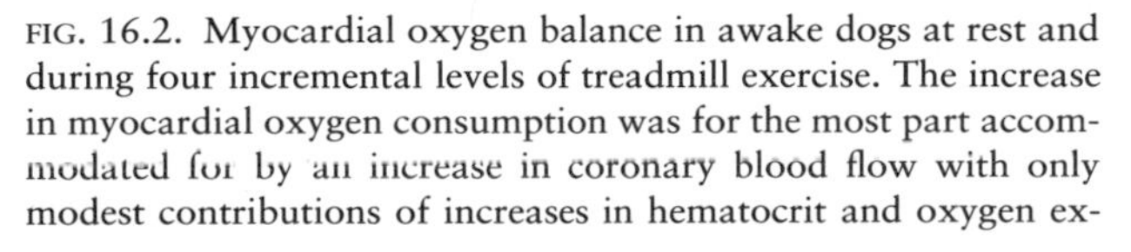

FIG. 16.2. Myocardial oxygen balance in awake dogs at rest and during four incremental levels of treadmill exercise. The increase in myocardial oxygen consumption was for the most part accommodated for by an increase in coronary blood flow with only modest contributions of increases in hematocrit and oxygen extraction. MVO_2, myocardial oxygen consumption; Hct, hematocrit; Art O_2 sat, arterial oxygen saturation; CVO_2 sat = coronary venous oxygen saturation. Data are mean SEM, and are from von Restorff et al. (557).

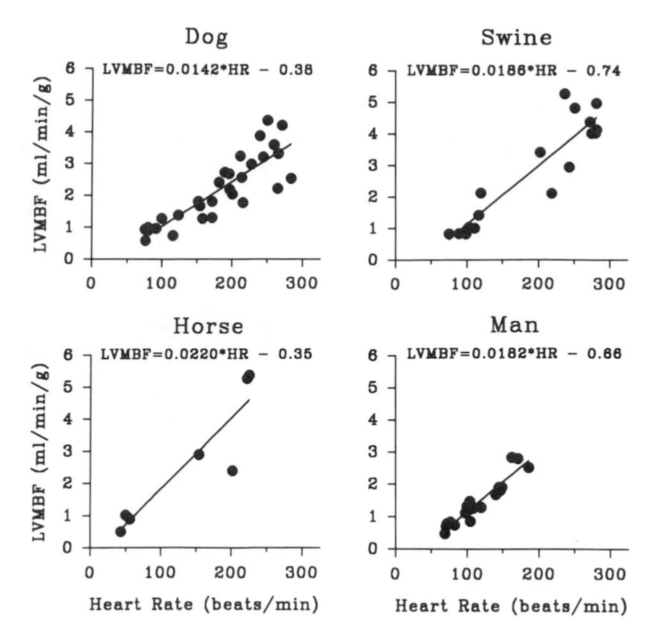

FIG. 16.3. Relationship between heart rate (HR) and left ventricular myocardial blood flow (LVMBF) at rest and during treadmill exercise in dogs (37, 38, 43, 46, 53, 406, 557), swine (75, 76, 136, 318, 393, 460, 461, 568), horses (22, 350, 410), and humans (150, 217, 236, 266, 268, 278, 392, 433).

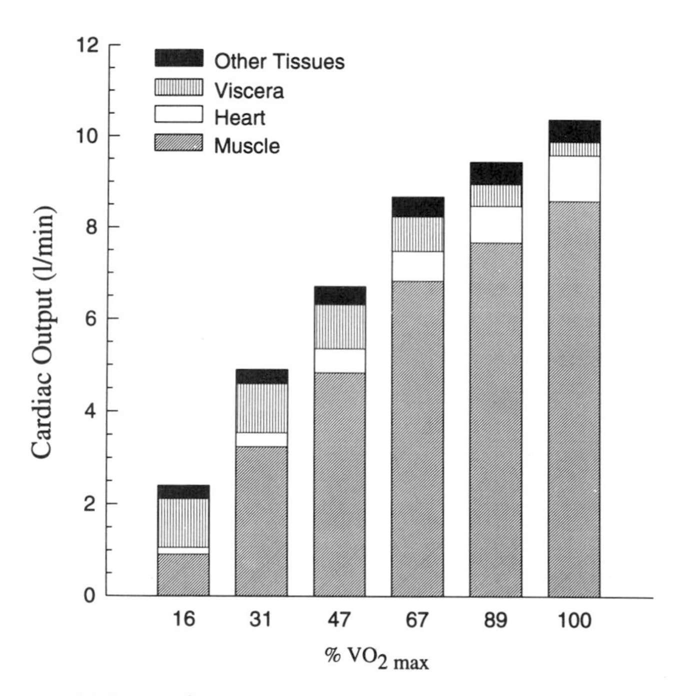

FIG. 16.4. Distribution of cardiac output to skeletal muscle (muscle), heart, visceral organs, and other tissues of miniature swine as a function of oxygen consumption, over the full range of oxygen uptake from rest to $\dot{V}O_{2max}$. Data are from Armstrong et al. (20). Note that blood flow to the heart and skeletal muscle increases with increases in exercise intensity, whereas visceral blood flows decrease.

muscle vascular beds and the control of vascular conductance in striated muscle tissues.

HEMODYNAMICS AND CONTROL OF BLOOD FLOW

Determinants of Vascular Resistance

The flow of blood in any tissue is governed by perfusion pressure (i.e., arterial minus venous pressure) and vascular resistance to blood flow. Since mean arterial and venous pressures are normally maintained within narrow limits, blood flow control is accomplished in large part by variations in vascular resistance. Alterations in vascular resistance are due to changes in the caliber of resistance vessels which, in turn, are regulated by the contractile activity of vascular smooth muscle (213, 379, 505, 506). Since vascular resistance is determined largely by the level of contraction in vascular smooth muscle in the wall of resistance vessels, it is often referred to as vascular or vasomotor tone. Vasomotor tone is influenced by a multitude of factors that can be divided into two general categories: central cardiovascular control mechanisms and local vascular control mechanisms. Central cardiovascular control mechanisms can be considered to be designed for the maintenance of systemic blood pressure and central cardiovascular homeostasis (Chapters 15 and 17). In contrast, local vascular control mechanisms can be considered to be designed for the maintenance of tissue homeostasis.

Skeletal muscle blood flow is low at rest (5–10 ml $\cdot$ min^{-1} $\cdot$ 100 g^{-1}) compared to coronary blood flow (Figs. 16.1 through 16.3) because of high vasomotor tone (Fig. 16.1). Vasomotor tone in the vasculature of resting skeletal muscle is determined by inherent myogenic activity of the resistance vessels and relatively high sympathetic nerve activity (171, 245, 247, 264, 310, 367, 451, 491, 494). Sympathetic tone results from the relatively constant discharge of norepinephrine by sympathetic postganglionic neurons that terminate near vascular smooth muscle cells in skeletal muscle resistance arteries (491, 494). The released norepinephrine binds to α-adrenergic receptors on vascular smooth muscle cells causing contraction and, therefore, increases in vascular resistance. The importance of sympathetic tone in determining basal vascular resistance in skeletal muscle is illustrated by the fact that interruption of sympathetic tone (by denervation or with α-adrenergic–blocking drugs) results in a 50%–100% increase in blood flow to resting skeletal muscle (171, 245, 247, 264, 310, 367, 451, 491, 494). This increase in flow is transient in that 12–24 h following denervation, resting blood flow returns to normal levels by currently unknown mechanisms (247). Although skeletal muscle blood flow is quite low at rest, it increases during exercise in proportion to exercise intensity (Figs. 16.1 and 16.4). Thus, in both skeletal and cardiac muscle, blood flow increases with increasing exercise intensity (Figs. 16.1 through 16.3). As described below, these increases in blood flow are the result of interactions of central control mechanisms, locally mediated vasodilation of resistance vessels, and the mechanical effects of muscle contraction.

Central Vascular Control Mechanisms

Central control of vascular resistance is mediated by neural control and hormonal control systems. Neural control of vascular resistance in skeletal muscle is mediated primarily by the sympathetic nervous system. Both the sympathetic and parasympathetic nervous systems can influence coronary vascular resistance. Although hormonal factors can influence vascular resistance in cardiac and skeletal muscle, as in responses to orthostasis and other systemic cardiovascular stresses, they do not appear to be foremost in importance in the phenomenon of exercise hyperemia in these tissues. Similarly, neural control mechanisms do not appear to be the cause of exercise hyperemia. However, sympathetic vasomotor tone is important in modulating regional coronary vascular resistance and coronary blood flow distribution. Also, sympathetic adrenergic vasoconstriction contributes to the milieu that regulates increases in vascular conductance in exercising skeletal muscle. Current information indicates that the increases in blood flow to cardiac and skeletal muscle that occur during exercise are the result of local vascular control systems within the muscle tissue. Central control mechanisms are responsible for regulating cardiac activity and regional vascular tone throughout the body to maintain systemic vascular homeostasis during exercise. During high-intensity exercise, central and local vascular control mechanisms within skeletal muscle vasculature can become antagonistic if the need for blood flow to the tissues exceeds the ability of the cardiovascular system to provide cardiac output. The interesting and important interplay between central and local control mechanisms under these conditions is discussed in detail in Chapter 17.

Local Vascular Control Mechanisms

There is a close relationship between myocardial metabolic rate (often measured as myocardial oxygen consumption) and coronary blood flow (164). In resting mammals, coronary blood flow is generally between 70 and 100 ml · min^{-1} · 100 g^{-1} because, even at rest, the heart must pump resting cardiac output. As the work of the heart increases during exercise, coronary blood flow increases in proportion (Figs. 16.2 and 16.3). Blood flow and oxygen consumption also appear to be tightly linked in skeletal muscle tissue. Blood flow is very low in resting skeletal muscle, in part because the muscle is inactive. The increase in blood flow observed with initiation of rhythmic contractile activity in skeletal muscle is called exercise hyperemia (also often referred to as functional or active hyperemia) (49, 180, 192, 206, 245–251, 310, 370, 449, 491, 508). It is possible that the mechanisms responsible for linking blood flow responses to metabolic rate are similar in cardiac and skeletal muscle. High vasomotor tone in resting skeletal muscle is important, since its presence makes possible the graded vasomotor responses required to exquisitely regulate capillary perfusion in proportion to the metabolic demand when muscular activity is increased. Indeed, the prevailing view is that skeletal muscle functional hyperemia and normal coronary blood flow are mediated primarily by local control mechanisms and that other control systems are superimposed on these dominant control mechanisms (49, 92, 193, 206, 370, 436, 491, 501, 509, 514). Local vascular control mechanisms involved in exercise hyperemia include metabolic control, myogenic control, endothelium-mediated control, propagated responses, and the muscle pump.

Metabolic Hypothesis. According to the metabolic hypothesis of vascular control, tissue metabolism and arteriolar smooth muscle constitute a local control system that provides the coupling between blood flow and tissue nutritional requirements (104, 375, 491, 508, 509). That is, the increased metabolic activity associated with striated muscle contraction results in an outpouring of metabolites into the interstitial fluid. These metabolites diffuse to the large and small arterioles and functional precapillary sphincters to cause vasodilation and capillary recruitment. It has also been proposed that metabolites initiate vasodilation in the smallest resistance arteries and that this vasodilation is propagated throughout the vascular tree (479–483). In skeletal muscle, metabolic vasodilators also appear to compete with sympathetic tone and/or to reduce norepinephrine release at sympathetic nerve terminals, producing what has been called functional sympatholysis (280, 281, 434, 548). The increased blood flow and oxygen extraction that result from metabolic vasodilation increase oxygen supply to a level compatible with tissue oxygen demand. Thus, the metabolic hypothesis predicts that oxygen delivery to the tissues, not blood flow per se, is the controlled variable producing exercise hyperemia. The importance of metabolic control in regulation of blood flow to striated muscle has been discussed in detail previously (49, 61, 128, 129, 132, 164, 190, 192, 206, 224, 245, 247, 275, 310, 369, 370, 374, 436, 480, 491, 501, 509, 514). Therefore, our discussion focuses on data and observations reported since 1986.

Myogenic Vascular Control. The myogenic theory of local blood flow control is based on the assumption that vascular resistance is determined in part by transmural pressure at the arteriolar level because of the effect of stretch on vascular smooth muscle tone (264, 275, 367, 377, 491). In essence, this theory proposes the existence of arteriolar tension receptors that modulate vascular smooth muscle tone in response to changes in transmural pressure. Because vascular wall tension is determined by the product of transmural pressure and vessel diameter, one would predict, on the basis of the myogenic theory, that a decrease in vascular transmural pressure will result in arteriolar vasodilation and reduced vascular resistance. The myogenic mechanism may contribute to the relaxation of vascular smooth muscle in arterioles and precapillary sphincters of contracting cardiac and skeletal muscle. Thus, muscle contraction elevates extravascular pressure, thereby reducing transmural pressure of blood vessels (222, 277, 282, 417). The ensuing reduction in wall tension may provide a stimulus for myogenic vasodilation. In skeletal muscle it appears that myogenic relaxation of vascular smooth muscle may play a more important role in the vascular responses to tetanic contractions than in the arteriolar vasodilation induced by twitch contractions (34, 187, 377).

Endothelium-Mediated Vascular Control. The revelation of the importance of the endothelium in regulating vascular smooth muscle has had a major impact on concepts of peripheral vascular control (114, 117, 142, 168, 292, 369, 373, 374). Evidence indicates that the endothelium mediates and/or participates in vasodilator responses, vasoconstrictor responses, and structural vascular adaptation in response to several simuli (1, 142, 172, 374). The endothelium is able to sense chemical substances within the blood as well as physical forces imparted to blood vessel walls, such as shear stress and vessel stretch, and is able to initiate responses to these chemical and/or physical signals by releasing substances that modulate vascular tone and/or blood vessel structure.

Vascular endothelium releases vasodilator substances in response to a variety of signals. At least two such endothelium-derived vasodilator substances have been established: prostacyclin (PGI_2) and endothelium-derived relaxing factor (EDRF), which appears to be nitric oxide (NO) or a nitroso compound. There is also evidence of other endothelium-derived vasodilator substances such as endothelium-derived hyperpolarization factor (113, 142, 148, 149, 168). It appears that one intracellular signal for release of PGI_2 and EDRF from endothelial cells is an increase in free Ca^{2+} in the endothelial cells. Intracellular free Ca^{2+} concentration may be increased either as a result of receptor/signal transduction pathways for various agents (113, 168) or due to shear stress–induced events (flow-induced vasodilation) (113, 115, 252, 270, 290, 292, 422). Evidence indicates that endothelium-mediated vascular control is important in the coronary circulation (6, 237, 298, 408, 564, 578) and in skeletal muscle vascular beds at rest (369) and during muscle contraction, perhaps through flow-induced vasodilation (218, 270, 290–292, 422, 452, 528). There is also evidence that the relative importance of endothelium-mediated vascular control may vary regionally throughout the vascular tree in skeletal muscle tissue (218, 369, 414).

An endothelium-dependent local control phenomenon that may be involved in the regulation of blood flow in cardiac and skeletal muscle is flow-induced vasodilation. Flow-induced vasodilation is the dilation observed in arteries that appears to be the direct result of increases in blood flow. It has been demonstrated in both coronary (237, 300) and femoral (252, 420) arteries and is believed to be caused by a local (within the blood vessel wall) mechanism. Most evidence indicates that flow-induced vasodilation is dependent on the presence of a normal endothelium in the artery (252, 300, 422, 452). Also, Kuo et al. (298) recently demonstrated flow-induced vasodilation in isolated coronary resistance vessels. It is possible that endothelium-dependent, flow-induced vasodilation is an integral and important mechanism in regulation of cardiac and skeletal muscle vascular beds.

Propagated Vasodilation and Coordination of Vasodilation. Hilton (223) observed dilation of cat femoral artery during contraction of the gastrocnemius muscle and proposed that vasodilator signals were propagated from the microcirculation by conduction of the response along smooth muscle cells of the arterial media. It now appears that such dilation of femoral arteries is likely endothelium-dependent flow-induced vasodilation as described above. However, Duling and Berne demonstrated propagation of dilation along arterioles of hamster cheek pouch microcirculation that was not mediated by changes in flow (131). More recently, Segal and co-workers (479–484) formulated the concept that conducted or propagated vasodilation may coordinate blood flow and red cell distribution, and decrease perfusion heterogeneity in skeletal muscle during conditions such as exercise. This concept is based on the observation that local application of vasodilator at discrete points along the arteriolar network elicits an increase in vascular caliber that is propagated along the arteriole to parent and daughter vessels. Since conducted vasodilation is inhibited by agents that uncouple cell–cell communication through gap junctions, these investigators proposed that the spread of vasodilation is related to electrotonic propagation across these points of communication between adjacent endothelial and/or vascular smooth muscle cells (479–484). This phenomenon serves to shift the locus of vascular control upstream from distal arterioles into feeding arteries and to minimize the potential for more dilated vessels to steal flow from less dilated vessels during increased metabolic demand (480, 482). The phenomenon of propagated vasodilation has not been clearly demonstrated in the coronary circulation.

The Muscle Pump Mechanism. An important difference between the determinants of vascular conductance in striated muscle and nonmuscle tissues is the effects of muscle contraction and the associated effects of extravascular compression on conductance. Extravascular compression expels blood from the venous vasculature and impedes inflow of blood into the arterial vasculature. In skeletal muscle the net effect of these forces appears to be enhanced perfusion of the muscle, while in the coronary circulation the net effect appears to be decreased conductance.

The phrase "muscle pump" refers to contraction-induced, rhythmic propulsion of blood from skeletal muscle vasculature that facilitates venous return to the heart and perfusion of skeletal muscle. Muscular contraction produces compression of the veins, causing blood to flow out of compressed segments. Blood can only flow out of compressed venous segments towards the heart due to the orientation of venous valves. Of course, if the muscle maintains a tetanic contraction, the net effect is increased resistance to blood flow. Therefore, the muscle pump mechanism only exists during rhythmic contractions. Rhythmic contraction produces a pumping action on the venous circulation in skeletal muscle, imparting energy to the blood, ejecting it out of the veins. The refilling of the "muscle pump" occurs during muscle relaxation (49, 169, 170, 307, 341, 424, 425, 492, 517, 521). It has been proposed, based largely on results of Folkow et al. (169) that, during relaxations of skeletal muscle, pressures in the venules and deep small veins are negative (307). This hypothesis is also consistent with the fact that the muscles relax rapidly (50–100 ms) so that the compressive force is suddenly removed. Because the walls of small veins are fused to surrounding muscle tissue, negative pressure has to occur when veins are pulled open by relaxing muscle. The magnitude of the pressure fall observed in these veins and the duration of the decrease should be determined by how rapidly blood flows from the arterial side through the capillaries into the empty venous segments. Since Folkow et al. (169) observed that arterial inflow continued throughout the relaxation period and there was no femoral venous outflow during relaxation, it appears that the venous segments do not refill instantaneously. It seems feasible that after contraction there is a wave of venous segment filling (and venous pressure increases) moving from the first venous valves in the small veins to the systemic veins. If sufficient time is allowed before the next contraction, the effect of the previous contraction would be dissipated. On the other hand, if another contraction occurs before venous refilling is complete, then venous pressures will remain depressed. Estimates indicate that during treadmill exercise in rats, the muscle pump provides as much as 30%–60% of the total energy for perfusion of the soleus and red portion of the gastrocnemius muscles, respectively (307). The muscle pump appears to provide a substantial amount of energy for muscle perfusion in exercising humans as well (341, 450, 517). Although many of the mechanical effects of contraction are similar in cardiac and skeletal muscle, the muscle pump effect has not been demonstrated to facilitate perfusion in the coronary circulation. The major effect of cardiac contraction appears to be increased resistance to blood flow in the coronary circulation. However, coronary venous flow occurs during systole and arterial inflow occurs primarily during diastole in a manner similar to that observed in rhythmically contracting skeletal muscle.

CORONARY VASCULAR RESPONSE TO EXERCISE

Over a wide range of cardiac activity, blood flow to the heart is regulated in response to changing myocardial demands to maintain a high level of oxygen extraction. Energy production in the normally functioning heart is primarily dependent on oxidative phosphorylation, with less than 10% of adenosine triphosphate (ATP) production resulting from glycolytic metabolism (402). Because of this dependence upon oxidative energy production, increases of cardiac activity are dependent on almost instantaneous parallel increases of oxygen availability. The hemodynamic adjustments that result in increased cardiac output and arterial pressure during exercise cause increases in each of the major determinants of myocardial oxygen demand including *(1)* heart rate, *(2)* systolic wall stress, and *(3)* contractility.

Effect of Exercise on Left Ventricular Blood Flow

Comparisons of myocardial oxygen consumption during heavy exercise with similar increases in heart rate produced by cardiac pacing indicate that 30%–40% of the increase in coronary blood flow that occurs during exercise can be attributed to the increased heart rate (266, 551). Systolic wall stress (force per unit cross-sectional area) increases during exercise in proportion to the increased arterial pressure and secondary to a modest increase of left ventricular end-diastolic volume associated with the increased central blood volume (242, 423, 549). Stroke volume is augmented, as the increased contractility during exercise causes the ventricle to eject to a smaller end-systolic volume (242, 423, 549). Increases in contractility also increase the rate of left ventricular ejection so that despite a greater stroke volume, the duration of systole decreases to accommodate the higher heart rates. The increase in contractility is due to β-adrenergic activation as well as the direct positive inotropic effect of heart rate (treppe) (288). Studies in which the inotropic effect produced by β-adrenergic nervous system was blocked with propranolol while heart rate was maintained constant by atrial pacing suggest that ~40% of the increased myocardial oxygen demands during exercise can be attributed to adrenergically mediated effects on contractility (56, 150, 386).

Increased myocardial oxygen demands during exercise are met principally by augmenting coronary blood flow. In some species such as the dog (276, 552), horse (153, 410) and sheep (385) oxygen delivery is facilitated by a prominent increase in hemoglobin (by up to 20%–50%). The hemoglobin concentration in swine (212, 318) and especially in man (447, 450) increases much less. Although myocardial oxygen extraction also increases during exercise (37, 63, 189, 217, 276, 278, 340, 371, 392, 556, 557), the high level of basal oxygen extraction (typically 70%–80% during resting conditions) limits further increases. In chronically instrumented dogs, von Restorff et al. (557) found that an increase of myocardial oxygen consumption from 0.09 ± 0.01 at rest to 0.57 ± 0.05 ml · min^{-1} · g^{-1} during heavy treadmill exercise was provided by a 434% increase of coronary blood flow, an increase of arterial oxygen content from 20 ± 1 to 23 ± 1 ml/dl, and an increase of myocardial oxygen extraction from $75 \pm 2\%$ to $93 \pm 1\%$ (Fig. 16.2). Thus, the principal mechanism for augmenting myocardial oxygen delivery is by increasing coronary blood flow and, as a result, coronary flow is strongly correlated with myocardial oxygen consumption. The increase in myocardial blood flow results from a combination of coronary vasodilation, with a decrease of coronary vascular resistance to 30%–50% of the resting level, and a higher coronary driving pressure that results from a 20%–30% increase in mean arterial pressure (46, 236, 276, 392, 410, 433, 556, 557).

Magnitude of the Increase in Coronary Blood Flow during Exercise. Left ventricular myocardial blood flow during resting conditions in chronically instrumented awake animals and in normal human subjects is generally reported in the range of 0.5–1.4 ml · min^{-1} · g^{-1} of myocardium (22, 37, 38, 43, 46, 53, 136, 278, 406, 410, 459–461, 557, 568). The values reported by Sanders et al. (459) are for total heart flow and thus are lower values than from other studies in which left ventricular flow is reported. The wide range of resting values of left ventricular flow in animals appears to be partially related to the state of alertness. Animals conditioned to rest quietly in the laboratory have the lowest reported values, whereas animals standing on a treadmill ready to run tend to have higher heart rates and higher coronary flow rates. Dynamic exercise increases coronary blood flow in proportion to the heart rate, with peak values during maximal exercise typically three to five times the resting level (350, 410, 459–461, 547, 557, 568). The strong correlation between coronary blood flow and heart rate occurs because heart rate is a common multiplier for the other determinants of myocardial oxygen demand, which are computed on a per-beat basis. Regression analysis of published myocardial blood flow data against heart rate demonstrate remarkably similar relationships between human, canine, equine, and porcine data during dynamic exercise (Fig. 16.3). All available studies of left ventricular blood flow in dogs, swine, and horses undergoing treadmill exercise were pooled for these regression analyses (22, 37, 38, 43, 46, 53, 75, 76, 136, 278, 318, 350, 393, 406, 410, 460, 461, 557, 568). Data from humans were obtained from young healthy male subjects performing upright bicycle exercise (150, 217, 236, 266, 268, 278, 392, 433).

Blood Oxygen-Carrying Capacity

Importance of splenic contraction. In the dog, horse, and sheep oxygen delivery to the myocardium (and skeletal muscle) is facilitated by prominent increases in hemoglobin concentration during exercise and the resultant increase in oxygen-carrying capacity of arterial blood. The hemoglobin concentration (or hematocrit) increases because exercise elicits splenic contraction that expresses erythrocyte-rich blood into the general circulation. Thus, dogs performing near maximal treadmill exercise have been reported to sustain a 12%–21% increase in hematocrit (276, 557). Similarly, Vatner et al. (552) reported a 23% increase in hematocrit during heavy free running exercise in dogs that was abolished by splenectomy. Manohar (350) reported that in ponies hemoglobin increased from 11.4 g/dl at rest to 16.9 g/dl at maximal exercise, a 48% increase. This increase in hemoglobin concentration resulted principally from splenic contraction, since in splenectomized ponies hemoglobin content increased from 12.3 g/dl at rest to 13.9 g/dl at maximal exercise, an increase of only 13%. Augmentation of the arterial oxygen content is an important response to exercise in normal ponies, since splenectomized ponies had diminished work capacity and higher myocardial blood flow rates at similar workloads. Furthermore, normal ponies had residual coronary vasodilator reserve in response to adenosine infusion even during maximal exercise, while in splenectomized ponies vasodilator reserve was exhausted in the subendocardium during heavy exercise (350). In sheep, hemoglobin concentration increased from 9.1 ± 0.4 g/dl at rest to 13.1 ± 0.8 g/dl during maximal exercise (385). Pretreatment with the nonselective α-adrenergic receptor blocker phenoxybenzamine blunted the increase from 8.9 ± 1.2 g/dl to 11.1 ± 0.7 g/dl, and this was associated with an attenuated maximum total-body oxygen consumption, indicating that contraction of the spleen is mediated by α-adrenergic receptor activation during exercise. In man (87) and swine (20, 212, 318) the hemoglobin concentration increases by no more than 15% in response to exercise. In man this is principally due to a decrease in plasma volume resulting from extravasation of fluid from the capillaries rather than to splenic contraction (210, 446).

Arterial desaturation. Arterial oxygen tension and saturation are unaltered during submaximal and maximal exercise in normal humans (87), but in endurance athletes with a higher maximum total body oxygen consumption, decreases in arterial oxygen tension have been reported (118, 536). Arterial oxygen tensions were not changed during maximal exercise in chronically instrumented dogs (212, 556) or ponies (350), but a 7–10 mm Hg decrease in arterial oxygen tension was reported in chronically instrumented swine (20, 212). Small changes in arterial oxygen tension would contribute very little to the arterial oxygen content, since the oxygen hemoglobin dissociation curve operates at its upper plateau in arterial blood even during resting conditions.

Myocardial Oxygen Extraction

Relation to myocardial oxygen consumption. Exercise results in an increase of myocardial oxygen extraction, with widening of the arteriovenous oxygen difference and a decrease in coronary venous oxygen content (37, 109, 217, 236, 278, 522, 557, 567). In young normal male human subjects who performed bicycle exercise to achieve heart rates of 171 bpm (approximately 85% of predicted maximum heart rate), coronary sinus oxygen content decreased from 8.5 ± 1.6 ml/dl at rest to 6.6 ± 0.7 ml/dl at peak exercise (22% decrease) (278). Similar findings have been reported from other groups during heavy exercise (217, 236), whereas studies in which lesser exercise loads were imposed have resulted in smaller or insignificant increases of myocardial oxygen extraction (63, 340, 433). It is possible that the relatively light levels of exercise used in the latter studies can account for the lesser increases of oxygen extraction. Von Restorff et al. (556) reported that heavy treadmill exercise in dogs, which increased heart rate to 284 bpm, increased myocardial oxygen extraction from $75 \pm 2\%$ at rest to $93 \pm 1\%$ during exercise. Bache and Dai (37) observed a decrease in coronary sinus oxygen tension from 21 ± 2 mm Hg to 13 ± 1 mm Hg over a similar exercise range. Heiss et al. (217) observed that coronary venous oxygen content decreased by 8% with no change in coronary venous oxygen tension, suggesting that a rightward shift of the hemoglobin oxygen dissociation curve may facilitate oxygen availability to the myocardium during exercise in man. A rightward shift can be caused by a decrease in blood pH in man and swine due to lactate production from working skeletal muscle (212). However, in dogs the blood pH did not change even during maximal exercise (212) and therefore cannot contribute to a rightward shift of the dissociation curve.

Vasodilator reserve. The increased oxygen extraction evident in coronary venous blood of exercising subjects indicates that the increase of myocardial blood flow during high-intensity exercise does not fully compensate for the increased oxygen demands. Failure of blood flow to fully meet the increase in myocardial oxygen consumption is not the result of exhaustion of coronary vasodilator reserve during exercise, since a further increase in coronary blood flow can be elicited with pharmacologic or ischemic vasodilator stimuli (557, 568). Thus, during maximal treadmill exercise in dogs and swine, a brief total coronary occlusion has been shown to result in reactive hyperemia, with a further increase in blood flow (557, 568). Furthermore, intravenous administration of adenosine to dogs and swine resulted in a 15%–26% increase in myocardial blood flow during maximum exercise, despite a significant drop in arterial pressure (76, 461, 568). When the results were expressed in terms of coronary resistance, adenosine resulted in a $20 \pm 1\%$ further decrease in coronary vascular resistance in swine during maximal exercise (568). Similarly, dipyridamole administered intravenously or into the left atrium of dogs or swine during near maximal or maximal treadmill exercise caused a 20%–46% further increase in myocardial blood flow (53, 314). These studies demonstrate that in the normal heart substantial vasodilator reserve exists even during maximal exercise.

Neural control. Adrenergic vasoconstrictor mechanisms restrain the increase in coronary blood flow during exercise, thereby contributing to the increased oxygen extraction. Thus, nonselective α-adrenergic blockade with phentolamine or selective α_1-adrenergic blockade with prazosin increased myocardial blood flow during exercise; this was accompanied by decreased myocardial oxygen extraction and increased coronary venous oxygen tension (39, 41, 110, 219). However, α-adrenergic blockade did not completely eliminate the increase in myocardial oxygen extraction that occurred during exercise; it is unclear whether this resulted from incomplete blockade, from other unidentified factors that restrain coronary vasodilation during exercise, or because generation of an error message for vasodilation necessitates a slight decrease in oxygen availability.

Relation to contractility. Although the increase in myocardial oxygen extraction indicates that coronary blood flow does not keep pace with the increased myocardial oxygen demands during exercise, there is no evidence to suggest that this disparity results in ischemia in the normal heart even during heavy exercise. Studies examining myocardial lactate metabolism for evidence of anaerobic glycolysis demonstrated continued lactate consumption even during heavy exercise (217, 236, 371). Nevertheless, Gwirtz et al. (200, 202) found that pharmacologically induced increases of coronary blood flow during exercise can enhance contractile function. Thus, intracoronary administration of the selective α_1-adrenergic blocker prazosin during treadmill exercise in dogs caused a $21 \pm 3\%$ increase in coronary blood flow that was associated with a $21 \pm 4\%$ increase in the maximal rate of regional myocardial segment shortening (total systolic shortening was unchanged). The increased velocity of shortening was not mediated by enhanced β-adrenergic activation, since a similar response to prazosin was observed after β-adrenergic blockade with propranolol (202). Similarly, intracoronary administration of adenosine during exercise caused a 26% increase in coronary blood flow, and this was associated with a 27% increase in the rate of systolic segment shortening (200). The effects on contractile function produced by both intracoronary adenosine and prazosin occurred with no change in heart rate, left ventricular systolic pressure, or myocardial end-diastolic segment length. The observed increase in the velocity of segment shortening in response to increasing coronary blood flow during exercise suggests that coronary flow may modulate the increase of myocardial contractility that occurs during exercise.

Distribution of Left Ventricular Blood Flow

Systolic compression of intramyocardial vessels. Cardiac contraction impedes myocardial blood flow during systole so that during basal conditions arterial inflow occurs predominantly during diastole. Measurements of proximal coronary artery flow in chronically instrumented dogs and swine demonstrate that during resting conditions only 15%–20% of left ventricular flow occurs during systole (276, 461). However, the high heart rates associated with exercise result in progressive encroachment of systole on the diastolic interval, while absolute blood flow rates during systole increase (276, 461). As a result, during heavy exercise 40%–50% of total coronary artery blood flow occurs during systole (276, 461). The increase in the fraction of coronary flow during systole has implications for the transmural distribution of left ventricular myocardial blood flow, because the throttling effect of cardiac contraction on the intramural coronary vessels is expressed nonuniformly across the left ventricular wall. Myocardial compressive force increases from intrathoracic pressure at the epicardial surface to equal or to exceed intraventricular pressure at the endocardial surface (19, 74). Interaction of this gradient of effective tissue pressure with the intravascular distending pressure acts to create an array of vascular waterfalls across the wall of the left ventricle that selectively impedes subendocardial blood flow during systole (127, 216). Nevertheless, in the normal heart a modest *net* transmural gradient of blood flow favoring the subendocardium exists, reflecting the higher systolic tension development and oxygen requirements of this layer (566). Maintenance of this normal pattern of transmural perfusion requires augmentation of subendocardial flow during diastole in proportion to the degree of systolic underperfusion. This diastolic gradient of blood flow favoring the subendocardium is dependent on a transmural gradient of vasomotor tone, with vascular resistance during diastole being lowest in the subendocardium (36).

Subendocardial/subepicardial blood flow ratio. The transmural distribution of myocardial blood flow during exercise has been measured with radioactive microspheres. In most cases, the left ventricular wall has been divided into three or four layers and the transmural distribution of perfusion expressed as the ratio of blood flow to the innermost layer (subendocardium) divided by blood flow to the outermost layer (subepicardium) (ENDO/EPI ratio). In chronically instrumented awake dogs and swine, ENDO/EPI blood flow ratios at rest have been reported from 1.18 to 1.45 (37, 38, 43, 46, 53, 75, 76, 136, 314, 406, 460, 461, 557, 568). ENDO/EPI ratios during exercise vary with the size of microspheres used. In early studies in which 7–10 μm diameter microspheres were used ENDO/EPI ratios decreased during exercise, with values near 1.0 during heavy exercise (46, 53, 568). In contrast, when 15 μm diameter microspheres were used, higher ENDO/EPI ratios have generally been reported, with values of 1.10–1.31 during heavy exercise (37, 38, 406, 460, 461), although some studies in swine reported values near 1.00 (75, 76, 393). The reason for this disparity in the transmural distribution of microspheres during exercise based on size of microspheres is uncertain, but could be the result of streaming of the larger microspheres into the penetrating arteries that deliver blood to the subendocardium, or to arteriovenous shunting of a small fraction of the 7–10 μm diameter microspheres from the tissue in the subendocardium. Size-dependent characteristics of microsphere measurements in the myocardium have been previously reviewed (545). Ponies and standardbred horses appear to have a more prominent decrease in ENDO/EPI ratio during exercise than either dogs or swine. Using 15 μm diameter microspheres, Manohar and associates (350, 410) reported decreases in ENDO/EPI ratio in ponies from 1.18–1.27 at rest to 0.97–0.99 during heavy treadmill exercise. Similarly, Armstrong et al. (22) reported a decrease in ENDO/EPI ratio from 1.24 at rest to 1.05 during exercise in standardbred horses. An explanation for these findings may be the marked increase in left ventricular end-diastolic pressure from 11±2 mm Hg at rest to 36±4 mm Hg during heavy exercise, which contrasts with increases in left ventricular end-diastolic or left atrial pressure from 2–5 mm Hg at rest to only 5–15 mm Hg during heavy exercise in dogs (6, 37, 38, 46, 139, 242, 406) and swine (461, 568).

Influence of vasomotor tone on myocardial blood flow distribution. Several studies suggest that coronary vasomotor tone is of importance in maintaining subendocardial blood flow during exercise. Thus, studies in swine have demonstrated that coronary vasodilation with adenosine or dipyridamole during heavy exercise caused the ENDO/EPI ratio to fall significantly below 1.0 (314, 461, 568). These findings suggest that at high heart rates during exercise, active vasomotion is required to maintain a gradient of vascular resistance favoring diastolic perfusion of the deeper myocardial layers. In contrast to these reports, Barnard et al. (53) reported that the ENDO/EPI ratio during heavy exercise in dogs increased from 1.03 during control conditions to 1.15 after the administration of dipyridamole. Intravenous adenosine had no effect on the ENDO/EPI ratio during maximal exercise in ponies (350, 410), and Breisch et al. (76) reported that during heavy exercise in swine the ENDO/EPI ratio was maintained near unity during vasodilation with adenosine. The reason for this disparity is unclear. Of greatest importance, however, is the finding that absolute subendocardial blood flow rates increased in response to exogenous adenosine or dipyridamole during heavy exercise (53, 76, 314, 350, 410, 461, 568), indicating that vasodilator reserve had not been exhausted.

Unique Responses to Exercise in Rodents. An inexpensive small-animal model that would reproduce the effects of exercise seen in larger animals would be extremely useful. However, the technical difficulty of measuring coronary blood flow in small animals is formidable. Flaim et al. (167) administered microspheres into the left ventricle of rats exercised by swimming or on a treadmill. In comparison with rest, swimming caused no changes of heart rate, cardiac output, or myocardial blood flow. Treadmill exercise at 70 ft/min for 5 min or until exhaustion increased heart rates from approximately 380 to 480 bpm and increased cardiac output, while arterial blood pressure was unchanged. Left ventricular myocardial blood flow was 5.9 ml · min^{-1} · g^{-1} at rest and increased to 7.8 ml · min^{-1} · g^{-1} during exercise, an approximately 30% increase. Thus, myocardial blood flow in the rat is much higher than in larger animals during resting conditions, while the relative increase in blood flow during exercise is much less than in larger animals. The lack of hemodynamic response to swimming indicates that this stress is likely to be of little value in examining coronary vascular responses to exercise (45). Furthermore, the response to treadmill exercise in the rat is so dissimilar to that of larger animals (including humans) that even treadmill exercise is likely to be of limited value in obtaining data that could be applicable to larger animal species or to humans.

Right Ventricular Blood Flow during Exercise

During quiet resting conditions, right ventricular blood flow in the dog expressed per gram of myocardium is typically 50%–60% of left ventricular blood flow, while the transmural distribution of perfusion is uniform or slightly favors the subendocardium (43, 46, 406). In resting swine, right ventricular blood flow per gram of myocardium is 70 to 90% of left ventricular blood flow, with an ENDO/EPI ratio of 1.10–1.50 (314, 460). During graded treadmill exercise in dogs and swine right ventricular blood flow increases as a direct function of heart rate. Right ventricular blood flow expressed per gram of myocardium is approximately 75%–90% of flow to the left ventricle during the heaviest levels of exercise. The transmural distribution of perfusion does not change from rest to exercise (43, 46, 314, 406, 460). Manohar (350) demonstrated substantial vasodilator reserve in the right ventricle of ponies during maximal treadmill exercise, with blood flow increasing from 4.80±0.31 ml · min^{-1} · g^{-1} during maximal exercise to 7.54±0.30 when adenosine was infused at a rate of 3 μmol · kg^{-1} · min^{-1} while maximal exercise continued. Right ventricular blood flow per gram of myocardium tended to be higher during maximal exercise in ponies than in swine or dogs, likely because of the exercise-induced pulmonary hypertension that is characteristic of horses (mean pulmonary pressure increased from 19±2 mm Hg at rest to 66±4 mm Hg during maximal exercise). During maximal exercise in ponies, vasodilator reserve existed in all transmural layers of the right ventricular wall; the right ventricular ENDO/EPI ratio during maximal exercise was 1.00± 0.02 and actually increased to 1.32±0.10 when adenosine was infused while exercise continued (350).

Mechanisms Of Coronary Vasodilation during Exercise

Metabolic Mechanisms

Adenosine. Adenosine has been proposed as a metabolite that couples myocardial oxygen demands to vasomotor tone of the coronary resistance vessels (61). Adenine nucleotides do not cross the cell membrane of cardiac myocytes, but adenosine formed from the action of nucleotide phosphorylase on adenosine monophosphate (AMP) can be transported out of myocytes into the interstitial space (510). Upon entering the interstitial space adenosine can interact with A_2 receptors on coronary vascular smooth muscle to produce vasodilation and increased myocardial blood flow (399). Adenosine release is enhanced during conditions of increased myocardial oxygen demands or decreased arterial oxygen supply (51, 152, 330, 364, 565).

McKenzie et al. (364) examined the relationship between tissue adenosine content and coronary blood flow by analyzing myocardial biopsies obtained during treadmill exercise in chronically instrumented dogs. Exercise sufficient to increase heart rates to 211 bpm increased myocardial adenosine content from 1.35±0.54 to 8.18±0.60 nmol/g. Arterial and coronary sinus plasma adenosine concentrations were similar during resting conditions; exercise caused no change in arterial adenosine concentration, but nearly doubled the coronary venous concentration. Watkinson et al. (565) and Ely et al. (152) sampled pericardial fluid to estimate myocardial interstitial adenosine concentrations. In dogs with chronically implanted pericardial catheters, these investigators found that pericardial fluid adenosine concentration increased to 279±23% of the resting value during moderate treadmill exercise (heart rate to 204 bpm). A significant positive relationship was found between coronary blood flow and pericardial fluid adenosine concentration, but not between coronary sinus adenosine concentration and coronary blood flow. Although adenosine in pericardial fluid does not fully equilibrate with interstitial concentrations, it likely reflects directional changes in interstitial fluid adenosine. Unlike blood adenosine, which has a short half-life owing to enzymatic degradation and uptake by endothelial cells and erythrocytes, little adenosine catabolism occurs in pericardial fluid. Bacchus et al. (35) reported that pericardial adenosine concentration increased from 91±9 pmol/ml at rest to 223±28 pmol/ml in dogs during heavy treadmill exercise. The increase in coronary blood flow during exercise was positively correlated with the pericardial fluid adenosine concentration (r = 0.88). However, this level of exercise increased myocardial blood flow to only 1.63±0.10 ml · min^{-1} · g^{-1}, which is approximately half of the expected increase based on other reports in the literature (see Fig. 16.3). The subnormal coronary artery flow rates raises concern that chronic instrumentation of the coronary artery may have restricted blood flow, thereby augmenting myocardial adenosine production.

Although these findings indicate that myocardial adenosine production increases during exercise, demonstration of an essential role for adenosine in mediating exercise-induced coronary vasodilation requires that interruption of the adenosine effect interfere with exercise-induced coronary vasodilation. Bache et al. (40) examined the effects of adenosine receptor blockade with 8-phenyltheophylline as well as augmented adenosine catabolism produced by intracoronary adenosine deaminase. Adenosine antagonism inhibited coronary vasodilation evoked by ischemia; adenosine deaminase caused a 33%–39% decrease in reactive hyperemia following coronary occlusions of 5–20 s duration, while 8-phenyltheophylline caused a 40%–62% decrease in reactive hyperemia. Neither agent significantly changed heart rate or arterial pressure during treadmill exercise. Furthermore, neither the absolute values for myocardial oxygen consumption and coronary blood flow nor the relationship between these variables were altered by either adenosine receptor blockade or adenosine deaminase (40). Edlund et al. (144) examined the effect of adenosine receptor blockade with theophylline on coronary sinus blood flow measured with the thermodilution technique during supine bicycle exercise in normal young adult human subjects. Theophylline (6 mg/kg intravenously) caused an increase in heart rate and the rate-pressure product, likely because of inhibition of phosphodiesterase by theophylline. Coronary vascular resistance was significantly higher after theophylline both at rest and during exercise, but the decrease in coronary resistance in response to exercise was not altered.

Although adenosine deaminase or adenosine receptor blockade does not prevent the normal increase of coronary blood flow during exercise, this does not exclude the possibility that adenosine normally contributes to coronary vasodilation. When the effects of adenosine are blocked other vasodilator mechanisms compensate to maintain normal coronary flow. This is supported by the finding that when exercise was performed in the presence of a flow-limiting coronary stenosis, blockade of the effects of adenosine resulted in a significant decrease of blood flow in the ischemic myocardial region (134, 330). In this experimental model, where hypoperfusion presumably caused other vasodilator mechanisms to be fully activated, interruption of the adenosine effect *did* impair vasodilation of the coronary resistance vessels. In contrast, in the normal coronary circulation loss of the adenosine effect appears to be fully compensated for by other vasodilator mechanisms during exercise.

K^+_{ATP} channels. Potassium channels sensitive to intracellular ATP content (K^+_{ATP} channels) have been identified in vascular smooth muscle cells (516). Opening of K^+_{ATP} channels results in an outward flux of potassium that increases the membrane potential of the sarcolemma. This leads to a decreased influx of extracellular calcium, thereby causing vascular relaxation. K^+_{ATP} channels have been implicated in metabolic regulation of coronary vasomotor tone (115, 293, 458), and their contribution to the increase in coronary blood flow produced by exercise has been evaluated in chronically instrumented dogs (137). The K^+_{ATP} channel blocker glibenclamide was infused into the coronary artery at a rate of 50 μg · kg^{-1} · min^{-1} to cause 90% inhibition of the increases in coronary blood flow produced by the K^+_{ATP} channel opener pinacidil. Glibenclamide decreased coronary blood flow at rest by 20% but did not block the increase in coronary flow produced by exercise, resulting in a parallel downward shift in the relationship between heart rate and coronary blood flow during exercise (137). This suggests either that K^+_{ATP} channels do not contribute to coronary vasodilation during exercise, or that in the presence of K^+_{ATP} channel blockade other vasodilator mechanisms are activated in response to further deterioration of the myocardial oxygen supply–demand balance. There is evidence that when K^+_{ATP} channels are inhibited, adenosine assumes greater importance as a metabolic coronary vasodilator during exercise (40, 139, 458). Thus, although neither glibenclamide nor the adenosine receptor blocker 8-phenyltheophylline alone inhibited the increase in coronary blood flow produced by exercise, vasodilation was inhibited when both agents were administered simultaneously [Fig. 16.5; (139)]. This suggests that K^+_{ATP} channels normally *do* contribute to coronary vasodilation during exercise, but that the decreased blood flow after K^+_{ATP} channel blockade elicits a compensatory release of adenosine that preserves the increase in coronary blood flow. This is analogous to the finding that adenosine does contribute to coronary vasodilation during exercise when an arterial stenosis prevents the normal increase in blood flow (134, 330). The modest residual increase in coronary blood flow during exercise in the presence of combined K^+_{ATP} channel and adenosine receptor blockade suggests that still other vasodilator mechanisms are active.

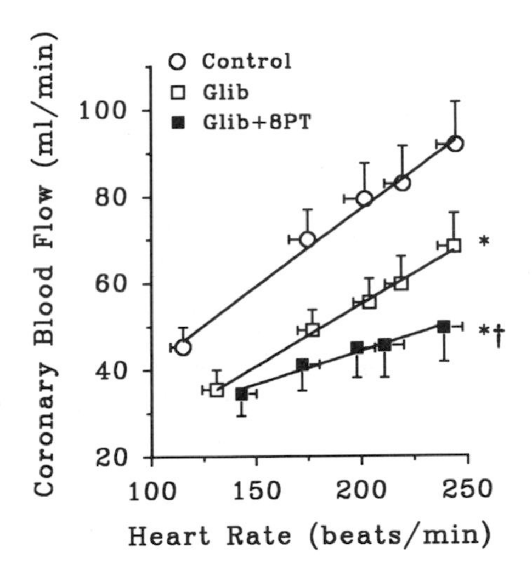

FIG. 16.5. Relationship between heart rate and coronary blood flow at rest and during four incremental levels of treadmill exercise in dogs, under control conditions (*Control, open circles*), during K^+_{ATP} channel blockade (glibenclamide, 50 μg · kg^{-1} · min^{-1}, intracoronary) (*Glib, open squares*), and during combined adenosine receptor blockade (8-phenyltheophylline, 5 mg/kg intravenously) and K^+_{ATP} channel blockade (*Glib+8PT, closed squares*). K^+_{ATP} channel blockade alone decreased coronary blood flow at rest but did not affect the exercise-induced increase in coronary flow. In contrast, combined adenosine receptor and K^+_{ATP} channel blockade decreased coronary blood flow at rest and markedly attenuated the increase in coronary flow produced by exercise. Data are mean ± SEM, *n* = 11. Data are from Duncker et al. (139).

Endothelium-Derived Vasodilators

Nitric oxide. Coronary artery vasodilation in response to agonists such as acetylcholine is mediated by endothelial production of nitric oxide (NO) or a nitrosyl compound produced from L-arginine (254, 407). Endothelial production of NO can be triggered by receptor-mediated mechanisms or in response to the increased shear force associated with increased blood flow (176, 237, 564). In addition to effects on coronary arteries, NO-dependent mechanisms also cause vasodilation of coronary resistance vessels in response to increased blood flow in vitro (298) and contribute to coronary reactive hyperemia in vivo (408, 578). Altman et al. (6) examined the contribution of NO to coronary vasodilation during treadmill exercise in dogs by intracoronary administration of N^G-nitro-L-arginine (LNNA), a competitive inhibitor of L-arginine that is the substrate for NO synthase. LNNA caused an 80±6% inhibition of the coronary vasodilation produced by intra-arterial administration of acetylcholine, but did not alter the response to the endothelium-independent vasodilator nitroprusside. LNNA caused a slight increase in arterial pressure at rest and during exercise. Graded treadmill exercise that produced peak heart rates of 225 bpm increased left circumflex coronary artery blood flow from 47±7 ml/min to 81±11 ml/min. Coronary blood flow rates during exercise were slightly higher after LNNA in parallel with a slight increase in myocardial oxygen consumption. LNNA caused a slight decrease of coronary sinus oxygen tension during exercise from 16±2 mm Hg to 14±2 mm Hg, indicating that coronary vasodilation in response to the increased myocardial oxygen demands was slightly blunted. However, this difference was small and not likely of physiologic significance. The findings do not support a critical role for endogenous NO in coronary vasodilation during exercise, possibly because other vasodilator mechanisms are able to compensate for the loss of NO-mediated vasodilation. This possibility is supported by the finding that when the increase in coronary blood flow in response to exercise was limited by a proximal coronary artery stenosis, LNNA impaired resistance vessel dilation and led to a 35±4% further decrease of blood flow in the ischemic myocardial region (133). This suggests that when metabolic vasodilator mechanisms have been exhausted, endogenous NO production *does* contribute to maintaining vasodilation of the resistance vessels in the hypoperfused region.

Prostaglandins. Coronary endothelium is capable of synthesizing vasodilator prostanoids from arachidonic acid that can act on coronary vascular smooth muscle to increase myocardial blood flow (66, 389, 473). Early investigations reported that cyclooxygenase inhibitors depressed physiologic vasodilator responses associated with coronary reactive hyperemia and myocardial hypoxia (4, 5), but more recent studies in intact animals have generally found little effect of these agents on ischemic or hypoxic coronary vasodilation (226, 403). These differences may be related to the experimental preparation, with less effect observed in preparations in which surgical trauma was minimized, as tissue trauma tends to activate the prostaglandin system (403). Dai and Bache (109) examined the effect of cyclooxygenase blockade with a dose of indomethacin (5 mg/kg intravenously) that caused marked blunting of the vasodilator response to intracoronary arachidonic acid and found no change in coronary blood flow during resting conditions and no change in the increase in coronary flow in response to exercise. Furthermore, indomethacin did not alter the relationship between coronary blood flow and myocardial oxygen consumption. Edlund et al. (144) used the coronary sinus thermodilution technique to measure the response of myocardial blood flow in healthy young human subjects during supine leg exercise that increased heart rate from 62±2 bpm to 96±4 bpm.

Cyclooxygenase blockade with oral ibuprofen did not alter either the decrease in coronary resistance or the increase in coronary blood flow during exercise. These studies do not support a significant contribution of the prostaglandin system to exercise-induced vasodilation of the coronary resistance vessels.

Integration of Coronary Vasodilator Mechanisms. Enhanced delivery of oxygen and metabolic substrate is critical for the cardiac response to exercise and appears to involve several parallel and independent mechanisms that contribute to exercise-induced coronary vasodilation. Presently available data suggest that opening of K^{+}_{ATP} channels plays a central role in coronary vasodilation. However, when activation of these channels is pharmacologically blocked, a compensatory increase in myocardial adenosine production acts to preserve coronary vasodilation. Redundant mechanisms for increasing coronary blood flow during exercise are likely of critical importance to the organism, but this redundancy confounds assessment of the contributions of individual vasodilator systems; that is, blocking one system leads to increased activation of other parallel vasodilator mechanisms. Thus, blockade of adenosine or NO-mediated vasodilation need not cause a discernible effect on coronary vasodilation in the normal heart. Only when myocardial ischemia (e.g., during exercise in the presence of a coronary stenosis) has caused all vasodilator mechanisms to become activated does interruption of the adenosine or NO effect inhibit dilation of the resistance vessels. However, the magnitude of the contribution of each of these individual mechanisms to exercise-induced coronary vasodilation in the presence of normal arterial inflow is unclear.

Autonomic Nervous System Influences

Autonomic influences have been studied by examining coronary blood flow during exercise after surgical or chemical cardiac denervation of the heart or in the presence of selective autonomic receptor antagonists.

Cardiac Neural Ablation. Techniques have been devised to produce effective denervation of the heart as demonstrated by lack of an inotropic response to cardiac sympathetic nerve stimulation or to administration of tyramine, which releases endogenous norepinephrine from adrenergic nerve terminals, as well as by depletion of myocardial norepinephrine stores (125, 272). However, the results obtained using these preparations are complicated by supersensitivity to circulating catecholamines, which develops after sympathetic neural ablation. This supersensitivity appears to be selective, in that an enhanced response of myocardial contractility to norepinephrine is regularly observed (90, 125), whereas α-adrenergic responses of the coronary vasculature do not appear to be enhanced (90, 121, 177).

The ability to maintain steady-state levels of exercise is not substantially impaired following surgical denervation of the heart, but the initial hemodynamic adjustment to exercise is delayed. For example, Gregg et al. (195) observed that in dogs with surgical cardiac denervation the onset of heavy treadmill exercise resulted in a 25% decrease in arterial blood pressure that did not return to control levels until 36–90 s after beginning exercise. In contrast, in normal dogs arterial pressure decreased only slightly and recovered within 3–6 s after beginning exercise. Similarly, the increase in coronary blood flow was delayed 10–30 s after the onset of treadmill exercise in animals with cardiac denervation, in contrast to the 3–6 s delay observed in normal dogs.

Gregg et al. (195) reported that myocardial oxygen consumption and coronary blood flow were decreased in denervated hearts. At rest, coronary blood flow rates were 46% lower in animals with denervated hearts than in a control group. During exercise, coronary flow increased in parallel with myocardial oxygen consumption in both groups, so that blood flows remained proportionately reduced in animals with cardiac denervation. Resting heart rates were increased in dogs with surgical cardiac neural ablation because of loss of vagal inhibitory tone, whereas heart rates during exercise were lower than in control animals. This decrease in heart rate could in part account for the lower levels of coronary blood flow during exercise. β-Adrenergic blockade with propranolol further attenuated the peak heart rate and coronary blood flow rates achieved, and further delayed responses at the onset of exercise. Myocardial oxygen extraction was similar in normal and denervated hearts both at rest and during exercise. Similarly, Gwirtz et al. (201) observed that cardiac sympathectomy decreased left ventricular peak systolic pressure and left ventricular dP/dt_{max}, suggesting that the reduction of myocardial oxygen consumption was due, at least in part, to decreased myocardial contractility. Myocardial oxygen extraction at rest was similar in control and denervated hearts, and increased similarly in both groups during exercise. Thus, sympathetic coronary vasoconstriction is not the exclusive cause of the increased oxygen extraction during exercise. Since Chilian et al. (90) reported that coronary α-adrenergic vasoconstriction does not exhibit postdenervation supersensitivity, the findings suggest that either the increased oxygen extraction during exercise is not dependent upon adrenergic mechanisms or that adrenergic tone is maintained via circulating catecholamines (90).

Schwartz and Stone (476) demonstrated that increases of heart rate and contractility during exercise were attenuated by ablation of the right but not the left stellate ganglion in dogs. In contrast, the increase in coronary blood flow in response to exercise was not altered after right stellate ganglionectomy but was slightly increased after left stellate ganglionectomy. Bilateral stellate ganglionectomy decreased heart rate and left ventricular dP/dt_{max} at equivalent exercise levels, but coronary blood flow was slightly increased. These findings suggest that both left and right stellate ganglia exert a coronary vasoconstrictor effect during exercise. DiCarlo et al. (120) ablated the left stellate ganglion in chronically instrumented dogs and reported that during submaximal exercise coronary blood flows were higher than in control dogs. In the animals that had undergone neural ablation, nonselective α-adrenergic blockade with intracoronary phentolamine (1 mg) had no effect on coronary blood flow. The authors concluded that sympathetic neural ablation removes tonic α-adrenergic vasoconstriction during submaximal exercise.

Furuya et al. (177) examined coronary blood flow during graded treadmill exercise in dogs with surgical cardiac denervation during control conditions and after nonselective α-adrenergic blockade with phentolamine. Left circumflex coronary artery blood flow was slightly higher in denervated than in normal hearts during exercise at comparable levels of myocardial oxygen demand (reflected by the heart rate $\times$ mean aortic pressure product), and α-adrenergic receptor blockade with phentolamine (2 mg/kg intravenously) caused a slight further increase in coronary flow (177). In contrast to the report of DiCarlo et al. (120), these findings suggested that adrenergic coronary vasoconstriction during exercise is mediated both by circulating catecholamines and by direct neural influences on the coronary vessels.

Chilian et al. (90) examined the effect on coronary blood flow of sympathetic denervation of the posterior left ventricular wall produced by epicardial application of phenol. They observed no difference in mean myocardial blood flow or in the transmural distribution of perfusion between normally innervated and sympathectomized left ventricular regions either at rest or during moderate treadmill exercise. This finding failed to support neurogenic α-adrenergic coronary vasoconstriction during exercise. After β-adrenergic blockade with propranolol, nonselective α-adrenergic blockade with phentolamine decreased coronary vascular resistance in both the innervated (28%) and sympathectomized (23%) regions. The decrease in resistance likely occurred at least in part to compensate for an 18% decrease in mean aortic pressure caused by the systemic α-adrenergic blockade. The authors concluded that α-adrenergic coronary vasoconstriction does occur during exercise, but is principally mediated by circulating catecholamines rather than by direct neural connections. A role for circulating catecholamines, rather than sympathetic nerve activity, is also suggested by the time course of the decrease in coronary venous oxygen saturation that occurs in dogs in response to exercise. Thus, von Restorff et al. (557) observed that the exercise-induced decrease in coronary venous oxygen saturation required 90–100 s to reach a stable plateau, whereas the increase in heart rate was almost instantaneous.

Bassenge et al. (55) examined the effect of whole-body chemical sympathectomy with 6-hydroxydopamine on exercise capacity in chronically instrumented dogs. 6-Hydroxydopamine causes degeneration of adrenergic nerve terminals in both the heart and peripheral vasculature, whereas adrenal medullary function remains intact or is enhanced (55). Because of peripheral adrenergic denervation, the circulatory response to exercise was markedly impaired; the onset of exercise was associated with a profound decrease of mean arterial pressure to 40–45 mm Hg, which required discontinuing exercise. Arterial pressure recovered after 90 s so that exercise could be resumed, but exercise tolerance was impaired. At comparable levels of total-body oxygen consumption, coronary blood flow was approximately 20% less in animals with chemical sympathectomy than in control animals. Myocardial oxygen consumption was not measured but, based on the lower heart rate and blood pressure, it is likely that the decrease in coronary blood flow was at least in part secondary to decreased oxygen requirement.

α-Adrenergic Activity during Exercise. Blockade of α-adrenergic receptors can influence coronary blood flow through two separate mechanisms. First, blockade of prejunctional α_2-adrenergic receptors interrupts the negative feedback control of norepinephrine release (221, 302). The resultant increase in norepinephrine levels augments cardiac β-adrenergic stimulation and increases coronary blood flow secondary to the increased myocardial oxygen consumption. Second, α-adrenergic blockade can increase coronary blood flow by interrupting postjunctional vasoconstriction of coronary resistance vessels, which competes with metabolic vasodilation (376). Postjunctional coronary vasoconstriction can be mediated by both α_1- (arteries and arterioles) and α_2-adrenoceptors (arterioles) on coronary vascular smooth muscle. Conversely, α_2-adrenergic receptors on coronary vascular endothelium stimulate release of EDRF, which can oppose the direct vasoconstrictor effect (96).

In chronically instrumented dogs, exercise produces a greater increase in coronary blood flow after systemic α-adrenergic blockade than during control conditions (39, 110, 204, 219, 336). Systemic nonselective α-adrenergic antagonists exaggerate the increases of heart rate, left ventricular systolic pressure, and dP/dt_{max} during exercise as the result of blockade of prejunctional α_2-adrenergic receptors that inhibit norepinephrine release. Thus, after nonselective or selective α_2-adrenergic blockade, plasma norepinephrine levels during exercise are elevated and there is evidence for increased β-adrenergic stimulation (221, 302). As anticipated, β-adrenergic blockade blocks the marked increase in hemodynamic determinants of myocardial oxygen consumption produced by nonselective α-adrenergic blockade. Even so, coronary blood flow during exercise was slightly higher after nonselective α-adrenergic blockade (386). When nonselective α-blockers were administered intracoronary to minimize systemic hemodynamic effects in chronically instrumented dogs, coronary blood flow during exercise was 10%–30% greater than during control exercise (111, 120, 202, 205, 244). At comparable levels of myocardial oxygen consumption, α-adrenergic blockade increases coronary venous oxygen tension and decreases coronary vascular resistance, indicating that α-adrenergic vasoconstriction competes with metabolic coronary vasodilation during exercise (39, 41, 110, 219).

Both α_1- and α_2-adrenoceptors can mediate coronary vasoconstriction, but adrenergic coronary vasoconstriction during exercise in the normal heart appears to involve principally α_1-adrenoceptors. At comparable levels of myocardial oxygen consumption during treadmill exercise in dogs, nonselective α-adrenergic blockade with phentolamine and selective α_1-adrenergic blockade with prazosin resulted in similar decreases of coronary vascular resistance and increases in coronary venous oxygen tension (39). Furthermore, selective α_1-adrenergic blockade with intracoronary prazosin resulted in higher levels of coronary blood flow and lower coronary vascular resistance during graded treadmill exercise (111, 524), whereas intracoronary administration of the selective α_2-adrenergic blockers yohimbine or idazoxan did not alter coronary blood flow or coronary vascular resistance during exercise (111, 524). Since the effect of increased release of norepinephrine produced by α_2-adrenoceptor blockade might be concealed by the α_1-adrenergic vasoconstriction, which it can produce, studies were repeated with the addition of α_1-adrenergic blockade. However, combined intra-arterial administration of α_1- and α_2-adrenergic blockers was not more effective in increasing coronary blood flow or coronary venous oxygen tension during exercise than was α_1-adrenergic blockade alone (111). These findings suggest that the α-adrenergic vasoconstrictor tone that opposes metabolically mediated coronary vasodilation in the normal heart during exercise is mediated principally by postjunctional α_1-adrenoceptor activity.

α-Adrenergic vasoconstriction also limits coronary vasodilation in regions of ischemic myocardium. Thus, when a coronary artery stenosis prevented the normal increase of myocardial blood flow, exercise resulted in subendocardial underperfusion and impairment of regional systolic segment shortening. Local α_1-adrenergic blockade with intracoronary prazosin significantly increased blood flow to the hypoperfused region with no change in coronary pressure distal to the stenosis and caused improved contractile performance; selective α_2-adrenergic blockade with intracoronary idazoxan caused no change in myocardial blood flow or contractile function (328). In contrast, Seitelberger et al. (485) reported that adrenergic coronary vasoconstriction in regions of hypoperfused myocardium during exercise was mediated by α_2-adrenoceptors. The difference may be related to the more severe coronary stenosis used by Seitelberger et al. (485); α_2-adrenoceptor stimulation may be of greater importance during more severe degrees of ischemia.

Several investigators have proposed that adrenergically mediated coronary vasoconstriction may contribute to maintenance of subendocardial blood flow during exercise. Huang and Feigl (244) observed that although total myocardial blood flow during exercise was less in regions where α-adrenoceptor activity was intact than where α-adrenoceptors were blocked with phenoxybenzamine (0.2 mg/kg intracoronary), the ENDO/EPI blood flow ratio was slightly higher in the region with α-adrenoceptors intact. In contrast, adrenergic coronary vasoconstriction caused transmurally uniform reduction of blood flow in myocardial regions perfused by a stenotic coronary artery (328), as well as in the pressure-overloaded hypertrophied left ventricles of dogs (141).

β-Adrenergic Activity during Exercise.

Direct β-adrenergic coronary vasodilation during exercise is difficult to study because of the overwhelming effect of metabolic vasodilation resulting from β-adrenergic inotropic and chronotropic effects on the myocardium. Nonselective β-adrenergic blockade with propranolol decreased coronary blood flow more than expected from the decrease in myocardial oxygen consumption, resulting in a significant increase in myocardial oxygen extraction (56, 220). These findings suggest that β-adrenergic stimulation during exercise acts on the coronary vessels to oppose α-adrenergic vasoconstriction; loss of this direct β-adrenergic vasodilator effect enhanced the exercise-induced coronary vasoconstriction.

During supine leg exercise in patients with angiographically normal coronary arteries, propranolol (5 mg/kg intravenously) significantly decreased myocardial oxygen consumption with no effect on myocardial oxygen extraction (575). Jorgensen et al. (268) examined the effect of β-adrenergic blockade with propranolol (0.25 mg/kg intravenously) on coronary blood flow in healthy young adult male human subjects performing upright bicycle exercise. Exercise loads were adjusted to achieve heart rates of 120 bpm during control conditions (63 W) and after propranolol (112 W). At matched heart rates myocardial oxygen consumption was similar during control conditions and after β-adrenergic blockade, but coronary blood flow was 25% less after β-adrenergic blockade and myocardial oxygen extraction was increased. Furthermore, β-adrenergic blockade with sotalol (10 mg intravenously) decreased myocardial blood flow during supine bicycle exercise out of proportion to the reduction of myocardial oxygen consumption, so that myocardial oxygen extraction rose and coronary sinus oxygen content fell (150).

Selective β_1-adrenergic blockade with intra-arterial atenolol and nonselective β-adrenergic blockade with intra-arterial propranolol produced similar reductions of both regional segment shortening and the rate of segment shortening in dogs during moderate treadmill exercise (359), indicating blockade of the positive inotropic effect of exercise; there was no effect on heart rate, left ventricular systolic pressure, or contractile function in the distant wall. Propranolol caused a 22±4% decrease in coronary artery blood flow, which was slightly but consistently greater than the 18±3% decrease produced by atenolol, suggesting a slight β_2-adrenergic vasodilator effect during exercise. In contrast, Gwirtz and Stone (205) reported that selective β_1-adrenergic blockade with intra-arterial atenolol produced an identical decrease in coronary blood flow as did nonselective blockade with intra-arterial propranolol. Intracoronary administration of the selective β_2-adrenoceptor blocker ICI 118,551 (250 μg) during exercise caused no change in contractile function but produced an 11%–14% decrease in coronary blood flow during moderate treadmill exercise in chronically instrumented dogs (120, 359). This response occurred despite lack of a significant effect on systemic hemodynamics or regional contractile function. The modest decrease in coronary blood flow produced by selective β_2-adrenergic receptor blockade persisted after local α-adrenergic blockade with phentolamine, and was also observed in animals with left stellate ganglionectomy (120). These findings indicate that β_2-adrenoceptor activation during exercise causes a small but significant degree of coronary resistance vessel dilation independent of the myocardial effects of β_1-adrenergic stimulation on coronary blood flow.

Parasympathetic Effects. Gwirtz and Stone (203) administered the muscarinic receptor antagonist atropine into a coronary artery of dogs during submaximal treadmill exercise that resulted in heart rates of 190–210 bpm. Atropine had no effect on heart rate or coronary blood flow, indicating that parasympathetic effects on both the myocardium and coronary bed were negligible. This is in accordance with the finding that vagal tone to the myocardium is progressively withdrawn during increasing levels of exercise to be completely abolished at heart rates of approximately 170 bpm (554).

Integration of Autonomic Nervous System Influences. Intact cardiac innervation is necessary for prompt initial cardiac adjustments to treadmill exercise. Cardiac denervation does not appear to affect the myocardial responses to sustained treadmill exercise, which suggests a greater dependence on circulating catecholamines. This may in part be facilitated by postdenervation β-adrenergic supersensitivity. Studies of the relative contributions of neuronal vs. circulating catecholamines for α-adrenergic control of coronary blood flow during exercise are inconclusive, which may suggest that both neuronal and humoral catecholamines are involved. During exercise in the normal heart α-adrenergic tone is mediated principally by the α_1-adrenoceptor subtype. Assessment of β-adrenergic control of coronary blood flow is complicated by the dramatic effects of β-adrenergic antagonists on the myocardium. Available data indicate the presence of β_2-adrenergic vasodilator influence during exercise, which appears mediated by circulating catecholamines. Parasympathetic control of the coronary circulation during exercise is negligible.

Extravascular Determinants of Coronary Blood Flow

Increases in the force of contraction and time spent in systole resulting from increased contractility and heart rate during exercise increase the extravascular compressive forces acting on the intramural coronary vessels. Study of the impeding effects of cardiac contraction on coronary blood flow requires elimination of active vasomotor influences by producing maximal pharmacological vasodilation of the coronary vascular bed. An early study in ponies reported that "minimum" coronary vascular resistance (calculated as aortic pressure/mean coronary blood flow during intravenous administration of adenosine) was lower during treadmill exercise than at rest (410). However, computation of vascular resistance from single measurements of pressure and flow do not fully characterize the effects of changes in extravascular forces in response to exercise.

Comprehensive analysis of mechanical effects of cardiac contraction on blood flow is provided by the pressure–flow relationship, obtained from multiple measurements of coronary blood flow over a range of perfusion pressures. During maximum vasodilation the pressure–flow relationship is determined by the maximum vascular conductance, represented by the slope of the relationship, and the x-intercept or pressure at which flow ceases [zero flow pressure (Pzf)]. In the maximally dilated circulation, changes in Pzf are determined principally by changes of the extravascular compressive forces (286). Duncker et al. (138) used this technique to study the effect of exercise on coronary blood flow in dogs. Maximum coronary vasodilation was maintained by intra-arterial infusion of adenosine (50 $\mu g \cdot kg^{-1} \cdot min^{-1}$); this dose was determined to cause maximum vasodilation, since larger doses caused no further increase in blood flow. As heart rate increased from 118 bpm at rest to 213 bpm during treadmill exercise, blood flow in the maximally vasodilated coronary circulation decreased from 5.66±0.41 $ml \cdot min^{-1} \cdot g^{-1}$ during resting conditions to 4.62±0.43 $ml \cdot min^{-1} \cdot g^{-1}$ of myocardium despite a significant increase in coronary artery pressure. The decrease of coronary blood flow resulted from an increase of Pzf from 13±1 mm Hg at rest to 23±2 mm Hg during exercise, as well as a decrease in the slope of the pressure–flow relationship from 12.3±0.9 to 10.9±0.9 ($ml \cdot min^{-1} \cdot g^{-1}$)/mm Hg during exercise. Several factors may contribute to the altered coronary pressure–flow relationship during exercise. First, the increase in heart rate decreases maximum coronary blood flow rates by increasing the total time spent in systole (36). Second, increased contractility increases systolic compression of intramural coronary vessels (295, 357, 507, 543). However, increased contractility simultaneously augments myocardial relaxation which, by itself, increases diastolic perfusion time (135, 428, 581). Finally, an increase of left ventricular diastolic filling pressure decreases maximum coronary blood flow (33, 140, 151). Analysis of the individual contributions of each of these variables to the exercise-induced changes in the coronary pressure–flow relationship demonstrated that heart rate and left ventricular diastolic pressure contributed to the increases in the Pzf, whereas the increase in contractility did not have a significant effect (133), likely because the impeding effect of the increased force of contraction was offset by an increase in the diastolic perfusion time.

The increase in extravascular compressive forces during exercise is unlikely to be of physiologic significance in the normal coronary circulation, because coronary vasodilator reserve capacity persists even during maximal exercise (53, 76, 314, 350, 410, 461, 568). However, when the oxygen-carrying capacity of the blood is reduced by anemia or hypoxia, or when atherosclerotic coronary artery disease reduces vascular caliber, then the increased extravascular forces produced by exercise could produce a functionally significant limitation of coronary blood flow rates during exercise.

Epicardial Coronary Arteries

The coronary arteries have generally been considered to be conduit vessels that have little influence on myocardial blood flow. However, detailed examination of the distribution of vascular resistance within the coronary system has demonstrated that during basal conditions approximately 25% of total resistance resides in arterial vessels larger than 200 μm in diameter, with approximately 50% of total resistance in vessels larger than 100 μm (89, 91). Vasomotor activity in these arterial vessels, which likely are not strongly influenced by the local metabolic factors that control the smaller arterioles, has potential for influencing total coronary vascular resistance and myocardial blood flow (164, 165). Although much information concerning coronary artery vasomotor responsiveness has been derived from studies using isolated vessel segments, measurements during exercise must be performed in the intact animal. These measurements have been facilitated by the development of ultrasonic techniques for measurement of epicardial coronary artery diameter in chronically instrumented awake animals

(555). Studies of the responses of the coronary arteries to exercise in human subjects have been performed using contrast angiography. Although intracoronary injection of radiopaque contrast material can be followed by arterial vasodilation, Gaglione et al. (179) demonstrated that repeated injections of contrast material caused no persistent change in coronary artery luminal cross-sectional area, so that valid comparisons of coronary artery dimensions can be obtained with this technique.

Dynamic Exercise. Moderate treadmill exercise causes a 3%–4% increase in coronary artery external diameter (approximately 8%–10% increase in luminal cross-sectional area) as measured with ultrasonic crystals affixed to opposing sides of the left circumflex coronary artery of chronically instrumented dogs (474, 564). In patients undergoing diagnostic coronary angiography, Gage and associates (178) observed a 23% increase in cross-sectional area of angiographically normal coronary artery segments in response to mild supine bicycle exercise (mean heart rate to 99 bpm). This exercise-induced vasodilation was approximately half of the maximal coronary artery vasodilation assessed with sublingual nitroglycerin (40% increase in cross-sectional area).

Endothelium-derived relaxing factor. Schwartz et al. (474) observed that exercise-induced coronary artery vasodilation is a flow-mediated response that was blocked when the normal increase in blood flow during exercise was prevented by partially inflating a hydraulic occluder on the coronary artery. Flow-induced vasodilation is typical of an endothelium-mediated response in which the increased blood flow causes release of an EDRF (176, 227, 237). This concept is supported by the finding that in human subjects bicycle exercise fails to cause dilation or even results in vasoconstriction in arteries with luminal irregularities indicative of atherosclerotic involvement (78, 178). Such atherosclerotic vessels have been demonstrated to have endothelial dysfunction, with loss of the normal production of EDRF in response to endothelium-dependent agonists or increased shear stress (188). Wang et al. (564) demonstrated that in chronically instrumented dogs exercise-induced coronary artery dilation was converted to a vasoconstrictor response by administration of nitro-L-arginine which acts as a competitive antagonist of L-arginine for NO synthase (378). Collectively, these findings implicate endothelial production of NO in the flow-mediated coronary artery vasodilation during exercise. In some vascular beds increased prostaglandin production also contributes to flow-mediated vasodilation (291), but the effect of inhibition of prostaglandin production on exercise-induced coronary artery vasodilation has not been studied.

Sympathetic influences. Sympathetic nerve fibers course along the epicardial arteries to innervate the myocardium and distal vasculature, and likely the coronary arteries themselves (164). Epicardial arteries possess both α-adrenergic (predominantly of the α_1-subtype) vasoconstrictor and β-adrenergic (predominantly β_1-subtype) vasodilator mechanisms, but in both isolated arteries and in the intact heart the response to sympathetic stimulation favors vasoconstriction (164, 165, 183, 274). Activation of the sympathetic nervous system during exercise appears to blunt the normal flow-mediated coronary artery dilation. Thus, α_1-adrenergic blockade with prazosin enhanced the normal exercise-induced coronary artery vasodilation, indicating that α_1-adrenergic vasoconstriction opposes exercise-induced vasodilation (47). Gaglione et al. (179) used contrast angiography to examine responses of epicardial coronary artery segments during supine bicycle exercise in patients undergoing coronary angiography to determine whether β-adrenergic blockade would result in unmasking of α-adrenergic vasoconstrictor activity. In angiographically normal coronary artery segments, exercise resulted in a 23% increase of computed coronary artery cross-sectional area. Intracoronary propranolol did not alter resting coronary artery cross-sectional area, but the vasodilator response to exercise (13% increase) was blunted, possibly because of attenuation of the myocardial blood flow response to exercise in the region under study. Intravenous propranolol did decrease the coronary artery luminal area during resting conditions, but exercise still caused coronary artery dilation. Since coronary blood flow was not measured, it is not possible to relate the degree of exercise-induced coronary artery vasodilation to coronary blood flow rates. These findings suggest that direct β-adrenergic activation does not contribute substantially to exercise-induced coronary artery vasodilation, and that β-adrenergic blockade does not result in unmasking of α-adrenergic vasoconstriction in the epicardial arteries.

Isometric Exercise. Coronary artery vasoconstriction is more prominent with static than with dynamic exercise. Thus, handgrip exercise for 4.5 min sustained at 25% of maximum grip strength resulted in vasoconstriction with a 14% decrease in mean cross-sectional area of angiographically normal coronary artery segments (78). Central and peripheral mechanisms elicit a vasoconstrictor reflex during isometric exercise. The efferent limb of this reflex includes sympathetic nerve fibers innervating the coronary arteries, likely with a contribution from increased circulating catecholamine. Thus, in contrast to dynamic exercise, which causes vasodilation of normal epicardial coronary arteries, isometric exercise results in vasoconstriction.

EFFECTS OF PHYSICAL CONDITIONING ON THE CORONARY CIRCULATION

Physical conditioning leads to adaptations in the heart that act to augment maximum cardiac output and maximum total body oxygen consumption. These adaptations also affect the major determinants of myocardial oxygen demand: heart rate, contractility, and left ventricular systolic wall stress. Dynamic exercise training lowers heart rate at rest and at any given level of submaximal exercise, and this is accompanied by parallel decreases of myocardial oxygen consumption (93, 217, 355, 557) and coronary blood flow (52, 217, 557). Myocardial contractility appears minimally affected by physical conditioning (83, 394, 453). Left ventricular systolic pressure is not significantly altered by exercise training in normal individuals, although in older or hypertensive subjects it may decrease slightly (472). Left ventricular end-diastolic internal diameter and wall thickness increase in parallel so that their ratio is not significantly altered (147, 351, 471, 567). Consequently, left ventricular systolic wall stress is minimally affected by exercise training. Thus, myocardial oxygen demand is decreased at rest or at any submaximal level of exercise in physically conditioned subjects mainly because of training bradycardia.

In addition to the decreased myocardial oxygen demands at rest and during submaximal exercise, physical conditioning causes adaptations that can augment myocardial oxygen supply. Oxygen supply can be increased by raising arterial oxygen-carrying capacity, by increasing oxygen extraction, or by augmenting blood flow. The oxygen-carrying capacity of the blood is generally not altered or is slightly decreased (<10%) following exercise training (87). Myocardial oxygen extraction does increase following exercise training (522, 557), but this effect is very modest, since oxygen extraction is already near maximum even in the untrained state. An enhanced ability to increase blood flow to the heart could result from adaptations within the coronary vessels or from a decrease in the extravascular forces that compress the intramural coronary vasculature. Coronary vascular adaptations in response to physical conditioning can be divided into structural (angiogenesis and vascular remodeling) and functional adaptations (alterations in vasomotor control) (305, 306, 316). Functional adaptations include changes in neurohumoral control or in local vascular control mechanisms (i.e. metabolic, myogenic, and endothelial control of vasomotor tone). The following section will consider each of these effects of exercise training.

Structural Adaptations

Epicardial Coronary Arteries. Two early studies using the corrosion cast technique reported an increase in coronary vascular volume (520, 535), which was mainly due to an increase in proximal coronary artery cross-sectional area (72, 211, 296, 332, 411, 576, 577). Swimming for 60 min/day increased proximal coronary artery luminal area in young male rats that underwent daily exercise and had cardiac hypertrophy, but not in rats that were exercised only twice each week and had no myocardial hypertrophy (332). Studies in dogs (576), atherosclerotic monkeys (296), and humans (211, 411) also suggest that the exercise-induced increase of proximal coronary artery dimensions parallels the increase in left ventricular weight, although coronary artery dimensions can sometimes increase out of proportion to the increment in myocardial mass (72, 296). A methodological limitation of the in vivo studies is that proximal coronary arteries were not maximally dilated at the time of study (e.g., with nitroglycerin), so that differing degrees of vasomotor tone between conditioned and sedentary animals could have influenced the results. In humans, resting heart rates are significantly lower following exercise training, likely resulting in lower basal blood flow per gram of myocardium. The lower shear stress in the proximal coronary arteries could lead to higher coronary artery tone, resulting in underestimation of the structural alterations as measured in vivo. This is supported by the finding that coronary artery cross-sectional area was not different between elite athletes and sedentary individuals under basal conditions, but was significantly greater in the athletes following arterial vasodilation with nitroglycerin (211). It must be kept in mind that an inherent problem with intergroup comparisons is the natural selection that may occur when comparing elite athletes with sedentary individuals. Additional longitudinal studies employing maximal coronary artery vasodilation (i.e., with nitroglycerin) are needed to determine whether exercise training increases coronary artery dimensions in humans beyond what would be expected from the degree of myocardial hypertrophy.

Coronary Arterioles. The effect of chronic treadmill exercise training on coronary arteriolar numerical density (i.e., the number of vessels per square millimeter) has been studied in domestic (76) and miniature swine (568). Arterioles were defined as vessels containing at least three layers of vascular smooth muscle with diameters between 35 and 75 μm. Arteriolar numerical density was 40%–60% greater in exercise-trained swine than in sedentary animals (76, 567, 568). Although the data included only coronary arterial microvessels with a limited range of diameters, the increase in arteriolar density provides a morphometric basis for the observed increase in peak coronary blood flow rates in exercise-trained animals (see later under Maximal Coronary Blood Flow).

Coronary Capillaries. Several investigations have examined the effects of physical conditioning on the capillary/fiber ratio (number of capillaries per myocyte), the capillary numerical density (number of capillaries per square millimeter), or capillary surface density (total capillary surface area per myocardial tissue volume). Early studies in which open capillaries were identified by erythrocyte staining (417, 418) suggested an increase in capillary numerical density and exercise-induced cardiac hypertrophy in young guinea pigs following treadmill exercise training. Similar results were obtained with hematoxylin-eosin staining in treadmill exercise–conditioned dogs (541). Capillary numerical density was found to be greater in wild than in domesticated rabbits or rats (558, 559), suggesting that greater physical activity of wild animals is associated with a higher capillary density. However, it is not clear to what extent natural selection vs. physical conditioning caused increased capillary densities in the wild animals. In contrast, adult guinea pigs subjected to swimming (174) or young guinea pigs subjected to running (207) had decreased capillary numerical densities compared to sedentary controls, as the capillary/fiber ratio failed to increase in the face of myocardial hypertrophy.

Subsequent studies examined genetically similar rats trained by either swimming or treadmill exercise. In the rat, the response of myocardial capillary density is critically dependent on age. In *young* rats trained by swimming or running, exercise-induced capillary angiogenesis occurs as indicated by an increase in [^{3}H]-thymidine labeling of capillary endothelial cells (85, 544) and an increase in the capillary/fiber ratio (60, 68, 259, 332, 363, 542). Angiogenesis outweighed myocyte hypertrophy in most of these studies, resulting in increased capillary numerical density (17, 68, 259, 538, 542) or relative capillary surface area (363). In *adult* rats 3–4 months of age, and in *old* rats 6–18 months of age, exercise training was also associated with enhanced formation of capillaries (68, 259, 333, 339, 542, 544). In contrast to the young rats, angiogenesis in adult (68, 259, 542) and old rats (68, 542) usually did not exceed the degree of cardiac hypertrophy, leaving capillary numerical density unchanged. Interestingly, swimming increased the capillary/fiber ratio because of a loss of myocardial fibers in old rats (68).

Evidence indicating that exercise training results in an increase in myocardial capillary density is derived mainly from studies of young male rats trained by swimming (60, 68, 85, 332, 363, 544). In contrast, studies of treadmill exercise–trained rats reported either an increase (17, 229, 259, 542) or no change in capillary density (15, 409, 537). Most studies in larger animals such as dogs (327, 576, 577) or swine (76) have failed to find an increase in capillary/fiber ratio (76, 327) or capillary numerical density (76, 327, 576, 577) following treadmill exercise training. A methodological concern is that several of the rat studies reported histologic data exclusively for the left ventricle (339, 363, 409, 542), while others reported data averaged for both ventricles (60, 68, 85, 259, 332, 333, 544). Anversa et al. (17) showed that a moderate treadmill exercise program increased capillary numerical density in the right but not the left ventricle. A more strenuous exercise program also failed to increase capillary numerical density in the left ventricle (16), and actually decreased capillary density in the right ventricle (15, 18). These findings raise concern that combined analysis of tissue from both ventricles might obscure differences in capillarization induced by exercise training in the individual ventricles.

In summary, most evidence that exercise training increases myocardial capillary density has been obtained from studies of young male rats trained by swimming. In larger animals trained by treadmill exercise, the formation of new capillaries occurs at a rate commensurate with the degree of myocardial hypertrophy. This does not imply a lack of effect of exercise on the formation of new capillaries, since capillary rarefaction often occurs in pathologic forms of hypertrophy secondary to hypertension or aortic stenosis (75, 320).

Adaptations of Neurohumoral Control

Alterations in neurohumoral control of the coronary vasculature can result from altered central autonomic activity, changes in the number or affinity of vascular receptors, or changes in postreceptor events. Several investigators have reported decreased circulating levels of catecholamines in exercise-trained humans and animals. These differences are most pronounced when similar absolute levels of submaximal exercise are compared before and after training, and suggest that sympathetic activity is decreased following training (67, 430, 472). Little information is available concerning adaptations at the adrenergic receptor level. Current evidence suggests that myocardial β-adrenergic receptor density and sensitivity are unchanged (208, 570), whereas decreased α-adrenergic receptor density has been found in rat myocardium following exercise training (570). Resting parasympathetic tone to the heart is increased following exercise conditioning; this is thought to arise from increased parasympathetic nerve activity rather than from changes at the muscarinic receptor level, since myocardial receptor density and sensitivity appear to be slightly decreased (70, 570). Studies of the effects of exercise training on adrenergic and muscarinic receptors in the coronary vasculature are lacking (570).

Epicardial Coronary Arteries. Using quantitative coronary angiography in closed-chest sedated adult dogs, Bove and Dewey (72) found that physical conditioning blunted the vasoconstrictor response of the proximal coronary arteries to α_1-adrenergic receptor stimulation with phenylephrine, but not to serotonin. Similarly, maximum vasoconstrictor responses to norepinephrine and phenylephrine were blunted in isolated endothelium-denuded proximal coronary artery rings of exercise-trained dogs (441) and swine (400). Steno-Bittel et al. (518, 519) suggested that the blunted vasoconstrictor responses might be the result of a decreased calcium content of sarcoplasmic reticulum in coronary vascular smooth muscle. However, vasoconstrictor responses of proximal coronary artery rings to KCl and prostaglandin $F_{2\alpha}$ were maintained (400, 441). These agonists act through different vasoconstrictor pathways: voltage-dependent calcium channels (KCl) and inositol trisphosphate (prostaglandin $F_{2\alpha}$), suggesting that exercise training has minimal effects on a variety of vasoconstrictor mechanisms. Since α_1-adrenergic receptor stimulation, like prostaglandin $F_{2\alpha}$, is believed to cause vasoconstriction via inositol trisphosphate–mediated release of calcium from the sarcoplasmic reticulum, this suggests that the attenuated α-adrenergic vasoconstriction observed in proximal coronary arteries following exercise training (72, 400) must involve altered α_1-adrenergic receptor density or coupling between the receptor and the second messenger system. Endothelium-dependent vasodilation produced by α_2-adrenergic receptor stimulation in precontracted coronary artery rings of dogs was not altered by exercise training (441). Blunting of the β-adrenergic vasodilator response was observed in isolated coronary arteries of dogs (441) but not swine (400).

In summary, in the proximal coronary artery exercise training results in reduced smooth muscle responsiveness to α_1-adrenergic receptor agonists, while endothelium-dependent α_2-adrenergic vasodilation is unaltered. Studies of the effects of training on β-adrenergic responsiveness are inconclusive.

Coronary Resistance Vessels

α-Adrenergic activity. Stone and co-workers (120, 205, 336) examined neurohumoral control in dogs subjected to 4–5 weeks of daily treadmill exercise. The nonselective α-adrenergic receptor antagonist phentolamine caused an increase in diastolic coronary blood flow during submaximal treadmill exercise in dogs, but this response was significantly less in exercise-trained animals than in sedentary dogs (336). In subsequent studies, phentolamine produced greater (205) or smaller (120) increases in mean coronary blood flow in partially trained dogs during submaximal exercise as compared to sedentary animals. The reason for these differing results is unclear, but in the latter study phentolamine produced identical increases in mean coronary flow in trained and sedentary dogs during submaximal exercise in the presence of β_2-adrenoceptor blockade (120). In open-chest dogs, α_1-adrenoceptor blockade caused a slightly greater increment of mean coronary blood flow in exercise-trained than in sedentary animals (306). Taken together, studies of mean coronary blood flow suggest that exercise training maintains or slightly increases α-adrenergic tone in coronary resistance vessels during submaximal exercise. The finding of maintained or increased α-adrenergic tone despite lower circulating levels of catecholamines implies increased α-adrenergic receptor responsiveness.

There is evidence in both peripheral (331, 348) and coronary vascular beds (121, 205) that resistance vessel constriction in response to α_1-adrenergic stimulation is enhanced after exercise training. Thus, the decreases in coronary blood flow in awake dogs produced by intracoronary injections of the α_1-adrenergic agonist phenylephrine or the nonselective agonist norepinephrine are greater following exercise training (121, 205). Left stellate ganglionectomy abolished the training-induced increase of α-adrenergic responsiveness during exercise, indicating the importance of intact sympathetic innervation for the coronary vascular adaptations to physical conditioning (121). Maintained or slightly increased α-adrenergic tone in coronary resistance vessels despite lower levels of circulating catecholamines may be an adaptation that results in an improved match of blood flow distribution and exchange area optimizing capillary diffusion (see later under Capillary Diffusion Capacity). This hypothesis is supported by the observation that myocardial oxygen extraction is enhanced following exercise training (522, 557).

β-Adrenergic activity. Several investigators have observed similar reductions of coronary blood flow during submaximal exercise in response to nonselective (205, 337), β_1-selective (205, 337), or β_2-selective (120) adrenoceptor blockade in exercise-trained dogs as compared to sedentary dogs. β_2-Adrenergic receptor responsiveness of the coronary resistance vessels is enhanced following exercise training (121, 209). This suggests that a decrease in sympathetic neuronal input during submaximal exercise is balanced by an increased vascular β-adrenergic receptor responsiveness, resulting in maintained vascular coronary β_2-adrenergic activity.

Parasympathetic activity. Muscarinic receptor blockade had no effect on coronary blood flow in exercising dogs before or after exercise training (205). This indicates that parasympathetic tone to the heart is absent during submaximal exercise at heart rates of 190–210 bpm both before and after exercise training (205).

In summary, exercise training maintains or slightly increases α-adrenergic coronary vasomotor tone but does not alter β-adrenergic tone in coronary resistance vessels during submaximal exercise. Maintenance of adrenergic tone in the presence of lower circulating catecholamine levels appears to be due to increased receptor responsiveness to adrenergic stimulation.

Local Coronary Vascular Control

Metabolic Control. Exercise-training has generally been reported to result in slightly decreased coronary blood flow rates per gram of myocardium at rest and during similar levels of submaximal exercise [Fig. 16.6*A*; (217, 557)]. However, at similar levels of *cardiac* work coronary blood flow is not altered by exercise training [Fig. 16.6*B*; (205, 217, 336, 522, 557)], suggesting minimal effect of exercise training on the coupling between myocardial metabolism and coronary blood flow. Von Restorff et al. (557) and Stone (522) reported a slight increase in myocardial oxygen extraction in exercise-trained dogs (Fig. 16.6*B*) that was not sufficient to result in a measurable decrease of coronary blood flow at any submaximal heart rate. The slightly increased myocardial oxygen extraction during treadmill exercise likely reflects improved capillary blood flow distribution and/or increased α-adrenergic tone in coronary resistance vessels.

The mechanisms involved in metabolic regulation of coronary blood flow likely include mediators released by the myocardium. Although adenosine does not play an essential role in regulation of coronary blood flow under conditions of normal arterial inflow (40), exercise-training was reported to increase resistance vessel sensitivity or maximal responsiveness to adenosine in dogs in vivo (121, 306, 327), and in miniature swine in vivo (324), but not in swine coronary resistance vessels in vitro (382).

Myogenic Control. Myogenic control has been implicated in autoregulation of coronary blood flow and coronary reactive hyperemia (61, 164). Muller et al. (383) studied the effect of exercise training on myogenic responses of small coronary arteries of swine (75–150 μm in diameter) in vitro. Active changes in vessel diameter measured in response to 10 mm Hg increments of distending pressure were similar in small arteries from exercise-trained and sedentary swine for intraluminal pressures below 40 mm Hg. However, for pressures above 40 mm Hg the myogenic response was significantly greater in vessels from exercise-trained swine.

Endothelium-Mediated Control

Large epicardial arteries. Wang et al. (564) exercised chronically instrumented awake dogs on a treadmill for 2 h/day for 7 days; this degree of training had no effect on heart rate, left ventricular mass, or coronary blood flow at rest or during exercise. Seven days of training enhanced proximal coronary artery vasodilation in response to acetylcholine and during reactive hyperemia; these vasodilator responses were abolished by inhibition of NO production with the arginine analog *N*-nitro-L-arginine. Since proximal coronary artery vasodilation by the endothelium-independent dilator nitroglycerin was not affected, the results could not be due to enhanced vascular smooth muscle sensitivity to NO. Thus, exercise training for as little as 1 week can increase receptor- and flow-mediated endothelium-dependent coronary artery dilation. Longer periods of exercise training (> 10 weeks) slightly attenuated the vasodilator response of the proximal coronary arteries to the endothelium-independent vasodilator nitroprusside in swine (401), but failed to enhance endothelium-dependent relaxation of proximal canine coronary artery rings in response to α_2-adrenergic stimulation, substance P, or vasoactive intestinal peptide (441).

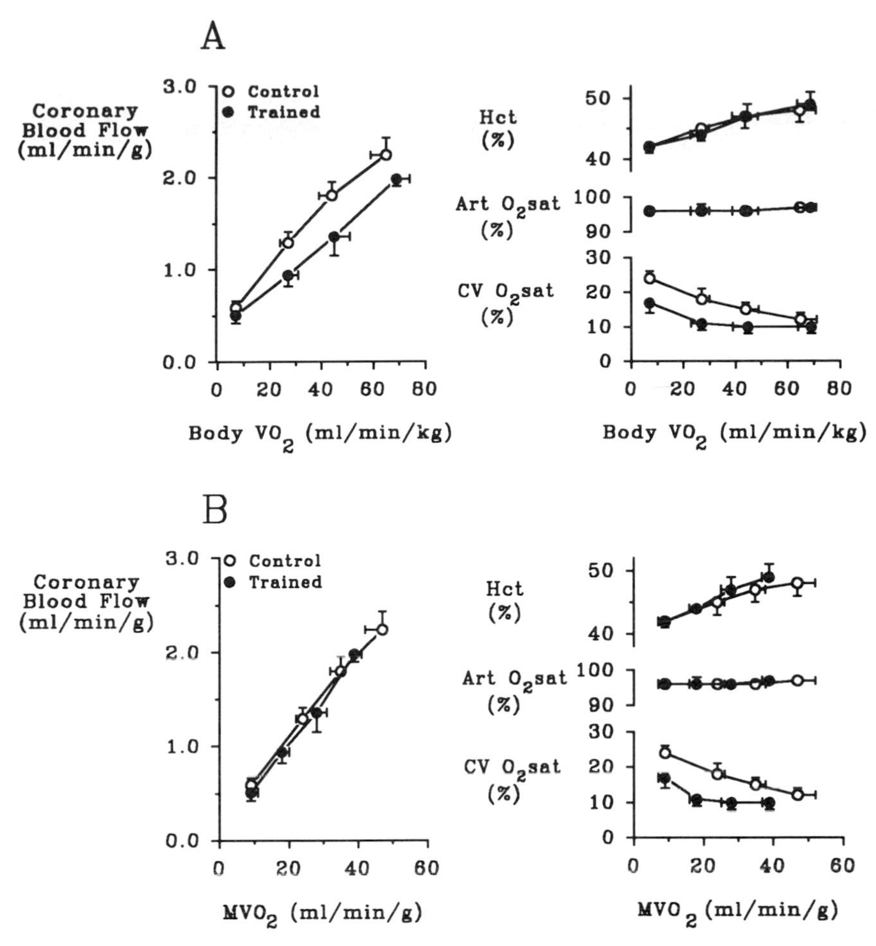

FIG. 16.6. Effects of exercise training on the myocardial oxygen balance in awake dogs at rest and during four incremental levels of treadmill exercise. *A*, Exercise training had no effect on the arterial oxygen-carrying capacity, but caused a small but significant increase in myocardial oxygen extraction and decreased coronary blood flow at comparable workloads during exercise (reflected by total-body oxygen consumption. *B*, However, the relationship between myocardial oxygen consumption and coronary blood flow was not altered by exercise training, as the increase in myocardial oxygen extraction was too small to result in a measurable decrease in coronary blood flow. Body $\dot{V}O_2$, total body oxygen consumption; MVO_2, myocardial oxygen consumption; Hct, hematocrit; Art O_2 sat, arterial oxygen saturation; CVO_2 sat, coronary venous oxygen saturation. Data are mean ± SEM, and are from von Restorff et al. (557).

Coronary resistance vessels. Bove and Dewey (72) observed that 8 weeks of exercise training enhanced the increases in myocardial blood flow produced by serotonin in closed-chest anesthetized dogs. Since coronary resistance vessel dilation by serotonin is mediated through endothelium-dependent S_1 receptors, the findings suggest that exercise training augmented endothelium-dependent coronary resistance vessel dilation. Similarly, Muller et al. (382) reported that vasodilation in response to the endothelium-dependent vasodilator bradykinin was enhanced in isolated coronary arterioles (64–157 μm in diameter) from exercise-trained compared to sedentary swine. Indomethacin decreased the vasodilator responses in both groups but did not alter the difference between the two groups. In contrast, N^G-monomethyl-L-arginine (L-NMMA) inhibited the bradykinin-induced vasodilation to a greater extent in the exercise-trained group and eliminated the difference between the two groups, suggesting that exercise training enhances bradykinin-induced vasodilation through increased NO production (382). Consistent with this interpretation, vasodilator responses to sodium nitroprusside were not different between sedentary and exercise-trained swine (382).

The available data thus indicate that exercise training can enhance endothelium-dependent vasodilation throughout the coronary vascular tree. This enhanced responsiveness may be due to increased expression of NO synthase (488).

Integrated Coronary Vascular Adaptations

To document a beneficial effect of exercise training on coronary vascular function, it is necessary to show that the structural or functional adaptations of the different vessel segments improve the myocardial oxygen supply. Increases in maximal coronary blood flow per gram of myocardium, capillary diffusion capacity, and/or coronary collateral circulation are mechanisms that could improve oxygen supply.

Maximal Coronary Blood Flow. Exercise training has been reported to cause either no change (52, 73, 76, 84, 97, 334, 468, 522, 580) or an increase (57, 82, 121, 316, 324, 327, 335, 412, 513) in maximal coronary blood flow capacity. Several factors may have contributed to the differing results, including differences in species, sex, and age of the experimental animals, as well as the type and intensity of the exercise training protocol. The method used to assess blood flow capacity can also influence the results. Studies in which increments in cardiac workload were used to increase coronary blood flow have found either no change (52, 73, 522) or an increased blood flow capacity (335, 412). Studies in which hypoxia was used to dilate the coronary vasculature in young rat hearts have also yielded divergent results, with increased blood flow in isolated buffer-perfused hearts from exercise-trained animals (57) but similar (580) or increased (513) flow rates in blood-perfused in situ hearts of exercise-trained rats. Laughlin et al. (316) reported an increase in peak reactive hyperemia flow following a 10 s coronary artery occlusion in exercise-trained dogs, whereas Stone (522) found no difference between sedentary and exercise-conditioned dogs. It should be noted that increased cardiac work, hypoxia, or a 10 s occlusion may not elicit maximal coronary vasodilation, nor is it certain that maximal coronary vasodilation was achieved when adenosine was infused intravenously (76, 84, 334). When maximal vasodilation was achieved by intracoronary infusion of adenosine, maximum coronary blood flow per gram of myocardium was generally increased following exercise training in swine (324), dogs (121, 306, 327), and rats (82). In only two studies in which maximal coronary vasodilation was documented and systemic hemodynamic variables were controlled (97, 468) was maximal blood flow not increased by exercise training. In the study of Scheel et al. (468), coronary blood flow was expressed as milliliters per minute without regard for the size of the perfusion bed, so that interanimal variability might have obscured a difference between the trained and sedentary dogs. The negative results obtained by Cohen (97) could have been influenced by differences between breeds (trained greyhounds vs. sedentary mongrel dogs). In addition, four of the five studies that reported an increase in maximal blood flow rates documented a training effect (82, 121, 306, 324, 327), whereas in neither of the two negative studies was a training effect reported (97, 468). Thus, the weight of evidence suggests that physical conditioning can increase maximal coronary blood flow per gram of myocardium if the exercise training program is of sufficient intensity.

Capillary Diffusion Capacity. Capillary exchange capacity is determined by the product of capillary permeability and total capillary surface area (PS product). Although exercise training does not increase capillary numerical density, an increase in PS product could result from optimization of the distribution of blood flow, so that all capillaries are perfused close to their exchange capacity. This would increase the effective capillary surface area without an increase in anatomical surface area. The PS product can be determined using indicator dilution techniques that incorporate a diffusible test substance and an intravascular reference agent. Laughlin and associates have shown an increase in PS product in exercise-trained dogs (306, 315, 327) and miniature swine (324). When the PS product and morphometric measurements of capillarization were compared in the same hearts, exercise was found to increase the PS product with no change in capillary numerical density (327). This suggests that the increase in PS product resulted from optimization of the distribution of blood flow, thereby increasing the effective surface area. In the maximally vasodilated bed the PS product is a function of the coronary flow rate, possibly because higher flows cause recruitment of additional capillaries, with an increase in the microvascular exchange area (327, 444). Although a higher PS product could be due to the higher maximal flow rates in trained animals when hearts are perfused at comparable coronary artery pressures, this cannot fully explain the reported results, since a higher PS product was also observed when exercise-trained and sedentary animals were compared at similar flow rates by using a lower coronary pressure in the trained animals (327). The findings suggest that exercise training alters the distribution of coronary vascular resistance so that more capillaries are recruited, resulting in an increase in the PS product without a change in capillary numerical density.

Coronary Collateral Circulation. There is considerable interest in whether chronic exercise is capable of stimulating the formation of coronary collateral vessels. Human studies using angiography to assess the collateral circulation in exercise-trained patients with coronary artery disease have generally yielded negative results (175). However, these studies are limited to visual assessment of coronary collateral vessels without measurement of collateral blood flow.

Native collateral vessels in the normal heart. The effect of exercise training on collateral function in normal hearts has been assessed by measuring retrograde blood flow from the cannulated collateral-dependent coronary artery opened to atmospheric pressure (81, 100, 468) or with radioactive microspheres (98, 124, 287, 289, 462, 469). Comparisons of collateral blood flow in trained and sedentary groups of animals have yielded exclusively negative results (81, 100, 124, 289, 462, 468, 469). To compensate for interanimal differences in native collaterals, Knight and Stone (287) measured collateral blood flow in chronically instrumented dogs before and after exercise training. Collateral blood flow was found to increase between early pre-exercise measurements and later measurements obtained after exercise conditioning. Cohen (98) also observed a tendency for collateral flow to increase in chronically instrumented dogs following exercise training, but a similar increase was also observed in sedentary animals, suggesting that the chronic instrumentation procedure stimulated the growth of coronary collateral vessels independent of exercise training. The preponderance of evidence suggests that physical conditioning does not enhance native collateral vascularity in the normal heart.

Exercise training with a coronary stenosis or occlusion. Eckstein (143) first reported a beneficial effect of exercise training on collateral formation in dogs with a fixed coronary artery stenosis. The increase in retrograde blood flow produced by exercise training was most striking in the presence of a mild stenosis that resulted in minimal collateral formation in the sedentary animals, suggesting that exercise produced ischemia, which then acted to stimulate collateral vessel growth. Cohen et al. (101) reported similar results in chronically instrumented dogs, further suggesting that exercise training that induces or aggravates ischemia in myocardium perfused by a stenotic coronary artery can stimulate collateral growth.

Studies of the effect of exercise training on collateral formation in response to a progressive coronary artery occlusion using the ameroid constrictor technique have yielded equivocal results. Heaton et al. (215) and Neill and Oxendine (390) reported no difference between sedentary and exercise-trained dogs in mean collateral blood flow measured 6–8 weeks after placement of an ameroid constrictor on a proximal coronary artery, although a slight improvement in the ENDO/EPI flow ratio in the collateralized region was observed after exercise training (215). Exercise training may have failed to exert an effect because the stimulus for collateral formation was nearly maximal even in the sedentary animals. Thus, at the time of study mean blood flow to the collateral-dependent region was equal to that in the normal zone even in the sedentary dogs, so that exercise training may not have induced ischemia (215, 390). In contrast, in swine, blood flow in the collateral-dependent region was less than 50% of blood flow in the normal myocardial region during exercise, so that exercise-induced ischemia might have further stimulated collateral vessel growth (69, 445). Moreover, differences in collateral blood flow between exercised and sedentary dogs might not have been detected because maximal dilation was not achieved (215, 390). This could explain why retrograde blood flow (which is not affected by resistance vessel tone) has been reported to be increased by exercise conditioning in trained dogs with ameroid occlusion of a coronary artery (390, 468). However, Schaper et al. (467) observed no effect of exercise training on collateral blood flow in isolated dog hearts in which maximal coronary resistance vessel dilation was produced with adenosine. In none of the above studies was an attempt made to maximally dilate the coronary collateral vessels (e.g., with nitroglycerin) so that differences in collateral vessel tone might have influenced the measured collateral blood flow rates (214).

In summary, exercise does not stimulate growth of coronary collateral vessels in the normal heart. However, if exercise produces myocardial ischemia that would be absent or minimal under resting conditions, there is evidence that collateral growth can be enhanced. Finally, if ischemia is present even under resting conditions, exercise may have only a modest additional effect on collateral vessel development. However, the concept that exercise-induced ischemia can enhance collateral vessel growth is not supported by two studies in which β-adrenergic blockade with propranolol was used to minimize the occurrence of myocardial ischemia during gradual coronary occlusion with an ameroid constrictor. In these studies, propranolol had no effect on the rate of collateral vessel growth in either swine (533) or dogs (99). These studies suggest that other factors such as the pressure gradient between adjacent vascular beds, which determines the flow rate and therefore endothelial shear stress, may be more important than ischemia in stimulating growth of collateral vessels.

Extravascular Determinants of Coronary Blood Flow

Alterations of systemic hemodynamic variables produced by exercise training can affect the extravascular compressive forces that influence coronary blood flow. For example, exercise training results in a lower heart rate at rest and during submaximal levels of exercise (32, 472). By reducing the time spent in systole, the net impedance to blood flow produced by systolic compression of the intramural coronary vessels is decreased (138). Exercise training slightly improves indices of global left ventricular systolic and diastolic function, mainly because of altered ventricular dimensions and loading conditions (102) with little change in intrinsic myocardial contractility (83, 394). Improvements of systolic and diastolic function have opposing effects on impedance to coronary blood flow, and tend to balance each other (138), with minimal net effect on impedance to blood flow. Dynamic exercise training increases both left ventricular end-diastolic internal diameter and wall thickness, with little change in their ratio (351, 567). Since left ventricular diastolic and systolic pressures are minimally affected by endurance exercise training in normal animals (52, 108, 567), it is likely that left ventricular diastolic and systolic wall stress are not altered by exercise conditioning. The available data thus indicate that physical conditioning causes a modest decrease of extravascular compressive forces at rest and at comparable absolute levels of exercise, principally because of a decrease in heart rate.

SKELETAL MUSCLE BLOOD FLOW DURING EXERCISE

During sustained exercise, the delivery of adequate blood flow through microvascular exchange vessels of muscle tissue is essential to provide nutrients, to maintain fluid balance, and to remove metabolites and heat from rhythmically contracting skeletal muscle. The amounts of blood flow provided to individual muscles at various intensities of exercise are illustrated in Figure 16.1 and the total amount of blood flow provided to skeletal muscle vascular beds during exercise at intensities that produce $\dot{V}O_{2max}$ is illustrated in Figure 16.4. This portion of the text discusses the mechanisms involved in increasing skeletal muscle vascular conductance allowing these amounts of blood flow during exercise. Although experiments that model exercise with various skeletal muscle preparations provide important insight into the mechanisms of exercise hyperemia (49, 180, 206, 245, 491), this portion of the text concentrates on studies of skeletal muscle blood flow during voluntary, whole-body exercise in humans and animals. The highest blood flows seen in skeletal muscle occur under these conditions [Fig. 16.1; (11, 307, 310, 319, 449, 450)].

Two general types of exercise are considered: isometric and dynamic. Since the cardiovascular response to these two types of exercise and their effects on skeletal muscle perfusion are different, we discuss them separately. Consistent with the theme of this *Handbook*, the primary focus is on dynamic exercise.

Skeletal Muscle Blood Flow during Isometric Contraction

Sustained, maximal, isometric contraction of skeletal muscle causes a rapid and transient expulsion of blood from its veins and an abrupt decrease in blood flow into its arteries (104). Relaxation of an isometric contraction permits a dramatic, though transient, increase in arterial inflow (104). If an isometric contraction is brief (100–300 ms), blood flow, after the contraction, reaches peak values immediately (within 1 s) and then decreases rapidly to resting levels over 15–20 s. The peak value of blood flow observed following such a contraction is proportional to the strength of the contraction (104). If an isometric contraction is maintained for more than a few seconds it is accompanied by a postexercise hyperemia (491) producing greater peak blood flows and more prolonged increases in blood flow than the brief contractions described above (104).

Isometric contractions that develop less than 15%–30% of the force developed by a maximal voluntary contraction (MVC) produce moderate increases in blood flow during contraction. Depending upon the muscle group examined, isometric contractions begin to interfere with blood flow when the contraction develops 15%–50% of MVC (491). Following such contractions, a transient postexercise hyperemia is observed, then blood flow slowly decreases to resting levels. It appears that, when muscles develop sufficient tension, extravascular forces compress the vasculature, increasing resistance so that blood flow is impeded. The degree of interference with blood flow produced by contraction is influenced by the fiber-type composition and location of the muscle within muscle groups. For example, fusiform muscles such as the soleus muscle appear to be designed such that blood flow can be maintained during sustained contraction. In contrast, contraction of pennate muscles generally produces decreases in vascular conductance. This effect is amplified in deep muscles within muscle groups (307, 491). The phenomenon of postexercise hyperemia and mechanisms responsible for it have been reviewed (49, 486, 491) and will not be discussed in detail here. Rather, we focus upon the blood flow response to dynamic, locomotory exercise. We acknowledge that many of the mechanisms responsible for exercise hyperemia and postexercise hyperemia appear to be similar. Indeed, in the hyperemia associated with rhythmic muscle contraction, most arterial inflow occurs between contractions, whereas most venous outflow occurs during contraction. In this regard, the pattern of skeletal muscle blood flow during normal dynamic exercise is similar to blood flow patterns observed in the coronary circulation.

Skeletal Muscle Exercise Hyperemia

The initiation of dynamic exercise produces immediate increases in blood flow to active skeletal muscle tissue. During rhythmic isometric contractions of various muscle groups (49, 50, 65, 546, 562) and in human subjects performing supine leg cycling exercise (154), blood flow increases following the first contraction. Although time-averaged arterial inflow and venous outflow are generally equal, it is important to keep in mind that during dynamic exercise and/or rhythmic contraction of skeletal muscle, venous outflow occurs during contractions and most arterial inflow occurs during relaxation of the muscle (169). These time-dependent changes in blood flow are important because they mean that durations of contraction and relaxation as well as frequency of contraction have effects on muscle perfusion not apparent in time-averaged flow measurements. The relationships among venous pressures, arterial pressures, venous outflow, and time during rhythmic tetanic contraction are illustrated in Figure 16.7, redrawn from the work of Folkow et al. (169). The effects of the physical forces produced by alternating contraction and relaxation on muscle hemodynamics are essential to our understanding of the mechanisms that determine muscle blood flow during exercise. Many studies of muscle blood flow during dynamic exercise have only measured time-averaged blood flow (mean blood flow), so that these pulsatile changes in muscle blood flow that occur with each contraction/relaxation cycle are obscured.

Antal was among the first to measure muscle blood flow during voluntary exercise in instrumented dogs (14). He observed rapid increases in mean skeletal muscle blood flow associated with commencement of locomotory exercise. Antal stated: "Simultaneously with the first locomotory movements of the hind extremity, blood flow starts to increase steeply and already during 2–3 s it reaches the maximal value, the magnitude of which is proportional to the rate of running." With the use of Doppler flow probes in dogs, Vatner et al. (554) also observed that commencement of exercise produced rapid increases in iliac artery blood flow in proportion to exercise

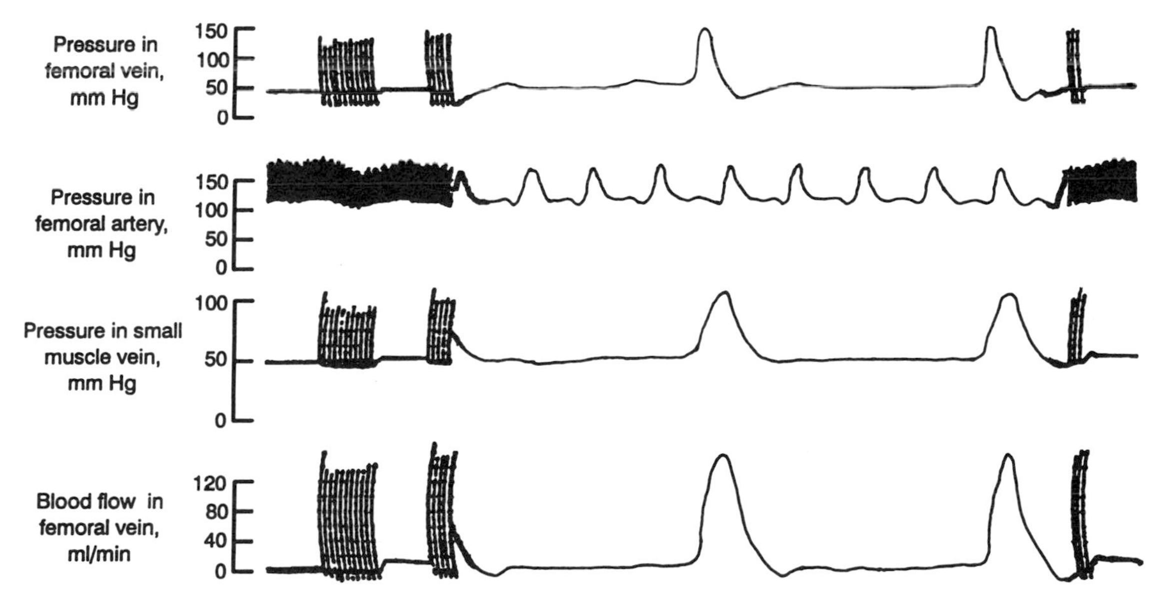

FIG. 16.7. Hemodynamic effects of rhythmic, 0.2 ms duration, tetanic contractions of cat calf muscle at a frequency of one tetanic contraction per second. Femoral venous pressure was increased to 50 mm Hg by elevations of outflow catheter as described by Folkow et al. (169). [Adapted from Folkow et al. (169).]

intensity. Also, terminal aortic blood flow in rats increases at the initiation of exercise and reaches peak values within 15–20 s of running (24). Thus, initiation of locomotory exercise produces rapid and substantial increases in skeletal muscle blood flow (14, 24, 25, 126, 184, 311, 434, 547, 550). During sustained low-intensity exercise, this rapid increase in blood flow has an "overshoot" during the first few seconds of exercise followed by a decrease in blood flow, towards resting flows, over the next 1–5 min (311, 346, 416, 495). This rapid, initial increase in blood flow has been referred to as an "on response" because it appears to be relatively independent of metabolic rate during walking and lower running speeds. A similar "on response" is observed at the start of running at faster speeds approaching and including maximal speeds (sprinting) (23). As illustrated in Figure 16.8, during initiation of low to moderate intensities of locomotory exercise, the rate of increase in vascular conductance is more related to frequency of contraction than work performed during this "on response" (495). Comparison of increments in hindlimb vascular conductance in response to locomotion at 2 mph and 4 mph (illustrated in Fig. 16.8) reveals that doubling the treadmill speed doubled the initial increase in vascular conductance. In contrast, the initial increases in vascular conductance (on response) were similar when work was increased by increasing treadmill grade from 0% to 10% at the same treadmill speed (4 mph). Thus the initial hyperemic response to locomotory exercise appears to be more related to the frequency of muscle contraction than to total metabolic rate. However, vascular conductance (blood flow) observed after 15–30 s of exercise appears to be more closely related to metabolic rate. Note vascular conductance is higher at 20 s of running at 4 mph up a 10% incline than for running at 4 mph with 0% incline in Figure 16.8. Thus, during sustained exercise, skeletal muscle blood flow is generally proportional to exercise intensity, showing only moderate or no increase with time of sustained exercise at this intensity (24, 25, 311, 434).

Regional Distribution of Skeletal Muscle Blood Flow

The increases in skeletal muscle blood flow observed during voluntary exercise do not occur uniformly throughout skeletal muscle [Fig. 16.1; (166, 167, 308–312)]. In fact, microsphere measurements of regional skeletal muscle blood flow reveal that flows range from 30–300 ml · min^{-1} · 100 g^{-1} during swimming and treadmill running (166, 167, 310–312, 316). Laughlin and Armstrong (310) examined relationships among fiber-type composition of skeletal muscle, patterns of muscle fiber recruitment, and regional patterns of muscle blood flow distribution in rats during various modes of exercise. They found

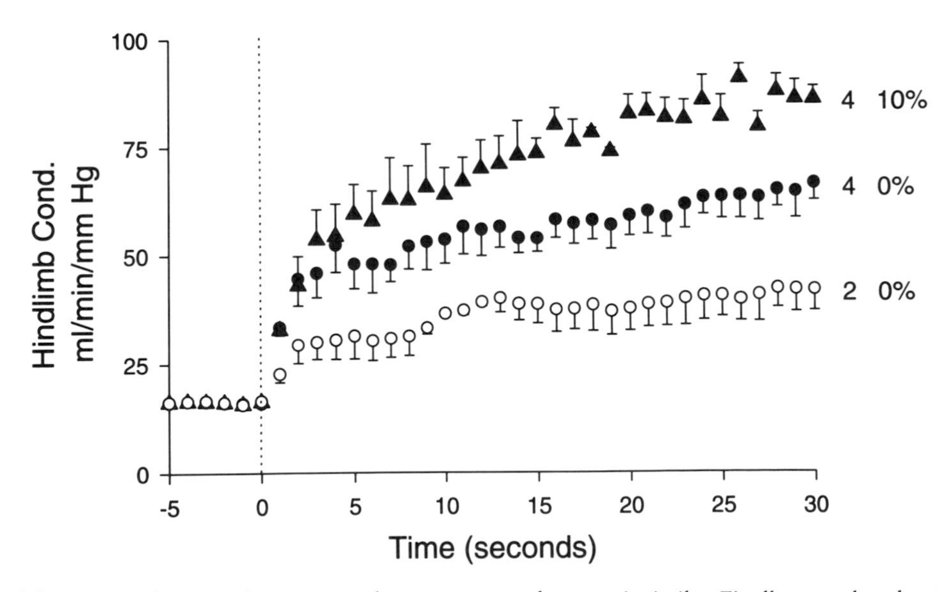

FIG. 16.8. Effects of frequency of contraction on vascular conductance of the dog hind limb. Data from Sheriff et al. (495). Note that doubling contraction frequency by increasing treadmill speed from 2 mph to 4 mph at 0% grade resulted in the initial rise in conductance to approximately double. In contrast, when the treadmill grade was increased from 0% to 10% and running speed held the same at 4 mph, the initial increase in vascular conductance is similar. Finally, note that the steady-state vascular conductance (15–30 s) appeared to be related to metabolic rate under all three conditions. These results were obtained from dogs in which cardiovascular reflex responses were blocked with hexamethonium (10 mg/kg, intravenously), atropine (0.2 mg/kg, intravenously), and captopril (1 mg/kg, intravenously) and during AV-linked ventricular pacing as described in Sheriff et al. (495).

that muscle blood flow within extensor muscles is preferentially distributed to active oxidative fibers under baseline conditions (310), as well as during different intensities (311), durations (23, 25, 312), and types of exercise (323). These and other studies reveal that blood flow appears to be directed to slow-twitch, oxidative (SO), postural muscles prior to exercise (310) (preexercise in Fig. 16.1). During exercise at various intensities, the magnitude of increase in blood flow in muscles, over resting, was found to be directly related to the percentage fast-twitch, oxidative-glycolytic (FOG) fiber type composition of the muscles and the intensity of exercise [Fig. 16.1; (311)]. In contrast, blood flow appeared to decrease in muscles like the VL_w (Fig. 16.1) composed largely of fast-twitch, glycolytic muscle fibers (FG) when low-intensity exercise commenced. Since blood flow increases in these muscles during exercise at higher running speeds (311, 388) when the FG fibers in them are recruited (526), it appears that blood flow did not increase in these muscles during low-intensity exercise because they are not recruited. Thus, the indication is that, in actively contracting skeletal muscles, blood flow is proportional to the oxidative capacities of muscle fibers (156, 309, 311, 388). During sustained exercise, blood flow continues to be directed to active fast- and slow-twitch, oxidative fibers within extensor muscles (20–23, 156, 312, 318, 388). In general, patterns of blood flow distribution within flexor muscles appear to be similar to those described above for extensor muscle groups. However, recruitment patterns and biochemical characteristics are not as well established for flexor muscle groups.

Mechanisms of Exercise Hyperemia

Barcroft, in his 1961 *Handbook* article, stated that understanding "the mechanisms of the increase in blood flow associated with exercise . . . is the most important problem in the field of skeletal muscle circulation" (49). As reflected in several excellent reviews, the search for mechanisms responsible for exercise hyperemia has remained a subject of great interest, and much has been learned about regulation of skeletal muscle vascular conductance since 1961 (129, 192, 206, 245, 247, 310, 369, 370, 375, 449, 491, 494, 508). Current thought in the field indicates that exercise hyperemia of skeletal muscle depends primarily on metabolic vasodilation and mechanical effects of contraction on muscle hemodynamics and secondarily on other control mechanisms. The essence of the metabolic control theory is that muscle vascular conductance is increased as the result of vasodilator, metabolic by-products (metabolites) released into the interstitial space of the active muscles. Many metabolic by-products have been demonstrated to be vasodilators. Indeed, nearly every substance known to be released into the interstitial space during skeletal muscle contraction has been shown to be vasoactive to some degree. The putative roles of each known metabolite in metabolic control of blood flow have been reviewed (129, 192, 206, 245, 310, 368–370, 375, 491). Although the magnitude of increase in vascular conductance measured in skeletal muscle during voluntary exercise has not been reproduced in vitro, this may be due largely to the inability to simulate voluntary muscle fiber recruitment during contraction (see later under *Muscle pump mechanism*).

There is evidence that the mechanisms responsible for initiating exercise hyperemia differ in relative importance or may be different from the mechanisms responsible for sustaining increases in blood flow during exercise. Therefore, we separately discuss initial hyperemic responses (0–1 min) and sustained (>1 min) increases in blood flow during exercise.

Initial Blood Flow Responses to Exercise

Direct neural linkage. Although the notion of a direct neural linkage between motor unit recruitment and the vascular supply of muscle fibers within the motor unit would be an attractive mechanism for matching blood flow to recruitment of muscle fibers, there is little experimental evidence to support the idea. The rapid increase in blood flow at onset of exercise led Gaskell (180) to propose that exercise hyperemia is initiated by vasodilator nerve fibers that are activated concomitantly with activation of the motor nerves to the muscles. Also, Antal concluded that: "The sudden appearance of changes in heart-rate and blood flow supports the view that at the beginning of exercise the co-innervation of skeletal and smooth muscles and muscle-visceral reflexes play a decisive role rather than metabolic changes" (14). The proposed neural pathways have not been identified. Honig et al. (238, 241) proposed that neuronal cell bodies located in the arteriolar walls were stimulated by α-motoneurons or muscle spindle afferents resulting in increases in vascular conductance and blood flow around activated muscle fibers. This interesting hypothesis has not gained general acceptance perhaps due to nonspecificity of the local anesthetics used to demonstrate the proposed effects of these intrinsic neurons (238, 241). Furthermore, the mechanisms for activating these nerve cell bodies during α-motoneuron activation in vivo have not been identified (491).

Sympathetic control. It has been proposed that sympathetic cholinergic stimulation and/or withdrawal of sympathetic nervous stimulation (tone) contribute to exercise hyperemia in skeletal muscle (238, 258, 447, 491, 494, 508). Although sympathetic cholinergic vasodilation appears to be one component of the defense reaction, it is not an inherent component of exercise hyperemia in skeletal muscle (26).

Chronic, cervical sympathectomy in humans had no effect on the magnitude or time of onset of the increase in blood flow following a 300 ms contraction of forearm muscles (104). Donald et al. (126) reported that unilateral lumbar sympathectomy had no effect on the iliac artery blood flow response to exercise in dogs. Also, Peterson et al. (416) examined the distribution of blood flow within and among rat skeletal muscles during locomotory exercise and found that lumbar sympathectomy had no effect on the rapid increase in muscle blood flow observed at the start of exercise. More recently, Sheriff et al. (495) reported that neither the magnitude nor the rate of rise of hindlimb vascular conductance measured at the initiation of exercise is altered by autonomic blockade in dogs. However, in both these studies (416, 495) sympathetic vasoconstriction appeared to cause moderate decreases in vascular conductance after 10–15 s of sustained exercise. Thus, the initial phase of exercise hyperemia does not appear to be dependent upon the sympathetic nervous system, but sympathetic control may contribute to modulation of skeletal muscle blood flow during sustained exercise.

Interactions of skeletal muscle metabolism and sympathetic vasoconstriction. The term "functional sympatholysis" refers to the concept that sympathetic vasoconstriction in active skeletal muscles may be overridden by local control factors, causing the vascular smooth muscle to be less sensitive to catecholamines (280, 434). A more recent interpretation is that release of norepinephrine from sympathetic adrenergic nerve endings in blood vessel walls is inhibited by certain metabolites (prejunctional inhibition) (72, 79, 449, 494). The notion that sympathetic activity is increased to all tissues during exercise, decreasing blood flow to most nonmuscular tissues and inactive skeletal muscle at the same time that blood flow is elevated in contracting muscle due to functional sympatholysis, emerged from the work of Remensnyder et al. (434) and Kjellmer (280). The decrease in forearm muscle blood flow observed during leg exercise (62, 65, 263) and the simultaneous increase in blood flow to red and decrease in blood flow to white portions of the same muscles during low-intensity exercise, as illustrated in Figure 16.1*A*, are consistent with this notion. However, Rowlands and Donald (451) reported that the attenuation of sympathetically mediated vasoconstrictor responses during sustained exercise was transient. Also, Peterson et al. (416) and Sheriff et al. (495) have reported a similar time dependency of the effects of sympathetic nerves on muscle blood flow during exercise. Thus, removal of sympathetic influences has no effect on the "on response" but does result in increases in blood flow measured during sustained exercise. If, as Sheriff et al. (495) propose, the rapid increase in blood flow at the initiation of exercise is caused by the muscle pump, this may explain why it appears that sympathetic effects are not as effective during the initiation of exercise.

Myogenic control. As discussed above, the myogenic mechanism is one major determinant of vasomotor tone in resting skeletal muscle. Contraction of skeletal muscle may increase vascular conductance via myogenic relaxation of vascular smooth muscle in response to extravascular compression (163, 264, 275, 377, 491). During contraction, pressure within skeletal muscle tissue is known to increase to 200–300 mm Hg (222, 277, 279, 307, 419). This increase in tissue pressure may decrease transmural pressure across the wall of intramuscular resistance arteries, leading to relaxation of vascular smooth muscle, so that vascular conductance and blood flow increase via the myogenic mechanism. In support of this concept, externally applied pressures of 100 mm Hg for 1 s resulted in about half as large an increase in skeletal muscle vascular conductance as produced by a 1 s tetanic contraction (377). The relative importance of the myogenic mechanism in skeletal muscle hyperemia remains in doubt because Bacchus et al. (34) demonstrated that simulations of twitch contractions with externally applied pressure do not produce increases in blood flow. Also, Sheriff et al. (495) recently initiated increases or decreases in transmural pressure in muscles of conscious dogs to determine whether myogenic responses were important in the initial hyperemic responses to dynamic exercise. Altering transmural pressure in this manner did not affect initial response of hindlimb vascular conductance in a manner consistent with myogenic control (495).

Metabolic control. A host of substances have been proposed as metabolites involved in modulating blood flow in proportion to metabolic activity, including decreased tissue and/or blood P_{O_2}, decreased pH, increased P_{CO_2}, increased osmolarity, increased adenosine and/or adenine nucleotides, potassium, histamine, kinins, phosphates, and prostaglandins (206, 375, 491, 494, 501, 508, 509). However, no one of these factors acting alone can produce the degree of vasodilation observed in skeletal muscle during exercise. Recognition of this has led to the development of the concept that there is an orchestration of several factors, each of which may contribute to a variable extent, depending on factors such as muscle fiber type, exercise intensity, and time after initiation of exercise. Two sets of observations indicate that metabolic control is not of primary importance in the blood flow "on response" at the start of exercise: (*1*) the time course of resistance vessel dilation is too slow, and (*2*) there is a poor relationship between metabolic rate and the initial hyperemia.

An abrupt increase in the concentration of vasodilator metabolites in interstitial spaces surrounding active muscle fibers could produce rapid increases in vascular conductance as proposed by Corcondilas et al. (104). However, direct measurements of diameters of arterioles in contracting skeletal muscle tissue indicate that vasodilation only becomes apparent 5–20 s after contraction begins and that arteriolar diameters do not reach steady-state values until 30–60 s of contraction (187, 352, 353). This time course of vasodilation is too slow to explain sudden increases in blood flow recorded after the first step of exercise or the rapid increases in conductance that occur within 2–4 s of the initiation of exercise (238, 241, 495). Simultaneous, direct measurements of tissue Po_2 indicate that arteriolar dilation precedes the fall in tissue Po_2, suggesting that early vasodilation is not related to changes in tissue oxygenation. However, steady-state arteriolar dilation correlates with steady-state values of tissue Po_2. In addition, arteriolar dilation is reduced in contracting skeletal muscle when tissue Po_2 is artificially maintained at normal levels (192). This latter observation suggests that tissue oxygenation is a critical factor in the regulation of steady-state microvessel relaxation in contracting skeletal muscle.

The poor correlation between exercise intensity and the magnitude of the initial hyperemic response also argues against a metabolic mechanism for the rapid increase in blood flow at the start of exercise. For example, Sheriff et al. (495) demonstrated that increasing exercise intensity by raising treadmill grade at a constant speed did little to the initial hyperemic response (Fig. 16.8). In contrast, vascular conductance was related to exercise intensity during sustained exercise after metabolic vasodilation had manifested itself. Thus, the "on response" appears to be independent of exercise intensity, suggesting a limited role for metabolic control.

In a unique study, partial neuromuscular blockade (tubocurarine) was used to selectively inhibit activity of oxidative skeletal muscle fibers during exercise. Results of this experiment support the notion that the "on response" of exercise hyperemia is poorly related to muscle metabolism (29, 186). Curare decreased glycogen depletion rate and electromyographic (EMG) activity of deep red skeletal muscle, indicating that the fibers in these muscles had less metabolic activity than fibers in the same muscles of control rats. Despite the lower metabolic rate in these muscle fibers, the initial increase in blood flow in the deep, high-oxidative skeletal muscle was the same in control and curare-treated rats. These results indicate that at the initiation of low- to moderate-intensity treadmill exercise, blood flow to high-oxidative muscle is not proportional to the activity or metabolism of the muscle fibers (29, 186). In contrast, in these same curare-treated rats, blood flow appeared to be matched to metabolic activity after 1–3 min of sustained exercise (186). Thus, it appears that at the initiation of low-intensity exercise, the "on response" is relatively independent of metabolic rate in skeletal muscle but largely determined by frequency of contraction. In contrast, muscle blood flow during sustained exercise appears to be consistently related to metabolic rate of the muscle (29, 186, 495). Although these findings indicate that metabolic control is not likely to be the sole cause of the rapid increases in blood flow at the initiation of exercise, as discussed below, metabolic control is of primary importance in maintaining blood flow during sustained exercise.

Muscle pump mechanism. Another possibility is that the muscle pump effect contributes to the dramatic increases in vascular conductance at the initiation of exercise. Rhythmical contractions cause a pumping action on the venous circulation in skeletal muscle, imparting both potential and kinetic energy to the blood, propelling it out of the veins during muscle contraction. Folkow et al. (169) first proposed that skeletal muscle has the ability to facilitate its own perfusion via the pumping action of contracting muscle fibers. Recently, Sheriff et al. (495) concluded that "the muscle pump actively assists the perfusion of muscle and accounts for much of the immediate rise in vascular conductance at the onset of exercise, before metabolic vasodilation."

The impact of the muscle pump on perfusion of active skeletal muscle is critically determined by the type of contractile activity (307, 391, 495, 521). Figure 16.9 presents the apparent vascular conductance in skeletal muscle during maximal vasodilation and during different forms of contractile activity. As illustrated in Figure 16.9, the muscle pump seems to be more effective in locomotory exercise than in various models of exercise such as twitch contractions and trains of tetanic contractions. This appears to

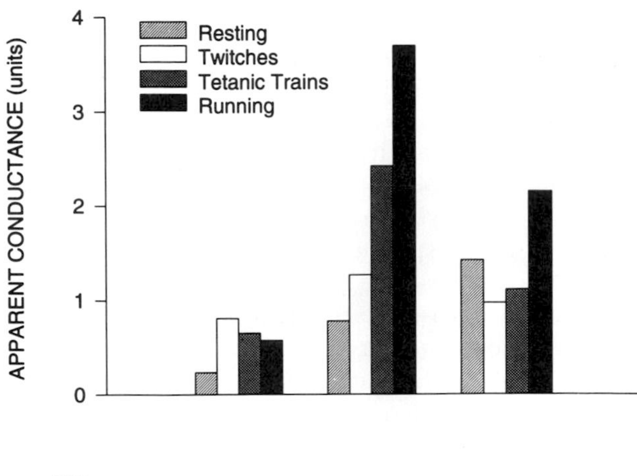

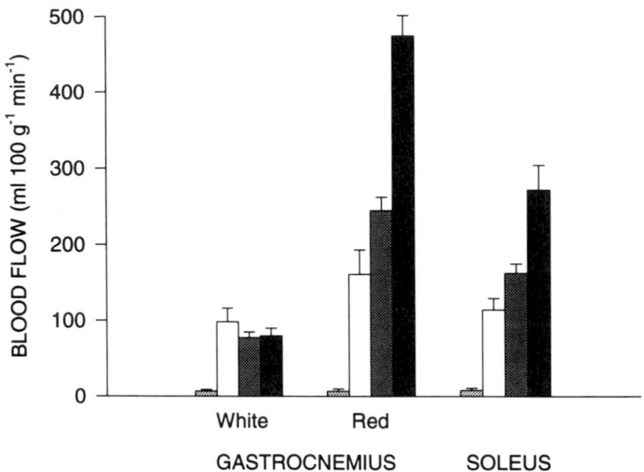

FIG. 16.9. Apparent vascular conductance and blood flows of rat skeletal muscle. [Adapted from Laughlin (304).] Vascular conductance was calculated for perfusion pressures of 130 mm Hg with equations derived from linear regression analysis of conductance (for each muscle) and perfusion pressure (corrected for effects of viscosity). Data for resting conditions are from Laughlin and Ripperger (325), data for twitch and tetanic conditions are from Mackie and Terjung (346), and data for running rats are from Armstrong and Laughlin (25). Data for twitch contractions were collected after 10 min of contraction and for tetanic contractions after 1 min of contractions.

result from the sequence of muscle fiber activation and type of contraction used in normal exercise activity. All muscle fibers are activated simultaneously in most in situ and in vitro models of exercise. In contrast, during locomotory exercise the time at which muscles are active during the stride cycle varies so that each muscle has a unique period of activity within each stride cycle (28, 80, 197, 310, 563). Furthermore, in locomotory exercise muscle fiber recruitment is sequential, not simultaneous (197). This sequential activation of skeletal muscles and fibers within muscle in exercising subjects may provide for a more effective pumping action on the veins of skeletal muscle in a manner similar to the wave of contraction that travels from the apex to the base of the heart. That is, the efficacy of the muscle pump is not only determined by the maximal pressure developed but also by the spatial and temporal sequence of pressure development and precontraction vascular volume (169, 170). Another potentially important characteristic of the type of contractile activity is whether changes in muscle length occur. During locomotory exercise the muscle pump mechanism may be more effective because muscle contractions consist of active lengthening and shortening as well as passive lengthening in different phases of the stride cycle (80, 197, 310). Thus, the finding that rhythmic isometric contractions produce lower peak vascular conductances than locomotory exercise may be due to the fact that the muscle pump mechanism is less effective in the absence of muscle length changes (compare tetanic trains to running in Fig. 16.9) (307). Other factors that are believed to influence the efficacy of the muscle pump include skeletal muscle fiber type and location within muscles or muscle groups, arrangement of the vasculature in the muscle (307), function of venous valves (62, 424), and the effects of gravity and/or venous filling pressures (169, 170).

The type (swimming, running, cycling) and intensity of exercise may also importantly influence the efficacy of the muscle pump (307). Pollack and Wood (425) observed that in humans the efficiency of the muscle pump, reflected in ankle venous pressures, was greatest at a treadmill speed of 1.7 mph and that this efficiency was not influenced by incline of the treadmill. Similarly, Sheriff et al. reported that the rapid increase in blood flow when dogs started to exercise on the treadmill (Fig. 16.8) was related to the frequency of contractions (speed) but not to treadmill incline (495). Available data do not allow a more rigorous analysis of the effects of stride frequency, stride length, and other gait-related factors on the muscle pump.

Although vascular "conductances" are presented in Figure 16.9, it is important to emphasize that they are as labeled, apparent because an ohmic conductance or resistance does not exist across a pump. That is, if the differences among conductance values are the result of the muscle pump, the apparent increase in conductance produced by contraction is actually the result of increased energy imparted to the blood by the pump and not due to relaxation of vascular smooth muscle and increased diameter of resistance vessels. The muscle pump may facilitate blood flow by at least two mechanisms: decreased venous pressures and increased total kinetic energy in the system (i.e., the total energy gradient available to force blood through the muscle vascular bed is increased). Because of the assumptions used to calculate the vascular conductances presented in Figure 16.9, this increased energy is translated to increased apparent conductance.

Endothelium-mediated vascular control. Endothelium-mediated vascular control has been shown to be important in skeletal muscle vascular beds at rest (369) and during muscle contraction, perhaps through flow-induced vasodilation (218, 270, 290–292). Endothelium-mediated vascular control may vary in skeletal muscle depending upon fiber type composition of the muscle (225) and regionally throughout the vascular tree in skeletal muscle tissue (218, 369, 415). Ekelund and Mellander (149) reported that in resting skeletal muscle, basal release of endothelium-derived nitric oxide (EDNO) is important in determining vascular resistance and that blockade of EDNO formation with L-NMMA produced greater vasoconstriction of large arteries than of resistance arteries. Hester et al. (218) presented evidence that EDNO is important in the initial (1 min) hyperemic response produced by twitch stimulation of the hamster cremaster muscle. Inhibition of EDNO production with N^G-nitro-L-arginine methyl ester (L-NAME) caused a significant decrease in the dilation of both the first- and second-order arterioles but not in the third-order arterioles. It may be that the rapid increase in blood flow produced by the muscle pump stimulates release of EDNO via flow-mediated changes in shear stress or other physical interactions with the endothelium. There is also preliminary evidence that EDNO plays a role in normal exercise hyperemia in conscious animals (228). On the other hand, Ekelund et al. (148) reported that blockade of EDNO production did not alter exercise hyperemia in cat skeletal muscle. Also, L-NMMA increased vascular resistance in resting rabbit tenuissimus muscle but did not alter exercise hyperemia in this muscle (414). Likewise, brachial arterial infusion of L-NMMA into human subjects produced decreases in resting forearm blood flow but had no effect on the blood flow response to forearm exercise (571). These studies imply either that exercise hyperemic responses are not endothelium dependent or that the endothelium releases an endothelium-derived vasodilator substance not blocked by arginine analogues during exercise hyperemia (148, 292, 369, 414, 571). There is currently insufficient data to allow definitive conclusions about the possible role of endothelium-mediated control phenomena in determining blood flow distribution within and among skeletal muscle during locomotory exercise.

Steady-State Exercise Hyperemia. Since there may be a limited number of primary vascular control mechanisms operative in skeletal muscle vascular beds, it seems likely that initial and steady-state exercise hyperemia are governed by the same vascular control mechanisms in skeletal muscle. If this is true, the relative contributions of vascular control mechanisms appear to be different in initial and steady-state hyperemia (206, 224, 237, 245, 416, 491, 495). Hudlická (245) concluded that "some control mechanisms may be initiators of exercise hyperemia and other mechanisms may be maintainers of exercise hyperemia." As described above, when exercise is initiated there is a rapid increase in blood flow that is not related to metabolic rate. Following the "on response," what happens to blood flow depends largely on the exercise intensity and the mass of active skeletal muscle. In general, during low intensities of exercise, blood flow will decrease from 30–120 s of sustained exercise. Muscle blood flow then remains relatively stable during sustained low-intensity exercise, settling at a level above resting flow, but below the initial hyperemia, showing only moderate increases as a function of time through 1–2 h (21, 312). In contrast, during exercise at moderate to high intensities, blood flow often does not decrease following the "on response" (Fig. 16.10). Rather, it will plateau within the first minute and/or increase gradually with time during sustained exercise. The primary cause of sustained exercise hyper-

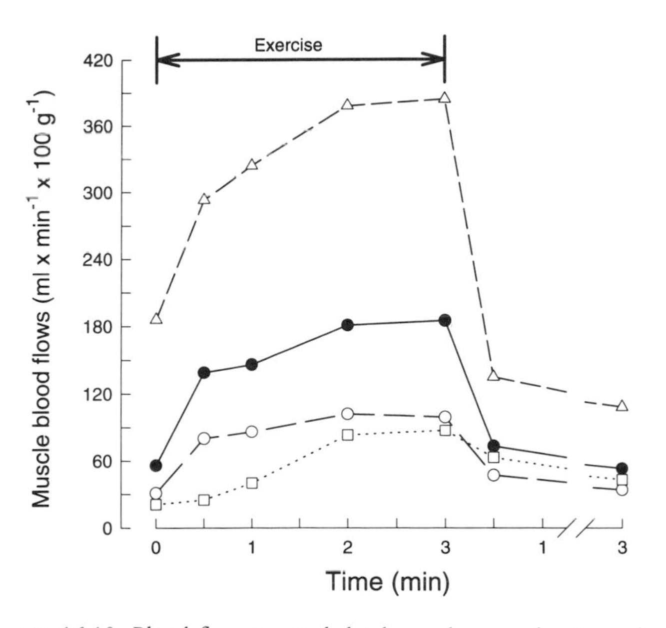

FIG. 16.10. Blood flow to rat skeletal muscles as a function of time during high-intensity treadmill exercise. Rats ran at 60 m/min from time 0 through 3 min. Recovery blood flows were measured at 30 s and 3 min following exercise. Data are presented for red (*triangles*) and white (*boxes*) vastus lateralis, biceps femoris (*open circles*), and total hindlimb muscle (*filled circles*). [Adapted from Armstrong and Laughlin (23).]

emia appears to be a combination of metabolic vasodilation and increased vascular conductance due to the muscle pump. However, as described below and in Chapter 17, neurohumoral control systems are important in regulating muscle blood flow during exercise.

Metabolic control mechanisms. Available data indicate that a primary determinant of skeletal muscle blood flow during sustained exercise is metabolic rate of the muscle (49, 129, 192, 206, 245, 247, 368, 375, 491). Over the past 30 years, many have sought substances that fulfill criteria that Mellander and Johansson stated should be "satisfied for a proposed metabolic factor to play an important causal role in exercise hyperemia" (370). Although this list of criteria has been refined and expanded over the years (245, 491), it continues to dominate thinking in this field. Implicit to these criteria is the assumption that exercise hyperemia is solely the result of relaxation of vascular smooth muscle in resistance vessels stimulated by one or more of these metabolites. This assumption, though reasonable and internally consistent with the metabolic hypothesis, may be the underlying reason why we have been unable to determine which substance or substances are the mediators of metabolic vasodilation. For example, one common criterion is that intra-arterial or interstitial infusion of the substance should be capable of causing an increase in vascular conductance that is as large as that occurring in exercise hyperemia (245, 370, 491). However, in resting skeletal muscle it appears to be impossible to increase vascular conductance to the levels measured during locomotory exercise. It is likely that the inability of vasodilator agents to increase vascular conductance in resting muscle to the levels of apparent vascular conductance calculated during exercise is that the muscle pump, aided possibly by abdominal and thoracic pumps, provides additional energy for muscle perfusion during normal exercise (307). Thus, even if the appropriate mediators are known, when applied in resting muscle, they will not be able to raise vascular conductances to the levels measured in locomotory exercise. The high skeletal muscle vascular conductance measured under these conditions is not due simply to relaxation of vascular smooth muscle in resistance vessels. The magnitude and time course of skeletal muscle exercise hyperemia during locomotory exercise appears not to be explained exclusively by metabolic control mechanisms (307).

ROLE OF ADENOSINE. Adenosine is a putative mediator of metabolic vasoregulation that has received a lot of attention over the past 10 years. Blockade of adenosine receptors with aminophylline was reported to blunt the ability of hindlimb vasculature of exercising dogs to adapt to decreases in hindlimb perfusion pressure, suggesting a role for adenosine in blood flow autoregulation in active skeletal muscle (372). Granger et al. (192) concluded that "most studies have failed to demonstrate a major role for adenosine in functional hyperemia." For example, infusion of adenosine deaminase (ADA) into rats did not alter resting skeletal muscle blood flow or blood flows measured during low-intensity exercise (285). If adenosine were essential for exercise hyperemia, ADA should have blunted the hyperemic response to exercise (285).

Dipyridamole increases blood flow in cardiac, respiratory, and SO skeletal muscle of miniature swine during submaximal treadmill exercise (318). Dipyridamole is believed to cause vasodilation by blocking adenosine uptake by various cells in the tissue. As a result, dipyridamole will cause adenosine to accumulate at a faster rate in tissues that release adenosine. The finding that dipyridamole increased blood flow to respiratory skeletal muscle, slow-twitch postural skeletal muscle, and cardiac muscle indicates that these types of muscle release more adenosine than skeletal muscle composed of other fiber types during submaximal exercise. These results also suggest that adenosine plays a role in exercise hyperemia in high-oxidative skeletal muscles. In contrast, these results indicate that adenosine does not play a major role in exercise hyperemia in fast-twitch glycolytic skeletal muscle (318). This differential control hypothesis is supported by the results of a study that compared the potential role of adenosine in exercise hyperemia in cat soleus muscle (SO) and gracilis muscle (FG) and found that ADA decreased exercise hyperemia in soleus muscle but had no effect in gracilis muscle (475).

There is also evidence that active mammalian skeletal muscle, irrespective of fiber-type composition, produces adenosine when perfused at constant flow, or with limited perfusion (192, 285, 318). During exercise at or above intensities producing maximal oxygen consumption, dipyridamole has been shown to produce vasodilation in all types of skeletal muscle (318). These data suggest that all skeletal muscle releases adenosine into the interstitium during maximal exercise, perhaps because blood flow is limited by maximal cardiac output under these conditions as discussed in more detail in Chapter 17.

IMPORTANCE OF MUSCLE FIBER TYPE. Experimental designs often ignored the importance of fiber type–related differences within and among skeletal muscles causing conflicting reports in the literature such as the adenosine results discussed above. There is a growing body of evidence suggesting that the relative importance of vascular control mechanisms varies as a function of skeletal muscle fiber type (224, 309, 318, 368, 539). For example, the vasculature of fast-twitch muscles is more sensitive to the vasodilator effects of epinephrine (313). On the other hand, the vasculature in slow-twitch oxidative (SO) skeletal muscle is less influenced by sympathetic α-adrenergic activity than is the vasculature of fast-twitch muscle (193). However, fast-twitch, glycolytic muscle appears to be more susceptible to functional sympatholysis (539). Thus, future studies need to be designed to enhance understanding the importance of various vascular control mechanisms in muscles composed of different fiber types.

RESPIRATORY SKELETAL MUSCLE. Manohar (349) reported that vascular resistance in the diaphragm and intercostal muscles of ponies was not changed by infusion of adenosine (3.0 μM · kg^{-1} · min^{-1}, into the pulmonary artery) during maximal exercise. He took these results as evidence that "vasodilator capacity was being completely utilized" during exercise at maximal intensities. However, blood flow and vascular resistance were not altered by adenosine, during maximal exercise, in any of the skeletal muscles examined by Manohar (349). Only the coronary circulation demonstrated vasodilation with adenosine infusion during exercise. These results may indicate that the vasodilation induced by adenosine was overcome by sympathetic vasoconstriction via mechanisms discussed in Chapter 17. On the other hand, in a similar study of respiratory muscle perfusion in swine during maximal exercise, it was found that dipyridamole increased vascular conductances of the diaphragm and intercostal muscles by 30%–50%. Thus, while there are data suggesting that vasodilator reserve is exhausted in respiratory muscles (349), in swine, vasodilator reserve was present, even during exercise at intensities sufficient to produce maximal oxygen consumption (318).

Role of the muscle pump. As described above, the rapid increases in blood flow observed at the initiation of exercise appear to be partly due to the action of the muscle pump. It is likely that the muscle pump continues to support perfusion of skeletal muscle during sustained exercise as well. Comparison of maximal blood flows measured during normal locomotory exercise, models of exercise, and during maximal pharmacological vasodilation as illustrated in Figure 16.9 supports the hypothesis that the muscle pump is important in sustaining muscle blood flow during exercise. Figure 16.9 depicts the apparent vascular conductances of rat muscle determined under four different conditions: (*1*) isolated, perfused hindquarters maximally vasodilated with papaverine; (*2*) performing isometric twitch-type contractions; (*3*) performing trains of isometric, tetanic contractions; and (*4*) running on a motor-driven treadmill. The reason that apparent vascular conductance in high-oxidative muscle tissue (soleus and red gastrocnemius muscles) is higher during normal exercise than during twitch and tetanic contraction may be that the type of muscle activity associated with voluntary exercise produces a more efficient pumping action. Also, one reason that trains of tetanic contractions appear to be less effective for increasing perfusion of white gastrocnemius muscle than of red gastrocnemius muscle could be that the white muscle is located superficially in the leg (277). That is, the muscle pump has less effect on the superficially located muscle tissue. It is also possible that the muscle pump component of perfusion in white muscle is less because of lower vascularity in this muscle tissue, resulting in a lower "stroke volume" (307). It is interesting that apparent vascular conductance is about the same during all three types of rhythmic muscle contraction in white, fast-twitch muscle. In contrast, in the red gastrocnemius muscle, apparent vascular conductance is much higher than in white gastrocnemius and increases from left to right (i.e., comparing resting to twitches, to tetanic trains, to running, in Fig. 16.9). Locomotory exercise produces the greatest value for apparent vascular conductance in the soleus and red gastrocnemius muscles. These data indicate that during treadmill exercise in rats, the muscle pump provides as much as 30%–60% of the total energy for perfusion of the soleus and red portion of the gastrocnemius muscles, respectively (307). Similar estimates indicate that the muscle pump provides substantial amounts of energy for muscle perfusion in exercising humans as well (341, 449, 517). The data summarized in Figure 16.9 suggest that the muscle pump is an important determinant of apparent vascular conductance (or blood flow) during locomotory exercise.

Neural control. Although the increases in muscle blood flow that occur during exercise are caused by the muscle pump and metabolic vasodilation, sympathetic adrenergic vasoconstriction appears to be involved in regulating these increases in vascular conductance in a manner similar to that which occurs in the coronary circulation described above (39). For example, during low-intensity exercise, the decrease in blood flow that is observed following the "on response" is abolished by removal of sympathetic influences, either with acute lumbar sympathectomy (416) or autonomic blockade with hexamethonium and atropine (495). These results indicate that, during low-intensity exercise, competition exists between sympathetic vasoconstriction and metabolic vasodilation. Indeed, it appears that increased sympathetic nerve activity to skeletal muscle vascular beds is part of the normal, generalized increase in sympathetic outflow during exercise.

MUSCLE SYMPATHETIC NERVE ACTIVITY. Recordings of muscle sympathetic nerve activity (MSNA) during dynamic exercise in humans indicate that MSNA increases only at or above moderate exercise intensities (478). That is, there appears to be a threshold exercise intensity below which MSNA is not changed. However, when exercise intensity increases sufficiently to raise heart rate above 100 bpm, there appears to be a generalized increase in sympathetic outflow that is proportional to exercise intensity (449). The relationships among regional visceral blood flows, heart rate, MSNA, and plasma norepinephrine concentrations are illustrated in Figure 16.11 (449). As described in detail in Chapter 7, current evidence indicates that the increase in MSNA during dynamic exercise can originate from muscle chemoreflex-stimulation associated with glycogenolysis and lactate production by active skeletal muscle tissue (449, 478). Increased MSNA and vasoconstriction of skeletal muscle vascular beds appears to be important for maintenance of blood pressure (416, 448, 449, 539, 550) and fluid balance in the muscle (358, 369). Thus, in a fascinating manner, during high intensities of dynamic exercise, muscle perfusion begins to have a major influence on the cardiovascular system. As described in Chapter 17, the interaction between the drive to provide adequate skeletal muscle blood flow (via local vascular control mechanisms and the skeletal muscle chemoreflex) and the drive to maintain arterial blood pressure (baroreceptor reflex) appear to come into conflict.

FUNCTIONAL SYMPATHOLYSIS. It is important to consider the question of whether there is a true functional sympatholysis in skeletal muscle vascular beds during sustained exercise. Remensnyder et al. (434) first reported evidence of functional sympatholysis during sustained exercise. In contrast, Thompson and Mohrman (540) reported that local metabolic mechanisms do not override sympathetic vasoconstriction in contracting skeletal muscle. Vatner et al. (550) demonstrated that carotid sinus nerve stimulation during exercise in conscious dogs caused profound increases in skeletal muscle blood flow and vascular conductance, indicating that sympathetic tone was limiting blood flow during exercise. Also, Peterson et al. (416) and Sheriff et al. (495) found that sympathetic activation decreased vascular conductance during sustained exercise. Recently, it was found that increased sympathetic activity, caused by orthostatic stress (upright posture), caused decreased blood flow and oxygen uptake in muscles of humans performing heavy rhythmic handgrip exercise (269). Thus, available of data indicate that the sympathetic nervous system retains the ability to decrease vascular conductance in active skeletal muscle.

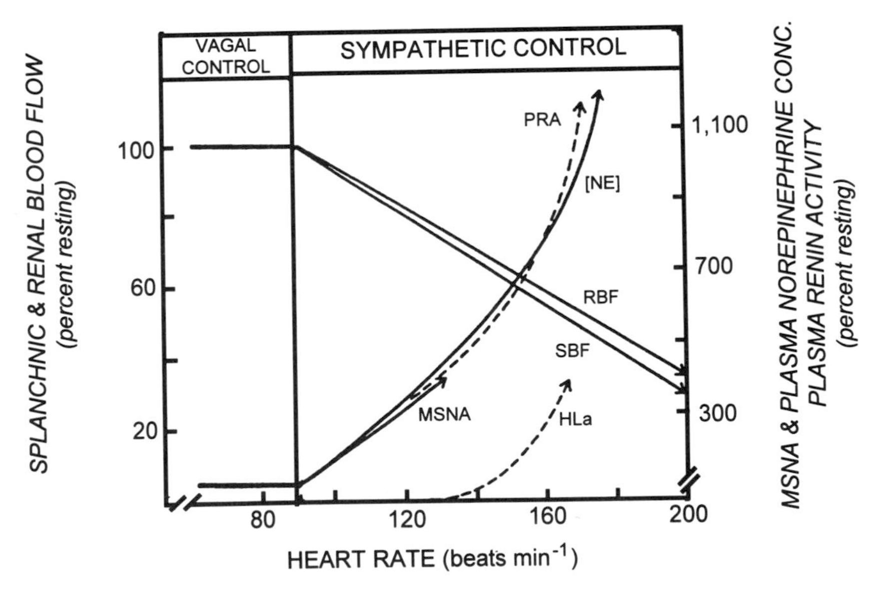

FIG. 16.11. Overview of changes in autonomic control of the cardiovascular system associated with increase intensity in humans. At rest, vagal control is important. Sympathetic nervous activity starts to increase as vagal control is withdrawn. Vagal control is negligible and sympathetic activity beginning to increase when exercise intensity produces heart rates of about 100 bpm. Indices of increased sympathetic nervous activity include: decreases in blood flow to splanchnic (SBF) and renal (RBF) vascular beds, increased plasma norepinephrine (NE) concentrations, increased plasma renin activity (PRA), and increased muscle sympathetic nerve activity (MSNA). Blood lactate concentration (HLa) does not increase until exercise intensity is 50%–60% of VO_{2max} (Heart rates of 130–140 bpm). [Adapted from Rowell et al. (449).]

Different approaches used to express and analyze data (e.g., change in blood flow, change in resistance, change in conductance) have caused some to conclude that exercise causes a functional sympatholysis in skeletal muscle and others to conclude that sympathetic vasoconstriction successfully overrides metabolic vasodilation during exercise. The problem is that changes in baseline blood flow (before sympathetic stimulation) can lead to difficulty in interpretation depending on how the data are analyzed. Sympathetic stimulation causes muscle blood flow to decrease by a similar absolute amount in contracting and resting skeletal muscle, but relative to baseline, the effect is slight during strenuous exercise because blood flows are higher (525, 540). Rowell demonstrated that recalculation of Kjellmer's (280) data reveals that steady-state changes in vascular conductance caused by sympathetic nerve stimulation are similar during exercise at various intensities, whereas Kjellmer had reported that the amount of increase in vascular resistance produced by sympathetic stimulation progressively decreased with increasing exercise intensity (449). Rowell stated that "when muscle blood flow is high, vasoconstriction causes large changes in vascular conductance . . . but only small changes in resistance" (449).

SENSITIVITY OF α_1- AND α_2-ADRENERGIC VASOCONSTRICTION TO METABOLIC VASODILATION. Adrenoreceptor-mediated vasoconstrictor mechanisms vary throughout the vascular tree of skeletal muscle (157, 397, 421). Adrenergic-induced constriction has been shown to be mediated through both α_1- and α_2-receptors in larger arterioles, but primarily through α_2-receptors in precapillary arterioles (157, 158). Differences in the spacial distribution of adrenergic-receptor subtypes could be functionally important, because the susceptibility of α-receptor-mediated constriction to interference by metabolic (12, 123), hormonal (123), myogenic (161, 421), and endothelium-derived (398) factors varies between the two α-receptor subtypes. For example, α_2-receptor-mediated constriction is more sensitive to metabolic inhibition than is α_1-mediated constriction (12). Anderson and Faber reported that a given concentration of metabolic vasodilator substances produced ten times greater opposition of α_2-mediated vasoconstriction than vasoconstriction mediated by α_1 receptors (12). Due to the differential distribution of postjunctional α_1- and α_2-adrenoceptors in the microcirculation of rat cremaster muscle [large resistance arterioles possessing both receptor types and small terminal arterioles possessing a predominance of α_2 receptors (157, 158)], these results suggest that low-intensity exercise specifically attenuates α_2 constriction in terminal arterioles producing increased capillary perfusion. As exercise intensity is increased, vasodilation is spread into the large resistance vessels (both receptor types), leading to increased blood flow. Thomas et al. reported that the relative importance of α_1- and α_2-adrenergic vasoconstriction during exercise may also differ between oxidative and glycolytic skeletal muscle as reflected in measurements of femoral artery blood flow during stimulation of the sciatic nerve and force produced by the soleus or gastrocnemius-plantaris muscles (539). They assumed that muscle blood flow only increased in the muscle attached to the force transducer (soleus or gastrocnemius-plantaris) and not to other leg muscles during stimulation of the sciatic nerve. Therefore, conclusions based on these results may be altered if these assumptions about blood flow distribution prove to be false. Their results indicate that lumbar sympathetic nerve stimulation produced similar decreases in vascular conductance at rest and during contraction of soleus muscle and during low-intensity contractile activity of gastrocnemius-plantaris muscles of rats (539). In contrast, during high-intensity contractile activity of gastrocnemius-plantaris muscle, sympathetic vasoconstriction was abolished (539). Thomas et al. concluded that the degree of functional sympatholysis observed in active skeletal muscle is dependent on fiber type and intensity of muscle contraction (539). Results suggest that the degree of sympatholysis produced within an active muscle is related to the severity of acidosis in the muscle. During voluntary exercise, increased muscle sympathetic nerve activity is generally associated with increases in arterial pressure (Chapter 17). Thus, reflex-mediated increases in arterial pressure coupled with functional sympatholysis may serve to limit acidosis within active glycolytic skeletal muscle. It is not yet possible to predict how the distribution of junctional and nonjunctional adrenergic receptors, adrenoceptor subtypes, and their activation throughout the skeletal muscle microcirculation interact with the differential effects of metabolic vasodilation to determine total and regional vascular resistance and the perfusion of exchange vessels throughout skeletal muscle vascular beds (12, 123, 192).

Regulation of Transcapillary Fluid and Solute Exchange in Skeletal Muscle

Rhythmic Contractions of Skeletal Muscle-Models of Exercise. This section has been written to summarize what is known from experiments with various contracting muscle preparations because detailed studies of transcapillary fluid and solute exchange have not been conducted with voluntary exercise, due to technical limitations. Current methods for stimulating skeletal muscle to contract do not adequately simulate the normal activation of muscle fibers that occurs in voluntary exercise (310, 346). Some have used stimulation parameters that are more similar to muscle stimulation associated with voluntary exercise such as rhythmic trains of tetanic contraction rather than trains of twitch contractions (346). To illustrate some of the problems, consider the common experiment involving stimulating muscle to twitch at various frequencies (171, 346). Advantages of this model of exercising skeletal muscle are that developed tension can be maintained for some time (depending on the type of muscle), and blood flow and capillary exchange are increased and stable so that a steady state is maintained, allowing quality measurements of hemodynamic parameters. However, skeletal muscles do not twitch during voluntary exercise. The hemodynamic effects of twitch contractions are dramatically different from those of rhythmic tetanic contractions and voluntary contractions (310, 346). Although experiments with these preparations have been used to improve our understanding of capillary exchange processes in contracting skeletal muscle, the often dramatic differences between muscle hemodynamics associated with voluntary exercise and these models of exercise must be kept in mind when interpreting results.

The rate of fluid filtration from blood to tissues is markedly elevated in muscle at the onset of rhythmic contraction (30, 44, 206, 260, 261, 279–282, 342, 344, 366, 431, 432). The increased transcapillary filtration rate results from an increase in capillary hydrostatic pressure (262, 263, 280, 281, 301), increased microvascular surface area that results from capillary recruitment (260, 261, 280, 281, 297, 342, 344, 356, 436, 438), and an increase in tissue osmotic pressure that results from the formation and release of metabolites from the exercising muscle cells (342, 344). However, measurements of venous blood and lymph osmolality obtained at various time points after the onset of muscular activity suggest that osmolality is only transiently increased (342, 523). These effects may also vary with muscle fiber type (342, 523).

Initially, the rate of fluid filtration exceeds the drainage capacity of the lymphatic system and fluid accumulates in active muscle. Indeed, transcapillary filtration rates can approach 1.5 ml $\cdot$ min^{-1} $\cdot$ 100 g^{-1} muscle tissue during intense rhythmic contractions, and measurements of fluid accumulation indicate that interstitial fluid volume can almost double during 15 min of contraction (260, 261, 342, 345). However, during sustained muscle activity, the rate of fluid filtration across the microcirculation slows such that lymphatic drainage and net filtration appear to be balanced and no further fluid accumulation occurs (260, 261).

The attainment of a new, steady-state, interstitial fluid volume implies that compensatory mechanisms act rapidly to limit the extent of fluid accumulation. While a large amount of evidence exists concerning the mechanisms of transcapillary fluid movement in active muscle, relatively little attention has been focused on the integrated interaction of capillary and interstitial forces and lymph flow to limit excessive accumulation of tissue fluid in exercising skeletal muscle. The increase in lymph flow during muscle contraction tends to limit the accumulation of excessive interstitial fluid by acting as a volume removal system (94, 260, 261, 342). In addition, the lymphatic system effectively opposes edema formation by removal or "washout" of tissue proteins, thereby decreasing interstitial oncotic pressure (431, 432). Several mechanisms contribute to the increase in lymph flow noted with muscle contraction. First, the accumulation of interstitial fluid during activity leads to increased tissue pressure which, in turn, provides the driving force for lymphatic filling and thus lymph flow (279, 282). In addition, since large collecting lymphatics encircle arterioles in skeletal muscle, the increase in the rate of arterial pulsation associated with exercise-induced tachycardia may propel lymph from active muscle (500). Contraction of active skeletal muscle fibers may compress the lymphatic vessels and pump lymph from the active muscle. Muscular contraction also limits edema formation by raising interstitial fluid pressure (277, 279, 282, 486, 521) as well as by pumping blood from the active skeletal muscle, thereby reducing the increment in capillary pressure (307). Increased sympathetic nerve stimulation in exercising muscle produces a modest flow restriction and, as a result, a dramatic decrease in capillary pressure (358). This effect of sympathetic tone during high-intensity exercise may be very important in maintaining fluid balance within active skeletal muscle (64, 358, 369).

Several other factors act to limit accumulation of interstitial fluid during exercise. For example, whereas metabolic vasodilation may provide for the necessary increase in muscle blood flow, myogenic mechanisms may function to limit edema formation by regulating functional exchange vessel surface area (344, 370, 491). This notion is supported by the observation that elevation of transmural pressure by 30 mm Hg during rhythmic muscle contraction reduces the increment in the capillary filtration coefficient (344). The contribution of this myogenic mechanism becomes inactive at higher exercise intensity due to metabolic vasodilation of functional precapillary sphincters. A final factor that limits edema formation during contraction of skeletal muscle relates to the decrease in postcapillary resistance associated with muscular activity (511). Even slight reductions in postcapillary resistance, which exert only minor influences on blood flow, can have a large impact on capillary pressure (due to changes in the precapillary/postcapillary resistance ratio).

It does not appear that barrier characteristics of the skeletal muscle microvasculature are altered during exercise. Although lymph flow increases with muscle contraction, lymph protein concentration remains unchanged or decreases. This observation is consistent with vasodilation and increased capillary pressure without altering capillary permeability (260, 261, 369). In addition, lymph/plasma dextran concentration ratios do not change during muscle contraction and there is little loss of labeled albumin from the blood as it passes through the microcirculation of active skeletal muscle (30, 44).

It may be argued that capillary permeability to filtered fluid could be increased in the absence of a detectable change in permeability to large solutes if only permeability to small solutes is increased during exercise. This hypothesis has not been systematically evaluated in the vasculature of exercising skeletal muscle. However, since measurements of the capillary diffusion coefficient [or permeability–surface area product (PS)] for small, lipid-insoluble solutes increases approximately twofold during rhythmic muscle contraction this possibility seems unlikely, (436–438). This is in agreement with the reported twofold increase in the capillary filtration coefficient obtained under similar conditions (279, 282). Since the capillary diffusion capacity varies with the square of pore radius, whereas the capillary filtration coefficient varies with the fourth power of radius, a twofold increase in the rate of diffusion secondary to increased small pore radius would require a fourfold increase in the capillary filtration coefficient. On the other hand, it is generally accepted that essentially the same pathways (small pore equivalents) across the microvascular wall are available for the net transport of water and small, lipid-insoluble substances (534). Therefore, an increase in capillary surface area stemming from capillary recruitment would be expected to produce equivalent changes in the capillary diffusion capacity (PS) and the capillary filtration coefficient, as has been reported in the references cited above.

Fluid Exchange in Voluntary Exercise. During whole-body exercise, the decrease in plasma volume is much less than would be predicted from in vitro studies (31, 457). There are a least three potential explanations for this apparent discrepancy. First, as discussed above, in vitro models of exercise using electrical stimulation of muscle do not truly simulate conditions within skeletal muscle during voluntary exercise. In addition, the isolation procedures involved in the preparation of muscles for ex vivo studies may impair the lymphatic drainage, whereas intact muscle would not suffer from this problem. Second, intact active muscle may accumulate fluid at a lesser rate than in isolated muscle preparations because capillary surface area may be less in intact muscle (where fewer fibers are active) (511). Third, the relatively small effect of voluntary exercise on plasma volume may relate to the mobilization of extravascular fluid from nonactive tissue to the plasma compartment (342).

Solute Exchange. It is clear that the primary function of exercise hyperemia is to increase capillary perfusion so that the transcapillary transport of oxygen, nutrients, and metabolites can be facilitated. It is clear that the transcapillary transport of small solutes is flow limited at low perfusion rates and only becomes limited by diffusion across capillaries at very high blood flows (106, 107, 404, 405, 436). Thus, during exercise, when blood flow is high, the transport of most small solutes becomes limited by diffusion rate and is, therefore, directly related to the capillary surface area available for exchange (435–437). The most efficient transport of solutes (adequate solute for the muscle with minimum blood flow) will occur when capillary exchange capacity and blood flows are matched, whereas maximal solute transport (with unlimited blood flow) may be seen only at very high blood flows (436).

Regulation of Tissue Oxygenation in Exercising Skeletal Muscles

At any given moment at rest or during muscular activity, the partial pressure of oxygen (P_{O_2}) in skeletal muscle myocytes reflects the prevailing balance between oxygen delivery and demand. Three processes govern the delivery of oxygen from arteries to skeletal muscle mitochondria: convective delivery of oxygen in the blood to exchange vessels, diffusion, and mitochondrial oxygen utilization (132, 190, 192).

Convective Delivery. The first process is convective delivery of oxygen in the stream of blood coursing through the microcirculation. Total oxygen delivery to capillaries within the muscle depends on blood flow rate and the concentration of oxygen carried in blood. Thus, regulation of convective oxygen delivery is accomplished by modulation of blood flow through adjustments in vascular tone and, in some mammals, increases in oxygen-carrying capacity of the blood by modulation of hematocrit via splenic contraction. The control of skeletal muscle blood flow was discussed earlier under *Mechanisms of Exercise Hyperemia* and the control of hematocrit was discussed earlier under *Magnitude of the Increase in Coronary Blood Flow during Exercise*. Matching of blood flow rate and oxygen-carrying capacity (convective oxygen supply) in the microcirculation to oxygen demand is central to homeostasis.

The microcirculatory parameters that have the most significant impact on oxygen delivery include: RBC transit time through exchange vessels; number of RBCs per length of capillary; the relationship between RBC transit time and surface area available for gas exchange; microvascular oxygen content; and functional capillary density. If exchange surface area is heterogeneously distributed, a matched, heterogeneous distribution of blood flow and RBC transit times is most efficient for oxygen transport (efficient in that the largest amount of O_2 can be transported with the smallest amount of blood flow). Capillaries with the greatest exchange surface area should receive relatively greater flow (436, 437). Thus, the presence of microvascular blood-flow heterogeneity is not necessarily a sign of poor vascular function.

RBC transit time is determined by both capillary length and by the route RBCs take through the bed (path length). If an RBC goes through branches or cross-connections between capillaries, its transit time and the capillary surface area to which the cell is exposed will be increased as compared to transit directly through the shortest path. Sarelius (463) measured RBC path lengths by following RBCs through skeletal muscle microvascular beds and determined that mean RBC path length is longer than would be predicted from anatomical measurements of capillary lengths and capillary RBC velocities. Thus RBC transit times are longer than capillary mean transit times estimated from the combination of indicator dilution techniques and histological estimates of capillarization. Indeed, Sarelius's measured RBC transit times (2–3 s) indicate that exchange-vessel transit time may be an order of magnitude greater than the minimal time required for unloading O_2 from RBCs (463).

Diffusion of Oxygen. The second process is the diffusive flux of oxygen from the capillaries to the mitochondria. The difference between capillary and cellular oxygen tension provides the driving force for diffusive flux of oxygen from blood to mitochondria. Since capillary surface area and capillary-to-cell diffusion distance are also determinants of diffusive flux of oxygen across capillaries, modulation of perfused capillary density by arterioles and precapillary sphincters is important (190). Estimates indicate that 25% of the total number of capillaries are open for flow at any given time in quiescent skeletal muscle, allowing for increased capillary surface area for exchange during exercise (44, 279–282, 342, 344, 436–438, 454). Capillary density varies greatly depending on muscle fiber type and appears to match the oxidative capacity of the respective fibers (7, 10, 13, 194, 245, 247, 347, 395, 396, 429, 442, 443, 454, 455). Red or slow-twitch oxidative fibers can be perfused by approximately three times as many capillaries/fiber as white or fast-twitch glycolytic fibers. The arrangement of capillaries in relation to muscle fibers also varies with fiber type (191, 192, 198). Although some capillaries encircle fibers in white muscle, the vast majority of these microvessels run parallel to the long axis of fibers. In red muscle, the capillaries follow a more tortuous route and form parallel loops that encircle the fibers. The net effect of this arrangement in red fibers is to provide more surface area for transcapillary exchange.

The importance of capillary density becomes even more apparent when one considers that the geometric organization of capillaries in relation to parenchymal cells in skeletal muscle not only allows for changes in surface area but also in diffusion distance when the number of open capillaries (N) is altered (192). In skeletal muscle, surface area changes in direct proportion to N, while diffusion distance is inversely proportional to the square root of N. Inasmuch as the diffusive flux of oxygen is proportional to $N^{3/2}$ in skeletal muscle, oxygen diffusion rate increases eightfold, for a fourfold increase in functional capillary density (192).

Although alterations in arteriolar tone govern vascular resistance and blood flow, the anatomic location of control sites for capillary exchange capacity in skeletal muscle is not certain. Careful intravital microscopic examination of the muscle microcirculation has failed to confirm the existence of sphincter-like structures at the capillary orifices (155). This has led some investigators to suggest that vascular resistance and capillary density are controlled by the same microvascular elements. However, this concept is difficult to reconcile with the observation that changes in vascular resistance and capillary exchange capacity can occur in opposite directions (95, 122, 191). These considerations have led to the proposal that terminal arterioles regulate functional capillary density and that larger arterioles regulate vascular resistance and blood flow. This notion is based on the observation that terminal arterioles exhibit vasomotion (159, 160, 338, 343, 380), which could account for changes in capillary patency with time. Moreover, terminal arterioles contribute very little to total microvascular resistance (360).

Recruitment (perfusion) of nonperfused capillaries (exchange vessels) occurs in association with the hyperemia observed at the initiation of exercise (191, 241). Capillary perfusion does not appear to be controlled on a single capillary basis. Rather, it appears that groups of capillaries are recruited as "units" at the initiation of exercise. The fundamental unit of capillary recruitment in the microcirculation of skeletal muscle appears to be a grouping of capillaries into small capillary networks (116, 187, 532). Sarelius (463) observed that hyperemia is associated with recruitment of such groups of capillaries, i.e., capillary networks, in hamster cremaster muscle. Similarly, Damon and Duling (112) concluded that microvascular units must be recruited during exercise because capillary perfusion heterogeneity did not decrease with increases in blood flow produced by vasodilation in hamster tibialis anterior muscles. Thus, microvascular units recruited via vasodilation have dispersions of capillary blood flows similar to the microvascular units perfused under resting conditions (prior to vasodilation).

It has been proposed that control of capillary perfusion is located in terminal arterioles (112, 132, 187, 241). However, Sweeney and Sarelius (532) found that feed vessels of terminal arterioles control cell flow in the capillary units of cremaster muscle. It appears that recruitment of these capillary units is spatially ordered and the arterioles controlling these units can respond to vasoactive signals differently from each other, in a spatially organized manner (173, 463). Analysis of flow heterogeneity of capillary segments sampled randomly across the muscle tissue tended to decrease with the transition from rest to exercise hyperemia whereas heterogeneity appeared to increase during hyperemia when distributions of flow were examined across complete capillary networks (464). These data support the hypothesis that functional capillary units consist of networks of non-uniform capillary path lengths. These observations highlight the fact that further progress in understanding matching of flow and exchange area in the microcirculation requires that the analyses include the fact that capillary perfusion is controlled via microvascular units, not single capillaries.

During exercise hyperemia, capillary blood flow, RBC distribution, and RBC concentrations may be coordinated, within and among microvascular units of muscle so that O_2 supply is equalized (465). Recent evidence indicates that conducted or propagated vasodilation contributes to the regulatory processes modulating flow distribution throughout the vasculature (480). Segal and co-workers (479–483) suggested that conducted or propagated vasodilation may also reduce perfusion heterogeneity during exercise by minimizing the potential for more dilated vessels to "steal" flow from less dilated vessels (482).

From the foregoing discussion, it is apparent that muscular activity elicits a complex vascular response that matches oxygen delivery to demand. For small increments in oxygen uptake associated with low twitch frequencies, increased oxygen extraction and capillary recruitment (functional precapillary sphincter dilation) predominate over arteriolar vasodilation (190, 192). When oxygen consumption is increased by nine- to tenfold, the capillary filtration coefficient is increased by fourfold, indicating a dramatic recruitment of capillaries. Oxygen delivery is facilitated by increases in blood flow and oxygen extraction (i.e., threefold increase in the arteriovenous oxygen content difference). These observations are consistent with the results of Anderson and Faber (12), who have reported that metabolic signals released during moderate exercise preferentially reduce α_2-adrenoceptor tone. As a consequence, small arterioles, subject to predominantly α_2-mediated tone, dilate resulting in capillary recruitment. On the other hand, the release of metabolic vasodilators associated with higher contraction frequencies inhibits both intrinsic myogenic tone and α_1-adrenoreceptor–mediated constriction in large arterioles so that both blood flow and functional capillary density increase to match oxygen delivery with demand.

Microvascular oxygen flux also occurs across precapillary arterioles (130, 487). Since the paired venule flows in a countercurrent direction, this may create a diffusion shunt (427) that decreases capillary P_{O_2} to a level lower than venous P_{O_2}. However, the high red cell velocity in arterioles associated with increased blood flow during exercise reduces the extent of precapillary diffusional shunting, thereby improving the effectiveness of oxygen delivery to the capillary level.

It must be emphasized that there is a fine balance between the increase in blood flow through the microcirculation of exercising skeletal muscle and the mean capillary red cell transit time required to maximize oxygen extraction (240). For example, if red cell transit time is shorter than the period required for oxygen release from hemoglobin, the capillary is perfused but the oxygen carried in red cell hemoglobin is not available for muscle oxygenation. Accordingly, a convective shunt can be created at high red cell velocities, the net effect of which is to limit tissue oxygenation despite increased oxygen delivery to the capillary by the bloodstream. However, the propensity for such convective shunting of oxygen associated with large increments in blood flow during exercise is reduced by concomitant opening of capillaries that increase vascular cross-sectional area and capillary volume, preventing dramatic reductions in red cell transit time.

Mitochondrial Oxygen Utilization. The third process that governs oxygen consumption of skeletal muscles and the final stage of oxygen delivery from the blood to the tissues is mitochondrial oxygen utilization (190). Once oxygen has diffused into mitochondria, it removes reducing equivalents from cytochrome a_3, the terminal oxidase in the respiratory chain. Thus, the rate of oxygen utilization in mitochondria is determined by cell Po_2 and the concentration of reduced cytochrome a_3. A consideration of reaction kinetics for the interaction of oxygen in the respiratory chain indicates that mitochondrial oxygen utilization is independent of cell Po_2 until oxygen tension falls below 0.5–1 mm Hg (265). Although it is generally accepted that mitochondrial Po_2 is maintained well above this level at rest and most levels of muscular activity, recent evidence suggests that tissue respiration during exercise may be modulated by mitochondrial oxygen levels at concentrations that are not considered rate limiting (233–235).

Determinants of Skeletal Muscle Arteriovenous Oxygen Difference

The extraction of oxygen from capillary blood in exercising skeletal muscle lowers venous oxygen content and thereby widens the arteriovenous oxygen difference (48, 128, 230–235). A limitation for oxygen diffusion from muscle capillaries to mitochondria has been proposed as a determinant of maximal oxygen consumption. The reasoning is that the relationship between maximal oxygen consumption and venous Po_2 is linear and passes through the origin (232–235, 439, 560, 561), as would be expected from a consideration of Fick's first law of diffusion. Moreover, this relationship remains linear and passes through the origin in the face of alterations in arterial Po_2 and oxygen content. According to this postulate, as venous Po_2 decreases, oxygen uptake decreases because the pressure gradient driving oxygen diffusion from the capillary to the mitochondria is reduced. The location of the limitation for oxygen diffusion is a subject of controversy.

Honig and co-workers (239) attempted to define the location of diffusion barriers to oxygen transport from red cells in the capillaries to muscle mitochondria. They used quick-freezing techniques during muscle contraction and determined myoglobin oxygen saturation spectrophotometrically in thin frozen sections of muscle biopsies. Their results indicate that the main diffusion barriers were represented by the thin layer of plasma between red blood cells and the capillary wall, the endothelium, and the interstitial space. Venous oxygen saturation fell with increasing muscle oxygen uptake and blood flow as rate of muscle contractions was increased from one to four twitches per second. However, twitch rates in excess of four per second were associated with increased oxygen consumption and blood flow but lower muscle myoglobin saturation and cell Po_2. High rates of twitch produced an increase in venous Po_2, suggesting that muscle capillaries can act as a functional diffusion barrier. Honig et al. (239) proposed that at the rates of flow associated with these twitch rates, red cell velocity is increased to a level that does not provide adequate time for unloading of oxygen from hemoglobin during capillary transit.

Recall that the presence of myoglobin serves to maximize the transcapillary Po_2 gradient but minimizes intracellular Po_2 gradients (181, 182, 239). This is related to the fact that the partial pressure of oxygen required to produce 50% saturation of this hemeprotein is only 5.3 mm Hg. As such, myoglobin serves to stabilize tissue Po_2 at a level that is well below capillary Po_2. This is supported by the observation that cell Po_2 and myoglobin saturation were low but remarkably uniform throughout a given muscle cell and were not related to the distance from nearby capillaries (239). The apparent stabilization of intracellular oxygen by myoglobin thus minimizes intracellular Po_2 gradients and suggests that diffusional limitations to oxygen transport within the cell are relatively small when compared to that offered in moving oxygen from the capillary blood to the muscle cell.

Oxygen uptake by active skeletal muscles may also be limited by the oxidative capacity of the contracting myocytes (103, 181, 243, 362, 515). However, the bulk of the experimental evidence supports the concept that there is not a metabolic limitation to maximal oxygen consumption in skeletal muscle in normal individuals (243, 446–449, 454, 456, 493). Perhaps the most compelling support for this concept is that increasing arterial oxygen concentration raises maximal oxygen consumption (162, 271). If maximal oxygen uptake had been limited by the metabolic capacity of the exercising muscles, oxygen consumption would not have increased.

Perfusional and diffusional shunting can also limit oxygen uptake by active muscle cells. While it is clear that muscle perfusion is heterogeneous (420, 512), the extent of mismatching between blood flow and oxygen consumption is not known. However, recent evidence suggests that such mismatching becomes less with increasing oxygen uptake, especially when arterial oxygen content or delivery is reduced (58, 234, 466).

EFFECTS OF PHYSICAL CONDITIONING ON SKELETAL MUSCLE VASCULAR BEDS

As described above for the coronary circulation, mechanisms for vascular adaptation induced by chronic exercise training in skeletal muscle can be grouped into two major categories: structural adaptations and adaptations in vascular control. Structural vascular adaptation in response to exercise training takes at least two forms: vascular remodeling and growth (i.e., growth of already-existing vessels such as increased length, cross-sectional area, and/or diameters of the existing large and small arteries and veins) and angiogenesis (i.e., increased numbers of capillaries and other microvessels per gram of muscle). Adaptive changes in vascular control can be the result of *(1)* altered neurohumoral control of the vascular bed; *(2)* altered local control via changes in metabolic control systems, altered myogenic responses to mechanical stimuli, intrinsic changes in vascular smooth muscle cells, and/or endothelial cells; or *(3)* the effects of structural changes on the distribution of resistance throughout the microcirculation (321, 322).

Skeletal Muscle Blood Flow Capacity

The increased maximal oxygen consumption characteristic of trained individuals has been attributed to increases in both maximal cardiac output and maximal arteriovenous oxygen difference (58, 67, 92, 185, 439, 448, 472). Since the increase in maximal cardiac output is largely directed to working skeletal muscle during exercise in trained subjects, skeletal muscle blood flow capacity is also thought to be increased by exercise training (58, 320, 387, 388, 439). Both cross-sectional (273, 354, 497, 503) and longitudinal (353, 499) studies suggest that limb muscle blood flow capacity is greater in trained individuals. Roca et al. (440) reported that 9 week endurance exercise training resulted in a 36.5% increase in maximal oxygen consumption, and a 19.2% increase in leg blood flow during exercise at $\dot{V}O_{2max}$. Also, Musch et al. (387) demonstrated that exercise training induces an increase in skeletal muscle blood flow during maximal exercise in dogs. Their results indicated that 80% of the training-induced increase in maximal cardiac output was directed to active skeletal muscle (387). Rowell (449) proposed that the increase in muscle blood flow during maximal exercise in trained subjects is the result of a combination of increased maximal cardiac output and decreased sympathetic vasoconstrictor outflow. Discussion of available evidence that training increases blood flow capacity of skeletal muscle requires that the terms "maximal blood flow" and "blood flow capacity" be carefully defined.

The terms "maximal blood flow," "maximal vasodilation," "minimal resistance," and "maximal conductance" are not used in a rigorous or uniform manner by all investigators (321, 324, 325, 327, 470). Precise definition of these terms and consideration of appropriate methods for assessing blood flow capacity are necessary (321). The term "maximal blood flow" should be used to refer to a specific blood flow value measured during maximal vasodilation at a defined, physiologic perfusion pressure (90–120 mm Hg). If maximal blood flow is to be estimated, it is essential to control perfusion pressure, because once maximal vasodilation has been produced, both blood flow and resistance (through distention of resistance vessels) are related to arterial pressure (324, 325). A truly maximal blood flow cannot be determined because blood vessels will continue to distend with increasing pressures until they burst. Therefore, blood flow capacity can best be estimated by measuring blood flow as a function of perfusion pressure, during maximal vasodilation. The mathematical expression describing the relationship between blood flow and perfusion pressure can then be compared between control and trained groups. Even the term "maximal vasodilation" is misused in the literature. Maximal correctly refers to the greatest possible response, such as that seen at (and beyond) the plateau in a dose–response curve. It is a unique, reproducible value for each vasodilator agent in a given vascular bed. In theory, maximal vasodilation exists when vascular smooth muscle is completely relaxed. However, this is difficult to control in vivo. Procedures utilized to estimate blood flow capacity should include control of key hemodynamic parameters to ensure that measurements are made under comparable conditions in trained and control animals so that differences in vascular resistance are the major determinant of differences in blood flow (307, 449).

The hypothesis that exercise training increases maximal skeletal muscle blood flow during exercise by increasing skeletal muscle blood flow capacity is supported by measurements of blood flow capacity of rat hindlimb musculature, in situ, during maximal vasodilation induced by metabolically demanding muscle contractions (346, 362) and by similar measurements in rat hindlimb musculature in situ during maximal vasodilation induced by infusion of papaverine (320, 324, 489). Results demonstrate that blood flow capacity of skeletal muscle vascular beds is increased by exercise training (325, 339, 346, 489, 490). Furthermore, the results suggest that these increases are accounted for by adaptations that are localized in and around muscle fibers having the greatest relative increases in activity during training bouts (154, 198, 320, 322, 325, 326, 489, 490). On the other hand, Silber et al. (496) report that leg exercise training increases peak forearm blood flow in humans, and Yasuda and Miyamura (579) reported cross-transfer of training effects on blood flow in ipsilateral and contralateral forearms. Thus, data currently available indicate that training-induced adaptations that influence skeletal muscle perfusion are restricted to the areas around muscle fibers that have the greatest relative increases in activity during training bouts [e.g., capillarization, blood flow capacity (structural vascular adaptation)]. Conversely, there is evidence that some vascular adaptations occur generally throughout the peripheral vasculature (e.g., some changes in vascular control mechanisms).

Skeletal Muscle Capillary Diffusion Capacity

Several animal studies reveal that training increases skeletal muscle capillary diffusion capacity (325, 439, 489, 490). Others find no change in capillary diffusion capacity (145, 325). One source of conflict is the failure to ensure maximal vasodilation during capillary exchange measurements (145, 325). In addition to these findings from nonhuman species, Roca et al. (440) reported that 9 weeks of endurance exercise training of human subjects increased oxygen-diffusing capacity in skeletal muscle by 33.5% during maximal exercise. Roca et al. used the ratio of maximal oxygen consumption divided by mean capillary PO_2 as an index of tissue diffusion capacity (439). They found that physical conditioning reduces diffusional limitations to oxygen transport, in that tissue diffusion capacities in individuals with maximal oxygen consumptions of approximately 70 $ml \cdot kg^{-1} \cdot min^{-1}$ were nearly twice values of individuals whose maximal oxygen consumption only approached 55 $ml \cdot kg^{-1} \cdot min^{-1}$. It is likely that the well-established increase in capillarity induced by exercise training, described below, largely accounts for this observation. Increased capillary density not only reduces diffusion distances but also increases total capillary volume and cross-sectional area. The increase in capillary volume reduces red cell velocity at a given capillary flow rate, thereby increasing mean residence time available for oxygen exchange.

Structural Vascular Adaptation

Small Arteries and Arterioles. Segal et al. (484) reported that treadmill exercise training in rats produced 12%–18% increases in the medial wall thickness in abdominal aorta and femoral, axillary, superior mesenteric, and coeliac arteries, and increased total wall area in aorta and femoral and axillary arteries. There were no differences between lumen diameter in any of these arteries (484). In contrast, Delp et al. (117) reported that an endurance training program of more moderate intensity did not alter lumen diameters or wall thickness of abdominal aorta of rats. Information concerning the effects of exercise training on the size and/or number of small arteries and arterioles in skeletal muscle vascular beds is limited. Lash and Bohlen (303) found that arteriolar density was unchanged in rat skeletal muscle following training. However, the finding that precapillary vascular resistance is decreased in hindquarters isolated from trained rats suggests that training induces changes in precapillary resistance vessels (145, 489, 490). There is a need for detailed analysis of the effects of exercise training on small arteries and arterioles of skeletal muscle vascular beds of other mammals.

Capillary (and/or Microvascular Exchange) Vessels. The effects of exercise training on the density of skeletal muscle capillary beds has been extensively investigated. Numerous cross-sectional and longitudinal studies in humans demonstrated increased capillarization in response to training (71, 77, 256, 257, 284, 322, 454). Results from animal studies have been less consistent. There is evidence that training either increases skeletal muscle capillarization (2, 3, 86, 347, 426) or causes no change (339, 384, 409). Causes for this controversy include: models of training and lack of rigorous documentation of training state, choice of muscle tissue to examine, and failure to appreciate potential differences among capillary beds in different types of skeletal muscle.

Surprisingly, some studies of the effects of training on skeletal muscle capillarization have not documented training efficacy with an independent measure of training-induced adaptation (339, 384, 426). Importantly, studies that ensured training efficacy by demonstrating increased skeletal muscle oxidative capacity consistently show that training increases capillarization in the conditioned muscles (198, 320, 325, 347, 488, 490).

Capillarization of muscle is greatest in muscle composed primarily of FOG fibers, followed in order by slow-twitch oxidative (SO) and fat-twitch, glycolytic (FG) fibers (86, 347). There are similar differences between SO and FOG fiber capillarization in human muscles, though the differences are less pronounced (454). Exercise training appears to modulate relationships among fiber-type composition and capillarization. Capillarization is increased by exercise training in muscles composed of FOG fibers but is not changed in SO or FG muscle tissue (347). This discrete increase in capillarization in FOG muscle may stem from the moderate intensity of the training program used in this study (347). This intensity of exercise would be expected to increase recruitment of FOG fibers and to increase blood flow to FOG fibers during training bouts (310). More recently, a systematic series of investigations of capillary adaptations to exercise training that compared interval sprint training to endurance training revealed that capillarization in fast-twitch muscle increased in the areas of muscle with the greatest relative increase in fiber activity during training bouts (198). Others have also observed that training-induced increases in capillarization are focused in the areas of muscle with the greatest relative increases in fiber activity during the training bouts (320, 325, 489, 490). The soleus muscle appears to be more resistant to training-induced signals for angiogenesis (198).

In contrast to these animal studies, in humans capillarization appears to increase in muscle composed of all three types of fiber rather than specifically in the areas of muscle expected to have the greatest relative increase in fiber activity as in other species (9, 255, 283). This is surprising because continuous, submaximal (requiring 70%–80% $\dot{V}O_{2max}$) exercise training was utilized in these human studies. Thus, during training bouts, little FG fiber recruitment would be expected.

Small Veins and Venules. There appears to be no information in the literature concerning the effect of exercise training on these skeletal muscle microvessels. However, the fact that postcapillary vascular resistance is decreased in hindquarters from exercise-trained rats (145, 489, 490) is consistent with the hypothesis that training alters the venous circulation of skeletal muscle.

Adaptations of Vascular Control

Neural Control. One important factor responsible for the increase in skeletal muscle blood flow during exercise in trained subjects could be less neurogenic vasoconstrictor tone (449). Alterations in sympathetic nerve activity (SNA) to skeletal muscle at rest and during exercise may be one component of an overall training-induced adaptation of sympathetic neural control of vascular resistance. Training-induced alterations in SNA have been investigated with measurements of: *(1)* plasma norepinephrine (NE) concentration, *(2)* skeletal and/or total vascular resistance, and *(3)* direct microneurographic recordings of SNA (449, 504, 529–531, 572, 573). Although plasma concentrations of NE in resting subjects are not altered by training (105, 196, 413, 569, 570, 572, 574), the increase in plasma NE associated with exercise at a given absolute intensity is attenuated (67, 413, 472, 569, 570, 572, 573). As expected, plasma NE concentrations are the same in trained and untrained subjects during exercise when responses to exercise of the same relative intensities are compared (105, 413, 572, 573). Plasma NE concentration has been reported to be greater during maximal exercise, after training (572).

There is no information concerning the effects of training on SNA in the skeletal muscle microcirculation. Thus, although there is clear evidence that cardiovascular control mechanisms are modified by exercise training (59, 67, 119, 253, 294, 361, 366, 503, 570), and that exercise training attenuates SNA to skeletal muscle during exercise, the impact of these changes on skeletal muscle microcirculation remains to be explored. In a related study, Lash et al. (304) reported that exercise training altered adrenergic and pressure-dependent vasoregulatory mechanisms in both skeletal muscle and intestinal tissues. These training-induced changes appeared to involve interactions among neurohumoral, myogenic, and metabolic control mechanisms (304).

Local Vascular Control in Skeletal Muscle. Lash and Bohlen (303) reported that arterioles from trained rats exhibit greater vasodilation during skeletal muscle contractions than those from sedentary control rats. These data were obtained from an in situ spinotrapezius muscle preparation, induced to contract with electrical stimulation. Arteriolar responses were measured with in vivo microscopy. The results of this study suggest that exercise training increases the exercise hyperemic response in skeletal muscle microcirculatory beds (303). Also, Wiegman et al. (569) reported decreased norepinephrine sensitivity in the microcirculation following exercise training. Such changes in vascular control could result from training-induced changes in function of vascular smooth muscle and/or endothelial cells. Conversely, training did not appear to alter norepinephrine dose–response relationships in helical strips of aorta, femoral artery, or renal artery of rat (146). Also, segments of femoral arteries isolated from sedentary and trained miniature swine had similar sensitivity and responsiveness to norepinephrine (199). Furthermore, no training-induced alterations were found in vasodilator responses induced by sodium nitroprusside or adenosine (199). In contrast, Delp et al. (117) found that rings of aorta isolated from exercise-trained rats were less sensitive to the vasoconstrictor effects of norepinephrine. The altered norepinephrine sensitivity produced by exercise training appeared to be the result of endothelium-mediated events rather than changes in smooth muscle reactivity, since removal of endothelium abolished the difference.

Endothelium-Mediated Control. As described above, there is evidence that training alters endothelium-mediated vascular control in the coronary circulation. Some recent results indicate that these changes are not limited to the coronary vascular endothelium. Delp et al. (117) reported that the vasodilator effects of the endothelium-dependent vasodilator, acetylcholine, were enhanced in aortas of trained rats. The notion that training can enhance endothelium-dependent vasodilation in skeletal muscle microcirculation is supported by the finding that exercise training can enhance NO synthesis in isolated arterioles from rat gracilis muscle (527). Furthermore, Miller et al. (373, 374) observed similar enhancement of endothelium-dependent vasodilation in dog femoral artery in response to the creation of a femoral arteriovenous fistula, which chronically increased femoral arterial blood flow through the artery proximal to the fistula. Endothelium-mediated vasodilation was enhanced in arterial rings isolated from the femoral artery proximal to the fistula.

In conclusion, aerobic exercise training induces an increase in vascular transport capacity in the conditioned skeletal muscles. This increased transport capacity is the result of increases in capacities for both blood flow and capillary exchange. These functional changes are the result of two major types of adaptive responses: structural vascular adaptation and altered vascular control. Vascular adaptation in skeletal muscle tissue is not uniformly distributed throughout the tissue. The most evident structural (increases in capillary density) and functional (increased vascular transport capacity) adaptations appear to occur in the skeletal muscle tissue with the greatest relative increase in activity during training bouts (i.e., around muscle fibers that experience the largest increase in activity during physical activity).

One bout of exercise induces a complex array of factors that may be involved in initiating training-induced adaptations. Vasodilation and increased blood flow in active skeletal muscle are always associated with exercise. Vasodilation produces one of the likely "signals" for vascular adaptation: an alteration in mechanical forces in the vessel wall. The other major effect of vasodilation is increased blood flow, which will produce a second potential signal for vascular adaptation: increased shear stress at the vascular wall. Repetitive exposure to these two mechanical stimuli (stretch and shear stress) and/or metabolic signals during exercise training bouts may initiate both structural vascular adaptation and altered vascular control (1, 321, 322, 381). Mechanical effects of increased contractile force during exercise and/or changes in concentrations of many hormones and peptides during exercise may also act as signals or modifiers for vascular adaptation. Additionally, exercise produces changes in many neurohumoral stimuli that could be involved in altered gene expression (1, 321, 322).

CONCLUSION

Blood flow is tightly coupled to metabolic rate in both cardiac and skeletal muscle during locomotory exercise. Blood flow is determined by the interactions among perfusion pressure, extravascular mechanical effects of muscle contraction, and the caliber of resistance vessels. Normally, perfusion pressure is maintained or slightly increased during exercise. The predominant effect of extravascular mechanical effects in the coronary vascular bed is to increase resistance to blood flow and influence the regional distribution of blood flow across the ventricular wall. In contrast, in skeletal muscle, the muscle pump effect appears to augment perfusion during dynamic exercise. The caliber of resistance vessels is regulated by central neurohumoral factors, and by local factors including metabolic, myogenic, and endothelial components. It is clear that the primary importance of the tight relationship between blood flow and metabolism in cardiac and skeletal muscle is the maintenance of adequate capillary perfusion so that transcapillary exchange of oxygen, nutrients, and metabolites is optimized. Relaxation of vascular smooth muscle in arteries and arterioles increases the convective delivery of oxygen and nutrients to the capillaries. Dilation of terminal arterioles and functional precapillary sphincters enhances diffusional exchange between capillary blood and mitochondria of active myocytes by reducing diffusion distance and increasing the surface area available for exchange. In skeletal muscle, diffusional exchange of oxygen is also enhanced by increased capillary-to-cell oxygen concentration gradient that occurs secondary to reductions in cellular PO_2 caused by increased oxygen consumption. As a consequence, the extraction of oxygen from capillary blood is enhanced and the arteriovenous oxygen concentration difference is increased during exercise. Thus, the mechanisms controlling blood flow within the coronary circulation and active skeletal muscle vascular beds tightly couple oxygen delivery and oxygen demand during exercise.

The fundamental mechanisms responsible for regulating the caliber of resistance vessels appear to be similar in cardiac and skeletal muscle tissue. However, the relative importance of these mechanisms is different in these two organs and also among types of skeletal muscle. Current evidence indicates that several of these independent mechanisms contribute, in parallel, to the maintenance of adequate blood flow in cardiac and skeletal muscle. As a consequence, the common experimental approach of blocking a specific putative mechanism of control to ascertain its importance to maintenance of adequate blood flow may lead to incorrect interpretations because of the redundant control mechanisms. When one vasodilator system is blocked, activation of other parallel vasodilator systems may be increased, masking the role of the blocked vasodilator mechanism. Although recent revelations of the potential for endothelium-mediated vascular control are exciting, the role of endothelium-dependent mechanisms and their functional significance in exercise hyperemia in cardiac and skeletal muscle has yet to be established. It is possible that integration of neurohumoral influences, metabolic vasodilation, endothelial vasodilator mechanisms, and the muscle pump mechanism may allow definitive identification of the determinants of blood flow in cardiac and skeletal muscle in the near future.

In skeletal muscle, contractile activity is associated with marked increases in transcapillary fluid filtration. This effect appears to be largely due to increased microvascular hydrostatic pressure and surface area that occurs secondary to dilation of arterioles and functional precapillary sphincters. Initially, the rate of fluid filtration exceeds the drainage capacity of the lymphatic system and fluid accumulates in active muscle. However, during sustained exercise, the rate of fluid filtration slows such that lymphatic drainage and net filtration are balanced and no further fluid accumulation occurs. The major compensatory mechanisms that limit fluid accumulation during sustained exercise include increased lymph flow (via the muscle pump effect), decreased interstitial oncotic pressure, and elevated tissue fluid pressure.

Chronic exposure to exercise training produces vascular adaptation in both cardiac and skeletal muscle. Two general forms of adaptation have been identified: structural adaptations and adaptations in vascular control. Structural vascular adaptation occurs in the form of vascular remodeling, vascular growth, and angiogenesis. Adaptive changes in vascular control can be the result of altered neural control as well as altered local control via changes in metabolic control systems, altered myogenic responses to mechanical stimuli, and intrinsic changes in vascular smooth muscle cells and/or endothelial cells. In addition, structural changes may alter the distribution of resistance throughout the microcirculation.

John T. Shepherd ended his review of *Circulation to Skeletal Muscle* by stating: "From basal tone to exercise hyperemia, from adrenergic reflexes to nonadrenergic control systems, there is a wealth of hidden information awaiting those with the ability to find it" (491). As detailed above, much has been revealed about regulatory mechanisms in the coronary circulation and skeletal muscle vascular beds during exercise since 1983. Some revelations have come in areas anticipated in 1983, other revelations have been less predictable. Although we do not yet fully understand exercise hyperemia in striated muscle, progress since 1983 sustains the dream that integration of neurohumoral influences, metabolic vasodilation, endothelial vasoregulatory processes, and the muscle pump mechanism with improved understanding of vascular smooth muscle and endothelium may yield definitive identification of how vascular transport is controlled in cardiac and skeletal muscle during exercise.

REFERENCES

1. Adair, T. H., W. J. Gay, and J. Montani. Growth regulation of the vascular system: evidence for a metabolic hypothesis. *Am. J. Physiol.* 259 (*Regulatory Integrative Comp. Physiol.* 28): R393–R404, 1990.
2. Adolfsson, J. The time dependence of training-induced increase in skeletal muscle capillarization and the spatial capillary to fibre relationship in normal and neovascularized skeletal muscle of rats. *Acta Physiol. Scand.* 128: 259–266, 1986.
3. Adolfsson, J., A. Ljungqvist, G. Tornling, and G. Unge. Capillary increase in the skeletal muscle of trained young and adult rats. *J. Physiol.* 310: 529–532, 1981.
4. Afonso, S., G. T. Bandow, and G. G. Rowe. Indomethacin and the prostaglandin hypothesis of coronary blood flow regulation. *J. Physiol. (Lond.)* 241: 299–308, 1974.
5. Alexander, R. W., K. M. Kent, J. J. Pasano, H. R. Keiser, and T. Cooper. Regulation of postocclusive hyperemia by endogenously synthesized prostaglandins in the dog heart. *J. Clin. Invest.* 55: 1174–1181, 1975.
6. Altman, J. D., J. Kinn, D. J. Duncker, and R. J. Bache. Effect of inhibition of nitric oxide formation on coronary

blood flow during exercise in the dog. *Cardiovasc. Res.* 28: 119–124, 1994.
7. Andersen, P. Capillary density in skeletal muscle of man. *Acta. Physiol. Scand.* 95: 203–205, 1975.
8. Andersen, P., and J. Henriksson. Capillary supply of the quadriceps femoris muscle of man: adaptive response to exercise. *J. Physiol. (Lond.)* 270: 670–690, 1977.
9. Andersen, P., and J. Henricksson. Training induced changes in the subgroups of human type II skeletal muscle fibres. *Acta Physiol. Scand.* 99: 123–125, 1977.
10. Andersen, P., and A. J. Kroese. Capillary supply in soleus and gastrocnemius muscles of man. *Pflugers Arch.* 375: 245–249, 1978.
11. Andersen, P., and B. Saltin. Maximal perfusion of skeletal muscle in man. *J. Physiol. (Lond.)* 366: 233–249, 1985.
12. Anderson, K. M., and J. E. Faber. Differential sensitivity of arteriolar α_1- and α_2-adrenoceptor constriction to metabolic inhibition during rat skeletal muscle contraction. *Circ. Res.* 69: 174–184, 1991.
13. Aniansson, A., G. Grimby, M. Hedberg, and M. Krotkiewski. Muscle morphology, enzyme activity and muscle strength in elderly men and women. *Clin. Physiol.* 1: 73–86, 1981.
14. Antal, J. Changes in blood flow during exercise in unanesthetized animals. *Circulation in Skeletal Muscle.* New York: Pergaman Press, 1968, p. 181–187.
15. Anversa, P., C. Beghi, V. Levicky, S. L. McDonald, and Y. Kikkawa. Morphometry of right ventricular hypertrophy induced by strenuous exercise in rat. *Am. J. Physiol.* 243 (*Heart Circ. Physiol.* 12): H857–H861, 1982.
16. Anversa, P., C. Beghi, V. Levicky, S. L. McDonald, Y. Kikkawa, and G. Olivetti. Effects of strenuous exercise on the quantitative morphology of left ventricular myocardium in rat. *J. Mol. Cell Cardiol.* 17: 587–595, 1985.
17. Anversa, P., V. Levicky, C. Beghi, S. L. McDonald, and Y. Kikkawa. Morphometry of exercise-induced right ventricular hypertrophy in the rat. *Circ. Res.* 52: 57–64, 1983.
18. Anversa, P., R. Ricci, and G. Olivetti. Effects of exercise on the capillary vasculature of the rat heart. *Circulation* 75(Suppl. I): I-12–I-18, 1987.
19. Archie, J. P., Jr. Transmural distribution of intrinsic and transmitted left ventricular diastolic intramyocardial pressure in dogs. *Cardiovasc. Res.* 12: 255–262, 1978.
20. Armstrong, R. B., M. D. Delp, E. F. Goljan, and M. H. Laughlin. Distribution of blood flow in muscles of miniature swine during exercise. *J. Appl. Physiol.* 62: 1285–1298, 1987.
21. Armstrong, R. B., M. D. Delp, E. F. Goljan, and M. H. Laughlin. Progressive elevations in muscle blood flow during prolonged exercise in swine. *J. Appl. Physiol.* 63: 285–291, 1987.
22. Armstrong, R. B., B. Essen-Gustavsson, H. Hoppeler, J. H. Jones, S. R. Kayer, M. H. Laughlin, A. Lindholm, K. E. Longsworth, C. R. Taylor, and E. R. Weibel. O_2 delivery at $\dot{V}O_2$ max and oxidative capacity in muscles of standardbred horses. *J. Appl. Physiol.* 73: 2274–2282, 1992.
23. Armstrong, R. B., and M. H. Laughlin. Blood flows within and among rat muscles as a function of time during high speed treadmill exercise. *J. Physiol. (Lond.)* 344: 189–208, 1983.
24. Armstrong, R. B., and M. H. Laughlin. Metabolic indicators of fiber recruitment in mammalian muscles during locomotion. *J. Exp. Biol.* 115: 201–231, 1985.
25. Armstrong, R. B., and M. H. Laughlin. Rat muscle blood flows during high speed locomotion. *J. Appl. Physiol.* 59: 1322–1328, 1985.
26. Armstrong, R. B., and M. H. Laughlin. Atropine: no effect on anticipatory or exercise muscle hyperemia in conscious rats. *J. Appl. Physiol.* 61: 679–692, 1986.
27. Armstrong, R. B., and M. H. Laughlin. Adrenoreceptor effects on rat muscle blood flow during treadmill exercise. *J. Appl. Physiol.* 62: 1465–1472, 1987.
28. Armstrong, R. B., P. Marum, C. W. Saubert, IV, H. W. Seeherman, and C. R. Taylor. Muscle fiber activity as a function of speed and gait. *J. Appl. Physiol.* 43: 672–677, 1977.
29. Armstrong, R. B., C. B. Vanderakker, and M. H. Laughlin. Muscle blood flow patterns during exercise in partially-curarized rats. *J. Appl. Physiol.* 58: 698–701, 1985.
30. Arturson, O., and I. Kjellmer. Capillary permeability in skeletal muscle during rest and activity. *Acta. Physiol. Scand.* 62: 41–49, 1964.
31. Åstrand, P., and B. Saltin. Plasma and red cell volume after prolonged severe exercise. *J. Appl. Physiol.* 19: 829–832, 1964.
32. Åstrand, P. O., and K. Rodahl. *Textbook of Work Physiology.* New York: McGraw-Hill, 1977, p. 681.
33. Aversano, T., F. J. Klocke, R. E. Mates, and J. M. Canty. Preload-induced alterations in capacitance-free diastolic pressure-flow relationships. *J. Appl. Physiol.* 259 (*Heart Circ. Physiol.* 28): H643–H647, 1984.
34. Bacchus, A., G. Gamble, D. Anderson, and J. Scott. Role of the myogenic response in exercise hyperemia. *Microvasc. Res.* 21: 92–102, 1981.
35. Bacchus, A. N., S. W. Ely, R. M. Knabb, R. Rubio, and R. M. Berne. Adenosine and coronary blood flow in conscious dogs during normal physiological stimuli. *Am. J. Physiol.* 243 (*Heart Circ. Physiol.* 12): H628–H633, 1982.
36. Bache, R. J., and F. R. Cobb. Effect of maximal coronary vasodilation on transmural myocardial perfusion during tachycardia in the awake dog. *Circ. Res.* 41: 648–653, 1977.
37. Bache, R. J., and X.-Z. Dai. Myocardial oxygen consumption during exercise in the presence of left ventricular hypertrophy secondary to supravalvular aortic stenosis. *J. Am. Coll. Cardiol.* 15: 1157–1164, 1990.
38. Bache, R. J., X.-Z. Dai, D. Alyono, T. R. Vrobel, and D. C. Homans. Myocardial blood flow during exercise in dogs with left ventricular hypertrophy produced by aortic banding and perinephritic hypertension. *Circulation* 76: 835–842, 1987.
39. Bache, R. J., X. Dai, C. A. Herzog, and J. S. Schwartz. Effects of non-selective and selective α_1-adrenergic blockade on coronary blood flow during exercise. *Circ. Res.* 61(Suppl. II): II-36–II-41, 1987.
40. Bache, R. J., X.-Z. Dai, J. S. Schwartz, and D. C. Homans. Role of adenosine in coronary vasodilation during exercise. *Circ. Res.* 62: 846–853, 1988.
41. Bache, R. J., D. C. Homans, J. S. Schwartz, and X.-Z. Dai. Differences in the effects of α-1 adrenergic blockade with prazosin and indoramin on coronary blood flow during exercise. *J. Pharmacol. Exp. Ther.* 245: 232–237, 1988.
42. Bache, R. J., and J. S. Schwartz. Effect of perfusion pressure distal to a coronary stenosis on transmural myocardial blood flow. *Circulation* 65: 928–935, 1982.
43. Bache, R. J., T. R. Vrobel, W. S. Ring, R. W. Emery, and R. W. Andersen. Regional myocardial blood flow during exercise in dogs with chronic left ventricular hypertrophy. *Circ. Res.* 48: 76–87, 1981.
44. Baker, C. H., and D. L. Davis. Isolated skeletal muscle blood flow and volume changes during contractile activity. *Blood Vessels* 11: 32–37, 1974.

45. Baldwin, K. M. Effects of chronic exercise on biochemical and functional properties of the heart. *Med. Sci. Sports Exerc.* 17: 522–528, 1985.
46. Ball, R. M., R. J. Bache, F. R. Cobb, and J. C. Greenfield, Jr. Regional myocardial blood flow during graded treadmill exercise in the dog. *J. Clin. Invest.* 55: 43–49, 1975.
47. Baran, K. W., R. J. Bache, X.-Z. Dai, and J. S. Schwartz. Effect of α-adrenergic blockade with prazosin on large coronary diameter during exercise. *Circulation* 85: 1139–1145, 1992.
48. Barclay, J. K., and W. N. Stainsby. The role of blood flow in limiting maximal metabolic rate in muscle. *Med. Sci. Sports Exerc.* 7: 116–119, 1975.
49. Barcroft, H. Circulation in skeletal muscle. *Handbook of Physiology*. Bethesda, MD: Am. Physiol. Soc., 1963, p. 1353–1385.
50. Barcroft, H., and A. C. Dornhorst. Blood flow through the human calf during rhythmic exercise. *J. Physiol. (Lond.)* 109: 402–411, 1949.
51. Bardenheuer, H., and J. Schrader. Supply-to-demand ratio for oxygen determine formation of adenosine by the heart. *Am. J. Physiol.* 250 (*Heart Circ. Physiol.* 19): H173–H180, 1986.
52. Barnard, R. J., H. W. Duncan, K. M. Baldwin, G. Grimditch and G. D. Buckberg. Effects of intensive exercise training on myocardial performance and coronary blood flow. *J. Appl. Physiol.* 49: 444–449, 1980.
53. Barnard, R. J., H. W. Duncan, J. J. Livesay, and G. D. Buckberg. Coronary vasodilator reserve and flow distribution during near-maximal exercise in dogs. *J. Appl. Physiol.* 43: 988–992, 1977.
54. Barr, D. P., H. E. Himwich, and H. P. Green. Studies in the physiology of muscular exercise. I. Changes in acid-base equilibrium following short periods of vigorous muscular exercise. *J. Biol. Chem.* 55: 459–515, 1923.
55. Bassenge, E., J. Holtz, W. Von Restorff, and K. Oversohl. Effect of chemical sympathectomy on coronary flow and cardiovascular adjustment to exercise in dogs. *Pflugers Arch.* 341: 285–296, 1973.
56. Bassenge, E., M. Kucharczyk, J. Holtz, and D. Stolan. Treadmill exercise in dogs under β-adrenergic blockade: adaptation of coronary and systemic hemodynamics. *Pflugers Arch.* 332: 40–55, 1972.
57. Baur, T. S., G. R. Brodowicz, and D. R. Lamb. Indomethacin suppresses the coronary flow response to hypoxia in exercise trained and sedentary rats. *Cardiovasc. Res.* 24: 733–736 1990.
58. Bebout, D. E., M. C. Hogan, S. C. Hempleman, and P. D. Wagner. Effects of training and immobilization on $\dot{V}O_2$ and DO_2 in dog gastrocnemius muscle in situ. *J. Appl. Physiol.* 74: 1697–1703, 1993.
59. Bedford, T. G., and C. M. Tipton. Exercise training and the arterial baroreflex. *J. Appl. Physiol.* 63: 1926–1932, 1987.
60. Bell, R. D., and R. L. Rasmussen. Exercise and the myocardial capillary-fiber ratio during growth. *Growth* 38: 237–244, 1974.
61. Berne, R. M., and R. Rubio. Regulation of coronary blood flow. *Adv. Cardiol.* 12: 303–317, 1974.
62. Bevegård, S. Studies on the regulation of the circulation in man. *Acta Physiol. Scand. Suppl.* 200: 1–36, 1963.
63. Binak, K., N. Harmanci, N. Sirmaci, N. Ataman, and H. Ogan. Oxygen extraction rate of the myocardium at rest and on exercise in various conditions. *Br. Heart J.* 29: 422, 1967.
64. Bjornberg, J., M. Maspers, and S. Mellander. Metabolic control of large-bore arterial resistance vessels, arterioles, and veins in cat skeletal muscle during exercise. *Acta Physiol. Scand.* 135: 83–94, 1989.
65. Blair, D. A., W. E. Gloves, and I. C. Roddie. Vasomotor response in the human arm during leg exercise. *Circ. Res.* 9: 264–274, 1961.
66. Block. A. J., S. Poole, and J. R. Vane. Modification of basal release of prostaglandins from rabbit isolated hearts. *Prostaglandins* 7: 473–486, 1974.
67. Blomquist, C., and B. Saltin. Cardiovascular adaptations to physical training. *Ann. Rev. Physiol.* 45: 169–189, 1983.
68. Bloor, C. M., and A. S. Leon. Interaction of age and exercise on the heart and its blood supply. *Lab. Invest.* 22: 160–165, 1970.
69. Bloor, C. M., F. C. White, and T. M. Sanders. Effects of exercise on collateral development in myocardial ischemia in pigs. *J. Appl. Physiol.* 56: 656–665, 1984.
70. Bolter, C. P., R. L. Hughson, and J. B. Critz. Intrinsic rate and cholinergic sensitivity of isolated atria from trained and sedentary rats. *Proc. Soc. Exp. Biol. Med.* 144: 364–367, 1973.
71. Booth, F. W., and D. B. Thomason. Molecular and cellular adaptation of muscle in response to exercise: perspectives of various models. *Physiol. Rev.* 71: 541–586, 1991.
72. Bove, A. A., and J. D. Dewey. Proximal coronary vasomotor reactivity after exercise training in dogs. *Circulation* 71: 620–625, 1985.
73. Bove, A. A., P. B. Hultgren, T. F. Ritzer, and R. A. Carey. Myocardial blood flow and hemodynamic responses to exercise training in dogs. *J. Appl. Physiol.* 46: 571–578, 1979.
74. Brandi, G., and M. McGregor. Intramural pressure in the left ventricle of the dog. *Cardiovasc. Res.* 3: 472–475, 1969.
75. Breisch, E. A., F. C. White, L. E. Nimmo, and C. M. Bloor. Cardiac vasculature and flow during pressure-overload hypertrophy. *Am. J. Physiol.* 251 (*Heart Circ. Physiol.* 20): H1031–H1037, 1986.
76. Breisch, E. A., F. C. White, L. E. Nimmo, M. D. McKirnan, and C. M. Bloor. Exercise-induced cardiac hypertrophy: a correlation of blood flow and microvasculature. *J. Appl. Physiol.* 60: 1259–1267, 1986.
77. Brodal, P., F. Ingjer, and L. Hermansen. Capillary supply of skeletal muscle fibers in untrained and endurance-trained men. *Am. J. Physiol.* 232 (*Heart Circ. Physiol.* 1): H705–H712, 1977.
78. Brown, B. G., A. B. Lee, E. L. Bolson, and H. T. Dodge. Reflex constriction of significant coronary stenosis as a mechanism contributing to ischemic left ventricular dysfunction during isometric exercise. *Circulation* 70: 18–24, 1984.
79. Burcher, E., and D. Garlick. Antagonism of vasoconstrictor responses by exercise in the gracilis muscle of the dog. *J. Pharmacol. Exp. Ther.* 187: 78–85, 1973.
80. Burke, R. E. Motor units: anatomy, physiology, and functional organization. *Handbook of Physiology, The Nervous System, Motor Control*, edited by V. B. Brooks. Bethesda, MD: Am. Physiol. Soc., 1981, p. 345–422.
81. Burt, J. J., and R. Jackson. The effects of physical exercise on the coronary collateral circulation of dogs. *J. Sports Med. Physiol.* 4: 203–206, 1965.
82. Buttrick, P. M., H. A. Levitye, T. F. Schaible, G. Ciambrone, and J. Scheuer. Early increases in coronary vascular reserve in exercised rats are independent of cardiac hypertrophy. *J. Appl. Physiol.* 59: 1861–1865, 1985.

83. Buttrick, P. M., and J. Scheuer. Physiologic, biochemical, and coronary adaptation to exercise conditioning. *Cardiol. Clin.* 5: 259–270, 1987.
84. Carey, R. A., W. P. Santamore, J. J. Michelle, and A. A. Bove. Effects of endurance training on coronary resistance in dogs. *Med. Sci. Sports Exerc.* 15: 355–359, 1983.
85. Carlsson, S., A. Ljungqvist, G. Tornling, and G. Unge. The myocardial vasculature in repeated physical exercise. *Acta Pathol. Microbiol. Scand.* 86: 117–119, 1978.
86. Carrow, R., R. Brown, and W. Van Huss. Fiber sizes and capillary to fiber ratios in skeletal muscle of exercised rats. *Anat. Rec.* 159: 33–40, 1967.
87. Cerretelli, P., and P. E. Di Prampero. Gas exchange in exercise. In: *Handbook of Physiology, The Respiratory System, Gas Exchange*, edited by L. E. Farhi and S. M. Tenney. Bethesda, MD: Am. Physiol. Soc., 1987.
88. Chang, P. C., E. Kreik, J. van der Krogt, and P. van Brummelen. Does regional norepinephrine spillover represent local sympathetic activity? *Hypertension* 18: 56–66, 1991.
89. Chilian, W. M., C. L. Eastham, M. L. Marcus. Microvascular distribution of coronary vascular resistance in beating left ventricle. *Am. J. Physiol.* 251 (*Heart Circ. Physiol.* 20): H779–H788, 1986.
90. Chilian, W. M., D. G. Harrison, C. W. Haws, W. D. Snyder, and M. L. Marcus. Adrenergic coronary tone during submaximal exercise in the dog is produced by circulating catecholamines. Evidence for adrenergic denervation supersensitivity in the myocardium but not in coronary vessels. *Circ. Res.* 58: 68–82, 1986.
91. Chilian, W. M., S. M. Lyne, E. C. Klausner, C. L. Eastham, and M. L. Marcus. Redistribution of coronary microvascular resistance produced by dipyridamole. *Am. J. Physiol.* 256 (*Heart Circ. Physiol.* 25): H383–H390, 1989.
92. Clausen, J. Circulatory adjustments to dynamic exercise and effect of physical training in normal subjects and in patients with coronary artery disease. *Prog. Cardiovasc. Dis.* 18: 459–495, 1976.
93. Clausen, J., O. Larsen, and J. Trap-Jensen. Physical training in the management of coronary artery disease. *Circulation* 40: 143–154, 1969.
94. Coates, G., H. O'Brodovich, and G. Goeree. Hindlimb and lung lymph flows during prolonged exercise. *J. Appl. Physiol.* 75: 633–638, 1993.
95. Cobbold, A., B. Folkow, I. Kjellmer, and S. Mellander. Nervous and local chemical control of pre-capillary sphincters in skeletal muscle as measured by changes in filtration coefficient. *Acta Physiol. Scand.* 57: 180–192, 1963.
96. Cocks, T. M., and J. A. Angus. Endothelium-dependent relaxation of coronary arteries by noradrenaline and serotonin. *Nature* 305: 627–630, 1983.
97. Cohen, M. V. Coronary vascular reserve in the greyhound with left ventricular hypertrophy. *Cardiovasc. Res.* 20: 182–194, 1986.
98. Cohen, M. V. Training in dogs with normal coronary arteries: lack of effect on collateral development. *Cardiovasc. Res.* 24: 121–128, 1990.
99. Cohen, M. V. Lack of effect of propranolol on canine coronary collateral development during progressive coronary collateral development during progressive coronary stenosis and occlusion. *Cardiovasc. Res.* 27: 249–254, 1993.
100. Cohen, M. V., T. Yipintsoi, A. Malhotra, S. Penpargkul, and J. Scheuer. Effect of exercise on collateral development in dogs with normal coronary arteries. *J. Appl. Physiol.* 45: 797–805, 1978.
101. Cohen, M. V., T. Yipintsoi, and J. Scheuer. Coronary collateral stimulation by exercise in dogs with stenotic coronary arteries. *Appl. Physiol.* 52: 664–671, 1982.
102. Colan, S. D. Mechanisms of left ventricular systolic and diastolic function in physiologic hypertrophy of the athletic heart. *Cardiol. Clin.* 10: 227–240, 1992.
103. Connett, R. J., and C. R. Honig. Regulation of $\dot{V}O_2$ in red muscle: do current biochemical hypotheses fit in vivo data? *Am. J. Physiol.* 256 (*Regulatory Integrative Comp. Physiol.* 25): R898–R906, 1989.
104. Corcondilas, A., G. T. Koroxenidis, and J. T. Shepherd. Effect of brief contraction of forearm muscles on forearm blood flow. *J. Appl. Physiol.* 19: 142–146, 1964.
105. Cousineau, D., R. J. Ferguson, J. de Champlain, P. Gauthier, P. Côté, and M. Bourassa. Catecholamines in coronary sinus during exercise in man before and after training. *J. Appl. Physiol.* 43: 801–806, 1977.
106. Crone, C. Does "restricted diffusion" occur in muscle capillaries? *Proc. Soc. Exp. Biol. Med.* 112: 453–455, 1963.
107. Crone, C. Permeability of capillaries in various organs as determined by use of the "indicator diffusion" method. *Acta Physiol. Scand.* 58: 292–305, 1963.
108. Cutilletta, A. F., K. Edmiston, and R. T. Dowell. Effect of a mild exercise program on myocardial function and the development of hypertrophy. *J. Appl. Physiol.* 46: 354–360, 1979.
109. Dai, X.-Z., and R. J. Bache. Effect of indomethacin on coronary blood flow during graded treadmill exercise in the dog. *Am. J. Physiol.* 247 (*Heart Circ. Physiol.* 16): H452–458, 1984.
110. Dai, X.-Z., C. A. Herzog, J. S. Schwartz, and R. J. Bache. Coronary blood flow during exercise following nonselective and selective alpha 1-adrenergic blockade with indoramin. *J. Cardiovasc. Pharm.* 8: 574–581, 1986.
111. Dai, X.-Z., E. Sublett, P. Lindstrom, J. S. Schwartz, D. C. Homans, and R. J. Bache. Coronary flow during exercise after selective alpha 1- and alpha 2-adrenergic blockade. *Am. J. Physiol.* 256 (*Heart Circ. Physiol.* 25): H1148–H1155, 1989.
112. Damon, D. H., and B. R. Duling. Evidence that capillary perfusion heterogeneity is not controlled in striated muscle. *Am. J. Physiol.* 248 (*Heart Circ. Physiol.* 18): H386–H392, 1986.
113. Daniel, T. O., and H. E. Ives. Endothelial control of vascular function. *News Physiol. Sci.* 4: 139–142, 1989.
114. Davies, P. F., and S. C. Tripathi. Mechanical stress mechanisms and the cell: an endothelial paradigm. *Circ. Res.* 72: 239–245, 1993.
115. Daut, J., W. M. Rudolph, N. von Beckerath, G. Meherke, K. Gunther, and L. G. Meinen. Hypoxic dilation of coronary arteries is mediated by ATP-sensitive potassium channels. *Science* 247: 1341–1344, 1990.
116. Delashaw, J. B., and B. R. Duling. A study of the functional elements regulating capillary perfusion in striated muscle. *Microvasc. Res.* 36: 162–180, 1988.
117. Delp, M. D., R. M. McAllister, and M. H. Laughlin. Exercise training alters endothelium-dependent vasoreactivity of rat abdominal aorta. *J. Appl. Physiol.* 75: 1354–1363, 1993.
118. Dempsey, J. A., P. Hanson, and K. Henderson. Exercise-induced arterial hypoxemia in healthy humans at sea-level. *J. Physiol. (Lond.)* 161–175, 1984.
119. DiCarlo, S. E., and V. S. Bishop. Regional vascular resistance during exercise: role of cardiac afferents and exercise training. *Am. J. Physiol.* 258 (*Heart Circ. Physiol.* 27): H842–H847, 1990.

120. DiCarlo. S. E., R. W. Blair, V. S. Bishop, H. L. Stone. Role of beta 2-adrenergic receptors on coronary resistance during exercise. *J. Appl. Physiol.* 64: 2287–2293, 1988.
121. DiCarlo, S. E., R. W. Blair, V. S. Bishop, and H. L. Stone. Daily exercise enhances coronary resistance vessel sensitivity to pharmacological activation. *J. Appl. Physiol.* 66: 421–428, 1989.
122. Djojosugito, A. M., B. Folkow, B. Lisander, and H. Sparks. Mechanisms of escape of skeletal muscle resistance vessels from the influence of sympathetic cholinergic vasodilator fibre activity. *Acta Physiol. Scand.* 72: 148–156, 1968.
123. Dodd, L. R., and P. C. Johnson. Antagonism of vasoconstriction by muscle contraction differs with alpha-adrenergic subtype. *Am. J. Physiol.* 264 (*Heart Circ. Physiol.* 33): H892–H900, 1993.
124. Dodd-o, J. M., and P. A. Gwirtz. Cardiac response to acute coronary artery occlusion in exercise-trained dogs. *Med. Sci. Sports Exerc.* 24: 1245–1251, 1992.
125. Donald, D. E. Myocardial performance after excision of the extrinsic cardiac nerves in the dog. *Circ. Res.* 34: 417, 1974.
126. Donald, D. E., D. J. Rowlands, and D. A. Ferguson. Similarity of blood flow in the normal and the sympathetectomized dog hind limb during graded exercise. *Circ. Res.* 46: 185–199, 1970.
127. Downey, J. M., and E. S. Kirk. Inhibition of coronary blood flow by a vascular waterfall mechanism. *Circ. Res.* 36: 753–760, 1975.
128. Duling, B. R., Coordination of microcirculatory function with oxygen demand in skeletal muscle. In: *Advances in Physiology. Cardiovascular Physiology: Microcirculation and Capillary Exchange.* Budapest: Akademiai Kaido, 1981, p. 1–16.
129. Duling, B. R. Control of striated muscle blood flow. *The Lung: Scientific Foundations.* New York: Raven Press, 1991, p. 1497–1505.
130. Duling, B. R., and R. M. Berne. Longitudinal gradients in periarteriolar oxygen tension. A possible mechanism for the participation of oxygen in local regulation of blood flow. *Circ. Res.* 27: 669–678, 1970.
131. Duling, B. R., and R. M. Berne, Propagated vasodilation in the microcirculation of the hamster cheek pouch. *Circ. Res.* 26: 163–170, 1970.
132. Duling, B. R., and B. Klitzman. Local control of microvascular function: role in tissue oxygen supply. *Ann. Rev. Physiol.* 42: 373–382, 1980.
133. Duncker, D. J., and R. J. Bache. Inhibition of nitric oxide production aggravates myocardial hypoperfusion during exercise in the presence of a coronary artery stenosis. *Circ. Res.* 74: 629–640, 1994.
134. Duncker, D. J., D. D. Laxson, P. Lindstrom, and R. J. Bache. Endogenous adenosine and coronary vasoconstriction in hypoperfused myocardium during exercise. *Cardiovasc. Res.* 27: 1592–1597, 1993.
135. Duncker, D. J., E. O. McFalls, R. Krams, and P. D. Verdouw. Pressure-maximal coronary flow relationship in regionally stunned porcine myocardium. *Am. J. Physiol.* 262 (*Heart Circ. Physiol.* 31): H1744–H1751, 1992.
136. Duncker, D. J., P. R. Saxena, and P. D. Verdouw. The effects of nisoldipine alone and in combination with beta-adrenoceptor blockade on systemic hemodynamics and myocardial performance in conscious pigs. *Eur. Heart J.* 8: 1332–1339, 1987.
137. Duncker, D. J., N. S. van Zon, J. D. Altman, T. J. Pavek, and R. J. Bache. Role of K^+ATP channels in coronary vasodilation during exercise. *Circulation* 88: 1245–1253, 1993.
138. Duncker, D. J., N. S. van Zon, M. Crampton, S. Herringer, D. C. Homans, and R. J. Bache. Coronary pressure-flow relationship and exercise: contributions of heart rate, contractility, and α1-adrenergic tone. *Am. J. Physiol.* 266 (*Heart Circ. Physiol.* 35): H795–H810, 1994.
139. Duncker, D. J., N. S. van Zon, T. J. Pavek, S. K. Herrlinger, and R. J. Bache. Endogenous adenosine mediates coronary vasodilation in response to exercise after K^+ATP channel blockade. *J. Clin. Invest.* 95: 285–295, 1995.
140. Duncker, D. J., J. Zhang, and R. J. Bache. Coronary pressure-flow relationship in left ventricular hypertrophy: importance of changes in back pressure versus changes in minimum resistance. *Circ. Res.* 72: 579–587, 1993.
141. Duncker, D. J., J. Zhang, T. Pavek, P. Lindstrom, and R. J. Bache. α1-adrenergic tone does not influence the transmural distribution of myocardial blood flow during exercise in dogs with pressure overload left ventricular hypertrophy. *Basic Res. Cardiol.* 90: 73–83, 1995.
142. Dzau, V. J., and G. H. Gibbons. The role of the endothelium in vascular remodeling. In: *Cardiovascular Significance of Endothelium-Derived Vasoactive Factors.* Mount Kisco, NY: Futura Publishing Co., Inc., 1991, p. 281–291.
143. Eckstein, R. W. Effect of exercise and coronary artery narrowing on coronary collateral circulation. *Circ. Res.* 5: 230–235, 1957.
144. Edlund, A., A. Sollevi, and A. Wennmalm. The role of adenosine and prostacyclin in coronary flow regulation in healthy man. *Acta Physiol. Scand.* 135: 39–46, 1989.
145. Edwards, M. T., and J. N. Diana. Effect of exercise on pre- and postcapillary resistance in the spontaneously hypertensive rat. *Am. J. Physiol.* 234 (*Heart Circ. Physiol.* 3): H439–H446, 1978.
146. Edwards, J. G., C. M. Tipton, and R. D. Matthes. Influence of exercise training on reactivity and contractility of arterial strips from hypertensive rats. *J. Appl. Physiol.* 58: 1683–1688, 1985.
147. Ehsani, A. A., J. M. Hagberg, and R. C. Hickson. Rapid changes in left ventricular dimensions and mass in response to physical conditioning and deconditioning. *Am. J. Cardiol.* 42: 52–56, 1978.
148. Ekelund, U., J. Bjornberg, U. Albert, P. O. Grande, and S. Mellander. Myogenic vascular regulation in skeletal muscle in vivo is not dependent on endothelium-derived nitric oxide. *Acta Physiol. Scand.* 144: 199–207, 1992.
149. Ekelund, U., and S. Mellander. Role of endothelium-derived nitric oxide in the regulation of tonus in large-bore arterial resistance vessels, arterioles and veins in cat skeletal muscle. *Acta Physiol. Scand.* 140: 301–309, 1990.
150. Ekstrom-Jodal, B., E. Haggendal, R. Malmberg, and N. Svedmyr. The effect of adrenergic β-receptor blockade on coronary circulation in man during work. *Acta Med. Scand.* 191: 245–248, 1972.
151. Ellis, A. K., and F. J. Klocke. Effects of preload on the transmural distribution of perfusion and pressure-flow relationships in the canine coronary vascular bed. *Circ. Res.* 46: 68–77, 1979.
152. Ely, S. W., R. M. Knabb, A. N. Bacchus, R. Rubio, and R. M. Berne. Measurements of coronary plasma and pericardial infusate adenosine concentrations during exercise in conscious dog: relationship to myocardial oxygen consumption and coronary blood flow. *J. Mol. Cell Cardiol.* 15: 673–683, 1983.

153. Engelhardt, W. V. Cardiovascular effects of exercise and training in horses. *Adv. Vet. Sci. Comp. Med.* 7: 173–205, 1977.
154. Eriksen, M., G. A. Waaler, L. Walloe, and J. Wesche. Dynamics and dimensions of cardiac output changes in humans at the onset and at the end of moderate rhythmic exercise. *J. Physiol. (Lond.)* 426: 423–437, 1990.
155. Eriksson, E., and B. Lisander. Changes in precapillary resistance in skeletal muscle vessels studied by intravital microscopy. *Acta Physiol. Scand.* 84: 295–305, 1972.
156. Essen, B., A. Lindholm, and J. Thornton. Histochemical properties of muscle fibre types and enzyme activities in skeletal muscles of standard bred trotters of different ages. *Equine Vet. J.* 12: 175–180, 1980.
157. Faber, J. E. In situ analysis of alpha-adrenoceptors on arteriolar and venular smooth muscle in rat skeletal muscle microcirculation. *Circ. Res.* 62: 37–50, 1988.
158. Faber, J. E. Effect of local tissue cooling on microvascular smooth muscle and postjunctional α-adrenoceptors. *Am. J. Physiol.* 255 (*Heart Circ. Physiol.* 24): H121–H130, 1988.
159. Faber, J. E., P. D. Harris, and I. G. Joshua. Microvascular response to blockade of prostaglandin synthesis in rat skeletal muscle. *Am. J. Physiol.* 243 (*Heart Circ. Physiol.* 12): H51–H60, 1982.
160. Faber, J. E., P. D. Harris, and F. N. Miller. Microvascular sensitivity to PGE2 and PGI2 in skeletal muscle of decerebrate rat. *Am. J. Physiol.* 243 (*Heart Circ. Physiol.* 12): H844–H851, 1982.
161. Faber, J. E., and G. A. Meininger. Selective interaction of α adrenoceptors with myogenic regulation of microvascular smooth muscle. *Am. J. Physiol.* 259 (*Heart Circ. Physiol.* 28): H1126–H1133, 1990.
162. Fagraeus, L. Cardiorespiratory and metabolic functions during exercise in the hyperbaric environment. *Acta Physiol. Scand. Suppl.* 414: 1–40, 1974.
163. Falcone, J. C., M. J. Davis, and G. A. Meininger. Endothelial independence of myogenic response in isolated skeletal muscle arterioles. *Am. J. Physiol.* 260 (*Heart Circ. Physiol.* 29): H130–H135, 1991.
164. Feigl, E. O. Coronary physiology. *Physiol. Rev.* 63: 1–205, 1983.
165. Feigl, E. O. The paradox of adrenergic coronary vasoconstriction. *Circulation* 75: 737–745, 1987.
166. Fixler, D. E., J. M. Atkins, J. H. Mitchell, and L. D. Horwitz. Blood flow to respiratory, cardiac and limb muscles in dogs during graded exercise. *Am. J. Physiol.* 231: 1515–1519, 1976.
167. Flaim, S. F., W. J. Minteer, D. P. Clark, and R. Zelis. Cardiovascular response to acute aquatic and treadmill exercise in the untrained rat. *J. Appl. Physiol.* 46: 302–308, 1979.
168. Flavahan, N. A. Atherosclerosis or lipoprotein-induced endothelial dysfunction: potential mechanisms underlying reduction in EDRF/nitric oxide activity. *Circulation* 85: 1927–1938, 1992.
169. Folkow, B., P. Gaskell, and B. A. Waaler. Blood flow through limb muscles during heavy rhythmic exercise. *Acta Physiol. Scand.* 80: 61–72, 1970.
170. Folkow, B., U. Haglund, M. Jodal, and O. Lundgren. Blood flow in the calf muscle of man during heavy rhythmic exercise. *Acta Physiol. Scand.* 81: 157–163, 1971.
171. Folkow, B., and H. D. Halicka. A comparison between red and white muscle with respect to blood supply, capillary surface area and oxygen uptake during rest and exercise. *Microvasc. Res.* 1: 1–14, 1968.
172. Folkman, J., and M. Klagsbrun. Angiogenic factors. *Science* 235: 442–447, 1987.
173. Frame, M. D. S., and I. H. Sarelius. Regulation of capillary perfusion by small arterioles is spatially organized. *Circ. Res.* 73: 155–163, 1993.
174. Frank, A. Experimentelle Herzhypertrophie. *Z. Ges. Exp. Med.* 115: 312–349, 1950.
175. Franklin, B. A. Exercise training and coronary collateral circulation. *Med. Sci. Sports. Exerc.* 23: 648–653, 1991.
176. Furchgott, R. F. Role of endothelium in responses of vascular smooth muscle. *Circ. Res.* 53: 557–573, 1983.
177. Furuya, F., H. Yoshitaka, H. Morita, and H. Hosomi. Neural, humoral, and metabolic control of coronary vascular resistance during exercise. *Jpn. J. Physiol.* 42: 117–130, 1992.
178. Gage, J. E., O. M. Hess, T. Murakami, M. Ritter, J. Grimm, and H. P. Krayenbuehl. Vasoconstriction of stenotic coronary arteries during dynamic exercise in patients with classic angina pectoris: reversibility by nitroglycerin. *Circulation* 73: 865–876, 1986.
179. Gaglione, A., O. M. Hess, W. J. Corin, M. Ritter, J. Grimm, and H. P. Krayenbuehl. Is there coronary vasoconstriction after intracoronary beta-adrenergic blockade in patients with coronary artery disease. *J. Am. Coll. Cardiol.* 10: 299–310, 1987.
180. Gaskell, W. H. On the changes of the blood stream in muscle through stimulation of their nerves. *J. Anat.* 11: 360–402, 1977.
181. Gayeski, T. E. J., R. J. Connett, and C. R. Honig. Minimum intracellular PO_2 for maximum cytochrome turnover in red muscle in situ. *Adv. Exp. Med. Biol.* 200: 487–494, 1987.
182. Gayeski, T. E. J., and C. R. Honig. Intracellular PO_2 in long axis of individual fibers in working dog gracilis muscle. *Am. J. Physiol.* 254 (*Heart Circ. Physiol.* 23): H1179–H1186, 1988.
183. Gerová, M., E. Barta, and J. Gero. Sympathetic control of major coronary artery diameter in the dog. *Circ. Res.* 44: 459–467, 1979.
184. Gleeson, T. T., and K. M. Baldwin. Cardiovascular response to treadmill exercise in untrained rats. *J. Appl. Physiol.* 50: 1206–1211, 1981.
185. Gleeson, T. T., W. J. Mullin, and K. M. Baldwin. Cardiovascular response to treadmill exercise in rats: effects of training. *J. Appl. Physiol.* 54: 789–793, 1983.
186. Glen, G. M., M. H. Laughlin, and R. B. Armstrong. Muscle blood flow and fiber activity in partially curarized rats during exercise. *J. Appl. Physiol.* 63: 1450–1456, 1987.
187. Gorczynski, R. J., B. Klitzman, and B. R. Duling. Interrelations between contracting striated muscle and precapillary microvessels. *Am. J. Physiol.* 235 (*Heart Circ. Physiol.* 4): H494–H504, 1978.
188. Gordon, J. B., P. Ganz, E. G. Nabel, R. D. Fish, J. Zebede, G. H. Mudge, R. W. Alexander, and A. P. Selwyn. Atherosclerosis influences the vasomotor response of epicardial coronary arteries to exercise. *J. Clin. Invest.* 83: 1946–1952, 1989.
189. Gorlin, R., N. Krasnow, H. J. Levine, and J. V. Messer. Effect of exercise on cardiac performance in human subjects with minimal heart disease. *Am. J. Physiol.* 13: 293–300, 1964.
190. Granger, H. J., J. L. Borders, G. A. Meininger, A. H. Goodman, and G. E. Barnes. Microcirculatory control systems. In: *Physiology and Pharmacology of the Microcirculation.* Bethesda, MD: Academic Press, 1983, p. 209–236.
191. Granger, H. J., A. H. Goodman, and D. N. Granger. Role of resistance and exchange vessels in local microvascular

control of skeletal muscle oxygenation in the dog. *Circ. Res.* 38: 379–385, 1976.
192. Granger, H. J., G. A. Meininger, J. L. Borders. R. J. Morff, and A. H. Goodman. Microcirculation of skeletal muscle. In: *Physiology and Pharmacology of the Microcirculation.* Bethesda, MD: Academic Press, 1984, p. 181–265.
193. Gray, S. D. Responsiveness of the terminal vascular bed in fast and slow skeletal muscle to adrenergic stimulation. *Angiologica* 8: 285–296, 1971.
194. Gray, S. D., and E. M. Renkin. Microvascular supply in relation to fiber metabolic type in mixed skeletal muscles of rabbits. *Microvasc. Res.* 16: 404–425, 1978.
195. Gregg, D. E., E. M. Khouri, D. E. Donald, H. S. Lowensohn, and S. Pasyk. Coronary circulation in the conscious dog with cardiac neural ablation. *Circ. Res.* 31: 129–144, 1972.
196. Grossman, E., P. C. Chang, A. Hoffman, M. Tamrat, I. J. Kopin, and D. S. Goldstein. Tracer norepinephrine kinetics: dependence on regional blood flow and the site of infusion. *Am. J. Physiol.* 260 (*Regulatory Integrative Comp. Physiol.* 29): R946–R952, 1991.
197. Gruner, J. A., and J. Altman. Swimming in the rat: analysis of locomotor performance in comparison to stepping. *Exp. Brain. Res.* 40: 374–382, 1980.
198. Gute, D. C., M. H. Laughlin, and J. F. Amann. Regional distribution of capillary angiogenesis in interval-sprint and low-intensity, endurance training. *Microcirculation* 1: 183–193, 1994.
199. Gute, D. C., J. Muller, R. McAllister, and M. H. Laughlin. Effects of exercise training on femoral arterial smooth muscle in miniature swine. *Med. Sci. Sports. Exerc.* 23: S88, 1991.
200. Gwirtz, P. A., J. M. Dodd-o, M. A. Brandt, and C. E. Jones. Augmentation of coronary flow improves myocardial function in exercise. *J. Cardiovasc. Pharmacol.* 15: 752–758, 1990.
201. Gwirtz, P. A., H. J. Mass, J. R. Strader, and C. E. Jones. Coronary and cardiac responses to exercise after chronic ventricular sympathectomy. *Med. Sci. Sports. Exerc.* 20: 126–135, 1988.
202. Gwirtz, P. A., S. P. Overn, H. J. Mass, and C. E. Jones. Alpha 1-adrenergic constriction limits coronary flow and cardiac function in running dogs. *Am. J. Physiol.* 250 (*Heart Circ. Physiol.* 19): H1117–H1126, 1986.
203. Gwirtz, P. A., and H. L. Stone. Coronary blood flow changes following activation of adrenergic receptors in the conscious dog. *Am. J. Physiol.* 243 (*Heart Circ. Physiol.* 12): H13–H19, 1982.
204. Gwirtz, P. A., and H. L. Stone. Coronary blood flow and myocardial oxygen consumption after alpha adrenergic blockade during submaximal exercise. *J. Pharmacol. Exp. Ther.* 217: 92–98, 1981.
205. Gwirtz, P. A., and H. L. Stone. Coronary vascular response to adrenergic stimulation in exercise-conditioned dogs. *J. Appl. Physiol.* 243: 315–320, 1984.
206. Haddy, F. J., and J. B. Scott. Metabolic factors in peripheral circulatory regulation. *Federation Proc.* 34: 2006–2011, 1975.
207. Hakkila, J. Studies on the myocardial capillary concentration in cardiac hypertrophy due to training. *Ann. Med. Exp. Biol. Fenn.* 33: 1–79, 1955.
208. Hammond, H. K., F. C. White, L. L. Brunton, and J. C. Longhurst. Association of decreased myocardial β-receptors and chronotropic response to isoproterenol and exercise in pigs following chronic dynamic exercise. *Circ. Res.* 60: 720–726, 1987.
209. Harri, M. N. E. Physical training under the influence of beta-blockade in rats. II. Effects on vascular reactivity. *Eur. J. Appl. Physiol.* 42: 151–157, 1979.
210. Harrison, M. H. Effect of thermal stress and exercise on blood volume in humans. *Physiol. Rev.* 65: 149–199, 1985.
211. Haskell, W. L., C. Sims, J. Myll, W. M. Bortz, F. G. Goar, and E. L. Alderman. Coronary artery size and dilating capacity in ultradistance runners. *Circulation* 87: 1076–1082, 1993.
212. Hastings, A. B., F. C. White, T. M. Sanders, and C. M. Bloor. Comparative physiological responses to exercise stress. *J. Appl. Physiol.* 52: 1077–1083, 1982.
213. Hathaway, D. R., K. L. March, J. A. Lash, L. P. Adam, and R. L. Wilensky. Vascular smooth muscle: a review of the molecular basis of contractility. *Circulation* 83: 382–390, 1991.
214. Hautamaa, P. V., X.-Z. Dai, D. C. Homans, and R. J. Bache. Vasomotor activity of moderately well-developed canine coronary collateral circulation. *Am. J. Physiol.* 256 (*Heart Circ. Physiol.* 25): H890–H897, 1989.
215. Heaton, W. H., K. C. Marr, N. L. Capurro, R. E. Goldstein, and S. E. Epstein. Beneficial effect of physical training on blood flow to myocardium perfused by chronic collaterals in the exercising dog. *Circulation* 57: 575–581, 1978.
216. Hess, D. S., and R. J. Bache. Transmural distribution of myocardial blood flow during systole in the awake dog. *Circ. Res.* 38: 5–15, 1976.
217. Heiss, H. W., J. Barmeyer, K. Wink, G. Hell, F. J. Cerny, J. Keul, and H. Reindell. Studies on the regulation of myocardial blood flow in man. I. Training effects on blood flow and metabolism of the healthy heart at rest and during standardized heavy exercise. *Basic Res. Cardiol.* 71: 658–675, 1976.
218. Hester, R. L., A. Eraslan, and Y. Saito. Differences in EDNO contribution to arteriolar diameters at rest and during functional dilation in striated muscle. *Am. J. Physiol.* 265 (*Heart Circ. Physiol.* 34): H146–H151, 1993.
219. Heyndrickx, G. R., P. Muylaert, and J. L. Pannier. α-Adrenergic control of oxygen delivery to myocardium during exercise in conscious dogs. *Am. J. Physiol.* 242 (*Heart Circ. Physiol.* 11): H805–H809, 1982.
220. Heyndrickx, G. R., J. L. Pannier, P. Muylaert, C. Mabilde, and I. Leusen. Alteration in myocardial oxygen balance during exercise after beta-adrenergic blockade in dogs. *J. Appl. Physiol.* 49: 28–33, 1980.
221. Heyndrickx, G. R., J. P. Vilaine, E. J. Moerman, and I. Leusen. Role of prejunctional α_2-adrenergic receptors in the regulation of myocardial performance during exercise in conscious dogs. *Circ. Res.* 54: 683–693, 1984.
222. Hill, A. V. The pressure developed in muscle during contraction. *J. Physiol. (Lond.)* 107: 518–526, 1948.
223. Hilton, S. M. A peripheral arterial conducting mechanism underlying dilatation of the femoral artery and concerned in functional vasodilation in skeletal muscle. *J. Physiol. (Lond.)* 149: 93–111, 1959.
224. Hilton, S. M. O. Hudlická, and J. M. Marshall. Possible mediators of functional hyperemia in skeletal muscle. *J. Physiol. (Lond.)* 282: 131–147, 1978.
225. Hilton, S. M., M. G. Jefferies, and G. Vrboba. Functional specialization of the vascular bed of soleus *J. Physiol. (Lond.)* 206: 131–147, 1970.
226. Hintze, T. H., and G. Kaley. Prostaglandins and the control of blood flow in the canine myocardium. *Circ. Res.* 40: 313–320, 1977.

227. Hintze, T. H., and S. F. Vatner. Reactive dilation of large coronary arteries in conscious dogs. *Circ. Res.* 54: 50–57, 1984.
228. Hirai, T., M. D. Visneski, K. J. Keams, R. Zelis, and T. I. Musch. Role of endothelial function in rat muscular blood flow response to submaximal treadmill exercise. *Circulation* 88: I-376, 1993.
229. Ho, K. W., R. R. Roy, R. Taylor, W. W. Heusner, and W. D. Van Huss. Differential effects of running and weightlifting on the rat coronary arterial tree. *Med. Sci. Sports. Exerc.* 6: 472–477, 1983.
230. Hogan, M. C., P. G. Arthur, D. E. Bebout, P. W. Hochachka, and P. D. Wagner. Role of O_2 in regulating tissue respiration in dog muscle working in situ. *J. Appl. Physiol.* 73: 728–736, 1992.
231. Hogan, M. C., D. D. Bebout, and P. D. Wagner. Effect of blood flow reduction on maximal O_2 uptake in canine gastrocnemius muscle in situ. *J. Appl. Physiol.* 74: 1742–1747, 1993.
232. Hogan, M. C., S. Nioka, W. F. Brechue, and B. Chance. A ^{31}P-NMR study of tissue respiration in working dog muscle during reduced O_2 delivery conditions. *J. Appl. Physiol.* 73: 1662–1670, 1992.
233. Hogan, M. C., J. Roca, P. D. Wagner, and J. B. West. Limitation of maximal O_2 uptake and performance by acute hypoxia in dog muscle in situ. *J. Appl. Physiol.* 65: 815–821, 1988.
234. Hogan, M. C., J. Roca, J. B. West, and P. D. Wagner. Dissociation of maximal O_2 uptake from O_2 delivery in canine gastrocnemius in situ. *J. Appl. Physiol.* 66: 1219–1226, 1989.
235. Hogan, M. C., D. C. Willford, P. E. Kiepert, N. S. Faithfull, and P. D. Wagner. Increased plasma O_2 solubility improves O_2 uptake of in situ dog muscle working maximally. *J. Appl. Physiol.* 73: 2470–2475, 1992.
236. Holmberg, S., W. Serzysko, and E. Varnauskas. Coronary circulation during heavy exercise in control subjects and patients with coronary heart disease. *Acta Med. Scand.* 190: 465–480, 1971.
237. Holtz, J., M. Giesler, and E. Bassenge. Two dilatory mechanisms of anti-anginal drugs on epicardial coronary arteries in vivo: indirect, flow-dependent, endothelium-mediated dilation and direct smooth muscle relaxation. *Z. Kardiol.* 72(Suppl. 3): 98–106, 1983.
238. Honig, C. R. Contributions of nerves and metabolites to exercise vasodilation: a unifying hypothesis. *Am. J. Physiol.* 236 (*Heart Circ. Physiol.* 5): H705–H719, 1979.
239. Honig, C. R., T. E. J. Gayeski, W. Federspeil, A. Clark, Jr., and P. Clark. Muscle O_2 gradients from hemoglobin to cytochrome: new concepts, new complexities. *Adv. Exp. Med. Biol.* 169: 23–38, 1984.
240. Honig, C. R., and C. L. Odoroff. Calculated dispersion of capillary transit times: significance for oxygen exchange. *Am. J. Physiol.* 240 (*Heart Circ. Physiol.* 9): H199–H208, 1981.
241. Honig, C. R., C. L. Odoroff, and J. L. Frierson. Active and passive capillary control in red muscle at rest and in exercise. *Am. J. Physiol.* 243 (*Heart Circ. Physiol.* 12): H196–H206, 1982.
242. Horwitz, L. D., J. M. Atkins, and S. J. Leshin. Role of the Frank-Starling mechanism in exercise. *Circ. Res.* 31: 868–875, 1972.
243. Houston, M. E., H. Bentzen, and H. Larsen. Interrelationships between skeletal muscle adaptations and performance as studied by detraining and retraining. *Acta. Physiol. Scand.* 105: 163–170, 1979.
244. Huang, A. H., and E. O. Feigl. Adrenergic coronary vasoconstriction helps maintain uniform transmural blood flow distribution during exercise. *Circ. Res.* 62: 286–298, 1988.
245. Hudlická, O. Regulation of muscle blood flow. *Clin. Physiol.* 5: 201–229, 1985.
246. Hudlická, O. Effect of training on macro- and microcirculatory changes in exercise. *Exerc. Sport Sci. Rev.* 5: 181–230, 1977.
247. Hudlická, O. *Muscle Blood Flow: Its Relation to Muscle Metabolism and Function.* Amsterdam: Swets and Zeitlinger, 1973.
248. Hudlická, O. Growth of vessels—historical review. *Prog. Appl. Microcirc.* 4: 1–8, 1984.
249. Hudlická, O. Capillary growth: role of mechanical factors. *News Physiol. Sci.* 3: 117–120, 1988.
250. Hudlická, O., and S. Price. The role of blood flow and/or muscle hypoxia in capillary growth in chronically stimulated fast muscles. *Pflugers Arch.* 417: 67–72, 1990.
251. Hudlická, O., and K. R. Tyler. *Angiogenesis.* New York: Academic Press, 1986.
252. Hull, S. S. Jr., L. Kaiser, M. D. Jaffe, and H. V. Sparks. Endothelium-dependent flow induced dilation of canine femoral and saphenous arteries. *Blood Vessels* 23: 183–198, 1986.
253. Hurley, B. F., D. R. Seals, A. A. Ehsani, L.-J. Cartier, D. P. Dalsky, J. M. Hagberg, and J. O. Holloszy. Effects of high-intensity strength training on cardiovascular function. *Med. Sci. Sports. Exerc.* 16: 483–488, 1984.
254. Ignarro, L. J., R. E. Byrns, G. M. Buga, and K. S. Wood. Endothelium-derived relaxing factor from pulmonary artery and vein possesses pharmacologic and chemical properties identical to those of nitric oxide radical. *Circ. Res.* 61: 866–879, 1987.
255. Ingjer, F. Effects of endurance training on muscle fiber ATP-ase activity, capillary supply and mitochondrial content in man. *J. Physiol. (Lond.)* 294: 419–432, 1979.
256. Ingjer, F. Maximal aerobic power related to the capillary supply of the quadriceps femoris muscle in man. *Acta Physiol. Scand.* 104: 238–240, 1978.
257. Ingjer, F., and P. Brodal. Capillary supply of skeletal muscle fibers in untrained and endurance-trained women. *Eur. J. Appl. Physiol.* 38: 291–299, 1978.
258. Iriuchijima, J., Y. Kawane, and Y. Teranishi. Blood flow distribution in transposition response of the rat. *Jpn. J. Physiol.* 32: 807–816, 1982.
259. Jacobs, T. B., R. O. Bell, and J. D. McClements. Exercise, age and the development of the myocardial vasculature. *Growth* 48: 148–157, 1984.
260. Jacobsson, S., and I. Kjellmer. Flow and protein content of lymph in resting and exercising skeletal muscle. *Acta Physiol. Scand.* 60: 278–285, 1964.
261. Jacobsson, S., and I. Kjellmer. Accumulation of fluid in exercising muscle. *Acta Physiol. Scand.* 60: 286–295, 1964.
262. Jennekens, F. G. I., B. E. Tomlinson, and J. N. Walton. Data on the distribution of fibre type in five human limb muscles. *J. Neurol. Sci.* 14: 245–257, 1971.
263. Johnson, J. M., and L. B. Rowell. Forearm skin and muscle vascular responses to prolonged leg exercise in man. *J. Appl. Physiol.* 39: 920–924, 1975.
264. Johnson, P. C. The myogenic response. In: *Handbook of Physiology, The Cardiovascular System, Vascular Smooth Muscle*, edited by D. F. Bohr, A. P. Somlyo, and H. V. Sparks, Jr. Bethesda, MD: Am. Physiol. Soc., 1980. p. 409–442.

265. Jones, D. P. Intracellular diffusion gradients of oxygen and ATP. *Am. J. Physiol.* 250 (*Cell Physiol.* 19): C663–C675, 1986.
266. Jorgensen, C. R., F. L. Gobel, H. L. Taylor, and Y. Wang. Myocardial blood flow and oxygen consumption during exercise. *Ann. N. Y. Acad. Sci.* 301: 213–223, 1977.
267. Jorgensen, C. R., K. Kitamura, F. L. Gobel, H. L. Taylor, and Y. Wang. Long-term precision of the N2O method for coronary flow during heavy upright exercise. *J. Appl. Physiol.* 30: 338–344, 1971.
268. Jorgensen, C. R., K. Wang, Y. Wang, F. L. Gobel, R. R. Nelson, and H. Taylor. Effect of propranolol on myocardial oxygen consumption and its hemodynamic correlates during upright exercise. *Circulation* 48: 1173–1182, 1973.
269. Joyner, M. J., L. A. Nauss, M. A. Warner, and D. O. Warner. Sympathetic modulation of blood flow and O_2 uptake in rhythmically contracting human forearm muscles. *Am. J. Physiol.* 263 (*Heart Circ. Physiol.* 32): H1078–H1083, 1992.
270. Kaley, G., A. Koller, J. M. Rodenburg, E. J. Messina, and M. S. Wolin. Regulation of arteriolar tone and responses via L-arginine pathway in skeletal muscle. *Am. J. Physiol.* 262 (*Heart Circ. Physiol.* 31): H987–H992, 1992.
271. Kanstrup, I., and B. Ekblom. Blood volume and hemoglobin concentration as determinants of maximal aerobic power. *Med. Sci. Sports. Exerc.* 16: 256–262, 1984.
272. Kaye, M. P., G. G. Brynjolfsson, and W. P. Geis. Chemical epicardiectomy: a method of myocardial denervation. *Cardiologia* 53: 139–149, 1968.
273. Kayer, B., H. Hoppeler, H. Claasen, and P. Cerretelli. Muscle structure and performance capacity of Himalayan Sherpas. *J. Appl. Physiol.* 70: 1938–1942, 1991.
274. Kelley, K. O., and E. O. Feigl. Segmental α-receptor-mediated vasoconstriction in the canine coronary circulation. *Circ. Res.* 43: 908–917, 1978.
275. Khayutin, V. M. Determinants of working hyperaemia in skeletal muscle. In: *Circulation in Skeletal Muscle*. New York: Permagon Press, 1968, p. 145–157.
276. Khouri, E. M., D. E. Gregg, and C. R. Rayford. Effect of exercise on cardiac output, left coronary flow and myocardial metabolism in the unanesthetized dog. *Circ. Res.* 17: 427–437, 1965.
277. Kirkebo, A., and A. Wisnes. Regional tissue fluid pressure in rat calf muscle during sustained contraction or stretch. *Acta Physiol. Scand.* 114: 551–556, 1982.
278. Kitamura, K., C. R. Jorgensen, F. L. Gobel, H. L. Taylor, and Y. Wang. Hemodynamic correlates of myocardial oxygen consumption during upright exercise. *J. Appl. Physiol.* 32: 516, 1972.
279. Kjellmer, I. An indirect method for estimating tissue pressure with special reference to tissue pressure in muscle during exercise. *Acta Physiol. Scand.* 62: 31–40, 1964.
280. Kjellmer, I. On competition between metabolic vasodilation and neurogenic vasoconstriction in skeletal muscle. *Acta Physiol. Scand.* 63: 450–459, 1965.
281. Kjellmer, I. Studies on exercise hyperemia. *Acta Physiol. Scand.* 224: 1–64, 1965.
282. Kjellmer, I. The effect of exercise on the vascular bed of skeletal muscle. *Acta Physiol. Scand.* 62: 18–30, 1964.
283. Klausen, K., L. Andersen, and I. Pelle. Adaptive changes in work capacity, skeletal muscle capillarization and enzyme levels during training and detraining. *Acta Physiol. Scand.* 113: 9–16, 1981.
284. Klausen, K., N. Secher, J. Clausen, O. Hartling, and J. Trap-Jensen. Central and regional circulatory adaptations to one-leg training. *J. Appl. Physiol.* 52: 976–983, 1982.
285. Klabunde, R. E., M. H. Laughlin, and R. B. Armstrong. Systemic adenosine deaminase administration does not reduce active hyperemia in running rats. *J. Appl. Physiol.* 64: 108–114, 1988.
286. Klocke, F. J., R. E. Mates, J. M. Canty, and A. K. Ellis. Coronary pressure-flow relationships: controversial issues and probable implications. *Circ. Res.* 56:310–323, 1985.
287. Knight, D. R., and H. L. Stone. Alteration of ischemic cardiac function in normal heart by daily exercise. *J. Appl. Physiol.* 55: 52–60, 1983.
288. Koch-Weser, J., and J. R. Blinks. Influence of the interval between beats on myocardial contractility. *Pharmacol. Rev.* 15: 610–652, 1963.
289. Koerner, J. E., and R. L. Terjung. Effect of physical training on coronary collateral circulation of the rat. *J. Appl. Physiol.* 52: 376–387, 1982.
290. Koller, A., and G. Kaley. endothelial regulation of wall shear stress and blood flow in skeletal muscle microcirculation. *Am. J. Physiol.* 260 (*Heart Circ. Physiol.* 29): H862–H868, 1991.
291. Koller, A., D. Sun, and G. Kaley. Role of shear stress and endothelial prostaglandins in flow- and viscosity-induced vasodilation of arterioles in vitro. *Circ. Res.* 72: 1276–1284, 1993.
292. Koller, A., M. S. Wolin, E. J. Messina, P. D. Cherry, and G. Kaley. Endothelium-derived vasodilator factors in skeletal muscle microcirculation. In: *Endothelium-Derived Vasoactive Factors*. Basel: Drager Press, 1990, p. 303–314.
293. Komaru, T., K. G. Lamping, C. L. Eastham, and K. C. Dellsperger. Role of ATP-sensitive potassium channels in coronary microvascular auto-regulatory responses. *Circ. Res.* 69: 1146–1151, 1991.
294. Kowalchuk, J. M., C. S. Klein, and R. L. Hughson. The effect of beta-adrenergic blockade on leg blood flow with repeated maximal contractions of the triceps surae muscle group in man. *Eur. J. Appl. Physiol.* 60: 360–364, 1990.
295. Krams, R., P. Sipkema, J. Zegers, and N. Westerhof. Contractility is the main determinant of coronary systolic flow impediment. *Am. J. Physiol.* 257 (*Heart Circ. Physiol.* 26): H1936–H1944, 1989.
296. Kramsch, D. M., A. J. Aspen, B. M. Abramowitz, T. Kreimendahl, and W. B. Hood, Jr. Reduction of coronary atherosclerosis by moderate conditioning exercise in monkeys on an atherogenic diet. *N. Engl. J. Med.* 305: 1483–1489, 1981.
297. Krogh, A. *The Anatomy & Physiology of Capillaries*. New Haven: Yale University Press, 1929, p. 30.
298. Kuo, L., M. J. Davis, and W. M. Chilian. Endothelium-dependent, flow-induced dilation of isolated coronary arterioles. *Am. J. Physiol.* 259 (*Heart Circ. Physiol.* 28): H1063–H1070, 1990.
299. Laine, G. A., E. E. Smith, and H. J. Granger. Transcapillary fluid balance in exercising skeletal muscle (Abstract). *Federation Proc.* 40: 406, 1981.
300. Lamping, K. G., and W. P. Dole. Flow-mediated dilation attenuates constriction of large coronary arteries to serotonin. *Am. J. Physiol.* 255 (*Heart Circ. Physiol.* 24): H1317–H1324, 1988.
301. Landis, E. M. Capillary pressure and permeability. *Physiol. Rev.* 14: 404–481, 1932.
302. Langer, S. Z. Presynaptic receptors and their role in the regulation of transmitter release. *Br. J. Pharmacol.* 60: 481–497, 1977.
303. Lash, J., and H. G. Bohlen. Functional adaptations of rat skeletal muscle arterioles to aerobic exercise training. *J. Appl. Physiol.* 72: 2052–2062, 1992.

304. Lash, J. M., T. Reilly, M. Thomas, and H. G. Bohlen. Adrenergic and pressure-dependent vascular regulation in sedentary and trained rats. *Am. J. Physiol.* 265 (*Heart Circ. Physiol.* 34): H1064–H1073, 1993.
305. Laughlin, M. H. Coronary transport reserve in normal dogs. *J. Appl. Physiol.* 57: 551–561, 1984.
306. Laughlin, M. H. Effects of exercise training on coronary transport capacity. *J. Appl. Physiol.* 58: 468–476, 1985.
307. Laughlin, M. H. Skeletal muscle blood flow capacity: role of muscle pump in exercise hyperemia. *Am. J. Physiol.* 253 (*Heart Circ. Physiol.* 22): H993–H1004, 1987.
308. Laughlin, M. H. Distribution of skeletal muscle blood flow during locomotory exercise. In: *Oxygen Transfer from Atmosphere to Tissues*. New York, Plenum Publishing, 1988, p. 87–102.
309. Laughlin, M. H. Heterogeneity of blood flow in striated muscle. *The Lung: Scientific Foundations*. New York: Raven Press, 1991, p. 1507–1516.
310. Laughlin, M. H., and R. B. Armstrong. Muscle blood flow during locomotory exercise. *Exerc. Sport Sci. Rev.* 13: 95–136, 1985.
311. Laughlin, M. H., and R. B. Armstrong. Muscular blood flow distribution patterns as a function of running speed in rats. *Am. J. Physiol.* 243 (*Heart Circ. Physiol.* 12): H296–H306, 1982.
312. Laughlin, M. H., and R. B. Armstrong. Rat muscle blood flow as a function of time during prolonged slow treadmill exercise. *Am. J. Physiol.* 244 (*Heart Circ. Physiol.* 13): H814–H824, 1983.
313. Laughlin, M. H., and R. B. Armstrong. Adrenoreceptor effects on rat muscle blood flow during treadmill exercise. *J. Appl. Physiol.* 62: 1465–1472, 1987.
314. Laughlin, M. H., J. W. Burns, J. Fanton, J. Ripperger, and D. F. Peterson. Coronary blood flow reserve during $+G_z$ stress and treadmill exercise in miniature swine. *J. Appl. Physiol.* 64: 2589–2596, 1988.
315. Laughlin, M. H., and J. N. Diana. Myocardial transcapillary exchange in the hypertrophied heart of the dog. *Am. J. Physiol.* 229: 838–846, 1975.
316. Laughlin, M. H., J. N. Diana, and C. M. Tipton. Effects of chronic exercise training on coronary reactive hyperemia and coronary blood flow in the dog. *J. Appl. Physiol.* 45: 604–610, 1978.
317. Laughlin, M. H., C. C. Hale, L. Novela, D. Gute, N. Hamilton, and C. D. Ianuzzo. Biochemical characterization of exercise-trained porcine myocardium. *J. Appl. Physiol.* 71: 229–235, 1991.
318. Laughlin, M. H., R. E. Klabunde, M. D. Delp, and R. B. Armstrong. Effects of dipyridamole on muscle blood flow in exercising miniature swine. *Am. J. Physiol.* 257 (*Heart Circ. Physiol.* 26): H1507–H1515, 1989.
319. Laughlin, M. H., and R. J. Korthuis. Control of muscle blood flow during sustained physiological exercise. *Can. J. Sport Sci.* 12: 77S–83S, 1987.
320. Laughlin, M. H., R. J. Korthuis, W. L. Sexton, and R. B. Armstrong. Regional muscle blood flow capacity and exercise hyperemia in high-intensity trained rats. *J. Appl. Physiol.* 64: 2420–2427, 1988.
321. Laughlin, M. H., and R. M. McAllister. Exercise training-induced coronary vascular adaptation. *J. Appl. Physiol.* 73: 2209–2225, 1992.
322. Laughlin, M. H., R. M. McAllister, and M. D. Delp. Physical activity and the microcirculation in cardiac and skeletal muscle. In: *Physical Activity, Fitness, and Health: International Proceedings and Consensus Statement*. Champaign, IL: Human Kinetics Publishes, Inc., 1994, p. 302–319.
323. Laughlin, M. H., S. J. Mohrman, and R. B. Armstrong. Muscular blood flow distribution patterns in the hind limb of swimming rats. *Am. J. Physiol.* 246 (*Heart Circ. Physiol.* 15): H398–H403, 1984.
324. Laughlin, M. H., K. A. Overholser, and M. Bhatte. Exercise training increases coronary transport reserve in miniature swine. *J. Appl. Physiol.* 67: 1140–1149, 1989.
325. Laughlin, M. H., and J. Ripperger. Vascular transport capacity of hind limb muscles of exercise-trained rats. *J. Appl. Physiol.* 62: 438–443, 1987.
326. Laughlin, M. H., W. Sexton, R. J. Korthuis, and R. B. Armstrong. Regional muscle blood flow capacity and exercise hyperemia in high-intensity trained rats. *J. Appl. Physiol.* 64: 2420–2427, 1988.
327. Laughlin, M. H., and R. J. Tomanek. Myocardial capillarity and maximal capillary diffusion capacity in exercise-trained dogs. *J. Appl. Physiol.* 63: 1481–1486, 1987.
328. Laxson, D. D., X.-Z. Dai, D. C. Homans, and R. J. Bache. The role of α1- and α2-adrenergic receptors in mediation of coronary vasoconstriction in hypoperfused ischemic myocardium during exercise. *Circ. Res.* 65: 1688–1697, 1989.
329. Laxson, D. D., X.-Z. Dai, D. C. Homans, and R. J. Bache. Coronary vasodilator reserve in ischemic myocardium of the exercising dog. *Circulation* 85: 313–322, 1992.
330. Laxson, D. D., D. C. Homans, and R. J. Bache. Inhibition of adenosine-mediated coronary vasodilation exacerbates myocardial ischemia during exercise. *Am. J. Physiol.* 265 (*Heart Circ. Physiol.* 34): H1471–H1477, 1993.
331. LeBlanc, J., M. Boulay, S. Dulac, M. Jobin, A. Labrie, and S. Rousseau-Migneron. Metabolic and cardiovascular responses to norepinephrine in trained and nontrained human subjects. *J. Appl. Physiol.* 42: 166–173, 1977.
332. Leon, A. S., and C. M. Bloor. Effects of exercise and its cessation on the heart and its blood supply. *J. Appl. Physiol.* 24: 485–490, 1968.
333. Leon, A. S., and C. M. Bloor. The effect of complete and partial deconditioning on exercise-induced cardiovascular changes in the rat. *Adv. Cardiol.* 18: 81–92, 1976.
334. Liang, I. Y. S., M. Hamara, and H. L. Stone. Maximum coronary blood flow and minimum coronary resistance in exercise trained dogs. *J. Appl. Physiol.* 56: 641–647, 1984.
335. Liang, I. Y. S., and H. L. Stone. Effect of exercise conditioning on coronary resistance. *J. Appl. Physiol.* 53: 631–636, 1982.
336. Liang, I. Y., and H. L. Stone. Changes in diastolic coronary resistance during submaximal exercise in conditioned dogs. *J. Appl. Physiol.* 54: 1057–1062, 1983.
337. Liang, I. Y., H. L. Stone, and P. A. Gwirtz. Effect of beta 1-receptor blockade on coronary resistance in partially trained dogs. *Med. Sci. Sports. Exerc.* 19: 382–388, 1987.
338. Lindbom, L., R. F. Tuma, and K. E. Arfors. Influence of oxygen on perfused capillary density and capillary red cell velocity in rabbit skeletal muscle. *Microvasc. Res.* 19: 197–208, 1980.
339. Ljungquist, A., and G. Unge. Capillary proliferative activity in myocardium and skeletal muscle of exercised rats. *J. Appl. Physiol.* 43: 306–307, 1977.
340. Lombardo, T. A., L. Rose, M. Taeschler, S. Tuluy, and R. J. Bing. The effect of exercise on coronary blood flow, myocardial oxygen consumption and cardiac efficiency in man. *Circulation* 7: 71–78, 1953.

341. Ludbrook, J. *Aspects of Venous Function in the Lower Limbs*. Springfield, IL: Charles C Thomas Publishers, Inc., 1966.
342. Lundvall, J. Tissue hyperosmolarity as a mediator of vasodilation and transcapillary fluid flux in exercising skeletal muscle. *Acta Physiol. Scand.* 379: 1–81, 1972.
343. Lundvall, J., and J. Hillman. Noradrenaline-evoked beta adrenergic dilation of precapillary sphincters in skeletal muscle. *Acta Physiol. Scand.* 102: 126–128, 1978.
344. Lundvall, J., S. Mellander, and H. Sparks. Myogenic response of resistance vessels and precapillary sphincters in skeletal muscle during exercise. *Acta Physiol. Scand.* 70: 257–268, 1967.
345. Lundvall, J., S. Mellander, H. Westling, and T. White. Fluid transfer between blood and tissues during exercise. *Acta Physiol. Scand.* 85: 258–267, 1972.
346. Mackie, B., and R. Terjung. Influence of training on blood flow to different skeletal muscle fiber types. *J. Appl. Physiol.* 55: 1072–1078, 1983.
347. Mai, J., V. R. Edgerton, and R. Barnard. Capillarity of red, white, and intermediate muscle fibers in trained and untrained guinea-pigs. *Experientia* 26: 1222–1223, 1970.
348. Mann, S. J., L. R. Krakoff, K. Felton, and K. Yeager. Cardiovascular responses to infused epinephrine: effect of the state of physical conditioning. *J. Cardiovasc. Pharmacol.* 6: 339–343, 1984.
349. Manohar, M. Vasodilator reserve in respiratory muscles during maximal exertion in ponies. *J. Appl. Physiol.* 60: 1571–1577, 1986.
350. Manohar, M. Transmural coronary vasodilator reserve and flow distribution during maximal exercise in normal and splenectomized ponies. *J. Physiol. (Lond.)* 387: 425–440, 1987.
351. Maron, B. J. Structural features of the athlete heart as defined by echocardiography. *J. Am. Coll. Cardiol.* 7: 190–203, 1986.
352. Marshall, J. M., and H. C. Tandon. Direct observations of muscle arterioles and venules following contraction of skeletal muscle fibers in the rat. *J. Physiol. (Lond.)* 350: 447–459, 1984.
353. Martin, W. H., W. M. Kohrt, M. T. Malley, E. Korte, and S. Stoltz. Exercise training enhances leg vasodilatory capacity of 65-yr-old men and women. *J. Appl. Physiol.* 69: 1804–1809, 1990.
354. Martin. W. H., T. Ogawa, W. M. Kohrt, W. T. Malley, E. Korte, P. S. Kieffer, and K. B. Schechtmann. Effects of aging, gender, and physical training on peripheral vascular function. *Circulation* 84: 654–664, 1991.
355. Martin. W. H., R. J. Spina, E. Korte, and T. Ogawa. Effects of chronic and acute exercise on cardiovascular β-adrenergic responses. *J. Appl. Physiol.* 71: 1523–1528, 1991.
356. Martin, E. G., E. C. Woolley, and M. Miller. Capillary counts in resting and active muscle. *Am. J. Physiol.* 100: 407–416, 1932.
357. Marzilli, M., S. Goldstein, H. N. Sabbah, T. Lee, and P. D. Stein. Modulating effect of regional myocardial performance on local myocardial perfusion in the dog. *Circ. Res.* 45: 634–641, 1979.
358. Maspers, M., U. Ekelund, J. Bjornberg, and S. Mellander. Protective role of sympathetic nerve activity to exercising skeletal muscle in the regulation of capillary pressure and fluid filtration. *Acta Physiol. Scand.* 141: 351–361, 1991.
359. Mass, H., and P. A. Gwirtz. Myocardial flow and function after regional beta-blockade in exercising dogs. *Med. Sci. Sports. Exerc.* 19: 443–450, 1987.
360. Mayrovitz, H. N., M. P. Wiedeman, and A. Noordergraaf. Microvascular hemodynamic variations accompanying microvessel dimensional changes. *Microvasc. Res.* 10: 322–329, 1975.
361. McAllister, R. M., and S. J. K. Lee. The effects of exercise training in patients with coronary artery disease taking beta-blockers. *J. Cardiopulmonary Rehab.* 6: 245–250, 1986.
362. McAllister, R. M., and R. L. Terjung. Training-induced muscle adaptations: increased performance and oxygen consumption. *J. Appl. Physiol.* 70: 1569–1574, 1991.
363. McElroy, C. L., S. A. Gissen, and M. C. Fishbein. Exercised-induced reduction in myocardial infarct size after coronary artery occlusion in the rat. *Circulation* 57: 958–962, 1978.
364. McKenzie, J. E., R. P. Steffen, and F. J. Haddy. Relationships between adenosine and coronary resistance in conscious exercising dogs. *Am. J. Physiol.* 242 (*Heart Circ. Physiol.* 11): H24–H29, 1982.
365. McLeod, A. A., W. E. Kraus, and R. S. Williams. Effects of beta$_1$-selective and nonselective beta-adrenoceptor blockade during exercise conditioning in healthy adults. *Am. J. Physiol.* 253 (*Heart Circ. Physiol.* 22): H1656–H1661, 1987.
366. McSorley, P. D., and P. J. Warren. Effects of propranolol and metoprolol and the peripheral circulation. *BMJ* 2: 1598–1600, 1978.
367. Meininger, G. A., and M. J. Davies. Cellular mechanisms involved in the vascular myogenic response. *Am. J. Physiol.* 263 (*Heart Circ. Physiol.* 32): H647–H659, 1992.
368. Mellander, S. Differentiation of fiber type composition, circulation and metabolism in limb muscles of dog cat and man. In: *Vasodilation*. New York: Raven Press, 1981, p. 243–254.
369. Mellander, S., and J. Bjornberg. Regulation of vascular smooth muscle tone and capillary pressure. *News Physiol. Sci.* 7: 113–119, 1992.
370. Mellander, S., and B. Johansson. Control of resistance, exchange, and capacitance functions in the peripheral circulation. *Pharmacol. Rev.* 20: 117–196, 1968.
371. Messer, J. V., R. J. Wagman, H. J. Levine, W. A. Neill, N. Krasnow, and R. Gorlin. Patterns of human myocardial oxygen extraction during rest and exercise. *J. Clin. Invest.* 41: 725–742, 1962.
372. Metting, P. J., D. L. Weldy, T. F. Ronau, and S. L. Britton. Effect of aminophylline on hind limb blood flow autoregulation during increased metabolism in dogs. *J. Appl. Physiol.* 60: 1857–1864, 1986.
373. Miller, V. M., L. A. Aarhus, and P. M. Vanhoutte. Modulation of endothelium-dependent responses by chronic alterations of blood flow. *Am. J. Physiol.* 251 (*Heart Circ. Physiol.* 20): H520–H527, 1986.
374. Miller, V. M., and P. M. Vanhoutte. Enhanced release of endothelium-derived factors by chronic increases in blood flow. *Am. J. Physiol.* 255 (*Heart Circ. Physiol.* 24): H446–H451, 1988.
375. Mohrman, D. E. Local metabolic influences on resistance vessels. In: *The Resistance Vasculature*. Totowa, NJ: Humana Press, 1991, p. 241–249.
376. Mohrman, D. E., and E. O. Feigl. Competition between sympathetic vasoconstriction and metabolic vasodilation in the canine coronary circulation. *Circ. Res.* 42: 79–86, 1978.
377. Mohrman, D. E., and H. V. Sparks. Myogenic hyperemia following brief tetanus of canine skeletal muscle. *Am. J. Physiol.* 227: 531–535, 1974.

378. Moncada, S., R. M. J. Palmer, and E. A. Higgs. Biosynthesis of nitric oxide from L-arginine. A pathway for the regulation of cell function and communication. *Biochem. Pharmacol.* 38: 1709–1715, 1989.
379. Moreland, R. S. *Regulation of Smooth Muscle Contraction.* New York: Plenum Press, 1991.
380. Morff, R. J., and H. J. Granger. Autoregulation of blood flow within individual arterioles in the rat cremaster muscle. *Circ. Res.* 51: 43–55, 1982.
381. Morrow, N. G., W. E. Kraus, J. W. Moore, R. S. Williams, and J. L. Swain. Increased expression of fibroblast growth factors in a rabbit skeletal muscle model of exercise conditioning. *J. Clin. Invest.* 85: 1816–1820, 1990.
382. Muller, J. M., P. R. Myers, and M. H. Laughlin. Vasodilator responses of coronary resistance arteries of exercise trained pigs. *Circulation* 89: 2308–2314, 1994.
383. Muller, J. M., P. R. Myers, and M. H. Laughlin. Exercise training alters myogenic responses in porcine coronary resistance arteries. *J. Appl. Physiol.* 75: 2677–2682, 1993.
384. Muller, W. Subsarcolemmal mitochondrial and capillarization of soleus muscle fibers in young rats subjected to endurance training. *Cell Tiss. Res.* 174: 367–389, 1976.
385. Mundie, T. G., A. J. Januszkiewicz, and G. R. Ripple. Effects of epinephrine, phenoxybenzamine, and propranolol on maximal exercise in sheep. *Lab. Anim. Sci.* 42: 486, 1992.
386. Murray, P. A., and S. F. Vatner. α-Adrenoceptor attenuation of coronary vascular response to severe exercise in the conscious dog. *Circ. Res.* 45: 654–660, 1979.
387. Musch, T. I., G. C. Haidet, G. A. Ordway, J. C. Longhurst, and J. H. Mitchell. Training effects on regional blood flow response to maximal exercise in fox hounds. *J. Appl. Physiol.* 62: 1724–1732, 1987.
388. Musch, T. I., C. T. Nguyen, H. V. Pham, and R. L. Moore. Training effects on the regional blood flow response to exercise in myocardial infarcted rats. *Am. J. Physiol.* 262 (*Heart Circ. Physiol.* 31): H1846–H1852, 1992.
389. Needleman, P. The synthesis and function of prostaglandins in the heart. *Federation Proc.* 35: 2376–2381, 1976.
390. Neill, W. A., and J. M. Oxendine. Exercise can promote coronary collateral development without improving perfusion of ischemic myocardium. *Circulation* 60: 1513–1519, 1979.
391. Neillsen, H. V. Effect of vein pump activation upon muscle blood flow and venous pressure in the human leg. *Acta Physiol. Scand.* 114: 481–485, 1982.
392. Nelson, R. R., F. L. Gobel, C. R. Jorgensen, K. Wang, Y. Wang, and H. L. Taylor. Hemodynamic predictors of myocardial oxygen consumption during static and dynamic exercise. *Circulation* 50: 1179–1189, 1974.
393. Norton, K. I., M. D. Delp, C. Duan, J. A. Warren, and R. B. Armstrong. Hemodynamic responses during exercise at and above $\dot{V}O_{2max}$ in swine. *J. Appl. Physiol.* 69: 1587–1593, 1990.
394. Nutter, D. O., and E. O. Fuller. The role of isolated cardiac muscle preparations in the study of training effects on the heart. *Med. Sci. Sports. Exerc.* 9: 239–245, 1977.
395. Nygaard, E. Skeletal muscle characteristics in young women. *Acta Physiol. Scand.* 112: 299–304, 1982.
396. Nygaard, E., and E. Neilsen. Skeletal muscle fiber capillarization with extreme endurance training in man. In: *Swimming Medicine IV.* Baltimore, MD: University Park Press, 1978, p. 282–293.
397. Ohyanagi, M., J. E. Faber, and K. Nishigaki. Differential activation of α_1- and α_2-adrenoceptors on microvascular smooth muscle during sympathetic nerve stimulation. *Circ. Res.* 68: 232–244, 1991.
398. Ohyanagi, M., K. Nishigaki, and J. E. Faber. Interaction between microvascular α_1- and α_2-adrenoceptors and endothelium-derived relaxing factor. *Circ. Res.* 71: 188–200, 1992.
399. Olsson, R. A., R. Bunger, and J. A. E. Spaan. Coronary circulation. In: *The Heart and Cardiovascular System.* New York: Raven Press, 1992, p. 1393–1426.
400. Oltman, C. L., J. L. Parker, H. R. Adams, and M. H. Laughlin. Effects of exercise training on vasomotor reactivity of porcine coronary arteries. *Am. J. Physiol.* 263 (*Heart Circ. Physiol.* 32): H372–H382, 1992.
401. Oltman, C. L., J. L. Parker, and M. H. Laughlin. Endothelium-dependent vasodilation of proximal coronary arteries from exercise-trained pigs. *J. Appl. Physiol.* 79: 33–72, 1995.
402. Opie, L. H. *The Heart: Physiology and Metabolism.* New York: Raven Press, 1991, p. 208–246.
403. Owen, T. L., I. C. Ehrhart, W. S. Weidner, J. B. Scott, and F. J. Haddy. Effects of indomethacin on local blood flow regulation in canine heart and kidney. *Proc. Soc. Exp. Biol. Med.* 149: 871–876, 1975.
404. Paaske, W. P. Capillary permeability in skeletal muscle. *Acta Physiol. Scand.* 101: 1–14, 1977.
405. Paaske, W. P., and P. Sejrsen. Transcapillary exchange of 14-C insulin by free diffusion in channels of fused vesicles. *Acta Physiol. Scand.* 100: 437–445, 1977.
406. Pagny, J. Y., F. Peronnet, L. Beliveau, F. Sestier, and R. Nadeau. Systemic and regional blood flows during graded treadmill exercise in dogs. *J. Physiol. (Paris)* 81: 368–373, 1986.
407. Palmer, R. M. J., A. G. Ferrige, and S. Moncada. Nitric oxide release accounts for the biological activity of endothelium-derived relaxing factor. *Nature* 327: 524–526, 1987.
408. Parent, R., R. Pare, and M. Lavallee. Contribution of nitric oxide to dilation of resistance coronary vessels in conscious dogs. *Am. J. Physiol.* 262 (*Heart Circ. Physiol.* 31): H10–H16, 1992.
409. Parizkova, J., M. Wachtlová, and M. Soukupova. The impact of different motor activity on body composition, density of capillaries and fibers in the heart and soleus muscles, and cell's migration in vitro in male rats. *Int. Z. Angew Physiol.* 30: 207–216, 1972.
410. Parks, C. M., and M. Manohar. Transmural coronary vasodilator reserve and flow distribution during severe exercise in ponies. *J. Appl. Physiol.* 54: 1641–1652, 1983.
411. Pelliccia, A., A. Spataro, M. Granata, A. Biffi, G. Caselli, and A. Alabiso. Coronary arteries in physiological hypertrophy: echocardiographic evidence of increased proximal size in elite athletes. *Int. J. Sports. Med.* 11: 120–126, 1990.
412. Penpargkul, S., and J. Scheuer. The effects of physical training upon the mechanical and metabolic performance of the rat heart. *J. Clin. Invest.* 49: 1859–1868, 1970.
413. Peronnêt, F., J. Cléroux, H. Perrault, D. Cousineau, J. De Champlain, and R. Nadeau. Plasma norepinephrine response exercise before and after training in humans. *J. Appl. Physiol.* 51: 812–815, 1981.
414. Persson, M. G., L. E. Gustafsson, N. P. Wiklund, P. Hedquist, and S. Moncada. Endogenous nitric oxide as a modulator of rabbit skeletal muscle microcirculation in vivo. *Br. J. Pharmacol.* 100: 463–466, 1990.
415. Persson, M. G., N. P. Wiklund, and L. E. Gustafsson. Nitric oxide requirement for vasomotor nerve-induced vasodila-

tion and modulation of resting blood flow in muscle microcirculation. *Acta Physiol. Scand.* 141: 49–56, 1991.

416. Peterson, D. F., R. B. Armstrong, and M. H. Laughlin. Sympathetic neural influences on muscle blood flow in rats during submaximal exercise. *J. Appl. Physiol.* 65: 434–440, 1988.
417. Petrén, T., T. Sjöstrand, and B. Sylvén. Der influss des trainings auf die häufigkeit der capillaren in herz- und skeletmuskulatur. *Arbeitsphysiologie* 9: 376–386, 1930.
418. Petrén T., and B. Sylvén. Weitere Untersuchungen uber den Einfluss des Traiings auf die Kapillarisierung der Herzuskulatur. *Morphol. Jahrb.* 80: 439–444, 1937.
419. Petrorfsky, J. S., and D. M. Hendershot. The interrelationship between blood pressure, intramuscular pressure, and isometric endurance in fast and slow twitch skeletal muscle in the cat. *Eur. J. Appl. Physiol.* 53: 106–111, 1984.
420. Piiper, J., and P. Haab. Oxygen supply and uptake in tissue models with unequal distribution of blood flow and shunt. *Respir. Physiol.* 84: 261–271, 1991.
421. Ping, P., and P. C. Johnson. Arteriolar network response to pressure reduction during sympathetic nerve stimulation in cat skeletal muscle. *Am. J. Physiol.* 266 (*Heart Circ. Physiol.* 35): H1251–H1259, 1994.
422. Pohl, U., J. Holtz, R. Busse, and E. Bassenge. Crucial role of endothelium in the vasodilation response to increased flow in vivo. *Hypertension* 8: 37–44, 1986.
423. Poliner, L. R., G. J. Dehmer, S. E. Lewis, R. W. Parkey, C. G. Blomqvist, and J. T. Willerson. Left ventricular performance in normal subjects: a comparison of the responses to exercise in the upright and supine positions. *Circulation* 62: 528–534, 1980.
424. Pollack, A. A., B. E. Taylor, T. T. Myers, and E. H. Wood. The effect of exercise and body position in patients having venous valvular defects. *J. Clin. Invest.* 23: 559–563, 1949.
425. Pollack, A. A., and E. H. Wood. Venous pressure in the saphenous vein at the ankle in man during exercise and changes in posture. *J. Appl. Physiol.* 1: 649–662, 1949.
426. Poole, D. C., O. Mathieu-Costello, and J. B. West. Capillary tortuosity in rat soleus muscle is not affected by endurance training. *Am. J. Physiol.* 256 (*Heart Circ. Physiol.* 25): H1110–H1116, 1989.
427. Popel, A. S. Oxygen diffusive shunts under conditions of heterogenous oxygen delivery. *J. Theor. Biol.* 96: 533–541, 1982.
428. Raff, W. F., F. Kosche, and W. Lochner. Extravascular coronary resistance and its relation to the microcirculation. *Am. J. Cardiol.* 29: 598–603, 1972.
429. Ranvier, L. Note sur les vaisseaux sanguine et la circulation dans muscles rouges. *C. R. Hebd. Seances Mem. Soc. Biol.* 26: 28–31, 1874. Cited in Saltin and Gollnick, 1983.
430. Raven, P. B., D. Rohm-Young, and C. G. Blomqvist. Physical fitness and cardiovascular response to lower body negative pressure. *J. Appl. Physiol.* 56: 138–144, 1984.
431. Reed, R. K. Interstitial fluid volume, colloid osmotic pressure and hydrostatic pressures in rat skeletal muscle. Effect of venous stasis and muscle activity. *Acta Physiol. Scand.* 112: 7–17, 1981.
432. Reed, R. K., S. Johansen, and H. Noddeland. Turnover rate of interstitial albumin in rat skin and skeletal muscle. Effects of limb movements and motor activity. *Acta Physiol. Scand.* 125: 711–718, 1985.
433. Regan, T. J., G. Timmis, M. Gray, K. Binak, and H. K. Hellems. Myocardial oxygen consumption during exercise in fasting and lipemic subjects. *Clin. Invest.* 40: 624–630, 1961.
434. Remensnyder, J. P., J. H. Mitchell, and S. J. Sarnoff. Functional sympatholysis during muscular activity. *Circ. Res.* 11: 370–380, 1962.
435. Renkin, E. M. Transport of potassium-42 from blood to tissue in isolated mammalian skeletal muscle. *Am. J. Physiol.* 197: 1205–1210, 1959.
436. Renkin, E. M. Control of Microcirculation and exchange. *Handbook of Physiology, Cardiovascular System, Microcirculation*, edited by E. M. Renkin and C. C. Michel. Bethesda, MD: Am. Physiol. Soc., 1984, p. 627–687.
437. Renkin, E. M., O. Hudlická, and R. M. Sheehan. Influence of metabolic vasodilation on blood-tissue diffusion in skeletal muscle. *Am. J. Physiol.* 211: 87–98, 1966.
438. Renkin, R. M., and S. Rosell. Effects of different types of vasodilator mechanisms on vascular tonus and on transcapillary exchange of diffusible material in skeletal muscle. *Acta. Physiol. Scand.* 54: 241–251, 1962.
439. Roca, J., A. G. N. Agusti, A. Alonso, D. C. Poole, C. Viegas, J. A. Barbera, R. Rodriguez-Roisin, A. Ferrer, and P. D. Wagner. Effects of training on muscle O_2 transport at $\dot{V}_{o2}$max. *J. Appl. Physiol.* 73: 1067–1076, 1992.
440. Roca, J., M. C. Hogan, D. Story, D. E. Bebout, P. Haab, R. Gonzales, O. Ueno, and P. D. Wagner. Evidence for tissue diffusion limitation of $\dot{V}O_{2max}$ in normal humans. *J. Appl. Physiol.* 67: 291–299, 1989.
441. Rogers, P. J., T. D. Miller, B. A. Bauer, M. M. Brum, A. A. Bove, and P. M. Vanhoutte. Exercise training and responsiveness of isolated coronary arteries. *J. Appl. Physiol.* 71: 2346–2351, 1991.
442. Romanul, F. C. A. Capillary supply and metabolism of muscle fibers. *Arch. Neurol.* 12: 497–509, 1965.
443. Romanul, F. C. A., and M. Pollock. The parallelism of changes in oxidative metabolism and capillary supply of skeletal muscle fibers. In: *Modern Neurology*. Boston, MA: Little, Brown, 1969, p. 204–214.
444. Rose, C. P., C. A. Goresky, P. Belanger, and M. Chen. Effect of vasodilation and flow rate on capillary permeability surface product and interstitial space size in the coronary circulation. *Circ. Res.* 47: 312–328, 1980.
445. Roth, D. M., F. C. White, M. L. Nichols, S. L. Dobbs, J. C. Longhurst, and C. M. Bloor. Effect of long term exercise on regional myocardial function and coronary collateral development after gradual coronary artery occlusion in pigs. *Circulation* 82: 1778–1789, 1990.
446. Rowell, L. B. Human cardiovascular adjustments to exercise and thermal stress. *Physiol. Rev.* 54: 75–159, 1974.
447. Rowell, L. B. Active neurogenic vasodilation in man. *Vasodilation*. New York: Raven Press, 1981, p. 1–17.
448. Rowell, L. B. Cardiovascular adaptations to chronic physical activity and inactivity. *Human Circulation*. New York: Oxford University Press, 1986, p. 257–286.
449. Rowell, L. B. *Human Cardiovascular Control*. New York: Oxford University Press, 1993, p. 1–483.
450. Rowell, L. B., B. Saltin, B. Kiens, and N. J. Christensen. Is peak quadriceps blood flow in humans even higher during exercise with hypoxemia? *Am. J. Physiol.* 251 (*Heart Circ. Physiol.* 20): H1038–H1044, 1986.
451. Rowlands, D. J., and D. E. Donald. Sympathetic vasoconstrictive responses during exercise- or drug-induced vasodilation. *Circ. Res.* 23: 45–60, 1968.
452. Rubanyi, G. M., J. C. Romero, and P. M. Vanhoutte. Flow-induced release of endothelium-derived relaxing factor. *Am. J. Physiol.* 250 (*Heart Circ. Physiol.* 19): H1145–H1149, 1986.
453. Sabel, D. L., H. L. Brammell, M. W. Sheehan, A. S. Nies, J. Gerber, and L. D. Horwitz. Attenuation of exercise con-

ditioning by beta-adrenergic blockade. *Circulation* 65: 679–684, 1982.

454. Saltin, B., and P. D. Gollnick. Skeletal muscle adaptability: significance for metabolism and performance. *Handbook of Physiology, Skeletal Muscle*, edited by L. D. Peachey, R. H. Adrian, and S. R. Geiger. Bethesda, MD: Am. Physiol. Soc., 1983, p. 555–631.
455. Saltin, B., J. Henriksson, E. Nygaard, E. Jansson, and P. Andersen. Fiber types and metabolic potentials of skeletal muscles in sedentary man and endurance runners. *Ann. N. Y. Acad. Sci.* 301: 3–29, 1977.
456. Saltin, B., and L. B. Rowell. Functional adaptations to physical activity and inactivity. *Federation Proc.* 39: 1506–1513, 1980.
457. Saltin, B., and J. Stenberg. Circulatory response to prolonged severe exercise. *J. Appl. Physiol.* 19: 833–838, 1964.
458. Samaha, F. F., F. W. Heineman, C. Ince, J. Fleming, and R. S. Balaban. ATP-sensitive potassium channel is essential to maintain basal coronary vascular tone in vivo. *Am. J. Physiol.* 262 (*Cell Physiol.* 31): C1220–C1227, 1992.
459. Sanders, M., F. White, and C. Bloor. Cardiovascular responses of dogs and pigs exposed to similar physiological stress. *Comp. Biochem. Physiol.* 58: 365–370, 1977.
460. Sanders, M., F. C. White, and C. M. Bloor. Myocardial blood flow distribution in miniature pigs during exercise. *Basic Res. Cardiol.* 72: 326–331, 1977.
461. Sanders, M., F. C. White, T. M. Peterson, and C. M. Bloor. Characteristics of coronary blood flow and transmural distribution in miniature pigs. *Am. J. Physiol.* 235 (*Heart Circ. Physiol.* 4): H601–H609, 1978.
462. Sanders, M., F. C. White, T. M. Peterson, and C. M. Bloor. Effects of endurance exercise on coronary collateral blood flow in miniature swing. *Am. J. Physiol.* 234 (*Heart Circ. Physiol.* 3): H614–H619, 1978.
463. Sarelius, I. H. Cell flow path influences transit time through striated muscle capillaries. *Am. J. Physiol.* 250 (*Heart Circ. Physiol.* 19): H899–H907, 1986.
464. Sarelius, I. H. An analysis of microcirculatory flow heterogeneity using measurements of transit time. *Microvasc. Res.* 40: 88–98, 1990.
465. Sarelius, I. H. Cell and oxygen flow in arterioles controlling capillary perfusion. *Am. J. Physiol.* 265 (*Heart Circ. Physiol.* 34): H1682–H1687, 1993.
466. Schaffartzik, W., E. D. Barton, D. C. Poole, K. Tsukimoto, M. C. Hogan, D. E. Bebout, and P. D. Wagner. Effect of reduced hemoglobin concentration on leg oxygen uptake during maximal exercise in humans. *J. Appl. Physiol.* 75: 419–498, 1993.
467. Schaper, W. Influence of physical exercise on coronary collateral blood flow in chronic experimental two-vessel occlusion. *Circulation* 65: 905–912, 1982.
468. Scheel, K. W., L. A. Ingram, and J. L. Wilson. Effects of exercise on the coronary and collateral vasculature of beagles with and without coronary occlusion. *Circ. Res.* 48: 523–530, 1981.
469. Scheffer, M. G., and P. D. Verdouw. Decreased incidence of ventricular fibrillation after an acute coronary artery ligation in exercised pigs. *Basic Res. Cardiol.* 78: 298–309, 1983.
470. Scheuer, J. Effects of physical training on myocardial vascularity and perfusion. *Circulation* 66: 491–495, 1982.
471. Scheuer, J., and S. W. Stezoski. Effect of physical training on the mechanical and metabolic response of the rat heart to hypoxia. *Circ. Res.* 30: 418–429, 1972.
472. Scheuer, J., and C. M. Tipton. Cardiovascular adaptations to physical training. *Ann. Rev. Physiol.* 39: 221–251, 1977.
473. Schrör, K., S. Moncada, F. B. Ubatuba, and J. R. Vane. Transformation or arachidonic acid and prostaglandin endoperoxides by the guinea pig heart. *Eur. J. Pharmacol.* 47: 103–114, 1978.
474. Schwartz, J. S., K. W. Baran, and R. J. Bache. Effect of stenosis on exercise-induced dilation of large coronary arteries. *Am. Heart J.* 119: 520–524, 1990.
475. Schwartz, L. M., and J. E. McKenzie. Adenosine and active hyperemia in soleus and gracilis muscle of cats. *Am. J. Physiol.* 259 (*Heart Circ. Physiol.* 28): H1295–H1304, 1990.
476. Schwartz, P. J., and H. L. Stone. Effects of unilateral stellectomy upon cardiac performance during exercise in dogs. *Circ. Res.* 44: 637–645, 1979.
477. Seals, D. R. Sympathetic neural adjustments to stress in physically trained and untrained humans. *Hypertension* 17: 36–43, 1991.
478. Seals, D. R., and R. G. Victor. Regulation of muscle sympathetic nerve activity during exercise in humans. *Exerc. Sports Sci. Rev.* 19: 313–349, 1991.
479. Segal, S. S. Microvascular recruitment in hamster striated muscle: role for conducted vasodilation. *Am. J. Physiol.* 261 (*Heart Circ. Physiol.* 30): H181–H189, 1991.
480. Segal, S. S. Communication among endothelial and smooth muscle cells coordinates blood flow control during exercise. *News Physiol. Sci.* 7: 152–156, 1992.
481. Segal, S. S., and J. L. Beny. Intracellular recording and dye transfer in arterioles during blood flow control. *Am. J. Physiol.* 263 (*Heart Circ. Physiol.* 32): H1–H7, 1992.
482. Segal, S. S., D. N. Damon, and B. R. Duling. Propagation of vasomotor responses coordinates arteriolar resistances. *Am. J. Physiol.* 256 (*Heart Circ. Physiol.* 25): H832–H837, 1989.
483. Segal, S. S., and B. R. Duling. Conduction of vasomotor responses in arterioles: a role for cell-to-cell coupling? *Am. J. Physiol.* 256 (*Heart Circ. Physiol.* 25): H838–H845, 1989.
484. Segal, S. S., D. T. Kurjiaka, and A. L. Caston. Endurance training increases arterial wall thickness in rats. *J. Appl. Physiol.* 74: 722–726, 1993.
485. Seitelberger, R., B. D. Guth, G. Heusch, J.-D. Lee, K. Katayama, and J. Ross, Jr. Intracoronary α_2-adrenergic receptor blockade attenuates ischemia in conscious dogs during exercise. *Circ. Res.* 62: 436–442, 1988.
486. Sejersted, O. M., A. R. Hargens, K. R. Kardel, P. Blom, O. Jensen, and L. Hermansen. Intramuscular fluid pressure during isometric contraction of human skeletal muscle. *J. Appl. Physiol.* 56: 287–295, 1984.
487. Sejrsen, P., and K. H. Tønnesen. Shunting by diffusion of inert gas in skeletal muscle. *Acta. Physiol. Scand.* 86: 82–91, 1972.
488. Sessa, W. C., K. Pritchard, N. Seyedi, J. Wang, and T. H. Hintze. Chronic exercise in dogs increases coronary vascular nitric oxide production and endothelial cell nitric oxide synthase gene expression. *Circ. Res.* 74: 349–353, 1994.
489. Sexton, W. L., R. J. Korthuis, and M. H. Laughlin. High-intensity exercise training increases vascular transport capacity of rat hindquarters. *Am. J. Physiol.* 254 (*Heart Circ. Physiol.* 23): H274–H278, 1988.
490. Sexton, W. L., and M. H. Laughlin. Influence of exercise intensity on distribution of vascular adaptations in skeletal muscle. *Am. J. Physiol.* 266 (*Heart Circ. Physiol.* 35): H483–H490, 1994.

491. Shepherd, J. T. Circulation to skeletal muscle. In: *Handbook of Physiology, The Cardiovascular System, Peripheral Circulation and Organ Blood Flow*, edited by J. T. Shepherd and F. M. Abboud. Bethesda, MD: Am. Physiol. Soc., 1983, p. 319–370.
492. Shepherd, J. T. Behavior of resistance and capacity vessels in human limbs during exercise. *Circ. Res.* 20(Suppl. 1): I70–I82, 1967.
493. Shepherd, R., and P. Gollnick. Oxygen uptake of rats at different work intensities. *Pflugers Arch.* 362: 219–222, 1976.
494. Shepherd, J. T., and P. M. Vanhoutte. Skeletal-muscle blood flow:neurogenic determinants. In: *The Peripheral Circulation*. New York: Grune & Stratten, 1975, p. 3–55.
495. Sheriff, D. D., L. B. Rowell, and A. M. Scher. Is rapid rise in vascular conductance at onset of dynamic exercise due to muscle pump? *Am. J. Physiol.* 265 (*Heart Circ. Physiol.* 34): H1227–H1234, 1993.
496. Silber, D., D. McLaughlin, and L. Sinoway. Leg exercise conditioning increases peak forearm blood flow. *J. Appl. Physiol.* 71: 1568–1573, 1991.
497. Sinoway, L. I., T. I. Musch, J. R. Minotti, and R. Zelis. Enhanced maximal metabolic vasodilation in the dominant forearms of tennis players. *J. Appl. Physiol.* 61: 673–678, 1986.
498. Sinoway, L., R. Rea, M. Smith, and A. Mark. Physical training induces desensitization of the muscle metaboreflex (Abstract). *Circulation* 80: II-290, 1989.
499. Sinoway, L. I., J. Shenberger, J. Wilson, D. McLaughlin, T. Musch, and R. Zelis. A 30 day forearm work protocol increases maximal forearm blood flow. *J. Appl. Physiol.* 62: 1063–1067, 1987.
500. Skalak, T. C., G. W. Schmid-Schonbein, and B. W. Zweifach. New morphological evidence for a mechanism of lymph formation in skeletal muscle. *Microvasc. Res.* 28: 9–112, 1984.
501. Skinner, N. S. Skeletal muscle blood flow: Metabolic determinants. In: *The Peripheral Circulations*. New York: Grune & Stratton, 1975, p. 57–79.
502. Smith, M. L., and P. B. Raven. Cardiovascular responses to lower body negative pressure in endurance and static exercise-trained men. *Med. Sci. Sports. Exerc.* 18: 545–550, 1986.
503. Snell, P. G., W. H. Martin, J. C. Buckey, and C. G. Blomqvist. Maximal vascular leg conductance in trained and untrained men. *J. Appl. Physiol.* 62: 606–610, 1987.
504. Somers, V. K., K. C. Leo, M. P. Green, and A. L. Mark. Forearm training attenuates the sympathetic nerve response to isometric handgrip (Abstract). *Circulation* 78: II-177, 1988.
505. Somlyo, A. Modulation of the Ca^{2+} switch: by G proteins, kinase and phosphatase. *News Physiol. Sci.* 8: 2, 1993.
506. Somlyo, A., and A. Somlyo. Vascular smooth muscle. *Pharmacol. Rev.* 20: 197–272, 1968.
507. Spaan, J. A. E. Coronary diastolic pressure-flow relations and zero flow pressure explained on the basis of intramyocardial compliance. *Circ. Res.* 56: 293–309, 1985.
508. Sparks, H. V. Skin and muscle. In: *Peripheral Circulation*. New York: John Wiley & Sons, 1978, p. 193–230.
509. Sparks, H. V. Effect of local metabolic factors on vascular smooth muscle. In: *Handbook of Physiology, The Cardiovascular System, Vascular Smooth Muscle*, edited by D. F. Bohr, A. P. Somlyo, and H. V. Sparks, Jr. Bethesda, MD: Am. Physiol. Soc., 1980.
510. Sparks, H. V., Jr., and H. Bardenheuer. Regulation of adenosine formation by the heart. *Circ. Res.* 58: 193–201, 1986.
511. Sparks, H. V., R. J. Korthuis, and J. B. Scott. *Pharmacology of Hemodynamic Factors in Fluid Balance*. Edema, NY: Raven Press, 1984, p. 425–439.
512. Sparks, H. V., and D. E. Mohrman. Heterogeneity of flow as an explanation of the multiexponential washout of inert gas from skeletal muscle. *Microvasc. Res.* 13: 181–184, 1977.
513. Spear, K. L., J. E. Koerner, and R. L. Terjung. Coronary blood flow in physically trained rats. *Cardiovasc. Res.* 12: 135–143, 1978.
514. Stainsby, W. N. Local control of regional blood flow. *Ann Rev. Physiol.* 35: 151–168, 1973.
515. Stainsby, W. N., W. F. Brechue, D. M. O'Drobinak, and J. K. Barclay. Oxidation reduction state of cytochrome oxidase during repetitive contractions. *J. Appl. Physiol.* 67: 2158–2162, 1989.
516. Standen, N. B., J. M. Quayle, N. W. Davies, J. E. Brayden, Y. Huang, and M. T. Nelson. Hyperpolarizing vasodilators activate ATP-sensitive K^+ channels in arterial smooth muscle. *Science* 245: 177–180, 1989.
517. Stegall, H. F. Muscle pumping in the dependent leg. *Circ. Res.* 19: 180–190, 1966.
518. Stehno-Bittel, L., M. H. Laughlin, and M. Sturek. Exercise training alters Ca release from coronary smooth muscle sarcoplasmic reticulum. *Am. J. Physiol.* 259 (*Heart Circ. Physiol.* 28): H643–H647, 1990.
519. Stehno-Bittel, L., M. H. Laughlin, and M. Sturek. Exercise training depletes sarcoplasmic reticulum calcium in coronary smooth muscle. *J. Appl. Physiol.* 71: 1764–1773, 1991.
520. Stevenson, J. A., V. Feleki, and P. Rechnitzer. Effect of exercise on coronary tree size in the rat. *Circ. Res.* 15: 265–269, 1964.
521. Stick, C., H. Jaeger, and E. Witzleb. Measurements of volume changes and venous pressure in the human lower leg during walking and running. *J. Appl. Physiol.* 72: 2063–2068, 1992.
522. Stone, H. L. Coronary flow, myocardial oxygen consumption and exercise training in dogs. *J. Appl. Physiol.* 49: 759–768, 1980.
523. Stowe, D. F., T. L. Owen, D. K. Anderson, and J. B. Scott. Interaction of O_2 and CO_2 in sustained exercise hyperemia of canine skeletal muscle. *Am. J. Physiol.* 229: 28–33, 1975.
524. Strader, J. R., P. A. Gwirtz, and C. E. Jones. Comparative effects of alpha-1 and alpha-2 adrenoceptors in modulation of coronary flow during exercise. *J. Pharm. Exp. Ther.* 246: 772–778, 1988.
525. Strandell, T., and J. T. Shepherd. The effect in humans of increased sympathetic activity on the blood flow to active muscles. *Acta Med. Scand.* 472: 146–167, 1967.
526. Sullivan, T. E. and R. B. Armstrong. Rat locomotory muscle fiber activity during trotting and galloping, *J. Appl. Physiol.* 44: 358–363, 1978.
527. Sun, D., A. Huang, A. Koller, and G. Kaley. Short-term daily exercise enhances endothelial nitric oxide synthesis in skeletal muscle arterioles of rats. *J. Appl. Physiol.* 76: 2241–2247, 1994.
528. Sun, D., G. Kaley, and A. Koller. Role of endothelium in function of isolated arterioles of rat mesentery and gracilis muscle. *Endothelium* 1: 115–122, 1993.

529. Svendenhag, J. The sympatho-adrenal system in physical conditioning. *Acta Physiol. Scand. Suppl.* 543: 1–73, 1985.
530. Svedenhag, J., A. Martinsson, B. Ekblom, and P. Hjemdahl. Altered cardiovascular responsiveness to adrenoceptor agonists in endurance-trained men. *J. Appl. Physiol.* 70: 531–538, 1991.
531. Svedenhag, J., B. G. Wallin, G. Sundlöf, and J. Henriksson. Skeletal muscle sympathetic activity at rest in trained and untrained subjects. *Acta Physiol. Scand.* 120: 499–504, 1984.
532. Sweeney, T. E., and I. H. Sarelius. Arteriolar control of capillary cell flow in striated muscle. *Circ. Res.* 64: 112–120, 1989.
533. Symons, J. D., K. F. Pitsillides, and J. C. Longhurst. Chronic reduction of myocardial ischemia does not attenuate coronary collateral development in miniswine. *Circulation* 86: 660–671, 1992.
534. Taylor, A. E., and D. N. Granger. Exchange of macromolecules across the microcirculation. *Handbook of Physiology, The Cardiovascular System, Microcirculation*, edited by E. M. Renkin and C. C. Michel. Bethesda, MD: Am. Physiol. Soc., 1984, p. 467–520.
535. Tepperman, J., and D. Pearlman. Effects of exercise and anemia on coronary arteries in small animals as revealed by the corrosion-cast technique. *Circ. Res.* 9: 576–584, 1961.
536. Terrados, N., M. Mizuno, and H. Andersen. Reduction in maximal oxygen uptake at low altitudes: role of training status and lung function. *Clin. Physiol.* 5: 75–79, 1985.
537. Tharp, G. D., and C. T. Wagner. Chronic exercise and cardiac vascularization. *Eur. J. Appl. Physiol.* 48: 97–104, 1982.
538. Thomas, D. P. Effects of acute and chronic exercise on myocardial ultrastructure. *Med. Sci. Sports. Exerc.* 17: 546–553, 1985.
539. Thomas, G. D., J. Hansen, and R. G. Victor. Inhibition of α_2-adrenergic vasoconstriction during contraction of glycolytic, not oxidative, rat hindlimb muscle. *Am. J. Physiol.* 266 (*Heart Circ. Physiol.* 35): H920–H929, 1994.
540. Thompson, L. P., and D. E. Mohrman. Blood flow and oxygen consumption in skeletal muscle during sympathetic stimulation. *Am. J. Physiol.* 245 (*Heart Circ. Physiol.* 14): H66–H71, 1983.
541. Thörner, W. Trainingsversuche an Hunden. III. Histologische Beobachtungen und Herz- und Skeletmuskeln. *Arbeitphysiologie* 8: 359–370, 1935.
542. Tomanek, R. J. Effects of age and exercise on the extent of the myocardial capillary bed. *Anat. Rec.* 167: 55–62, 1970.
543. Trimble, J., and J. Downey. Contribution of myocardial contractility to myocardial perfusion. *Am. J. Physiol.* 236 (*Heart Circ. Physiol.* 5): H121–H126, 1979.
544. Unge, G., S. Carlsson, A. Ljungqvist, G. Tornling, and J. Adolfsson. The proliferative activity of myocardial capillary wall cells in variously aged swimming-exercised rats. *Acta Pathol. Microbiol. Scand.* 87: 15–17, 1979.
545. Utley, J., E. L. Carlson, J. I. E. Hofman, H. H. Martinez, and G. D. Buckberg. Total and regional myocardial blood flow measurements with 25μ, 15μ, 9μ and filtered 1-10 μm diameter microspheres and antipyrine in dogs and sheep. *Circ. Res.* 34: 391–405, 1974.
546. Van Leeuwen, B. E., G. J. Barendsen, J. Lubbers, and L. De Pater. Calf blood flow and posture: Doppler ultrasound measurements during and after exercise. *J. Appl. Physiol.* 72: 1675–1680, 1992.
547. Van Citters, R. B., and D. L. Franklin. Cardiovascular performance of Alaska sled dogs during exercise. *Circ. Res.* 24: 33–42, 1969.
548. Vanhoutte, P. M., T. J. Verbeuren, and R. C. Webb. Local modulation of adrenergic neuroeffector interaction in the blood vessel wall. *Physiol. Rev.* 61: 151–247, 1981.
549. Vatner, S. F., D. Franklin, C. B. Higgins, T. Patrick, and E. Braunwald. Left ventricular response to severe exertion in untethered dogs. *J. Clin. Invest.* 51: 3052–3060, 1972.
550. Vatner, S. F., D. Franklin, R. C. Van Citters, and E. Braunwald. Effects of carotid sinus nerve stimulation on blood flow distribution in conscious dogs at rest and during exercise. *Circ. Res.* 27: 495–503, 1970.
551. Vatner, S. R., C. B. Higgins, D. Franklin, and E. Braunwald. Role of tachycardia in mediating the coronary hemodynamic response to severe exercise. *J. Appl. Physiol.* 32: 380–385, 1972.
552. Vatner, S. F., C. B. Higgins, R. W. Millard, and D. Franklin. Role of the spleen in the peripheral vascular response to severe exercise in untethered dogs. *Cardiovasc. Res.* 8: 276–282, 1974.
553. Vatner, S. F., C. B. Higgins, S. White, T. Patrick, and D. Franklin. The peripheral vascular response to severe exercise in untethered dogs before and after complete heart block. *J. Clin. Invest.* 50: 1950–1960, 1971.
554. Vatner, S. F., and M. S. Pagani. Cardiovascular adjustments to exercise: hemodynamics and mechanisms. *Prog. Cardiovasc. Dis.* 19: 91–108, 1976.
555. Vatner, S. F., M. Pagani, and W. T. Manders, and A. D. Pasipoularides. Alpha adrenergic vasoconstriction and nitroglycerin vasodilation of large coronary arteries in the conscious dog. *J. Clin. Invest.* 65: 5–14, 1980.
556. von Restorff, W., B. Hofling, J. Holtz, and E. Bassenge. Effect of increased blood fluidity through hemodilution on coronary circulation at rest and during exercise in dogs. *Pflügers Arch.* 357: 15–24, 1975.
557. von Restorff, W., J. Holtz, and E. Bassenge. Exercise induced augmentation of myocardial oxygen extraction in spite of normal coronary dilatory capacity in dogs. *Pflügers Arch.* 372: 181–185, 1977.
558. Wachtlová, M., K. Rakusan, and O. Poupa. The coronary terminal vascular bed in the heart of the hare and the rabbit. *Physiol. Biochem.* 14: 328–331, 1965.
559. Wachtlová, M., K. Rakusan, Z. Roth, and O. Poupa. The terminal vascular bed of the myocardium in the wild rat (*Rattus norvegicus*) and the laboratory rat (*Rattus norvegicus lab*). *Physiol. Bohemoslov.* 16: 548–554, 1967.
560. Wagner, P. D. An integrated view of the determinants of maximum oxygen uptake. *Adv. Exp. Med. Biol.* 227: 245–256, 1988.
561. Wagner, P. D. Central and peripheral aspects of oxygen transport and adaptations with exercise. *Sports Med.* 11: 133–142, 1991.
562. Walloe, L., and J. Wesche. Time course and magnitude of blood flow changes in the human quadriceps muscles during and following rhythmic exercise. *J. Physiol. (Lond.)* 405: 257–273, 1988.
563. Walmsley, B., J. A. Hodgson, and R. E. Burke. Forces produced by medial gastrocnemius and soleus muscles during locomotion in freely moving cats. *J. Neurophysiol.* 41: 1103–1216, 1978.
564. Wang, J., M. S. Wolin, and T. H. Hintze. Chronic exercise enhances endothelium-mediated dilation of epicardial coronary artery in conscious dogs. *Circ. Res.* 73: 829–838, 1993.

565. Watkinson, W. P., D. H. Foley, R. Rubio, and R. M. Berne. Myocardial adenosine formation with increased cardiac performance in the dog. *Am. J. Physiol.* 236 (*Heart Circ. Physiol.* 5): H13–H21, 1979.
566. Weiss, H. R. Regional oxygen consumption and supply in the dog heart; effect of atrial pacing. *Am. J. Physiol.* 236 (*Heart Circ. Physiol.* 5): H231–H237, 1979.
567. White, F. C., M. D. McKirnan, E. A. Breisch, B. D. Guth, Y. Liu, and C. M. Bloor. Adaptation of the left ventricle to exercise-induced hypertrophy. *J. Appl. Physiol.* 62: 1097–1110, 1987.
568. White, F. C., M. Sanders, and C. M. Bloor. Coronary reserve at maximal heart rate in the exercising swine. *Cardiac. Rehab.* 1: 31–39, 1981.
569. Wiegman, D. L., P. D. Harris, I. G. Joshua, and F. N. Miller. Decreased vascular sensitivity to norepinephrine following exercise training. *J. Appl. Physiol.* 51: 282–287, 1981.
570. Williams, R. S. Role of receptor mechanisms in the adaptive response to habitual exercise. *Am. J. Cardiol.* 55: 68D–73D, 1985.
571. Wilson, J. R., and S. Kapoor. Contribution of endothelium-derived relaxing factor to exercise-induced vasodilation in humans. *J. Appl. Physiol.* 75: 2740–2744, 1993.
572. Winder, W. W., J. M. Hagberg, R. C. Hickson, A. A. Ehsani, and J. A. McLane. Time course of sympathoadrenal adaptation to endurance exercise training in man. *J. Appl. Physiol.* 45: 370–374, 1978.
573. Winder, W. W., R. C. Hickson, J. M. Hagberg, A. A. Ehsani, and J. A. McLane. Training-induced changes in hormonal and metabolic responses to submaximal exercise. *J. Appl. Physiol.* 46: 766–771, 1979.
574. Wolfel, E. E., W. R. Hiatt, H. L. Brammell, V. H. Travis, and L. D. Horwitz. Plasma catecholamine responses to exercise after training with beta-adrenergic blockade. *J. Appl. Physiol.* 68: 586–593, 1990.
575. Wolfson S., and R. Gorlin. Cardiovascular pharmacology of propranolol in man. *Circulation* 40: 501–511, 1969.
576. Wyatt, H. L., and J. H. Mitchell. Influences of physical training on the heart of dogs. *Circ. Res.* 35: 883, 1974.
577. Wyatt, H. L., and J. Mitchell. Influences of physical conditioning and deconditioning on coronary vasculature of dogs. *J. Appl. Physiol.* 45: 619–625, 1978.
578. Yamabe, H., K. Okumura, H. Ishizaka, T. Tsuchiya, and H. Yasue. Role of endothelium-derived nitric oxide in myocardial reactive hyperaemia. *Am. J. Physiol.* 263 (*Heart Circ. Physiol.* 32): H8–H14, 1992.
579. Yasuda, Y., and M. Miyamura. Cross transfer effects of muscular training on blood flow in the ipsilateral and contralateral forearms. *Eur. J. Appl. Physiol.* 51: 321–329, 1983.
580. Yipintsoi, T., J. Rosenkrantz, M. A. Codini, and J. Scheuer. Myocardial blood flow responses to acute hypoxia and volume loading in physically trained rats. *Cardiovasc. Res.* 14: 50–57, 1980.
581. Zhang, J., G. Path, D. C. Homans, V. Chepuri, H. Merkle, K. Hendrich, M. M. Meyn, R. J. Bache, K. Ugurbil, and A. H. L. From. Bioenergetic and functional consequences of dobutamine infusion in tachycardic, blood flow limited myocardium. *Circulation* 86(Suppl. I): I-338, 1992.

17. Integration of cardiovascular control systems in dynamic exercise

LORING B. ROWELL | Departments of Physiology and Biophysics and of Medicine (Cardiology), University of Washington School of Medicine, Seattle, Washington

DONAL S. O'LEARY | Department of Physiology, Wayne State University School of Medicine, Detroit, Michigan

DEAN L. KELLOGG, JR. | Departments of Physiology and of Medicine, University of Texas Health Science Center at San Antonio, San Antonio, Texas

CHAPTER CONTENTS

I. INTRINSIC PROPERTIES OF THE CARDIOVASCULAR SYSTEM: HOW THEY PERMIT THE RISE IN CARDIAC OUTPUT

THE AIM OF THIS CHAPTER IS TO INTEGRATE the basic mechanisms of cardiovascular control into a coherent scheme of overall control during dynamic exercise. Some intrinsic properties of the heart and blood vessels that maintain or raise ventricular end-diastolic volume (EDV) and permit the rise in cardiac output provide the foundation for Part I of this chapter.

Paradoxically, cardiac output is a determinant of EDV because of the positive effect of increased blood flow on peripheral vascular volume—coupled with the negative effect of increased vascular volume on EDV; conversely, EDV is a determinant of stroke volume (SV) and cardiac output. A central theme of this chapter is that the heart cannot by itself increase its outflow without adjustments in the peripheral circulation that translocate blood from the vasculature back to the heart. Two adjustments in the peripheral circulation are crucial to the ability to raise EDV and cardiac output. The first is mechanical and depends both on the effectiveness of muscle pumps in displacing peripheral vascular volume back to the heart and also on the force these pumps impart to venous return. The second adjustment requires that the sympathetic nervous system control the distribution of cardiac output between compliant and noncompliant vascular beds. Without a balance between mechanical and neural effects on blood flow and blood volume distribution, neither adequate cardiac output nor mean systemic arterial pressure (SAP) can be maintained during dynamic exercise.

Part I provides the background required in Part II, which deals with those reflexes that initiate the neural control of the heart and vasculature. The questions to be answered in Part 2 are: What is sensed and what is regulated, how, and how well?

THE HEART

Intrinsic Properties of the Heart

Overall Cardiac Performance. When heart rate (HR) reaches 195 bpm in humans during severe exercise, ventricular diastolic filling time is only 0.12 s compared to 0.55 s at rest (HR = 70 bpm). Nevertheless, adjustments in cardiac performance normally keep SV constant up to maximal HR and cardiac output (8, 118, 238, 273, 364). The factors that determine ventricular SV (in addition to heart size) are ventricular preload or ventricular afterload, and the inotropic state of the myocardium.

Myocardial Contractile Force

In young adults. The strength or vigor of cardiac contraction can be altered by factors that are independent of myocardial fiber length (length–tension relationship) or the ventricular afterload (force–velocity relationship). The intrinsic myocardial contractile or inotropic state is increased during dynamic exercise by shortening the interval between beats, by increased circulating epinephrine, and by increased norepinephrine (NE) release from cardiac sympathetic nerves. All of these factors act ultimately by affecting the availability of Ca^{2+} to the myocardial cell by increasing Ca^{2+} influx across the sarcolemma (see Chapter 15). This effect on the heart is revealed by the more complete emptying of the left ventricle and the greater fraction of blood ejected.

Radionuclide angiographic measurements of technetium-labeled red blood cells have permitted the evaluation of ventricular performance in measures of EDV, end-systolic volume, and ejection fraction of the left ventricle in response to exercise. With these techniques, the measurement of ejection fraction is the least subject to errors in measuring absolute ventricular volumes caused by influences of background, tissue attenuation, and movement by exercise (98, 118). Errors in absolute volume measurements are approximately 25% for normal EDV and 50% for normal end-systolic volume. Ejection fraction, which is ~65% at rest, is commonly measured within approximately 5%–10%. Ejection fraction can reach or exceed 85% during severe upright exercise (29, 32, 118, 238, 249).

Ejection fractions do not always reach the high values described above. For example, Higgenbotham et al. (118) found averages rising from 59% to only 76% during severe exercise in a heterogeneous subject population that ranged in age between 20 and 50 years. Data were averaged from all 24 men irrespective of age or exercise capacity. Flamm et al. (79) also observed somewhat lower values. Surprisingly, their radionuclide angiographic measurements of ejection fraction and EDV showed little increase with rising exercise intensity despite marked increases in thoracic, cardiac, and lung volumes.

Changes with aging. The effects of advanced age on cardiovascular function have been reviewed by Lakatta (172) and Folkow and Svanborg (82). Lakatta's group utilized radionuclide imaging to uncover an age-related increase in EDV during exercise [note that in contrast to investigations using direct Fick or dye-dilution techniques, maximal SV and cardiac output were highest in the oldest people (65–80 years) (255) rather than lowest (126, 305)]. A point to recognize is that when cardiac output is measured by conventional direct Fick or indicator dye dilution techniques, SV is calculated by dividing cardiac output by HR so that the error in measuring cardiac output is *divided by* HR. Conversely, when cardiac output is determined from radioangiographically measured SV, SV is multiplied by HR. This means that errors in SV determination are *multiplied by* HR when cardiac output is derived in this manner, so the error is much greater. Such technical differences may account for the controversy discussed later concerning how aging affects cardiac function in exercise (9, 172).

Despite the rise in EDV with advancing age, left ventricular end-systolic volume decreased less with exercise than it did in younger people (see 94). Thus ejection fraction was lower in older than in younger people during heavy exercise. In one study (94), the lower ejection fraction was not attributed to greater left ventricular afterload because SAP was not higher in the elderly subjects. Usually, however, the end-systolic afterload tends to be greater in older people. In addition, at a given HR the diastolic period is slightly reduced and systolic time is increased with age (82).

In aging animals, human and nonhuman, β-adrenoceptor–mediated cardiac responses to catecholamines are attenuated (56, 82). β-Adrenoceptor binding affinity on human white blood cells declines with increasing age (82, 94), suggesting that a generalized decrease in β-adrenergic modulation of cardiac function accompanies aging. Gerstenblith et al. (94) suggested that hemodynamic responses of older people resemble those of younger subjects who have received β-adrenoceptor blockade.

In general, radionuclide angiographic measurements of ventricular volumes indicate that approximately two-thirds of the increase in SV from seated upright rest to peak upright exercise is achieved by increased EDV; increased ejection fraction accounts for the remaining one-third (see 238). Ejection fraction appears to decline after midlife (172).

Stroke Volume: Importance of Frank-Starling Mechanism. In addition to the inotropic state of the myocardium, the mechanical interaction between right and left ventricles, the volume of blood available to them to provide filling pressure (preload), and the pressure against which the heart must pump blood (afterload) all determine left ventricular SV. These determinants of cardiac performance are in turn determined by the effectiveness of the regulation of resistance and capacitance elements of the peripheral vascular system.

Historically, controversy once centered on the relative importance of the Frank-Starling or length–tension relationship vs. the inotropic state of the myocardium as primary determinants of SV during exercise. Proponents of the primacy of the Frank-Starling mechanism pointed to the marked rise in SV accompanied by increased ventricular filling pressure and EDV at the onset of upright exercise in humans. In upright posture, central venous pressure (CVP) or ventricular filling pressure, EDV, and SV are reduced by gravitational shifts of blood volume into dependent regions. As soon as muscle contraction begins, EDV and SV are restored by muscle pumping (see below). Of course, if one compared SV in exercising humans with SV measured during supine rest when it would be close to maximal, a far less convincing argument could be ventured for the importance of length–tension effects (see 238). Or if one compared the relevant variables during normal standing rest vs. exercise in the quadruped (e.g., a dog), which has much of its total blood volume at or above heart level, again one might argue for the primacy of inotropic effects in maintaining SV. Indeed, the observations of Rushmer and co-workers (281) suggested reductions in EDV with exercise in dogs. These observations supported their view that "Starling's law of the heart is applicable to exposed or isolated hearts but not to the intact hearts of animals and man." The question therefore became: Can the heart by itself provide the cardiac output required for exercise by simply increasing the rate and force of contraction? Guyton et al. (103) concluded it could not and stated:

> The normal [i.e., at rest] circulatory system operates near this limit [i.e., collapse of central veins owing to increased cardiac output] so that an increase in efficacy of the heart as a pump cannot by itself increase the cardiac output more than a few percent, unless some simultaneous effect takes place in the peripheral circulatory system at the same time to translocate blood from the peripheral vessels to the heart."

The importance of this concept is repeatedly reinforced in Chapter 15 and in this chapter.

The potential importance of the Frank-Starling mechanism is most dramatically demonstrated in the denervated heart. The classic experiments of Donald and Shepherd (60) showed that after cardiac denervation the rise in cardiac output with mild to moderately heavy exercise in dogs was achieved mainly by increased SV with relatively small increments in HR. That is, the responses of HR and SV were the reverse of their normal patterns. Similar results have been obtained from humans with surgical atrioventricular (A-V) block and chronically implanted ventricular pacemakers that permit ventricular rate to be held constant during rest and exercise (268). Therefore, a normal rise in cardiac output can be achieved, within limits, entirely by increased SV paralleled by rising EDV and pulmonary wedge pressure (reflecting left atrial filling pressure). In addition to the length-tension effects on SV, end-systolic volume fell markedly at peak levels of exercise and ejection fraction approached 90%. In these patients, and in the experiments of Donald and Shepherd (60), the surgery required that the pericardium be cut so that the marked increases in SV were permitted by release of pericardial constraints (see below) on ventricular expansion.

Ventricular Filling Pressure (Preload). Ventricular filling pressure in humans, in contrast to quadrupeds, varies markedly owing to gravitational shifts in blood volume with changing posture (cf. 123, 268). Conversely, filling pressures in the dog rise markedly with increasing work intensity (314, 316). Note also that dogs, unlike humans, have a strong Bainbridge reflex so that cardiac output can increase not only through length-tension effects on SV but also by a direct effect of atrial expansion on HR [approximately 5–8 bpm per mm Hg increase in right atrial pressure (245)]. The Bainbridge reflex acts as a partial self-correction for increased filling pressure inasmuch as increased cardiac output, with all else constant, will decrease right atrial pressure.

Atrial transmural pressure is difficult to quantify. Inasmuch as measurements of right atrial pressure and pulmonary wedge pressure are referred to atmospheric pressure rather than to the intrathoracic pressures surrounding the heart and thoracic vessels, transmural or effective filling pressures are unknown. Intrathoracic pressures become increasingly negative as the rate and tidal volume of respiration increase during exercise. Furthermore, the phase and amplitude of pressure pulsations are important to atrial filling; these are not shown in the filtered "mean" pressure that is commonly measured. In his detailed investigation of right atrial pressure during mild to severe supine and upright exercise (cycling), Holmgren (123) found no consistent increase, even when he took into account simultaneously determined intraesophageal pressures. The latter are assumed to reflect intrathoracic pressure, although this assumption has been questioned (see 123).

Pulmonary wedge pressure, which presumably reflects left atrial pressure, increases with exercise intensity [Fig. 17.1; (72, 118, 247)]. This pressure is

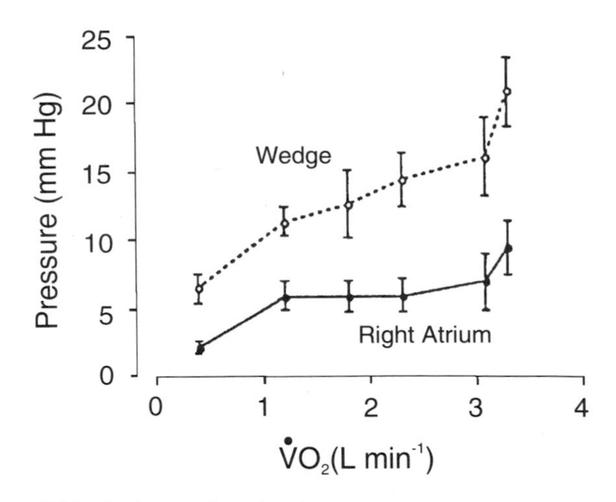

FIG. 17.1. Right atrial and pulmonary wedge pressures during seated rest and five levels of upright dynamic leg exercise (cycling). Note relationship between wedge and right atrial pressure and abrupt rise in both pressures at peak exercise. [Adapted from Reeves et al. (247) with permission.]

determined by differences between intrathoracic and alveolar pressures and pressures in any small collateral vessels that connect the wedge site to adjoining small arteries and veins.

Pulmonary wedge pressure and right atrial pressure appear to be linked so that for each mm Hg increase in right atrial pressure (see Fig. 17.1), pulmonary wedge pressure rises ~1.5 mm Hg (247). Right atrial pressure remains almost constant during exercise (Fig. 17.1), except for the abrupt rise at the highest oxygen uptake ($\dot{V}O_2$). Such an abrupt rise could be interpreted as a transient failure to match precisely the increased cardiac output with the augmented return of blood to the heart by the muscle pump. To our knowledge, no sudden rise in right atrial pressure at or near maximal exertion has been reported previously in normal people.

Right atrial pressure and/or CVP (referred to atmospheric pressure) vary markedly among individuals. During severe to maximal exercise, values ranged from 2–22 mm Hg (247). Pulmonary wedge pressure ranged from 11–35 mm Hg in the same individuals. Robinson et al. (253) reported a sudden rise in right atrial pressure and/or CVP values ranging from −4 to +10 mm Hg during maximal exercise (Fig. 17.2). This range was +0.5 to +19.5 mm Hg after acute expansion of blood volume by 1 liter.

The striking variation in CVP is consistent with the idea that CVP is not regulated by reflexes but is instead governed by both passive and mechanical properties of the cardiovascular system. The sudden rise in CVP at the onset of exercise (Fig. 17.2) (explained later) is a mechanical effect of the muscle pump (see also Chapter 15). These variations might

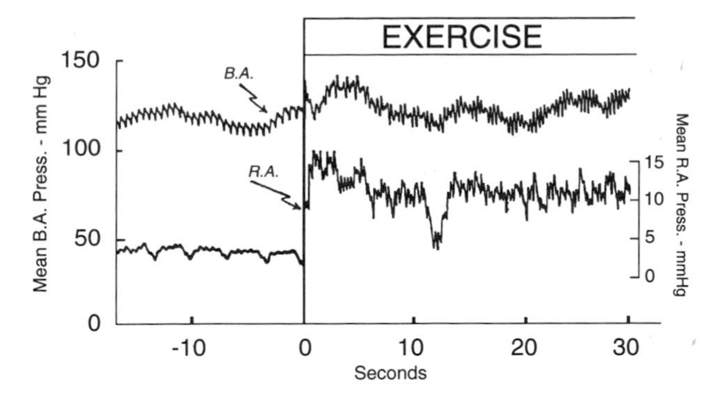

FIG. 17.2. Abrupt rise in mean right atrial (R.A.) pressure at onset of upright treadmill exercise. Sudden return of blood to the heart by skeletal muscle pump transiently exceeds left ventricular output [mean brachial arterial pressure (B.A.) also shown]. [Adapted from Robinson et al. (253).]

also argue against the primacy of the Frank-Starling mechanism in determining ventricular SV during exercise. Two points refute this thinking. First, ventricular transmural pressures are unknown. They could actually be rising at a time when right atrial pressure, referred to atmospheric pressure, is falling in relation to increasing negativity of intrathoracic pressure. Second, a very small increase in ventricular transmural pressure is required to increase ventricular stroke work because of the initial steepness of the ventricular function curve in upright posture. Also, the tendency for SV to remain relatively constant across increasing intensities of exercise suggests that ventricular filling pressure need only be maintained at a level that counteracts the decline in CVP associated with rising cardiac output.

Ventricular Afterload. The rise in SAP from rest to maximal dynamic exercise is only about 25 mm Hg (e.g., from 90 to 115 mm Hg). When pulsatile pressures are measured in the aortic arch, the increments in peak systolic pressure and pulse pressure are only about one-half those observed in peripheral arteries (269). These small changes in left ventricular afterload have little influence on ventricular function during dynamic exercise (12, 118, 238, 253) (see Chapter 15).

Pericardial Constraints

The skeletal muscle pump provides ample ventricular filling pressure at all levels of exercise and can clearly increase EDV and pulmonary blood volume (e.g., 79, 314). Perhaps the failure of right and left ventricular SV to rise in parallel with increased ventricular filling pressure is due to pericardial constraints (note again the terminal rise in CVP in Fig. 17.1).

Acute volume loading raises CVP, but in some cases maximal cardiac output and SV are not increased, whereas in others they are (29, 83, 143, 144). Robinson et al. (253) raised CVP by 7 mm Hg in five unconditioned young men by reinfusing 1 liter of their own blood withdrawn 2 weeks earlier. Resting cardiac output rose with increases in CVP and SV, but in "maximal" exercise the additional rise in CVP affected neither cardiac output nor SV. Failure to increase SV could be explained by a pericardial constraint.

In humans, SV can rise markedly when the heart is paced at a low rate during dynamic exercise after the pericardium has been cut (268). More surprising is the effect of pericardiectomy in the foxhound, a high-endurance animal (338). Pericardiectomy enabled the heart to respond to a high filling pressure at maximal exercise with a 14% increase in SV and a 17% increase in cardiac output above the maximal values established before pericardiectomy. Intensity of maximal exercise (and thus muscle pumping action) were the same before and after pericardiectomy. In pigs, pericardiectomy permitted percentage increments in SV and cardiac output that were nearly twice as large [Fig. 17.3; (108)]. Thus, the muscle pump appears to provide a ventricular filling pressure sufficient to raise SV by the Frank-Starling mechanism whenever pericardial constraints are removed. It is consistent with the view that skeletal muscle and left ventricular pumps are similarly effective in generating blood flow (in these examples, approximately 85% of cardiac output was perfusing active muscles).

THE VASCULAR SYSTEM

The main problem considered here concerns those intrinsic physical properties of the vascular system that necessitate neural and humoral vasomotor control coupled with mechanical alteration of the system in order to maintain or raise EDV so that cardiac output can increase.

Distribution of Resistance, Conductance, and Compliance

Resistance and Conductance. The principal site for control of vascular resistance is in arterioles, or resistance vessels. More than 50% of total peripheral vascular resistance lies in arterioles approximately 250–100 μm in diameter. The peripheral regions having the greatest vascular conductance at rest and

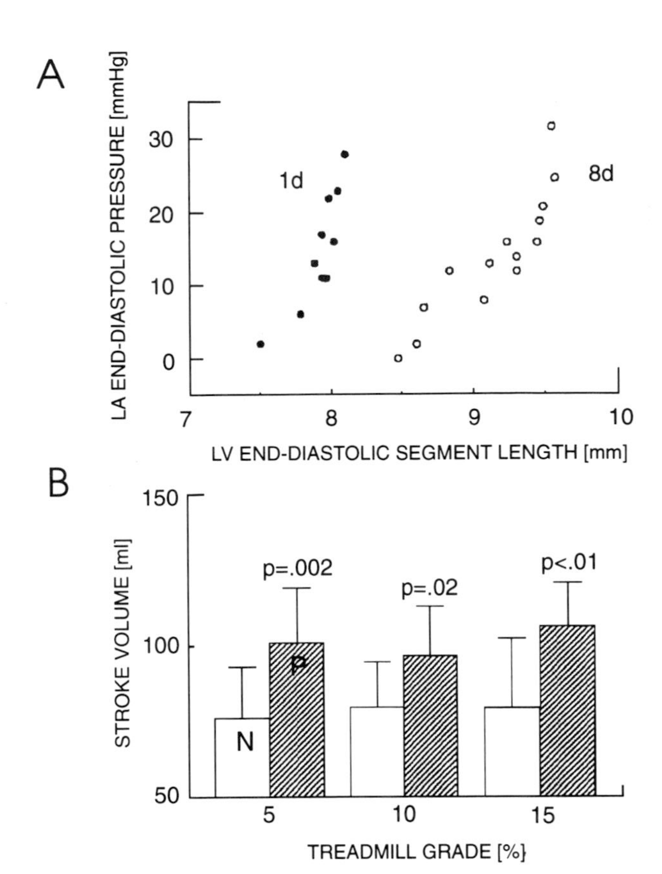

FIG. 17.3. *A*, Relationship between left atrial pressure (LA) and left ventricular (LV) segment length at end-diastole in one pig at 1 day (1d) and 8 days (8d) after thoracotomy without (*solid circles*) and with (*open circles*) pericardiectomy. *B*, Average stroke volumes before (*open bars, N*) and after (*hatched bars, P*) pericardiectomy. Data averaged from five pigs during three levels of treadmill exercise shown as percentage grade at 80–91 m/min. [Adapted from Hammond et al. (108) with permission.]

under normal environmental conditions are those that receive the greatest fraction of cardiac output. In most mammals, these organs are *(1)* splanchnic (27% of cardiac output), *(2)* kidneys (22%), *(3)* skeletal muscle (~18%), and *(4)* skin (~10%). Much of this chapter is about the enormous potential for vascular conductances in skeletal muscle and skin to rise.

Compliance. The distribution of blood volume among organs is determined by their vascular compliance, their size and transmural pressure, and the fraction of cardiac output they receive (for thorough reviews, see 99, 258).

Compliance of the arterial system is 0.05 ml · mm Hg^{-1} · kg^{-1} of body weight or only about 3% of that of the venous system. Estimates of total vascular compliance for dogs and humans vary between 2 and 3 ml · mm Hg^{-1} · kg^{-1} of body weight. Total venous compliance is about 30–50 times greater than arterial compliance.

Vascular compliances of different organs differ by orders of magnitude. These values are expressed in terms of milliliters of volume contained per millimeter of mercury of transmural pressure per kilogram of animal or organ weight. The latter is called specific compliance and permits comparisons between organs in which compliance may vary only as a function of organ size rather than distensibility of their vessels. The most compliant region is the liver at 20.0 ml · mm Hg^{-1} · kg^{-1} of tissue weight. The liver receives ~27% of cardiac output and, in humans, its blood volume is approximately 500–600 ml (10% of total blood volume). Total splanchnic blood volume is approximately (1500 ml, or about 27% of total blood volume in humans. Both the total and specific compliance of skin in humans are thought to be high as well, based on the marked increase in limb blood volume when cutaneous blood flow is increased (265).

In contrast to splanchnic organs and the skin, the specific compliance of canine skeletal muscle is low at only 0.48 ml · mm Hg^{-1} · kg^{-1} of tissue weight (258; see also 45, 194). A key point is that in humans, two of the largest vascular beds, splanchnic and cutaneous, also have the highest total and specific compliances, meaning that their blood flows have major effects on the distribution of blood volume. The largest vascular bed with the highest range of vascular conductance has the lowest total and specific compliance. At rest, the 30 kg of skeletal muscle in a 75 kg human, for example, contains only ~750 ml of blood.

The functional consequences of a compliant vascular system become most obvious when humans stand up. Blood volume moves into those dependent organs having greatest capacitance, which relates organ transmural pressure to its total intravascular volume. Volume shifts into splanchnic organs and approximately 500–600 ml move into capacious leg veins and another 200–300 ml shift into veins of buttocks and the pelvic area. Much of this volume is assumed to be translocated out of thoracic vessels. If total systemic vascular compliance is about 2.5 ml·mm Hg^{-1}·kg^{-1} of body weight, then the commonly observed 5 mm Hg fall in CVP would mean that approximately 940 ml of blood was translocated out of the central circulation in a 70 kg human (268). This calculation is valid only if cardiac output remains constant (see below).

Dependency of CVP on Cardiac Output

Rest. The interaction between the heart and the vasculature was analyzed thoroughly in Chapter 15. It is useful to review here those physical properties of the vascular system that prevent the heart by itself from increasing its output during dynamic exercise. The integration must deal with those mechanical and neural adjustments that counteract this crucial limitation.

At rest, an increase in cardiac output would increase blood flow to all organs in proportion to their vascular conductance. Then blood volume of each region will increase in proportion to its blood flow and its capacitance. The peripheral translocation of central venous volume reduces CVP. The converse occurs when cardiac output is reduced; the fall in blood flow to compliant regions causes a passive release and central translocation of their blood volume. Therefore, cardiac output and its distribution between compliant and noncompliant regions determines the distribution of blood volume and ventricular filling pressure (12, 43, 99, 171, 265, 316, 324).

Historically, Guyton's famous experiments on "venous return" show how changes in right atrial pressure can act in a *retrograde* direction to alter blood flow (or venous return) from the left ventricle through the systemic circulation and back to the right atrium (103). Our focus here is on how right atrial pressure responds in an *anterograde* direction when left ventricular output is varied (see 177, 268, 348).

Figure 15.15 (Chapter 15) and Figure 17.4 show that at rest, a fall in cardiac output raises CVP and a rise in cardiac output lowers it (24, 316). The fall in CVP with rising cardiac output is a purely passive, self-limiting feature of cardiac control; the rise in cardiac output is limited by the decline in SV with decreased filling pressure and, finally, by the collapse of the cavae when central venous transmural pressure reaches zero (see 234). Neither sinoaortic baroreceptor denervation (245) nor sympathetic ganglionic blockade by hexamethonium (316) fundamentally alter the cardiac output–CVP relationship (i.e., the effects are not neurally mediated).

Exercise. When humans stand at rest, the translocation of blood volume into dependent veins and the

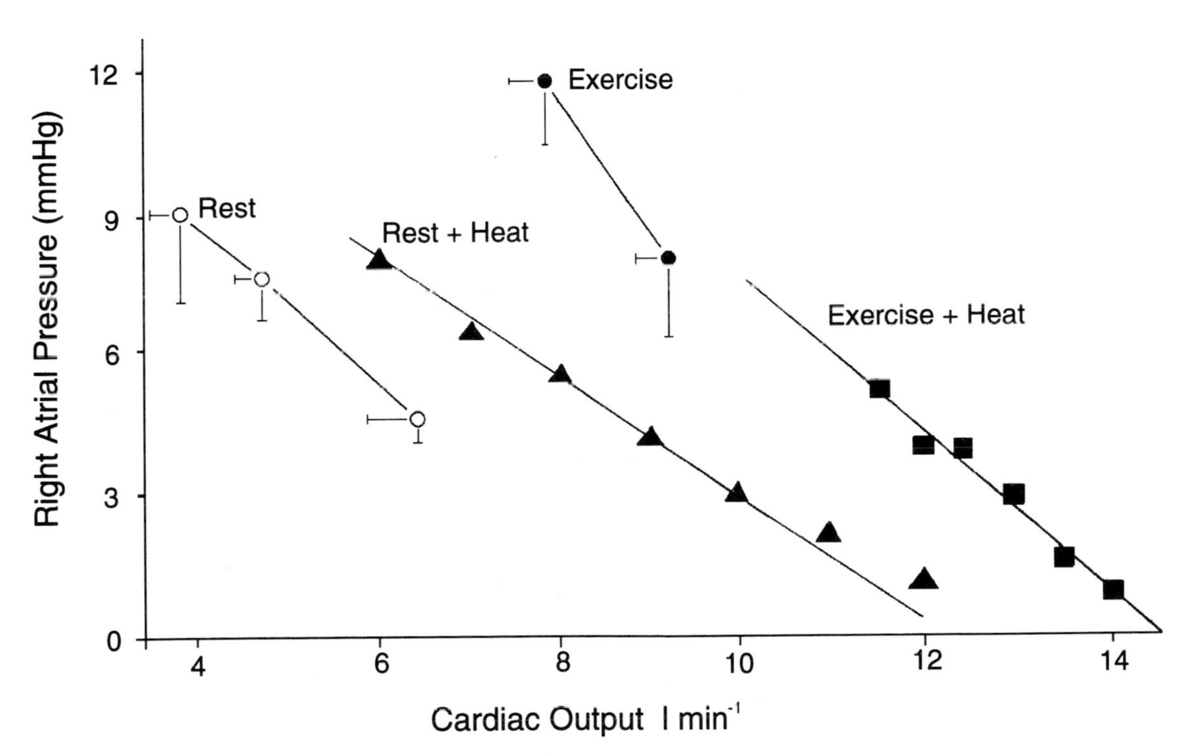

FIG. 17.4. Effects of changing cardiac output by ventricular pacing on right atrial pressure in supine human subjects during rest (*open circles*) and exercise (cycling) (*solid circles*) [From Bevegard et al. (24).] Results were similar to those of Sheriff et al. (316) on resting and exercising dogs (see Chapter 15). Increments in cardiac output at rest caused by raising skin blood flow [Rest + Heat (*solid triangles*) from Rowell (262, 264)], or further increments in cardiac output during exercise also caused by raising skin blood flow [Exercise + Heat (solid squares) from Rowell et al. (274)] also reduced right atrial pressure in proportion to the rise in cardiac output. Slopes during heating with and without exercise were obtained from different subjects in separate studies.

fall in CVP to nearly zero mean that the rise in HR and cardiac contractility can cause only a small initial rise in left ventricular output. This rise cannot be sustained after pulmonary blood volume, the sump for the left ventricle, has been depleted. Right ventricular output is reduced by the fall in CVP and cannot be restored owing to collapse of the central veins when CVP is close to zero.

Returning to the earlier quotation from Guyton et al. (103), because of the effect of raising cardiac output on CVP and central blood volume, increases in the rate and force of contraction cannot by themselves raise cardiac output significantly at the onset of upright exercise. An event in the peripheral circulation must at the same time translocate blood from the peripheral vasculature to the heart. Guyton et al. (103) showed in stop-flow experiments on anesthetized dogs with right heart bypass that electrical stimulation of the spinal cord immediately raised cardiac output by 40% and CVP by 7.5 mm Hg when this stimulation contracted hindlimb and abdominal muscles. These contractions expelled blood volume from muscle veins. Additionally, abdominal contractions forced blood from splanchnic veins as a result of their compression. Sympathetic blockade with hexamethonium did not block these responses, whereas spinal cord stimulation in animals paralyzed with decamethonium caused no immediate rise in cardiac output. These observations underscore the importance of muscle contraction.

Figures 17.4 and 15.14 show that even during dynamic exercise, changes in cardiac output caused by ventricular pacing have the same effect on the cardiac output–CVP relationship as at rest; similar slopes are shifted rightward and upward to higher cardiac output and CVP. This rightward shift in the curves with increased work rate is mainly an effect of the muscle pump, which decreases peripheral vascular volume and raises CVP (316). Also, as the fraction of cardiac output perfusing the noncompliant muscles increases (and the fraction to compliant regions decreases), the negative effect of increased cardiac output on CVP is reduced. Thus, if the entire increase in cardiac output with ventricular pacing during exercise were directed to muscle, the slope would be zero (i.e., because muscle vascular volume does not increase along with blood flow). The negative slope reveals that some of the increase in cardiac output with pacing goes to compliant organs, and as their vascular volume increases, CVP decreases.

Subsequent sections explore the mechanical and reflex modifications of the cardiovascular system that permit 400%–700% increases in cardiac output during exercise without the self-limiting reductions in CVP and SV.

Mechanical Effects on the Circulation—Auxiliary Pumps

The Skeletal Muscle Pump: The Second Heart. The muscle pump is a major determinant of "venous return," thoracic blood volume, and ventricular filling pressure during exercise (103, 314, 316). The muscle pump can be viewed as a second heart on the venous return portion of the circuit, having a capacity to generate blood flow rivaling that of the left ventricle. If the two pumps were not similar in pumping capacity, CVP would not rise when cardiac output rises in response to exercise. The flow-dependent accumulation of blood volume in compliant peripheral vasculature, which causes CVP to fall when cardiac output rises at rest, must be counteracted by the muscle pump (103, 314, 316). Figure 17.2 shows the immediate and marked rise in right atrial pressure at the onset of treadmill exercise in humans shown to be an effect of the muscle pump (103, 314, 316).

The muscle pump is a true pump and has central importance to circulatory regulation during both upright posture (265, 268) and exercise (80, 81, 174, 314, 333). Three key requirements for the effective operation of the muscle pump are: (*1*) intact venous valves; (*2*) it must maintain a low volume of blood within the muscle veins (see Chapter 15) (80, 314); and (*3*) it must be an effective *pump* doing more than simply compressing and emptying veins—it must increase the driving pressure for blood flow through the muscle (81, 174, 314) (see Chapter 16).

Contracting leg muscles can generate a driving force for blood flow that overcomes a venous outflow pressure (raised by venous occlusion) of 90–100 mm Hg (311, 333). The effectiveness of the muscle pump in the dependent legs is most clearly seen in tall animals by its momentary lowering of the muscle venous hydrostatic pressure to zero (or less, see below) while the added and height-related hydrostatic effect on the arterial driving pressure persists (e.g., as in humans or giraffes) (81, 111, 353). This added effect of gravity on driving pressure explains why peak blood flows to exercising legs are greater during upright than in supine posture (81).

Laughlin (174) proposed that the muscle pump could also work effectively without the high venous hydrostatic pressures that are seen in humans. The fast (50–100 ms) release of high compressive force when muscle relaxes should pull open, by elastic recoil, the collapsed veins, making the transmural pressure *negative*. Inasmuch as these veins are securely tethered to the surrounding muscle tissue (11), their rapid stretching is virtually ensured to generate a negative venous transmural pressure as long as venous valves remain closed. Evidence of negative intramuscular venous pressures comes from films showing contrast medium being rapidly drawn from superficial to deep veins via the small interconnecting perforating veins (with high resistance) immediately following each contraction (1). To be effective, the next muscle contraction must precede complete venous refilling so that repeated frequent contractions will maintain a low muscle venous pressure with an actual, maintained increase in arterial-venous driving pressure across the muscle. This action by the muscle pump not only increases muscle blood flow (MBF) above what could be provided by left ventricular force alone, but it will also displace blood volume back toward the heart, thereby maintaining CVP. Finally, the muscle pump exerts an edema-preventing effect owing to its reductions in muscle venous and capillary transmural pressures and enhancement of lymph flow (335).

Both Laughlin (174) and Stegall (333) estimated that approximately one-third of the calculated energy for muscle perfusion is generated by this muscle pump. This estimate assumes that muscle venous pressure remains positive throughout a contraction cycle. Depending on how negative muscle venous pressure actually goes immediately following contraction (this has not been measured), the actual contribution could be substantially higher than one-third. Also, Sheriff et al. (314) demonstrated that the sudden increases in cardiac output, CVP, and calculated vascular conductance at the onset of exercise could be attributed to the muscle pump (see also 74) (the problem of specifying a "conductance" across a pump is discussed below). These changes were too fast to be explained by metabolic vasodilation (97, 179, 198), and they were not affected by sympathetic blockade with hexamethonium (314).

The Abdominal Pump. The effects of the abdominal "pump" are complex, partly because of their interaction with the respiratory pump (below). The aforementioned experiments of Guyton et al. (103) showed that compression of intra-abdominal vessels by abdominal muscle contraction caused almost as much rise in cardiac output and CVP as did contraction of hindlimb muscles.

In studies of man running in place, Stegall (333) observed a 22–25 mm Hg rise in rectal pressure (reflecting intra-abdominal cavity pressure) and a similar rise in inferior vena caval pressure. The latter suggest an impedance to venous return from the legs, although this is a degree of back-pressure easily overcome by the muscle pump. On the other hand, muscle compression of compliant visceral organs that contain approximately 25% of total blood volume could translocate a substantial volume to the thorax irrespective of the changes in inferior vena caval pressure. For example, the 35% decrease in splanchnic blood volume reported by Wade et al. (363) occurred during mild supine exercise with splanchnic blood flow reduced only slightly (i.e., passive translocation of blood volume out of veins by arteriolar constriction would be small). Two possibilities are that compression by contracting abdominal muscles reduced splanchnic blood volume during supine cycling or, alternatively, splanchnic veins may have constricted.

The Respiratory Pump. The abdominal and respiratory pumps interact mechanically, but neither their interaction nor their effectiveness during exercise is well understood. An early view was that the decrease in intrathoracic pressure could not influence the flow of blood into the right atrium because of the collapse of the great veins at the point where they enter the chest (see 33). Another view was that the augmentation of venous return by inspiration would be canceled by the corresponding reduction in flow during expiration so that the respiratory pump provided no net gain of venous return (33). The early recordings of Brecher (33) and Wexler et al. (374), however, demonstrated the net gain in venous return during inspiration. Brecher showed the collapse with inspiration to be a time-dependent phenomenon that would reduce caval flow only if the downstream fall in intravascular pressure was too prolonged or unusually deep. Breathing changes transmural pressure in the cavae and other large veins passing through the thoracic cavity. Deepening inspiration lowers intrathoracic pressure and increases the pressure gradient between the right atrium and that point where the inferior vena cava enters the thoracic cavity. Wexler et al. (374) measured the acceleration of vena caval flow in humans during inspiration and found this acceleration to be augmented by exercise.

Several factors influence the effectiveness of the respiratory pump. For example, the descent of the diaphragm during inspiration lowers intrathoracic pressure. Inspiration also raises intra-abdominal pressure, increasing the pressure gradient between the abdomen and thorax, thus causing the inferior vena cava to expel blood centrally. Also, the inferior vena cava is shortened by inspiration and the consequent decrease in its volume shifts blood centrally toward the heart (33). Near the end of inspiration this increase in intra-abdominal pressure momentarily impedes venous blood flow from the quiescent legs into abdominal veins (for references, see 33).

Expiration reduces intra-abdominal pressure and releases blood from the resting legs when the relaxed diaphragm descends. Intrathoracic pressure then rises, approaching atmospheric pressure as tension within the inflated lungs is released so that inflow to the heart is retarded (33).

Another factor described by Moreno et al. (214) is the function of the liver as a pre–right ventricular sump that diminishes oscillations in venous return caused by breathing. When the diaphragm descends during inspiration it compresses hepatic veins and stops their flow. While hepatic venous outflow is arrested, inflow of blood into the liver continues and hepatic volume increases. During expiration, the ascent of the diaphragm releases hepatic venous compression and the expanded hepatic blood volume is rapidly discharged toward the right atrium by the elastic recoil of distended hepatic vasculature. This mechanical effect of inspiration and expiration on hepatic venous outflow is 180 degrees out of phase with the inspiratory and expiratory effects of caval inflow to the thorax, so that respiratory oscillations in venous return are smoothed out (cf. 341).

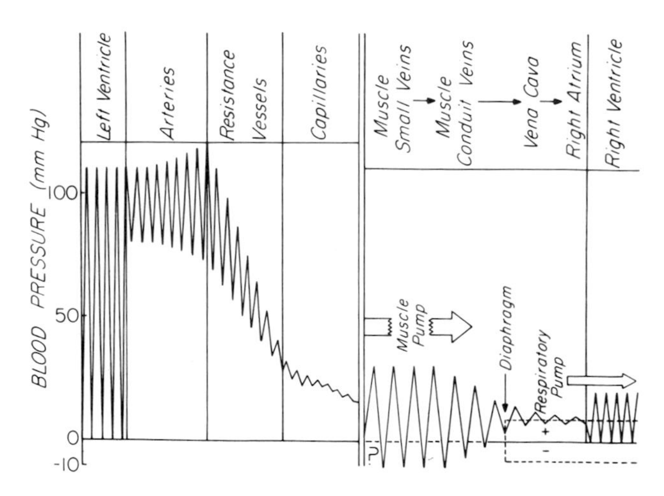

FIG. 17.5. Schematic illustration of the pressure profile across the vascular system. Up to the capillaries pressure oscillations characterize only the changing magnitudes of pulse pressure and not cardiac frequency. The circuit is broken in the muscle by the muscle pump, and pressure oscillations show external effects of muscle pumping and then respiratory pumping—four pumps in series. Blood flow from the left ventricle to the muscle is determined by the pressure difference between the heart and some unknown point in the muscle, whereas blood flow from active muscle to the right ventricle is determined by the force provided by the muscle pump. [Reproduced from Rowell (268) with permission.]

Pumps and "Virtual" Conductance. It is common to speak of vascular conductance of active muscles as if all of the energy driving blood flow through them were provided by the left ventricle and as if vascular conductance increased as a simple function of increased vascular diameter associated with metabolic vasodilation. The active muscles are, however, true pumps that provide most of the energy needed to drive blood back to the right ventricle. Figure 17.5 summarizes the effects of muscle and respiratory pumps on the pressure profile across the circulation (268). Inasmuch as the circulation is essentially broken by a second pump (skeletal muscle), the aortic–right atrial pressure difference is not determined by a simple ohmic resistance, so we speak of a "virtual" conductance between the aorta and the right atrium during dynamic exercise. This so-called conductance has two determinants: (*1*) metabolic vasodilators, and (*2*) reduction in muscle venous pressure by the muscle pump. Inasmuch as muscle venous pressures are unknown, the relative contributions of pumping and metabolic vasodilation to calculated "conductance" remain unknown. Parenthetically, this raises questions concerning the extent to which the known metabolic vasodilators of muscle might account for the magnitude of actual vasodilation during exercise uncomplicated by the influence of muscle pumping (see 312).

Total Mobilization of Blood Volume during Exercise. Can muscle compression of veins counteract the blood flow–dependent fall in CVP when cardiac output rises at the onset of exercise? Inasmuch as CVP rises or remains constant rather than falling when cardiac output rises at the onset of exercise, muscle contraction must prevent any blood flow–dependent fall in CVP. In fact, CVP rises immediately at the onset of dynamic exercise in dogs (314) and humans (253) (see Fig. 17.2), indicating that return of blood to the right ventricle transiently exceeds the output of the left ventricle. Sheriff et al. (316) calculated that 9.5 ml/kg body weight, or 19 ml/kg muscle weight, is translocated by the muscle pump in dogs. If these numbers were extrapolated to a 75 kg human, 712 ml of blood would be mobilized mechanically (note that relative to body mass, dogs have more muscle than humans).

Flamm et al. (79) used radionuclide imaging to estimate regional changes in the volume of technetium-99m–labeled red blood cells during zero-load cycling and cycling at loads requiring 50%, 75%, and 100% of $\dot{V}O_{2max}$. The relative blood volume of the legs fell by 32% due to the effect of the muscle pump during zero-load cycling at 60 rpm (seated upright) (cf. 184). Total thoracic volume and individual volumes of heart and lungs all rose 20%–30%, but abdominal volume was unchanged. If we assume that total blood volume of each leg was 700 ml (400 ml per leg at supine rest with a shift of 300 ml into dependent leg veins on assumption of upright posture), then approximately 450 ml would be expelled from the leg veins by zero-load contractions. This would include some expulsion not only from deep intramuscular veins but from superficial cutaneous veins as well (184, 239).

At the three higher work rates, total abdominal blood volumes fell progressively, reaching 20% at the highest work rate with reductions of 46%, 18%, and 24% in splenic, hepatic, and renal volumes, respectively, at $\dot{V}O_{2max}$. Muscle blood volume was reduced by 24%, 22%, and 23% at the three higher loads of exercise. If we assume the 20% decrease in total abdominal volume is about 300 ml (0.2 × 1500 ml), then combined with that from muscle total volume translocated could be as high as 750 ml at $\dot{V}O_{2max}$ and as low as 390 ml at 50% of $\dot{V}O_{2max}$. Estimation of splanchnic blood volume by dye techniques showed greater reductions in volume, 30%–40%, during relatively mild exercise in humans (31, 48, 363). Increments in cardiac volume (24%) and in total lung blood volume (50%) are somewhat greater than those determined from proximal aortic blood flow and mean transit time between the right atrium and the aortic arch by dye dilution (273).

Clearly, during the first few heart beats after the onset of exercise, before reflexes can be effective, the extracardiac pumps must return as much to the left ventricle as it puts out (or more), otherwise CVP would fall. Again, the abrupt rise in CVP (Fig. 17.2) means that venous return momentarily exceeded left ventricular output.

Does Exercise Reduce Systemic Vascular Compliance?

Some assume that dynamic exercise reduces systemic vascular compliance both as a consequence of compression of the vasculature by muscle contractions as well as by the sympathetic vasoconstriction discussed later (and possibly by venoconstriction as well). Such changes would increase the rise in CVP caused by any given volume of blood forced centrally by muscle pumps. This concept has not been directly tested by comparing the effects of a rapid infusion of a large volume of blood during rest with what the effects might be during exercise. In early studies (for references, see 184) rapid infusion into resting humans of 1–1.5 liters of whole blood or plasma gave no hint that limits of vascular distensibility had been approached. When Robinson et al. (253) infused 1–1.2 liters of subjects' own blood (drawn 2 weeks previously) as the subjects rested, their CVP rose only 1.9 mm Hg above normal. Subsequently, CVP rose 7.4 mm Hg higher than normal during maximal exercise. The infusion increased cardiac output at rest from 5.3 to 6.8 liters/min, but it had no effect on cardiac output and SV during maximal exercise. Presumably, the rise in cardiac output at rest lessened the rise in CVP. The point is that one cannot examine effects of altered blood volume on CVP if cardiac output changes; since it changed at rest and not during maximal exercise, no comparison between the two states was possible (for further discussion, see Chapter 15).

Neural Control of the Vascular System during Exercise: How Important?

Will the initial mechanical effects on the distribution of blood volume in response to dynamic exercise suffice to maintain ventricular filling pressure, cardiac output, and SAP throughout exercise, or does neural control become essential? Sympathetic nervous activity (SNA) increases in a highly predictable manner in relation to the intensity of dynamic exercise (262, 265, 268). What does this rise in SNA achieve? Our goal is to show that the maintenance of SV, cardiac output, and SAP during dynamic exercise requires a close balance between the purely mechanical effects of muscle pumps and the sympathetic control of blood vessels. Without the latter, even with the muscle pump, regulation fails.

Characteristics of Sympathetic Vasoconstrictor Outflow during Dynamic Exercise

Patterns of SNA to major organs. Figure 17.6 summarizes human sympathetic responses to mild to maximal dynamic exercise. A highly consistent finding is that regional vasoconstriction (splanchnic and renal) does not begin until HR approaches 100 bpm. Up to this point, autonomic control is mainly directed to raising cardiac output by vagal withdrawal; as HR progresses toward 100 bpm, sympathetic control begins to dominate [*vertical dashed line*, Fig. 17.6; (70, 191, 230, 252)]. Other indices of increased SNA, in addition to regional vasoconstriction, are the progressive increments in muscle sympathetic nerve activity (MSNA), plasma renin activity (PRA), and plasma NE concentration. Cutaneous arterioles and even coronary vessels (see below and Chapter 16) constrict, suggesting a generalized or diffuse sympathetic outflow (119) unlike the more discrete distribution seen during other stresses [e.g., hyperthermia (318)].

Spillover of sympathetic neurotransmitters. An increased plasma concentration of NE is a useful qualitative index of SNA under many conditions (46, 75, 95, 271, 308). In humans, plasma NE is derived from neuronal leakage into plasma along with neu-

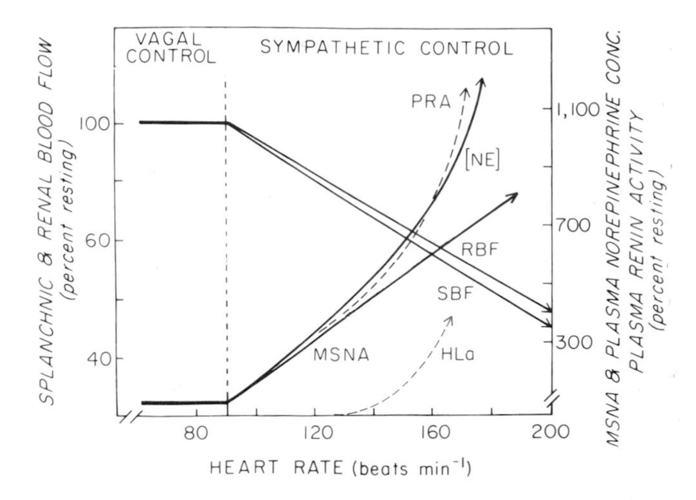

FIG. 17.6. Summary of human sympathetic responses to mild to maximal dynamic exercise. Response pattern was unaffected by ambient temperature, active muscle mass, or physical conditioning (47, 262, 264, 265, 270, 271). Sympathetic nervous activity begins to rise when vagal withdrawal is nearly complete and heart rate approaches 100 bpm. The indices of increased SNA are splanchnic and renal vasoconstriction (decline in RBF and SBF), increased plasma norepinephrine (NE) concentration, and plasma renin activity (PRA). Cutaneous, coronary, and skeletal muscle arterioles also constrict, suggesting diffuse sympathetic outflow. Also, MSNA (burst frequency) rises with HR up to near maximal values (see Fig. 17.10). Lactic acid (HLa) does not rise until HR reaches 130–140 bpm (50%–60% of $\dot{V}O_{2max}$) or much higher in athletes. [Adapted from Rowell and O'Leary (275).]

ropeptides and other putative neurotransmitters [see Figs. 17.7 and 17.8; (41, 235, 236, 347)]. Only 10%–20% of the neuronally released NE diffuses from the synaptic cleft into interstitial fluid, and from there it spills into plasma where it is degraded by monamine oxidases (75). The remainder of the NE is either taken up by sympathetic neurons or by vascular smooth muscle cells.

Close correlations between plasma NE concentration and NE spillover during exercise are observed but are partly due to the derivation of NE spillover from its plasma concentration (176). Some data suggest that NE clearance rate is minimally affected by exercise intensity and duration (at least up to 30 min) (176). Minor reductions in NE clearance in severe exercise may stem from the effects of marked reductions in hepatic and renal blood flows on their NE clearance rates (114). Figures 17.7 and 17.8 show changes in HR and NE spillover in relation to HR that are generally consistent with the summary in Figure 17.6. An additional effect of exercise duration on NE spillover presumably stems from the declining SAP associated with skin vasodilation during prolonged exercise (71, 136, 265, 274).

Sources of NE. In humans at rest, organ spillover of NE is greatest from skeletal muscle and kidneys. Skeletal muscle contributes 20%–50% of total NE spillover; kidneys, about 25%; splanchnic region, approximately 10%; skin, possibly 5%; and the heart contributes only 2%–3% (75).

Total NE spillover rose ~340% above resting baseline values in normal human subjects during 10–15 min of *supine* dynamic exercise at 60%–70% of "maximal" working capacity, whereas spillover from the heart, kidneys, and exercising muscle rose 1778%, 340%, and 300%, respectively (114). Because of its large mass, skeletal muscle contributed most of the NE to plasma despite its smaller percentage increases relative to the other regions. Furthermore, spillover from one active muscle increases in proportion to the mass of other muscles that become simultaneously active (295). Together these findings point to active muscle as the dominant source of circulating NE during exercise (296). Parenthetically, only a small percentage of the NE spillover from active muscles is likely to stem from a flow-dependent washout of the neurotransmitter rather than its release by increased sympathetic activity (106, 296).

The kidney also contributes significantly to the total spillover of NE, despite the reduction in renal blood flow in proportion to exercise intensity [Fig. 17.6; (114, 347)]. Figure 17.7 shows the abrupt rise in renal spillover of NE and release of renin when HR reached 100 bpm. During heavy exercise (HR = 175 bpm), NE concentration increased tenfold and NE spillover increased 13-fold (347). Dynamic exercise is a far more potent stimulus to renal SNA than stresses such as isometric contraction, orthostasis, or mental stress (347). Tidgren et al. (347) also found marked outpouring of neuropeptide Y (NPY) into the renal vein at the highest work rates (Fig. 17.7). NPY, a co-transmitter released by sympathetic nerves along with NE at high rates of nerve firing (64, 235, 236), is a more potent and longer acting vasoconstrictor than NE and may contribute importantly to renal vasoconstriction when SNA is highest during severe exercise.

Sympathetic nerve activity. Microneurographic techniques permit continuous registration of firing in sympathetic axons within fascicles containing efferent fibers that innervate either skeletal muscle or skin of a limb (e.g., 349, 369). This technique can provide unambiguous evidence of increased SNA directed to muscle and potentially allows vasomotor effects of sympathetic origin to be separated from those of humoral origin (see 307, 349, 369). It cannot, however, distinguish among types of sympathetic efferent fibers (i.e., sudomotor, vasoconstrictor, or vasodilator).

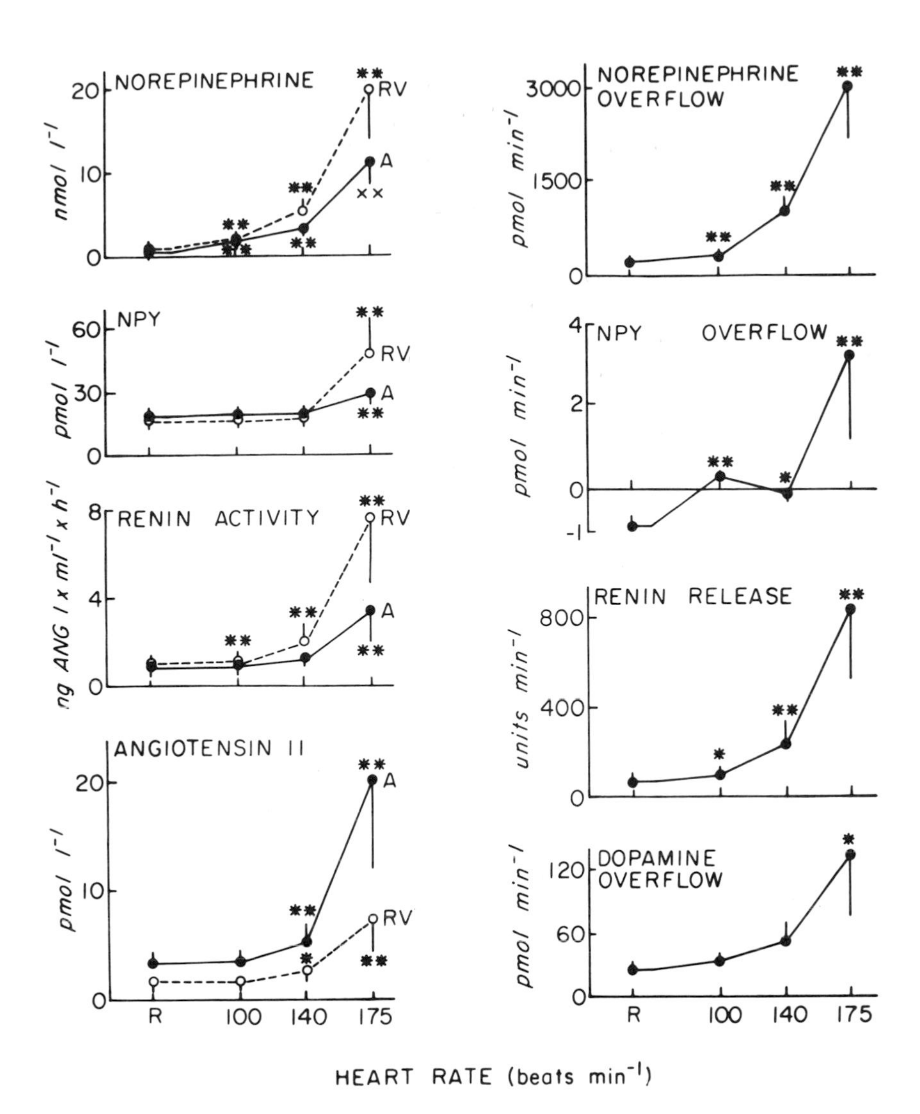

FIG. 17.7. Renal neurohormonal responses to graded dynamic exercise (supine posture) in eight normal young humans. Exercise levels were 69, 132, and 188 W. Arteriovenous differences across the kidney (*left column*) and renal overflows (*right column*) of norepinephrine, immunoreactive neuropeptide Y, renin, and dopamine are related to the average heart rates during exercise. The renal arteriovenous differences for angiotensin (*lower left*) and also for epinephrine (*not shown*) were positive, showing net renal uptake of these hormones. The average values for renal blood flow at the three heart rates fall on the regression line for RBF vs. HR shown in Figure 17.6. Note the similar response pattern among all indices of RSNA. [Redrawn from Tidgren et al. (347) and reproduced from Rowell (268) with permission)]

In humans, measurements of SNA, which have been confined to muscle (MSNA) and skin of resting limbs, have been made mostly during isometric contractions of a contralateral limb because the measurements are extremely sensitive to motion (307). Nevertheless, MSNA has been successfully measured during rhythmic handgrip exercise and dynamic arm cycling (361), and recently during dynamic leg exercise (244, 287). Recently, activity has also been measured in sympathetic fibers that were supplying active muscle (110).

Figure 17.9 shows the rise in MSNA recorded from the peroneal nerve during arm cranking of an ergometer at the loads shown (361). Three important features are as follows: (*1*) There is a threshold below which MSNA is not increased by intensity of rhythmic arm exercise; (*2*) above this threshold, MSNA increases in proportion to work rate; and (*3*) onset of increased MSNA has a delay that becomes shorter as work intensity increases. The relationship between HR and the rise in MSNA was the same as for other measures of SNA shown in Figure 17.6; MSNA rose when HR reached 100 bpm [this was also observed by Ray and Mark (243)].

Saito et al. (287) recently measured MSNA burst frequency from a median nerve at the elbow during leg exercise requiring 20%, 40%, 60%, and 75% of $\dot{V}O_{2max}$. Figure 17.10 reiterates for MSNA the typical pattern for SNA in general; that is, MSNA did not rise above resting (seated) control values until HR reached 100 bpm and work rate required approximately 40% of $\dot{V}O_{2max}$. MSNA fell below baseline levels measured during upright seated rest in response to mild upright exercise. The importance of activation of the muscle pump during upright rest to counteract the fall in both CVP and arterial pulse pressure is well known. Even gentle muscle contractions counteract the fall in CVP and arterial pulse pressure, which cause the rise in SNA that is initiated by cardiopulmonary and arterial baroreflexes. Ray et al. (244) also observed the fall in MSNA in response to mild dynamic one-legged exercise in up-

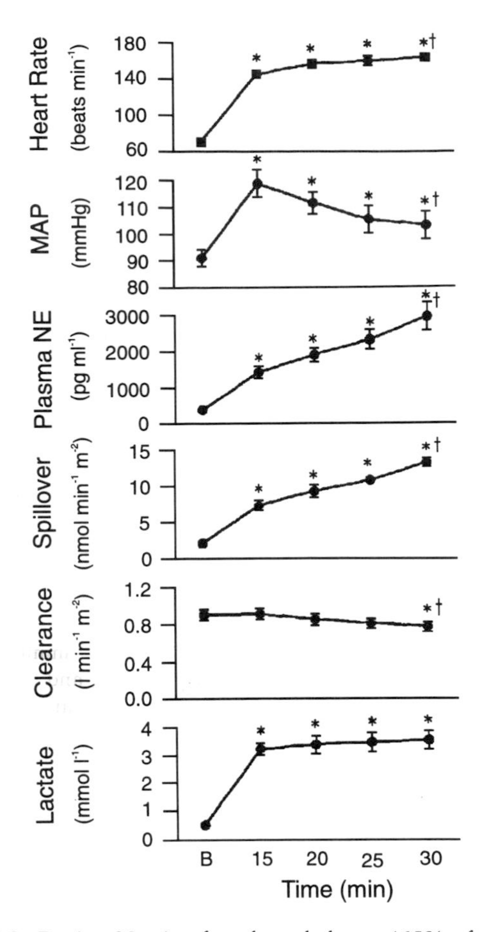

FIG. 17.8. During 20 min of moderately heavy (65% of maximal workrate) leg exercise (upright cycling), HR, plasma NE concentration, and NE spillover rate rose continuously, whereas NE clearance was reduced slightly and significantly only at 30 min (176). $^*P < 0.05$ compared with resting and $^{\dagger}P < 0.05$ compared with 5 min exercise value. The increments in plasma NE and NE spillover are probably associated with the decline in mean arterial pressure (MAP). [From Leuenberger et al. (176) with permission.]

right but not in supine posture. Nor does MSNA fall in response to mild dynamic arm exercise, owing to less significant muscle pumping [Fig. 17.9; (361)]. In short, the fall in MSNA during very mild exercise is a response to the reversal of venous pooling. The rise in SNA attributable to "exercise-related reflexes" occurs at higher levels of exercise.

DIFFUSE VS. PUNCTATE ACTIVATION OF THE SYMPATHETIC NERVOUS SYSTEM. Two concerns are (*1*) that MSNA in resting limbs may not represent that directed to active muscles, and (*2*) that MSNA does not necessarily parallel the changes in SNA to other organs. Clearly, sympathetic outflow can be quite discrete (349). Although quantitative comparisons are extremely difficult to make, it appears that different organs may not only receive different magnitudes of SNA, but that changes in SNA can even be of the opposite sign. Good examples are responses to hyperthermia and hypoxemia (318).

These newer findings conflict with W.B. Cannon's original notion that the entire sympathetic nervous system is activated en masse. Any differential effects of SNA among organs were seen as stemming from local modulation of sympathetic effects. However, the regional specificity, as well as the unfolding revelation of differences in neurotransmitters noted in the sympathetic control of the human cutaneous circulation, may not be evident in other regions during exercise (286, 303, 362). For example, the generalized vasoconstriction in the exercising baboon signifies that SNA during exercise must be quite diffuse (119). The increases in MSNA to resting muscle appear to parallel the increases in SNA (by other measures) to many regions including active muscle (see NE spillover), the heart (10, 104), kidneys (347) and visceral organs (268), and possibly even respiratory muscle [Fig. 17.6; (340)].

Seals and Victor (307) point to the consistent burst pattern of MSNA measured at different sites in several studies (246, 339) as suggestive evidence that (*1*) MSNA is uniform throughout the body—at least under resting conditions, and (*2*) the activity represents a centrally driven SNA to muscle rather than regionally determined activity.

NE SPILLOVER VS. SYMPATHETIC RECORDINGS. The most direct measures of SNA are microneurographic recordings and the determination of H3-NE spillover rate. NE spillover into the venous drainage from an organ is assumed to be proportional to sympathetic nerve firing rate to that organ. Although this is generally the case, quantitative relationships between nerve firing and NE spillover can vary greatly from organ to organ (75) and even within a specific organ (232, 278).

Among the most important problems with direct measurements of SNA is the nonlinear and nonpredictable relationship between sympathetic discharge rate and vasomotor responses (373). For measurements of MSNA, impulses are recorded from a small fraction of the potentially active sympathetic fibers in a nerve fascicle. Nevertheless, measurements of SNA and NE spillover are valuable in that they provide evidence that the sympathetic nervous system is contributing to the vasomotor responses. The only quantitative alternative to these measures, however, is the measurement of the vascular response (which could include humoral effects as well).

Changes with aging. The α_1-adrenoceptor–mediated neural control seems to be well maintained with aging; essentially normal receptor populations have normal antagonist affinity, but α_2-adrenoceptor–mediated responses may be somewhat attenuated (56,

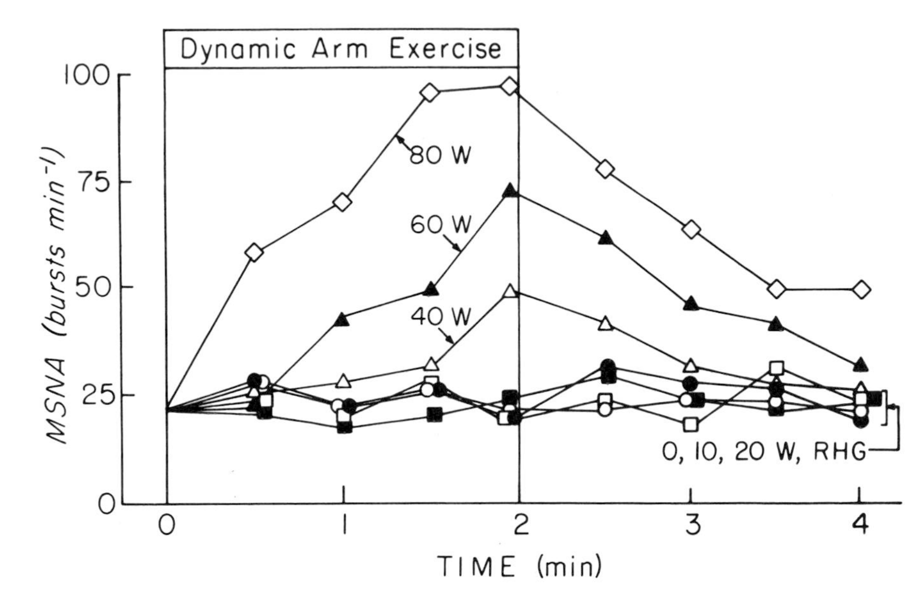

FIG. 17.9. Muscle sympathetic nerve activity (MSNA) in resting legs increases in proportion to intensity of dynamic arm exercise (cycling). Data are unillustrated from a subject-coauthor studied by Victor et al. (361). This subject could exercise at 80 W before body motion made microneurographic measurements of MSNA from a peroneal nerve impossible. Two important features are (*1*) there was a threshold for the rise in MSNA at 40 W (for all subjects), and (*2*) the delay in the rise in MSNA decreased with increasing work intensity and may have been almost absent at 80 W. [From original data kindly provided by D. R. Seals and reproduced from Rowell (268) with permission.]

82). The latter may explain the increase in NE spillover in response to increased SNA in the aged; negative feedback from prejunctional α_2-adrenoceptors on neuronal release of NE may be diminished. In addition to these α-adrenergic changes, vascular responsiveness to β_2-adrenoceptor agonists is also attenuated in old age (82).

Throughout the remainder of Part I and the discussion of reflex control of cardiovascular system in Part II, no comparisons are made relative to age or gender because it is assumed that the mechanisms underlying control of blood flow, SAP, and SNA during exercise are basically the same across groups. The old and young are simply viewed as being functionally similar but operating over widely differing scales of $\dot{V}O_{2max}$. This thinking is supported by studies revealing that healthy, noninstitutionalized old people have virtually normal control of SAP during orthostasis (172, 182) and during mild to maximal exercise (82, 172). These two stresses demand the utmost of reflex sympathetic adrenergic control of the vascular system.

Overall Importance of Increased SNA in Dynamic Exercise

Redistribution of oxygen from inactive regions to active muscle. In humans the pattern of flow reduction shown in Figure 17.6 can provide an additional 500–600 ml of oxygen each minute for active muscle (262). Because of the low resting oxygen extraction of kidneys, splanchnic organs, inactive muscle, and skin, these regions could withstand the 70%–80% reduction in blood flow at $\dot{V}O_{2max}$ without compromising their own oxygen needs. In other species, redistribution of oxygen to active muscle by vasoconstriction of visceral organs is much less pronounced. However, dogs and horses, for example, constrict the spleen and exhibit marked decreases in splenic volume (15, 79, 90, 93, 139, 173, 292). A 46% reduction in human splenic volume (79) and a 34% decrease in splenic erythrocyte content (173) suggests a role for splenic contraction in raising hematocrit during exercise. However, earlier experiments showed that increased capillary filtration during exercise caused the rise in hematocrit (55, 156). In healthy subjects with or without spleens, hematocrit rose in proportion to the increase in serum protein concentration (55). In contrast to humans, the spleens of dogs and horses release large quantities of red blood cells into the circulation during exercise (see 15, 139).

Systemic arterial pressure regulation. The decrease in regional vascular conductance caused by the vasoconstriction in nonactive regions during severe exercise (Fig. 17.6) has a trivial effect on SAP in endurance athletes with high maximal cardiac outputs. In contrast, the same degree of regional vasoconstriction and reduction in vascular conductance has highly significant effects on SAP in cardiac patients with low maximal cardiac outputs, because total vascular conductance is low and the conductance of nonmuscular regions is a larger fraction of the total (for details, see 262, 265).

Maintenance of ventricular filling pressure. The maintenance of CVP depends on the distribution of cardiac output, as already discussed. In this context, the importance of regional vasoconstriction goes far beyond the calculated effect on SAP based simply on Ohm's law. In part, this is because of the additional capacitive functions of regions like the splanchnic

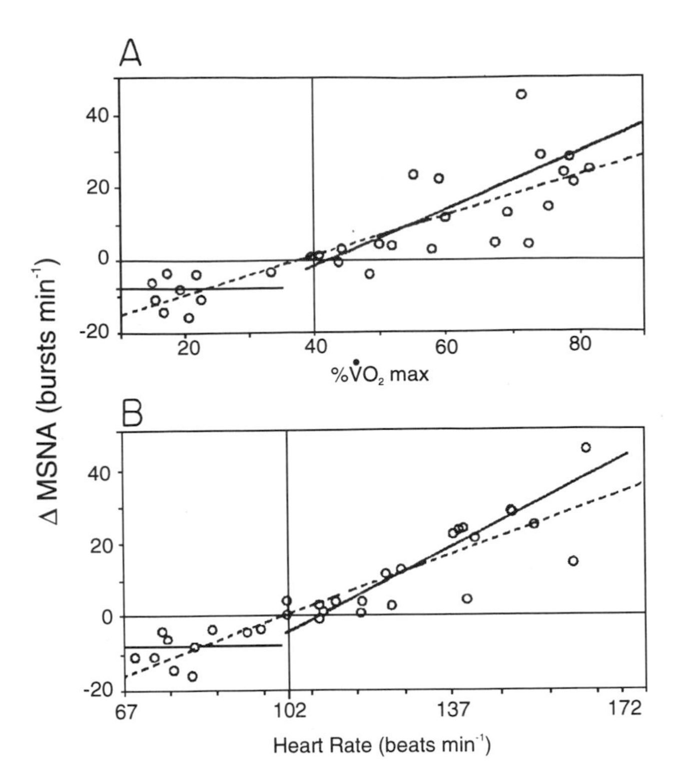

FIG. 17.10. *A*, Relationship between MSNA (expressed as Δburst frequency from the median nerve) and percentage of $\dot{V}O_{2max}$ during dynamic leg exercise (cycling) at approximately 20%, 40%, 60%, and 75% $\dot{V}O_{2max}$. Disagreement with interpretation of Saito et al. (287) is revealed by two sets of regression lines: *dashed line* by Saito et al., *solid line* by us. The ΔMSNA was calculated from "baseline" values (Δ = 0) that had been elevated by orthostatic stress (seated upright rest). Mild exercise and muscle pump restored CVP and aortic pulse pressure, thus lowering MSNA to supine resting values. MSNA appeared not to rise until work required 40% $\dot{V}O_{2max}$ (*rising solid line*) (*horizontal solid line* illustrates our assumption that the slope of MSNA response is zero below 40% $\dot{V}O_{2max}$). *B*, Relationship between MSNA and HR based on our interpretation (*solid lines*) is consistent with other findings and with Figure 17.6 [see also Victor et al. (361)]. *Dashed line* of Saito et al. shows no HR threshold for MSNA. [Adapted from Saito et al. (287).]

bed and skin and the marked passive effects exerted by vasoconstriction on the volume of blood they contain. The ability to maintain adequate SAP and blood flow during exercise is lost if vasoconstriction in these capacious regions is blocked, thereby unleashing their deleterious effects on blood volume distribution.

The negative relationship between cardiac output and CVP shown in Figure 17.4 is demonstrated when blood flow to a nonmuscular, compliant region (skin) is *increased* during exercise with heat stress. Heat vasodilates the skin and not muscle (219, 294) or other regions (262, 264) so that the additional rise in cardiac output is directed to skin, and CVP falls in proportion to this rise. Similarly, even a passive rise in blood flow to the relatively noncompliant paralyzed legs of paraplegic individuals during arm exercise reduces SV (124, 125). In contrast, increments in cardiac output are unaccompanied by any decrease in SV and presumably in CVP when MBF is raised by hypoxemic vasodilation, at a constant level of exercise (334, 364). In this case the rise in cardiac output is directed to noncompliant skeletal muscle.

THE IMPORTANCE OF SPLANCHNIC VASOCONSTRICTION. The splanchnic region is the largest and most compliant blood reservoir in the body; consequently, the passive effects of splanchnic vasoconstriction on CBV and CVP should be large. Estimates of splanchnic blood volume by radionuclide images (79, 90, 292) and by indicator dilution techniques (which measure splanchnic blood flow plus mean transit time) (31), both reveal that large reductions in splanchnic blood flow in dogs cause similarly large decreases in splanchnic blood volume (e.g., 58). The data of Rothe and Gaddis (259) suggest that a 70%–80% reduction in splanchnic blood flow (depending on the prevailing central venous backpressure on hepatic venous outflow) could passively expel as much as 35%–50% of total splanchnic blood volume, or 350–500 ml if these percentage changes are extrapolated to humans. Some additional reduction might be achieved by active constriction of splanchnic veins as well.

Selective loss of splanchnic vasomotor control is rare, but effects of unrestricted blood flow into this capacious region should be large. Experimentally, surgical denervation of the splanchnic vasculature and adrenal medulla by thoracic sympathectomy markedly reduced the rise in cardiac output with voluntary dynamic exercise in chronically instrumented dogs (7). A marked fall in SV with exercise caused the diminished rise in cardiac output. The interpretation was that after splanchnic denervation, both splanchnic blood flow and splanchnic blood volume rose passively along with increased SAP during exercise. As a consequence, thoracic blood volume, CVP, and SV all fell. Similar consequences were observed in an athletic young woman who had received a series of surgical ganglionectomies to prevent hyperhydrosis (354). Removal of celiac and superior mesenteric ganglia in her final surgery precipitated a disabling orthostatic intolerance and greatly reduced her exercise tolerance. Up to a point her response to exercise (cycling) was aided by normal vagal control of HR and by muscle and respiratory pumps plus the abdominal compression associated with cycling. Her limited ability to raise cardiac output was presumably caused at least in part by splanchnic denervation and passive expansion of splanchnic blood volume (354).

Balance between Mechanical and Neural Effects on Blood Flow and Blood Volume Distribution

The preceding discussion reveals that the translocation of blood volume to central vasculature by muscle, respiratory, and abdominal pumps cannot maintain an adequate level of CVP and cardiac output after splanchnic vasomotor control is lost. The following findings reveal the additional importance of overall sympathetic vasomotor outflow.

Autonomic Dysfunction. When control of the sympathetic nervous system is disrupted by disease, two sequelae are severe orthostatic hypotension and marked exercise intolerance. Loss of sympathetic vasomotor control in skeletal muscle and in other regions adds significantly to the regulatory problems attending splanchnic denervation described above.

Individuals with autonomic dysfunction experience progressive hypotension in response to mild *supine* exercise (23, 199). Hypotension occurred even when the supine body was tilted head downward by 15 degrees. Supine exercise and head-down tilt minimized gravitational forces on the circulation and facilitated venous return to the heart so that CVP was maintained (199). Bevegård et al. (23) confirmed that the fall in SAP was caused by failure of vasoconstriction in such dysfunctional patients. Their rise in cardiac output in relation to $\dot{V}O_2$ was normal during supine cycling with legs elevated above the heart. Their exercise performance was limited by severe hypotension rather than by reduced CVP caused by "pooling" of blood in splanchnic organs to which blood flow (and volume) must have been reduced passively by the fall in SAP.

When these individuals exercised while tilted head-up by 30–40 degrees, SAP fell markedly, owing to insufficient rise in cardiac output relative to the excessive rise in total vascular conductance (23). The cardiac output response was impaired by the low thoracic blood volume and SV, owing to gravitational expansion of blood volume in dependent veins.

The principal defect in SAP regulation was thought to be inadequate vasoconstriction in *nonactive regions* to compensate for metabolic vasodilation in active muscle. However, during supine exercise with a normal cardiac output of 11 liters/min and SAP at approximately 100 mm Hg (23), had both splanchnic and renal conductances risen from 50% of resting values (6% of total conductance) up to normal resting values (now 12% of total conductance), SAP would have fallen only by ~10 mm Hg rather than by the 30–40 mm Hg often observed.

Importance of Vasoconstriction in Active Muscle. A dominant cause of hypotension during exercise without autonomic control must be the loss of tonic vasoconstriction in active muscles. The vascular conductance of active muscles comprises most of the total; therefore, changes will alter SAP most significantly. Conversely, the vascular conductances of inactive and nonmuscular regions are a small fraction of the total, so that even if vasoconstriction reduced their conductances to zero, the effect on SAP would be small (224, 262, 265, 268).

Evidence for tonic sympathetic vasoconstriction in active muscles, based on measurements of NE spillover, is indirect and is still sometimes opposed by a view that NE is rendered ineffective by metabolites in active muscle; that is, a putative "functional sympatholysis" inhibits vasoconstriction in dogs (e.g., 248) and in cats (159) (see Chapter 16).

Competition between Neural and Metabolic Control. The idea that metabolic vasodilation can prevent adrenergic vasoconstriction, either by blocking the postjunctional actions of NE or by prejunctional inhibition of NE release from sympathetic varicosities, has been challenged by numerous findings (59, 162, 228, 280, 346). Nevertheless, in sufficient concentrations, potassium and hydrogen ions, adenosine, and hyperosmolarity can impede neuronal release of NE (312, 352).

High rates of metabolism in canine muscle (predominantly red, oxidative fibers) do not override vasoconstriction caused either by direct electrical stimulation of sympathetic nerves (e.g., 59, 346), or by reflex activation of these nerves (228). For example, carotid sinus occlusion in exercising dogs (baroreflex) reduced hindlimb vascular conductance, and this reduction increased with severity of exercise even though the pressure stimulus at the carotid sinus appeared to be constant (228). Also, the degree of vasoconstriction caused by NE infusion is also increased by exercise (280). Presumably, tension developed by vascular smooth muscle increases as its initial fiber length increases with vasodilation. Nevertheless, during *severe exercise*, a slight blunting of sympathetic vasoconstriction may occur in dogs (162). Beaty and Donald (16) also showed that the initial potassium release from active muscle can cause some transient suppression of vasoconstriction early during exercise. Nevertheless, vasoconstriction was far from being abolished [for review, see Britton and Metting (39) and Shepherd (312)].

Some causes of disagreement concerning the blunting of vasoconstriction by metabolites have recently surfaced. Although Burcher and Garlick (40) found no blunting of vasoconstrictor responses to either neurogenically released or infused NE in dog muscle perfused with blood at a Po_2 of 17 mm Hg, elevation of blood potassium levels by infusion abolished the neurogenic vasoconstriction but not the response to infused NE. The presumption was that potassium suppressed NE release from sympathetic varicosities but the infused NE could still act normally on the α-adrenoceptors. This conclusion rested on the assumption that neuronally released NE acts on the same α-adrenoceptors as NE carried in blood. Subsequently, a counterview was that the different effects of neuronally released NE and exogenous NE stem from the fact that NE from the two sources acts on different subtypes of α-adrenoceptors (for references, see 3, 57, 77, 223).

Although the resistance vessels of skeletal muscle contain both α_1- and α_2-adrenoceptors, small terminal arterioles that serve as "precapillary sphincters" have predominantly α_2-adrenoceptors (77, 223). The larger arterioles that control vascular resistance are preferentially stimulated to vasoconstrict by neuronally released NE, which acts primarily on their α_1-adrenoceptors to cause vasoconstriction. These receptors are less susceptible to metabolic inhibition than are α_2-adrenoceptors, which dominate control of terminal arteriolar diameter and thus regulate capillary perfusion rather than total vascular resistance. Thus, the ideal site for any "sympatholysis" would be on these terminal arteriolar α_2-adrenoceptors and not on the α_1-adrenoceptors of the major resistance vessels.

A recent finding is that sympathetic innervation of resistance vessels in white (glycolytic) fibers of rat gastrocnemius muscle acts mainly via α_2-adrenoceptors; vasoconstriction in this muscle is blunted by increased metabolism, as shown in Figure 17.11 (345). Vasoconstriction persisted in red (oxidative) soleus muscle in which NE acts on the predominant population of α_1-adrenoceptors. Canine muscle is dominated by oxidative fibers and α_1-adrenoceptor control of vascular resistance, so that "sympatholysis" probably does not occur in this species. Note that Thomas et al. (345) assumed that MBF rose only in the muscle attached to the force transducer and not in the unattached muscle when both were activated by sciatic nerve stimulation. Their conclusions may only be correct if this assumption is true.

A major problem in assessing the effects of metabolism on vasoconstriction stems from the misleading effects of changing baselines (175, 224, 280). Vascular conductance reflects the magnitude of active changes in blood flow and vascular tone, whereas resistance does not. When MBF is high, the same degree of vasoconstriction causes large changes in vascular conductance and only small changes in resistance, but of course the effect on SAP is the same. Kjellmer (159) observed a diminishing rise in muscle vascular resistance in response to sympathetic nerve stimulation during exercise; however, the same data replotted as vascular conductance reveal no effect of exercise on the reduction in conductance (see Fig. 10 in 267).

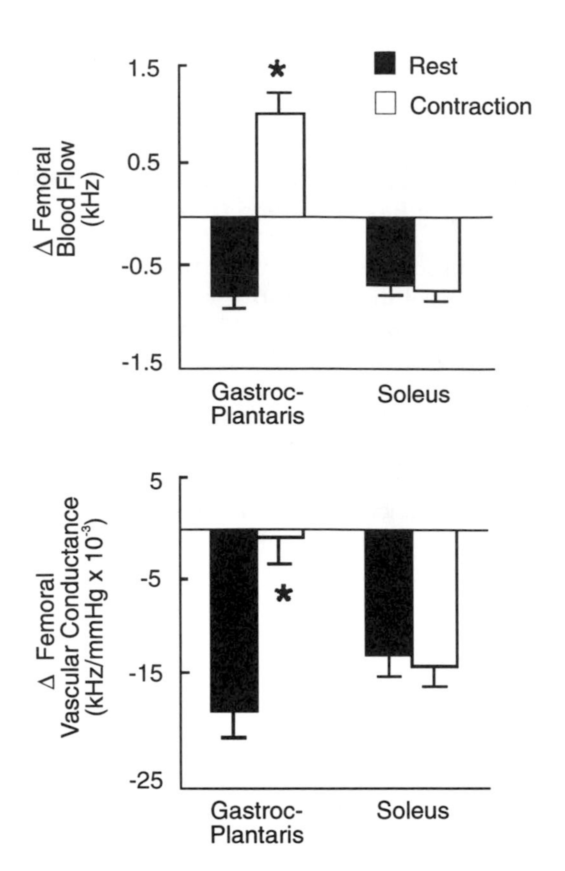

FIG. 17.11. Differential responses to lumbar sympathetic nerve stimulation during rest and maximal contractions of rat gastrocnemius-plantaris and soleus muscles. During contractions of the gastrocnemius-plantaris, sympathetic stimulation had no effect on femoral vascular conductance so that blood flow rose passively with a sympathetically mediated rise in SAP. Vasoconstriction was prevented by the dominance of metabolite-sensitive α_2-adrenoceptors in this glycolytic muscle. Conversely, the dominance of metabolite-insensitive α_1-adrenoceptors in oxidative soleus muscle is revealed in the maintained vasoconstriction and fall in femoral vascular conductance during sympathetic stimulation combined with muscle contraction. A potential problem in interpreting these results is noted in the text. [From Thomas et al. (345) with permission.]

The fact that vasoconstrictor control of MBF is effective and persists at all levels of exercise [accepting that there can be marked inhibition in muscle with predominantly white, glycolytic muscle during severe exercise (345)] is of paramount importance to understanding what is regulated and how in Part II.

Experimental Blockade of Sympathetic Nerve Supply to Active Muscle. Generalized loss of sympathetic control due to dysautonomia (23, 199), systemic ganglionic blockade with hexamethonium (314), and reflex inhibition by carotid sinus hypertension (355) all lead to marked vasodilation of active muscle during mild to heavy exercise. This is in conflict with one study in which acute ablation of sympathetic nerve supply to a limb had no effect on muscle vascular conductance during exercise (59).

Effects of acute surgical ablation of sympathetic nerves supplying active muscle. Donald et al. (59) denervated acutely the sympathetic nerve supply to one hindlimb in dogs. Denervation did not change blood flow to that limb in comparison to the flow in the intact contralateral limb during five 3 min periods of mild to severe graded exercise. Thus, vascular conductance of working muscle in dogs appeared to be closely regulated by local factors in proportion to metabolic demands but not by sympathetic nerves. In contrast, Peterson et al. (237) found that after acute sympathectomy of hindlimbs in rats, hindlimb MBF (microsphere technique) was about the same in both normal and denervated states for the first 2 min of exercise. After MBF reached a peak value, the flow then fell to a lower level in the innervated leg, but in the denervated leg MBF never fell and remained at the peak value throughout exercise (15 min).

Reflex inhibition of SNA. When Vatner et al. (355) reflexly inhibited SNA by electrical stimulation of the carotid sinus nerve, iliac vascular conductance in dynamically exercising dogs rose markedly. The interpretation was that mimicking carotid sinus hypertension reflexly withdrew sympathetic vasoconstrictor outflow to active muscles.

Strange et al. (336) conducted a similar experiment on humans during exercise requiring 40%–88% of $\dot{V}O_{2max}$ to assess the potential importance of arterial baroreceptors in maintaining vasoconstriction in active muscle during moderate to severe exercise. They applied pulsatile negative pressure (−50 mm Hg) over the carotid sinus to simulate carotid sinus hypertension. Sympathetic vasoconstriction competed with local vasodilation over the entire range of $\dot{V}O_2$, and this vasoconstrictor tone is withdrawn by arterial baroreceptor stimulation during moderate to heavy exercise (but not peak exercise, for unknown reasons).

With the exception of one study (59) the above experiments all point to the existence of tonic sympathetic vasoconstrictor outflow to active muscle during exercise. The source of conflict with Donald and colleagues' (59) results remains a puzzle.

Anesthetic blockade of SNA. Figure 17.12 reveals the magnitude of vasoconstrictor bias during rest and graded rhythmic exercise with small (forearm) muscle groups before and after stellate ganglion blockade (see also 190). Initially, the higher blood flow after blockade could simply result from the loss of tonic vasoconstriction normally present in muscle at rest (and probably not in skin at neutral temperatures) (e.g., 257, 311). The lower levels of blood flow in the sympathetically intact limbs at high rates of work (which even appear to reduce $\dot{V}O_2$) suggest that additional vasoconstrictor tone was introduced by exercise. The effect on $\dot{V}O_2$ shown in Figure 17.12 is unexpected and puzzling (141).

Pharmacological blockade of SNA. Recent studies of adrenoceptor types and location in skeletal muscle

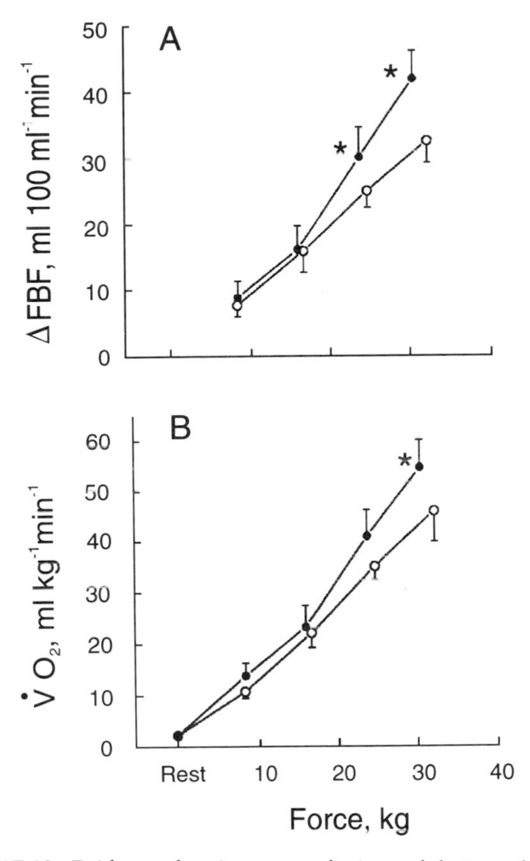

FIG. 17.12. Evidence showing sympathetic modulation of both muscle blood flow and $\dot{V}O_2$ in rhythmically contracting human forearm muscles. *A*, Forearm blood flow (FBF) before (*open circles*) and after (*solid circles*) stellate ganglion block, measured as changes from resting flow before and after nerve block. *B*, Forearm $\dot{V}O_2$ (from calculated arterial and measured deep venous O_2 contents and FBF) also rose with higher forearm blood flow, suggesting that $\dot{V}O_2$ had also been depressed by tonic SNA before blockade. $^*P < 0.05$. [Adapted from Joyner et al. (141) with permission.]

microvasculature (e.g., 3) reveal why use of traditional α-adrenoceptor blockers has not clarified the importance of sympathetic vasoconstriction in active muscle. Figure 17.13 shows that autonomic blockade with hexamethonium and atropine has an effect on total vascular conductance in exercising dogs that is similar to that observed in humans with dysautonomia (23, 199, 314). Despite the mimicking of normal cardiac output by electrical stimulation of the ventricles (the mimicking was imperfect during only the first 20–30 s in Fig. 17.13), SAP fell markedly while both total and hindlimb vascular conductance rose. Another surprise was that muscle vascular conductance rose more during mild exercise (4 mph, 0% grade) with autonomic blockade than it rose duiring exercise at 4 mph, 20% grade without blockade [some have clearly been wrong about the lack of tonic vasoconstriction in exercising dogs (e.g., 262, 265)].

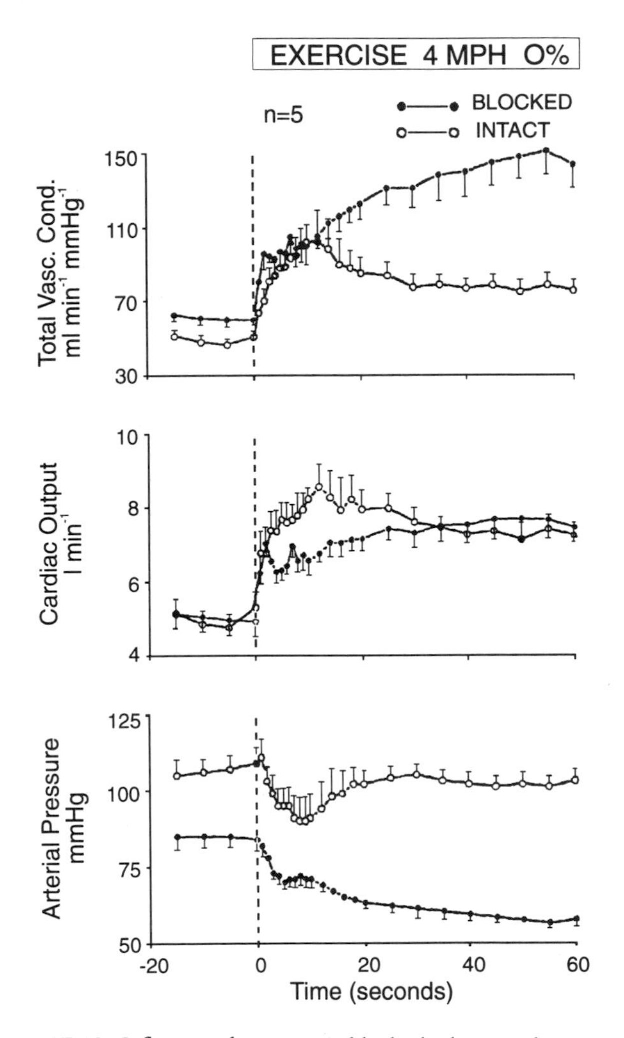

FIG. 17.13. Influence of autonomic blockade (hexamethonium + atropine) on the hemodynamic responses to mild treadmill exercise in dogs. Despite the maintenance of normal cardiac output by ventricular pacing (after ~30 s), arterial pressure fell to 55 mm Hg during mild treadmill exercise after autonomic blockade (*solid circles*). Total vascular conductance (and hindlimb vascular conductance, not shown) continued to rise 60 s after blockade. Conversely, conductance fell after reaching a peak near 10 s when sympathetic nerves were not blocked (*open circles*). [From Sheriff et al. (314) with permission.]

Additional evidence for significant vasoconstriction in active muscle of dogs, even during mild exercise, is the fall in vascular conductance at approximately 10–15 s after the onset of mild exercise (note the recovery of SAP at the same time) (Fig. 17.13). This fall in conductance, or vasoconstriction, is reversed to vasodilation by autonomic blockade (see Fig. 3 in 237).

To summarize, Figure 17.13 reveals two things: (*1*) The fall in muscle vascular conductance ~10 s after an initial overshoot at the onset of exercise must have been mediated by sympathetic vasoconstriction because autonomic blockade prevented it; and (*2*) there was significant tonic sympathetic vasoconstriction in active muscles even during mild exercise (see also 227). Without this constraint, muscle vascular conductance rises to levels observed during much heavier exercise. The cause of the continued vasodilation of active muscle after removal of sympathetic restraint is presumably not an accumulation of metabolites because exercise was mild and cardiac output (and presumably MBF) was maintained by pacing. Also, this vasodilation appears to progress over a period of minutes in dysautonomia patients based on the time course of SAP (23, 199). Recently, MSNA (peroneal nerve) was observed to rise ~100% over 30 min of rhythmic isotonic forearm exercise without any indication of a metabolic stimulus based on ^{31}P-NMR spectroscopy (14).

Role of endothelial relaxing factors. Does tonic sympathetic vasoconstriction normally restrain endothelial-mediated vasodilation? Are the actions of endothelial-derived relaxing factors (EDRF) so great that their effects on muscle vascular conductance must be counteracted by sympathetic vasoconstriction in order to maintain SAP? Bear in mind that if this is the case, the sympathetic nervous system is correcting a mismatch between blood flow and vascular conductance—a pressure error—during exercise and not a mismatch between blood flow and metabolism—a metabolic error.

An increase in blood flow velocity and shear stress on the vascular endothelium elicits release from the endothelial cells of factors that relax vascular smooth muscle (115, 164, 166, 213). The rise in shear force during the early seconds of exercise might activate release of nitric oxide and prostaglandins. Without subsequent opposition to these relaxing factors by neuronally released NE, muscle vascular conductance might simply continue to rise. In dogs, the rise in vascular conductance shown in Figure 17.13 was not affected by blockade of nitric oxide formation by L-nitroarginine methyl ester (L-NAME) (226 and D.D. Sheriff, unpublished observations), suggesting that nitric oxide (or a related nitroso compound) did not contribute to vasodilation of active muscle. Recent evidence indicates that when shear stress releases EDRF, it relaxes not only the larger conducting arteries, but also the small arterioles that dominate regulation of muscle vascular conductance as well (167).

In canine skeletal muscle, this flow-mediated vasodilation can be blocked by inhibitors of prostaglandin synthesis (165). Continual endothelial release of both nitric oxide and prostaglandins in rabbit femoral arteries is increased by shear stress, but higher shear rates may be required to release prostaglandins (115). Both endothelial factors apparently counteract neurogenic and myogenic vasoconstriction in vivo. The issue is whether this local vasodilation is unmasked by autonomic blockade in exercising dogs.

Attempts to uncover significant participation of nitric oxide in regulation of MBF in humans and dogs revealed that *N*-monomethyl-L-arginine (L-NMMA) approximately halved resting forearm blood flow (FBF) during postexercise hyperemia immediately after rhythmic forearm contractions (377). When these investigators blocked prostaglandin production with indomethacin in the same basic experimental design, human FBF was reduced by 10%–20% during postexercise hyperemia (376). In dogs, L-NAME lowered hindlimb blood flow during mild exercise but not during more severe exercise (sympathetic nerves intact). Nevertheless, hindlimb vascular conductance was reduced by a small but constant amount across work rates (226).

The rise in total and hindlimb vascular conductance after autonomic blockade is not simply due to the loss of resting sympathetic vasoconstrictor tone but must also involve the elevated MSNA in exercise. The effect on total vascular conductance, although large at rest (190), can explain neither the entire rise in conductance nor its gradual increase during exercise after autonomic blockade. Furthermore, the effect of sympathetic blockade on MBF increases with severity of exercise [see Fig. 17.12; (141)].

Summary: Importance of Balance between Neural and Mechanical Factors

Defective venous valves. With neural control of the circulation intact, loss of effective pumping action in muscle due to either damaged or absent venous valves leads to well-known loss of exercise tolerance (22, 102). This stems mainly from marked reductions in SV and cardiac output. When exercising patients with absence of valves in deep veins of the legs shifted from supine to sitting position, SV fell 35% below the value during supine exercise (undoubtedly it was also subnormal during supine exercise as well). In persons with normal venous valves, the postural difference in SV during exercise is only about 10% (20).

Absence of vasoconstriction. The absence of splanchnic vasoconstriction to oppose passive increases in blood flow and blood volume of this region associated with increased SAP depletes central or thoracic blood volume and lowers CVP and SV. The ability to raise cardiac output is diminished.

In skeletal muscle, absence of vasoconstriction during exercise allows muscle vascular conductance to rise unopposed and thereby becomes the main cause of hypotension after normal sympathetic function is lost. Skeletal muscle, respiratory, and abdominal "pumps" can delay and diminish the ensuing hypotension somewhat but cannot prevent it. The defect is evident in both supine and upright exercise, but the magnitude and speed of onset of hypotension are greatest in upright posture.

Balance between vasoconstriction and compliant vs. noncompliant regions. How is it possible to increase cardiac output four- to sevenfold without depletion of thoracic blood volume and reduction in left ventricular filling? The muscle and respiratory pumps have to increase thoracic blood volume and ventricular filling pressure, while the sympathetic nervous system acts to control the distribution of blood flow and therefore blood volume between active muscle and compliant regions (e.g., splanchnic and cutaneous). In effect, the sympathetic nervous system must optimize the ratio of blood flows through noncompliant circuits (C_2 in Fig. 17.14) to flows through compliant regions (C_1 in Fig. 17.14). Therefore, the maintenance of SV and cardiac output during exercise requires a balance between mechanical actions of the muscle pump and sympathetic control of blood vessels; the maintenance of SAP depends critically on tonic sympathetic control of blood vessels in active skeletal muscle.

Concepts regarding reflex control of the circulation during exercise have traditionally centered mainly on reflexes thought to increase MBF so as to prevent accumulation of metabolites within the muscle owing to deficient washout. Thinking has not focused on reflexes that are required to prevent excessive vasodilation in active muscle—particularly during mild to moderate exercise. In Part II, we ad-

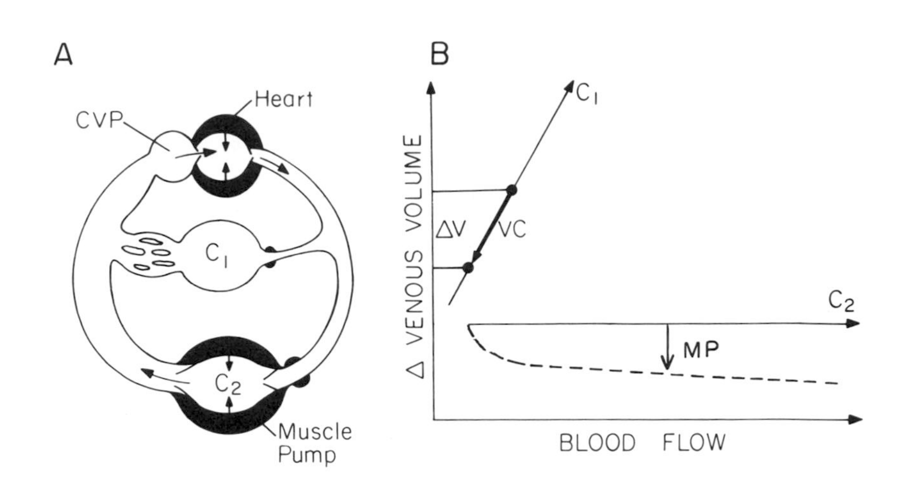

FIG. 17.14. *A*, The volume of blood available to fill the heart depends on the distribution of blood flow between compliant (C_1) and noncompliant (C_2) circuits. In exercise, active muscle [noncompliant circuit (C_2)] becomes another pump actively returning blood to the heart. Cardiac filling pressures are determined by effectiveness of muscle pumping and sympathetic control of other circuits (e.g., C_1); that is, in effect the ratios of blood flows through C_1 and C_2. *B*, The relationship between venous volume and blood flow in a compliant (C_1) region (e.g., splanchnic or skin) and a noncompliant region (C_2) (e.g., muscle). Line C_2 shows no increase in venous volume with increased perfusion of resting muscle. *Dashed line with arrow* shows that muscle pump (MP) reduces venous volume. [Adapted from Rowell (268) with permission.]

dress the question: Does the autonomic nervous system normally correct primarily "flow errors" or "pressure errors" or both, during dynamic exercise?

II. REFLEX CONTROL OF THE CARDIOVASCULAR SYSTEM DURING DYNAMIC EXERCISE

WHAT VARIABLES ARE SENSED AND THEN REGULATED BY THE AUTONOMIC NERVOUS SYSTEM DURING DYNAMIC EXERCISE?

Part I described basic properties of the cardiovascular system and their modulation by mechanical and neural factors. Part II analyzes how these neural factors are controlled and how their control modifies the cardiovascular responses to exercise. A key issue concerns the reflexes that might control sympathetic vasoconstrictor outflow to active muscle and other organs. What is regulated, SAP or blood flow? What regulatory errors are detected and how are they sensed? How are they corrected and how well are they corrected? Perhaps these are the most basic questions one can ask about how the entire cardiovascular system works.

The above questions are specifically directed to how an entire system functions when demands placed upon it are the greatest ever experienced (i.e., in exercise). Sir Joseph Barcroft (1934) emphasized the great importance of forcing a system to perform its function at high levels in order to understand better how it works. These are also the kinds of fundamental questions that typify integrative systems physiology. They are unanswerable at cellular or molecular levels at which different classes of important problems are addressed.

Questions concerning what might be the primary errors sensed and corrected by the autonomic nervous system will distill down to two main potential errors, "flow errors," caused by mismatches between blood flow and metabolism (or body temperature), and "pressure errors," caused by mismatches between cardiac output and vascular conductance. Another error discussed in Chapter 10 is similar to the flow error above, but the mismatch may be between blood flow or oxygen delivery and muscle force development (which is proportional to oxygen demands). In addition to the correction of these "errors," the central command hypothesis has stimulated thinking about a feedforward control that is modulated by feedback from synergistic reflexes.

Central Command

A centrally generated motor command signal that simultaneously activates somatomotor and cardiovascular motor systems at the beginning of exercise was examined in Chapter 9. Three main points are summarized below.

A Central Hypothesis. Central command has been hypothesized to act through cortical and spinal motor systems and "to set the basic patterns of effector activity, which are in turn modulated by baroreceptors, muscle mechanoreceptors, and muscle chemoreceptors [actually chemosensitive afferent fibers] as error signals may develop" (263).

Parasympathetic vs. Sympathetic Actions. Current evidence attributes the initial major cardiovascular effect of a central command signal to the parasympathetic nervous system. This generalization originates from the observed responses to an attempted static handgrip contraction when the forearm muscles were either paralyzed by succinylcholine (88) or tubocurarine (358). Attempts to contract were accompanied by increases in HR, cardiac output, and SAP. This initial rise in HR and SAP during the first few seconds of the attempt (whether contractions occurred or not) was blocked by atropine and was unaffected by propranolol (88, 192, 200, 358).

The idea that central command signals do not significantly raise SNA originates from observations that MSNA shows little or no increase during a mild voluntary static contraction (197, 307) or an attempted contraction after neuromuscular blockade (358). In these studies the duration of the contraction and the attempted contraction (which ended with "near-maximal" motor effect) was ~2 min. Overall, these studies suggested that central command exerts its primary influence (at least in the first 2 min of static contraction) on parasympathetic outflow to the heart rather than on SNA to blood vessels. Presumably the increase in HR and cardiac output by vagal withdrawal produces the initial increase in SAP. If these generalizations are correct, and apply as well to dynamic exercise, then the control of SNA during dynamic exercise may best be sought in reflexes providing feedback rather than feedforward control of SAP and/or blood flow. Note, however, in our later discussion of central command and baroreflexes (see later under ROLE OF CARDIOPULMONARY BARORECEPTORS IN DYNAMIC EXERCISE) that renal SNA rises immediately at the onset of dynamic exercise (54, 221) suggesting that the rise may be initiated by central command [others have suggested a muscle mechanoreflex (359)].

Feedforward Control with Feedback Control. Although central command provides a classic example of "feedforward control," its primary mode of action could still depend on a conventional feedback controller (127, 265, 268). Motor system signals, used to initiate both locomotion and feedforward actions on the cardiovascular system, could coordinate with feedback control by sending the feedforward command to a feedback controller (Fig. 17.15; (127)]. This latter command could, for example, "reset" the operating point of a major homeostatic reflex such as the arterial baroreflex. This idea has been reinforced by the observation that central command no longer raises SAP at the onset of exercise if baroreflexes are absent (see below).

Reflexes from Active Muscles

Muscle Chemoreflexes (Metaboreflexes). The term "chemoreflexes" is used here rather than "metaboreflexes" because a link between these reflexes and normal metabolism under free-flow, nonischemic conditions is not yet established.

The concept that underlies the muscle chemoreflex hypothesis is that any mismatch between blood flow and metabolism would change the intramuscular concentration of metabolites, which would be detected by chemosensitive afferent nerve fibers within the muscle. Through their afferent input into the central nervous system (CNS), this "flow" error would be corrected through autonomic nervous effects on cardiac output, vascular conductance, and SAP.

Chapter 10 presents the basic neurophysiological evidence supporting the concept that the group III

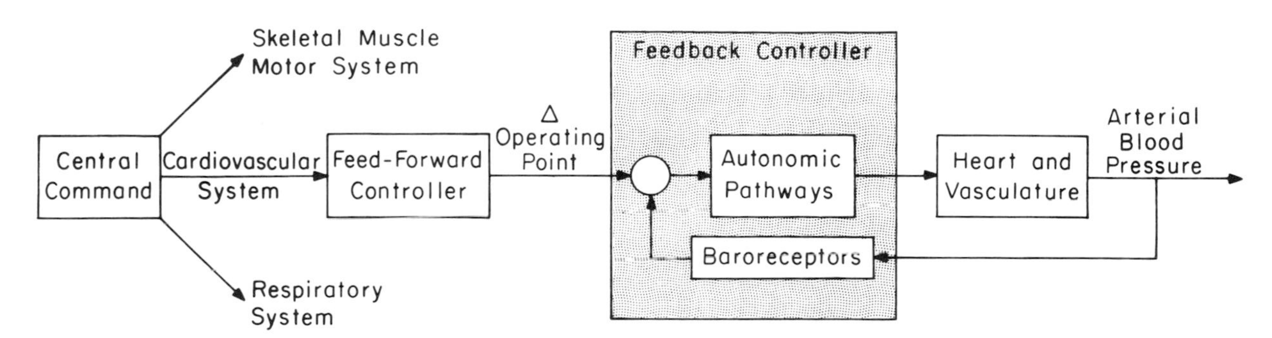

FIG. 17.15. A scheme for coordination of feedforward and feedback control of the cardiovascular system during exercise. Motor system signals used to initiate locomotion initiate feedforward actions (central command) on the cardiovascular system. Coordination with feedback control (the arterial baroreflex) is accomplished by sending the feedforward command to the feedback controller, which resets the operating point for arterial pressure regulation during exercise. [Adapted from Houk (127) and reproduced from Rowell (268) with permission.]

and IV afferent fibers in skeletal muscle are activated by substances generated by muscles whenever their blood flow is restricted during contraction so that delivery of oxygen and washout of metabolites are reduced. The reflex they cause is often referred to as the ischemic muscle pressor reflex. A major review of this topic was also published in 1983 (210).

Activators of group III and IV afferents. Infusions containing lactic acid (rather than sodium or lithium lactate), arachidonic acid, or potassium activate group III and IV afferents (260, 344). Effects of potassium are only transient even when interstitial levels are elevated and maintained by infusion (282). Lactic acid and some cyclooxygenase products along with bradykinin, which also releases prostaglandins from the vascular endothelium, can activate group III and IV afferents during electrically induced contractions (331). When the production of lactic acid was reduced by dichloroacetate in electrically stimulated cat muscle, discharge of group III afferents was reduced in proportion to the fall in venous lactate concentration (319).

Reflexes. Both chemical and mechanical stimuli activate group III and IV afferent fibers and raise SAP; the response is abolished by cutting the ventral roots (210). The rise in SAP appears to be achieved mainly by sympathetic vasoconstriction; effects on HR appear relatively small. The small effect on HR has been interpreted to mean that HR and sympathetic vasomotor activity are controlled differently during exercise [a view recently challenged (225)—see below].

The chemical changes in venous blood that best correlate with changing SAP during electrically induced static contraction are increases in lactic acid concentration and in P_{CO_2}, and decreased pH. Bradykinin and prostaglandins may also contribute (331, 332).

Caveats regarding interpretation. The value of the mechanistic studies, briefly outlined above, is unquestioned. They provide information about chemoreflexes uncontaminated by any influence of central command or reflexes of nonmuscle origin. However, there is room for misinterpretation. For example, the abnormal patterns of motor unit recruitment, of muscle contraction, and of force development caused by electrical stimulation can cause minor tissue injury. Release of bradykinin, prostaglandins, and other substances could be related to tissue injury and would explain the pain and soreness often experienced by humans after abnormal muscle contractions. Also, abnormal contraction can produce local regions of severe ischemia (266).

Release of "pressor substances" from active muscles is normally observed under conditions of restricted blood flow (i.e., during either electrically induced or voluntary static contractions). This is in contrast to the small (if any) changes in putative pressor substances normally seen during mild to moderate dynamic exercise with free flow. Restriction of blood flow not only raises venous concentration of muscle metabolites, it can also increase their production and thus their effects. This is especially true for substances that might be diffusion limited in free-flow conditions (the higher blood flow and shorter capillary mean transit time reduces time for diffusion out of the muscle into venous blood).

Mechanoreflexes. Substantial fractions of mechanosensitive afferents in muscle are also chemosensitive (210; see also Chapter 10). Conversely, many primarily chemosensitive afferents also respond to mechanical stimuli (146). Thus, group III and IV fibers (which are also temperature sensitive) are polymodal (161, 208).

Nonnoxious mechanical stimulation of receptor fields in the muscles activated most group III afferents and approximately one-third of the group IV afferents (147). Either stretch or compression of muscle will raise SAP by stimulation of group III and IV afferents (330). Furthermore, either compression or venous occlusion of the human forearm during static contractions raises MSNA during contraction, but not during postcontraction ischemia, suggesting the mechanoreceptor stimulation and not reduced blood flow was the stimulus (203, 204). A fraction of group III and IV afferents are also activated by electrically induced muscle contraction (146). The sensitivity of group III mechanosensitive afferents appears to be raised by contraction-induced increases in both cyclooxygenase and lipooxygenase products of arachidonic acid (261). Thus, prostaglandin and bradykinin described above could exert their reflex effects on SAP through their actions on either mechanosensitive or chemosensitive afferent fibers.

Firing pattern of group III and IV afferents during electrically induced static contractions suggest that group III afferents are only transiently active during the early seconds of contraction, whereas group IV afferents remain active throughout contraction (145). This is consistent with a predominantly mechanosensitive role of group III afferents and a predominantly chemosensitive role for the group IV fibers during static contraction. So far, insurmountable recording difficulties have prevented the registration of group III and IV nerve impulses during rhythmic contractions under free-flow conditions.

Hollander and Bouman (122) proposed the existence of a "muscle-heart reflex" mediated by mechanosensitive afferents that initiate a rise in HR at the onset of dynamic exercise in humans. Within 550 ms after beginning either a voluntary or electrically induced contraction (no central command), HR suddenly increased by vagal withdrawal. Yet anesthetic blockade of muscle afferents that is sufficiently complete to block the ischemic pressor reflex (and presumably mechanoreflexes) does not prevent the sudden rise in HR with exercise (87).

Muscle Thermoreflexes? Group III and IV afferents are thermosensitive, responding to increases in muscle temperature over a physiological range between 24° and 44°C; firing rates of both group III and IV fibers rose more than 50% over this temperature range (161). Muscle temperature is normally below 35°C in resting human limbs and can exceed 40°C during dynamic exercise. The rise in muscle temperature is proportional to muscle metabolic rate; accordingly, changes in muscle temperature could in theory bear a closer relationship to muscle's metabolic rate than would its interstitial metabolite concentration. The importance of muscle afferent thermosensitivity has not been studied. A key experimental problem is to manipulate the temperature in exercising muscle without the obscuring effects of high blood flow through warm muscle on central body temperature. This problem is solvable.

The Problem of Redundancy. More than one means of raising HR and SAP exists. This introduces the sometimes overwhelming problem of redundant control systems. Coactivation of multiple control systems during exercise may so far have masked the important role of any one system. Participation of any one system might be observed when all others are inoperative, or when extreme conditions such as muscle ischemia, or hypotension, call forth a dominant contribution from one controller. This offers a highly stimulating challenge for creative experimental design.

ISOMETRIC CONTRACTIONS: TESTING HYPOTHESES

Isometric contractions have been applied productively to the investigation of central command, but less so to understanding how muscle reflexes might function during dynamic exercise. An assumption underlying use of isometric contractions is that the dramatic rise in SAP they cause can be explained *(1)* by central command, which triggers the initial rise in HR and cardiac output (see Chapter 9 and above); *(2)* by chemoreflexes originating from contracting muscle made ischemic by muscular compression of blood vessels; and *(3)* by the growing indirect evidence for a contribution from muscle mechanoreceptors as well (14, 203, 204).

Extrapolation of concepts about regulation from responses to isometric contractions vs. responses to rhythmic isotonic contractions has caused confusion. This section uses isometric contractions as a framework to unravel differences caused by: *(1)* free-flow vs. obstructed or zero-flow conditions; *(2)* open-loop vs. closed-loop conditions, and *(3)* positive vs. negative feedback.

Isometric Contractions vs. Dynamic Exercise

Isometric contractions are characterized by a failure of the cardiovascular system to secure adequate blood flow to the muscle and consequently also by a mismatch among blood flow, vascular conductance, and metabolism. The sympathetic nervous system can correct the regulatory problems associated with dynamic exercise but not those associated with isometric contractions (268).

The striking differences in responses to these two forms of muscle activation are ascribable in part to their effects on MBF. Whereas the pumping action of rhythmic isotonic contractions increases blood flow at any given perfusion pressure, in isometric contractions MBF is reduced by twisting and shearing of vessels along with narrowing by compression of larger arteries and especially of veins as they exit the muscle (100).

The cardiovascular response to isometric contraction is exaggerated in relation to the small increase in $\dot{V}O_2$ (181). In contrast to earlier findings (180, 181), the rise in cardiac output appears to serve no useful purpose once contraction force exceeds ~15% of MVC and MBF is reduced by vascular compression (109). In isometric contractions, changes in cardiac output and/or blood flow, metabolism, and vascular conductance are not matched, whereas in dynamic exercise, they are well matched. During isometric contractions, the autonomic nervous system raises SAP by an exaggerated rise in cardiac output usually with little or no accompanying rise in total vascular conductance (see 180). The rise in SAP does not raise MBF in contracting muscles (109).

In marked contrast, during dynamic exercise the autonomic nervous system must prevent a fall in SAP in response to an enormous rise in total vascular conductance both by raising cardiac output and by vasoconstricting most major organs, especially active muscle. In short, the vasoconstriction in active muscle during dynamic exercise is essential to regulation of SAP and/or blood flow, whereas any vasoconstriction in isometrically active muscles (see below) would constitute a failure of regulation.

Open-Loop vs. Closed-Loop Conditions

Qualitative evaluation of the sensitivity, or "gain," of reflexes (see below) comes from experiments employing open-loop conditions. The term "open-loop" means that the primary feedback loop of the reflex has been eliminated, or opened, so that its receptors are isolated from and deprived of the feedback that counteracts the stimulus. In "closed-loop" conditions, the primary feedback loop is intact, or closed, so that the receptors are affected by the feedback that then counteracts the stimulus.

A common example of an open-loop experiment (described in detail later) is the isolation of the carotid sinus to study the gain of the carotid sinus baroreflex. The rise in SAP in response to a decreased pressure within the isolated carotid sinuses can do nothing to restore carotid sinus pressure. Similarly, the rise in SAP in response to occlusion of the muscle circulation by isometric contraction can do little to restore MBF—the conditions are "open-loop."

Cushing Reflex and Muscle Chemoreflex. A revealing analogy exists between the Cushing reflex and a muscle chemoreflex activated by isometric contractions (268). The Cushing reflex supposedly guards cerebral perfusion when intracranial pressure rises and reduces cerebral blood flow, as with bleeding into the cerebral spinal fluid (CSF) after head injury. The analogy is with the reflex that supposedly guards muscle perfusion when intramuscular pressure rises and reduces MBF during an isometric contraction. The two reflexes are the two most powerful blood pressure–raising reflexes known.

The stimulus for the extreme sympathetic activation and hypertension in the Cushing reflex is ischemia of vasomotor "centers" of the medulla. The hypertension increases cerebral perfusion pressure, which in turn increases bleeding into the CSF, and further raises CSF pressure and so on, around a vicious cycle of *positive feedback* ending in death. The feedback is positive because the correction for the "error" in cerebral blood flow winds up increasing the error.

The strength of the pressure-raising reflex initiated by isometric contraction is unknown because neither the input, muscle perfusion pressure past the obstruction to blood flow, nor the change in MBF is known. Experimental control of perfusion pressure and MBF to see the effect on SAP during isometric contraction to our knowledge has not been achieved.

The putative stimulus for the hypertension caused by isometric contraction is muscle ischemia. At moderate to high contraction forces mechanical impedance to MBF cannot be overcome by increased SAP. This describes an open-loop condition. If the reflex that presumably serves to restore MBF originates from chemosensitive afferents in the muscle, these afferents (i.e., "receptors") are isolated from any feedback (i.e., increased blood flow) that counteracts the stimulus.

The muscle chemoreflex is also a positive feedback reflex if, like the Cushing reflex, the response exacerbates the condition that initiated it. Evidence indicates that the rise in MSNA causes vasoconstriction within the isometrically contracting muscles (91, 110, 375). This potentially worsens the muscle ischemia and increases further the stimulus.

Does the Pressor Response to Voluntary Isometric Contraction have Chemoreflex or Mechanoreflex Origin?

When isometric contractions are voluntary, central command, chemoreflexes, and mechanoreflexes become factors in the responses. Increased SNA is directed to inactive muscle after a substantial delay [Fig. 17.9; (307, 361)]. MSNA to active muscle also increases as indicated by the parallel increments in both left and right peroneal nerve firing (MSNA) during static contractions of the ischemic left toes (110). Also, there appears to be vasoconstriction in active muscle (91, 375).

The rise in skin SNA at the onset of contraction appears to be primarily in sudomotor fibers (286, 362); skin blood flow increases (158). SNA to the heart must also increase to provide the marked elevations in cardiac output observed by Lind et al. (180). The mystery is how cardiac output could rise so much when the heart is essentially unassisted by a muscle pump during a static contraction and further, compliant regions are not vasoconstricted (158, 268). Even the most marked increase in ejection fraction should be unable to counteract the flow-induced fall in CVP. CVP was not measured but must have fallen eventually in these experiments because SV fell at the high cardiac outputs (see 180). Parenthetically, this fall in SV may provide a negative feedback that eventually limits the rise in SAP during severe isometric contractions (268).

Figure 17.16 summarizes how central command and muscle reflexes are thought to combine and exert their effects on the cardiovascular system during a powerful isometric contraction. The main hypotheses are as follows:

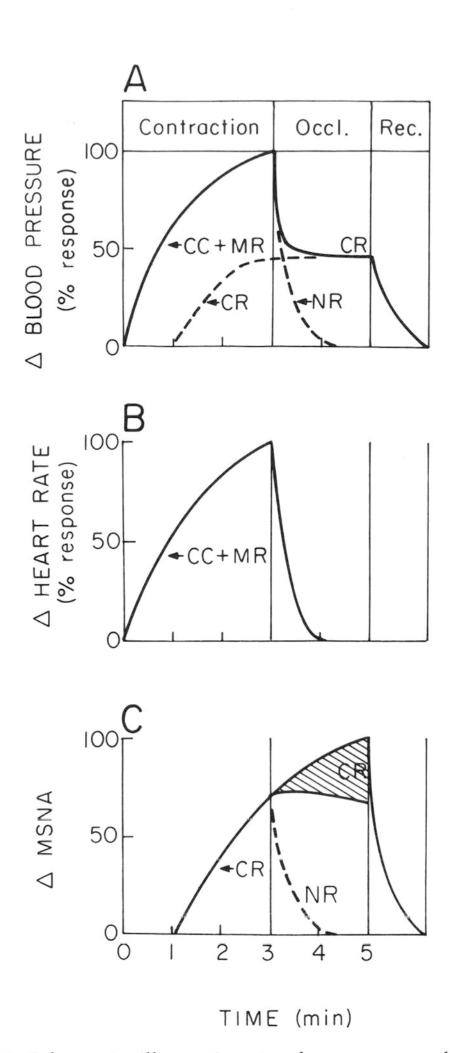

FIG. 17.16. Schematic illustration to demonstrate relative responses to central command (CC), muscle chemoreflex (CR), and muscle mechanoreflex (MR) during a powerful isometric contraction. *A*, Normal rise in arterial pressure is achieved initially by CC and some MR component. After about 1 min, CR may contribute to rise in pressure. Time course of CR is derived from ΔMSNA (arbitrary units) in bottom panel. Vascular occlusion (Occl.) of active limb at end of contraction prevents normal recovery (NR) of pressure. This is the test for a muscle chemoreflex. Pressure drops approximately 50% when CC ceases and is kept elevated by CR as long as ischemia persists. *B*, Heart rate is raised by CC (some MR?) via vagal withdrawal. C, MSNA is presumably increased by CR and remains elevated during postexercise ischemia (*shaded region* reveals variations in response). [Adapted from Rowell and O'Leary (275).]

1. The immediate rise in SAP and HR is initiated by central command (CC), which suddenly reduces tonic vagal outflow. Muscle mechanoreflexes (MR) could also play a role at this time. The rise in SAP appears to be caused by the increase in cardiac output (88, 180, 181, 192, 200, 358).

2. After a delay ranging from 30 s to 2 min, depending on force of contraction, MSNA, and also SNA to the heart rise [cardiac SNA rises a bit sooner (192, 200)] and contribute to the continuing rise in SAP. The rise in SNA, which is assumed to be caused by a muscle chemoreflex (CR), is presumably delayed by a gradual accumulation of metabolites brought on by obstruction of blood flow by the contraction.

3. Alam and Smirk's original test for a muscle chemoreflex in 1937 (see 181, 268) was a demonstration that SAP remained elevated after exercise stopped if blood and metabolites were trapped in the muscle by total vascular occlusion (see Chapter 10). During postexercise occlusion there is no longer central command; the rise in SAP is kept at 50% of peak value by increased SNA, presumably originating from muscle chemoreflex. Note in Figure 17.16 the recovery of HR and not SAP during occlusion.

It originally appeared that the HR response to isometric contraction was governed by central command, whereas SNA was governed by the chemoreflex (181, 210). However, after parasympathetic blockade with atropine, HR remains elevated along with SAP during postexercise ischemia as opposed to the rapid fall normally seen (Fig. 17.16). Furthermore, this rise in HR with atropine was reversed by β-adrenergic blockade (225). This signifies that SNA to both heart and blood vessels is under control of the muscle chemoreflex. Parenthetically, if this were not so, the chemoreflex could not function adequately during dynamic exercise because a rise in cardiac output is needed to restore a deficient MBF, as described below. HR normally fell during postexercise ischemia because sympathetic activation of the heart is normally overpowered by the dominance of vagal control of cardiac pacemaker activity (178). That is, when contraction (or exercise) stops, and both central command and its reduction of vagal activity end, the sudden restoration of vagal outflow lowers HR and overpowers the sympathetic activation of the heart by the chemoreflex. In short, when the vagus nerve is turned on, sympathetic effects disappear, and they reappear when the vagus is turned off (225).

Further evidence for chemoreflex origin of MSNA in humans comes from examination of isometrically contracting forearm muscles with phosphorous-31 nuclear magnetic resonance (^{31}P-NMR) spectroscopy (241, 320, 356). The rise in MSNA was closely associated with increments in intramuscular hydrogen ion activity presumably linked with lactic acid formation. Furthermore, MSNA did not rise during isometric contractions in patients who could not break down muscle glycogen and form lactic acid, owing to myophosphorylase deficiency (McArdle's disease) (241), or when lactic acid production was inhibited by dichloroacetate (76). Also, the human pressor response to postexercise muscle ischemia was blunted by glycogen depletion (323). The cause of the rise in MSNA may not actually be release of hydrogen ion per se, but rather the conversion of monoprotonated phosphate to its diprotonated form ($H_2PO_4^-$) (322).

In summary, hemodynamic conditions during isometric contractions do not permit the muscle chemoreflex to counteract the reductions in MBF that initiate this reflex. The chemoreflex cannot overcome the mechanical restriction of muscle perfusion and raise MBF; in fact, this reflex appears to vasoconstrict the active muscle and potentially worsen the ischemia. Alternately, when MBF is lowered during the normal, free-flow condition of dynamic exercise, the muscle chemoreflex presumably has the potential to restore MBF partially (depending on reflex gain) and correct the metabolic error signal. The next section examines this potential.

FUNCTIONAL IMPORTANCE OF MUSCLE CHEMOREFLEXES DURING DYNAMIC EXERCISE

The focus shifts here to the reflexes initiated during dynamic exercise, with and without restricted blood flow, from large masses of muscle. The two most important questions are: *(1)* Is the muscle chemoreflex a tonically active controller of the circulation during dynamic exercise under free-flow conditions? *(2)* Alternatively, is this reflex active only when MBF falls below a "critical level" defined in terms of adequate oxygen delivery?

Basic Concepts and Theory

One conceptual scheme has the muscle chemoreflex inactive during mild exercise, but MBF is so closely matched to metabolism that even a small decrease in MBF might reduce intramuscular P_{O_2} below a critical level. The consequent accumulation of lactic acid and other metabolites would constitute an error signal and initiate a chemoreflex. This reflex would correct this imbalance within limits permitted by the gain of the chemoreflex and the gains of any reflexes that reinforce or oppose it (e.g., baroreflexes). As exercise intensity approaches maximum, the margin for any flow error may be extremely small, and may even disappear, so that a persistent metabolic error signal could generate a tonically active chemoreflex (263). The basic hypothesis is that the muscle chemoreflex keeps MBF above a certain critical level that maintains an adequate supply of oxygen.

Changes in MSNA as Evidence for Chemoreflex Activity in Dynamic Exercise

Characteristics of MSNA during exercise in humans were recently reviewed by Seals and Victor (307). The changes in MSNA in response to dynamic exercise, with small (Fig. 17.9) and with large muscle groups (Fig. 17.10), are consistent with overall effects of whole-body exercise on the various indexes of SNA described in Figure 17.6. MSNA during dynamic exercise (cycling) appears not to increase above resting baseline levels until most vagal activity is withdrawn and HR approaches 100 bpm (176, 243, 287, 308, 361). Thereafter, MSNA (and NE spillover) rises in proportion to exercise intensity (308, 361), and also increases with exercise duration (14, 176). MSNA also rises in parallel with progressive degrees of forearm venous occlusion during rhythmic arm exercise (360).

As with isometric contractions, MSNA commonly rises only after a *delay* of about 1–2 min, depending on work intensity. This delay is reduced to less than 30 s during the most severe exercise at 80 W (Fig. 17.9). MSNA remains elevated during postexercise ischemia (Fig. 17.16) and the rise is proportional to muscle mass (302, 304). This latter feature plus the delayed increase in MSNA are assumed to signify that the muscle chemoreflex raised SNA, just as in static contractions.

The initial decline in MSNA found by Saito et al. [Fig. 17.10; (287)] and Ray et al. (244) appears not to be at odds with data shown in Figure 17.9. Before exercise, MSNA is elevated by orthostasis (seated upright); activation of leg muscle pumps during mild exercise immediately increases CVP, SV, and arterial pulse pressure [preference has been to attribute the decrease in SNA to a cardiopulmonary baroreflex (e.g., 244, 287)], but restoration of arterial pulse pressure is just as important (128, 138)]. This effect on MSNA was seen when one-leg dynamic exercise was initiated in upright (seated) posture, but not in supine position with CVP at normal resting levels (244). Furthermore, MSNA did not decrease in response to arm exercise in which muscle pumping has a much smaller effect on CVP [Fig. 17.9; (361)].

Saito et al. (287) placed their regression line through all data points relating delta MSNA to percentage, $\dot{V}O_{2max}$, and by so doing, argued there is no threshold for the rise in MSNA. They included in their analysis all points below 40% $\dot{V}O_{2max}$ at which MSNA was below preexercise control levels owing to the reversal of the orthostatic effects on CVP and MSNA by the muscle pump [as discussed above (see Fig. 17.10)]. Below this "threshold" point, the slope for the cluster of points could be zero, as would be expected after counteracting venous pooling, and as drawn in their revised figure (Fig. 17.10). A threshold for the rise in lactic acid could not be determined from their data [the authors estimated it was close to 45% $\dot{V}O_{2max}$, which is an unusually low threshold (e.g., see 202)].

In summary, during mild dynamic exercise, before HR reaches ~100 bpm and before SNA exceeds resting baseline values, control of the circulation could be dominated by central command signals that may act mainly on vagal outflow to the heart. Presumably, when exercise intensity becomes sufficient to raise muscle metabolite concentration and initiate a chemoreflex, SNA increases. This presumption is more or less an outgrowth of the control scheme proposed for isometric contractions; namely, central command dominates vagal control of HR and the muscle chemoreflex controls SNA. Note, however, that Fig. 17.6 reveals that all indicators of increased SNA during dynamic exercise first become apparent at work rates well below those that generate the putative stimulus for the chemoreflex (hydrogen ion or $H_2PO_4^-$).

Several important questions remain unanswered. Most measurements of MSNA have come from exercise with small muscle groups. Circulatory responses to dynamic exercise are much greater with small active muscles than with large ones at the same absolute $\dot{V}O_2$ (20). Saito and colleagues' (287) experiments are an exception (Fig. 17.10) and there is disagreement on what they show. Answers to the following questions are needed (275): *(1)* Is the delay in onset of MSNA related to active muscle mass as well as work rate? *(2)* Are the time courses of the rise in MSNA and SNA to other organs the same? *(3)* Does the rise in SNA to muscle have a stimulus that differs from that stimulating the rise in SNA to other regions?

Does the Muscle Chemoreflex Initiate Increased SNA during Dynamic Exercise with Unimpaired Flow?

Experiments Employing Anesthetic Blockade. It is possible to block the ascending traffic from muscle afferents to the CNS in humans by spinal or epidural anesthesia in order to discover any tonic influence of muscle reflexes on circulatory control during dynamic exercise. If the anesthetic blockade totally blocks the reflex, are the cardiovascular responses to exercise significantly altered?

Two types of experiments have been carried out with epidural anesthesia and only the main points are summarized here (see 209, 268, 272). In the initial study (87) two criteria were applied to discern complete blockade of the chemoreflex: *(1)* No pain in response to intramuscular injection of KCl in order to test complete group IV afferent fiber blockade, in addition to the standard criteria for sensory blockade; and *(2)* complete abolishment of the pressor response to postexercise ischemia. Unfortunately, it required total blockade of all motor and sensory fibers followed by several hours of recovery to satisfy criteria 1 and 2. Nevertheless the muscle chemoreflex could be completely blocked in only one-half of the subjects and only their data were reported. When motor function returned and sensory function and the pressor response remained blocked, cardiovascular responses to mild dynamic exercise were essentially normal. This suggested that the sensory fibers that mediate the chemoreflex are not essential for normal cardiovascular responses during mild exercise. However, the price of full blockade of chemoreflexes was marked motor weakness, meaning that the hypothesis could not be tested at higher levels of exercise where tonic effects of chemoreflex feedback should be more likely, and more obvious.

Examination of the role of chemoreflexes during higher rates of work was undertaken in a series of experiments by Secher's group in Denmark, reviewed by Mitchell (209). In their efforts to preserve motor strength, the muscle chemoreflex was only partially blocked despite the satisfaction of several standard criteria of sensory blockade (criterion 1 above was not used). Therefore, it was not possible to assess the importance of its effects without observing the responses when the reflex was totally absent. In short, both approaches were hampered by serious problems, not the least of which was blockade or reduction of SNA to the exercising legs by the anesthetic (the potential importance of these effects on muscle vascular conductance was not appreciated at that time). For example, this could explain the lower SAP observed by Fernandes et al. (78) during moderately heavy exercise (see also 337).

Experiments on dogs suggested that reflexes from active muscles are either not tonically active or exert no important influence during mild to moderate exercise (169). Lesions were made in the lateral funiculus of the lumbar spinal cord that avoided descending sympathetic and somatomotor pathways and selectively cut the ascending spinal pathway carrying afferent nerve traffic from the exercising hindlimbs (dogs were trained to exercise on a treadmill using only their hindlegs). Inasmuch as this lesion essentially eliminated the pressor response to hindlimb ischemia during exercise (occlusion of the left external iliac artery), but had no effect on responses to exercise without ischemia, reflexes from active muscles were not required for a normal circulatory response.

Functional Tests of the Chemoreflex Hypothesis and the Question of Tonic Feedback Control

Experimental approach. Returning to the analogy between the Cushing reflex and the muscle chemoreflex, Sagawa et al. (285) estimated the open-loop gain of the Cushing reflex by isolating cerebral arterial supply from the systemic circulation and by eliminating baroreflex opposition to the rise in SAP by sinoaortic denervation. Cerebral input pressure could be controlled at any level and be independent of the output, which was the effect of the reflex on systemic SAP. Open-loop gain was calculated as the change in SAP (the response) divided by the change in cerebral perfusion pressure (the stimulus).

Similarly, open-loop gain of the muscle chemoreflex was determined by reducing perfusion pressure and blood flow to active hindlimb muscles by graded partial terminal aortic occlusion and observing the extent to which the reflex raises SAP and restores hindlimb perfusion pressure (225, 227, 313, 315, 378). The findings are schematically illustrated and summarized in Figure 17.17, which shows effects of graded reductions in terminal aortic flow and in hindlimb perfusion pressure (femoral arterial pressure) on SAP during mild and moderate dynamic exercise. In the studies of both the Cushing reflex and the muscle chemoreflex, the determination of gain followed the convention in which input and output are the same physical variables expressed in the same units (e.g., 284, 298).

Open- and closed-loop gain of the muscle chemoreflex. The open-loop gain (G_{OL}) of the muscle chemoreflex was calculated as the change in SAP (ΔSAP) (the output or response) (less the increase in SAP due to mechanical effect of occlusion) divided by the change in femoral arterial pressure (ΔFAP) (the input or stimulus), as shown in the equation below.

$$G_{OL} = \Delta SAP/\Delta FAP \quad (1)$$

The maximal open-loop gain of this reflex is commonly found to be close to −2.0 (227, 313, 315). This gain can also be expressed as a closed-loop gain (G_{CL}), which represents the gain in the presence of feedback that counteracts the stimulus, as follows:

$$G_{CL} = G_{OL}/1 - G_{OL} = -0.67 \quad (2)$$

Gains are negative because the slope of output vs. input is negative. A G_{CL} of −0.67 indicates that with feedback, the muscle chemoreflex would correct by 67% the fall in femoral arterial perfusion pressure beyond the threshold for the reflex (Fig. 17.17). By comparison, the G_{OL} of the Cushing reflex is −7.7 with G_{CL} of −0.89, whereas G_{OL} of the carotid sinus reflex, for example, is also approximately −2.0 (e.g., 206, 313).

The Cushing reflex has a distinct threshold (285); beyond a particular decrease in perfusion pressure and cerebral blood flow, SAP rises markedly. As with the Cushing reflex, the chemoreflex in mild exercise has a wide margin for "flow error" and a distinct threshold beyond which SAP rises markedly. The rise in SAP in response to muscle ischemia is four times greater than that attributable to a simple mechanical effect of hindlimb occlusion on SAP (378). Also, the depictions in Figure 17.17*B* and *C* show that the "prevailing" terminal aortic flow (*point F*) and femoral AP were on the flat zero-gain portion of the chemoreflex stimulus–response curves, meaning that the reflex was not tonically active.

After sinoaortic denervation, when the muscle chemoreflex was unopposed by the arterial baroreflex, the open-loop gain of the muscle reflex approximately doubled, reaching values of −4 to −6 (G_{CL} = −0.8 to −0.86) (313) and rivaled that of the Cushing reflex (G_{CL} = −0.89) [see dashed lines (DNX) in Figure 17.17*B* and *C*).

Calculation of chemoreflex gain based on changes in SAP in order to estimate the sensitivity of a flow-raising reflex is not ideal. For example, both the Cushing reflex and the reflex from isometrically contracted muscle raise SAP but appear not to restore blood flow to the brain or active muscle, respectively (109). Inasmuch as dynamically active muscles are also vasoconstricted by the reflex (211), the gain, based on changes in SAP and femoral arterial pressure, does not reflect the ability of this reflex to restore MBF [the rationale for basing gain calculation on changes in SAP and in femoral arterial pressure, [i.e., in the same units (284, 298), was discussed further by Wyss et al. (378)].

The extent to which these increments in SAP can restore MBF in the dynamically exercising dog hindlimb rendered ischemic by partial occlusion was calculated as closed-loop gain (G_{CL}) with the following equation:

$$G_{CL} = [(TAQ_0 - TAQ_P)/(TAQ_I - TAQ_P)] \quad (3)$$

where TAQ_0 is steady-state flow during occlusion; TAQ_P is predicted flow during occlusion; and TAQ_I is initial steady-state flow before occlusion (231). During very mild exercise G_{CL} was zero. Once the threshold for the reflex was reached, closed-loop gain was −0.4 to −0.5 and remained there with increasing work rate (231). Thus, the reflex provided a 40–50% correction of the flow error when all baroreflexes were intact.

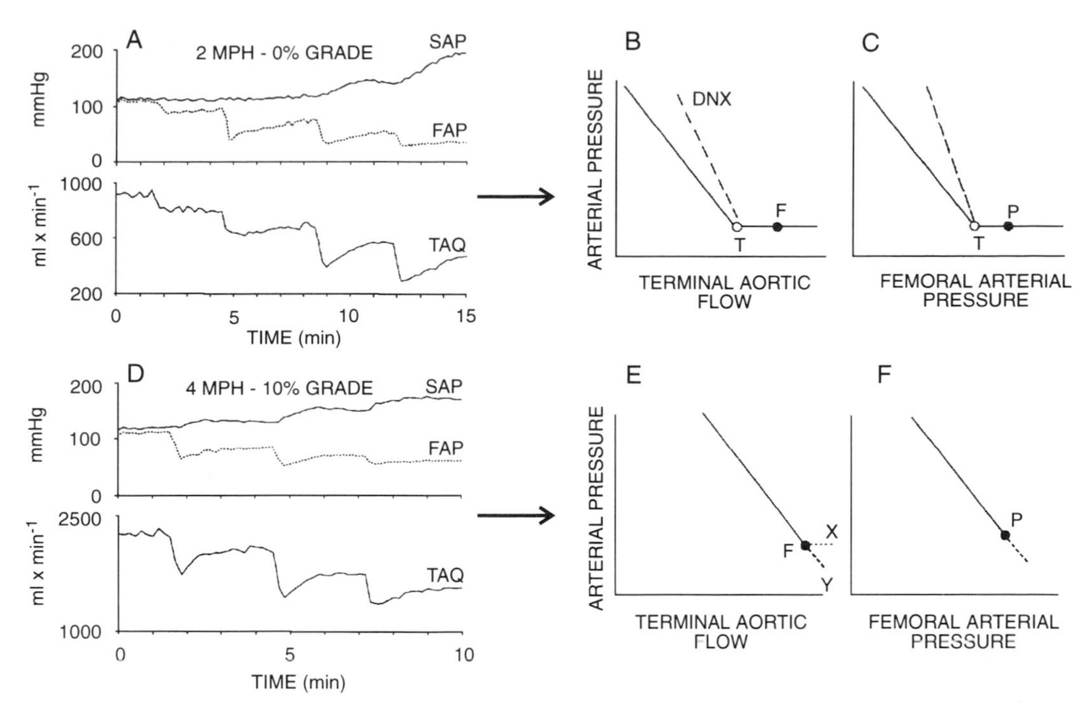

FIG. 17.17. Schematic illustration of responses to the muscle chemoreflex during mild and moderate dynamic exercise. *A*, Mild exercise. Graded partial occlusions of the terminal aorta of an exercising dog generate graded decrements in terminal aortic flow (TAQ) and femoral arterial pressure, but arterial pressure (SAP) will not rise, and TAQ will not be partially restored until the chemoreflex becomes active—which happens at the second through fourth occlusions. The rise in SAP causes an ~50% recovery of TAQ and femoral arterial pressure. *B* and *C*, Stimulus–response curves for the chemoreflex show that the reflex has a threshold (T). "Prevailing" TAQ (*F*, in *panel B*) and femoral arterial pressure (*P*, in *panel C*) represent their normal operating levels in exercise—which are on the flat (low-gain) parts of the curves. Therefore, the chemoreflex is not tonically active and SAP does not rise until TAQ and/or femoral arterial pressure fall below some critical level (at *T*). *D*, Moderate dynamic exercise. Shows characteristic responses of a tonically active muscle chemoreflex. *E* and *F* show prevailing TAQ and *P* are on (or just at) the steep (high-gain) portion of the stimulus–response curves and there is no threshold. Proof of tonic activity would require raising TAQ and observing if SAP fell (*line Y, panel E*) or stayed constant (*line X*). The *dashed lines* (DNX) (*B* and *C*) show the effect of arterial baroreceptor denervation on the gain (slope) of the chemoreflex. [Adapted from Rowell and Sheriff (279) and Rowell and O'Leary (275).]

During moderate exercise (Fig. 17.17*D*, *E*, and *F*) there was no apparent margin for flow error and thus no threshold for the reflex, but reflex gain was the same as for milder exercise (i.e., above levels where G_{CL} = 0) (313, 315, 378). Panel *E* suggests that the reflex could be tonically active but this is not established. *Point F* in panel *E* could be at the threshold and therefore not active until a slight decrease in terminal aortic flow occurs. If so, any rise in terminal aortic flow would abolish tonic activity and move *point F* off the reflex response slope and back on to a horizontal, zero-response line (shown by *dashed horizontal line x* in panel *E*), and SAP would be unaffected. Conversely, if the reflex were tonically active, a rise in terminal aortic flow would lower SAP along the steep stimulus–response curve (*dashed line y*). Therefore, the crucial (and difficult) test to show tonic activity is to *raise* terminal aortic flow during exercise.

Joyner and Wieling (142) tested for tonic action of the muscle chemoreflex on MSNA and SAP by raising human forearm blood flow. They applied suction (−50 mm Hg) to the forearm during rhythmic handgripping (30/min) at 40%–50% of MVC. The rise in forearm deep venous oxygen saturation, which suggested that MBF rose by ~20%, was accompanied by an attenuated rise in MSNA but no change in SAP. This attenuation persisted during postexercise occlusion (for normal response to occlusion, see Fig. 17.16*C*). These findings suggest that the chemoreflex was active during rhythmic forearm exercise so that when reflex feedback was reduced by higher MBF, the drive to raise MSNA was lessened, but the effect was too small to alter SAP.

Reflex gain and muscle mass. Open-loop gain of the muscle chemoreflex (based on the rise in SAP) appears to be a function of muscle mass. For example, the rise in SAP during muscle ischemia generated by postexercise occlusion is proportional to the mass of ischemic muscle (86). Also, increases in SAP and in MSNA are both roughly proportional to the mass of statically contracted muscle (302, 304), even when the contraction is taken to an end-point of fatigue (304). If one assumes that SAP and MSNA were increased by chemoreflexes in these experiments, then the reflex gain might be a function of muscle mass during dynamic exercise as well. The estimated open-loop gain of about −2 during dynamic exercise is based on experiments in which only about one-third of the total muscle mass (i.e., the dogs' hindlimbs) was made ischemic (225, 227, 231, 313, 315, 378). It is not known if this gain increases with severity of exercise, possibly as a consequence of the involvement of greater muscle mass. A direct proportionality to muscle mass could raise its open-loop gain to as high as −6 to −9 (with the baroreflex intact).

What Stimuli Elicit the Muscle Chemoreflex and what Explains its Threshold?

Dynamic exercise with restricted blood flow. The threshold for the pressor response (Fig. 17.17) was reached when oxygen delivery rate (terminal aortic flow times arterial oxygen content) fell below a critical level attended by increments in femoral venous hydrogen ion activity, lactate, and CO_2 concentration plus low oxygen content (315). That is, the metabolic events were the same as those later shown to raise SAP and MSNA during isometric contractions (241, 320, 356). When oxygen delivery was experimentally reduced by reducing arterial oxygen content, pressor responses and the rise in lactate and fall in pH occurred at higher blood flows, but at the same oxygen delivery rate as in control experiments. This constant threshold for oxygen delivery, irrespective of blood flow, suggests that the appearance of the "pressor substance" does not depend simply on flow-dependent washout of metabolites such as potassium, the femoral venous concentration of which was unrelated to the pressor response (315). Rather, rate of production and release of the substance depends on oxygen delivery and not blood flow per se. Furthermore, the rise in SAP in humans during partial occlusion of the working legs (supine cycling) by lower body positive pressure was well correlated with femoral venous pH and lactate concentration, and also with femoral venous P_{O_2} and O_2 content (277).

Dynamic exercise with unrestricted blood flow. Does the generalization that central command determines parasympathetic outflow, whereas the muscle chemoreflex determines SNA (as proposed for static contractions), apply to dynamic exercise? Lactate concentration normally does not rise in venous blood during dynamic exercise in humans until work intensity far exceeds that at which SNA starts to rise above resting levels [Fig. 17.6; (268, 275)]; that is, not until $\dot{V}O_2$ exceeds 50%–60% of VO_{2max} (202) or until HR exceeds 130–140 bpm. In physically well-conditioned individuals, whose sympathetic responses are also represented in Figure 17.6, blood lactate may not rise until exercise requires 80% or more of $\dot{V}O_{2max}$ and HR is above 160 bpm.

Another problem is that lactate appearance in humans during heavy dynamic exercise with unrestricted blood flow does not normally reflect deficient delivery of oxygen as it may in dogs. Because of the low oxidative capacity of human muscle (related to that of dogs), lactic acid is produced as soon as muscle glycolysis and glucose oxidation become a significant part of total oxidative metabolism (96). The appearance of lactate reflects the increased production of pyruvate and our limited ability to oxidize it, owing to low oxidative enzyme activity rather than to inadequate oxygen delivery (96).

It appears that some stimulus (or reflex) other than one indexed by H^+ or lactate activates the increase in SNA once HR approaches 100 bpm in humans during whole-body dynamic exercise. At least a metabolic error signal is not evident (268, 275).

Does Activation of the Muscle Chemoreflex Correct Blood Flow Errors, and if so, How?

Mild to Moderate Dynamic Exercise. There are two lines of evidence, one favoring a correction of blood flow by a chemoreflex, and the other arguing against it. Experiments on dogs have followed the experimental design shown in Figure 17.17.

Evidence for correction. Figure 17.17 shows little or no recovery of terminal aortic flow during initial occlusions, but after a threshold was reached, increases in SAP and cardiac output restore blood flow by approximately 50% (see equation 3). Wyss et al. (378) found that in mild exercise (at the threshold for the reflex), most of the rise in SAP was attributable to the increase in cardiac output. In moderate exercise SAP was elevated by similar contributions of vasoconstriction and increased cardiac output. Accordingly, the contribution of cardiac output to the restoration of MBF diminishes as the severity of exercise increases. Also, when the cardiac contribution to the rise in SAP during moderate exercise was prevented by β-adrenoceptor blockade, the gain of the reflex was reduced by 41% (225) [this is in contrast to the lack of effect of β-blockade on the pressor response to static contraction, at least one-half of which is attributed to central command (see 181)].

Mittlestadt et al. (211) observed a fall in the vascular conductance of exercising forelimbs in response to reduction in hindlimb blood flow in exercising dogs. Nevertheless, despite this vasoconstriction forelimb blood flow was greater after occlusion because the rise in SAP was proportionally greater than the fall in forelimb vascular conductance. Thus, vasoconstriction in active muscle need not reduce MBF below what it was before the reflex occurred—as long as cardiac output can rise.

In humans, graded reductions in leg blood flow were introduced by steps of lower body positive pressure at 25, 35, 45, and 50–60 mm Hg at levels of supine exercise requiring 1.0, 1.5, and 2.0 liters/min of oxygen. Reductions in leg blood flow were calculated from increments in femoral A-V_{O_2} difference (whole-body $\dot{V}_{O_2}$ was unaffected by the positive pressure). Inasmuch as percentage reductions in leg vascular conductance during occlusion exceeded by twofold reductions in leg blood flow, the muscle chemoreflex appeared to correct by approximately 50% the reductions in blood flow (but it was not possible to calculate the contribution of the purely mechanical effect of partial occlusion on SAP) (277). Approximately 50% of the correction of leg blood flow could be explained by the rise in HR (and in cardiac output assuming constant SV—see 265). The activation of sympathetic vasoconstriction by the chemoreflex was indicated by the rise in femoral venous NE concentrations along with rising SAP and falling leg blood flow (277).

Evidence against correction. Joyner (140) applied positive pressure (50 mm Hg) to the rhythmically contracting forearm muscles and reduced calculated forearm blood flow by 20%–25% based on the reductions in deep venous oxygen saturation. The resultant 20 mm Hg rise in SAP did not restore venous oxygen saturation, suggesting that any rise in SNA presumably elicited by the chemoreflex vasoconstricted the active muscles enough to prevent a rise in MBF. The crucial assumption was that the positive pressure did not decrease forearm $\dot{V}_{O_2}$.

Subsequently, Joyner et al. (141) blocked sympathetic nerves supplying the forearm and observed a rise in forearm blood flow above that of the intact forearm; this rise became progressively greater during higher rates of forearm exercise (Fig. 17.12). This release of vasoconstriction could signify that the muscle chemoreflex had been maintaining increased MSNA (and presumably causing the vasoconstriction) in exercising muscle as well as in resting muscle. They cautiously suggested, however, that a reflex that would reduce MBF so as to lower forearm $\dot{V}_{O_2}$ probably originates from a pressure-control system (arterial baroreflex?) rather than a flow-control system.

Severe Exercise—Positive Feedback? The muscle chemoreflex is more likely to be tonically active during severe whole-body dynamic exercise when venous oxygen content and P_{O_2} are low and lactate concentration is high. How can this reflex raise MBF when cardiac output approaches its maximum, and when active muscle comprises 85% of total vascular conductance, and also when vascular conductance of nonmuscle regions is minimum owing to maximal sympathetic vasoconstriction? In this setting the chemoreflex can only raise SAP by vasoconstricting active muscle because no other region has sufficient vascular conductance to influence SAP significantly.

Is the reflex a flow-sensitive, pressure-raising reflex with positive feedback because of its curtailment of MBF and its augmentation of the metabolic error signal? At present the only conceptual escape from this dilemma is to propose a chemoreflex that vasoconstricts the least active muscle so as to raise SAP enough to increase blood flow to the most active muscles (268, 275, 279). However, there is no known way to redistribute MBF in accordance with local metabolic needs by reflex control of MSNA. Nevertheless, the same effect might be achieved by local modulation of α_1- and α_2-adrenoceptor function within the muscle (as discussed above; see Fig. 17.11). An increase in MSNA during exhaustive exercise might curtail flow to oxidative muscle in which metabolite-insensitive α_1-adrenoceptors are dominant, whereas flow to glycolytic fibers in which metabolite-sensitive α_2-adrenoceptors dominate might be augmented despite constant or reduced total MBF [this would be unlikely in dogs because of the dominance of oxidative fibers (cf. 345)].

Another perspective concerning a hypothetical role for the chemoreflex centers on the potential for serious mismatches between cardiac output and total vascular conductance caused by outstripping the pumping capacity of the heart by muscle vasodilation (2, 250, 276, 370). This could happen in two ways, the first of which we have seen in people whose deficient vasoconstrictor control of MBF causes severe hypotension. The second way is to vasodilate more muscle than the heart can supply. In both cases active muscle must vasoconstrict to maintain SAP. Does the muscle chemoreflex initiate the vasoconstriction in active muscle necessary to maintain SAP?

Some have hypothesized that SAP and not MBF may be the primary variable that is sensed and regulated during severe exercise (268, 275). Although the muscle chemoreflex is effective in counteracting a restriction in MBF during mild to moderate exercise, its effectiveness as a reflex that keeps muscle vascular conductance from rising too high during exercise by initiating vasoconstriction is questioned. The error signal for a mismatch between blood flow and vascular conductance is pressure. The next section deals with control of SAP during exercise.

BAROREFLEX REGULATION OF ARTERIAL PRESSURE (SAP) AND VASCULAR CONDUCTANCE IN DYNAMIC EXERCISE

Does the Arterial Baroreflex Control SAP During Exercise?

The mechanisms by which SAP is controlled during exercise have been reviewed (65, 185, 268, 275, 298, 367). The perceived importance of baroreflex control of the autonomic nervous system during exercise continues to vary among investigators. This section examines some conflicting views and points out that both sides of a dispute may argue from the same data.

Perspective. In Part I of this chapter, it was indicated that one major function of the autonomic nervous system during mild to heavy exercise is to restrict muscle vasodilation so that its conductance does not rise enough to lower SAP. In Part II, we have analyzed the potential of the muscle chemoreflex to restore MBF (or SAP) when MBF is reduced below a critical level. But what reflex vasoconstricts active muscle, keeping it from either being overperfused or excessively vasodilated? This section offers the arterial baroreflex as a solution.

Ideas about the role of baroreflexes in circulatory control during exercise have oscillated between their having a central role to having no role (see 185). At one time the arterial baroreflex was thought to provide the stimulus for autonomic control of cardiac output and vascular conductance during exercise. The thinking was that sudden vasodilation of active muscle at the onset of exercise caused total vascular conductance to rise more rapidly than cardiac output. The consequent fall in SAP initiated the cardiac and vasomotor responses via the arterial baroreflex. This reflex was seen as being essential not only in restoring SAP but also in maintaining SAP during exercise in the face of an enormous and sustained elevation in total vascular conductance.

Arguments offered against this thinking were as follows: First, SAP does not always fall at the onset of exercise (cf. 269, 327) and does not fall during a transition from one severity of exercise to a higher one (123, 269), yet cardiac output and SAP still rise in proportion to work intensity. Second, when SAP does fall at the onset of exercise, it is somehow restored to levels exceeding those present before exercise began. Open-loop gain of the reflex would have to be infinite to correct by 100% the fall in SAP. Third, the observations that SAP rises above the preexercise level and that cardiac output and HR continue to rise along with SAP suggested that the baroreflex (which should oppose the rise in cardiac output) is turned off or greatly suppressed by exercise. One way around this third objection has been to propose that the stimulus–response curve for the baroreflex is shifted (or "reset") by exercise to a higher operating pressure so that the baroreflex now becomes the stimulus to raise HR, cardiac output, and SNA and SAP—in contrast to its "normal" role of opposing a rise in SAP. This idea has, until recently, been justifiably viewed with skepticism, because complete stimulus–response curves for the reflex had not been constructed in intact animals during both rest and exercise.

In general, these arguments have for decades offered a legacy of skepticism concerning the importance of the arterial baroreflex during exercise.

Evidence Indicating Reduced Baroreflex Sensitivity. In humans, the slope of the relationship of R-R interval to SAP is reduced by exercise in proportion to work intensity (38, 51). A recent reanalysis of these data also revealed some attenuation of the HR response as well by exercise (230). In addition, the lengthening of R-R interval was found to be greatly reduced during direct bilateral electrical situation of the carotid sinus nerves in humans during treadmill exercise (63); however, reductions in SAP were unaffected, as also noted by others (73). Staessen et al. (329) observed a progressive decline in the changes in SAP in response to positive pressure over the carotid sinus during graded supine exercise. Exercise intensity had much less effect on the change in SAP in response to positive than to negative neck pressure (329).

In dogs, sinoaortic denervation caused no obvious defect in the overall cardiovascular responses to moderate exercise; neither the level to which SAP rose nor its stability throughout moderate exercise were much affected (5, 170, 205, 351). Further, changes in SAP, HR, and cardiac output in response to sinusoidal changes in carotid sinus pressure in rabbits (aortic baroreceptors were denervated) were reduced slightly by exercise (185).

Evidence Indicating Unchanged Baroreflex Sensitivity. Many of those who have evaluated baroreflex sensitivity by examining the steady-state relationship between HR and SAP during mild to moderate exercise find that baroreflex control of HR is not affected (19, 230, 252). The transient effects of bolus drug injection or rapid neck suction on either HR or R-R interval miss the steady-state effects of maintained changes in SAP on the slower sympathetically mediated changes in HR (230) [the HR response to baroreceptor stimulation does appear to be blunted during severe exercise; see below (65, 233, 329, 336)].

Studies on either side of the argument that examined only the sensitivity of the HR response ignored the sensitivity of the vasomotor response that determines total peripheral resistance. The point is that:

baroreflex gain ∝ HR gain + total vascular resistance gain

As stated by Sagawa (283):

> control of HR does not reveal the quantitative or under some circumstances [e.g., exercise] even the qualitative ability of the baroreceptor reflex to control arterial pressure.

Note also that the substitution of HR for cardiac output in the above expression for gain assumes constant SV. The gains of the components do not simply add when cardiac output does not change in proportion to HR (186). Thus, determination of sensitivity or gain of the entire reflex response requires examination of both of its components, or more simply, the change in SAP (which includes both components) in response to a change in carotid sinus pressure. Also, the stimulus must be applied long enough to include sympathetic as well as parasympathetic effects on the heart.

In both humans and dogs, application of positive and negative pressure to the neck over the carotid sinus inhibits and activates, respectively, the carotid sinus baroreflex, and the reflex changes SAP by similar amounts during rest and mild to heavy dynamic exercise (19, 206, 233, 240, 336, 367) and even during isometric contractions (61, 185).

Finally, direct electrical stimulation of the carotid sinus nerves in dogs (355) and in humans (73) during rest and exercise elicited similar reductions in SAP (see also 63), HR, and regional vascular resistances. Thus, a preponderance of evidence points toward maintained baroreflex sensitivity.

Characterization and Analysis of Arterial Baroreflex Function

Baroreflex Stimulus–Response Curves—Definitions and Characteristics. This concise treatment of the characteristics underlying any quantitative description of baroreflex function cannot substitute for the superb review of this topic by Sagawa (283). The goal is to set the stage for discussion of how the arterial baroreflex might be modified by exercise and how this modification might permit the reflex to control the circulation during this stress.

Gain. The concept of open- and closed-loop gains was discussed earlier in a comparison of the muscle chemoreflex, the Cushing reflex, and the carotid sinus baroreflex. The carotid sinus reflex was used as a prototype to illustrate how open- and close-loop gains are determined experimentally—an approach brilliantly pioneered by Eberhard Koch in 1931 (see 65, 298). The value of gain derived from the change in SAP (output) caused by an isolated change in pressure within the carotid sinus (input) will be reduced substantially by aortic baroreceptors which will oppose the change in SAP. These baroreceptors must be denervated before maximum open-loop gain of the carotid sinus reflex can be determined.

Sensitivity. Sensitivity, like gain, also defines the slope of a curve relating independent and dependent variables, but often with input and output not being the same physical variable nor having the same units. For example, the change in heart interval, in milliseconds (output), in response to a change in SAP (input) caused by drug injection is used by some to estimate the HR sensitivity of the baroreflex in units of milliseconds per millimeter of mercury.

Sigmoidal Stimulus–Response Curves. The relationship between SAP and the pressure within the isolated carotid sinus over the full range of receptor firing is conveniently shown as a sigmoidal stimulus–response curve schematically illustrated in Figure 17.18. The curve has a *threshold* (*T*) and *operating point* (*OP*), which is the pressure at the receptor around which the reflex is regulating SAP, and finally there is a *saturation point* (*S*) at which further elevations in carotid sinus pressure cause no further lowering of SAP.

Data for baroreceptor function curves are traditionally fitted to a sigmoidal logistic function, although it is not clear that any units in the reflex, either separately or in combination, consistently show sigmoidal behavior (see 62, 283, 298). Plotting logistic functions does provide a means to evaluate baroreflex function curves according to theoretical schemes such as those presented in Figure 17.18. The sigmoidal curves represent a model of the system; however, a model is an hypothesis—it does not mean that the data actually take that form.

The Concepts of Set Point, Operating Point, and Resetting. "Set point" is a term borrowed from engineering and applies to a feedback system with on–

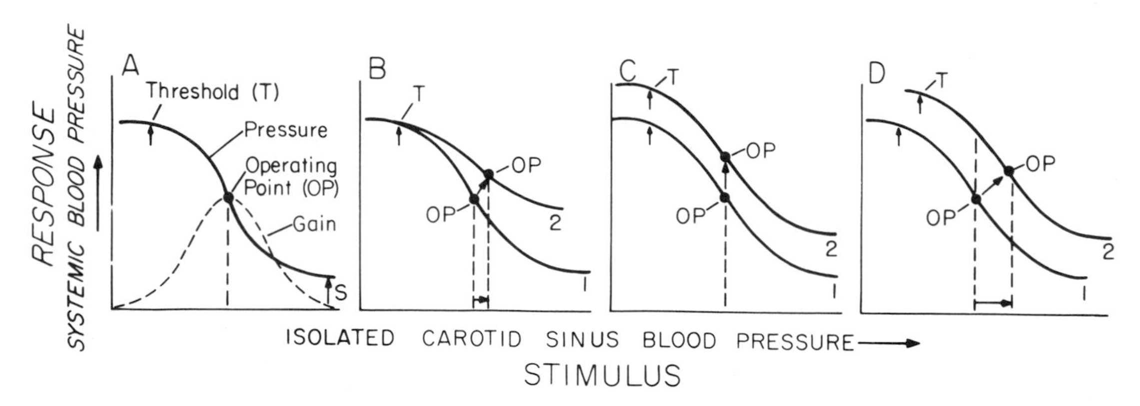

FIG. 17.18. Hypothetical stimulus–response curves (or baroreflex function curves) for the carotid sinus baroreflex. *A*, Important landmarks on the curves are defined (*S* marks point of saturation). *Dashed line* in *panel A* shows the gain or sensitivity of the reflex over the slope of the curve. Point of maximum gain is sometimes taken as putative baroreflex operating point. *B*, Illustrates decrease in the baroreflex gain or sensitivity (curve 1 to curve 2) in which operating point (*OP*) and systemic pressure are also shifted upward with no change in threshold. *C*, Shows upward shift in response (systemic pressure) with no change in threshold, gain, *OP*, or saturation point (*S*) of the baroreflex. *D*, shows a shift in threshold and OP to a higher carotid sinus and systemic pressure; this is the classical picture of so-called baroreceptor resetting. [Adapted from Korner (168) and reproduced from Rowell (268) with permission.]

off control that controls a variable close to some set reference value (set point). The arterial baroreflex is not an on–off control system and has no fixed set point. Rather, it has an operating point around which SAP is regulated. The operating point of the reflex (*OP* in Fig. 17.18) can be continuously variable over a wide range of SAP. This operating point may or may not coincide with the point of maximal slope (or maximal gain) on a sigmoidal stimulus–response curve (283). As noted by Sagawa (283) and later emphasized by Scher et al. (298) the slope relating SAP or R-R interval and carotid sinus pressure, for example, can be *linear* between threshold and saturation levels (cf. 62, 65).

Technically, the term "resetting" does not apply to a feedback control system without a set point. Nevertheless, we continue to use this term for concise description of a mainly lateral shift in the baroreflex stimulus–response curve as in Figure 17.18*D*. Such a shift would put the point of maximum gain of the function curve at a higher carotid sinus pressure. Stated differently, the higher firing frequency of the baroreceptor is no longer translated by the CNS to be an error signal that reflexly alters SAP—the entire reflex has been "reset."

Determination of Gain or Sensitivity and Operating Points for the Arterial Baroreflex. Figure 17.18*B* illustrates a reduction in baroreflex sensitivity as the lower slope of curve 2 compared to curve 1 (a shift in operating point need not occur). The reduction in sensitivity means that the baroreflex opposition to a change in SAP would be lessened. An acute change in baroreflex sensitivity is commonly initiated centrally by some perturbation that acts on the central neuron pool controlling the reflex. For example, sensitivity of reflex control might be altered by central command or by emotion (168).

Figure 17.18*D* illustrates baroreflex resetting in which the operating point of the reflex shifts rightward to a higher carotid sinus pressure. Reflex sensitivity can remain constant, but threshold, maximum gain, and saturation pressures move to higher carotid sinus pressures. Here the perturbation that causes resetting is again, as in Figure 17.18*B*, presumed to act on the central neuron pool receiving baroreceptor afferents. This lateral shift is usually combined with an upward shift as well, meaning that the perturbation could also act on the motor neurons governing the efferent arms of the reflex (increased HR and sympathetic vasoconstriction), which in turn raise SAP (168).

In contrast, Figure 17.18*C* shows a vertical shift in the entire stimulus–response curve to a higher SAP at every point with no change in the carotid sinus threshold, operating point, saturation point, or sensitivity. In contrast to the central neural influences that alter baroreflex sensitivity or cause "resetting," a vertical shift is presumably attributable to a tonic elevation in sympathetic vasoconstrictor activity, or in cardiac output, with neither being of baroreflex origin (168, 283).

Closed-Loop vs. Open-Loop Experiments: Interpretation and Problems. In their excellent monograph on human baroreflexes, Eckberg and Sleight (65) review the methods used to evaluate baroreflex function in humans. The two most commonly used techniques to alter pressure at the receptors are bolus injection of vasoactive drugs and positive and negative neck pressure.

Bolus injection of vasoactive drugs—the Oxford method. This approach evaluates the changes in HR or heart interval in response to a sudden rise in SAP caused by injection of an α-agonist (usually phenylephrine). The baroreceptor stimulation is physiological (i.e., a change in the normal arterial pulse wave). The sudden rise in SAP is caused by the drug-induced vasoconstriction; thus, the sympathetic vasomotor component of the reflex is abolished by the drug. The baroreflex can therefore act only on HR via the rapid parasympathetically mediated responses, and the analysis misses the additional but slower sympathetic control (230). In addition to the problems of using HR alone to assess baroreflex sensitivity, there is also the analytical ambiguity caused by using R-R interval rather than HR. For any given increase in HR with exercise, the corresponding change in R-R interval becomes less and less even though HR, and particularly its steady-state response to changes in SAP, might be unaffected by mild to moderate exercise (185, 230, 265, 275, 367).

Positive and negative neck pressure. Eckberg and his co-workers developed a simple collar to tightly encircle the anterior and lateral aspects of the neck over the carotid sinus (62, 65). Application of negative and positive pressure to the neck collar raises and lowers carotid sinus transmural pressure, respectively. The technique has as advantages a wide range over which carotid sinus transmural pressure can be altered plus the ability to control accurately the rate, timing, intensity, and duration of the pressure stimulus (62). An advantage over the bolus injection of a pressor drug is that neck pressure changes SAP by activating or inhibiting both the cardiac and vasomotor arms of the baroreflex arch. Thus one can examine the reflex in its entirety. Sensitivity of the reflex will not be underestimated as a consequence of its greater effect on vascular resistance than on HR during severe exercise. However, aortic baroreceptors still oppose the carotid sinus reflex and reduce its calculated gain.

Baroreceptors adapt rapidly to maintained static pressure and, as a consequence, reflex responses decrease quickly (44, 207). More sustained cardiac and vasomotor responses are obtained when positive or negative pulsatile pressure is applied suddenly on each electrocardiographic (ECG) R wave and maintained through only a portion of the R-R interval (62, 233, 336).

The two main disadvantages of the neck pressure technique are first, that although experiments may be essentially open-loop for the carotid sinus reflex, they are closed-loop for the aortic baroreflex. Reflex responses to changes in carotid sinus transmural pressure are partially counteracted by negative feedback from the aortic baroreceptors. So far, all who have used this or similar approaches, in humans and other animals, during dynamic exercise have had this problem to some degree. The second disadvantage is that the transmission of neck chamber pressure to the carotid sinus may not be complete, as indicated by measurements of underlying tissue pressure. However, tissue pressure measurement has many pitfalls and all transmission data have been questioned (see 65, 233).

Incomplete transmission of neck pressures may not invalidate comparisons of arterial baroreflex function during rest vs. exercise (65, 233). First, any transmission defect should be constant between rest and exercise and incomplete transmission should reduce apparent gain equally in both states. Second, if gains of both aortic and carotid sinus baroreflexes are similar over the range of pressures studied, uniform opposition of the carotid sinus reflex by the aortic baroreflex would be expected (233, 283). Stimulus–response curves for the two baroreflexes were virtually superimposable (in anesthetized dogs) when both receptors were forced with pulsatile pressures (4). If these data apply as well to conscious exercising dogs and humans, the sensitivity of the carotid sinus reflex should be reduced by the aortic baroreflex to the same degree across interventions.

Isolated carotid sinus. Vascular isolation of the carotid sinus has enabled control of intrasinus pressure separately from pressures existing at other sites. Again, the experiments approximate open-loop conditions for the carotid sinus but closed-loop for the aortic baroreceptors. In the 1980s two important series of experiments, one by Donald and his colleagues in the United States and the other by Ludbrook and his co-workers in Australia, provided the first detailed look at the functional characteristics of the carotid sinus reflex in exercising animals (for reviews, see 185, 268, 275, 367).

Melcher and Donald (206) surgically prepared carotid sinuses so that they could be isolated from the rest of the circulation by inflation of implanted occlusion cuffs around the common and external carotid arteries. When cuffs were inflated, intrasinus pressure could be clamped at any desired static pressure via a nonocclusive implanted catheter.

Baroreflex Sensitivity in Dynamic Exercise

Conclusions about the sensitivity have often been based on a limited range of forcings of carotid sinus transmural pressure via neck chambers (e.g., 19,

329, 336). The preceding discussion of baroreflex characteristics reveals the difficulty in quantifying reflex sensitivity without examining the reflex function curve over most of its operating range.

Dogs with Vascularly Isolated Carotid Sinuses. Isolation of the carotid sinuses permitted the first detailed investigations of how exercise might alter the entire baroreflex function curve in conscious dogs (206, 366, 367). In dogs with intact aortic baroreflexes, mild to heavy dynamic exercise displaced the baroreflex curves vertically and had no effect on the apparent threshold, slope (or gain), or saturation levels of the curves relating SAP to carotid sinus transmural pressure over a range of intrasinus pressures from 50–250 mm Hg (these portions of the curves were not specifically identified by the authors). These results are typified in Figure 17.18C. Presumably, such a shift would be caused by the effect of increased SNA on SAP, and not by a change in the functional characteristics of the carotid sinus reflex per se (168, 283).

Unfortunately, attempts to raise carotid sinus pressure in dogs with the aortic baroreflex interrupted by vagotomy (this also interrupted vagal control of HR) caused precipitous hypotension and collapse during exercise (see 367). The inability to eliminate the aortic receptors and the nonpulsatile pressures used to force the carotid sinus may have altered the characteristics of the reflex (4).

Carotid Sinus Pressure Forcings in Humans. Papelier et al. (233) showed that the sensitivity of the carotid sinus baroreflex in humans was not altered between rest and graded dynamic exercise up to levels requiring 87% of $\dot{V}O_{2max}$ (average 75% $\dot{V}O_{2max}$). They determined sensitivity of the reflex by linear regression of SAP against carotid sinus pressure, because it fitted their data better than a sigmoidal logistic function (Fig. 17.19*A*). Slopes of the relationship between steady-state SAP and carotid sinus pressure were the same during rest and exercise. These responses were obtained during the last 3 min of 6 min periods of exercise. Pulsatile pressure forcings were electronically triggered 40 ms after the ECG R wave and maintained for 200–500 ms, depending on R-R interval. Each 20 mm Hg step in neck pressure, from −80 mm Hg to +60 mm Hg, was applied for 20 s so as to include both the fast vagal responses (<1 s) and the much slower sympathetic cardiac and vasomotor responses (10–15 s) (371). On the other hand, the 20 s of neck pressure also gave ample time for full expression of aortic baroreceptor opposition, which could make carotid sinus sensitivity appear low. Adaptation of carotid sinus mechanoreceptors to superimposed static pressures from the neck collar was lessened by pulsatile application of neck pressure (see also 4, 13).

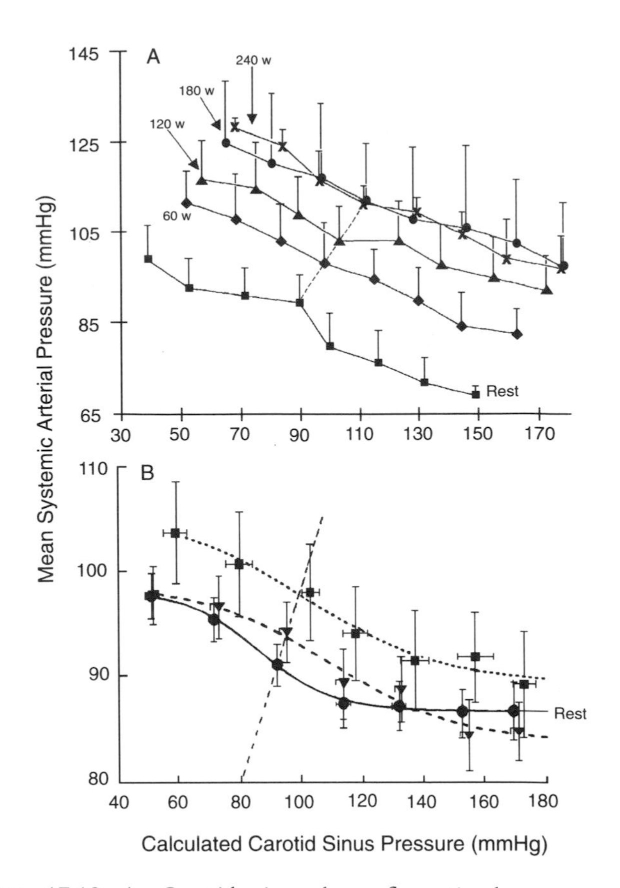

FIG. 17.19. *A*, Carotid sinus baroreflex stimulus–response curves at rest and levels of dynamic exercise (cycling) requiring 25%–75% of $\dot{V}O_{2max}$. Calculated carotid sinus transmural pressure was increased or decreased by 20 s applications of pulsatile negative or positive neck collar pressure applied at each ECG R wave and lasting 500–200 ms (at each calculated sinus pressure) depending on HR. Data were best described by linear fit with no difference in slope among rest and the levels of exercise. *Dashed line* connects prevailing systemic arterial and carotid sinus pressures (no external neck pressure) at rest and exercise. [Adapted from Papelier et al. (233).] *B*, Responses (as in *A*) to changes in neck collar pressures steadily applied for 5 s periods during rest and dynamic exercise requiring 25% and 50% of peak $\dot{V}O_2$. Intersection of *dashed line* with *curves* shows prevailing pressure at rest and 50% peak exercise; prevailing pressure was taken as the operating point. Fitting of curves to logistic function provided threshold and saturation levels and supported the conclusion that the baroreflex had been "reset" by exercise. [Adapted from Potts et al. (240) with permission.]

Potts et al. (240) obtained similar results to those of Papelier et al. (233) but used a different strategy. Static positive and negative neck pressures were applied randomly for only 5 s in an attempt to lessen negative feedback from the aortic baroreceptors. However, the short stimulus duration would minimize the sympathetic component in HR control and especially the vasomotor component. Figure 17.19*B* shows their fit of data to logistic function curves from which they derived maximum gains for the reflex at rest and 25% and 50% of peak $\dot{V}O_2$. Surprisingly, gains in the two studies were similar except at 50% peak $\dot{V}O_2$ where gains were higher in the study by Potts et al. (240). Exercise shifted the relation between SAP and carotid sinus pressure upward and to the right in both studies (see below).

All of these studies indicate that when aortic baroreceptors are intact, the operating point of the carotid sinus reflex is displaced by dynamic exercise to a higher pressure, but the sensitivity of this reflex over its full range of function is not significantly altered by such exercise. Computed closed-loop gains for the reflex in humans ($G_{CL} = -0.3$ to -0.6) (233, 240) were somewhat lower than to those reported from dogs ($G_{CL} = -0.6$ to -0.7) (206, 313) (owing perhaps to the methodological differences) (206, 275).

Importance of Arterial Baroreflexes at the Onset of Exercise

Activation of the muscle pump at the onset of dynamic exercise immediately withdraws blood from the arterial system and forces it through muscle and into the venous system, raising CVP immediately (314). Volume and compliance are much less in arteries than in veins, so that a sudden reduction in arterial volume will reduce SAP until it is restored by increased cardiac output and constriction of arterioles. The fall in SAP at the onset of exercise is immediate, and reaches a nadir at ~5–10 s; metabolic vasodilation does not begin until after a delay of 5–20 s (97, 198). Figure 17.13 shows the time course of the changes in SAP, cardiac output, and total vascular conductance in dogs with or without autonomic blockade during the first 60 s of mild dynamic exercise. With the sympathetic nervous system intact, SAP begins to recover from its nadir within ~10 s. With autonomic blockade (hexamethonium) SAP does not recover but continues to fall. These events in intact animals are too rapid (<1 s) to be explained by reflex vasodilation elicited by a cardiopulmonary baroreflex response to the sudden rise in CVP as proposed by Sprangers (327; cf. 268).

Effects of Sinoaortic Denervation. Several studies suggested that sinoaortic denervation had no significant effect on cardiovascular responses to exercise in the steady state (170, 205, 351). However, Krasney et al. (170) observed that this denervation exaggerated the sudden transient fall in SAP at the onset of exercise. This observation was confirmed in subsequent studies (5, 54, 107, 206, 366).

The exaggerated fall in SAP in baroreceptor-denervated dogs was accompanied by a recovery back toward resting SAP during moderate to heavy exercise (5, 206), whereas during mild exercise, SAP remained depressed and very unstable. Recovery and improved stability of SAP during heavier exercise (366) probably originates from reflexes activated in hypoperfused active muscles; for example, muscle chemoreflex (268, 275) (there are redundant controllers of SAP as pointed out earlier).

Some discrepancies among the studies just described may stem from different periods of recovery after denervation and the potential for adaptation to loss of receptors (188); that is, plasticity can occur in the control of autonomic output (229). Complete denervation deprives the CNS of neural feedback from the baroreceptors, and this appears to profoundly alter responses (188). An advantage of controlling pressure within the isolated carotid sinus is that neural feedback to the CNS is not only preserved but controllable (206, 366). With this approach, the carotid sinus reflex could be reversibly interrupted by holding intrasinus pressure below the threshold of receptor firing while responses to exercise were studied at various stages of denervation of remaining receptor groups. The initial rise in SAP at the onset of exercise required either an intact carotid sinus or the combination of intact aortic and cardiopulmonary baroreflexes. If the latter reflexes were not intact and the carotid sinus was hydraulically isolated from the rest of the circulation, the rise in SAP in response to exercise was abolished. Therefore, the rise in SAP at the onset of exercise requires functioning arterial baroreflexes.

Why does Arterial Baroreceptor Denervation Cause Hypotension at the Onset of Exercise? Walgenbach and Donald (366) concluded that the fall in SAP accompanying acute lack of baroreceptor input to the CNS is caused by an abnormally large rise in total vascular conductance; cardiac output rose normally. This suggests that the arterial baroreflex supports, rather than opposes, the rise in SAP at the onset of exercise by initiating vasoconstriction and opposing the increase in total vascular conductance. In rabbits, DiCarlo and Bishop (54) found that the sudden and large rise in renal SNA at the onset of exercise was abolished (it actually fell) after sinoaortic denervation. Note also in Figure 17.13 that after sympathetic blockade, even when cardiac output was controlled at normal levels, SAP fell markedly owing to increased total vascular conductance. Thus, acute elimination of either the arterial baroreflex or its vasomotor arm can suppress or even reverse the rise in SAP during exercise, even when HR and cardiac output are raised to normal levels by ventricular pacing (313).

The studies by Ludbrook's group differed from those of Donald and his colleagues by focusing on the mechanisms causing hypotension during the first 10 s of exercise in sinoaortic denervated rabbits (107, 187, 188), rather than on the steady-state conditions later in exercise (206, 366). Ludbrook's group proposed that at the onset of exercise the arterial baroreflex normally ceases to exert its tonic inhibitory effects on HR and systemic vascular resistance. As a consequence, these variables increase suddenly, causing SAP to rise. When Ludbrook et al. (188) performed bilateral carotid occlusion (all of the remaining baroreceptors were denervated) at the onset of exercise, the normal increases in HR and systemic vascular resistance were suppressed and SAP fell. Thus, the arterial baroreflex appeared to be essential for these variables to increase at the onset of the mild dynamic exercise.

Hales and Ludbrook (107) examined the distribution of radioactive microspheres at the onset of mild exercise before and after sinoaortic denervation of their rabbits. They estimated that normally ~40% of the initial rise in MBF was contributed by vasoconstriction in splanchnic organs, kidneys, and skin which diverted their blood flows to active muscle. Presumably, this vasoconstriction in rabbits is necessitated by the long time required for a rise in cardiac output to a stable level (~40 s). Exercise was very mild and rabbits have small hearts (per kilogram body weight) with small outputs. This diversion of regional blood flow to muscle was lost after sinoaortic denervation and, as a result, SAP fell markedly when exercise began. This initial vasoconstrictor response at the onset of exercise was interpreted by the authors to be a momentary loss of tonic baroreceptor restraint of sympathetic vasoconstriction (107).

These above findings and those from dogs (e.g., 206) at the onset of exercise support the proposition that the baroreflex had shifted rightward to higher baroreceptor pressure so that the baroreflex not only suppresses any initial fall in SAP but actually becomes the stimulus to raise SNA and SAP. Figure 17.20*A* illustrates why such a lateral shift of the baroreflex to a higher pressure would momentarily have the same effect as a sudden reduction of reflex sensitivity; that is, if carotid sinus pressure had not yet shifted from the flat (insensitive) portion of the reset curve (above OP_1), to its higher operating pressure on the steep portion at OP_2. In short, the findings just described (107, 188) could be explained by "resetting" of the baroreflex as illustrated in Figure 17.20*A*.

Evidence Indicating "Resetting" of the Arterial Baroreflex

The central question is if the stimulus–response curve for the entire baroreflex (baroreceptors, central neuron pool, and reflex effector mechanisms) is altered during exercise so that SAP is regulated by the reflex at a higher value during exercise than at rest. Is this why SAP is higher during exercise than rest and why active muscle is vasoconstricted during exercise?

The proposition that the increase in SAP and SNA at the onset of exercise depends on a rapid resetting of the arterial baroreflex to a higher operating pressure has fundamental importance. It means that cardiovascular control during exercise could be explained by continuous corrections, via the baroreflex, of small "errors" in SAP, with errors being defined as differences between SAP and baroreflex operating point. In this scheme, the primary function of the autonomic nervous system during exercise would be correction of any mismatches between cardiac output and vascular conductance (i.e., pressure errors). Opponents justifiably argue that this hypothesis simply shifts the question to what stimulus resets the reflex. Furthermore, the pressure to which the reflex is reset is extremely difficult to determine (e.g., 206, 233, 240, 366).

Studies on Nonhuman Species. So far, the indirect evidence suggesting baroreceptor resetting during exercise is as follows:

1. Cardiac output, HR, and SAP rise together during exercise despite maintained sensitivity (gain) of the arterial baroreflex.
2. A functioning arterial baroreflex is essential for the rise in SAP at the onset of exercise. SAP does not rise in response to exercise or in proportion to work intensity if feedback from the baroreceptors is eliminated either by denervation or by keeping transmural pressure of the isolated intact baroreceptor below a threshold level.
3. The rise in SAP at the onset of exercise requires sympathetic vasoconstriction to oppose the rise in total vascular conductance. Sinoaortic denervation prevents the rise in SNA.

Although the results of Melcher and Donald (206), typified by Figure 17.20*B*, appear to argue against baroreceptor resetting, the presence of intact aortic baroreceptors and forcings with nonpulsatile pressures may have affected position as well as slope of the carotid sinus function curve (366, 367).

An experiment providing convincing but indirect support for arterial baroreflex resetting is summa-

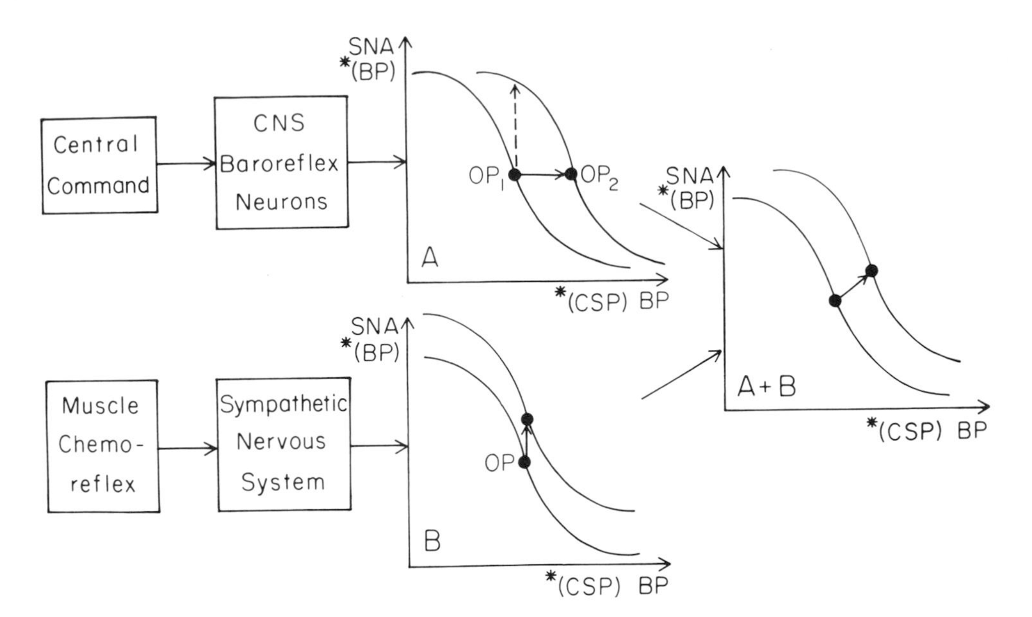

FIG. 17.20. Hypothetical baroreflex–function curves illustrate contrasting effects of central command and muscle chemoreflexes on curve position and operating points. Function curves can be expressed as the relationship between systemic arterial pressure (BP) and sympathetic nervous activity (SNA) or as carotid sinus pressure *(CSP) substituted for BP on the x axis vs. systemic arterial pressure *(BP), substituted for SNA on the y axis. *A*, In theory, central command "resets" the baroreflex to OP_2 by acting on the neuron pool receiving baroreceptor afferents. The *vertical dashed arrow* from OP_1 (initial operating point) to the reset curve shows that any perturbation of pressure around the original OP is poorly corrected because this pressure falls on the least sensitive region of the new curve (i.e., the baroreflex appears momentarily insensitive at the onset of exercise). *B*, A vertical shift in the baroreflex function curve signifies that the muscle chemoreflex could raise BP or SNA without changing OP because the stimulus acts only on the efferent arm of the reflex and not the central neurons controlling the reflex. A + B illustrates the combined predicted effects of both stimuli on the baroreflex–function curve during exercise. [From Rowell and O'Leary (275) with permission.]

rized in Figure 17.21 (366). In a preparation like that of Melcher and Donald (206), a static intrasinus pressure in dogs was held constant at 140 mm Hg, a level required to maintain normal resting SAP (366). The remaining baroreceptors had been denervated so as dogs exercised, the CNS received only a constant level of "resting" afferent nerve traffic from the isolated sinus, the only remaining baroreceptor. Figure 17.21 shows that the increases in cardiac output were essentially the same in these dogs before and after surgery, but after an initial fall, the increments in SAP were extreme when the sinuses were isolated. Surprisingly, after the initial rise in total vascular conductance between rest and exercise at 0% grade, conductance rose no further as intensity of exercise increased. A powerful vasoconstrictor outflow opposed any further vasodilation in active muscle; also, other regions had to be maximally vasoconstricted as well to explain the extreme rise in SAP. Presumably the baroreflex was reset to progressively higher pressures at each increase in work rate. A "resting" carotid sinus pressure appears to have been interpreted by the CNS as a progressively increasing hypotensive stimulus as the severity of exercise increased. At each work rate the reflex reset, and when pressure within the isolated carotid sinus failed to increase, the CNS initiated extreme vasoconstriction in an attempt to raise carotid sinus pressure to the reset level it was seeking but could never attain.

DiCarlo and Bishop (54) tested the hypothesis that the increase in SNA and SAP at the onset of exercise depends on a rapid shift of the operating point of the arterial baroreflex to a higher pressure. They attenuated the normal rise in SAP attending exercise in rabbits by infusing nitroglycerin as shown in Figure 17.22. Exercise was accompanied by abnormally large and rapid increases in renal SNA and in HR. Figure 17.22 reveals a marked upward shift in the relationship between renal SNA vs. SAP and in HR vs. SAP when the rise in SAP was suppressed by nitroglycerin infusion.

An analogous study was carried out in humans by pharmacologically suppressing the rise in SAP in response to an isometric forearm contraction (299). Increases in HR and especially MSNA were greatly increased above those during normal contractions when the rise in SAP was suppressed. These authors argued that something (e.g., muscle chemoreflex or mechanoreceptor?) normally produces this increase

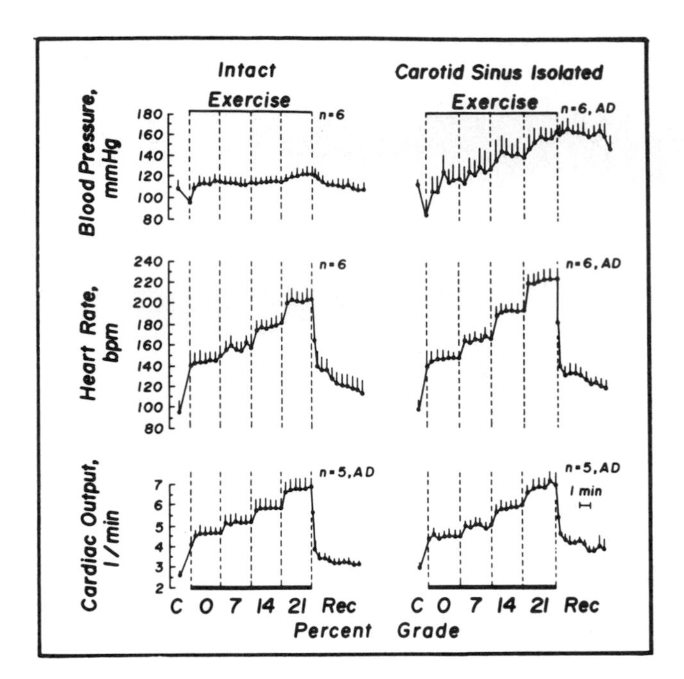

FIG. 17.21. Evidence for stepwise "resetting" of the arterial baroreflex with graded increases in work intensity. Responses are from intact dogs (*left*) and after denervation of aortic baroreceptors (AO) and surgical isolation of carotid sinuses, with sinus pressure maintained constant at "resting" level. In dogs with isolated sinuses, HR and cardiac output rose normally, but elevations in SAP were extreme. After an initial rise in total vascular conductance between rest and exercise at 0% grade, total vascular conductance increased little thereafter with work intensity because of intense vasoconstriction, largely in working muscle. "Resting" carotid sinus pressure must have been interpreted centrally as a hypotensive stimulus that became greater with work intensity as a result of stepwise resetting of the baroreflex. [From Walgenbach and Donald (366), with permission from the American Heart Association.]

in MSNA and that it is reduced by arterial baroreflexes. A finding that argues against this view is that when graded exercise was carried out in dogs with chronic sinoaortic denervation, SAP remained constant at ~110 mg Hg across the four work rates (366); presumably SNA (and thus SAP) did not rise when there was no baroreflex. Therefore, as in the dogs with isolated carotid sinuses and the rabbits (54), these responses in humans appear to reflect an attempt by the CNS and the arterial baroreflex to raise SAP to a reset operating point, rather than suppress a rise in SNA from some other source.

Studies on Humans. Two recent studies on humans have provided function curves for the carotid sinus reflex that are consistent with resetting by exercise (233, 240). Both studies showed that the carotid sinus function curve is changed by exercise so that at any given carotid sinus pressure, SAP is higher (Fig. 17.19). Also, sensitivity of the carotid sinus reflex remained constant during mild to severe exercise. This upward shift in the function curves was increased relative to work rate. The use of a linear function by Papelier et al. (233) (Fig. 17.19*A*) to relate SAP to carotid sinus pressure precluded selection of the point of maximum slope or gain, which is sometimes defined as the "operating point" of the reflex. By this criterion and without threshold and saturation levels defined, there was no certainty regarding the degree to which the shift in curves is horizontal (i.e., "resetting") or vertical (no "resetting"). However, if the prevailing pressure, or observed SAP prior to changing intrasinus pressure, was assumed to represent the baroreflex operating point, then resetting, or a lateral shift in the curves was evident [this latter approach was recently defended by Bishop (25)].

Potts et al. (Fig. 17.19*B*) fit their data to a sigmoidal logistic function curve that obligatorily provides threshold and saturation pressures, and also a centering point (as illustrated in Fig. 17.20*A* and *B*) around which SAP rose or fell by equal amounts. The operating point was assumed to be the prevailing pressure (shown as *dashed line* in Fig. 17.19*B*). All derived points on these function curves were shifted rightward to higher carotid sinus pressures by mild to moderate exercise. Their detailed analysis provides a theoretical basis (based on the sigmoidal model) for arguing that the carotid sinus reflex had been reset to a higher operating pressure. Their findings and those of Papelier et al. (233) were clearly consistent with some previous observations from dogs and rabbits (discussed above), suggesting resetting of the reflex.

Central Command and Resetting of the Arterial Baroreflex—An Hypothesis

Centrally generated motor command signals are putative feedforward activators of circulatory responses to exercise. The hypothesis is that central command might achieve its effect on the circulation by changing the operating point of a feedback controller of the circulation (127, 268).

If central command raises SAP by raising HR and cardiac output at the onset of exercise, why does SAP fall markedly in animals with intact central command after sinoaortic denervation? An hypothetical answer is that central command exerts its effects on SAP by resetting the arterial baroreflex (54, 127, 268, 275). Presumably, central command and the CNS cannot reset the baroreflex without afferent signals from the baroreceptors (i.e., central

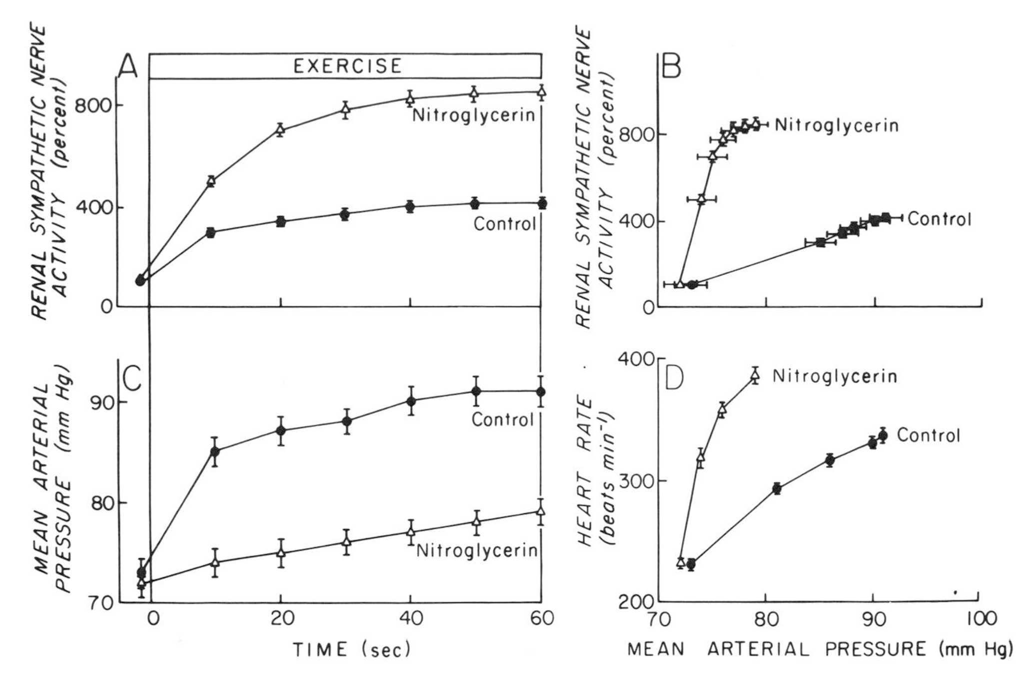

FIG. 17.22. Further evidence that onset of exercise shifts arterial baroreflex operating point to higher pressures. Delaying the rise in arterial pressure (in rabbits) during exercise by infusing nitroglycerin (*C*) markedly increased renal sympathetic nerve activity (*A*) and also heart rate. *B* and *D*, The exaggerated increases in sympathetic outflow and heart rate at any given arterial pressure when the rise in pressure was delayed by nitroglycerin. [Redrawn from DiCarlo and Bishop (54) and reproduced from Rowell (268) with permission.]

command cannot reset the baroreflex if there is no reflex).

The rise in SAP at the beginning of exercise requires a functioning arterial baroreflex. At exercise onset, central command could suddenly reset the baroreflex to a higher operating point, as shown in Figure 17.20. However, a finite period of time is required for SAP to reach its new operating point. Presumably, the error signal that elicits the vasoconstriction is the centrally preceived "hypotension" caused by the time lag between the shift in the operating point and the actual rise in SAP (268, 275).

Simultaneous with the initiation of central command, arterial baroreflex control of renal SNA appears to be reset. Renal SNA rises immediately at the onset of exercise (54, 221). Surprisingly, renal blood flow also falls sharply without perceptible delay (120) and certainly far faster than predicted from the normal time constant for sympathetic responses (371). Because of their sudden onset, these results may be more consistent with a rapid central origin of increased SNA, rather than a mechanoreflex, for example. [Victor et al. (359) saw a 0.8 s delay when they electrically induced static contractions and proposed that muscle mechanosensitive afferents may govern the rise in renal SNA.]

Although the reduced vagal outflow to the heart attributed to central command appears to be independent of the arterial baroreflex (52); the rise in HR attributed to cardiac SNA appears to depend on an intact baroreflex (54). The increase in cardiac and renal SNA at the onset of exercise could therefore be secondary to resetting of the arterial baroreflex—presumably by central command.

Houk (127) proposed that a feedforward controller like central command could also achieve close regulation of a variable (e.g., SAP) by working in combination with feedback controllers such as the arterial baroreflex. His scheme, summarized in Figure 17.15, proposes that coordination of feedback control (the arterial baroreflex) with feedforward control (central command) is accomplished by directing feedforward command to the baroreflex or feedback controller, where it resets its operating point.

ROLE OF CARDIOPULMONARY BARORECEPTORS IN DYNAMIC EXERCISE

The Cardiopulmonary, or Low-Pressure, Baroreflex

Mechanoreceptors in the atria, ventricles, pulmonary artery, and pulmonary veins alter their firing rates in response to changes in pressure within these chambers and vessels (for reviews, see 26, 27, 196). At rest, when CVP and cardiopulmonary receptor activity decrease from normal levels, this reflex increases SNA. Conversely, an increased CVP will decrease SNA. A notable exception, the rabbit, was found to lack any tonic cardiopulmonary receptor activity during rest (53) in that removal of this activity (intrapericardial procaine) did not alter renal or mesenteric vascular resistance or SAP [as it normally does in other species (26, 27)]. Only after rabbits were physically conditioned did removal of tonic cardiopulmonary afferent activity elicit reflex increases in SNA (53). This may be due to an expansion of blood volume sufficient to generate tonic activity. Thus, in the normal rabbit, which has a limited cardiac pumping capacity relative to dogs, or even humans, these receptors contribute little to tonic restraint of SNA.

The relative importance of cardiopulmonary vs. arterial baroreflexes in the control of HR and peripheral vascular resistance was quantitatively assessed in conscious dogs (245). Cardiopulmonary receptors have a much greater effect on vascular resistance than does the arterial baroreflex based on per-mm Hg changes in CVP vs. arterial pressure (245). This comparison is deceptive, however, inasmuch as there is a 20-fold difference between CVP and SAP. Changes in HR evoked by CVP were attributable to the Bainbridge effect. Although chemical activation of vagal afferents can induce bradycardia (26), physiological changes in cardiopulmonary receptor activity (i.e., changes in CVP) appear to cause little if any change in HR. Nevertheless, two factors complicate interpretation. First, perturbations causing large changes in CVP will also change aortic pulse pressure and perhaps SAP as well, so that it is difficult, if not impossible, to determine whether responses are caused by arterial or cardiopulmonary baroreflexes (128, 138). Second, inasmuch as the majority of cardiopulmonary afferents travel in the vagus, interruption of vagal activity (to mimic unloading of cardiopulmonary receptors) also removes a major efferent source of reflex changes in HR (via changes in parasympathetic tone). Parenthetically, Öberg and White (220) observed that section of cardiac afferents or vagal cooling in atropinized cats without a functioning arterial baroreflex raised HR by only 3.5%–4.5%. Effects on regional vascular resistances were much greater (30%–70%) than on HR.

Interaction between the Cardiopulmonary and Arterial Baroreflexes at Rest

The response to cardiopulmonary baroreceptor inhibition at rest depends on the level of activity of the arterial baroreceptors (21, 28, 116, 195, 196). If, for example, static pressure within the isolated carotid sinus is maintained at high levels (aortic baroreceptors denervated), the pressor responses to elimination of cardiopulmonary receptor afferent feedback to the CNS is abolished (28, 116, 195). Conversely, the pressor response to vagal block is enhanced by a reduction in intrasinus pressure or arterial baroreceptor denervation. This interaction between the two reflexes may also explain some disparate conclusions about the role of cardiopulmonary baroreflexes during exercise. Thus, the ability of the cardiopulmonary baroreflex to change SNA may depend on the extent to which the arterial baroreflex is simultaneously active (21, 28, 116, 195, 196).

Role of Cardiopulmonary Baroreflex during Dynamic Exercise

Ventricular filling pressure during exercise appears to be determined primarily by the match between left ventricular pumping and muscle pumping. A more negative pleural pressure could contribute as well (see Chapter 15). Figure 17.14 illustrates the concept that the maintenance of CVP during exercise requires a balance between mechanical effects of muscle pumping and sympathetic control of regional blood flow between noncompliant and compliant organs. Inasmuch as cardiopulmonary baroreflexes are activated by changes in CVP at rest, the same activation might be expected during exercise (there are no data indicating cardiopulmonary baroreflexes are "reset" during exercise by the CNS, which reinterprets the higher CVP as being optimal).

This section examines the importance of cardiopulmonary baroreflexes in the control of regional vascular resistance during exercise. Is regional vasoconstriction somehow optimized so that the balance illustrated in Figure 17.14 is preserved, or is this function dominated by the arterial baroreflex either through its interactive effects on the cardiopulmonary reflex or as a consequence of its initiation of high tonic SNA to most organs? Bear in mind the necessity of tonic vasoconstriction in active skeletal muscle at a time when CVP is elevated. Does the cardiopulmonary baroreflex oppose this vasoconstriction?

Evidence Supporting a Role for the Cardiopulmonary Baroreflex. Blockade of cardiopulmonary (vagal) afferents in unconditioned rabbits exaggerated reflex vasoconstriction in inactive areas (53) and the increase in renal SNA (222) during exercise. Importantly, cardiopulmonary afferent blockade did not alter hindlimb vasodilation during exercise (53). Inasmuch as blockade of these afferents at rest has no effect on regional vascular resistance, exercise must have increased their tonic sympathoinhibitory effect. Conversely, blockade of vagal afferents increased tonic sympathetic vasoconstriction during both rest and exercise after rabbits were endurance conditioned (again, blood volume may have increased) (53).

Endurance conditioning attenuates sympathetic vasoconstriction at a given level of exercise in rabbits (53), as in other species, including humans (262, 265). Blockade of vagal afferents restored sympathetic vasoconstriction to levels observed in unconditioned rabbits. Accordingly, the attenuation of regional vasoconstriction at a given level of submaximal exercise, such as commonly observed in humans after physical conditioning (262, 265), could be achieved by raising cardiopulmonary baroreceptor activity. The unanswered question is what would raise cardiopulmonary baroreceptor firing—the effect of conditioning on CVP is not established (see later under HOW DOES PHYSICAL CONDITIONING ALTER CARDIOVASCULAR FUNCTION?). Possibly CVP rose because of an unusually large increase in blood volume of the rabbits.

Reductions in CVP and presumably in cardiopulmonary baroreceptor firing during supine dynamic exercise by simultaneous application of low levels of lower body negative pressure (LBNP) (e.g., 10 mm Hg) increased forearm vasoconstriction (193). At rest, this low level of LBNP decreases CVP without changing HR, mean SAP, or aortic pulse pressure (138). If the same applies with LBNP during supine exercise, then it was presumably the cardiopulmonary baroreflex that increased vascular resistance rather than the arterial baroreflex (128).

SNA is reduced when CVP and cardiopulmonary baroreceptor firing are increased by activating the muscle pump at the onset of mild exercise in upright position (244, 287). Both CVP and aortic pulse pressure fall during quiet upright posture, and activation of the muscle pump at the beginning of exercise immediately restores CVP, SV, and aortic pulse pressure (268). This returns MSNA to resting values (i.e., as though posture became supine) (244, 287). For example, the dominance of the postural influence on MSNA is revealed by the lack of effect of supine exercise on this variable (244). Inasmuch as mild supine exercise does not increase CVP, nor does it change SV or aortic pulse pressure, MSNA is unchanged. From these findings it was assumed that the increase in CVP at the onset of mild upright exercise inhibited SNA by increasing cardiopulmonary receptor firing (244, 287). It is equally plausible, however, that the sympathoinhibitory effects stemming from sudden restoration of reduced aortic pulse pressure also contribute to the fall in MSNA.

Evidence Against a Role for the Cardiopulmonary Baroreflex. Interruption of the cardiopulmonary baroreflex in dogs by bilateral vagotomy had no significant effect on SAP during mild to heavy exercise when the carotid sinus reflex was intact (206). This is the principal evidence against a role for this reflex in cardiovascular control during exercise. Also, after progressive interruption of carotid and aortic baroreflexes, the subsequent elimination of the cardiopulmonary baroreflex did not further alter SAP in response to graded exercise (365). After sinoaortic arterial baroreceptor denervation, however, vagotomy reduced cardiac output at moderate to heavy work rates; therefore, inasmuch as cardiac output was reduced and SAP was unchanged, total peripheral resistance was increased by vagotomy (52). This suggests that cardiopulmonary baroreceptors do tonically inhibit SNA during exercise in dogs. These results also underscore the importance of analysis based on factors in addition to SAP [i.e., in the latter study (52) SAP was not different before and after vagotomy, but analysis of cardiac output and total peripheral resistance indicate that vasomotor responses were altered].

Interaction between Cardiopulmonary Baroreflex and Muscle Chemoreflex

The powerful opposition of the arterial baroreflex to the pressor response to muscle ischemia (313) is indicated in Figure 17.17. A corollary question is whether a similar interaction exists between the cardiopulmonary baroreflex and the muscle chemoreflex. This has been examined in several studies and conclusions differ (6, 49, 300, 301, 368).

When a muscle chemoreflex was elicited by mild isometric contractions (10% MVC) (6, 368), vasoconstriction in the inactive forearm was greater when CVP was reduced by a low level of LBNP (−5 mm Hg). Inasmuch as the vasoconstriction during the combined stresses exceeded the algebraic sum of the responses to stresses when applied separately, a facilitation of the muscle chemoreflex by the cardiopulmonary baroreflex was assumed; however, a second assumption was that the responses add linearly. This putative facilitatory interaction was not observed with higher levels of handgrip or LBNP (6).

No evidence for facilitatory interaction between these reflexes was found when the increases in MSNA (peroneal nerve) were evaluated during LBNP of −5 or −10 mm Hg (300, 301) over contraction forces of 15%–30% MVC. Increments in MSNA (burst frequency) in response to combined LBNP and handgrip were not different from the sum of the increments in MSNA when stresses were applied separately. Furthermore, MSNA during combined LBNP and handgrip at 30% MVC was less than the sum of the responses to separate application of the two stresses. Again, the summation assumes the responses add linearly. Also, LBNP did not alter the sustained elevation of MSNA caused by the muscle chemoreflex during posthandgrip ischemia (300).

The potential consequences of elevated SAP during isometric contractions may bear importantly on the above results. The increases in arterial baroreceptor activity caused by contraction-induced hypertension could significantly attenuate changes in SNA induced by unloading cardiopulmonary baroreceptors. This assumes that SAP has actually exceeded the new operating point of the baroreflex. Thus, a blunted rise in SNA could stem from inhibition of the cardiopulmonary baroreflex by the arterial baroreflex (28, 116, 195). The minimal hypertension during handgrip at low force may lessen or eliminate arterial baroreflex inhibition of the cardiopulmonary baroreflex.

In only one study has the interaction between the cardiopulmonary baroreflex and the muscle chemoreflex during dynamic exercise been examined (49). Vagal afferents from cardiopulmonary baroreceptors could modulate changes in SAP during progressive muscle ischemia induced by partial terminal aortic occlusion during exercise. The experimental approach in rats was modeled after that applied to exercising dogs [see Fig. 17.17; (315, 378)]. Inhibition of cardiac efferent and afferent nerve fibers by intrapericardial administration or procainamide markedly increased the rise in SAP (>200%) in response to muscle ischemia compared to the responses observed with only cardiac efferent blockade. Presumably, after inhibition of cardiac vagal afferents, reflex vasoconstriction in response to muscle ischemia was augmented; the rise in SAP was the same with or without cardiac nerve blockade despite elimination of most of the tachycardia by the combined blockade of both the efferent and afferent fibers. Furthermore, the elevation of cardiopulmonary receptor discharge by modest blood volume expansion reduced muscle chemoreflex control of SAP and HR by 40% (49). Although these results suggest that the cardiopulmonary baroreflex can modulate pressor response to muscle ischemia, they do not rule out the potential effects of volume expansion on arterial baroreflex via changes in pulse pressure.

Interaction between Cardiopulmonary and Arterial Baroreflexes in Exercise

Complete examination of the interaction between arterial and cardiopulmonary baroreflex during exercise is exceedingly difficult (if not impossible) in many preparations, especially in humans. As discussed above, except for very mild loading/unloading of cardiopulmonary baroreceptors, any perturbation designed to affect cardiopulmonary baroreceptor activity will also change SAP or aortic pulse pressure. With activity changing simultaneously in both sets of receptors one cannot ascribe the afferent origin of the reflex response to one of them. Thus, to a large extent the interaction between arterial and cardiopulmonary baroreflexes during exercise remains unknown.

Cardiovascular responses to supine exercise do differ from those during upright exercise (20). Central blood volume, cardiac output, CVP, and SV are all higher in supine than in upright exercise, whereas SAP is the same. Therefore, total vascular conductance is higher during supine exercise. This could be due to increased cardiopulmonary baroreceptor activity (due to the increased CVP) or increased arterial baroreceptor activity (due to the increased SV and greater aortic pulse pressure). In addition, the increased level of cardiopulmonary baroreceptor activity may attenuate arterial baroreflex–mediated vasoconstriction, as has been shown to occur during supine rest (21).

A pivotal question is whether the cardiopulmonary baroreflex responds to the rising filling pressure during upright exercise by buffering vasoconstriction. As pointed out earlier, withdrawal of sympathetic vasoconstrictor outflow to skeletal muscle and other organs, particularly during severe exercise, would not only reduce SV and CO (7) but severe hypotension would accompany the unrestrained vasodilation in muscle (23, 199, 314). In sinoaortic-denervated rabbits with intact cardiopulmonary reflexes, renal sympathetic nerve activity (RSNA), HR, and SAP decreased at the initiation of exercise (54). After 1 min, HR and RSNA recovered or exceeded resting levels; however, SAP remained low. It is possible that the inhibition of RSNA (and decrease in SAP and HR) at the initiation of exercise in these denervated rabbits was caused by activation of an intact cardiopulmonary baroreflex (due to an increase in CVP via the muscle pump). Inasmuch as RSNA and HR recovered over time to near resting levels, any sympathoinhibition induced by the cardiopulmonary baroreflex must have been overridden by other mechanisms (muscle chemoreflex/mechanoreflex?). Ray et al. (244) and Saito et al. (287) also concluded that in humans the cardiopulmonary baroreflex is activated and reduces MSNA at the initiation of mild exercise in the upright posture. However, in sinoaortic-denervated dogs a sudden large fall in SAP at the initiation of mild exercise was not affected by acute cardiopulmonary baroreceptor denervation by vagotomy. At higher workloads, total vascular conductance was reduced after vagotomy, suggesting that cardiopulmonary baroreceptors do tonically inhibit SNA during moderate to heavy steady-state exercise (52).

There is evidence from human subjects that the cardiopulmonary baroreflex may elicit the cutaneous vasoconstriction that accompanies the fall in CVP caused by cutaneous vasodilation during exercise (193) (these experiments are discussed below).

Importance of Cardiopulmonary Baroreflexes during Dynamic Exercise

Despite the preceding documentation of effects of putative changes in cardiopulmonary baroreceptor activity (i.e., based mainly on changes in CVP), their importance during dynamic exercise remains unclear. The preceding sections have emphasized the need for the autonomic nervous system to match cardiac output and total vascular conductance via the arterial baroreflex to maintain SAP, and to match blood flow to metabolism via the muscle chemoreflex in order to minimize changes in interstitial chemical composition of active muscles. In what fashion do we express the matching of functions by the cardiopulmonary baroreflex, since it acts on a part of the circulation from which is it hydraulically separated? The reflex response to changes in CVP by lowering or increasing SNA does little to restore CVP. Parenthetically, this could be done by raising and lowering HR and cardiac output, but these adjustments appear not to attend physiological changes in cardiopulmonary receptor activity.

Cardiac performance during exercise is enhanced by the increases in CVP and EDV, and in myocardial contractility, all of which increase cardiopulmonary baroreceptor discharge. Although a reduction in myocardial contractility by the cardiopulmonary baroreflex might decrease SV by reducing ejection fraction, the consequent fall in cardiac output would increase rather than lower CVP and EDV. Will the combination of reduced contractility and elevated CVP increase or decrease cardiopulmonary activity? A fundamental question is whether the cardiopulmonary baroreflex is a negative feedback reflex that acts to maintain afferent activity of its receptors within a specific range as is presumed to occur with the arterial baroreflex (283). One need ask what change the initiation of a cardiopulmonary reflex makes in the firing of its receptors.

The severity of hypotension that would be the consequence of losing tonic vasoconstriction in active skeletal muscle during dynamic whole-body exercise is emphasized throughout this chapter. Does the cardiopulmonary baroreflex attenuate regional vasoconstriction during exercise and thus inhibit increases in SAP via the arterial baroreflex or the muscle chemoreflex? Is the cardiopulmonary baroreflex important when CVP is reduced by excessive vasodilation in compliant regions such as the skin during exercise? The cardiopulmonary baroreflex might act before an arterial baroreflex is initiated in this setting by raising SNA prior to any change in SAP, thereby delaying the fall in SAP. In this sense the reflex might serve as a feedforward auxiliary to sinoaortic baroreflexes, analogous to the feedforward aspect of central command.

CONTROL OF THE CIRCULATION DURING EXERCISE AND HEAT STRESS: COMPETING REFLEXES

In addition to corrections of mismatches between MBF and muscle metabolism and mismatches between cardiac output and total vascular conductance, there is a third important correction: mismatches between cardiac output and skin blood flow or ultimately between skin flow and core temperature (T_c). These lead to "temperature errors." During heavy dynamic exercise, or exercise in hot environments, the demands on the cardiovascular system to maintain SAP, MBF, and T_c are competing. Of course, correction of "temperature errors" depends critically on sweating and evaporative cooling; however, here the focus will be on competitive control of skin blood flow. The goal of this section is to contrast the unique control of the cutaneous circulation, potentially the second largest vascular bed in exercising humans, with control of blood flow to skeletal muscle and visceral organs during dynamic exercise. Indeed, the thermogenic aspect of dynamic exercise introduces a thermoregulatory reflex that competes with baroreflexes and possibly with muscle chemoreflexes in cardiovascular control during exercise.

Cardiovascular Demands of Heat Stress

Severe heat stress combined with exercise makes the greatest demands voluntarily imposed on the human cardiovascular system (264, 265). The importance of the cutaneous circulation is that humans can protect the CNS from hyperthermia only by raising skin blood flow and sweating (35). Unlike panting mammals, humans have no heat exchange mechanisms in the head to minimize selectively the rise in brain temperature when T_c reaches deleterious levels. This requires that brain and whole-body temperatures be controlled together as a single unit. (Note, there is controversy regarding this point—see 34, 218, 242, 317, 372.)

Heat stress during exercise introduces two fundamental regulatory problems. First, the skeletal muscle and skin circulations must compete for blood flow because their combined demands could potentially exceed the pumping capacity of the heart, even during moderate exercise. The second problem is that a rise in cardiac output directed to skin lowers both CVP and SV because of translocation of blood volume into cutaneous veins. Unlike muscle veins, cutaneous veins lack the direct pumping action of contracting muscle to aid venous return to the heart. The inverse relationship between cardiac output and CVP during heat stress at rest and exercise is shown in Figure 17.4. When the reduced ventricular filling and consequently lower SV can no longer be compensated for by tachycardia, cardiac pumping capacity is diminished; this at a time when total demands for blood flow are the greatest (273).

The main compensation for inadequate cardiac output is greater vasoconstriction and diversion of blood flow and blood volume from visceral organs and other regions (273). Unfortunately, regional vasoconstriction by itself cannot meet the needs for increased skin blood flow during severe exercise (264, 265). Much of the evidence argues against the proposal (130, 136, 262, 264) that active muscle also vasoconstricts further to increase the fraction of cardiac output directed to skin (217, 219, 294), although it appears to occur in sheep (17). On the other hand, heat stress has been observed to increase markedly plasma NE levels during dynamic exercise (271). Inasmuch as active muscle is normally the major site of NE spillover (75, 176, 295), this observation indirectly supports the proposal that SNA to active muscle (110) has increased further. The unanswered question is whether the greater rise in MSNA is sufficient to reduce MBF further.

Overall Neural Control of the Cutaneous Circulation

Control of the cutaneous resistance vessels originates from thermoregulatory and also from nonthermoregulatory reflexes. The latter include the arterial and cardiopulmonary baroreflexes (133) and the reflex adjustments to dynamic exercise (129–133). Often these reflexes compete for control of skin blood flow. For example, during exercise, a time of high metabolic heat production, the need for increased MBF to active muscle conflicts with the thermoregulatory role of the cutaneous circulation. Thus, there is an inherent competition for control of the cutaneous circulation during dynamic exercise that requires well-integrated cardiovascular responses. These integrated responses are effected by the unique dual control of the skin circulation: a sympathetic vasoconstrictor system and a sympathetic active vasodilator system.

Cutaneous arterioles in all regions of the body receive sympathetic noradrenergic innervation (257). Released NE acts on both α_1- and α_2-receptors (30, 84, 154). In nonapical areas of skin (i.e., limbs, head, and trunk) cutaneous resistance vessels are also controlled by an active vasodilator mechanism that is sympathetically mediated, but is not adrenergic (66, 257). The neurotransmitter causing active vasodilation is unknown; however, it appears to be linked to sweat gland activation (36, 183, 257) possibly via a sympathetic cotransmitter system (121, 153, 293).

Thermoregulatory Reflex Control. In palmar and plantar skin cutaneous resistance vessels receive primarily vasoconstrictor fiber innervation (189, 257). In those regions, skin vasodilation is predominantly passive—that is, primarily, if not entirely, due to withdrawal of vasoconstrictor tone (257).

Over the rest of the body, skin blood flow is controlled by both noradrenergic fibers and the active vasodilator system. Here, blockade of cutaneous sympathetic nerves reverses or prevents most of the cutaneous vasodilator response to heat stress. Reversal or prevention of vasodilation by sympathetic nerve blockade signifies an active process (66, 257).

Reflex modulation of sympathetic vasoconstrictor tone can provide a range of heat elimination that exceeds basal heat production by three- to fourfold (see Brengelmann in 132). Although adequate in conditions of rest, this is clearly inadequate for exercise and the attendant 10- to 20-fold (or more) increments in heat production (35, 132, 135). Therefore, regulation of heat exchange via skin blood flow also calls on activation of the neurogenic vasodilator system.

Nonthermoregulatory Reflex Control. The cutaneous circulation is also on the efferent arm of reflexes that regulate SAP and regional blood flow during exercise (130, 131, 264). Furthermore, control of skin blood flow by these reflexes is modified by simultaneous activation of thermoregulatory reflexes (130, 131, 135). The site of the interaction or integration of thermoregulatory and nonthermoregulatory reflexes is unclear, partly because of the dual sympathetic control of cutaneous blood vessels.

The traditional view has been that nonthermoregulatory reflexes modulate only cutaneous vasoconstrictor outflow whereas the thermoregulatory reflexes modulate both vasoconstrictor and vasodilator systems (130, 131, 264). However, the presumption that active vasodilation is exclusively controlled by centrally initiated thermoregulatory reflexes no longer stands (150). Figure 17.23 incorporates recent evidence for the modulation of cutaneous vasodilator outflow by nonthermoregulatory reflexes, including the arterial and cardiopulmonary baroreflexes.

Reflex Control of the Cutaneous Circulation during Exercise

Control by Sympathetic Noradrenergic Nerves: Isometric Contraction

Direct recordings of skin SNA. Direct measures of skin SNA in humans have only been made during isometric contraction (responses may differ with dynamic exercise). Skin SNA increases at or just before the onset of a static contraction (286, 362). This is in contrast to the delay of up to 1–2 min in the rise in MSNA (307). This delay in MSNA is presumed to indicate its activation by an accumulation of metabolites (i.e., a muscle chemoreflex), whereas the immediate or anticipatory rise in skin SNA has been presumed to be caused by central command (362). However, the increase in skin SNA appears to be mainly sudomotor (i.e., sympathetic cholinergic fibers) (286, 303, 362). In contrast to recordings from noradrenergic nerves supplying muscle, recordings from cutaneous nerves show an irregular burst pattern that varies markedly with emotion or arousal, and with ambient temperature (369). The immediate rise in skin SNA at the onset of muscle contraction could simply reflect arousal. The presence of multiple nerve types in mixed cutaneous nerves and the statistical bias for recording sudomotor activity limit inferences about sympathetic vasomotor activity.

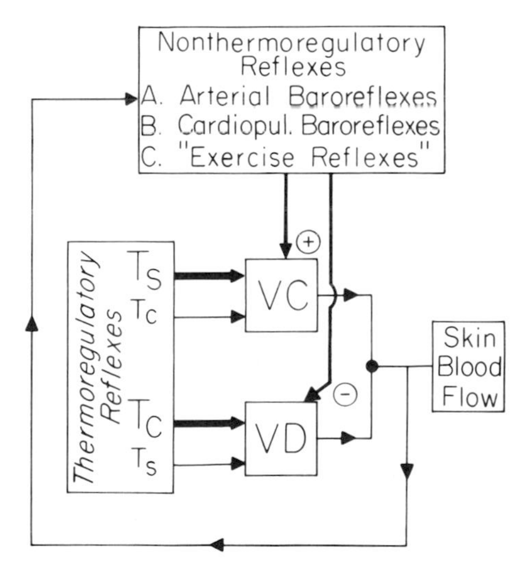

FIG. 17.23. Schematic representation of control of skin blood flow via thermoregulatory and nonthermoregulatory reflex control of vasoconstrictor (VC) and vasodilator (VD) outflow to skin. Thermoregulatory reflexes turn vasoconstriction and active vasodilation on (or off). Traditionally, nonthermoregulatory reflexes were thought to modulate only vasoconstrictor tone, but current evidence also indicates inhibition (−) of active vasodilation as well (150, 151). [From Rowell (268) with permission.]

Cutaneous vasoconstriction in response to dynamic exercise. Currently, vasoconstriction can only be unambiguously discerned from changes in skin blood flow (by laser-Doppler flowmetry or plethysmography). Evidence from investigations employing this approach also provide no support for an obvious role for central command in the cutaneous vasomotor response to the onset of dynamic exercise (89). In normothermic humans, cutaneous resistance vessels in apical and nonapical regions constrict at the initiation of exercise (18, 129, 134, 137, 343). The vasoconstriction is graded in relation to work rate (131, 342, 343), being transient at lower work rates and sustained only as maximal levels of exercise are performed (325, 343). The vasoconstriction in skin is only apparent when large muscle groups are performing moderate or higher levels of dynamic exercise (342, 343).

Competing vasoconstriction and vasodilation. As T_c rises during exercise, cutaneous vasoconstriction comes into conflict with competing thermoregulatory demands for skin blood flow. It is not known how or where the interaction between these two control systems occurs. Both central modulation (168) and peripheral modulation at receptor site (350) are probable. A key question has been whether cutaneous vasodilator outflow can be centrally modulated by nonthermoregulatory reflexes such as those attending exercise so that reduced or delayed vasodilator activity might complement cutaneous vasoconstriction to reduce skin blood flow during exercise (264). This dual vasomotor control provides at least three ways by which exercise might limit the cutaneous vasodilator response. *First*, increased noradrenergic (vasoconstrictor) activity could simply counteract active vasodilator activity. *Second*, a limit could stem from reduced or delayed active vasodilator activity without affecting the vasoconstrictor system. *Third*, exercise could both enhance vasoconstrictor activity and inhibit vasodilator activity.

Kellogg et al. (148–152) investigated the preceding possibilities by using local iontophoresis of bretylium tosylate to abolish norepinephrine release and thus noradrenergic active vasoconstriction selectively without altering active vasodilator control in human forearm skin. Laser-Doppler flowmetry was used to index skin blood flow at a treated and an adjacent untreated site. Once the cutaneous vasodilator response to heat stress was fully developed, initiation of dynamic exercise significantly reduced skin blood flow, but only at the untreated site (151). Inasmuch as skin blood flow did not fall at the site pretreated by bretylium, an increase in sympathetic vasoconstriction must have reduced skin blood flow at the untreated site. Some data suggest that this initial vasoconstriction is mediated by α_2-adrenoreceptors (155). Thus, in this setting, a net cutaneous vasoconstriction must stem from a summation of constrictor (exercise-induced) and dilator (heat stress–induced) actions. Inasmuch as the initiation of exercise did not affect the dilator system, the site of the competitive interaction between thermoregulatory reflexes and the exercise-induced reflexes appears to have been at the cutaneous arterioles rather than in the CNS.

Reflex Control of Active Vasodilation during Dynamic Exercise. Although the cutaneous vasoconstriction at the onset of dynamic exercise appears to be solely due to enhanced adrenergic vasoconstrictor activity in both cool and warm environments (151), reflexes associated with exercise also can affect the neurogenic vasodilator system.

Relationship between skin blood flow and T_c. Figure 17.24 shows the relationship between the index of cutaneous vascular conductance and T_c at rest and during exercise, with and without presynaptic sym-

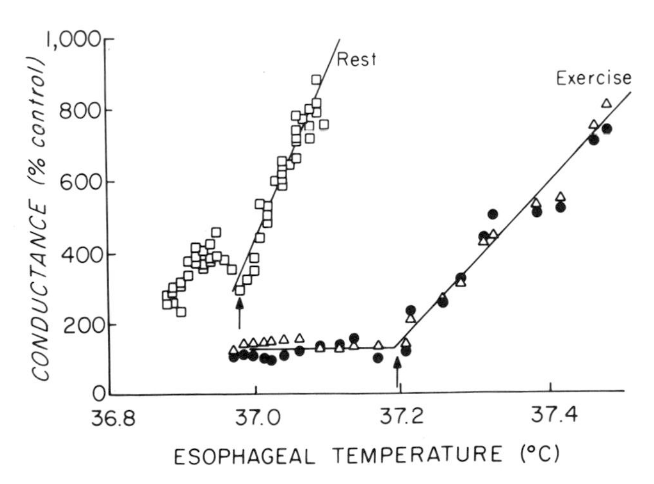

FIG. 17.24. Increase in vasodilator threshold (rise in skin vascular conductance) from ~37°C at rest to 37.2°C during moderate exercise. *Open squares* are normal skin at rest; *solid circles* are normal skin at exercise; *open triangles* are for skin with sympathetic adrenergic blockade by bretylium tosylate. [Adapted from Kellogg et al. (152).]

pathetic noradrenergic blockade (152). In relation to T_c, the threshold for increased skin blood flow is displaced rightward to higher T_c during exercise (134, 343) through a delay in the onset of active vasodilation (152). Thus, the mechanism for the lower skin blood flow at any given T_c during exercise as compared to rest is not attributable to a competing tonic vasoconstrictor outflow, but instead is due largely if not entirely to lower vasodilator activity.

The rightward shift in the skin blood flow–T_c relationship is caused by an exercise-induced delay in the activation of the vasodilator system in relation to T_c (152). Inasmuch as the slope relating skin blood flow to T_c appears not to be changed significantly by exercise (134), the elevated threshold for cutaneous vasodilation can explain part of the rise in T_c. This shift might be considered analogous to the shift in the relationship between SNA and carotid sinus pressure in response to exercise; the higher carotid sinus pressure threshold for inhibition of sympathetic vasoconstrictor outflow is responsible for part of the rise in SAP with exercise (Fig. 17.20). In both cases, the shifts in these relationships have been viewed as reflecting a centrally integrated reflex response to exercise. Inasmuch as "exercise reflexes" also act on the active vasodilator system, this suggests that these reflexes and thermoregulatory reflexes are integrated neurally (centrally or peripherally) and are not the result of local interactions at vascular receptor sites, for example. If interaction were at local sites, the T_c thresholds at sites with and without functional vasoconstrictor systems would have differed; they did not (152).

Active vasodilation and the reduced upper limit for skin blood flow in exercise. During moderate upright exercise the rate of rise of human forearm skin blood flow falls off suddenly, typically when T_c is at about 38°C. This fall-off occurs at levels of skin blood flow that are only 50%–60% of maximal in the forearm (37, 154, 155). Also, when body skin is directly heated during exercise, cardiac output rises further, but, as with forearm skin blood flow, the rate of rise falls off when T_c is near 38°C (274) [the rise in cardiac output is directed to the skin circulation (136, 262, 270)]. This decline in the rates of rise of skin blood flow and of cardiac output was previously thought to be caused by an abrupt increase in sympathetic vasoconstrictor outflow to skin, originating from the baroreflex, raising SNA in order to prevent further decline in SAP (37, 274). The same arguments were applied to explain how and why the vasodilator potential of active skeletal muscle was restricted by sympathetic vasoconstriction (2, 266, 276, 295). This argument appears not to be applicable to the cutaneous circulation during submaximal exercise.

The studies of Kellogg et al. (148) and Kenny et al. (154, 155) showed that the initial increase in skin blood flow with rising T_c is mediated by active vasodilation. Attenuation of the rate of rise in skin blood flow when T_c exceeded 38°C was not reversed by either pre- or postsynaptic adrenergic blockade. The reflex that initiated this response, presumably the arterial or cardiopulmonary baroreflex, appears to suppress cutaneous vasodilation by inhibiting sympathetic active vasodilator outflow (148, 150, 154). Alternatively, skin blood flow might have been restricted by a potent circulating vasoconstrictor substance acting on skin. However, the fact that postsynaptic α-blockade does not alter the pattern (154, 155) together with the data from Kellogg et al. (148) suggest that sympathetic vasoconstrictor activity may have been slowly withdrawn during this stage of exercise.

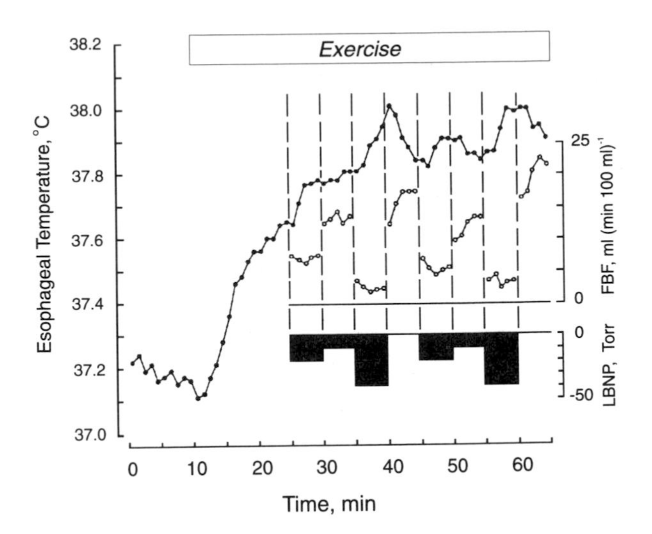

FIG. 17.25. Influence of lower body negative pressure (LBNP) on forearm blood flow (FBF) (*open circles*) and esophageal temperature (*solid circles*) during supine dynamic leg exercise. Data are from one representative experiment. [From Mack et al. (193) with permission.]

Baroreflex v. Thermoregulatory Reflex Control of the Cutaneous Circulation during Exercise

Figure 17.24 illustrates, in part, the extent to which control of skin blood flow is changed by exercise; it does not show the continuing rise in skin blood flow as T_c exceeds 38°C at rest nor the leveling off of skin blood flow at this T_c during exercise. These changes as well as the threshold shift depicted in Figure 17.24 favor regulation of SAP rather than T_c during exercise.

Cardiopulmonary Baroreflexes. When the fraction of cardiac output distributed to skin increases during exercise, CVP falls and causes SV to fall, often before there is any decline in SAP (264). Potentially, the fall in CVP and/or a fall in aortic pulse pressure initiate vasoconstriction. When Mack et al. (193) applied LBNP of −10, −20, and −40 mm Hg during mild supine exercise (HR = 100 bpm), negative pressures of −10 and −20 mm Hg had no effect on HR or SAP. The lack of HR response suggested that an arterial baroreflex was not elicited (138, 196). Rather, forearm vasoconstriction (dominated in this setting by the response in vasodilated skin) appears to have been initiated by a cardiopulmonary baroreflex. Figure 17.25 shows that cutaneous vasoconstriction reduced heat loss, leading to an increase in T_c. Presumably, the vasoconstriction in skin was attributable to inhibition of active vasodilation (150). Clearly, cutaneous vasoconstriction in this setting was defending SAP rather than T_c. Inasmuch as cardiopulmonary receptors do not sense SAP, arterial baroreceptors or possibly left ventricular receptors were probably also involved.

Interaction between Cardiopulmonary and Arterial Baroreflexes. The level of activity of one baroreflex changes the sensitivity of the other by unknown mechanisms (21, 196, 357). This interaction may be especially important in upright humans at rest because of the simultaneous reduction in firing by both groups of receptors. Decrements in CVP and thoracic blood volume by gravity (or LBNP) appear to increase the sensitivity of the arterial baroreflex; the converse applies when CVP is raised (21, 196, 357).

The impairment of cardiopulmonary baroreflex control of forearm vascular resistance (212) and MSNA (128), in resting patients with orthotopically transplanted hearts suggests that ventricular receptors may also play a role in these reflexes. The transplanted ventricles are without afferent connections, whereas atrial afferents should be largely intact.

At this time it is not clear if the additional vasoconstriction to visceral organs and skeletal muscle during exercise (262, 264) that accompany the decline in CVP caused by heat stress is initiated by cardiopulmonary and/or arterial baroreflexes or, alternatively, if it could be a direct effect of increased T_c on SNA (264). Figure 17.6 suggests that the adrenergic control of SNA (relative to HR but not to $\dot{V}O_2$) is essentially the same during exercise with heat stress and during exercise under other conditions. This, however, appears not to apply to skin (e.g., 148).

Importance of Upright Posture. In upright posture, gravity imposes an increase in vascular transmural pressure that is roughly equivalent to an application of LBNP to −50 mm Hg below the iliac crest. CVP is close to zero, arterial pulse and/or mean pressure is reduced, and the sensitivity of the arterial baroreflex is increased by the fall in thoracic volume and pressure (21). Activation of the muscle pump immediately restores CVP, arterial pressure, and SNA back toward levels prevailing at supine rest. However, when heat stress is also imposed, the effectiveness of the muscle pump is reduced because dependent cutaneous veins in the legs are only partially emptied by contractions of underlying muscle (117, 264). Although after each contraction the low or negative pressure in skeletal muscle veins draws cutaneous venous blood through perforating veins with high resistance into veins draining muscle (1), there is nevertheless slower emptying of cutaneous veins: CVP and SV fall, whereas HR and SNA are elevated and SAP may be well maintained, at least for a while (262, 264). The sudden decrease in the rate of rise of skin blood flow when T_c reaches 38°C (mild hyperthermia) could be associated with a further decline in CVP (274). Also, a more highly sensitive arterial baroreflex, due to reduced CVP, could detect small decrements in aortic pulse or mean pressure and this could initiate a withdrawal of cutaneous vasodilation guarding against falling SAP. This hypothesis could be tested by manipulation of carotid sinus transmural pressure (which does not change CVP) when the upper limit of skin blood flow is approached.

HOW DOES PHYSICAL CONDITIONING ALTER CARDIOVASCULAR FUNCTION?

Physical conditioning for endurance increases the capacity of the cardiovascular system to transport oxygen to the active muscles. Is autonomic control of the circulation during exercise changed by physical conditioning, and if so, how? What cardiac and peripheral circulatory adjustments permit the further increase in cardiac performance attending physical conditioning? The mechanisms that enhance greater oxygen extraction by the muscles are treated in Chapter 16.

Range of Adjustment in Overall Cardiovascular Function

The $\dot{V}O_{2max}$ (the product of maximal cardiac output and maximal A-VO_2 difference) provides the best measure of cardiovascular functional capacity. Physical conditioning increases $\dot{V}O_{max}$, and neither gender (157) nor age (68, 69, 113, 163, 290, 305, 306) appears to have much influence on the magnitude of adaptation (82, 172, 262). The percentage increase in $\dot{V}O_{2max}$ depends on the initial value, with the lowest $\dot{V}O_{2max}$ being associated with the largest increase (288, 289). Bear in mind that the increase in older people is measured from a baseline $\dot{V}O_{2max}$ that declines at a rate of ~0.4–0.5 ml · kg^{-1} · min^{-1} · year^{-1} after age 20 in men and ~0.2–0.35 ml · kg^{-1} · min^{-1} · year^{-1} in women (42). Conditioning lessens this decline in $\dot{V}O_{2max}$ (105).

What Cardiovascular Adjustments Explain the Rise in $\dot{V}O_{2max}$?

In normally active and sedentary young people, ~50% of the increase in $\dot{V}O_{2max}$ caused by physical conditioning is attributable to increased SV (maximal HR does not increase) and ~50% is explained by the increase in systemic A–VO_2 difference (68, 69, 262, 289). In physically active people whose preconditioning level of $\dot{V}O_{2max}$ was high, the small (a few percent) rise in $\dot{V}O_{2max}$ was due almost entirely to increased SV (289). The same adjustment was observed in middle-aged men (113) and middle-aged to elderly women (157) and also in foxhounds (216). Any failure to observe a rise in systemic A–VO_2 difference is puzzling because any rise in maximal cardiac output appears to be directed to active muscle where oxygen extraction is greatest (47, 254, 291).

How does Maximal SV Increase with Physical Conditioning?

Four mechanisms by which SV could increase during conditioning are briefly reviewed here: *(1)* increases in myocardial contractility, *(2)* reduction in ventricular afterload, *(3)* increase in ventricular preload, and *(4)* altered geometry and mechanical (pericardial) constraints (for more details, see Chapter 15).

Increases in Myocardial Contractility. Left ventricular ejection fraction is a reasonable index of myocardial contractility in this setting. It is already so high at ~80%–85% at peak exercise in unconditioned young people that further improvement would be difficult to observe (29, 32, 238, 328), owing to limited resolution of radionuclide imaging (98) and inability to detect the small effects on cardiac performance that would result (29).

In older subjects, an 18% increase in SV after conditioning was attributable to a reduction in end-systolic volume and a rise in ejection fraction (67). Enhanced ejection fraction reflected increases in myocardial contractility (SAP was unaffected) and possibly in myocardial muscle mass (which may or may not increase with endurance conditioning). If reduced cardiac performance with aging is attributable to a down-regulation of cardiac β_1-adrenoceptors (94), improvement after conditioning could stem, at least in part, from an up-regulation of these receptors, inasmuch as β-receptor density appears not to change with age (172).

Reduction in Ventricular Afterload. There is a close relationship between $\dot{V}O_{2max}$ and total vascular conductance so that when physical conditioning raises $\dot{V}O_{2max}$ and maximal cardiac output, total vascular conductance increases and SAP at any given fraction of $\dot{V}O_{2max}$ remains unchanged (29, 47). Thus, at maximal cardiac outputs of 20 liters/min in the sedentary individual and 40 liters/min in the endurance athlete, SAP is virtually the same. Physical conditioning is accompanied by a precise adjustment in SNA that matches total vascular conductance to maximal cardiac output (262, 265) (thus giving the appearance that SAP might be the primary regulated variable).

Increased Ventricular Preload. Part I of this chapter emphasizes that the autonomic nervous system can do little by itself to increase cardiac output beyond the small contribution of increased ejection fraction, unless, there is a way to maintain or increase ventricular filling pressure. The rise in SV is often assumed to originate from a rise in ventricular filling pressure. It has been more instructive to look for changes in EDV; an increase would suggest either that ventricular filling pressure had increased or some mechanical constraint on the heart had been removed (or less likely, myocardial compliance increased). Either way, a rise in ventricular volume means that ventricular wall tension increases at any given ventricular filling pressure (law of Laplace). Also, the heart functions on the steep portion of the curve relating SV to end-diastolic pressure; therefore, even small changes in ventricular filling pressure could exert large effects on SV (Chapter 15).

Changes in EDV. EDV, determined by radionuclide imaging, is higher in well-conditioned than in sedentary individuals when the separate groups are compared cross-sectionally (32, 215, 256) or when the same individuals are compared before and after physical conditioning (249).

Changes in blood volume. Historically, expansion of blood volume by physical conditioning has been credited for the rise in SV (50, 112), presumably secondary to a rise in CVP and EDV. However, the findings are not consistent in that others find small (101) to functionally insignificant increased in blood volume (289). The effect of blood volume expansion on CVP during exercise is not easily predicted. Exercise changes cardiac output and its distribution, both of which affect CVP irrespective of blood volume (see Chapter 15).

Altered Geometry and Pericardial Constraints. Simply cutting the pericardium without affecting control of HR permits increases in maximal SV and cardiac output that can equal or exceed those afforded by physical conditioning [see Figure 17.3; (338)]. Therefore, it could be argued that before physical conditioning, ventricular filling pressure was already higher than needed to raise SV, suggesting that EDV and therefore SV had been limited by the pericardium (268). Also, acute expansion of blood volume in humans raised their right atrial pressure by 7 mm Hg without effect on maximal SV and cardiac output (or on $\dot{V}O_{2max}$) (253). This idea of pericardial constraint is not supported by findings of others (83, 143, 144), who found only small (but statistically significant) increases in presumably "maximal" SV after volume loading. Blomqvist and Saltin (29) observed that people with larger than average SV appeared to respond more to volume loading than those with average SV. Possibly some adaptation had already occurred in those with larger SV. Also, the larger the heart to start with, the smaller the rise in filling pressure needed for any given increase in pericardial and ventricular wall tensions (law of Laplace). In short, a rise in EDV might originate from reduced pericardial restrictions on SV rather than alterations in either ventricular filling pressure or in blood volume.

Pericardial constraints on SV are markedly reduced by increasing ventricular filling pressure over time [e.g., by a chronic A-V fistula (85)]. Once the pericardium has expanded, the rise in filling pressure needed to raise SV becomes smaller. Therefore, the measurement of CVP before and after conditioning may tell nothing about adjustments in effective ventricular filling pressure or cardiac dimensions. It is conceivable that the rise in SV that attends physical conditioning may simply be the consequence of the chronic bradycardia that temporarily lowers cardiac output (47, 69) and raises CVP during submaximal exercise, and this in turn enlarges the pericardium.

Does Physical Conditioning Change Autonomic Control of the Circulation?

Physical conditioning increases both maximal cardiac output and total vascular conductance, whereas at maximal cardiac output, SAP is unchanged. Inasmuch as 85% of cardiac output is directed to active muscles at $\dot{V}O_{2max}$ and peak blood flow to exercising legs increases in proportion to the rise in $\dot{V}O_{2max}$ caused by conditioning, all of the rise in total vascular conductance must be in active muscle (47, 160, 291). Also, the major inactive regions are maximally vasoconstricted at $\dot{V}O_{2max}$ both before and after conditioning.

The rise in muscle vascular conductance must be attributable to inhibition of tonic vasoconstrictor outflow to muscle rather than to an increased capacity for muscles to vasodilate. Greater vasodilator capacity is observed in young (321, 326) and old (201), but presumably does not affect conductance during exercise involving a large muscle mass because the capacity of muscle to vasodilate is already so great that it must be tonically vasoconstricted to prevent hypotension (47, 160, 265). Active muscle is the major site of NE spillover in exercise (75, 295, 296), and this spillover is decreased by physical conditioning (92).

Physical conditioning reduces vasoconstriction in inactive regions at any absolute $\dot{V}O_2$, but the degree of vasoconstriction remains unchanged and is presumably at a maximum at $\dot{V}O_{2max}$. The degree of vasoconstriction at any given percentage of $\dot{V}O_{2max}$ required also remains unchanged before and after the adaptation (47, 262). The negative slope relating the reduction in regional blood flow to $\dot{V}O_2$ simply shifts rightward to higher $\dot{V}O_2$, just as does the slope relating the rise in HR to $\dot{V}O_2$. As a consequence, the relationships of splanchnic and renal blood flows to both the percentage of $\dot{V}O_{2max}$ required (i.e., relative $\dot{V}O_2$) and to HR remain constant throughout conditioning. Figure 17.6 shows that relationships among visceral organ blood flow, PRA, plasma NE concentration (all indices of SNA) remain constant when plotted against HR (plotted against percentage of $\dot{V}O_{2max}$, data would appear the same).

Control of HR. Physical conditioning changes the balance between parasympathetic and sympathetic control of HR by expanding the range of HR over which vagal control tends to dominate (230, 265, 268). The lowering of HR, both at rest and at submaximal levels of exercise expands both the range of $\dot{V}O_2$ and the range of HR over which cardiac output is raised predominantly by vagal withdrawal. Blockade of vagal control of HR with atropine reveals that in humans most of the HR response to exercise is attributable to withdrawal of tonic vagal outflow until HR approaches 100 bpm (70, 191, 252).

Two important points are first, that vagal withdrawal causes very rapid increases in HR (<1 s) and cardiac output. This means that by expanding the range of predominantly vagal control, we increase the range of $\dot{V}O_2$ over which HR and cardiac output can be raised rapidly. Second, above an HR of 100 bpm, the more slowly responding (~10–15 s) sympathetic system begins to dominate control of HR and cardiac output up to maximal values (70, 191, 252). The range of $\dot{V}O_2$ (but not the range of HR) over which sympathetic control of cardiac output dominates is also expanded by conditioning.

Control of SNA. As HR approaches 100 bpm, an increasing role for sympathetic control of the cardiovascular system first becomes obvious as summarized in Figure 17.6. Neither a chronic adjustment over months, such as in physical conditioning (which reduces SNA at a given $\dot{V}O_2$), nor an acute stress such as excessive heat during exercise (which increases SNA at a given $\dot{V}O_2$) alters the basic relationship between HR and any of the indices of SNA used so far (47, 262, 265, 268). The lower HR at any given $\dot{V}O_2$ after conditioning simply means that regional vasoconstriction and augmented release of NE and renin began at a higher absolute $\dot{V}O_2$ (but the same HR). In short, the scale of $\dot{V}O_2$ (and of work rate) over which the sympathetic nervous system operates during exercise is expanded, but its functions at any particular fraction of full scale (i.e., $\dot{V}O_{2max}$) are virtually constant (265; see also 310).

SYNTHESIS

What is the Autonomic Nervous System Controlling during Exercise?

This integration of cardiovascular control in dynamic exercise begins with an apparent paradox revealed in Guyton's seminal work on the mechanical coupling between the heart and peripheral circulation. The paradox is that when cardiac output is increased during rest the consequent decrease in CVP reduces SV and thereby self-limits the rise in cardiac output. Conversely, cardiac output cannot be increased without increasing or at least maintaining CVP. These observations constitute the keystone of Guyton's concepts presented graphically in his "venous return curves" and "cardiac function curves."

The limited ability to increase cardiac output at rest stems from the relatively high compliance of the peripheral circulation; when blood flow rises, the consequent increase in peripheral vascular volume lowers CVP, EDV, and SV, thus restricting further increases in cardiac output. Therefore, despite the availability of full autonomic control of its rate and contractile force, the heart cannot *by itself* raise its output substantially.

In contrast, cardiac output can increase by five to sevenfold during exercise without decrements (and usually with increases) in CVP, EDV, and SV. This reversal of the negative effect of increased peripheral vascular volume on EDV and cardiac output is achieved by adjustments in the peripheral circulation. Two events can counteract the interaction between blood flow and vascular volume, by translocating peripheral vascular volume back to the heart so as to restore its filling pressure. The first event is mechanical. It is the compression of veins by muscle contraction that reduces peripheral venous volume and, consequently, raises CVP and EDV. The second event that permits cardiac output and CVP to rise together during exercise requires the autonomic nervous system and, specifically, sympathetically mediated vasoconstriction. Although an adequate rise in cardiac output can be achieved during dynamic exercise by length–tension effects on SV if pericardial constraints on EDV are surgically eliminated, sympathetic vasomotor control is essential nevertheless. Without it, neither SAP nor CVP can be maintained, especially in upright humans.

The first requirement of the sympathetic nervous system is to control the distribution of cardiac output between compliant and noncompliant vascular beds by vasoconstriction. Vasoconstriction of large, highly compliant regions like the splanchnic and cutaneous reduces venous transmural pressure along with blood flow of the region. Blood volume is thereby passively expelled from capacious veins and translocated to the central circulation where it contributes to the maintenance of CVP and EDV, and consequently SV. Limited evidence suggests that splanchnic veins may actively constrict as well, but the main effects on splanchnic blood volume appear to be passive. In general, the translocation of blood volume by the muscle pumps (skeletal, abdominal, and respiratory muscles) and by the passive effects of vasoconstriction on peripheral venous volume appears to supersede any effects of venoconstriction.

Failure to maintain adequate sympathetic vasoconstriction in compliant regions (as, for example, in patients with dysautonomias or in normal people under heat stress) has as its main initial effect a lowering of SV rather than SAP. (Eventually, however, SAP will decline as well owing to the inevitable decline in cardiac output.) Therefore, the autonomic nervous system must counteract any tendency for increased blood flow to compliant regions by increasing tonic vasoconstriction.

Sympathetic vasoconstriction of the splanchnic region during exercise also increases the fraction of cardiac output directed to active muscle. In general, the maintenance of adequate ventricular filling pressure during dynamic exercise requires a balance between the purely mechanical effects of the muscle pumps and the sympathetic control of blood vessels. The negative relationship between cardiac output and CVP, intrinsic to the resting state, can still be observed during exercise whenever cardiac output is increased further to supply needs for additional blood flow to compliant regions such as the skin. That is, the additional rise in cardiac output lowers CVP just as it does at rest. This can be counteracted by vasoconstricting cutaneous vessels, by matching the vasodilation and the rise in cutaneous blood flow (and blood volume) with vasoconstriction and a fall in splanchnic blood flow (and blood volume), or by withdrawal of sympathetic vasodilator outflow to the skin. All three autonomic responses have now been observed during heat stress.

A second requirement of the autonomic nervous system, and one of equal importance to the first, is the control of SAP by sympathetic vasoconstriction. Inasmuch as the large compliant regions (splanchnic, cutaneous) normally comprise only a small fraction of total vascular conductance, their direct influence on SAP is small—even when vasoconstriction is abolished. Conversely, active skeletal muscle accounts for most of the total vascular conductance during exercise; therefore, its influence on SAP is great. Bear in mind this is in contrast to the lack of direct influence of changes in MBF on CVP and EDV because muscle vascular volume is essentially unaffected by flow per se.

Until recently, the special importance of sympathetic vasoconstriction in active muscles to the maintenance of SAP tended to pass unnoticed. Failure to increase (above resting levels) vasoconstriction in active muscle, even during submaximal exercise, causes hypotension due to the mismatch between cardiac output and total vascular conductance. Even when cardiac output is maintained in exercising humans with dysautonomia by body positioning or in dogs with sympathetic blockade by ventricular pacing, SAP falls markedly owing primarily to the unopposed rise in muscle vascular conductance. Muscle vasodilation can gradually outstrip the pumping capacity of the heart.

What Errors Are Sensed and then Corrected by the Autonomic Nervous System during Exercise?

This question quickly distills down to the choice between *flow errors* caused by mismatches between blood flow and metabolism and *pressure errors* caused by mismatches between blood flow and vascular conductance. There are, however, also temperature errors stemming from mismatches between cutaneous blood flow and body temperatures, and these demand additional blood flow.

Blood Flow Errors. In addition to metabolic stimuli such as lactic acid, which activate muscle afferent fibers, the same fibers respond to mechanical forces generated by muscle contraction and also changes in muscle temperature. Neither of these latter two variables, despite their potential importance, has yet been incorporated into a scheme of overall cardiovascular control during dynamic exercise.

The original and still viable hypothesis concerning blood flow errors is that they become manifest in an accumulation of metabolites within the interstitium of active muscles whenever MBF falls below some critical level. These accumulated metabolites increase the firing of muscle afferent nerve fibers. Their increased traffic to the CNS acts on neurons that control sympathetic nervous outflow to the cardiovascular system. The presumed role of the sympathetic nervous system is to restore MBF and the intramuscular concentration of metabolites to some optimal level by raising cardiac output and SAP. The reflex is called the muscle chemoreflex, and a still unanswered question is if this reflex is *ever* a tonically active controller of the normal circulation during exercise.

The critical level of MBF at which the muscle chemoreflex is evoked appears to be reached when oxygen delivery to muscle cells no longer suffices. The muscle chemoreflex is more than two times stronger than the arterial baroreflex when unopposed by the baroreflex. Normally, the rise in SAP caused by the chemoreflex is reduced by 50% by the arterial baroreflex. If exercise is mild, a substantial reduction in MBF is required to elicit the chemoreflex; the margin for flow error is large, meaning that this reflex is not tonically active. In mild to moderate dynamic exercise, the chemoreflex raises both cardiac output and SAP to partially restore MBF when the latter falls enough to make oxygen supply inadequate. The rise in cardiac output plus regional vasoconstriction can correct the error in MBF by approximately 50%. When exercise becomes increasingly severe and approaches maximal, the chemoreflex can no longer raise cardiac output or MBF; it raises SAP by vasoconstricting active muscle, and as such converts from a flow-sensitive, MBF-raising reflex to an SAP-raising reflex and thus one with apparent positive feedback. That is, the vasoconstriction in active muscle may augment the signal that initiates the reflex. Another possibility is that different distribution of α_1- and α_2-adrenoceptors within a muscle may redistribute MBF during sympathetic stimulation so as to lessen any positive feedback. The reflex clearly plays a role under conditions of severe muscle ischemia as, for example, in atherosclerosis obliterans.

Blood Pressure Errors. Arterial blood pressure errors are sensed as changes in either mean or pulsatile pressures at the carotid sinus and aortic baroreceptors. During exercise these errors commonly originate from either too little or too much vasoconstriction. The arterial baroreflex is viewed as protecting SAP by vasoconstricting not only inactive regions but especially active skeletal muscle as well. In addition, changes in CVP are sensed by cardiopulmonary baroreceptors, but the changes in SNA initiated by these receptors do little to restore CVP. We have a problem discussing the matching of functions by the cardiopulmonary baroreflex, since it acts on a part of the circulation from which it is hydraulically separated (i.e., the arteries). Another problem is the passive interaction between CVP, SV, and aortic pulse pressure can sometimes make it impossible to determine which reflex, cardiopulmonary or arterial baroreflex, initiates a response.

Three observations favor the arterial baroreflex as the primary controller for the cardiovascular system during exercise. First, strong evidence suggests that the arterial baroreflex is rapidly reset to a higher operating pressure at the onset of exercise. Second, the baroreflex is a tonically active controller of SNA in exercise and its function is necessary for a normal cardiovascular response. Third, skeletal muscle appears to be a major target of a reflex that maintains nearly constant SAP during dynamic exercise before and after physical conditioning.

One hypothesis is that the increase in SAP and SNA at the onset of exercise depends on a rapid resetting of the arterial baroreflex to a higher operating point (275). If such resetting occurs, autonomic control during exercise could originate from the arterial baroreflex, making continuous corrections of errors in SAP, with those errors being any difference between actual SAP and the reset baroreflex operating point.

We hypothesize that the most important function of central command, or feedforward control, is to reset the operating point of a feedback controller, the arterial baroreflex, at the onset of exercise. Then in turn, central command raises cardiac output and SAP by sudden withdrawal of cardiac vagal tone. The sudden increase in CVP by the muscle pump permits the immediate rise in cardiac output and in SAP. If exercise is mild (HR <100 bpm), the rise in cardiac output and SAP are presumably so rapid that

SAP is immediately raised to the new operating point of the reset arterial baroreflex. Because of the speed of response, no pressure error is perceived by the CNS; speed of response is the key to this hypothesis. In theory, this part of a broader scheme (below) could apply only up to the highest level of exercise at which the rise in HR and cardiac output is dominated by rapid vagal withdrawal. In humans this would mean that HR would rise only to ~100 bpm before a more slowly responding sympathetic outflow would begin to dominate the control of HR and cardiac output.

Figure 17.6 reveals that when HR approaches 100 bpm, the effects of increased SNA become manifest. Although all major inactive regions, including skin, initially vasoconstrict, the major source of NE is active muscle. As the sympathetic nervous system becomes the dominant controller of HR, the rise in HR and cardiac output at the onset of exercise becomes slower (sympathetic response time is 10–15 s as compared to <1 s for the vagus nerve). As a consequence, the rise in cardiac output cannot compensate fully for the rise in total vascular conductance stemming from the muscle vasodilation and SAP falls below, or does not rise up to, the new operating point of the baroreflex. For example, if we assume resetting of the arterial baroreflex is virtually instantaneous, then SAP can no longer be raised immediately to its new "reset" operating point. This is translated as a "pressure error" by the CNS. Sympathetically mediated constriction in renal, splanchnic, cutaneous, and skeletal muscle (both resting and active) vasculature would be initiated by the CNS to minimize this pressure error. Recall that in dogs and rabbits when the baroreflex was absent, SNA did not increase and SAP fell rather than rose at onset of exercise (i.e., the baroreflex was needed to raise SAP). Again, in this scheme it is the speed of the cardiovascular responses that would dictate the presence of a pressure error [the range of HR over which rapid vagal control dominates varies among species (297)].

This hypothesis is consistent with the effects of physical conditioning and heat stress and other stresses that change the relationship between HR and $\dot{V}O_2$ during dynamic exercise. In these cases the relationship between HR and all indices of SNA remains fixed. SNA increases only when vagal control of HR appears to be no longer dominant (i.e., HR exceeds 100 bpm). These stresses, and the adjustments to them, alter the range of parasympathetic control of HR and, therefore, at the same time, the level of exercise (but not the HR) at which sympathetic control becomes important.

As the severity of exercise increases, control shifts from predominantly cardiac control of SAP to combined cardiac and vasomotor control, and finally as maximal cardiac output is approached, to predominantly vasoconstrictor control of active skeletal muscle. This vasoconstriction in active muscle increases with work rate so that when work rate is augmented by raising muscle mass, muscle vascular conductance is reduced, presumably in order to raise SAP to its higher operating point (see 251, 309). Neither the arterial baroreflex nor the muscle chemoreflex can do much to alter SAP without vasoconstricting active muscle when that vascular bed comprises 85% of total vascular conductance.

Conclusions. The apparent precision with which SAP is regulated encourages speculation that it is the major variable being controlled during dynamic exercise; but constancy does not prove active regulation. A more compelling argument is the tight control of muscle vascular conductance by the sympathetic nervous system during exercise. This control has been shown to be critical to the regulation of SAP; that is, muscle vascular conductance appears to be the dominant variable in SAP regulation during dynamic exercise and its dominance increases with severity of exercise. To place control of muscle vascular conductance with the muscle chemoreflex could be tantamount to placing control of SAP with a flow-sensitive reflex that is SAP-*raising*, not SAP-regulating. In contrast, the arterial baroreflex is a pressure-sensitive reflex that is pressure-*regulating* and this difference is fundamental.

Rather than disputing which reflex might be *the* controller of the circulation during exercise, perhaps it suffices to say that mammals benefit from a muscle chemoreflex that guards against hypoperfusion of active muscle. In humans and dogs, it is most effective when exercise is mild to moderate; in that setting it can counteract muscle ischemia by raising cardiac output and redistributing blood flow by vasoconstriction, thereby partially restoring MBF.

Mammals also benefit from an arterial baroreflex that protects against hypo- or hypertension and is therefore likely to control total vascular conductance and SAP when muscle is adequately perfused. This reflex is tonically active, and is effective during mild through severe exercise. The likelihood that the two reflexes might act synergistically during severe exercise has been postulated but not yet explored experimentally. The next paragraph suggests a possibility.

Although vasoconstriction within the working muscle must be maintained to protect SAP, is there also, during severe exercise, local modulation of vasoconstriction within the muscle so that its blood flow is redistributed from the most active to the least active motor units? Could this be achieved perhaps via the different sensitivities of the α_1- vs. α_2-adrenoceptors to the surrounding concentrations of metabolites? Does the greater sensitivity of α_2-adrenoceptors to metabolites minimize vasoconstriction in fast-fatiguing, glycolytic fibers, at the expense of greater α_1-adrenoceptor (metabolite-insensitive) vasoconstriction is slowly fatiguing oxidative fibers? Intuitively, however, one might prefer that the vasoconstriction be manifest in the fast-fatiguing glycolytic fibers instead—but perhaps we evolved to make sudden bursts of effort for escapes rather than to run marathons.

We are grateful to Pam Stevens for invaluable assistance. We thank the investigators who sent reprints of their most recent work.

Investigations from our laboratories were supported by grants from the National Heart, Lung, and Blood Institute grants HL-16910 (L.B.R.); HL-45038 and HL-02844 (D.S.O'L.); and HL-20663 and HL-36080 (D.L.K.).

REFERENCES

1. Almen T., and G. Nylander. Serial phlebography of the normal lower leg during muscular contraction and relaxation. *Acta Radiol. (Stockh.)* 57: 264–272, 1962.
2. Andersen, P., and B. Saltin. Maximal perfusion of skeletal muscle in man. *J. Physiol. (Lond.)* 366: 233–249, 1985.
3. Anderson, K. M., and J. E. Faber. Differential sensitivity of arteriolar α_1- and α_2-adrenoceptor constriction to metabolic inhibition during rat skeletal muscle contraction. *Circ. Res.* 69: 174–184, 1991.
4. Angell-James, J. E., and M. De B. Daly. Effects of graded pulsatile pressure on the reflex vasomotor responses elicited by changes of mean pressure in the perfused carotid sinus-aortic arch of the dog. *J. Physiol. (Lond.)* 214: 51–64, 1971.
5. Ardell, J. L., A. M. Scher, and L. B. Rowell. Effects of baroreceptor denervation on the cardiovascular response to dynamic exercise. In: *Arterial Baroreceptors and Hypertension*, edited by P. Sleight. Oxford, UK: Oxford University Press, 1980, p. 311–317.
6. Arrowood, J. A., P. K. Mohanty, C. McNamara, and M. D. Thames. Cardiopulmonary reflexes do not modulate exercise pressor reflexes during isometric exercise in humans. *J. Appl. Physiol.* 74: 2559–2565, 1993.
7. Ashkar, E. Effects of bilateral splanchnicectomy on circulation during exercise in dogs. *Acta Physiol. Lat. Am.* 23: 171–177, 1973.
8. Åstrand, P.-O., T. E. Cuddy, B. Saltin, and J. Stenberg. Cardiac output during submaximal and maximal work. *J. Appl. Physiol.* 19: 268–274, 1964.
9. Åstrand, P.-O., and G. Grimby. Physical activity in health and disease. *Acta Med. Scand. Suppl.* 711: 1–244, 1986.
10. Bache, R. J., D. C. Homans, and X.-Z. Dai. Adrenergic vasoconstriction limits coronary blood flow during exercise in hypertrophied left ventricle. *Am. J. Physiol.* 260 (*Heart Circ. Physiol.* 29): H1489–H1494, 1991.
11. Bader, H. The anatomy and physiology of the vascular wall. In: *Handbook of Physiology, Circulation*, edited by W. F. Hamilton and P. Dow. Washington, DC: Am. Physiol. Soc., 1963, p. 865–889.
12. Barcroft, H., and S. Samaan. Explanation of the increase in systemic flow caused by occluding the descending thoracic aorta. *J. Physiol. (Lond.)* 85: 47–61, 1935.
13. Båth, E., L. E. Lindblad, and B. G. Wallin. Effects of dynamic and static neck suction on muscle nerve sympathetic activity, heart rate and blood pressure in man. *J. Physiol. (Lond.)* 311: 551–564, 1981.
14. Batman, B. A., J. C. Hardy, U. A. Leuenberger, M. B. Smith, Q. X. Yang, and L. I. Sinoway. Sympathetic nerve activity during prolonged rhythmic forearm exercise. *J. Appl. Physiol.* 76: 1077–1081, 1994.
15. Bayly, W. M., D. R. Hodgson, D. A. Schultz, J. A. Dempsey, and P. D. Gollnick. Exercise-induced hypercapnia in the horse. *J. Appl. Physiol.* 67: 1958–1966, 1989.
16. Beaty, O., III, and D. E. Donald. Role of potassium in the transient reduction in vasoconstrictive responses of muscle resistance vessels during rhythmic exercise in dogs. *Circ. Res.* 41: 452–460, 1977.
17. Bell, A. W., J. R. S. Hales, R. G. King, and A. A. Fawcett. Influence of heat stress on exercise-induced changes in regional blood flow in sheep. *J. Appl. Physiol. Respir. Environ. Exerc. Physiol.* 55: 1916–1923, 1983.
18. Bevegård, B. S., and J. T. Shepherd. Reaction in man of resistance and capacity vessels in forearm and hand to leg exercise. *J. Appl. Physiol.* 21: 123–132, 1966.
19. Bevegård, B. S., and J. T. Shepherd. Circulatory effects of stimulating the carotid arterial stretch receptors in man at rest and during exercise. *J. Clin. Invest.* 45: 132–142, 1966.
20. Bevegård, B. S., and J. T. Shepherd. Regulation of the circulation during exercise in man. *Physiol. Rev.* 47: 178–213, 1967.
21. Bevegård, S., J. Castenfors, L. E. Lindblad, and J. Tranesjo. Blood pressure and heart rate regulating capacity of the carotid sinus during changes in blood volume distribution in man. *Acta Physiol. Scand.* 99: 300–312, 1977.
22. Bevegård, S., and A. Lodin. Postural circulatory changes at rest and during exercise in five patients with congenital absence of valves in the deep veins of the legs. *Acta Med. Scand.* 172: 21–29, 1962.
23. Bevegård, S., B. Jonsson, and I. Karlof. Circulatory response to recumbent exercise and head-up tilting in patients with disturbed sympathetic cardiovascular control (postural hypotension). *Acta Med. Scand.* 172: 623–636, 1962.
24. Bevegård, S., B. Jonsson, I. Karlof. H. Lagergren, and E. Sowton. Effect of changes in ventricular rate on cardiac output and central pressures at rest and during exercise in patients with artificial pacemakers. *Cardiovasc. Res.* 1: 21–33, 1967.
25. Bishop, V. S. Invited editorial on "carotid baroreflex control of blood pressure and heart rate in men during dynamic exercise. *J. Appl. Physiol.* 77: 491–492, 1994.
26. Bishop, V. S., and S. E. DiCarlo. Role of vagal afferents in cardiovascular control. In: *Vagal Control of the Heart: Experimental Basis and Clinical Implications*, edited by M. N. Levy and P. J. Schwartz. Mount Kisco, NY: Futura Publishing Co., Inc., 1993, p. 1–20.
27. Bishop, V. S., A. Malliani, and P. Thorén. Cardiac Mechanoreceptors. In: *Handbook of Physiology, The Cardiovascular System, Peripheral Circulation and Organ Blood Flow*, edited by J. T. Shepherd and F. M. Abboud. Bethesda, MD: Am. Physiol. Soc., 1983, p. 497–555.

28. Bishop, V. S., and D. F. Peterson. The circulatory influences of vagal afferents at rest and during coronary occlusion in conscious dogs. *Circ. Res.* 43: 840–847, 1978.
29. Blomqvist, C. G., and B. Saltin. Cardiovascular adaptations to physical training. *Annu. Rev. Physiol.* 45: 169–189, 1983.
30. Borbujo, J., A. L. Garcia-Villalon, J. Valle, B. Gomez, and G. Diequez. Postjunctional α_1- and α_2-adrenoceptors in human skin arteries. An in vitro study. *J. Pharmacol. Exp. Ther.* 249: 284–287, 1989.
31. Bradley, S. E., P. A. Marks, P. C. Reynell, and J. Meltzer. The circulating splanchnic blood volume in dog and man. *Trans. Assoc. Am. Phys.* 66: 294–302, 1953.
32. Brandao, M. U. P., M. Wajngarten, E. Rondon, M. C. P. Giorgi, F. Hironaka, and C. E. Negrao. Left ventricular function during dynamic exercise in untrained and moderately trained subjects. *J. Appl. Physiol.* 75: 1989–1995, 1993.
33. Brecher, G. A. *Venous Return*. New York: Grune & Stratton, 1956.
34. Brengelmann, G. L. Specialized brain cooling in man? *FASEB J.* 7: 1148–1153, 1993.
35. Brengelmann, G. L. Temperature regulation. In: *Scientific Foundations of Sports Medicine*, edited by C. C. Teitz. Philadelphia. B. C. Decker, Inc., 1989, p. 77–116.
36. Brengelmann, G. L., P. R. Freund, L. B. Rowell, J. E. Olerud, and K. K. Kraning. Absence of active cutaneous vasodilation associated with congenital absence of sweat glands in humans. *Am. J. Physiol.* 240 (*Heart Circ. Physiol.* 9): H571–H575, 1981.
37. Brengelmann, G. L., J. M. Johnson, L. Hermansen, and L. B. Rowell. Altered control of skin blood flow during exercise at high internal temperature. *J. Appl. Physiol. Respir. Environ. Exerc. Physiol.* 43: 790–794, 1977.
38. Bristow, J. D., E. B. Brown, Jr., D. J. C. Cunningham, M. G. Howson, E. S. Petersen, T. G. Pickering, and P. Sleight. Effect of bicycling on the baroreflex regulation of pulse interval. *Circ. Res.* 28: 582–592, 1971.
39. Britton, S. L., and P. J. Metting. Reflex regulation of skeletal muscle blood flow. In: *Reflex Control of the Circulation*, edited by I. H. Zucker, and J. P. Gilmore. Boca Raton, FL: CRC Press, Inc., 1991, p. 737–764.
40. Burcher, E., and D. Garlick. Effects of exercise metabolites on adrenergic vasoconstriction in the gracilis muscle of the dog. *J. Pharmacol. Exp. Ther.* 192: 149–156, 1975.
41. Burnstock, G. The changing face of autonomic neurotransmission. *Acta Physiol. Scand.* 126: 67–91, 1986.
42. Buskirk, E. F., and J. L. Hodgson. Age and aerobic power: the rate of change in men and women. *Federation Proc.* 46: 1824–1829, 1987.
43. Caldini, P., S. Permutt, J. A. Waddell, and R. L. Riley. Effect of epinephrine on pressure, flow, and volume relationships in the systemic circulation of dogs. *Circ. Res.* 34: 606–623, 1974.
44. Chapleau, M. W., G. Hajduczok, and F. M. Abboud. Peripheral and central mechanisms of baroreflex resetting. *Clin Exp. Pharmacol. Physiol. Suppl.* 15: 31–43, 1989.
45. Chihara, E., T. Morimoto, K. Shigemi, T. Natsuyama, and S. Hashimoto. Vascular viscoelasticity of perfused rat hindquarters. *Am. J. Physiol.* 260 (*Heart Circ. Physiol.* 29): H1834–H1840, 1991.
46. Christensen, N. J. Plasma noradrenaline and adrenaline measured by isotope-derivative assay. *Dan Med. Bull.* 26: 17–56, 1979.
47. Clausen, J.-P. Effect of physical training on cardiovascular adjustments to exercise in man. *Physiol. Rev.* 57: 779–815, 1977.
48. Clausen, J.-P., and J. Trap-Jensen. Arteriohepatic venous oxygen difference and heart rate during initial phases of exercise. *J. Appl. Physiol.* 37: 716–719, 1974.
49. Collins, H. L., and S. E. Dicarlo. Cardiac afferents attenuate the muscle metaboreflex in the rat. *J. Appl. Physiol.* 75: 114–120, 1993.
50. Convertino, V. A., G. W. Mack, and E. R. Nadel. Elevated central venous pressure: a consequence of exercise training-induced hypervolemia? *Am. J. Physiol.* 260 (*Regulatory Integrative Comp. Physiol.* 29): R273–R277, 1991.
51. Cunningham, D. J. C., E. Strange Petersen, R. Peto, T. C. Pickering, and P. Sleight. Comparison of the effect of different types of exercise on the baroreflex regulation of heart rate. *Acta Physiol. Scand.* 86: 444–455, 1972.
52. Daskalopoulos, D. A., J. T. Shepherd, and S. C. Walgenbach. Cardiopulmonary reflexes and blood pressure in exercising sinoaortic-denervated dogs. *J. Appl. Physiol.* 57: 1417–1421, 1984.
53. DiCarlo, S. E., and V. S. Bishop. Regional vascular resistance during exercise: role of cardiac afferents and exercise training. *Am. J. Physiol.* 258 (*Heart Circ. Physiol.* 27): H842–H847, 1990.
54. DiCarlo, S. E., and V. S. Bishop. Onset of exercise shifts operating point of arterial baroreflex to higher pressures. *Am. J. Physiol.* 262 (*Heart Circ. Physiol.* 31): H302–H307, 1992.
55. Dill, D. B., J. H. Talbott, and H. T. Edwards. Studies in muscular activity. VI. Responses of several individuals to a fixed task. *J. Physiol. (Lond.)* 69: 267–305, 1930.
56. Docherty, J. R. Cardiovascular responses in aging. *Pharmacol. Rev.* 42: 103–126, 1990.
57. Dodd, L. R., and P. C. Johnson. Antagonism of vasoconstriction by muscle contraction differs with α-adrenergic subtype. *Am. J. Physiol.* 264 (*Heart Circ. Physiol.* 33): H892–H900, 1993.
58. Donald, D. E. Splanchnic circulation. In: *Handbook of Physiology, The Cardiovascular System, Peripheral Circulation and Organ Blood Flow*, edited by J. T. Shepherd and F. M. Abboud. Bethesda, MD: Am. Physiol. Soc., 1993, p. 219–240.
59. Donald, D. E., D. J. Rowlands, and D. A. Ferguson. Similarity of blood flow in the normal and the sympathectomized dog hind limb during graded exercise. *Circ. Res.* 26: 185–199, 1970.
60. Donald, D. E., and J. T. Shepherd. Response to exercise in dogs with cardiac denervation. *Am. J. Physiol.* 205: 393–400, 1963.
61. Ebert, T. Baroreflex responsiveness is maintained during isometric exercise in humans. *J. Appl. Physiol.* 61: 797–803, 1986.
62. Eckberg, D. L. Baroreflex inhibition of the human sinus node: importance of stimulus intensity, duration and rate of pressure change. *J. Physiol. (Lond.)* 269: 561–577, 1977.
63. Eckberg, D. L., G. F. Fletcher, and E. Braunwald. Mechanism of prolongation of the R-R interval with electrical stimulation of the carotid sinus nerves in man. *Circ. Res.* 30: 131–138, 1972.
64. Eckberg, D. L., R. F. Rea, O. K. Andersson, T. Hedner, J. Pernow, J. M. Lundberg, and B. G. Wallin. Baroreflex modulation of sympathetic activity and sympathetic neurotransmitters in humans. *Acta Physiol. Scand.* 133: 221–231, 1988.

65. Eckberg, D. L., and P. Sleight. *Human Baroreflexes in Health and Disease*. Oxford, UK and New York: Oxford University Press, 1992.
66. Edholm, O. G., R. H. Fox, and R. K. MacPherson. Vasomotor control of the cutaneous blood vessels in the human forearm. *J. Physiol. (Lond.)* 139: 455–465, 1957.
67. Ehsani, A. A., T. Ogawa, T. R. Miller, R. J. Spina, and S. M. Jilka. Exercise training improves left ventricular systolic function in older men. *Circulation* 83: 96–103, 1991.
68. Ekblom, B. Effect of physical training on oxygen transport system in man. *Acta Physiol. Scand. Suppl.* 328: 5–45, 1969.
69. Ekblom, B., P.-O. Åstrand, B. Saltin, J. Stenberg, and B. Wallstrom. Effect of training on circulatory response to exercise. *J. Appl. Physiol.* 24: 518–528, 1968.
70. Ekblom, B., A. N. Goldbarg, A. S. A. Kilbom, and P. O. Åstrand. Effects of atropine and propranolol on the oxygen transport system during exercise in man. *Scand. J. Clin. Lab. Invest.* 30: 35–42, 1972.
71. Ekelund, L.-G. Circulatory and respiratory adaptation during prolonged exercise. *Acta Physiol. Scand.* 70 (Suppl. 292): 1–38, 1967.
72. Eklund, L.-G., and A. Holmgren. Central hemodynamics during exercise. *Circ. Res.* 21 (Suppl. 1): I-33–I-43, 1967.
73. Epstein, S. E., G. D. Beiser, R. E. Goldstein, M. Stampfer, A. S. Wechsler, G. Glick, and E. Braunwald. Circulatory effects of electrical stimulation of the carotid sinus nerves in man. *Circulation* 40: 269–276, 1969.
74. Eriksen, M., B. A. Waaler, L. Walløe, and J. Wesche. Dynamics and dimensions of cardiac output changes in humans at the onset and at the end of moderate rhythmic exercise. *J. Physiol. (Lond.)* 426: 423–437, 1990.
75. Esler, M., G. Jennings, G. Lambert, I. Meredith, M. Horne, and G. Eisenhofer. Overflow of catecholamine neurotransmitters to the circulation: source, fate, and functions. *Physiol. Rev.* 70: 963–985, 1990.
76. Ettinger, S., K. Gray, S. Whisler, and L. Sinoway. Dichloroacetate reduces sympathetic nerve responses to static exercise. *Am. J. Physiol.* 261 (*Heart Circ. Physiol.* 30): H1653–H1658, 1991.
77. Faber, J. E. In situ analysis of α-adrenoceptors on arteriolar and venular smooth muscle in rat skeletal muscle microcirculation. *Circ. Res.* 62: 37–50, 1988.
78. Fernandes, A., H. Galbo, M. Kjaer, J. H. Mitchell, N. H. Secher, and S. N. Thomas. Cardiovascular and ventilatory responses to dynamic exercise during epidural anesthesia in man. *J. Physiol. (Lond.)* 420: 281–293, 1990.
79. Flamm, S. D., J. Taki, R. Moore, S. F. Lewis, F. Keech, F. Maltais, M. Ahmad, R. Callahan, S. Dragotakes, N. Alpert, and H. W. Strauss. Redistribution of regional and organ blood volume and effect on cardiac function in relation to upright exercise intensity in healthy human subjects. *Circulation* 81: 1550–1559, 1990.
80. Folkow, B., P. Gaskell, and B. A. Whaler. Blood flow through limb muscles during heavy rhythmic exercise. *Acta Physiol. Scand.* 80: 61–72, 1970.
81. Folkow, B., U. Haglund, M. Jodal, and O. Lundgren. Blood flow in the calf muscle of man during heavy rhythmic exercise. *Acta Physiol. Scand.* 81: 157–163, 1971.
82. Folkow, B., and A. Svanborg. Physiology of cardiovascular aging. *Physiol. Rev.* 73: 725–764, 1993.
83. Fortney, S. M., E. R. Nadel, C. B. Wenger, and J. R. Bove. Effect of acute alterations of blood volume on circulatory performance in humans. *J. Appl. Physiol. Respir. Environ. Exerc. Physiol.* 50: 292–298, 1981.
84. Freedman, R. R., S. C. Sabharwal, M. Moten, and P. Migaly. Local temperature modulates α_1- and α_2-adrenergic vasoconstriction in men. *Am. J. Physiol.* 263 (*Heart Circ. Physiol.* 32): H1197–H1200, 1992.
85. Freeman, G. L., and M. M. LeWinter. Pericardial adaptations during chronic cardiac dilation in dogs. *Circ. Res.* 54: 294–300, 1984.
86. Freund, P. R., S. F. Hobbs, and L. B. Rowell. Cardiovascular responses to muscle ischemia in man—dependency on muscle mass. *J. Appl. Physiol. Respir. Environ. Exerc. Physiol.* 45: 762–767, 1978.
87. Freund, P. R., L. B. Rowell, T. M. Murphy, S. F. Hobbs, and S. H. Butler. Blockade of the pressor response to muscle ischemia by sensory nerve block in man. *Am. J. Physiol.* 236 (*Heart Circ. Physiol.* 6): H433–H439, 1979.
88. Freyschuss, U. Elicitation of heart rate and blood pressure increase on muscle contraction. *J. Appl. Physiol.* 28: 758–761, 1970.
89. Friedman, D. B., J. M. Johnson, J. H. Mitchell, and N. H. Secher. Neural control of the cutaneous vasoconstrictor response to dynamic exercise. *J. Appl. Physiol.* 71: 1892–1896, 1991.
90. Froelich, J. W., H. W. Strauss, R. H. Moore, and K. A. McKusick. Redistribution of visceral blood volume in upright exercise in healthy volunteers. *J. Nucl. Med.* 29: 1714–1718, 1988.
91. Gaffney, F. A., G. Sjogaard, and B. Saltin. Cardiovascular and metabolic responses to static contraction in man. *Acta Physiol. Scand.* 138: 249–258, 1990.
92. Galbo, H. *Hormonal and Metabolic Adaptation to Exercise*. New York: Thieme-Stratton, 1983.
93. Gates, G. F., and A. W. Ames. Splenic "disappearance" during gated exercise nuclear angiocardiography. *Clin. Nucl. Med.* 11: 683–687, 1986.
94. Gerstenblith, G., D. S. Renlund, and E. G. Lakatta. Cardiovascular response to exercise in younger and older men. *Federation Proc.* 46: 1834–1839, 1987.
95. Goldstein, D. S., R. McCarty, R. J. Polinsky, and I. J. Kopin. Relationship between plasma norepinephrine and sympathetic neural activity. *Hypertension* 5: 552–559, 1983.
96. Gollnick, P. D., M. Riedy, J. J. Quintinskie, and L. A. Bertocci. Differences in metabolic potential of skeletal muscle fibres and its significance for metabolic control. *J. Exp. Biol.* 115: 191–199, 1985.
97. Gorczynski, R. J., B. Klitzman, and B. R. Duling. Interrelations between contracting striated muscle and precapillary microvessels. *Am. J. Physiol.* 235 (*Heart Circ. Physiol.* 4): H494–H504, 1978.
98. Gould, K. L. Quantitative imaging in nuclear cardiology. *Circulation* 66: 1141–1146, 1982.
99. Gow, B. S. Circulatory correlates: vascular impedance, resistance, and capacity. In: *Handbook of Physiology, The Cardiovascular System, Vascular Smooth Muscle*, edited by D. F. Bohr, A. P. Somlyo, and H. V. Sparks, Jr. Bethesda, MD: Am. Physiol. Soc., 1980, p. 353–408.
100. Gray, S. D., E. Carlsson, and N. C. Staub. Site of increased vascular resistance during isometric muscle contraction. *Am. J. Physiol.* 213: 683–689, 1967.
101. Green, H. J., J. R. Sutton, G. Coates, M. Ali, and S. Jones. Response of red cell and plasma volume to prolonged training in humans. *J. Appl. Physiol.* 70: 1810–1815, 1991.
102. Grimby, G. N., J. Nilsson, and H. Sanne. Cardiac output during exercise in patients with varicose veins. *Scand. J. Clin. Lab. Invest.* 16: 21–30, 1964.
103. Guyton, A. C., B. H. Douglas, J. B. Langston, and T. Q. Richardson. Instantaneous increase in mean circulatory

pressure and cardiac output at onset of muscular activity. *Circ. Res.* 11: 431–441, 1962.

104. Gwirtz, P. A., S. P. Overn, J. H. Mass, and C. E. Jones. α-Adrenergic constriction limits coronary flow and cardiac function in running dogs. *Am. J. Physiol.* 250 (*Heart Circ. Physiol.* 19): H1117–H1126, 1986.
105. Hagberg, J. M. Effect of training on the decline of $\dot{V}O_2$ max with aging. *Federation Proc.* 46: 1830–1833, 1987.
106. Haggendal, J. Some further aspects on the release of the adrenergic transmitter. In: *New Aspects of Storage and Release Mechanisms of Catecholamines*. Bayer Symposium II. New York: Springer-Verlag, 1970, p. 100–109.
107. Hales, J. R. S., and J. Ludbrook. Baroreflex participation in redistribution of cardiac output at onset of exercise. *J. Appl. Physiol.* 64: 627–634, 1988.
108. Hammond, H. K., F. C. White, V. Bhargava, and R. Shabetai. Heart size and maximal cardiac output are limited by the pericardium. *Am. J. Physiol.* 263 (*Heart Circ. Physiol.* 32): H1675–H1681, 1992.
109. Hansen, J., T. N. Jacobsen, and A. Amtorp. The exercise pressor response to sustained handgrip does not augment blood flow in the contracting forearm skeletal muscle. *Acta Physiol. Scand.* 149: 419–425, 1993.
110. Hansen, J., G. D. Thomas, T. N. Jacobsen, and R. G. Victor. Muscle metaboreflex triggers parallel sympathetic activation in exercising and resting human skeletal muscle. *Am. J. Physiol.* 266 (*Heart Circ. Physiol.* 35): H2508–H2514, 1994.
111. Hargens, A. R., R. W. Millard, K. Pettersson, and K. Johansen. Gravitational haemodynamics and oedema prevention in the giraffe. *Nature* 329: 59–60, 1987.
112. Harrison, M. H. Effects of thermal stress and exercise on blood volume in humans. *Physiol. Rev.* 65: 149– 209, 1985.
113. Hartley, L. H., G. Grimby, A. Kilbom, N. J. Nilsson, I. Åstrand, J. Bjure, B. Ekblom, and B. Saltin. Physical training in sedentary middle-aged and older men. III. Cardiac output and gas exchange at submaximal and maximal exercise. *Scand. J. Clin. Lab. Invest.* 24: 335–344, 1969.
114. Hasking, G. J., M. D. Esler, G. L. Jennings, E. Dewar, and G. Lambert. Norepinephrine spillover to plasma during steady-state supine bicycle exercise. Comparison of patients with congestive heart failure and normal subjects. *Circulation* 78: 516–521, 1988.
115. Hecker, M., A. Mulsch, E. Bassenge, and R. Busse. Vasoconstriction and increased flow: two principal mechanisms of shear stress-dependent endothelial autacoid release. *Am. J. Physiol.* 265 (*Heart Circ. Physiol.* 34): H828–H833, 1993.
116. Heesch, C. M., and V. S. Bishop. Cardiovascular reflex modulation of plasma catecholamine concentrations in the anesthetized cat. *Circ. Res.* 52: 391–399, 1982.
117. Henry, J. P., and O. H. Gauer. The influence of temperature upon venous pressure in the foot. *J. Clin. Invest.* 29: 855–861, 1950.
118. Higginbotham, M. B., K. G. Morris, R. S. Williams, P. A. McHale, R. E. Coleman, and F. R. Cobb. Regulation of stroke volume during submaximal and maximal upright exercise in normal man. *Circ. Res.* 58: 281–291, 1986.
119. Hohimer, A. R., J. R. S. Hales, L. B. Rowell, and O. A. Smith. Regional distribution of blood flow during mild dynamic leg exercise in the baboon. *J. Appl Physiol. Respir. Environ. Exerc. Physiol.* 55: 1173–1177, 1983.
120. Hohimer, A. R., and O. A. Smith. Decreased renal blood flow in the baboon during mild dynamic leg exercise. *Am. J. Physiol.* 236 (*Heart Circ. Physiol.* 5): H141–H150, 1979.
121. Hökfelt, T., O. Johansson, A. Ljungdahl, J. M. Lundberg, and M. Schultzberg. Peptidergic neurons. *Nature* 284: 515–521, 1980.
122. Hollander, A. P., and L. N. Bouman. Cardiac acceleration in man elicited by a muscle-heart reflex. *J. Appl. Physiol.* 38: 272–278, 1975.
123. Holmgren, A. Circulatory changes during muscular work in man: with special reference to arterial and central venous pressures in the systemic circulation. *Scand. J. Clin. Lab. Invest.* 8 (Suppl. 24): 1–97, 1956.
124. Hopman, M. T. E., B. Oeseburg, and R. A. Binkhorst. The effect of an anti-G suit on cardiovascular responses to exercise in persons with paraplegia. *Med. Sci. Sports. Exerc.* 24: 987–990, 1992.
125. Hopman, M. T. E., P. H. E. Verheijen, and R. A. Binkhorst. Volume changes in the legs of paraplegic subjects during arm exercise. *J. Appl Physiol.* 75: 2079–2083, 1993.
126. Hossack, K. F., and R. A. Bruce. Maximal cardiac function in sedentary normal men and women: comparison of age-related changes. *J. Appl. Physiol.* 53: 799–804, 1982.
127. Houk, J. C. Control strategies in physiological systems. *FASEB J.* 2: 97–107, 1988.
128. Jacobsen, T. N., B. J. Morgan, U. Scherrer, S. F. Vissing, R. A. Lange, N. Johnson, W. S. Ring, P. S. Rahko, P. Hanson, and R. G. Victor. Relative contributions of cardiopulmonary and sinoaortic baroreflexes in causing sympathetic activation in the human skeletal muscle circulation during orthostatic stress. *Circ. Res.* 73: 367–378, 1993.
129. Johnson, J. M. Responses of forearm blood flow to graded leg exercise in man. *J. Appl. Physiol.* 46: 457–462, 1979.
130. Johnson, J. M. Nonthermoregulatory control of human skin blood flow. *J. Appl. Physiol.* 61: 1613–1622, 1986.
131. Johnson, J. M. Exercise and the cutaneous circulation. *Exerc. Sports Sci. Rev.* 20: 59–97, 1992.
132. Johnson, J. M., G. L. Brengelmann, J. R. S. Hales, P. M. Vanhoutte, and C. B. Wenger. Regulation of the cutaneous circulation. *Federation Proc.* 45: 2841–2850, 1986.
133. Johnson, J. M., M. Niederberger, L. B. Rowell, M. M. Eisman, and G. L. Brengelmann. Competition between cutaneous vasodilator and vasoconstrictor reflexes in man. *J. Appl. Physiol.* 35: 798–803, 1973.
134. Johnson, J. M., and M. K. Park. Effect of upright exercise on the threshold for cutaneous vasodilation and sweating. *J. Appl. Physiol.* 50: 814–818, 1982.
135. Johnson, J. M., and D. W. Proppe. Cardiovascular adjustments to heat stress. *Handbook of Physiology, Environmental Physiology*, edited by C. Blatteis and M. Fregly. Bethesda, MD: Am. Physiol. Soc., 1996 (in press).
136. Johnson, J. M., and L. B. Rowell. Forearm skin and muscle vascular responses to prolonged leg exercise in man. *J. Appl. Physiol.* 39: 920–924, 1975.
137. Johnson, J. M., L. B. Rowell, and G. L. Brengelmann. Modification of the skin blood flow-body temperature relationship by upright exercise. *J. Appl. Physiol.* 37: 880–886, 1974.
138. Johnson, J. M., L. B. Rowell, M. Niederberger, and M. M. Eisman. Human splanchnic and forearm vasoconstrictor responses to reduction of right atrial and aortic pressure. *Circ. Res.* 34: 515–524, 1974.
139. Jones, J. H., K. E. Longworth, A. Lindholm, K. E. Conley, R. H. Karas, S. R. Kayer, and C. R. Taylor. Oxygen transport during exercise in large mammals. I. Adaptive variation in oxygen demand. *J. Appl. Physiol.* 67: 862–870, 1987.

140. Joyner, M. J. Does the pressor response to ischemic exercise improve blood flow to contracting muscles in humans? *J. Appl. Physiol.* 71: 1496–1501, 1991.
141. Joyner, M. J., L. A. Nauss, M. A. Warner, and D. O. Warner. Sympathetic modulation of blood flow and O_2 uptake in rhythmically contracting human forearm muscles. *J. Appl. Physiol.* 263 (*Heart Circ. Physiol.* 32): H1078–H1083, 1992.
142. Joyner, M. J., and W. Wieling. Increased muscle perfusion reduces muscle sympathetic nerve activity during handgripping. *J. Appl. Physiol.* 75: 2450–2455, 1993.
143. Kanstrup, I., and B. Ekblom. Acute hypervolemia, cardiac performance, and aerobic power during exercise. *J. Appl. Physiol. Respir. Environ. Exerc. Physiol.* 52: 1186–1191, 1982.
144. Kanstrup, I. L., J. Marving, and P. F. Høilund-Carlsen. Acute plasma expansion: left ventricular hemodynamics and endocrine function during exercise. *J. Appl. Physiol.* 73: 1791–1796, 1992.
145. Kaufman, M. P., J. C. Longhurst, K. J. Rybicki, J. H. Wallach, and J. H. Mitchell. Effects of static muscular contraction on impulse activity of groups III and IV afferents in cats. *J. Appl. Physiol. Respir. Environ. Exerc. Physiol.* 55: 105–112, 1983.
146. Kaufman, M. P., D. M. Rotto, and K. J. Rybicki. Pressor reflex response to static muscular contraction: its afferent arm and possible neurotransmitters. *Am. J. Cardiol.* 62: 58E–62E, 1988.
147. Kaufman, M. P., and K. J. Rybicki. Discharge properties of group III and IV muscle afferents: their responses to mechanical and metabolic stimuli. *Circ. Res.* 61 (Suppl. I): 60–65, 1987.
148. Kellogg, D. L., Jr., J. M. Johnson, W. L. Kenny, P. E. Pérgola, and W. A. Kosiba. Mechanisms of control of skin blood flow during prolonged exercise in humans. *Am. J. Physiol.* 265 (*Heart Circ. Physiol.* 34): H562–H568, 1993.
149. Kellogg, D. L., Jr., J. M. Johnson, and W. A. Kosiba. Selective abolition of adrenergic vasoconstrictor responses in skin by local iontophoresis of bretylium. *Am. J. Physiol.* 257 (*Heart Circ. Physiol.* 26): H1599–H1606, 1989.
150. Kellogg, D. L., Jr., J. M. Johnson, and W. A. Kosiba. Baroreflex control of the cutaneous active vasodilator system in humans. *Circ. Res.* 66: 1420–1426, 1990.
151. Kellogg, D. L., Jr., J. M. Johnson, and W. A. Kosiba. Competition between cutaneous active vasoconstriction and active vasodilation during exercise in humans. *Am. J. Physiol.* 261 (*Heart Circ. Physiol.* 30): H1184–H1189, 1991.
152. Kellogg, D. L., Jr., J. M. Johnson, and W. A. Kosiba. Control of internal temperature threshold for active cutaneous vasodilation by dynamic exercise. *J. Appl. Physiol.* 71: 2476–2483, 1991.
153. Kellogg, D. L., Jr., P. E. Pérgola, K. L. Piest, W. A. Kosiba, C. G. Crandall, M. Grossman, and J. M. Johnson. Cutaneous active vasodilation in humans is mediated by cholinergic nerve co-transmission. *Circ. Res.* 77: 1222–1228, 1995.
154. Kenny, W. L., C. G. Tankersley, D. L. Newswanger, and S. M. Puhl. α_1-Adrenergic blockade does not alter control of skin blood flow during exercise. *Am. J. Physiol.* 260 (*Heart Circ. Physiol.* 29): H855–H861, 1991.
155. Kenney, W. L., D. H. Zappe, C. G. Tankersley, and J. A. Derr. Effect of systemic yohimbine on the control of skin blood flow during local heating and dynamic exercise. *Am. J. Physiol.* 266 (*Heart Circ. Physiol.* 35): H371–H376, 1994.
156. Keys, A., and H. Taylor. The behavior of the plasma colloids in recovery from brief severe work and the question as to the permeability of the capillaries to proteins. *J. Biol. Chem.* 109: 55–67, 1935.
157. Kilbom, A. Physical training in women. *Scand. J. Clin. Lab. Invest.* 28 (Suppl. 119): 7–34, 1971.
158. Kilbom, A., and T. Brundin. Circulatory effects of isometric muscle contractions, performed separately and in combination with dynamic exercise. *Eur. J. Appl. Physiol.* 36: 7–17, 1976.
159. Kjellmer, I. On the competition between metabolic vasodilation and neurogenic vasoconstriction in skeletal muscle. *Acta Physiol. Scand.* 63: 450–459, 1965.
160. Klausen, J., M. H. Secher, J. P. Clausen, O. Hartling, and J. Trap-Jensen. Central and regional circulatory adaptations to one-leg training. *J. Appl. Physiol.* 52: 976–983, 1982.
161. Kniffki, K.-D., S. Mense, and R. F. Schmidt. Muscle receptors with fine afferent fibers which may evoke circulatory reflexes. *Circ. Res.* 48 (Suppl. 1): 25–31, 1981.
162. Koch, L. G., D. M. Strick, S. L. Britton, and P. J. Metting. Reflex versus autoregulatory control of hindlimb blood flow during treadmill exercise in dogs. *Am. J. Physiol.* 260 (*Heart Circ. Physiol.* 29): H436–H444, 1991.
163. Kohrt, W. M., M. T. Malley, A. R. Coggan, R. J. Spina, T. Ogawa, A. A. Ehsani, R. E. Bourey, W. H. Martin, III, and J. O. Holloszy. Effects of gender, age, and fitness level on response of $\dot{V}O_2$ max to training in 60–71 yr olds. *J. Appl. Physiol.* 71: 2004–2011, 1991.
164. Koller, A., and G. Kaley. Endothelium regulates skeletal muscle microcirculation by a blood flow velocity sensing mechanism. *Am. J. Physiol.* 258 (*Heart Circ. Physiol.* 27): H916–H920, 1990.
165. Koller, A., and G. Kaley. Prostaglandins mediate arteriolar dilation to increased blood flow velocity in skeletal muscle microcirculation. *Circ. Res.* 67: 529–534, 1990.
166. Koller, A., and G. Kaley. Endothelial regulation of wall shear stress and blood flow in skeletal muscle microcirculation. *Am. J. Physiol.* 260 (*Heart Circ. Physiol.* 29): H862–H868, 1991.
167. Koller, A., D. Sun, A. Huang, and G. Kaley. Corelease of nitric oxide and prostaglandins mediates flow-dependent dilation of rat gracilis muscle arterioles. *Am. J. Physiol.* 267 (*Heart Circ. Physiol.* 36): H326–H332, 1994.
168. Korner, P. I., Central nervous control of autonomic cardiovascular function. In: *Handbook of Physiology, The Cardiovascular System, The Heart*, edited by R. M. Berne and N. Sperelakis. Bethesda, MD: Am. Physiol. Soc., 1979, p. 691–739.
169. Kozelka, J. W., G. W. Christy, and R. D. Wurster. Ascending pathways mediating somatoautonomic reflexes in exercising dogs. *J. Appl. Physiol.* 62: 1186–1191, 1987.
170. Krasney, J. A., M. G. Levitzky, and R. C. Koehler. Sinoaortic contribution to the adjustment of systemic resistance in exercising dogs. *J. Appl. Physiol.* 36: 679–685, 1974.
171. Krogh, A. Regulation of the supply of blood to the right heart (with a description of a new circulation model). *Scand. Arch. Physiol.* 27: 227–248, 1912.
172. Lakatta, E. G. Cardiovascular regulatory mechanisms in advanced age. *Physiol. Rev.* 73: 413–467, 1993.
173. Laub, M., K. Hvid-Jacobsen, P. Hovind, I. L. Kanstrup, N. J. Christensen, and S. L. Nielsen. Spleen emptying and venous hematocrit in humans during exercise. *J. Appl. Physiol.* 74: 1024–1026, 1993.

174. Laughlin, M. H. Skeletal muscle blood flow capacity: role of muscle pump in exercise hyperemia. *Am. J. Physiol.* 253 (*Heart Circ. Physiol.* 22): H993–H1004, 1987.
175. Lautt, W. W. Resistance or conductance for expression of arterial vascular tone. *Microvasc. Res.* 37: 230–236, 1989.
176. Leuenberger, U., L. Sinoway, S. Gubin, L. Gaul, D. Davis, and R. Zelis. Effects of exercise intensity and duration on norepinephrine spillover and clearance in humans. *J. Appl. Physiol.* 75: 668–674, 1993.
177. Levy, M. N. The cardiac and vascular factors that determine systemic blood flow. *Circ. Res.* 44: 739–746, 1979.
178. Levy, M. N., and H. Zieske. Autonomic control of cardiac pacemaker activity and atrioventricular transmission. *J. Appl. Physiol.* 27: 465–470, 1969.
179. Leyk, D., D. Essfeld, K. Baum, and J. Stegemann. Influence of calf muscle contractions on blood flow parameters measured in the arteria femoralis. *Int. J. Sports Med.* 13: 588–593, 1992.
180. Lind, A. R., S. H. Taylor, P. W. Humphreys, B. M. Kennelly, and K. W. Donald. The circulatory effects of sustained voluntary muscle contraction. *Clin. Sci.* 27: 229–244, 1964.
181. Lind, A. R. Cardiovascular adjustments to isometric contractions: static effort. In: *Handbook of Physiology, The Cardiovascular System, Peripheral Circulation and Organ Blood Flow*, edited by J. T. Shepherd and F. M. Abboud. Bethesda, MD: Am. Physiol. Soc., 1983, p. 947–966.
182. Lipsitz, L. A. Orthostatic hypotension in the elderly. *N. Engl. J. Med.* 321: 952–957, 1989.
183. Love, A. H. G., and R. G. Shanks. The relationship between the onset of sweating and vasodilation in the forearm during body heating. *J. Physiol.* (*Lond.*) 162: 121–128, 1962.
184. Ludbrook, J. *Aspects of Venous Function in the Lower Limbs*. Springfield, IL: Charles C Thomas, 1966.
185. Ludbrook, J. Reflex control of blood pressure during exercise. *Annu. Rev. Physiol.* 45: 155–168, 1983.
186. Ludbrook, J. Concern about gain: is this the best measure of performance of cardiovascular reflexes? *Clin. Exp. Pharmacol. Physiol.* 11: 385–389, 1984.
187. Ludbrook, J., and W. F. Graham. Circulatory responses to onset of exercise: role of arterial and cardiac baroreflexes. *Am. J. Physiol.* 248 (*Heart Circ. Physiol.* 17): H457–H467, 1985.
188. Ludbrook, J., W. F. Graham, and S. M. Potocnik. Effects of acute versus chronic deletion of arterial baroreceptor input on the cardiovascular responses to exercise in the rabbit. *Clin. Exp. Pharmacol. Physiol.* 13: 25–37, 1986.
189. Lundberg, J., L. Norgren, E. Ribbe, I. Rosen, S. Steen, J. Thorne, and B. G. Wallin. Direct evidence of active sympathetic vasodilation in the skin of the human foot. *J. Physiol.* (*Lond.*) 417: 437–446, 1989.
190. Lundvall, J., and H. Edfeldt. Very large range of baroreflex sympathetic control of vascular resistance in human skeletal muscle and skin. *J. Appl. Physiol.* 76: 204–211, 1994.
191. Maciel, B. C., L. Gallo, J. A. Marin Neio, E. C. Lima Filho, and L. E. B. Martins. Autonomic nervous control of the heart rate during dynamic exercise in normal man. *Clin. Sci. Lond.* 71: 457–467, 1986.
192. Maciel, B. C., L. Gallo, Jr., J. A. Marin Neto, and L. E. B. Martins. Autonomic nervous control of the heart rate during isometric exercise in normal man. *Pflugers Arch.* 408: 173–177, 1987.
193. Mack, G. W., H. Nose, and E. R. Nadel. Role of cardiopulmonary baroreflexes during dynamic exercise. *J. Appl. Physiol.* 65: 1827–1832, 1988.
194. Magder, S. Vascular mechanics of venous drainage in dog hindlimbs. *Am. J. Physiol.* 259 (*Heart Circ. Physiol.* 38): H1789–H1795, 1990.
195. Mancia, G., J. T. Shepherd, and D. E. Donald. Interplay among carotid sinus, cardiopulmonary, and carotid body reflexes in dogs. *Am. J. Physiol.* 230: 19–24, 1976.
196. Mark, A. L., and G. Mancia. Cardiopulmonary baroreflexes in humans. In: *Handbook of Physiology, The Cardiovascular System, Peripheral Circulation and Organ Blood Flow*, edited by J. T. Shepherd, and F. M. Abboud. Bethesda, MD: Am. Physiol. Soc., 1983, p. 795–813.
197. Mark, A. L., R. G. Victor, C. Nerhed, and B. G. Wallin. Microneurographic studies of the mechanisms of sympathetic nerve responses to static exercise in humans. *Circ. Res.* 57: 461–469, 1985.
198. Marshall, J. M., and H. C. Tandon. Direct observations of muscle arterioles and venules following contraction of skeletal muscle fibres in the rat. *J. Physiol.* (*Lond.*) 350: 447–459, 1984.
199. Marshall, R. J., A. Schirger, and J. T. Shepherd. Blood pressure during supine exercise in idiopathic orthostatic hypotension. *Circulation* 24: 76–81, 1961.
200. Martin, C. E., J. A. Shaver, D. F. Leon, M. E. Thompson, P. S. Reddy, and J. J. Leonard. Autonomic mechanisms in hemodynamic responses to isometric exercise. *J. Clin. Invest.* 54: 104–115, 1974.
201. Martin, W. H., III, W. M. Kohrt, M. T. Malley, E. Korte, and S. Stoltz. Exercise training enhances leg vasodilatory capacity of 65-yr-old men and women. *J. Appl. Physiol.* 69: 1804–1809, 1990.
202. Mazzeo, R. S., and P. Marshall. Influence of plasma catecholamines on the lactate threshold during graded exercise. *J. Appl. Physiol.* 67: 1319–1322, 1989.
203. McClain, J., C. Hardy, B. Enders, M. Smith, and L. Sinoway. Limb congestion and sympathoexcitation during exercise. Implications for congestive heart failure. *J. Clin. Invest.* 92: 2353–2359, 1993.
204. McClain, J., J. C. Hardy, and L. I. Sinoway. Forearm compression during exercise increases sympathetic nerve traffic. *J. Appl. Physiol.* 77: 2612–2617, 1994.
205. McRitchie, R. J., S. F. Vatner, D. Boettcher, G. R. Heyndrickx, T. A. Patrick, and E. Braunwald. Role of arterial baroreceptors in mediating cardiovascular response to exercise. *Am. J. Physiol.* 230: 85–89, 1976.
206. Melcher, A., and D. E. Donald. Maintained ability of carotid baroreflex to regulate arterial pressure during exercise. *Am. J. Physiol.* 241 (*Heart Circ. Physiol.* 10): H838–H849, 1981.
207. Mendelowitz, D., and A. M. Scher. Pulsatile sinus pressure changes evoke sustained baroreflex responses in awake dogs. *Am. J. Physiol.* 255 (*Heart Circ. Physiol.* 24): H673–H678, 1988.
208. Mense, S. Effects of temperature on the discharges of muscle spindles and tendon organs. *Pflugers Arch.* 374: 159–166, 1978.
209. Mitchell, J. H. Neural control of the circulation during exercise. *Med. Sci. Sports Exerc.* 22: 141–154, 1990.
210. Mitchell, J. H., and R. F. Schmidt. Cardiovascular reflex control by afferent fibers from skeletal muscle receptors. In: *Handbook of Physiology, The Cardiovascular System, Peripheral Circulation and Organ Blood Flow*, edited by J. T. Shepherd and F. M. Abboud. Bethesda, MD: Am. Physiol. Soc., 1983, p. 623–658.
211. Mittelstadt, S. W., L. B. Bell, K. P. O'Hagan, and P. S. Clifford. Muscle chemoreflex alters vascular conductance in

nonischemic exercising skeletal muscle. *J. Appl. Physiol.* 77: 2761–2766, 1994.
212. Mohanty, P. K., M. D. Thames, J. A. Arrowood, J. R. Sowers, C. McNamara, and S. Szentpetery. Impairment of cardiopulmonary baroreflex after cardiac transplantation in humans. *Circulation* 75: 914–921, 1987.
213. Moncada, S., R. M. J. Palmer, and E. A. Higgs. Nitric oxide: physiology, pathophysiology, and pharmacology. *Pharmacol. Rev.* 43: 109–142, 1991.
214. Moreno, A. H., A. R. Burchell, R. van der Woude, and J. H. Burke. Respiratory regulation of splanchnic and systemic venous return. *Am. J. Physiol.* 213: 455–465, 1967.
215. Morganroth, J., B. J. Maron, W. L. Henry, and S. E. Epstein. Comparative left ventricular dimensions in trained athletes. *Ann. Intern. Med.* 82: 521–524, 1975.
216. Musch, T. I., G. C. Haidet, G. A. Ordway, J. C. Longhurst, and J. H. Mitchell. Dynamic exercise training in foxhounds. I. Oxygen consumption and hemodynamic responses. *J. Appl. Physiol.* 59: 183–189, 1985.
217. Nielsen, B., J. R. S. Hales, S. Strange, N. J. Christensen, J. Warberg, and B. Saltin. Human circulatory and thermoregulatory adaptations with heat acclimation and exercise in a hot, dry environment. *J. Physiol. (Lond.)* 460: 467–485, 1993.
218. Nielsen, B., and C. Jessen. Evidence against brain stem cooling by face fanning in severely hyperthermic humans. *Pflugers Arch.* 422: 168–172, 1992.
219. Nielsen, B., G. Savard, E. A. Richter, M. Hargreaves, and B. Saltin. Muscle blood flow and muscle metabolism during exercise and heat stress. *J. Appl. Physiol.* 69: 1040–1046, 1990.
220. Öberg, B., and S. White. Circulatory effects of interruption and stimulation of cardiac vagal afferents. *Acta Physiol. Scand.* 80: 383–394, 1970.
221. O'Hagan, K. P., L. B. Bell, S. W. Mittelstadt, and P. S. Clifford. Effect of dynamic exercise on renal sympathetic nerve activity in conscious rabbits. *J. Appl. Physiol.* 74: 2099–2104, 1993.
222. O'Hagan, K. P., L. B. Bell, S. W. Mittelstadt, and P. S. Clifford. Cardiac receptors modulate the renal sympathetic response to dynamic exercise in rabbits. *J. Appl. Physiol.* 76: 507–515, 1994.
223. Ohyanagi, M., J. E. Faber, and K. Nishigaki. Differential activation of α_1- and α_2-adrenoceptors on microvascular smooth muscle during sympathetic nerve stimulation. *Circ. Res.* 68: 232–244, 1991.
224. O'Leary, D. S. Regional vascular resistance vs. conductance: which index for baroreflex responses? *Am. J. Physiol.* 260 (*Heart Circ. Physiol.* 29): H632–H637, 1991.
225. O'Leary, D. S. Autonomic mechanisms of muscle metaboreflex control of heart rate. *J. Appl. Physiol.* 74: 1748–1754, 1993.
226. O'Leary, D. S., R. C. Dunlap, and K. W. Glover. Role of endothelium-derived relaxing factor in hindlimb reactive and active hyperemia in conscious dogs. *Am. J. Physiol.* 266 (*Regulatory Integrative Comp. Physiol.* 35): R1213–R1219, 1994.
227. O'Leary, D. S., N. F. Rossi, and P. C. Churchill. Muscle metaboreflex control of vasopressin and renin release. *Am. J. Physiol.* 264 (*Heart Circ. Physiol.* 33): H1422–H1427, 1993.
228. O'Leary, D. S., L. B. Rowell, and A. M. Scher. Baroreflex-induced vasoconstriction in active skeletal muscle of conscious dogs. *Am. J. Physiol.* 260 (*Heart Circ. Physiol.* 29): H37–H41, 1991.
229. O'Leary, D. S., A. M. Scher, and J. E. Bassett. Effects of steps in cardiac output and arterial pressure in awake dogs with AV block. *Am. J. Physiol.* 256 (*Heart Circ. Physiol.* 25): H361–H367, 1989.
230. O'Leary, D. S., and D. P. Seamans. Effect of exercise on autonomic mechanisms of baroreflex control of heart rate. *J. Appl. Physiol.* 75: 2251–2257, 1993.
231. O'Leary, D. S., and D. D. Sheriff. Is the muscle metaboreflex important in control of blood flow to active skeletal muscle? *Am. J. Physiol.* 268 (*Heart Circ. Physiol.* 37): H980–H986, 1995.
232. Oliver, J. A., J. Pinto, R. R. Sciacca, and P. J. Cannon. Basal norepinephrine overflow into the renal vein: effect of renal nerve stimulation. *Am. J. Physiol.* 239 (*Renal Fluid Electrolyte Physiol.* 8): F371–F377, 1980.
233. Papelier, Y., P. Escourrou, J. P. Gauthier, and L. B. Rowell. Carotid baroreflex control of blood pressure and heart rate in man during dynamic exercise. *J. Appl. Physiol.* 77: 502–506, 1994.
234. Permutt, S., and P. Caldini. Regulation of cardiac output by the circuit: venous return. In: *Cardiovascular System Dynamics*, edited by J. Baan, A. Noordergraaft, and J. Raines. Cambridge, MA: MIT Press, 1978, p. 465–479.
235. Pernow, J., T. Kahan, P. Hjemdahl, and J. M. Lundberg. Possible involvement of neuropeptide Y in sympathetic vascular control of canine skeletal muscle. *Acta Physiol. Scand.* 132: 43–50, 1988.
236. Pernow, J., A. Ohlen, T. Hökfelt, O. Nillson, and J. M. Lundberg. Neuropeptide Y: presence in perivascular noradrenergic neurons and vasoconstrictor effects on skeletal muscle blood vessels in experimental animals and man. *Regul. Pept.* 19: 313–324, 1987.
237. Peterson, D. F., R. B. Armstrong, and M. H. Laughlin. Sympathetic neural influences on muscle blood flow in rats during submaximal exercise. *J. Appl. Physiol.* 65: 434–440, 1988.
238. Poliner, L. R., G. J. Dehmer, S. E. Lewis, R. W. Parkey, C. G. Blomqvist, and J. T. Willerson. Left ventricular performance in normal subjects: a comparison of the responses to exercise in the upright and supine positions. *Circulation* 62: 528–534, 1980.
239. Pollack, A. A., and E. H. Wood. Venous pressure in the saphenous vein at the ankle in man during exercise and changes in posture. *J. Appl. Physiol.* 1: 649–662, 1949.
240. Potts, J. T., S. R. Shi, and P. B. Raven. Carotid baroreflex responsiveness during dynamic exercise in humans. *Am. J. Physiol.* 265 (*Heart Circ. Physiol.* 34): H1928–H1938, 1993.
241. Pryor, S. L., S. F. Lewis, R. G. Haller, L. A. Bertocci, and R. G. Victor. Impairment of sympathetic activation during static exercise in patients with muscle phosphorylase deficiency (McArdle's disease). *J. Clin. Invest.* 85: 1444–1449, 1990.
242. Rasch, W., and M. Cabanac. Selective brain cooling is affected by wearing headgear during exercise. *J. Appl. Physiol.* 74: 1229–1233, 1993.
243. Ray, C. A., and A. L. Mark. Augmentation of muscle sympathetic nerve activity during fatiguing isometric leg exercise. *J. Appl. Physiol.* 75: 228–232, 1993.
244. Ray, C. A., R. F. Rea, M. P. Clary, and A. L. Mark. Muscle sympathetic nerve responses to dynamic one-legged exercise: effect of body posture. *Am. J. Physiol.* 264 (*Heart Circ. Physiol.* 33): H1–H7, 1993.
245. Raymundo, H., A. M. Scher, D. S. O'Leary, and P. D. Sampson. Cardiovascular control by arterial and cardiopulmonary baroreceptors in awake dogs with atrioventric-

ular block. *Am. J. Physiol.* 257 (*Heart Circ. Physiol.* 26): H2048–H2058, 1989.
246. Rea, R. F., and B. G. Wallin. Sympathetic nerve activity in arm and leg muscles during lower body negative pressure in humans. *J. Appl. Physiol.* 66: 2778–2781, 1989.
247. Reeves, J. T., B. M. Groves, A. Cymerman, J. R. Sutton, P. D. Wagner, D. Turkevich, and C. S. Houston. Operation Everest II: cardiac filling pressures during cycle exercise at sea level. *Respir. Physiol.* 80: 147–154, 1990.
248. Remensnyder, J. P., J. H. Mitchell, and S. J. Sarnoff. Functional sympatholysis during muscular activity. *Circ. Res.* 11: 370–380, 1962.
249. Rerych, S. K., P. M. Scholz, D. C. Sabiston, and R. H. Jones. Effects of exercise training on left ventricular function in normal subjects: a longitudinal study by radionuclide angiography. *Am. J. Cardiol.* 45: 244–252, 1980.
250. Richardson, R. S., D. C. Poole, D. R. Knight, S. S. Kurdak, M. C. Hogan, B. Grassi, E. C. Johnson, K. F. Kendrick, B. K. Erickson, and P. D. Wagner. High muscle blood flow in man: is maximal O_2 extraction compromised? *J. Appl. Physiol.* 75: 1911–1916, 1993.
251. Richter, E. A., B. Kiens, M. Hargreaves, and J. Kjaer. Effect of arm-cranking on leg blood flow and noradrenaline spillover during leg exercise in man. *Acta Physiol. Scand.* 144: 9–14, 1992.
252. Robinson, B. F., S. E. Epstein, G. D. Beiser, and E. Braunwald. Control of heart rate by the autonomic nervous system: studies in man on the interrelation between baroreceptor mechanisms and exercise. *Circ. Res.* 19: 400–411, 1966.
253. Robinson, B. R., S. E. Epstein, R. L. Kahler, and E. Braunwald. Circulatory effects of acute expansion of blood volume: studies during maximal exercise and at rest. *Circ. Res.* 19: 26–32, 1966.
254. Roca, J., A. G. N. Agusti, A. Alonso, D. C. Poole, C. Viegas, J. A. Barbera, R. Rodriguez-Roisin, A. Ferrer, and P. D. Wagner. Effects of training on muscle O_2 transport at $\dot{V}O_2$ max. *J. Appl. Physiol.* 73: 1067–1076, 1992.
255. Rodeheffer, R. J., J. G. Gerstenblith, L. C. Becker, J. L. Fleg, M. L. Weisfeldt, and E. G. Lakatta. Exercise cardiac output is maintained with advancing age in healthy human subjects: cardiac dilatation and increased stroke volume compensate for a diminished heart rate. *Circulation* 69: 203–213, 1984.
256. Roeske, W. R., R. A. O'Rourke, A. Klein, G. Leopold, and J. S. Karliner. Noninvasive evaluation of ventricular hypertrophy in professional athletes. *Circulation* 53: 286–292, 1975.
257. Roddie, I. C. Circulation to skin and adipose tissue. In: *Handbook of Physiology, The Cardiovascular System, Peripheral Circulation and Organ Blood Flow*, edited by J. T. Shepherd and F. M. Abboud. Bethesda, MD: Am. Physiol. Soc. 1983, p. 285–317.
258. Rothe, C. F. Venous system: physiology of the capacitance vessels. In: *Handbook of Physiology, The Cardiovascular System, Peripheral Circulation and Organ Blood Flow*, edited by J. T. Shepherd and F. M. Abboud. Bethesda, MD: Am. Physiol. Soc., 1983, p. 397–452.
259. Rothe, C. F., and M. L. Gaddis. Autoregulation of cardiac output by passive elastic characteristics of the vascular capacitance system. *Circulation* 81: 360–368, 1990.
260. Rotto, D. M., and M. P. Kaufman. Effect of metabolic products of muscular contraction on discharge of group III and IV afferents. *J. Appl. Physiol.* 64: 2306–2313, 1988.
261. Rotto, D. M., H. D. Schultz, J. C. Longhurst, and M. P. Kaufman. Sensitization of group III muscle afferents to static contraction by arachidonic acid. *J. Appl. Physiol.* 68: 861–867, 1990.
262. Rowell, L. B. Human cardiovascular adjustments to exercise and thermal stress. *Physiol. Rev.* 54: 75–159, 1974.
263. Rowell, L. B. What signals govern the cardiovascular responses to exercise? *Med. Sci. Sports* 12: 307–315, 1980.
264. Rowell, L. B. Cardiovascular adjustments to thermal stress. In: *Handbook of Physiology, The Cardiovascular System, Peripheral Circulation and Organ Blood Flow*, edited by J. T. Shepherd and F. M. Abboud. Bethesda, MD: Am. Physiol. Soc., 1983, p. 967–1023.
265. Rowell, L. B. *Human Circulation. Regulation During Physical Stress*. New York: Oxford University Press, 1986.
266. Rowell, L. B. Muscle blood flow in humans: how high can it go? *Med. Sci. Sports. Med.* 20: S97–S103, 1988.
267. Rowell, L. B. Control of the circulation during exercise. In: *Reflex Control of the Circulation*, edited by J. P. Gilmore and I. H. Zucker. Boca Raton, FL: CRC Press, 1991, p. 795–828.
268. Rowell, L. B. *Human Cardiovascular Control*. New York: Oxford University Press, 1993.
269. Rowell, L. B., G. L. Brengelmann, J. R. Blackmon, R. A. Bruce, and J. A. Murray. Disparities between aortic and peripheral pulse pressures induced by upright exercise and vasomotor changes in man. *Circulation* 37: 954–964, 1968.
270. Rowell, L. B., G. L. Brengelmann, J. R. Blackmon, and J. A. Murray. Redistribution of blood flow during sustained high skin temperature in resting man. *J. Appl. Physiol.* 28: 415–420, 1970.
271. Rowell, L. B., G. L. Brengelmann, and P. R. Freund. Unaltered norepinephrine: heart rate relationship in exercise with exogenous heat. *J. Appl. Physiol.* 62: 646–650, 1987.
272. Rowell, L. B., P. R. Freund, and S. F. Hobbs. Cardiovascular responses to muscle ischemia in humans. *Circ. Res.* 48 (Suppl. 1): 37–47, 1981.
273. Rowell, L. B., H. J. Marx, R. A. Bruce, R. D. Conn, and F. Kusumi. Reductions in cardiac output, central blood volume, and stroke volume with thermal stress in normal men during exercise. *J. Clin Invest.* 45: 1801–1816, 1966.
274. Rowell, L. B., J. A. Murray, G. L. Brengelmann, and K. K. Kraning, II. Human cardiovascular adjustments to rapid changes in skin temperature during exercise. *Circ. Res.* 24: 711–724, 1969.
275. Rowell, L. B., and D. S. O'Leary. Reflex control of the circulation during exercise: chemoreflexes and mechanoreflexes. *J. Appl. Physiol.* 69: 407–418, 1990.
276. Rowell, L. B., B. Saltin, B. Kiens, and N. J. Christensen. Is peak quadriceps blood flow in humans even higher during exercise with hypoxemia? *Am. J. Physiol.* 251 (*Heart Circ. Physiol.* 20): H1038–H1044, 1986.
277. Rowell, L. B., M. V. Savage, J. Chambers, and J. R. Blackmon. Cardiovascular responses to graded reductions in leg perfusion in exercising humans. *Am. J. Physiol.* 271 (*Heart Circ. Physiol.* 30): H1545–H1553, 1991.
278. Rowell, L. B., and D. R. Seals. Sympathetic activity during graded central hypovolemia in hypoxemic humans, *Am. J. Physiol.* 259 (*Heart Circ. Physiol.* 28): H1197–H1206, 1990.
279. Rowell, L. B., and D. D. Sheriff. Are muscle "chemoreflexes" functionally important? *News Physiol. Sci.* 3: 250–253, 1988.
280. Rowlands, D. J., and D. E. Donald. Sympathetic vasoconstrictive responses during exercise- or drug-induced vasodilation. *Circ. Res.* 23: 45–60, 1968.

281. Rushmer, R. F., O. Smith, and D. Franklin. Mechanisms of cardiac control in exercise. *Circ. Res.* 7: 602–627, 1959.
282. Rybicki, K. J., T. G. Waldrop, and M. P. Kaufman. Increasing gracilis muscle interstitial potassium concentrations stimulate group III and IV afferents. *J. Appl. Physiol.* 58: 936–941, 1985.
283. Sagawa, K. Baroreflex control of systemic arterial pressure and vascular bed. In: *Handbook of Physiology, The Cardiovascular System, Peripheral Circulation and Organ Blood Flow*, edited by J. T. Shepherd and F. M. Abboud. Bethesda, MD: Am. Physiol. Soc., 1983, p. 453–496.
284. Sagawa, K. Editorial: Concerning "gain." *Am. J. Physiol.* 235 (*Heart Circ. Physiol.* 4): H117, 1978.
285. Sagawa, K., J. M. Ross, and A. C. Guyton. Quantitation of cerebral ischemic pressor response in dogs. *Am. J. Physiol.* 200: 1164–1168, 1961.
286. Saito, M., M. Naito, and T. Mano. Different responses in skin and muscle sympathetic nerve activity to static muscle contraction. *J. Appl. Physiol.* 69: 2085–2090, 1990.
287. Saito, M., A. Tsukanaka, D. Yanagihara, and T. Mano. Muscle sympathetic nerve responses to graded leg cycling. *J. Appl. Physiol.* 75: 663–667, 1993.
288. Saltin, B. Physiological effects of physical conditioning. *Med. Sci. Sports* 1: 50–56, 1969.
289. Saltin, B., G. Blomqvist, J. H. Mitchell, R. L. Johnson, Jr., K. Wildenthal, and C. B. Chapman. Response to exercise after bed rest and after training. *Circulation* 38 (Suppl. 7): 1–78, 1968.
290. Saltin, B., L. H. Hartley, A. Kilbom, and I. Åstrand. Physical training in sedentary middle-aged and older men. II. Oxygen uptake, heart rate, and blood lactate concentrations at submaximal and maximal exercise. *Scand. J. Clin. Lab. Invest.* 24: 323–334, 1969.
291. Saltin, B., and L. B. Rowell. Functional adaptations to physical activity and inactivity. *Federation Proc.* 39: 1506–1513, 1980.
292. Sandler, M. P., M. W. Kronenberg, M. B. Forman, O. H. Wolfe, J. A. Clanton, and C. L. Partain. Dynamic fluctuations in blood and spleen radioactivity: splenic contractions and relation to clinical radionuclide volume calculations. *J. Am. Col. Cardiol.* 3: 1205–1211, 1984.
293. Savage, M. V., G. L. Brengelmann, A. M. J. Buchan, and P. R. Freund. Cystic fibrosis, vasoactive intestinal polypeptide, and active cutaneous vasodilation. *J. Appl. Physiol.* 69: 2149–2154, 1990.
294. Savard, G. K., B. Nielsen, I. Laszczynska, B. E. Larsen, and B. Saltin. Muscle blood flow is not reduced in humans during moderate exercise and heat stress. *J. Appl. Physiol.* 64: 649–657, 1988.
295. Savard, G., E. A. Richter, S. Strange, B. Kiens, N. J. Christensen, and B. Saltin. Norepinephrine spillover from skeletal muscle during exercise in humans: role of muscle mass. *Am. J. Physiol.* 257 (*Heart Circ. Physiol.* 26): H1812–H1818, 1989.
296. Savard, G., S. Strange, B. Kiens, E. A. Richter, N. J. Christensen, and B. Saltin. Noradrenaline spillover during exercise in active versus resting skeletal muscle in man. *Acta Physiol. Scand.* 131: 507–515, 1987.
297. Scher, A. M., W. W. Ohm, K. Bumgarner, R. Boynton, and A. C. Young. Sympathetic and parasympathetic control of heart rate in the dog, baboon and man. *Federation Proc.* 31: 1219–1225, 1972.
298. Scher, A. M., D. S. O'Leary, and D. D. Sheriff. Arterial baroreceptor regulation of peripheral resistance and of cardiac performance. In: *Baroreceptor Reflexes*, edited by P. Persson and H. Kirchheim. Heidelberg: Springer-Verlag, 1991.
299. Scherrer, U., S. L. Pryor, L. A. Bertocci, and R. G. Victor. Arterial baroreflex buffering of sympathetic activation during exercise-induced elevations in arterial pressure. *J. Clin. Invest.* 86: 1855–1861, 1990.
300. Scherrer, U., S. F. Vissing, and R. G. Victor. Effects of lower-body negative pressure on sympathetic nerve responses to static exercise in humans. *Circulation* 78: 49–59, 1988.
301. Seals, D. R. Cardiopulmonary baroreflexes do not modulate exercise-induced sympathoexcitation. *J. Appl. Physiol.* 64: 2197–2203, 1988.
302. Seals, D. R. Influence of muscle mass on sympathetic neural activation during isometric exercise. *J. Appl. Physiol.* 67: 1801–1806, 1989.
303. Seals, D. R. Influence of force on muscle and skin sympathetic nerve activity during sustained isometric contractions in humans. *J. Physiol. (Lond.)* 462: 147–159, 1993.
304. Seals, D. R. Influence of active muscle size on sympathetic nerve discharge during isometric contractions in humans. *J. Appl. Physiol.* 75: 1426–1431, 1993.
305. Seals, D. R. Influence of aging on autonomic-circulatory control at rest and during exercise in humans. In: *Perspectives in Exercise Science and Sports Medicine*, edited by D. R. Lamb, and C. V. Gisolfi. Dubuque, IA: Wm. C. Brown Publishers, 1993, p. 257–304.
306. Seals, D. R., J. M. Hagberg, B. F. Hurley, A. A. Ehsani, and J. O. Holloszy. Endurance training in older men and women. I. Cardiovascular responses to exercise. *J. Appl. Physiol. Respir. Environ. Exerc. Physiol.* 57: 1024–1029, 1984.
307. Seals, D. R., and R. G. Victor. Regulation of muscle sympathetic nerve activity during exercise in humans. In: *Exercise and Sport Sciences Reviews*, edited by J. O. Holloszy. Baltimore: Williams & Wilkins, 1990, p. 313–349.
308. Seals, D. R., R. G. Victor, and A. L. Mark. Plasma norepinephrine and muscle sympathetic discharge during rhythmic exercise in humans. *J. Appl. Physiol.* 65: 940–944, 1988.
309. Secher, N. H., J. P. Clausen, K. Klausen, K. Noer, and J. Trap-Jensen. Central and regional circulatory effects of adding arm exercise to leg exercise. *Acta Physiol. Scand.* 100: 288–297, 1977.
310. Sheldahl, L. M., T. J. Ebert, B. Cox, and F. Tristani. Effect of aerobic training on baroreflex regulation of cardiac and sympathetic function. *J. Appl. Physiol.* 76: 158–165, 1994.
311. Shepherd, J. T. *Physiology of the Circulation in Human Limbs in Health and Disease*. Philadelphia: W. B. Saunders Company, 1963.
312. Shepherd, J. T. Circulation to skeletal muscle. In: *Handbook of Physiology, The Cardiovascular System, Peripheral Circulation and Organ Blood Flow*, edited by J. T. Shepherd and F. M. Abboud. Bethesda, MD: Am. Physiol. Soc., 1983, p. 319–370.
313. Sheriff, D. D., D. S. O'Leary, A. M. Scher, and L. B. Rowell. Baroreflex attenuates pressor response to graded muscle ischemia in exercising dogs. *Am. J. Physiol.* 258 (*Heart Circ. Physiol.* 27): H305–H310, 1990.
314. Sheriff, D. D., L. B. Rowell, and A. M. Scher. Is the rapid rise in vascular conductance at onset of dynamic exercise due to the muscle pump? *Am. J. Physiol.* 265 (*Heart Circ. Physiol.* 34): H1227–H1234, 1993.
315. Sheriff, D. D., C. R. Wyss, L. B. Rowell, and A. M. Scher. Does inadequate O_2 delivery trigger the pressor response

to muscle hypoperfusion during exercise? *Am. J. Physiol.* 253 (*Heart Circ. Physiol.* 22): H1199–H1207, 1987.

316. Sheriff, D. D., X. P. Zhou, A. M. Scher, and L. B. Rowell. Dependence of cardiac filling pressure on cardiac output during rest and dynamic exercise in dogs. *Am. J. Physiol.* 265: (*Heart Circ. Physiol.* 34): H316–H322, 1993.
317. Shiraki, K., S. Sagawa, F. Tajima, A. Yokota, M. Hashimoto, and G. L. Brengelmann. Independence of brain and tympanic temperatures in an unanesthetized human. *J. Appl. Physiol.* 65: 482–486, 1988.
318. Simon, E., and W. Riedel. Diversity of regional sympathetic outflow in integrative cardiovascular control: patterns and mechanisms. *Brain Res.* 87: 323–333, 1975.
319. Sinoway, L. I., J. M. Hill, J. G. Pickar, and M. P. Kaufman. Effects of contraction and lactic acid on the discharge of group III muscle afferents in cats. *J. Neurophysiol.* 69: 1053–1059, 1993.
320. Sinoway, L. I., S. Prophet, I. Gorman, T. Mosher, J. Shenberger, M. Dolecki, R. Briggs, and R. Zelis. Muscle acidosis during static exercise is associated with calf vasoconstriction. *J. Appl. Physiol.* 66: 429–436, 1989.
321. Sinoway, L. I., J. Shenberger, J. Wilson, D. McLaughlin, T. Musch, and R. Zelis. A 30-day forearm work protocol increases maximal forearm blood flow. *J. Appl. Physiol.* 62: 1063–1067, 1987.
322. Sinoway, L. I., M. B. Smith, B. Enders, U. Leuenberger, T. Dzwonczyk, K. Gray, S. Whisler, and R. L. Moore. The role of diprotonated phosphate in evoking muscle reflex responses in cats and humans. *Am. J. Physiol.* 267 (*Heart Circ. Physiol.* 36): H770–H778, 1994.
323. Sinoway, L. I., K. J. Wroblewski, S. A. Prophet, S. M. Ettinger, K. S. Gray, S. K. Whisler, G. Miller, and R. L. Moore. Glycogen depletion-induced lactate reductions attenuate reflex responses in exercising humans. *Am. J. Physiol.* 263 (*Heart Circ. Physiol.* 32): H1499–H1505, 1992.
324. Skokland, O. Factors contributing to acute blood pressure elevation. *J. Oslo City Hosp.* 33: 81–95, 1983.
325. Smolander, J., J. Saalo, and O. Korhonen. Effect of work load on cutaneous vascular responses to exercise. *J. Appl. Physiol.* 71: 1614–1619, 1991.
326. Snell, P. G., W. H. Martin, J. C. Buckey, and C. G. Blomqvist. Maximal vascular leg conductance in trained and untrained men. *J. Appl. Physiol.* 62: 606–610, 1987.
327. Sprangers, R. L. H., K. H. Wesseling, A. L. T. Imholz, B. P. M. Imholz, and W. Wieling. Initial blood pressure fall on stand up and exercise explained by changes in total peripheral resistance. *J. Appl. Physiol.* 70: 523–530, 1991.
328. Spina, R. J., T. Ogawa, A. R. Coggan, J. O. Holloszy, and A. A. Ehsani. Exercise training improves left ventricular contractile response to β-adrenergic agonist. *J. Appl. Physiol.* 72: 307–311, 1992.
329. Staessen, J., R. Fiocchi, R. Fagard, P. Hespel, and A. Amery. Progressive attenuation of the carotid baroreflex control of blood pressure and heart rate during exercise. *Am. Heart J.* 114: 765–772, 1987.
330. Stebbins, C. L., B. Brown, D. Levin, and J. C. Longhurst. Reflex effect of skeletal muscle mechanoreceptor stimulation on the cardiovascular system. *J. Appl. Physiol.* 65: 1539–1547, 1988.
331. Stebbins, C. L., and J. C. Longhurst. Bradykinin-induced chemoreflexes from skeletal muscle: implications for the exercise reflex. *J. Appl. Physiol.* 59: 56–63, 1985.
332. Stebbins, C. L., and J. C. Longhurst. Potentiation of the exercise pressor reflex by muscle ischemia. *J. Appl. Physiol.* 66: 1046–1053, 1989.
333. Stegall, H. F. Muscle pumping in the dependent leg. *Circ. Res.* 19: 180–190, 1966.
334. Stenberg, J., B. Ekblom, and R. Messin. Hemodynamic response to work at simulated altitude, 4,000 m. *J. Appl. Physiol.* 21: 1589–1594, 1966.
335. Stick, C., H. Jaeger, and E. Witzleb. Measurements of volume changes and venous pressure in the human lower leg during walking and running. *J. Appl. Physiol.* 72: 2063–2068, 1992.
336. Strange, S., L. B. Rowell, N. J. Christensen, and B. Saltin. Cardiovascular responses to carotid sinus baroreceptor stimulation during moderate to severe exercise in man. *Acta Physiol. Scand.* 138: 145–153, 1990.
337. Strange, S., N. H. Secher, J. A. Pawelczyk, J. Karpakka, N. J. Christensen, J. H. Mitchell, and B. Saltin. Neural control of cardiovascular responses and of ventilation during dynamic exercise in man. *J. Physiol. (Lond.)* 470: 693–704, 1993.
338. Stray-Gunderson, J., T. I. Musch, G. C. Haidet, D. P. Swain, G. A. Ordway, and J. H. Mitchell. The effect of pericardiectomy on maximal oxygen consumption and maximal cardiac output in untrained dogs. *Circ. Res.* 58: 523–530, 1986.
339. Sundlöf, G., and B. G. Wallin. The variability of muscle nerve sympathetic activity in resting recumbent man. *J. Physiol. (Lond.)* 272: 383–397, 1977.
340. Supinski, G. S., D. Stofan, E. Nashawati, and A. F. DiMarco. Failure of vasodilator administration to increase blood flow to the fatiguing diaphragm. *J. Appl. Physiol.* 74: 1178–1185, 1993.
341. Takata, M., and J. L. Robotham. Effects of inspiratory diaphragmatic descent on inferior vena caval venous return. *J. Appl. Physiol.* 72: 597–607, 1992.
342. Taylor, W. F., J. M. Johnson, and W. A. Kosiba. Roles of absolute and relative load in skin vasoconstrictor responses to exercise. *J. Appl. Physiol.* 69:1131–1136, 1990.
343. Taylor, W. F., J. M. Johnson, W. A. Kosiba, and C. M. Kwan. Graded cutaneous vascular responses to dynamic leg exercise. *J. Appl. Physiol.* 64: 1803–1809, 1988.
344. Thimm, F., M. Carvalho, M. Babka, and E. Meier zu Verl. Reflex increases in heart rate induced by perfusing the hind leg of the rat with solutions containing lactic acid. *Pflugers Arch.* 400: 286–293, 1984.
345. Thomas, G. D., J. Hansen, and R. G. Victor. Inhibition of α_2-adrenergic vasoconstriction during contraction of glycolytic, not oxidative, rat hindlimb muscle. *Am. J. Physiol.* 266 (*Heart Circ. Physiol.* 35): H920–H929, 1994.
346. Thompson, L. P., and D. E. Mohrman. Blood flow and oxygen consumption in skeletal muscle during sympathetic stimulation. *Am. J. Physiol.* 245 (*Heart Circ. Physiol.* 14): H66–H71, 1983.
347. Tidgren, B., P. Hjemdahl, E. Theodorsson, and J. Nussberger. Renal neurohormonal and vascular responses to dynamic exercise in humans. *J. Appl. Physiol.* 70: 2279–2286, 1991.
348. Tyberg, J. V. Venous modulation of ventricular preload. *Am. Heart J.* 123: 1098–1104, 1992.
349. Vallbo, A. B., K.-E. Hagbarth, H. E. Torebjork, and B. G. Wallin. Somatosensory, proprioceptive, and sympathetic activity in human peripheral nerves. *Physiol. Rev.* 59: 919–957, 1979.
350. Vanhoutte, P. M. Physical factors of regulation. In: *Handbook of Physiology, The Cardiovascular System, Vascular Smooth Muscle*, edited by D. F. Bohr, A. P. Somlyo, and H. V. Sparks, Jr. Bethesda, MD: Am. Physiol. Soc., 1980, p. 443–474.

351. Vanhoutte, P. M., E. Lacroix, and I. Leusen. The cardiovascular adaptation of the dog to muscular exercise: role of the arterial pressoreceptors. *Arch. Int. Physiol. Biochim.* 74: 201–222, 1966.
352. Vanhoutte, P. M., T. J. Verbeuren, and R. C. Webb. Local modulation of adrenergic neuroeffector interaction in the blood vessel wall. *Physiol. Rev.* 61: 151–247, 1981.
353. van Leeuwen, B. E., G. J. Barendsen, J. Lubbers, and L. de Pater. Calf blood flow and posture: Doppler ultrasound measurements during and after exercise. *J. Appl. Physiol.* 72: 1675–1680, 1992.
354. van Lieshout, W. Wieling, K. H. Wesseling, E. Endert, and J. M. Karemaker. Orthostatic hypotension caused by sympathectomies performed for hyperhidrosis. *Neth. J. Med.* 36: 53–57, 1990.
355. Vatner, S. F., D. Franklin, R. L. Van Citters, and E. Braunwald. Effects of carotid sinus nerve stimulation on blood flow distribution in conscious dogs at rest and during exercise. *Circ. Res.* 27: 495–503, 1970.
356. Victor, R. G., L. A. Bertocci, S. L. Pryor, and R. L. Nunnally. Sympathetic nerve discharge is coupled to muscle cell pH during exercise in humans. *J. Clin. Invest.* 82: 1301–1305, 1988.
357. Victor, R. G., and A. L. Mark. Interaction of cardiopulmonary and carotid baroreflex control of vascular resistance in humans. *J. Clin. Invest.* 76: 1592–1598, 1985.
358. Victor, R. G., S. L. Pryor, N. H. Secher, and J. H. Mitchell. Effects of partial neuromuscular blockade on sympathetic nerve responses to static exercise in humans. *Circ. Res.* 65: 468–476, 1989.
359. Victor, R. G., D. M. Rotto, S. L. Pryor, and M. P. Kaufman. Stimulation of renal sympathetic activity by static contraction: evidence for mechanoreceptor-induced reflexes from skeletal muscle. *Circ. Res.* 64: 592–599, 1989.
360. Victor, R. G., and D. R. Seals. Reflex stimulation of sympathetic outflow during rhythmic exercise in humans. *Am. J. Physiol.* 257 (*Heart Circ. Physiol.* 26): H2017–H2024, 1989.
361. Victor, R. G., D. R. Seals, and A. L. Mark. Differential control of heart rate and sympathetic nerve activity during dynamic exercise. *J. Clin. Invest.* 79: 508–516, 1987.
362. Vissing, S. F., U. Scherrer, and R. G. Victor. Stimulation of skin sympathetic nerve discharge by central command. *Circ. Res.* 69: 228–238, 1991.
363. Wade, O. L., B. Combes, A. W. Childs, H. O. Wheeler, A. Cournand, and S. E. Bradley. The effects of exercise on the splanchnic blood flow and splanchnic blood volume in normal man. *Clin. Sci.* 15: 457–463, 1956.
364. Wagner, P. D., G. E. Gale, R. E. Moon, J. R. Torre-Bueno, B. W. Stolp, and H. A. Saltzman. Pulmonary gas exchange in humans exercising at sea level and simulated altitude. *J. Appl. Physiol.* 61: 260–270, 1986.
365. Walgenbach, S. C., and D. E. Donald. Cardiopulmonary reflexes and arterial pressure during rest and exercise in dogs. *Am. J. Physiol.* 244 (*Heart Circ. Physiol.* 13): H362–H369, 1983.
366. Walgenbach, S. C., and D. E. Donald. Inhibition by carotid baroreflex of exercise-induced increases in arterial pressure. *Circ. Res.* 52: 253–262, 1983.
367. Walgenbach-Telford, S. Arterial baroreflex and cardiopulmonary mechanoreflex function during exercise. In: *Reflex Control of the Circulation*, edited by J. P. Gilmore and I. H. Zucker. Boca Raton, FL: CRC Press, 1991, p. 765–793.
368. Walker, J. L., F. M. Abboud, A. L. Mark, and M. D. Thames. Interaction of cardiopulmonary and somatic reflexes in humans. *J. Clin. Invest.* 65: 1491–1497, 1980.
369. Wallin, B. G., and J. Fagius. Peripheral sympathetic neural activity in conscious humans. *Annu. Rev. Physiol.* 50: 565–576, 1988.
370. Walløe, L., and J. Wesche. Time course and magnitude of blood flow changes in the human quadriceps muscles during and following rhythmic exercise. *J. Physiol. (Lond.)* 405: 257–273, 1988.
371. Warner, H. R., and A. Cox. A mathematical model of heart rate control by sympathetic and vagus efferent information. *J. Appl. Physiol.* 17: 349–355, 1962.
372. Wenger, C. B. More comments on "keeping a cool head" by M. Cabanac. *News Physiol. Sci.* 2: 150, 1987.
373. Wennergren, G. Aspects of central integrative and efferent mechanisms in cardiovascular reflex control. *Acta Physiol. Scand. Suppl.* 428: 5–53, 1975.
374. Wexler, L., D. H. Bergel, I. T. Gabe, G. S. Makin, and C. J. Mills. Velocity of blood flow in normal human venae cavae. *Circ. Res.* 23: 349–359, 1968.
375. Williams, C. A., J. G. Mudd, and A. R. Lind. The forearm blood flow during intermittent hand-grip isometric exercise. *Circ. Res.* 48 (Suppl. 1): 110–117, 1981.
376. Wilson, J. R., and S. Kapoor. Contribution of prostaglandins to exercise-induced vasodilation in humans. *Am. J. Physiol.* 265 (*Heart Circ. Physiol.* 34): H171–H175, 1993.
377. Wilson, J. R., and S. Kapoor. Contribution of endothelium-derived relaxing factor to exercise-induced vasodilation in humans. *J. Appl. Physiol.* 75: 2740–2744, 1993.
378. Wyss, C. R., J. L. Ardell, A. M. Scher, and L. B. Rowell. Cardiovascular responses to graded reductions in hindlimb perfusion in exercising dogs. *Am. J. Physiol.* 245 (*Heart Circ. Physiol.* 14): H481–H486, 1983.

III

Control of Energy Metabolism during Exercise

Associate Editor Ronald Terjung

18. Cellular processes integrating the metabolic response to exercise

RONALD A. MEYER | *Departments of Physiology and Radiology, Michigan State University, East Lansing, Michigan*

JEANNE M. FOLEY | *Departments of Physiology, and Physical Education and Exercise Science, Michigan State University, East Lansing, Michigan*

CHAPTER CONTENTS

THE REMARKABLE FEATURE OF skeletal muscle compared to other tissues is its ability to cope with rapid and dramatic increases in metabolic rate. For example, in rat fast-twitch muscle, the adenosine triphosphatase (ATPase) rate increases by over tenfold from rest during steady-state twitch contractions, and by over 200-fold from rest, or to near 10 μmol $\cdot$ g^{-1} $\cdot$ s^{-1}, during a short tetanus. The adenosine triphosphate (ATP) content of mammalian fast muscle is only about 7 μmol/g. Nonetheless, these changes in ATP turnover rate are accomplished with only insignificant changes in muscle ATP concentration. Although heart muscle can maintain higher ATPase rates in the steady state for prolonged periods, only skeletal muscle undergoes repeated transitions between ATPase rates over such a broad range. It is apparent that skeletal muscles have evolved a sensitive and accurate metabolic control system, one effect of which is to maintain nearly constant cellular ATP. The aim of this chapter is to summarize some key features of this control system.

The study of muscle metabolism has a long and rich history (131). Many key concepts in biochemistry, including recognition of the central role of ATP in energy transduction, arose from studies of muscle. We now know in detail both the molecular mechanisms of muscle contraction and the enzymatic pathways by which ATP is generated to support contraction. Several excellent reviews and monographs about muscle energetics and metabolism have been published over the last two decades (e.g., 73, 77, 96, 138, 200). Furthermore, several chapters in this volume will discuss specific topics in greater depth. Therefore, the goals of this chapter are to provide a perspective on the metabolic events that occur in muscle cells during exercise, and to identify some areas in which further research is clearly needed. We cannot exhaustively review all the cellular aspects of muscle metabolism, or even provide an overview that fairly covers the whole field.

THE CENTRAL ROLE OF ADENINE NUCLEOTIDES

Our perspective begins with the fact that ATP is the direct energetic link between muscle force development and catabolic metabolism (Fig. 18.1). While seemingly trivial, this simple view immediately leads

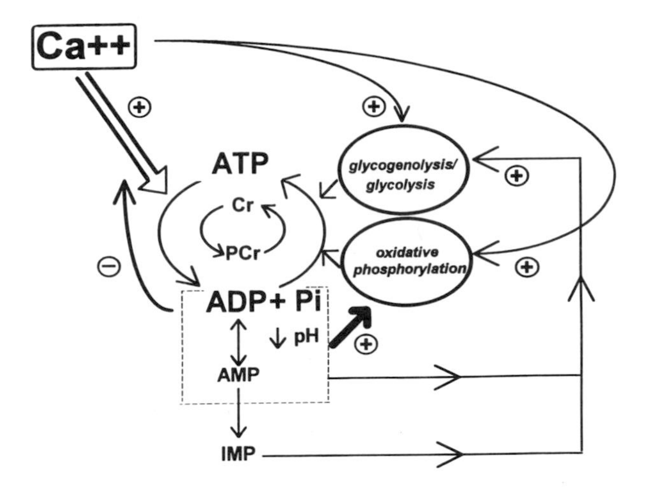

FIG. 18.1. Schematic illustrating the key roles of calcium and phosphate metabolites in regulating force and ATP production in skeletal muscle.

TABLE 18.1. *Consensus Estimates of Metabolite Levels in Mammalian Skeletal Muscles**

	Fast-Twitch	Slow-Twitch
pH	7.0–7.1	7.0–7.1
PCr (μmol/g)	24–30	15–20
Cr (μmol/g)	3–12	5–10
Pi (μmol/g)	1–3	3–10
ATP (μmol/g)	6–8	3.5–5
Total ADP (μmol/g)	0.4–0.6	0.4–0.6
Total AMP (μmol/g)	0.05–0.1	0.05–0.1
[ADP] (μM)†	5–41	7–34
[AMP] (μM)†	0.003–0.16	0.01–0.18
ΔG_{ATP} (kJ/mole)	−60 to −69	−56 to −64

*Composite estimates from measurements in rodent (26, 31, 41, 124), cat (121), and human (41) muscles. These are approximations only. Single-fiber measurements show considerable variance in metabolite levels among rat fast fibers (69). On the other hand, single fiber studies found similar ATP content in human fast vs. slow fibers (168). †Calculated from equations 2 and 3, assuming 75% of tissue volume is intracellular fluid.

to an important conceptual point. As noted by Hochachka and Matheson (71), one cannot study the regulation of ATP synthesis pathways in intact muscle independently of the regulation of ATP hydrolysis. For example, what if one observed that during intense exercise, muscle fatigue coincided with a fall in glycolytic flux? It is impossible to determine from this observation alone either that the fatigue was due to reduced glycolytic ATP supply, or that glycolytic flux decreased because of reduced ATP demand. The main determinant of the ATP turnover rate in muscle is activation of the contractile apparatus by calcium. If ATP does not significantly change, and if the stoichiometry of ATP-generating pathways is fixed, then the summed flux through those pathways is ultimately set by the contractile apparatus. Therefore, in most studies that examine the regulation of ATP synthesis in muscle, ATP hydrolysis and synthesis rates are the variables that are experimentally manipulated by muscle stimulation or exercise, and potential regulatory metabolites such as adenosine diphosphate (ADP) are the dependent variables (71). It is difficult (but not impossible) to vary these metabolites independently of the ATPase rate in intact muscle. As another example, consider the commonly posed question, What determines the steady-state rate of oxidative phosphorylation in working muscle? The simple answer is: the contractile apparatus! The harder question is: What are the coupling mechanisms that coordinate the response of aerobic ATP synthesis to changes in ATPase rate?

Components of the High-Energy Phosphate System

We will argue that changes in the adenine nucleotides, and in other metabolites directly coupled to adenine nucleotide levels by near-equilibrium reactions, are key signals that regulate skeletal muscle metabolism during exercise (see Table 18.1). These include, first, the hydrolysis products of ATP itself, ADP and inorganic phosphate (Pi):

$$ATP \rightarrow ADP + Pi + 0.6\ H^+ \text{ (at pH 7)}$$

ATP hydrolysis per se is far from equilibrium in the cytosol, and proceeds only when coupled to other reactions or processes such as force generation. The Gibbs free energy available to drive such coupled reactions from ATP hydrolysis is

$$\Delta G_{ATP} = \Delta G^{o}_{ATP} + RT \ln([ADP] \cdot [Pi]/[ATP]) \quad (1)$$

where the metabolite concentrations are the total concentrations in solution (i.e., the sum of all various ionic species) and ΔG^{o}_{ATP} is the standard free energy (= RT ln K_{eq}) under defined conditions of pH, pMg, ionic strength, and so forth. The adenine nucleotides are largely complexed with Mg^{2+} in vivo, and the distribution of various ionic species (e.g., $MgATP^{2-}$, $MgHATP^{1-}$, $HATP^{3-}$, $KATP^{3-}$) depends on pH. Note, however, that equation 1 does not explicitly include [H^+], [Mg^{2+}], or [K^+], because these are implicit in the definition of ΔG^{o}_{ATP}. At pH = 7, pMg = 3, and [K^+] = 100 mM, ΔG^{o}_{ATP} is −32 kJ/mole (187). At pH 6.5 and pMg 3, ΔG^{o}_{ATP} decreases (i.e., is less negative) by about 2 kJ/mole (3).

All vertebrate skeletal muscles also contain creatine (Cr) and phosphocreatine (PCr), which are coupled to ATP and ADP levels by the creatine kinase reaction:

$$PCr + ADP + H^+ \leftrightarrow Cr + ATP$$

Skeletal muscle contains very high activity of the MM cytoplasmic isoform of the enzyme, and direct nuclear magnetic resonance (NMR) measurements of unidirectional flux through the reaction in intact muscle confirm that it must be close to equilibrium under all but the most extreme conditions (125). At pMg = 3, $[K^+]$ = 100 mM, the equilibrium constant of the reaction is (102):

$$K_{eq} = [Cr]/[PCr] \cdot [ATP]/[ADP] \cdot 1/[H^+] = 1.66 \cdot 10^9 M^{-1} \quad (2)$$

where again the concentrations are the totals of all ionic species. However, in this case it is convenient to explicitly include a hydrogen ion term, because the stoichiometry of proton uptake by the reaction in vivo is close to 1 (102).

Because of the high enzyme activity, the high equilibrium constant, and the high ATP/ADP ratio in muscle at rest, PCr hydrolysis is the net reaction observed during a short contraction, or during more prolonged series of contractions if oxidative and glycolytic ATP generation are inhibited:

$$ATP \rightarrow ADP + Pi + \alpha H^+$$
$$ADP + PCr + H^+ \leftrightarrow ATP + Cr$$
$$\text{net: } PCr + \beta H^+ \rightarrow Cr + Pi$$

This net reaction consumes protons, and thus a brief alkaline shift of up to 0.1 pH units is observed in muscle at the onset of contraction, and a corresponding acid shift coinciding with PCr resynthesis is observed after contraction (2, 119). The stoichiometric coefficient β is pH dependent, and ranges from about 0.4–0.8 at pH 7.0 and 6.0, respectively.

A useful consequence of the creatine kinase (CK) equilibrium is that it provides a way to calculate the free, metabolically active cytoplasmic ADP concentration in muscle. This is necessary because measurements of total ADP in extracts of frozen muscle include about 0.5 μmol/g, which is known to be tightly bound to f-actin and other proteins in vivo. On the other hand, ATP, creatine, and PCr are present in millimolar amounts and are probably not significantly bound to proteins in vivo. Thus, equation 2 is commonly used to calculate [ADP] in muscle.

Muscle also contains high levels of adenylate kinase (myokinase), so adenosine monophosphate (AMP) levels are also coupled to ATP and ADP levels (102):

$$2ADP \leftrightarrow ATP + AMP$$
$$K_{eq} = [ATP] \cdot [AMP]/[ADP]^2 = 1.05 \text{ at pH=7, pMg=3} \quad (3)$$

In this case, the evidence for equilibrium in vivo rests entirely on the high total enzyme activity, insofar as the free levels of both ADP and AMP in muscle are very low and difficult to measure, and direct NMR measurements of flux have not been possible. Nonetheless, equation 3 is commonly used to calculate free AMP concentration in muscle. The result (Table 18.1) is about 1000-fold less than the total AMP typically measured in extracts of muscle. Unfortunately, almost nothing is known about the location of this large bound pool of AMP.

Finally, because all of the above reactions are pH dependent, intracellular pH must be taken into account when considering the regulatory roles of these metabolites. Fortunately, the cytoplasmic pH in muscle can now be routinely measured by phosphorus NMR (52, 128). In mammalian muscles, pH at rest is 7.0–7.1 (34, 144, 154), but can decrease to below 6.2 during series of fatiguing contractions (121).

Phosphate Metabolites are a Linked Network

By assuming equilibrium of the myokinase and creatine kinase reactions and constant pH, and by using initial metabolite concentrations similar to those in Table 18.1, it is possible to calculate changes in all of the above metabolites as a function of net high-energy phosphate depletion, or Pi production. This calculation was most recently performed by Connett (26), who reported the results for each metabolite as a fraction of its maximum possible level and as a function of the fractional decrease in total high-energy phosphate (PCr + 2ATP + ADP). The calculation, shown in Figure 18.2*A*, illustrates the well-known buffering effect of ATP levels by the creatine kinase system. Significant depletion of ATP occurs only when PCr is substantially depleted. However, in intact muscles, ADP and AMP never rise to the level depicted in the "depletion zone" of Figure 18.2*A*. Instead, increases in AMP are limited by AMP deamination to inosine monophosphate (IMP) and dephosphorylation to adenosine. The former reaction predominates in skeletal muscle, so that decreases in ATP and total adenine nucleotide (TAN) are largely accounted for by IMP and ammonia accumulation (124):

$$AMP \rightarrow IMP + NH_3$$

This reaction is essentially irreversible in vivo. Although the enzyme AMP deaminase shows a pH

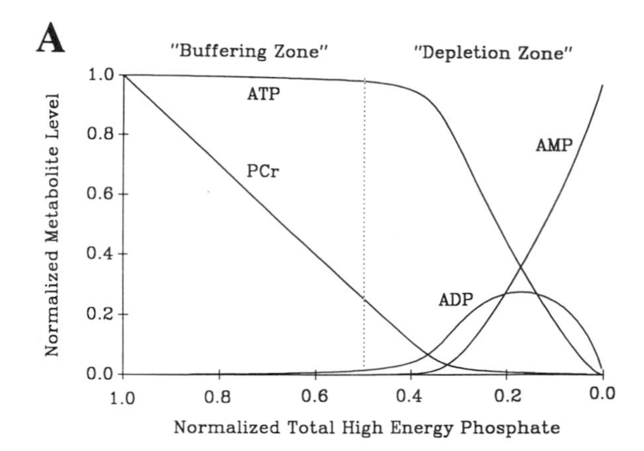

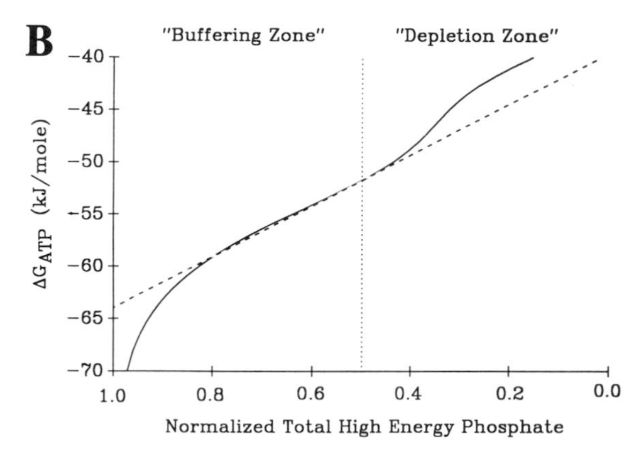

FIG. 18.2. *A*, Calculated changes in normalized metabolite levels as a function of high-energy phosphate depletion assuming constant pH = 7. PCr is normalized as a fraction of the total creatine pool (TCr), adenine nucleotides as fractions of the total adenine nucleotide pool (TAN), and high-energy phosphate (PCr + 2ATP + ADP) as a fraction of (TCr + 2TAN). [Recalculated from Connett (26).] *B*, Changes in ΔG_{ATP} as a function of high-energy phosphate depletion, assuming constant pH = 7, TCr = 40 mM, TAN = 10 mM, and Pi = 0 at PCr/TCr = 1.

optimum at 6.5, and is allosterically regulated by Pi, GTP, AMP, and ADP (197), most evidence suggests that the rate is limited at least in part by AMP availability (37). The effect of the reaction, along with the myokinase reaction, is to preserve a high ATP/ADP ratio, and hence ΔG_{ATP}, at the cost of depletion of the TAN pool (106, 126).

It is important to note that the "buffering zone" of Figure 18.2*A* is the region over which changes in ATP are minimal. Nonetheless, Pi (from net PCr hydrolysis) and ADP (proportional to Cr/PCr) are changing in this zone. Therefore, the free energy available from ATP hydrolysis changes over this region. In fact, to a good approximation, the change in ΔG_{ATP} over much of this region is directly proportional to the change in PCr (26, 117). Thus, in the buffering zone there is a roughly linear relationship between the extent of phosphagen depletion and ΔG_{ATP} (Fig. 18.2*B*). On the other hand, in the absence of ADP and AMP removal by myokinase and AMP deaminase, ΔG_{ATP} would fall dramatically in the depletion zone.

The view that emerges from the above is of a network of metabolites, coupled via near-equilibrium reactions, the state of which is defined by the cytoplasmic free energy of ATP hydrolysis, by pH, and by the TAN and total creatine pools. Net phosphagen hydrolysis results, first, in a roughly linear drop in ΔG_{ATP}, and ultimately, in depletion of total adenine nucleotides. Changes in this network of metabolites, along with changes in intracellular pH and calcium, can explain many but not all of the control processes that stabilize ATP during exercise in skeletal muscle. As illustrated in Figure 18.1, such control can in principle occur by two mechanisms: *(1)* by increasing flux through the pathways of ATP synthesis, and *(2)* by decreasing the rate of ATP hydrolysis. The second mechanism can be accomplished either by changing the economy of force generation or, more obviously, by decreasing force. Thus, decreased force, or fatigue, can be viewed as an important aspect of a control system designed to preserve cytoplasmic ΔG_{ATP}, rather than as an undesirable or pathological result of repeated contractions.

APPROACHES TO UNDERSTANDING METABOLIC CONTROL

Classic Enzyme Kinetics

Before proceeding, it is useful to summarize briefly the conditions under which net flux through an enzymatic reaction can change. Consider a simple enzymatic reaction

$$S + E \leftrightarrow ES \leftrightarrow EP \leftrightarrow E + P \text{ , where } K_{eq} = [P]/[S]$$

Assume that the enzyme, E, is a simple one, with no allosteric control sites and no potential for covalent modification. In general, the net flux through the reaction depends on the kinetic properties of the enzyme, and on the total concentrations of S, P, and E. If the concentration of P is negligible, if [E]<< [S], and if the binding steps are relatively fast, then the net flux, J, will behave in the classic Michaelis-Menton fashion (163); that is,

$$J = J_{max} \cdot [S]/(K_{ms} + [S]) \tag{4}$$

where K_{ms} is the binding constant for S, and J_{max} is proportional to total [E] (Fig. 18.3*A*). This description is commonly taught by biochemists to physiologists, and hence forms the starting point for many discussions of metabolic control in muscle. Equation 4 immediately suggests three possible mechanisms

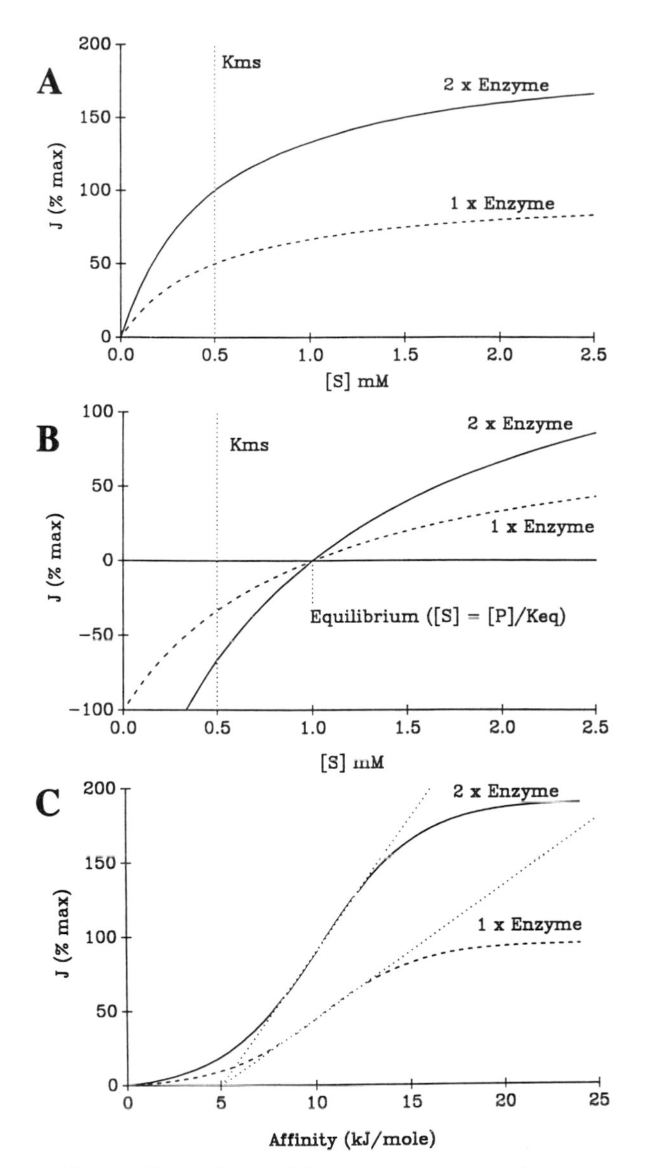

FIG. 18.3. *A*, Dependence of the net reaction rate of an enzyme-catalyzed reaction on substrate concentration, [S], assuming classic Michaelis-Menton kinetics with K_{ms} = 0.5 mM, and [P] = 0. *B*, Dependence of net reaction rate on substrate concentration assuming K_{eq} = 1, K_{ms} = 0.5 mM, K_{mp} = 1 mM, and [P] = 1 mM. *C*, Dependence of net reaction rate on reaction affinity, assuming K_{eq} = 100, K_{ms} = 0.5 mM, K_{mp} = 1 mM, [S] + [P] = 10 mM.

for increasing net flux: increase the substrate concentration, decrease K_{ms} by some allosteric or covalent modification, or increase J_{max} by increasing the effective enzyme concentration. As noted above, the AMP deaminase reaction may be an example of the first mechanism, inasmuch as both AMP and IMP levels are very low at rest, and AMP increases sharply when PCr is depleted (Fig. 18.2*A*).

Unfortunately, the classic Michaelis-Menton equation is not always applicable in vivo. Typically [P] is not negligible, and the reaction may be near equilibrium; that is, $[P]/[S] \approx K_{eq}$. In this case, the dependence of the net flux on [S] is quite different (Fig. 18.3*B*; (163)]:

$$J = \frac{J_{max} \cdot ([S] - [P]/K_{eq})}{K_{ms} \cdot (1 + [P]/K_{mp}) + [S]} \tag{5}$$

When [S] equals its equilibrium concentration (=[P]/K_{eq}), there is no net flux, and changes in K_{ms} or J_{max} have no effect. On the other hand, even small deviations from equilibrium can result in large changes in net flux, particularly when the enzyme concentration is high.

Attempts to apply the classic Michaelis-Menton equation when [P] is not negligible can lead to conceptual errors. For example, suppose one measured the substrate concentration and net flux through some simple enzyme in vivo and found that [S] was approximately equal to K_{ms}. From equation 4, one might be tempted to conclude that the measured flux was equal to half the maximum possible flux, and hence could only be increased by a maximum of twofold. Consideration of equation 5 or Figure 18.3*B* demonstrates that this is not the case. If the reaction is anywhere near equilibrium, the net flux could still increase enormously, even if [S] is already far in excess of K_{ms}. Similarly, large increases in net flux could be induced by decreasing P, even if it is above its K_m. Finally, increases in total [E] result in proportional increases in flux, even if the displacement from equilibrium is small. Thus, adaptations that alter enzyme concentrations [e.g., increased mitochondrial enzymes with endurance training (56)] can have physiologically significant effects even if the catalyzed reaction never approaches J_{max} in vivo.

Nonequilibrium Thermodynamics

Nonequilibrium thermodynamics (NET) offers another approach to describing the behavior of enzymatic reactions (19, 185, 148, 195). Although formally correct for simple chemical reactions only when close to equilibrium, this approach turns out to be more generally applicable and conceptually simpler than equation 5. The basic idea is that the net flux, J, through a reaction or sequence of reactions is the product of the net reaction affinity, *A* ($A = -\Delta G$), and a conductance coefficient, *L*:

$$J = L \cdot A \tag{6}$$

This relation is exactly analogous to Ohm's law; that is, a flow (current or reaction flux) equals a conductance coefficient times a driving force (voltage or reaction affinity). For a simple enzyme-catalyzed reaction, assuming constant total [S] + [P] = C, and

K_{eq} near 1, L can be solved analytically (185):

$$L = (V_s/(K_{ms}/C + 1) + V_p/(K_{mp}/C + 1))/4RT \quad (7)$$

where V_s and V_p are the maximum forward and reverse rates, which depend directly on [E]. If $K_{eq}>>1$, the relationship between A and J is sigmoidal, but still shows a very broad region of linearity (e.g., Fig. 18.3C), which can be approximated by

$$J = L \cdot A - b \quad (8)$$

where b also depends on C, and on the kinetic properties of the enzyme (185). The useful feature of this approach is that it can be applied even to complicated vectorial chemical systems, (e.g. oxidative phosphorylation and other transmembrane reactions), even if the detailed reaction steps are unknown (19). In such cases, L is a measure of the flux capacity or conductance of the overall reaction.

Regulated Enzymes and the Role of Calcium

Of course, some enzymatic reactions are always far from equilibrium in vivo. By definition, an abundant enzyme catalyzing such a reaction must be tightly regulated, either allosterically or by covalent modifications such as phosphorylation; otherwise, the reaction would run to equilibrium. The role of allosterically regulated enzymes in controlling flux through the pathways of intermediary metabolism has received considerable attention, and elaborate mathematical models have been developed to describe flux in complex metabolic networks based on the "control strength" of such enzymes (30). For our purposes, it is sufficient to point out that, in the extreme case, such an enzyme can behave as a metabolic switch, in which flux increases from near zero to near maximum very rapidly. A multisite enzyme with high cooperativity might behave this way even in the absence of covalent activation, if exposed to a sufficiently large and rapid rise in substrate concentration. More commonly, such a transition between low and high flux is induced by changes in calcium, cyclic AMP, or some other allosteric messenger that alters K_{ms} or J_{max}.

In muscle, the most prevalent allosterically regulated enzyme is the actomyosin ATPase, which is activated by calcium. Figure 18.4 summarizes the key steps of calcium cycling during muscle cell activation (for reviews, see 92, 135, 179). The kinetics of calcium release from the sarcoplasmic reticulum (SR), as well as its resequestration by the SR Ca^{2+} ATPase, are extremely rapid, at least on the time scale of many of the subsequent metabolic events. Moreover, in unfatigued skeletal muscle, calcium release is sufficient to fully activate the contractile apparatus during a short tetanus. Thus, the calcium transient in muscle can be considered a metabolic switch that triggers bursts of ATP hydrolysis.

DETERMINANTS OF MUSCLE CELL ATPase RATE

The total ATP hydrolysis rate in muscle varies with the nature and frequency of contraction, as well as

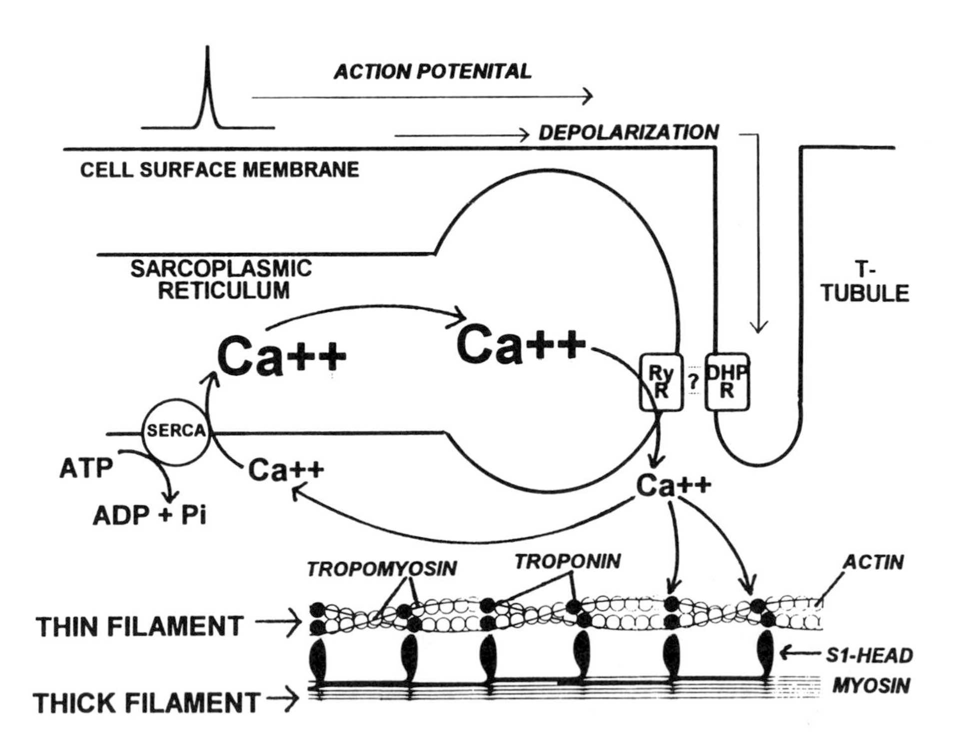

FIG. 18.4. Schematic illustrating some important features of excitation-contraction coupling and calcium cycling in skeletal muscle. DHP-R, dihydropyridine-sensitive voltage-gated calcium channel; RY-R, ryanodine-sensitive SR calcium release channel; SERCA, sarcoplasmic/endoplasmic reticulum calcium ATPase.

with the muscle type. These variations result from the kinetic properties of the sarcomeric actomyosin ATPase and SR Ca^{2+}-ATPase, and from fiber type and species variations in these proteins.

The Basal ATPase

The basal ATP turnover rate in resting muscle can be estimated from the rate of oxygen consumption ($\dot{Q}O_2$). Resting whole-body $\dot{Q}O_2$ varies across mammalian species roughly in proportion to the two-thirds power of body size (191), and this difference is reflected in the resting $\dot{Q}O_2$ of isolated muscles. For example, in perfused rat mixed muscle resting oxygen consumption is 0.37 $\mu mol \cdot g^{-1} \cdot min^{-1}$ at 37°C (75), while in cat and dog muscle, resting QO_2 is about 0.1 $\mu mol \cdot g^{-1} \cdot min^{-1}$ (27, 55, 99). Assuming the optimum ATP/O_2 ratio of 6, this corresponds to resting ATP turnover rates of 0.037 and 0.01 $\mu mol \cdot g^{-1} \cdot s^{-1}$ for rat and cat muscles, respectively. These estimates ignore the potential contribution of glycolysis, which may contribute up to 10% of the ATP generated at rest (75). Furthermore, studies of isolated liver mitochondria (14) and intact heart muscle (184) suggest that the mitochondrial ATP/O_2 ratio is less than 6. On the other hand, direct comparison of chemical changes during short contractions with recovery oxygen consumption in mouse muscle are consistent with an ATP/O_2 ratio close to 6 (31). Similarly, comparison of steady-state oxygen consumption during twitch contractions with PCr transients during the approach to steady state yield an ATP/O_2 ratio close to 6 in both rat (117) and cat muscle (S. J. Harkema and R. A. Meyer, unpublished observations). While the lower ATP/O_2 ratio in isolated mitochondria might be attributed to damage during the extraction process, the apparent discrepancy between ATP/O_2 ratio in heart vs. skeletal muscle deserves further attention.

The specific ATPases responsible for ATP turnover in resting skeletal muscle are not quantitatively identified. The basal rate of sodium influx in resting muscle is low [~4 $\mu Eq \cdot g^{-1} \cdot h^{-1}$ (11)], so the estimated contribution of the sarcolemal Na^+/K^+ ATPase to resting ATP turnover is less than 5%. This inference is confirmed by the observation that ouabain has little immediate effect on basal heat production (23), or on the rate of PCr hydrolysis in ischemic muscle (11). Although the T tubule membrane also contains a ouabain-insensitive Ca^{2+}-ATPase, its basal activity and function are not known (9, 59, 134). Based on the similarities between the temperature dependence of myosin ATPase in vitro and resting $\dot{Q}O_2$ of frog muscle, it was suggested that much of the basal ATPase is due to residual actomyosin ATPase activity (138). However, the peculiar temperature dependence of actomyosin in vitro is probably due to actin dissociation in dilute solutions (7), and could not occur in sarcomeres of intact muscle. Furthermore, resting $\dot{Q}O_2$ is the same in slow- and fast-twitch mammalian muscles (31, 121), despite their very different maximum myosin ATPase activities. We are left with the unsatisfying conclusion that the basal ATPase reflects the sum of the above, plus many other ATPases involved in protein synthesis and other "cell maintenance" functions.

The Contractile ATPase

In contrast to the basal ATPase, the increase in energy use during contractions is known in quantitative detail from classic myothermic and chemical studies. These studies and their importance to understanding the molecular mechanism of muscle contraction have been thoroughly reviewed by others (73, 96, 200). We summarize here some key points needed for discussion of the subsequent metabolic events.

Of the total increase in ATP hydrolysis during an isometric contraction, about 70% is due to actomyosin ATPase, and most of the remaining 30% is due to the SR Ca^{2+}-ATPase (138, 140). Although maintenance of transcellular sodium and potassium gradients during contraction is necessary for normal excitation, the Na^+/K^+-ATPase accounts for an insignificant fraction of contractile ATP use. The fraction of ATP use that is not due to actomyosin can be estimated by stretching muscles to lengths at which the thin and thick filaments do not overlap. The result is quite consistent across species, muscle types, contraction modes, and measurement methods. For example, the nonactomyosin fraction of ATP hydrolysis is similar during a twitch and a tetanus (140, 166), and tetanus duration seems to have little effect (74). This fraction is similar in mouse fast- and slow-twitch muscles (32), rat fast muscle (193), and various amphibian muscles (166). Stretch experiments have been criticized on the grounds that calcium release may be decreased in stretched muscles (73), or that residual myosin ATPase activity may be significant at long lengths (79). However, measurements of intracellular calcium with fluorescent indicators do not always support the first criticism (e.g., 10), and in any case, the above errors would tend to cancel each other.

During isometric contractions of a few seconds' duration, total ATP hydrolysis is proportional to the force·time integral [Fig. 18.5; (31)]. However, the

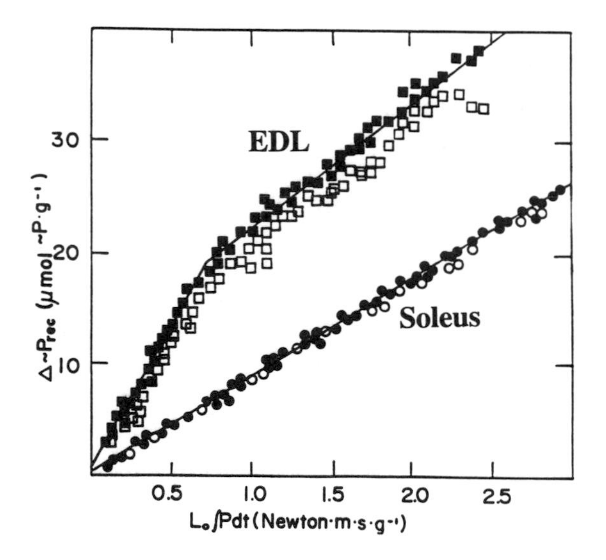

FIG. 18.5. High-energy phosphate utilization (~P) as a function of tetanus tension–time integral in mouse soleus and EDL muscle at 20°C. [From Crow and Kushmerick (31).]

ATP cost, or economy of isometric contraction (d∫fdt/dATP), varies by over 200-fold across the animal kingdom (including smooth and invertebrate muscles), and by over threefold between slow- and fast-twitch skeletal muscles within a single mammalian species. For example, the ATP cost of a 1 s tetanus at 20°C in mouse fast EDL is 4.3 μmol/g, vs. 1.3 μmol/g in mouse soleus (31). Similarly, cat biceps consumes four times more ATP during a single twitch than cat soleus muscle (99). These differences largely reflect differences in the kinetic properties of specific myosin isozymes between various fiber types and species. Such differences also underlie the classic observation by Bárány (7) that the maximum shortening velocity of muscles depends linearly on the specific activity of their actomyosin ATPase measured in vitro.

The molecular basis for the relationship between myosin isozyme composition and shortening velocity or ATPase rate is currently an active research area (for review, see 137, 196). Myosin consists of a heavy chain (MHC) homodimer, with two pairs of light chains bound to the globular head: the alkali or essential light chains, and the regulatory or phosphorylatable light chains. Two major classes of alkali light chains (LC1 and LC3) and one of regulatory light chains (LC2) have been identified, with subclasses and fast and slow variants within each of these major classes. Most evidence indicates that variations in MHC are the major determinant of ATPase rate (107), but changes in light chains alone have up to a twofold effect on shortening velocity in skinned fibers (176, 177). Mixed expression of the various alkali light chains can occur in vivo, and fast light chains can mix with slow heavy chains, and vice versa (137). It follows that the traditional classification of mammalian fibers into three categories on the basis of histochemical stains is inadequate. Mammalian muscle may include a continuum of fibers with a substantial range of mechanical and metabolic characteristics (see Chapter 24). Nonetheless, for our purposes we will continue to refer to the extremes of this continuum; that is, slow-twitch aerobic muscle, typified by rodent and cat soleus, and fast-twitch muscle with variable mitochondrial content, typified by rodent EDL and lateral gastrocnemius muscle and cat biceps brachii muscle.

Total sarcoplasmic/endoplasmic reticulum calcium ATPase (SERCA) activity is about sixfold greater in fast- compared to slow-twitch mammalian fibers (44, 202). About half this difference is accounted for by the greater total SR surface area in fast-twitch fibers (15, 104). The remainder reflects the faster kinetics of the SERCA-1 isoform that is expressed in fast-twitch fibers (80, 202). The slower SERCA-2a isoform is predominant in slow-twitch fibers, while both fiber types also express the SERCA-2b isoform found in the endoplasmic reticulum of most tissues.

Active shortening increases the rate of ATP hydrolysis in frog muscle by about 50% compared to the rate during an isometric contraction (97). The peak ATPase rate occurs at about the velocity of peak mechanical power output, and drops off at higher velocities. [The extra ATP hydrolysis during rapid shortening is less than expected from heat measurements (the Fenn effect)—a problem considered in detail by Rall (139).] On the other hand, lengthening of active muscle (eccentric contraction) decreases total ATP hydrolysis by up to 70%, implying nearly complete suppression of the actomyosin ATPase component (138, 200). Unfortunately, the ATP cost of lengthening and shortening contractions is not as well characterized in mammalian as in frog muscles. However, extrapolating from various measurements of the ATP cost of isometric contractions in rodent (31, 49, 75, 165, 193) and cat fast-twitch muscle (5.3 μmol/g during 1 s isometric tetanus; S. J. Harkema, G. R. Adams, and R. A. Meyer, unpublished observations) an upper limit for the ATPase rate at peak mechanical power at 37°C must be on the order of 15 and 7 $\mu mol \cdot g^{-1} \cdot s^{-1}$, respectively. In human mixed muscle, the maximum is probably around 2.0 $\mu mol \cdot g^{-1} \cdot s^{-1}$ (170).

Finally, during the fatigue that develops after repetitive contraction, contractile ATP use decreases in proportion to the decrease in peak force or tension–time integral (36). In some mammalian fast-twitch muscles, the economy of contraction appears to increase during prolonged tetani or after repeated contractions (31), further reducing ATP used per contraction (EDL in Fig. 18.5). In mouse EDL muscle this change in economy coincides with a reduction in maximum shortening velocity (32), implying a reduced rate of cross-bridge cycling. The mechanism for this effect is not known. It is not due to phosphorylation of myosin LC2 (176), but does seem to coincide with the accumulation of IMP (48).

METABOLITE CHANGES DURING MUSCLE STIMULATION

Methodology

We now turn to a description of the changes in high-energy phosphates and coupled metabolites that are observed during repetitive series of contractions, or during exercise. These changes have been observed by two basic methodologies: chemical assay of rapidly-frozen muscles or biopsies, and NMR spectroscopy. Unfortunately, each method has limitations.

Freezing and the subsequent acid extraction process can result in artifactual hydrolysis of PCr and other labile metabolites (121). Furthermore, acid extraction liberates partially bound metabolites such as ADP and AMP, and precipitates some other metabolites of potential interest. For example, it appears that a fraction of the total adenine nucleotide pool of heart and slow-twitch muscle exists in a polymeric form that precipitates during acid extraction (78, 103, 183). Of course, freezing also destroys the sample, so determination of the time course of metabolic changes by chemical assay can be tedious and expensive.

^{31}P-NMR spectroscopy is completely noninvasive, and thus is ideally suited for studies of the time course of changes in phosphorus metabolites (for reviews, see 52, 123, 162). However, the method is very insensitive, so relatively large samples are needed, and signal averaging is usually required. Furthermore, as commonly practiced, NMR yields only relative metabolite levels, which must be scaled in reference to chemical assays of ATP or some other observed metabolite. Metabolites that are tightly bound to structural proteins are not observed in high-resolution NMR spectra so, in principle, the method is well suited for measuring soluble, metabolically active metabolite concentrations. Unfortunately, the free concentrations of key metabolites such as ADP and AMP are below the practical minimum sensitivity of in vivo ^{31}P-NMR (about 0.2 μmol/g). Finally, even relative quantification of large peaks in NMR spectra is subject to various errors (122).

Muscle heterogeneity is a major limitation shared by both NMR and chemical assay. This heterogeneity has two related components: first, the intrinsic variability in fiber-type metabolism within a muscle, and second, variations in recruitment and fatigue rates among the fibers. The latter component seriously complicates the interpretation of data acquired during voluntary exercise in humans. It is well known that increases in force or work rate during voluntary exercise are accomplished by recruitment of additional motor units, as well as by increasing motor unit frequency. It follows that changes in global muscle metabolite levels measured as a function of workload could reflect changes in motor unit recruitment at least as much as events in individual cells. Thus, attempts to quantitatively relate metabolite changes during voluntary exercise with cellular regulatory events should be viewed with skepticism. This problem is diminished by direct muscle stimulation, or by nerve stimulation under conditions in which transmission failure does not occur. However, even in this case, at higher workloads fatigue is likely to occur in some fibers before others (24). Therefore, it is also difficult to quantitatively relate global metabolic changes with the decline in force during fatigue in muscles with mixed fiber type. Finally, even during nonfatiguing stimulation, global measurements from mixed muscle ignore the fact that the different fiber types have different resting metabolite contents (Table 18.1), different contractile ATPase rates, and respond at different rates at the onset of stimulation (see below). If the metabolic relationships under study are not linear, then the global metabolic response will not necessarily be a simple function of the averaged metabolic changes in individual fibers.

Despite all these problems, the basic metabolic events observed by both methods in animal and human skeletal muscles are remarkably consistent. In describing these events, it is useful to consider two distinct domains: *(1)* during contraction at low rates which can be maintained in the steady state for many minutes without force decrement, and *(2)* during contraction at high rates, which results in substantial force decline within a few minutes.

The Low-Rate, Nonfatiguing Domain

At the onset of twitch contractions at low rates, PCr declines along an approximately exponential time course toward a steady-state level that depends linearly on stimulation rate [see Fig. 18.6*A* and *B*; (20,

117)]. The initial rate of PCr decline also depends on stimulation rate, and in rat fast-twitch muscle this was shown to be a good measure of the ATP cost of the contractions (49). To a good approximation, the recovery of PCr after stimulation follows the inverse time course of that at the onset of stimulation, and the time constant for PCr recovery does not vary with stimulation rate within a given muscle in the low-rate domain (117). Similar results have been obtained in various animal muscles and in human muscle, although the time constant for the PCr changes varies widely between muscles and species (8, 99). In rat fast muscle, the PCr time constant depends linearly on total creatine content (Fig. 18.6*C*), and inversely on mitochondrial content (Fig. 18.6*D*). In perfused cat soleus muscle, there is some evidence for nonexponential behavior of PCr changes as stimulation rate is increased (99). However, this behavior was not evident in a recent study of cat soleus muscles stimulated at low to moderate rates in situ (64).

There is abundant evidence that oxidative phosphorylation accounts for most of the ATP generated in the steady state at low stimulation rates. Similarly, in mammalian muscles, PCr recovery after stimulation depends almost entirely on aerobic metabolism (31, 155, 159). Unfortunately, measurement of the kinetics of cellular $\dot{Q}O_2$ in intact muscle is difficult, because it requires consideration of blood or perfusate distribution, oxygen diffusion and binding to myoglobin, mitochondrial distribution, and so forth. Nonetheless, the time constant for the approach of $\dot{Q}O_2$ toward steady state is reported to be comparable to that for PCr in isolated frog muscle (110), perfused hearts (40, 61), and dog (28) and human (8, 114) skeletal muscle during exercise. The implication of this for theories of control of oxidative phosphorylation in muscle is discussed later.

The substrate supporting oxidative phosphorylation in the low-rate domain depends on substrate supply, on the hormonal milieu, and on the fiber's mitochondrial content and glycolytic enzyme capacity. In intact animals, fibers with high mitochondrial

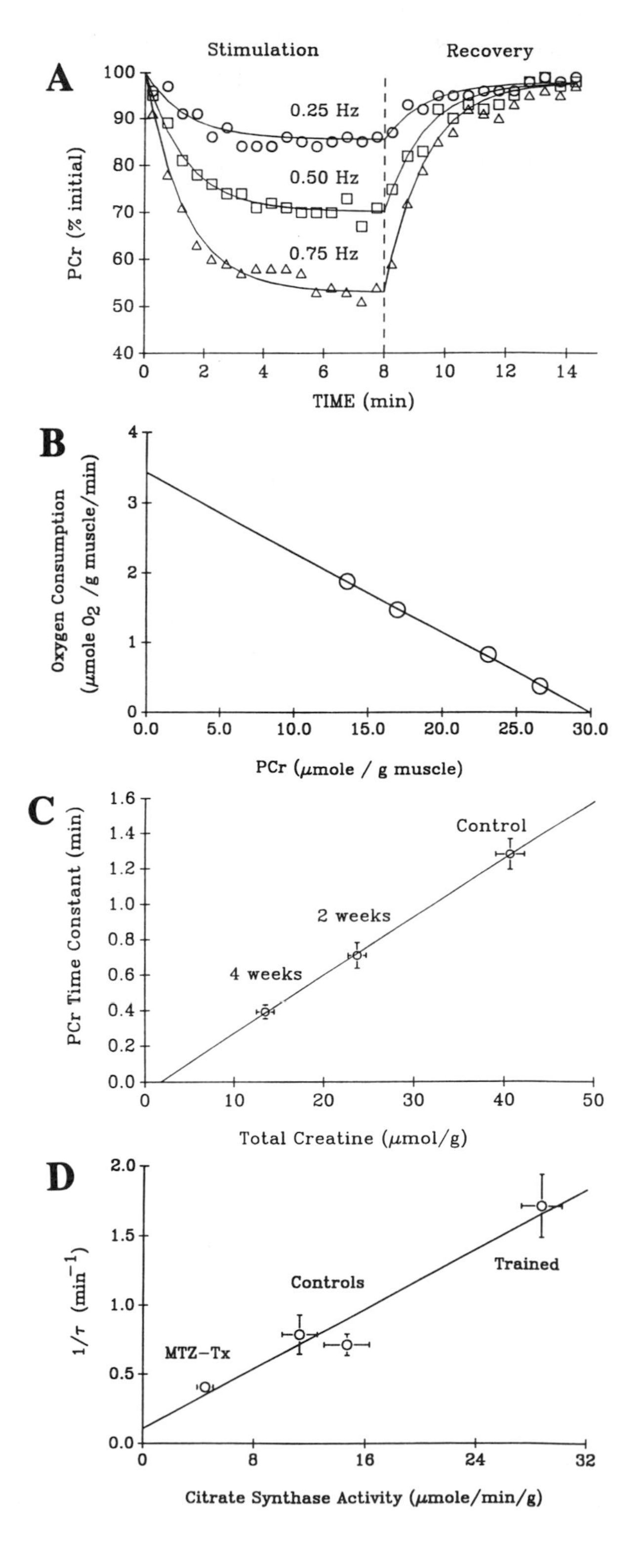

FIG. 18.6. *A*, Time course of PCr changes in rat gastrocnemius muscle during and after nonfatiguing twitch stimulation. [From Meyer (117).] *B*, Relationship between steady-state PCr and oxygen consumption in rat gastrocnemius muscle during nonfatiguing stimulation. [From Meyer (117).] C, Relationship between time constant for PCr changes (τ) and muscle total creatine content. Total creatine content of rat gastrocnemius muscle was depleted by 2 or 4 weeks feeding the creatine analog, β-guanidinopropionate. [From Meyer (118).] *D*, Relationship between rate constant for PCr recovery ($1/\tau$) and muscle mitochondrial content. Mitochondrial content of rat gastrocnemius muscle was increased by endurance training (10 weeks' duration, 1 h/day on a running wheel, final mean speed 38 m/min). Mitochondrial content was decreased by chemical thyroidectomy (0.025% methiamizole in drinking water for 8 weeks). (From Paganini, Foley, and Meyer, unpublished observations.)

content typically rely on triglyceride during low-intensity steady-state exercise (17). On the other hand, both fast and slow muscles can contract at moderate rates without fatigue for many minutes while oxidizing only carbohydrate (31, 99). (See Chapters 21, 22, and 23 for details on fat, carbohydrate, and amino acid oxidation in muscle.)

Intracellular pH is relatively stable in both fast- and slow-twitch muscles during low-intensity contraction (99). However, as noted earlier, net PCr hydrolysis causes transient alkalininzation at the onset of contraction, and PCr resynthesis causes transient acidosis during recovery. The pH transients associated with PCr changes can be used to estimate the buffer capacity of intact muscle, which is about 25–30 slykes (sl) at rest, but is effectively increased during stimulation due to the rise in Pi (2). It should be noted that failure to observe muscle acidification in this low-rate, steady-state domain does not rule out net lactic acid production (27). Nonetheless, most data indicate that this anaerobic component makes a minor contribution to total ATP production in the low-rate domain.

There is no evidence for significant changes in TAN, total creatine, or total phosphate during steady-state series of nonfatiguing contractions. There is also little doubt that both the creatine kinase and myokinase reactions are close to equilibrium in this low-rate domain. (The possibility that cytoplasmic metabolites are not freely diffusible will be considered later.) Therefore, mean cytoplasmic ADP, AMP, and ΔG_{ATP} can be estimated from the observed PCr changes, as depicted in Figure 18.2.

The High-Rate, Fatiguing Domain

In contrast to the low-rate domain, the observable metabolic events during contraction in the high-rate, fatiguing domain are dramatically different (e.g., Fig. 18.7). The decline in PCr is much more rapid, and is not adequately described by a single exponential. However, in rat mixed fast muscle with intact circulation, PCr does not fall to less than 10% of initial, even under the most fatiguing stimulation conditions [e.g., 5–10 Hz twitch stimulation (76, 98, 120, 126), or repetitive tetani with duty cycle more than 5–10% (48, 124)]. In fact, during more prolonged stimulation under these conditions, PCr begins to recover (Fig. 18.7), although force generation does not (76). Thus, the maintenance of some PCr in mixed muscle in the high-rate domain probably reflects two consequences of fiber heterogeneity. First, the decline in PCr is attenuated in the most highly aerobic fibers, a few of which may still be

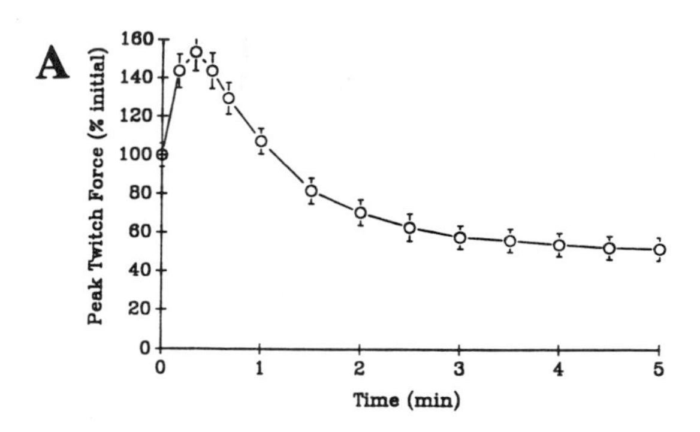

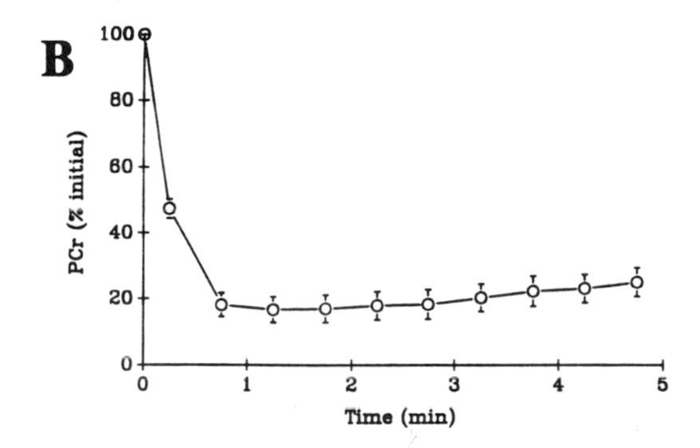

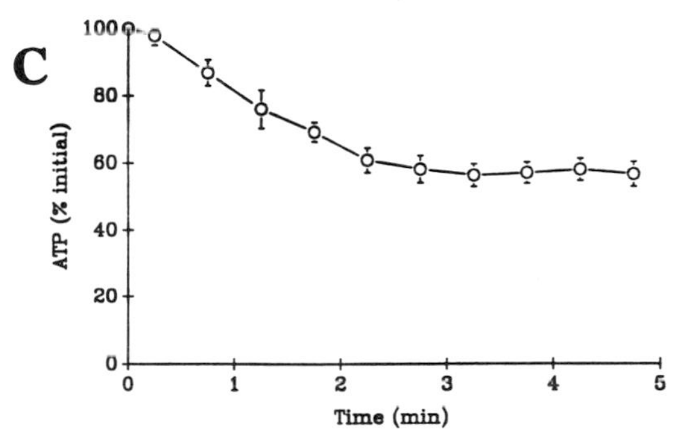

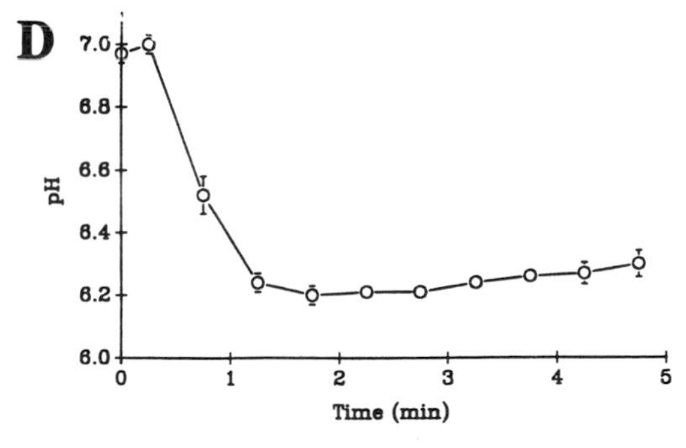

FIG. 18.7. Time course of changes in peak twitch force (*A*), PCr (*B*), ATP (*C*), and intracellular pH (*D*) during fatiguing (5 Hz) stimulation. PCr, ATP, and pH measured by ^{31}P-NMR as described in Meyer et al. (120). (From Paganini and Meyer, unpublished observations.)

operating in their low-rate domain (38). Second, force generation quickly drops in the less aerobic, easily fatiguable fibers, resulting in dramatically decreased ATP hydrolysis and significant net PCr resynthesis.

In predominantly fast-twitch muscle, profound intracellular acidosis occurs in the high-rate domain (Fig. 18.7). Overwhelming evidence confirms the conventional belief that this acidosis is due to net glycogenolysis and lactic acid production in the fibers. Under these conditions, anaerobic glycolysis can account for about 50%–70% of the total ATP production, with most of the remainder due to net PCr and ATP depletion (48, 169).

It is possible to lose sight of this simple explanation for the pH change during intense exercise by focusing on mechanistic details. For example, when considered in isolation, the net glycogen/glycolytic reaction is

$$\text{Glucose}_{(n)} + 3\text{ADP} + 3\text{Pi} \rightarrow \text{glucose}_{(n-1)} + 2\ \text{lactate} + 3\text{ATP} + \alpha\text{H}^{+}$$

where the nucleotides are again the total of all ionic species, and the stoichiometric coefficient α depends on pMg and pH, just as for the reactions described earlier. From this, one might be tempted to conclude that proton production by "glycolysis" is variable, or even that under some conditions, the process could consume protons (72). While semantically correct, this observation is not very relevant to understanding pH changes in intact muscle, because in muscle the reaction is always balanced by ATP hydrolysis. Compared to the change in lactic acid content, which can be over 30 μmol/g (e.g., 120, 124), the net changes in adenine nucleotides are small, and occur independently of glycolysis. Therefore, with respect to its effect on intracellular pH, the observed net glycolytic reaction in mammalian muscle is just:

$$\text{Glucose} \rightarrow 2\ \text{lactate} + 2\ \text{H}^{+}$$

More recently, the mathematical analysis developed by Stewart (173) was applied to estimate the pH changes observed in human muscle during intense exercise (94). The analysis confirmed that lactic acid is by far the dominant source of hydrogen ion production during intense exercise. However, while chemically correct, the Stewart analysis requires estimations of intracellular ion activity and dissociation constants that are likely to be much less reliable than measurements of PCr, lactate, or pH. This may explain why the resting intracellular pH yielded by the calculation was 6.87, or 0.1–0.2 pH units below the pH measured by all other methods. We conclude that there is no advantage to this analysis over the more conventional view, by which pH changes *during* intense exercise are estimated from the net changes in PCr and lactic acid, along with the measured buffer capacity of the muscle (158, 160). Conversely, during intense, short-duration exercise, lactic acid accumulation can be estimated from the observed pH and PCr changes (2, 48, 120).

The recovery of intracellular pH after high-rate stimulation is slower than PCr recovery, and more complicated (48, 91). There are many potential mechanisms for proton extrusion [or equivalently, restoration of the intracellular strong ion difference (173)] including the Na^{+}/H^{+} and HCO_3^{-}/Cl^{-} transporters (91, 144), lactate transport (147), lactic acid and ammonia diffusion, and so forth. Overlaid on these processes is the resynthesis of PCr, which contributes an additional acid load, particularly at low pH. The time course of PCr recovery after high-rate stimulation or exercise has been extensively reported, but the results are not very consistent. Some studies suggest that PCr recovery includes a fast component (time constant <1 min in human muscle), and a much slower component that has been attributed to low pH driving the creatine kinase reaction toward ATP production (67). However, this behavior is not always observed (90, 98), and the explanation is not satisfying, because muscle acidification due to hypercapnia does not decrease PCr (1, 119).

Depletion of up to 50% of both ATP (e.g., Fig. 18.7) and the TAN pool (48, 124) can occur in mammalian fast muscle during high-rate stimulation. Most of this depletion can be accounted for by IMP accumulation, although adenosine, inosine, and purine bases are produced in much lower amounts (12). The time course of IMP formation has not been carefully studied. In rat mixed fast muscle, IMP accumulation is evident before PCr is depleted (124), but as noted above, this may reflect fiber heterogeneity rather than true cellular events. This is an important issue, because if IMP formation occurs at high cellular PCr levels, it would suggest that local AMP concentrations near the AMP deaminase enzyme are higher than calculated from the assumed equilibrium of the creatine kinase and myokinase reactions (155). This could have implications for understanding control of glycogenolysis as well as AMP deamination (see below). The reamination of IMP is much slower than PCr recovery, and can be prevented by inhibiting either of the two enzymes involved [i.e., adenylosuccinate synthase (126), and adenylosuccinate lyase (47)]. Together, the deamination and reamination of IMP comprise the purine nucleotide cycle (106). The net effect of the cycle is to generate fumarate from aspartate, thus providing a mechanism for amino acid deamination during exercise.

The metabolic events in slow-twitch muscle in the high-rate domain are markedly different compared to fast muscle in two respects: first, the degree of acidosis and lactate accumulation is much less (1, 124), and second, IMP accumulation is negligible (124, 183). These differences cannot be explained entirely on the basis of the lower glycolytic capacity or AMP deaminase activity in slow-twitch muscle. For example, substantial lactic acid and IMP formation can be induced in slow-twitch muscle by ischemic stimulation (198). Instead, the differences may depend on the very different fatigue pattern observed in slow compared to fast mammalian muscles (24, 70). During repetitive stimulation in the high domain, fast muscle maintains relatively high force for tens of seconds, and then force falls precipitously. In contrast, if the circulation is intact, force in slow-twitch muscle rapidly falls to a level that depends on stimulation rate, and then is maintained at this level for many minutes (70). Conversely, if blood flow or perfusion pressure are varied, force rises and falls with these variations (70). Thus, there appears to be a mechanism that closely couples muscle activation to energy balance in mammalian slow-twitch muscle. Unfortunately, this phenomenon has received little attention in the literature on muscle fatigue.

The Transitional Domain

Of course, the above distinction between high and low contraction rate domains is artificial, because muscle fibers operate along a continuum, which must include some transitional domain. From the above discussion, it should be evident that this transitional domain depends on the ATPase rate relative to the aerobic capacity of the fiber. More highly aerobic fibers can sustain steady-state contraction at higher rates than less aerobic fibers without lactic acid accumulation and nucleotide depletion (38), and slower contracting fibers can sustain contraction at higher rates than fast fibers (99, 124). Although the transition can be induced by decreased oxygen delivery, it occurs in perfused muscle when oxygen delivery is not limiting (75, 124), so it is not simply due to muscle hypoxia. The situation in intact animals and humans is more complex. For example, cardiac output, and hence muscle oxygen delivery, may become limited during whole-body exercise in humans, but probably not during exercise of small muscle groups (150). Insofar as muscle capillarity and mitochondrial content adapt together in response to chronic exercise and other environmental challenges (191), the transitional domain probably depends on both factors in vivo. In any case, we have purposely avoided the transitional domain in our own metabolic studies, because we feel that it is hopelessly confounded in intact muscles by the heterogeneity problems discussed above. Therefore, until methods for studying the time course of metabolic events in single fibers, or phenotypically uniform muscles become available, we leave discussion of the "anaerobic threshold" and related issues to others (e.g., 16, 29, 81, 87). Instead, we now consider to what extent the regulation of ATP synthesis can be explained by metabolic changes in the two extremes.

CONTROL OF OXIDATIVE PHOSPHORYLATION IN MUSCLE

Mitochondria are complex organelles with an array of membrane transport and matrix enzymes (Fig. 18.8). ATP synthesis in mitochondria is driven by the electrochemical energy of the proton gradient across the inner membrane, which is in turn generated by membrane components of the electron transport chain. The mitochondrial ATP synthase is a proton ATPase pump, structurally and conceptually analogous to the proton pump in cytoplasmic vesicles, but operating in the direction of net ATP synthesis (45). The inner membrane also contains transport systems for adenine nucleotides, inorganic phosphate, calcium, and other metabolites. In view of this complexity, it is not surprising that there have been many studies of respiratory control in isolated mitochondria and various intact cells and tissues. Several recent reviews of respiratory control are available (6, 66, 82, 116, 178, 199), so we will focus only on the situation in intact skeletal muscle.

Kinetic Control by [ADP]

The most commonly presented scheme of respiratory control in skeletal muscle is kinetic limitation by cytoplasmic [ADP]. This idea evolved from Chance's classic studies of isolated mitochondria (21), in which the rate of oxygen consumption is low in the absence of ADP but in the presence of oxygen, substrate, and phosphate. In this "state 4" condition, mitochondrial NADH is fully reduced, the terminal cytochrome a_3 is oxidized, and oxygen consumption rate varies with [ADP] in the classic Michaelis-Menton fashion. There is no doubt that this condition can be achieved in isolated mitochondria (83). However, it is not clear that this is the condition in intact muscle at rest or in the low-rate domain described above.

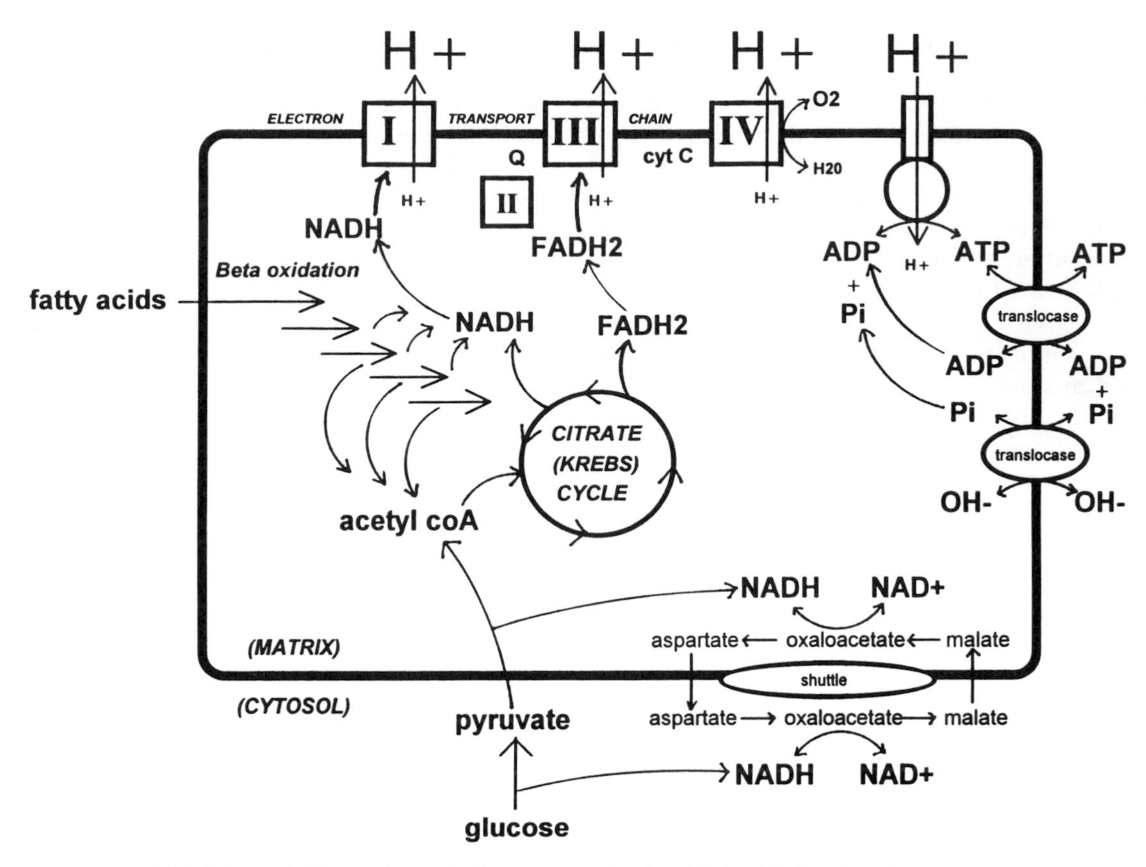

FIG. 18.8. Schematic illustrating main features of mitochondrial oxidative phosphorylation.

The first problem with the simple ADP model is that it requires [ADP] in resting muscle to be less than 10% of its apparent K_m. If [ADP] is not less than 10% of the K_m, then the model cannot explain the tenfold or greater increase in steady-state respiration rate observed in active muscle (71). The estimated [ADP] in resting mammalian muscles, calculated from the creatine kinase reaction, varies from 5μM to 25 μM, depending on the muscle; assay methods; and assumptions about reaction equilibrium constants, intracellular ions, and intracellular fluid volume (see Table 18.1). On average, this is more than 25% of the apparent K_m measured in isolated mitochondria [3–30 μM, (e.g., 60, 83)]. This problem becomes evident in various studies in which the apparent K_m for ADP was estimated by fitting the observed steady-state relationship between $\dot{Q}O_2$ vs. [ADP] to the Michaelis-Menton equation. Generally, as the range of respiratory rates studied increases, the fitted K_m increases (e.g., 13). For example, in perfused cat soleus muscle, which can be studied at steady-state respiratory rates over tenfold above rest, the apparent K_m is twice as high as in biceps muscle, which can only be studied in the steady state at rates up to sixfold above rest because of heterogeneity problems (99). Still, it can be argued that these discrepancies are due to errors in the various measurements, or to difficulty in estimating the true maximum $\dot{Q}O_2$ of intact muscle. Therefore, on this basis alone, the ADP model cannot be ruled out.

The second problem with the simple ADP control model is that the concentration of the product ATP in muscle is not negligible, and [Pi] is relatively low at rest, particularly in fast-twitch muscles (100). Furthermore, the calculated cytoplasmic ΔG_{ATP} in resting muscle is comparable to that calculated for the reactions of sites I and II of the respiratory chain (43, 199), as well as to that of the electrochemical proton gradient across the inner membrane of isolated mitochondria in state 4 (45). At respiratory rates near state 4, the backward flux through ATP synthase in isolated mitochondria is comparable to the forward flux (101). Therefore, it is likely that the ATP synthase reaction in resting muscle is not extremely far from equilibrium, as is required for application of the classic Michaelis-Menton equation. Unfortunately, a more general rate equation analogous to equation 5, but which applies to the entire process of oxidative phosphorylation, is not available. Even if such an equation were available, it would probably not be very helpful from the conceptual point of view. In such situations, the simple NET concepts introduced above can be useful.

Thermodynamic Control by Cytoplasmic Phosphates

Rigorous applications of NET to oxidative phosphorylation and other complex vectorial reactions have been developed by Westerhoff and van Dam (195), Jeneson et al. (84), and others (148, 174). The basic result, stripped of many interesting details, is that over a considerable range, the steady-state ATP synthesis rate, J, is a linear function of the cytoplasmic free energy of ATP hydrolysis, and of the redox potential ($\Delta G_r = \Delta G_r^o + RT\ln([NADH]/[NAD])$:

$$J = Lp \cdot (\Delta G_{ATP} - \Delta G^*_{ATP}) + L_r \cdot (\Delta G_r - \Delta G_r^*) \quad (9)$$

In the more complete treatment by Westerhoff (195) and Jeneson et al. (84), the L coefficients explicitly depend on proton coupling coefficients, on the mitochondrial substrate translocases, and so on. The ΔG^*'s are complex constants that define the onset of the linear domain, as illustrated previously by parameter b in equation 8. Assuming for the moment that all these coefficients are constant, and that the redox potential does not significantly change during moderate stimulation, the conclusion is that the rate of oxidative phosphorylation ought to depend linearly on ΔG_{ATP} over some range.

It should be noted that this NET analysis is conceptually different from the kinetic respiratory model of Wilson and colleaques (43, 199). That model assumes complete equilibrium of sites I and II of the respiratory chain, such that the terminal cytochrome oxidase step is always rate limiting. A recent study of the effect of chloramphenicol on respiration rate in muscle is not consistent with this view (111). However, the predictions of the Wilson model are superficially similar to those of the NET analysis, in that both predict dependence of respiration on the "phosphorylation potential" [i.e., [ATP]/([ADP]·[Pi])] and on [NADH]/[NAD] ratio.

As pointed out above, in the low-rate domain, steady-state PCr level is proportional to stimulation or ATP turnover rate. As depicted in Figure 18.2, ΔG_{ATP} is also proportional to PCr level over much of the ATP buffering zone. Thus, the observed near-linear relationship between steady-state PCr and $\dot{Q}O_2$ that has been observed in rat (117), cat (99), and human (20) muscles during moderate stimulation or exercise is consistent with the NET analysis of respiration. Furthermore, this coincidence of quasi-linear relationships between PCr vs. ΔG_{ATP} and ΔG_{ATP} vs. $\dot{Q}O_2$ nicely explains the exponential nature of the observed PCr changes in the low-rate domain. If decreasing PCr linearly activates high-energy phosphate synthesis, and if ATP hydrolysis is independently stepped between constant rates, $\dot{Q}$, by muscle stimulation, then

$$d[PCr]/dt = k \cdot [PCr] - \dot{Q} \quad (10)$$

that is, a simple first-order system. Further analysis (117) shows that the rate constant k ($=1/\tau$, where τ is the observed time constant of PCr changes during the approach to a steady state) should be proportional to mitochondrial capacity (i.e, to the lumped coefficient, L_p, of the NET analysis), and inversely proportional to the total creatine content. To a good approximation, both relationships hold in rat fast muscle (see Figs. 18.6*C* and *D*). Finally, as required by this linear approximation, the time course of changes in muscle $\dot{Q}O_2$ is probably comparable to that of changes in PCr (8, 28, 51, 110, 114).

Experimental Tests of Control Models

Observation of a quasi-linear relationship between PCr or ΔG_{ATP} and $\dot{Q}O_2$ does not by itself favor the NET model over the ADP model. As pointed out by Connett (26), the changes in high-energy phosphates predicted by the two models during moderate steady-state stimulation are experimentally almost indistinquishable. Although the ADP control model does predict slightly different kinetics during the approach to steady state, the difference is small, and depends on the assumed K_m for ADP (51). The solution to this experimental dilemma may lie in the point made at the start of this chapter. In studies of intact muscle, we typically control only the ATPase rate. The metabolites are the dependent variables, and they all change in concert during stimulation. To experimentally distinguish these models of respiratory control, we need to change metabolite levels independently of ATPase rate. Recall that the state of the high-energy phosphate system depends on the TAN and total creatine pools, and on intracellular pH. To some degree, each of these variables can be independently manipulated in intact muscle. However, in each case, the interpretation of the experiments is complicated by additional and sometimes surprising effects.

Depletion of up to 90% of the total creatine content of muscle can be induced by chronically feeding animals slowly metabolized creatine analogs such as β-guanidinopropionate (βGPA). However, the creatine depletion occurs over several weeks (120, 165), and is accompanied by other changes, including accumulation of phosphorylated analog (βGPAP), decreased TAN, increased mitochondrial content (164), and a variable shift toward slower myosin isoforms (127, 175). Remarkably similar enzyme adaptations occur in muscles of transgenic mice in which muscle expression of MM creatine kinase is eliminated (186). These adaptations provide strong evidence for a link between energetic parameters and muscle gene expression (see Chapter 25).

Despite the chronic adaptations, study of the time course of high-energy phosphate recovery in βGPAP-loaded muscles after prolonged low-rate stimulation provided evidence against simple ADP control of respiration (118). During moderate stimulation, the phosphorylated analog was partially hydrolyzed. Because the resynthesis of βGPAP is very slow, extra Pi was available during recovery compared to at rest, before stimulation. The result was that PCr recovered to higher levels than before stimulation. This result is consistent with the NET, but not the simple ADP control model, insofar as it demonstrates sensitivity of recovery metabolism to cytoplasmic Pi levels.

The TAN content of rat fast muscle can be partially depleted by high-rate stimulation, followed by inhibition of IMP reamination during recovery (48). After this manipulation, the calculated [ADP] in resting muscles with depleted TAN was half of that in control muscles, while ΔG_{ATP} was the same in both groups. During subsequent low-rate stimulation, calculated [ADP] in TAN-depleted muscles barely rose above the resting [ADP] in control muscles, despite similar force generation. Again, however, the results were complicated by another surprising effect of TAN depletion: the apparent ATP cost of isometric contractions was decreased.

Acidosis can be easily induced in isolated muscles by perfusion or superperfusion with hypercapnic media. Many such experiments have been performed in order to examine the effect of acidosis on force (46), but few studies have examined the effect of acidosis on respiratory control. Nioka et al (132) recently found that the relationship between calculated [ADP] and steady-state tension–time integral was not altered by hypercapnia in rabbit mixed muscle in situ. In contrast, a recent study in our laboratory (65) of the effect of hypercapnia on oxygen consumption in perfused cat soleus muscle was not at all consistent with respiratory control by [ADP]. First, we found that hypercapnia, which decreased intracellular pH from 7.1 to 6.5, had no effect on resting $\dot{Q}O_2$, but reduced peak steady-state $\dot{Q}O_2$ during twitch stimulation by over half (Fig. 18.9*A*). PCr content at rest was unchanged by hypercapnia (Fig. 18.9*B*), but calculated [ADP] was much less than during normocapnic perfusion (Fig. 18.9*C*). As expected from the decrease in peak $\dot{Q}O_2$, steady-state PCr decreased more during hypercapnic compared to normocapnic stimulation at similar absolute $\dot{Q}O_2$. However, calculated [ADP] during hypercapnic stimulation barely exceeded [ADP] in normocapnic muscles at rest.

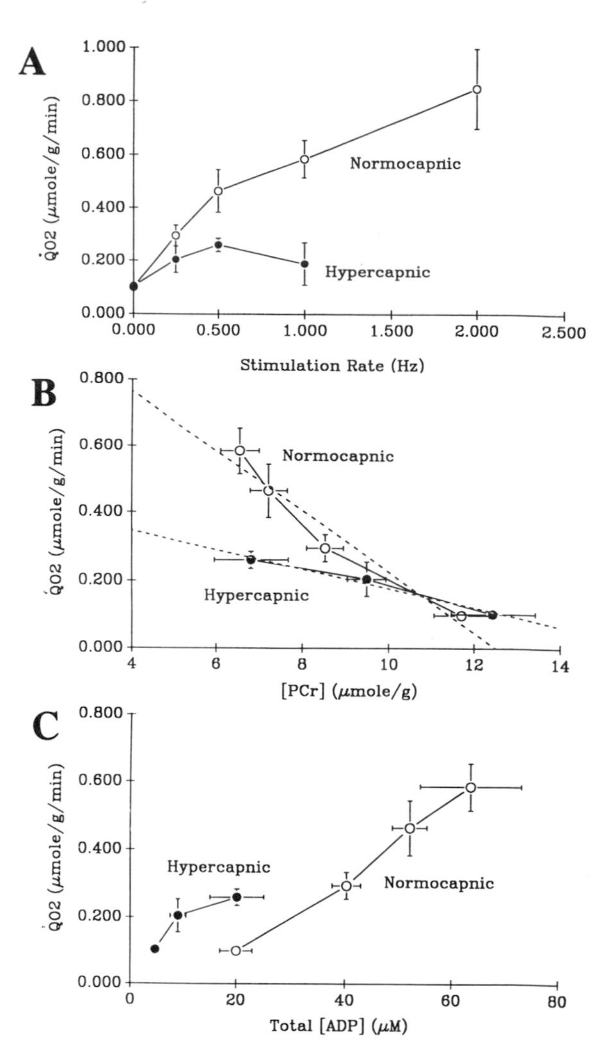

FIG. 18.9. *A*, Steady-state $\dot{Q}O_2$ as a function of stimulation rate in cat soleus muscles perfused at 37°C with red cell suspension in Krebs-Hensleit solution equilibrated with 5% CO_2 (perfusate pH 7.4) and 70% CO_2 (perfusate pH 6.7). Intracellular pH was 7.1 and 6.5, respectively. [From Harkema and Meyer (65).] *B*, Relationship between steady-state PCr and $\dot{Q}O_2$ in cat soleus muscles during normocapnic and hypercapnic perfusion. *C*, Relationship between steady-state calculated [ADP] and $\dot{Q}O_2$.

Taken together, the results of these experiments in which phosphate metabolites were manipulated independently of stimulation are not consistent with simple control of muscle respiration by cytoplasmic [ADP]. The results are generally consistent with the NET analysis. Unlike the simple ADP model, the

NET analysis also accounts for the effect of NADH changes on respiratory rate. Many studies of isolated mitochondria show that respiratory rate depends on intramitochondrial [NADH]/[NAD] ratio, as well as on extramitochondrial nucleotides and phosphate (e.g., 93). Furthermore, several mitochondrial dehydrogenases are activated by calcium (62, 63, 113, 115). Therefore, it is plausible that increased intramitochondrial [NADH]/[NAD] occurs during exercise, and that this change is important for increasing respiratory rate. Testing this idea requires estimation of mitochondrial [NADH]/[NAD] ratio in intact muscle. Unfortunately, the literature in this area is not very enlightening.

Estimates of mitochondrial [NADH]/[NAD] ratio in skeletal muscle have been made by NADH fluorescence, by direct assay of NADH and NAD in extracts, and by calculation of [NADH]/[NAD] from the assumed equilibrium of the mitochondrial glutamate dehydrogenase reaction. Each of these methods has been effectively criticized by proponents of the others (e.g., 58, 86, 89), with the result that there is no consensus on the direction or extent of changes in mitochondrial [NADH]/[NAD] in muscle during exercise. In general, studies in the high-rate domain report increased [NADH]/[NAD] (161, 180, 192), while studies at low rates report decreased [NADH]/[NAD] (85, 146, 192, 201). However, this generalization is complicated by the fact that most studies in the low-rate domain were done by fluorescence, while most studies in the high-rate domain were by the biopsy methods, and these methods have different flaws. It is not even clear what fraction of the total nicotinamide dinucleotide measured in skeletal muscle is cytoplasmic, with estimates ranging from 1% to 40% (95, 133, 156). The cytoplasmic [NADH]/[NAD] ratio, which can be reliably estimated from the lactate/pyruvate ratio, dramatically increases at high workloads (57, 88), and this change may contribute to both the fluorescence and direct assay results. Furthermore, because the total muscle content of dinucleotides is low, a significant fraction may be bound to proteins in vivo. In principle, the glutamate dehydrogenase method avoids these compartmentation and binding problems, inasmuch as the enzyme is confined to the mitochondrial matrix, and the reaction equilibrium depends only on free metabolite activities. Unfortunately, skeletal muscle mitochondria contain relatively little glutamate dehydrogenase activity, and there is no proof that the reaction is near equilibrium during exercise (86, 89).

The NET analysis of respiration does raise a potential problem. In muscles with high mitochondrial content, the mitochondrial ATP synthase reaction could run close to equilibrium at rest (84), since in these muscles the resting rate of oxygen consumption is a small fraction of the maximum rate. Therefore, during hypoxia, when the mitochondrial proton gradient must fall, the synthase could act as an ATPase. In fact, this does not occur in heart muscle (149) because of an F1-ATPase inhibitor protein, IF1 (66). It has been proposed that IF1 plays a crucial role in regulation of respiration in the heart (66). However, there is as yet no evidence that IF1 is involved in respiratory control in well-oxygenated skeletal muscle.

In summary, respiratory control in skeletal muscle contracting in the low-rate domain can be accounted for by a NET analysis, in which the fall in cytoplasmic ΔG_{ATP} is the main drive for increased oxidative rate. Additional respiratory drive can be provided by increased redox potential, mediated by calcium activation of mitochondrial dehydrogenase reactions. In heart muscle, the latter changes may dominate, inasmuch as two- to fourfold changes in respiratory rate can occur with no change in cytoplasmic high-energy phosphates (6). In intact skeletal muscle, the quantitative role of calcium and redox changes is uncertain.

The Importance of Muscle Aerobic Capacity

As noted above, the transition between the low- and high-rate domains is determined in part by the muscle's "aerobic capacity." This term is commonly taken to mean the maximum possible $\dot{Q}O_2$ of a muscle, although the true maximum $\dot{Q}O_2$ is in fact hard to measure in intact muscle because of the heterogeneity problems mentioned above. Aerobic capacity can also be operationally defined by the L parameters of the NET analysis, or ignoring redox changes, by the slope of the relationship between $\dot{Q}O_2$ vs. ΔG_{ATP} or PCr. By either definition, What limits aerobic capacity? Obviously, respiratory rate can be diminished by limiting either oxygen or substrate availability. However, in well-perfused muscles, aerobic capacity appears to be determined largely by mitochondrial content, and in particular, by activity at sites I to II of the electron transport chain. This is nicely demonstrated by the study of McAllister and Terjung (112), in which peak $\dot{Q}O_2$ of perfused rat muscle was titrated downward by progressive inhibition of mitochondrial NADH–cytochrome c reductase with myxothiazol (Fig. 18.10).

It is important to note that higher muscle mitochondrial content or aerobic capacity enables higher steady-state $\dot{Q}O_2$ in intact muscles, even if the mitochondrial enzymes never approach their maximum

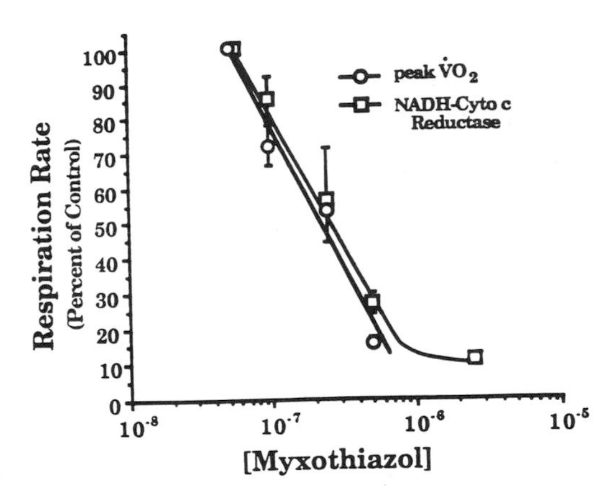

FIG. 18.10. Parallel dose-dependent effects of perfusion with myxothiazol on peak $\dot{Q}O_2$ and NADH–cytochrome reductase activity in rat hindlimb muscle. [From McAllister and Terjung (112).]

possible flux in vivo. This follows from the fact that if aerobic capacity is increased, less change in ΔG_{ATP} is required to drive oxidative phosphorylation (39). In intact muscles, large decreases in ΔG_{ATP} are associated with two related effects that effectively limit steady-state ATP turnover: lactic acidosis and fatigue. In addition to contributing to fatigue, intracellular acidosis may decrease maximum $\dot{Q}O_2$, both in intact muscle (Fig. 18.9*A*), and in isolated mitochondria (68). Thus, the maximum observed $\dot{Q}O_2$ in intact muscle may be less than predicted from in vitro measurements of mitochondrial enzyme activities (56).

This volume includes detailed chapters on the control of muscle glycogenolysis and on the metabolic bases of fatigue. Therefore, we will only briefly discuss these processes in the context of the scheme shown in Figure 18.1.

CONTROL OF GLYCOGENOLYSIS/GLYCOLYSIS IN MUSCLE

The Conventional View

Unlike respiration, glycolysis cannot be modeled as a first-order system with flux proportional to ΔG_{ATP}. This is demonstrated by the occurrence of oscillations in glycolytic flux even in relatively simple cell-free glycolytic systems (54). This higher order behavior arises from the combined feedforward and feedback regulatory properties of phosphofructokinase (PFK; see Fig. 18.11). As noted above, such nonlinear behavior further exacerbates the effect of muscle heterogeneity on studies of glycolysis in intact muscle. Nonetheless, even a semiquantitative consideration of the events in intact muscle during

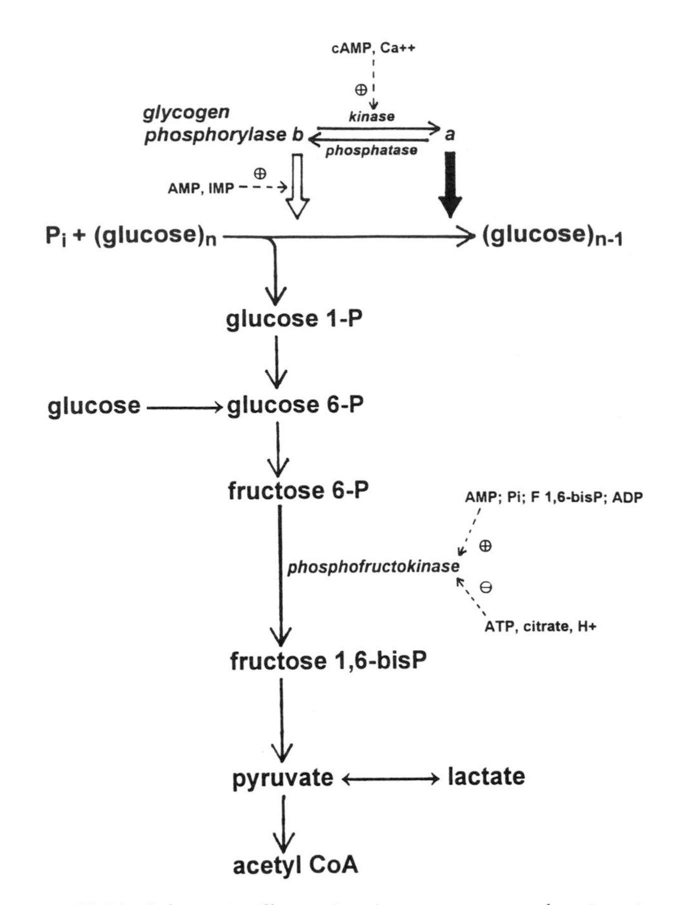

FIG. 18.11. Schematic illustrating important control points in muscle glycogenolysis and glycolysis.

high-rate stimulation shows that the conventional view of glycogenolytic/glycolytic control is inadequate (155).

Glycogen breakdown starts with the reaction catalyzed by glycogen phosphorylase (GP):

$$(\text{glucose})_n + \text{Pi} \rightarrow \text{glucose-1-P} + (\text{glucose})_{(n-1)}$$

The enzyme is covalently activated by phosphorylase kinase, which is in turn activated by calcium, as well as by the well-known cyclic AMP cascade (18, 22, 172). The phosphorylated, *a*, form of GP is active at low [AMP], while the unphosphorylated, *b*, form requires allosteric activation by AMP or IMP [in vitro K_a 50–100 μM and 1–5 mM, respectively (4, 108, 129)]. In addition, the reaction may be limited by Pi at rest, inasmuch as the K_m of GP for Pi (7–26 mM) is above the Pi level at rest (22, 100). The PFK step is also activated by AMP and Pi, as well as by fructose bisphosphates, ADP, and ammonium ion, and inhibited by ATP, citrate, and low pH (172, 181). Thus, the conventional view of glycogenolytic/glycolytic control in muscle during high-rate stimulation is that calcium and Pi activate GP, and changes in adenine nucleotides, phosphate, and possibly fructose bisphosphate activate PFK. The whole process is presumably limited by decreased pH inhibiting PFK.

Problems with the Conventional View

There are at least three problems with the conventional view. First, the activity of muscle PFK in vitro is almost completely suppressed at pH below 6.5 (181). However, the intracellular pH of mammalian fast muscles can fall to below pH 6.2 during high-rate stimulation (121), and this acidosis is due to lactic acid production. Second, the conversion of GP *b* to *a* that occurs at the onset of stimulation is apparently reversed after 1–2 min, but glycogenolysis can continue (25). Conversely, in resting muscle, the rate of glycogenolysis is still low after epinephrine stimulation, which results in nearly complete conversion of GP to the *a* form (141). Third, glycogenolysis and net lactic acid production decrease immediately after a bout of high-rate stimulation, even though PCr, Pi, ATP, pH, and calculated ADP and AMP are similar to that immediately before the end of the stimulation. Thus, in mammalian muscles, PCr recovery requires oxidative phosphorylation, even in fast glycolytic fibers in which glycolytic capacity vastly exceeds aerobic capacity (67, 155, 157). The same problem occurs in explaining the regulation of AMP deaminase; that is, net deamination virtually stops with contraction, but calculated [AMP] and [ADP] must remain high for some time afterward (157). Taken together, these observations show that the rates of glycogenolysis, lactate production, and AMP deamination are all tightly coupled to contractile ATP hydrolysis. This tight coupling cannot easily be explained from the known in vitro behavior of the enzymes involved.

There are four classes of explanation for this dilemma. First, it may be that the reactions catalyzed by creatine kinase and myokinase are not near equilibrium during contraction, and therefore, that [ADP] and [AMP] levels rise to much higher levels than calculated. Second, it may be that intracellular diffusion is restricted, such that local concentrations of Pi, AMP, and other metabolites around the enzymes in vivo are much different than calculated from the global measurements. Third, it may be that the kinetic properties of the enzymes in vivo are different than in vitro (e.g., due to binding or other interactions with neighboring proteins). Fourth, there may be other regulatory mechanisms (e.g., calcium-calmodulin–mediated events) that remain to be discovered. Obviously, the last of these explanations is difficult to discuss.

Reaction Disequilibria and Metabolite Diffusion

We find little evidence in favor of the first two explanations. First, the steady-state unidirectional flux through the creatine kinase reaction has been measured by NMR spin-transfer methods (123). In rat fast-twitch muscle, the flux at rest is 7.5 $\mu mol \cdot g^{-1} \cdot s^{-1}$ (120). This is over tenfold higher than the ATP turnover rate that can be maintained in the steady state during low-rate twitch stimulation [~ 0.4 $\mu mol \cdot g^{-1} \cdot s^{-1}$, assuming mitochondrial ATP/O_2 = 6 (75)]. Therefore, there is little doubt that the creatine kinase reaction is, on average, near equilibrium in the low-rate domain. On the other hand, during a short isometric tetanus, the ATP hydrolysis rate in rat fast muscle may be as high as 10 $\mu mol \cdot g^{-1} \cdot s^{-1}$ (49, 75). Therefore, the creatine kinase reaction must be somewhat displaced from equilibrium during a tetanus.

It is possible to model the displacement of the creatine kinase reaction from equilibrium during contractions, since the mechanism of the reaction (130) and the in vivo equilibrium fluxes at rest are known. Such modeling assumes that the cytoplasm is a uniform, well-mixed solution, and requires estimates of substrate-binding constants that may not be precisely correct. Nonetheless, the results are instructive. Figure 18.12 shows the estimated changes in [ADP] during idealized twitch and tetanic contractions of rat fast muscle at high and low PCr level. Also shown is the [ADP], assuming complete equilibrium of the creatine kinase reaction. During a 100 ms tetanus (mean ATPase rate 15 mM/s), [ADP] rises two- to threefold above the equilibrium value. When PCr is low, the [ADP] may be transiently as high as 760 μM, vs. 490 μM assuming complete equilibrium. However, this displacement from equilibrium is rapidly reversed after the contraction. The displacement from equilibrium is less extensive during a twitch because of the shorter duration (30 ms), and relatively lower mean ATPase rate (10 mM/s).

Can these transient increases in [ADP] during contractions explain the high glycolytic and AMP deaminase flux during, but not immediately after, repetitive stimulation? We think not, for the following reason. According to the above calculations, the ADP transients must be higher during repetitive tetanic compared to twitch stimulation. For example, we ran the calculation depicted in Figure 18.12 over a 20 s interval during tetanic stimulation (100 ms duration at 1 Hz), and during twitch stimulation at a rate (5 Hz) that required the same total net phosphagen hydrolysis (30 mM). The peak ADP during tetani was always 15–200 μM higher than that during twitches. The mean difference between [ADP]

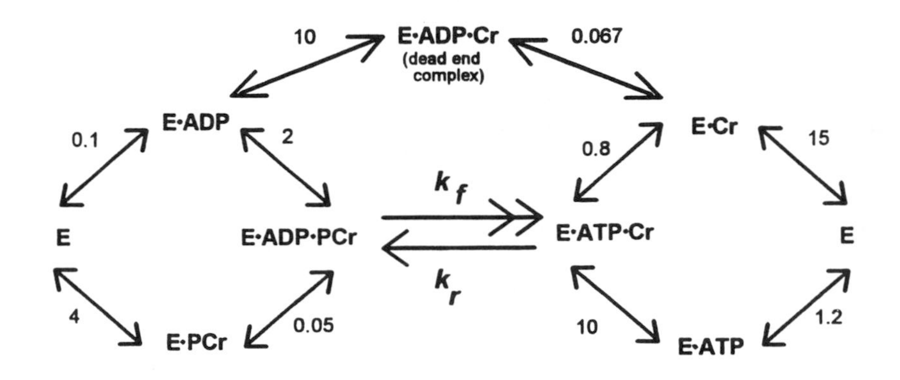

$$k_{eq} = \frac{[ATP]\,[Cr]}{[ADP]\,[PCr]} = 166 \qquad k_f \cdot E_{total} = 0.21\ M/s$$

$$dADP/dt = [E\ ATP\ Cr]\ k_r - [E\ ADP\ PCr]\ k_f + Q$$

$$dATP/dt = [E\ ADP\ PCr]\ k_r - [E\ ATP\ Cr]\ k_f - Q$$

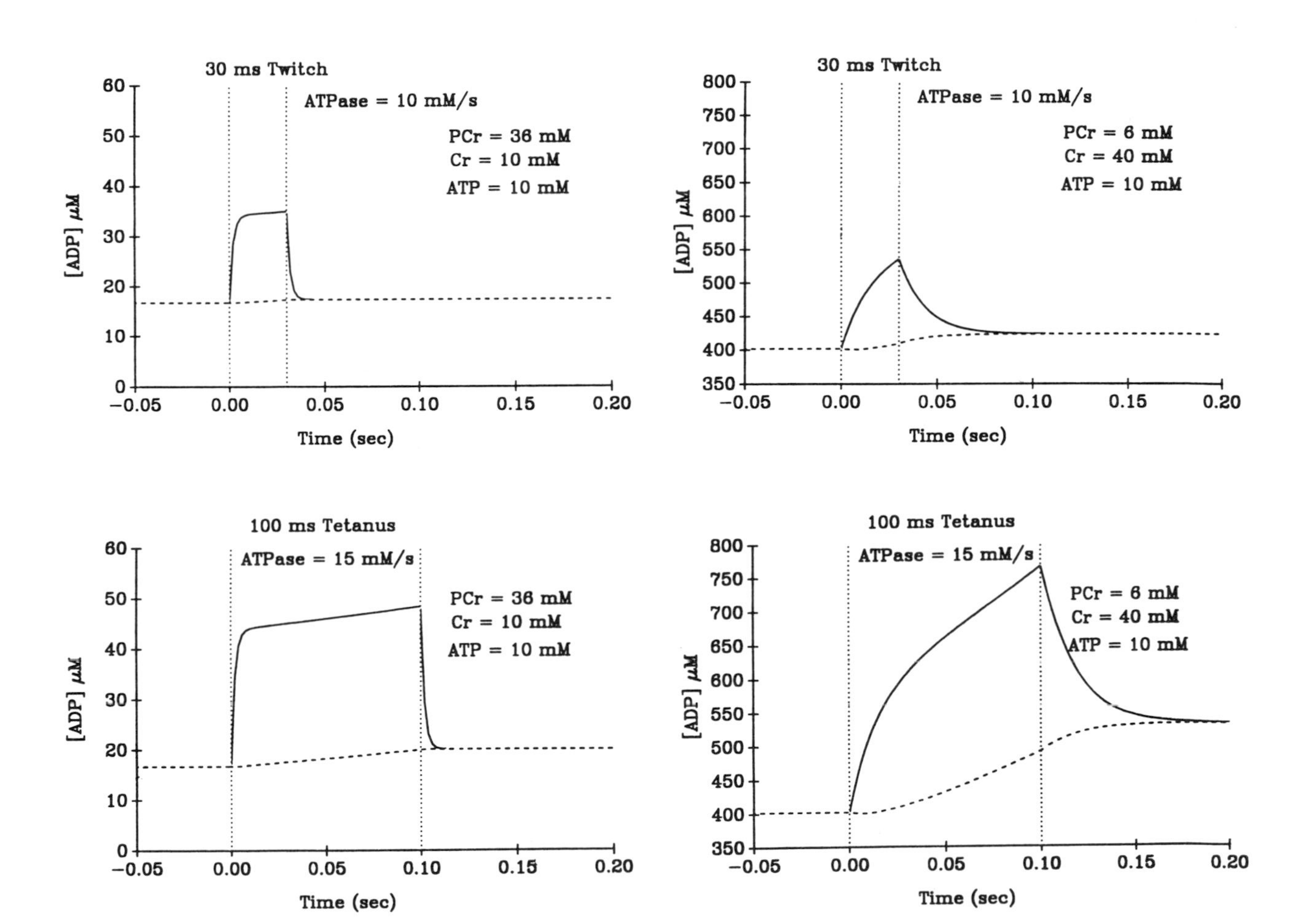

FIG. 18.12. *Top*, Kinetic model for the creatine kinase reaction (130). The assumed equilibrium constants for the depicted substrate binding reactions are given in mM. The rate constants k_f and k_r were selected so that model yielded equilibrium unidirectional fluxes of 10 mM/s for [ATP] = 10 mM, [PCr] = 36 mM, and [Cr] = 10 mM. pH was held constant at 7. ADP changes during tetani and twitches were computed by Euler's method (dt = 10 μs) assuming step changes in ATPase rate, Q. *Bottom*, Calculated [ADP] during tetanic and twitch contractions using the above model with high and low initial [PCr]/[Cr] ratio. Total phosphagen use was assumed to be 1.5 mM and 0.3 mM for single tetani and twitches, respectively (49, 75). *Solid lines* are [ADP] calculated from the kinetic model, and *dashed lines* are [ADP] calculated from the same PCr levels assuming instantaneous equilibrium of the net creatine kinase reaction.

and the equilibrium [ADP], averaged over all the contraction periods, was twofold higher for tetanic compared to twitch stimulation. Therefore, if transient increases in [ADP] due to disequilibrium of the CK reaction are responsible for activation of glycolysis and AMP deamination, then these processes ought to occur to a greater extent during tetanic compared to twitch stimulation. In fact, the extent and time course of lactic acid accumulation and AMP deamination in rat fast muscle are similar during both high-rate twitch [5 Hz (38, 126)] and tetanic (100 ms, 1 Hz (48, 124)] stimulation. Of course, the above model ignores the acidosis and fatigue that occur in real muscles during such intense stimulation. However, inasmuch as these changes also occur to a similar extent during twitch and tetanic contractions, incorporating these changes in the model should not change the overall conclusion.

Transient disequilibrium of the myokinase reaction is more difficult to model, because no measurement of the in vivo flux is available. However, if myokinase undergoes transient disequilibrium similar to creatine kinase, then the rise in AMP during contractions might well be smaller than predicted from the equilibrium equation, despite the transiently higher [ADP]. Therefore, it is hard to see how this solves the overall problem.

The second class of explanation for high glycolytic and deamination rates is that key regulating metabolites are compartmentalized around the myofibrils, and hence rise to locally higher levels then calculated, even if local equilibrium is maintained. Direct measurements of the diffusion coefficients of Pi, PCr, and ATP are not consistent with this idea. The diffusion coefficients of these metabolites in muscle are roughly 1×10^{-6} cm^2/s (125). Thus, the root-mean-square diffusion path length ($d = \sqrt{6Dt}$) in a 100 ms interval is about 8 μm, or four times greater than the diameter of a myofibril. It has been calculated that net diffusion of these metabolites even over the dimensions of a large myofibrillar bundle (20 μm diameter) requires only a trivial gradient (<3%) relative to the total concentrations of these metabolites (125, 175).

Of course, ADP and AMP are present in much lower amounts than PCr, ATP, and Pi, and so it might be argued that the same absolute gradient would be significant for these metabolites. However, because changes in ADP and AMP are coupled to changes in PCr by the creatine kinase and myokinase reactions, direct diffusion of ADP and AMP over distances greater than a micron or so is not necessary. Assuming that creatine kinase and myokinase activities are available near every site where changes in ADP and AMP might occur, these changes must be rapidly transmitted throughout the cell by diffusion of PCr and Cr (125, 175). Thus, the creatine kinase system functions as a "spatial buffer," as well as a "temporal buffer" of changes in adenine nucleotide levels. The result is that very little ΔG_{ATP} is lost in driving the diffusive flux of nucleotides between various sites inside the cell (Fig. 18.13).

It has been argued that direct coupling between creatine kinase and various other enzymes (e.g., mitochondrial nucleotide translocase, myosin, Na^+/K^+-ATPase) is critical to intracellular energy transport (82, 145, 188–190). Certainly, substrate channeling between coupled enzymes can significantly alter the kinetic properties of the net reaction compared to that when the enzymes are in dilute solution (171).

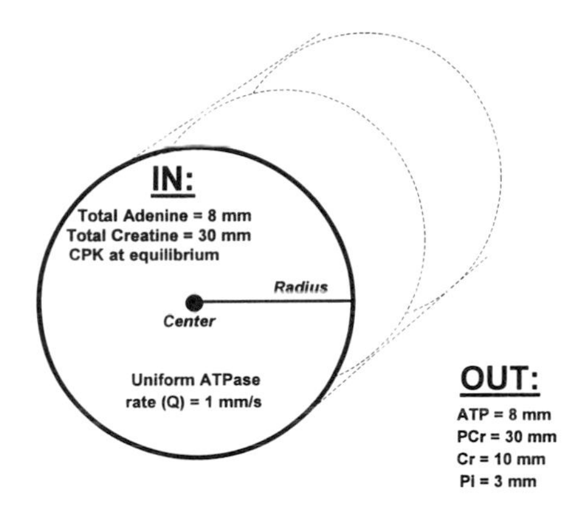

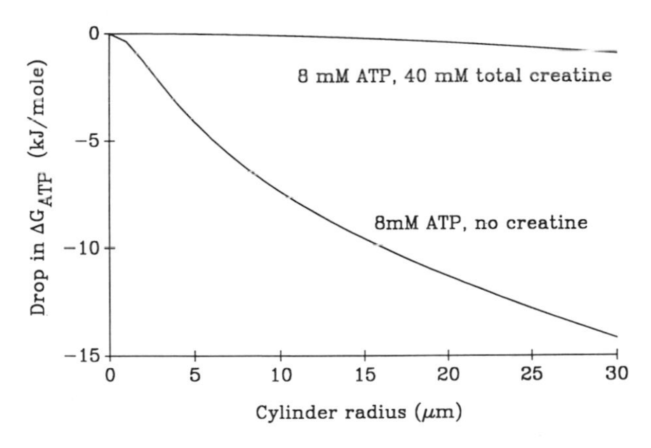

FIG. 18.13. Calculated drop in ΔG_{ATP} at the center of a cylinder in which ATP is consumed at a constant, steady-state rate (Q = 1 mM/s), as a function of cylinder radius, and in the presence or absence of the creatine kinase reaction at equilibrium ($K_{eq} = 1.66 \times 10^9$ M^{-1}, pH 7). Metabolites outside the cylinder were assumed to be constant at the indicated levels. Diffusion coefficients of Pi, adenine nucleotides, and PCr and creatine were assumed to be 3×10^{-6}, 1×10^{-6}, and 2×10^{-6} cm^2/s, respectively (125). Even over the dimensions of a large cyclindrical cell (radius 30 μm) the creatine kinase reaction virtually abolishes any radial gradient in ΔG_{ATP}.

However, although substrate channeling can provide a mechanism for faster approach toward equilibrium, it cannot alter the final equilibrium of the net reaction. Therefore, if substrate channeling between creatine kinase and other reactions does occur, this does not alter, and in fact reinforces, the overall conclusion drawn by us earlier (125): In the presence of the CK system, direct diffusion of high-energy phosphates is almost entirely due to PCr and creatine. The experimental evidence for substrate channeling between CK and other enzymes in intact muscle or organelles is not very convincing, because most tracer studies of the phenomenon fail to consider the facilitating effect of the CK reaction on nucleotide diffusion (125). In any case, coupling of myosin to CK is clearly not required for muscle contraction, because muscles of transgenic mice that express no detectable MM isozyme contract normally during moderate stimulation (186). Further studies of AMP deamination and lactate production in muscles of these mice should be interesting.

Enzyme Organization

The third possible explanation for tight coupling between contractile ATP hydrolysis and lactate and IMP production is that the intracellular binding or organization of the enzymes alters their regulatory properties compared to those observed in dilute solution in vitro. There is evidence for this, particularly in the case of glycogenolysis (42, 153, 171). GP, phosphorylase kinase, and phosphatase 1 (which dephosphorylates GP) are all associated together with glycogen particles in vivo. Therefore, the effective local concentrations *of the enzymes* are much higher than their average cellular concentrations. Under these conditions, the sensitivity of GP activation to changes in kinase or phosphatase activity is manyfold higher than predicted from study of dilute solutions (42). Conversely, the sensitivity of GP-*b* to AMP activation is less when the enzyme is complexed with synthetic glycogen particles (42). In addition, there is evidence that GP also binds to the SR Ca^{2+}-ATPase, suggesting a link between glycogenolysis and calcium sequestration (33). Together, these observations suggest relatively greater dependence of glycogenolysis rate on calcium than on nucleotide changes, which is consistent with the results in intact muscle.

There is also evidence that binding of AMP deaminase to myofibrils occurs coincident with IMP accumulation in rat muscle (151). In this case, the molecular details are even less clear. Binding apparently decreases the K_m for AMP (152), but there is no evidence to suggest how binding might be linked to contractile ATP hydrolysis. Nonetheless, the observation is intriguing, insofar as it highlights the possible importance of enzyme organization in control of nucleotide depletion in vivo.

In sum, the rates of both glycogenolysis and AMP deamination in muscle working in the high-rate domain are tightly coupled to contractile ATP hydrolysis. The precise mechanism by which this coupling is achieved is not known in any detail, but all indications are that the key link is calcium. Presumably, changes in nucleotides and phosphate are necessary, but not sufficient, for activation of these processes. Further studies of the time course of events in homogeneous muscles during intense stimulation, and of experimental interventions that alter the amount or organization of the enzymes in vivo, are clearly needed.

CONTROL OF FORCE GENERATION

The idea that muscle fatigue is the result of metabolic changes has been prevalent for at least 150 years. Fitts recently provided a comprehensive review of this literature (46; see also Chapter 26), so we need not repeat any of the details here. We will, however, reiterate a few simple points in the context of Figure 18.1.

First, it is clear that fatigue, defined here as the decrease in peak force during repetitive high-domain stimulation, cannot be explained by lack of ATP per se, since even during the most extreme fatigue, muscle ATP content is still at least 50-fold above the K_m of myosin and other ATPases. Fatigue also cannot be due simply to product inhibition of myosin ATPase by ADP and Pi, because when caffeine or other agents that enhance calcium release are administered, contracture and additional ATP hydrolysis occur (46). Therefore, fatigue and the associated decrease in ATP hydrolysis are regulated responses, the effect of which is to preserve cytoplasmic ΔG_{ATP}. This makes teleological sense, because the rate of calcium sequestration decreases when cytoplasmic ΔG_{ATP} falls (35). Failure to sequester calcium after a contraction would lead to continued ATP hydrolysis, and ultimately to rigor and cell death.

Second, there is overwhelming evidence that decreased force during stimulation or exercise in the high-rate domain correlates with changes in the phosphagen pool and pH (46). Unfortunately, just as for studies of the control of ATP synthesis, these correlations provide little insight into the precise mechanism for the link between fatigue and metabolism, because during repetitive stimulation of intact muscle, all the metabolites are changing together. For example, many studies of both skinned fibers and intact muscle suggested that intracellular acidosis could explain fatigue by a direct effect on the contractile apparatus. However, recent studies of intact mammalian muscles found little direct effect of hypercapnic acidosis on peak tetanic force (1, 119), despite the good correlation between pH and force during repetitive stimulation in normocapnic conditions (Fig. 18.14). In any case, acidosis is clearly not necessary for fatigue, because subjects with glycogen phosphorylase deficiency (McArdle's disease), who do not develop lactic acidosis during exercise, fatigue rapidly during intense exercise (105).

Third, there is good evidence that calcium release is decreased after stimulation in the high-rate domain, and that this decrease can explain much of the decrease in force (5, 194). Considering this, along with the above two points, it seems inescapable that there must exist a mechanism by which decreased ΔG_{ATP}, or something coupled to it, results in decreased calcium release. Such a mechanism could also explain the ability of mammalian slow-twitch muscle to quickly down-regulate steady-state force under conditions when ATP synthesis is compromised (70). Unfortunately, the nature of this metabolic link is not known.

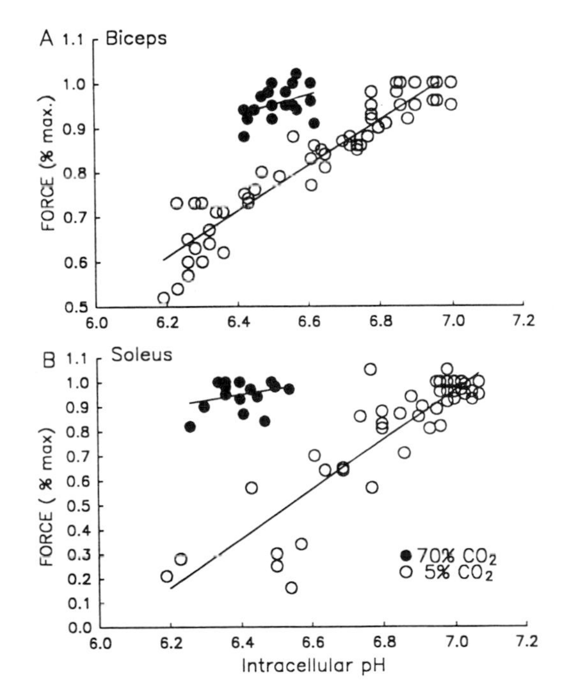

FIG. 18.14. Relationship between intracellular pH and peak tetanic force during repetitive tetanic stimulation (*open circles*) and during perfusion with hypercapnic media (*closed*), in cat biceps brachii (*top*) and soleus (*bottom*) muscles. [From Adams et al. (1).]

The molecular details of excitation-contraction coupling and calcium release are just beginning to be understood (143). There are two calcium channel proteins in the triad of muscle fibers: the SR calcium release channel, or ryanodine receptor protein, and the T-tubule voltage-sensitive calcium channel, or dihydropyridine (DHP) sensitive channel (Fig. 18.4). The SR channel is itself activated by calcium, and in heart muscle, calcium release from the channel is primarily triggered by influx of extracellular calcium. In skeletal muscle, the exact mechanism of signal transmission between these two channels is not yet clear, but it does depend on their intimate proximity to each other. Over a dozen endogenous modulators have been found that act on the SR release channel, including ATP (136), phosphate (50), IP3, cyclic AMP, H^+, and a newly discovered metabolite, cyclic-ADP-ribose (53). It does not appear that the sensitivity of the channel to ATP can explain decreased calcium release during fatigue, because ATP remains above the 1 mM needed to activate the channel (167). Conversely, although the probability of channel opening is optimal at pH 7.1 (109, 203), in intact mammalian muscle acidosis has little direct effect on peak tetanic force (Fig. 18.14). On the other hand, acidosis does decrease peak twitch force (1), which should be more sensitive to the initial rate of calcium release. Clearly, we need more studies of the effects of metabolites on these calcium channels, along with quantitative comparison to results from intact muscle.

SUMMARY AND FUTURE DIRECTIONS

We have described a simple view of the relation between metabolic changes and the regulatory events in muscle cells during exercise. The key players in this simple view are calcium and the adenine nucleotide pool, including its links to PCr, Pi, and pH. Calcium provides the initial trigger for force development and ATP hydrolysis, and contributes to the activation of glycogenolysis and possibly oxidative phosphorylation. Changes in the phosphagen pool provide the main stimulus for increased oxidative phosphorylation, and are necessary, but not sufficient, for full activation of glycolytic ATP synthesis during more intense exercise. Finally, changes in the phosphagen pool, or other metabolites linked to it, provide feedback modulation of calcium release, and hence ATP hydrolysis.

Of course, this simple view raises as many questions as it answers. For example, What is the exact mechanistic link between phosphagen changes and fatigue, or between ATP hydrolysis and AMP deamination? How crucial is the intracellular organization of "soluble" metabolic enzymes to their function? We believe that studies of intact muscle will be required to answer such questions. However, we also believe that the field cannot be advanced much further by simple correlative measurements of metabolite changes during stimulation or exercise. Fortunately, recent advances in molecular biology will enable experimental manipulations of intact muscle that could only be imagined before now (182). The MM creatine kinase–deficient mouse referred to above is one example of the power of these techniques (186). Another example is provided by the recent work of Ren et al. (142), who increased glucose transporter expression in mouse skeletal muscle, and thus clearly demonstrated that glucose transport normally limits basal glucose consumption. In the near future, it may be possible to replace specific native enzymes with engineered mutants, in order to study the effects on metabolism. For example, if muscle glycogen phosphorylase were replaced by mutants that could not be phosphorylated, or which did not bind AMP, what would be the effects on glycogenolysis rate during intense stimulation? Someday it will be feasible to perform these and many similar experiments.

The authors' work has been supported by National Institutes of Health grant AR38972.

REFERENCES

1. Adams, G. R., M. J. Fisher, and R. A. Meyer. Hypercapnic acidosis and increased $H_2PO_4^-$ concentration do not decrease force in cat skeletal muscle. *Am. J. Physiol.* 260 (*Cell Physiol.* 29): C805–C812, 1991.
2. Adams, G. R., J. M. Foley, and R. A. Meyer. Muscle buffer capacity estimated from pH changes during rest-to-work transitions. *J. Appl. Physiol.* 69: 968–972, 1990.
3. Alberty, R. A. Effect of pH and metal ion concentration on the equilibrium hydrolysis of adenosine triphosphate to adenosine diphosphate. *J. Biol. Chem.* 243: 1337–1343, 1968.
4. Aragon, J. J., K. Tornheim, and J. M. Lowenstein. On the possible role of IMP in the regulation of phosphorylase activity in skeletal muscle. *FEBS Lett.* 117: K56–K64, 1980.
5. Baker, A. J., M. C. Longuemare, R. Brandes, and M. W. Weiner. Intracellular tetanic calcium signals are reduced in fatigue of whole skeletal muscle. *Am. J. Physiol.* 264 (*Cell Physiol.* 33): C577–C582, 1993.
6. Balaban, R. S. Regulation of oxidative phosphorylation in the mammalian cell. *Am. J. Physiol.* 258 (*Cell Physiol.* 27): C377–C389, 1990.
7. Bárány, M. ATPase activity of myosin correlated with speed of shortening. *J. Gen. Physiol.* 50: 197–216, 1967.
8. Barstow, T. J., S. Buchthal, S. Zanconato, and D. M. Cooper. Muscle energetics and pulmonary O2 uptake kinetics during moderate exercise. *J. Appl. Physiol.* 77: 1742–1749, 1994.
9. Benders, A., T. van Kuppevelt, A. Oseterhof, R. A. Wevers, and J. H. Veerkamp. Adenosine triphosphatases during maturation of cultured human skeletal muscle cells and in adult human muscle. *Biochim. Biophys. Acta* 1112: 89–98, 1992.
10. Blinks, J. R., R. Rudel, and S. R. Taylor. Calcium transients in isolated amphibian skeletal muscle fibres: detection with aequorin. *J. Physiol. (Lond.)* 277: 291–323, 1978.
11. Blum, H., M. D. Schnall, B. Chance, and G. P. Buzby. Intracellular sodium flux and high-energy phosphorus metabolites in ischemic skeletal muscle. *Am. J. Physiol.* 255 (*Cell Physiol.* 24): C377–C384, 1988.
12. Bockman, E. L., and J. E. McKenzie. Tissue adenosine content in active soleus and gracilis muscles of cats. *Am. J. Physiol.* 244 (*Heart Circ. Physiol.* 13): H555–H559, 1983.
13. Boska, M. ATP production rate as a function of force level in the human gastrocnemius/soleus using 31P MRS. *Magn. Reson. Med.* 32: 1–10, 1994.
14. Brand, M. D., M. E. Harper, and H. C. Taylor. Control of the effective P/O ratio of oxidative phosphorylation in liver mitochondria and hepatocytes. *Biochem. J.* 291: 739–748, 1993.
15. Briggs, F. N., J. L. Poland, and R. J. Solaro. Relative capabilities of sarcoplasmic reticulum in fast and slow mammalian skeletal muscles. *J. Physiol. (Lond.)* 266: 587–594, 1977.
16. Brooks, G. A. Anaerobic threshold: review of the concept and directions for future research. *Med. Sci. Sports Exerc.* 17: 22–34, 1985.
17. Brooks, G. A., and J. Mercier. Balance of carbohydrate and lipid utilization during exercise: the "crossover" concept. *J. Appl. Physiol.* 76: 2253–2261, 1994.
18. Brown, D. H., and C. F. Cori. Animal and plant phosphorylases. In: *The Enzymes V*, edited by P. D. Boyer, H. Lardy, and K. Myrback. New York: Academic Press, 1961, p. 207–228, 1961.
19. Caplan, S. R., and A. Essig. *Bioenergetics and Linear Non-Equilibrium Thermodynamics: The Steady State.* Cambridge, MA: Harvard University Press, 1983.
20. Chance, B., J. S. Leigh, Jr., B. J. Clark, J. Maris, J. Kent, S. Nioka, and D. Smith. Control of oxidative metabolism and oxygen delivery in human skeletal muscle: a steady-state analysis of the work/energy cost transfer function. *Proc. Natl. Acad. Sci. U.S.A.* 82: 8384–8388, 1985.
21. Chance, B., and C. M. Williams. The respiratiory chain and oxidative phosphorylation. *Adv. Enzymol.* 17: 65–134, 1956.
22. Chasiotis, D. The regulation of glycogen phosphorylase and glycogen breakdown in human skeletal muscle. *Acta Physiol. Scand. Suppl.* 518: 1–68, 1983.
23. Chinet, A., T. Clausen, and L. Girardier. Microcalorimetric determination of energy expenditure due to active sodium-potassium transport in soleus muscle and brown adipose tissue of the rat. *J. Physiol. (Lond.)* 256: 43–61, 1977.
24. Close, R. Dynamic properties of mammalian skeletal muscle. *Ann. Rev. Physiol.* 52: 129–196, 1972.
25. Conlee, R. K., J. A. McLane, M. J. Rennie, W. W. Winder, and J. O. Holloszy. Reversal of phosphorylase activation in muscle despite continued contractile activity. *Am. J. Physiol.* 237 (*Regulatory Integrative Comp. Physiol.* 6): R291–R296, 1979.
26. Connett, R. J. Analysis of metabolic control: new insights using a scaled creatine kinase model. *Am. J. Physiol.* 254 (*Regulatory Integrative Comp. Physiol.* 23): R949–R959, 1988.

27. Connett, R. J., E. J. Gayeski, and C. R. Honig. Lactate accumulation in fully aerobic, working dog gracilis muscle. *Am. J. Physiol.* 246 (*Heart Circ. Physiol.* 15): H120–H128, 1984.
28. Connett, R. J., T. Gayeski, and C. R. Honig. Energy sources in fully aerobic rest-work transitions. *Am. J. Physiol.* 248 (*Heart Circ. Physiol.* 17): H922–H929, 1985.
29. Connett, R. J., C. R. Honig, T. E. J. Gayeski, and G. A. Brooks. Defining hypoxia: a systems view of VO2, glycolyis, energetics, and intracellular PO2. *J. Appl. Physiol.* 68: 833–842, 1990.
30. Cornish-Bowden, A., and M. L. Cardenas (Eds.). *Control of Metabolic Processes. NATO ASI Series A: Life Sci. 190.* New York: Plenum Press, 1989.
31. Crow, M. T., and M. J. Kushmerick. Chemical energetics of slow and fast twitch muscles of the mouse. *J. Gen. Physiol.* 79: 147–166, 1982.
32. Crow, M. T., and M. J. Kushmerick. Correlated reduction of velocity of shortening and the rate of energy utilization in mouse fast-twitch muscle during a continuous tetanus. *J. Gen. Physiol.* 82: 703–720, 1983.
33. Cuenda, A., F. Centeno, and C. Gutierrez-Merino. Modulation of phosphorylation of glycogen phosphorylase-sarcoplasmic reticulum interaction. *FEBS Lett.* 283: 273–276, 1991.
34. Curtin, N. A. Buffer power and intracellular pH of frog sartorius muscle. *Biophys. J.* 50: 837–841, 1986.
35. Dawson, M. J., D. G. Gadian, and D. R. Wilkie. Mechanical relaxation rate and metabolism studied in fatiguing muscle by phosphorus nuclear magnetic resonance. *J. Physiol. (Lond.)* 299: 456–585, 1980.
36. Dawson, M. J., D. G. Gadian, and D. R. Wilkie. Muscular fatigue investigated by phosphorus nuclear magnetic resonance. *Nature* 274: 861–866, 1978.
37. Dudley, G. A., and R. L. Terjung. Influence of acidosis on AMP deaminase activity in contracting fast-twitch muscle. *Am. J. Physiol.* 248 (*Cell Physiol.* 17): C43–C50, 1985.
38. Dudley, G. A., and R. L. Terjung. Influence of aerobic metabolism on IMP accumulation in fast-twitch muscle. *Am. J. Physiol.* 248 (*Cell Physiol.* 17): C37–C42, 1985.
39. Dudley, G. A., P. C. Tullson, and R. L. Terjung. Influence of mitochondrial content on the sensitivity of respiratory control. *J. Biol. Chem.* 262: 9109–9114, 1987.
40. Echteld, C. J. A., J. H. G. M. van Beek, J. H. Kirkels, P. van der Meer, T. J. C. Ruigrok, and N. Westerhof. *31P NMR study of the response of myocardial energy metabolism to heart rate steps.* Yufuin, Japan: International Congress on Muscle Energetics: 1989.
41. Edstrom, L., E. Hultman, K. Sahlin, and H. Sjoholm. The contents of high-energy phosphates in different fibre types in skeletal muscles from rat, guinea-pig, and man. *J. Physiol. (Lond.)* 332: 47–58, 1982.
42. Edstrom, R. D., M. H. Meinke, M. E. Gurnack, D. M. Steinhorn, X. Yang, R. Yang, and D. F. Evans. Regulation of muscle glycogenolysis. In: *Control of Metabolic Processes. NAT0 ASI Series A: Life Sci. 190.* edited by A. Cornish-Bowden and M. L. Cardenas. New York: Plenum Press, 1989, p. 209–217.
43. Erecinska, M., D. F. Wilson, and K. Nishiki. Homeostatic regulation of cellular energy metabolism: experimental characterization in vivo and fit to a model. *Am. J. Physiol.* 234 (*Cell Physiol.* 3): C82–C89, 1978.
44. Everts, M. E., J. P. Andersen, T. Clausen, and O. Hansen. Quantitative determination of Ca^{2+}-dependent Mg^{2+}-ATPase from sarcoplasmic reticulum in muscle biopsies. *Biochem. J.* 260: 443–448, 1989.
45. Ferguson, S. J., and M. C. Sorgato. Proton electrochemical gradients and energy transduction processes. *Ann. Rev. Biochem.* 51: 185–217, 1982.
46. Fitts, R. H. Cellular mechanisms of muscle fatigue. *Physiol. Rev.* 74: 49–94, 1994.
47. Foley, J. M., G. R. Adams, and R. A. Meyer. Utility of AICAr for metabolic studies is diminished by systemic effects in situ. *Am. J. Physiol.* 257 (*Cell Physiol.* 26): C488–C494, 1989.
48. Foley, J. M., S. J. Harkema, and R. A. Meyer. Decreased ATP cost of isometric contractions in ATP-depleted rat fast-twitch muscle. *Am. J. Physiol.* 261 (*Cell Physiol.* 30): C872–C881, 1991.
49. Foley, J. M., and R. A. Meyer. Energy cost of twitch and tetanic contractions of rat muscle estimated in situ by gated 31P NMR. *NMR Biomed.* 5: 32–38, 1993.
50. Fruen, B. R., J. R. Michelson, N. H. Shomer, T. J. Roghair, and C. F. Louis. Regulation of the sarcoplasmic reticulum ryanodine receptor by inorganic phosphate. *J. Biol. Chem.* 269: 192–198, 1994.
51. Funk, C. I., A. Clark, Jr., and R. J. Connett. A simple model of aerobic metabolism: applications to work transitions in muscle. *Am. J. Physiol.* 258 (*Cell Physiol.* 27): C995–C1005, 1990.
52. Gadian, D. G. *Nuclear Magnetic Resonance and Its Applications to Living Systems.* London: Oxford University Press, 1982.
53. Galione, A. Cyclic ADP-ribose: a new way to control calcium. *Science* 259: 325–326, 1993.
54. Garcia-Tejedor, A. J., J. M. Riol-Cimas, F. Morani, E. Melendez-Hevia, and F. Montero. Transition state of the glycolytic pathway under FDP saturating conditions: experimental studies and a theoretical model. *Int. J. Biochem.* 20: 421–426, 1988.
55. Gladden, L. B., W. N. Stainsby, and B. R. MacIntosh. Norepinephrine increases canine skeletal muscle Vo_2 during recovery. *Med. Sci. Sports Exerc.* 14: 471–478, 1982.
56. Gollnick, P., and B. Saltin. Significance of skeletal muscle oxidative enzyme enhancement with endurance training. *Clin. Physiol.* 2: 1–12, 1992.
57. Graham, T. E., J. K. Barclay, and B. A. Wilson. Skeletal muscle lactate release and glycolytic intermediates during hypercapnia. *J. Appl. Physiol.* 60: 568–575, 1986.
58. Graham, T. E., and B. Saltin. Estimation of the mitochondrial redox state in human skeletal muscle during exercise. *J. Appl. Physiol.* 66: 561–566, 1989.
59. Green, N. M. Evolutionary relationships within the family of P-type cation pumps. *Ann. N. Y. Acad. Sci.* 671: 104–112, 1992.
60. Gyulai, L., J. Z. Roth, J. S. Leigh, Jr., and B. Chance. Bioenergetic studies of mitochondrial oxidative phosphorylation using 31-phosphorus NMR. *J. Biol. Chem.* 260: 3947–3954, 1985.
61. Hak, J. B., J. H. G. M. van Beek, M. H. van Wijhe, and N. Westerhof. Influence of temperature on the response time of mitochondrial oxygen consumption in isolated rabbit heart. *J. Physiol. (Lond.)* 447: 17–31, 1992.
62. Hansford, R. G. Relation between mitochondrial calcium transport and control of energy metabolism. *Rev. Physiol. Biochem. Pharmacol.* 102: 1–72, 1985.
63. Hansford, R. G. Role of calcium in respiratory control. *Med. Sci. Sports Exerc.* 26: 44–51, 1994.
64. Harkema, S. J., and R. A. Meyer. Control of oxidative metabolism by cytosolic phosphorylation potential in slow twitch muscle in situ. *Physiologist* 35: 206, 1992.

65. Harkema, S. J., and R. A. Meyer. Evidence that ADP does not control respiration in acidotic skeletal muscle. *Proceedings of the Society of Magnetic Resonance* (2nd meeting), 1994, p. 358.
66. Harris, D. A., and A. M. Das. Control of mitochondrial ATP synthesis in the heart. *Biochem. J.* 280: 561–573, 1991.
67. Harris, R. C., R. H. T. Edwards, E. Hultman, and L. O. Nordesto. The time course of phosphorylcreatine resynthesis during recovery of the quadriceps muscle in man. *Pflugers Arch.* 367: 137–142, 1976.
68. Hillered, L., L. Ernster, and B. K. Siesjo. Influence of in vitro lactic acidosis and hypercapnia on respiratory activity of isolated rat brain mitochondria. *J. Cereb. Blood Flow Metab.* 4: 430–437, 1984.
69. Hintz, C. S., M. M.-Y. Chi, R. D. Fell, J. L. Ivy, K. K. Kaiser, C. V. Lowry, and O. H. Lowry. Metabolite changes in individual rat muscle fibers during stimulation. *Am. J. Physiol.* 242 (*Cell Physiol.* 11): C218–C228, 1982.
70. Hobbs, S. F., and D. I. McCloskey. Effects of blood pressure on force production in cat and human muscle. *J. Appl. Physiol.* 63: 834–839, 1987.
71. Hochachka, P. W., and G. O. Matheson. Regulating ATP turnover rates over broad dynamic work ranges in skeletal muscles. *J. Appl. Physiol.* 73: 1697–1703, 1992.
72. Hochachka, P. W., and T. P. Mommsen. Protons and anaerobiosis. *Science* 219: 1391–1397, 1983.
73. Homsher, E., and C. J. Kean. Skeletal muscle energetics and metabolism. *Ann. Rev. Physiol.* 40: 93–131, 1978.
74. Homsher, E., W. F. H. M. Mommaerts, N. V. Ricchiuti, and A. Wallner. Activation heat, activation metabolism and tension-related heat in frog semitendinosis muscles. *J. Physiol. (Lond.)* 220: 601–625, 1972.
75. Hood, D. A., J. Gorski, and R. L. Terjung. Oxygen cost of twitch and tetanic isometric contractions in rat skeletal muscle. *Am. J. Physiol.* 250 (*Endocrinol. Metab.* 13): E449–E456, 1986.
76. Hood, D. A., and G. Paren. Metabolic and contractile responses of rat fast-twitch muscle to 10-Hz stimulation. *Am. J. Physiol.* 260 (*Cell Physiol.* 29): C832–C840, 1991.
77. Horton, E. S., and R. L. Terjung (Eds.). *Exercise, Nutrition, and Energy Metabolism*. New York: Macmillan Publishing Company, 1988.
78. Hutchinson, W. L., P. G. Morris, and J. Mowbray. The molecular structure of a rapidly formed oligomeric adenosine tetraphosphate derivative from rat heart. *Biochem. J.* 234: 623–627, 1986.
79. Huxley, H.E. Cross-bridge movement and filament overlap. *Biophys. J.* 11: 235a, 1971.
80. Inesi, G., and M. R. Kirtley. Structural features of cation transport ATPases. *J. Bioenerg. Biomembr.* 24: 271–283, 1992.
81. Ivy, J. L., R. T. Withers, P. J. Van Handel, D. H. Elger, and D. L. Costill. Muscle respiratory capacity and fiber type as determinants of the lactate threshold. *J. Appl. Physiol.* 48: 523–527, 1980.
82. Jacobus, W. E. Respiratory control and the integration of heart high-energy phosphate metabolism by mitochondrial creatine kinase. *Ann. Rev. Physiol.* 47: 707–725, 1985.
83. Jacobus, W. E., R. W. Moreadith, and K. M. Wandegaer. Mitochondrial respiratory control: evidence against the regulation of respiration by extramitochondrial phosphorylation potential or ATP/ADP ratios. *J. Biol. Chem.* 257: 2397–2402, 1982.
84. Jeneson, J. A. L., H. V. Westerhoff, T. R. Brown, C. J. A. van Echteld, and R. Berger. Quasi-linear relationship between Gibbs free energy of ATP hydrolysis and power-output in human forearm muscle. *Am. J. Physiol.* 268 (*Cell Physiol.* 37): C1474–C1484, 1995.
85. Jobsis, F. F., and W. N. Stainsby. Oxidation of NADH during contractions of circulated skeletal muscle. *Respir. Physiol.* 4: 291–300, 1968.
86. Katz, A. Mitochondrial redox state in skeletal muscle cannot be estimated with glutamate dehyrogenase system (letter). *Am. J. Physiol.* 254 (*Cell Physiol.* 23): C587–C590, 1988.
87. Katz, A., and K. Sahlin. Regulation of lactic acid production during exercise. *J. Appl. Physiol.* 65: 509–518, 1988.
88. Katz, A., and K. Sahlin. Effect of decreased oxygen availablity on NADH and lactate contents in human skeletal muscle during exercise. *Acta Physiol. Scand.* 131: 119–127, 1987.
89. Katz, A., M. K. Spencer, and K. Sahlin. Failure of glutamate dehydrogenase system to predict oxygenation state of human skeletal muscle. *Am. J. Physiol.* 259 (*Cell Physiol.* 28): C26–C28, 1990.
90. Kemp, G. J., D. J. Taylor, and G. K. Radda. Control of phosphocreatine synthesis during recovery from exercise in human skeletal muscle. *NMR Biomed.* 6: 66–72, 1993.
91. Kemp, G. J., C. H. Thompson, A. L. Sanderson, and G. K. Radda. pH control in rat skeletal muscle during exercise, recovery from exercise, and acute respiratory acidosis. *Magn. Reson. Med.* 31: 103–109, 1994.
92. Klug, G. A., and G. F. Tibbits. The effect of activity on calcium-mediated events in striated muscle. *Exerc. Sport Sci. Rev.* 16: 1–60, 1988.
93. Koretsky, A. P., and R. S. Balaban. Changes in pyridine nucleotide levels alter oxygen consumption and extramitochondrial phosphates in isolated mitochondria: a ^{31}P NMR and NAD(P)H fluorescence study. *Biochim. Biophys. Acta* 893: 398–408, 1987.
94. Kowalchuk, J. M., G. J. F. Heigenhauser, M. I. Lindinger, J. R. Sutton, and N. L. Jones. Factors influencing hydrogen ion concentration in muscle after intense exercise. *J. Appl. Physiol.* 65: 2080–2089, 1988.
95. Kunz, W. S., A. V. Kuznetsov, W. Schulze, K. Eichorn, L. Schild, F. Stiggow, R. Bohnensack, S. Neuhof, H. Grasshoff, and H. W. Neumann. Functional characterization of mitochondrial oxidative phosphorylation in saponin-skinned human muscle fibers. *Biochim. Biophys. Acta* 1144: 46–53, 1993.
96. Kushmerick, M. J. Energetics of muscle contraction. In: *Handbook of Physiology, Skeletal Muscle, Skeletal Muscle,* edited by L. D. Peachey, R. H. Adrian, and S. R. Gieger. Bethesda, MD: Am. Physiol. Soc., 1983, p. 189–236, 1983.
97. Kushmerick, M. J., and R. E. Davies. The chemical energetics of muscle contraction. II. The chemistry, efficiency, and power of maximally working sartorius muscles. *Proc. R. Soc. Lond. B* 174: 315–353, 1969.
98. Kushmerick, M. J., and R. A. Meyer. Chemical changes in rat leg muscle by phosphorus nuclear magnetic resonance. *Am. J. Physiol.* 248 (*Cell Physiol.* 13): C542–C549, 1985.
99. Kushmerick, M. J., R. A. Meyer, and T. R. Brown. Regulation of oxygen consumption in fast- and slow-twitch muscle. *Am. J. Physiol.* 263 (*Cell Physiol.* 32): C598–C606, 1992.
100. Kushmerick, M., T. S. Moerland, and R. W. Wiseman. Mammalian skeletal muscle fibers distinguished by contents of phosphocreatine, ATP, and Pi. *Proc. Natl. Acad. Sci. U. S. A.* 89: 7521–7525, 1992.

101. LaNoue, K. F., F. M. H. Jeffries, and G. K. Radda. Kinetic control of mitochondrial ATP systhesis. *Biochemistry* 25: 7667–7675, 1986.
102. Lawson, J. W. R., and R. L. Veech. Effects of pH and free Mg^{2+} on the Keq of the creatine kinase reaction and other phosphate hydrolyses and phosphate transferases. *J. Biol. Chem.* 254: 6528–6537, 1979.
103. Lawson, R., and J. Mowbray. Purine nucleotide metabolism: the discovery of a major new oligomeric adenosine tetraphosphate derivative in rat heart. *Int. J. Biochem.* 18: 407–412, 1986.
104. Leberer, E., and D. Pette. Immunochemical quantification of sarcoplasmic reticulum Ca-ATPase, of calsequestrin and of parvalbumin in rabbit skeletal muscles of defined fiber composition. *Eur. J. Biochem.* 156: 489–496, 1986.
105. Lewis, S. F., and R. G. Haller. The pathophysiology of McArdle's disease: clues to regulation in exercise and fatigue. *J. Appl. Physiol.* 61: 391–401, 1986.
106. Lowenstein, J. M. Ammonia production in muscle and other tissues: the purine nucleotide cycle. *Physiol. Rev.* 52: 382–414, 1972.
107. Lowey, S., G. S. Waller, and K. M. Trybus. Function of skeletal muscle myosin heavy chain and light chain isoforms by an in vitro motility assay. *J. Biol. Chem.* 268: 20414–20418, 1993.
108. Lowrey, O. H., D. W. Schulz, and J. V. Passonneau. Effects of adenylic acid on the kinetics of muscle phosphorylase a. *J. Biol. Chem.* 239: 1947–1953, 1964.
109. Ma, J., M. Fill, C. M. Knudson, K. P. Campbell, and R. Coronado. Ryanodine receptor of skeletal muscle is a gap junction-type channel. *Science* 242: 99–102, 1988.
110. Mahler, M. First-order kinetics of muscle oxygen consumption, and an equivalent proportionality between $\dot{Q}O_2$ and phosphorylcreatine level. *J. Gen. Physiol.* 86: 135–165, 1985.
111. McAllister, R. M., R. W. Ogilvie, and R. L. Terjung. Impact of reduced cytochrome oxidase activity on peak oxygen consumption of muscle. *J. Appl. Physiol.* 69: 384–389, 1990.
112. McAllister, R. M., and R. L. Terjung. Acute inhibition of respiratory capacity of muscle reduces peak oxygen consumption. *Am. J. Physiol.* 259 (*Cell Physiol.* 28): C889–C896, 1990.
113. McCormack, J. G., A. P. Halestrap, and R. M. Denton. Role of calcium ions in regulation of mammalian intramitochondrial metabolism. *Physiol. Rev.* 70: 391–425, 1990.
114. McCully, K. K., S. Iotti, K. Kendrick, Z. Wang, J. D. Posner, J. Leigh, Jr., and B. Chance. Simultaneous in vivo measurements of HbO_2 saturation and PCr kinetics after exercise in normal humans. *J. Appl. Physiol.* 77: 5–10, 1994.
115. McMillin, J. B., and M. C. Madden. The role of calcium in the control of respiration by muscle mitochondria. *Med. Sci. Sports Exerc.* 21: 406–410, 1989.
116. McMillin, J. B., and D. F. Pauly. Control of mitochondrial respiration in muscle. *Mol. Cell. Biochem.* 81: 121–129, 1988.
117. Meyer, R. A. A linear model of muscle respiration explains monoexponential phosphocreatine changes. *Am. J. Physiol.* 254 (*Cell Physiol.* 23): C548–C553, 1988.
118. Meyer, R. A. Linear dependence of muscle phosphocreatine kinetics on total creatine content. *Am. J. Physiol.* 257 (*Cell Physiol.* 26): C1149–C1157, 1989.
119. Meyer, R. A., G. R. Adams, M. J. Fisher, P. F. Dillon, J. M. Krisanda, T. R. Brown, and M. J. Kushmerick. Effect of decreased pH on force and phosphocreatine in mammalian skeletal muscle. *Can. J. Physiol. Pharmacol.* 69: 305–310, 1991.
120. Meyer, R. A., T. R. Brown, B. L. Krilowicz, and M. J. Kushmerick. Phosphagen and intracellular pH changes during contraction of reatine depleted rat muscle. *Am. J. Physiol.* 250 (*Cell Physiol.* 19): C264–C274, 1986.
121. Meyer, R. A., T. R. Brown, and M. J. Kushmerick. Phosphorus nuclear magnetic resonance of fast- and slow-twitch muscle. *Am. J. Physiol.* 248 (*Cell Physiol.* 17): C279–C287, 1985.
122. Meyer, R. A., M. J. Fisher, S. J. Nelson, and T. R. Brown. Evaluation of manual methods for integration of in vivo phosphorus NMR spectra. *NMR Biomed.* 1: 131–135, 1988.
123. Meyer, R. A., M. J. Kushmerick, and T. R. Brown. Application of 31P-NMR spectroscopy to the study of striated muscle metabolism. *Am. J. Physiol.* 242 (*Cell Physiol.* 11): C1–C11, 1982.
124. Meyer, R. A., and R. L. Terjung. Differences in ammonia and adenylate metabolism in contracting fast- and slow-twitch muscle. *Am. J. Physiol.* 237 (*Cell Physiol.* 6): C111–C118, 1979.
125. Meyer, R. A., H. L. Sweeney, and M. J. Kushmerick. A simple analysis of the "phosphocreatine shuttle". *Am. J. Physiol.* 246 (*Cell Physiol.* 15): C365–C377, 1984.
126. Meyer, R. A., and R. L. Terjung. AMP deamination and IMP resamination in working skeletal muscle. *Am. J. Physiol.* 239 (*Cell Physiol.* 8): C32–C38, 1980.
127. Moerland, T. S., N. G. Wolf, and M. J. Kushmerick. Administration of a creatine analogue induces isomyosin transitions in muscle. *Am. J. Physiol.* 257 (*Cell Physiol.* 26): C810–C816, 1989.
128. Moon, R. B., and J. H. Richards. Determination of intracellular pH by 31P magnetic resonance. *J. Biol. Chem.* 248: 7276–7278, 1973.
129. Morgan, H. E., and A. Parmeggiani. Regulation of glycogenolysis in muscle III: control of muscle glycogen phosphorylase activity. *J. Biol. Chem.* 239: 2440–2445, 1964.
130. Morrison, J. F., and W. W. Cleland. Isotope exchange studies of the mechanism of the reaction catalyzed by adenosine triphosphate: creatine phosphotransferase. *J. Biol. Chem.* 241: 673–683, 1966.
131. Needham, D. M. Machina Carnis: *The Biochemistry of Muscular Contraction and its Historical Development.* Cambridge: Cambridge University Press, 1971.
132. Nioka, S., Z. Argov, G. P. Dobson, R. E. Forster, H. V. Subramanian, R. L. Veech, and B. Chance. Substrate regulation of mitochondrial oxidative phosphorylation in hypercapnic rabbit muscle. *J. Appl. Physiol.* 72: 521–528, 1992.
133. Paddle, B. M. A cytoplasmic component of pyridine nucleotide flouresence in rat diaphragm: evidence from comparisons with flavoprotein flourescence. *Pflugers Arch.* 404: 326–331, 1985.
134. Parkhouse, W. S. Regulation of skeletal muscle metabolism by enzyme binding. *Can. J. Physiol. Pharmacol.* 70: 150–156, 1992.
135. Peachey, L. D. Excitation-contraction coupling: the link between the surface and the interior of a muscle cell. *J. Exp. Biol.* 115: 91–98, 1985.
136. Pessah, I. N., R. A. Stambuk, and J. E. Casida. Ca^{2+}-activated ryanodine binding: mechanisms of sensitivity and intensity modulation by Mg^{2+}, caffeine, and adenine nucleotides. *Mol. Pharmacol.* 31: 232–238, 1987.

137. Pette, D., and R. S. Staron. Cellular and molecular diversities of mammalian skeletal muscle fibers. *Rev. Physiol. Biochem. Pharmacol.* 116: 1–76, 1990.
138. Rall, J. A. Energetic aspects of skeletal muscle contraction: implication of fiber types. *Exerc. Sport Sci. Rev.* 13: 33–74, 1985.
139. Rall, J. A. Sense and nonsense about the Fenn effect. *Am. J. Physiol.* 242 (*Heart Circ. Physiol.* 11): H1–H6, 1982.
140. Rall, J. A. Energetics of Ca^{2+} cycling during skeletal muscle contraction. *Federation Proc.* 41: 155–160, 1982.
141. Ren, J. M., and E. Hultman. Regulation of glycogenolysis in human skeletal muscle. *J. Appl. Physiol.* 67: 2243–2248, 1989.
142. Ren, J. M., B. A. Marshall, E. A. Gulve, J. Gao, D. W. Johnson, J. O. Holloszy, and M. Mueckler. Evidence from transgenic mice that glucose transport is rate-limiting for glycogen deposition and glycolysis in skeletal muscle. *J. Biol. Chem.* 268: 16113–16115, 1993.
143. Rios, E., and G. Pizarro. Voltage sensor of excitation-contraction coupling in skeletal muscle. *Physiol. Rev.* 71: 849–908, 1991.
144. Roos, A., and W. F. Boron. Intracellular pH. *Physiol. Rev.* 61: 296–434, 1981.
145. Rossi, A. M., H. M. Eppenberger, P. Volpe, R. Cutrofo, and T. Wallimann. Muscle-type MM creatine kinase is specifically bound to sarcoplasmic reticulum and can support Ca^{2+} uptake and regulate local ATP/ADP ratios. *J. Biol. Chem.* 265: 5258–5266, 1990.
146. Rossini, L., P. Rossini, and B. Chance. Continuous readout of cytochrome b, flavin and pyridine nucleotide oxidoreduction processes in the perfused frog heart and contracting skeletal muscle. *Pharm. Res.* 22: 349–365, 1991.
147. Roth, D. A., and G. A. Brooks. Lactate transport is mediated by a membrane-bound carrier in rat skeletal muscle sarcolemmal vesicles. *Arch. Biochem. Biophys.* 944: 213–222, 1988.
148. Rottenberg, H. The thermodynamic description of enzyme-catalyzed reactions. *Biophys. J.* 13: 503–511, 1973.
149. Rouslin, W. The mitochondrial adenosine 5′-triphosphatase in slow and fast rate hearts. *Am. J. Physiol.* 252 (*Heart Circ. Physiol.* 21): H622–H637, 1987.
150. Rowell, L. B. Muscle blood flow in humans: how high can it go? *Med. Sci. Sports Exerc.* 20: S97–S103, 1988.
151. Rundell, K. W., P. C. Tullson, and R. L. Terjung. AMP deaminase binding in contracting rat skeletal muscle. *Am. J. Physiol.* 263 (*Cell Physiol.* 32): C287–C293, 1992.
152. Rundell, K. W., P. C. Tullson, and R. L. Terjung. Altered kinetics of AMP deaminase by myosin binding. *Am. J. Physiol.* 263 (*Cell Physiol.* 32): C294–C299, 1992.
153. Sabbadini, R. A., and A. S. Dahms. Biochemical properties of isolated transverse tubular membranes. *J. Bioenerg. Biomembr.* 21: 163–213, 1989.
154. Sahlin, K. Intracellular pH and energy metabolism in skeletal muscle of man. *Acta Physiol. Scand.* 455: 1–56, 1978.
155. Sahlin, K. Control of energetic processes in contracting human skeletal muscle. *Biochem. Soc. Trans.* 19: 353–358, 1991.
156. Sahlin, K. NADH and NADPH in human skeletal muscle at rest and during ischaemia. *Clin. Physiol.* 3: 477–485, 1983.
157. Sahlin, K., J. Gorski, and L. Edstrom. Influence of ATP turnover and metabolite changes on IMP formation and glycolysis in rat skeletal muscle. *Am. J. Physiol.* 259 (*Cell Physiol.* 28): C409–C412, 1990.
158. Sahlin, K., R. C. Harris, and E. Hultman. Creatine kinase equilibrium and lactate content compared with muscle pH in tissue samples obtained after isometric exercise. *Biochem. J.* 152: 173–180, 1975.
159. Sahlin, K., R. C. Harris, and E. Hultman. Resynthesis of creatine phosphate in human muscle after exercise in relation to intramuscular pH and availability of oxygen. *Scand. J. Clin. Lab. Invest.* 39: 551–558, 1979.
160. Sahlin, K., R. C. Harris, B. Nylind, and E. Hultman. Lactate content and pH in muscle samples obtained after dynamic exercise. *Pflugers Arch.* 367: 143–149, 1976.
161. Sahlin, K., A. Katz, and J. Henriksson. Redox state and lactate accumulation in human skeletal muscle during dynamic exercise. *Biochem. J.* 245: 551–556, 1987.
162. Sapega, A. A., D. P. Sokolow, T. J. Graham, and B. Chance. Phosphorus nuclear magnetic resonance: a non-invasive technique for the study of muscle bioenergetics during exercise. *Med. Sci. Sports Exerc.* 19: 410–420, 1987.
163. Segel, I. H. *Enzyme Kinetics: Behavior and Analysis of Rapid Equilibrium and Steady-State Enzyme Systems.* New York: John Wiley & Sons, 1975.
164. Shoubridge, E. A., R. A. J. Challiss, D. J. Hayes, and G. K. Radda. Biochemical adaptation in the skeletal muscle of rats depleted of creatine with the substrate analogue β-guanidinopropionic acid. *Biochem. J.* 232: 125–131, 1985.
165. Shoubridge, E. A., and G. K. Radda. A gated 31P-NMR study of tetanic contraction in rat muscle depleted of phosphocreatine. *Am. J. Physiol.* 252 (*Cell Physiol.* 21): C532–C542, 1987.
166. Smith, I. C. H. Energetics of activation in frog and toad muscle. *J. Physiol. (Lond.)* 220: 583–599, 1972.
167. Smith, J. S., R. Coronado, and G. Meissner. Sarcoplasmic reticulum contains adenine nucleotide-activated calcium channels. *Nature* 316: 446–449, 1985.
168. Soderlund, K., and E. Hultman. ATP and phosphocreatine changes in single human muscle fibers after intense electrical stimulation. *Am. J. Physiol.* 261 (*Endocrinol. Metab.* 25): E737–E741, 1991.
169. Spriet, L. L. Anaerobic metabolism in human skeletal muscle during short-term, intense activity. *Can. J. Physiol. Pharmacol.* 70: 157–165, 1992.
170. Spriet, L. L., K. Soderlund, and E. Hultman. Energy cost and metabolic regulation during intermittent and continuous tetanic contractions in human skeletal muscle. *Can. J. Physiol. Pharmacol.* 66: 134–139, 1988.
171. Srere, P. A. Complexes of sequential metabolic enzymes. *Ann. Rev. Biochem.* 56: 89–124, 1987.
172. Stanley, W. C., and R. J. Connett. Regulation of muscle carbohydrate metabolism during exercise. *FASEB J.* 5: 2155–2159, 1991.
173. Stewart, P. A. Modern quantitative acid-base chemistry. *Can. J. Physiol. Pharmacol.* 61: 1444–1461, 1983.
174. Stoner, C. D. An investigation of the relationships between rate and driving force in simple uncatalyzed and enzyme-catalyzed reactions with appplications of the findings to chemiosmotic reactions. *Biochem. J.* 283: 541–552, 1992.
175. Sweeney, H. L. The importance of the creatine kinase reaction: the concept of metabolic capacitance. *Med. Sci. Sports Exerc.* 26: 30–36, 1994.
176. Sweeney, H. L., B. Bowman, and J. T. Stull. Myosin light chain phosphorylation in vertebrate striated muscle: regulation and function. *Am. J. Physiol.* 264 (*Cell Physiol.* 33): C1085–C1095, 1993.
177. Sweeney, H. L., M. J. Kushmerick, K. Mabuchi, F. A. Streter, and J. Gergely. Myosin alkali light chain and heavy chain variations correlate with altered shortening velocity of isolated skeletal muscle muscle fibers. *J. Biol. Chem.* 263: 9034–9039, 1988.

178. Tamura, M., O. Hazeki, S. Nioka, and B. Chance. In vivo study of tissue oxygen metabolism using optical and nuclear magnetic resonance spectroscopies. *Ann. Rev. Physiol.* 51: 813–834, 1989.
179. Tate, C. A., and G. E. Taffet. The regulatory role of calcium in striated muscle. *Med. Sci. Sports Exerc.* 21: 393–398, 1989.
180. Teodosiu, D. C., G. Cederblad, and E. Hultman. PDC activity and acetyl group accumulation in skeletal muscle during isometric contraction. *J. Appl. Physiol.* 74: 1712–1718, 1993.
181. Trevida, B., and W. H. Danforth. Effect of pH on the kinetics of frog muscle phosphofructokinase. *J. Biol. Chem.* 241: 4110–4114, 1966.
182. Tsika, R. W. Transgenic animal models. *Exerc. Sport Sci. Rev.* 22: 361–388, 1994.
183. Tullson, P. C., D. M. Whitlock, and R. L. Terjung. Adenine nucleotide degradation in slow-twitch red muscle. *Am. J. Physiol.* 258 (*Cell Physiol.* 27): C258–C265, 1990.
184. Ugurbil, K., P. B. Kingsley-Hickman, E. Y. Sako, S. Zimmer, P. Mohanakrishnan, P. M. L. Robitaille, W. J. Thoma, A. Johnson, J. E. Foker, and A. H. L. From. 31P NMR studies of the kinetics and regulation of oxidative phosphorylation in the intact myocardium. *Ann. N. Y. Acad. Sci.* 508: 265–286, 1987.
185. Van der Meer, R., H. V. Westerhoff, and K. van Dam. Linear relation between rate and thermodynamic force in enzyme-catalyzed reactions. *Biochim. Biophys. Acta* 591: 488–493, 1980.
186. Van Deursen, J., A. Heerschap, F. Oerlemans, W. Ruttenbeek, P. Jap, H. ter Leak, and B. Wieringa. Skeletal muscles of mice deficient in muscle creatine kinase lack burst activity. *Cell* 74: 621–631, 1993.
187. Veech, R. L., J. W. R. Lawson, N. W. Cornell, and H. A. Krebs. Cytosolic phosphorylation potential. *J. Biol. Chem.* 254: 6538–6547, 1979.
188. Wallimann, T., and H. M. Eppenberger. The subcellular compartmentation of creatine kinase isozymes as a precondition for a proposed phosphoryl-creatine circuit. *Prog. Clin. Biol. Res.* 344: 877–889, 1990.
189. Wallimann, T., and H. M. Eppenberger. Localization and function of M-line-bound creatine kinase: M-band model and creatine phosphate shuttle. *Cell Muscle Motil.* 6: 239–285, 1985.
190. Wallimann, T., T. Schlosser, and H. M. Eppenberger. Function of M-line-bound creatine kinase as intramyofibrillar ATP regenerator at the receiving end of the phosphorylcreatine shuttle in muscle. *J. Biol. Chem.* 259: 5238–5246, 1984.
191. Weibel, E. R. *The Pathway for Oxygen.* Cambridge, MA: Harvard University Press, 1984.
192. Wendt, I. R., and J. B. Chapman. Flourometric studies of recovery metabolism of rat fast- and slow-twitch muscles. *Am. J. Physiol.* 230: 1644–1649, 1976.
193. Wendt, I. R., and C. L. Gibbs. Energy production of rat extensor digitorum longus muscle. *Am. J. Physiol.* 224: 1081–1086, 1973.
194. Westerblad, H., J. A. Lee, J. Lannergren, and D. G. Allen. Cellular mechanisms of fatigue in skeletal muscle. *Am. J. Physiol.* 261 (*Cell Physiol.* 30): C195–C209, 1991.
195. Westerhoff, H. V., and K. van Dam. *Thermodynamics and Control of Biological Free-Energy Transduction.* Amsterdam: Elsevier, 1987.
196. Whalen, R. G. Myosin isozymes as molecular markers for muscle physiology. *J. Exp. Biol.* 115: 43–53, 1985.
197. Wheeler, T. J., and J. M. Lowenstein. Adenylate deaminase from rat muscle. Regulation by purine nucleotides and orthophosphate in the presense of 150mM KCl. *J. Biol. Chem.* 254: 8994–8999, 1979.
198. Whitlock, D. M., and R. L. Terjung. ATP depletion in slow-twitch red muscle of rat. *Am. J. Physiol.* 253 (*Cell Physiol.* 22): C426–C432, 1987.
199. Wilson, D. F. Factors affecting the rate and energetics of mitochondrial oxidative phosphorylation. *Med. Sci. Sports Exerc.* 26: 37–43, 1994.
200. Woledge, R. C., N. A. Curtin, and E. Homsher. Energetic aspects of muscle contraction. *Monogr. Physiol. Soc.*, Vol. 41, London: Academic Press, 1985.
201. Wolfe, B. R., T. E. Graham, and J. K. Barclay. Hyperoxia, mitochondrial redox state, and lactate metabolism of in situ canine muscle. *Am. J. Physiol.* 253 (*Cell Physiol.* 22): C263–C268, 1987.
202. Wu, K. D., and J. Lytton. Molecular cloning and quantification of sarcoplasmic reticulum Ca^{2+}-ATPase isoforms in rat muscles. *Am. J. Physiol.* 264 (*Cell Physiol.* 33): C333–C341, 1993.
203. Zamanyi, I., and I. N. Pessah. Comparison of $[^3H]$ryanodine receptors and Ca^{++} release from rat cardiac and rabbit skeletal muscle sarcoplasmic reticulum. *J. Pharmocol. Exp. Ther.* 256: 938–946, 1991.

19. Control of glycolysis and glycogen metabolism

RICHARD J. CONNETT | *Department of Physiology, University of Rochester School of Medicine and Dentistry, & Department of Biological Sciences, Monroe Community College, Rochester, New York*

KENT SAHLIN | *Department of Physiology and Pharmacology, Karolinska Institute and Department of Sports and Health Sciences, University College of Physical Education, Stockholm, Sweden*

CHAPTER CONTENTS

IMPORTANCE OF GLYCOLYSIS IN SKELETAL MUSCLE AT REST AND DURING EXERCISE.

Carbohydrate (CHO) is the major energy source during intense exercise and is stored primarily as glycogen in muscle and liver. Free glucose is present in only a small amount, mainly in the extracellular fluid, corresponding to less than 5% of total CHO. The chemically stored energy of glycogen is liberated through degradation by well-defined metabolic pathways involving glycogenolysis, glycolysis, and mitochondrial oxidation of pyruvate. Oxidation of muscle glycogen may have energetic advantages over fat because of the greater ATP yield per oxygen (O_2) consumed, the higher maximal rate of adenosine triphosphate (ATP) formation, and the more rapid recruitment of the pathway. In contrast to fat and protein, degradation of CHO (to lactic acid) can also provide energy at a high rate, but for a short period of time during anaerobic conditions. Thus, during conditions of rapid changes in ATP turnover rate, when circulatory delivery of O_2 is approaching a limit, or energy demand is very high relative to capacity (e.g., during heavy exercise), one would predict that degradation of glycogen should be the preferred pathway.

In contrast to fat, CHO is stored with water [2.7 g H_2O/g glycogen (9)]. Together with the higher energy density of fat, the energy yield per gram stored fuel is about seven times higher for fat than for CHO. Considering the extra weight to be carried, there is a conflict between the superiority of CHO as a fuel and the poor energy yield per gram stored fuel. The animal kingdom has solved this dilemma by having relatively small stores of CHO used primarily during conditions of high-power output. Depletion of CHO will severely limit the rate of ATP formation and the power output. In contrast, fat is stored in abundancy and is not considered to be limiting for endurance.

Because of the unique ability to dramatically change its metabolic demands, skeletal muscle is faced with intricate problems related to fuel homeostasis and metabolic regulation. Transition between rest and exercise involves a drastic increase in the energy demand, and during maximal exercise the cellular ATP content would be depleted within 2–3 s if there were no resynthesis of ATP. To maintain muscle ATP constant, which is necessary for cellular homeostasis, the rate of ATP regeneration must equal the rate of ATP utilization. The precision of adjusting the rate of the ATP generating processes to the energy requirements during exercise is remarkable (133) and is achieved by both feedforward and feedback control. Glycolysis and carbohydrate oxidation are of major importance for ATP regeneration; therefore precise control of these processes is required.

Glycolysis is part of the metabolic system in muscle (see Fig. 19.1). The regulatory goal of this system during exercise appears to be to keep the ATP supply equal to the ATP consumption by the contractile machinery and various ion pumps that are required for muscle activity. In addition to controlling glycolysis the system must coordinate it with controls on mitochondrial functions (see Chapter 18), membrane transport, circulatory delivery of substrate and, potentially, controls on ATP demand. In this chapter we will focus only on glycogen metabolism and glycolysis. Since this pathway is part of the whole metabolic system, it serves not only to produce ATP but also to support other parts of the integrated system. Some control signals and mechanisms are clearly related to the phosphorylation state of the cytosol. Other effects (e.g., redox interactions, citrate on Phosphofructokinase) serve to keep glycolysis coordinated with the mitochondria and other parts of the metabolic system. Finally, there are endocrine controls that serve to keep local metabolic activity coordinated with the needs of the rest of the body.

GENERAL OVERVIEW OF THE GLYCOLYTIC PATHWAY

ATP Supply

Traditionally, glycolysis has been thought to be important primarily as a backup source of ATP to supplement or replace mitochondrial oxidative phosphorylation. Thus, glycolysis should be activated when mitochondrial ATP production is inadequate to meet the demands of muscle adenosine triphosphatase (ATPase) activity. There are two types of exercise situations where one would expect glycolytic ATP production:

1. Conditions where mitochondrial capacity is inadequate to meet the ATP demand. This could occur in heavily recruited fibers within a muscle (near $V_{O_{2max}}$ for the muscle fiber) or during heavy exercise with a small muscle mass. This level of ATP turnover will of course vary from fiber to fiber depending on the mitochondrial content which in turn depends on fiber type, training state, and so forth. Another situation of this type would occur when the availability of substrates for the mitochondria (especially O_2) become limiting (148). This could happen when competing physiological demand for blood flow limits local flow (e.g., during heavy exercise with large muscle groups and high heat loads).

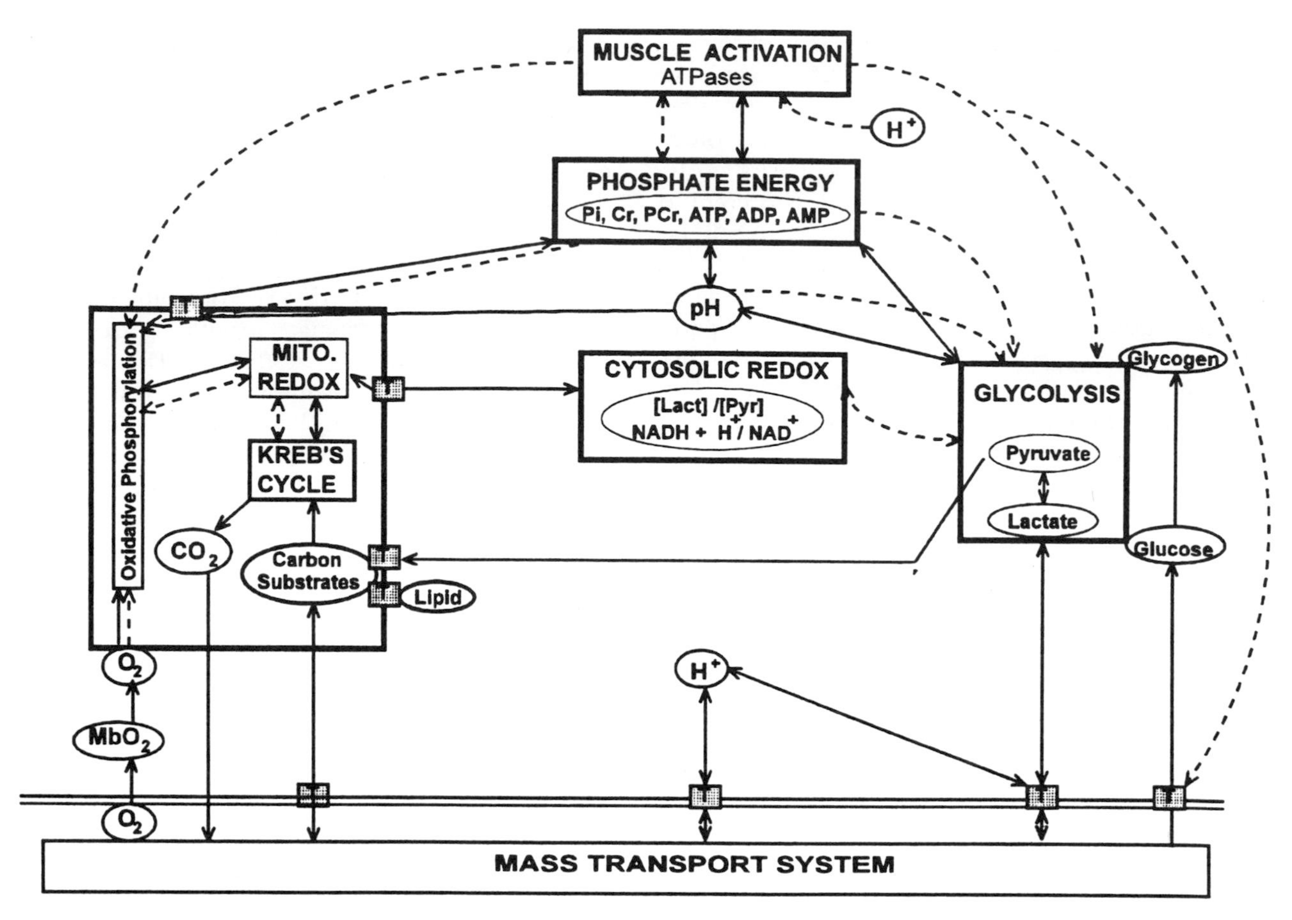

FIG. 19.1. Schematic diagram of biochemical system in muscle. Subsystems are indicated by *rectangles*. Those with a *T* indicate specialized transport systems. Important reactant pools are shown in *ellipses*. *Solid arrows* indicate material flow; *dashed arrows*, flow of information.

2. Conditions of rapid changes in energy turnover such as from rest to work or transitions between work levels. The ATP demand can change almost instantaneously ($t_{1/2}$ on the order of milliseconds), whereas mitochondrial activation takes a longer time to reach a new steady state. The activation of V_{O_2} appears to be directly related to changes in cytosolic high-energy phosphorylation state (63, 105) and therefore has a relatively long half-time. In in situ stimulated muscles, values on the order of 15 s have been measured (61). In human studies, values consistent with this ($t_{1/2}$ = 18–30 s) have been measured (39, 198, 87). The $t_{1/2}$ for glycolysis is very small. As discussed below, activation of critical enzymes involves signals related to muscle activation independent of the energy state and therefore can respond in milliseconds. Many studies have demonstrated significant accumulations of lactate within 15 s of muscle activity in all fiber types (110). The red fibers of dog gracilis muscle showed a mean flux of 10 μmole lactate · g^{-1} · min^{-1} in the first 5 s of submaximal stimulation, with declining values after that (54, 211). Activation of individual enzymes occurs on the time scale of chemical binding.

Support of Other Metabolic Needs

These three exercise conditions (rapid transition in work, turnover near max, or oxygen supply limits on mitochondria) all require glycolysis as a supplier of ATP. There seems to be an additional role for glycolysis during sustained moderate to heavy exercise at levels where the mitochondrial capacity should be adequate to supply the ATP needed. The evidence for this includes observations that when the muscle glycogen supply is exhausted the sustainable energy turnover in working muscle decreases (112, 257). This is supported by data obtained from individuals having inactive glycolytic enzymes (14, 22, 98, 168, 200, 228). In every case of inadequate glycolytic activity the individual cannot sustain normal muscle activity above ~50% of the aerobic capacity (22, 80). The defining symptom is usually pain or the inability to sustain normal levels of work output even though the mitochondrial capacity is normal or even above normal. When glycogen phosphorylase cannot be activated, increased glucose supply can ameliorate the problem (168). Thus, glycolysis is required for adequate aerobic production of ATP by the mitochondria. The system illustrated in Figure 19.1 shows that the glycolytic pathway can interact with mitochondrial metabolism in a number of ways. It produces ATP, thus changing the phosphorylation state signal to the mitochondrion. It produces cytosolic reducing equivalents that may serve to stabilize (buffer) mitochondrial redox, thereby permitting control to be dominated by the phosphorylation state (61, 58, 233). It produces pyruvate which can serve as a substrate or as a source for Krebs cycle intermediates (5, 232, 248).

In summary, it appears that glycolysis plays a role in supplying ATP during rapid transients in energy turnover and as a supplement to mitochondrial ATP production during high levels of activity, but also plays other roles in support of mitochondrial function. Thus, we see mechanisms that respond to muscle activation and cytosolic high-energy phosphorylation state as well as those responding to delivery of redox potential and/or pyruvate to the mitochondrion. Finally, there are endocrine controls that make the muscle system respond to the state of glucose metabolism in the whole body. Glycolysis is one of the best studied biochemical pathways. Many control signals have been identified and the changes of these during exercise described. However, in the absence of a model that incorporates our current knowledge and quantitatively accounts for glycolytic flux under conditions ranging from rest-work transitions through steady moderate work to heavy exercise, there may still be unidentified control mechanisms operating.

PROPERTIES OF GLYCOGEN AND ASSOCIATED ENZYMES

Structure of Glycogen

Glycogen is a polymer of glucose, and in muscle the molecule contains about 10,000 glycosyl units linked by α-1,4 (93%) and α-1,6 (7%) glycosidic linkages. The two types of linkage constitute the basis of the branched structure of glycogen. Storage of CHO in the form of glycogen avoids the problem with the otherwise large osmotic pressure that would be created by storage of a similar amount of free glucose. Simultaneously, the branched structure of glycogen leads to exposure of a large number of the glycosyl units (7%–10%) to the metabolizing enzymes (13) and thus provides the potential for rapid metabolism.

Glycogen particles have a diameter of 15–50 nm (33) and, after appropriate preparation, are clearly visible with the electron microscope. The glycogen particle contains, in addition to glycogen, a covalently bound protein (glycogenin), which is the priming protein for de novo synthesis of glycogen (241). The number of glycogenin molecules will determine the number of glycogen particles and is therefore of direct importance for tissue glycogen content. Whether glycogenin content varies under different physiological conditions is currently not known. The enzymes involved in the metabolism of glycogen are noncovalently bound to the glycogen particle. Most of the glycogen particles are located close to the sarcoplasmic reticulum (SR) bound to the membrane. Evidence exists that the SR-glycogen-protein complex is a functional compartment controlled by SR calcium flux (92). Glycogen particles are also located close to the sarcolemma and to a minor extent in the intramyofibrillar space. The different pools of glycogen appear to be utilized to different extents during exercise (102). There is evidence that the close interaction between proteins and glycogen in the glycogen particle affects the kinetic characteristics and the control sensitivity of the enzymes (23, 127, 167). Data from in vitro studies of enzymes in dilute concentration may therefore not always be pertinent to in vivo conditions.

Glycogen synthesis and degradation occur in vivo by two separate pathways (Fig. 19.2). Degradation is catalyzed by two enzymes in parallel: glycogen phosphorylase [(GP) transfer of a glucose unit to inorganic phosphate and formation of glucose 1-phosphate (G1P)] and debranching enzyme or amylo-1,6-glucosidase, which is a bifunctional enzyme (oligoglucan transferase and cleavage of exposed 1,6-glycosidic linkages and formation of free glucose). Since about 7% of the linkages between glycosyl units are 1,6-glycosidic linkages, 7% of glycogen will theoretically be released as glucose. However, there is evidence that the initial breakdown of glycogen can occur without formation of glucose (229) (i.e., without activation of debranching enzyme). This may be explained by the fact that normally about 50% of glycogen is in the outer branches (191) and can be degraded without the action of debranching enzyme (i.e., until a limit dextrin is reached).

Glycogen synthesis from G1P is catalyzed by two enzymes in series: UDP-glucose pyrophosphorylase and glycogen synthase (GS), where GS is considered to be the rate-limiting reaction. The branched struc-

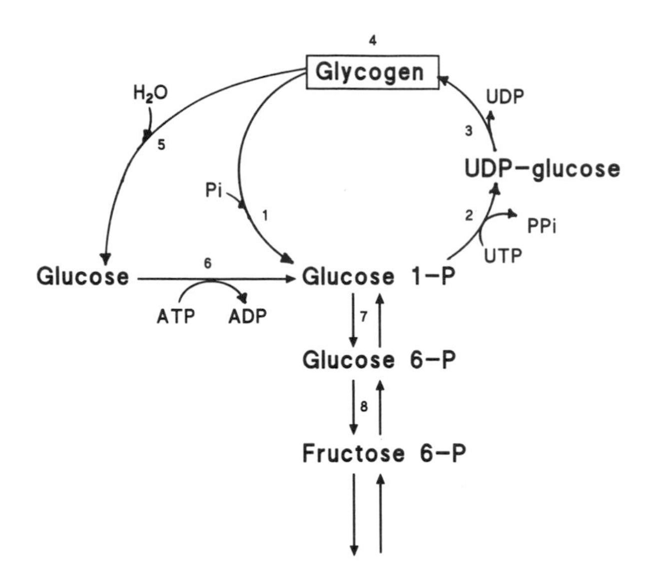

FIG. 19.2. Metabolic pathways of glycogen metabolism. Numbers refer to the following enzymes: *1*, glycogen phosphorylase; *2*, UDP-glucose pyrophosphorylase; *3*, glycogen synthase; *4*, branching enzyme; *5*, debranching enzyme; *6*, hexokinase; *7*, phosphoglucomutase; *8*, phosphoglucose isomerase.

ture of glycogen is due to the activity of branching enzyme (α-1,4-glucan:α-1,4-glucan 6-glucosyltransferase) acting on the glycogen molecule when the chains have reached a certain length. Both GP and GS exist in two interconvertible forms, being regulated by phosphorylation-dephosphorylation mechanisms. These two forms of GP and GS exhibit different kinetic characteristics of high complexity that will be discussed below.

Control of GP

Glycogen phosphorylase is a flux-generating enzyme and is rate-limiting for glycogenolysis. The discovery that GP exists in two enzymatically interconvertible forms initiated extensive studies of the control mechanisms. GP is the classic control enzyme, exhibiting both allosteric and substrate regulation, as well as covalent modification (phosphorylation). There are three basic mechanisms known to be involved in the control of GP activity:

1. Interconversion between the nonphosphorylated, less active form (GPb) and the phosphorylated, more active form (GPa).
2. Control by changes in substrate availability.
3. Allosteric control.

Interconversion between GPb and GPa. GP was one of the first enzymes shown to be activated by a second messenger like cyclic adenosine monophosphate (cAMP) and to have phosphorylation involved (32). The basic steps involved in the epinephrine-induced covalent modification of GP have been covered in numerous reviews (33, 76, 49, 96, 97, 100, 164, 181) and are outlined in Figure 19.3. The cascade mechanism of interconversion starts with epinephrine-mediated increases in cAMP, which activates cAMP-dependent protein kinase (cAMP-PK). cAMP-PK then phosphorylates phosphorylase kinase *b* (PKb) to PKa. Phosporylase kinase phosphorylates GP*b* at one site to GP*a*. Both PKa and PKb are activated by Ca^{2+} but with different sensitivities. PKa is active at the concentration of Ca^{2+} prevailing in resting muscle (0.1 μM), whereas PKb requires a higher Ca^{2+} concentration, similar to that found in contracting muscle, for activity. The Ca^{2+} sensitivity of PK*b* is influenced by the concentration of H^+ (160), glycogen (160), and troponin (49). Increases in pH and glycogen will increase the sensitivity (i.e., for a given Ca^{2+} concentration, the activity of PKb will be higher). Protein phosphatase (PP) catalyzes the dephosphorylation of GP*a* and PKa to the less active forms GPb and PKb. Phosphorylation of one site of PP by cAMP-dependent protein kinase inhibits the enzyme, whereas phosphorylation of another site by insulin-dependent protein kinase (49) activates the enzyme.

The cAMP-mediated conversion of PKb to PK*a* provides a link between circulating epinephrine and glycogenolysis, whereas activation of PKb by Ca^{2+} couples glycogenolysis during exercise to the contraction process (70, 90). The exercise-induced increase in GPa is only transient, and within some minutes of exercise GPa is converted back to or below the initial level (6, 44, 51). The regulatory mechanisms underlying reconversion of GPa to GPb during exercise are not fully understood. Suggested mechanisms are: release of phosphorylase from the glycogen-protein-SR complex when glycogen is degraded (92), increases in G6P which affect the converter enzymes (for references, see 6), or decrease in pH which would decrease the activity of PKb (160). However, the blunting of GPa formation is independent of the degree of glycogen depletion and persists for 25 min after cessation of exercise (66) at which time both G6P and pH are expected to be restored to basal levels. Thus, additional unknown mechanisms are likely to be involved in the reversal of GP*a* transformation.

Allosteric Control. The activity of GPb is sensitive to several allosteric modulators, of which adensine monophosphate (AMP) and inosine monophosphate (IMP) are activators and ADP, ATP, and G6P are inhibitors. GPb activity is dependent on the relative

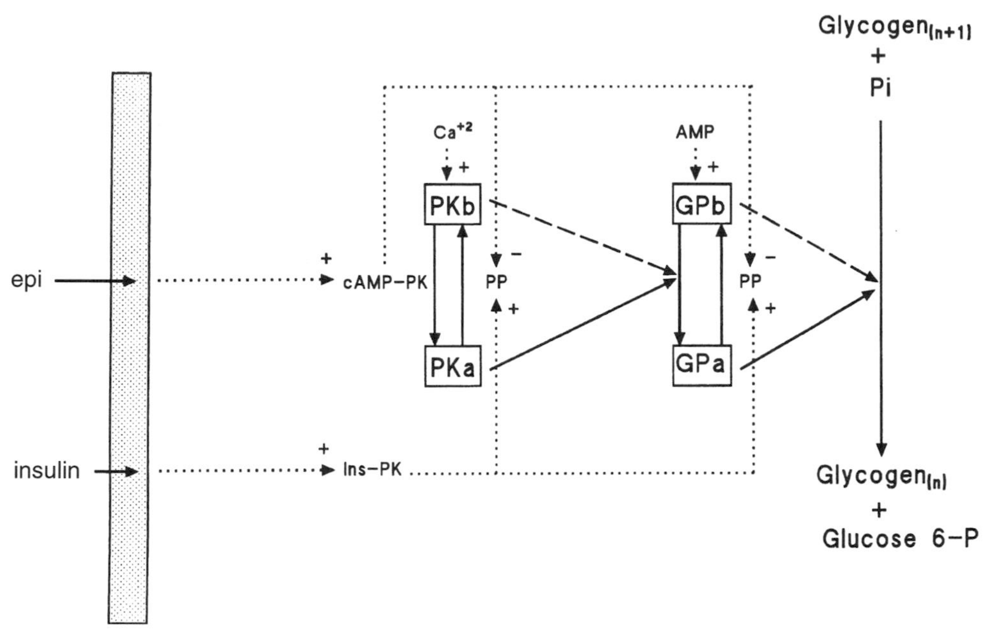

FIG. 19.3. Control of glycogenolysis by phosphorylation/dephosphorylation of glycogen phosphorylase. cAMP-PK, cAMP-dependent protein kinase; Epi, epinephrine; Ins-PK, insulin-dependent protein kinase; PKb, unphosphorylated protein kinase; PKa, phosphorylated protein kinase; PP, protein phosphatase; GPa, glycogen phosphorylase *a*; GPb, glycogen phosphorylase *b*. *Filled arrows* denote enzymatic reaction or connect active enzyme with catalyzed reaction. *Dashed arrows* connect enzyme, which can be active under some conditions with catalyzed reaction. *Dotted arrows* denote activation (+) or inhibition (-) of indicated enzyme. All substrates and products in metabolic reactions are not shown.

concentration of the allosteric modulators, and the sensitivity for each factor is dependent on the concentration of other allosteric factors, substrates (Pi and glycogen), and product (G1P). Models describing GP activity will therefore be complex. When the AMP level increases sufficiently the inhibition of GPb by G6P, ATP, and ADP is overcome and GPb becomes active. The effect of AMP appears to be mediated by an increased sensitivity of GPb for Pi (41, 44, 188, 213). The K_a of GPb for AMP is between 0.05 and 0.9 mM, depending on the concentration of the other modulators (6, 119, 172, 188, 269). In the absence of G6P, K_a is 0.05 mM and in the presence of 20 mM G6P K_a is 0.7 mM (269). However, studies in human muscle extracts have shown that the affinity of GP to Pi is considerably increased at 0.01 mM AMP (213). The total concentration of AMP (determined by chemical methods) is about 0.03 mM in relaxed muscle and increases threefold during maximal exercise. For a discussion of the potential role of AMP as a regulator of GP see later under CARBOHYDRATE UTILIZATION AT REST AND DURING EXERCISE. GPb is inhibited by ATP [K_i = 2 mM (188)] and G6P [K_i = 0.3 mM (189)]. Since the in vivo concentrations of ATP and G6P are above or within this region, the inhibition is likely to be of physiological importance.

GPa is active in the absence of AMP, but the activity is augmented by low concentrations of AMP (K_a <5 μM) (6, 169) and by IMP at 50 times higher concentrations (6). The other allosteric modulators of GPb have only a minor influence on GPa activity (188).

Substrate Control. Reported K_m values for glycogen are 1–2 mM (32), 1–14 mM [or 0.05–0.8 mM glycosylic end groups (188)] or less than 0.3 mM (GPa) (170). The concentration of glycogen in resting muscle is about 100 mM and GP is thus under most conditions saturated with glycogen. However, since muscle glycogen is stored in the form of glycogen particles (protein-glycogen complex), it is uncertain whether in vitro determined K_m reflects the conditions in vivo.

Studies of human muscle homogenates have shown that in the absence of AMP the K_m value of GPa for Pi is 27 mM and in the presence of 2 mM AMP K_m for both GPa and GPb is 7 mM (44). Further studies (213) showed that an increase in AMP to 0.01 mM is sufficient to decrease the K_m value from 27 mM to 12 mM in control muscles and to 6 mM after treatment with epinephrine (i.e., most of GP in the GPa form). The in vivo concentration of Pi changes from 1 mM at rest to about 20 mM after heavy exercise and changes in Pi are therefore of major physiological importance for in vivo control of GP activity (see later under CARBOHYDRATE UTILIZATION AT REST AND DURING EXERCISE).

Control of GS

The control of GS has been reviewed in detail (48, 49, 163). GS exists in two interconvertible forms (Fig. 19.4): one less active (GSd) and dependent on G6P concentration and one more active (GSi) and independent of G6P under physiological conditions. Interconversion between the two forms is, as for GP, controlled by phosphorylation-dephosphorylation reactions. In contrast to GP, the phosphorylated form of GS (GSd) is the less active form of the enzyme. GSi can be phosphorylated at more than ten sites (218) and thus several intermediary forms of GS exist. The activity of GS is usually expressed as the fractional activity of GSi; that is, GSi/(GSi + GSd), where GSi is the activity in the absence of G6P and GSi + GSd is the activity at saturating concentrations of G6P and UDP-glucose. The intermediary forms of GS exhibit different sensitivities towards G6P and measurements of GSi and GSi + GSd will therefore only represent an average value for the phosphorylation state of GS and will not reveal the whole diversity of the system control. Alternative methods have therefore been developed where the sensitivity of GS for G6P is determined at a lower, more physiological concentration of UDP-glucose (120, 156).

GS and the interconverting enzymes are bound to the glycogen particle in a glycogen-protein complex. The enzymes involved in interconversion of GS are to a large extent identical to those involved in GP interconversion. Thus, phosphorylation of GS is catalyzed by several kinases including cAMP-dependent protein kinase and Ca^{2+}-dependent kinase PK*b*. Furthermore, as for GP, dephosphorylation of GS is catalyzed by PP, which is activated by insulin and inhibited by epinephrine (49). GS can also be dephosphorylated by phosphatases other than PP (48). The percentage of GS present as GSi is inversely proportional to the glycogen content (20, 77). The relationship is generally considered to be an effect of glycogen on the converter enzymes where high glycogen inhibits the dephosphorylation of GS (26) and activates phosphorylation of GS (160). However, later studies with more purified systems have failed to detect these effects of glycogen concentration on the converter enzymes (for references, see 48). Dephosphorylation of GSd to GSi is stimulated by physiological concentrations of G6P, and the mechanism is considered to be binding of G6P to GSd and subsequent configuration change of the enzyme thus enhancing the activity of phosphatase (265).

Allosteric and Substrate Control. The phosphorylated form, GS*d*, is activated by G6P and the major effect is an increase in V_{max} (163, 222). There are a number of potent allosteric inhibitors of GS*d* (ATP, ADP, AMP, and UDP), and the enzyme is considered to be inactive in vivo under most physiological conditions. The unphosphorylated form of GS (GSi) remains ac-

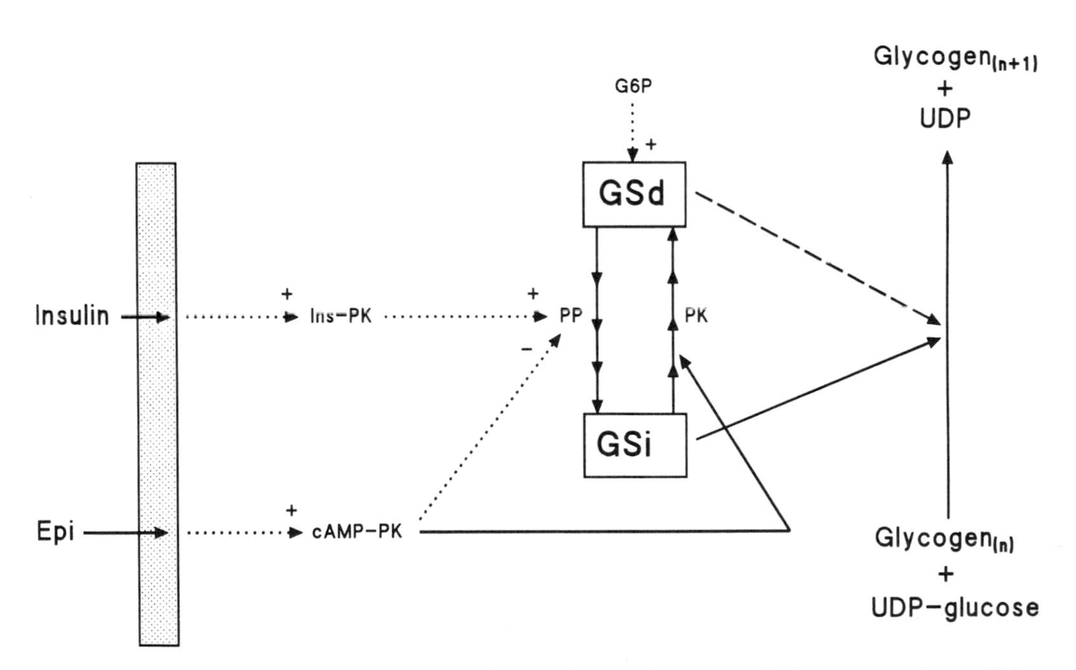

FIG. 19.4. Control of glycogen synthesis by covalent modification of glycogen synthase. GSd, phosphorylated glycogen synthase (G6P dependent form); GSi, unphosphorylated glycogen synthase; PK, Ca^{2+}-dependent and other protein kinases; G6P, glucose 6-phosphate. See legend of Figure 19.3 for further details.

tive at low G6P levels, and increases in G6P will decrease the K_m for UDP-glucose (163, 222). The different intermediary phosphorylated forms of GS exhibit different sensitivities to G6P and the concentration of G6P required to achieve 50% of maximum activity varies from 0.2 mM to 1.8 mM (191). Since the concentration of G6P in human muscle varies between 0.3 mM in resting muscle to about 3 mM after maximal exercise, it is clear that G6P will be an important parameter for control of GS activity in vivo.

The K_m for UDP-glucose in rat skeletal muscle varies between 0.2 and 1.0 mM and is dependent both on the phosphorylation state of GS and on the level of G6P (163, 222). In rat skeletal muscle the concentration of UDP-glucose (0.03 mM) is far below the K_m value (238), whereas the concentration in relaxed human skeletal muscle is higher (~0.3 mM) (209). Since UDP-glucose concentration is lower or within the range of the K_m, it seems likely that changes in UDP-glucose concentration and G6P (which both may be influenced by glucose transport) will play a role for the rate of glycogen synthesis.

Integrated Control of GP and GS During Exercise

The various factors of importance for control of glycogen metabolism during exercise are schematically depicted in Figure 19.5. The system will adequately respond to increased energy demand during exercise by mobilizing glycogen. The control will be exerted both by feedforward control (covalent control of both GP and GS by increases in Ca^{2+} and adrenaline) and by feedback activation of GP (increases in AMP and Pi). Modulation of the glycogenolytic response will be achieved by product concentration (G6P and lactic acid through changes in H^+). The concentration of glycogen will in itself affect the metabolism, and high glycogen will promote glycogen degradation and retard glycogen synthesis. The maximal activity of GP is much higher than that for GS (tenfold higher in human skeletal muscle) and is related to the requirement of high rates of fuel mobilization during exercise. Phosphorylation of GP will activate glycogenolysis, whereas phosphorylation of GS will inhibit glycogen synthesis. Thus, the system is arranged in a way that will minimize simultaneous degradation and buildup of glycogen.

OTHER SPECIFIC GLYCOLYTIC ENZYME CONTROLS

Figure 19.6 illustrates the steps in the glycolytic pathway between glucose 1-phosphate and lactate. Most of the individual glycolytic enzymes have been well studied. The contribution of each to the overall operation of the pathway has been postulated, but a detailed accounting for the changes in flux during exercise has not been done. The maximal capacity (V_{max}) of most of the enzymes in the pathway is much higher than documented flux through the pathway (10–15 μmol · g wet^{-1} · min^{-1}); see Table 19.1). Thus, it has been postulated that near-equilibrium conditions operate throughout much of the pathway except for well-defined allosterically controlled steps. The content of the glycolytic enzymes in the cell appear to be regulated in a coordinated manner so that the relative capacity of the individual steps in the pathway is always the same even though the total throughput capacity can vary over a wide range (202, 249). This means that a model describing the kinetic behavior of the pathway will only need scaling to be transferred from red slow muscle fibers with low glycolytic capacity to fast white fibers with a very high glycolytic capacity. That is, coordinated control of the individual steps in the pathway may be universal.

There are two clear allosteric control points (glycogen phosphorylase, discussed above, and phosphofructokinase) that probably dominate the control of flux through the glycolytic pathway. The kinetic operation of several other steps in the pathway can contribute to the overall rate of production of ATP, reducing equivalents, and pyruvate and/or lactate. Three enzymes have a very high V_{max} and appear to always be essentially at equilibrium, even at high glycolytic fluxes.

Equilibrium Group

1. Phosphoglucomutase, which catalyzes the reaction:

Glucose 1-phosphate (G1P)

$\leftrightarrow$ glucose 6-phosphate (G6P)

It has a catalytic requirement for glucose 1,6-bisphosphate. This latter compound appears to be tightly bound to the enzyme and a role in glycolytic control at this step has not been documented. The equilibrium at this point (17:1 in favor of G6P) helps maintain glycolytic flux via glycogen phosphorylase.

2. Glucose isomerase (Fig. 19.6, 2), which catalyzes the reaction:

Glucose 6-phosphate (G6P)

$\leftrightarrow$ fructose 6-phosphate (F6P)

The equilibrium constant is ~0.3 (145). Although there are some studies suggesting that this reaction

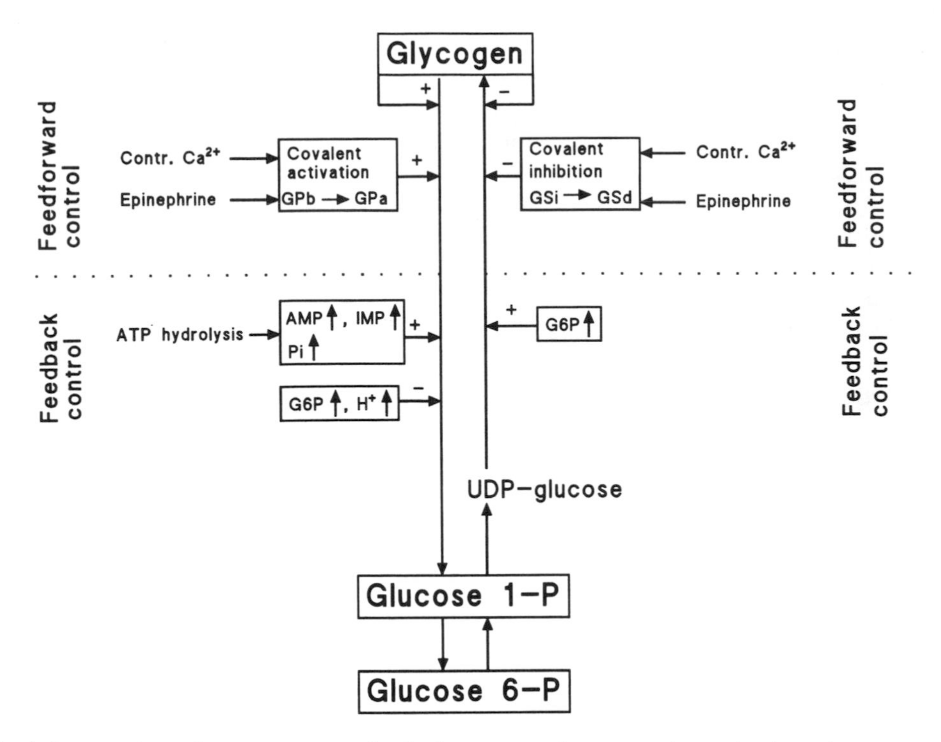

FIG. 19.5. Control of glycogenolysis during exercise. The feedback inhibition of GP by increases in H^+ may involve both reduced covalent activation of GP, decreased availability of active substrate (HPO_4^{2-}), and allosteric inhibition of Gpb by increases in G6P occurring secondary to inhibition of PFK. See text for further details. cAMP-Pk, cAMP-dependent protein kinase; Epi, epinephrine; Ins-Pk, insulin-dependent protein kinase; PP, protein phosphatase; GPa, glycogen phosphorylase *a*; GPb, glycogen phos-phorylase *b*; Pkb, unphosphorylated protein kinase; Pka, phosphorylated protein kinase; Gsd, phosphorylated glycogen synthase; GSi, unphosphorylated gycogen synthase; Pk, Ca^{2+}-dependent and other protein kinase si GGP, glucose G-phosphate.

may deviate from equilibrium during very rapid glycolytic flux, most data under physiological conditions support an essentially equilibrium state for this reaction in vivo. This step connects control of the production of G6P via glycogen phosphorylase or glucose transport and hexokinase to the availability of substrate for phosphofructokinase.

3. Triosephosphate isomerase (Fig 19.6, *5*) which catalyzes the reaction:

Glyceraldehyde 3-phosphate (GAP)
↔ dihydroxyacetonephosphate (DHAP)

Triosephosphate isomerase has the highest capacity of all the enzymes in the glycolytic pathway and is thought to always be near equilibrium. The equilibrium constant of the reaction in vitro is 20 in favor of DHAP (263). There is considerable evidence that under in vivo conditions it may be shifted to 12 (57, 259).

Phosphofructokinase

Phosphofructokinase (PFK) (Fig 19.6, *3*) has long been known to be a major regulatory point for glycolysis. It was one of the first allosteric enzymes identified and thus one of the most intensively studied. Despite the considerable energy spent on study there is still controversy over the control of this enzyme activity in vivo. It catalyzes the reaction:

Fructose 6-phosphate (F6P) + ATP
→ fructose 1,6-bisphosphate (F16P) + ADP

Kinetics. The activity in vitro responds to a number of ligands (see Table 19.2). The active enzyme appears to be a tetramer that easily dissociates into a relatively inactive dimer. The equilibrium between the dimer and tetramer depends on the protonation of the proteins and thus the pK of the enzyme (see below). In the absence of other modulators, the enzyme shows near maximal activity at pH >8.0 and has progressively lower activity as the pH falls. The effect of many of the allosteric modulators is to affect the position of the equilibrium between the dimer and tetramer. Because the enzyme is relatively unstable in the dilute solutions normally used for assay, much of the kinetic information is not useful for quantitative analysis of the behavior of the enzyme in vivo, where protein concentrations are high and interaction with other proteins is possible (e.g.,

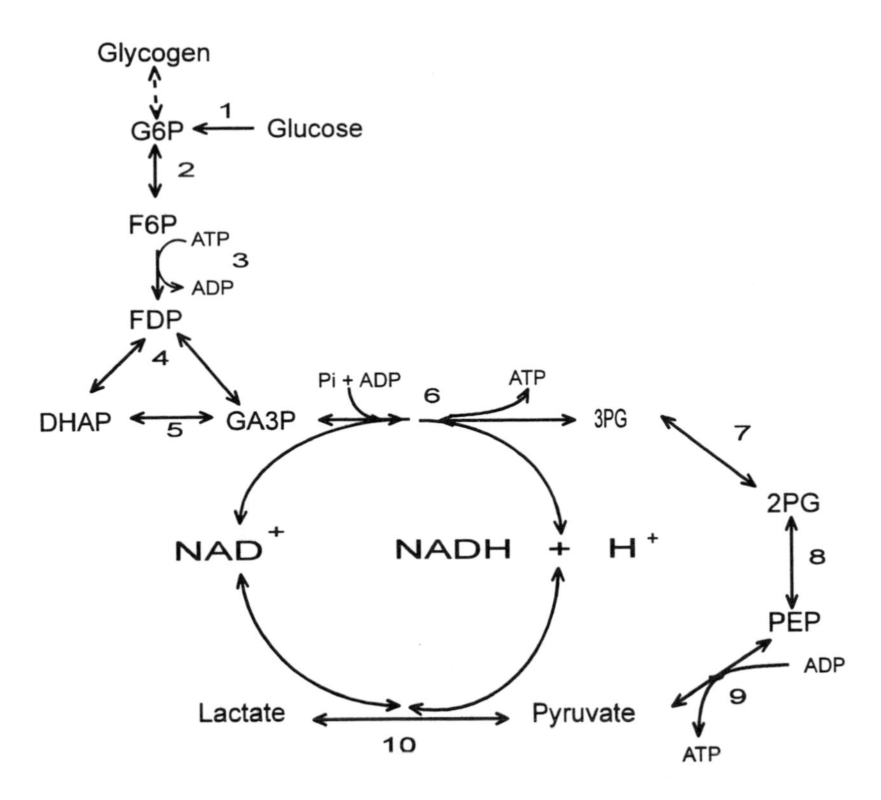

FIG. 19.6. Outline of the glycolytic pathway from G6P to lactate. *Solid lines* show reactions. *Dashed line* indicates pathways included in Figure 19.2. G6P, glucose 6-phosphate; F6P, fructose 6-phosphate; FDP, fructose 1,6-bisphosphate; DHAP, dihydroxyacetone phosphate; GA3P, glyceraldehyde 3-phosphate; 3PG, 3-phosphoglycerate; 2PG, 2-phosphoglycerate; PEP, phosphoenolpyruvate. Numbers refer to enzymes: *1*, hexokinase; *2*, phosphoglucoisomerase; *3*, phosphofructokinase (PFK); *4*, aldolase; *5*, triosephosphate isomerase; *6*, combined glyceraldehyde phosphate dehydrogenase (GAPDH) and phosphoglycerate kinase (PGK) steps; *7*, phosphoglycerate mutase; *8*, enolase; *9*, pyruvate kinase; *10*, lactate dehydrogenase (LDH).

TABLE 19.1. *Reported V_{max} for Glycolytic Enzymes in Human Vastus Muscles*

	Estimated V_{max} U · g^{-1} wet · min^{-1} @ 37 °C*		
Enzymes	Mixed Fibers†	Type I‡	Type II
Phosphoglucomutase	64.5 (27)		
Hexokinase	3.0 (25, 239), 7 (192)		
Hexoseisomerase	209 (27)		
Phosphofructokinase	38 (27), 63 (25, 142, 201), 126 (239)	7	21
Aldolase	72 (27, 201)		
Triosephosphate isomerase	431 (27, 201)		
Glyceraldehydephosphate dehydrogenase	250–300 (15, 27, 201), 502 (192)	56	174
Phosphoglycerate kinase	281 (27, 201)		
Phosphoglycerate mutase	545 (27)		
Enolase	146–170 (27, 123)		
Pyruvate kinase	183 (27)	70	244
Lactate dehydrogenase	109 (15), 340–378 (27, 192, 201, 239)	35	349
Creatine kinase	609 (239)	174	174
Adenylate kinase		14	140
Glycerolphosphate dehydrogenase	11 (192)	6	17

*Used Q_{10} = 2.0 and 1 g dry = 4.3 g wet to normalize values. †Numbers in parentheses represent references. ‡Based on analysis of single fibers (169).

TABLE 19.2. *Ligand Binding to Phosphofructokinase*

Name of Site	Ligand and Order of Binding Affinities
ATP (catalytic)	MgATP
Fructose 6-phospate (catalytic)	F6P > sedoheptulose 7-P >> F1P, G1P
ATP (inhibitory)	ATPH > ATP > MgATP >> MgADP
Adenine nucleotide (activating)	cAMP > AMP > ADP > ADPR > NAD, NADH, NADP, NADPH, ATP
Other binding (activating)	Pi > F2,6-P_2 > F1,6-P_2 > G1,6-P_2
Other binding (inhibitory)	citrate > 3-P-glycerate > PEP H^+

26). This protein–protein interaction seems to stabilize the tetrameric form and significantly change the quantitative response to modulators. In addition, much of the data have been collected in buffers containing unphysiologically high levels of phosphate. This compound stabilizes the enzyme and appears to act as an allosteric modulator. As a result, much of the kinetic analysis is of limited value for understanding control of PFK activity in vivo. There are a number of studies that have focused on the number and specificity of binding sites of the protomers that make up the tetrameric form. These are useful in identifying potential modulators. There appear to be four interacting sites per protomer (203):

1. A site specific for AMP, cAMP, and ADP that is an activating site. The affinity of this site appears to depend primarily on the presence of the adenine and phosphoribose structure. Thus adenosine diphosphoribose, nicotinamide-adenine dinucleotide (NAD), reduced form of NAD (NADH), nicotinamide-adenine-dinucleotide phosphate (NADP, and reduced form of NADP (NADPH) can bind to this site. They are not activators but block the effect of AMP or cAMP binding. The affinities are on the order of 0.5–50 μM (110). Binding to this site appears to decrease the affinity for the protonated form of ATP (ATPH) at the inhibitory site, stabilizes the active form of the enzyme, and decreases the pK of the enzyme. Thus, binding of modulators like AMP not only activate the enzyme but decrease the inhibitory effect of lower pH.

2. A site specific for ATP that may be dominated by binding of the ATPH. This is an inhibitory site. Binding increases the pK, thus increasing the inhibitory effect of pH <8.0 and decreases the affinity for nucleotide binding at the activating site. At pH >8.0 in the absence of other modulators the affinity at this site is ~0.1 μM. In vivo levels of ATPH are on this order of magnitude and vary significantly with changes in both H^+ and Mg^{2+} concentrations.

3. A substrate site relatively specific for MgATP. The affinity for this site in the absence of other modulators and at pH >8.0 is 79–200 μM depending on the level of F6P and hence order of binding (see below). At in vivo levels of ATP this site should remain saturated.

4. Another substrate site relatively specific for F6P. The affinity at this site varies from ~50 μM to 500 μM, which is within the range of observed concentrations in vivo at rest and during exercise. F6P concentration will depend on the level of glycogenolytic flux and will determine the order of substrate binding and thus the kinetic pattern of PFK independent of other modulators (see below).

The sites for binding of hexose bisphosphates, citrate, and ammonium ion are not well defined. There is evidence that these ligands are only active in the presence of ATP inhibition. That is, citrate enhances binding to the inhibitory site, while Pi and the hexosebisphosphates decrease the affinity for binding at this site (26). While there is some indication in the kinetic analyses that HPO_4^{-2} rather than $H_2PO_4^-$ is the active form, the currently available data are insufficent to resolve this issue. The enzyme appears to interact with calmodulin, opening the possibility of a Ca^{2+}-dependent control mechanism. The effects are not large and there is some question as to whether this interaction is related to the strong propensity of PFK to interact with other proteins, especially in dilute solution. Separation of this effect in vivo would be very difficult, since shifts in Ca^{2+} levels in muscle are always associated with changes in pH and the adenine nucleotides. These latter changes have a much larger quantitative effect on PFK activity than the demonstrated calmodulin effects.

In addition to other ligands, PFK activity is very sensitive to pH, with the protonated form having less activity. The pK for protonation is interactive with binding at most of the sites, with the highest sensitivity to binding at sites 1 and 2 (203). Thus, the pK of the enzyme and the K_m's for substrates are interdependent. To complete the complications, the mechanism of substrate binding and reaction may be a random-order mechanism that leads to sigmoidal kinetics for one substrate (F6P) and substrate inhibition for the other substrate (MgATP) independent of allosteric and enzyme dissociation effects (12, 122). In spite of the complicated kinetic interactions, models of PFK kinetics have been made and used to see if our current state of knowledge accounts for the observed changes in glycolytic flux in skeletal muscle. Initial attempts led to the conclusion that glycolysis could not occur at pH values near 7.0 and below. With increasingly sophisticated models that include the binding interactions and the levels of all ligands expected under physiological conditions, it is clear that PFK flux will be significant under these acid conditons. Transitions in flux during muscle activation are also accurately predicted in terms of direction and timing, although not quantitatively (see discussion of exercise, below) (56, 88, 245). These changes in flux reflect the coordinated effects of ATP, ADP, AMP, Pi, and pH as well as the substrate F6P, and cannot be accounted for by changes in any single variable. This is discussed further under INTEGRATIVE ASPECTS OF GLYCOLYTIC CONTROL AND FUTURE DIRECTIONS (R. CONNETT).

Studies of cell-free glycolyzing systems from heart, skeletal muscle, or yeast, as well as kinetic model analysis led to the conclusion that primary control resides in the energy state as reflected in the adenine nucleotides (56, 101, 157, 190, 260). With the discovery of the effects of citrate and the hexose bisphosphates and the realization that in heart and skeletal muscle the adenine nucleotide levels are quite stable due to the buffering effects of creatine kinase and phosphocreatine, it was suggested that control is independent of the adenine nucleotides under normal physiological conditions. These concerns have led to a situation where one study in 1987 on heart (165) was interpreted as indicating that fructose 2,6-bisphosphate had a permissive action, but control rested with the adenine nucleotides; another study (28) concluded that control rested in the activator fructose 2,6-bisphosphate and the substrate (F6P) and not in citrate or the adenine nucleotides. The effect of citrate has been cited as responsible for the inhibition of glycolysis in heart when the tissue is metabolizing fatty acids (197). This fatty acid inhibition is not universally seen (e.g., 153, 271). Concerns have been raised that all conclusions were based on whole tissue citrate concentrations and we do not have any solid data on the distribution between the mitochondrial and cytosolic compartments. PFK may "see" no citrate concentration changes. It is generally agreed that in vivo the activation of glycolysis and PFK must be related in some fashion to the match between energy supply and demand or, in other words, to the "energy state" of the tissue. It has been argued that the observed changes in known effectors are insufficient to account for the glycolytic flux (81, 185, 186, 207, 216) and the trigger is unknown. There may be signals related to the substrate supply in the mitochondrion, such as redox (59, 157). It is generally agreed that concerted action by several effectors is required to account for the observed activity in working muscles (55, 88, 157, 203, 256, 272). The quantitative responses to all known effectors have not been accurately modeled, and other "unknown" signals may contribute to the control of PFK kinetics in vivo.

Aldolase

Aldolase (Fig 19.6, *4*) is a well-studied enzyme with defined kinetic constants. It catalyzes the reaction after PFK in the pathway:

Fructose 1,6-bisphosphate
$\leftrightarrow$ dihydroxyacetonephosphate
+ glyceraldehyde 3 phosphate

It does not appear to have significant allosteric kinetic effects. The substrate for the reaction appears to be the β-anomeric and/or the acyclic form of F16P (183, 220). At equilibrium in free solution without Mg^{2+} the β-form accounts for ~80% of the total F16P and the acyclic form 2%. The anomeric equilibrium is sensitive to pH and Mg^{2+} and lowered pH and elevated Mg^{2+} would tend to raise the concentration of the β-anomer and slow the interconversion. Thus the in vivo fraction of the β-anomer might be expected to be lower than 80%. However, PFK appears to produce the β-anomer exclusively (220). Aldolase does associate with PFK in vitro. The kinetic effects of this association seem to be some slowing of the PFK reaction and perhaps an increase in the throughput from F6P to triosephosphates (30). This might reflect an effect of the substrate anomerization. There are a number of studies suggesting that in vivo observations cannot be accounted for simply by kinetic calculations based on measured substrate and product concentrations and kinetic constants determined in vitro. These can be grouped into two observations: equilibrium measurements and modeling studies. Mass-action ratios ([GA3P][DHAP]/[F16P]) are relatively constant in vivo, suggesting a near-equilibrium condition. However, the ratio is ~50 times smaller than the measured equilibrium in vitro (57). This is the opposite direction expected from a flux-limited approach to equilibrium but is consistent with a change in the anomer distribution toward more of the active substrate. When glycolysis is blocked, the ratio approaches the equilibrium value measured in vitro (57). Again, this is consistent with an anomer redistribution. Attempts to account for glycolytic fluxes using kinetic models have consistently failed unless aldolase flux is coupled to PFK flux rather than to the measured F16P concentrations (2). Thus, it appears that there is a strong kinetic interaction between PFK and aldolase. The mechanism is currently unknown, but current information suggests the anomer distribution of F16P, enzyme–enzyme interaction, or some combination of both effects might account for the observations.

Glyceraldehydephosphate Dehydrogenase and Phosphoglycerate Kinase (PGK)

These enzymes (Fig 19.6, *6*) catalyze the reactions involved in the first production of ATP in the glycolytic pathway:

$$\text{Glyceraldehyde 3-phosphate} + \text{Pi} + \text{NAD}^+ \leftrightarrow \text{1,3-diphosphoglycerate} + \text{NADH} + \text{H}^+ \quad (1)$$

$$\text{1,3 diphosphoglycerate} + \text{ADP} \leftrightarrow \text{3-phosphoglycerate} + \text{ATP} \quad (2)$$

The kinetics of the two enzymes have been well studied in vitro. The activities of the two enzymes in skeletal muscle are very similar and are much higher than the glycolytic flux. A number of studies have suggested that the combined reaction is near equilibrium in vivo, and the value of the mass action ratio is consistent with the equilibrium constant measured in vitro (57, 71). Attempts to model glycolytic flux using measured substrate concentrations indicate that the measured 1,3-glycerate phosphate levels are too low by at least an order of magnitude to account for the observed fluxes. It has been suggested that these two enzymes physically associate so that this intermediate is channeled between them (249), and the free concentration does not reflect the value "seen" by PGK (249). Although this interpretation has been questioned (31), the mass action studies suggest a close kinetic association and maintenance of near-equilibrium conditions. Studies on enzyme binding suggest that any interaction of these enzymes with each other or with the contractile machinery increases the flux through these steps. This in turn would help promote a near-equilibrium condition.

The combined GAPDH-PGK step is a critical point in the pathway. It is at this point that the phosphorylation state and the redox state of the cytosol interacts with the glycolytic pathway and each other. As discussed in the following section, the next two steps along the pathway appear to be almost entirely governed by mass-action considerations. That is, the delivery of substrate to them determines the ultimate rate of the glycolytic flux as well as ATP and pyruvate production. If The GAPDH-PGK steps are maintained near equilibrium, the phosphorylation and redox states of the cytosol will set the level of 3-phosphoglycerate and hence the flux through the rest of the pathway.

Phosphoglycerate Mutase and Enolase

$$\text{3-Phosphoglycerate} \leftrightarrow \text{2-phosphoglycerate} \quad (3)$$

$$\text{2-Phosphoglycerate} \leftrightarrow \text{2-phosphoenolpyruvate} \quad (4)$$

In most analyses of glycolytic flux, phosphoglycerate mutase (Fig. 19.6, *7*) and enolase (Fig. 19.6, *8*) are treated as being essentially at equilibrium. Their activity levels are high relative to the glycolytic flux. However, phosphoglycerate mutase has a very high K_m under in vivo conditions (1–5 mM), leading to operation at a small fraction of V_{max} (118, 221). Thus, any sharp transition in flux above this step should result in a transient disequilibrium and a lag until the 3-phosphoglycerate levels could increase adequately to match the flux. The lag would help promote equilibrium at the GAPDH-PGK step. The mutase disequilibrium has been observed during rest-work transitions in dog gracilis muscles in situ (54). A lag (phase shift) at this level that forces the adenine nucleotide and redox changes to be out of phase has also been observed in oscillating glycolytic systems (101).

Pyruvate Kinase

Pyruvate kinase (Fig. 19.6, *9*) catalyzes the reaction:

$$\text{Phosphoenolpyruvate (PEP)} + \text{ADP} \rightarrow \text{ATP} + \text{pyruvate (PYR)}$$

Both divalent (Mg^{2+}) and monovalent (K^+) cations are required for this reaction (180). There are several isozymes found in the body and all appear to be tetrameric and can form hybrids with each other (35, 36, 86). The liver form (L) shows sigmoidal kinetics with PEP and an allosteric activation by F16P and inhibition by ATP and alanine. These compounds have no effect on the muscle (M1) isozyme found in skeletal muscle and heart. Kinetic studies show hyperbolic kinetics with respect to both substrates and reversibility with high concentrations of ATP and pyruvate and very low concentrations of PEP (86, 91, 180). A pH-sensitive allosteric inhibition of the muscle enzyme has been demonstrated with phenylalanine (65). While this probably does not have a physiological role, it does indicate the possibility of an unknown allosteric modulator. The reaction appears to be far from equilibrium in vivo and flux should therefore be dominated by the concentrations of the substrates, ADP and PEP. Attempts to model glycolytic flux in heart required some activation related to the phosphorylation state of the tissue to be present in order to account for the data (1). Although a phosphorylation state-dependent control of the PEP level as discussed in above may account for this observation, there does appear to be some uncertainty about the mechanism regulating flux through this enzyme in vivo.

Lactate Dehydrogenase

Lactate dehydrogenase (LDH) (Fig. 19.6, *10*) catalyzes the reaction:

$$\text{Pyruvate (PYR)} + \text{NADH} + \text{H}^+ \leftrightarrow \text{lactate (LAC)} + \text{NAD}^+$$

There are several isozymes of LDH found in the body. All forms appear as tetramers, and the subunits will randomly associate. Heart and skeletal muscle have the most kinetically extreme isozymes (H and M1 forms, respectively). While the heart form is inhibited by pyruvate, the muscle form shows simple hyperbolic kinetics in both directions and will rapidly reduce pyruvate. All types of muscle have a high capacity of LDH relative to the overall glycolytic flux, and this enzyme is thought to be at equilibrium with the cytosolic redox. That this equilibrium occurs in the glycolytic pathway is reinforced by the observation that GAPDH and LDH react with the opposite sides of the nucleotide and can associate and directly transfer the nucleotide substrate (250). Although the direct transfer conclusion has been called into question (31), it is clear that there is a potential for rapid equilibrium between the glycolytic dehydrogenases and the cytosolic NAD/NADH pools. Because of this equilibrium, lactate/pyruvate ratios provide a good method for estimating the redox state of the cytosol ($[\text{NADH}][\text{H}^+]/[\text{NAD}^+]$), especially as it affects glycolysis.

CARBOHYDRATE UTILIZATION AT REST AND DURING EXERCISE

Diurnal Variations of Body Stores at Rest

Liver glycogen is used primarily for maintaining a stable blood glucose value. This is accomplished by the presence of glucose 6-phosphatase, which catalyzes the conversion of G6P to glucose, a high intracellular glucose level similar to that in blood and a high gluconeogenic capacity. In line with its function as a controller of the blood glucose level, liver glycogen demonstrates large diurnal variations and a high dependence on dietary CHO. After a 24 h fast, liver glycogen is almost completely depleted (121) and maintenance of stable blood glucose is then dependent on gluconeogenesis and a down-regulation of whole-body glucose utilization.

Muscle glycogen concentration in the postprandial state is lower than in the liver, but due to the large amount of muscle tissue, more than 80% of total CHO is located in skeletal muscle. In contrast to the liver, muscle glycogen cannot be released to blood as glucose. This is due to the absence of glucose 6-phosphatase in skeletal muscle and to the fact that the intracellular concentration of glucose is lower than in the extracellular space. Intracellular glucose in relaxed muscle is less than 0.3 mM but increases during intense exercise, mainly due to an increased uptake from the blood (147). Although muscle glucose levels of about 2.8 mM have been observed after maximal dynamic exercise (147), it is still considerably lower than plasma glucose (4–6 mmol/liter). Thus, although a small part of glycogen can be transformed to glucose by the debranching enzyme, a net release of glucose to blood is unlikely to be of physiological significance.

There is no major difference in glycogen content between human muscle fibers at rest (95). Glycogen content in human skeletal muscle at rest shows only small diurnal variations (134) and is influenced to a small extent by dietary intake of CHO. Total starvation for 3 and 4 days decreased muscle glycogen by 15% (38) and 40% (135), respectively, and another 5 days of CHO-rich diet restored muscle glycogen to the basal level (135). Basal glycogen content in rodent skeletal muscle is much lower than that in humans and shows more pronounced diurnal variations. This may have implications for the control of CHO metabolism, and extrapolations from studies in rodents to humans may not always be relevant.

CHO Utilization during Exercise

Methodological Considerations. Lactate accumulation is often taken as an index of increased glycolysis. In a closed system (circulatory occlusion and/or sustained isometric contraction) the rate of lactate formation is approximately equal to the rate of glycolysis, since accumulation of other glycolytic intermediates are small and pyruvate oxidation is negligible. Glycolytic and glycogenolytic rates can then be estimated from accumulation of lactate, pyruvate and G6P (glycogenolysis). Measurements in humans demonstrate that the rate of muscle lactate accumulation and thus the glycolytic rate is linearly related to the contraction force during sustained isometric contraction (4), with a maximal rate of glycogenolysis of 45 mmol · kg dry^{-1} · min^{-1}.

In an open system (dynamic exercise), large increases in glycolysis can occur without lactate accumulation (Fig. 19.7). For instance, during exercise at 40% of $\dot{V}O_{2max}$ the rate of lactate formation is negligible, but the glycolytic flux increases 20- to 30-fold over that at rest, and nearly all of the formed pyruvate is oxidized. Increases in muscle and blood lactate may therefore be related to, but are not measures of, glycolysis. In an open system the rate of glycolysis during steady state can be quantified by measurements of changes in muscle glycogen and muscle glucose uptake. Total body CHO oxidation can be derived from measurements of the respiratory exchange ratio (RER = CO_2 produced/O_2 consumed) and $\dot{V}O_2$. RER is a valid measure of relative CHO and fat oxidation under steady-state submaximal exercise when expired CO_2 equals CO_2 formation in mitochondria, but the method can give erroneous data during high-intensity exercise or when some of the expired CO_2 is derived from decreases in the CO_2 stores due to hyperventilation or acidosis.

Influence of Workload on CHO Utilization. Measurements of RER give evidence that the relative contribution of CHO to total fuel oxidation increases in relation to workload and that at high exercise intensities nearly all substrate oxidation is derived from CHO (9, 47).

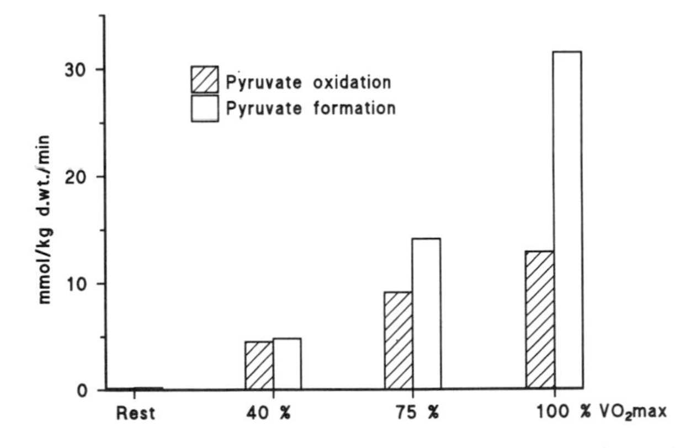

FIG. 19.7. Rate of pyruvate formation and pyruvate oxidation in muscle at rest and during exercise in muscle at different workloads. Rate of pyruvate oxidation was calculated from O_2 consumption and estimated or measured respiratory exchange ratio. Rate of pyruvate production was calculated from the accumulation in muscle of lactate, pyruvate, alanine, and acetylcarnitine + release of lactate + rate of pyruvate oxidation. (Data are from 147, 232, 233.)

With the needle biopsy technique introduced by Bergström (16), consecutive samples can be taken from the active muscle in humans during exercise. Direct measurements in muscle samples demonstrated that muscle glycogen was a major substrate during exercise (17). In accordance with previous measurements of RER, the rate of muscle glycogen utilization increased when the workload increased (235). The rate of glycogen utilization was 0.6 and 3.6 mmol glycosyl units · kg^{-1} · min^{-1} at 50% and 100% of $\dot{V}O_{2max}$, respectively (235), and the increase in glycogen utilization was thus more pronounced than the increase in workload. During maximal dynamic exercise the rate of glycogen breakdown can increase to 30–50 mmol · kg^{-1} · min^{-1}, which is similar to that during maximal isometric contraction (Table 19.3). The high glycogen utilization during heavy exercise is due to an increased fraction of total fuel oxidation, due to CHO oxidation as well as to an increased formation of lactate (Fig. 19.7).

Influence of Muscle Glycogen Concentration. It has long been known that a CHO-poor diet following glycogen-depleting exercise results in decreased RER and thus CHO oxidation compared with a normal or CHO-rich diet (47, 176). In one study, a difference in initial glycogen content between the legs was produced by a combination of exercise and diet (107). During two-legged submaximal exercise the normal glycogen leg released lactate and the low glycogen leg extracted lactate despite similar power output. Furthermore, measurements of local respiratory exchange ratio indicated a larger CHO oxidation in the normal glycogen leg than in the low glycogen leg. It was concluded that the magnitude of the local glycogen store has an impact on substrate utilization during exercise (107). The data suggested that the rate of glycogenolysis was controlled by local factors rather than by humoral factors. The importance of initial muscle glycogen content on glycogenolysis has also been studied in perfused isolated contracting rat muscle (215). The initial glycogen content in some rats was increased above that in control rats (57 vs. 39 mmol/kg wet) by exercise followed by a normal diet. The rate of glycogen utilization was higher in muscles with high preexercise glycogen levels despite identical modes of exercise and perfusate composition. Again, the data indicate that the concentration of muscle glycogen may influence the rate of glycogenolysis during submaximal exercise. Subsequent studies have shown that during submaximal contractions the percentage of phosphorylase *a* is higher in perfused rat muscles with high glycogen than in glycogen-depleted muscles (132). The higher rate of glycogenolysis at high gly-

TABLE 19.3. *Rate of Glycogen Degradation during Maximal Exercise and In Vitro Maximal Activity of Glycogen Phosphorylase**

Rate of Glycogen Breakdown, mmol · kg wet^{-1} · min^{-1}	Conditions†	V_{max} of GP, mmol · kg wet^{-1} · min^{-1}	Conditions†
Human m. quadriceps femoris (mean ± SD):			
45	Maximal isometric contraction (4)	38 ± 5	pH = 6.8; 35°C (125)
28	Continuous electrical stimulation at 20 Hz (137)	33 ± 8	pH = 7.0; 35°C (44)
32	Maximal 30 s sprint (46)		
38	Maximal 30 s sprint (115)		
Rat fast-twitch muscle (mean ± SD):			
23	50 Hz for 10 s; 20°C (42)	32 ± 3	pH = 7.0; 35°C (42)
86	100 Hz for 5 s; 37°C (51)	37 ± 1	pH = 7.5; 30°C (212)

*A factor of 4.3 kg wet weight per kilogram dry weight has been used for conversion from dry weight to wet weight. GP was measured in the direction of glycogenolysis. †Numbers in parentheses represent references.

cogen concentration may thus be explained by an increased conversion of GP*b* to GP*a*.

Paradoxically, the interaction between glycogen concentration and rate of glycogenolysis is less evident during heavy exercise than during submaximal exercise. Maximal lactate accumulation in blood (7, 175) and muscle (141) is reduced during high-intensity exercise following prolonged exercise. However, a number of studies have shown that a low preexercise glycogen concentration has no influence on the rate of glycogenolysis (11, 210, 246) or on the rate of blood lactate increase (175, 254). The preexercise glycogen levels in some of these studies (210, 254) were lower or within the same range as the glycogen level where, during submaximal exercise, a reduced CHO oxidation was observed (107, 215). In contrast to submaximal contractions (132), GPa increased to a similar extent during heavy exercise in muscles with low and high glycogen (210) and is consistent with the unchanged glycogenolytic rate.

Muscle Fiber-Type Differences. Due to fiber type differences in contractile and metabolic properties, a heterogeneous metabolic response between muscle fibers during exercise is expected. Measurements of lactate in the two fiber types of human muscle demonstrate that lactate content after high-intensity isometric and dynamic exercise was higher in type II fibers (94, 258) than in type I fibers. The difference was maximally 44% and was abolished or diminished when the exercise was prolonged (258), suggesting transport of lactate between neighboring fibers. More reliable information about interfiber differences in glycogenolytic rate will therefore be obtained with glycogen measurements. High rates of glycogen breakdown have been observed in both fiber types after high-intensity exercise. The rate of glycogenolysis was about twofold higher in type II fibers (1.0 mmol glycosyl units · kg^{-1} · s^{-1}) than in type I fibers (0.5 mmol · kg^{-1} · s^{-1}) during electrical stimulation under circulation occlusion (114) and during maximal sprinting of 30 s duration (115). During cycling to exhaustion at about 200% of $\dot{V}O_{2max}$ (30 s), glycogen breakdown estimated by histochemical methods (266) was lower but the fiber-type differences remained (type II 0.52 mmol · kg^{-1} · s^{-1} and type I 0.35 mmol · kg^{-1} · s^{-1}). No significant difference in the rate of glycogenolysis was observed between the subgroups of type II fibers (266). The approximate twofold higher rate of glycogenolysis in type II fibers than in type I fibers during maximal exercise is in agreement with the higher activity of GP observed in vitro in type II fibers (125).

During submaximal light and moderate exercise, glycogen depletion is more pronounced in type I than in type II fibers (108), whereas at higher workloads type II fibers are glycogen depleted before type I fibers. The differences in glycogen depletion between fiber types during voluntary submaximal exercise are consequences both of differences in metabolic characteristics and of selective fiber-type recruitment. Glycogen depletion has been used as an index of fiber recruitment during exercise, but since the energy requirement can be met by other processes (e.g., oxidation of fat or blood-borne substrates), usage of this technique may be questionable under aerobic conditions.

The energy demand is thus a major factor determining the rate of glycogen utilization. However, during submaximal exercise there is a complex interaction between the metabolic pathways, and substrate utilization will be influenced by a number of other factors such as oxygen availability, training status influencing muscle oxidative capacity, muscle glycogen concentration, blood-borne substrate availability (i.e., plasma free fatty acids and plasma glucose), plasma hormone levels, and exercise duration.

Control of Glycogenolysis during Heavy Exercise

Maximal GP Activity and Glycogenolytic Rate. The rates of glycogenolysis in human skeletal muscle observed during heavy exercise (4, 46, 137, 115) are similar to the maximal activity of GP measured in vitro under optimal conditions (Table 19.3). In fast-twitch skeletal muscle of rats, the observed maximal rates of glycogenolysis were similar or higher than maximal GP activity measured in vitro. Although it is possible that some GP activity is lost during the muscle sample preparation, it is evident that the observed in vivo flux requires near maximal activation of GP, which implies that both GP*a* and GP*b* are active.

Control of Glycogenolysis through Enzymatic Interconversion of GP. In the classic experiments in isolated frog muscle (78, 187) it was shown that GPa in resting muscle was less than 5% of total GP activity and increased up to 100% within 3 s during tetanic contraction. Upon cessation of contraction, GPa rapidly reverted back to the b form, with a half-time of 12 s. Experiments with isolated glycogen particles linked to sarcoplasmic reticulum showed an even more rapid activation and was termed "flash activation" (127–129). From these and other results the initial model for control of glycogenolysis during contraction was established (transformation of inactive GPb to active GPa) and is still the information conveyed in current textbooks of physiology. Transformation of GPb to GPa has also been observed in humans during exercise (44), although the degree of transformation to GPa was less pronounced (30%–50% GPa). The model is attractive, since it links the energy-yielding processes to the energy-requiring processes through a common denominator (increases in cytosolic Ca^{2+}). However, a number of experimental findings cannot be reconciled with the basic concept that GPa is fully active and GPb inactive.

There is substantial experimental evidence that GPb is also active during exercise. The similarity between glycogenolytic activity, observed in vivo, and total GPb + GPa activity, observed in vitro (Table 19.3), despite a substantial amount of the enzyme being in the GPb form implies that GPb is active during exercise. Further evidence for activation of GPb comes from a rat strain deficient in phosphorylase *b* kinase and with low GPa activity (79, 208) and experiments in anoxic heart (188), where high rates of glycogenolysis were observed during exercise despite low GPa activity.

It also appears that under some conditions GPa may not be fully active. First, the fractional activity of phosphorylase *a* in relaxed mammalian muscle has been shown to be considerably higher than what was originally reported for isolated frog muscle (78). Artifactual increases in GPa during tissue sampling and analysis may explain part but not all of the high GPa activity (51, 117). The low rate of glycogenolysis in relaxed muscle cannot be reconciled with the high fractional activity of GPa, provided this is fully active. Second, administration of epinephrine induces conversion of GPb to GPa independently of contraction. GPa increases to 60% in isolated frog muscle (78) and to 80%–90% of total activity in human muscle (43). Despite nearly complete transformation of GPb to GPa, the glycogenolytic rate was increased only to a minor extent. The basic concept of glycogenolysis being controlled solely by phosphorylation/dephosphorylation of GP is thus untenable.

Control of Glycogenolysis by Substrate Availability. To explain the anomalous findings reported above, the control theories of glycogenolysis were reexamined (43, 117). From phosphate-31 nuclear magnetic resonance (^{31}P-NMR) studies it appears as if the concentration of Pi in relaxed muscle is much lower (1–3 mM) than previous measurements by chemical analysis (~ 10 mM) (for references, see 43). Since the affinity of GP for Pi is comparatively low [K_m = 27 in the absence and 7 mM in the presence of AMP (44, 213)], it was suggested that the low glycogenolytic rate in relaxed muscle and after epinephrine stimulation was due to substrate limitation of GP (43, 117). Contractile activity will liberate Pi in proportion to the breakdown of phosphocreatine, due to the coupling between ATP hydrolysis and ATP resynthesis by the creatine kinase reaction. Cytosolic Pi can increase to 20 mM or more during exercise, which together with a small increase in AMP should be sufficient for complete activation of GPa. The decrease in PCr (and corresponding increase in Pi) is maintained during steady-state exercise and is related to the workload and to the glycogenolytic rate. Increases in Pi can thus be a link between breakdown of PCr and activation of glycogenolysis and serve to adjust the glycogenolytic flux to the energetic demands.

Allosteric Activation of GP during Exercise. GPb is allosterically activated by increases in AMP. However, the adenine nucleotides are under most cellular conditions buffered by PCr (52, 104), and calculations based on the equilibria of the creatine kinase (Ck) and adenylate kinase (Ak) reactions demonstrate that the free AMP concentration varies between 1 μM at rest and 13 μM after maximal exercise (178), which implies that 90% or more of AMP is sequestered in the cell. The calculated increase in AMP concentration during exercise is sufficient to activate GPa (K_a <5 M (6, 169)] but considering the inhibition of GPb by G6P probably insufficient to activate GPb. It has been suggested that more pronounced increases in ADP and AMP may occur at the ATP-utilizing site during high rates of ATP turnover (150). However, provided the CK and AK reactions are at equilibrium and the PCr content is maintained above 10% of the initial level, the PCr-creatine system was considered to act as a potent buffer of the adenine nucleotides, preventing major temporal and spatial gradients of ATP. However, under non–steady-state conditions such as at the onset of exercise and intense exercise there may be reasons to question the assumption of the CK reaction being at equilibrium (see below); considering the uncertainties involved in the calculations of free AMP, the possibility that sequestered AMP may be released during exercise (117) and uncertainties of the applicability of GP kinetic properties determined in vitro to in vivo conditions, activation of GPb by AMP may very well occur.

The concentration of IMP required to attain 50% activation of GPb is about 5 mM (5, 269). The IMP level is very low in relaxed muscle (0.03 mM) but increases during heavy exercise up to about 1 mM (229). Activation of GPb by IMP may thus be of importance during the later stages of exercise but is unlikely to play a role at the onset of exercise. Furthermore, since the disappearance of IMP is relatively slow and only occurs during the recovery phase, IMP is unlikely to play a role for rapid on/off switch of glycogenolysis during exercise.

Potential Factors Involved in the On/Off Switch of Glycogenolysis. Although transformation of GPb to GPa, increases in Pi, and allosteric activation of GPb are important clues for the understanding of how glycogenolysis is controlled during exercise, the model is unable to account for the close coupling between glycogenolysis and muscle contraction. For instance, when high-intensity exercise is followed by anaerobic recovery, glycolysis is immediately switched off and PCr and Pi are maintained at, respectively, low and high levels similar to those during the contraction (81, 82, 207). Despite elevated values of Pi and free AMP (calculated from the AK and CK equilibrium), both of which are factors that should stimulate GP and PFK, glycolytic rate is maintained low. This anomaly was further accentuated when exercise was combined with epinephrine-induced elevation of GPa (213). The paradox of an extensive transformation to GPa, high levels of Pi, and elevated AMP levels but low rates of glycogenolysis and glycolysis during the anaerobic recovery period indicates that some additional factor (or factors) closely related to the contraction process is (are) involved in the rapid switching between on and off. The identity of this (these) factor(s), which should affect both GP and PFK activity, is unknown but several candidates have been proposed.

Cytosolic Ca^{2+} changes rapidly in concert with the initiation/termination of contraction and has been suggested to act as a metabolic switch (81; see also Chapter 18). However, because glycogenolysis is switched off after contraction, despite high GPa levels (213), the regulatory mechanism must be different than interconversion between GPb and GPa. Such a mechanism, triggered by Ca^{2+} transients, is possible but remains to be identified. An increase in Ca^{2+} has in some studies been shown to activate PFK (see above) (177) but the effect during physiological conditions is small and the physiological significance of Ca^{2+} activation of PFK has been questioned (262). AMP is a potent activator of both GP and PFK (see above) and fluctuating AMP levels may function as a metabolic switch. During non–steady-state conditions, such as at the onset of exercise and during heavy exercise, there is a progressive decrease in PCr, and the assumption of the CK reaction being at equilibrium may be questioned. To drive the CK reaction in the direction of ATP synthesis an increase in ADP above that at equilibrium is required and a disequilibrium in the CK reaction is thus expected. By using data on CK fluxes obtained from saturation transfer NMR studies, kinetic analysis showed that during a tetanus the concentration of ADP should be twofold higher than that calculated from the CK equilibrium (106). Due to the stoichiometry of the AK reaction, the relative increase in AMP will be in proportion to the square of that of ADP and may be of a sufficient magnitude to activate both GPb and PFK. When the PCr store becomes depleted the function of PCr as a buffer of high-energy phosphates will diminish and substantial temporal fluctuations of ADP and AMP are expected to occur during the contraction cycle (105). This will be further accentuated during acidotic conditions, since the activity of CK in the direction of ATP synthesis is sharply reduced when pH is lower than 6.5 (270) and when the PCr level is reduced. AMP deaminase catalyzes the dea mination of AMP to IMP and the reaction is activated by increases in AMP and ADP (223). A close coupling between contractile activity and IMP formation has been observed in energy-depleted muscle (230). The high rate of AMP deamination that occurs in concert with the contraction in energy-depleted muscle supports the hypothesis of AMP transients (230). The high rates of glycolysis at the onset of exercise and during heavy exercise may thus be explained by transient increases in AMP above that predicted from the CK and AK equilibrium (150, 236). Since AMP transients are intimately coupled to the high rate of ATP turnover that occurs during exercise, they may function as a contraction-induced trigger of glycolysis and glycogenolysis.

Another possible explanation for the observed coupling between glycogenolysis/glycolysis and the contraction process could be conformation changes of regulatory enzymes by binding to cellular structural proteins during the contraction process. Evidence of augmented activity of PFK (increased F6P affinity) when bound to components in the cytomatrix have been presented (174). Furthermore, several glycolytic enzymes exhibit an increased binding to proteins during stimulation (174, 268) that is reversed during the recovery period (280). However, it is uncertain whether the degree of contraction-induced binding is of sufficient magnitude (twofold increase) to explain the large changes in glycolytic rates or if the kinetics is sufficiently rapid to explain the instantaneous on/off switch of glycolysis during exercise. Finally, there is a question as to whether the binding changes the overall pathway kinetics in the correct direction (30, 31). Further studies to elucidate these possibilities are required.

Changes in pH and Control of Glycogenolysis. Changes in pH may influence glycogenolysis by a number of mechanisms. Transformation of GPb to GPa by both the contraction- and the epinephrine-mediated mechanisms has been shown to be influenced by changes in pH. GPa conversion during con traction is attenuated under acidotic conditions (43, 77) and augmented under alkalotic conditions (77). The effect of pH on GP transformation seems to be exerted both at the phosphorylase kinase (see above) and at the adenylcyclase reaction (43). The true substrate of GP is the dibasic form of Pi (HPO_4^{2-}) (146) and since $H_2PO_4^-$ has a pK_a of 6.8, substrate concentration and the activity of GP will be sensitive to changes in pH. By this effect a decrease in pH will decrease substrate level and GP activity and vice versa, with an increase in pH. A decrease in pH could also affect glycogenolysis secondarily to a primary inhibition of PFK through increased levels of F6P and G6P, of which the latter will allosterically inhibit GPb and activate GSd. At the onset of exercise, an increase in pH from 7.0 at rest to 7.1 has been observed in some studies (3, 55), whereas the alkalotic phase was lower or absent in other studies (184, 255). The alkalotic phase may be explained by an uptake of H^+ in the CK reaction during PCr breakdown. During sustained exercise, muscle pH decreases linearly with lactate accumulation (224) and reaches about 6.5 at fatigue. With ^{31}P-NMR cytosolic pH values as low as 6.0–6.3 have been reported (184, 255). A decrease in pH from 7.0 to 6.5 will decrease the amount of Pi present as HPO_4^{2-} by about 50% compared with that at rest and and an increase in pH from 7.0 to 7.1 will increase HPO_4^{2-} by 8%.

Concluding Remarks. The current state of knowledge is that the increased rate of glycogenolysis during exercise is a consequence of *(1)* conversion of GPb to GPa, *(2)* increased concentration of substrate (Pi), *(3)* allosteric activation by AMP of GPb and GPa, and *(4)* activation by an unknown factor closely associated with the contraction process. Evidence exists that GPb under some conditions can be active during exercise and that changes in the cellular concentration of AMP, IMP, and G6P may be of importance for allosteric control. Changes in pH will have a modulating effect on GP activity. The increase in cytosolic pH at the onset of exercise is on the order of 0.1 units and the stimulating effect on glycogenolysis will be small. However, the decrease in cytosolic pH during sustained muscular activity with up to 1 pH unit may be a potent feedback inhibitor of both GP and PFK.

POSTEXERCISE GLYCOGEN SYNTHESIS AND ITS CONTROL

Resynthesis of Muscle Glycogen After Exercise

Since muscle glycogen is of primary importance for exercise performance, repletion of glycogen constitutes an important part of the postexercise recovery processes. After cessation of exercise and with adequate CHO intake, muscle glycogen is rapidly resynthesized. The rate of postexercise glycogen resynthesis is negatively correlated to glycogen concentration (23, 206). The highest rate of glycogenesis is observed during the first hour of recovery. After 24 h of recovery with adequate supply of CHO, glycogen is restored to near preexercise levels and following another 2–3 days muscle glycogen can exceed the preexercise levels by more than twofold. Repletion of glycogen has been shown to occur only in glycogen-depleted muscles (18, 205). Thus, after one-leg exercise, glycogen repletion occurred only in the glycogen-depleted leg, which after 3 days reached a muscle glycogen level two to three times above the level in the nonexercised leg (18). Glycogen repletion can also occur during the actual exercise, provided that the intensity is low (67, 205). In the first studies of glycogen supercompensation, a combination of prolonged exercise and a CHO-free diet was followed by a CHO-rich diet (17). Subsequent studies showed that supercompensated muscle glycogen levels can be obtained without a period of CHO-free diet (237) and that trained athletes can reach supercompensated glycogen levels by reduced training and high CHO intake.

The substrate for glycogen resynthesis is primarily blood-borne glucose. Glycogen repletion is thus dependent on an adequate muscle glucose uptake. Analysis of human muscle biopsies showed that when exercise-induced glycogen depletion was followed by fasting or a CHO-free diet a marked attenuation of glycogen resynthesis was observed (135, 136, 139, 171) and preexercise muscle glycogen levels were not reached even after 5–6 days (135). The rate of postexercise glycogen repletion increases with the amount of CHO consumed, and when intake is 0.7 g glucose $\cdot$ kg^{-1} $\cdot$ h^{-1} there is a leveling off at 0.1 mmol $\cdot$ kg^{-1} $\cdot$ min^{-1} [Table 19.4; (24)]. With intravenous glucose infusion the rate of glycogen repletion increased further to 0.42 mmol $\cdot$ kg^{-1} $\cdot$ min^{-1} (19). The higher rate of glycogen repletion during glucose infusion than during oral glucose intake was considered to be an effect of limitation in gastric emptying that is bypassed during glucose infusion, resulting in higher plasma glucose and insulin values (139). A large CHO intake during the early recovery period is thus essential for obtaining maximal values of glycogen repletion. In contrast to these biopsy studies, a much higher rate of glycogen repletion (0.7 mmol $\cdot$ kg wet^{-1} $\cdot$ min^{-1}) has been observed during the early recovery period (30 min) when glycogen was measured with the noninvasive ^{13}C-NMR technique (206). This high rate of glycogen repletion occurred in fasting subjects when muscle glycogen decreased to less than 25% of the initial value. The difference between rates of glycogen repletion measured with these two technique is large and it is at present unclear whether glycogenesis measured by the biopsy technique is falsely too low [impaired glycogen synthesis due to the induced trauma of biopsy (74)) or whether glycogenesis measured by the ^{13}C-NMR technique is overestimated at low glycogen levels.

From experiments on perfused isolated rat hindlimb, direct incorporation of (^{14}C) lactate into muscle glycogen was demonstrated in the fast-twitch plantaris muscle (179). Repeated high-intensity exercise with high intramuscular and blood lactate indicated that glycogenesis from lactate can occur also in vivo (8, 131). Measurements of substrate exchange over the leg and of intramuscular glycogen and metabolites showed that the rate of glycogen repletion during the immediate postexercise period was similar to the rate of lactate disappearance and could not be explained by glucose uptake. It was suggested that glyconeogenesis occurred in human muscle in vivo during conditions of high intramuscular lactate. However, direct evidence for conversion of lactate to glycogen in vivo is lacking, and alternative explanations such as heterogeneous rates of glucose uptake and lactate release within the leg between different muscle groups cannot be excluded.

Regulatory Mechanisms

It is well documented that the fraction of GS present in the active form (GSi) increases during the recovery period after prolonged exercise. The conversion of GSd to GSi is stimulated by insulin, and since both insulin sensitivity and responsiveness in muscle tissue is increased after exercise (103, 217, 273) the postexercise increase in GSi may partially be an effect of insulin stimulation. The percentage of GSi is inversely related to muscle glycogen (20, 77) and glycogen concentration is thus in itself an important regulator of the rate of glycogenesis. The underlying mechanism for the inverse relationship between glycogen and GSi is unclear. It has been suggested that during the process of glycogen degradation both GS and phosphatase are released from the glycogen-protein complex, enabling a dephosphorylation of GSd to GSi (139). Glycogen has also been shown to be an activator of phosphatase and an inhibitor of phosphorylase kinase (see earlier under GLYCOGEN AND PROPERTIES OF INVOLVED ENZYMES) and low glycogen would thus favor conversion of GS to GSi. The effect of glycogen depletion on the conversion of GSd to Gsi appears to be additive to the effect of insulin (77), and the effect of low glycogen and insulin on the converting enzymes are therefore likely to be independent. Furthermore, dephosphorylation of GSd is stimulated by G6P (265). The postexercise increase in GSi may thus be explained by depleted muscle glycogen stores, increases in G6P, and insulin stimulation.

Postexercise glycogen repletion is associated with an increased GSi activity, and a linear relation has been observed between glycogenesis and the activity of GSi in different muscles (50). The relation between GSi and glycogen repletion was, however, time dependent, with a higher rate of glycogenesis in the immediate postexercise period than after 1 h despite similar GSi activities. A similar time dependence has been observed in humans (139, 206).

TABLE 19.4. *Rates of Postexercise Glycogen Repletion and In Vitro Maximal Glycogen Synthase Activity*

Rate of Glycogen Repletion, mmol · kg wet^{-1} · min^{-1}	Conditions*	V_{max} of GS (% GSi), mmol · kg wet^{-1} · min^{-1}	Conditions*
Human muscle (mean ± SD):			
0.10	VL; Oral glucose; 0–6 h postexercise (24)	3.4 ± 0.2 (75%)	VL; 15–30 min postexercise; 30°C (20)
0.13	VL; Oral glucose; 0–2 h postexercise (140)	2.8 ± 0.1 (50%)	VL; 30 min postexercise; 30°C (155)
0.04	VL; Oral glucose; 2–4 h postexercise (140)		
0.42	VL; Glucose infusion; 0–2 h postexercise (19)		
0.7	G; Glycogen <30 mM; 0–0.5 h postexercise; ^{13}C-NMR (206)		
Rat muscle (mean ± SD):			
0.27	VL; Oral glucose; 0–1 h postexercise (50)	4.5 ± 0.1 (38%)	VL; 0–60 min postexercise; 30°C (50)
0.09	VL; Oral glucose; 1–2 h postexercise (50)	3.1 (83%)	G; 10 min postexercise; 37°C (23)
0.46	G; 0–0.5 h postexercise; ^{13}C-NMR (23)		
0.11	G: 1.3–1.7 h postexercise; ^{13}C-NMR (23)		

*Numbers in parentheses represent references. VL, vastus lateralis; G, gastrocnemius; ^{13}C-NMR, measurements of glycogen with nuclear magnetic resonance detection of natural enriched ^{13}C.

Studies in normal subjects (206) demonstrate that glycogen repletion during the early recovery period is independent of insulin but negatively correlated to glycogen, whereas during the later phase of recovery glycogen repletion is insulin dependent. This may reflect different temporal influence of glycogen, G6P, and insulin on GSi activity, although other factors may also be involved. In Table 19.4 the total activity of GS and the percentage of the enzyme present as GSi have been compared with the observed rates of glycogen synthesis during the recovery period after exercise. It is evident that only a small fraction of the in vitro activity of GSi is utilized. The rapid glycogen repletion during the early postexercise recovery period corresponds only to about 2%–13% of the reported GSi activity. This is in contrast to liver, where the maximal in vitro activity of GS was insufficient to account for the rate of glycogenesis observed in vivo (195). The comparable low rate of glycogen repletion in muscle could, in theory, be due to breakdown and synthesis of glycogen occurring simultaneously. Evidence for a glycogen/glucose 1-P cycle has been presented (40), but the rate (<0.02 mmol · kg^{-1} · min^{-1}) is about 100 times less than the activity of GSi (Table 19.4). A glycogen/glucose 1-P cycle would consume one UTP per turn (equivalent to one ATP), and a high rate of cycling was considered unlikely due to the high ATP requirement (44). The low rate of glycogenesis in comparison with GSi activity is probably explained by the low concentration of GS substrate (UDP-glucose) in comparison with the K_m value (see earlier under GLYCOGEN AND PROPERTIES OF INVOLVED ENZYMES). Evidence from rats indicates that when GS is measured at a physiological nonsaturating concentration of UDP-glucose, postexercise glycogen repletion can be quantitatively accounted for by an increased phosphorylation of GS (i.e., GSi formation) and allosteric activation of GS by G6P (23).

The mechanism for supercompensation of muscle glycogen is unclear. The postexercise increase in GSi and the augmented insulin-stimulated glucose transport is reversed after 24 h when preexercise glycogen levels are reached and thus before the period of supercompensation (20). The further slow rise in muscle glycogen can thus not be explained by increased activity of GSi, nor by an augmented insulin-stimulated glucose transport (37). An increased sensitivity of GS towards G6P despite unchanged percentage of GSi has been observed, and it was suggested that supercompensation was in part explained by this mechanism (155). The increased G6P sensitivity is likely related to intermediary forms of GS with different degrees of phosphorylation and with different sensitivities to G6P.

The dependence of glycogen repletion on the amount and time of CHO intake (see above) suggests that substrate availability influences the rate of glycogen synthesis. Glucose transport across the cell membrane is a regulated process influenced independently by contractile activity and insulin and there is indirect evidence that glycogen repletion is controlled by glucose transport (for a review, see 103). Experiments in transgenic mice demonstrate that muscle glycogen can be elevated tenfold when the glucose transporter is overexpressed (214) and provide evidence that glucose transport may control glycogen synthesis. The transgenic mice had lower GSi activity, normal GPa activity, and normal G6P. The mechanism by which an increased glucose transport augments glycogenesis can therefore not be related to covalent or allosteric activation of GS by G6P. However, since measurements of GSi and G6P were done after an augmented glycogen level had been reached (214), one cannot exclude that the mechanism for the enhanced glycogenesis was mediated by increases in G6P or GSi.

If changes occur in the concentration of UDP-glucose they will directly influence the rate of glycogen synthesis. The concentration of UDP-glucose in rat muscle appears to remain constant despite large differences in the rate of glycogen synthesis (204). In human skeletal muscle UDP-glucose has been found to increase under certain conditions (209). The possibility that an increased glucose transport influences glycogen synthesis via increased UDP-glucose has not been fully explored. Glucose utilization and glucose transport is covered in detail in Chapter 20 this *Handbook*.

Additional Factors of Importance for Muscle Glycogenesis. Epinephrine is known to result in impaired glucose tolerance and increased peripheral insulin resistance (85). The effect may be explained in part by an activation of the AMP-dependent protein kinase, which influences the activity of the converter enzymes [Figs. 19.3 and 19.4; (49)], resulting in a decrease in GSi and an increase in GPa (209). The effect of epinephrine on glucose metabolism may also be related to the fact that the insulin-induced glucose transport is impaired by epinephrine (reviewed in 267).

Glycogen repletion has been found to be impaired after eccentric exercise (73, 196). Eccentric exercise is associated with mechanical damage of the muscle ultrastructure. Infiltration with inflammatory cells and associated alteration of glucose metabolism was considered to be the explanation for the reduced rate of glycogen resynthesis (73). The reduced rate of glycogen repletion could in part be overcome by excessive CHO intake (73).

In summary, the increased postexercise rate of glycogen repletion is determined by an increased dephosphorylation of GS (conversion to GSi) and allosteric activation of GS by G6P. The increase in GSi during the recovery period is a consequence of low glycogen, insulin stimulation, and increases in G6P. The mechanism of several aspects of glycogen synthesis is unclear (e.g., supercompensation of glycogen, influence of glycogen on the GSi/GSd ratio, and the link between increased glucose transport and increased glycogenesis).

MUSCLE GLYCOGEN METABOLISM AND FATIGUE

Muscle fatigue has been the subject of numerous studies and reviews and a full discussion can be found in Fitts (99; see also Chapter 26 of this *Handbook*). There is considerable evidence that muscle glycogen stores are essential for endurance during prolonged exercise. Glycogen content in the working muscle is known to be nearly completely depleted at fatigue during cycling at intensities between 60% and 85% of $\dot{V}O_{2max}$ (17, 235). These findings have been confirmed in a number of studies that used different types of exercise and experimental protocols. With work rates above 90% of $\dot{V}O_{2max}$ working muscles contain considerable amounts of glycogen at exhaustion (235), and fatigue is related to factors other than glycogen depletion (e.g., accumulation of end products such as lactic acid, ADP, or Pi). Furthermore, with work rates below 60% of $\dot{V}O_{2max}$ exhaustion is less well defined and central fatigue influenced by hypoglycemia and other factors will probably increase in importance.

Importance of CHO during Prolonged Exercise

The importance of CHO for exercise capacity was demonstrated in an early study where a carbohydrate-rich diet 3–7 days prior to exercise increased endurance time two to three times compared with a fat-rich diet (47). In later studies, direct measurements in muscle biopsy samples demonstrated that the enhanced endurance was related to increased local stores of glycogen. By combinations of exercise and diet, muscle glycogen could be varied within a range of 30–300 mmol glycosyl units/kg muscle, and it was shown that endurance at 75% of $\dot{V}O_{2max}$ was linearly related to preexercise glycogen content (17). Exhaustion at this workload coincided with muscle glycogen depletion irrespective of prior diet and verifies the requirement of endogenous glycogen for exercise capacity. Supercompensation of glycogen is now widely used in sport events where endurance is essential (e.g., marathon running, cross-country skiing, cycling). High glycogen levels will improve endurance at moderate exercise intensities but will not enhance $\dot{V}O_{2max}$ and thus the capacity for high-intensity exercise. High glycogen levels could in fact reduce performance during high-intensity exercise due to the extra weight to be carried (up to 2–3 kg).

The rate of glycogen utilization and endurance can be influenced by the use of alternative fuels (i.e., oxidation of fat or/and glucose). Glucose administration during exercise has, in a number of studies, been shown to improve exercise capacity (for references, see 75). In most but not all studies glucose ingestion is associated with a reduced rate of glycogen depletion. Exogenous glucose can thus partially replace endogenous glycogen as a fuel. However, at higher work intensities (>75% of $\dot{V}O_{2max}$) muscle glycogen appear to be an essential substrate. Despite increased uptake, utilization is blocked and there is an accumulation of glucose within the muscle (147). The decreased utilization of glucose at high exercise intensities was considered to be caused by inhibition of hexokinase by accumulating G6P. The preferential use of glycogen at high work intensities is advantageous, since the ATP yield per amount of consumed O_2 is higher for glycogen combustion than for fat and glucose.

An increased reliance on fat oxidation will also spare muscle glycogen and improve endurance. An increase in plasma fatty acids by prior high-fat diet and heparin reduced the rate of glycogenolysis during submaximal exercise in humans (72). Similarly, endurance training will increase muscle aerobic capacity and enhance fat oxidation. The endurance at a certain relative workload will be considerably longer for the trained subjects, and the improvement is at least partially due to a lower rate of glycogen depletion. Studies of patients with GP deficiency (McArdle's disease) who are unable to utilize muscle glycogen demonstrate a work capacity of only 35%–50% of the expected normal value (151, 168). Some improvement of their exercise capacity can be achieved by administration of glucose (168) or elevation of plasma fatty acids (200). Evidence from normal subjects demonstrates that exclusive dependency on fat combustion can only sustain a metabolic rate corresponding to 50% of $\dot{V}O_{2max}$ (80), and oxidation of fat can only partially replace CHO oxidation. There are a number of other factors that will affect the rate of glycogen depletion (e.g., training status, oxygen availability, hormonal factors, temperature, fiber-type recruitment, diet). In general, factors that will affect the rate of glycogen utilization will also affect endurance. Formation and release of lactate corresponds to a rapid loss of endogenous CHO from the working muscle where only a small amount (8%) of the potential energy is utilized. Lactic acid formation can thus be related to fatigue not only during high-intensity exercise but also during prolonged exercise. The latter will be related to glycogen depletion and may explain the observed relation between lactate threshold intensity and endurance (240).

Mechanisms Involved. Although the importance of CHO availability for exercise capacity is accepted and documented in numerous descriptive reports, the mechanism by which muscle glycogen depletion is linked to fatigue is under debate. The most commonly held view is that glycogen depletion impairs the rate of ATP regeneration and that energetic failure is the cause of fatigue. If the rate of ATP utilization exceeds ATP regeneration, an increased catabolism of the adenine nucleotide pool to NH3 and IMP is expected. Prolonged exercise to fatigue leading to low intramuscular levels of glycogen is associated with increased accumulation of IMP and NH_3 (29, 109, 193). Formation of IMP occurred in both fiber types and was inversely related to the glycogen content (193). Furthermore, exercise with low initial glycogen levels resulted in a rapid development of fatigue and in more pronounced formation of IMP and NH_3 compared with exercise with normal preexercise glycogen levels (29, 243). When CHO was administered during exercise, the duration of exercise was prolonged and accumulation of IMP was attenuated after equal times of exercise (244). These studies support the hypothesis that glycogen depletion results in a reduced rate of aerobic ATP production and that fatigue is related to energetic deficiency at the adenine nucleotide level.

Although there is evidence that glycogen depletion is associated with fatigue, it is unclear why fat oxidation is unable to completely replace CHO oxidation. The most commonly held hypothesis is that metabolism of fat to acetyl-CoA is limited either by a low rate of sarcolemma transport of fatty acids (189) or by limitation in β-oxidation. The increased endurance and the lower rate of muscle glycogen degradation when plasma fatty acid concentration is increased (72, 200) support the hypothesis of substrate limitation. However, after prolonged exercise to glycogen depletion and energy crisis, muscle content of mitochondrial substrate (acetyl-CoA or acetylcarnitine) is maintained elevated (68, 225). These findings speak against the idea that fatigue is related to a shortage of mitochondrial substrate and that transport of exogenous fuel into muscle is a limiting step. An alternative hypothesis is that high rates of mitochondrial substrate oxidation require expansion of the concentration of tricarboxylic cycle intermediates (TCAI) and that CHO availability is necessary for these processes (34, 166). Experimental evidence in favor of this hypothesis is that the initial increase in TCAI is partially reverted during the latter phase of prolonged exercise (225) and that CHO supplementation retards the reversion (243).

Despite signs of energy crisis (i.e., impaired rate of ATP generation), cellular ATP at fatigue is only slightly decreased (10%–30%). A number of alternative nonmetabolic causes of fatigue have been suggested (99, 112). The relevance of these must be considered in light of findings that endurance is closely related to the availability of muscle glycogen under a variety of conditions.

Importance of Glycogen during High-Intensity Exercise

In contrast to prolonged exercise, a substantial part of the ATP supply is derived from the anaerobic processes during high-intensity exercise. Depletion of glycogen could, in theory, severely limit lactate formation and thus the work capacity. The decrease in maximal lactate accumulation and work capacity after prolonged exercise supports this hypothesis (7, 73, 141, 175), whereas other studies demonstrate no effect of low muscle glycogen on glycolytic rate (see earlier under CARBOHYDRATE UTILIZATION AT REST AND DURING EXERCISE). The observed decrease in lactate formation after prolonged exercise may be related to factors other than substrate limitations such as an impaired ability to activate muscle phosphorylase (66), or to failure of excitation contraction coupling in certain muscle fibers.

Lactic Acid Accumulation and Fatigue. Formation of lactic acid is generally implicated in the mechanisms of fatigue. During high-intensity exercise, lactic acid formation is considered to lead to fatigue via accumulation of metabolic products (e.g., lactic acid and Pi). The lactate ion is not known to adversely affect muscle function, whereas acidosis could impair the contraction process through various mechanisms (e.g., 130). One possibility is that increased hydrogen ion concentration interferes with the energy-yielding processes, which secondarily affect one or several steps in the contraction process. The effect of acidosis on GP and glycogenolysis has been discussed in earlier under GLYCOGEN AND PROPERTIES OF INVOLVED ENZYMES. Inhibition of PFK by H^+ has been recognized for a long time (261), and almost complete inhibition was observed at pH values close to that observed in muscle at fatigue. The physiological importance of this inhibition has been questioned, since high rates of glycolysis can be maintained at low pH values (88, 116, 247). However, allosteric activation of both GP and PFK can counterbalance the inhibitory effects of H^+. The allosteric PFK activators AMP, ADP, fructose 6-phosphate, fructose 1,6-diphosphate, and Pi are known to increase during conditions of high ATP turnover rates and acidosis and are probably of importance to overcome acidotic inhibition of PFK. The increases in ADP and Pi may be the cellular signals that link energetic deficiency to muscle fatigue. Increases in Pi and ADP are known to impair the contractile function (69, 194, 227). The ionic form of Pi that has the most potent inhibitory effect is $H_2PO_4^-$ (194), and increases in H^+ will thus enhance the inhibitory effect of Pi accumulation. An alternative mechanism by which H^+ accumulation could be linked to fatigue is direct interference with the contractile machinery (69, 89) or with excitation-contraction coupling. Although muscle fatigue during short-term exercise under many situations is associated with acidosis, there is yet no conclusive evidence that there is a cause-and-effect relationship in vivo. In fact, contractile function after exhaustive exercise can be restored despite high concentrations of H^+. During recovery from isometric contraction (234) and short-term dynamic exercise (236), maximal force or power output were rapidly restored, with a time course similar to that of PCr resynthesis but considerably faster than H^+ removal. The data suggest that fatigue is related more to an impaired capacity to generate ATP than to acidosis per se. The increased catabolism of ATP to IMP during a variety of conditions of fatigue (e.g., acidosis, glycogen depletion, phosphorylase deficiency, β-adrenoceptor blockade) supports this concept (229). Muscle fatigue is a powerful brake of glycolysis and could be regarded as an appropriate event by which irreversible damage of muscle is prevented.

INTEGRATIVE ASPECTS OF GLYCOLYTIC CONTROL AND FUTURE DIRECTIONS (K. SAHLIN)

Experimental evidence and theoretical considerations support the notion that the major control of glycolysis from glycogen resides at the nonequilibrium reactions catalyzed by GP and PFK. The potential importance of glucose transport and hexokinase for control of glycolysis from glucose is covered in Chapter 20 of this *Handbook* and will not be discussed here. Maintenance of the flux through post-PFK reactions is to a major extent determined by changes in the pathway substrate concentration occurring secondary to activations of GP and PFK. Many of the control signals are similar for GP and PFK, but the control strength is likely to be different. Changes in the hexose monophosphates, products of GP and substrates of PFK and GS, appear to have a crucial role in coordinating the net rate of glycogenolytic flux to that of glycolysis (and the converse). Increases in hexose monophosphates will thus reduce the activity of GPb and increase the activity of GSd and PFK. The following discussion will focus on the central role of GP and PFK in metabolic control and has been separated into three conditions:

rest-work transition, continuous submaximal exercise, and intense exercise.

Rest-Work Transition

In relaxed muscle a considerable proportion of GP is still in the "active" form (GPa). The low glycogenolytic rate is a consequence of the low concentration of Pi, which is far below the K_m of GPa at the prevailing low AMP level. The small increase in glycogenolytic rate that occurs in relaxed muscle during hypoxia can be explained by increases in Pi and AMP, which are of sufficient magnitude to increase the activity of GPa but inadequate to activate GPb (212). During epinephrine stimulation, transformation of GPb to GPa will augment glycogenolysis, but the low Pi and AMP levels will prevent large increases in flux rate. The low glycogenolytic rate in relaxed muscle results in low levels of fructose 6-phosphate which together with inhibition of PFK by ATP (increases the K_m for fructose 6-phosphate), results in a low PFK flux. Theoretical considerations of metabolic control demonstrate that considerable difficulties exist in switching off a metabolic pathway (191). There is evidence that substrate cycling occurs between glycogen-glucose 1-P-glycogen and between fructose 6-P-fructose 1,6-diP-fructose 6-P (40), which in addition to the above-mentioned factors can explain the low net rate of glycogenolysis and glycolysis in relaxed muscle.

Transition to work involves a transient transformation of GPb to GPa and a progressive decrease in PCr. The decrease in PCr corresponds to increases in Pi, pH, ADP, and AMP. Since PCr decreases progressively until a steady-state value is reached, the increases in ADP-AMP will be higher than that predicted from the CK and AK equilibrium (see earlier under Control of Glycogenolysis during Heavy Exercise). The increases in Pi and ADP-AMP will activate both glycolysis (GP and PFK) and oxidative phosphorylation. The initial burst of lactate formation at the onset of exercise may be explained by transient increases in GPa, pH, and in ADP-AMP above the equilibrium state. Additional factors of importance for the initial burst of lactate formation are the lag in oxidative phosphorylation and initial recruitment of fast-twitch glycolytic fibers. The lag in attaining a steady state in the rate of oxidative phosphorylation will play a role since, lactate formation is the difference between formation and oxidation of pyruvate.

Continuous submaximal exercise (<60% $\dot{V}O_{2max}$) is a near-steady-state condition and is characterized by ATP demand being matched by oxidative ATP generation. The rate of pyruvate formation is nearly equal to that of pyruvate oxidation, and lactate formation occurs at a low rate. The increase in GPa at the onset of exercise is during continuous exercise reversed to or even below the value at rest. PCr is decreased but maintained constant at a level that is inversely related to work intensity and thus to energy demand. Since PCr is stable, the increase in ADP-AMP will be determined by the CK and AK equilibrium. The increases in Pi and ADP-AMP are the major feedback signals that control both glycolysis (GP and PFK) and oxidative phosphorylation and ensure that formation and oxidation of pyruvate are matched and adjusted to the energy demands. The increases in AMP and Pi during steady-state exercise are probably of a sufficient magnitude to activate GPa but not GPb.

Exercise at intensities of 60%–80% of whole-body $\dot{V}O_{2max}$ correspond to a transitional metabolic state where pyruvate formation exceeds that of pyruvate oxidation. The increased lactate formation is not related to an O_2-limited mitochondrial ATP formation. Nevertheless, there is an abundance of evidence (148, 149, 233, 271) that metabolism is O_2 dependent at these exercise intensities. Thus, submaximal exercise during hypoxemia result in a number of metabolic changes such as decreases in muscle PCr and increases in muscle NADH, lactate, IMP, and free ADP (148). This O_2 dependency of metabolism (before reaching O_2-limited ATP formation) is explained on the basis that mitochondrial $\dot{V}O_2$ and ATP formation are controlled by the O_2 tension, the phosphorylation drive, and the redox drive (93, 149, 233, 271). A decrease in O_2 tension will adjust the other parameters (mitochondrial redox state and phosphorylation state) until mitochondrial VO_2 is restored and ATP demand is covered by mitochondrial oxidative processes (93, 64, 149, 233, 271). Since both glycolysis, PCr breakdown, and oxidative phosphorylation are controlled by the phosphorylation state, the adapative change to a decrease in oxygen tension will activate PCr breakdown and glycolysis. The increase in cytosolic NADH/NAD$^+$, which is related to the increase in mitochondrial redox drive, will add to the response in pushing the LDH reaction to lactate (233). The oxygen tension at which metabolism is affected is dependent on the ATP demand in relation to oxidative capacity of the fiber (i.e., the fraction of fiber $\dot{V}O_{2max}$ that is utilized). The glycolytic response to a change in the phosphorylation state will be influenced by the maximal glycolytic capacity of the fiber and the control strength.

Lactate formation during submaximal exercise will produce a relatively small amount of ATP. The primary mechanism for lactate formation under these conditions seems more related to the integrative control of metabolic pathways as outlined above than to quantitative glycolytic ATP formation. This simplified model may be the primary explanation for the increased lactate formation during the transitional state, although other factors such as diet, glycogen levels, temperature, fiber-type recruitment, and epinephrine stimulation will add to the metabolic response. The term "anaerobic threshold," although correct in denoting a work intensity where an increased proportion of ATP formation is derived from non–oxygen-dependent processes (113), may be misleading, since it has been used synonymously for O_2-limited metabolism by some investigators.

Intense exercise is a non–steady-state condition and is characterized by a progressive decrease in PCr and a progressive increase in muscle and blood lactate. The progressive decrease in PCr corresponds to increases in ADP and AMP above that predicted from the CK and AK equilibria. Since the rate of the CK reaction in the forward direction is reduced by low pH (270) and by low PCr, the extent of displacement from equilibrium and thus the increase in ADP-AMP will be further accentuated during the late stage of intense exercise. The increased catabolism of adenine nucleotides to IMP during intense exercise may be taken as evidence of elevated AMP levels above that predicted from the CK and AK equilibria. The increases in AMP-ADP and Pi are probably sufficient to activate both GPa and GPb as well as PFK. The decrease in muscle pH to 6.5 or lower based on in vitro studies be sufficient to reduce the activity of both PFK and GP. However, since AMP-ADP and Pi increase progressively in parallel to the decrease in pH, these activating signals are likely to counteract the pH inhibition. The increase in fructose 6-phosphate is a further contributing factor for maintenance of a high PFK flux at low pH. During intense exercise, pyruvate formation is much higher than pyruvate oxidation probably because glycolytic pathway has a higher maximal rate than that of oxidative phosphorylation. At high rates of ATP turnover oxidative phosphorylation approaches the maximal rate and the control strength of ADP-AMP and Pi is much higher for glycolysis than for pyruvate oxidation.

Future Directions

Although the knowledge of how glycogenolysis and glycolysis are controlled has increased substantially during recent years, it is clear from this review that a number of major issues remain to be solved. One is to identify the trigger of GP and PFK. Our present knowledge from modeling and system analyses would predict a high glycolytic rate when changing from exercise to anaerobic recovery but, as discussed above, glycolysis is turned on and off in concert with the contraction. The hypothesis of Ca^{2+} being the trigger can be tested experimentally by comparing the metabolic response during conditions when Ca^{2+} is maintained high but the ATP demand is varied. Considering the importance of adenine nucleotides for the control of energy metabolism, it is crucial to know the concentrations of ADP and AMP in different cellular compartments under various conditions. The currently used method of calculating ADP and AMP from the CK and AK equilibria are based on a number of assumptions, the validity of which may be questioned during intense exercise. The hypothesis of AMP transients being the trigger of glycolysis may be tested by using specific inhibitors of AK. Our understanding of system control is to a large extent based on in vitro studies of dilute enzymes. The in vivo control is likely to be more complex and involve other parameters such as interaction between enzymes and between enzymes and other cellular components (e.g., cellular organelles and glycogen). This may change the structure of and thus the catalytic activity and the regulatory properties of enzymes. One example is the protein-glycogen-sarcoplasmic reticulum complex where the in vivo control encompasses additional dimensions. More information is required about how and to what extent exercise alters the regulatory properties of enzymes in vivo.

INTEGRATIVE ASPECTS OF GLYCOLYTIC CONTROL AND FUTURE DIRECTIONS (R. J. CONNETT)

The glycolytic pathway is one of the most studied biochemical pathways. It was one of the first to have identified allosterically controlled "rate-limiting" enzymes. As described above, individual enzymes have been studied and attempts to account for control have been carried out in cell-free glycolyzing systems. In spite of all this attention there is still considerable uncertainty about control under conditions of exercise. To date no comprehensive model has been developed that quantitatively accounts for its behavior under physiological conditions. Part of the limitation involves the difficulty in obtaining appropriate data for systems analysis. Current approaches can be used to clarify the system structure and focus attention for future studies.

Systems Analysis

Recent developments in control theory have made it clear that metabolic pathways are very seldom controlled at one location, although one step may dominate under certain conditions. System control is generally distributed over several enzymes including near-equilibrium steps, and this distribution can change with time during transients or with conditions in other pathways (e.g. 260). Quantitative understanding of the control requires knowledge of the kinetic behavior of each step and all inputs to and outputs from the system. Until models are put together and tested against appropriate data, we don't know if we even have all the parameters involved in control of glycolysis. Such a complete analysis has not been done in exercising skeletal muscle, although a fairly complete model has been developed for the palmitate-perfused heart (157–159). In this case control was considerably distributed, but one clear conclusion arose: most of the control of lactate production rested in the mitochondria (157). In spite of the limitation on a full quantitative understanding, a number of studies have qualitatively identified some important parameters under various exercise conditions. These allow us to begin testing our understanding of integrated control in vivo.

General Considerations. One useful approach to studying system behavior is to divide the complete system into subsystems that can be formally analyzed and then reintegrated in a stepwise fashion. We will use that approach here and relate the predicted behavior with that seen in various exercise conditions. The most obvious subsystems of the glycolytic pathway are the allosterically regulated enzymes (glycogen phosphorylase and phosphofructokinase) with *near-equilibrium* steps that only transiently deviate from near-equilibrium conditions in between. In addition, the section between the triosephosphates and pyruvate seem to behave as a coordinated unit. These have been analyzed in detail above. The more complex ones involving several enzymes and intermediates that serve to couple glycolysis to the rest of the metabolic systems of the cell are discussed below.

Phosphate Energy Subsystem. This subsystem has been analyzed in detail and initial steps in reintegrating it with phosphofructokinase and other metabolic subsystems has been carried out (52 56 105).

Creatine kinase and adenylate kinase appear to be essentially at equilibrium under most conditions in vivo (52). Since the cytosolic pools of creatine, adenine nucleotides, and total phosphate are nearly constant for most exercise conditions, these components form a subsystem in the muscle (see Fig. 19.1). Changes in PCr, ATP, ADP, AMP, and Pi are tightly coupled so that it is characterized by two variables: the total high energy phosphate bonds and the pH (52). Thus, in vivo control must reflect the coordinated response to simultaneous changes in all of the components of the system. These changes can be quantitatively defined by the total pool sizes, the equilibrium constants of the enzymes, and the phosphate energy state of the system (PE state) (52). The most sensitive and easiest measure of this phosphate energy state is a measure of the fractional phosphorylation of creatine or the *creatine charge* (PCr/Cr_{total}). In skeletal muscle (and perhaps in most creatine-containing tissues) the relative sizes of the total adenine nucleotide, phosphate, and creatine pools appears to be constant. This constancy is maintained through various muscle fiber types. When this is factored in, a simple measure of the creatine charge and pH defines the state of this whole subsystem (52).

Analysis. Figure 19.8 illustrates the adenine nucleotide pool changes as a function of the state of the phosphate energy subsystem. As ATP turnover increases, the activators ADP and AMP slowly increase while ATP levels are maintained (buffering region). With further increase in turnover rates and depletion of high-energy phosphate, a point is reached where ATP begins to decrease and the rise in ADP and AMP accelerates (depleting region). This gives a very strong activation to glycogen phosphorylase and phosphofructokinase. Pi levels change almost linearly with changes in high-energy phosphate

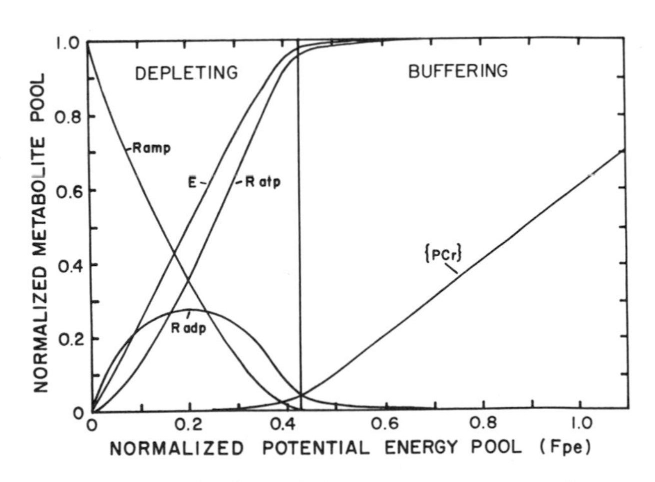

FIG. 19.8. Normalized metabolite concentrations as a function of high-energy phosphate. All values were computed using pH = 7.0, $[Mg^{2+}]$ = 1 mM, and total free adenine nucleotide pool (ADt) = 0.2 × total creatine pool. Fc, [PCr]/[total creatine]; R_{atp}, [ATP]/[ADt]; R_{adp}, [ADP]/[ADt]; R_{amp}, [AMP]/[ADt]; Fpe, ([PCr] + 2[ATP] + ADP])/[total creatine]. [After Connett (52).]

levels in the buffering region. Thus, changes in Pi probably dominate control at low to moderate work rates, with AMP and ADP playing a more significant role when turnover is high relative to ATP production capacity. Although, as discussed above, there is uncertainty about the detailed quantitative responses of PFK to its various effectors, we can ask how the various models of its behavior respond to the changes in the PE state it would see in vivo. This analysis has been done (66). Three insights came from the study:

1. It was clear that this model could better account for the glycolytic flux seen in working skeletal muscle when the cytosolic pH was low. Previous analyses that focused on changes in one or two of the adenine nucleotides predicted negligible flux under these conditions.

2. Most models showed an almost linear response to the PE state as reflected in the creatine charge until the very low values seen in maximally working or anoxic muscles were reached. At this point phosphofructokinase was maximally activated and the flux was determined by substrate alone. Up to this point both the PE state and the concentration of F6P determined the net flux. The F6P levels will of course be determined by glycogen phosphorylase and perhaps hexokinase (see above).

3. The fractional activation of the enzyme was almost independent of the absolute concentration of the effectors but rather responded to the ratio of the inhibitors and activators. The consequence of this observation is that there will not be a qualitative difference in the control of PFK between type I and type II muscle fibers in spite of the almost twofold difference in the total pool sizes (161, 162, 182). The flux through this enzyme will reflect only the energy state of the tissue, the level of F6P, and the total enzyme concentration. Although there are few studies where the appropriate measurements have been made, some confirmation of this prediction can be found. The ratio of PFK activity for type II/type I fibers is ~5:1 (10, 242). Measurement of the PE state in rat EDL and soleus muscles after a 10 s stimulation at 50 Hz showed that the values were almost identical (42). If F6P concentrations and pH were not different between the two muscles, the flux through PFK should have been about five times faster in the EDL than in the soleus. If one uses the glycogenolytic rate as an estimate of this flux, one finds that indeed the ratio is ~5. Further studies are certainly necessary to confirm and extend this observation, especially in human muscles, where the ratio of enzyme activities appears to be closer to 3: 1. It does suggest that we have a reasonable method for analyzing the quantitative behavior of PFK in response to changes in energy turnover. The fractional recruitment of flux through PFK in all fiber types can, in the first approximation, be accounted for by three variables: the PE state, cytosolic pH, and F6P concentrations. Because type II fibers have a higher total Pi pool and GP is stimulated with increasing Pi, it would be expected that in type II fibers increased F6P would lead to a slightly greater fraction of PFK capacity being used at any given state of the PE system. The absolute rate will depend on the amount of enzyme present in that fiber. Preliminary analyses based on data from rest-work transitions in dog muscle (see below) are consistent with this conclusion.

Limitations and future studies. The system analysis to date has assumed equilibrium at both creatine kinase and adenylate kinase. Although this may be a reasonable assumption under many conditions, it may not always be true in exercising muscle, especially at very high ATP turnover rates and during the early period of transients. A kinetic model of the phosphate energy subsystem may be required under these conditions. This is important in dealing with the interaction between GP and PFK, since the control strengths of Pi and pH are very different at these two steps (see earlier under Control of GP, Phosphofructokinase, and POSTEXERCISE GLYCOGEN SYNTHESIS AND ITS CONTROL) and coupling will be tied to changes in G6P (and F6P).

Although application of the equilibrium phosphate energy subsystem to current PFK kinetic models shows qualitative fits with some of the data in exercising muscle, there is a need for further study. As discussed earlier under Phosphofructokinase, the current kinetic models of PFK probably do not deal adequately with the quantitative effects of Pi and pH on the kinetics in vivo. Analysis of rest-work transitions in dog muscle indicate that, while the time course of kinetic transitions is reasonably predicted, the measured lactate accumulation is less than the model would predict (53, R. J. Connett unpublished obsdervations). Furthermore, during fatigue and recovery from exercise the energetic signals would suggest a high PFK and glycolytic flux whereas the observations indicate that it is very low (see earlier under MUSCLE GLYCOGEN METABOLISM AND FATIGUE). These observations suggest that two lines of inquiry need to be pursued: study of PFK kinetics with a view to in vivo conditons and more simultaneous measurement of changes in system parameters beyond the phosphate energy system under conditions of extreme exercise stress and recovery.

Redox State Subsystem. The cytosolic redox state, defined as {[NADH][H^+]/[NAD^+]}, can be treated as another interactive subsystem, comparable to the PE state. Note it includes [H^+], since this term is part of the redox reactions in the cell. Due to buffering in the cell, the redox reactions probably play a negligible role in determining the cytosolic pH. However, because of the participation of H^+ in the redox reactions, pH can play a large role in mass action effects at redox reactions. It is not simple to develop a quantitative model for the redox subsystem. It involves more reactions than the PE system, some with poorly defined states in the cell. Nonetheless, a qualitative analysis of its operation and effects on glycolysis can be developed. A simplified diagram illustrating the "sources" and "sinks" affecting cytosolic redox as related to glycolysis in a working muscle is shown in Figure 19.9. The major reducing input shown is the production of NADH by the GAPDH reaction, although the mitochondrial transport steps and other reactions affecting cytosolic pH may be important sources. The major oxidizing "sinks" include the following:

1. *Lactate production from pyruvate.* By itself, this is a limited capacity sink. If LDH is at equilibrium with the cytosolic redox pool (see above), then with continued glycolytic production of NADH, lactate will accumulate, lactate/pyruvate (L/P) ratios will increase, and the pool of NADH + NAD^+ will gradually be converted to NADH and H^+ will accumulate. The production will stop through mass-action effects of the increasing [NADH] and [H^+] and falling [NAD^+] on GAPDH. This puts an absolute limit on glycolysis in the absence of other "sinks." This has been observed repeatedly in cell-free glycolyzing systems and in ischemic muscle.

2. *Transport of reducing equivalents across the mitochondrial membrane via the "shuttle systems."* In skeletal muscle this seems to be dominated by the "aspartate-malate" system and may operate near an equilibrium that is coupled to the mitochondrial membrane potential (152). This process serves to couple glycolysis to mitochondrial function. Mitochondria can also be a source of reducing equivalents for the cytosol via the same " shuttle" systems. When there is a nonglycolytic source of substrate for production of mitochondrial reducing equivalents such as fatty acids, export of reducing equivalents to the cytosol will serve to limit glycolysis independent of an effect of citrate on PFK (see above).

3. *Lactate efflux from the muscle.* The loss of a reduced compound from the system is equivalent to consumption of a reducing equivalent. Thus, lactate transport may be an important variable in permit-

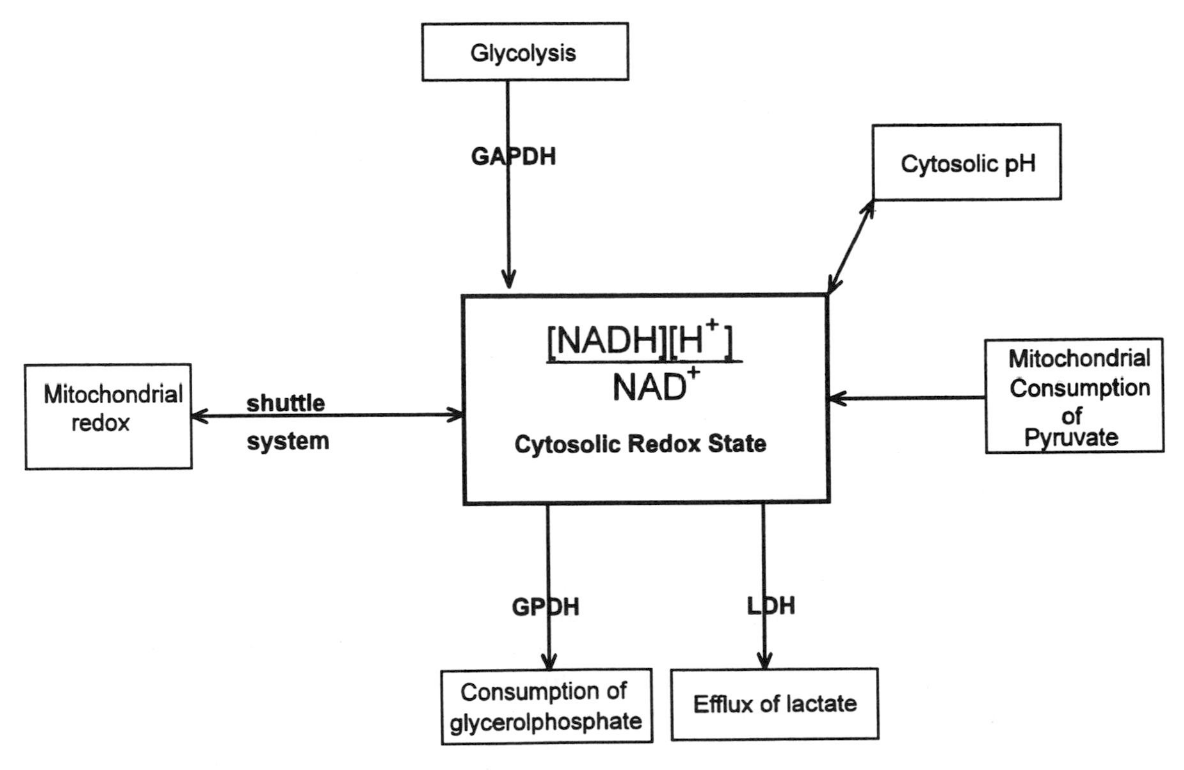

FIG. 19.9. Schematic of cytosolic redox subsystem. GAPDH, glyceraldehydephosphate dehydrogenase; GPDH, glycerolphosphate dehydrogenase; LDH, lactate dehydrogenase.

ting sustained glycolysis under conditions where the consumption of reducing equivalents by mitochondria is limited. This consumption may be limited either by substrate availability (e.g., oxygen supply) or by capacity limitations (e.g., limited mitochondrial content in white muscle fibers or near maximal exercise where turnover capacity is reached). Studies of this process are still in the early stages and there may be as yet unknown controls operating (83, 84, 219).

4. *Changes in cellular pH and H^+ efflux from the muscle.* Since $[H^+]$ is part of the redox reactions, loss of H^+ from the cytosol is, like loss of lactate, identical to consuming reducing equivalents in this system. Production of acidic products (like lactate) is production of reducing equivalents. Finally, changes in cellular buffering capacity (variations in P_{CO_2} and bicarbonate) will also affect the cytosolic redox state.

5. *Production of glycerolphosphate from DHAP by glycerolphosphate dehydrogenase.* This is usually relegated to a minor role in the operation of glycolysis, but there is evidence that glycerolphosphate can and does accumulate under exercising conditions (126, 233). This may contribute to the overall regulation of glycolytic flux, especially since muscle may dephosphorylate the glycerolphosphate and export it (138, 199). It, like lactate export, is equivalent to the consumption of reducing equivalents.

The final consideration of the redox system is its interaction with the phosphate energy subsystem. This certainly occurs at the near-equilibrium reactions catalyzed by GAPDH-PGK (see earlier under Glyceraldehydephosphate Dehydrogenase and Phosphoglycerate Kinase). Changes in either PE state or redox can cause parallel changes in the other signal. Another point of interaction is at the mitochondrial membrane. The PE state signal appears to be the dominating control on recruitment of mitochondrial ATP production. However, it is clear that this must interact with the mitochondrial redox state (93) and via the shuttle system the cytosolic redox state (21). The cytosolic pH affects both the PE state and the redox state. This is another factor resulting in interaction between the two subsystems.

The PE state appears to dominate control by allosteric mechanisms at PFK and via both substrate (Pi) and allosteric (AMP) at glycogen phosphorylase, whereas redox considerations dominate control by mass-action effects in the lower section. The coupling of these two signals permits control of the two sections of glycolysis to be tightly coordinated at all times (231).

Analysis. While a quantitative analysis of the effects of this subsystem have not been carried out in the detail possible for the phosphate energy system, certain consequences of its action can be identified.

Consumption of pyruvate by the mitochondria must be accompanied by parallel consumption of reducing equivalents by the shuttle system. If this doesn't happen, the cytosolic NADH levels will increase and ultimately limit flux through GAPDH, slowing or halting glycolytic flux. The effect of this requirement can be seen in several conditions.

1. A limit to the oxygen supply in the absence of lactate efflux may reflect such a state. The correlation between the redox state and the PE state should remain the same. Preliminary studies in ischemic muscles support this conclusion. Under these conditions, glycerolphosphate and glycerol concentrations should also increase. As a corollary to this, if lactate and/or H^+ can be exported, the elevation of the redox state is limited and glycolytic production of ATP can continue longer and faster. This accounts for a major difference in glycolytic flux between ischemic and hypoxemic-dysoxic conditions in working muscle (e.g., see 251).

2. Glycolytic flux and cytosolic redox are sensitive to mitochondrial content, giving rise to differences in lactate production between fiber types and training effects when mitochondrial contents are increased. If mitochondrial contents are increased, the capacity to transport and consume reducing equivalents is increased as well as the rate of production of ATP. At the same ATP turnover rate the fractional utilization of mitochondrial capacity is less and therefore the shift in the PE state necessary to recruit it is less, leading to a smaller change in PE state and thus lower recruitment of glycolysis via this signal. Similarly, the transmembrane redox gradient is less and thus cytosolic redox as reflected in the L/P is less. This results in lower lactate accumulation and export. Consequently, there is a shift in the observed lactate threshold in the blood. The prediction is that L/P ratios still are related to $\dot{V}_{O_2}$ but that the actual lactate concentration is decreased by the same fraction as the increase in mitochondrial capacity.

3. Internal production of reducing equivalents in the mitochondrion with export to the cytosol. When fatty acid oxidation dominates in the mitochondria, reducing equivalents may be exported to the cytosol. In fact, this may be required when the mitochondrial membrane potential changes as the rate of ATP turnover increases (58, 59). The result would be an elevation in the cytosolic redox state. However, if the coupling between PE state and the redox state occurs primarily via glycolytic enzymes, small changes in both PE and redox states might occur. Glycolytic flux will then be restrained by both changes. This

has been observed in both heart and liver (154, 157, 252). Limited data from resting rat soleus did not show a significant change in redox as measured by L/P, but the glycolytic rate decreased in response to palmitate loading (199). More information relating these variables is necessary to clarify this issue.

The net flux through glycolysis and the production of lactate appears to decline with sustained muscle activity. During sustained aerobic exercise lactate production occurs at a lower rate than during the rest-work transition, but the levels of lactate in the muscle and blood rise as a function of the fractional turnover leading to the so-called lactate threshold phenomenon. The lactate levels in both blood and muscle appear to be closely tied to the fraction of $\dot{V}O_{2max}$ being used by the working muscle, which is in turn related to the PE state (see above). When mitochondrial contents are increased by training, the concentration of lactate found in the muscle at a given $\dot{V}O_2$ decreases; but when expressed as a fraction of mitochondrial capacity, the levels are similar. Pyruvate levels in the tissue are nearly stable; thus, changes in lactate concentration reflect a change in the L/P ratio and hence the cytosolic redox state. Glycolytic control under conditions of sustained exercise appears to be more dependent on the state of the redox system and its interaction with the PE state (58). This in turn is dominated by the mitochondrial membrane potential and redox shuttle, which depend on the flux density of transport across the mitochondrial membrane (i.e., the fraction of the oxidative phosphorylation capacity being used). Several lines of information and analysis support this hypothesis:

1. Data from muscles stimulated in situ show a linear relationship between the cytosolic redox (as reflected in the L/P ratio) and V_{O_2} [see Fig. 19.10; (59, 60)]. Data from exercising humans do not show as linear a relationship between L/P ratio and V_{O_2} (233).
2. In a cell free system containing mitochondria, the enzymes involved in transport of reducing equivalents across the mitochondrial membrane, and a complete glycolyzing system, the L/P ratio is coupled to the rate of ATP turnover only when the mitochondria are coupled (143).
3. Sensitivity analysis of models incorporating both mitochondrial and cytosolic systems show that control of glycolysis at steady-state is dominated by redox considerations (157).

Control dominated by redox considerations focuses attention on the issues of the sinks in the redox system (Fig 19.9). These include lactate and H^+ efflux mechanisms as well as the mitochondrial shuttle system (144). A redox-dominated control also requires that glyceraldehyde phosphate dehydrogenase and phosphoglycerate kinase play a critical role during sustained exercise. This suggests a need for more quantitative exploration of the coupling between the redox and PE state systems, especially will respect to effects on PFK.

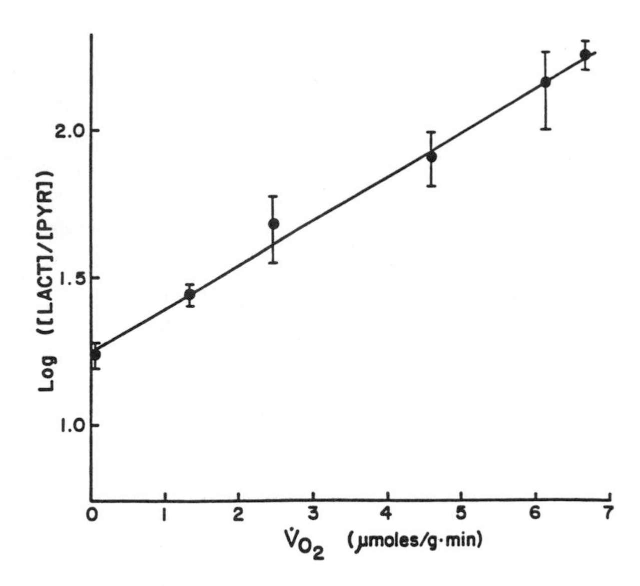

FIG. 19.10. Relationship between cytosolic redox potential and $\dot{V}O_2$. Correlation between cytosolic redox potential as estimated from the [lactate]/[pyruvate] ratio and oxygen consumption in dog gracilis muscle. [From Connett and Gayeski (59).]

Cytosolic pH Subsystem. The pH of the cytosol is a central control parameter (see Fig. 19.11). It directly affects the major allosterically controlled enzymes of glycolysis and it is a component of both the phosphate energy and redox subsystems as well as potentially interacting with ATP production in the mitochondrion. Its value is affected by the balance between the production of acidic compounds such as lactate and CO_2 and the consumption and export of these compounds. Shifts in the creatine kinase equilibrium will change it. Finally, changes in the buffering capacity of the cell due to shifts in the HCO_3^-/Cl^- and P_{CO_2} across the cell membrane will contribute to the final value. Our current quantitative understanding of the dynamics of pH changes in relation to other system components has been limited by our ability to directly measure cytosolic pH values. Modern NMR methods are helping in this respect, but further analysis of this subsystem in relation to the many factors affecting it needs to be done.

System Mass-Action Considerations. While the mass-action effects on rate resulting from changes in sub-

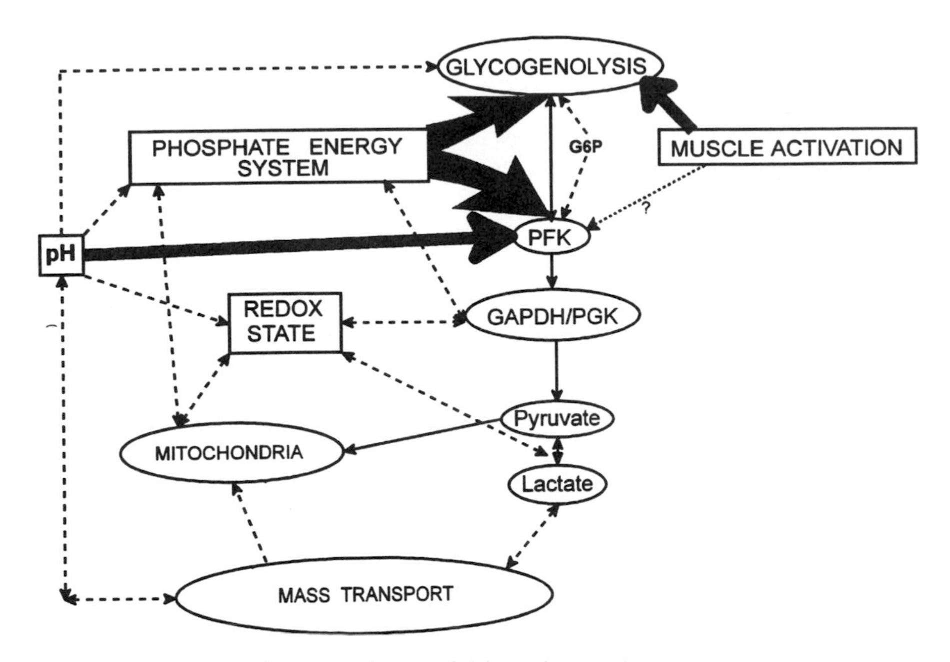

FIG. 19.11. System controls on glycolysis. *Solid lines* show carbon flow in pathway. Other lines indicate control interactions either allosteric or substrate effects. Details are given in the text.

strate and product concentrations at a single enzyme are well understood, there are system effects when inhibition downstream results in an increase in intermediates throughout the pathway. All enzymes will be operating at a different point relative to their K_m's, and the distribution of control strengths at each step can change dramatically (157). In addition, there may be other changes in behavior. Although F16diP has been shown to be an activator of PFK in vitro (see earlier under Phosphofructokinase), there appears to be a special relationship between PFK and aldolase. There is some evidence that these two enzymes may be physically associated. If this is true, mass-action effects may play a more important role than expected in the control of PFK. Accumulation of triosphosphates will slow flux through aldolase. If there is flux coupling via F16diP, then PFK will be slowed independent of the PE state or [F6P]. This could serve as another mechanism for increasing reduction of the cytosol that slows flux through GAPDH-PGK and increases triosephosphate concentrations, to slow flux through PFK. A similar effect via G6P on phosphorylase would serve to keep the whole glycolytic pathway coordinated in response to mitochondrial induced changes in redox and/or pyruvate levels.

Cellular Oxygen Tension and Lactate Formation

Oxygen-limited ATP formation. As indicated earlier under GENERAL OVERVIEW OF THE GLYCOLYTIC PATHWAY, glycolysis will serve a primary purpose of ATP supply *(1)* when the ATP demand exceeds the fiber $\dot{V}O_{2max}$ and mitochondrial capacity is inadequate or *(2)* when O_2 supply is limiting. Condition 1) may be reached during heavy dynamic exercise with small muscle groups when O_2 supply is not limited by the circulatory system, but may be a rare condition during in vivo exercise. Condition 2) will occur when exercise intensity exceeds or is near the whole-body $\dot{V}O_{2max}$ or alternatively when muscle blood flow is impaired (e.g., by the high intramuscular pressure during static contractions). The increase in the rate of glycolysis during conditions of O_2-limited ATP formation will be related to the energy demand and thus to the ATP turnover. The mechanism by which the rate of glycolysis is matched to the ATP turnover is unclear. The changes in the PE state including increases in Pi are large and there is evidence that both GPb and GPb are activated. The rate of glycolysis during sustained maximal exercise will not increase in proportion to the change in PE state, probably due to feedback inhibition of PFK and GP by accumulating H^+, augmented by the feedback of the redox system state on GAPDH. The capacity of lactate formation appears to be limited by H^+ accumulation, although it is unclear whether the effect is mediated by a direct inhibition of the contractile process (decrease in ATP demand) or if a feedback inhibition of glycolysis impairs ATP formation and the contractile process.

Summary

The major influences regulating glycolytic flux can be summarized as reflecting the influence of a few major and some minor or transient sytem variables (see Fig. 19.11).

State of the Phosphate Energy System

1. Glycogen synthetase and phosphorylase are sensitive to changes in Pi and AMP.
2. Phosphofructokinase is strongly influenced by all components of this system except PCr and creatine.

Any change in the rate of energy turnover will change the state of this system and thus the flux through these major glycolytic control points. This probably is the major site coupling energy demand during exercise to glycolytic flux. Since mitochondria also respond to the state of this system, this is a major point of interaction between glycolysis and aerobic metabolism.

Cytosolic pH

1. PFK is exquisitely sensitive to pH below 8.0 and strongly interacts with the state of the phosphate energy system. This, coupled with the phosphate energy system, is the dominating control on this step.
2. Glycogenolysis is affected via titration of Pi and its effect on phosphorylase kinase activity.
3. pH affects both the position of the creatine kinase equilbrium and its kinetics during transients. Thus, changes in pH will operate via changes in the phosphate energy system.
4. Due to its role in redox reactions, pH will affect both mitochondrial activity and the state of the GAPDH-PGK couple. This again will influence the phosphate energy system.

An alkaline shift may play an activating role on both glycogenolysis and phosphofructokinase during the onset of muscle activity, and decreased pH will restrict flux during activity with sustained glycolytic flux and acid accumulation.

Redox State

1. Cytosolic redox influences and is influenced by mitochondrial activity. Thus redox state will modify the mitochondrial role in the state of the phosphate energy system.
2. The redox state also interacts with the phosphate energy state at the GAPDH-PGK couple and modifies the position of the near-equilibrium thus affecting glycolytic flux directly.

This may be a significant area of coupling between the glycolytic and mitochondrial pathways at steady state and during high rates of turnover. As discussed above, there is indirect evidence, but more study on the role of this system variable needs to be carried out.

Muscle Activation. Other than the obvious effect due to increased ATP consumption, other results of muscle activation can play a role in the control of glycolysis.

1. Ca^{2+} has a direct effect on phosphorylase kinase. This probably has a critical role in glycolytic activation during the onset of exercise, but its role is less clear during sustained activity.
2. Membrane potential changes during muscle activation can affect cell levels of Cl^- and HCO_3^-. These changes in turn will affect cell buffering, pH, and lactate transport. While these may be minor effects, they have not been adequately explored.
3. Activation of the contractile machinery can affect enzyme binding and hence sensitivy to the other controls. While this is thought to be insignificant in the overall control, it may play an important role under some conditions.

Substrate Effects

1. G6P is a point of direct interaction between glycogenolysis and phosphofructokinase. As discussed earlier under Control of GP and under Phosphofructokinase both feedforward from glycogenolysis and feedback from phosphofructokinase will occur. This serves to keep the fluxes through these two steps coupled and coordinated with glucose uptake.
2. Glycogen levels affect the glycogenolytic capacity.
3. The supply of O_2 and other mitochondrial substrates affects mitochondrial metabolic turnover. This will function via the phosphate energy and redox states.

Further direct interaction with the cytosolic redox state will result from the effect of the relative rates of glycolytic pyruvate production and mitochondrial consumption. The importance of this in the overall regulation is poorly understood at this time.

Other Mass Transport Considerations. Transport of lactate and H^+ affect the pH and redox state. Furthermore, transport of lactate can affect the availability of pyruvate as mitochondrial substrate. Controls on lactate transport are poorly understood at this time and the role of this variable on control of glycolysis can only be indirectly inferred. This will be strongly influenced by whole-body considerations.

Future Directions

While much is known about the factors that influence the recruitment and rate of glycolysis, we cannot at this time account quantitatively for the changes in glycolytic flux either during exercise or recovery. The failures include both activation of glycolysis with the onset of exercise and the slowing of glycolysis when our current models suggest that both GP and PFK should be activated. Two lines of inquiry appear to be fruitful at this time.

Modeling. Quantitative models that take into account all of the known enzyme behavior of both the glycolytic pathway and its integration with the phosphate energy and redox subsystems need to be developed. While these may be limited by current knowledge of enzyme kinetic parameters of the complex GP and PFK systems, exploration of model behavior in response to changes in redox (as influenced by mitochondria and lactate efflux) may significantly add to our understanding. While the phosphate energy subsystem seems to be well understood, a fraction of the total measured adenine nucleotide pool does not appear to be involved. A model can be used to explore the consequences of changes in this pool. Finally, if the models cannot quantitatively account for the observations in tissue, that analysis can be used to identify those modifications necessary to make them describe the events and help focus future enzyme and tissue studies.

System Based Experiments. Since it is increasingly clear that single control variables and single enzymes are not responsible for the regulation of glycolysis, experiments must take these system concerns into account. This can be done by focusing on parts of the system that may be conceptually isolated (e.g., phosphate energy, or redox subsystems) or by doing multiparameter measurements that permit correlations between changes in critical system variables that act at several points. Many previous studies have been limited by the application of one or two methodologies at a time. More direct testing of quantitative system-based hypotheses are needed. This is especially important in dealing with coordination of the redox system with mitochondrial behavior and the PE state. It is also important in identifying the coupling parameters between whole-body concerns such as blood flow, pH control, lactate efflux and turnover, and substrate delivery.

Identify Possible New Controllers. Our present knowledge from modeling and system analysis would predict a high glycolytic rate when changing from exercise to anaerobic recovery but, as discussed above, glycolysis is turned off in concert with the contraction. It is possible that unknown controllers play a dominating role in the on/off switch of glycolysis. Alternatively, the concentrations of some of the known controllers at the active site of the enzymes are different from the measured or estimated concentrations.

It is clear that in spite of our knowledge, our understanding of system control in vivo is limited. To establish the *quantitative role* of known variables and/or identify new controllers will be a future challenge.

This work was supported in part by Swedish Medical Research Council (No. 08671), National Institutes of Health grant HL-03290, and Monroe Communty College, New York.

REFERENCES

1. Achs, M. J., and D. Garfinkel. Computer simulation of energy metabolism in anoxic perfused rat heart *Am. J. Physiol.* 232 (*Regulatory Integrative Comp. Physiol.* 1): R164–R174, 1977.
2. Achs, M. J., and D. Garfinkel. Computer simulation of rat heart metabolism after adding glucose to the perfusate. *Am. J. Physiol.* 232 (*Regulatory Integrative Comp. Physiol.* 1): R175–R184, 1977.
3. Adams, G. R., J. M. Foley, and R. A. Meyer. Muscle buffer capacity estimated from pH changes during rest-to-work transitions. *J. Appl. Physiol.* 69: 968–972, 1990.
4. Ahlborg, B., J. Bergström, L.-G. Ekelund, G. Guarnieri, R. C. Harris, E. Hultman, and L.-O. Nordesjö. Muscle metabolism during isometric exercise performed at constant force. *J. Appl. Physiol.* 33: 224–228, 1972.
5. Aragon, J. J., and J. M. Lowenstein. The purine-nucleotide cycle. Comparison of the levels of citric acid cycle intermediates with the operation of the purine nucleotide cycle in rat skeletal muscle during exercise and recovery from exercise. *Eur. J. Biochem.* 110: 371–377, 1980.
6. Aragon, J. J., K. Tornheim, and J. M. Lowenstein. On a possible role of IMP in the regulation of phosphorylase activity in skeletal muscle. *Fed. Eur. Biochem. Soc. Lett.* 117: K56–K64, 1980.
7. Astrand, P.-O., J. Hallbäck, R. Hedman, and B. Saltin. Blood lactates after prolonged severe exercise. *J. Appl. Physiol.* 18: 619–622, 1963.
8. Astrand, P.-O., E. Hultman, A. Juhlin-Dannfelt, and G. Reynolds. Disposal of lactate during and after strenous exercise in humans. *J. Appl. Physiol.* 61: 338–343, 1986.
9. Astrand, P.-O., and K. Rodahl. *Textbook of Work Physiology*, 3rd edition. New York: McGraw-Hill, 1986.
10. Baldwin, K. M., W. W., Winder, R. L. Terjung, and J. O. Holloszy. Glycolytic enzymes in different types of skeletal muscle: adaptation to exercise. *Am. J. Physiol.* 225: 962–966, 1973.
11. Bangsbo, J., T. E. Graham, B. Kiens, and B. Saltin. Elevated muscle glycogen and anaerobic energy production during

exhaustive exercise in man. *J. Physiol. (Lond.)* 451: 205–227, 1992.

12. Bar-Tana, J., and Cleland, W. W. Rabbit muscle phosphofructokinase II. Product and dead end inhibition *J. Biol. Chem.* 249: 1271–1276, 1974.
13. deBarsy, T., and H.-G. Hers. Normal metabolism and disorders of carbohydrate metabolism. *Baillieres Clin. Endocrinol. Metab.* 4: 499–522, 1990.
14. Bardosi, A., Eber, S. W., and Roessmann, U. Ultrastructural and histochemical abnormalities of skeletal muscle in a patient with a new variant (type Homburg) of glucosephosphate isomerase (GPI) deficiency. *Clin. Neuropathol.* 4: 72–76, 1985.
15. Bass, A., A. Brdiczka, P. Eyer, S. Hofer, and D. Pette. Metabolic differentiation of distinct muscle types at the level of enzymatic organization. *Eur. J. Biochem.* 10: 198–206, 1969.
16. Bergström, J. Muscle electrolytes in man. *Scand. J. Clin. Lab. Invest.* 14(Suppl. 68): 1–110, 1962.
17. Bergström, J., L. Hermansen, E. Hultman, and B. Saltin. Diet, muscle glycogen and physical performance. *Acta. Physiol. Scand.* 71: 140–150, 1967.
18. Bergström, J., and E. Hultman. Muscle glycogen synthesis after exercise: an enhancing factor localized to the muscle cells in man. *Nature* 1210: 309–310, 1966.
19. Bergström, J., and E. Hultman. Synthesis of muscle glycogen in man after glucose and fructose infusion. *Acta Med. Scand.* 182: 93–107, 1967.
20. Bergström, J., E. Hultman, and A. E. Roch-Norlund. Muscle glycogen synthetase in normal subjects. *Scand. J. Clin. Lab. Invest.* 29: 231–236, 1972.
21. Berry, M. N., A. R. Grivell, and P. G. Wallace. Energy-dependent regulation of the steady-state concentrations of the components of the lactate dehydrogenase reaction in liver. *FEBS Lett.* 119: 317–322, 1980.
22. Bertocci, L. A., R. G. Haller, S. F. Lewis, J. L. Fleckenstein, and R. L. Nunnally. Abnormal high-energy phosphate metabolism in human muscle phosphofructokinase deficiency. *J. Appl. Physiol.* 70: 1201–1207, 1991.
23. Bloch, G., J. R. Chase, D. B. Meyer, M. J. Avison, G. I. Shulman, and R. G. Shulman. In vivo regulation of rat muscle glycogen resynthesis after intense exercise. *Am. J. Physiol.* 266 (*Endocrinol. Metab.* 29): E85–E91, 1994.
24. Blom, P. C. S., N. K. Vollestad, and D. L. Costill. Factors affecting changes in muscle glycogen concentration during and after prolonged exercise. *Acta Physiol. Scand.* 128 (Suppl. 556): 67–74, 1986.
25. Blomstrand, E., B. Ekblom, and E. A. Newsholme. Maximum activities of key glycolytic and oxidative enzymes in human muscle from differently trained individuals. *J. Physiol. (Lond.)* 381: 111–118, 1986.
26. Bosá, L., J. J. Aragón, and A. Sols. Modulation of muscle phosphofructokinase at physiological concentration of enzyme. *J. Biol. Chem.* 260: 2100–2107, 1985.
27. Bresolin, N., Y. I. Ro, M. Reyes, A. F. Miranda, and D. Maura. Muscle phosphoglycerate mutase (PGAM) deficiency: A second case. *Neurology* 33: 1049–1053, 1983.
28. Bristow, J., D. M. Bier, and L. G. Lange. Regulation of adult and fetal myocardial phosphofructokinase relief of cooperativity and competition between fructose 2,6-bisphosphate, ATP, and citrate. *J. Biol. Chem.* 262: 2171–2175, 1987.
29. Broberg, S., and K. Sahlin. Adenine nucleotide degradation in human skeletal muscle during prolonged exercise. *J. Appl. Physiol.* 67: 116–122, 1989.
30. Brooks, S. P., and K. B. Storey. The effect of enzyme-enzyme complexes on the overall glycolytic rate in vivo. *Biochem. Int.* 25: 477–489, 1991.
31. Brooks, S. P., and K. B. Storey. Where is the glycolytic complex? A critical evaluation of present data from muscle tissue. *FEBS Lett.* 278: 135–138, 1991.
32. Brown, D. H., and C. F. Cori. Animal and plant polysaccharide phosphorylase. In: *The Enzymes,* edited by L. M. Boyer. New York: Academic Press, 1961.
33. Busby, S. J. W., and G. K. Radda. Regulation of the glycogen phosphorylase system—from physical measurements to biological speculations. *Curr. Top. Cell. Regul.* 10: 89–160, 1976.
34. Canela, E. I., I. Ginesta, and R. Franco. Simulation of the purine nucleotide cycle as an anaplerotic process in skeletal muscle. *Arch. Biochem. Biophys.* 254: 142–155, 1987.
35. Cardenas, J. M., and R. D. Dyson. Bovine pyruvate kinases. II. Purification of the liver isozyme and its hybridization with skeletal muscle pyruvate kinase. *J. Biol. Chem.* 248: 6938–6944, 1973.
36. Cardenas, J. M., R. D. Dyson, and J. J. Strandholm. Bovine pyruvate kinases. I. Purification and characterization of the skeletal muscle isozyme. *J. Biol. Chem.* 248: 6931–6937, 1972.
37. Cartee, G. D., D. A. Young, M. D. Sleeper, J. Zierath, H. Wallberg-Henriksson, and J. O. Holloszy. Prolonged increase in insulin-stimulated glucose transport in muscle after exercise. *Am. J. Physiol.* 256 (*Endocrinol. Metab.* 19): E494–E499, 1989.
38. Castillo, C. E., A. Katz, M. K. Spencer, Z. Yan, and B. L. Nyomba. Fasting inhibits insulin-mediated glycolysis and anaplerosis in human skeletal muscle. *Am. J. Physiol.* 261 (*Endocrinol. Metab.* 24): E598–E605, 1991.
39. Ceretelli, P., D. Pendergast, W. C. Paganelli, and D. W. Rennie. Effects of specific muscle training on VO2 on-response and early blood lactate. *J. Appl. Physiol.* 47: 761–769, 1979.
40. Chaliss, R. A. J., B. Crabtree, and E. A. Newsholme. Hormonal regulation of the rate of the glycogen/glucose-1-phosphate cycle in skeletal muscle. *Eur. J. Biochem.* 163: 205–210, 1987.
41. Chasiotis, D. The regulation of glycogen phosphorylase and glycogen breakdown in human skeletal muscle. *Acta Physiol. Scand. Suppl.* 518: 1–68, 1983.
42. Chasiotis, D., L. Edstrom, K. Sahlin, and H. Sjoholm. Activation of glycogen phosphorylase by electrical stimulation of isolated fast-twitch and slow-twitch muscles from rat. *Acta Physiol. Scand.* 123: 43–47, 1985.
43. Chasiotis, D., E. Hultman, and K. Sahlin. Acidotic depression of cyclic AMP accumulation and phosphorylase b to a transformation in skeletal muscle of man. *J. Physiol (Lond).* 335: 197–204, 1983.
44. Chasiotis, D., K. Sahlin, and E. Hultman. Regulation of glycogenolysis in human muscle at rest and during exercise. *J. Appl. Physiol.* 53: 708–715, 1982.
45. Chasiotis, D., K. Sahlin, and E. Hultman. Regulation of glycogenolysis in human muscle in response to epinephrine infusion. *J. Appl. Physiol.* 54: 45–50, 1983.
46. Cheetham, M. E., L. H. Boobis, L. Brooks, and C. Williams. Human muscle metabolism during sprint running. *J. Appl. Physiol.* 61: 54–60, 1986.
47. Christensen, E. H., and O. Hansen. Arbeitsfähigkeit undernährung. IV. Hypoglykemie, Arbeitsfähigkeit und Ermudung. *Scand. Arch. Physiol.* 81: 160–181, 1939.
48. Cohen, P. Muscle glycogen synthase. *Enzymes* 17: 461–497, 1986.

49. Cohen, P. Signal integration at the level of protein kinases, protein phosphatases and their substrates. *Trends Biochem. Sci.* 17: 408–413, 1992.
50. Conlee, R. K., R. C. Hickson, W. W. Winder, J. M. Hagberg, and J. O. Holloszy. Regulation of glycogen resynthesis in muscles of rats following exercise. *Am. J. Physiol.* 235 (*Regulatory Integrative Comp. Physiol.* 4): R145–R150, 1978.
51. Conlee, R. K., J. A. McLane, M. J. Rennie, W. W. Winder, and J. O. Holloszy. Reversal of phosphorylase activation in muscle despite continued contractile activity. *Am. J. Physiol.* 237 (*Regulatory Integrative Comp. Physiol.* 6): R291–R296, 1979.
52. Connett, R. J. Analysis of metabolic control: new insights using a scaled creatine kinase model. *Am. J. Physiol.* 254 (*Regulatory Integrative Comp. Physiol.* 23): R949–R959, 1988.
53. Connett, R. J. Cytosolic pH during a rest-to-work transition in red muscle: application of enzyme equilibria. *J. Appl. Physiol.* 63: 2360–2365, 1987.
54. Connett, R. J. Glycolytic regulation during an aerobic rest-to-work transition in dog gracilis muscle. *J. Appl. Physiol.* 63: 2366–2374, 1987.
55. Connett, R. J. Glycolytic regulation during rest-to-work transition in dog gracilis muscle. *J. Appl. Physiol.* 63: 2370–2374, 1987.
56. Connett, R. J. In vivo control of phosphofructokinase: system models suggest new experimental protocols. *Am. J. Physiol.* 257 (*Regulatory Integrative Comp. Physiol.* 26): R878–R888, 1989.
57. Connett, R. J. In vivo glycolytic equilibria in dog gracilis muscle. *J. Biol. Chem.* 260: 3314–3320, 1985.
58. Connett, R. J. The cytosolic redox is coupled to VO2: a working hypothesis. *Adv. Exp. Med. Biol.* 222: 133–142, 1988.
59. Connett, R. J., T. E. J. Gayeski, and C. R. Hong. Does energy demand have an additional control in ischemia or are current models of metabolic control adequate at extremes? *Adv. Exp. Med. Biol.* 361: 509–520, 1994.
60. Connett, R. J., T. E. J. Gayeski, and C. R. Honig. Lactate accumulation in fully aerobic, working dog gracilis muscle. *Am. J. Physiol.* 246 (*Heart Circ. Physiol.* 15): H120–H128, 1984.
61. Connett, R. J., T. E. J. Gayeski, and C. R. Honig. Energy sources in fully aerobic rest-work transitions: a new role for glycolysis. *Am. J. Physiol.* 248 (*Heart Circ. Physiol.* 17): H922–H929, 1985.
62. Connett, R. J., T. E. J. Gayeski, and C. R. Honig. Lactate efflux is unrelated to intracellular PO2 in a working red muscle in situ. *J. Appl. Physiol.* 61: 402–408, 1986.
63. Connett, R. J., and C. R. Honig. Regulation of VO2 in red muscle: do current biochemical hypotheses fit in vivo data? *Am. J. Physiol.* 256 (*Regulatory Integrative Comp. Physiol.* 25): R898–R906, 1989.
64. Connett, R. J., C. R. Honig, T. E. J. Gayeski, and G. A. Brooks. Defining hypoxia: a systems view of VO2, glycolysis, energetics, and intracellular PO2. *J. Appl. Physiol.* 68: 833–842, 1990.
65. Consler, T. G., M. J. Jennewein, G. Z. Cai, and J. C. Lee. Synergistic effects of proton and phenylalanine on the regulation of muscle pyruvate kinase. *Biochemistry* 29: 10765–10771, 1990.
66. Constable, S. H., R. J. Favier, and J. O. Holloszy. Exercise and glycogen depletion: effects on ability to activate muscle phosphorylase. *J. Appl. Physiol.* 60: 1518–1523, 1986.
67. Constable, S. H., J. C. Young, M. Higuchi, and J. O. Holloszy. Glycogen resynthesis in leg muscles of rats during exercise. *Am. J. Physiol.* 247 (*Regulatory Integrative Comp. Physiol.* 16): R880–R883, 1984.
68. Constantin-Teodosiu, D., G. Cederblad, and E. Hultman. Pyruvate dehydrogenase complex activity and acetyl group accumulation in skeletal muscle during prolonged exercise. *J. Appl. Physiol.* 74: 1712–1718, 1993.
69. Cooke, R., and E. Pate. The effects of ADP and phosphate on the contraction of muscle fibers. *Biophys. J.* 48: 789–798, 1985.
70. Cori, G. T. The effect of stimulation and recovery on the phosphorylase a content of muscle. *J. Biol. Chem.* 151: 31–38, 1945.
71. Cornell, N. W., M. Leadbetter, and R. L. Veech. Effects of free magnesium concentration and ionic strength on equilibrium constants for the glyceraldehyde phosphate dehydrogenase and phosphoglycerate kinase reactions. *J. Biol. Chem.* 254: 6522–6527, 1979.
72. Costill, D. L., E. Coyle, G. Dalsky, W. Evans, W. Fink, and D. Hoopes. Effects of elevated plasma FFA and insulin on muscle glycogen usage during exercise. *J. Appl. Physiol.* 43: 695–699, 1977.
73. Costill, D. L., D. D. Pascoe, W. J. Fink, R. A. Robergs, S. I. Barr, and D. Pearson. Impaired muscle glycogen resynthesis after eccentric exercise. *J. Appl. Physiol.* 69: 46–50, 1990.
74. Costill, D. L., D. R. Pearson, and W. L. Fink. Impaired muscle glycogen storage after muscle biopsy. *J. Appl. Physiol.* 64: 2245–2248, 1988.
75. Coyle, E. F. Carbohydrate supplementation during exercise. *J. Nutr.* 122 (Suppl. 3): 788–795, 1992.
76. Danforth, W. H. Activation of glycolytic pathway in muscle. In: *Control of Energy Metabolism*, edited by B. Chance and R. W. Estabrook. New York: Academic Press, 1965, p. 287–296.
77. Danforth, W. H. Glycogen synthetase activity in skeletal muscle: interconversion of two forms and control of glycogen synthesis. *J. Biol. Chem.* 240: 588–593, 1965.
78. Danforth, W. H., E. Helmreich, and C. F. Cori. The effect of contraction and of epinephrine on the phosphorylase activity of frog sartorius muscle. *Biochemistry* 48: 1191–1199, 1962.
79. Danforth, W. H., and J. B. Lyon. Glycogenolysis during tetanic contraction of isolated mouse muscles in the presence and absence of phosphorylase a. *J. Biol. Chem.* 239: 4047–4050, 1964.
80. Davies, C. T. M., and M. W. Thompson. Aerobic performance of female marathon and male ultramarathon athletes. *Eur. J. Appl. Physiol.* 41: 233–245, 1979.
81. Dawson, M. J., D. G. Gadian, and D. R. Wilkie. Studies of the biochemistry of contracting and relaxing muscle by the use of 31P n.m.r. in conjunction with other techniques. *Phil. Trans. R. Soc. Lond.* 3289: 445–455, 1980.
82. Dawson, M. J., D. G. Gadian, and D. R. Wilkie. Contraction and recovery of living muscles studied by 31P nuclear magnetic resonance. *J. Physiol. (Lond.)* 267: 703–735, 1977.
83. de Bruijne, A. W., H. Vreeburg, and J. van Steveninck. Alternate-substrate inhibition of L-lactate transport via the monocarboxylate-specific carrier system in human erythrocytes. *Biochim. Biophys. Acta* 812: 841–844, 1985.
84. deBarsy, T., and H.-G. Hers. Normal metabolism and disorders of carbohydrate metabolism. *Baillieres Clin. Endocrinol. Metab.* 4: 499–522, 1990.

85. Deibert, D. C., and R. A. DeFronzo. Epinephrine-induced insulin resistance in man. *J. Clin. Invest.* 65: 717–721, 1980.
86. Denton, R. M., and A. P. Halestrap. Regulation of pyruvate metabolism in mammalian tissues. *Essays Biochem.* 15: 37–77, 1979.
87. Di Prampero, P. E., C. T. M. Davies, P. Cerretelli, and R. Margaria. An analysis of O_2 debt contracted in submaximal exercise. *J. Appl. Physiol.* 29: 547–551, 1970.
88. Dobson, G. P., E. Yamamoto, and P. W. Hochachka. Phosphofructokinase control in muscle: nature and reversal of pH dependent ATP inhibition. *Am. J. Physiol.* 250 (*Regulatory Integrative Comp. Physiol.* 19): R71–R76, 1986.
89. Donaldson, S. K. B., L. Hermansen, and L. Bolles. Differential direct effects of H^+ on Ca^{2+} activated force of skinned fibers from the soleus, cardiac and adductor magnus muscles of rabbits. *Pflugers Arch.* 376: 55–65, 1978.
90. Drummond, G. I., J. P. Harwood, and C. A. Powell. Studies on the activation of phosphorylase in skeletal muscle by contraction and by epinephrine. *J. Biol. Chem.* 244: 4235–4240, 1969.
91. Dyson, R. D., J. M. Cardenas, R. J. Barsotti. The reversibility of skeletal muscle pyruvate kinase and an assessment of its capacity to support glyconeogenesis. *J. Biol. Chem.* 250: 3316–3321, 1975.
92. Entman, M. L., S. S. Keslensky, A. Chu, and W. B. Van Winkle. The sarcoplasmic reticulum-glycogenolytic complex in mammalian fast twitch skeletal muscle. *J. Biol. Chem.* 255: 6245–6252, 1980.
93. Erecinska, M., R. L. Veech, and D. F. Wilson. Thermodynamic relationships between oxidation-reduction reactions and the ATP synthesis in suspensions of isolated pigeon heart mitochondria. *Arch. Biochem. Biophys.* 160: 412–421, 1974.
94. Essén, B., and T. Häggmark. Lactate concentration in type I and type II fibres during muscular contractions in man. *Acta Physiol. Scand.* 95: 344–346, 1975.
95. Essén, B., E. Jansson, J. Henriksson, A. W. Taylor, and B. Saltin. Metabolic characteristics of fibre types in human skeletal muscle. *Acta Physiol. Scand.* 95: 153–165, 1975.
96. Fischer, E. H., L. M. G. Heilmeyer, Jr., and R. H. Haschke. Phosphorylase and the control of glycogen degradation. *Curr. Top. Cell. Reg.* 4: 211–251, 1971.
97. Fischer, E. H., and E. G. Krebs. Commentary on "the phosphorylase b to a converting enzyme of rabbit skeletal muscle." *Biochem. Biophys. Acta* 1000: 297–301, 1989.
98. Fishbein, W. N. Lactate transporter defect: a new disease of muscle. *Science* 234: 1254–1256, 1986.
99. Fitts, R. H. Cellular mechanisms of muscle fatigue. *Physiol. Rev.* 74: 49–94, 1994.
100. Fletterick, R. J. The structures and related functions of phosphorylase a. *Annu. Rev. Biochem.* 49: 31–61, 1980.
101. Frenkel, R. Control of reduced diphosphopyridine nucleotide oscillations in beef heart extracts. *Arch. Biochem. Biophys.* 125: 151–165, 1968.
102. Fridén, J., J. Seger, and B. Ekblom. Topographical localization of muscle glycogen: an ultrahistochemical study in the human vastus lateralis. *Acta Physiol. Scand.* 135: 381–391, 1989.
103. Friedman, J. E., P. D. Neufer, and G. L. Dohm. Regulation of glycogen resynthesis following exercise. Dietary considerations. *Sports Med.* 11: 232–243, 1991.
104. Funk, C., A. Clark, Jr., and R. J. Connett. How phosphocreatine buffers cyclic changes in ATP demand in working muscle. *Adv. Exp. Med. Biol.* 248: 687–692, 1989.
105. Funk, C. I., A. Clark, Jr., and R. J. Connett. A simple model of aerobic metabolism: applications to work transitions in muscle. *Am. J. Physiol.* 258 (*Regulatory Integrative Comp. Physiol.* 27): R949–R959, 1990.
106. Gadian, D. G., G. K. Radda, T. R. Brown, E. M. Chance, M. J. Dawson, and D. R. Wilkie. The activity of creatine kinase in frog skeletal muscle studied by saturation-transfer nuclear magnetic resonance. *Biochem. J.* 194: 215–228, 1981.
107. Gollnick, P. D., B. Pernow, B. Essén, E. Jansson, and B. Saltin. Availability of glycogen and plasma FFA for substrate utilization in leg muscle of man during exercise. *Clin. Physiol.* 1: 27–42, 1981.
108. Gollnick, P. D., K. Piehl, and B. Saltin. Selective glycogen depletion pattern in human muscle fibres after exercise of varying intensity and at varying pedalling rates. *J. Physiol.* 241: 45–57, 1974.
109. Goodman, M. N., and J. M. Lowenstein. The purine nucleotide cycle. Studies of ammonia production by skeletal muscle in situ and in perfused preparations. *J. Biol. Chem.* 252: 5054–5060, 1977.
110. Gottschalk, M. E., and R. G. Kemp. Interaction of dinucleotides with muscle phosphofructokinase. *Biochemistry* 20: 2245–2251, 1981.
111. Graham, T. E., D. G. Sinclair, and C. K. Chapler. Metabolic intermediates and lactate diffusion in active dog skeletal muscle. *Am. J. Physiol.* 231: 766–771, 1976.
112. Green, H. J. How important is endogenous muscle glycogen to fatigue in prolonged exercise? *Can. J. Physiol. Pharm.* 69: 290–297, 1991.
113. Green, H. J., R. L. Hughson, G. W. Orr, and D. A. Ranney. Anaerobic threshold, blood lactate, and muscle metabolites in progressive exercise. *J. Appl. Physiol. Respir. Environ. Exer. Physiol.* 54: 1032–1038, 1983.
114. Greenhaff, P. L., E. Hultman, and R. C. Harris. Carbohydrate metabolism. In: *Principles of Exercise Biochemistry in Medicine and Sport Sciences*, edited by J. R. Poortmans. Basel: Karger, 1993, p. 89–136.
115. Greenhaff, P. L., M. E. Nevill, K. Söderlund, K. Bodin, L. H. Boobis, C. Williams, and E. Hultman. The metabolic responses of human type I and type II fibres during maximal treadmill sprinting. *J. Physiol. (Lond.)* 1994 (in press).
116. Greenhaff, P. L., K. Söderlund, J. M. Ren, and E. Hultman. Energy metabolism in single human muscle fibres during intermittent contraction with occluded circulation. *J. Physiol. (Lond.)* 460: 443–453, 1993.
117. Griffiths, J. R. A fresh look at glycogenolysis in skeletal muscle. *Biosci. Rep.* 1: 595–610, 1981.
118. Grisolia, S., and W. W. Cleland. Influence of salt, substrate, and cofactor concentrations on the kinetic and mechanistic behavior of phosphoglycerate mutase. *Biochemistry* 7: 1115–1121, 1968.
119. Gross, S. R., K. Bromwell, and I. V. Baanante. Comparison of the mechanism of isoproterenol-stimulated glycogenolysis in skeletal muscle of normal and phosphorylase kinase-deficient mice (I strain). *J. Pharmacol. Exp. Ther.* 205: 732–742, 1978.
120. Guinovart, J. J., A. Salavert, J. Massague, C. J. Ciudad, E. Salsas, and E. Itarte. Glycogen synthase: a new activity ratio expressing a high sensitivity to the phosphorylase state. *FEBS Lett.* 106: 284–288, 1979.
121. H:son Nilsson, L., and E. Hultman. Liver glycogen in man—the effect of total starvation or a carbohydrate-poor diet followed by carbohydrate refeeding. *Scand. J. Clin. Lab. Invest.* 32: 325–330, 1973.

122. Hanson, R. L., F. R. Rudolph, and H. A. Lardy. Rabbit muscle phosphofructokinase. The kinetic mechanism of action and the equilibrium constant. *J. Biol. Chem.* 248: 7852–7859, 1973.
123. Haralambie, G., and H. Reinartz. Human skeletal muscle enolase factors influencing its activity. *Enzyme* 23: 404–409, 1978.
124. Hargreaves, M., and E. A. Richter. Regulation of skeletal muscle glycogenolysis during exercise. *Can. J. Sport Sci.* 13: 197–203, 1988.
125. Harris, R. C., B. Essén, and E. Hultman. Glycogen phosphorylase activity in biopsy samples and single muscle fibres of muscle quadriceps femoris of man at rest. *Scand. J. Clin. Lab. Invest.* 36: 521–526, 1976.
126. Harris, R. C., E. Hultman, and K. Sahlin. Glycolytic intermediates in human muscle after isometric contraction. *Pflugers Arch.* 389: 277–282, 1981.
127. Haschke, R. H., K. W. Grätz, and L. M. G. Heilmeyer. Control of phosphorylase activity in a muscle glycogen particle. *J. Biol. Chem.* 247: 5351–5356, 1972.
128. Haschke, R. H., L. M. G. Heilmeyer, Jr., F. Meyer, and F. Fischer. Control of phosphorylase activity in a muscle glycogen particle III. Regulation of phosphorylase phosphatase. *J. Biol. Chem.* 245: 6657–6663, 1970.
129. Heilmeyer, L. M. G., F. Meyer, R. H. Haschke, and E. H. Fischer. Control of activity in a muscle glycogenparticle. *J. Biol. Chem.* 245: 6649–6656, 1970.
130. Hermansen, L. Effect of metabolic changes on force generation in skeletal muscle during maximal exercise. In: *Human Muscle Fatigue: Physiological Mechanisms*, edited by R. Porters and J. Whelan. London: Pitman Medical, 1981, p. 75–88.
131. Hermansen, L., and O. Vaage. Lactate disappearance and glycogen synthesis in human muscle after maximal exercise. *Am. J. Physiol.* 233 (*Endocrinol. Metab. Gastrointest. Physiol.* 2): E422–E429, 1977.
132. Hespel, P., and E. A. Richter. Mechanism linking glycogen concentration and glycogenolytic rate in perfused contracting rat muscle. *Biochem. J.* 284: 777–780, 1992.
133. Hochachka, P. W., and G. O. Matheson. Regulating ATP turnover rates over broad dynamic work ranges in skeletal muscles. *J. Appl. Physiol.* 73: 1697–1703, 1992.
134. Hultman, E. Muscle glycogen in man determined in needle biopsy specimens. *Scand. J. Clin. Lab. Invest.* 19: 209–217, 1967.
135. Hultman, E., and J. Bergström. Muscle glycogen in relation to diet studied in normal subjects. *Acta Med. Scand.* 182: 109–117, 1967.
136. Hultman, E., J. Bergström, A. E. Roch-Norlund. Glycogen storage in human skeletal muscle. *Adv. Exp. Med. Biol.* 2: 273–288, 1971.
137. Hultman, E., and H. Sjöholm. Energy metabolism and contraction force of human skeletal muscle in situ during electrical stimulation. *J. Physiol. (Lond.)* 345: 525–532, 1983.
138. Issekutz, B., Jr., W. S. Shaw, and T. B. Issekutz. Effect of lactate on glycerol turnover in resting and exercised dogs. *J. Appl. Physiol.* 39: 349–353, 1975.
139. Ivy, J. L. Muscle glycogen synthesis before and after exercise. *Sports Med.* 11: 6–19, 1991.
140. Ivy, J. L., A. L. Katz, C. L. Cutler, W. M. Sherman, and E. F. Coyle. Muscle glycogen synthesis after exercise: effect of time of carbohydrate ingestion. *J. Appl. Physiol.* 64: 1480–1485, 1988.
141. Jacobs, I. Lactate concentrations after short, maximal exercise at various glycogen levels. *Acta Physiol. Scand.* 111: 465–469, 1981.
142. Jansson, E., and C. Sylven. Activities of key enzymes in the energy metabolism of human myocardial and skeletal muscle. *Clin. Physiol.* 6: 465–471, 1986.
143. Jong, Y. A., and E. J. Davis. Reconstruction of steady state in cell free systems. *Arch. Biochem. Biophys.* 222: 179–191, 1983.
144. Juel, C., and F. Wibrand. Lactate transport in isolated mouse muscles studied with tracer technique—kinetics, stereospecificity, pH dependency, and maximal capacity. *Acta Physiol. Scand.* 137: 33–39, 1989.
145. Kahana, S. E., O. H. Lowry, D. W. Schulz, J. V. Passonneau, and E. J. Crawford. The kinetics of phosphoglucoisomerase. *J. Biol. Chem.* 235: 2178–2184, 1960.
146. Kasvinsky, P. J., and W. L. Meyer. The effect of pH and temperature on the kinetics of native and altered glycogen phosphorylase. *Arch. Biochem. Biophys.* 181: 616–631, 1977.
147. Katz, A., S. Broberg, K. Sahlin, and J. Wahren. Leg glucose uptake during maximal dynamic exercise in humans. *Am. J. Physiol.* 251 (*Endocrinol. Metab.* 14): E65–E70, 1986.
148. Katz, A., and K. Sahlin. Effect of decreased oxygen availability on NADH and lactate contents in human skeletal muscle during exercise. *Acta Physiol. Scand.* 131: 119–127, 1987.
149. Katz, A., and K. Sahlin. Regulation of lactic acid production during exercise. *J. Appl. Physiol.* 65: 509–518, 1988.
150. Katz, A., K. Sahlin, and J. Henriksson. Muscle ammonia metabolism during isometric contraction in humans. *Am. J. Physiol.* 250: C834–C840, 1986.
151. Katz, A., M. K. Spencer, S. Lillioja, Z. Yan, D. M. Mott, R. G. Haller, and S. Lewis. Basal and insulin-mediated carbohydrate metabolism in human muscle deficient in phosphofructokinase 1. *Am. J. Physiol.* 261 (*Endocrinol. Metab.* 24): E473–E478, 1991.
152. Kauppinen, R. A., J. K. Hiltunen, and I. E. Hassinen. Mitochondrial membrane potential, transmembrane difference in the NAD^+ redox potential and the equilibrium of the glutamate-aspartate translocase in the isolated perfused rat heart. *Biochim. Biophys. Acta* 725: 425–433, 1983.
153. Kauppinen, R. A., J. K. Hiltunen, and I. E. Hassinen. Compartmentation of citrate in relation to the regulation of glycolysis and the mitochondrial transmembrane proton electrochemical potential gradient in isolated perfused rat heart. *Arch. Biochem. Biophys.* 120: 542–546, 1967.
154. Kobayashi, K., and J. R. Neely. Control of maximum rates of glycolysis in rat cardiac muscle. *Circ. Res.* 44: 166–175, 1979.
155. Kochan, R. G., D. R. Lamb, S. A. Lutz, C. V. Perill, E. M. Reimann, and K. K. Schlender. Glycogen synthase activation in human skeletal muscle: effects of diet and exercise. *Am. J. Physiol.* 236 (*Endocrinol. Metab. Gastrointest. Physiol.* 5): E660–E666, 1979.
156. Kochan, R. G., D. R. Lamb, E. M. Reimann, and K. K. Schlender. Modified assays to detect activation of glycogen synthase following exercise. *Am. J. Physiol.* 240 (*Endocrinol. Metab.* 3): E197–E202, 1981.
157. Kohn, M. C. Computer simulation of metabolism in palmitate-perfused rat heart. III. Sensitivity analysis. *Ann. Biomed. Eng.* 11: 533–549, 1983.
158. Kohn, M. C., and D. Garfinkel. Computer simulation of metabolism in palmitate perfused rat heart. II. Behavior of complete model. *Ann. Biomed. Eng.* 11: 511–531, 1983.
159. Kohn, M. C., and D. Garfinkel. Computer simulation of metabolism in palmitate-perfused rat heart. I. Palmitate oxidation. *Ann. Biomed. Eng.* 11: 361–384, 1983.

160. Krebs, E. G., D. S. Love, G. E. Bratvold, K. A. Trayser, W. L. Meyer, and E. H. Fischer. Purification and properties of rabbit skeletal muscle phosphorylase b kinase. *Biochemistry* 3: 1022–1033, 1964.
161. Kushmerick, M. J., and R. A. Meyer. Chemical changes in rat leg muscle by phosphorus nuclear magnetic resonance. *Am. J. Physiol.* 248 (*Cell Physiol.* 17): C542–C549, 1985.
162. Kushmerick, M. J., R. A. Meyer, and T. R. Brown. Phosphorus NMR spectroscopy of cat biceps and soleus muscle. *Adv. Exp. Med. Biol.* 159: 303–325, 1983.
163. Larner, J., and C. Villar-Palasi. Glycogen synthase and its control. In: *Current Topics in Cell Regulation*, edited by E. R. Hoerecker and E. Stadtmen. New York: Academic Press, 1971, p. 195–236.
164. Lawrence, J. C., and R. L. Smith. Phosphorylase kinase isozymes and phosphorylase in denervated skeletal muscles. *Muscle Nerve* 13: 133–137, 1990.
165. Lawson, J. W. R., and K. Uyeda. Effects of insulin and work on fructose 2,6-bisphosphate content and phosphofructokinase activity in perfused rat hearts. *J. Biol. Chem.* 262: 3165–3173, 1987.
166. Lee, S.-H., and E. J. Davis. Carboxylation and decarboxylation reactions. Anaplerotic flux and removal of citric acid cycle intermediates in skeletal muscle. *J. Biol. Chem.* 254: 420–430, 1979.
167. Leijendekker, W. J., P. Edauw, C. van Hardeveld, and W. S. Simonides. Phosphorylase a formation in protein-glycogen particles isolated from fast-twitch muscle of euthyroid and hypothyroid rats. *Arch. Biochem. Biophys.* 274: 120–129, 1989.
168. Lewis, S. F., and R. G. Haller. The pathophysiology of McArdle's disease: clues to regulation in exercise and fatigue. *J. Appl. Physiol.* 61: 391–401, 1986.
169. Lowry, C. V., J. S. Kimmey, S. Felder, M. M.-Y. Chi, K. K. Kaiser, P. N. Passonneau, K. A. Kirk, and O. H. Lowry. Enzyme patterns in single muscle fibers. *J. Biol. Chem.* 253: 8269–8277, 1978.
170. Lowry, O. H., D. W. Schulz, and J. V. Passonneau. Effects of adenylic acid on the kinetics of muscle phosphorylasea. *J. Biol. Chem.* 239: 1947–1953, 1964.
171. Maehlum, S., and L. Hermansen. Muscle glycogen concentration during recovery after prolonged severe exercise in fasting subjects. *Scand. J. Clin. Lab. Invest.* 38: 557–560, 1978.
172. Martin, J. L., L. N. Johnson, and S. G. Withers. Comparison of the binding of glucose and glucose 1-phosphate derivatives to T-state glycogen phosphorylase b. *Biochemistry* 29: 10745–10757, 1990.
173. Mason, M. J., and R. C. Thomas. A microelectrode study of L-lactate entry into and release from frog sartorius muscle. *J. Physiol. (Lond.)* 400: 459–479, 1988.
174. Masters, C. Interactions between glycolytic enzymes and components of the cytomatrix. *J. Cell Biol.* 99: 222S–225S, 1984.
175. Maughan, R. J., and D. C. Poole. The effects of a glycogen-loading regimen on the capacity to perform anaerobic exercise. *Eur. J. Appl. Physiol.* 46: 211–219, 1981.
176. Maughan, R. J., C. Williams, D. M. Campbell, and D. Hepburn. Fat and carbohydrate metabolism during low intensity exercise: effects of the availability of muscle glycogen. *Eur. J. Appl. Physiol.* 39: 7–16, 1978.
177. Mayr, G. W. Interaction of calmodulin with muscle phosphofructokinase. Interplay with metabolic effectors of the enzyme under physiological conditions. *Eur. J. Biochem.* 143: 521–529, 1984.
178. McGilvery, R. W., and T. W. Murray. Calculated equilibria of phosphocreatine and adenosine phosphates during utilization of high energy phosphate by muscle. *J. Biol. Chem.* 249: 5845–5850, 1974.
179. McLane, J. A., and J. O. Holloszy. Glycogen synthesis from lactate in the three types of skeletal muscle. *J. Biol. Chem.* 254: 6548–6553, 1979.
180. McQuate, J. T., and M. F. Utter. Equilibrium and kinetic studies of the pyruvic kinase reaction. *J. Biol. Chem.* 234: 2151–2157, 1959.
181. Meinke, M. H., and R. D. Edstrom. Muscle glycogenolysis. Regulation of the cyclic interconversion of phosphorylase a and phosphorylase b. *J. Biol. Chem.* 266: 2259–2266, 1991.
182. Meyer, R. A., T. R. Brown, and M. J. Kushmerick. Phosphorus nuclear magnetic resonance of fast- and slow-twitch muscle. *Am. J. Physiol.* 248 (*Cell Physiol.* 17): C279–C287, 1985.
183. Midelfort, C. F., R. K. Gupta, and I. A. Rose. Fructose 1,6-bisphosphate: isomeric composition, kinetics, and substrate specificity for the adolases. *Biochemistry* 15: 2178–2185, 1976.
184. Miller, R. G., M. D. Boska, R. S. Moussavi, P. J. Carson, and M. W. Weiner. 31P nuclear magnetic resonance studies of high energy phosphates and pH in human muscle fatigue. *J. Clin. Invest.* 81: 1190–1196, 1988.
185. Minatogawa, Y., and L. Hue. Fructose 2,6-bisphosphate in rat skeletal muscle during contraction. *Biochem. J.* 223: 73–79, 1984.
186. Mole, P. A., R. L. Coulson, J. R. Caton, B. G. Nichols, and T. J. Barstow. In vivo 31P-NMR in human muscle: transient patterns with exercise. *J. Appl. Physiol.* 59: 101–104, 1985.
187. Mommaerts, W. F. H. M., K. Vegh, and E. Homsher. Activation of phosphorylase in frog muscle as determined by contractile activity. *J. Gen. Physiol.* 66: 657–669, 1975.
188. Morgan, H. E., and A. Parmeggiani. Regulation of glycogenolysis in muscle. In: *Control of Glycogen Metabolism*, edited by W. J. Whelan. London: Churchill Livingstone, 1964, p. 254–272.
189. Newsholme, E. A. Control of metabolism and the integration of fuel supply for the marathon runner. In: *Biochemistry of Exercise*, edited by H. G. Knuttgen, J. A. Vogels, and J. Poortmans. Champaign, IL: Human Kinetics, 1983, p. 144–150.
190. Newsholme, E. A. *Essays in Cell Metabolism*, edited by W. Bartley, H. L. Kornberg, and J. R. Quayle. New York: John Wiley & Sons, 1970, p. 144–150.
191. Newsholme, E. A., and A. R. Leech. *Biochemistry for the Medical Sciences*. New York: John Wiley & Sons, 1984.
192. Nolte, J., D. Pette, B. Bachmaier, P. Kiefhofer, H. Schneider, and P. C. Scriba. Enzyme response to thyrotoxicosis and hypothyroidism in human liver and muscle: comparative aspects. *Eur. J. Clin. Invest.* 2: 141–149, 1972.
193. Norman, B., A. Sollevi, and E. Jansson. Increased IMP content in glycogen-depleted muscle fibres during submaximal exercise in man. *Acta Physiol. Scand.* 133: 97–100, 1988.
194. Nosek, T. M., K. Y. Fender, and R. E. Godt. It is diprotonated inorganic phosphate that depresses force in skinned skeletal muscle fibers. *Science* 236: 191–193, 1987.
195. Nuttall, F. Q., and M. C. Gannon. Allosteric regulation of glycogen synthase in liver. A physiological dilemma. *J. Biol. Chem.* 268: 13286–13290, 1993.

196. O'Reilly, K. P., M. J. Warhol, R. A. Fielding, W. R. Fontera, C. N. Meredith, and W. J. Evans. Eccentric exercise-induced muscle damage impairs muscle glycogen repletion. *J. Appl. Physiol.* 63: 252–256, 1987.
197. Opie, L. H., K. R. L. Mansford, and P. Owen. Effects of increased heart work on glycolysis and adenine nucleotides in the perfused heart of normal and diabetic rats. *Biochem. J.* 124: 475–490, 1971.
198. Paganelli, W., D. R. Pendergast, J. Koness, and P. Cerretelli. The effect of decreased muscle energy stores on the VO2 kinetics at the onset of exercise. *Eur. J. Appl. Physiol.* 59: 321–326, 1989.
199. Pearce, F. J., and R. J. Connett. Effect of lactate and palmitate on substrate utilization of isolated rat soleus. *Am. J. Physiol.* 238 (*Cell Physiol.* 7): C149–C159, 1980.
200. Pernow, B. B., R. J. Havel, and D. B. Jennings. The second wind phenomenon in McArdle's syndrome. *Acta Med. Scand. Suppl.* 472: 294–307, 1967.
201. Pette, D., and G. Dolken. Some aspects of regulation of enzyme levels in muscle energy-supplying metabolism. *Adv. Enzyme Regul.* 13: 355–377, 1975.
202. Pette, D., W. Luh, and T. H. Bucher. A constant-proportion group in the enzyme activity pattern of the Embden-Myerhof chain. *Biochem. Biophys. Res. Commun.* 7: 419–424, 1962.
203. Pettigrew, D. W., and C. Frieden. Rabbit muscle phosphofructokinase. A model for regulatory kinetic behavior. *J. Biol. Chem.* 254: 1896–1901, 1979.
204. Piras, R., and R. Staneloni. In vivo regulation of rat muscle glycogen synthetase activity. *Biochemistry* 8: 2153–2160, 1969.
205. Price, T. B., D. L. Rothman, M. J. Avison, P. Buonamico, and R. G. Shulman. C-NMR measurements of muscle gly cogen during low-intensity exercise. *J. Appl. Physiol.* 70: 1836–1844, 1991.
206. Price, T. B., D. L. Rothman, R. Taylor, M. J. Avison, G. I. Shulman, and R. G. Shulman. Human muscle glycogen resynthesis after exercise: insulin-dependent and independent phases. *J. Appl. Physiol.* 76: 104–111, 1994.
207. Quistorff, B., L. Johansen, and K. Sahlin. Absence of phosphocreatine resynthesis in human calf muscle during ischaemic recovery. *Biochem. J.* 291: 681–686, 1992.
208. Rahim, Z. H. A., D. Perrett, G. Lutaya, and J. R. Griffiths. Metabolic adaptation in phosphorylase kinase deficiency. *Biochem. J.* 186: 331–341, 1980.
209. Raz, I., A. Katz, and M. K. Spencer. Epinephrine inhibits insulin-mediated glycogenesis but enhances glycolysis in human skeletal muscle. *Am. J. Physiol.* 260 (*Endocrinol. Metab.* 23): E430–E435, 1991.
210. Ren, J. M., S. Broberg, K. Sahlin, and E. Hultman. Influence of reduced glycogen level on glycogenolysis during short-term stimulation in man. *Acta Physiol. Scand.* 139: 467–474, 1990.
211. Ren, J.-M., D. Chasiotis, M. Bergstrom, and E. Hultman. Skeletal muscle glucolysis, glycogenolysis and glycogen phosphorylase during electrical stimulation in man. *Acta Physiol. Scand.* 133: 101–107, 1988.
212. Ren, J. M., E. A. Gulve, G. D. Cartee, and J. O. Holloszy. Hypoxia causes glycogenolysis without an increase in percent phosphorylase a in rat skeletal muscle. *Am. J. Physiol.* 263 (*Endocrinol. Metab.* 26): E1086–E1091, 1992.
213. Ren, J. M., and E. Hultman. Regulation of phosphorylase activity in human skeletal muscle. *J. Appl. Physiol.* 69: 919–923, 1990.
214. Ren, J.-M., B. A. Marshall, E. A. Gulve, J. Gao, D. W. Johnson, H. O. Holloszy, and M. Mueckler. Evidence from transgenic mice that glucose transport is rate-limiting for glycogen deposition and glycolysis in skeletal muscle. *J. Biol. Chem.* 268: 16113–16115, 1993.
215. Richter, E. A., and H. Galbo. High glycogen levels enhance glycogen breakdown in isolated contracting skeletal muscle. *J. Appl. Physiol.* 61: 827–831, 1986.
216. Richter, O., A. Betz, and C. Giersch. The response of oscillating glycolysis to perturbations in the NADH/NAD system: a comparison between experiments and a computer model. *Biosystems* 7: 137–146, 1975.
217. Richter, E. A., K. J. Mikines, H. Galbo, and B. Kiens. Effect of exercise on insulin action in human skeletal muscle. *J. Appl. Physiol.* 66: 876–885, 1989.
218. Roach, P. J. Control of glycogen synthase by hierarchal protein phosphorylation. *FASEB J.* 4: 2961–2968, 1990.
219. Roos, A. Intracellular pH and distribution of weak acids across cell membranes. A study of D- and L-lactate and of DMO in rat diaphragm. *J. Physiol. (Lond.)* 249: 1–25, 1975.
220. Rose, I. A., and E. L. O'Connell. Specificity of fructose-1,6-P2 aldolase (muscle) and partition of the enzyme among catalytic intermediates in the steady state. *J. Biol. Chem.* 252: 479–482, 1977.
221. Rose, Z. B., and S. Dube. Phosphoglycerate mutase. Kinetics and effects of salts on the mutase and bisphosphoglycerate phosphatase activities of the enzyme from chicken breast muscle. *J. Biol. Chem.* 253: 8583–8592, 1978.
222. Rosell-Perez, M., C. Villar Palasi, and J. Larner. Uridine diphosphate glucose (UDPG)-glycogentransglucosylase. 1. Preparation and differentiation of two activities of UDP-glycogen transglucosylase from ratskeletal muscle. *Biochemistry* 1: 763–768, 1962.
223. Sabina, R. L., J. L. Swain, C. W. Olanow, W. G. Bradley, W. N. Fishbein, S. DiMauro, and E. W. Holmes. Myoadenylate deaminase deficiency. Functional and metabolic abnormalities associated with disruption of the purine nucleotide cycle. *J. Clin. Invest.* 73: 720–730, 1984.
224. Sahlin, K. Muscle fatigue and lactic acid accumulation. *Acta Physiol. Scand.* 128: 83–91, 1986.
225. Sahlin, K. Muscle carnitine metabolism during incremental dynamic exercise in humans. *Acta Physiol. Scand.* 138: 259–262, 1990.
226. Sahlin, K. Control of energetic processes in contracting human skeletal muscle. *Biochem. Soc. Trans.* 19: 353–358, 1991.
227. Sahlin, K. Metabolic aspects of fatigue in human skeletal muscle. *Med. Sport Sci.* 34: 54–68, 1992.
228. Sahlin, K., N.-H. Areskog, P. G. Haller, K. G. Henriksson, L. Jorfeldt, and S. F. Lewis. Impaired oxidative metabolism increases adenine nucleotide breakdown in McArdle's disease. *J. Appl. Physiol.* 69: 1231–1235, 1990.
229. Sahlin, K., S. Broberg, and A. Katz. Glucose formation in human skeletal muscle-influence of glycogen level. *Biochem. J.* 258: 911–913, 1989.
230. Sahlin, K., J. Gorski, and L. Edström. Influence of ATP turnover and metabolite changes on IMP formation and glycolysis in rat skeletal muscle. *Am. J. Physiol.* 259 (*Cell Physiol.* 28): C409–C412, 1990.
231. Sahlin, K., R. C. Harris, and E. Hultman. Creatine kinase equilibrium and lactate content compared with muscle pH in tissue samples obtained after isometric exercise. *Biochem. J.* 152: 173–180, 1975.
232. Sahlin, K., A. Katz, and S. Broberg. Tricarboxylic acid cycle intermediates in human muscle during prolonged exer-

cise. *Am. J. Physiol.* 259 (*Cell Physiol.* 28): C834–C841, 1990.
233. Sahlin, K., A. Katz, and J. Henriksson. Redox state and lactate acccumulation in human skeletal muscle during dynamic exercise. *Biochem. J.* 245: 551–556, 1987.
234. Sahlin, K., and J. M. Ren. Relationship of contraction capacity to metabolic changes during recovery from a fatiguing contraction. *J. Appl. Physiol.* 67: 648–654, 1989.
235. Saltin, B., and J. Karlsson. Muscle glycogen utilization during work of different intensities. In: *Muscle Metabolism During Exercise*, edited by B. Pernow and B. Saltin. New York: Plenum Press, 1972, p. 289–299.
236. Sargeant, A. J., and P. Dolan. Effect of prior exercise on maximal short-term power output in humans. *J. Appl. Physiol.* 63: 1475–1480, 1987.
237. Sherman, W. M., L. E. Armstrong, T. M. Murray, F. C. Hagerman, D. L. Costill, R. C. Staron, and J. L. Ivy. Effect of 42.2-km footrace and subsequent rest or exercise on muscular strength and work capacity. *J. Appl. Physiol.* 57: 1668–1673, 1984.
238. Shikama, H., J. Chiasson, and J. H. Exton. Studies on the interaction between insulin and epinephrine in the control of skeletal muscle glycogen metabolism. *J. Biol. Chem.* 256: 4450–4454, 1981.
239. Simoneau, J.-A., and C. Bouchard. Human variation in skeletal muscle fiber-type proportion and enzyme activies. *Am. J. Physiol.* 257 (*Endocrinol. Metab.* 20): E567–E572, 1989.
240. Sjödin, B., and J. Svedenhag. Applied physiology of marathon running. *Sports Med.* 2: 83–99, 1985.
241. Smythe, C., and P. Cohen. The discovery of glycogenin and the priming mechanism for glycogen biogenesis. *Eur. J. Biochem.* 200: 625–631, 1991.
242. Spamer, C., and D. Pette. Activity patterns of phosphofructokinase, glyceraldehyde dehydrogenase, lactate dehydrogenase, and malate dehydrogenase in microdissected fast and slow fibers from rabbit psoas and soleus muscle. *Histochemistry* 52: 201–216, 1977.
243. Spencer, M. K., and A. Katz. Role of glycogen in control of glycolysis and IMP formation in human muscle during exercise. *Am. J. Physiol.* 260 (*Endocrinol. Metab.* 23): E859–E864, 1991.
244. Spencer, M. K., Z. Yan, and A. Katz. Carbohydrate supplementation attenuates IMP accumulation in human muscle during prolonged exercise. *Am. J. Physiol.* 261 (*Cell Physiol.* 30): C71–C76, 1991.
245. Spriet, L. L. Phosphofructokinase activity and acidosis during short-term tetanic contractions. *Can. J. Physiol. Pharmacol.* 69: 298–304, 1991.
246. Spriet, L. L., L. Berardinucci, D. R. Marsh, C. B. Campbell, and T. E. Graham. Glycogen content has no effect on skeletal muscle glycogenolysis during short-term tetanic stimulation. *J. Appl. Physiol.* 68: 1883–1888, 1990.
247. Spriet, L. L., M. I. Lindinger, R. S. McKelvie, G. J. F. Heigenhauser, and N. L. Jones. Muscle glycogenolysis and H^+ concentration during maximal intermittent cycling. *J. Appl. Physiol.* 66: 8–13, 1989.
248. Spydevold, O., E. J. Davis, and J. Bremer. Replenishment and depletion of citric acid cycle intermediates in skeletal muscle. *Eur. J. Biochem.* 71: 155–165, 1976.
249. Srivastava, D. K., and S. A. Bernhard. Enzyme-enzyme interactions and the regulation of metabolic reaction pathways. *Curr. Top. Cell. Regul.* 28: 1–68, 1986.
250. Srivastava, D. K., and S. A. Bernhard. Mechanism of transfer of reduced nicotinamide adenine dinucleotide among dehydrogenases. *Biochemistry* 24: 623–628, 1985.
251. Stainsby, W. N., W. F. Brechue, D. M. O'Drobinak, and J. K. Barclay. Effects of ischemic and hypoxic hypoxia on VO_2 and lactate acid output during tetanic contractions. *J. Appl. Physiol.* 68: 574–579, 1990.
252. Stubbs, M., R. L. Veech, and H. A. Krebs. Control of the redox state of the nicotinamide-adenine dinucleotide couple in rat liver cytoplasm. *Biochem. J.* 126: 59–65, 1972.
253. Stura, E. A., G. Zanotti, Y. S. Babu, M. S. Sansom, D. I. Stuart, K. S. Wilson, L. N. Johnson, and G. Van de Werve. Comparison of AMP and NADH binding to glycogen phosphorylase b. *J. Mol. Biol.* 170: 529–565, 1983
254. Symons, J. D., and I. Jacobs. High-intensity exercise performance is not impaired by low intramuscular glycogen. *Med. Sci. Sports Exerc.* 21: 550–557, 1989.
255. Taylor, D. J., P. J. Bore, P. Styles, D. G. Gadian, and G. K. Radda. Bioenergetics of intact human muscle. A 31P nuclear magnetic resonance study. *Mol. Biol. Med.* 1: 77–94, 1983.
256. Tejwani, G. A., A. Ramaiah, and M. Ananthanarayanan. Regulation of glycolysis in muscle. The role of ammonium and synergism among the positive effectors of phosphofructokinase. *Arch. Biochem. Biophys.* 158: 195–199, 1973.
257. Terblanche, S. E., R. D. Fell, A. C. Juhlin-Dannfelt, B. W. Craig, and J. O. Holloszy. Effects of glycerol feeding before and after exhausting exercise in rats. *J. Appl. Physiol. Respir. Environ. Exer. Physiol.* 50: 94–101, 1981.
258. Tesch, P., B. Sjödin, A. Thorstensson, and J. Karlsson. Muscle fatigue and its relation to lactate accumulation and LDH activity in man. *Acta Physiol. Scand.* 103: 413–420, 1978.
259. Tornheim, K., and J. M. Lowenstein. Purine nucleotide cycle. Study of interactions with oscillations of the glycolytic pathway in muscle extracts. *J. Biol. Chem.* 247: 162–169, 1974.
260. Tornheim, K., and J. M. Lowenstein. The purine nucleotide cycle. Control of phosphofructokinase and glycolytic oscillations in muscle extracts. *J. Biol. Chem.* 250: 6304–6314, 1975.
261. Trivedi, B., and W. H. Danforth. Effect of pH on the kinetics of frog muscle phosphofructokinase. *J. Biol. Chem.* 241: 4110–4114, 1966.
262. Vaughan, H., S. D. Thornton, and E. A. Newsholme. The effects of calcium ions on the activities of trehalase, hexokinase, phosphofructokinase, fructose diphosphatase and pyruvate kinase from various muscles. *Biochem. J.* 132: 527–535, 1973.
263. Veech, R. L., L. Raijman, K. Dalziel, and H. A. Krebs. Disequilibrium in the triose phosphate isomerase system in rat liver. *Biochem. J.* 115: 837–842, 1969.
264. Villar-Palasi, C. Oligo- and polysaccharide inhibition of muscle transferase D phosphatase. *Ann. N.Y. Acad. Sci.* 166: 719–730, 1969.
265. Villar-Palasi, C. Substrate specific activation by glucose-6-phosphate of the dephosphorylation of muscle glycogen synthase. *Biochim. Biophys. Acta* 1095: 261–267, 1991.
266. Vøllestad, N. K., I. Tabata, and J. I. Medbö. Glycogen breakdown in different human muscle fibre types during exhaustive exercise of short duration. *Acta Physiol. Scand.* 144: 135–141, 1992.
267. Wallberg-Henriksson, H. Glucose transport into skeletal muscle. Influence of contractile activity, insulin, catecholamines and diabetes mellitus. *Acta Physiol. Scand. Suppl.* 564: 7–80, 1987.

268. Walsh, T. P., C. J. Masters, D. J. Morton, and F. M. Clarke. The reversible binding of glycolytic enzymes in bovine skeletal muscle in response to tetanic stimulation. *Biochem. Biophys. Acta* 675: 29–39, 1981.
269. Wang, J. H., J.-I. Tu, and F. M. Lo. Effects of glucose 6-phosphate on the nucleotide site of glycogen phosphorylase b. *J. Biol. Chem.* 245: 3115–3121, 1970.
270. Williams, G. D., B. Enders, and M. B. Smith. Effect of pH and inorganic phosphate on creatine kinase inactivation: an in vitro 31P NMR saturation-transfer study. *Biochem. Int.* 26: 35–42, 1992.
271. Wilson, D. F., M. Erecinska, C. Drown, and I. A. Silver. The oxygen dependence of cellular energy metabolism. *Arch. Biochem. Biophys.* 195: 485–493, 1979.
272. Wilson, J. E., B. Sacktor, and C. G. Tiekert. In situ regulation of glycolysis in tetanized cat skeletal muscle. *Arch. Biochem. Biophys.* 120: 542–546, 1967.
273. Zorzano, A., T. W. Balon, M. N. Goodman, and N. B. Ruderman. Glycogen depletion and increased insulin sensitivity and responsiveness in muscle after exercise. *Am. J. Physiol.* 251 (*Endocrinol. Metab.* 19): E664–E669, 1986.

20. Glucose utilization

ERIK A. RICHTER | *Copenhagen Muscle Research Centre, August Krogh Institute, University of Copenhagen, Copenhagen, Denmark*

CHAPTER CONTENTS

IN HIGHER ANIMALS, SOME CELL TYPES (e.g., nerve cells, erythrocytes) under normal conditions are almost totally dependent upon glucose utilization as a source of energy. Most other cell types can utilize a variety of fuels, and skeletal muscle provides an example of this ability to use diverse fuels both at rest and during exercise. The major fuel sources for muscle during exercise are lipids and carbohydrates. Whereas the body's stores of lipid are large and in effect unlimited, carbohydrate stores are limited to 300–500 g glycogen in skeletal muscle, 60–100 g glycogen in the liver, and 15–20 g glucose in the blood and extracellular space (254). Of the total body stores of carbohydrate, the liver and blood stores can be used directly as glucose. The muscle glycogen store can be directly utilized in the working muscles, and even stored glycogen in nonexercising muscle to some degree may become available as a fuel for those muscles that are working. However, this is not in the form of glucose, since skeletal muscle, unlike liver, lacks the glucose-6-phosphatase needed for hydrolysis of glucose 6-phosphate to glucose (254). Rather, resting muscle may release appreciable amounts of lactate during exercise with other muscles (3, 4, 6), some of which is taken up by exercising muscle (332) and some of which can be converted to glucose via hepatic gluconeogenesis. This glucose can then be taken up by the exercising muscles. Thus, glucose and glycogen are the two major sources of carbohydrate for muscle during exercise, and the relative importance of the two sources varies according to the exercise conditions.

More than 100 years ago it was first suggested that exercise increases glucose utilization in the working muscles. Thus, by measuring arterial and venous blood glucose concentration and the rate of venous outflow from the masseter muscle of the horse, Chauveau and Kaufmann showed that masseter muscle glucose uptake was increased during chewing compared with rest (65). Then, in the 1950s, studies in rats (133) and perfused dog hindlimb (168) confirmed that contractions increase muscle glucose uptake. However, the quantitative aspects of glucose utilization in man during exercise were first studied in the 1960s and 1970s. It was found that glucose oxidation could account for 16%–37% of leg oxidative metabolism during light to heavy bicycling exercise (152, 357). In turn, glucose utilization proved to account for 75%–89% of total leg carbohydrate oxidation during light to heavy exercise (357). During prolonged exercise, when glycogen stores become depleted, glucose uptake can even account for close to 100% of carbohydrate metabolism (5, 87, 357). In contrast, during very intense, short-term exercise glucose utilization may be quantitatively unimportant (185), glycogen being the major fuel.

Fueled by intense research into glucose transport in adipocytes and cell lines during the last one to two decades, rapid progress has been made in understanding the molecular mechanisms behind stimulation of glucose transport by insulin (27, 131, 221). In skeletal muscle, less is known about the molecular mechanisms involved in insulin and especially contraction induced increase in glucose transport, primarily because differentiated skeletal muscle is a much more difficult tissue to work with than adipocytes or various cell lines. Nevertheless, the last decades have been characterized by rapid growth in research aiming at elucidating the regulatory mechanisms involved in glucose utilization in muscle during contractions and especially with elucidating the molecular mechanisms behind the increase in glucose transport in contracting muscle, as discussed below.

MOLECULAR BASIS FOR GLUCOSE TRANSPORT

Family of Glucose Transporters

Under most physiological conditions glucose transport is the rate-limiting step in glucose utilization in muscle (125, 213, 284). Therefore, the glucose transport step is an important determinant of rate of glucose utilization in muscle and is consequently under tight regulation.

In the various cell types in the body, glucose transport is tailored to the particular needs of the cells in question. This has resulted in the evolutionary development of different glucose transporters with distinct cellular expression and kinetic characteristics (Table 20.1). Except for the sodium-dependent glucose transporters located in the apical cell surface of the small intestine and the kidney (22), the family of glucose transporters includes only transporters that transport glucose via facilitated diffusion. These transporters allow the movement of glucose across the plasma membrane in or out of cells according to the chemical gradient of glucose without coupling to energy-utilizing processes such as adenosine triphosphate (ATP) hydrolysis.

The favored model for the glucose transporter is based on studies using human erythrocytes (20, 140) and studies using expression of mutated GLUT1 in chinese hamster ovary cells (261). It is suggested that the glucose transporter functions as a gated channel (Fig. 20.1). The outer and inner gates alternate between an open and a closed state so that the transporter changes its conformation between an outward open and an inward open state. After binding of glucose to the binding site, transport of glucose is then carried out by a conformational change between these two forms. This model has been worked out on the GLUT1 isoform, but due to the high degree of homology between the isoforms (22), it is

TABLE 20.1. *The Facilitative Glucose Transporter Family**

Isoform	Tissue Distribution	Function
GLUT1	Ubiquitous; high expression in brain endothelial cells and human erythrocytes	Basal glucose transport located in plasma membrane Low K_m(~2–3 mM)
GLUT2	Liver, kidney, and small intestinal epithelial cells; β-cells	High K_m (~15–20 mM) Glucose transport in and out of hepatocytes and β-cells
GLUT3	Neurons, placenta	Low K_m (~2–3 mM) Transport into central nervous system
GLUT4	Skeletal muscle, brown and white adipose tissue, heart	Mediates insulin and (in muscle) contraction regulated glucose transport K_m ~ 5 mM
GLUT5	Small intestine, kidney, skeletal muscle	Fructose transporter
GLUT7	Liver	Part of the glucose-6-phosphatase complex in endoplasmic reticulum

*For extensive review of the tissue distribution and characteristics of the facilitative glucose transporters see 22, 23, 27, 141, 184, 247, 343. GLUT6 is not indicated because it encodes a pseudogene.

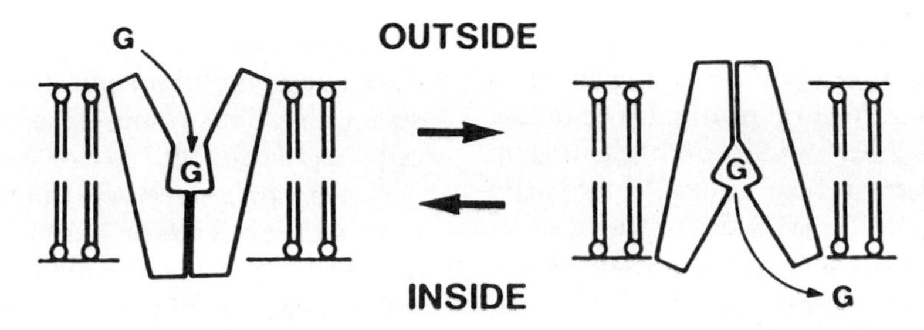

FIG. 20.1. Proposed mechanism of glucose transport. The glucose transporter alternates from an outward to an inward facing conformation. For details, see Oka et al. (261).

likely that this mechanism is also valid for the other isoforms.

GLUT1 is the ubiquitous transporter thought to be responsible for basal rates of glucose tranport in many cells, including muscle. Studies using subcellular fractionation of rat muscle have shown that GLUT1 in muscle is located mainly in the plasma membrane (107, 109). However, when subcellular fractionation was combined with immunohistochemistry, it was found that a large part of the GLUT1 found in the so-called plasma membrane fraction in fact stems from perineural sheaths (148, 230). Thus, it was estimated that approximately 60% of GLUT1 in cell fractions termed plasma membrane stems from the perineurium and only 40% from the plasma membrane (148). In giant sarcolemmal vesicles prepared by collagenase treatment of rat skeletal muscle, no GLUT1 was detectable (275). Furthermore, in single rat muscle fibers (presumably devoid of nervous tissue), GLUT1 was barely detectable (207). However, chronic electrical stimulation markedly increased muscle GLUT1 expression (207). In giant sarcolemmal vesicles prepared from human muscle GLUT1 protein was barely detectable (Kristiansen, Hargreaves, and Richter, unpublished observations). Taken together, these results suggest that in muscle GLUT1 protein is found mainly in nervous tissue and little if any GLUT1 is present in the actual sarcolemma.

In accordance with its function as a transporter providing basal glucose transport, the GLUT1 transporter in muscle is not translocated to the plasma membrane in response to insulin stimulation and/or contractions (107, 109, 137, 230, 271). This is in contrast to findings in the adipocyte in which insulin stimulation does increase GLUT1 in the plasma membrane two- to fivefold (164, 367, 396).

GLUT2 and GLUT3 are expressed mainly in the liver and pancreatic β-cell as well as the brain, respectively (Table 20.1), and these transporters are well adapted to their functions by having high and low K_m, respectively, because the high K_m of GLUT2 makes glucose transport in the liver and β-cells almost linearly dependent upon plasma glucose concentration so that transport does not become rate limiting for glucose flux. The low K_m of GLUT3 secures an almost constant glucose supply to the brain in spite of fluctuations in plasma glucose concentration (22, 23, 184, 343).

GLUT4 is expressed almost exclusively in cardiac and skeletal muscle and brown and white fat (Table 20.1) and is known as the insulin-regulatable glucose transporter. Furthermore, in rat muscle, GLUT4 is also translocated by muscle contractions (107, 109, 136, 137, 275) and should therefore be named the "insulin-and-contraction regulatable glucose transporter." In contrast to observations using subcellular fractionation (107, 109, 136, 137), immunocytochemical studies (43, 310, 328) and surface labeling of GLUT4 with exofacial photolabeling (111, 224, 378) suggest that the majority of GLUT4 in unstimulated rat muscle is located intracellularly in tubulovesicular elements that are clustered either in the trans-Golgi reticulum (Fig. 20.2), or in the cytoplasm, but mostly close to the cell membrane (310). Furthermore, T tubules also seem to contain GLUT4 [Fig. 20.2); (43, 55, 104, 111, 122)]. This intracellular sequestration is mediated by internalization motifs apparently located both in the amino terminal end of GLUT4 (130, 270) as well as in the carboxy terminus (352).

GLUT5 is expressed mainly in the small intestine (Table 20.1). The main function of GLUT5 may be as a fructose transporter (23, 53). Interestingly, GLUT5 is also expressed in small quantities in human skeletal muscle (167), but is undetectable in rat skeletal muscle (279). In muscle GLUT5 may also function as a fructose transporter, but its precise physiological role remains to be determined, since the fructose concentration in blood usually is very low and, due to its hepatic conversion to glucose, does not increase to high plasma levels even after large oral intakes. For instance, when ingesting 52.5 g fructose per hour during exercise, the arterial fruc-

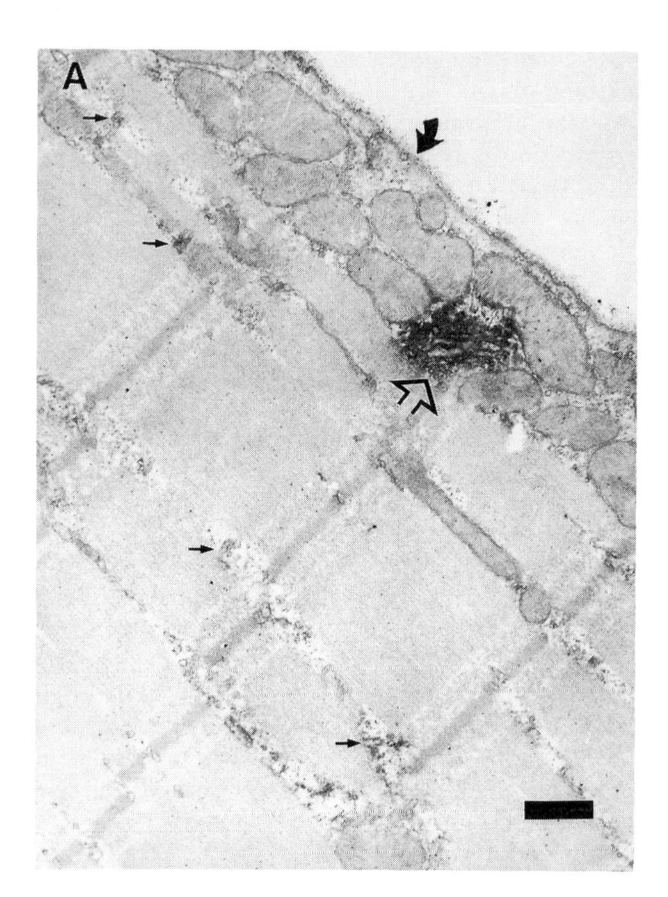

FIG. 20.2. Low-power electron micrograph of nonstimulated soleus muscle fibers immunostained with anti-GLUT4 showing subsarcolemmal aggregation of mitochondria. A stack of flattened cirsternae (*open arrows*) resembling Golgi apparatus is stained. Plasma membrane (*curved arrow*) is unstained. Note weak staining of several triadic junctions (*small arrows*). [Reproduced from Bornemann et al. (43), with permission.]

tose concentration only increased to around 0.5 mM (29).

GLUT7 is expressed in liver. When glucose is formed by gluconeogenesis or glycogenolysis, the last step is removal of phosphate from glucose 6-phosphate. Glucose 6-phosphatase is a multicomponent enzyme, and the glucose produced by the action of this phosphatase is initially confined to the lumen of the endoplasmic reticulum. In order to leave the hepatocytes, the glucose first has to be transported out of the endoplasmic reticulum, and this is performed by GLUT7 (356).

Translocation of Glucose Transporters

Upon stimulation with insulin, glucose transporters (GLUT4) are translocated from the interior of the cell to the plasma membrane (Fig. 20.3). This was first shown in rat adipocytes using cytochalasin B binding and subcellular fractionation (90, 340) and shortly thereafter in rat muscle (368). When measured with exofacial photolabeling, the concentration of GLUT4 in the plasma membrane increases 15- to 20-fold in the adipocyte (164) and six to eight fold in the incubated soleus muscle (224, 378) when stimulated by insulin. This increase in GLUT4 content is accompanied by a similar increase in glucose transport (164, 224, 378), suggesting that the insulin-stimulated increase in glucose transport is due entirely to translocation of GLUT4 from the interior of the cell to the plasma membrane. Large insulin-induced [rat brown adipocytes and cardiac muscle (326, 327)] and insulin- and contraction-induced [rat skeletal muscle (310)] increases in plasma membrane GLUT4 concentration have also been reported in studies using immunocytochemistry and electron microscopy. These findings are in contrast to those found in studies using sub-cellular fractionation of rat muscle in which much more modest insulin-induced increases in plasma membrane glucose transporter number have been reported. These increases are usually in the order of 1.3–3 (107, 109, 136, 137, 230), which more or less closely matches a decrease in GLUT4 protein in intracellular membranes (109, 160, 230). The effect of insulin on translocation of GLUT4 in human muscle has been investigated in two studies using subcellular fractionation. In one study no translocation could be demonstrated upon insulin stimulation (224) whereas in a more recent one, insulin induced a 1.6 fold increase in GLUT4 protein in a surface membrane fraction and a 50% decrease in an internal membrane pool (146). Because the increase in number of membrane glucose transporters measured with the fractionation technique in rat muscle is much less than the concomitant increase in muscle glucose transport, these findings have led to the indirect conclusion that the intrinsic activity of the individual transporter is increased by insulin (230, 271, 334, 335). This conclusion, however, does not seem to be supported by the aforementioned studies using surface labeling or immunohistochemistry. Furthermore, fractionation techniques are problematic due to low recovery of membranes and cross-contamination among membrane subfractions (108, 135, 138, 137, 146, 160, 230, 271, 334, 335). Therefore, quantitative aspects of glucose transporter distribution are probably not correct when subcellular fractionation techniques are used, especially not in muscle, which is a difficult tissue from which to obtain pure membrane fractions.

When it comes to muscle contractions, the picture is less clear, in part because there have been no studies, except for subcellular fractionation studies, of the pure effect of contractions. Nevertheless, available data indicate that muscle contractions, similarly to insulin stimulation, also increase glucose transport by increasing the number of glucose transporters (GLUT4) in the plasma membrane (108, 109, 135, 136, 138, 271, 275, 335). There is controversy regarding whether the intracellular pool of GLUT4 that is translocated with muscle contractions is identical to or distinct from the intracellular pool translocated in response to insulin stimulation (117, 136, 137, 335) The studies show a small increase (twofold) in plasma membrane GLUT4 concentration, suggesting that the intrinsic activity of the transporters is also increased, since glucose transport increases several times more. For instance, in perfused rat muscle maximal contractile activity increases glucose transport ~10- to 40-fold in white and red muscle, respectively (273). However, to date no data directly show that muscle contractions lead to an increase in intrinsic activity of GLUT4. Thus, at this time it seems prudent to state that in the rat, muscle contractions increase sarcolemmal GLUT4 concentration and this mechanism is probably the main mechanism responsible for the increase in glucose transport. Whether intrinsic activity is changed or not is still uncertain. In humans, we have recently shown that 5-6 min of maximal bicycle ergometer exercise increases giant sarcolemmal vesicle glucose transport 2.5 fold and vesicle GLUT4 protein 1.6 fold (Kristiansen, Hargreaves and Richter, unpublished observations). Thus, these data show that translocation of GLUT4 to the sarcolemma occurs with exercise in humans. Furthermore, they suggest that intrinsic activity of GLUT4 is increased at least with maximal exercise.

T tubules may contain five times more glucose transporters (measured by binding of cytochalasin B) than the plasma membrane in rat muscle (55), and GLUT4 has also been found in T tubules and triadic junctions by immunohistochemistry [Fig. 20.2; (43, 122)] and by surface labeling combined with autoradiography (111). Furthermore, biochemical methods involving subcellular fractionation (229), immunohistochemistry (122), and surface labeling (111) reveal that GLUT4 labeling of T tubules increases with insulin stimulation. It is not known whether contractions change the distribution of GLUT4 in T tubules. Nevertheless, the presence of GLUT4 in T tubules extending deep into the muscle fibers could provide a mechanism for efficient delivery of glucose into the muscle fiber. Whether glucose in fact can diffuse at a sufficiently fast rate in the narrow T tubules to make transport efficient or in addition may be pumped by some peristaltic-like pumping action during muscle contraction/relaxation is at present not well established but could be possible (104).

The mechanisms involved in regulation of GLUT4 translocation in response to insulin and contractions are not well understood. Nevertheless, progress stems from the idea that this translocation may resemble exocytosis in secretory cells and neurotransmitter release from synaptosomes. Thus, GLUT4 in the unstimulated state resides in intracellular vesicles, and its movement to the surface is thought to involve a complex exocytotic machinery involving vesicle docking and membrane fusion. The control of this machinery is in the process of being unraveled, as discussed below.

Rapid changes in the concentration of GLUT4 at the cell surface can be affected by two processes: *(1)* rate of exocytosis of GLUT4-containing vesicle from the intracellular pool and *(2)* rate of internalization of GLUT4 from the cell surface to the intracellular pool. Several groups have worked on determining whether insulin affects the rate of exocytosis or internalization of GLUT4. Strong evidence suggests that the exocytotic pathway is the important regulated one (181, 277, 316, 327), although insulin may also regulate the rate of endocytosis (91). It is not known whether contractions alter the rate of exo- or endocytosis of GLUT4 in muscle (Fig. 20.3).

Several important proteins, originally shown to be involved in neurotransmitter release from synaptic vesicles, seem to be involved in the cellular machinery controlling exocytosis. In rat adipocytes, GLUT4 co-localizes with synaptobrevin (58), a synaptic vesicle protein [vesicle associated membrane protein (VAMP)] and also with secretory carrier membrane proteins (SCAMPs) (218). Apparently, SCAMPs are ubiquitously localized to secretory and endocytotic vesicles that are involved in transport to and from the cell surface and therefore can be regarded as markers of a general recycling system (45). VAMPs apparently participate in storage and release of neurotransmitters (93). Furthermore, GLUT4, VAMPs, and to a lesser extent SCAMPs translocate upon insulin stimulation in rat adipocytes (218) indicating that the translocation process can be likened to exocytosis/endocytosis. Recently, the synaptic vesicle proteins (VAMPs) synaptobrevin 1 and 2 have also been identified in rat muscle tissue (278) and we have recently shown that VAMP-2 (synaptobrevin 2) translocates to the sarcolemma with 5–6 min of maximal exercise in humans (Kristiansen, Hargreaves, and Richter, unpublished observations). Furthermore, it has been hypothesized that low-molecular-weight GTP-binding Rab proteins, belonging to the growing superfamily of *ras*-related proteins (147) are involved in exocytosis (15). GTP-binding

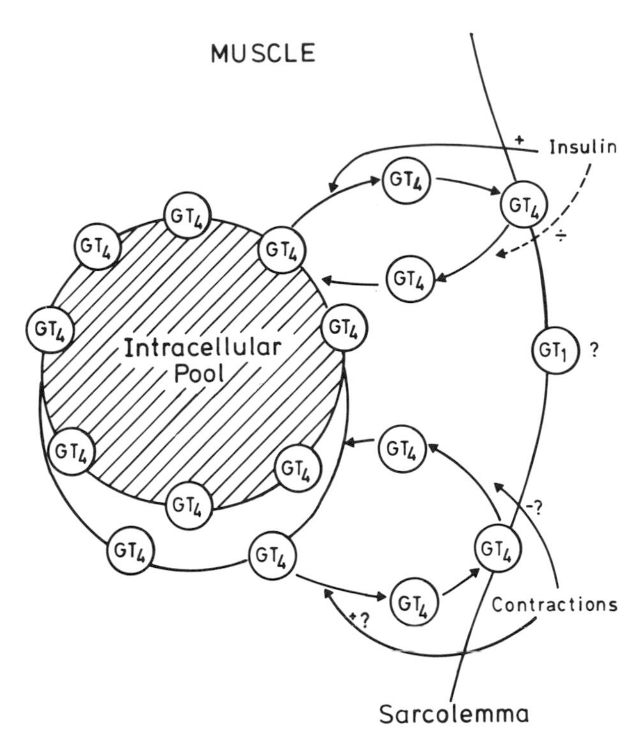

FIG. 20.3. Schematic drawing of a muscle cell showing distribution of GLUT1 and GLUT4 and effect of insulin and contractions. It is indicated that the intracellular pool of GLUT4 may possibly be divided into an insulin-sensitive and a contraction-sensitive pool, but this is not certain. GLUT4 recycles between intracellular pool and sarcolemma, and insulin has in adipocytes been shown to increase mainly the exocytotic rate and may or may not decrease the internalization rate constant (91, 181, 316, 327). Thus, a similar effect of insulin in muscle is hypothesized. Whether contractions affect the exocytotic and/or endocytotic pathway is unknown. If present in myocytes, GLUT1 resides mainly in the plasma membrane. GT_1, GLUT1; GT_4, GLUT4.

proteins have a size of 21–30 kd and are weak GTPases that are active in the GTP-bound state and inactive in the GDP-bound state (266). Several proteins appear to control the transition from one state to the other (56, 57). Recent evidence suggests that GTP binding proteins of the Rab family are involved in the translocation of GLUT4-containing vesicles in adipocytes (16, 84). For instance, Rab4 co-localizes with GLUT4 in the basal state and apparently upon insulin stimulation redistributes to the cytosol (84). This event of leaving the GLUT4-containing vesicle may be important for translocation (84). Furthermore, in rat skeletal muscle, GLUT4 and GTP-binding Rab proteins (the type of Rab proteins was not specified) were found to be translocated by insulin to a similar extent from a microsomal fraction to the sarcolemma (117), suggesting a functional relationship between these proteins. Contractions also increased sarcolemmal GLUT4 and GTP-binding protein concentration but did not decrease it in the microsomal fraction (117). Moreover, the nonhydrolizable GTP analogue GTPτS, which activates GTP-binding proteins, stimulates GLUT4 protein translocation in adipocytes (17, 306) and glucose transport in cardiac myocytes (227). Because Rab3a, originally described in the brain, dissociates from synaptic vesicle after Ca^{2+}-mediated neurotransmitter release and reassociates after recovery (245) Rab3a may have a role in Ca^{2+}-mediated neurotransmitter release. Recently it was shown that although Rab3a is not essential for synaptic vesicle exocytosis, it does play a role in the recruitment of synaptic vesicles during repetitive nerve stimulation (132). By analogy, other Rab proteins in muscle may be involved in translocation of GLUT4 during contractions during which cytosolic Ca^{2+} is increased (Fig. 20.4).

When a maximally effective concentration of insulin is added to a muscle that has contracted shortly beforehand, the effects of insulin and contractions on glucose transport are additive (129, 273, 274, 294, 364, 395). This suggests that the mechanisms by which insulin and contractions increase glucose transport are different. In terms of glucose transporters, these findings suggest *(1)* the existence of two intracellular pools of GLUT4, each sensitive to

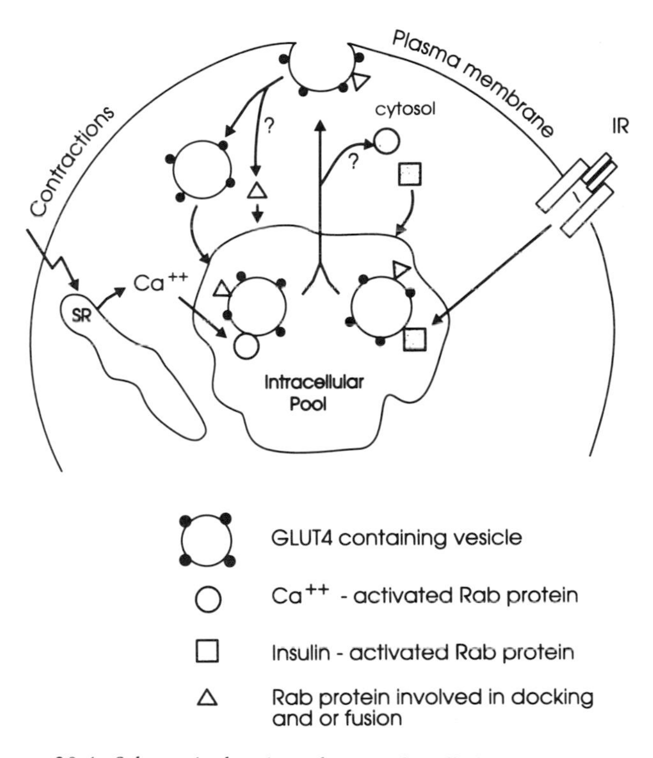

FIG. 20.4. Schematic drawing of a muscle cell showing *hypothesized* effect of insulin and contractions on GLUT4 translocation and Rab protein participation. The subtypes of Rab proteins in muscle associated with GLUT4-containing vesicles are yet unidentified. SR, sarcoplasmic reticulum; IR, insulin receptor.

either insulin or contractions, or *(2)* that only one pool of GLUT4 exists but insulin as well as contractions are each unable to translocate more than a fraction of the common pool. Another possibility is the existence of a distinct "exercise transporter isoform," but there is no evidence for such a contention.

Intrinsic Activity

Using subcellular fractionation—with its inherent pitfalls—it has been suggested that both insulin and contractions increase the intrinsic activity of GLUT4 (136, 138, 196, 335). Until recently, mechanisms that change glucose transporter intrinsic activity were not known. In erythrocytes expressing large numbers of GLUT1, three nucleotide-binding sites have been identified (60), and binding to these sites decreases transporter activity. However, only one of these sites is conserved in GLUT4 (60). Nevertheless, dibutyryl cyclic adenosine monophosphate decreases GLUT4 intrinsic activity by an unidentified mechanism unrelated to changes in phosphorylation status of the transporter but possibly by direct binding to the transporter (269). By analogy, intrinsic activity of GLUT4 could be decreased by binding of nucleotides (e.g., ATP), and contraction-induced decrease of muscle ATP might thus increase glucose transporter activity and thereby appropriately provide increased glucose transport to the energy-depleted muscle cell. The problem with this speculation is that muscle ATP stores are not markedly depleted even during strenous exercise (46, 47). However, it is not inconceivable that other nucleotides and metabolites may influence GLUT4 intrinsic activity. For instance, it has been suggested that glucose transport is decreased in adipocytes by glucose 6-phosphate (120), a metabolite that accumulates in muscle during some types of exercise. However, glucose 6-phosphate did not alter GLUT4 intrinsic activity in sarcolemmal vesicles from rat muscle (212).

Another possibility for changing intrinsic activity of GLUT4 is by changing its phosphorylation state. It is suggested that increasing the phosphorylation state of the transporter decreases its intrinsic activity (21, 220, 257, 269, 288). Furthermore, studies in adipocytes combining exofacial labeling of GLUT4 with 2-*N*-4(1-azi-2,2,2-trifluoro ethyl)benzoyl1,3-bis (D-mannos-4-yloxy)-2-propylamine (ATB-BMPA), Western blotting against GLUT4, and glucose transport measurements suggest that treatment with isoproterenol and adenosine can change the accessibility of insulin-stimulated GLUT4 to extracellular substrate (350). Thus, it was concluded that the insulin-stimulated GLUT4 transporters can exist in two distinct states within the plasma membrane: one that is functional and accessible to extracellular substrate and one that is nonfunctional (occluded) and unable to bind extracellular substrate (350). Thus, it could be hypothesized that GLUT4 during muscle contractions was also transformed from a nonfunctional to a functional state, possibly by altering the phosphorylation status of the transporter and in turn increasing its intrinsic activity. This is undetermined, however.

Fiber-Type Specific Expression of GLUT4

The glucose transporters GLUT1 and GLUT4 are expressed differently in the various muscle fiber types of the rat. Thus, expression of GLUT1 and GLUT4 protein is greater in homogenates of red than of white muscle (137, 155, 230). This might at first glance seem strange, since white muscle is more glycolytic than red muscle. Nevertheless, GLUT4 expression correlates with indices of muscle oxidative capacity such as citrate synthase activity (156, 166) and malate dehydrogenase (207), indicating that GLUT4 expression is related to the activity pattern of the various muscle fiber types. This assumption is supported by the finding that denervation decreases muscle GLUT4 protein (30, 156) and that red muscle is more afflicted than white (238). In contrast, training (19, 99, 121, 169, 189, 274) and chronic electrical stimulation (207) increase muscle GLUT4 protein. With endurance training of rats, a single bout of exercise transiently increases GLUT4 transcription in red muscle (252) and this increase is larger after 1 week of training. Interestingly, after 1 week of training muscle GLUT4 protein content was increased but GLUT4-mRNA was not. This suggests that the early increase in GLUT4 protein in red muscle is due to translational or post-translational mechanisms and that it takes prolonged training before GLUT4-mRNA is increased (274, 360). In the predominantly white epitrochlearis muscle, however, increases in GLUT4 protein and mRNA content have been found already 16 h after a 2 h bout of swimming (285).

Chronic electrical stimulation of white rat muscle with a stimulation pattern resembling nerve activity in a nerve innervating a red muscle increases GLUT4 expression as well as the activity of citrate synthase (116) and malate dehydrogenase (207), suggesting that the activity pattern of the motor nerve is decisive for GLUT4 expression. However, studies of tail-suspended rats with unweighted hindlimbs suggest that it may not only be the nerve activity as such that regulates GLUT4 expression. Thus, unweighting of the hindlimbs drastically decreases the nerve activity to red muscle as shown by a 50% decrease in muscle electromyography (EMG) (237). Nevertheless, muscle GLUT4 content increases and so does insulin sensitivity (36, 154). These findings suggest that the expression of GLUT4 in muscle is determined not only by nerve activity per se but also by some other factor related to innervation of muscle. The nature of this mechanism is not known but could be related to neurotrophic factors known to influence expression of muscle enzymes (265). Direct evidence that neurotrophic factors are important for GLUT4 expression is provided by findings in rat muscle in which the speed at which denervation decreases GLUT4 protein content is slowed if a long nerve stump is attached to the muscle compared to when the stump is short (239).

ROLE OF GLUT4 IN CONTRACTION-INDUCED SKELETAL MUSCLE GLUCOSE TRANSPORT

Augmentation of glucose transport during maximal stimulation with both insulin and contractions might be related to the GLUT4 content of the muscles (155). Thus, muscles composed mainly of oxidative fibers, which possess a high concentration of GLUT4 protein, increased glucose transport in response to insulin more than muscles composed mainly of glycolytic fibers with a low concentration of GLUT4 (155, 238). Furthermore, during insulin stimulation there is a fairly good correlation between muscle GLUT4 content and glucose uptake, [Fig. 20.5; (11, 19, 99, 155, 209, 238)]. Muscle contractions alone increase glucose transport, and the maximal effect of contractions also correlates to GLUT4 content (155). The best correlation between increase in glucose transport and GLUT4 content in muscle is found when muscle is stimulated by both insulin and contractions [Fig. 20.5; (155)]. However, the rat soleus muscle, which is usually used to study the properties of slow-twitched muscle, often does not increase its glucose transport very much in response to contractions. It requires extensive electrical stimulation to achieve maximal increase in glucose transport (272, 273). Furthermore, when stimulation ceases, the half-life of recovery of glucose transport is approximately 8 min. This means that when measurements of glucose transport are carried out even a few minutes after electrical stimulation of the soleus, a significant reversal of increased glucose transport has occurred (273). However, when measured immediately after intense electrical stimulation, glucose transport in the soleus is at least as high as it

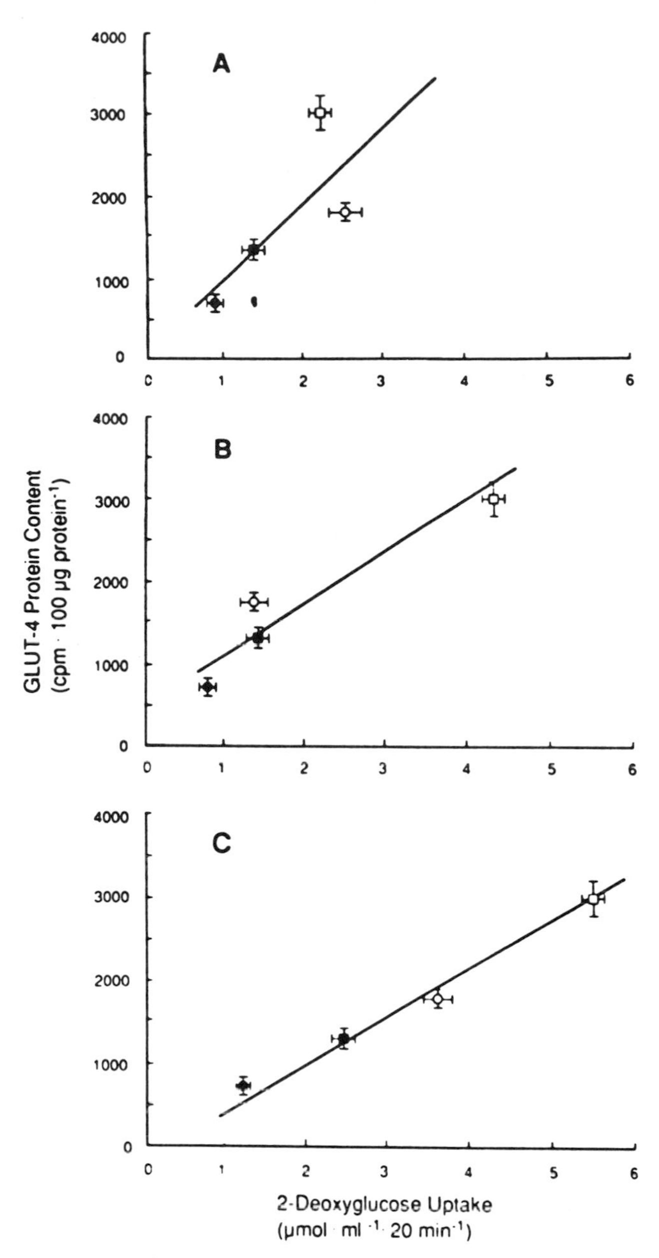

FIG. 20.5. Relationship between stimulated glucose transport and GLUT4 protein content in epitrochlearis (●), soleus (○), EDL (■), and FDB (□) muscles. Glucose transport (2-Deoxyglucose uptake) was stimulated by insulin alone (A), contractions alone (B), and insulin and contractions in combination (C). [Adapted from Henriksen et al. (155) with permission.]

is in fast-twitch red muscle (273). These two fiber types have approximately the same GLUT4 protein concentration (137, 155, 238). Further evidence for a role of GLUT4 concentration in contraction-induced glucose transport comes from studies of rat muscle reversibly damaged by eccentric exercise. In these muscles GLUT4 concentration is decreased by ~50% and so is contraction-induced glucose transport (S. Kristiansen, S. Asp, and E. A. Richter, unpublished observations). The conclusion thus seems to be that muscle GLUT4 content is important for glucose transport both during insulin stimulation and during contractions in vitro. However, as will be discussed later, the GLUT4 content is by no means the only factor of importance to the magnitude of increase in muscle glucose transport elicited by insulin and especially not by exercise in vivo.

Glucose transport must increase in order to increase glucose utilization during exercise, because glucose transport during most conditions is rate limiting for glucose uptake in resting muscle (125, 213, 284). However, metabolism of the transported glucose is also accelerated during contractions. Glucose is metabolized via glycolysis and subsequent oxidation, and a minor fraction is released as lactate. The question is to what extent and by which mechanisms is the enzymatic apparatus necessary for glucose metabolism accelerated during exercise. For details, the reader is referred to Chapter 19 which deals with regulation of glycolysis. For the present, it will suffice to mention that the hexokinase step, the phosphofructokinase step, and the pyruvate dehydrogenase step controlling pyruvate entry to the Krebs cycle seem to be important regulators of glucose metabolism. For instance, hexokinase is inhibited by glucose 6-phosphate, and under some conditions when intramuscular glucose 6-phosphate concentrations are elevated, glucose phosphorylation, and not glucose transport, becomes limiting for glucose uptake, because some of the transported glucose is not phosphorylated but accumulates as free glucose inside the muscle fiber (158, 185). In a similar manner, inhibition of phosphofructokinase and/or pyruvate dehydrogenase may cause glucose metabolism rather than transport to be rate limiting, as discussed later.

SIGNALING MECHANISMS INVOLVED IN CONTRACTION-INDUCED INCREASE IN GLUCOSE TRANSPORT

The cellular signaling mechanism involved in contraction-induced increased membrane transport of glucose is poorly understood. The first step in initiating muscle contractions is depolarization of the sarcolemma with subsequent release of Ca^{2+} from the sarcoplasmic reticulum. Ca^{2+} is required for cross-bridge formation between actin and myosin, but increasing evidence also points to Ca^{2+} as mediating the increase in glucose transport in muscle. The original studies were performed in frog sartorius muscle incubated with caffeine. Caffeine causes muscle contractures by directly releasing Ca^{2+} from the sarcoplasmic reticulum, and it also causes a large increase in glucose transport, providing evidence that the increase in glucose transport activity is not dependent on membrane depolarization (161). Furthermore, increasing the amount of isotonic work done per contraction did not influence the magnitude of increase in glucose transport (161). Together, these findings indicate that the increase in glucose transport during muscle contractions is not dependent on membrane depolarization nor on the ATP utilization rate. Rather, these findings point to an important role for the increase in cytosolic Ca^{2+} in increasing glucose transport. Support for this contention is found in studies showing that, within limits, the increase in glucose transport is greater the more Ca^{2+} enters the muscle during contractures elicited by increased extracellular K^+ (161, 349). Further support for the role of Ca^{2+} in increasing glucose transport comes from studies of incubated contracting frog muscle in which Cl^- in the incubation medium was substituted with NO_3^-, which impairs the uptake of Ca^{2+} by the sarcoplasmic reticulum. Thus, this approach would tend to augment the contraction-induced increase in intracellular Ca^{2+}. It was found that NO_3^- increased glucose transport elicited by a submaximal stimulus even when twitch potentiation was prevented (163).

Amphibian muscle may not always be representative of mamalian muscle; however, evidence for an important role of Ca^{2+} has also been found in mamalian muscle. Thus, in incubated rat epitrochlearis muscle, low concentrations (50–100 μM) of the compound *N*-(6-aminohexyl)-5-chloro-1-naphtalenesulfonamide (W-7) increased the efflux of preloaded $^{45}Ca^{2+}$, suggesting an increase in cytoplasmic Ca^{2+}. At this low concentration of W-7 the increase in Ca^{2+} was not sufficient to cause muscle contraction; still, an increase of six to eight times in transport of 3-O-methylglucose (3-O-MG) was observed (384). Similar findings were obtained when muscles were incubated with concentrations of caffeine (2.5–3.0 mM) that were too low to cause muscle contractions. Furthermore, the increase in transport of 3-O-MG was blocked by cytochalasin B, providing evidence that the increase in transport was due to specific glucose transport (384).

Older studies in the incubated rat soleus muscle also support the notion that increased cytosolic Ca^{2+} increases glucose transport (72, 73). Finally, results from studies using incubation of rat epitrochlearis muscle with phospholipase C suggest that phospholipase C causes release of Ca^{2+} from the sarcoplasmic reticulum, which in turn increases glucose transport (153). The fact that in neuronal tissue Ca^{2+} seems to be involved in neurotransmitter exocytosis via activation of Rab proteins (245) supports an analogous role for Ca^{2+} in GLUT4 translocation in muscle as discussed above (see Fig 20.3).

Protein kinase C, the Ca^{2+} dependent protein kinase (258), may also be involved in stimulation of glucose transport in various tissues. For instance, protein kinase C activation by phorbol esters increases glucose transport in adipocytes (69, 71, 169, 264), and insulin apparently also activates protein kinase C (by stimulating the translocation of protein kinase C from the cytosol to the membrane fraction) in adipocytes (69, 71, 83, 169, 264). In muscle, the picture may be more complex. Results of experiments with the cell line BC3H-1 suggest that insulin activates glucose transport in muscle through diacylglycerol generation and activation of protein kinase C (2, 81, 331). Also, insulin has in incubated muscle been implicated in stimulation of glucose transport via protein kinase C activation (170, 330, 342, 361), although there is also evidence against a role for protein kinase C in insulin activation of glucose transport (153, 202). During muscle contractions, protein kinase C is activated by translocation to the membrane fraction and by diacylglycerol production (75, 290) in addition to activation by the increase in cytosolic Ca^{2+} during contractions. Therefore, by analogy with the proposed role of protein kinase C for insulin stimulation of glucose transport, activation of protein kinase C might be involved in contraction-induced stimulation of glucose transport in muscle. The fact, that down-regulation of protein kinase C activity by prolonged incubation of soleus muscles with phorbol esters led to loss of contraction-induced glucose transport as well as diminished insulin-stimulated glucose transport (74) favors such a hypothesis. Furthermore, treatment of rats with polymyxin B, an inhibitor of protein kinase C, decreased enhancement of muscle glucose transport by muscle contractions in rats (388). It is not known whether protein kinase C activation during contractions is involved in GLUT4 translocation or changes in intrinsic activity, but the evidence mentioned earlier would seem to justify cautious support for a role for protein kinase C in contraction-induced increased glucose transport in muscle.

Findings from the perfused rat hindlimb suggest that glycogen depletion in some way is involved in stimulation of glucose transport. Thus, intermittent subtetanic electrical stimulation of the sciatic nerve increased glucose transport in fast-twitch red and white portions of the gastrocnemius muscle that were glycogen depleted but not in the slow-twitch red fibers of the soleus muscle, which by this stimulation protocol was not glycogen depleted (272). More intense electrical stimulation with longer stimulation trains both depletes glycogen and also increases glucose transport in the soleus (272, 273). Alternatively, these findings may suggest that the stimulation pattern was sufficient for increasing neither glycogenolysis nor glucose transport in this slow-twitch aerobic muscle even though in fast-twitch red and white fibers the same stimulation pattern caused marked glycogenolysis as well as increased glucose transport. Nevertheless, such observations indicate that large differences in the stimulation of glucose transport exist in the various muscle fiber types when they contract. One such difference could stem from the the amount of sarcoplasmic reticulum present in the various muscle fiber types. Fast-twitch muscle has much more abundant sarcoplasmic reticulum than slow-twitch muscle (314), hence during contractions cytosolic Ca^{2+} may well be higher in fast-twitch than in slow-twitch muscle. This could be the reason for the less marked increase in glucose transport in slow-twitch muscle. Nevertheless, slow-twitch fibers do possess the capacity for a marked increase in glucose transport during muscle contractions [at least as high as in fast-twitch red muscle (273)]. This was demonstrated during stimulation with longer stimulation trains resulting in tetanic contractions (273).

REGULATION OF GLUCOSE UTILIZATION IN VIVO

In muscle, like other tissues, glucose utilization is a function of three factors that usually, but not always, vary in concert: *(1)* supply (arterial concentration × blood flow), *(2)* membrane glucose transport capacity, and *(3)* metabolism.

Glucose Supply

The rate of transmembrane glucose transport at any given glucose transport capacity is dependent upon the transmembrane glucose gradient. Therefore, the rate of glucose transport is critically dependent upon glucose supply to the outside of the muscle membrane. The concentration at the outside of the muscle membrane is the interstitial glucose concentration; accordingly, the transfer of glucose from the capillaries to the interstitium and diffusion through the interstitium is important. Glucose leaves the capillaries in muscle by simple diffusion through the capillary pores or slits (89) because the glucose molecule (molecular radius 4.4 Å) is much smaller than the average pore size (50–200 Å) (89). Diffusion through the interstitial space is facilitated by the aqueous environment in the space; however, a glucose gradient exists from the "capillary end" to the "sarcolemmal end" of the interstitium. The magnitude of such a gradient probably varies with the diffusion distance from capillary to sarcolemma, the arterial glucose concentration, the capillary perfusion, and the actual sarcolemmal glucose transport capacity.

The interstitial space is not easily accessible experimentally, but recent developments in microdialysis techniques have suggested that the average interstitial glucose concentration in adipose tissue (123, 179) and resting rat muscle tissue (123) is very close to the venous *blood* glucose concentration. However, in the rat, unlike in humans, the *plasma* glucose concentration is ~50%–75% higher than the *blood* glucose concentration, and one should expect the interstitial concentration of glucose to be similar to the venous *plasma* glucose concentration if no significant gradient between capillary and interstitium exists. Therefore, similarity between the interstitial and *blood* glucose concentration in the rat in fact suggests the existence of a rather marked glucose gradient between capillary and interstitium. Also, local gradients within the interstitial space may occur as may gradients from the "arterial" to the "venous" end of the interstitium. Local gradients may be increased if muscle glucose transport capacity is increased without a corresponding decrease in diffusion distance and/or increased capillary flow. Preliminary data obtained with the microdialysis technique in human muscle during dynamic exercise suggest that the interstitial glucose concentration is close to the venous plasma concentration (D. McLean and J. Bangsbo, personnal communication).

The critical role of glucose supply for glucose utilization during exercise has been shown in studies examining the kinetics of glucose uptake and oxidation in dog muscle during moderate-intensity exercise. Leg glucose uptake and oxidation followed Michaelis-Menten kinetics (390) with K_m ~5 mM when plasma insulin was clamped at basal levels with somatostatin and replacement insulin infusion. In humans, we determined thigh glucose uptake during knee-extensor exercise of a moderate intensity at four different glucose concentrations with insulin clamped at basal levels by somatostatin and replacement insulin infusion (Fig. 20.6). Although the K_m in our experiment (~10 mM) was somewhat higher than in the dog, taken together these experiments indicate that glucose uptake, at least during moderate-intensity exercise, where phosphorylation is not limiting, is very dependent upon the arterial glucose concentration. This has also been shown in humans, where arm cranking added to leg bicycling increased the arterial glucose concentration and with it leg glucose uptake (201). Similarly, in cyclist exercising at 73% of $\dot{V}O_{2max}$, whole-body glucose utilization increased markedly when plasma glucose was increased from 4.2 mM to 10 mM (88). Furthermore, during prolonged exercise when plasma glucose concentration decreases, leg glucose uptake decreases too (4, 5).

Membrane Glucose Transport Capacity

Muscle glucose transport capacity sets the rate of membrane glucose transport at any transmembrane glucose gradient. As described earlier, membrane glucose transport capacity depends upon the number—and possibly intrinsic activity—of the GLUT4 transporter proteins in the sarcolemma. The two physiologically relevant stimuli of membrane glucose transport capacity in muscle are insulin and contractions (79, 108, 109, 135, 136, 155, 161, 162, 251, 271, 273, 274, 300, 365). The reader is referred to the previous section of this chapter dealing with regulation of glucose transport.

Glucose Metabolism

In most cases, glucose transport is the rate-limiting step in glucose utilization in muscle (125, 213, 284). However, during certain conditions glucose metabolism may be slower than the rate of glucose transport, resulting in glucose metabolism becoming the rate-limiting step in glucose utilization. Such cases include hyperglycemia and hyperinsulinemia at rest (186, 213) and inhibition of glucose phosphoryla-

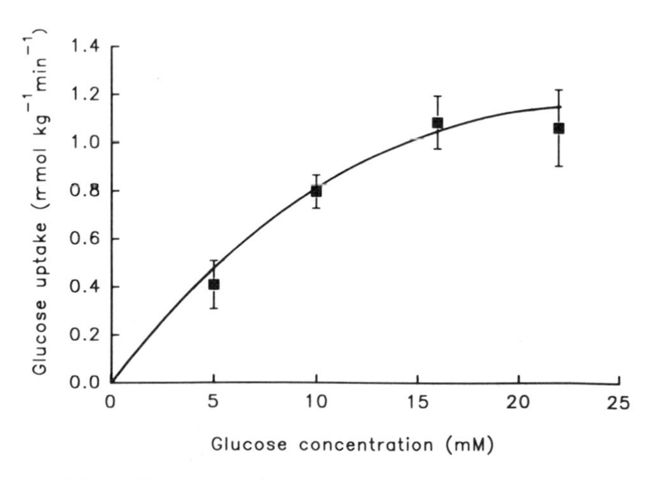

FIG. 20.6. Glucose uptake across the human thigh during dynamic knee-extensor exercise at moderate intensity. Glucose uptake was measured after 30 min exercise at each plasma glucose concentration and plasma insulin concentration was clamped at basal levels by infusion of somatostatin and replacement insulin. Values are means ±SE of four observations. K_m was calculated to 10.5 mM and V_{max} to 1.67 mmol · kg^{-1} · min^{-1}.

tion by glucose 6-phosphate during exercise (158, 187), as discussed below.

REGULATION OF GLUCOSE UTILIZATION AT REST

At rest in the postabsorptive state muscle glucose utilization is low (5, 190, 298, 346) and lipids are the predominant fuel as indicated by a local respiratory quotient (RQ) close to 0.70 (92, 182). In this situation, whole-body glucose utilization is mainly due to utilization in nonmuscle tissues, primarily the brain (262). Nevertheless, in accordance with glucose transport being the rate-limiting step for glucose uptake in resting muscle at basal insulin concentrations, the kinetics of glucose uptake in resting muscle in vivo can be described by Michaelis-Menten kinetics in man (383) and dog (390) with K_m values in the range of 5 to 8 mM. This means that variations of plasma glucose concentration in the physiological range in healthy man (~3.5–7 mM) will cause ~100% change in glucose uptake in muscle simply due to variations in plasma glucose concentrations. Still, because of the low V_{max} at basal insulin concentrations the absolute rate of uptake in muscle will be small even at a plasma glucose concentration of 7 mM, unless plasma insulin concentration is increased concomitantly by the increase in plasma glucose concentration.

At rest, by far the most important physiological stimulator of muscle glucose uptake is insulin. The actual molecular mechanisms involved in insulin-signalling mechanisms are at the moment not clarified but under intense investigation. The reader is referred to recent reviews on insulin-signaling mechanisms (66, 131, 221, 378). In terms of glucose utilization, the most important effect of insulin is to increase glucose transport in muscle. This has been demonstrated in humans (34) and in rat muscle (79, 251, 273, 366), and is accomplished mainly by increasing the V_{max} of the transport (251, 273), although a decrease in K_m has also been described (273). In vivo insulin stimulation is in fact accompanied by an increase in muscle perfusion (123, 297, 299). This increase in perfusion is probably important for maintenance of interstitial glucose concentrations during insulin stimulation. However, during euglycemic hyperinsulinemia in man glucose extraction across the legs increases markedly in comparison with the basal state (243, 297, 299). This suggests that the interstitial glucose concentration may be markedly lower than the arterial plasma concentration. This further suggests that interstitial glucose concentration and hence sarcolemmal glucose transport could be increased even more if capillary perfusion during hyperinsulinemia was increased more than it is.

Another important effect of insulin is stimulation of the glycogen storage pathway, primarily by increasing the activity of glycogen synthase (228, 382), thus increasing the ability of the cell to dispose of the transported glucose. At high insulin concentrations the rate-limiting step in glucose uptake may change from transport to disposal (213), thereby changing the kinetic characteristics (383). Thus, at plasma insulin concentrations of 50, 160, and 1700 μU/ml, respectively, K_m for glucose across the human forearm increased to average values of 18.1 $\pm$ 7.5, 16.2 $\pm$ 9.2, and 37.7 $\pm$ 20.7 mM (mean $\pm$ SE for five or six experiments), respectively, from the basal value of 7.4 $\pm$ 1.4 mM (383). This change in kinetic characteristics was interpreted as meaning that the rate-limiting step with insulin stimulation changed from transport to a step beyond transport. This step was not identified but is likely to be glucose phosphorylation.

The effect of insulin on muscle glucose metabolism may be altered by the activity level of the muscle. Thus, decreased muscle activity (223, 243, 297, 323, 339) and denervation (52, 217, 348) cause various degrees of insulin resistance, whereas increased activity level (100, 175, 192, 193, 242, 246, 308) augments insulin action. The decrease in insulin action with denervation is as rapid as 3 h in rat soleus muscle (348). This rapid effect of denervation seems to be due to decreased insulin-receptor signaling (52) rather than decreased muscle GLUT4 content, because muscle GLUT4 content is reduced only if denervation has existed for more than 1 day (30, 156, 238). The nature of this decrease in insulin signaling is not understood. It does not seem to involve decreased insulin receptor binding (52, 54), decreased insulin receptor kinase activation (54), or defective activation of the PI_3-kinase (68). Another model of decreased activity is the hindlimb suspension model, in which EMG activity to the rat hindlimb decreases by $\approx$50% (237) yet muscle GLUT4 content and insulin sensitivity increase (36, 156). This suggests that not only activity but also neurotrophic factors are of importance for insulin action in muscle as it is for expression of several muscle enzymes and GLUT4 protein (239, 265, 322).

The mechanism responsible for increased insulin action in trained muscle is also not well understood. However, training is associated with increased muscle GLUT4 content (10, 19, 99, 114, 115, 121, 166, 189, 325) whereas effects of training on insulin binding and insulin receptor tyrosine kinase activity have not been persuasive (35, 99, 103, 143, 341). As discussed previously, GLUT4 protein concentration in muscle may correlate with insulin action, but conditions can certainly be found in which GLUT4 concentration and glucose transport do not seem to be causally related. Another factor relates to the larger capillarization in trained muscle compared with untrained muscle (314). This results in shorter average diffusion distances from capillary to muscle cell for glucose and perhaps more importantly for insulin as well. Shorter average diffusion distances should make it possible to maintain higher interstitial concentrations of glucose as well as of insulin. Changes in the interstitial insulin concentration as measured by lymph insulin concentration has recently been shown to correlate closely with changes in glucose uptake rates in dogs (381) and humans (64). In agreement with an important role of diffusion distance for insulin sensitivity, a significant correlation (r = 0.63) between muscle capillarization and insulin sensitivity has been observed (222). Although exercise training is usually not found to increase resting muscle blood flow (100, 190, 346), it has been reported that athletes (bandy players) both at rest and during insulin infusion have higher blood flow per volume forearm than untrained controls (114). Together with increased capillarization this would probably provide conditions for better maintenance of interstitial glucose concentrations during insulin stimulation than in the untrained.

Diet may also influence insulin action in muscle. In rats, high-fat feeding with safflower oil and linoleic acid induces a state of insulin resistance (210, 336) that can be ameliorated by feeding fish oil (337) or by exercise training (211). In insulin-resistant non–insulin-dependent diabetics, however, addition of fish oil to the diet did not improve insulin action (41). However, in normal men insulin sensitivity was positively correlated to the average degree of fatty acid unsaturation in the phospholipid fraction of skeletal muscle (42). The extent to which variation in phospholipid composition of muscle in humans is determined by diet or genes is, however, not yet known but in rats diet can markedly affect muscle phospholipid composition (338). The actual mechanism explaining the relation between membrane phospholipid composition and insulin action is not known (42). In humans, a high-carbohydrate diet (68% of total energy vs. 43% in the control diet) increased average glucose disposal rate by 26% during an euglycemic clamp (124). However, other studies have been unable to show any significant effect of a high-carbohydrate diet on insulin action (40, 206). Thus, whether in humans realistic variations in dietary carbohydrate intake affect insulin action is controversial. Recently, it was shown that within the normal carbohydrate intake in a Western diet (approximately 45 energy percent), the type of carbohydrates (low vs. high glycemic index) may affect insulin action in man (191).

Glucose utilization at rest may also be influenced by hormones other than insulin such as epinephrine, growth hormone, and cortisol. Effects of these hormones will be described in the section below, REGULATION OF GLUCOSE UTILIZATION DURING EXERCISE.

Finally, insulin action is decreased in a number of pathological conditions, among which non–insulin-dependent diabetes and obesity are the most prevalent. For discussion of these states the reader is referred to other reviews (95, 131, 283, 319).

REGULATION OF GLUCOSE UTILIZATION DURING EXERCISE

During exercise, any one of the three factors—supply, transport, and metabolism—may be limiting for glucose uptake. Hence, when examining regulation of glucose utilization in vivo it is helpful to consider which of the three regulatory factors are affected by any intervention or perturbation of the system. For the maximal increase in glucose utilization to occur all three factors have to be increased simultaneously.

Exercise increases whole-body glucose utilization compared with the resting state (59, 76, 199, 201, 329, 392), and the majority of the increase is due to an increase in skeletal muscle glucose utilization (201). Whole-body glucose utilization during exercise can be measured from isotopic tracer infusion studies using stable or radioactive tracers, and if the label is on carbon molecules (^{14}C or ^{13}C) it is possible to follow glucose oxidation, provided there exists steady-state labeling of the bicarbonate pool, a condition that takes time to accuire. The advantage of using tracer technology is the noninvasive nature of the technique, whereas the drawbacks are problems with lack of steady state during short-term experiments and inability to provide metabolic information in specific tissues, unless combined with catheterization. The method of choice for studying local metabolism is by combining arterial and venous catheterization with measurements of blood flow. A disadvantage is that arteriovenous (A-V) differences of glucose are small during exercise at euglycemia (in the range of 0.05–0.4 mmol/liter) (5, 96, 185, 187, 298) and hence sometimes not easy to measure accurately. A direct comparison between isotopic turnover studies and local catheterization has been done during submaximal exercise in humans (201), and the two measures agreed well (Fig. 20.7) when considering that the majority of glucose disposal at rest takes place in nonmuscle tissues. Thus, the rise

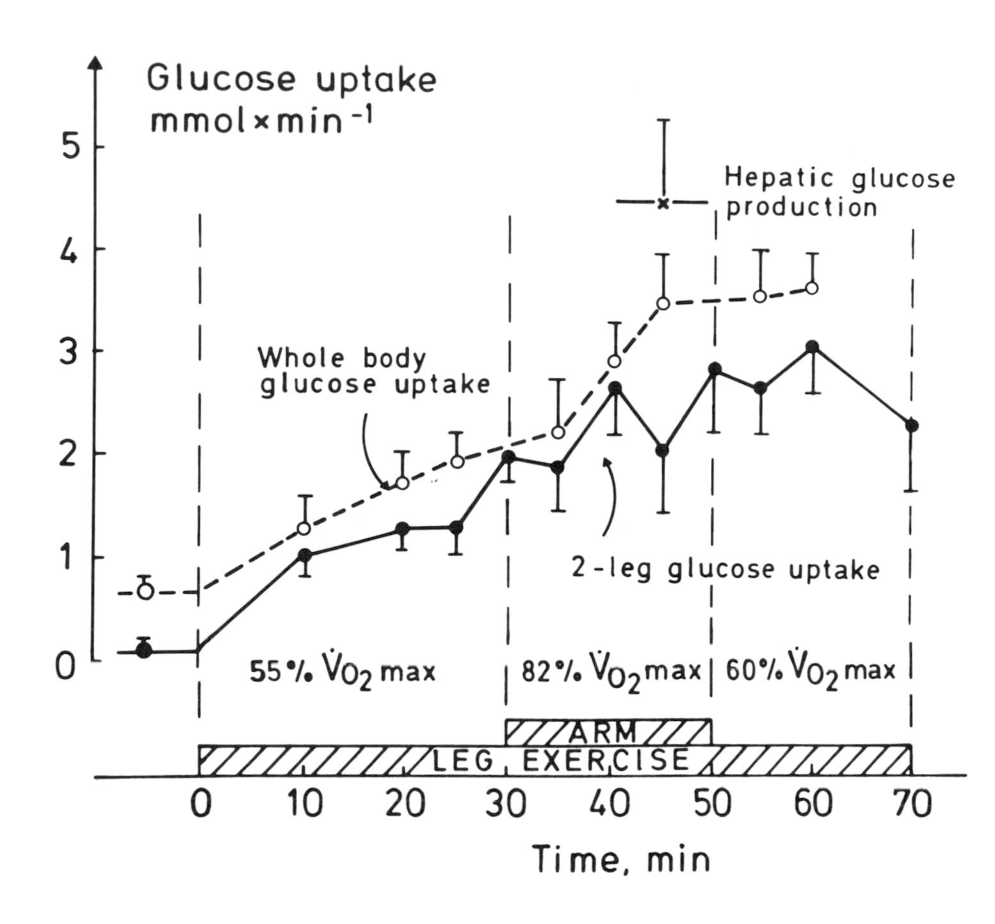

FIG. 20.7. Isotopically measured whole-body glucose disappearance (*dotted line*) and directly measured two-leg glucose uptake (*solid line*) in man at rest and during ergometer cycling with legs only and with added arm cranking from 30–50 min exercise. Values are means ±SE of seven observations. [Reproduced from Kjaer et al. (201), with permission.]

in glucose disposal with exercise was of the same magnitude when measured with catheterization as with isotopes (Fig. 20.7).

Effect of Exercise Intensity

In general, glucose utilization of a given muscle or muscle group increases with increasing exercise intensity (Fig 20.8.) (185, 357). However, at the onset of intense exercise, glucose may actually be released from contracting muscle (182), probably because rapid glycogenolysis results in significant formation of free glucose by the glycogen debranching enzyme. This free glucose formation together with the glucose transported into the muscle may exceed the capacity of the hexokinase reaction (which furthermore is inhibited by the high intramuscular concentrations of glucose 6-phosphate that prevail during such conditions), resulting in a transient reversal of the glucose gradient and consequent net efflux of glucose. An additional factor that may contribute to inhibition of hexokinase activity during heavy exercise is a change in the degree of binding to mitochondria. In horse muscle, approximately 38% of hexokinase is bound to mitochondria at rest, whereas after heavy exercise at maximal oxygen uptake only 7% is bound. This shift in binding is pos-

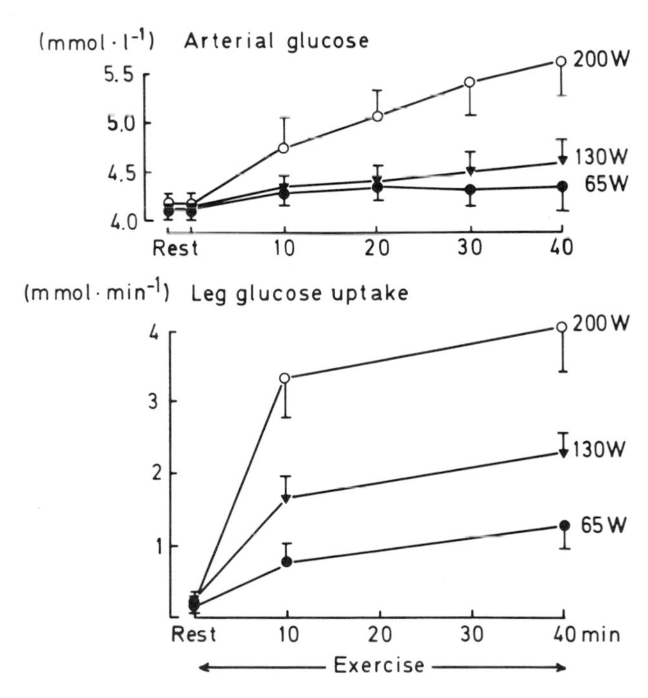

FIG. 20.8. Arterial blood glucose concentration and leg glucose uptake at rest and during ergometer cycling with the legs. [Adapted from Wahren et al. (358), with permission.]

sibly due to glucose 6-phosphate displacing hexokinase from mitochondria (67). At any rate, a decrease in binding to mitochondria apparently increases the K_m for ATP and decreases the K_i for glucose 6-phosphate (235).This increases the ability of glucose 6-phosphate to inhibit the enzyme. Thus, glucose 6-phosphate apparently inhibits hexokinase activity by a dual mechanism. This involves both direct enzyme inhibition but also redistribution of hexokinase to a nonmitochondrial-bound form that is more sensitive to inhibition by glucose 6-phosphate. The phenomenon of glucose release only lasts a couple of minutes, after which it reverts to glucose uptake, possibly because the rate of glycogenolysis and glucose 6-phosphate accumulation decreases and rate of glycolysis increases.

Blood Flow. During dynamic exercise blood flow increases linearly with increasing workload (9), and when intensity increases beyond 70%–80% of VO_{2max}, arterial glucose concentration usually increases too (199, 201, 132, 379). This means that supply of glucose increases markedly with increasing exercise intensity and sets the stage for a high rate of glucose transport that can feed the metabolic machinery (Fig 20.9). When considering that glucose uptake is the product of blood flow and A-V glucose difference, the increase in blood flow emerges as the largest contributor to the exercise-induced increase in glucose uptake. Blood flow may increase up to about 20-fold from rest to intense dynamic exercise. For instance, in the resting leg, blood flow is ~300–600 ml/min (4, 5, 97, 201, 243, 357) and increases linearly with increasing intensity to values around 5–7 liters/min during maximal dynamic exercise (7, 185, 307). In contrast, the A-V difference only increases by two- to fourfold at a constant arterial glucose concentration [Fig. 20.9; (185, 357)]. Thus, although the cellular events that increase muscle membrane glucose transport capacity with muscle contractions are important, the increase in muscle perfusion accompanying exercise is of quantitatively larger importance for glucose utilization. Direct evidence for the importance of blood flow for muscle glucose uptake comes from studies in perfused muscle in which an increase in flow (up to a certain level) at a given glucose concentration proportionally increased glucose uptake in resting muscle (144, 159, 321). In perfused contracting hindlimb muscle the increase in glucose uptake with contractions also is dependent upon the concomitant increase in perfusate flow [Fig. 20.10; (159, 320, 351)]. The mechanism for this effect of perfusion rate probably relates to maintenance of the interstitial glucose concentration and possibly to increased

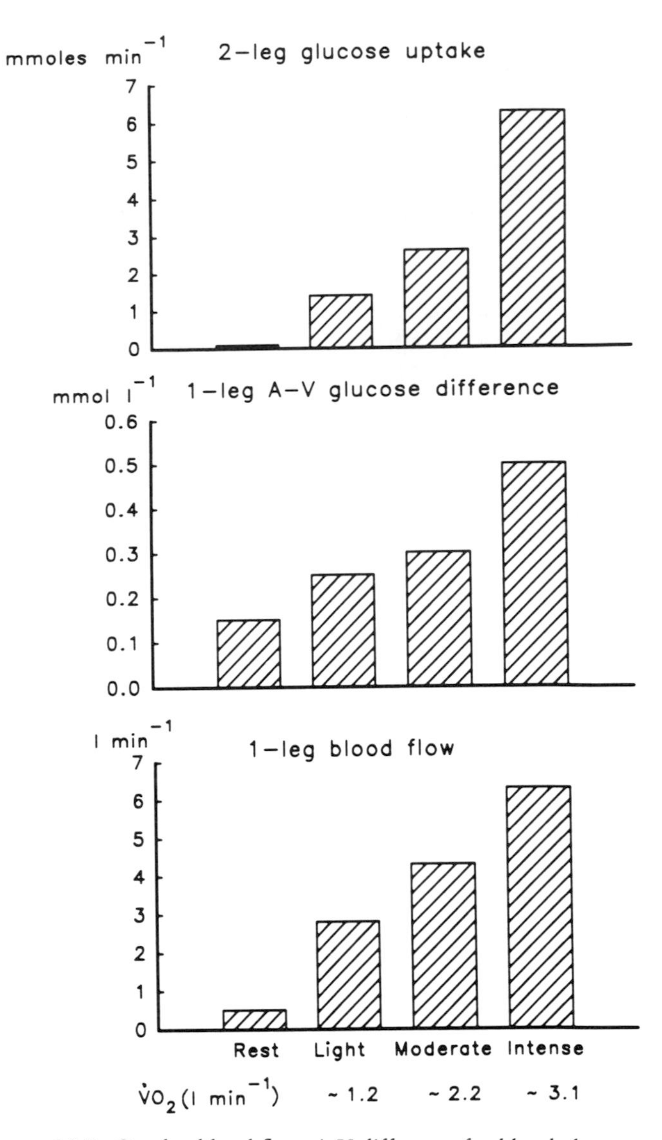

FIG. 20.9. One-leg blood flow, A-V difference for blood glucose, and two-leg glucose uptake in man at rest and during bicycling at light, moderate, and heavy exercise. Each workload corresponds to a pulmonary oxygen uptake of ~1.2, 2.2, and 3.3 liters/min, respectively. Values are from references (4, 5, 185) and are recorded after 40 min of exercise except at the highest workload, which was sustained for only 3.5 min but preceded by 15 min submaximal exercise (185).

interstitial insulin concentration. With increasing membrane glucose transport capacity with muscle contractions, the interstitial glucose concentration would decrease if glucose delivery was not increased. Hence, increased perfusion plus the opening of more capillaries during contractions decreases the average diffusion distance from capillary to muscle fiber and probably alleviates decreases in interstitial muscle glucose concentration. Estimates of the increase in capillary surface area in muscle with contractions range from four- to tenfold (89). A fourfold increase

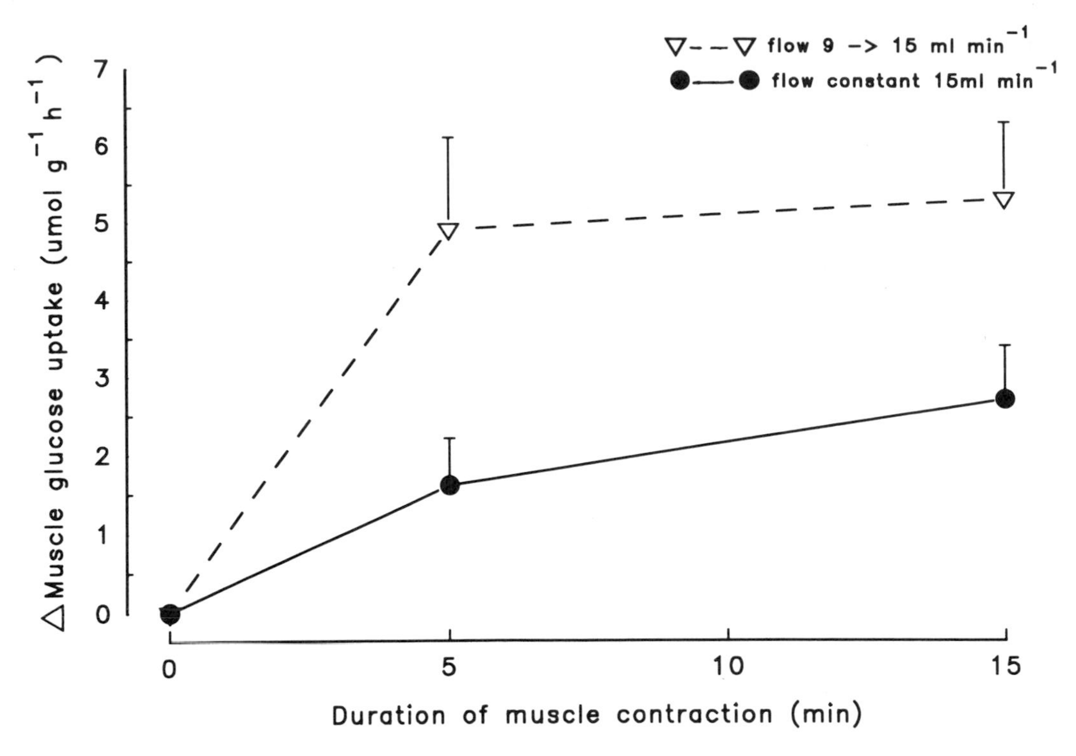

FIG. 20.10. Increase in hindlimb glucose uptake with electrical stimulation. Perfusate flow was either increased from 9 ml/min to 15 ml/min at the onset of contractions (*broken line*) or was constant at 15 ml/min both at rest and during contractions (*full line*). Values are means ±SE of 11–12 observations.

decreases the average diffusion distance by half (89). The low extraction of glucose during exercise (1%–10%) (5, 151, 185, 298, 357) suggests that interstitial glucose concentrations are maintained well during exercise. As indicated earlier, preliminary data obtained with the microdialysis technique agree with this conclusion (D. McLean and J. Bangsbo, personal communication).

Blood flow within a muscle both at rest and during electrically induced muscle contractions apparently exhibits rather marked spatial heterogeneity (173, 268). Glucose uptake apparently does so as well (173). The correlation between blood flow and glucose uptake within the muscle is nonsignificant at rest, but during muscle contractions the correlation coefficient was 0.51 ($P < 0.05$) (173). The mechanism behind this inhomogeneity in blood flow and glucose uptake as well as their partial covariation is not known and remains to be demonstrated in humans during exercise.

At the cellular level the increase in firing frequency associated with increased exercise intensity (314) probably increases the glucose uptake of the individual muscle fiber (251), but the recruitment of more fibers within the muscle is also expected to increase whole-muscle glucose utilization. However, with increasing exercise intensity more and more type IIa and eventually type IIb fibers are recruited (314). Type IIb fibers have a lower GLUT4 protein content than type IIa and type I fibers (137, 155, 230, 289) and have also been shown to have a lower glucose transport during maximal electrical stimulation (51, 273). Thus, recruitment of type IIb fibers will be expected to increase glucose utilization less than type I and type IIa fibers of the same mass.

Glucose utilization of the whole body increases with increasing exercise intensity. Because most of the glucose is utilized in nonmuscle tissues at rest, however, the magnitude of the increase with exercise is much smaller than when measuring directly across a muscle with catheters according to the Fick principle (blood flow × A-V glucose difference). Thus, at rest whole-body glucose disposal (Rd) is typically around 0.8 mmol/min and may increase to maximal values of ~3 mmol/min at exercise at 100% $\dot{V}O_{2max}$ (199, 232). This is in fact only about 50% of two-leg glucose uptake during exercise at 100% $\dot{V}O_{2max}$ when measured via the Fick principle (185) and suggests that because of problems with steady state during the short exercise bouts at maximal exercise, isotope-derived figures on whole-body glucose utilization are quite inaccurate at high exercise intensities.

Another way of increasing exercise intensity on the whole-body level is by adding more active muscle mass (e.g., adding arm exercise to leg exercise). The effect of adding arm exercise to leg exercise at a constant workload was in one study found to be a slight inhibition of leg glucose uptake (298) without any changes in limb flow. In another study, the interpretation was complicated by an increase in plasma glucose concentration when arm exercise was added to leg exercise (201). Teleologically it makes sense that utilization of a limited fuel source like glucose is decreased per kilogram of active muscle when a large muscle mass is engaged in exercise. The mechanism probably involves increased sympathoadrenal activity (201, 298, 317) which, by increasing plasma free fatty acid (FFA) concentration and muscle glycogenolysis, can limit glucose uptake in muscle during exercise (28, 151, 158, 369)

Fate of Glucose. It is generally assumed that most of the glucose taken up by muscle during exercise is oxidized, at least during moderately intense exercise (76, 185, 390, 391). During high intensity exercise, however, it has been reported that the glucose taken up is mostly just accumulating in the muscle rather than being oxidized because of strong inhibition of glucose phosphorylation (185). But these findings are based on glucose assay of muscle homogenates, and the intracellular concentration is computed by subtraction of an amount assumed to reside in the extracellular space. Without proper estimation of the extracellular space and the interstitial glucose concentration, such measurements are fraught with inaccuracy. Furthermore, possible compartmentalization of glucose inside the cell could make even rather large changes in small compartments difficult to detect in a homogenate. Nevertheless, a large increase in the glucose concentration of muscle homogenate in the absence of increased plasma glucose concentration (185) can hardly be interpreted other than as due to an increase in intracellular glucose. The origin of this glucose is, however, uncertain and might as well originate from activity of the glycogen debranching enzyme as from extracellular glucose. In the quoted study (185), the free intracellular glucose concentration was estimated to be 8.5 mmol/kg dry weight at the end of maximal exercise. Assuming a water content of the muscle fibers alone of 60% means that the average glucose concentration in intracellular water would be ~3.4 mmol/liter (8.5 × 40/100). Given that the arterial plasma glucose concentration was ~4.9 mmol/liter, the glucose gradient during maximal exercise was ~1.5 mmol/liter compared to ~4.9 mmol/liter during moderate-intensity exercise, during which no glucose accumulated in muscle. From these numbers, it thus appears almost incomprehensible that the A-V difference of glucose was only ~0.35mmol/liter during moderate-intensity exercise, whereas it was ~0.60 mmol/liter at maximal exercise (185). Nevertheless, the study does show a marked increase in muscle glucose and glucose 6-phosphate concentration, which is compatible with the idea that during intense exercise phosphorylation may be rate limiting for glucose utilization in muscle.

Effect of Exercise Duration

When one is exercising at a constant power output, the blood flow to the working muscles increases to reach a plateau within the first 4–5 min and is maintained remarkably constant for the duration of exercise (5, 151, 201, 345, 357). Thus, one component of glucose supply (namely, blood flow) does not vary much except for the first few minutes. Glucose supply during exercise at a fixed power output therefore varies directly with plasma glucose concentration. During most submaximal exercise, plasma glucose is quite constant until hepatic glucose production, because of glycogen depletion, cannot keep pace with glucose utilization (370, 371). Thus, during prolonged exercise, glucose supply is characterized by being fairly constant during the first part, and it declines thereafter. During exercise of intensities requiring more than 70%–80% of maximal aerobic capacity, plasma glucose may increase [Fig. 20.8; (199, 201, 232, 379)]. This increases the supply above that which can be accounted for by increased flow.

With onset of contractions, membrane glucose transport capacity probably increases quite fast. In contracting perfused rat skeletal muscle, glucose transport as measured by the uptake of radiolabeled 3-O-methylglucose was similar when measured over the first 5 min and over 10–15 min of contractions (158) even though glucose uptake as measured as A-V glucose difference × perfusate flow was higher in the 10–15 min period. This suggests that the increase in membrane glucose transport capacity occurs rapidly and that other factors limit glucose uptake in the beginning of exercise. It has been suggested that such a factor may be glucose phosphorylation. Thus, during the initial stages of exercise, accumulation of glucose 6-phosphate in muscle may inhibit hexokinase and cause accumulation of free glucose in muscle (187). However, as exercise continues, glucose 6-phosphate concentrations decrease toward resting levels, which presumably gradually relieves hexokinase from inhibition and shifts the rate-limiting step in glucose utilization from metabolism to transport (187). However, recent data in sarcolemmal giant vesicles obtained from human muscle suggest that the sarcolemmal glucose transport capacity is only slightly increased after 5 min bicycling at 75% of Vo_{2max} but markedly increased after 40 min. These new findings therefore suggest that the gradual increase in leg glucose uptake during such submaximal exercise (186) is due not only to a lessening of inhibition of glucose metabolism but also to a gradual increase in glucose transport capacity of the muscle membrane (S. Kristiansen, M. Hargreaves and E. A. Richter, unpublished observations).

During very prolonged exercise (>4 h) not much is known about muscle glucose utilization. However, glucose utilization might eventually decrease because of a marked increase in FFA (25, 151), as discussed later. In a study employing 3 h of cycling followed by 5 h of treadmill running, glucose appearance increased to a maximum after 4 h of exercise and then declined to resting values. Since plasma glucose was apparently maintained, glucose disappearance must also have decreased after 4 h of exercise (333). At the end of exercise, carbohydrate oxidation was close to resting values and entirely due to oxidation of plasma glucose (333).

Together, the changes in supply, transport, and metabolism of glucose explain that glucose utilization generally increases with time during prolonged exercise (Fig. 20.8; see also Fig. 20.12 below) until glucose supply decreases. The increase in plasma concentrations of FFA during prolonged exercise is also expected to limit glucose utilization.

Concerning differences in glucose utilization by the different fiber types with exercise, no information is available in humans. Much probably depends on the specific fiber types recruited. Thus, recruitment of the more oxidative type I and type IIa fibers is expected to favor glucose utilization compared to recruitment of type IIb fibers. Besides differences in GLUT 4 protein content (137, 155, 230, 289), hexokinase activity is also higher in type I and type IIa than in type IIb fibers (314).

Effect of Exercise Type

In general, studies on glucose utilization in humans have utilized dynamic exercise. Static exercise is from the point of glucose utilization less interesting, since it is usually of much shorter duration. However, much of the literature on glucose utilization in animal muscles is from studies using intermittent isometric (static) contractions.

In man, glucose utilization seems to vary according to whether dynamic arm or leg exercise is performed. Thus, at the same oxygen uptake, which corresponds to a 25% lower absolute workload in arm exercise than in leg exercise (8), or at the same relative work rate, which during arm exercise corresponds to ~55%–60% of the corresponding leg workload (7, 180), R-values are higher during arm than during leg exercise. This greater carbohydrate reliance is partly due to an increased reliance on glucose utilization (8). The mechanism behind these differences remains a subject of speculation. Since fiber-type composition and oxidative capacity of arm muscles are fairly similar to leg muscles (314, 318), these factors cannot provide the explanation. The catecholamine response is larger in arm exercise when performed at the same oxygen uptake than leg exercise (8) but similar when performed at the same relative exercise intensity (180). If anything, a larger catecholamine response should decrease glucose uptake via hexokinase inhibition by glucose 6-phosphate. Therefore, differences in catecholamine concentrations during exercise with arms and legs cannot explain the difference in regional glucose metabolism during exercise either. Whatever mechanism elicits the greater muscle perfusion per unit muscle during arm than during leg exercise at the same relative intensity (180) may also be responsible for the higher glucose utilization.

Concentric exercise is the usual mode of exercise, and essentially all exercise studies have used either pure concentric exercise (bicycling) or combined concentric/eccentric exercise such as running. However, eccentric exercise may affect glucose utilization differently than concentric exercise, given the fact that the metabolic cost of eccentric exercise is much lower than the cost of comparable concentric exercise (12) and that the mechanical strain is larger in eccentric exercise. However, to date, no study has been published in which glucose utilization is measured during pure eccentric exercise. However, preliminary data from our laboratory show that during 60 min submaximal eccentric exercise (resisting a motordriven knee-flexion device) glucose uptake in the eccentric working thigh is very low as is oxygen uptake compared to if a similar number of Watts had been performed concentrically. Even when glucose uptake was expressed as a function of oxygen used, glucose uptake was roughly half of what is usually measured during concentric knee-extensor exercise (D. A. MacLean, B. Kiens, B. K. Pedersen, T. Rohde, B. Saltin and E. A. Richter, unpublished observations). These observations suggest that eccentric exercise may activate glucose uptake less than concentric exercise at a comparable oxygen uptake, possibly indicating that the actual shortening of skeletal muscle is of importance for stimulation of glucose uptake. Alternatively, since the neuromuscular recruitment pattern is different in concentric and eccentric exercise, this factor alone may also be responsible for at least part of the difference in glucose uptake between concentric and eccentric exercise.

Alternative Substrates

Glucose utilization in muscle during exercise is influenced by availability of other substrates, primarily glycogen and FFA. Whether availability of intramuscular triglycerides influences glucose utilization is unknown.

Glycogen. The metabolism of glycogen and glucose share the same pathway from conversion to glucose 6-phosphate (Fig. 20.11). Most of the glycogen is degraded by phosphorylase, which cleaves the α-1,4 bonds of the glycogen molecule to form glucose 1-phosphate, which is rapidly converted to glucose 6-phosphate. In addition, some of the glycogen is degraded to glucose via action of the debranching enzyme cleaving the α-1,6 bonds at branch points in the glycogen molecule. On the average, 6%–7% of glycogen is degraded to glucose, but this percentage may vary according to the glycogen concentration. Thus, because the glycogen molecule has a finite size and because at high glycogen concentrations relatively more glycosyl units are located in the outer, less-branched chains where α-1,4 bonds predominate, it is conceivable that glycogen degradation at high glycogen concentrations initially occurs mainly by the action of phosphorylase giving rise to glucose 6-phosphate. This has been shown in vitro in protein-glycogen particles isolated from rabbit muscle (250). Also, in man, glucose formation during exercise may be higher at low than at high initial muscle glycogen concentrations (312). The model used was static exercise, but the findings probably apply to dynamic exercise as well. No matter whether glucose formation is significant or not, breakdown of glycogen ultimately leads to formation of glucose 6-phosphate, which is a powerful inhibitor of hexokinase (254). Thus, rapid glycogenolysis may directly, by action of the debranching enzyme or indirectly via hexokinase inhibition, lead to accumulation of free glucose. This will decrease the concentration gradient driving glucose transport. Thus, glycogenolysis may inhibit glucose uptake and utilization. In perfused contracting rat muscle that had been preconditioned with high glycogen concentrations, rate of glycogenolysis was increased and

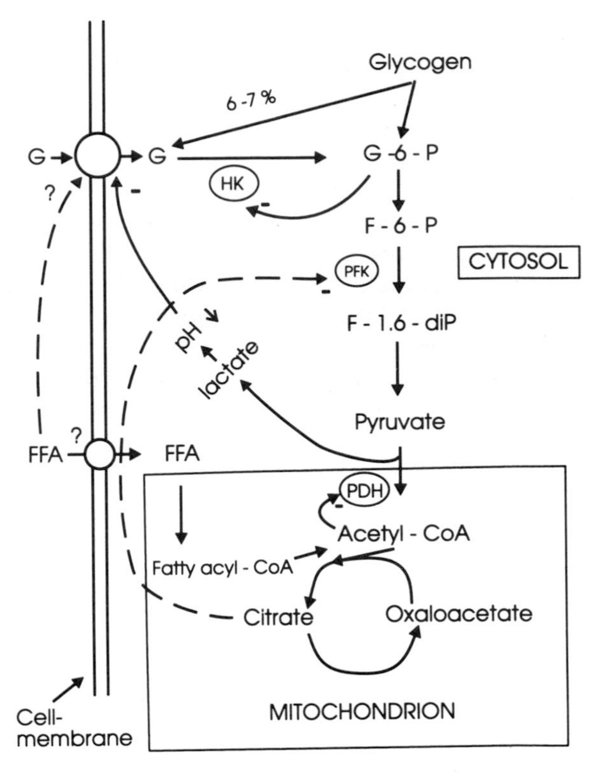

FIG. 20.11. Schematic presentation of possible biochemical mechanisms involved in regulation of glucose utilization by the alternative substrates glycogen and free fatty acids (FFA) in muscle during exercise. Glycogen breakdown may inhibit glucose phosphorylation via production of glucose 6-phosphate in turn inhibiting hexokinase. In addition, rapid glycogenolysis may by virtue of lactate production decrease pH, which decreases intrinsic activity of GLUT4 (212). Finally, 6%–7% of glycogen is broken down to free glucose via activity of the debranching enzyme. In concert with hexokinase inhibition this may lead to decreased glucose gradient from interstitium to cytosol. FFA is proposed to inhibit glucose utilization via pyruvatedehydrogenase and phosphofructokinase inhibition, again leading to build-up of glucose 6-phosphate and hexokinase inhibition. However, evidence for this mechanism in contracting muscle is weak. FFA may possibly have direct inhibitory effects on glucose transport. G, glucose; G-6-P, glucose 6-phosphate; FFA, free fatty acids; HK, hexokinase; PFK, phosphofructokinase; PDH, pyruvatedehydrogenase.

rate of glucose uptake was decreased compared with muscles preconditioned with normal or low glycogen concentrations (158, 292). Contractions in muscle with high initial muscle glycogen concentrations elicited much larger increases in muscle glucose 6-phosphate and free glucose concentrations than did contractions in muscle with low initial glycogen concentrations (158). This suggests that the inhibition of glucose uptake occured via inhibition of hexokinase and accumulation of intracellular glucose. These findings are supported by results from humans in which glucose uptake during cycling exercise was higher in the glycogen-depleted leg than in the contralateral control leg (134). Furthermore, glucose uptake correlated positively with the percentage of glycogen-depleted muscle fibers and inversely with the muscle glucose 6-phosphate concentration (134). At the end of exercise, muscle glucose concentration was also higher in the normal than in the glycogen-depleted leg (134). Thus, there is little doubt that glycogenolysis and glucose uptake are inversely related in muscle during exercise and that the predominant mechanism is through glucose 6-phosphate inhibition of hexokinase. However, in contracting perfused rat muscle glucose transport as measured by accumulation of the glucose analogue 3-0-methylglucose was decreased by 25% in muscles with high initial glycogen concentrations compared with muscles with low glycogen concentrations (158). This finding seems to indicate that muscle membrane glucose transport capacity was also affected by the glycogen concentration either directly or indirectly. One possibility could be a direct inhibition of glucose transporter intrinsic activity by glucose 6-phosphate, as suggested in adipocytes (120). However, incubation of rat sarcolemmal vesicles with glucose 6-phosphate did not influence GLUT4 intrinsic activity (212). On the other hand, decreases or increases in pH from an optimal value of 7.2 decreases GLUT4 intrinsic activity (212, 334). Therefore, in muscles with a high rate of glycogenolysis and ensuing lactate production (134, 158, 292) pH may decrease and in turn decrease muscle glucose transporter activity.

Free fatty acids. During exercise, FFA constitute the major alternative circulating fuel to glucose. In the early 1960s, Randle and co-workers proposed the "glucose–free fatty acid cycle" based on experiments mainly in the rat heart (281, 282). According to their findings, an increased supply and in turn greater oxidation of FFA lead to inhibition of pyruvate dehydrogenase (PDH) and phophofructokinase (PFK), with the latter occuring because of increased citrate formation. Inhibition of these key enzymes in glycolysis and in glucose oxidation would then lead to decreased glucose utilization. A major prerequisite for this scheme to work is that inhibition of these enzymes leads to the subsequent accumulation of glucose 6-phosphate in turn inhibiting hexokinase. Inhibition of hexokinase then again leads to accumulation of glucose inside the cell, decreasing the net driving concentration gradient for glucose transport. However, it was later proposed that FFA might also directly decrease membrane glucose transport capacity (282). Although there is little doubt that the glucose–free fatty acid cycle operates in heart and in skeletal muscle at rest during insulin stimulation (31, 33, 259, 267, 280, 362), the bulk of evidence argues against its operation in skeletal muscle during exercise, as discussed below.

In rats, fat feeding before exercise decreases the exercise-induced muscle glycogen breakdown (287). In one study in the perfused rat hindlimb, muscle glycogenolysis as well as glucose uptake during electrical stimulation was decreased by 1.8 mM oleate in the perfusate (286). Analysis of muscle samples showed that oleate caused accumulation of citrate and glucose 6-phosphate and free glucose in the red muscle fibers, supporting that the effect of oleate was through operation of the glucose–free fatty acid cycle. However, in other studies in the perfused hindlimb muscle glucose uptake during electrical stimulation was not inhibited by palmitate (24, 302), oleate (113), or octanoate (24).

Fasting (203, 263) or ingestion of a fat-rich diet for a few days (177) have been used as methods to study the effect of fatty acids on carbohydrate metabolism. Fasting decreased glucose utilization during exercise compared to the control condition, whereas ingestion of a fat-rich diet in fact tended to increase glucose utilization even though arterial FFA concentrations were increased compared with a carbohydrate-rich diet (177). This unexpected effect of the fat-rich diet was likely due to the lower muscle glycogen concentrations observed after fat feeding (177). This study shows how difficult it is to isolate an effect of a single factor such as FFA in whole-body studies involving major perturbations in glucose and glycogen concentrations as well as glucoregulatory hormones.

To isolate more clearly the effect of FFA on glucose metabolism, techniques have been used with the aim of acutely altering FFA concentrations without concomitant changes in other substrates or in hormone concentrations. Infusion of triglycerides (Intralipid) and heparin acutely increase whereas nicotinic acid acutely decreases arterial FFA concentrations. Intralipid and heparin infusion decreased leg glucose uptake before, during, and after exercise [Fig. 20.12; (151)], whereas administration of nicotinic acid had no clear effect on leg glucose uptake during cycle ergometer exercise (25, 134). The decrease in leg glucose utilization with Intralipid and heparin was, however, not accompanied by increases in muscle concentrations of glucose 6-phosphate or free glucose (151). Thus, the operation of the classic glucose–fatty acid cycle was not supported, but rather a direct inhibiting effect of FFA on glucose transport might explain the findings. A direct effect of FFA on rat muscle glucose transport has previously been reported (282). Recently, basal glucose transport was found to be unaffected in rat

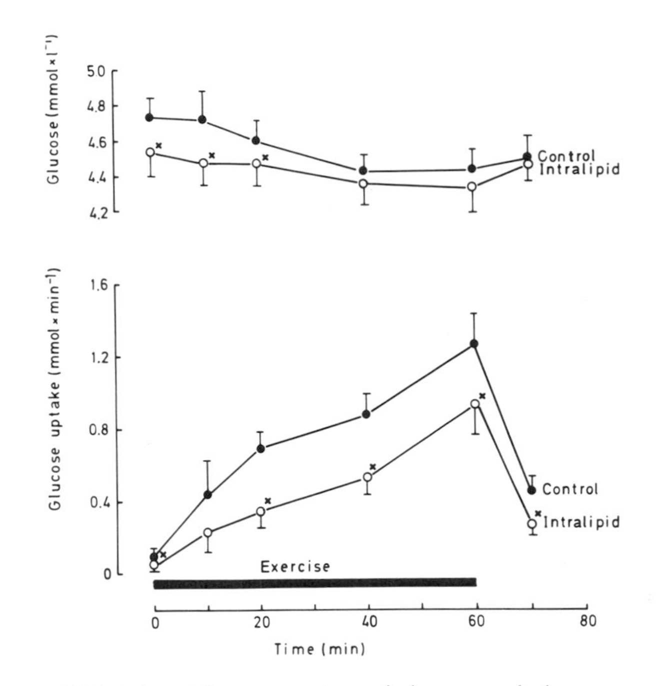

FIG. 20.12. Arterial concentrations of glucose, and glucose uptake before, during, and after 1 h of one-legged dynamic knee extensions. Subjects exercised with one leg during control conditions (plasma FFA ~0.50 mM) and with the other leg during intralipid infusion (plasma FFA ~1.1 mM). Values are means ±SE of seven observations. [Adapted from Hargreaves et al. (151) with permission.] $^*P < 0.05$ compared with values during control conditions.

muscle by 1–2 mM palmitate, but glucose transport stimulated by insulin was inhibited in slow-twitch muscle but not in fast-twitch muscle by palmitate (150). Effects of FFA on glucose transport in human muscle during exercise have, however, not been directly shown. In incubated human muscle strips, 1.0 mM oleate did not decrease insulin-stimulated glucose transport (389).

Several studies have examined the effect of elevated plasma concentrations of FFA on glycogen breakdown during exercise in humans. Although not directly pertinent to this review, these studies may be useful in understanding the possible mechanisms by which FFA affect carbohydrate metabolism. Three studies have found that elevated plasma FFA decreased muscle glycogen breakdown during exercise (85, 112, 355), whereas one did not (151). Of the three studies reporting an effect of FFA on muscle glycogen breakdown, only one study elucidated the biochemical mechanism (112) and reported no FFA-induced accumulation of citrate or acetyl-CoA as would be expected if the classic glucose–fatty acid cycle was operating. Thus, the available evidence suggests that elevated plasma concentrations of FFA may under some conditions decrease muscle glucose uptake as well as glycogen breakdown during exercise in man, but the underlying mechanism does not seem to be the classic glucose–fatty acid cycle.

Glucose Utilization During Exercise in Adverse Environment

Hypoxia. During acute exposure to hypoxia, glucose utilization during moderate-intensity exercise in man is modestly increased (49, 50, 82). After 3 weeks of chronic altitude exposure at 4300 m, however, whole-body glucose utilization was twice as high as during exercise at the same absolute workload at sea level before acclimation (49), mostly due to increased leg glucose utilization (50). The mechanism behind this increase in glucose utilization with acute and especially chronic exposure to altitude is not clear. Apparently, it is not due to changes in plasma insulin concentrations (49, 50).

Heat. Exercise in the heat compared to exercise in thermoneutral environments does not seem to cause marked changes in leg glucose utilization (256). After acclimation to heat (39.6°C) for 8 days a small increase in leg glucose utilization during exercise in the heat was reported (197) compared to exercise in the heat before acclimation. However, in another study, 9–12 days acclimation to heat (40°C) did not change leg glucose utilization during exercise in the heat (255). Thus, neither acute heat exposure nor exposure after acclimation seems to induce any substantial changes in glucose utilization during exercise.

Humoral Regulation of Glucose Utilization During Exercise

Insulin. In the total absence of insulin, muscle contractions in vitro elicit an increase in glucose uptake (251, 272, 300, 365). Thus, no humoral factors are necessary. In the face of decreasing plasma insulin concentrations during exercise (126), the autonomy of muscle glucose uptake during contractions is almost a necessity. However, it has been repeatedly demonstrated in vivo that muscle glucose uptake during exercise increases less in the insulin-deficient pancreatectomized dog than in controls (28, 354). Furthermore, in insulin-deficient diabetic man, leg glucose clearance during exercise was markedly lower than in nondiabetic controls (359). Moreover, a synergistic effect of insulin and exercise has been demonstrated in man (96, 372). These findings thus suggest that although insulin is not necessary for muscle contractions to elicit an increase in glucose uptake, a larger response to contractions is obtained in the presence than in the absence of insulin even at the low concentration normally found during exercise in the postprandial state (374). Part of this effect no doubt is found in the antilipolytic effect of insulin, since insulinopenia is associated with increased plasma FFA (28, 369), which, as described above, may lead to decreased glucose uptake. Furthermore, in the insulin-deficient dog, increased catecholamine secretion acts in concert with the lack of insulin in further increasing plasma FFA and probably also by increasing glycogenolysis in muscle, which in turn decreases glucose utilization (373, 380).

Apart from the indirect effects of insulin on glucose utilization during exercise, there are direct effects too. Obviously, a high plasma insulin concentration will increase glucose utilization during exercise, but the interesting aspect is that the interaction between insulin and exercise apparently is of a synergistic nature (96, 351, 372). This may be related in part to the exercise-induced increase in insulin delivery due to the high blood flow and increased number of open capillaries during exercise (96, 351). This shortens diffusion distances from capillary to sarcolemma for insulin as well as for glucose, thus creating conditions for increased insulin binding and maintenance of interstitial glucose concentrations close to the plasma concentration. Combined with the increased membrane glucose transport capacity induced by contractions, this creates optimal conditions for glucose uptake. It is in keeping with this interpretation that isolated increased loads (arterial concentrations × flow) of either glucose or insulin to the resting dog limb, simulating the increased loads during exercise, do not create nearly the increase in glucose utilization that is observed during exercise (391).

Adenosine. Adenosine produced in contracting muscle augments the effect of insulin on glucose uptake and transport in perfused rat muscle [Fig. 20.13; (351)]. Adenosine is also important for insulin-stimulated glucose uptake in the heart (219). Interestingly, this adenosine-induced increase in insulin-mediated glucose transport in contracting muscle was only demonstrable in the insulin-sensitive slow-twitch and fast-twitch red fibers (351). Although the molecular mechanism behind the effect of adenosine on insulin action is not well characterized, the demonstration of metabolic effects in addition to the known vascular effects of adenosine (139, 276) makes adenosine production in contracting muscle potentially important. Thus, adenosine might play a dual enhancing role in glucose metabolism during

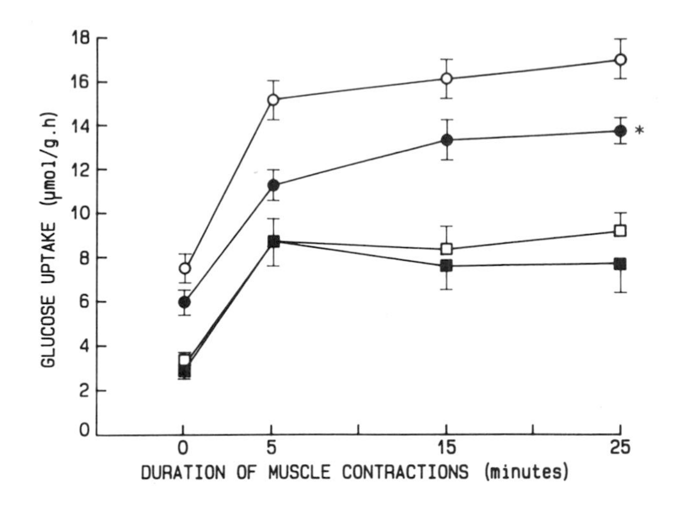

FIG. 20.13. Glucose uptake at rest and during electrical stimulation in perfused rat hindlimb. Perfusate contained no insulin (*squares*) or insulin at 100 μ/ml (*circles*). *Filled symbols* denote addition of caffeine at 77 μM. *Values in the presence of caffeine are significantly lower than in the absence during muscle contractions. Values are means ±SE of 13–27 observations. [Adapted from Vergauen et al. (351), with permission.]

exercise: it apparently increases insulin action and, at least during some types of exercise (139, 204, 276), may also be important for increasing blood flow and hence insulin and glucose delivery to contracting muscle. The role of adenosine in glucose metabolism during exercise in man, however, remains to be established.

Epinephrine. Glucose utilization during exercise can also be modulated by epinephrine. In vitro studies provide no clear picture regarding the effect of catecholamines on glucose utilization during muscle contractions. Most studies describing the effects of catecholamines on glucose transport in muscle have been performed at rest. Some investigators find that α-adrenergic stimulation may increase glucose transport (313), whereas β-adrenergic stimulation may inhibit it (26). However, in vitro, the effect of β-adrenergic stimulation in resting muscle apparently varies with the albumin concentration in the incubation medium, being inhibitory in the absence and stimulatory in the presence of albumin (26, 313, 385). Furthermore, in the perfused resting rat hindlimb, epinephrine increased glucose uptake via β-adrenergic mechanisms in the absence of insulin but decreased glucose uptake in the presence of maximally stimulating insulin concentrations (70). In the perfused *contracting* rat hindlimb, epinephrine at a concentration of 2.4×10^{-8} M increased glucose uptake (302), and this effect was elicited by α-adrenergic stimulation (301). Pure β-adrenergic stimulation with epinephrine and phentolamine (an α-adrenergic blocker) did not significantly decrease glucose uptake (301). However, in recent experiments, a low concentration of the β-adrenergic agonist isoproterenol (1.5×10^{-9} M) decreased glucose uptake by ~40% in the perfused hindquarter during muscle contractions (P. Hespel and E. A. Richter, unpublished observations).

In the resting rat (37, 174) and in man (98, 215, 303), epinephrine decreases insulin-stimulated peripheral glucose utilization via β-adrenergic mechanisms. Interestingly, in the rat epinephrine was found to translocate GLUT4 to the plasma membrane in spite of a decrease in 2-deoxyglucose uptake (37). These findings suggest that epinephrine markedly reduces GLUT4 intrinsic activity, but the mechanism behind was not explored.

Few studies have been carried out in vivo evaluating the role of epinephrine for glucose uptake during exercise. Infusion of epinephrine to the running dog decreased glucose clearance (172), and in man intra-arterial infusion of epinephrine into one leg decreased its glucose uptake compared to that of the contralateral leg during two-leg ergometer cycling (176). The mechanism for this decrease seems to be related to an increase in intramuscular glycogenolysis, which increases muscle glucose 6-phosphate concentrations, thereby inhibiting hexokinase activity. However, direct effects of epinephrine on intrinsic activity of GLUT4 cannot be excluded. Furthermore, because epinephrine stimulates lipolysis, increased epinephrine concentrations during exercise will contribute to raise plasma FFA concentration, which in turn probably will decrease glucose utilization, as discussed earlier. In accordance with this view, β-adrenergic blockade decreased plasma FFA concentrations and muscle glycogenolysis, and increased glucose clearance in running dogs (171). Also, in man, β-adrenergic blockade increased whole-body glucose clearance during exercise (231). Therefore, it can be concluded that during exercise epinephrine decreases muscle glucose utilization by β-adrenergic mechanisms that increase lipolysis and muscle glycogenolysis. The latter increases formation of glucose 6-phosphate and thereby inhibits hexokinase. In addition, epinephrine may possibly decrease intrinsic activity of GLUT4.

Cortisol, Growth Hormone. During exercise, plasma concentrations of both cortisol and growth hormone (GH) are elevated in relation to both intensity and duration of exercise (126). The question is whether increased plasma concentrations of cortisol and GH affect muscle glucose metabolism during exercise. This cannot be readily answered because the appropriate experiments have not been performed. However, it is well documented that at rest, infusion of cortisol (323) as well as GH (94, 248, 304, 397), raising the plasma concentration to values seen during exercise, decrease whole-body (94, 304, 324, 397) and forearm (248) glucose utilization. Whereas the action of cortisol seems to be rapid (324), the effect of GH is more slowly developed (248). Nevertheless, these findings at rest may not be applicable to contracting muscle. Accordingly, it cannot be concluded whether exercise-induced elevations in plasma concentrations of cortisol and GH have any effects on glucose utilization during exercise.

Effect of Physical Training Status

Both longitudinal and cross-sectional exercise training studies in man reveal that glucose utilization during exercise is decreased compared to the untrained state at the same absolute (76, 190, 240) or same relative (178, 346) exercise intensity. The decrease in glucose utilization has been reported to occur already after 10 days of training (240). The magnitude of the effect has been variable but, more often than not, (157, 315) detectable. In rats, no decreased glucose turnover during exercise with training has been shown (48, 106); in fact, an increased glucose utilization after training was found in one study (106). In the rat, endurance training also increased muscle GLUT4 content and contraction-induced glucose transport in perfused soleus muscle compared with transport and GLUT4 content in the nontrained soleus (274). Furthermore, in incubated muscles endurance training also increased insulin- combined with contraction-stimulated glucose transport (309, 325).

Contraction-induced glucose transport is thought to occur via translocation of GLUT4 to the plasma membrane and possibly by increased intrinsic activity of GLUT4 (108, 109, 135, 136, 138, 271, 275, 335). Furthermore, in rat skeletal muscle the total GLUT4 content correlates reasonably well with contraction-induced glucose transport [Fig. 20.5; (155)]. Because endurance training of man (99, 166) and rat (19, 121, 189, 274, 309, 325) increases total muscle GLUT4 protein content, one might expect training to increase rather than decrease transport and utilization of glucose during exercise.

Muscle glucose *transport* has never been measured in humans *during* exercise; therefore, it cannot be totally excluded that *membrane glucose transport capacity* increases more during exercise in the trained state than in the untrained state. If this were true, however, decreased glucose utilization during exercise (as found in the trained state) could only occur if glucose disposal was much inhibited in the trained muscle, giving rise to high intramuscular concentrations of glucose 6-phosphate and free glucose. In fact, during exercise glucose 6-phosphate and glucose are not elevated in trained muscle (346) and have even been reported to be decreased compared to that in untrained individuals (78, 178). Thus, it is unlikely that the exercise-induced increase in membrane glucose transport capacity is higher in trained than in untrained individuals.

We are thus faced with the fact that training increases muscle GLUT4 protein content but decreases glucose utilization during exercise because of decreased glucose transport. Actually, a significant *negative* correlation ($r = -0.89$) between muscle GLUT4 and the rate of isotopically measured whole-body glucose disappearence (Rd) during the final stage of 40 min submaximal bicycle exercise has been reported [Fig. 20.14; (236)]. This indicates that factors other than total muscle GLUT4 content are involved in the regulation of glucose uptake during submaximal voluntary exercise. It also indicates that even if the degree of training covaries with total muscle GLUT4 content, training apparently also decreases the ability of muscle contractions to increase glucose transport be it either by decreased translocation or activation of GLUT4. Any training-induced decrease in glucose transport during exercise is not inherent in the muscles themselves, because the in vitro studies mentioned above showed a positive correlation between muscle GLUT4 content and contraction-induced glucose transport. Rather, the effect of training on glucose uptake during exercise may hypothetically be sought in the neuromuscular activation pattern. Changes could be in the firing frequency or firing pattern of the individual motor neurones. The effect of training is probably not directly due to changed motorneuron recruitment after training, since this would favor recruitment of more oxidative than glycolytic fibers after training, at least if exercising at the same absolute intensity (190), and oxidative fibers have been shown to contain more GLUT4 than glycolytic fibers (19, 137, 166, 207, 238).

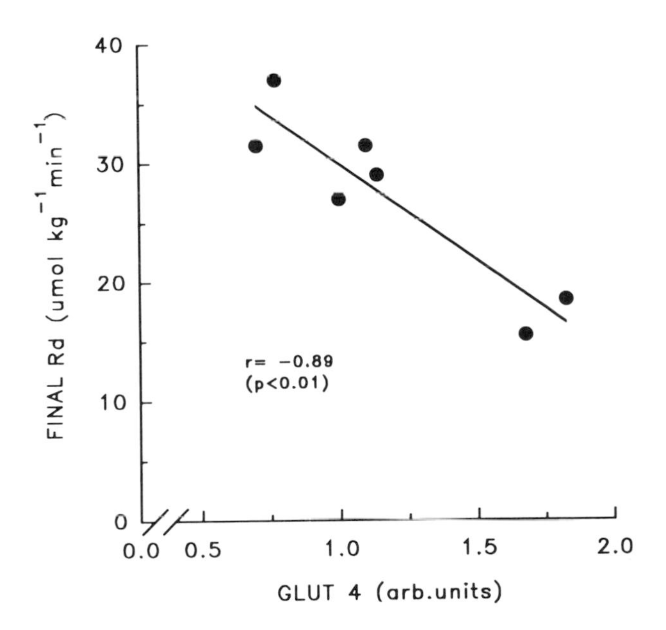

FIG. 20.14. Relationship between GLUT4 concentration in vastus lateralis muscle and whole-body glucose disappearence after 40 min of bicycle exercise at 72% of peak oxygen uptake. $r = -0.89$, $P < 0.01$. [Adapted from McConnell et al. (236), with permission.]

No comparison between muscle GLUT4 content and glucose uptake has been performed during maximal exercise. It is possible that maximal exercise more closely resembles electrical stimulation in vitro; therefore, a positive correlation between GLUT4 and glucose uptake might be revealed during this type of exercise.

The interesting thing is that total GLUT4 protein content in muscle correlates rather closely with insulin-stimulated glucose uptake in humans (11, 99, 209) and rats (19, 155, 238), although in insulin resistant states such as denervation, fat feeding, obesity, or non–insulin-dependent diabetes mellitus this correlation is offset completely (11, 30, 51, 149, 156, 183, 214, 238). These findings therefore confirm the view that insulin and muscle contractions activate glucose transport by at least partially different mechanisms. Furthermore, teleologically it seems that for the endurance trained muscle, increased GLUT4 content is not important for metabolism during exercise but maybe rather *after* exercise, at which time the high GLUT4 concentration makes rapid glucose transport and thereby rapid restoration of glycogen stores possible.

It could be argued that the reduction in glucose utilization during exercise after training might be due to enhanced fat oxidation and operation of the glucose fatty acid cycle. In keeping with such a notion, a significant inverse correlation ($r = -0.85$) between percentage of total energy derived from glucose oxidation during exercise and muscle citrate synthase activity has been described (77). However, direct evidence for this theory is weak. If the theory was true, one would expect to find higher citrate and (via PFK inhibition) also higher glucose 6-phosphate and glucose concentrations in trained compared with nontrained muscle. Although one study found higher muscle citrate concentrations in trained cyclists as opposed to untrained subjects working at the same relative intensity (178), increased muscle glucose 6-phosphate and glucose have never been demonstrated in trained compared with untrained muscle during exercise (78, 178, 346) nor in electrically stimulated rat muscle (80).

Exercise in States of Altered Glucose Utilization

In type I diabetes [insulin-dependent diabetes mellitus (IDDM)], the plasma insulin concentration is not well regulated, as it stems almost exclusively from the subcutaneous injection. Accordingly, in type I diabetes plasma insulin concentrations are mostly either too low or too high, and are seldom appropriate. Since muscle contractions and insulin have synergistic effects on glucose uptake (96, 351, 372), it follows that muscle glucose uptake during exercise in type I diabetes is either inappropriately high, leading to decreases in plasma glucose concentrations, at times even hypoglycemia; or it is inappropriately low, leading to exaggerated hyperglycemia, because in the latter condition secretion of insulin-antagonistic hormones and hepatic glucose production are exaggerated (165, 291). Furthermore, when plasma insulin concentration is high, its inhibiting effect on lipolysis tends to increase the direct insulin effects on muscle glucose metabolism (291). In type I diabetes the muscle GLUT4 protein concentration is normal (183, 205) and so is whole-body glucose turnover during exercise when plasma insulin is normalized by infusion (392).

Type II diabetes, non–insulin-dependent diabetes mellitus (NIDDM), is characterized by insulin resistance as well as by deficient β-cell function (95). Despite the insulin resistance, muscle GLUT4 concentrations are mostly normal in NIDDM (149, 183) except for findings in one study in which severely insulin-resistant subjects were reported to have decreased muscle GLUT4 concentrations (105). During moderate exercise at 60% of maximal oxygen consumption, plasma glucose concentrations decreased in subjects with NIDDM due to a normal increase in peripheral glucose clearance but impaired increase in hepatic glucose production (244). In heavy exercise, peripheral glucose disposal was impaired in patients with NIDDM (200). Direct measurements of glucose uptake over the leg (determined from arterial and femoral venous glucose concentrations and blood flow) during exercise at 60% of maximal oxygen uptake in patients with NIDDM revealed normal glucose uptake at rest. However, the increase with exercise was twice as high in the patients as in healthy controls (234). Blood glucose was higher in patients with NIDDM (~9.5 mM) than in controls (~5.7 mM). Thus, the clearance of glucose during exercise was fairly similar in the two groups. These findings suggest that the metabolic machinery that is activated by muscle contractions and responsible for increasing glucose utilization is normal in patients with NIDDM. This is in agreement with studies in rodent models of insulin resistance. In the insulin-resistant state 3 days after denervation, contraction-induced increase in muscle glucose transport was normal in the plantaris and gastrocnemius muscles but subnormal in the soleus (347). After hindlimb immobilization in the rat for 2 days, resting glucose clearance in the soleus and red gastrocnemius was decreased, but was normal during running (353). Thus, at least in the early stages of denervation and immobilization, insulin resistance is not accompanied by resistance to the effects of contractions. Also, in the obese insulin-resistant Zucker rat, contraction-induced glucose transport and translocation of glucose transporters is similar to nonobese control rats (51, 195). Furthermore, in the running fat-fed insulin-resistant rat glucose uptake in individual muscles was similar to controls (214). Thus, these studies indicate that on the whole, exercise-induced glucose uptake is much less (if at all) affected than insulin-stimulated glucose uptake in a variety of insulin-resistant states. This supports the view that the mechanisms involved in insulin- and contraction-induced glucose uptake are dissimilar.

For further information on exercise in patients with diabetes mellitus or other endocrine diseases the reader is referred to other recent reviews (e.g., 1, 127, 165, 249, 291, 311).

REGULATION OF GLUCOSE UTILIZATION IN THE POSTEXERCISE STATE

In the postexercise period, orally ingested glucose is diverted toward storage in muscle rather than in the liver (226). Thus, after exercise a greater part of an oral glucose load escapes hepatic retention, allowing muscle glycogen to be replenished with a higher priority than liver glycogen.

Membrane Glucose Transport Capacity Induced by Contraction

Compared to rest, muscle membrane glucose transport capacity is increased during contractions due to an increased number and possibly increased activity of GLUT4 in the sarcolemma and probably t tubules as discussed previously (43, 108, 109, 122, 135, 136, 138, 271, 275, 335). Furthermore, muscle blood flow is tremendously increased (151, 185, 201, 307). Moreover, in addition to increasing the non–insulin-stimulated glucose transport, contractions that deplete the muscles of glycogen increase the activity of glycogen synthase (294). This provides a mechanism for diverting the transported glucose into glycogen (294). The question is: For how long a time after cessation of exercise is membrane glucose transport capacity and blood flow increased?

In perfused rat muscle, the effects of muscle contractions on muscle membrane glucose transport capacity wear off according to a monoexponential decay, with markedly different time courses in the different muscle fiber types (273). The half-life of the glucose transport rate increased by contractions was 8 min in the slow-twitch red soleus muscle and 18 min in the fast-twitch red part of the gastrocnemius (273). In fast-twitch white muscle, the rate was much slower but could not be estimated accurately (273). The decay of glucose transport toward basal levels was unrelated to glycogen synthesis because in these particular experiments the perfusate contained no glucose and therefore no net glycogen synthesis occurred (273). In the incubated epitrochlearis muscle, increased glucose transport after in vitro electrical stimulation wears off in 2–2.5 h (145, 386). Since this is a muscle consisting of 10%–20% fast-twitch red and 70%–80% fast-twitch white fibers (363), this rate of decay agrees fairly well with the data obtained in the perfused muscle (273).

The above-mentioned studies (145, 273, 386) show that complete reversal of the increase in glucose transport induced by contractions can occur in vitro in the absence of glycogen resynthesis, in the absence of humoral factors, and also in the absence of protein synthesis (386). In contrast to these findings, however, are findings obtained in rats allowed to recover from exercise in vivo with subsequent measurement of muscle glucose transport in vitro. If rats after exercise are fed a carbohydrate-rich diet, complete reversal of increased glucose transport in the incubated epitrochlearis muscle is observed, whereas when fasted or fed a fat-rich diet, modestly increased glucose transport rates persists for 18 h (61, 387). The reason for the persistent increase in non–insulin-stimulated glucose transport in fast-twitch muscle from rats in which carbohydrate availability is low during recovery is not known and sharply contrasts with the complete reversal of contraction-induced glucose transport in vitro in the absence of glucose. It is not known whether recovery from exercise in the carbohydrate-deprived state also can inhibit complete reversal of contraction-induced increase in glucose transport in slow-twitch muscle.

At the termination of high-intensity muscle contractions, muscle blood flow decreases rapidly (18, 96, 151) and reaches preexercise values after 15–45 min of recovery, depending on the workload (18). Thus, glucose supply is diminishing rapidly after exercise, and this is expected to contribute to the rapid decrease in muscle glucose uptake after exercise (96, 151, 214, 390).

Insulin Sensitivity

In addition to increasing non–insulin-stimulated glucose transport, contractions also increase insulin sensitivity. Thus, as originally shown in the perfused rat hindquarter [Fig. 20.15; (293)], exercise in vivo shifts the dose–response curve for glucose uptake vs. insulin concentration to the left and thereby causes a decrease in the concentration of insulin that half-maximally stimulates glucose uptake. Subsequent experiments have shown that the increase in insulin sensitivity after exercise includes the glucose transport step (61, 293, 294, 364) as well as glycogen synthesis (216, 293, 294) and amino acid transport (393, 395). An increase in insulin sensitivity has also

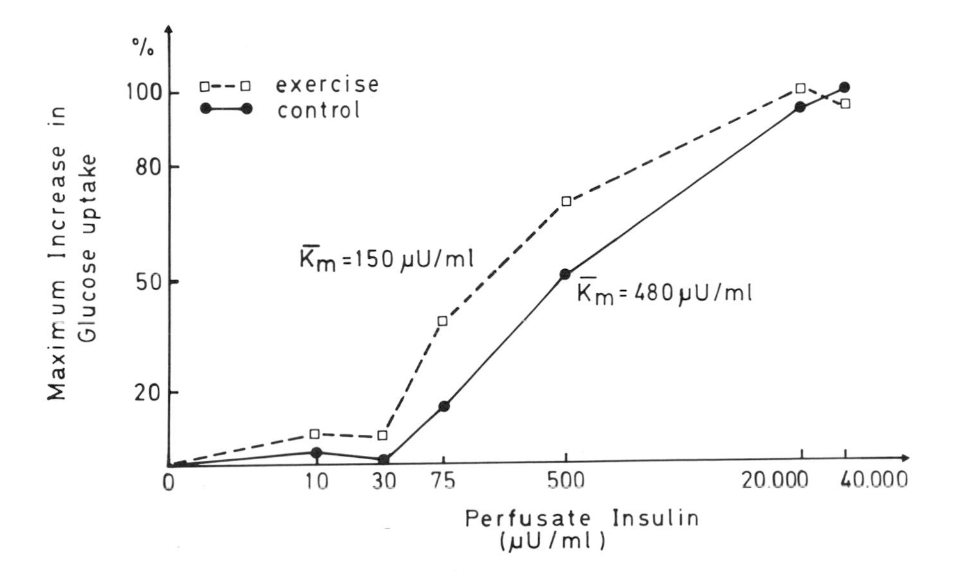

FIG. 20.15. Dose–response curve for insulin-stimulated glucose uptake in perfused rat hindquarters. Rats were either rested or exercised on a treadmill for 45 min before perfusion. [Adapted from Richter et al. (293), with permission.]

been demonstrated after exercise in humans (32, 102, 241, 299). The effect of a single exercise bout on whole-body glucose uptake persists for 48 h but has disappeared after 5 days in humans (241). However, recent studies determining leg glucose uptake (a better indicator of *muscle* uptake) in response to insulin found no effect of exercise on insulin action 16 h after exercise (100). In the fed rat the effect of a single bout of exercise was present 4 h but not 24 h after treadmill running (293). The duration of the increased sensitivity to insulin seems to depend on carbohydrate availability, at least in the rat. Thus, in the incubated epitrochlearis muscle, increased insulin sensitivity was not found 18 h after swimming when the rats were fed carbohydrate, whereas it persisted for at least 48 h in carbohydrate-deprived rats (61). Furthermore, reversal of increased insulin sensitivity depends on glucose uptake and metabolism and cannot be reproduced by a large uptake of 2-deoxyglucose that is transported by GLUT4 but not metabolized (145). Thus, some aspect of glucose metabolism seems to terminate the exercise-induced state of increased insulin sensitivity. This step has not been identified, but in adipocytes, perfused and incubated muscle, exposure to high glucose concentrations and insulin induces a state of insulin resistance (233, 295, 296, 305) due to the production of glucosamine from glucose (233, 305). Of the total glucose transported into the cell, a few percent are channeled into production of glucosamine, a substance that decreases insulin action, possibly by interfering with GLUT4 translocation (233). Thus, a bout of exercise might increase insulin sensitivity by decreasing glucosamine production from the transported glucose due to its preferential channeling into the glycogen synthesis pathway. If true, then as glycogen depots are repleted, glycogen synthesis rate would decrease and a larger fraction of the transported glucose would be diverted through the glucosamine pathway and thereby decrease insulin sensitivity at the glucose transport step.

Studies in the incubated epitrochlearis muscle have indicated that increased sensitivity to insulin does not develop when incubated muscle is stimulated directly to contractions in vitro (63) in contrast to when exercise or electrical stimulation are carried out in vivo (61, 128, 129, 145, 293, 294, 364, 387). It was also reported that a serum protein was responsible for the induction of increased insulin sensitivity by contractions (128). These findings are in contrast to a study in the perfused rat hindquarter in which electrical stimulation of the muscles via the sciatic nerve during perfusion increased insulin sensitivity determined after contractions (300). Together, these findings suggest that a neurotrophic factor (probably a protein) released from the motor nerve during stimulation may be necessary for the development of increased sensitivity of muscle to insulin. If correct, this mechanism does not necessarily exclude that the above described glucosamine hypothesis is valid too.

As to the mechanism involved in increased insulin sensitivity after exercise, considerable attention has been focused on insulin receptor binding. Hypothetically, the affinity of the insulin receptor toward insulin could be increased by exercise. Investigations aimed at resolving this question have yielded considerably divergent results, with reports of increased (375), unchanged (39, 344, 393) or decreased (38) insulin binding to skeletal muscle after exercise. These discrepancies probably reflect both the considerable technical difficulties in determining insulin binding to intact skeletal muscle and the probability that there is no effect of exercise on insulin binding. Furthermore, some have suggested that exercise also does not increase insulin receptor tyrosine kinase activity in muscle (344), but it is questionable whether conditions for isolating the insulin receptor preserved the full in vivo phosphorylation status. In agreement with the notion that increased insulin sensitivity after exercise is due to amplification of a postreceptor step, exercise in vivo increased the response of the epitrochlearis muscle to insulin mimetic agents such as vanadate and hydrogen peroxide (63), substances known to affect postreceptor steps in the insulin-signaling mechanism (142, 208). Interestingly, exercise was also shown to amplify the action of a submaximal hypoxic stimulus on glucose transport (63), suggesting that the exercise effect is not limited to the insulin-sensitive pathway but also affects the contraction-sensitive pathway, since hypoxia and contractions seem to activate the same signaling pathway (62). However, it has not yet been demonstrated that an exercise bout increases the effect of a second exercise bout on muscle glucose transport.

The maximal effect of insulin (insulin responsiveness) may also be increased by exercise in the rat (61, 293, 300, 394) but seems to be a more short-lived phenomenon (61) than the increase in sensitivity because it seems to require glycogen-depleted muscles (61, 394). In humans, an increase in insulin responsiveness after exercise has not been convincingly shown (44, 100, 198), since the one study claiming an effect in fact used a submaximal insulin concentration (241).

The concept of increased sensitivity to insulin after exercise does not always hold true but depends on the type of exercise performed and the time after termination of exercise. Thus, when exercise is intense, large elevations in plasma concentrations of catecholamines and maybe FFA as well may decrease insulin action in the immediate postexercise period (199, 200, 379). However, when these changes wear off, increased insulin action can in fact be demonstrated (200). In agreement with this interpretation, insulin sensitivity in nonexercised muscle actually seems to be decreased early after exercise with other muscle groups (101). This is possibly due to the altered hormonal and metabolic milieu after exercise, especially if no carbohydrate is taken (101).

Another factor relates to whether concentric or eccentric exercise is performed. In contrast to concentric exercise, a bout of eccentric exercise (downhill running) decreased *whole-body* glucose uptake during a euglycemic hyperinsulinemic clamp procedure (198), although a recent hyperglycemic clamp study found no effect of eccentric exercise on whole-body insulin action (194). However, after eccentric exercise which induces muscle damage (119, 253), glycogen repletion is impaired (86, 107, 260, 377). A possible explanation for this phenomenon might be that eccentric exercise induces a state of insulin resistance that is responsible for the impaired postexercise glycogen repletion. In accordance with such a view, it was recently reported in man that eccentric exercise causes a transient decrease in muscle GLUT4 protein content of 30%–35% [Fig. 20.16; (13)] and that this decrease coincides with low muscle glycogen concentrations (13). In rats, eccentric contractions also caused a transient decrease in muscle GLUT4 protein content (14). This decrease was fiber type specific such that the decrease was largest in the fast-twitch white fibers, smaller in the fast-twitch red fibers and absent in the slow-twitch red fibers (14). Preliminary data indicate that the 30%–35% reduction in muscle GLUT4 protein in man 2 days after eccentric exercise causes decreased maximally insulin stimulated glucose uptake but unaltered submaximally stimulated glucose uptake in muscle (S. Asp, J. Daŭgaard, S. Kristiansen, B. Kiens, and E. A. Richter, unpublished observations).

When the decrease in muscle GLUT 4 protein is more pronounced (~60% in the fast-twitch white fibers of rats) both submaximally and maximally insulin stimulated glucose transport is decreased (S. Asp and E. A. Richter, unpublished observations). Together these data suggest that submaximally insulin stimulated glucose transport is decreased only when muscle GLUT4 is markedly decreased (>35%) which in turn suggests that decreased insulin–stimulated glucose transport may not be the most important factor in the sustained decrease in muscle glycogen after eccentric exercise. Thus, attention also has to be directed toward possible activation of the glycogen degrading pathway after eccentric exercise.

The author is supported by the Danish Natural Sciences Research Council grant 11-0082, the Danish Medical Research Council grant 12-9535, the Novo-Nordisk Research Foundation, and the Danish National Research Foundation grant 504-14. Erika Nielsen is thanked for computerizing the references, and Bente Kiens and Peter Hespel are thanked for constructive criticism and inspiration throughout.

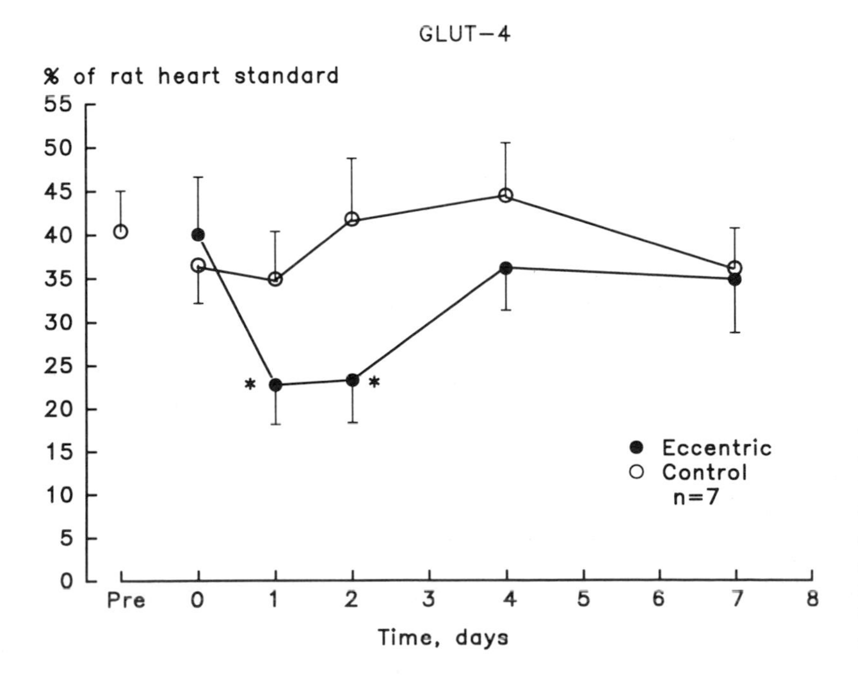

FIG. 20.16. Concentration of GLUT4 protein in eccentrically exercised and in the nonexercised control vastus lateralis muscle immediately after exercise and 1, 2, 4, and 7 days later. Before exercise, GLUT4 was only measured in the control leg. Values are means ±SE of seven observations and are expressed as concentration relative to a rat heart standard.* $P < 0.05$ compared to contralateral control leg. [Reproduced from Asp et al. (13), with permission.]

REFERENCES

1. Anonymous. *Diabetes Mellitus and Exercise*, edited by J. T. Devlin, E. S. Horton, and M. Vranic. London: Smith-Gordon, 1992, p. 1–258.
2. Acevedo-Duncan, M., D. Cooper, M. Standaert, and R. Farese. Immunological evidence that insulin activates protein kinase C in BC3H-1 myocytes. *FEBS Lett.* 244: 174–176, 1989.
3. Ahlborg, G. Mechanism for glycogenolysis in nonexercising human muscle during and after exercise. *Am. J. Physiol.* 248 (*Endocrinol. Metab.* 11): E540–E545, 1985.
4. Ahlborg, G., and P. Felig. Lactate and glucose exchange across the forearm, legs and splanchnic bed during and after prolonged leg exercise. *J. Clin. Invest.* 69: 45–54, 1982.
5. Ahlborg, G., P. Felig, L. Hagenfeldt, R. Hendler, and J. Wahren. Substrate turnover during prolonged exercise in man. Splanchinc and leg metabolism of glucose, free fatty acids and amino acids. *J. Clin. Invest.* 53: 1080–1090, 1974.
6. Ahlborg, G., L. Hagenfeldt, and J. Wahren. Substrate utilization by the inactive leg during one-leg or arm exercise. *J. Appl. Physiol.* 39: 718–723, 1975.
7. Ahlborg, G., and M. Jensen-Urstad. Metabolism in exercising arm vs. leg muscle. *Clin. Physiol.* 11: 459–468, 1991.
8. Ahlborg, G., J. Wahren, and P. Felig. Splanchnic and peripheral glucose and lactate metabolism during and after prolonged arm exercise. *J. Clin. Invest.* 77: 690–699, 1986.
9. Andersen, P., and B. Saltin. Maximal perfusion of skeletal muscle in man. *J. Physiol. (Lond.)* 366: 233–249, 1985.
10. Andersen, P. H., S. Lund, O. Schmitz, S. Junker, B. B. Kahn, and O. Pedersen. Increased insulin-stimulated glucose uptake in athletes: the importance of GLUT 4 mRNA, GLUT 4 protein and fibre type composition of skeletal muscle. *Acta Physiol. Scand.* 149: 393–404, 1993.
11. Andersen, P. H., S. Lund, H. Vestergaard, S. Junker, B. B. Kahn, and O. Pedersen. Expression of the major insulin regulatable glucose transporter (GLUT4) in skeletal muscle of noninsulin-dependent diabetic patients and healthy subjects before and after insulin infusion. *J. Clin. Endocrinol. Metab.* 77: 27–32, 1993.
12. Asmussen, E. Positive and negative muscular work. *Acta Physiol. Scand.* 28: 364–382, 1952.
13. Asp, S., J. R. Daùgaard, and E. A. Richter. Eccentric exercise decreases GLUT4 protein in human skeletal muscle. *J. Physiol. (Lond.)* 482: 705–712, 1995.
14. Asp S., S. Kristiansen, and E. A. Richter. Eccentric muscle damage transiently decreases rat skeletal muscle GLUT4 protein. *J. Appl. Physiol.* 79: 1338–1345, 1995.
15. Balch, W. E. Small GTP-binding proteins in vesicular transport. *Trends Biochem. Sci.* 15: 473–477, 1990.
16. Baldini, G., T. Hohl, H. Y. Lin, and H. F. Lodish. Cloning of a Rab3 isotype predominately expressed in adipocytes. *Proc. Natl. Acad. Sci. U. S. A.* 89: 5049–5052, 1992.
17. Baldini, G., R. Hohman, M. J. Charron, and H. F. Lodish. Insulin and nonhydrolyzable GTP analogs induce translocation of GLUT 4 to the plasma membrane in alpha-toxin-permeabilized rat adipose cells. *J. Biol. Chem.* 266: 4037–4040, 1991.
18. Bangsbo, J., P. Gollnick, T. Graham, C. Juel, B. Kiens, M. Mizuno, and B. Saltin. Anaerobic energy production and O2 deficit-debt relationship during exhaustive exercise in humans. *J. Physiol. (Lond.)* 422: 539–559, 1990.
19. Banks, E. A., J. T. Brozinick, Jr., B. B. Yaspelkis, III, H. Y. Kang, and J. L. Ivy. Muscle glucose transport, GLUT-4 content and degree of exercise training in obese Zucker rats. *Am. J. Physiol.* 263 (*Endocrinol. Metab.* 26): E1010–E1015, 1992.
20. Barnett, J. E. G., G. D. Holman, R. A. Chalkley, and K. A. Munday. Evidence for two asymmetric conformational states in the human erythrocyte sugar-transport system. *Biochem. J.* 145: 417–426, 1975.
21. Begum, N., W. Leitner, J. E.-B. Reusch, K. E. Sussman, and B. Draznin. GLUT-4 phosphorylation and its intrinsic activity. *J. Biol. Chem.* 268: 3352–3356, 1993.
22. Bell, G., T. Kayano, J. Buse, C. Burant, J. Takeda, D. Lin, H. Fukumoto, and S. Seino. Molecular biology of mammalian glucose transporters. *Diabetes Care* 13: 198–208, 1990.
23. Bell, G. I., C. F. Burant, J. Takeda, and G. W. Gould. Structure and function of mammalian facilitative sugar transporters. *J. Biol. Chem.* 268: 19161–19164, 1993.
24. Berger, M., S. Hagg, M. Goodman, and N. Ruderman. Glucose metabolism in perfused skeletal muscle. *Biochem. J.* 158: 191–202, 1976.
25. Bergström, J., E. Hultman, L. Jorfeldt, B. Pernow, and J. Wahren. Effect of nicotinic acid on physical working capacity and on metabolism of muscle glycogen in man. *J. Appl. Physiol.* 26: 170–176, 1969.
26. Bihler, I., P. Sawh, and I. Sloan. Dual effect of adrenalin on sugar transport in rat diaphragm muscle. *Biochim. Biophys. Acta* 510: 349–360, 1978.
27. Birnbaum, M. The insulin-sensitive glucose transporter. *Int. Rev. Cytol.* 137A: 239–297, 1992.
28. Björkman, O., P. Milles, D. Wasserman, L. Lickley, and M. Vranic. Regulation of glucose turnover during exercise in pancreatectomized, totally insulin-deficient dogs. *J. Clin. Invest.* 81: 1759–1767, 1988.
29. Björkman, O., K. Sahlin, L. Hagenfeldt, and J. Wahren. Influence of glucose and fructose ingestion on the capacity for long-term exercise in well-trained men. *Clin. Physiol.* 4: 483–494, 1984.
30. Block, N. E., D. R. Menick, K. A. Robinson, and M. G. Buse. Effect of denervation on the expression of two glucose transporter isoforms in rat hindlimb muscle. *J. Clin. Invest.* 88: 1546–1552, 1991.
31. Boden, G., F. Jadali, J. White, Y. Liang, M. Mozzoli, X. Chen, E. Coleman, and C. Smith. Effects of fat on insulin-stimulated carbohydrate metabolism in normal men. *J. Clin. Invest.* 88: 960–966, 1991.
32. Bogardus, C., P. Thuillez, E. Ravussin, B. Vasquez, M. Narimiga, and S. Azhar. Effect of muscle glycogen depletion on in vivo insulin action in man. *J. Clin. Invest.* 72: 1605–1610, 1983.
33. Bonadonna, R., K. Zych, C. Boni, E. Ferrannini, and R. DeFronzo. Time dependence of the interaction between lipid and glucose in humans. *Am. J. Physiol.* 257 (*Endocrinol. Metab.* 20): E49–E56, 1989.
34. Bonadonna, R. C., M. P. Saccomani, L. Seely, K. S. Zych, E. Ferrannini, C. Cobelli, and R. A. DeFronzo. Glucose transport in human skeletal muscle. *Diabetes* 42: 191–198, 1993.
35. Bonen, A., P. A. Clune, and M. H. Tan. Chronic exercise increases insulin binding in muscles but not liver. *Am. J. Physiol.* 251 (*Endocrinol. Metab.* 14): E196–E203, 1986.
36. Bonen, A., G. C. Elder, and M. Tan. Hindlimb suspension increases insulin binding and glucose metabolism. *J. Appl. Physiol.* 65: 1833–1839, 1988.
37. Bonen, A., L. A. Megeney, S. C. McCarthy, J. C. McDermott, and M. H. Tan. Epinephrine administration stimulates GLUT 4 translocation but reduces glucose transport

in muscle. *Biochem. Biophys. Res. Commun.* 187: 685–691, 1992.

38. Bonen, A., M. Tan, P. Clune, and R. Kirby. Effects of exercise on insulin binding to human muscle. *Am. J. Physiol.* 248 (*Endocrinol. Metab.* 11): E403–E408, 1985.
39. Bonen, A., M. Tan, and W. Watson-Wright. Effects of exercise on insulin binding and glucose metabolism in muscle. *Can. J. Physiol. Pharmacol.* 62: 1500–1504, 1984.
40. Borkman, M., L. V. Campbell, D. J. Chisholm and L. H. Storlien. Comparison of the effects on insulin sensitivity of a high carbohydrate and high fat diets in normal subjects. *J. Clin. Endocrinol. Metab.* 28: 731–736, 1991.
41. Borkman, M., D. Chisholm, S. Furler, L. Storlien, E. Kraegen, L. Simons, and C. Chesterman. Effects of fish oil supplementation on glucose and lipid metabolism in NIDDM. *Diabetes* 38: 1314–1319, 1989.
42. Borkman, M., L. H. Storlien, D. A. Pan, A. B. Jenkins, D. J. Chisholm, and L. V. Campbell. The relation between insulin sensitivity and the fatty-acid composition of skeletal-muscle phospholipids. *N. Engl. J. Med.* 328: 238–244, 1993.
43. Bornemann, A., T. Ploug, and H. Schmalbruch. Subcellular localization of GLUT4 in nonstimulated and insulin-stimulated soleus muscle of the rat. *Diabetes* 41: 215–221, 1992.
44. Bourey, R. E., A. R. Coggan, W. M. Kohrt, J. P. Kirwan, D. S. King, and J. O. Holloszy. Effect of exercise on glucose disposal: response to a maximal insulin stimulus. *J. Appl. Physiol.* 69: 1689–1694, 1990.
45. Brand, S. H., and J. D. Castle. Scamp-37, a new marker within the general cell-surface recycling system. *EMBO J.* 12: 3753–3761, 1993.
46. Broberg, S., A. Katz, and K. Sahlin. Propranolol enhances adenine nucleotide degradation in human muscle during exercise. *J. Appl. Physiol.* 65: 2478–2483, 1988.
47. Broberg, S., and K. Sahlin. Hyperammoniemia during prolonged exercise: an effect of glycogen depletion? *J. Appl. Physiol.* 65: 2475–2477, 1988.
48. Brooks, G., and C. Donovan. Effect of endurance training on glucose kinetics during exercise. *Am. J. Physiol.* 244 (*Endocrinol. Metab.* 7): E505–E512, 1983.
49. Brooks, G. A., G. E. Butterfield, R. R. Wolfe, B. M. Groves, R. S. Mazzeo, J. R. Sutton, E. E. Wolfel, and J. T. Reeves. Increased dependence on blood glucose after acclimatization to 4,300 m. *J. Appl. Physiol.* 70: 919–927, 1991.
50. Brooks, G. A., E. E. Wolfel, B. M. Groves, P. R. Bender, G. E. Butterfield, A. Cymerman, R. S. Mazzeo, J. R. Sutton, R. R. Wolfe, and J. T. Reeves. Muscle accounts for glucose disposal but not blood lactate appearance during exercise after acclimatization to 4,300 m. *J. Appl. Physiol.* 72: 2435–2445, 1992.
51. Brozinick, J. T. J., G. J. J. Etgen, B. B. Yaspelkis, III, and J. L. Ivy. Contraction-activated glucose uptake is normal in insulin-resistant muscle of the obese Zucker rat. *J. Appl. Physiol.* 73: 382–387, 1992.
52. Burant, C., S. Lemmon, M. Treutelaar, and M. Buse. Insulin resistance of denervated rat muscle: a model for impaired receptor-function coupling. *Am. J. Physiol.* 247 (*Endocrinol. Metab.* 10): E657–E666, 1984.
53. Burant, C. F., J. Takeda, E. Brot-Laroche, I. Graeme, B. Davidson, and N. O. Davidson. Fructose transporter in human spermatozoa and small intestine is GLUT5. *J. Biol. Chem.* 267: 14523–14526, 1992.
54. Burant, C. F., M. K. Treutelaar, and M. G. Buse. In vitro and in vivo activation of the insulin receptor kinase in control and denervated skeletal muscle. *J. Biol. Chem.* 261: 8985–8993, 1986.
55. Burdett, E., T. Beeler, and A. Klip. Distribution of glucose transporters and insulin receptors in the plasma membrane and transverse tubules of skeletal muscle. *Arch. Biochem. Biophys.* 253: 279–286, 1987.
56. Burstein, E. S., W. H. Brondyk, I. G. Macara, and Y. Takai. Regulation of the GTPase cycle of the neuronally expressed ras-like GTP-binding protein rab3a. *J. Biol. Chem.* 268: 22247–22250, 1993.
57. Burstein, E. S., and I. G. Macara. Characterization of a guanine nucleotide-releasing factor and a GTPase-activating protein that are specific for the ras-related protein p25 super(rab3A). *Proc. Natl. Acad. Sci. U. S. A.* 89: 1154–1158, 1992.
58. Cain, C. C., W. S. Trimble, and G. E. Lienhard. Members of the VAMP family of synaptic vesicle proteins are components of glucose transporter-containing vesicles from rat adipocytes. *J. Biol. Chem.* 267: 11681–11684, 1992.
59. Calles, J., J. Cunningham, L. Nelson, N. Brown, and E. Nadel. Glucose turnover during recovery from intensive exercise. *Diabetes* 32: 734–738, 1983.
60. Carruthers, A., and A. Helgerson. The human erythrocyte sugar transporter is also a nucleotide binding protein. *Biochemistry* 28: 8337–8346, 1989.
61. Cartee, G., D. Young, M. Sleeper, J. Zierath, H. Wallberg-Henriksson, and J. Holloszy. Prolonged increase in insulin-stimulated glucose transport in muscle after exercise. *Am. J. Physiol.* 256 (*Endocrinol. Metab.* 19): E494–E499, 1989.
62. Cartee, G. D., A. G. Douen, T. Ramlal, A. Klip, and J. O. Holloszy. Stimulation of glucose transport in skeletal muscle by hypoxia. *J. Appl. Physiol.* 70: 1593–1600, 1991.
63. Cartee, G. D., and J. O. Holloszy. Exercise increases susceptibility of muscle glucose transport to activation by various stimuli. *Am. J. Physiol.* 258 (*Endocrinol. Metab.* 21): E390–E393, 1990.
64. Castillo, C., C. Bogardus, R. Bergman, P. Thuillez, and S. Lillioja. Interstitial insulin concentrations determine glucose uptake rates but not insulin resistance in lean and obese men. *J. Clin. Invest.* 93: 10–16, 1994.
65. Chauveau, M. A., and M. Kaufmann. Experiences pour la determination du coefficient de l'activite nutritive et respiratoire des muscles en repos et en travail. *C. R. Acad. Sci.* 104: 1126–1132, 1887.
66. Cheatham, B., and C. R. Kahn. Insulin action and the insulin signaling network. *Endocr. Rev.* 16: 117–142, 1995.
67. Chen, J., and P. D. Gollnick. Effect of exercise on hexokinase distribution and mitochondrial respiration in skeletal muscle. *Pflugers Arch.* 427: 257–263, 1994.
68. Chen, K. S., J. C. Friel, and N. B. Ruderman. Regulation of phosphatidylinositol 3-kinase by insulin in rat skeletal muscle. *Am. J. Physiol.* 265 (*Endocrinol. Metab.* 28): E736–E742, 1993.
69. Cherqui, G., M. Caron, D. Wicek, O. Lascols, J. Capeau, and J. Picard. Insulin stimulation of glucose metabolism in rat adipocytes: possible implication of protein kinase C. *Endocrinology* 118: 1759–1769, 1986.
70. Chiasson, J.-L., H. Shikama, D. T. W. Chu, and J. H. Exton. Inhibitory effect of epinephrine on insulin-stimulated glucose uptake by rat skeletal muscle. *J. Clin. Invest.* 68: 706–713, 1981.
71. Christensen, R., D. Shade, C. Graves, and J. McDonald. Evidence that protein kinase c is involved in regulating glucose transport in the adipocyte. *Int. J. Biochem.* 19: 259–265, 1987.

72. Clausen, T. The role of calcium in the activation of the glucose transport system. *Cell Calcium* 1: 311–325, 1980.
73. Clausen, T., J. Elbrink, and A. B. Dahl-Hansen. The relationship between the transport of glucose and cations across cell membranes in isolated tissues. IX. The role of cellular calcium in the activation of the glucose transport system in rat soleus muscle. *Biochem. Biophys. Acta* 375: 2392–2408, 1975.
74. Cleland, P. J., K. Abel, S. Rattigan, and M. Clark. Long-term treatment of isolated rat soleus muscle with phorbol ester leads to loss of contraction-induced glucose transport. *Biochem. J.* 267: 659–663, 1990.
75. Cleland, P. J., G. Appleby, S. Rattigan, and M. Clark. Exercise-induced translocation of protein kinase C and production of diacylglycerol and phosphatidic acid in rat skeletal muscle in vivo. *J. Biol. Chem.* 264: 17704–17711, 1989.
76. Coggan, A., W. Kohrt, R. Spina, D. Bier, and J. Holloszy. Endurance training decreases plasma glucose turnover and oxidation during moderate-intensity exercise in men. *J. Appl. Physiol.* 68: 990–996, 1990.
77. Coggan, A. R., W. M. Kohrt, R. J. Spina, J. P. Kirwan, D. M. Bier, and J. O. Holloszy. Plasma glucose kinetics during exercise in subjects with high and low lactate thresholds. *J. Appl. Physiol.* 73: 1873–1880, 1992.
78. Coggan, A. R., R. J. Spina, W. M. Kohrt, and J. O. Holloszy. Effect of prolonged exercise on muscle citrate concentration before and after endurance training in men. *Am. J. Physiol.* 264 (*Endocrinol. Metab.* 27): E215–E220, 1993.
79. Constable, S., R. Favier, G. Cartee, D. Joung, and J. Holloszy. Muscle glucose transport: interactions of in vitro contractions, insulin and exercise. *J. Appl. Physiol.* 64: 2329–2332, 1988.
80. Constable, S., R. Favier, J. McLane, R. Fell, M. Chen, and J. Holloszy. Energy metabolism in contracting rat skeletal muscle: adaption to exercise training. *Am. J. Physiol.* 251 (*Cell Physiol.* 22): C3l6–C322, 1987.
81. Cooper, D., T. Konda, M. Standaert, J. Davis, R. Pollet, and R. Farese. Insulin increases membrane and cytosolic protein kinase c activity in BC3H-1 myocytes. *J. Biol. Chem.* 262: 3633–3639, 1987.
82. Cooper, D. M., D. H. Wasserman, M. Vranic, and K. Wasserman. Glucose turnover in response to exercise during high- and low-FIO2 breathing in man. *Am. J. Physiol.* 251 (*Endocrinol. Metab.* 14): E209–E214, 1986.
83. Cooper, D. R., J. E. Watson, H. Hemandez, B. Yu, M. L. Standaert, D. K. Ways, T. T. Arnold, T. Ishizuka, and R. Farese. Direct evidence for protein kinase c involement in insulin-stimulated hexose uptake. *Biochem. Biophys. Res. Commun.* 188: 142–148, 1992.
84. Cormont, M., J.-F. Tanti, A. Zahraoui, E. Van Obberghen, A. Tavitian, and Y. Le Marchand-Brustel. Insulin and okadaic acid induce Rab4 redistribution in adipocytes. *J. Biol. Chem.* 268: 19491–19497, 1993.
85. Costill, D. L., E. Coyle, G. Dalsky, W. Evans, W. Fink, and D. Hoopes. Effects of elevated plasma FFA and insulin on muscle glycogen usage during exercise. *J. Appl. Physiol.* 43: 695–699, 1977.
86. Costill, D. L., D. D. Pascoe, J. Fink, R. A. Robergs, S. I. Barr, and D. Pearson. Impaired muscle glycogen resynthesis after eccentric exercise. *J. Appl. Physiol.* 69: 46–50, 1990.
87. Coyle, E., A. Coggan, M. Hemmert, and J. Ivy. Muscle glycogen utilization during prolonged strenuous exercise when fed carbohydrate. *J. Appl. Physiol.* 61: 165–172, 1986.
88. Coyle, E. F., M. T. Hamilton, J. G. Alonso, S. J. Montain, and J. L. Ivy. Carbohydrate metabolism during intense exercise when hyperglycemic. *J. Appl. Physiol.* 70: 834–840, 1991.
89. Crone, C., and D. G. Levitt. Capillary permeability to small solutes. In: *Handbook of Physiology, Cardiovascular System, Microcirculation*, edited by E. M. Renkin and C. C. Michel. Bethesda, MD: Am. Physiol. Soc., 1984, p. 411–466.
90. Cushman, S. W., and L. J. Wardzala. Potential mechanism of insulin action on glucose transport in the isolated rat adipose cell. *J. Biol. Chem.* 255: 4758–4762, 1980.
91. Czech, M. P., and J. M. Buxton. Insulin action on the internalization of the GLUT4 glucose transporter in isolated rat adipocytes. *J. Biol. Chem.* 268: 9187–9190, 1993.
92. Dagenais, G., R. Tancredi, and K. Zierler. Free fatty acid oxidation by forearm muscle at rest and evidence for an intramuscular lipid pool in the human forearm. *J. Clin. Invest.* 58: 421–431, 1976.
93. De-Camilli, P., and R. Jahn. Pathways to regulated exocytosis in neurons. *Ann. Rev. Physiol.* 52: 625–645, 1990.
94. DeFeo, P., G. Perriello, E. Torlone, M. Ventura, and F. Santeusanio. Demonstration of a role for growth hormone in glucose counterregulation. *Am. J. Physiol.* 256 (*Endocrinol. Metab.* 19): E835–E843, 1989.
95. DeFronzo, R. The triumvirate: β-cell, muscle, liver. A collusion responsible for NIDDM. *Diabetes* 37: 667–687, 1988.
96. DeFronzo, R., E. Ferrannini, Y. Sato, P. Felig, and J. Wahren. Synergistic interaction between exercise and insulin on peripheral glucose uptake. *J. Clin. Invest.* 68: 1468–1474, 1981.
97. DeFronzo, R., R. Gunnarsson, O. Björkman, M. Olsson, and J. Wahren. Effects of insulin on peripheral and splanchnic glucose metabolism in noninsulin-dependent (type II) diabetes mellitus. *J. Clin. Invest.* 76: 149–155, 1985
98. Deibert, D. C., and R. A. DeFronzo. Epinephrine-induced insulin resistance in man. *J. Clin. Invest.* 65: 717–721, 1980.
99. Dela, F., A. Handberg, K. J. Mikines, J. Vinten, and H. Galbo. GLUT 4 and insulin receptor binding and kinase activity in trained human muscle. *J. Physiol. (Lond.)* 469: 615–624, 1993.
100. Dela, F., K. J. Mikines, M. von Linstow, N. H. Secher, and H. Galbo. Effect of training on insulin-mediated glucose uptake in human muscle. *Am. J. Physiol.* 263 (*Endocrinol. Metab.* 26): E1134–E1143, 1992.
101. Devlin, J., J. Barlow, and E. Horton. Whole body and regional fuel metabolism during early postexercise recovery. *Am. J. Physiol.* 256 (*Endocrinol. Metab.* 19): E167–E172, 1989.
102. Devlin, J., M. Hirshman, and E. Horton. Enhanced peripheral and splanchnic insulin sensitivity in NIDDM men after single bout of exercise. *Diabetes* 36: 434–439, 1987.
103. Dohm, G., M. Sinha, and J. Caro. Insulin receptor binding and protein kinase activity in muscles of trained rats. *Am. J. Physiol.* 252 (*Endocrinol. Metab.* 15): E170–E175, 1987.
104. Dohm, G. L., P. L. Dolan, W. R. Frisell, and R. W. Dudek. Role of transverse tubules in insulin stimulated muscle glucose transport. *J. Cell. Biochem.* 52: 1–7, 1993.
105. Dohm, G. L., C. W. Elton, J. E. Friedman, P. F. Pilch, W. J. Pories, S. M. J. Atkinson, and J. F. Caro. Decreased expression of glucose transporter in muscle from insulin-resistant patients. *Am. J. Physiol.* 260 (*Endocrinol. Metab.* 23): E459–E463, 1991.

106. Donovan, C., and K. Sumida. Training improves glucose homeostasis in rats during exercise via glucose production. *Am. J. Physiol.* 258 (*Regulatory Integrative Comp. Physiol.* 27): R770–R776, 1990.
107. Douen, A., T. Ramlal, G. Cartee, and A. Klip. Exercise modulates the insulin-induced translocation of glucose transporters in rat skeletal muscle. *FEBS Lett.* 261: 256–260, 1990.
108. Douen, A., T. Ramlal, A. Klip, D. Young, G. Cartee, and J. Holloszy. Exercise-induced increase in glucose transporters in plasma membranes of rat skeletal muscle. *Endocrinology* 124: 449–454, 1989.
109. Douen, A., T. Ramlal, S. Rastogi, P. Bilan, G. Cartee, M. Vranic, J. Holloszy, and A. Klip. Exercise induces recruitment of the "insulin-responsive glucose transporter." *J. Biol. Chem.* 265: 13427–13430, 1990.
110. Doyle, J. A., W. M. Sherman, and R. L. Strauss. Effects of eccentric and concentric exercise on muscle glycogen replenishment. *J. Appl. Physiol.* 74: 1848–1855, 1993.
111. Dudek, R. W., G. L. Dohm, G. D. Holman, S. W. Cushman, and C. M. Wilson. Glucose transporter localization in rat skeletal muscle. Auto-radiographic study using ATB-(2–3H)BMPA photolabel. *FEBS Lett.* 339: 205–208, 1994.
112. Dyck, D. J., C. T. Putman, G. J. F. Heigenhauser, E. Hultman, and L. L. Spriet. Regulation of fat-carbohydrate interaction in skeletal muscle during intense aerobic cycling. *Am. J. Physiol.* 265 (*Endocrinol. Metab.* 28): E852–E859, 1993.
113. Dyck, D. J., and L. L. Spriet. Elevated muscle citrate does not reduce carbohydrate utilization during tetanic stimulation. *Can. J. Physiol. Pharmacol.* 72: 117–125, 1994.
114. Ebeling, P., R. Bourey, L. Koranyi, J. A. Tuominen, L. C. Groop, J. Henriksson, M. Mueckler, A. Sovijärvi, and V. A. Koivisto. Mechanism of enhanced insulin sensitivity in athletes. *J. Clin. Invest.* 92: 1623–1631, 1993.
115. Etgen, G. J. J., J. T. J. Brozinick, H. Y. Kang, and J. L. Ivy. Effects of exercise training on skeletal muscle glucose uptake and transport. *Am. J. Physiol.* 264 (*Cell Physiol.* 33): C727–C733, 1993.
116. Etgen, G. J. J., R. P. Farrar, and J. L. Ivy. Effect of chronic electrical stimulation on GLUT-4 protein content in fast-twitch muscle. *Am. J. Physiol.* 264 (*Regulatory Integrative Comp. Physiol.* 33): R816–R819, 1993.
117. Etgen, G. J. J., A. R. Memon, G. A. Thompson, and J. L. Ivy. Insulin- and contraction-stimulated translocation of GTP-binding proteins and GLUT4 protein in skeletal muscle. *J. Biol. Chem.* 268: 20164–20169, 1993.
118. Ferrannini, E., E. Barrett, B. Bevilacqua, and R. DeFronzo. Effect of fatty acids on glucose production and utilization in man. *J. Clin. Invest.* 72: 1737–1747, 1983.
119. Fielding, R. A., T. J. Manfredi, W. Ding, M. A. Fiatarone, W. J. Evans, and J. G. Cannon. Acute phase response in exercise III. Neutrophil and IL-1β accumulation in skeletal muscle. *Am. J. Physiol.* 265 (*Regulatory Integrative Comp. Physiol.* 34): R166–R172, 1993.
120. Foley, J., and T. Huecksteadt. Glucose 6-phosphate effects on deoxyglucose, glucose and methylglucose transport in rat adipocytes. *Biochim. Biophys. Acta* 805: 313–316, 1984.
121. Friedman, J., W. Sherman, M. Reed, C. Elton, and G. Dohm. Exercise training increases glucose transport protein GLUT-4 in skeletal muscle of obese Zucker (fa/fa) rats. *FEBS Lett.* 268: 13–16, 1990.
122. Friedman, J. E., R. W. Dudek, D. S. Whitehead, D. L. Downes, W. R. Frisell, J. F. Caro, and G. L. Dohm. Immunolocalization of glucose transporter GLUT4 within human skeletal muscle. *Diabetes* 40: 150–154, 1991.
123. Fuchi, T., H. Rosdahl, R. C. Hickner, U. Ungerstedt, and J. Henriksson. Microdialysis of rat skeletal muscle and adipose tissue: dynamics of the interstitial glucose pool. *Acta Physiol. Scand.* 151: 249–260, 1994.
124. Fukagawa, N. K., J. W. Anderson, G. Hageman, V. R. Young, and K. L. Minaker. High-carbohydrate, high-fiber diets increase peripheral insulin sensitivity in healthy young and old adults. *Am. J. Clin. Nutr.* 52: 524–528, 1990.
125. Furler, S. M., A. B. Jenkins, L. H. Storlien, and E. W. Kraegen. In vivo location of the rate-limiting step of hexose uptake in muscle and brain tissue of rats. *Am. J. Physiol.* 261 (*Endocrinol. Metab.* 24): E337–E347, 1991.
126. Galbo, H. *Hormonal and Metabolic Adaptation to Exercise.* New York: Georg Thieme, 1983, p. 1–116.
127. Galbo, H. Integrated endocrine responses and exercise. In: *Endocrinology*, edited by L. J. De Groot. Philadelphia: W.B. Saunders Company, 1995, p. 2692–2701.
128. Gao, J., E. A. Gulve, and J. O. Holloszy. Contraction-induced increase in muscle insulin sensitivity: requirement for a serum factor. *Am. J. Physiol.* 266 (*Endocrinol. Metab.* 29): E186–E192, 1994.
129. Garetto, L. P., E. A. Richter, M. N. Goodman, and N. B. Ruderman. Enhanced muscle glucose metabolism after exercise in the rat: the two phases. *Am. J. Physiol.* 246 (*Endocrinol. Metab.* 9): E471–E475, 1984.
130. Garippa, R. J., T. W. Judge, D. E. James, and T. E. McGraw. The amino terminus of GLUT4 functions as an internalization motif but not an intracellular retention signal when substituted for the transferrin receptor cytoplasmic domain. *J. Cell Biol.* 124: 705–715, 1994.
131. Garvey, W. T., and M. J. Birnbaum. Cellular insulin action and insulin resistance. In: *Bailliere's Clinical Endocrinology and Metabolism*, edited by E. Ferrannini. London: Bailliere Tindal, 1993, p. 785–874.
132. Geppert, M., V. Y. Bolshakov, S. A. Siegelbaum, K. Takei, P. De Camilli, R. E. Hammer, and T. C. Südhof. The role of Rab3A in neurotransmitter release. *Nature* 369: 493–497, 1994.
133. Goldstein, M. S., V. Mullick, B. Huddlestun, and R. Levine. Action of muscular work on transfer of sugars across cell barriers: comparison with action of insulin. *Am. J. Physiol.* 173: 212–216, 1953.
134. Gollnick, P., B. Pernow, B. Essén, E. Jansson, and B. Saltin. Availability of glycogen and plasma ffa for substrate utilization in leg muscle of man during exercise. *Clin. Physiol.* 1: 27–42, 1981.
135. Goodyear, L., M. Hirshman, P. King, E. Horton, and C. Thompson. Skeletal muscle plasma membrane glucose transport and glucose transporters after exercise. *J. Appl. Physiol.* 68: 193–198, 1990.
136. Goodyear, L. J., M. F. Hirshman, and E. S. Horton. Exercise-induced translocation of skeletal muscle glucose transporters. *Am. J. Physiol.* 261 (*Endocrinol. Metab.* 24): E795–E799, 1991.
137. Goodyear, L. J., M. F. Hirshman, R. J. Smith, and E. S. Horton. Glucose transporter number, activity and isoform content in plasma membranes of red and white skeletal muscle. *Am. J. Physiol.* 261 (*Endocrinol. Metab.* 24): E556–E561, 1991.
138. Goodyear, L. J., P. A. King, M. F. Hirshman, C. M. Thompson, E. D. Horton, and E. S. Horton. Contractile activity increases plasma membrane glucose transporters in absence of insulin. *Am. J. Physiol.* 258 (*Endocrinol. Metab.* 21): E667–E672, 1990.

139. Goonewardene, I. P., and F. Karim. Attenuation of exercise vasodilatation by adenosine deaminase in anaesthetized dogs. *J. Physiol. (Lond.)* 442: 65–79, 1991.
140. Gorga, F. R., and G. E. Lienhard. Equilibria and kinetics of ligand binding to the human erythrocyte glucose transporter. Evidence for an alternating conformational model for transport. *Biochemistry* 20: 5108–5133, 1981.
141. Gould, G. W., and G. D. Holman. The glucose transporter family: structure, function and tissue-specific expression. *Biochem. J.* 295: 329–341, 1993.
142. Green, A. The insulin-like effect of sodium vanadate on adipocyte glucose transport is mediated at a post-insulin-receptor level. *Biochem. J.* 238: 663–669, 1986.
143. Grimditch, G., R. J. Barnard, S. A. Kaplan, and E. Sternlicht. Effect of training on insulin binding to rat skeletal muscle sarcolemmal vesicles. *Am. J. Physiol.* 250 (*Endocrinol. Metab.* 13): E570–E575, 1986.
144. Grubb, B., and J. Snarr. Effect of flow rate and glucose concentration on glucose uptake rate by the rat limb. *Proc. Soc. Exp. Biol. Med.* 154: 33–36, 1977.
145. Gulve, E. A., G. D. Carter, J. R. Zierath, V. M. Corpus, and J. O. Holloszy. Reversal of enhanced muscle glucose transport after exercise: roles of insulin and glucose. *Am. J. Physiol.* 259 (*Endocrinol. Metab.* 22): E685–E691, 1990.
146. Guma, A., J. R. Zierath, H. Wallberg-Henriksson, and A. Klip. Insulin induces translocation of GLUT-4 glucose transporters in human skeletal muscle. *Am. J. Physiol.* 268 (*Endocrinol. Metab.* 31): E613–E622, 1995.
147. Hall, A. Ras-related proteins. *Curr. Opin. Cell. Biol.* 5: 265–268, 1993.
148. Handberg, A., L. Kayser, P. E. Høyer, and J. Vinten. A substantial part of GLUT-1 in crude membranes from muscle originates from perineurial sheaths. *Am. J. Physiol.* 262 (*Endocrinol. Metab.* 25): E721–E727, 1992.
149. Handberg, A., A. Vaag, P. Damsbo, H. Beck-Nielsen, and J. Vinten. Expression of insulin regulatable glucose transporters in skeletal muscle from type 2 (non-insulin-dependent) diabetic patients. *Diabetologia* 33: 625–627, 1990.
150. Hardy, R. W., J. H. Ladenson, E. J. Henriksen, J. O. Holloszy, and J. M. McDonald. Palmitate stimulates glucose transport in rat adipocytes by a mechanism involving translocation of the insulin sensitive glucose transporter (GLUT 4). *Biochem. Biophys. Res. Commun.* 177: 343–349, 1991.
151. Hargreaves, M., B. Kiens, and E. A. Richter. Effect of increased plasma free fatty acid concentrations on muscle metabolism in exercising men. *J. Appl. Physiol.* 70: 194–201, 1991.
152. Havel, R. J., B. Pernow, and N. L. Jones. Uptake and release of free fatty acids and other metabolites in the legs of exercising men. *J. Appl. Physiol.* 23: 90–99, 1967.
153. Henriksen, E., K. J. Rodnick, and J. O. Holloszy. Activation of glucose transport in skeletal muscle by phospholipase C and phorbol ester. *J. Biol. Chem.* 264: 21536–21543, 1989.
154. Henriksen, E., M. Tischler, and D. Johnson. Increased response to insulin of glucose metabolism in the 6-day unloaded rat soleus muscle. *J. Biol. Chem.* 261: 10707–10712, 1986.
155. Henriksen, E. J., R. E. Bourey, K. J. Rodnick, L. Koranyi, M. A. Permutt, and J. O. Holloszy. Glucose transporter protein content and glucose transport capacity in rat skeletal muscles. *Am. J. Physiol.* 259 (*Endocrinol. Metab.* 22): E593–E598, 1990.
156. Henriksen, E. J., K. J. Rodnick, C. E. Mondon, D. James, and J. O. Holloszy. Effect of denervation or unweighting on GLUT-4 protein in rat soleus muscle. *J. Appl. Physiol.* 70: 2322–2327, 1991.
157. Henriksson, J. Training induced adaptations of skeletal muscle and metabolism during submaximal exercise. *J. Physiol. (Lond.)* 270: 661–675, 1977.
158. Hespel, P., and E. A. Richter. Glucose uptake and transport in contracting, perfused rat muscle with different pre-contraction glycogen concentrations. *J. Physiol. (Lond.)* 427: 347–359, 1990.
159. Hespel, P., L. Vergauen, K. Vandenberghe, and E. A. Richter. Important role of insulin and flow in stimulating glucose uptake in contracting skeletal muscle. *Diabetes* 44: 210–215, 1995.
160. Hirshman, M., L. Goodyear, L. Wardzala, and E. Horton. Identification of an intracellular pool of glucose transporters from basal and insulin-stimulated rat skeletal muscle. *J. Biol. Chem.* 265: 987–991, 1990.
161. Holloszy, J., and H. Narahara. Enhanced permeability to sugar associated with muscle contraction. *J. Gen. Physiol.* 50: 551–562, 1967.
162. Holloszy, J. O., and H. T. Narahara. Studies of tissue permeability. *J. Biol. Chem.* 240: 3493–3500, 1965.
163. Holloszy, J. O., and H. T. Narahara. Nitrate ions: potentiation of increased permeability to sugar associated with muscle contractions. *Science* 155: 573–575, 1967.
164. Holman, G. D., I. J. Kozka, A. E. Clark, C. J. Flower, J. Saltis, A. D. Habberfield, I. A. Simpson, and S. W. Cushman. Cell surface labeling of glucose transporter isoform GLUT4 by bis-mannose photolabel. *J. Biol. Chem.* 265: 18172–18179, 1990.
165. Horton, E. Exercise and diabetes mellitus. *Med. Clin. North Am.* 72: 1301–1321, 1988.
166. Houmard, J. A., M. H. Shinebarger, P. L. Dolan, N. Legget-Frazier, R. K. Bruner, M. R. McCammon, R. G. Israel, and G. L. Dohm. Exercise training increases GLUT-4 protein concentration in previously sedentary middle-aged men. *Am. J. Physiol.* 264 (*Endocrinol. Metab.* 27): E896–E901, 1993.
167. Hundal, H. S., A. Ahmed, A. Guma, Y. Mitsumoto, A. Marette, M. J. Rennie, and A. Klip. Biochemical and immunocytochemical localization of the "GLUT5 glucose transporter" in human skeletal muscle. *Biochem. J.* 286: 339–343, 1992.
168. Huycke, E., and P. Kruhøffer. Effects of insulin and muscular exercise upon the uptake of hexoses by muscle cells. *Acta Physiol. Scand.* 34: 231–249, 1955.
169. Ishizuka, T., D. Cooper, and R. Farese. Insulin stimulates the translocation of protein kinase C in rat adipocytes. *FEBS Lett.* 257: 337–340, 1989.
170. Ishizuka, T., D. Cooper, H. Hernandez, D. Buckley, M. Standaert, and R. Farese. Effects of insulin on diacylglycerol-protein kinase c signaling in rat diaphragm and soleus muscles and relationship to glucose transport. *Diabetes* 39: 181–190, 1990.
171. Issekutz, B. Role of beta-adrenergic receptors in mobilization of energy sources in exercising dogs. *J. Appl. Physiol.* 44: 869–876, 1978.
172. Issekutz, B. Effect of epinephrine on carbohydrate metabolism in exercising dogs. *Metabolism* 34: 457–464, 1985.
173. Iversen, P. O., and G. Nicolaysen. Local blood flow and glucose uptake within resting and exercising rabbit skeletal muscle. *Am. J. Physiol.* 260 (*Heart Circ. Physiol.* 29): H1795–H1801, 1991.

174. James, D., K. Burleigh, and E. Kraegen. In vivo glucose metabolism in individual tissues of the rat. *J. Biol. Chem.* 261: 6366–6374, 1986.
175. James, D., E. Kraegen, and D. Chisholm. Effects of exercise training on in vivo insulin action in individual tissues of the rat. *J. Clin. Invest.* 76: 657–666, 1985.
176. Jansson, E., P. Hjemdahl, and L. Kaijser. Epinephrine-induced changes in muscle carbohydrate metabolism during exercise in male subjects. *J. Appl. Physiol.* 60: 1466–1470, 1986.
177. Jansson, E., and L. Kaijser. Effect of diet on muscle glycogen and blood glucose utilization during short-term exercise in man. *Acta Physiol. Scand.* 115: 341–347, 1982.
178. Jansson, E., and L. Kaijser. Substrate utilization and enzymes in skeletal muscle of extremely endurance-trained men. *J. Appl. Physiol.* 62: 999–1005, 1987.
179. Jansson, P., J. Fowelin, U. Smith, and P. Lönnroth. Characterization by microdialysis of intercellular glucose level in subcutaneous tissue in humans. *Am. J. Physiol.* 255 (*Endocrinol. Metab.* 18): E218–E220, 1988.
180. Jensen-Urstad, M., and G. Ahlborg. Is the high lactate release during arm exercise due to a low training status? *Clin. Physiol.* 12: 487–496, 1992.
181. Jhun, B. H., A. L. Rampal, H. Liu, M. Lachaal, and C. Y. Jung. Effects of insulin on steady state kinetics of GLUT4 subcellular distribution in rat adipocytes. *J. Biol. Chem.* 267: 17710–17715, 1992.
182. Jorfeldt, L., and J. Wahren. Human forearm muscle metabolism during exercise. V. Quantitative aspects of glucose uptake and lactate production during exercise. *Scand. J. Clin. Lab. Invest.* 26: 73–81, 1970.
183. Kahn, B. B., A. S. Rosen, J. F. Bak, P. H. Andersen, P. Damsbo, S. Lund, and O. Pedersen. Expression of GLUT 1 and GLUT 4 glucose transporters in skeletal muscle of humans with insulin-dependent diabetes mellitus: regulatory effects of metabolic factors. *J. Clin. Endocrinol. Metab.* 74: 1101–1109, 1992.
184. Kasanicki, M., and P. Pilch. Regulation of glucose-transporter function. *Diabetes Care* 13: 219–227, 1990.
185. Katz, A., S. Broberg, K. Sahlin, and J. Wahren. Leg glucose uptake during maximal dynamic exercise in humans. *Am. J. Physiol.* 251 (*Endocrinol. Metab.* 14): E65–E70, 1986.
186. Katz, A., I. Raz, M. K. Spencer, R. Rising, and D. M. Mott. Hyperglycemia induces accumulation of glucose in human skeletal muscle. *Am. J. Physiol.* 260 (*Regulatory Integrative Comp. Physiol.* 29): R698–R703, 1991.
187. Katz, A., K. Sahlin, and S. Broberg. Regulation of glucose utilization in human skeletal muscle during moderate dynamic exercise. *Am. J. Physiol.* 260 (*Endocrinol. Metab.* 23): E411–E415, 1991.
188. Kelley, D. E., M. Mokan, J. Simoneau, and L. J. Mandarino. Interaction between glucose and free fatty acid metabolism in human skeletal muscle. *J. Clin. Invest.* 92: 91–98, 1993.
189. Kern, M., P. L. Dolan, R. S. Mazzeo, J. A. Wells, and G. L. Dohm. Effect of aging and exercise on GLUT-4 glucose transporters in muscle. *Am. J. Physiol.* 263 (*Endocrinol. Metab.* 26): E362–E367, 1992.
190. Kiens, B., B. Essen-Gustavsson, N. J. Christensen, and B. Saltin. Skeletal muscle substrate utilization during submaximal exercise in man: effect of endurance training. *J. Physiol. (Lond.)* 469: 459–478, 1993.
191. Kiens, B., and E. A. Richter. Types of carbohydrate in an ordinary diet affect insulin action and muscle substrates in humans. *Am. J. Clin. Nutr.* 1996 (in press).
192. King, D., G. Dalsky, W. Clutter, D. Young, and M. Staten. Effects of exercise and lack of exercise on insulin sensitivity and responsiveness. *J. Appl. Physiol.* 64: 1942–1946, 1988.
193. King, D., G. Dalsky, M. Staten, W. Clutter, D. vanHouten, and J. Holloszy. Insulin action and secretion in endurance-trained and untrained humans. *J. Appl. Physiol.* 63: 2247–2252, 1987.
194. King, D. S., T. L. Feltmeyer, P. J. Baldus, R. L. Sharp, and J. Nespor. Effects of eccentric exercise on insulin secretion and action in humans. *J. Appl. Physiol.* 75: 2151–2156, 1993.
195. King, P. A., J. J. Betts, E. D. Horton, and E. S. Horton. Exercise, unlike insulin, promotes glucose transporter translocation in obese Zucker rat muscle. *Am. J. Physiol.* 265 (*Regulatory Integrative Comp. Physiol.* 34): R447–R452, 1993.
196. King, P. A., M. F. Hirshman, E. D. Horton, and E. S. Horton. Glucose transport in skeletal muscle membrane vesicles from control and exercised rats. *Am. J. Physiol.* 257 (*Cell Physiol.* 26): C1128–C1134, 1989.
197. Kirwan, J., D. Costill, H. Kuipers, M. Burrell, and W. Fink. Substrate utilization in leg muscle of men after heat acclimation. *J. Appl. Physiol.* 63: 31–35, 1987.
198. Kirwan, J. P., R. C. Hickner, K. E. Yarasheski, W. M. Kohrt, B. V. Wiethop, and J. O. Holloszy. Eccentric exercise induces transient insulin resistance in healthy individuals. *J. Appl. Physiol.* 72: 2197–2202, 1992.
199. Kjær, M., P. Farrell, N. Christensen, and H. Galbo. Increased epinephrine response and inaccurate glucoregulation in exercising athletes. *J. Appl. Physiol.* 61: 1693–1700, 1986.
200. Kjær, M., C. Hollenbeck, B. Frey-Hewitt, H. Galbo, W. Haskell, and G. Reaven. Glucoregulation and hormonal responses to maximal exercise in non-insulin-dependent diabetes. *J. Appl. Physiol.* 68: 2067–2074, 1990.
201. Kjær, M., B. Kiens, M. Hargreaves, and E. A. Richter. Influence of active muscle mass on glucose homeostasis during exercise in humans. *J. Appl. Physiol.* 71: 552–557, 1991.
202. Klip, A., and T. Ramlal. Protein kinase C is not required for insulin stimulation of hexose uptake in muscle cells in culture. *Biochem. J.* 242: 131–136, 1987.
203. Knapik, J., C. Meredith, B. Jones, L. Suek, V. Young, and W. Evans. Influence of fasting on carbohydrate and fat metabolism during rest and exercise in men. *J. Appl. Physiol.* 64: 1923–1929, 1988.
204. Koch, L. G., S. L. Britton, and P. J. Metting. Adenosine is not essential for exercise hyperaemia in the hindlimb in conscious dogs. *J. Physiol. (Lond.)* 429: 63–75, 1990.
205. Koivisto, V. A., R. E. Bourey, H. Vuorinen-Markkola, and L. Koranyi. Exercise reduces muscle glucose transport protein (GLUT-4) mRNA in type 1 diabetic patients. *J. Appl. Physiol.* 74: 1755–1760, 1993.
206. Kolterman, O. G., M. Greenfield, G. M. Reaven, M. Saekow, and J. M. Olefsky. Effect of a high carbohydrate diet on insulin binding to adipocytes and on insulin action in vivo in man. *Diabetes* 28: 731–736, 1979.
207. Kong, X., J. Manchester, S. Salmons, and J. C. Lawrence, Jr. Glucose transporters in single skeletal muscle fibers. *J. Biol. Chem.* 269: 12963–12967, 1994.
208. Kono, T., F. W. Robinson, T. L. Blevins, and O. Ezaki. Evidence that translocation of the glucose transport activity is the major mechanism of insulin action on glucose transport in fat cells. *J. Biol. Chem.* 257: 10942–10947, 1982.

209. Koranyi, L. I., R. E. Bourey, H. Vuorinen-Markkola, V. A. Koivisto, M. Mueckler, M. A. Permutt, and H. Yki-Järvinen. Level of skeletal muscle glucose transporter protein correlates with insulin-stimulated whole body glucose disposal in man. *Diabetologia* 34: 763–765, 1991.
210. Kraegen, E., D. James, L. Storlien, K. Burleigh, and D. Chisholm. In vivo insulin resistance in individual peripheral tissues of the high fat fed rat: assessment by euglycaemic clamp plus deoxyglucose administration. *Diabetologia* 29: 192–198, 1986.
211. Kraegen, E., L. Storlien, A. Jenkins, and D. James. Chronic exercise compensates for insulin resistance induced by a high-fat diet in rats. *Am. J. Physiol.* 256 (*Endocrinol. Metab.* 19): E242–E249, 1989.
212. Kristiansen, S., J. Wojtaszewski, C. Juel, and E. A. Richter. Effect of glucose-6-phosphate and pH on glucose transport in muscle giant vesicles. *Acta Physiol. Scand.* 150: 227–233, 1994.
213. Kubo, K., and J. Foley. Rate-limiting steps for insulin-mediated glucose uptake into perfused rat hindlimb. *Am. J. Physiol.* 250 (*Endocrinol. Metab.* 13): E100–E102, 1986.
214. Kusunoki, M., L. H. Storlien, J. MacDessi, N. D. Oakes, C. Kennedy, D. J. Chisholm, and E. W. Kraegen. Muscle glucose uptake during and after exercise is normal in insulin-resistant rats. *Am. J. Physiol.* 264 (*Endocrinol. Metab.* 27): E167–E172, 1993.
215. Laakso, M., S. V. Edelman, G. Brechtel, and A. D. Baron. Effects of epinephrine on insulin-mediated glucose uptake in whole body and leg muscle in humans: role of blood flow. *Am. J. Physiol.* 263 (*Endocrinol. Metab.* 26): E199–E204, 1992.
216. Langfort, J., L. Budohoski, H. Kaciuba-Uscilko, K. Nazar, J. R. A. Challiss, and E. A. Newsholme. Effect of endurance and sprint exercise on the sensitivity of glucose metabolism to insulin in the epitrochlearis muscle of sedentary and trained rats. *Eur. J. Appl. Physiol.* 62: 145–150, 1991.
217. Langfort, J., D. Czarnowski, L. Budohoski, J. Górski, H. Kaciuba-Uscilko, and K. Nazar. Electrical stimulation partly reverses the muscle insulin resistance caused by tenotomy. *FEBS Lett.* 315: 183–186, 1993.
218. Laurie, S. M., C. C. Cain, G. E. Lienhard, and J. D. Castle. The glucose transporter GLUT4 and secretory carrier membrane proteins (SCAMPs) colocalize in rat adipocytes and partially segregate during insulin stimulation. *J. Biol. Chem.* 268: 19110–19117, 1993.
219. Law, W., M. McLane, and R. Raymond. Adenosine is required for mycocardial insulin responsiveness in vivo. *Diabetes* 37: 842–845, 1988.
220. Lawrence, J. C., Jr., J. F. Hiken, and D. E. James. Stimulation of glucose transport and glucose transporter phosphorylation by okadaic acid in rat adipocytes. *J. Biol. Chem.* 265: 19768–19776, 1990.
221. Lee, J., and P. F. Pilch. The insulin receptor: structure, function, and signaling. *Am. J. Physiol.* 266 (*Cell Physiol.* 35): C319–C334, 1994.
222. Lillioja, S., A. Young, C. Culter, J. Ivy, W. G. Abbott, J. K. Zawadzki, H. Yki-Järvinen, L. Christin, T. W. Secomb, and C. Bogardus. Skeletal muscle capillary density and fiber type are possible determinants of in vivo insulin resistance in man. *J. Clin. Invest.* 80: 415–424, 1987.
223. Lipman, R., J. Schnure, E. Bradley, and F. Lecocq. Impairment of peripheral glucose utilization in normal subjects by prolonged bed rest. *J. Lab. Clin. Med.* 76: 221–230, 1970.
224. Lund, S., G. D. Holman, O. Schmitz, and O. Pedersen. Glut 4 content in the plasma membrane of rat skeletal muscle: comparative studies of the subcellular fractionation method and the exofacial photolabelling technique using ATB-BMPA. *FEBS Lett.* 330: 312–318, 1993.
225. Lund, S., H. Vestergaard, P. H. Andersen, O. Schmitz, L. B. H. Gøtzsche, and O. Pedersen. GLUT-4 content in plasma membrane of muscle from patients with non-insulin-dependent diabetes mellitus. *Am. J. Physiol.* 265 (*Endocrinol. Metab.* 28): E889–E897, 1993.
226. Maehlum, S., P. Felig, and J. Wahren. Splanchnic glucose and muscle glycogen metabolism after glucose feeding during postexercise recovery. *Am. J. Physiol.* 235 (*Endocrinol. Metab. Gastrointest. Physiol.* 4): E255–E260, 1978.
227. Manchester, J., X. Kong, O. H. Lowry, and J. C. Lawrence, Jr. Ras signalling in the activation of glucose transport by insulin. *Proc. Natl. Acad. Sci. U. S. A.* 91: 4644–4648, 1994.
228. Mandarino, L., K. Wright, L. Verity, J. Nichols, and J. Bell. Effects of insulin infusion on human skeletal muscle pyruvate dehydrogenase, phosphofructokinase and glycogen synthase. *J. Clin. Invest.* 80: 655–663, 1987.
229. Marette, A., E. Burdett, A. Douen, M. Vranic, and A. Klip. Insulin induces the translocation of GLUT 4 from a unique intracellular organelle to transverse tubules in rat skeletal muscle. *Diabetes* 41: 1562–1569, 1992.
230. Marette, A., J. M. Richardson, T. Ramlal, T. W. Balon, M. Vranic, J. E. Pessin, and A. Klip. Abundance, localization, and insulin-induced translocation of glucose transporters in red and white muscle. *Am. J. Physiol.* 263 (*Cell Physiol.* 32): C443–C452, 1992.
231. Marker, J. C., I. B. Hirsch, L. J. Smith, C. A. Parvin, J. O. Holloszy, and P. E. Cryer. Catecholamines in the prevention of hypoglycemia during exercise in humans. *Am. J. Physiol.* 260 (*Enddocrinol. Metab.* 23): E705–E712, 1991.
232. Marliss, E. B., E. Simantirakis, P. D. G. Miles, C. Purdon, R. Gougeon, C. J. Field, J. B. Halter, and M. Vranic. Glucoregulatory and hormonal responses to repeated bouts of intense exercise in normal male subjects. *J. Appl. Physiol.* 71: 924–933, 1991.
233. Marshall, S., W. T. Garvey, and R. R. Traxinger. New insights into the metabolic regulation of insulin action and insulin resistance: role of glucose and amino acids. *FASEB J.* 5: 3031–3036, 1991.
234. Martin, I. K., A. Katz, and J. Wahren. Enhanced leg glucose uptake and normal hepatic glucose output during exercise in patients with NIDDM. *Diabetes* 42 (Suppl. 1): 107A, 1993 (Abstract).
235. Mayer, S. E., A. C. Mayfield, and J. A. Hass. Heart muscle hexokinase: subcellular distribution and inhibition by glucose-6-phosphate. *Mol. Pharmacol.* 2: 393–405, 1966.
236. McConnel, G., M. McCoy, J. Proietto, and M. Hargreaves. Skeletal muscle GLUT4 and glucose uptake during exercise in humans. *J. Appl. Physiol.* 77: 1565–1568, 1994.
237. Megeney, L. A., G. C. B. Elder, M. H. Tan, and A. Bonen. Increased glucose transport in nonexercising muscle. *Am. J. Physiol.* 262 (*Endocrinol. Metab.* 25): E20–E26, 1992.
238. Megeney, L. A., P. D. Neufer, L. G. Dohm, M. H. Tan, C. A. Blewett, G. C. B. Elder, and A. Bonen. Effects of muscle activity and fiber composition on glucose transport and GLUT-4. *Am. J. Physiol.* 264 (*Endocrinol. Metab.* 27): E583–E593, 1993.
239. Megeney, L. A., M. A. Prasad, M. H. Tan, and A. Bonen. Expression of the insulin regulatable transporter GLUT4 in muscle is influenced by neurogenic factors. *Am. J. Physiol.* 266 (*Endocrinol. Metab.* 29): E813–E816, 1994.
240. Mendenhall, L. A., S. C. Swanson, D. L. Habash, and A. R. Coggan. Ten days of exercise training reduces glucose production and utilization during moderate-intensity exer-

cise. *Am. J. Physiol.* 266 (*Endocrinol. Metab.* 29): E136–E143, 1994.
241. Mikines, K., B. Sonne, P. Farrell, B. Tronier, and H. Galbo. Effect of physical exercise on sensitivity and responsiveness to insulin in humans. *Am. J. Physiol.* 254 (*Endocrinol. Metab.* 17): E248–E259, 1988.
242. Mikines, K., B. Sonne, P. Farrell, B. Tronier, and H. Galbo. Effect of training on the dose-response relationship for insulin action in men. *J. Appl. Physiol.* 66: 695–703, 1989.
243. Mikines, K. J., E. A. Richter, F. Dela, and H. Galbo. Seven days of bed rest decrease insulin action on glucose uptake in leg and whole body. *J. Appl. Physiol.* 70: 1245–1254, 1991.
244. Minuk, H. L., M. Vranic, E. B. Marliss, A. K. Hanna, A. M. Albisser, and B. Zinman. Glucoregulatory and metabolic response to exercise in obese noninsulin-dependent diabetes. *Am. J. Physiol.* 240 (*Endocrinol. Metab.* 3): E458–E464, 1981.
245. Mollard, G. F., G. A. Mignery, M. Baumert, M. S. Perin, T. J. Hanson, P. M. Burger, R. Jahn, and T. C. Suedhof. Rab3 is a small GTP-binding protein exclusively localized to synaptic vesicles. *Proc. Natl. Acad. Sci. U. S. A.* 87: 1988–1992, 1990.
246. Mondon, C. E., C. B. Dolkas, and G. M. Reaven. Site of enhanced insulin sensitivity in exercise-trained rats. *Am. J. Physiol.* 239 (*Endocrinol. Metab.* 8): E169–E177, 1980.
247. Mueckler, M. Facilitative glucose transporters. *Eur. J. Biochem.* 219: 713–725, 1994.
248. Mǿller, N., P. Butler, M. Antsiverov, and K. G. M. Alberti. Effects of growth hormone on insulin sensitivity and forearm metabolism in normal man. *Diabetologia* 32: 105–110, 1989.
249. National Institutes of Health. Consensus development conference on diet and exercise in non-insulin-dependent diabetes mellitus. *Diabetes Care* 10: 639–644, 1987.
250. Nelson, T. E., R. C. White, and T. E. Watts. The action of the glycogen debranching enzyme system in a muscle protein particle. *Biochem. Biophys. Res. Commun.* 47: 254–259, 1972.
251. Nesher, R., I. Karl, and D. Kipnis. Dissociation of effects of insulin and contraction on glucose transport in rat epitrochlearis muscle. *Am. J. Physiol.* 249 (*Cell Physiol.* 18): C226–C232, 1985.
252. Neufer, P. D., and L. G. Dohm. Exercise induces a transient increase in transcription of the GLUT-4 gene in skeletal muscle. *Am. J. Physiol.* 265 (*Cell Physiol.* 34): C1597–C1603, 1993.
253. Newham, D., D. Jones, and P. Clarkson. Repeated high-force eccentric exercise: effects on muscle pain and damage. *J. Appl. Physiol.* 63: 1381–1386, 1987.
254. Newsholme, E. A., and A. R. Leech. *Biochemistry for the Medical Sciences.* Chichester: John Wiley & Sons, 1983.
255. Nielsen, B., J. R. S. Hales, S. Strange, N. J. Christensen, J. Warberg, and B. Saltin. Human circulatory and thermoregulatory adaptions with heat acclimation and exercise in a hot, dry environment. *J. Physiol. (Lond.)* 460: 467–485, 1993.
256. Nielsen, B., G. Savard, E. A. Richter, M. Hargreaves, and B. Saltin. Muscle blood flow and muscle metabolism during exercise and heat stress. *J. Appl. Physiol.* 69: 1040–1046, 1990.
257. Nishimura, H., J. Saltis, A. D. Haberfield, N. B. Garty, A. S. Greenberg, S. W. Cushman, C. Londos, and I. A. Simpson. Phosphorylation state of the GLUT4 isoform of the glucose transporter in subfractions of the rat adipose cell: Effects of insulin, adenosine and isoproterenol. *Proc. Natl. Acad. Sci. U. S. A.* 88: 11500–11504, 1991.
258. Nishizuka, Y. Intracellular signaling by hydrolysis of phospholipids and activation of protein kinase c. *Science* 258: 607–614, 1992.
259. Nuutila, P., V. A. Koivisto, J. Knuuti, U. Ruotsalainen, M. Teräs, M. Haaparanta, J. Bergman, O. Solin, L. Voipio-Pulkki, U. Wegelius, and H. Yki-Järvinen. Glucose-free fatty acid cycle operates in human heart and skeletal muscle in vivo. *J. Clin. Invest.* 89: 1767–1774, 1992.
260. O'Reilly, K., M. Warhol, R. Fielding, W. Frontera, C. Meredith, and W. Evans. Eccentric exercise-induced muscle damage impairs muscle glycogen repletion. *J. Appl. Physiol.* 63: 252–256, 1987.
261. Oka, Y., T. Asano, Y. Shibasaki, J.-L. Lin, K. Tsukuda, H. Katagiri, Y. Akanuma, and F. Takaku. C-terminal truncated glucose transporter is locked into an inward-facing form without transport activity. *Nature* 345: 550–553, 1990.
262. Owen, O. E., A. P. Morgan, H. G. Kemp, J. M. Sullivan, M. G. Herrera, and G. F. Cahill. Brain metabolism during fasting. *J. Clin. Invest.* 46: 1589–1595, 1967.
263. Owen, O. E., and G. A. Reichard. Human forearm metabolism during progressive starvation. *J. Clin. Invest.* 50: 1536–1545, 1971.
264. Pershadsingh, H., D. Shade, and J. McDonald. Insulin-dependent alterations of phorbol ester binding to adipocyte subcellular constituents. Evidence for the involvement of protein kinase c in insulin action. *Biochim. Biophys. Acta* 145: 1384–1389, 1987.
265. Pette, D., and G. Vrbova. Invited review: neural control of phenotypic expression in mammalian muscle fibers. *Muscle Nerve* 8: 676–689, 1973.
266. Pfeffer, S. R. GTP-binding proteins in intracellular transport. *Trends Cell Biol.* 2: 41–46, 1992.
267. Piatti, P. M., L. D. Monti, M. Pacchioni, A. E. Pontiroli, and G. Pozza. Forearm insulin- and non-insulin-mediated glucose uptake and muscle metabolism in man: role of free fatty acids and blood glucose levels. *Metabolism* 40: 926–933, 1991.
268. Piiper, J., D. R. Pendergast, C. Marconi, M. Meyer, N. Heisler, and P. Cerretelli. Blood flow distribution in dog gastrocnemius muscle at rest and during stimulation. *J. Appl. Physiol.* 58: 2068–2074, 1985.
269. Piper, R. C., D. E. James, J. W. Slot, C. Puri, and J. C. Lawrence. GLUT4 phosphorylation and inhibition of glucose transport by dibutyryl cAMP. *J. Biol. Chem.* 268: 16557–16563, 1993.
270. Piper, R. C., C. Tai, P. Kulesza, S. Pang, D. Warnock, J. Baenzinger, J. W. Slot, H. J. Geuze, C. Puri, and D. E. James. GLUT-4NH2 terminus contains a phenylalanine-based targeting motif that regulates intracellular sequestration. *J. Cell Biol.* 121: 1221–1232, 1993.
271. Ploug, T., H. Galbo, T. Ohkuwa, J. Tranum-Jensen, and J. Vinten. Kinetics of glucose transport in rat skeletal muscle membrane vesicles: effects of insulin and contractions. *Am. J. Physiol.* 262 (*Endocrinol. Metab.* 25): E700–E711, 1992.
272. Ploug, T., H. Galbo, and E. A. Richter. Increased muscle glucose uptake during contractions: no need for insulin. *Am. J. Physiol.* 247 (*Endocrinol. Metab.* 10): E726–E731, 1984.
273. Ploug, T., H. Galbo, J. Vinten, M. Jørgensen, and E. A. Richter. Kinetics of glucose transport in rat muscle: effects of insulin and contractions. *Am. J. Physiol.* 253 (*Endocrinol. Metab.* 16): E12–E20, 1987.

274. Ploug, T., B. M. Stallknecht, O. Pedersen, B. B. Kahn, T. Ohkuwa, J. Vinten, and H. Galbo. Effect of endurance training on glucose transport capacity and glucose transporter expression in rat skeletal muscle. *Am. J. Physiol.* 259 (*Endocrinol. Metab.* 22): E778–E786, 1990.
275. Ploug, T., J. Wojtaszewski, S. Kristiansen, P. Hespel, H. Galbo, and E. A. Richter. Glucose transport and transporters in muscle giant vesicles: differential effects of insulin and contractions. *Am. J. Physiol.* 264 (*Endocrinol. Metab.* 27): E270–E278, 1993.
276. Poucher, S. M., C. G. Nowell, and M. G. Collis. The role of adenosine in exercise hyperaemia of the gracilis muscle in anaesthetized cats. *J. Physiol. (Lond.)* 427: 19–29, 1990.
277. Quon, M. J. Advances in kinetic analysis of insulin-stimulated GLUT-4 translocation in adipose cells. *Am. J. Physiol.* 266 (*Endocrinol. Metab.* 29): E144–E150, 1994.
278. Ralston, E., S. Beushausen, and T. Ploug. Expression of the synaptic vesicle proteins VAMPs/synaptopbrevins 1 and 2 in non-neural tissues. *J. Biol. Chem.* 269: 15403–15406, 1994.
279. Rand, E. B., A. M. Depaoli, N. O. Davidson, G. I. Bell, and C. F. Burant. Sequence, tissue distribution and functional characterization of the rat fructose transporter GLUT5. *Am. J. Physiol.* 264 (*Gastrointest. Liver Physiol.* 27): G1169–G1176, 1993.
280. Randle, P., A. Kerbey, and J. Espinal. Mechanisms decreasing glucose oxidation in diabetes and starvation: role of lipid fuels and hormones. *Diabetes Metab. Rev.* 4: 623–638, 1988.
281. Randle, P. J., R. B. Garland, C. N. Hales, and E. A. Newsholme. The glucose-fatty acid cycle: its role in insulin sensitivity and the metabolic disturbances of diabetes mellitus. *Lancet* i: 785–789, 1963.
282. Randle, P. J., E. A. Newsholme, and P. B. Garland. Regulation of glucose uptake by muscle. *Biochem. J.* 93: 652–665, 1964.
283. Reaven, G. Role of insulin resistance in human disease. *Diabetes* 37: 1595–15607, 1988.
284. Ren, J.-M., B. A. Marshall, E. A. Gulve, J. Gao, D. W. Johnson, J. O. Holloszy, and M. Mueckler. Evidence from transgenic mice that glucose transport is rate-limiting for glycogen deposition and glycolysis in skeletal muscle. *J. Biol. Chem.* 268: 16113–16115, 1993.
285. Ren, J.-M., C. F. Semenkovich, E. A. Gulve, J. Gao, and J. O. Holloszy. Exercise induces rapid increases in GLUT4 expression, glucose transport capacity, and insulin-stimulated glycogen storage in muscle. *J. Biol. Chem.* 269: 14396–14401, 1994.
286. Rennie, M., and J. Holloszy. Inhibition of glucose uptake and glycogenolysis by availability of oleate in well-oxygenated perfused skeletal muscle. *Biochem. J.* 168: 161–170, 1977.
287. Rennie, M. J., W. W. Winder, and J. O. Holloszy. A sparing effect of increased plasma fatty acids on muscle and liver glycogen content in the exercisning rat. *Biochem. J.* 156: 647–655, 1976.
288. Reusch, J. E.-B., K. E. Sussman, and B. Draznin. Inverse relationship between GLUT-4 phosphorylation and its intrinsic activity. *J. Biol. Chem.* 268: 3348–3351, 1993.
289. Richardson, J. M., T. W. Balon, J. L. Treadway, and J. E. Pessin. Differential regulation of glucose transporter activity and espression in red and white skeletal muscle. *J. Biol. Chem.* 266: 12690–12694, 1991.
290. Richter, E. A., P. J. F. Cleland, S. Rattigan, and M. G. Clark. Contraction-associated translocation of protein kinase C in rat skeletal muscle. *FEBS Lett.* 217: 232–236, 1987.
291. Richter, E. A., and H. Galbo. Diabetes, insulin and exercise. *Sports Med.* 3: 275–288, 1986.
292. Richter, E. A., and H. Galbo. High glycogen levels enhance glycogen breakdown in isolated contracting skeletal muscle. *J. Appl. Physiol.* 61: 827–831, 1986.
293. Richter, E. A., L. P. Garetto, M. N. Goodman, and N. B. Ruderman. Muscle glucose metabolism following exercise in the rat. *J. Clin. Invest.* 69: 785–793, 1982.
294. Richter, E. A., L. P. Garetto, M. N. Goodman, and N. B. Ruderman. Enhanced muscle glucose metabolism after exercise: modulation by local factors. *Am. J. Physiol.* 246 (*Endocrinol. Metab.* 9): E476–E482, 1984.
295. Richter, E. A., B. F. Hansen, and S. A. Hansen. Glucose-induced insulin resistance of skeletal-muscle glucose transport and uptake. *Biochem. J.* 252: 733–737, 1988.
296. Richter, E. A., S. A. Hansen, and B. F. Hansen. Mechanisms limiting glycogen storage in muscle during prolonged insulin stimulation. *Am. J. Physiol.* 255 (*Endocrinol. Metab.* 18): E621–E628, 1988.
297. Richter, E. A., B. Kiens, M. Mizuno, and S. Strange. Insulin action in human thighs after one-legged immobilization. *J. Appl. Physiol.* 67: 19–23, 1989.
298. Richter, E. A., B. Kiens, B. Saltin, N. J. Christensen, and G. Savard. Skeletal muscle glucose uptake during dynamic exercise in humans: role of muscle mass. *Am. J. Physiol.* 254 (*Endocrinol. Metab.* 17): E555–E561, 1988.
299. Richter, E. A., K. J. Mikines, H. Galbo, and B. Kiens. Effect of exercise on insulin action in human skeletal muscle. *J. Appl. Physiol.* 66: 876–885, 1989.
300. Richter, E. A., T. Ploug, and H. Galbo. Increased muscle glucose uptake after exercise. *Diabetes* 34: 1041–1048, 1985.
301. Richter, E. A., N. B. Ruderman, and H. Galbo. Alpha and beta adrenergic effects on metabolism in contracting, perfused muscle. *Acta Physiol. Scand.* 116: 215–222, 1982.
302. Richter, E. A., N. B. Ruderman, H. Gavras, E. R. Belur, and H. Galbo. Muscle glycogenolysis during exercise: dual control by epinephrine and contractions. *Am. J. Physiol.* 242 (*Endocrinol. Metab.* 5): E25–E32, 1982.
303. Rizza, R. A., P. E. Cryer, M. W. Haymond, and J. E. Gerich. Adrenergic mechanisms for the effects of epinephrine on glucose production and clearance in man. *J. Clin. Invest.* 65: 682–689, 1980.
304. Rizza, R. A., L. J. Mandarino, and J. E. Gerich. Effects of growth hormone on insulin action in man. Mechanisms of insulin resistance, impaired suppression of glucose production, and impaired stimulation of glucose utilization. *Diabetes* 31: 663–669, 1982.
305. Robinson, K. A., D. A. Sens, and M. G. Buse. Pre-exposure to glucosamine induces insulin resistance of glucose transport and glycogen synthesis in isolated rat skeletal muscles. *Diabetes* 42: 1333–1346, 1993.
306. Robinson, L. J., S. Pang, J. Harris, J. Heuser, and D. E. James. Translocation of the glucose transporter (GLUT4) to the cell surface in permeabilized 3T3-L1 adipocytes: effects of ATP, insulin, and GTP-gammaS and localization of GLUT4 to clathrin lattices. *J. Cell Biol.* 117: 1181–1196, 1992.
307. Roca, J., A. G. N. Agusti, A. Alonso, D. C. Poole, C. Viegas, J. A. Barbera, R. Rodriguez-Roisin, A. Ferrer, and P. D. Wagner. Effects of training on muscle 0 2 transport at VO 2max. *J. Appl. Physiol.* 73: 1067–1076, 1992.
308. Rodnick, K., W. Haskell, A. L. Swislocki, J. Foley, and G. Reaven. Improved insulin action in muscle, liver and adi-

pose tissue in physically trained human subjects. *Am. J. Physiol.* 253 (*Endocrinol. Metab.* 16): E489–E495, 1987.

309. Rodnick, K. J., E. J. Henriksen, D. E. James, and J. O. Holloszy. Exercise training, glucose transporters and glucose transport in rat skeletal muscles. *Am. J. Physiol.* 262 (*Cell Physiol.* 31): C9–C14, 1992.
310. Rodnick, K. J., J. W. Slot, D. R. Studelska, D. E. Hanpeter, L. J. Robinson, H. J. Geuze, and D. E. James. Immunocytochemical and biochemical studies of GLUT 4 in rat skeletal muscle. *J. Biol. Chem.* 267: 6278–6285, 1992.
311. Ruderman, N. B., A. McCall, and S. Schneider. Exercise and endocrine disorders. *Scand. J. Sports Sci.* 8: 43–50, 1986.
312. Sahlin, K., S. Broberg, and A. Katz. Glucose formation in human skeletal muscle. *Biochem. J.* 258: 911–913, 1989.
313. Saitoh, Y., K. Itaya, and M. Ui. Adrenergic α-receptor-mediated stimulation of the glucose utilization by isolated rat diaphragm. *Biochim. Biophys. Acta* 343: 492–499, 1974.
314. Saltin, B., and P. Gollnick. Skeletal muscle adaptability: significance for metabolism and performance. In: *Handbook of Physiology, Skeletal Muscle, Skeletal Muscle,* edited by L. D. Peachey. Bethesda, MD: Am. Physiol. Soc., 1983, p. 555–631.
315. Saltin, B., K. Nazar, D. L. Costill, E. Stein, and E. Jansson. The nature of the training response: peripheral and central adaptations to one-legged exercise. *Acta Physiol. Scand.* 96: 289–305, 1976.
316. Satoh, S., H. Nishimura, A. E. Clark, I. J. Kozka, S. J. Vannucci, I. A. Simpson, M. J. Quon, S. W. Cushman, and G. D. Holman. Use of bismannose photolabel to elucidate insulin-regulated GLUT4 subcellular trafficking kinetics in rat adipose cells. Evidence that exocytosis is a critical site of hormone action. *J. Biol. Chem.* 268: 17820–17829, 1993.
317. Savard, G. K., E. A. Richter, S. Strange, B. Kiens, N. J. Christensen, and B. Saltin. Norepinephrine spillover from skeletal muscle during exercise in humans: role of muscle mass. *Am. J. Physiol.* 257 (*Heart Circ. Physiol.* 26): H1812–H1818, 1989.
318. Schantz, P., J. Henriksson, and E. Jansson. Adaptation of human skeletal muscle to endurance training of long duration. *Clin. Physiol.* 3: 141–151, 1983.
319. Schneider, S. H. and N. B. Ruderman. Exercise and NIDDM. *Diabetes Care* 13: 785–789, 1990.
320. Schultz, T., S. Lewis, D. Westbie, J. Wallin, and J. Gerich. Glucose delivery: a modulator of glucose uptake in contracting skeletal muscle. *Am. J. Physiol.* 233 (*Endocrinol. Metab. Gastrointest. Physiol.* 2): E514–E518, 1977.
321. Schultz, T. A., S. B. Lewis, D. K. Westbis, J. E. Gerich, R. J. Rushakoff, and J. D. Wallin. Glucose delivery—a clarification of its role in regulating glucose uptake in rat skeletal muscle. *Life Sci.* 20: 733–736, 1977.
322. Seedorf, U., E. Leberer, B. Kirschbaum, and D. Pette. Neural control of gene expression in skeletal muscle. *Biochem. J.* 239: 115–120, 1986.
323. Seider, M., W. Nicholson, and F. Booth. Insulin resistance for glucose metabolism in disused soleus muscle of mice. *Am. J. Physiol.* 242 (*Endocrinol. Metab* 5): E12–E18, 1982.
324. Shamoon, H., V. Soman, and R. Sherwin. The influence of acute physiological increments of cortisol on fuel metabolism and insulin binding to monocytes in normal humans. *J. Clin. Endocrinol. Metab.* 50: 495–501, 1980.
325. Slentz, C. A., E. A. Gulve, K. J. Rodnick, E. J. Henriksen, J. H. Youn, and J. O. Holloszy. Glucose transporters and maximal transport are increased in endurance-trained rat soleus. *J. Appl. Physiol.* 73: 486–492, 1992.
326. Slot, J. W., H. J. Geuze, S. Gigengack, D. E. James, and G. E. Lienhard. Translocation of the glucose transporter GLUT4 in cardiac myocytes of the rat. *Proc. Natl. Acad. Sci. U. S. A.* 88: 7815–7819, 1991.
327. Slot, J. W., H. J. Geuze, S. Gigengack, G. E. Lienhard, and D. E. James. Immuno-localization of the insulin regulatable glucose transporter in brown adipose tissue of the rat. *J. Cell Biol.* 113: 123–135, 1991.
328. Slot, J. W., R. Moxley, S. Geuze, and D. E. James. No evidence for expression of the insulin-regulatable glucose transporter in endothelial cells. *Nature* 346: 369–371, 1990.
329. Sonne, B., K. Mikines, and H. Galbo. Glucose turnover in 48-hour-fasted running rats. *Am. J. Physiol.* 252 (*Regulatory Integrative Comp. Physiol.* 21): R587–R593, 1987.
330. Sowell, M. O., K. P. Boggs, K. A. Robinson, S. L. Dutton, and M. G. Buse. Effects of insulin and phospholipase C in control and denervated rat skeletal muscle. *Am. J. Physiol.* 260 (*Endocrinol. Metab.* 23): E247–E256, 1991.
331. Standaert, M., R. Farese, D. Cooper, and R. Pollet. Insulin-induced glycerolipid mediators and the stimulation of glucose transport in BC3H-1 Myocytes. *J. Biol. Chem.* 263: 8696–8705, 1988.
332. Stanley, W., E. Gertz, J. Wisneski, R. Neese, D. Morris, and G. Brooks. Lactate extraction during net lactate release in legs of humans during exercise. *J. Appl. Physiol.* 60: 1116–1120, 1986.
333. Stein, T., R. Hoyt, M. O'Toole, M. Leskiw, M. Schluter, R. Wolfe, and W. D. Hiller. Protein and energy metabolism during prolonged exercise in trained athletes. *Int. J. Sports Med.* 10: 311–316, 1989.
334. Sternlicht, E., R. Barnard, and G. Grimditch. Mechanism of insulin action on glucose transport in rat skeletal muscle. *Am. J. Physiol.* 254 (*Endocrinol. Metab.* 17): E633–E638, 1988.
335. Sternlicht, E., R. Barnard, and G. Grimditch. Exercise and insulin stimulate skeletal muscle glucose transport through different mechanisms. *Am. J. Physiol.* 256 (*Endocrinol. Metab.* 19): E227–E230, 1989.
336. Storlien, L., D. James, K. Burleigh, D. Chisholm, and E. Kraegen. Fat feeding causes widespread in vivo insulin resistance, decreased energy expenditure and obesity in rats. *Am. J. Physiol.* 251 (*Endocrinol. Metab.* 14): E576–E583, 1986.
337. Storlien, L., E. Kraegen, D. Chisholm, G. Ford, D. Bruce, and W. Pascoe. Fish oil prevents insulin resistance induced by high-fat feeding in rats. *Science* 237: 885–888, 1987.
338. Storlien, L. H., A. B. Jenkins, D. J. Chisholm, W. S. Pascoe, S. Khouri, and E. W. Kraegen. Influence of dietary fat composition on development of insulin resistance in rats: relationship to muscle triglyceride and ω-3 fatty acids in muscle phospholipid. *Diabetes* 40: 280–289, 1991.
339. Stuart, C., R. Shangraw, M. Prince, E. Peters, and R. Wolfe. Bed-rest-induced insulin resistance occurs primarily in muscle. *Metabolism* 37: 802–806, 1988.
340. Suzuki, K., and T. Kono. Evidence that insulin causes translocation of glucose transport activity to the plasma membrane from an intracellular storage site. *Proc. Natl. Acad. Sci. U. S. A.* 77: 2542–2545, 1980.
341. Tan, M., and A. Bonen. Effect of exercise training on insulin binding and glucose metabolism in mouse soleus muscle. *Can. J. Physiol. Pharmacol.* 65: 2231–2234, 1987.

342. Tanti, J., N. Rochet, T. Grémeaux, E. vanObberghen, and Y. LeMarchand-Brustel. Insulin-stimulated glucose transport in muscle. *Biochem. J.* 258: 141–146, 1989.
343. Thorens, B., M. Charron, and H. Lodish. Molecular physiology of glucose transporters. *Diabetes Care* 13: 209–218, 1990.
344. Treadway, J., D. James, E. Burcel, and N. Ruderman. Effect of exercise on insulin receptor binding and kinase activity in skeletal muscle. *Am. J. Physiol.* 256 (*Endocrinol. Metab.* 19): E138–E144, 1989.
345. Turcotte, L. P., B. Kiens, and E. A. Richter. Saturation kinetics of palmitate uptake in perfused skeletal muscle. *FEBS Lett.* 279: 327–329, 1992.
346. Turcotte, L. P., E. A. Richter, and B. Kiens. Increased plasma FFA uptake and oxidation during prolonged exercise in trained vs. untrained humans. *Am. J. Physiol.* 262 (*Endocrinol. Metab.* 25): E791–E799, 1992.
347. Turinsky, J. Glucose and amino acid uptake by exercising muscles in vivo: effect of insulin, fiber population, and denervation. *Endocrinology* 121: 528–535, 1987.
348. Turinsky, J. Dynamics of insulin resistance in denervated slow and fast muscles in vivo. *Am. J. Physiol.* 252 (*Regulatory Integrative Comp. Physiol.* 2): R531-R537, 1987.
349. Valant, P., and D. Erlij. K^+-stimulated sugar uptake in skeletal muscle: role of cytoplasmic Ca^{++}. *Am. J. Physiol.* 245 (*Cell Physiol.* 14): C125–C132, 1983.
350. Vannucci, S. J., H. Nishimura, S. Satoh, S. W. Cushman, G. D. Holman, and I. A. Simpson. Cell surface accessibility of GLUT4 glucose transporters in insulin-stimulated rat adipose cells. *Biochem. J.* 288: 325–330, 1992.
351. Vergauen, L., P. Hespel, and E. A. Richter. Adenosine receptors mediate synergistic stimulation of glucose uptake and transport by insulin and by contractions in rat skeletal muscle. *J. Clin. Invest.* 93: 974–981, 1994.
352. Verhey, K. J., and M. J. Birnbaum. A Leu-Leu sequence is essential for COOH-terminal targetting signal of GLUT4 glucose transporter in fibroblasts. *J. Biol. Chem.* 269: 2353–2356, 1994.
353. Vissing, J., T. Ohkuwa, T. Ploug, and H. Galbo. Effect of prior immobilization on muscular glucose clearance in resting and running rats. *Am. J. Physiol.* 255 (*Endocrinol. Metab.* 18): E456–E462, 1988.
354. Vranic, M., R. Kawamori, S. Pek, N. Kovacevic, and G. A. Wrenshall. The essentiallity of insulin and the role of glucagon in regulating glucose utilization and production during strenuous exercise in dogs. *J. Clin. Invest.* 57: 245–256, 1976.
355. Vukovich, M. D., D. L. Costill, M. S. Hickey, S. W. Trappe, K. J. Cole, and W. J. Fink. Effect of fat emulsion infusion and fat feeding on muscle glycogen utilization during cycle exercise. *J. Appl. Physiol.* 75: 1513–1518, 1993.
356. Waddell, I. D., A. G. Zomershoe, and A. Burchell. *Biochem. J.* 286: 173–177, 1992.
357. Wahren, J., P. Felig, G. Ahlborg, and L. Jorfeldt. Glucose metabolism during leg exercise in man. *J. Clin. Invest.* 50: 2715–2725, 1971.
358. Wahren, J., P. Felig, and L. Hagenfeldt. Physical exercise and fuel homeostasis in diabetes mellitus. *Diabetologia* 14: 213–222, 1978.
359. Wahren, J., L. Hagenfeldt, and P. Felig. Splanchnic and leg exchange of glucose, amino acids and free fatty acids during exercise in diabetes mellitus. *J. Clin. Invest.* 55: 1303–1314, 1975.
360. Wake, S. A., J. A. Sowden, L. H. Storlien, D. E. James, P. W. Clark, J. Shine, D. J. Chisholm, and E. W. Kraegen. Effects of exercise training and dietary manipulation on insulin-regulatable glucose-transporter mRNA in rat muscle. *Diabetes* 40: 275–279, 1991.
361. Walaas, S., R. Horn, A. Adler, K. Albert, and O. Walaas. Insulin increases membrane protein kinase activity in rat diaphragm. *FEBS Lett.* 220: 311–318, 1987.
362. Walker, M., G. Fulcher, C. Catalano, G. Petranyi, H. Orskov, and K. G. M. Alberti. Physiological levels of plasma non-esterified fatty acids impair forearm glucose uptake in normal man. *Clin. Sci.* 79: 167–174, 1990.
363. Wallberg-Henriksson, H. Glucose transport into skeletal muscle. Influence of contractile activity, insulin, catecholamines and diabetes mellitus. *Acta Physiol. Scand. Suppl.* 564: 1–80, 1987.
364. Wallberg-Henriksson, H., S. Constable, D. Young, and J. Holloszy. Glucose transport into rat skeletal muscle: interaction between exercise and insulin. *J. Appl. Physiol.* 65: 909–913, 1988.
365. Wallberg-Henriksson, H., and J. Holloszy. Contractile activity increases glucose uptake by muscle in severely diabetic rats. *J. Appl. Physiol.* 57: 1045–1049, 1984.
366. Wallberg-Henriksson, H., and J. Holloszy. Activation of glucose transport in diabetic muscle: responses to contraction and insulin. *Am. J. Physiol.* 249 (*Cell Physiol.* 18): C233–C237, 1985.
367. Wang, C. The D-glucose transporter is tissue-specific. *J. Biol. Chem.* 262: 15689–15695, 1987.
368. Wardzala, L. J., and B. Jeanrenaud. Potential mechanism of insulin action on glucose transport in the isolated rat diaphragm—apparent translocation of intracellular transport units to the plasma membrane. *J. Biol. Chem.* 256: 7090–7093, 1981.
369. Wasserman, D., D. Lacy, R. Goldstein, P. Williams, and A. Cherrington. Exercise-induced fall in insulin and increase in fat metabolism during prolonged muscular work. *Diabetes* 38: 484–490, 1989.
370. Wasserman, D., D. Lacy, D. Green, P. Williams, and A. Cherrington. Dynamics of hepatic lactate and glucose balances during prolonged exercise and recovery in the dog. *J. Appl. Physiol.* 63: 2411–2417, 1987.
371. Wasserman, D. H., and A. D. Cherrington. Hepatic fuel metabolism during muscular work: role and regulation. *Am. J. Physiol.* 260 (*Endocrinol. Metab.* 23): E811–E824, 1991.
372. Wasserman, D. H., R. J. Geer, D. E. Rice, D. Bracy, P. J. Flakoll, L. L. Brown, J. O. Hill, and N. N. Abumrad. Interaction of exercise and insulin action in humans. *Am. J. Physiol.* 260 (*Endocrinol. Metab.* 29): E37–E45, 1991.
373. Wasserman, D. H., H. Lavina, A. Lickley, and M. Vranic. Role of β-adrenergic mechanisms during exercise in poorly controlled diabetes. *J. Appl. Physiol.* 59: 1282–1289, 1985.
374. Wasserman, D. H., T. Mohr, P. Kelly, D. B. Lacy, and D. Bracy. Impact of insulin deficiency on glucose fluxes and muscle glucose metabolism during exercise. *Diabetes* 41: 1229–1238, 1992.
375. Webster, B., S. Vigna, and T. Paquette. Acute exercise, epinephrine and diabetes enhance insulin binding to skeletal muscle. *Am. J. Physiol.* 250 (*Endocrinol. Metab.* 13): E186–E197, 1900.
376. White, M. F., and C. R. Kahn. The insulin signaling system. *J. Biol. Chem.* 269: 1–4, 1994.
377. Widrick, J. J., D. L. Costill, G. K. McConnel, D. E. Anderson, D. R. Pearson, and J. J. Zachweieja. Time course of glycogen accumulation after eccentric exercise. *J. Appl. Physiol.* 72: 1999–2004, 1992.

378. Wilson, C. M., and S. W. Cushman. Insulin stimulation of glucose transport activity in rat skeletal muscle: increase in cell surface GLUT4 assessed by photolabelling. *Biochem. J.* 299: 755–759, 1994.
379. Yale, J., L. Leiter, and E. Marliss. Metabolic responses to intense exercise in lean and obese subjects. *J. Clin. Endocrinol. Metab.* 68: 438–445, 1989.
380. Yamatani, K., Z. Q. Shi, A. Giacca, R. Gupta, S. Fisher, H. Lavina, A. Lickley, and M. Vranic. Role of FFA-glucose cycle in glucoregulation during exercise in total absence of insulin. *Am. J. Physiol.* 263 (*Endocrinol. Metab.* 26): E646–E653, 1992.
381. Yang, Y., I. Hope, M. Ader, and R. Bergman. Insulin transport across capillaries is rate limiting for insulin action in dogs. *J. Clin. Invest.* 84: 1620–1628, 1989.
382. Yki-Järvinen, H., D. Mott, A. Young, K. Stone, and C. Bogardus. Regulation of glycogen synthase and phosphorylase activities by glucose and insulin in human skeletal muscle. *J. Clin. Invest.* 80: 95–100, 1987.
383. Yki-Järvinen, H., A. Young, C. Lamkin, and J. Foley. Kinetics of glucose disposal in whole body and across the forearm in man. *J. Clin. Invest.* 79: 1713–1719, 1987.
384. Youn, J. H., E. A. Gulve, and J. O. Holloszy. Calcium stimulates glucose transport in skeletal muscle by a pathway independent of contraction. *Am. J. Physiol.* 260 (*Cell Physiol.* 29): C555–C561, 1991.
385. Young, D., H. Wallberg-Henriksson, and J. Cranshaw. Effect of catecholamines on glucose uptake and glycogenolysis in rat skeletal muscle. *Am. J. Physiol.* 248 (*Cell Physiol.* 17): C406–C409, 1985.
386. Young, D., H. Wallberg-Henriksson, M. Sleeper, and J. Holloszy. Reversal of the exercise-induced increase in muscle permeability to glucose. *Am. J. Physiol.* 253 (*Endocrinol. Metab.* 16): E331–E335, 1987.
387. Young, J., S. Garthwaite, J. Bryan, L. Cartier, and J. Holloszy. Carbohydrate feeding speeds reversal of enhanced glucose uptake in muscle after exercise. *Am. J. Physiol.* 245 (*Regulatory Integrative Comp. Physiol.* 14): R684–R688, 1983.
388. Young, J. C., T. G. Kurowski, A. M. Maurice, R. Nesher, and N. B. Ruderman. Polymyxin B inhibits contraction stimulated glucose uptake in rat skeletal muscle. *J. Appl. Physiol.* 70: 1650–1654, 1991.
389. Zierath, J. R., D. Galuska, A. Thörne, L. Nolte, J. Smedegaard Kristensen, and H. Wallberg-Henriksson. Elevated oleate levels have no effect on insulin-stimulated glucose transport in human skeletal muscle. *Acta Physiol. Scand.* 146 (Suppl. 608): 88, 1992.
390. Zinker, B. A., D. B. Lacy, D. Bracy, J. Jacobs, and D. H. Wasserman. Regulation of glucose uptake and metabolism by working muscle. *Diabetes* 42: 956–965, 1993.
391. Zinker, B. A., D. B. Lacy, D. P. Bracy, and D. H. Wasserman. Role of glucose and insulin loads to the exercising limb in increasing glucose uptake and metabolism. *J. Appl. Physiol.* 74: 2915–2921, 1993.
392. Zinman, B., E. Marliss, A. Hanna, H. Minuk, and M. Vranic. Exercise in diabetic man: glucose turnover and free insulin responses after glycemic normalization with intravenous insulin. *Can. J. Physiol. Pharmacol.* 60: 1236–1240, 1982.
393. Zorzano, A., T. Balon, L. Garetto, M. Goodman, and N. Ruderman. Muscle alpha-aminoisobutyric acid transport after exercise: enhanced stimulation by insulin. *Am. J. Physiol.* 248 (*Endocrinol. Metab.* 11): E546–E552, 1985.
394. Zorzano, A., T. Balon, M. Goodman, and N. Ruderman. Glycogen depletion and increased insulin sensitivity and responsiveness in muscle after exercise. *Am. J. Physiol.* 251 (*Endocrinol. Metab.* 14): E664–E669, 1986.
395. Zorzano, A., T. Balon, M. Goodman, and N. Ruderman. Additive effects of prior exercise and insulin on glucose and AIB uptake by rat muscle. *Am. J. Physiol.* 251 (*Endocrinol. Metab.* 14): E21–E26, 1986.
396. Zorzano, A., W. Wilkinson, N. Kotliar, G. Thoidis, and B. Wadzinkski. Insulin-regulated glucose uptake in rat adipocytes is mediated by two transporter isoforms present in at least two vesicle populations. *J. Biol. Chem.* 264: 12358–12663, 1989.
397. Ørskov, L., O. Schmitz, J. O. Jørgensen, J. Arnfred, N. Abildgaard, J. Christiansen, K. G. M. Alberti, and H. Ørskov. Influence of growth hormone on glucose-induced glucose uptake in normal men as assessed by the hyperglycemic clamp technique. *J. Clin. Endocrinol. Metab.* 68: 276–283, 1989.

21. Lipid metabolism in muscle

GER J. VAN DER VUSSE
ROBERT S. RENEMAN | *Departments of Physiology and Motion Sciences, Cardiovascular Research Institute Maastricht, University of Limburg, Maastricht, The Netherlands*

CHAPTER CONTENTS

SKELETAL MUSCLES are able to use fatty acids, carbohydrates, ketone bodies, and some amino acids as substrates to fulfil their energy requirements during rest and exercise (92, 120, 131, 278). Under normal conditions fatty acids and glucose are quantitatively the most important oxidizable substrates for muscle cells. The relative contribution of these substrates to aerobic energy conversion depends on a variety of factors, including the type of skeletal muscle cell, the intensity and duration of exercise, the training status, the availability of extra- and intracellular substrates, diet, and blood concentration of regulatory hormones.

Although our knowledge of fatty acid metabolism sin skeletal muscles has expanded considerably during the past three decades, the significance of fat as energy-delivering substrate to exercising muscles has been appreciated since the turn of the century. Pioneering studies of Chaveau and co-workers, reviewed in detail by Zierler (319), showed that in addition to carbohydrate, body fat furnishes the energy required to perform muscular activity. Initially, it was uncertain whether fat was used directly or after conversion to carbohydrates. Krogh and Lindhard (158) provided evidence for direct utilization of fat in energy-converting processes. As pointed out in an extensive review by Gollnick and Saltin (96) of the role of lipids as fuel for muscle cells during exercise, at the end of the nineteenth century explorers such as Nansen already realized that fat is an essential component in the diet for both men and animals performing prolonged strenuous exercise. A host of experimental findings has confirmed the notion that lipids are substrates for resting and exercising muscles (120).

Among the lipids present in the human body, fatty acids are the most important metabolic fuel. (Throughout this chapter the term "fatty acids" refers to fatty acids present in the unesterified form.) Skeletal muscle cells can derive fatty acids from both extracellular and intracellular sources (98, 278). Extracellular sources are fatty acids complexed to albumin or present in the esterified form as triacylglycerols in the core of circulating lipoproteins. Triacylglycerols accumulated in lipid droplets in the cytoplasm of skeletal muscle fibers represent the major intracellular source of fatty acids (98). Neutral fat in adipocytes, interlaced between muscle cells, may also serve as source of fatty acids. In general, the triacylglycerol content in muscle contains twice as much energy as the muscle carbohydrate pool (26). The bulk of fat, however, is sequestered in adipose tissue localized in various parts of the body.

In this chapter we review the utilization of fatty acids as oxidizable substrates in skeletal muscle. In particular, the supply, uptake, and intracellular fate of fatty acids (i.e., storage in intramuscular triacylglycerols and subsequent release of fatty acid residues from the endogenous lipid pool) and mitochondrial and peroxisomal oxidation will be discussed. The effect of intensity and duration of exercise and the influence of training and diet on skeletal muscle lipid metabolism will be addressed as well. Attention will be paid to differences in lipid handling between various muscle fiber types. Finally, some aspects of deficiencies of fatty acid oxidation in human skeletal muscles will be reviewed.

SUPPLY AND CELLULAR UPTAKE OF LIPIDS IN SKELETAL MUSCLES

Because the capacity of muscle fibers to synthesize fatty acids de novo is limited (232), the bulk of fatty acids has to be supplied from extracellular sources. In the human body, fat is made available to the skeletal muscle cells via blood either as fatty acids bound to albumin or as triacylglycerols that form the lipid core of circulating very-low-density lipoprotein (VLDL) and chylomicrons. Albumin-bound fatty acids are released from adipocytes when the body is in need of these substrates (36, 118, 120). Part of the circulating fatty acids is derived from lipoprotein-triacylglycerols after hydrolysis by lipoprotein lipase (LPL) (see later under Hydrolysis of Circulating Triacylglycerols by Lipoprotein).

We have attempted to calculate roughly the amount of fatty acids supplied to muscle tissue in rest and during submaximal exercise. Assuming in resting conditions a blood flow of 0.05 ml/g skeletal muscle per minute, an arterial plasma fatty acid concentration of 0.4 μmol/ml and a hematocrit of 40%, arterial fatty acid supply will be on the order of 12 nmol $\cdot$ g^{-1} $\cdot$ min^{-1}. Owen and Reichard (204) calculated that resting human muscle utilizes ~5 nmol fatty acids $\cdot$ g^{-1} $\cdot$ min^{-1}, indicating that in rest less than half of the amount of fatty acids supplied will be extracted during one transit of blood through the muscular capillaries. During strenuous exercise, the supply of albumin-bound fatty acids to muscle tissue will increase to about 600–900 nmol $\cdot$ g^{-1} $\cdot$ min^{-1}. Hagenfeldt and colleagues (108) demonstrated that the uptake of fatty acids by exercising muscles was on the order of 10%–20% of the amount supplied. The arterial supply of plasma triacylglycerol–fatty acids to muscle tissue exceeds by far the supply of fatty acids bound to albumin. Calculations indicate that on the order of 90 and 1800–2700 nmol triacylglycerol–fatty acids are delivered to resting and working skeletal muscles per gram and per minute, respectively. As indicated later under Circulating Lipoprotein-triacylglycerols as Potential Source of Fatty Acids during Exercise, only a minor part of the fatty acid residues present in circulating triacylglycerols will be extracted during one single capillary transit of blood.

Albumin-Bound Fatty Acids

After release of fatty acids from adipose tissue, albumin is required to transport the fatty acyl moieties to the muscles via blood because of the low solubility of fatty acids in an aqueous medium. Up to eight fatty acid molecules can be accommodated by high-affinity binding sites on the albumin molecule. The nature of the interaction between fatty acids and albumin has been described in detail elsewhere (157). The concentration of albumin in human plasma is ~0.6 mmol/liter, while in normal conditions the fatty acid concentration varies between 0.2 and 1.0 mmol/liter, indicating that under physiological circumstances the fatty acid binding sites on albumin are only partially occupied.

Fatty Acids in Circulating Lipoproteins

Because the vascular endothelium is virtually impermeable for circulating lipoproteins, the fatty acid residues have to be released from the triacylglycerol core before transendothelial transport of fatty acids occurs. Hydrolysis of lipoprotein-triacylglycerol is achieved by LPL. This enzyme is attached to the luminal surface of the endothelial cells (32).

Origin of Lipoprotein Lipase. There is convincing evidence that endothelium-bound LPL is synthesized de novo in the parenchymal cells (32). In muscle tissue, the gene expressing LPL appears to be exclusively located in the myocytes (37). After synthesis as an inactive proenzyme in the rough endoplasmic reticulum, the protein is glycosylated, which involves the transfer of a lipid-linked oligosaccharide to specific arginine residues of the proenzyme (32). Dimers of the protein are transported via vesicles to the *cis*-Golgi network inside the myocyte, where the proenzyme is further processed. The fully active LPL is stored in the trans-Golgi system. A proportion of the secretable LPL is subsequently packed in secretory vesicles and transferred through the cytoplasmic space to the sarcolemma. The vesicles fuse with the cellular membrane, and their protein content is released into the interstitial compartment. The enzymes are subsequently transported across the endothelial cells by an incompletely elucidated mechanism. When the vascular side of the endothelium is reached, the enzymes are positioned near the luminal extent of the glycocalyx, a structure that is anchored in the endothelial basement membrane. Attachment to the glycocalyx is achieved by association of the protein with the glucosaminoglycan chain of the heparan sulfate proteoglycans of the glycocalyx. The enzyme exerts its hydrolytic action on circulating triacylglycerols, most likely in the dimer configuration (32). Binding of VLDL and chylomicrons to the endothelium occurs in a specific and saturable way. The two lipid particles compete for the same binding site(s) (56).

Hydrolysis of Circulating Triacylglycerols by Lipoprotein Lipase. VLDL and chylomicrons are the two most important carriers of esterified fatty acyl moieties in blood plasma. Chylomicrons, transported to the vascular compartment from the intestinal cells via the thoracic lymphatic duct, deliver fatty acids from nutrition to the skeletal muscles. VLDLs are synthesized in hepatocytes and secreted into the vascular compartment. In this way excess carbohydrates supplied to the body in carbohydrate-rich meals are converted to lipids and supplied to, among others, skeletal muscle cells.

In addition to the ability to hydrolyze the bonds between fatty acyl residues and glycerol in the triacylglycerol molecule, LPL displays phospholipase A_2 activity (291). Hydrolysis of phospholipids composing the lipid layer that encloses the triacylglycerol core of lipoproteins renders the neutral lipids accessible to the active site of LPL. Neutral to alkaline pH, apoprotein C-II (i.e., a protein embedded in the surface of the lipoprotein particle), and phospholipids are needed for optimal enzymatic activity of LPL (56). Lipoprotein triacylglycerols are hydrolyzed to fatty acids, monoacylglycerol, and free glycerol. Approximately 50% of the fatty acid liberated is immediately extracted by the skeletal muscle cells. The remaining part is bound to plasma albumin and carried away via the bloodstream (20). Glycerol is transported to the liver for de novo synthesis of glucose or for resynthesis of triacylglycerol.

LPL is present in significant quantities in the microvascular compartment of most organs studied so far, with the exception of matured liver (32). Expressed per gram of tissue, the activity of the enzyme is high in adipose tissue, lactating mammary glands, and myocardium. LPL has also been detected in appreciable quantities in skeletal muscles (30, 37, 217, 271, 279).

Detailed studies on LPL activity in various skeletal muscles in rat (162, 271) revealed that in muscles with predominantly red fibers LPL activity is considerably higher than in muscles consisting of glycolytically white fibers. The differences in LPL activity obviously constitute one of many functional adaptations related to the oxidative and glycolytic capacity of red and white muscle fibers (162, 178).

Taking into account that total skeletal muscle mass is on the order of 40% of body mass, it can be inferred that skeletal muscle may play an important role in the removal of lipoprotein triacylglycerols from blood. In fasted rats the total activity of LPL in skeletal muscles exceeds that in adipose tissue (271). Interestingly, fasting lowers the activity of LPL in adipose tissue but does not affect (271) or even increases LPL activity in skeletal muscles (102, 156, 162, 194, 270). This observation suggests that in the fasting state skeletal muscles are more apt to utilize circulating lipoproteins for energy conversion than adipose tissue to extract the triacylglycerol–fatty acids for intracellular storage.

In rats, high-fat diet results in four- to sevenfold higher activity of LPL in red and white skeletal muscles, as compared to animals fed a carbohydrate-rich diet (217). This indicates that the capacity of skeletal muscles to utilize circulating triacylglycerols is governed by the proportion of fat in the diet. This notion is in line with the observation that rats fed a high-fat diet show a greater acceptance and oxidation of fat than animals fed a high-carbohydrate diet (224). Interestingly, changes in diet do not influence the activity of LPL in rat myocardium (217).

In both rat heart and skeletal muscles LPL activity showed diurnal variations. In fed animals, peak activities are on the average 80% higher than the lowest activity. The difference between the highest and the lowest values is considerably greater in fasted than in fed animals. The fluctuation in LPL activity was found to be independent of the light and dark cycle (155). The effect of exercise and training on muscle LPL activity is discussed later under *(1)* Contribution of Intramuscular Triacylglycerols to Fatty Acid Oxidation during Exercise and *(2)* Circulating Lipoproteins as Additional Source of Lipids for Trained Muscles.

The activity of skeletal muscle LPL is under hormonal control. Adrenaline, noradrenaline, and adrenocorticotrophic hormone (ACTH) display a stimulating effect on the total activity of the enzyme in rat skeletal muscles. Insulin exerts a strong negative effect on the activity of the enzyme in both red and white muscles (102, 150). Inhibition of the enzyme is most likely caused by alterations in the rate of synthesis of LPL, because insulin treatment results in decreased myocytal levels of LPL-specific mRNA (72). In thyroidectomized rats, LPL activity is significantly increased in red vastus muscle (142). In the same muscle, hyperthyroidism causes a decrease in LPL activity. The observation that sequestration of radiolabeled fatty acids, derived from circulating triacylglycerols, in red muscle cells is increased in the hyperthyroid animals led the authors to conclude that an inverse relationship exists between LPL activity and circulating triacylglycerol utilization in cases of high levels of plasma thyroid hormones (143).

Compounds like heparin are found to be potent agents to remove LPL from its binding to the glycocalyx (32). In experimental studies, the LPL-releasing property of heparin is used to separate endothelium-bound LPL from enzymes located inside the skeletal muscle cells. With the use of this technique, the activity of LPL in the vasculature of human muscles with predominantly red oxidative fibers, was found to be 15–40 nmol $\cdot$ g^{-1} $\cdot$ min^{-1} (149, 164).

Skeletal Muscle Fatty Acid Uptake

Blood Plasma–Cytoplasmic Fatty Acid Gradient as Driving Force of Fatty Acid Uptake. In skeletal muscle, uptake of fatty acids from the vascular compartment either supplied as albumin–fatty acid complex or released from the triacylglycerol core of circulating lipoproteins occurs via an incompletely elucidated process (96, 291). Fatty acids have to cross the endothelium, the interstitial space, the plasmalemma, and the cytoplasm of the myocytes to reach the intracellular sites of conversion located in mitochondria, sarcoplasmic reticulum, and peroxisomes (Fig. 21.1). It is generally believed that the driving force of muscle fatty acid extraction is the arterial concentration of fatty acids or, more precisely formulated, the concentration gradient of fatty acids from the vascular space to the intramyocytal compartment (107). This notion implies that under normal conditions the fatty acid content in blood should exceed that of muscle tissue. Górski (98) has pointed out that in most studies in which tissue levels of fatty acids were measured, very high values are reported. In dog and man, up to 8600 and 4800 nmol fatty acid per gram muscle mass, respectively, has been monitored (98). Taking into account that under normal conditions blood plasma levels of fatty acids range from 150–1000 nmol/ml, the conclusion has to be drawn that in the above-mentioned studies a fatty acid gradient exists from tissue to blood plasma rather than the reverse. However, measurements of the content of fatty acids in tissue are often marred by technical imperfections, leading to erroneously high levels of fatty acids. This subject has been extensively explored in cardiac tissue (292). It is now generally accepted that in normal cardiac tissue the endogenous level of fatty acids does not exceed 50–150 nmol/g wet weight (291). Recent attempts to monitor the content of fatty acids in dog vastus lateralis muscle with the use of a gas chromatographic technique, taking all precautions to prevent hydrolysis of endogenous esterified lipids during the assay procedure, indicated a value of 31 ± 7 nmol fatty acid per gram wet weight of muscle tissue whereas the arterial plasma concentration of fatty acids in the same dogs amounted to 511 ± 108 nmol/ml (293). When this value of muscular fatty acid levels reflects the true physiological cellular content, the data suggest that also in skeletal muscles a gradient of fatty acids exists from blood plasma to myocyte.

It is rather unlikely that the fatty acid molecules present in muscular tissue are homogeneously distributed over all (sub)cellular compartments. Due to their lipophilic nature, fatty acids readily dissolve in

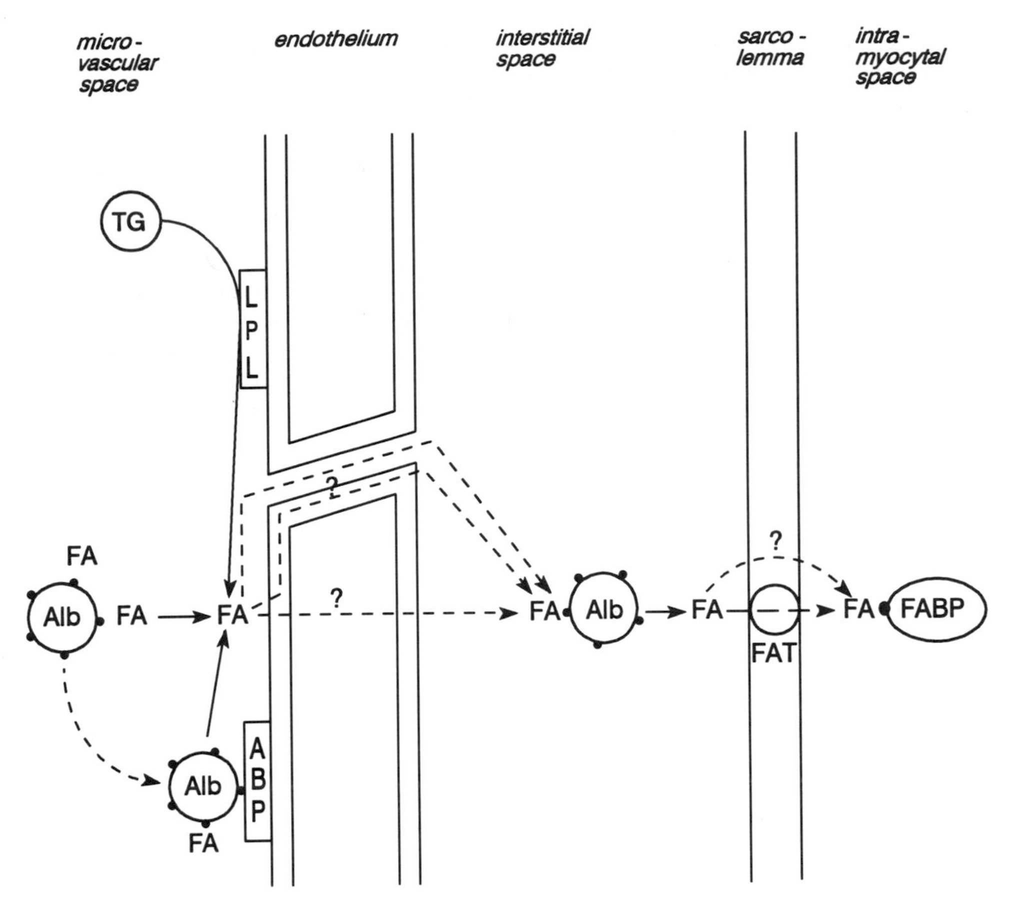

FIG. 21.1. Schematic representation of fatty acid uptake by skeletal muscle cells. TG, triacylglycerols (very-low-density lipoprotein and chylomicrons); LPL, lipoprotein lipase; FA, fatty acids; Alb, albumin; ABP, albumin-binding protein; FAT, fatty acid–transporter; FABP, fatty acid–binding protein; ?, route or mechanism of uptake incompletely understood.

a lipid matrix. In cardiac tissue the bulk of fatty acids is localized in the cellular membranes (301), which is most likely also true for skeletal muscles. This distribution of tissue fatty acids over membranes and the intracellular aqueous space will make the blood plasma–cytoplasmic gradient more steep. The cytoplasmic concentration of fatty acyl moieties is kept at low levels by a rapid conversion of fatty acid to fatty acyl CoA by fatty acyl CoA synthetase (see later under The Action of Fatty Acyl CoA Synthetase).

As extensively discussed by Zierler (319), a large number of studies failed to demonstrate an arterio-venous difference of plasma fatty acids in muscles at rest, suggesting that circulating fatty acids do not serve as oxidizable substrates for resting muscle fibers. However, extraction of fatty acids by muscle cells is most likely masked by a concomitant release of fatty acids from adipocytes, interlaced between muscle fibers, into the same venous blood draining muscles (319). Infusions of radiolabeled fatty acids in pioneering studies of Friedberg and colleagues (83) convincingly demonstrated that at rest human forearm muscles extract plasma fatty acids. Arterio–local venous differences of labeled fatty acids were always found to be positive, even under conditions where the differences between the arterial and local venous concentrations of unlabeled fatty acids were zero (319).

Transendothelial and Interstitial Transport of Fatty Acids. Information on the mechanism by which fatty acids pass the endothelium lining the microvascular compartment in skeletal muscle is scarce. Because most studies on transendothelial fatty acid transport are performed on hearts, the hypothesis discussed below is mainly based on experimental findings in cardiac tissue (291).

Due to the presence of closed fenestrae between the endothelial cells in muscles, the transport of fatty acids from the vascular compartment to the parenchymal cells is more complicated than, for instance, in liver. Diffusion of fatty acids complexed to albumin through the endothelial clefts will contribute very little to overall transendothelial transport because diffusion of proteins through the clefts is hampered (18). Diffusion of fatty acids through the clefts, after release from the albumin–fatty acid complex in the vascular compartment, will also be limited, since the surface area for diffusion is very small and free diffusion of fatty acids will be slowed down by proteins, such as albumin, trapped in the endothelial clefts. Hence, it has been postulated that the bulk of fatty acids is transported across the endothelial cells (Fig. 21.1).

Membranous albumin-binding proteins are thought to be involved in transendothelial transport of albumin and, hence, fatty acids (7, 241). After attachment of the albumin–fatty acid complex to the albumin-binding protein, the fatty acid–carrying albumin can be internalized by the endothelial cell and transported to the abluminal membrane in a vesicle-mediated process. Although the capacity of vesicle-mediated transport is most likely sufficient to replenish the albumin pool in the interstitial compartment, the transport rate is too slow to account for the bulk transfer of fatty acids from the luminal to abluminal site of the endothelial cells (18). This implicates that fatty acids are released from the albumin carrier prior to transendothelial transport. Hypothetical binding sites for albumin on the luminal endothelial cell membrane are supposed to accelerate the release of fatty acids from the albumin–fatty acid complex (291). Especially under conditions of high blood flow rate, when capillary transit time is short, the apparent dissociation rate of fatty acids from albumin might be rate limiting in the overall uptake rate of fatty acids by cardiac tissue (291). Whether the liberation of fatty acids from circulating albumin poses also a constraint on skeletal muscle fatty acid utilization warrants detailed analysis, because the inverse relation between fatty acid extraction fraction and muscular blood flow during exercise (115) suggests that the rate-limiting step in overall fatty acid might be localized in the microvascular compartment.

Lateral diffusion of fatty acids through the cell membrane from the vascular site of delivery to the interstitial space has been proposed as a mechanism of transendothelial fatty acid transport (249). However, calculations indicate that the contribution of this kind of transport to the overall transendothelial trafficking of fatty acids is minor (18). The most likely transport route for fatty acids is diffusion through the endothelial cytoplasmic space from the luminal to abluminal membrane, either as unbound fatty acids or complexed to specific endothelial fatty acid–binding proteins (FABP).

The presence of physiologically significant concentrations of FABP in the cytoplasm of muscle endothelial cells, however, is a matter of continuous debate. In cardiac endothelium, several investigators have reported the presence of a substantial amount of FABP, ranging from 8–26 μg/mg cytosolic protein (80, 209). These findings could not be confirmed by studies performed in our laboratory using sensitive and specific biochemical, molecular biological, and immunohistochemical techniques (163, 294). Only minute amounts of FABP—that is, on the order of 3–8 ng/mg of tissue protein—could be detected in endothelial cells. The latter observation supports the hypothesis that most fatty acids diffuse through the endothelial cytoplasmic space as free, non–protein bound molecules. The very short diffusion distance in the endothelial cell from luminal to abluminal membrane (i.e., 0.2–0.5 μm) makes the latter transport mechanism physically possible.

Albumin present in the interstitial compartment most likely acts as carrier for fatty acids crossing the space between endothelial and muscle cells (291).

Transsarcolemmal Transport of Fatty Acids. The sarcolemma of skeletal muscle cells represents the last membrane barrier for fatty acids on their way to the cell interior (Fig. 21.1). In cardiac myocytes transmembrane fatty acid transport has been proposed to be partially mediated by a membranous 40 kDa fatty acid–binding protein (267). Preliminary observations (286) suggest that this 40 kDa protein is also present in skeletal muscle. Recent studies (111) have identified an 88 kDa protein in the plasmalemma of adipocytes with putative fatty acid transporting properties. This protein has been named FAT. Molecular biological investigations disclosed the presence of mRNA of the protein in a variety of tissues, including skeletal muscle, which suggests that FAT is also localized in the sarcolemma of muscle cells (2). The precise biological function and the mechanism of action of this protein are incompletely understood. If we assume a crucial role for the 88 kDa protein in transsarcolemmal fatty acid transport, it may be part of a functional membrane-spanning complex constituting a vectorial transport system for fatty acid molecules (2). Alternatively, FAT might play a role in sequestering fatty acids within hydrophobic segments of the extracellular part of the protein, giving rise to high fatty acid levels on the interstitial side of the sarcolemma. This hypothetical property would create a steeper gradient of fatty acids across the membrane and stimulate the cellular uptake of fatty acid moieties (2). The observation that fatty acid uptake in rat and human skeletal muscle shows saturation kinetics might favor the notion that membrane carriers are instrumental in fatty acid transport (147, 285). Beside protein-mediated transport, a considerable part of fatty acids is thought to pass cellular membranes without involvement of specific membranous proteins, because of the lipophilic nature of fatty acids.

Transport of Fatty Acids Inside the Muscle Cell. Cytoplasmic FABP are likely candidates to transfer fatty acids from the sarcolemma to the intracellular sites of conversion, such as mitochondria, sarcoplasmic reticulum, and peroxisomes (Fig. 21.1). While experimental evidence for an intracellular transport role of FABP is circumstantial, recent calculations strongly suggest that sarcoplasmic FABP is required to facilitate the transport of the bulk of fatty acids from the sarcolemma through the interior of the muscle cell (301). When the flux of fatty acids exceeds ~40 nmol/g wet weight of tissue per minute for a diffusional distance of 1.5 μm, free diffusion of fatty acids is too low to account for the transport of all fatty acid moieties in the cytoplasm of the muscle cell. The intracellular presence of FABP will enhance the aqueous solubility of fatty acids more than 700-fold. The maximal diffusion capacity of fatty acids will be increased ~17-fold by the concentration of FABP observed in oxidative muscle fibers, indicating that the transsarcoplasmic fatty acid transport capacity is most likely not rate limiting in overall intramuscular fatty acid utilization (301). Due to the specific kinetic properties of FABP, the whole FABP–fatty acid complex diffuses through the cytoplasmic space rather than fatty acids jumping from one FABP to another (301).

The dissociation of fatty acids from FABP appears to be pH sensitive; that is, the rate of dissociation increases with decreasing pH (152). This particular property of FABP might be important for the regulation of the supply of fatty acids to the mitochondria, because it is well known that under conditions such as exercise, in which the need for fatty acids in muscle cells increases, cytoplasmic pH drops. Moreover, self-aggregation of the FABP molecule in the vicinity of the mitochondrial membrane has been thought to play an essential role in regulating mitochondrial fatty acid utilization and, hence, the energy made available to the cardiac muscle cell (81). It remains to be established whether skeletal muscle FABP is also involved in such a fine tuning of cellular fatty acid handling and energy conversion.

FABP is a 15 kDa protein ubiquitously present in the cytoplasm of most tissues examined (17, 91, 182, 295, 297). At least ten different members of the FABP family have been identified thus far (90, 295). The family also includes the retinol and retinoic acid-binding proteins, gastrotropin, and mammary-derived growth inhibitor. Molecular biological studies have revealed that heart and skeletal muscle type FABP are identical (45, 116, 211, 214). This notion is supported by immunohistochemical studies (304) showing a high cross-reactivity between heart and skeletal muscles towards antibodies raised against cardiac FABP.

FABP appears to be abundantly present in cardiac myocytes. Although the absolute values reported for the level of FABP in cardiac tissue show considerable variation (Table 21.1), accurate and sensitive enzyme-linked immunosorbent assay (ELISA) techniques have revealed that the amount of FABP in rat heart is on the order of 500–750 μg/g wet weight of tissue, which corresponds with ~15–20 μg/mg soluble cytosolic protein (289, 300). On a molar basis, ~5% of all soluble cytoplasmic proteins in cardiomyocytes appears to be FABP. In general, the FABP content in skeletal muscle cells is lower than in heart (297). Slow-twitch soleus muscle and fast-twitch red fibers (vastus lateralis red muscle) contain a higher amount of FABP than fast-twitch white fibers (vastus lateralis white muscle) (Table 21.1). These data suggest a functional relationship between the fatty acid–binding capacity and the degree of oxidative energy metabolism in the muscle fiber (38, 212, 213, 297, 300). In this respect it is also note-

TABLE 21.1. *The Content of FABP in Rat Heart and Skeletal Muscles**

Tissue	FABP, μg/g wet weight	References
Heart	500–2200	(55, 179, 208, 289, 300)
Gastrocnemius (red)	280	(55)
Soleus	250–1240	(55, 208, 300)
Diaphragm	246–590	(55, 179, 208, 289, 300)
Vastus lateralis (red)	222–680	(179, 300)
Extensor digitorum longus	53–840	(55, 208, 289, 300)
Gastrocnemius (white)	30	(55, 300)
Vastus lateralis (white)	13–132	(179, 300)

*The assumption was made that heart and skeletal muscles contain 40 mg soluble cytosolic protein per gram of wet weight tissue.

worthy that insect flight muscles, being among the most active muscles known and heavily depending on fatty acid oxidation for energy conversion, contain very large amounts of FABP (113, 290). Human heart and skeletal muscles contain generally lower amounts of FABP than comparable types of tissue in rat (208, 209).

The cytoplasmic fatty acid–binding protein possesses a clam-like tertiary structure formed by two β-sheets (17, 296). The three-dimensional configuration creates one ligand-binding site that can accommodate one or two fatty acid molecules. Muscle-type FABP is thought to bind maximally one fatty acid moiety. The apparent dissociation constant (K_d) is on the order of 10^{-7}–10^{-6} M, which is significantly less than that of the highest affinity site of albumin for fatty acids (i.e., an apparent K_d of 10^{-8} M) (291). The affinity of FABP for saturated fatty acids is somewhat less than that for unsaturated fatty acids (17).

The regulation of the amount of FABP in the cytoplasm of skeletal muscle cells is not yet completely elucidated. Hormonal control mechanisms have to be considered because in female rats testosterone treatment increased the FABP content in soleus and in extensor digitorum longus muscles (289). Physical training of the animals failed to increase the soleus muscle content of FABP (288, 289). In contrast, exercise training of rats 5 and 13 months of age induced an ~80% increase in the FABP content of plantaris muscle (63). However, no training effect on muscle FABP was observed in old animals (25 months of age) (298). In rat, chronic low-frequency electrostimulation of the fast-twitch tibialis anterior muscle significantly increased the cytoplasmic FABP content (145). It is interesting to note that the latter change was found to be accompanied by a shift from white to red characteristics of the muscle fibers.

Under conditions such as high-fat diets, diabetes, and fasting, in which skeletal muscle fatty acid oxidation has been shown to be enhanced, the muscle content of FABP increased only in diabetic and fasting rats (38), not in animals fed diets containing up to 40 en% fat (298). Carey and colleagues (38) observed that at least two mechanisms of control can be employed in the regulation of muscular FABP expression: one at the level of transcription, as was found during fasting, and one at the level of mRNA stability, as might occur in diabetic animals.

The majority of mammalian cells contain in addition to FABP a distinct 10 kDa protein with a relatively high affinity for long-chain fatty acyl CoA (154). The cardiac content of this acyl CoA–binding protein (ACBP) is ~25 times lower than that of FABP. The same holds most likely also for skeletal muscles (154, 176). Although the precise physiological role of ACBP is still unresolved, the protein is thought to play a specific role in transporting fatty acyl CoA moieties from their site of production (i.e., the mitochondrial outer membrane, sarcoplasmic reticulum, and peroxisomes) to intracellular sites of conversion. It remains to be established to what extent ACBP is involved in governing the rate of fatty acid utilization in skeletal muscle fibers.

FATTY ACID METABOLISM IN THE SKELETAL MUSCLE CELL

Inside skeletal muscle cells, the bulk of fatty acids is utilized for oxidative energy conversion in the mitochondrial compartment to generate adenosine triphosphate (ATP). Transport of fatty acid moieties across the mitochondrial inner membrane is mediated by carnitine. A relatively small proportion of fatty acids is oxidized in peroxisomes. Part of the fatty acids extracted from plasma is used to replenish the intracellular lipid pool (i.e., triacylglycerols predominantly stored in cytoplasmic lipid droplets). Fatty acids are also substrates for the synthesis of phospholipids, the important building blocks of cellular membranes.

Activation and Oxidation of Fatty Acids

The Action of Fatty Acyl CoA Synthetase. Prior to intracellular utilization, fatty acids are "activated" (i.e., esterified to coenzyme A). This condensation step is catalyzed by fatty acyl CoA synthetase (Fig. 21.2), present at three distinct intracellular locations. The bulk of the enzyme is attached to the cytoplasmic side of the mitochondrial outer membrane (291). The sarcoplasmic reticulum (SR) and peroxisomes also contain acyl CoA synthetase activity. In contrast to heart, where the specific activity of acyl CoA synthetase in mitochondrial and SR fractions is on the same order of magnitude (61), in rat skeletal muscle the specific activity of the SR enzyme is ~15% that of mitochondria (205). Taking into account the small amount of total SR protein in the skeletal muscle cell, the contribution of the SR acyl CoA synthetase to overall fatty acyl activation is quantitatively of minor importance. The energy required for the formation of the fatty acyl CoA ester is derived from hydrolysis of ATP to adenosine monophosphate (AMP). The apparent affinity constant for fatty acids is ~2–40 μM. The cytoplasmic ratio of acyl CoA to CoA effectively controls the activity of the enzyme. The reaction is inhibited by inorganic phosphate, AMP, and adenosine (104).

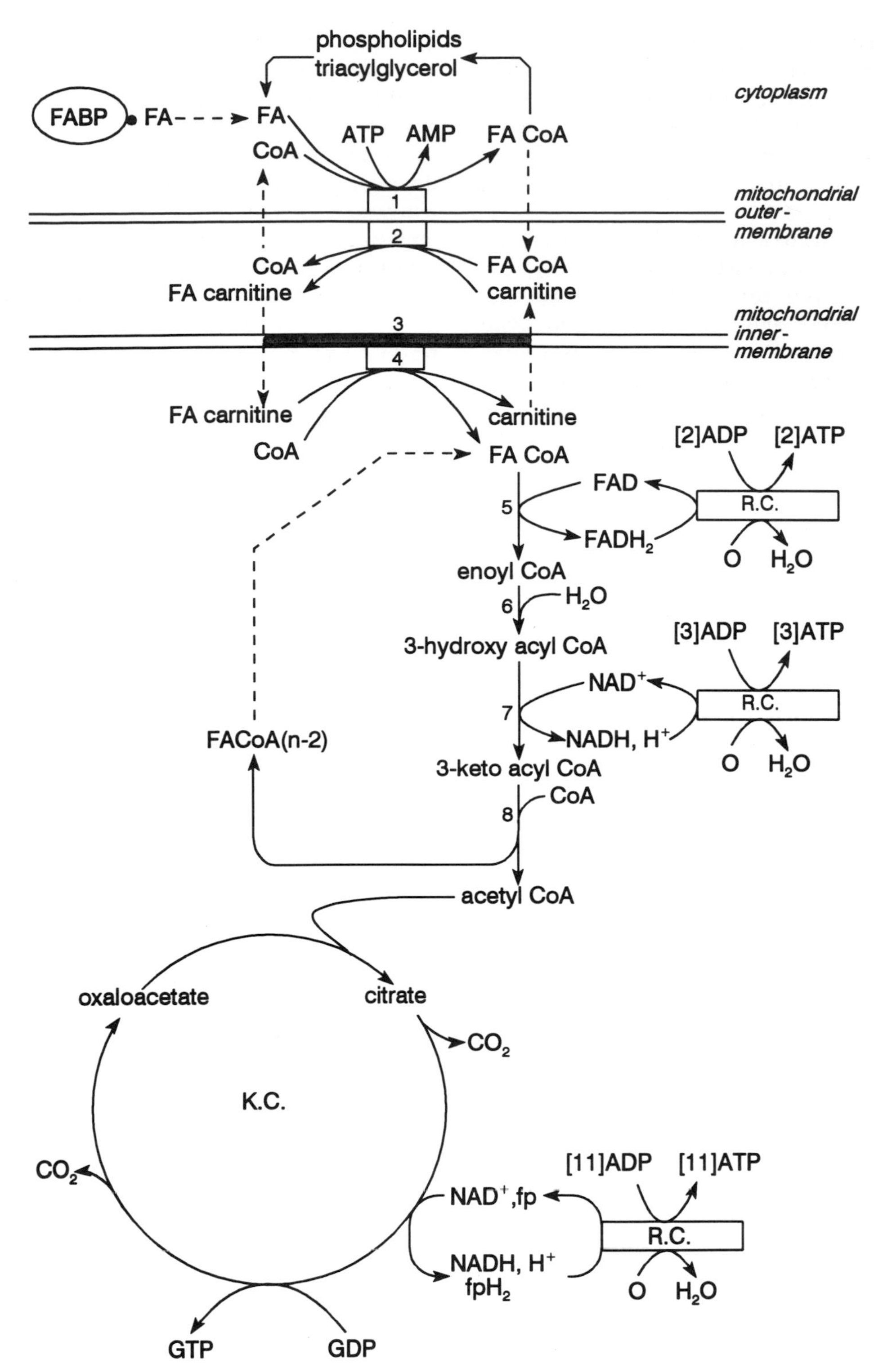

FIG. 21.2. Mitochondrial activation, transport and oxidation of fatty acids. FABP, fatty acid–binding protein; FA, fatty acyl moieties; CoA, coenzyme A; ATP, adenosine triphosphate; AMP, adenosine monophosphate; R.C., respiratory chain; O, oxygen; fp, flavoprotein; K.C., Krebs cycle; GTP, guanosine triphosphate; GDP, guanosine diphosphate; *numbers in brackets*, number of ADP converted to ATP; *1*, fatty acyl CoA synthetase; *2*, carnitine acyl transferase I; *3*, carnitine-acyl carnitine translocase; *4*, carnitine acyl transferase II; *5*, fatty acyl CoA dehydrogenase; *6*, enoyl CoA hydratase; *7*, 3-hydroxyacyl CoA dehydrogenase; *8*, 3-ketothiolase.

Carnitine-Mediated Mitochondrial Uptake of Fatty Acyl Residues. To reach the mitochondrial oxidative machinery, the fatty acyl CoA moiety has to pass the mitochondrial inner membrane (Fig. 21.2). Because this membrane is virtually impermeable for long-chain fatty acyl-CoA esters, nature has designed a specific carnitine-dependent shuttle mechanism to overcome the membrane barrier (33). The acyl CoA ester is converted to acyl carnitine by carnitine acyltransferase I, an enzyme attached to the inner side of the mitochondrial outer membrane (24, 187). Acyl carnitine crosses the mitochondrial inner membrane in a 1:1 exchange with a molecule free carnitine. This specific transport step is controlled by the transmembrane protein carnitine-acyl carnitine translocase. At the inner surface of the mitochondrial inner membrane, carnitine acyltransferase II is located to promote the exchange of the carnitine residue of acyl carnitine with CoA giving yield to intramitochondrial fatty acyl CoA. Although questioned by Zierz and Engel (321), carnitine acyltransferase I and II are most likely distinct enzymes (309).

The enzymes involved in the mitochondrial fatty acid transport pathway display a high specificity for the L-isomer of carnitine. The rate of the carnitine-mediated transport is basically energy independent and is governed mainly by the concentration of the metabolites involved. Because malonyl CoA, an intermediate in the fatty acid biosynthetic pathway, inhibits carnitine acyltransferase I (175, 233), it has been hypothetized that this substance is also involved in the regulation of the overall rate of fatty acid oxidation (31, 33, 175). Winder and colleagues (306) have provided evidence that in rat the muscular content of malonyl CoA significantly decreases during submaximal exercise. The reduced intramuscular levels of the inhibitor of carnitine acyltransferase I is thought to play a role in enhancing fatty acid oxidation during prolonged muscular activity. Consequent to the shift from glucose to fatty acid oxidation, reduced cellular malonyl CoA levels most likely exert a sparing effect on the limited stores of carbohydrates in the body (29). Moreover, increased fatty acyl CoA levels are most likely mitigating the inhibitory effect of malonyl CoA on carnitine acyltransferase I (269). The regulatory role of malonyl CoA will be discussed in more detail later under A Role for Malonyl CoA in Fuel Selection in Skeletal Muscle Cells.

Medium- and short-chain fatty acids can freely diffuse into the mitochondrial matrix, where they are converted to their respective CoA esters. Therefore, these substrates do not require a carnitine-dependent shuttle mechanism to allow for transport across the mitochondrial inner membrane (106).

Intramitochondrial Fatty Acid Oxidation. Inside the mitochondrial matrix, the fatty acid residue of fatty acyl CoA is degradated stepwise to form acetyl CoA via β-oxidation (Fig. 21.2). The final step in the β-oxidative pathway is cleavage of the end-standing two-carbon fragment connected to the CoA residue by 3-ketothiolase. In this reaction step a second CoA molecule is esterified to the carbon atom originally present at position 3. This metabolic conversion gives yield to one molecule of acetyl CoA and a new fatty acyl CoA shortened by two carbon atoms. The shortened fatty acyl CoA, on its turn, serves again as substrate for the enzymes in the β-oxidative pathway.

Acetyl CoA condenses with oxaloacetate, giving rise to the formation of citrate. Citrate is subsequently converted to oxaloacetate in a stepwise decarboxylation process called the tricarboxylic acid (TCA) cycle, or Krebs cycle. The reducing equivalents (hydrogen atoms) released during the conversion of long-chain acyl CoA to acetyl CoA and in the carboxylic acid cycle are transferred via NAD or FAD to the respiratory chain, localized in the mitochondrial inner membrane (305). Finally, the hydrogen atoms react with molecular oxygen and ~50% of the chemical energy liberated by the overall oxidation of fatty acids is used for the conversion of adenosine diphosphate (ADP) to ATP. The remaining part of the energy dissipates as heat.

The overall rate of β-oxidation is most likely regulated by the availability of fatty acyl CoA, the level of malonyl CoA, and the ratios of NAD^+/NADH and oxidized/reduced flavoprotein (248). Because under normal conditions accumulation of fatty acyl derivatives in the overall process of fatty acid activation, mitochondrial transport, and β-oxidation does not readily occur, the conclusion has to be drawn that all steps in the catabolic pathway are mutually very well tuned.

Slow-twitch red fibers are high in enzymes involved in β-oxidation, such as 3-hydroxyacyl-CoA dehydrogenase, while white fibers contain low levels of enzymes catalyzing fatty acid oxidation (167), confirming the observation that oxidative conversion of fatty acids in red muscles significantly exceeds that of white muscle preparations (197).

Peroxisomal Fatty Acid Oxidation. The major role of muscle peroxisomal fatty acid oxidation is the catabolism of fatty acyl moieties that are poorly oxidized by mitochondria, such as very-long-chain fatty acids (160). Peroxisomes or microbodies are spherical, single-membrane organelles ranging in size from ~0.5–1.0 μm (60). Fatty acids are activated to fatty acyl CoA by fatty acyl CoA synthetase, an integral membrane protein, the catalytic site of which faces the cytoplasmic compartment. Although the peroxisomal membrane seems to contain pore-forming proteins allowing free access of newly formed fatty acyl CoA into the cell organelle without the need of a carnitine-mediated transport system like in mitochondria (203), fatty acid–binding proteins are thought to be involved in directing the fatty acid residues from the cytoplasm into the peroxisomal interior (9).

Inside the peroxisomes, fatty acyl CoA is subsequently metabolized in a stepwise fashion comparable with mitochondrial β-oxidation. In contrast to the mitochondrial pathway, degradation in the peroxisomes is incomplete because the enzymes involved are relatively inactive towards medium-chain acyl CoA esters. The latter substances are transferred from the peroxisomes through the cytoplasm to the mitochondria for further processing to acetyl CoA. Unlike mitochondrial β-oxidation, the reducing equivalents derived in the peroxisomal pathway are directly transferred to molecular oxygen to yield H_2O_2. This biologically active oxygen derivative is inactivated by catalase inside the peroxisomal matrix.

In rat quadriceps muscle homogenates, the contribution of peroxisomal fatty acid utilization to overall oxidation, as measured under optimal in vitro conditions, was found to be ~15% (299). Extrapolation to the in vivo situation suggests that in skeletal muscle, in contrast to liver, only a relatively minor proportion of fatty acids is oxidized in the peroxisomal pathway.

It is of interest to note that mitochondria contain a second carnitine-dependent transferase-translocase system that displays specificity to short-chain acyl and acetyl CoA (24). This transport system might be involved in the transfer of peroxisomal-generated fatty acyl CoA intermediates from the cytoplasm into the mitochondrial matrix and in regulation of the overall fatty oxidation rate by modulating the availability of free CoA, required for the formation of fatty acyl CoA esters (24).

Intramuscular Triacylglycerols

Although the intramuscular triacylglycerol content is relatively small compared with the total-body triacylglycerol pool, muscle neutral lipids constitute quantitatively an important source of oxidizable substrates during prolonged, submaximal exercise (see later under Contribution of Intramuscular Triacylglycerols to Fatty Acid Oxidation during Exercise). Inside the skeletal muscle fibers, triacylglycerols are stored in lipid droplets in close vicinity to mitochondria. Muscular triacylglycerols are also present in adipocytes, which are interlaced between the muscle cells (250).

Incorporation of Fatty Acids in the Intramuscular Triacylglycerol Pool. Radiolabeled fatty acid moieties extracted by skeletal muscle cells from the extracellular space are readily incorporated in the cytoplasmic triacylglycerol pool (319). The first step of this metabolic process is the reaction of glycerol 3-phosphate with fatty acyl CoA (Fig. 21.3). Condensation of glycerol 3-phosphate with one fatty acyl CoA molecule yields 1-acylglycerol-3-phosphate. This reaction step, controlled by glycerol-3-phosphate acyltransferase, is followed by a second acylation step (i.e., the formation of phosphatidic acid from 1-acylglycerol-3-phosphate and fatty acyl CoA by catalytic action of 1-acylglycerol-3-phosphate acyltransferase).

Phosphatidic acid is at a crossroad of two important metabolic pathways. It can be converted to 1,2-diacylglycerol by phosphatidic acid phosphatase or used as substrate for the biosynthesis of phospholipids. In heart muscle, phosphatidic acid phosphatase is most likely present at various intracellular loci, since enzymatic activity has been monitored in mitochondrial, microsomal, and cytosolic fractions. It has been hypothesized that the actual activity of the enzyme and, hence, the rate of endogenous triacylglycerol formation is regulated by translocation of the enzyme between the cytosol and intracellular membranes (247).

Triacylglycerol is formed after condensation of 1,2-diacylglycerol with a third molecule of fatty acyl CoA, a reaction step catalyzed by diacylglycerol acyltransferase (Fig. 21.3).

Enzymatic Hydrolysis of Intramuscular Triacylglycerols. When the cellular need of oxidizable substrates increases (see later under Contribution of Intramuscular Triacylglycerols to Fatty Acid Oxidation during Exercise), intramuscular triacylglycerols can be enzymatically hydrolyzed to supply fatty acids (98). Moreover, in both resting and exercising skeletal muscles, the endogenous triacylglycerol pool is subject to a continuous turnover process (319). Both net degradation and triacylglycerol cycling require the presence of an active triacylglycerol lipase.

Three distinct enzymes are involved in complete hydrolysis of triacylglycerol into one glycerol and three fatty acid molecules. Triacylglycerol lipase promotes the hydrolytic removal of the first fatty acyl chain covalently bound to one of the end-standing carbon atoms of the glycerol backbone of triacylglycerol. Diacylglycerol lipase and monoacylglycerol lipase catalyze the removal of the second and third

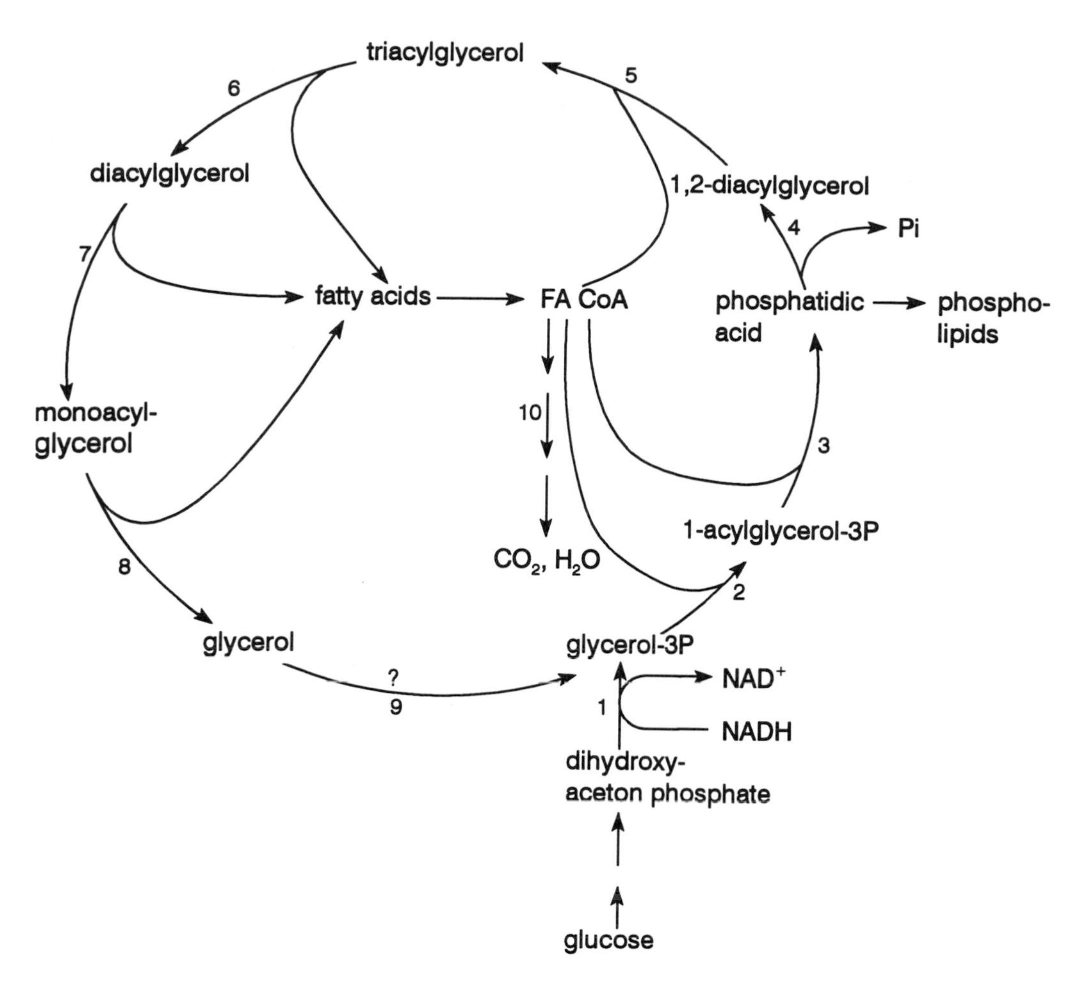

FIG. 21.3. Triacylglycerol–fatty acid cycle in skeletal muscle cells. FA, fatty acyl moieties; CoA, coenzyme A; Pi, inorganic phosphate; *1*, glycerol 3-phosphate dehydrogenase; *2*, glycerol 3-phosphate acyltransferase; *3*, 1-acylglycerol-3-phosphate acyltransferase; *4*, phosphatidic acid phosphatase; *5*, diacylglycerol acyltransferase; *6*, triacylglycerol lipase; *7*, diacylglycerol lipase; *8*, monoacylglycerol lipase; *9*, glycerol kinase; ?, indicates most likely insignificant in skeletal muscle.

fatty acid residues, respectively (Fig. 21.3). The activity of the latter two enzymes, located at the sarcoplasmic reticulum (251, 260), exceeds by far the hydrolytic activity of triacylglycerol lipase, which governs the rate-limiting step in overall triacylglycerol hydrolysis.

Skeletal muscles contain three different types of triacylglycerol lipase with distinct pH optima. Acid, neutral, and alkaline lipases with optimal activities in vitro at pH 5.0, 7.0, and 8.5, respectively, have been identified. Acid lipase is most likely identical to lysosomal lipase. Strohfeldt and Heugel (268) provided convincing evidence that alkaline lipase is identical to LPL, which is located at the luminal membrane of the endothelium as well as inside the myocyte in the Golgi system and transport vesicles. Muscle mainly composed of slow-twitch red fibers displays the highest activity of acid, neutral, and alkaline triacylglycerol lipase (98). In general, the neutral lipase possesses a considerably lower catalytic activity than acid and alkaline lipases in all muscle types studied (98).

It is far from clear which lipase is responsible for triacylglycerol hydrolysis inside the muscle cell. Oscai and co-workers (202) originally suggested that muscular alkaline LPL serves two functions. Attached to the luminal surface of the endothelial membrane, the enzyme catalyzes the release of fatty acids from circulating lipoprotein-triacylglycerols. The proportion of the enzyme residing in the parenchymal cells was thought to be involved in hydrolyzing intramuscular neutral lipids. Various theoretical considerations argue, however, against LPL as a candidate for liberating fatty acids from the intramuscular triacylglycerol pool (98). First, at an intracellular pH of 7.0 for the resting muscle cell and a considerably lower pH during mechanical work, the enzymatic activity of alkaline lipase or LPL is virtually zero. Second, experimental evidence is lacking that the enzyme, localized in the Golgi system and transport vesicles, has free access to the intramuscular triacylglycerol stores. Third, LPL requires apoprotein C-II for maximal activity. This protein is a constituent of the coating of lipoproteins in blood plasma and is absent inside parenchymal cells such as skeletal myocytes.

Nowadays, it is generally agreed that LPL does not play a role of importance in hydrolyzing the intramuscular triacylglycerol pool, but is indispensable for the muscular utilization of circulating triacylglycerols (201). Neutral lipase is presumably the enzyme responsible for intracellular triacylglycerol hydrolysis (Fig. 21.4). In myocardial tissue the enzyme was found to be present, and its activity is most likely under hormonal control (254). In heart, cyclic AMP (cAMP) mediates the lipolytic effects of hormones, such as catecholamines and glucagon (219). Immunological and molecular biological evidence has been provided in favor of the notion that also in skeletal muscle a hormone-sensitive neutral lipase is present (122, 314). Although neutral lipase is a likely candidate for intramuscular triacylglycerol degradation, further studies are required to definitely prove its role in this catabolic pathway. In heart, lysosomal (acid) triacylglycerol lipase most likely partakes in endogenous neutral lipid degradation. In cardiac cells, engulfment of lipid droplets by lysosomes was found to initiate the hydrolysis of the endogenous triacylglycerol pool (247). It remains to be established whether acid lipase serves the same role in skeletal muscle tissue.

Although the enzyme responsible for skeletal muscle triacylglycerol degradation awaits definite identification, experimental findings indicate that hydrolysis of the intramuscular triacylglycerol pool is under hormonal control. In human volunteers, infusion of noradrenaline caused a substantial decline in skeletal muscle content of triacylglycerols (86). In vitro studies on rat diaphragm showed that noradrenaline promotes hydrolytic degradation of muscle

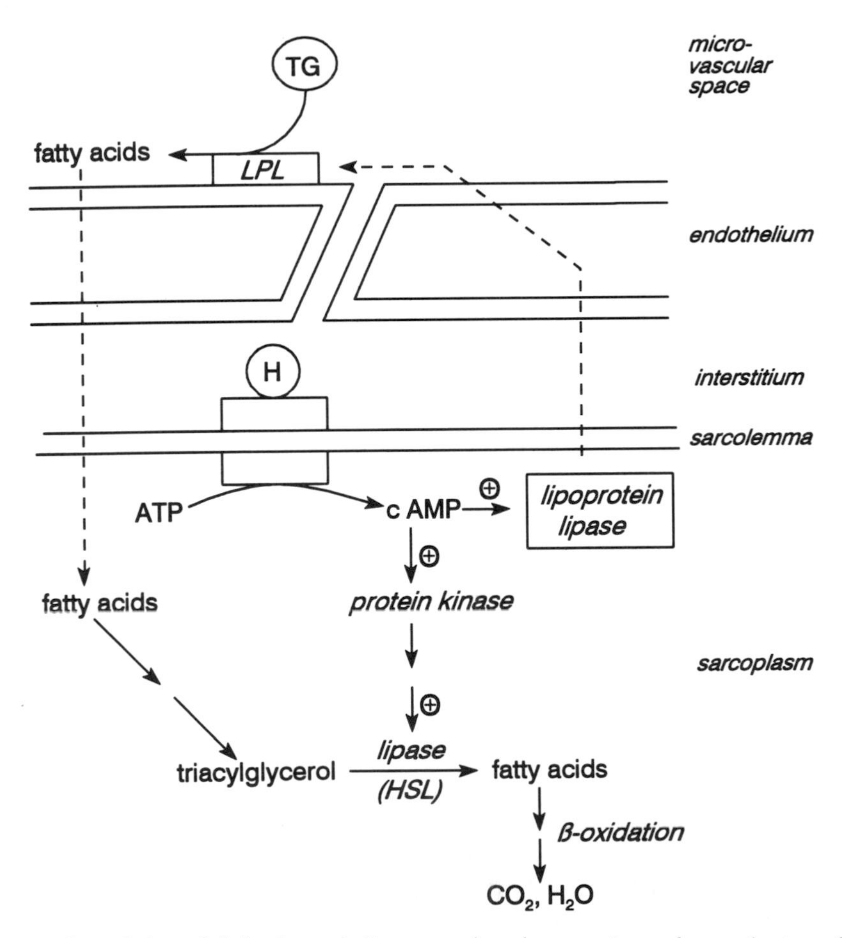

FIG. 21.4. Putative hormonal regulation of skeletal muscle lipase (201). Raised intracellular cAMP levels by hormone (H) is assumed to activate hormone-sensitive neutral triacylglycerol lipase (HSL). Triacylglycerol is hydrolyzed and fatty acids are utilized for oxidative energy conversion (β-oxidation). cAMP is also thought to activate the synthesis and transport of lipoprotein lipase (LPL) to the luminal surface of the endothelium, making more fatty acids available from circulatory triacylglycerols (TG) for replenishment of the depleted intramuscular triacylglycerol pool after exercise.

neutral lipids (98). Moreover, in the vastus lateralis of swimming rats (262) propranolol was found to maintain muscle triacylglycerols at their preexercise level, indicating that β-adrenocepter blockade effectively inhibits hormone-stimulated intramuscular neutral lipid degradation during strenuous physical activity. Insulin partially prevented catecholamine-induced depletion of the muscle triacylglycerol pool (3). A cAMP-dependent protein kinase is most likely involved via phosphorylation of an intracellular lipase in enhanced triacylglycerol degradation.

Conversely, in dogs, administration of noradrenaline over 4 h did not affect the muscle triacylglycerol content, whereas prolonged catecholamine infusion (i.e., up to 24 h) resulted in a significant increase of the muscle triacylglycerol pool (40). In this particular species the highly elevated plasma fatty acid levels, as have been observed in the dogs used in their experiments, might cause a dramatic increase in the number of fatty acyl moieties diffusing into the cell interior and, hence, promote by mass action excess formation of endogenous triacylglycerols as long as the uptake of exogenous fatty acids exceeds intramuscular oxidation.

Other experimental findings suggest that muscle triacylglycerol degradation is also under nonhormonal control. In skeletal muscles forced to contract either by direct electrical stimulation (54, 124) or via the efferent nerve (257), the triacylglycerol content significantly declined during the excercise bout, indicating that excercise-induced alterations inside the muscle cells are involved in the regulation of endogenous triacylglycerol hydrolysis. Górski (98) hypothesized that cytoplasmic Ca^{2+} released from intracellular stores may exert a stimulating effect, although the mechanisms of action of Ca^{2+} on endogenous lipases were not clarified.

Intramuscular Neutral Lipids: Content under Various Physiological Conditions. Dog and human muscles contain on the order of 7–17 μmol triacylglycerols per gram wet weight of tissue (98). The fat content in skeletal muscles of rat and monkey was found to be lower than in dog and man (98).

Human slow-twitch red oxidative (type I) fibers contain more triacylglycerols than fast-twitch red oxidative (type IIa) fibers. Type IIb fibers (i.e., fast-twitch white glycolytic fibers) display the lowest level of endogenous triacylglycerols (75, 76). Distribution of neutral fat among rat muscle fibers is similar (77, 98). From a metabolic point of view these differences are advantageous inasmuch as oxidative fibers rely more on fatty acids as a source of chemical energy than white glycolytic fibers.

The actual content of triacylglycerols in muscle is determined by a variety of factors, including the activity of the triacylglycerol synthesizing and hydrolyzing enzymes, the exogenous supply of fatty acids, the cellular need of oxidative substrates, composition of diet, and the hormonal and training status of the experimental animal or human subject.

In diabetic animals and human patients insensitive to insulin or with low levels of circulating insulin, the triacylglycerol content of muscle cells is increased (65, 261). The accumulation of neutral fat can be caused by either an increased supply of fatty acids from the extracellular environment due to elevated blood plasma levels of fatty acids or to specific intracellular changes in the enzymatic machinery caused by lack of insulin (98).

The chronic effect of thyroid hormones and catecholamines on human muscle triacylglycerol levels is unclear. For example, in human red vastus lateralis muscle, both hyper- and hypothyroidism cause a decline in tissue triacylglycerol content (142, 143). In rats, removal of the adrenal glands increased the muscle triacylglycerol level (170) or failed to affect the tissue content of neutral lipids (100).

Fasting does not cause consistent changes in muscle triacylglycerol content (98). Both increases and decreases have been reported (98, 173), whereas in rats subjected to 48 h of food deprivation the triacylglycerol level of fast-twitch red and white muscle fibers and diaphragm remained unchanged (196).

Cross-sectional studies performed on highly trained and nontrained subjects revealed that the volume density of lipid droplets in muscle fibers of the middle part of vastus lateralis muscle was 2.5-fold higher in the former than in the latter group (127). In human volunteers, physical training was found to enhance the triacylglycerol pool of the vastus lateralis muscle (185). In contrast, others observed no effect of endurance training on the neutral lipid store in the same muscle group (132). The deviant findings can most likely be ascribed to differences in training protocols applied. In humans, 6 weeks of endurance exercise training increased the volume density of intracellular lipid droplets significantly in fast-twitch red and white fibers (129). In male volunteers, the increase in fast-twitch white fibers was more pronounced than in female subjects. No significant increase of the volume density of the neutral lipid pool in slow-twitch fibers could be detected (129).

It should be stressed that biochemical data obtained in biopsies of muscle tissue have to be interpreted with caution. When individual muscle fibers are not dissected out, it remains unclear as to whether triacylglycerol values measured reflect true intramyocytal neutral lipid levels or pertain (in part) to adipocytes interlaced between the muscle fibers (82, 98, 250).

Turnover of the Intramuscular Triacylglycerol Pool. At rest, fatty acids extracted from the extracellular compartment are incorporated in the cytoplasmic triacylglycerol pool prior to utilization in energy-converting processes (319). Moreover, the intramuscular triacylglycerol pool is subject to a continuous turnover process. It is, however, doubtful whether the precise turnover rate of the neutral lipid pool can be calculated, because intramuscular lipids do not form a homogeneous pool (319).

While in resting muscular tissue almost all fatty acids originating from extracellular sources seem to be incorporated first in the endogenous triacylglycerol pool, experimental findings suggest that during exercise the metabolic fate of fatty acids newly entering the muscle cells is different. Studies on exercising human subjects suggest that almost all fatty acids extracted by the working muscle cells are directly oxidized in the mitochondrial degradative pathway or after entering triacylglycerol pools, which have a turnover time of only a few minutes (115). The analytical techniques employed, however, do not allow for discrimination between the latter two possibilities.

Bahr and co-workers (12) reported that the turnover rate of the intramuscular triacylglycerol pool was appreciably increased after termination of the exercise bout. They calculated that enhanced triacylglycerol–fatty acid cycling may account for approximately half of the prolonged increase of oxygen consumption in the postexercise period.

The process of continuous incorporation and release of fatty acids in and from the cytoplasmic triacylglycerol pool is commonly referred to as the "futile triacylglycerol–fatty acid cycle." Assuming that a particular fatty acid molecule is only once incorporated in intracellular triacylglycerol before entering the oxidative pathway, it can be calculated that ~2% of the energy converted during complete oxidation is lost in the futile cycle. At first glance, the physiological significance of a futile cycle in general and of a triacylglycerol–fatty acid cycle in particular may be obscure. In this respect, Newsholme (190) has proposed that (f)utile cycling in metabolic pathways offers the cell a powerful tool to rapidly adjust metabolic flux rates to acutely changing demands of oxidizable substrates by increasing the sensitivity in control mechanisms. Moreover, triacylglycerol–fatty acid cycling might be of utmost importance in mammalian cells to efficiently remove fatty acids from the cytoplasmic space to prevent toxic effects exerted by high concentrations of these amphiphilic compounds (291).

SUPPLY AND UTILIZATION OF LIPIDS DURING EXERCISE

In general, over 50% of the energy requirement of resting muscle tissue is derived from fatty acid oxidation (36, 96). During exercise, lipids remain important substrates for the muscle cells when the intensity of exercise does not exceed 80%–90% of $\dot{V}O_{2max}$ (92, 96, 109, 278). However, the relative contribution of lipids rapidly declines and that of carbohydrate increases as exercise intensity exceeds 90% $\dot{V}O_{2max}$ (1, 92, 278). Muscle cells recruited during partially anaerobic exercise, such as sprinting and weight lifting, rely heavily on the cellular content of high-energy phosphates (ATP, phosphocreatine) and glycogen-derived glucose to fulfill the energy requirement. Under such conditions, fatty acids are less suitable substrates because the chemical energy stored in the lipid molecule can only be utilized for ATP regeneration when sufficient amounts of molecular oxygen are available. Moreover, the maximum rate of high-energy phosphate (~P) formation from lipid oxidation is too low to match the rate of utilization of ~P during exercise of high intensity (Table 21.2). The data also indicate that the maximum anaerobic rate of ~P formation from endogenous glycogen stores is on the order of 2.4 mol/min (131). This value is just below the rate of ~P utilization during 100 m sprint, indicating that also net utilization of phosphocreatine occurs during the race. Aerobic glycogen-derived glucose utilization supplies ~P at a rate of 1.0 mol/min. When glucose is derived from extracellular sources, the maximum aerobic rate of ~P formation is considerably lower, which suggests that the rate-limiting step in glucose oxidation resides in the transport of glucose from the vascular to intracellular compartment (see also Chapter 20 of this *Handbook*).

The maximum aerobic rate of ~P production from fatty acid degradation is on the same order of magnitude as that of blood-borne glucose but appreciably lower than the maximum rate from aerobic utilization of endogenous glycogen. Because metabolic steps beyond the formation of acetyl CoA are similar in carbohydrate and fatty acid oxidation, the rate-limiting step in overall fatty acid utilization by skeletal muscle is located in the β-oxidation pathway, the activation of fatty acid to fatty acyl CoA, and subsequent carnitine-mediated intramitochondrial transport or in the transport route of fatty acids from the intracapillary space to the intracellular site

TABLE 21.2. *Maximum Rate of High-Energy Phosphate (~P) Regeneration from Carbohydrate and Lipid Substrates Compared to Utilization of ~P during Various Types of Exercise**

Maximum Rate of ~P Regeneration	Maximum Rate of Formation	
	μmol ~P · g^{-1} · min^{-1}	mol ~P · min^{-1}
Substrate utilized		
Endogenous glycogen (anaerobic)	84	2.4
Endogenous glycogen (aerobic)	35	1.0
Blood-borne glucose (aerobic)	13	0.37
Blood-borne fatty acids (aerobic)	14	0.40
Rate of ~P Utilization	**Rate of Utilization**	
	μmol ~P · g^{-1} · min^{-1}	mol ~P · min^{-1}
Type of exercise		
Rest	2.5	0.07
100 m sprint	93	2.6
800 m sprint	71	2.0
1500 m sprint	60	1.7
42,200 m marathon	36	1.0

*Modified from Hultman and Harris (131); μmol ~P · g^{-1} · min^{-1} refers to μmol high-energy phosphates formed or utilized per gram wet weight of skeletal muscles per minute. To calculate total ~P rate formation (mol · min^{-1}) the assumption was made that on the average 28 kg muscles of a 70 kg subject is used during the exercise bout. The same holds for ~P utilization.

of activation. At present, the question as to which part of overall fatty acid utilization harbors the rate-limiting step remains unsolved. Indirect evidence suggests that the transport of fatty acids from blood to the sarcoplasm determines the maximum rate of skeletal muscle fatty acid consumption (190). As discussed earlier under Transport of Fatty Acids Inside the Muscle Cell, it is unlikely that sarcoplasmic transport is rate limiting because of the relatively high abundancy of fatty acid–binding protein (301).

Data in Table 21.2 also indicate that during a marathon race, blood-borne fatty acids and glucose are equally important. Utilization of both substrates at maximum rates is insufficient to fulfill the maximum energy requirements of the exercising muscles. Endogenous substrate stores such as glycogen and triacylglycerols have to be recruited to generate aerobically high-energy phosphates to complete the race. During prolonged exercise bouts at a lower intensity than a marathon run, which requires the athlete to perform at 80%–90% of $\dot{V}O_{2max}$, fat utilization can contribute with a relatively higher proportion to overall aerobic energy conversion (36, 109). Earlier studies have shown that up to 80% of the energy requirement can be met by fat oxidation during prolonged light to moderate exercise (~50% of $\dot{V}O_{2max}$) (96, 239). Recently, O'Brien and colleagues (195), however, challenged the notion that lipids are important substrates during a marathon run at 73% of $\dot{V}O_{2max}$, and suggested that carbohydrates are the prime fuel.

During the exercise bout, three major lipid sources can be used by skeletal muscle cells. First, fatty acids complexed to albumin in the blood compartment; second, fatty acids present in the triacylglycerol core of circulating lipoproteins; and third, fatty acids stored in triacylglycerols in the cytoplasm of the myocytes, whereas fatty acids from adipocytes interlaced between the skeletal muscle fibers can contribute as well. The relative significance of the different fatty acid sources will be discussed below.

Albumin-Bound Fatty Acids in Plasma during Exercise

In a resting person, the concentration of fatty acids in blood plasma is on the order of 0.2–0.5 mmol/liter. As discussed earlier, the bulk of the fatty acids is derived from triacylglycerols stored in adipose tissue. In 1961, Carlson and Pernow (41) showed that plasma fatty acid levels drop during the first 20 min of endurance exercise. This is most likely caused by an imbalance between mobilization of fatty acids from adipose tissue and the increased fatty acid extraction by skeletal muscle cells. Hydrolysis of the triacylglycerol pool in adipocytes is accelerated during prolonged moderate and relatively heavy exercise, resulting in a progressive rise of the fatty acid concentrations in plasma after the initial decline (36). The extent of these changes is, among others, dependent on the training status of the exercising person (see later under Utilization of Plasma-Borne

Fatty Acids by Trained Muscles). The mechanisms underlying the release of fatty acids from adipose tissue are discussed in Chapter 23 of this *Handbook*.

The increased plasma levels of fatty acids during prolonged exercise will promote the flux of fatty acids to the exercising muscle cells (4, 133). The driving force of the flux of fatty acid from the vascular space to the intracellular site of conversion is assumed to be the concentration gradient of fatty acids between the two compartments under consideration (see earlier under Blood Plasma—Cytoplasmic Fatty Acid Gradient as Driving Force of Fatty Acid Uptake). Enhanced plasma fatty acid levels will promote the net diffusion of the substrates to the skeletal myocytes. Blood flow through muscles dramatically increases during submaximal exercise as a consequence of spatial and/or temporal capillary recruitment. The latter phenomenon causes an increase in the permeability–surface area for fatty acids at the endothelial level, which will also contribute to the enhanced flux of fatty acids from plasma to muscle cells until the release of fatty acids from the albumin complex becomes rate limiting because of a too-low transit time.

Circulating Lipoprotein-Triacylglycerols as a Potential Source of Fatty Acids during Exercise

Although the plasma content of fatty acyl units incorporated in the circulating lipoprotein-triacylglycerol pool generally exceeds the concentration of albumin-bound fatty acids, the actual contribution of plasma triacylglycerol-derived fatty acids to lipid utilization during exercise is a matter of continuous debate (278). Gollnick and Saltin (96) concluded that only a minor fraction, if any, of circulating triacylglycerol–fatty acids are oxidized in the exercising muscle cells. In contrast, Terjung and colleagues (279) concluded that lipoprotein-triacylglycerols represent a potentially rich source of plasma fatty acid substrates for the working muscle. Results of attempts to quantify the contribution of circulating triacylglycerols to energy conversion in the exercising muscle cells are, however, not unequivocal (279, 318).

Indirect evidence is available that plasma triacylglycerols are consumed during physical exercise (279). The observation that the level of circulating triacylglycerols decreases during prolonged exercise (188) suggests that the muscular utilization is increased. Terjung and colleagues (277) have addressed this issue in a study with ^{14}C-fatty acid–labeled chylomicrons in dogs and observed that the turnover of circulating chylomicrons is enhanced during exercise. Deviant findings are reported by Young and co-workers (318), who found in exercising man no significant alteration in the removal rate constant of circulating triacylglycerols. The difference in outcome might be caused by imperfections in the experimental set-up of Young and colleagues (318) as argued by Terjung and co-workers (279), so that enhanced removal of circulating triacylglycerols could indeed account for the lower blood triacylglycerol content observed in exercising humans (192, 279).

Low circulating triacylglycerol levels during submaximal exercise may also result from a reduced release of chylomicrons or VLDL by enterocytes or hepatocytes, respectively. Indeed, experimental findings suggest that the secretion of lipoproteins into the vascular compartment is decreased, which might be caused by a decline in production and/or reduced removal of lipoproteins from the site of production due to underperfusion of the splanchnic area during the exercise bout (253).

The activity of LPL, responsible for removal of triacylglycerol–fatty acids from blood, was found to be enhanced from 18 to 58 nmol · g^{-1} · min^{-1} in vastus lateralis muscle during an 85 km skiing race. The highest increment was observed in the less trained individuals (166). Taskinen and colleagues (273) observed a substantial increase in the microvascular activity of LPL in well-trained, overnight-fasted male subjects running a distance of 20 km. The enhanced activity of capillary LPL suggests that the capacity of exercising muscle to utilize circulating triacylglycerol is increased during the course of the exercise bout. The stimulatory effect of exercise on muscle LPL has also been observed in rat (11, 35). Since the increase in LPL activity was only observed in fasted animals but not in rats fed a mixed fat-rich meal, circulating insulin and/or fatty acids are thought to be involved in the up-regulation of muscle LPL activity during acute submaximal exercise (35). The observation that LPL activity is increased during exercise, most likely as a consequence of enhanced cAMP-dependent protein kinase activity, has led Oscai and colleagues (201) to hypothesize that a greater proportion of the enzyme is transferred to the microvascular compartment to hydrolyze circulating triacylglycerols in order to replenish the intracellular triacylglycerol pool, which most likely becomes depleted during exercise (Fig. 21.4). The exercise-induced increase of tissue LPL activity seems to be dependent on the duration of the exercise bout. Physical exercise shorter than 1 h does not result in measurable increments of intravascular and heparin-releasable muscle LPL activity (149, 166).

Direct evidence for utilization of circulating chylomicrons by exercising muscles stems from rat studies by Mackie and colleagues (168). The utilization of ^{14}C-palmitate–labeled chylomicron-triacylglycerols was found to be increased by 30%–40% in stimulated hindlimb muscles. The highest uptake was observed in slow-twitch red fibers, while deposition of label in fast-twitch white fibers was minor. Intermediate values were found for fast-twitch red fibers. This pattern follows the activity of LPL in the three different muscle fiber types (142, 279). The increased uptake of radiolabeled fatty acids might be caused by enhanced activity of the enzyme on the luminal endothelial membrane of the muscle capillary, as found in exercising human subjects (166), or a greater number of LPL enzymes exposed to circulating substrates due to spatial and/or temporal capillary recruitment in the stimulated hindlimb (279). The uptake of radiolabeled triacylglycerol-derived fatty acids by stimulated muscles has been confirmed in dogs running on a treadmill (277, 279). During exercise, the deposition of radiolabeled fatty acids in the working muscle cell increased from 2.4% to 4.0% of the chylomicrons injected. The authors calculated that during exercise and rest, per-minute and per-gram muscle tissue approximately 65 and 50 nmol triacylglycerol–fatty acids were incorporated in the endogenous lipid pool, respectively. These values most likely represent the lower limits of net utilization, because oxidation of labeled fatty acyl units extracted from the extracellular compartment was not taken into account (277–279).

Nikkilä and Konttinen (192) estimated that in exercising army recruits circulating triacylglycerols provided about 4% of the energy converted during the exercise bout. This number is in line with the conclusion of Rowell and colleagues (231) that during exercise net splanchnic lipid release provides at most 5% of the total energy in fasted subjects.

Direct measurements of skeletal muscle exogenous triacylglycerol utilization in human were made by Olsson and co-workers (198). In a carefully conducted study they assessed the arteriovenous (A-V) differences of triacylglycerol, both unlabeled and radiolabeled, and albumin-bound fatty acids in volunteers subjected to forearm exercise. A-V differences of fatty acids amounted to 56 μmol/liter, corresponding to ~10% of the arterial concentration. The A-V differences of triacylglycerols did not exceed the level of error of the analytical methods used in their study. The authors calculated that the extraction of plasma triacylglycerol–fatty acids must be higher than ~3% of the arterial triacylglycerol level to be statistically significant. In their study, this value corresponds with a triacylglycerol–fatty acid A-V difference of ~64 μmol/liter, which is on the same order of magnitude as the A-V difference of (free) fatty acids; that is, 56 μmol/liter. These findings and theoretical considerations may lead to the conclusion that, due to uncertainties inherent in the methods available for the assessment of triacylglycerol extraction from blood, at present no definitive answer can be given to the question as to whether and to what extent circulating triacylglycerols contribute to skeletal muscle energy conversion during rest and exercise.

Contribution of Intramuscular Triacylglycerols to Fatty Acid Oxidation during Exercise

As indicated earlier under Intramuscular Neutral Lipids: Content Under Various Physiological Conditions, skeletal muscle cells contain fatty acids stored in cytoplasmic lipid droplets. Although opinions differ concerning the importance of endogenous triacylglycerols as energy reserve for the exercising muscle cells (98), many studies indicated that sarcoplasmic triacylglycerols are involved in the conversion of energy in working skeletal muscles (96, 210). Havel and co-workers (115) concluded from studies with radiolabeled palmitate in human volunteers that during bicycle exercise about half of the fatty acids utilized was derived from local triacylglycerol stores. Martin and colleagues (172) reported comparable findings in exercising human subjects with the use of ^{13}C-labeled fatty acids.

Direct evidence for muscle triacylglycerol mobilization in human working muscles (87, 78, 98) reveals that, in general, 25%–40% of the skeletal muscle triacyglycerol content was consumed during a 60–147 min exercise test (Table 21.3). Histological support for the notion that intramuscular triacylglycerols are consumed during exercise is the observation that the size of fat vacuoles in muscle cells is appreciably reduced (96).

Unfortunately, in some studies on humans, muscle fibers were not separated from interlacing adipocytes, making it impossible to conclude how much of the decline in tissue triacylglycerol content could be ascribed to intramyocytal neutral lipid utilization. Finally, it is doubtful that all fatty acids released from endogenous triacylglycerol stores are used in the oxidative pathway during exercise. Jansson and Kaijser (139) found that exercising leg muscles of human volunteers release ~70 μmol fatty acids per liter plasma into the vascular space. This value corresponded with a release rate of ~75 nmol/g wet weight of tissue per minute. Part of the fatty acids released may be derived from circulating triacylglyc-

TABLE 21.3. *Utilization of Muscle Triacylglycerols during Aerobic Exercise**

Species	Exercise Conditions	Muscle	Muscle Triacylglycerol Consumption		References
			μmol · g^{-1} wet	%	
Human	Submaximal (55%–70% $\dot{V}O_{2max}$) exercise for 0.5–2 h	Mixed	0–35	0–41	(39, 75, 132, 137, 147)
	Prolonged running/skiing	Mixed	2.2–8.7	30–50	(53, 87)
Dog	Running until exhaustion	Mixed	4.4	58	(280)
Rat	Prolonged running/swimming (usually until exhaustion)	Slow-twitch red	0–3.6	0–50	(15, 99, 226, 259, 263)
		Fast-twitch red	0.7–1.6	33–70	(15, 99, 226, 259, 263)
		Fast-twitch white	0	0	(15, 99, 263)

*Modified from Górski (98).

erols hydrolyzed by LPL on the luminal surface of the microvascular endothelium (see earlier under Hydrolysis of Circulating Triacylglycerols by Lipoprotein Lipase). The remaining and as yet unquantified part is most likely released from muscular triacylglycerol stores.

Contrasting observations were made by Jansson and Kaijser (137), who could not detect a significant decline in the triacylglycerol content of quadriceps femoris muscle in human volunteers subjected to a submaximal leg exercise test (65% of VO_{2max}) during 25 min. Gollnick and colleagues (94) and Kiens and co-workers (147) also failed to observe a significant decrease in the muscle triacylglycerol pool in exercising man.

Additional evidence in favor of endogenous triacylglycerol utilization is derived from animal studies with electrically stimulated muscles in situ and in vitro (98). Although most studies revealed intramuscular triacylglycerol consumption (98, 124, 257), some experimental protocols failed to induce a net decline in tissue triacylglycerols (124, 257). In general, the triacylglycerol pool in fast-twitch white fibers does not respond to exercise (Table 21.3), supporting the notion that in this particular fiber type fatty acid oxidation is not important for energy conversion (98, 197). A consistent decline in tissue triacylglycerols has been reported for exercising fast-twitch red fibers (Table 21.3). On average, the rate of utilization amounted to 20 nmol triacylglycerol–fatty acids per gram wet weight of fast-twitch red fibers per minute, assuming that triacylglycerol hydrolysis is linear in time. Inconclusive findings were made in slow-twitch red fibers. Some studies reported a significant decline of the intramuscular triacylglycerol pool (226, 259), whereas other investigators failed to observe a significant change (98).

Deviating observations have been published concerning the time course of endogenous triacylglycerol utilization in skeletal muscle. Baldwin and colleagues (15) observed a fast decline of the intramuscular neutral lipid pool during the first 15 min of exercise. Thereafter, the tissue content of triacylglycerols remained stable until the end of the exercise bout of 2 h duration. In contrast, Stankiewicz-Choroszucha and Górski (263) reported a steady decline of the rat muscle triacylglycerol pool during a 3 h strenuous swimming test.

Relative Contribution of Various Sources of Lipids to Overall Fatty Acid Utilization during Exercise

A variety of studies have been performed to estimate the contribution of circulating fatty acids and lipoprotein-triacylglycerols, and of muscle triacylglycerols to overall energy conversion during submaximal exercise. Earlier investigations indicated that lipid oxidation contributed 40%–50% to overall energy conversion in human subjects exercising at 65%–67% $\dot{V}O_{2max}$ for 60–100 min (39, 139). The contribution of plasma fatty acid oxidation was found to be 15%–18% of total energy conversion. Intramuscular triacylglycerols were estimated to contribute 15% (139) or 35% (39).

Recently, Martin and co-workers (172) have reinvestigated this issue in human volunteers subjected to a prolonged exercise protocol (90–120 min cycling at ~63% of $\dot{V}O_{2max}$). During the final 30–60 min of the exercise bout, ~40% of the energy utilized was derived from fat oxidation. The contribution of plasma fatty acids to total energy conversion was found to be on the order of 17%. In quantitative terms, ~11 μmol plasma fatty acids were oxidized per kilogram body weight per minute. Assuming that 10 kg active skeletal muscle (i.e., about 40% of total muscle mass) is responsible for all plasma fatty acids oxidized, the oxidation rate of plasma fatty acids amounted to ~75 nmol/g muscle per minute. Since the total rate of fatty acid oxidation was calculated to be ~175 nmol fatty acids per gram of muscle per minute, other lipid sources, capable of supplying ~100 nmol fatty acids · g^{-1} · min^{-1}, are also mobilized. The authors concluded that intramuscular fatty acyl units stored in the sarcoplasmic triacylglycerol pool will provide the missing fatty acids used in the oxidative pathway (172). The authors neglected, however, the potential contribution of circulating triacylglycerols. Assuming a circulating triacylglycerol plasma level of 1.0 mmol triacylglycerols (corresponding with 3 mmol fatty acyl units) per liter and a skeletal muscle plasma flow of 0.9 ml/g wet weight of tissue per minute, the supply of triacylglycerol–fatty acids amounts to 2.7 μmol · g^{-1} · min^{-1}. When 3% of this amount is extracted by the skeletal muscle cells after intramicrovascular hydrolysis of triacylglycerols, an additional 80 nmol exogenous fatty acids becomes available for oxidative energy conversion. This amount is almost sufficient to cover the missing part of fatty acids oxidized. It should be recalled that 3% consumption of circulating triacylglycerols is within the analytical error of the chemical assay of plasma triacylglycerol (198). In support of the conclusion of Martin and colleagues (172) that intramuscular triacylglycerols contribute to a significant extent to overall fatty acid oxidation is the observation made by a variety of investigators that the endogenous triacylglycerol content substantially decreases during strenuous exercise (see Table 21.3). When only studies with a significant decline in tissue triacylglycerol content were taken into account, the calculated average rate of triacylglycerol depletion amounted to 86 nmol fatty acyl units · g^{-1} · min^{-1}, a value that also perfectly matches the calculated rate of endogenous fatty acid oxidation in the study of Martin and colleagues (172).

Kiens and colleagues (147) calculated that thigh muscles of untrained volunteers derived 8% of total energy conversion from oxidation of plasma fatty acids during knee extensor exercise. Oxidation of plasma glucose and tissue glycogen contributed 53%. Because in the latter study intramuscular triacylglycerols were not mobilized during the exercise bout, other lipid sources have to be considered. The authors concluded on the basis of inconsistent experimental results that the contribution of plasma triacylglycerols would be minor and that intercellular fat, that is, lipid stored in adipocytes interlaced between the muscle fibers, is most likely utilized during knee extensor exercise.

Gender Differences in Lipid Utilization during Exercise

Experimental findings obtained in carefully designed studies strongly suggest the existence of gender differences in substrate utilization during prolonged submaximal exercise. Tarnapolsky and colleagues (272) investigated the fuel consumption in male and equally trained female athletes performing at ~65% of the subjects' VO_{2max} for 90 min. The respiratory exchange ratio was consistently lower in the female than in the male group (0.87 vs. 0.94). It was calculated that male athletes consumed in toto 27 and 240 g fat and carbohydrates, respectively, during the race, whereas female subjects utilized 48 and 137 g fat and carbohydrates, respectively (272). Moreover, at the end of the exercise bout skeletal muscle glycogen stores were more depleted in the male than in the female runners. The relatively greater reliance on fat than on carbohydrate oxidation in female athletes was also observed by Blatchford and colleagues and Fröberg and Pedersen (27, 84), but not by others (52, 103, 216).

Enhanced lipid utilization in exercising females, as observed in the study of Tarnapolsky and co-workers (272), was not accompanied by higher plasma fatty acid and glycerol levels as compared with men, suggesting that probably more muscular triacylglycerols were consumed by women during the exercise bout. This possibility is in line with data indicating that the neutral lipid pool is greater in muscles of female than of male subjects (126). The enhanced consumption of fat by females would also offer an explanation for the finding that in female subjects muscle glycogen is more spared during the submaximal exercise test than in male athletes (272). The higher insulin and lower epinephrine plasma levels in the female group as compared with male subjects might partially explain the reduced consumption of muscular carbohydrates in the former group. Moreover, it cannot be excluded that sex hormones are involved in the differences in fuel selection during prolonged submaximal exercise in female and male athletes (272). The enhanced propensity of female athletes to use fat during submaximal exercise is most likely not caused by a difference in capacity of male and female muscles to handle fatty acyl moieties (52). Costill and colleagues (52) found a higher succinate dehydrogenase activity (marker for mitochondrial density), carnitine acyltransferase activity, and capacity to oxidize fatty acyl CoA in muscle specimen of male endurance-trained athletes than in that of female subjects.

EFFECT OF TRAINING ON SKELETAL MUSCLE LIPID UTILIZATION

Numerous investigations conducted during the past decades have demonstrated that endurance training substantially enhances the capacity to oxidize fatty acids in exercising muscles (28, 96, 121, 132, 234). In pioneering studies performed in the 1930s by Bang, Christensen, and Hansen [reviewed by Gollnick and Saltin (96)], a significantly lower respiratory exchange ratio was found in trained than in nontrained volunteers, indicating that a greater proportion of the energy is supplied by oxidation of lipids. This training-induced difference in respiratory exchange ratio was confirmed by a number of later studies (47, 96, 147).

Advantages of Enhanced Lipid Utilization by Trained Muscles during Exercise

The specific advantages of a shift to greater reliance on fat as a substrate during prolonged strenuous exercise are summarized by Gollnick and Saltin (96). In biological systems, lipids are a more efficient storage form of energy than carbohydrates, so that a relatively greater contribution of fat to overall energy conversion increases the capacity to utilize chemically stored energy, while increased utilization of fat has a "glycogen-sparing" effect. The latter is of utmost importance during prolonged exercise at relatively high work intensity (in the range of 50%–90% $\dot{V}O_{2max}$). Under these conditions, carbohydrates are required as oxidizable substrate to maintain exercise intensity at the desired level. Early depletion of tissue glycogen forces the athlete to stop the race or to continue at an appreciably lower intensity (96). A shift from carbohydrate to fat utilization will conserve the glycogen stores in the body and, hence, increase the capacity of the athlete to perform at high work intensities for a longer period of time (237).

Possible Causes of Increased Lipid Consumption by Trained Muscles during Exercise

Although the advantages of a greater usage of lipids in the exercising muscles are clear, the cellular and molecular mechanisms underlying the beneficial effect of training on muscle energy conversion are incompletely understood. A shift from carbohydrate to lipid oxidation in the endurance-trained muscles may be caused by a variety of specific adaptations of the body to endurance training (96, 119). In theory, the following mechanisms may be involved (95). First, enhanced muscular lipid utilization can be explained by an increase in the capacity of the mitochondria in the muscle cell to oxidize fatty acids. Second, increased capacity to transport fatty acids from the vascular space to the mitochondrial compartment will add to a training-induced shift from carbohydrate to lipid utilization. Third, elevation of the intramuscular triacylglycerol content will also contribute to the enhanced propensity of trained subjects to rely more on fatty acid oxidation. Fourth, subtle changes in the mutual control mechanisms of fatty acid and glucose utilization on the cellular level, as discussed below under INTERRELATIONSHIP BETWEEN MUSCULAR CARBOHYDRATE AND LIPID METABOLISM, will be instrumental in making lipids the substrates of choice in trained muscles.

Endurance training increases the oxidative capacity of skeletal muscles (95). In relatively young subjects, this increase is associated with an augmented number and volume of mitochondria in the skeletal muscle cell, which most likely form the basis for the greater potential for oxidative energy conversion (93, 184). In rats in particular the subsarcolemmal mitochondria responded to chronic changes in the level of contractile activity. This finding prompted Hoppeler and associates (126) to postulate that this specific adaptation brings the fatty acid–converting organelles closer to the poorly diffusable blood-borne fatty acids. The authors, however, overlooked the fact that skeletal muscle cells contain sufficient amounts of FABP to facilitate intracellular transport of fatty acids to mitochondria localized in the interior of the cell (301). Recent studies (289) demonstrated that endurance training of rats does not affect the soleus muscle content of FABP, indicating that the maximal capacity to transport fatty acids from the sarcolemma to the mitochondrial outer membrane is not increased. Furthermore, training of muscles of middle-aged man did not increase the volume of skeletal muscle mitochondria despite increased oxidative capacity (151).

On the basis of Michaelis-Menten kinetics, Gollnick and Saltin (95) have proposed that enhanced activity of fatty acid–handling enzymes might be the prime cause for the shift from carbohydrate to fatty acid oxidation in endurance-trained muscles during submaximal exercise. A variety of investigators has shown that endurance training increases, in addition to an augmented number and volume of mitochondria, the maximal activity (V_{max}) of mitochondrial enzymes involved in lipid oxidation [Table 21.4; (59, 95, 132, 139, 181)]. It is very likely that the enhanced enzymatic activity will accelerate the removal of fatty acyl moieties from the cytoplasmic space and, hence, enlarge the contribution of fatty acid oxidation to overall energy conversion in the skeletal muscle cell. Furthermore, due to the augmented mitochondrial density, an increased sensitivity of mitochondrial respiratory control in the trained state will result in alterations in substrate selection. In muscle tissue this

TABLE 21.4. *Effect of Training on Enzymes/Proteins Involved in Skeletal Muscle Lipid Handling*

Enzyme/Protein	Activity*/Content		Species	Muscle	References
	Untrained	Trained			
Fatty acyl CoA synthetase	0.03 ± 0.0	0.07 ± 0.01	Rat	Gastrocnemius/quadriceps	(181)
Carnitine acyltransferase	0.63 ± 0.07	1.20 ± 0.05	Rat	Soleus	(14)
	0.07 ± 0.00	0.13 ± 0.01	Rat	Gastrocnemius/quadriceps	(181)
	0.10 ± 0.01†	0.34 ± 0.04	Rat	Soleus	(105)
Fatty acyl CoA dehydrogenase	0.41 ± 0.06	0.97 ± 0.11	Rat	Gastrocnemius/quadriceps	(181)
3-Hydroxyacyl CoA dehydrogenase	30.6 ± 9.6	58.2 ± 8.6	Human	Vastus lateralis	(132)
	12.4	12.4	Human	Vastus lateralis	(240)
	6.2	12.2	Human	Triceps bracchi	(240)
	30.6 ± 2.4	48.8 ± 3.7	Horse	Semitendinosus	(255)
	0.86 ± 0.06	1.08 ± 0.08	Rat	Plantaris	(63)
FABP	58 ± 12	50 ± 18	Rat	Soleus	(289)
	255 ± 50	255 ± 21	Rat	Plantaris	(289)
	250 ± 17	429 ± 16	Rat	Soleus	(63)

*Enzyme activity is expressed as μmol · g^{-1} wet weight · min^{-1}; FABP as μg · g^{-1} wet weight. The assumption was made that mitochondria contribute 25% to total tissue protein. †Refers to carnitine acyltransferase I.

change leads most likely to less stimulated glycolysis and a higher metabolic flux in the fatty acid oxidative pathway (70). It can, however, not be ignored that enhanced mitochondrial oxidation of fatty acids has to be accompanied by a quantitatively similar increase in supply of fatty acyl units to the mitochondria. Since circumstantial evidence indicates that delivery of lipid substrates rather than oxidative metabolism might be the rate-limiting factor, an explanation for the effect of training should also be sought for in altered supply rates of fatty acids.

Endurance training results in augmented capillarization of skeletal muscles, characterized by a greater number of capillaries per muscle fiber (237), which reduces the average diffusion distance for blood-borne substrates and enhances the permeability–surface area of the endothelium constituting the microvascular wall (6, 147, 149). Since plasma fatty acids have to cross the endothelial barrier before entering the muscle cells, an increase in the permeability-surface area will favor the fatty acid flux from the vascular compartment to the muscle fibers. In addition, the increase in total surface area of the mitochondrial outer and inner membrane per unit of skeletal muscle cells (6, 184) offers a possibility for elevated activation of fatty acids and subsequent transport of fatty acyl residues into the mitochondrial matrix. Recent calculations demonstrated that in cardiac tissue the mitochondrial surface area is a determinant in the overall flux of fatty acids from the vascular space to the intracellular site of utilization (301).

Gollnick and Saltin (96) calculated that the capillary transit time of blood will increase as a consequence of enhanced capillary volume per unit of muscle mass at a given flow rate. The effect of this phenomenon can be substantial because the release rate of fatty acids from albumin might be rate-limiting in overall fatty acid uptake when blood is flowing too fast through the muscle capillaries (291). Finally, an increase in the surface of the endothelium offers the possibility to anchor more LPL enzymes to the glycocalyx covering the endothelial cell membrane, which enhances the capacity to utilize fatty acids from circulating lipoproteins.

Training-induced increases in intramuscular lipid stores have the practical advantage that the diffusion distance for fatty acids liberated from the triacylglycerol-containing lipid droplet to the mitochondrial outer membrane is extremely short because lipid droplets are located in close vicinity to the mitochondria present in the muscular cytoplasm. As summarized later under Utilization of Intramuscular Triacylglycerols in Endurance-Trained Muscles, the effect of endurance training on the muscular triacylglycerol content is inconclusive. Both increased (147, 172, 184) and unaffected triacylglycerol levels (132, 184) have been reported. As will be discussed in detail later under INTERRELATIONSHIP BETWEEN MUSCULAR CARBOHYDRATE AND LIPID METABOLISM, carbohydrates and lipids mutually control their rate of utilization in the exercising muscle cell. It cannot be excluded that subtle changes in concentration and/or availability of regulating factors in the cytoplasmic compartment of the trained muscle cell favor the utilization and oxidation of fatty acids above glucose during strenuous exercise bouts.

Utilization of Plasma-Borne Fatty Acids by Trained Muscles

Gollnick and Saltin (96) have argued that plasma fatty acid extraction is higher in trained than in untrained muscles when the same amount of fatty acids is delivered. The earlier studies of Keul and co-workers in 1970 (146) demonstrated that in trained subjects the circulating level of fatty acids is significantly higher than in untrained persons. During exercise, consumption of plasma fatty acids was also found to be higher at a given $\dot{V}O_{2max}$ in trained than in untrained subjects (146, 147, 234–236). Strenuous endurance training significantly increases the rate of total body triacylglycerol–fatty acid cycling at rest, which enhances the potential to supply fatty acids as oxidizable substrates rapidly at the onset of exercise (230). This finding underlines the notion that triacylglycerol–fatty acid cycling plays an important role in enabling a fast and adequate response of fatty acid metabolism to major changes in substrate demand (311). Paul (207) observed that in trained dogs a higher percentage of carbon dioxide production was derived from circulating fatty acids than in untrained animals during exercise. A substantial number of other studies, however, failed to confirm these observations. In plasma of human volunteers, after training the fatty acid levels were found to be significantly reduced during prolonged exercise at a given intensity (58, 132, 172, 308). The decline in circulating fatty acid concentration could be due to either enhanced consumption by the working muscles or reduced release from fat tissue. Hurley and co-workers (132) reported that in exercising subjects the blood concentration of glycerol was lower after than before training, which favors the notion that the triacylglycerol pool in adipocytes is mobilized to a lesser extent, since circulating glycerol can be taken as a rough index of triacylglycerol hydrolysis in fat tissue. A feasible explanation for decreased mobilization of fatty acids from adipose tissue is a training-induced blunting of the plasma catecholamine response to submaximal exercise and reduced activity of the sympathetic nervous system in trained subjects (112, 308). As a consequence, catecholamine-stimulated lipolysis in adipocytes is reduced and release of fatty acids into blood is lower during exercise in trained than in untrained subjects. Furthermore, endurance training may enhance the antilipolytic effect of insulin on adipocytes, which also results in a reduced release of fatty acids from adipose tissue into the blood compartment (159).

In general, a linear relationship exists between the plasma concentration of fatty acids and the uptake and utilization of the lipid substrates by resting muscle (206). A lower uptake of fatty acids during exercise in trained athletes has to be anticipated, when the rate of fatty acid extraction in trained muscles also is governed by the arterial concentration of this substrate. It is noteworthy that the increased endothelial permeability–surface area may compensate for the lower circulating fatty acid concentration, which might theoretically lead to an equal or enhanced flux of fatty acids from the vascular space to the skeletal muscle fibers. However, as stated previously, recent experimental evidence shows that endurance training reduces the utilization and oxidation rate of circulating fatty acids during prolonged submaximal exercise (172). In exercising subjects, the contribution of plasma fatty acid oxidation to overall energy conversion dropped from 18% to 14% after a 12 week training protocol. These findings clearly indicate that despite an increased endothelial permeability–surface area, shortened diffusion distance, and augmented mitochondrial outer membrane surface area, the net flux of plasma fatty acids is lower in trained than in untrained muscles during strenuous exercise. Low circulating fatty acid levels may be the main cause of this intriguing effect of training on muscle lipid handling. Although uptake of plasma fatty acids was reduced, the contribution of total lipid oxidation to overall energy conversion increased from 40% to 60% (172). Comparable changes in the proportion of the caloric expenditure derived from fat oxidation during strenuous exercise tests have been published by Hurley and co-workers (132), indicating that sources other than plasma albumin-bound fatty acids, such as circulating lipoprotein-triacylglycerols and muscular neutral lipids, are mobilized to a greater extent in trained muscles during the exercise bout.

The complexity of this issue is illustrated by findings in a recent study performed by Kiens and colleagues (147) on human volunteers performing knee extensor exercise at 65% $\dot{V}O_{2max}$ for 120 min. They failed to observe a difference in arterial fatty acid level between trained and untrained subjects during exercise. Moreover, fatty acid uptake by trained muscles during 60–120 min exercise was significantly greater than by untrained muscles, despite the fact that the arterial delivery of fatty acids to trained and untrained muscles was comparable. The latter observations suggest that the kinetics of fatty acid uptake by trained and untrained muscles are different. Due to the increased capillary density, diffusion distances are shorter and mean plasma transit time is longer in trained than in untrained muscle at the same blood flow rate. An increase in dwelling time of blood plasma in the microvascular space might allow for more fatty acids to be released from the albumin–fatty acid complex per unit of time because the dissociation rate of the albumin–fatty acid complex might pose a constraint on the overall transport rate of fatty acids from the microvascular compartment to the intramuscular space (291). The differences in experimental outcomes of several studies (132, 147, 172) might be explained by the fact that in the model of one study (147) exercise and training were confined to only one muscle group, whereas other studies involved whole body exercise.

Circulating Lipoproteins as an Additional Source of Lipids for Trained Muscles

Theoretically, increased capillarization of skeletal muscle may enhance the lipolytic capacity of LPL connected to the luminal side of the endothelial membrane, since the increase in surface area will provide more space for LPL enzymes to attach to the glycocalyx covering the endothelial membrane. Indeed, the LPL activity of skeletal muscle of highly trained male athletes was found to be significantly higher than that in untrained control males (193). Moreover, significant increase in the activity of microvascular LPL of quadriceps femoris muscle after 8 weeks of training consisting of knee extensor exercise was observed (149). The increment of enzymatic activity was linearily related to the increase in capillarization of the trained muscle. Under resting conditions, the extraction ratio of circulating triacylglycerols was found to be 8% and 15% in untrained and trained thigh muscles, respectively (149). However, utilization of plasma triacylglycerols during exercise was relatively small and inconsistent. Data in their reports suggest that no difference between untrained and trained muscle was present during the exercise bout (147, 149). In addition, Oscai and co-workers (200) were unable to demonstrate in rats a training-induced effect on the activity of LPL recovered from the capillary bed of both soleus muscle and the deepest portion of the quadriceps muscle (fast-twitch red fibers) after an intensive 12 week training program, confirming earlier studies (11). Moreover, exercise training significantly reduces the production and release of VLDL by hepatocytes (101), which suggests that during exercise in trained subjects the availability of circulating triacylglycerols is decreased rather than increased.

Utilization of Intramuscular Triacylglycerols in Endurance-Trained Muscles

A number of studies on humans have suggested that in trained subjects the major contribution to enhanced lipid oxidation in the exercising muscles is delivered by triacylglycerols present in the mechanically active muscles. Cross-sectional studies (139) showed that in untrained and trained subjects intramuscular triacylglycerols contributed, respectively, 15% and 34% to total energy conversion during 60 min exercise at 60% of $\dot{V}O_{2max}$. Endurance training for 12 weeks increased the relative contribution of muscle triacylglycerols to oxidative energy conversion from 22% to 37% during an exercise bout of 90–120 min at 63% of $\dot{V}O_{2max}$ (172). The utilization rate of muscle triacylglycerols amounted to 64 and 131 nmol triacylglycerol-derived fatty acids per gram wet weight per minute before and after the training protocol, respectively (132). Since muscle fibers were cleared from adipocytes prior to chemical lipid determination, these data reflect depletion rates of triacylglycerols inside the skeletal muscle cells. The utilization of plasma-borne fatty acids decreased slightly after the training period, indicating that muscle triacylglycerols were used instead of carbohydrates. This phenomenon stresses the notion that endurance training results in a glycogen-sparing effect during exercise.

In the trained state the enhanced mobilization of the muscular neutral lipid pool during the first couple of hours of submaximal exercise might be an intrinsic mechanism to compensate for the reduced availability of circulating fatty acids resulting from the lower level of sympathoadrenal response to exercise resulting in a decreased fatty acid liberation from the adipose triacylglycerol pool (172). This hypothesis is supported by recent findings (316), which suggest that a reciprocal relation exists between plasma concentration of fatty acids and utilization of intramuscular lipids. When work at a relatively high intensity continues for a period of time longer than 90–120 min, sympathoadrenal activity will increase, leading to an enhanced plasma level of adipose tissue-derived fatty acids that will likely permit the working muscle to extract more circulating fatty acids to compensate for the depleted intracellular neutral lipid pool (172).

In addition to an enhanced capacity to oxidize endogenous fatty acids in the endurance-trained skeletal muscles, tissue triacylglycerol levels were found to be higher in trained that in untrained leg muscles of male volunteers (185). The triacylglycerol content in vastus lateralis muscle increased by about 20% after approximately 39 days of training. Eight weeks of knee extensor training increased the intramuscular triacylglycerol content in thigh muscles from 4.3 to 6.6 μmol/g wet weight (147). Hoppeler and colleagues (126) observed a ~250% increase in intramuscular lipid volume in male subjects who underwent a 6 week endurance-training program. In female volunteers, no change in the lipid volume of vastus lateralis muscle could be detected. Pretraining lipid volume was already significantly higher in female that in male subjects (126). In contrast, Hurley and co-workers (132) failed to observe a significant change in the triacylglycerol content of the vastus lateralis muscle in male subjects after a strenuous training program for 12 weeks, confirming earlier findings (85). Moreover, in rats the content of triacylglycerols was found to be decreased in fast-twitch red, slow-twitch red, and fast-twitch white fibers after endurance training (143, 200). At present, no satisfactory explanation for the deviating findings can be offered (98).

A preferential use of fatty acids derived from intramuscular triacylglycerols has certain advantages over the utilization of circulating fatty acids. As previously discussed, transport of fatty acids from the vascular compartment to the cytoplasmic space most likely poses a constraint on overall fatty acid consumption of the working muscle cells. Release of fatty acids from the intracellular lipid pool offers a fatty acid supply in close vicinity of the mitochondrial membrane, circumventing the relatively long diffusion route from the vascular space.

Contrary to the contention that training stimulates oxidation of muscular lipids, it was postulated that subjects with higher capacity to perform aerobic work derive more fatty acids from extramuscular sources than from local stores in the muscle cells (39). This notion is in agreement with the apparently higher contribution of plasma fatty acids to carbon dioxide production in athletes than in untrained subjects (114). It is, however, doubtful whether the differences can be fully ascribed to the effect of training, because exercise conditions were not identical for the untrained volunteers and highly trained athletes (114). Later studies performed by Kiens and coworkers (147) confirmed the hypothesis of Carlson and collcagucs (39). They failed to detect a significant decline in the tissue triacylglycerol content in thigh muscles of both untrained and trained subjects during 120 min of strenuous knee extensor exercise, while the contribution of fat oxidation to overall energy conversion was significantly increased in the trained volunteers.

Regulation of Fatty Acid Release from Intramuscular Triacylglycerols in Trained Muscles

The mechanism underlying enhanced hydrolytic degradation of the intramuscular triacylglycerol pool in trained subjects, as observed in a variety of studies (see above), is incompletely understood. Theoretically, enhanced utilization of the intramuscular triacylglycerol stores can be caused by increased activity of triacylglycerol lipase, decreased capacity to resynthesize triacylglycerols, or a combination of both. Enhanced lipolytic capacity may result from allosteric and/or covalent changes of triacylglycerol lipase present in the exercising muscle cell or an increase in the number of enzymes with lipolytic activity. When the hormone-sensitive neutral lipase plays a crucial role in the release of fatty acids from the cytoplasmic lipid droplets, it remains to be established to which extent the enzymatic activity is controlled by catecholamines, since the sympathoadrenal response to exercise was found to be blunted after endurance training (276). It has been suggested that the activity of skeletal muscle lipase is better sustained at low levels of circulating catecholamines as that occurring in the trained state because skeletal muscle lipolysis was found to be more sensitive to β-adrenoceptor blockade than lipolysis in adipocytes (46, 172). Moreover, in rat, adenylate cyclase is more active in skeletal muscle of trained than untrained animals (34), whereas the β-adrenoceptor density in both slow-twitch and fast-twitch fibers remains unaffected by endurance training (171). It cannot be excluded that factors other than cAMP-mediated protein phosphorylation are involved in the regulation of intramuscular triacylglycerol lipase.

Alternatively, decreased capacity of triacylglycerol resynthesis in the exercising muscle cells of trained subjects will favor a more rapid net depletion of the endogenous neutral lipid store. The mechanism underlying a possible decline in rate of triacylglycerol formation might be multifactorial. First, due to a greater uptake of fatty acyl units by muscle mitochondria, less fatty acyl CoA moieties will be available for triacylglycerol synthesis. The increased mitochondrial volume in muscle cells of trained subjects (93) most likely favors the mitochondrial uptake of fatty acyl moieties at the expense of cytoplasmic reincorporation in the neutral lipid pool. The elevated activity of carnitine palmitoyltransferase, as observed in muscle in hightly trained rats (181), might also favor the mitochondrial uptake of fatty acyl units by converting the newly formed fatty acyl CoA into fatty acyl carnitine, which permits the uptake of the fatty acyl residue in the mitochondrial matrix and prevents incorporation of the fatty acyl residue of fatty acyl CoA in the triacylglycerol pool.

Endurance training causes a reduction in the net amount of lactate produced in subjects exercising at the same intensity as untrained subjects (139, 238). The driving force for lactate formation in prolonged submaximally exercising muscles is most likely an increase in the cytoplasmic NADH/NAD$^+$ ratio. Enhanced intracellular NADH levels also force the equilibrium between dihydroxyacetone phosphate and glycerol 3-phosphate into the direction of the latter compound, which is an indispensible substrate for triacylglycerol resynthesis. Assuming that in highly trained subjects as compared to untrained volunteers the production of both lactate and glycerol 3-phosphate is less pronounced during strenuous exercise consequent to a lower cytoplasmic NADH/NAD$^+$ ratio, low intracellular glycerol 3-phosphate levels will hamper reincorporation of fatty acyl moieties in the neutral lipid pool, which results in a faster net depletion of intramuscular triacylglycerols. The cytoplasmic NADH/NAD$^+$ ratio in trained muscles might be decreased due to a training-induced increase in the capacity to shuttle reducing equivalents across the mitochondrial membrane. Finally, in heart, high levels of lactate have been found to slow down fatty acid oxidation by blocking carnitine acyl transferase (25), giving rise to elevated levels of fatty acyl CoA, which in turn favor resynthesis of triacylglycerols. If extrapolation of findings of cardiac muscle to skeletal muscles is allowed, mitigation of the inhibition of carnitine acyltransferase by low tissue levels of lactate in the trained state might also favor net depletion of the cellular triacylglycerol pool.

EFFECT OF DIET ON MUSCLE LIPID METABOLISM

Pioneering studies of Christensen and Hansen (44) have demonstrated that consumption of a diet with a restricted amount of fat exerts a negative effect on the working capacity of the body. Their studies also showed that the relative amounts of lipids and carbohydrates utilized in both the resting and exercising state is influenced by the type of nutrition. In general, persons consuming a high-fat diet have a lower respiratory exchange ratio than individuals fed a high-carbohydrate diet, which indicates that the body can be conditioned by diet to select carbohydrates or lipids for aerobic energy conversion (96, 174, 274).

High-Carbohydrate vs. High-Fat Diets in Relation to Physical Performance

For many years, the traditional view was held that a high-carbohydrate diet exerts a beneficial effect on endurance during moderate- to high-intensity exercise (130, 144). This view is in line with the generally accepted contention that muscle fatique is correlated with glycogen depletion in liver and muscle cells (21, 130, 144). Moreover, during prolonged exercise at relatively high intensity the supply and consumption of fatty acyl units were found to be insufficient to fulfill the energy requirements of the muscles, and glycogen-derived glucose was required to maintain physical exercise at the desired level of intensity (see earlier under SUPPLY AND UTILIZATION OF LIPIDS DURING EXERCISE). These observations have provided the basis for the notion that administration of high-carbohydrate diets is advantageous for athletes to enhance the body glycogen stores to (supraphysiologically) high levels and consequently to result in improved performance at relatively high workloads (48). However, other studies have provided evidence that argues against the idea that tissue glycogen stores are the primary factor limiting the endurance performance of athletes (48, 169, 215, 252).

The knowledge that fatty acids to a substantial extent contribute to overall energy conversion in exercising muscle prompted some researchers to reinvestigate this subject matter. Phinney and colleagues (215) observed that elite bicyclists prolonged their endurance (i.e., duration of exercise until exhaustion) by 4 min after consuming a high-fat diet. Moreover, highly trained athletes increased their endurance running time from 76 min to 91 min when the composition of their diet was changed from 15 en% to 38 en% fat while the contribution of carbohydrates was reduced from 73 en% to 50 en% (186).

Animal studies confirmed the observations in humans that the diet composition exerts a strong influence on endurance during strenuous exercise (177). Rats were fed either a low-fat diet (17 en% fat and 69 en% carbohydrate) or a high-fat diet (78 en% fat and 2 en% carbohydrate). After 5 weeks of diet feeding, endurance time was found to be 47 min and 36 min in the high-fat and low-fat groups, respectively. The significant improvement occurred despite lower muscle and liver glycogen levels prior to the exercise bout. During exercise, the utilization rate of glycogen and the production rate of lactate were significantly reduced in animals fed the high-fat diet, indicating a glycogen-sparing effect of high-fat feeding.

Shift from Carbohydrate to Lipid Utilization by High-Fat Diet

The high-fat diet–induced increase in endurance is most likely related to the significant shift from carbohydrate to lipid utilization. Phinney and co-workers (215) observed a drop in respiratory exchange ratio (RER) of 0.83 to 0.72 during exercise at 62%–64% of $\dot{V}O_{2max}$ when the composition of the eucaloric diet was changed from low fat to high fat. The change in RER, reflecting a greater contribution of fat oxidation to overall energy conversion, is in line with the observation that glucose oxidation declined significantly with a concomitant decrease in the rate of muscle glycogen utilization. During the exercise bout, approximately 70% more lipid was utilized when the high-fat diet was consumed compared to high-carbohydrate conditions (215). Muoio and co-workers (186), however, failed to detect a significant change in RER in highly trained runners when the composition of the diet was changed from low fat to high fat, despite a 20% increase of endurance time. This discrepancy may be due to the fact that the differences in dietary conditions in the study of Muoio and colleagues (186) were not as extreme as those in other investigations, in which RER was found to be reduced in the high-fat diet group (136, 137, 215).

Source of Lipid for Muscles during High-Fat Diet Feeding

Critical analysis of data available in the literature reveals that no definite answer can be given to the question regarding the most important lipid source for resting and exercising muscles in animals or human subjects fed a high-fat diet. The great variation in diets supplied and exercise tests employed is most likely the cause of the deviant findings.

Gross extraction of plasma fatty acids was on the average 80% greater after a high-fat than after a high-carbohydrate diet, which explains the reduction in RER (136, 137). Plasma glycerol concentration was found to be lower and circulating fatty acid levels higher in subjects fed high-fat diets than in subjects fed low-fat diets, suggesting that mobilization of adipose triacylglycerols was blunted and the utilization of plasma fatty acids was decreased by the exercising muscles in high-fat diet conditions as compared to low-fat diet conditions (186). Because RER did not change in this study, intramuscular neutral lipids are most likely compensating for the assumed reduced uptake of circulating fatty acids (186).

The observation that intramuscular neutral lipid represents a substantial source of fatty acid moieties during relatively high-intensity, submaximal exercise (132, 265) stresses the notion that high preexercise intramuscular triacylglycerol levels may be critical to overall performance of the exercising muscles. This is particularly true for trained athletes, because in some studies they were found to rely more on intramuscular triacylglycerol–fatty acid oxidation than were untrained subjects (132, 172).

Jansson and Kaijser (136, 137) observed an increase in preexercise intramuscular triacylglycerol content from 10 to 19 μmol/g wet weight when the composition of diet changed from low fat to high fat. However, no decline in tissue triacylglycerols could be monitored during exercise irrespective of the type of diet consumed. A feasible explanation might be that the exercise time employed was too short (25 min) to provoke a sufficiently great decline in the muscle triacylglycerol pool that could be reliably measured with the chemical techniques used (136, 137). The fatty acid composition of the high-fat diet has a strong influence on the amount of triacylglycerol accumulating in skeletal muscle (266). Rats fed a diet containing 59 en% fat stored 9.1 μmol triacylglycerol per gram wet weight of soleus muscle when the nutritional fat consisted of saturated fatty acids. When a considerable proportion of the diet lipids consisted of polyunsaturated long-chain ω-3 fatty acids, abundantly present in fish oil, the soleus muscle content of triacylglycerols was found to be 5.6 μmol/g (266).

Indirect evidence is available that high-fat diets might alter the rate of utilization of circulating lipoprotein-triacylglycerols, because the activity of muscular LPL was found to be controlled by the composition of the diet (148). A 3-day high-carbohydrate diet decreased significantly skeletal muscle LPL and increased the circulating level of triacylglycerols (135). When well-trained human subjects were fed a high-fat diet followed by a high-carbohydrate diet for 4 weeks each, LPL activity in vastus lateralis muscle increased from 59 to 106 mU/g after the high-fat diet and returned to 57 mU/g following the subsequent high-carbohydrate diet (148). Interestingly, tissue triacylglycerol content increased from 6 to 9 μmol/g wet weight after 4 weeks of the high-fat diet and slightly declined after 4 weeks of the high-carbohydrate diet, reaching a value of 8 μmol/g wet weight of muscle tissues (148). In contrast to short-term administration of high-carbohydrate diet, the tissue activity of LPL did not decline below normal levels during long-term feeding on a high-carbohydrate diet. Moreover, circulating insulin and triacylglycerol levels were not significantly different from those found in subjects on an ordinary mixed diet (148), suggesting pancreatic and hepatic adaptation of the body to long-term alterations in nutrition.

It is doubtful whether the increase in skeletal muscle LPL activity can be fully ascribed to the increase in proportion of lipids in the diet consumed. Renal patients fed a diet consisting of 28 en% protein, 31 en% carbohydrates, and 41 en% fat for 2 weeks showed a significantly higher muscle LPL activity than patients fed a high-carbohydrate diet (11 en% protein, 48 en% carbohydrate, and 41 en% fat). Fat tissue LPL was found to be unaffected. The fractional removal rate constant of circulatory triacylglycerols was significantly higher in patients on a low-carbohydrate diet. These data indicate that carbohydrates in combination with proteins rather than lipids in the diet influence the capacity of skeletal muscle to utilize circulating triacylglycerols for energy conversion (165).

Possible Mechanisms Underlying Increased Muscular Lipid Utilization during High-Fat Feeding

The improved capacity for endurance exercise might be partially caused by muscular adaptations to the diet, since the activity of 3-hydroxyacyl-CoA dehydrogenase, a key enzyme in the β-oxidative pathway, almost doubled in both soleus muscle and red vastus lateralis muscle of rats on the high-fat diet for 5 weeks (177). The fact that the changes in the activity of citrate synthase were inconsistent indicates that the adaptation to a high-fat diet does not pertain to the total mitochondrial enzymatic machinery, but might be restricted to enzymes specifically involved in fatty acid handling. Other investigators, however, failed to detect a diet-induced change in the activity of 3-hydroxyacyl-CoA dehydrogenase in muscle tissue of training individuals (148). It remains to be elucidated whether other enzymes catalyzing fatty acid oxidation and proteins facilitating fatty acid transport are also affected by diets high in fat and low in carbohydrates. In this respect, it is noteworthy that no significant change in FABP content of rat muscle could be detected when the contribution of fat in the diet was increased to 40 en% (298).

The possible interaction between lipid and carbohydrate metabolism in muscles at rest and during submaximal exercise has been further explored by Jansson and Kaijser (138). Human volunteers were subjected to an exercise bout of 65% of the individual $\dot{V}O_{2max}$ for 25 min after a diet consisting of either 75 en% carbohydrate and 8 en% fat or 4 en% carbohydrate and 70 en% fat. Citrate release and muscle tissue citrate concentration were found to be significantly higher during the first 5 min of exercise in the high-fat diet group as compared to subjects on the low-fat diet. No differences could be observed 25 min after the onset of the exercise bout. This observation led the authors to hypothesize that intramuscular glycolysis was inhibited during the initial stage of exercise by citrate at the level of phosphofructokinase (138) according to the regulatory model originally proposed by Randle and colleagues (220) (see later under The Glucose–Fatty Acid or Randle Cycle). Because the amount of exogenous glucose utilized did not differ between the two diets, whereas the consumption rate of intramuscular glycogen was lower in the high-fat diet group than in the low-fat diet subjects (137), it was concluded that glycolysis from glycogen, but not glycolysis from exogenous glucose was inhibited by citrate (138). Moreover, it is very unlikely that citrate plays a role in the regulation of carbohydrate consumption during prolonged exercise, although respiration exchange ratios were still lower in the high-fat diet than in the low-fat diet individuals (138).

Orfali and associates (199) have explored in some detail the effect of high-fat diet on fuel selection in cardiac myocytes. They observed that in hearts of rats fed a high-fat diet the active form of pyruvate dehydrogenase was significantly reduced, with a concomitant increase in pyruvate dehydrogenase kinase activity. Their findings indicate that an increased availability of fatty acids modulates the phosphorylation state of pyruvate dehydrogenase and, hence, suppresses the supply of glucose-derived acetyl CoA moieties to the mitochondrial tricarboxylic acid cycle. Comparable effects of high-fat diet on the active form of pyruvate dehydrogenase activity were observed in resting skeletal muscles of human volunteers (218). Moreover, relief of the malonyl CoA–dependent inhibition of carnitine acyltransferase I during high-fat feeding will promote fatty acid oxidation in the muscle fibers. In this regard, the observation of Chen and colleagues (43), that the concentration of fatty acyl CoA in muscle tissue of rats fed a high-fat diet is significantly increased, is noteworthy. Fatty acyl CoA possesses the capability of mitigating the inhibitory effect of malonyl CoA on the activation of carnitine acyltransferase I (269) (see later under A Role for Malonyl CoA in Fuel Selection in Skeletal Muscle Cells).

INTERRELATIONSHIP BETWEEN MUSCULAR CARBOHYDRATE AND LIPID METABOLISM

The Glucose–Fatty Acid, or Randle, Cycle

In the preceding sections of this chapter a great number of examples of fuel selection by resting and exercising muscle fibers have been presented. In general, enhanced supply of lipid depresses the utilization of carbohydrates as oxidizable substrates, while increased glucose oxidation exerts a negative effect on fatty acid utilization (13, 22, 36, 51, 141). Three decades ago, Randle and co-workers (89, 220, 221) observed in rat heart and diaphragm that enhanced oxidation of fatty acids inhibits the anaerobic and aerobic utilization of glucose. The underlying mechanism was thought to be that oxidation of fatty acids gives rise to enhanced acetyl CoA and/or reduced free CoA levels in the muscle cell. The increase in acetyl CoA/CoA ratio will inhibit pyruvate dehydrogenase by phosphorylation of the enzyme by pyruvate dehydrogenase kinase, which in turn slows down the conversion of glycolytically derived pyruvate to acetyl CoA (222). Moreover, accumulation of citrate, also consequent to increased fatty acid oxidation, hampers the activity of phosphofructokinase, which results in elevated cytoplasmic glucose 6-phosphate levels (Fig. 21.5). The latter substance inhibits hexokinase. The overall effect, commonly referred to as the glucose–fatty acid cycle, or Randle cycle, is reduced utilization of glucose as oxidizable substrate.

The Existence of the Randle Cycle in Skeletal Muscle

Although many investigators have published data in favor of the occurrence of fuel selection in skeletal muscle cells, both the existence and the underlying mechanism of the Randle cycle in resting and exercising myocytes have been matters of continuous debate (36, 71, 287, 315, 316, 323).

In vitro studies on cell-free systems support the concept that the activity of pyruvate dehydrogenase and phosphofructokinase is regulated by the acetyl CoA/CoA ratio and citrate, respectively (10, 50, 67, 88, 89, 191). The results obtained in studies on intact muscles were less consistent (36). In soleus muscle preparations of mice and rats the Randle cycle was found to be operative (57, 161). Other investigators, however, were unable to detect an inhibitory effect of fatty acids on glucose uptake in rat skeletal muscle at rest (19, 97, 225, 246).

Rennie and Holloszy (227) have argued that the negative results can be (in part) attributed to technical imperfections of the experimental protocol, the choice of muscle type studied, and the resting state of the muscles under investigation. They showed that in perfused rat hindlimbs an adequate supply of oxygen to the preparation was an absolute requirement to demonstrate an inhibitory effect of oleate on both glucose uptake and intramuscular glycogen utilization. Moreover, the regulatory effect of oleate was most marked when the muscles were forced to

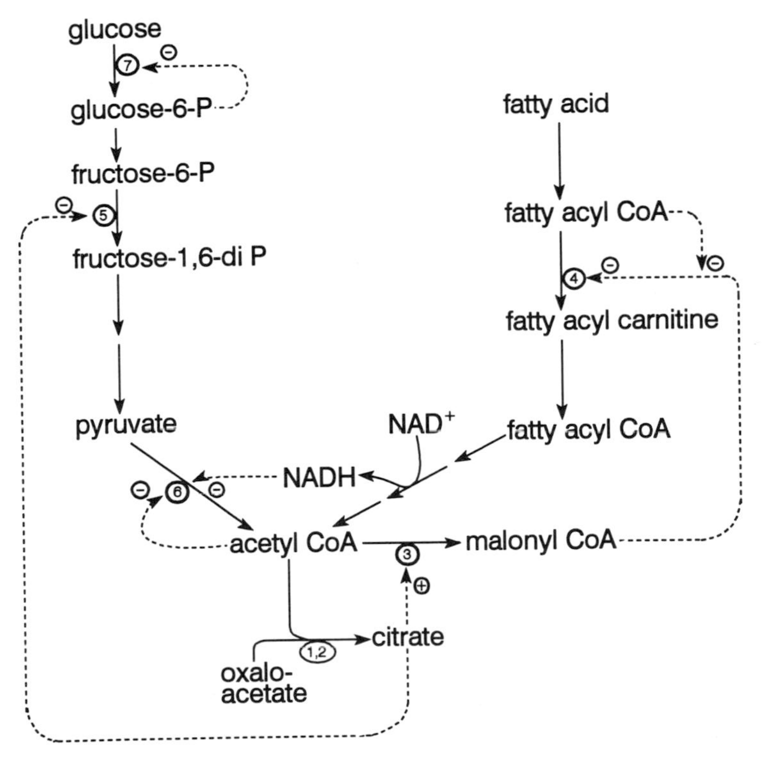

FIG. 21.5. Schematic description of the glucose–fatty acid cycle and malonyl CoA inhibition of fatty acid oxidation. *Solid* and *broken lines/arrows* refer to metabolic conversions and modes of action, respectively. ⊖ and ⊕ refer to inhibition and stimulation, respectively. *1*, citrate synthase; *2*, ATP, citrate lyase; *3*, acetyl CoA carboxylase; *4*, carnitine acyltransferase I; *5*, phosphofructokinase; *6*, pyruvate dehydrogenase; *7*, hexokinase.

contract. No effect of exogenous fatty acids could be demonstrated on glycogen utilization of the muscles at rest. The rate of glucose uptake in resting muscle was reduced by 0.11 μmol · g^{-1} · min^{-1}, while in exercising muscles glucose uptake rate dropped by 0.25 μmol · g^{-1} · min^{-1}. The regulatory effect of fatty acids was found to be confined to slow-twitch and fast-twitch red fibers. Carbohydrate metabolism in fast-twitch white fibers was insensitive to high levels of fatty acids in the perfusion medium, suggesting that the glucose–fatty acid cycle is only operative in muscle cells with a relatively high rate of oxidative metabolism and densely packed mitochondria. Citrate and glucose 6-phosphate significantly increased in slow-twitch and fast-twitch red fibers. The increments were appreciably greater in exercising than in resting muscle cells, favoring the notion that the two intermediates are instrumental in regulating the rate of the glycolytic pathway during muscle contraction. No change in citrate and glucose 6-phosphate content could be detected in fast-twitch white fibers. These findings prompted the authors (227) to conclude that, as in the heart, the glucose–fatty acid cycle is also operative in well-oxygenated red voluntary muscles. The observation that in exercising skeletal muscle the degree of citrate and glucose 6-phosphate accumulation is less marked than in myocardial tissue (89, 227), on the one hand, and that glycogen depletion is only partially inhibited in skeletal muscle and completely blocked in heart, on the other, also supports the hypothesis that in skeletal muscle tissue citrate and glucose 6-phosphate play a regulatory role in the glucose–fatty acid cycle.

In intact rats, increased plasma fatty acid levels by a high-fat meal prior to exercise caused a decrease in the utilization of glycogen in slow-twitch and fast-twitch red fibers, but not in fast-twitch white muscle cells (228), which corroborates the findings in the hindlimb perfusion experiments (228). Moreover, enhanced circulating fatty acid levels in rats improved endurance and spared muscle glycogen during physical exercise (117). A more recent study demonstrated that in rat skeletal muscle, inhibition of glucose uptake is not only dependent on the circulating level of fatty acids but also on the plasma concentration of insulin (140). This finding indicates that hormonal influences on muscle fuel selection cannot be ignored.

In studies on man aiming at unraveling the regulatory action of lipid oxidation on glucose uptake and intramuscular carbohydrate utilization, at least four different approaches were chosen to elevate plasma fatty acid levels, including fasting, moderate- and high-intensity exercise, feeding high-fat diets, and infusion of triacylglycerols plus heparin. As recently summarized by Dyck and colleagues (71), fat-feeding and fasting have the disadvantage of altering plasma hormone concentrations in addition to elevated circulating fatty acid levels, which may confound the experimentally obtained results. In contrast, infusion of a mixture of triacylglycerols (Intralipid) and heparin acutely elevates the plasma fatty acid concentration without additional hormone and substrate alterations (71). The majority of the studies performed on humans support the contention that enhanced availability of fatty acids affects the consumption of extracellular and intramuscular carbohydrates (71, 287, 315).

Increased levels of fatty acids by Intralipid and heparin administration inhibited insulin-mediated total-body glucose utilization at rest (16). Later studies demonstrated that the inhibitory effect of fatty acids on insulin-mediated glucose uptake specifically occurred in (resting) skeletal muscles (315). However, at normal ambient insulin levels high plasma fatty acid concentrations were found to promote glucose uptake in the resting forearm (315). The excess glucose is most likely used for production of glycerol 3-phosphate, a compound needed for the incorporation of fatty acids in the muscular triacylglycerol pool (315). Other studies showed that high plasma fatty acids did not affect peripheral glucose utilization during low insulin blood levels (79, 287) , while insulin-mediated glucose utilization was significantly depressed. In euglycemic resting subjects, Intralipid and heparin caused a reduction in total-body glucose uptake, oxidation, and storage in the intracellular carbohydrate pool (281). Conversely, Wolfe and coworkers (310) found that enhanced plasma fatty acid levels do not inhibit total-body blood-borne glucose oxidation, but significantly suppress the oxidation of glycogen. Glucose uptake and oxidation in resting forearm muscles were inhibited by high plasma fatty acid levels after Intralipid and heparin administration in euglycemic volunteers (302). In the hyperglycemic state glucose extraction was found to be unaffected despite decreased glucose oxidation rates (302).

Fasting resulted in high circulating fatty acid levels associated with reduced glucose utilization and oxidation rates at rest and a lower intramuscular glycogen depletion rate during exercise at 45% $\dot{V}O_{2max}$ until exhaustion than that observed in controls (153). Intramuscular glycogen utilization was also reduced in exercising subjects after a fat-rich meal and heparin injection (51).

Yki-Järvinen and associates (316) have explored in more detail the relationship between elevated plasma fatty acid levels and glucose utilization in human forearm muscles. They observed that exogenous fatty acids suppressed muscle glucose consumption when the circulating level of fatty acids was elevated to a supraphysiological concentration of greater than 1.5 mM. When the plasma fatty acid level was moderately increased by administration of heparin alone (~0.6–1.2 mM fatty acids), at a given insulin concentration carbohydrate oxidation was found to remain unchanged, while the oxidation of fatty acids from sources other than plasma fatty acids was significantly depressed. The latter observation led the authors to conclude that they demonstrated a novel feedback mechanism between fatty acid oxidation from intracellular and intravascular sources (316). The investigators, however, ignored the fact that heparin releases LPL from the luminal surface of the endothelium and, hence, reduces the capacity of the muscle to utilize plasma triacylglycerol–fatty acids as oxidizable substrates, which offers a feasible explanation for the observed decline in oxidation of fatty acids recruited from sources other than circulating albumin-bound fatty acids.

A relatively small number of investigators were unable to demonstrate an effect of fatty acids on glucose and/or glycogen metabolism. A single meal of medium-chain triacylglycerols did not affect the relative contribution of carbohydrates to overall energy conversion in exercising subjects, while the depletion rate of glycogen in vastus lateralis muscle was not different between subjects fed with medium-chain triacygylcerols and controls (62). Their findings are in line with earlier observations demonstrating an effect of diets containing long-chain triacylglycerols on fuel selection during 60 min of endurance exercise at 70% $\dot{V}O_{2max}$ (134). Ravussin and colleagues (223) increased plasma fatty acid concentration by infusion of Intralipid and heparin and were unable to detect an effect of increased availability of fatty acids on the relative contribution of carbohydrate and lipids to total energy expenditure in subjects exercising at 44% $\dot{V}O_{2max}$ for 2.5 h. Interestingly, only during the first 30 min of exercise could a carbohydrate sparing effect be observed, which disappeared when the exercise bout was prolonged. Ahlborg and Hagenfeldt (5) observed no effect of increased fatty acid utilization on glucose uptake and oxidation in exercising human leg muscles. Raised circulating fatty acid levels by administration of Intralipid and heparin inhibited glucose uptake both during rest and after 1 h of dynamic knee extension at 80% of knee-extensor maximal work capacity (110). The rate of intramuscular glycogen utilization, however, was found to be unchanged, while the relative contribution of carbohydrate and lipid oxidation to total energy conversion in the exercising muscles was also unaffected by high circulating levels of fatty acids.

Possible Mechanisms Underlying the Glucose–Fatty Acid Cycle in Skeletal Muscle

Detailed studies on the mechanism underlying the above-mentioned sparing effect of fatty acids on glucose and glycogen handling are inconclusive. According to Hargreaves and colleagues (110), who were unable to detect a change in muscle release of citrate and tissue content of glucose 6-phosphate, fatty acids have a direct effect on glucose transport into the muscular cell rather than a regulating influence on intracellular carbohydrate metabolism as suggested by Randle and co-workers (220). It is noteworthy that in subjects with high plasma fatty acid levels, citrate release from exercising muscles was initially (i.e., during the first 5 min of strenuous exercise) elevated, but not at 25 min of exercise (138). Glucose 6-phosphate showed a consistent drop from elevated tissue levels during the preexercise period to significantly lower levels at 25 min after the onset of physical work as compared to controls. Recently, Dyck and colleagues (71) demonstrated that tissue citrate, being increased at rest in subjects with high plasma fatty acids (Intralipid and heparin), did not differ from that in controls during 3 and 15 min of exercise at 85% $\dot{V}O_{2max}$ despite a significantly reduced rate of intramuscular glycogen consumption. Pyruvate dehydrogenase activity and acetyl CoA levels increased during exercise to the same extent in the Intralipid and control groups. These findings suggest that in human muscles citrate and acetyl CoA are not responsible for reduced glycogen utilization in exercising subjects with increased availability of plasma fatty acids as proposed by the classic glucose–fatty acid cycle theory. Similar observations concerning the relationship between acetyl CoA and pyruvate dehydrogenase activity were made in isometric contracting rat muscles (256), and in exercising muscle of human subjects fed a low- or high-carbohydrate diet (218). Constantin-Teodosiu and co-workers (49) hypothesized that in exercising muscles increased concentrations of Ca^{2+}, pyruvate, and ADP most likely override the inhibitory effect of a concomitantly elevated acetyl CoA/CoA ratio on pyruvate dehydrogenase. It has been proposed (71) that fatty acids exert a regulatory action at the level of muscle glycogen phosphorylase, possibly by decreased cytoplasmic levels of AMP, being a potent stimulator of glycogen phosphorylase *a* and *b* (42, 183). In favor of the classic glucose–fatty acid cycle theory is the observation that prolonged fasting, which is associated with enhanced plasma fatty acid levels and decreased muscle glucose utilization, causes a decrease in the proportion of active pyruvate dehydrogenase in muscle tissue (88, 123).

A variety of investigators have used caffeine ingestion to manipulate fuel selection during strenuous exercise. High concentrations of caffeine inhibit phosphodiesterase in adipocytes, giving rise to elevated cAMP levels (48). Caffeine administered at concentrations tolerated by human subjects most likely exerts its biological action by binding to the adenosine receptor. Consequent to the former process, lipolysis of triacylglycerols and release of fatty acids into the vascular compartment are enhanced. Increased availability of fatty acids should spare glycogen and improve endurance (48). Although earlier reports provided data for and against this concept, a recent study (258) indicates that caffeine ingestion prior to exercise decreases muscle glycogen utilization only during the first 15 min of exercise at ~80% $\dot{V}O_{2max}$. The spared glycogen was available later during the exercise bout, resulting in an improvement of endurance time. It is of interest to note that the muscle acetyl CoA/CoA ratio and citrate level are significantly increased at the onset of exercise, suggesting that pyruvate dehydrogenase and phosphofructokinase inhibition early during the exercise bout is involved in reduced utilization of the endogenous carbohydrate store. Plasma fatty acids were not increased. Since the turnover of the fatty acid pool in plasma and the intramuscular triacylglycerol pool were not measured, it remains to be established whether this study provides additional evidence that muscle carbohydrate and lipid metabolism share mutual control mechanisms.

A Role for Malonyl CoA in Fuel Selection in Skeletal Muscle Cells

From the above, it can be concluded that a substantial number of experiments indicate fuel selection is a real existing phenomenon in resting and exercising muscles. Recent findings strongly suggest that other factors than proposed in the classic glucose–fatty acid cycle are also involved in the selection of either fat or carbohydrates as prime fuel in skeletal muscle fibers. One likely candidate is malonyl CoA regulating carnitine acyltransferase I activity (31, 123, 232).

It has been firmly established that malonyl CoA exerts an inhibitory action on the enzyme responsible for the conversion of fatty acyl CoA in fatty acyl carnitine (i.e., carnitine acyltransferase I) located at the inner surface of the mitochondrial outer membrane [Fig. 21.2; (232, 306)]. Malonyl CoA is generated in the cytoplasm by the highly regulated acetyl CoA carboxylase [Fig. 21.5; (232, 284)]. In liver, malonyl CoA is an important intermediate in the de novo synthesis of fatty acids from carbohydrates. Because skeletal muscles lack lipogenic properties, the endogenous synthesis of malonyl CoA has to serve other purposes, such as controlling the rate of fatty acid oxidation. Malonyl CoA completely inhibits carnitine acyltransferase I activity in vitro at concentrations present in skeletal muscle fibers under normal physiological conditions (232). The affinity of muscle carnitine acyltransferase for malonyl CoA was found to be at least ten times higher than that of the liver enzyme. At first sight, the high sensitivity of the fatty acid–handling enzyme in muscle for physiological concentrations of malonyl CoA might be a puzzling observation, since muscle cells rely heavily on fatty acid oxidation for energy conversion. In this respect it is noteworthy that skeletal muscle mitochondria possess a substantial amount of malonyl CoA–binding proteins with high- and low-affinity binding sites for the malonyl derivative. These binding proteins are thought to play a crucial role in modulating the availability of malonyl CoA to carnitine acyltransferase I and, hence, the rate of fatty acid oxidation. The muscle tissue level of malonyl CoA is dependent on the concentration of plasma insulin and glucose. Elevated circulating levels of the two compounds keep the intracellular concentration of malonyl CoA high (69). This phenomenon might offer a mechanistic explanation for the depressive effect of carbohydrates on muscle fat oxidation (73). Submaximal physical exercise evokes a significant decline in the muscular content of malonyl CoA (68, 306, 307), which allows for an increased flux of fatty acyl units through the β-oxidative pathway by relieving the inhibition of carnitine acyltransferase I. Enhanced supply of fatty acids to skeletal muscle mitochondria is also thought to be instrumental in mitigating the inhibitory effect of malonyl CoA on fatty acid oxidation, because increased levels of fatty acyl CoA render carnitine acyltransferase I less sensitive to malonyl CoA [Fig. 21.5; (269)]. As a consequence, fatty acid oxidation increases with a concomitant increment of the NADH/NAD$^+$ and acetyl CoA/CoA ratios, theoretically resulting in inactivation of pyruvate dehydrogenase and depression of glucose utilization according to the classic Randle cycle theory. The observation that citrate promotes the acetyl CoA carboxylase–mediated production of malonyl CoA (232) might create a feedback mechanism for the exercising muscle cell to control effectively the flux of fatty acyl units through the catabolic pathway.

DEFECTS IN THE SKELETAL MUSCLE FATTY ACID OXIDATIVE PATHWAY

Detailed biochemical and molecular biological research has revealed that mitochondrial defects can be the cause of impaired functioning of skeletal muscles (242). In addition to defects in enzymes and/or proteins required for respiratory chain and citric acid cycle activity, an increasing number of defects of enzymes of the fatty acid oxidative pathway have been detected (242). The loss of proper fatty acid handling can have a primary or secondary cause. A primary cause is characterized by a genetic defect in a mitochondrial enzyme or translocator involved in the fatty acid degradative pathway. The genetic mutation can occur in the primary transcript, in enzymes regulating post-translational modification of the enzyme under consideration, or in proteins governing the translocation of the enzyme to the mitochondrial site of operation (242). A defect is considered to be secondary in all other cases (i.e., genetic defects or environmental conditions resulting in an impairment of normal mitochondrial functioning by shortage of cofactors or accumulation of inhibiting substances inside the affected cell). As summarized by Scholte (242), adverse conditions such as impaired blood supply, malnutrition, pathological changes in circulating levels of hormones and neurotransmitters, viral infections, poisoning by exogenous compounds like alcohol and a variety of drugs, and extramitochondrial or extracellular inborn or required errors of metabolism can negatively affect proper mitochondrial functioning.

Impaired fatty acid oxidation in skeletal muscle fibers is often accompanied by muscle weakness or exercise intolerance, depending on the nature and degree of the defect. For instance, muscular carnitine palmitoyl transferase deficiency is characterized by recurrent attacks of rhabdomyolysis (cellular release of myoglobin as index of loss of muscle cell integrity) after strenuous and/or prolonged exercise, long-term fasting, or exposure to cold (66, 322). Carnitine deficiency is characterized by permanent muscle weakness (322).

Until now, defects in the activity of a variety enzymes and proteins playing a significant role in mitochondrial fatty acid oxidation have been reported. Hostetler and colleagues (128) and Hoppel and coinvestigators (125) demonstrated the existence of carnitine acyltransferase I deficiency. This defect was found to be associated with intramuscular lipid accumulation. Defects in carnitine–acylcarnitine translocase and carnitine acyltransferase II were also demonstrated (64, 264). Under the latter conditions, accumulation of neutral lipids was absent.

In skeletal muscles of patients with impaired carnitine acyltransferase activity, the total activity of the enzyme measured under optimal in vitro conditions did not differ from the activity measured in muscle preparations of healthy controls (322). Palmitoyl carnitine was found to inhibit completely carnitine acyltransferase of patients but only about half of the activity in controls. Because in controls the fraction of the enzyme sensitive to palmitoyl carnitine appeared to be identical to the fraction blocked by malonyl CoA, it has been suggested that in patients with carnitine acyltransferase deficiency the defect is caused by abnormal inhibition of carnitine acyltransferase II, localized in the mitochondrial matrix, by high intracellular levels of fatty acid metabolites. This condition is most likely created when fatty acid supply to skeletal muscle is significantly enhanced, such as during fasting and strenuous exercise (322). Earlier studies indicated already that apparent carnitine acyltransferase deficiency might be caused by altered regulatory properties of the mutant enzyme or altered interaction between the enzyme and the membranous environment rather than loss of catalytically active enzymes (320). These findings are in agreement with earlier observations of Scholte and colleagues (243).

Pathophysiologically low levels of carnitine inside the myocytes readily result in impaired skeletal muscle functioning. Carnitine deficiency can be caused by primary defects in the transport of carnitine from extracellular sources into the muscle cytoplasm (74) and by primary systemic defects in uptake by a host of organs including intestines, kidneys, heart, and muscles (180, 244, 275, 282). Secondary systemic or muscular defects have also been described (242). Among others, the transport capacity of fatty acyl residues from the intermembrane space to the mitochondrial matrix will be appreciably depressed by a shortage of carnitine. Carnitine deficiency is often associated with accumulation of neutral lipids in the affected cells.

Defects in the β-oxidative pathway due either to deficiencies in the electron-transferring flavoprotein or in one or more of the enzymes constituting the fatty acid degradation pathway (Fig. 21.2) have been demonstrated (242). Short-chain, medium-chain, long-chain, and very-long-chain acyl CoA dehydrogenase deficiencies have been reported in the recent literature (8, 23, 189, 245, 283, 312, 313, 317). Moreover, patients with defects in the activity of 3-hydroxyacyl-CoA dehydrogenase have been described (229, 303). Until now, no cases have been identified with defects in proteins involved in fatty acid transport across cellular membranes or through the cytoplasmic space. Defects in FABP, for instance, might shed light on the physiological significance of this protein, abundantly present in the intracellular compartment of cardiac and red muscle fibers.

CONCLUDING REMARKS

In this chapter, an attempt was made to present an overview of the current knowledge of skeletal muscle lipid metabolism. From the wealth of scientific papers published in the literature, only a selection has been included in the reference list, highlighting the most important topics of this subject matter.

In summary, both albumin-bound fatty acids and triacylglycerol–fatty acids, present in circulating lipoproteins, can serve as lipid fuel for resting and exercising muscle fibers. Fatty acids, extracted from the extracellular compartment, are partly stored in the cytoplasmic triacylglycerol pool and subsequently used for oxidative energy conversion. During submaximal exercise, lipids are in most cases more favorable substrates than carbohydrates to fulfill the energy requirement of the muscle fibers.

The transport of fatty acids from the intravascular space, either released from the albumin–fatty acid complex or liberated from the triacylglycerol core of circulating lipoproteins by lipoprotein lipase, via endothelium, interstitital space, sarcolemma, and muscle cytosol to the intracellular site of conversion, is most likely in part mediated by fatty acid–binding and –translocating proteins. Mitochondrial lipid oxidation occurs after carnitine-mediated transport of the fatty acyl moieties across the mitochondrial inner membrane. The rate of fatty acid oxidation is regulated at various steps in the route of transport and the oxidative metabolic pathway. Endurance training and prolonged high-fat diet feeding increase the relative proportion of fat used for energy conversion in the red oxidative skeletal muscle cells, which results in a sparing effect on glycogen utilization. White glycolytic fibers are low in fatty acid oxidation.

Although our knowledge of muscle fatty acid handling has been dramatically increased during the past 30 years, many gaps in our understanding of essential parts of muscle lipid metabolism still exist. Information on the nature and regulation of rate-limiting steps in fatty acid transport is, for instance, incomplete. The same holds for many details of the interrelationship between carbohydrate and fat metabolism in the resting and working muscle cell. Moreover, the physiological significance of circulating and intramuscular triacylglycerols to muscle energy conversion is still a matter of debate. It is expected that in the near future, with the introduction of new, specific, and sensitive biochemical and molecular biological techniques, most of the questions posed today will be answered and undoubtedly replaced by other intriguing questions concerning skeletal muscle lipid metabolism.

The authors are greatly indebted to Mrs. C. Bollen, Mr. W.A. Coumans, and Mr. Th. Roemen for their help in preparing the manuscript. Prof. Dr. H.R. Scholte is thanked for his contribution to the last section of the chapter.

REFERENCES

1. Abernethy, P. J., R. Thayer, and A. W. Taylor. Acute and chronic responses of skeletal muscle to endurance and sprint exercise. *Sports Med.* 10: 365–389, 1990.
2. Abumrad, N. A., M. R. El-Maghrabi, E.-Z. Amri, E. Lopez, and P. A. Grimaldi. Cloning of a rat adipocyte membrane protein implicated in binding or transport of long-chain fatty acids that is induced during preadipocyte differentiation. *J. Biol. Chem.* 268: 17665–17668, 1993.
3. Abumrad, N. A., H. M. Tepperman, and J. Tepperman. Control of endogenous triglyceride breakdown in the mouse diaphragm. *J. Lipid Res.* 21: 149–155, 1980.
4. Ahlborg, G., P. Felig, L. Hagenfeldt, R. Hendler, and J. Wahren. Substrate turnover during prolonged exercise in man. Splanchnic and leg metabolism of glucose, free fatty acids, and amino acids. *J. Clin. Invest.* 53: 1080–1090, 1974.
5. Ahlborg, G., and L. Hagenfeldt. Effect of heparin on the substrate utilization during prolonged exercise. *Scand. J. Clin. Lab. Invest.* 37: 619–624, 1977.
6. Andersen, P., and J. Henriksson. Capillary supply of the quadriceps femoris muscle of man: adaptive response to exercise. *J. Physiol. (Lond.)* 270: 677–690, 1977.
7. Antohe, F., L. Dobrila, C. Heltianu, N. Simionescu, and M. Simionescu. Albumin-binding proteins function in the receptor-mediated binding and transcytosis of albumin across cultured endothelial cells. *Eur. J. Cell Biol.* 60: 268–275, 1993.
8. Aoyama, T., Y. Uchida, R. I. Kelley, M. Marble, K. Hofman, J. H. Tonsgard, W. J. Rhead, and T. Hashimoto. A novel disease with deficiency of mitochondrial very-long-chain acyl-CoA dehydrogenase. *Biochem. Biophys. Res. Commun.* 191: 1369–1372, 1993.
9. Appelkvist, E. L., and G. Dallner. Possible involvement of fatty acid binding protein in peroxisomal β-oxidation of fatty acids. *Biochim. Biophys. Acta.* 617: 156–160, 1980.
10. Ashour, B., and R. G. Hansford. Effect of fatty acids and ketones on the activity of pyruvate dehydrogenase in skeletal-muscle mitochondria. *Biochem. J.* 214: 725–736, 1983.
11. Askew, E. W., G. L. Dohm, R. L. Huston, T. W. Sneed, and R. P. Dowdy. Response of rat tissue lipases to physical training and exercise. *Proc. Soc. Exp. Biol. Med.* 141: 123–129, 1972.

12. Bahr, R., P. Hansson, and O. M. Sejersted. Triglyceride/fatty acid cycling is increased after exercise. *Metabolism* 39: 993–999, 1990.
13. Balasse, E. O., and M. A. Neef. Operation of the "glucose-fatty acid cycle" during experimental elevations of plasma free fatty acid levels in man. *Eur. J. Clin. Invest.* 4: 247–252, 1974.
14. Baldwin, K. M., G. H. Klinkerfuss, R. L. Terjung, P. A. Molé, and J. O. Holloszy. Respiratory capacity of white, red, and intermediate muscle: adaptative response to exercise. *Am. J. Physiol.* 222: 373–378, 1972.
15. Baldwin, K. M., J. S. Reitman, R. L. Terjung, W. W. Winder, and J. O. Holloszy. Substrate depletion in different types of muscle and in liver during prolonged running. *Am. J. Physiol.* 225: 1045–1050, 1973.
16. Baron, A. D., G. Brechtel, and S. V. Edelman. Effects of free fatty acids and ketone bodies on in vivo non-insulin-mediated glucose utilization and production in humans. *Metabolism* 38: 1056–1061, 1989.
17. Bass, N. M. The cellular fatty acid binding proteins: aspect of structure, regulation and function. *Int. Rev. Cytol.* 3: 143–184, 1988.
18. Bassingthwaighte, J. B., L. Noodleman, G. J. Van der Vusse, and J. F. C. Glatz. Modeling of palmitate transport in the heart. *Mol. Cell. Biochem.* 88: 51–59, 1989.
19. Beatty, C. H., and R. M. Bocek. Interrelation of carbohydrate and palmitate metabolism in skeletal muscle. *Am. J. Physiol.* 220: 1928–1934, 1971.
20. Bergman, E. N., R. J. Havel, B. M. Wolfe, and T. Bøhmer. Quantitative studies of the metabolism of chylomicron triglycerides and cholesterol by liver and extrahepatic tissues of sheep and dogs. *J. Clin. Invest.* 50: 1831–1839, 1971.
21. Bergström, J., L. Hermansen, E. Hultman, and B. Saltin. Diet, muscle glycogen and physical performance. *Acta Physiol. Scand.* 71: 140–150, 1967.
22. Bergström, J., E. Hultman, L. Jorfeldt, B. Pernow, and J. Wahren. Effect of nicotinic acid on physical working capacity and on metabolism of muscle glycogen in man. *J. Appl. Physiol.* 26: 170–176, 1969.
23. Bertrand, C., C. Largillière, M.-T. Zabot, M. Mathieu, and C. Vianey-Saban. Very long chain acyl-CoA dehydrogenase deficiency: identification of a newborn error of mitochondrial fatty acid oxidation in fibroblasts. *Biochim. Biophys. Acta* 1180: 327–329, 1993.
24. Bieber, L. L. Carnitine. *Annu. Rev. Biochem.* 57: 261–283, 1988.
25. Bielefeld, D. R., T. C. Vary, and J. R. Neely. Inhibition of carnitine palmitoyl-CoA transferase activity and fatty acid oxidation by lactate and oxfenicine in cardiac muscle. *J. Mol. Cell. Cardiol.* 17: 619–625, 1985.
26. Bjorkman, O. Fuel utilization during exercise. In: *Biochemical Aspects of Physical Exercise*, edited by G. Benzi, L. Packer, and N. Siliprandi. Amsterdam, Elsevier, 1986, p. 245–260.
27. Blatchford, F. K., R. G. Knowlton, and D. A. Schneider. Plasma FFA responses to prolonged walking in untrained men and women. *Eur. J. Appl. Physiol.* 53: 343–347, 1985.
28. Blomqvist, C. G., and B. Saltin. Cardiovascular adaptations to physical training. *Annu. Rev. Physiol.* 45: 169–189, 1983.
29. Booth, F. W., and D. B. Thomason. Molecular and cellular adaptation of muscle in response to exercise: perspectives of various models. *Physiol. Rev.* 71: 541–585, 1991.
30. Borensztjan, J., M. S. Rone, S. P. Babirak, J. A. McGarr, and L. B. Oscai. Effect of exercise on lipoprotein lipase activity in rat heart and skeletal muscle. *Am. J. Physiol.* 229: 394–397, 1975.
31. Brady, P. S., R. R. Ramsay, and L. J. Brady. Regulation of the longchain carnitine acyltransferases. *FASEB J.* 7: 1039–1044, 1993.
32. Braun, J. E. A., and D. L. Severson. Regulation of the synthesis, processing and translocation of lipoprotein lipase. *Biochem. J.* 287: 337–347, 1992.
33. Bremer, J. Carnitine-metabolism and functions. *Physiol. Rev.* 63: 1420–1480, 1983.
34. Buckenmeyer, P. J., A. H. Goldfarb, J. S. Partilla, M. A. Pineyro, and E. M. Dax. Endurance training, not acute exercise, differentially alters β-receptors and cyclase in skeletal fiber types. *Am. J. Physiol.* 258 (*Endocrinol. Metab.* 21): E71–E77, 1990.
35. Budohoski, L., S. Kozlowski, R. L. Terjung, H. Kaciuba-Uscilko, K. Nazar, and I. Falecka-Wieczorek. Changes in muscle lipoprotein lipase activity during exercise in dogs fed on a mixed fat-rich meal. *Pflugers Arch.* 394: 191–193, 1982.
36. Bülow, J. Lipid mobilization and utilization. In: *Principles of Exercise Biochemistry. Med. Sports Sci.*, edited by J. R. Poortmans. Basel: Karger, 1986, p. 140–163.
37. Camps, L., M. Reina, M. Lobera, S. Villard, and T. Olivecrona. Lipoprotein lipase: cellular origin and functional distribution. *Am. J. Physiol.* 258 (*Cell Physiol.* 27): C673–C681, 1990.
38. Carey, J. O., P. D. Neufer, R. P. Farrar, J. H. Veerkamp, and G. L. Dohm. Transcriptional regulation of muscle fatty acid-binding protein. *Biochem. J.* 298: 613–617, 1994.
39. Carlson, L. A., L.-G. Ekelund, and S. O. Fröberg. Concentration of triglycerides, phospholipids and glycogen in skeletal muscle and of free fatty acids and β-hydroxybutyric acid in blood in man in response to exercise. *Eur. J. Clin. Invest.* 1: 248–254, 1971.
40. Carlson, L. A., S.-O. Liljedahl, and C. Wirsén. Blood and tissue changes in the dog during and after excessive free fatty acid mobilization. *Acta Med. Scand.* 178: 81–102, 1965.
41. Carlson, L. A., and B. Pernow. Studies on blood lipids during exercise. II. The arterial plasma free fatty acid concentration during and after exercise and its regulation. *J. Lab. Clin. Med.* 58: 673–681, 1961.
42. Chasiotis, D., K. Sahlin, and E. Hultman. Regulation of glycogenolysis in human muscle at rest and exercise. *J. Appl. Physiol.* 53: 708–715, 1982.
43. Chen, M. T., L. N. Kaufman, T. Spennetta, and E. Shrago. Effects of high fat-feeding to rats on the interrelationship of body weight, plasma insulin, and fatty acyl-coenzyme A esters in liver and skeletal muscle. *Metabolism* 41: 564–569, 1992.
44. Christensen, E. H., and O. Hansen. Arbeitsfähigkeit und Ernährung. *Scand. Arch. Physiol.* 81: 160–171, 1939.
45. Claffey, K. P., V. L. Herrera, P. Brecher, and N. Ruiz-Opazo. Cloning and tissue distribution of rat heart fatty acid binding protein mRNA: identical forms in heart and skeletal muscle. *Biochem. J.* 26: 7900–7904, 1987.
46. Cleroux, J., P. Van Nguyen, A. W. Taylor, and F. H. H. Leenen. Effects of β_1- vs. $\beta_1 + \beta_2$-blockade on exercise endurance and muscle metabolism in humans. *J. Appl. Physiol.* 66: 548–554, 1989.
47. Coggan, A. R., D. L. Habash, L. A. Mendenhall, S. C. Swanson, and C. L. Kien. Isotopic estimation of CO_2 production during exercise before and after endurance training. *J. Appl. Physiol.* 75: 70–75, 1993.

48. Conlee, R. K. Muscle glycogen and exercise endurance: a twenty-year perspective. *Exerc. Sport Sci. Rev.* 15: 1–28, 1987.
49. Constantin-Teodosiu, D., G. Cederblad, and E. Hultman. PDC activity and acetyl group accumulation in skeletal muscle during prolonged exercise. *J. Appl. Physiol.* 73: 2403–2407, 1992.
50. Constantin-Teodosiu, D., G. Cederblad, and E. Hultman. PDC activity and acetyl group accumulation in skeletal muscle during isometric contraction. *J. Appl. Physiol.* 74: 1712–1718, 1993.
51. Costill, D. L., E. Coyle, G. Dalsky, W. Evans, W. Fink, and D. Hoopes. Effects of elevated plasma FFA and insulin on muscle glycogen usage during exercise. *J. Appl. Physiol.* 43: 695–699, 1977.
52. Costill, D. L., W. J. Fink, L. H. Getchell, J. L. Ivy, and F. A. Witzmann. Lipid metabolism in skeletal muscle of endurance-trained males and females. *J. Appl. Physiol.* 47: 787–791, 1979.
53. Costill, D. L., P. D. Gollnick, E. D. Jansson, B. Saltin, and E. M. Stein. Glycogen depletion pattern in human muscle fibers during distance running. *Acta Physiol. Scand.* 89: 374–383, 1973.
54. Côté, C., T. P. White, and J. A. Faulkner. Intramuscular depletion and fatigability of soleus grafts in rats. *Can. J. Physiol. Pharmacol.* 66: 829–832, 1988.
55. Crisman, T. S., K. P. Claffey, R. Saouaf, J. Hanspal, and P. Brecher. Measurement of rat heart fatty acid binding protein by ELISA. Tissue distribution, developmental changes and subcellular distribution. *J. Mol. Cell. Cardiol.* 19: 423–431, 1987.
56. Cryer, A. The role of the endothelium in myocardial lipoprotein dynamics. *Mol. Cell. Biochem.* 88: 7–15, 1989.
57. Cuendet, G. S., E. G. Loten, and A. E. Renold. Evidence that glucose-fatty acid cycle is operative in isolated skeletal (soleus) muscle. *Diabetalogica* 12: 336, 1975.
58. Dalsky, G., W. Martin, B. Hurley, D. Matthews, D. Bier, J. Hagberg, and J. O. Holloszy. Oxidation of plasma FFA during endurance exercise. *Med. Sci. Sports Exerc.* 16: 202, 1984.
59. Davies, K. J. A., L. Packer, and G. A. Brooks. Biochemical adaptation of mitochondria, muscle, and whole-animal respiration to endurance training. *Arch. Biochem. Biophys.* 209: 539–554, 1981.
60. De Duve, C. Peroxisomes and related particles in historical perspective. *Ann. N. Y. Acad. Sci.* 386: 1–4, 1982.
61. De Jong, J. W., and W. C. Hülsmann. Effects of Nagarse, adenosine and hexokinase on palmitate activation and oxidation. *Biochim. Biophys. Acta* 210: 499–501, 1970.
62. Décombaz, J., M.-J. Arnaud, H. Milon, H. Moesch, G. Philippossian, A.L. Thélin, and H. Howald. Energy metabolism of medium-chain triglycerides versus carbohydrates during exercise. *Eur. J. Appl. Physiol.* 52: 9–14, 1983.
63. Degens, H., J. H. Veerkamp, H. T. B. Van Moerkerk, Z. Turek, L. J. C. Hoofd, and R. A. Binkhorst. Metabolic capacity, fibre type area and capillarization of rat plantaris muscle. Effects of age, overload and training and relationship with fatigue resistance. *Int. J. Biochem.* 25: 1141–1148, 1993.
64. Demaugre, F., J.-P. Bonnefont, M. Colonna, C. Cepanec, J.-P. Leroux, and J.-M. Saudubray. Infantile form of carnitine palmitoyltransferase II deficiency with hepatomuscular symptoms and sudden death. Physiopathological approach to carnitine palmitoyltransferase II deficiencies. *J. Clin. Invest.* 87: 859–864, 1991.
65. Denton, R. M., and P. J. Randle. Concentrations of glycerides and phospholipids in rat heart and gastrocnemius muscle. Effects of Alloxandiabetes and perfusion. *Biochem. J.* 104: 416–422, 1967.
66. Di Donato, S., A. Castiglione, M. Rimoldi, F. Cornelio, F. Vendemia, G. Cardace, and B. Bertagnolio. Heterogeneity of carnitine-palmitoyltransferase deficiency. *J. Neurol. Sci.* 50: 207–215, 1981.
67. Dobson, G. P., E. Yamamoto, and P. W. Hochachka. Phosphofructokinase control in muscle: nature and reversal of pH-dependent ATP inhibition. *Am. J. Physiol.* 250 (*Regulatory Integrative Comp. Physiol.* 19): R71–R76, 1986.
68. Duan, C., and W. W. Winder. Nerve stimulation decreases malonyl-CoA in skeletal muscle. *J. Appl. Physiol.* 72: 901–904, 1992.
69. Duan, C., and W. W. Winder. Control of malonyl-CoA by glucose and insulin in perfused skeletal muscle. *J. Appl. Physiol.* 74: 2543–2547, 1993.
70. Dudley, G. A. Influence of mitochondrial content on the sensitivity of respiratory control. *J. Biol. Chem.* 262: 9109–9114, 1987.
71. Dyck, D. J., C. T. Putman, G. J. F. Heigenhauser, E. Hultman, and L. L. Spriet. Regulation of fat-carbohydrate interaction in skeletal muscle during intense aerobic cycling. *Am. J. Physiol.* 265 (*Endocrinol. Metab.* 28): E852–E859, 1993.
72. Eckel, R. H. Lipoprotein lipase: a multifunctional enzyme relevant to common metabolic diseases. *N. Engl. J. Med.* 320: 1060–1068, 1989.
73. Elayan, I. M., and W. W. Winder. Effect of glucose infusion on muscle malonyl-CoA during exercise. *J. Appl. Physiol.* 70: 1495–1499, 1991.
74. Engel, A. G., and C. Angelini. Carnitine deficiency of human skeletal muscle with associated lipid storage myopathy: a new syndrome. *Science* 179: 899–901, 1973.
75. Essén, B. Intramuscular substrate utilization during prolonged exercise. *Ann. N. Y. Acad. Sci.* 301: 30–44, 1977.
76. Essén, B., L. Hagenfeldt, and L. Kaijser. Utilization of blood-borne and intramuscular substrates during continuous and intermittent exercise in man. *J. Physiol. (Lond.)* 265: 489–506, 1977.
77. Essén, B., E. Jansson, J. Henriksson, A. W. Taylor, and B. Saltin. Metabolic characteristics of fibre types in human skeletal muscle. *Acta Physiol. Scand.* 95: 153–165, 1975.
78. Essén-Gustavsson, B., and P. A. Tesch. Glycogen and triglyceride utilization in relation to muscle metabolic characteristics in men performing heavy-resistance exercise. *Eur. J. Appl. Physiol.* 61: 5–10, 1990.
79. Ferrannini, E., E. J. Barrett, S. Bevilacqua, and R. A. DeFronzo. Effects of fatty acids on glucose production and utilization in man. *J. Clin. Invest.* 72: 1737–1747, 1983.
80. Fournier, N. C., and M. Rahim. Control of energy production in the heart: a new function for fatty acid binding protein. *Biochemistry* 24: 2387–2396, 1985.
81. Fournier, N. C., and M. A. Richard. Role of fatty acid-binding protein in cardiac fatty acid oxidation. *Mol. Cell. Biochem.* 98: 149–159, 1990.
82. Frayn, K. N., and P. F. Maycock. Skeletal muscle triacylglycerol in the rat: methods for sampling and measurement, and studies of biological variability. *J. Lipid Res.* 21: 139–144, 1980.
83. Friedberg, S. J., R. F. Klein, D. L. Trout, M. D. Bogdonoff, and E. H. Estes. The characteristics of the peripheral transport of C^{14}-labeled palmitic acid. *J. Clin. Invest.* 39: 1511–1515, 1960.

84. Fröberg, K., and P. K. Pedersen. Sex differences in endurance capacity and metabolic response to prolonged, heavy exercise. *Eur. J. Appl. Physiol.* 52: 446–450, 1984.
85. Fröberg, S. O. Effects of training and of acute exercise in trained rats. *Metabolism* 20: 1044–1051, 1971.
86. Fröberg, S. O., E. Hultman, and L. H. Nilsson. Effect of noradrenaline on triglyceride and glycogen concentrations in liver and muscle from man. *Metabolism* 24: 119–125, 1975.
87. Fröberg, S. O., and F. Mossfeldt. Effect of prolonged strenuous exercise on the concentration of triglycerides, phospholipids and glycogen in muscle of man. *Acta Physiol. Scand.* 82: 167–171, 1971.
88. Fuller, S. J., and P. J. Randle. Reversible phosphorylation of pyruvate dehydrogenase in rat skeletal-muscle mitochondria. Effects of starvation and diabetes. *Biochem. J.* 219: 635–646, 1984.
89. Garland, P. B., and P. J. Randle. Regulation of glucose uptake by muscle. 10. Effects of alloxan-diabetes, starvation, hypophysectomy and adrenalectomy, and of fatty acids, ketone bodies and pyruvate, on the glycerol output and concentrations of free fatty acids, long-chain fatty acylcoenzyme A, glycerol phosphate and citrate-cycle intermediates in rat heart and diaphragm muscles. *Biochem. J.* 93: 678–687, 1964.
90. Glatz, J. F. C., and G. J. van der Vusse. Cellular fatty acid-binding proteins: current concepts and future directions. *Mol. Cell. Biochem.* 98: 247–251, 1990.
91. Glatz, J. F. C., G. J. van der Vusse, and J. H. Veerkamp. Fatty acidbinding proteins and their physiological significance. *News Physiol. Sci.* 3: 41–43, 1988.
92. Gollnick, P. D. Metabolism of substrates: energy substrate metabolism during exercise and as modified by training. *Federation Proc.* 44: 353–357, 1985.
93. Gollnick, P. D., D. Ianuzzo, and D. W. King. Ultrastructural and enzyme changes in muscles with exercise. In: *Muscle Metabolism During Exercise*, edited by B. Pernow and B. Saltin. New York, London: Plenum Press, 1971, p. 69–81.
94. Gollnick, P. D., C. D. Ianuzzo, C. Williams, and T. R. Hill. Effect of prolonged, severe exercise on the ultrastructure of human skeletal muscle. *Int. Z. Angew. Physiol.* 27: 257–265, 1969.
95. Gollnick, P. D., and B. Saltin. Significance of skeletal muscle oxidative enzyme enhancement with endurance training. *Clin. Physiol.* 2: 1–12, 1982.
96. Gollnick, P. D., and B. Saltin. Fuel for muscular exercise: role of fat. In: *Exercise, Nutrition and Energy Metabolism*, edited by E. S. Horton and R. L. Terjung. New York: Macmillan Publishing Company, 1988, p. 71–88.
97. Goodman, M. N., M. Berger, and N. B. Ruderman. Glucose metabolism in rat skeletal muscle at rest. Effect of starvation, diabetes, ketone bodies and free fatty acids. *Diabetes* 23: 81–88, 1974.
98. Górski, J. Muscle triglyceride metabolism during exercise. *Can. J. Physiol. Pharmacol.* 70: 123–131, 1992.
99. Górski, J., and T. Kiryluk. The post-exercise recovery of triglycerides in rat tissue. *Eur. J. Appl. Physiol.* 45: 33–41, 1980.
100. Górski, J., M. Nowacka, Z. Namiot, and T. Kiryluk. Effect of exercise on energy substrates metabolism in tissues of adrenalectomized rats. *Acta Physiol. Pol.* 38: 331–337, 1987.
101. Górski, J., L. B. Oscai, and W. K. Palmer. Hepatic lipid metabolism in exercise and training. *Med. Sci. Sports Exerc.* 22: 213–221, 1990.
102. Górski, J., and B. Stankiewicz-Choroszucha. The effect of hormones on lipoprotein lipase activity in skeletal muscles of the rat. *Horm. Metab. Res.* 14: 189–191, 1982.
103. Graham, T. E., J. P. Van Dijk, M. Viswanathan, K. A. Giles, A. Bonen, and J. C. George. Exercise metabolic responses in men and eumenorrheic and amenorrheic women. In: *Biochemistry of Exercise, VI (Inter. Ser. Sports. Sci.), edited by B. Saltin. Champaign, IL: Human Kinetics Publishing Company, p. 227–228, 1986.*
104. Groot, P. H. E., H. R. Scholte, and W. C. Hülsmann. Fatty acid activation: specificity, localization and function. In: *Advances in Lipid Research*, edited by R. Paoletti and D. Kritchevsky. New York: Academic Press, 1976, p. 75–119.
105. Guzmán, M., and J. Castro. Effects of endurance exercise on carnitine palmitoyltransferase I from rat heart, skeletal muscle and liver mitochondria. *Biochim. Biophys. Acta* 963: 562–565, 1988.
106. Guzmán, M., and M. J. H. Geelen. Regulation of fatty acid oxidation in mammalian liver. *Biochim. Biophys. Acta* 1167: 227–241, 1993.
107. Hagenfeldt, L., and J. Wahren. Metabolism of free fatty acids and ketone bodies in skeletal muscle. In: *Muscle Metabolism during Exercise*, edited by B. Pernow and B. Saltin. New York, London: Plenum Press, 1971, p. 153–163.
108. Hagenfeldt, L., and J. Wahren. Human forearm muscle metabolism during exercise. VII. FFA uptake and oxidation at different work intensities. *Scand. J. Clin. Lab. Invest.* 30: 429–436, 1972.
109. Hagerman, F. C. Energy metabolism and fuel utilization. *Med. Sci. Sports Exerc.* 24: S309–S314, 1992.
110. Hargreaves, M., B. Kiens, and E. A. Richter. Effect of increased plasma free fatty acid concentrations on muscle metabolism in exercising men. *J. Appl. Physiol.* 70: 194–201, 1991.
111. Harmon, C. M., and N. A. Abumrad. Binding of sulfosuccinimidyl fatty acids to adipocyte membrane proteins: isolation and amino-terminal sequence of an 88-kD protein implicated in transport of long-chain fatty acids. *J. Membr. Biol.* 133: 43–47, 1993.
112. Hartley, L. H., J. W. Mason, R. P. Hogan, L. G. Jones, T. A. Kotchen, E. H. Mougey, F. E. Wherry, L. L. Pennington, and P. T. Ricketts. Multiple hormonal responses to prolonged exercise in relation to physical training. *J. Appl. Physiol.* 33: 607–610, 1972.
113. Haunerland, N. H., and J. M. Chisholm. Fatty acid binding protein in flight muscle of the locust, Schistocerca gregaria. *Biochim. Biophys. Acta.* 1047: 233–238, 1990.
114. Havel, R. J., L. A. Carlson, L.-G. Ekelund, and A. Holmgren. Turnover rate and oxidation of different free fatty acids in man during exercise. *J. Appl. Physiol.* 19: 613–618, 1964.
115. Havel, R. J., B. Pernow, and N. L. Jones. Uptake and release of free fatty acids and other metabolites in the legs of exercising men. *J. Appl. Physiol.* 23: 90–99, 1967.
116. Heuckeroth, R. O., E. H. Birkenmeier, M. S. Levin, and J. I. Gordon. Analysis of the tissue-specific expression, developmental regulation, and linkage relationships of a rodent gene encoding heart fatty acid binding protein. *J. Biol. Chem.* 262: 9709–9717, 1987.
117. Hickson, R. C. Effects of increased plasma fatty acids on glycogen utilization and endurance. *J. Appl. Physiol.* 43: 829–833, 1977.
118. Hodgetts, V., S. W. Coppack, K. N. Frayn, and T. D. R. Hockaday. Factors controlling fat mobilization from human subcutaneous adipose tissue during exercise. *J. Appl. Physiol.* 71: 445–451, 1991.

119. Holloszy, J. O. Biochemical adaptations in muscle. Effects of exercise on mitochondrial oxygen uptake and respiratory enzyme activity in skeletal muscle. *J. Biol. Chem.* 242: 2278–2282, 1967.
120. Holloszy, J. O. Utilization of fatty acids during exercise. In: *Biochemistry of Exercise VII (Int. Series Sports Sci.), edited by A. W. Taylor, 1990, p. 319–327.*
121. Holloszy, J. O., and E. F. Coyle. Adaptations of skeletal muscle to endurance exercise and their metabolic consequences. *J. Appl. Physiol.* 56: 831–838, 1984.
122. Holm, C., P. Belfrage, and G. Fredrikson. Immunological evidence for the presence of hormone-sensitive lipase in rat tissues other than adipose tissue. *Biochem. Biophys. Res. Commun.* 148: 99–105, 1987.
123. Holness, M. J., Y.-L. Liu, and M. C. Sugden. Time courses of the responses of pyruvate dehydrogenase activities to short-term starvation in diaphragm and selected skeletal muscle of the rat. *Biochem. J.* 264: 771–776, 1989.
124. Hopp, J. F., and W. K. Palmer. Effect of electrical stimulation on intracellular triacylglycerol in isolated skeletal muscle. *J. Appl. Physiol.* 68: 348–354, 1990.
125. Hoppel, C., S. Genuth, E. Brass, R. Fuller, and K. Hostetler. *Carnitine Biosynthesis, Metabolism and Function.* New York: Academic Press, 1980, p. 287–305.
126. Hoppeler, H., H. Howald, K. Conley, S. L. Lindstedt, H. Claasen, P. Vock, and E. R. Weibel. Endurance training in humans: aerobic capacity and structure of skeletal muscle. *J. Appl. Physiol.* 59: 320–327, 1985.
127. Hoppeler, H., P. Lüthi, H. Claassen, E. R. Weibel, and H. Howald. The ultrastructure of the normal human skeletal muscle. A morphometric analysis on untrained men, women and well-trained orienteers. *Pflugers Arch.* 344: 217–232, 1973.
128. Hostetler, K. Y., C. L. Hoppel, J. S. Romine, J. C. Sipe, S. R. Gross, and P. A. Higginbottom. Partial deficiency of muscle carnitine palmitoyltransferase with normal ketone production. *N. Engl. J. Med.* 298: 553–557, 1978.
129. Howald, H., H. Hoppeler, H. Claassen, O. Mathieu, and R. Straub. Influences of endurance training on the ultrastructural composition of the different muscle fiber types in humans. *Pflugers Arch.* 403: 369–376, 1985.
130. Hultman, E. Physiological role of muscle glycogen in man, with special reference to exercise. *Circ. Res.* 21/22 (Suppl.): I-99–I-112, 1967.
131. Hultman, E., and R. C. Harris. Carbohydrate metabolism. In: *Principles of Exercise Biochemistry. Med. Sports Sci.*, edited by J. R. Poortman. Basel: Karger, 1988, p. 78–119.
132. Hurley, B. F., P. M. Nemeth, W. H. Martin, III, J. M. Hagberg, G. P. Dalsky, and J. O. Holloszy. Muscle triglyceride utilization during exercise: effect of training. *J. Appl. Physiol.* 60: 562–567, 1986.
133. Issekutz, B., and H. Miller. Plasma free fatty acids during exercise and the effect of lactic acid. *Proc. Soc. Exp. Biol. Med.* 110: 237–239, 1962.
134. Ivy, J. L., D. L. Costill, W. J. Fink, and E. Maglischo. Contribution of medium and long chain triglyceride intake to energy metabolism during prolonged exercise. *Int. J. Sports Med.* 1: 15–20, 1980.
135. Jacobs, I., H. Lithell, and J. Karlsson. Dietary effects on glycogen and lipoprotein lipase activity in skeletal muscle in man. *Acta Physiol. Scand.* 115: 85–90, 1982.
136. Jansson, E. Diet and muscle metabolism in man. *Acta Physiol. Scand. Suppl.* 487: 3–24, 1980.
137. Jansson, E., and L. Kaijser. Effect of diet on the utilization of bloodborne and intramuscular substrates during exercise in man. *Acta Physiol. Scand.* 115: 19–30, 1982.
138. Jansson, E., and L. Kaijser. Leg citrate metabolism at rest and during exercise in relation to diet and substrate utilization in man. *Acta Physiol. Scand.* 122: 145–153, 1984.
139. Jansson, E., and L. Kaijser. Substrate utilization and enzymes in skeletal muscle of extremely endurance-trained men. *J. Appl. Physiol.* 62: 999–1005, 1987.
140. Jenkins, A. B., L. H. Storlien, D. J. Chisholm, and E. W. Kraegen. Effects of nonesterified fatty acid availability on tissue-specific glucose utilization in rats in vivo. *J. Clin. Invest.* 82: 293–299, 1988.
141. Johnson, A. B., M. Argyraki, C. J. Thow, B. G. Cooper, G. Fulcher, and R. Taylor. Effect of increased free fatty acid supply on glucose metabolism and skeletal muscle glycogen synthase activity in normal man. *Clin. Sci.* 82: 219–226, 1992.
142. Kaciuba-Uscilko, H., G. A. Dudley, and R. L. Terjung. Influence of thyroid status on skeletal muscle LPL activity and TG uptake. *Am. J. Physiol.* 238 (*Endocrinol. Metab.* 1): E518–E523, 1980.
143. Kaciuba-Uscilko, H., G. A. Dudley, and R. L. Terjung. Muscle LPL activity, plasma and muscle triglycerides in trained thyroidectomized rats. *Horm. Metab. Res.* 13: 688–689, 1981.
144. Karlsson, J., and B. Saltin. Diet, muscle glycogen, and endurance performance. *J. Appl. Physiol.* 31: 203–206, 1971.
145. Kaufmann, M., J.-A. Simoneau, J. H. Veerkamp, and D. Pette. Electrostimulation-induced increases in fatty acid-binding protein and myoglobin in rat fast-twitch muscle and comparison with tissue levels in heart. *FEBS Lett.* 245: 181–184, 1989.
146. Keul, J., E. Doll, and G. Haralambie. Freie Fettsäure, Glycerin und Triglyceride im arteriellen und femoralvenösen Blut vor und nach einem vierwöchigen körperlichen Training. *Pflugers Arch.* 316: 194–204, 1970.
147. Kiens, B., B. Éssen-Gustavsson, N. J. Christensen, and B. Saltin. Skeletal muscle substrate utilization during submaximal exercise in man: effect of endurance training. *J. Physiol. (Lond.)* 469: 459–478, 1993.
148. Kiens, B., B. Éssen-Gustavsson, P. Gad, and H. Lithell. Lipoprotein lipase activity and intramuscular triglyceride stores after long-term highfat and high-carbohydrate diets in physically trained men. *Clin. Physiol.* 7: 1–9, 1987.
149. Kiens, B., and H. Lithell. Lipoprotein metabolism influenced by traininginduced changes in human skeletal muscle. *J. Clin. Invest.* 83: 558–564, 1989.
150. Kiens, B., H. Lithell, K. J. Mikines, and E. A. Richter. Effects of insulin and exercise on muscle lipoprotein lipase activity in man and its relation to insulin action. *J. Clin. Invest.* 84: 1124–1129, 1989.
151. Kiessling, K.-H., L. Pilström, A.-C. Bylund, B. Saltin, and K. Piehl. Enzyme activities and morphometry in skeletal muscle of middle-aged men after training. *Scand. J. Clin. Lab. Invest.* 33: 63–69, 1974.
152. Kim, H.-K., and J. Storch. Mechanism of free fatty acid transfer from rat heart fatty acid-binding protein to phospholipid membranes. Evidence for a collisional process. *J. Biol. Chem.* 267: 20051–20056, 1992.
153. Knapik, J. J., C. N. Meredith, B. H. Jones, L. Suek, V. R. Young, and W. J. Evans. Influence of fasting on carbohydrate and fat metabolism during rest and exercise in men. *J. Appl. Physiol.* 64: 1923–1929, 1988.
154. Knudsen, J., P. Højrup, H. O. Hansen, H. F. Hansen, and P. Roepstorff. Acyl-CoA-binding protein in the rat. Purification, binding characteristics, tissue concentrations and amino acid sequence. *Biochem. J.* 262: 513–519, 1989.

155. Kotlar, T. J., and J. Borensztajn. Oscillatory changes in muscle lipoprotein lipase activity of fed and starved rats. *Am. J. Physiol.* 233 (*Endocrinol. Metab. Gastrointest. Physiol.* 2): E316–E319, 1977.
156. Kozlowski, S., L. Budohoski, E. Pohoska, and K. Nazar. Lipoprotein lipase activity in the skeletal muscle during physical exercise in dogs. *Pflugers Arch.* 382: 105–107, 1979.
157. Kragh-Hansen, U. Molecular aspects of ligand binding to serum albumin. *Pharmacol. Rev.* 33: 17–53, 1981.
158. Krogh, A., and J. Lindhard. The relative value of fat and carbohydrate as sources of muscular energy. *Biochem. J.* 14: 290–363, 1920.
159. Lavoie, J.-M., J. Bongbêlé, S. Cardin, M. Bélisle, J. Terettaz, and G. Van de Werve. Increased insulin suppression of plasma free fatty acid concentration in exercise-trained rats. *J. Appl. Physiol.* 74: 293–296, 1993.
160. Lazarow, P. B. The role of peroxisomes in mammalian cellular metabolism. *J. Inherit. Metab. Dis.* 10 (Suppl. 1): 11–22, 1987.
161. Li, J., J. S. Stillman, J. N. Clore, and W. G. Blackard. Skeletal muscle lipids and glycogen mask substrate competition (Randle cycle). *Metabolism* 42: 451–456, 1993.
162. Linder, C., S. S. Chernick, T. R. Fleck, and R. O. Scow. Lipoprotein lipase and uptake of chylomicron triglyceride by skeletal muscle of rats. *Am. J. Physiol.* 231: 860–864, 1976.
163. Linssen, M. C. J. G., M. M. Vork, Y. F. De Jong, J. F. C. Glatz, and G. J. van der Vusse. Fatty acid oxidation capacity and fatty acid-binding protein content of different cell types isolated from rat heart. *Mol. Cell. Biochem.* 89: 19–26, 1990.
164. Lithell, H., and J. Boberg. Determination of lipoprotein-lipase activity in human skeletal muscle tissue. *Biochim. Biophys. Acta* 528: 55–68, 1978.
165. Lithell, H., B. Karlström, I. Selinus, B. Vessby, and B. Fellström. Is muscle lipoprotein lipase inactivated by ordinary amounts of dietary carbohydrates? *Hum. Nutr. Clin. Nutr.* 39C: 289–295, 1985.
166. Lithell, H., J. Örlander, R. Schéle, B. Sjödin, and J. Karlsson. Changes in lipoprotein-lipase activity and lipid stores in human skeletal muscle with prolonged heavy exercise. *Acta Physiol. Scand.* 107: 257–261, 1979.
167. Lowry, C. V., J. S. Kimmey, S. Felder, M. M.-Y. Chi, K. K. Kaiser, P. N. Passonneau, K. A. Kirk, and O. H. Lowrey. Enzyme patterns in single human muscle fibers. *J. Biol. Chem.* 253: 8269–8277, 1978.
168. Mackie, B. G., G. A. Dudley, H. Kaciuba-Uscilko, and L. Terjung. Uptake of chylomicron triglycerides by contracting skeletal muscle in rats. *J. Appl. Physiol.* 49: 851–855, 1980.
169. Madsen, K., P. K. Pedersen, P. Rose, and E. A. Richter. Carbohydrate supercompensation and muscle glycogen utilization during exhaustive running in highly trained athletes. *Eur. J. Appl. Physiol.* 61: 467–472, 1990.
170. Maling, H. M., D. N. Stern, P. D. Altland, B. Highman, and B. B. Brodie. The physiologic role of the sympathetic nervous system in exercise. *J. Pharmacol. Exp. Ther.* 154: 35–45, 1966.
171. Martin, W. H., A. R. Coggan, R. J. Spina, and J. E. Saffitz. Effects of fiber type and training on β-adrenoreceptor density in human skeletal muscle. *Am. J. Physiol.* 257 (*Endocrinol. Metab.* 20): E736–E742, 1989.
172. Martin, W. H., G. P. Dalsky, B. F. Hurley, D. E. Matthews, D. M. Bier, J. M. Hagberg, M. A. Rogers, D. S. King, and J. O. Holloszy. Effect of endurance training on plasma free fatty acid turnover and oxidation during exercise. *Am. J. Physiol.* 265 (*Endocrinol. Metab.* 28): E708–E714, 1993.
173. Masoro, E. J., L. B. Rowell, and R. M. McDonald. Intracellular muscle lipids as energy sources during muscular exercise and fasting. *Federation Proc.* 25: 1421–1424, 1966.
174. Maughan, R. J., C. Williams, D. M. Campbell, and D. Hepburn. Fat and carbohydrate metabolism during low intensity exercise: effects of the availability of muscle glycogen. *Eur. J. Appl. Physiol.* 39: 7–16, 1978.
175. McGarry, J. D., S. E. Mills, C. S. Long, and D. W. Foster. Observations on the affinity for carnitine, and malonyl-CoA sensitivity, of carnitine palmitoyltransferase I in animal and human tissues. *Biochem. J.* 214: 21–28, 1983.
176. Mikkelsen, J., and J. Knudsen. Acyl-CoA-binding protein from cow. Binding characteristics and cellular and tissue distribution. *Biochem. J.* 248: 709–714, 1987.
177. Miller, W. C., G. R. Bryce, and R. K. Conlee. Adaptations to a high-fat diet that increase exercise endurance in male rats. *J. Appl. Physiol.* 56: 78–83, 1984.
178. Miller, W. C., J. Górski, L. B. Oscai, and W. K. Palmer. Epinephrine activation of heparin-nonreleasable lipoprotein lipase in 3 skeletal muscle fiber types of the rat. *Biochem. Biophys. Res. Commun.* 164: 615–619, 1989.
179. Miller, W. C., R. C. Hickson, and N. M. Bass. Fatty acid binding proteins in the three types of rat skeletal muscle. *Proc. Soc. Exp. Biol. Med.* 189: 183–188, 1988.
180. Mitchell, G., F. Demaugre, A. Pelet, J. P. Bonnefont, J. M. Paturneau, and J. M. Saudubray. Defective palmitate oxidation and lack of carnitine accumulation in intact fibroblasts from two patients with primary systemic carnitine deficiency. In: *Clinical Aspects of Human Carnitine Deficiency*, edited by P. R. Borum. New York: Pergamon Press, 1986, p. 148–149.
181. Molé, P. A., L. B. Oscai, and J. O. Holloszy. Adaptation of muscle to exercise. Increase in levels of palmityl CoA synthetase, carnitine palmityltransferase, and palmityl CoA dehydrogenase, and in the capacity to oxidize fatty acids. *J. Clin. Invest.* 50: 2323–2330, 1971.
182. Moore, K. K., P. J. Cameron, P. A. Ekeren, and S. B. Smith. Fatty acidbinding protein in bovine *longissimus dorsi* muscle. *Comp. Biochem. Physiol.* 104B: 259–266, 1993.
183. Morgan, H. E., and A. Parmeggiani. Regulation of glycogenolysis in muscle. III. Control of muscle glycogen phosphorylase activity. *J. Biol. Chem.* 239: 2440–2445, 1964.
184. Morgan, T. E., L. A. Cobb, F. A. Short, R. Ross, and D. R. Gunn. Effects of long-term exercise on human muscle mitochondria. In: *Muscle Metabolism During Exercise*, edited by B. Pernow and B. Saltin. New York, London: Plenum Press, 1971, p. 87–95.
185. Morgan, T. E., F. A. Short, and L. A. Cobb. Effect of long-term exercise on skeletal muscle lipid composition. *Am. J. Physiol.* 216: 82–86, 1969.
186. Muoio, D. M., J. J. Leddy, P. J. Horvath, A. B. Awad, and D. R. Pendergast. Effect of dietary fat on metabolic adjustments to maximal VO_2 and endurance in runners. *Med. Sci. Sports Exerc.* 26: 81–88, 1994.
187. Murthy, M. S. R., and S. V. Pande. Malonyl-CoA binding site and the overt carnitine palmitoyltransferase activity reside on the opposite sides of the outer mitochondrial membrane. *Proc. Natl. Acad. Sci. U. S. A.* 84: 378–382, 1987.
188. Nagel, D., D. Seiler, H. Franz, C. Leitzmann, and K. Jung. Effects of an ultra-long-distance (1000 km) race on lipid metabolism. *Eur. J. Appl. Physiol.* 59: 16–20, 1989.
189. Naito, E., Y. Indo, and K. Tanaka. Identification of two variant short chain acyl-coenzyme A dehydrogenase alleles,

each containing a different point mutation in a patient with short chain acyl-coenzyme A dehydrogenase deficiency. *J. Clin. Invest.* 85: 1575–1582, 1990.
190. Newsholme, E. A. Application of knowledge of metabolic integration to the problem of metabolic limitations in sprints, middle distance and marathon running. In: *Principles of Exercise Biochemistry. Med. Sport Sci.*, edited by J. R. Poortmans. Basel: Karger, 1988, p. 194–211.
191. Newsholme, E. A., P. H. Sugden, and T. Williams. Effect of citrate on the activities of phosphofructokinase from nervous and muscle tissues from different animals and its relationship to the regulation of glycolysis. *Biochem. J.* 166: 123–129, 1977.
192. Nikkilä, E. A., and A. Konttinen. Effect of physical activity on postprandial levels of fats in serum. *Lancet* i: 1151–1154, 1962.
193. Nikkilä, E. A., R. Taskinen, S. Rehunen, and M. Härkönen. Lipoprotein lipase activity in adipose tissue and skeletal muscle of runners: relation to serum lipoproteins. *Metabolism* 27: 1661–1671, 1978.
194. Nikkilä, E. A., P. Torsti, and O. Penttilä. The effect of exercise on lipoprotein-lipase activity of rat heart, adipose tissue and skeletal muscle. *Metabolism* 12: 863–865, 1963.
195. O'Brien, M. J., C. A. Viguie, R. S. Mazzeo, and G. A. Brooks. Carbohydrate dependence during marathon running. *Med. Sci. Sports Exerc.* 25: 1009–1017, 1993.
196. Okano, G., H. Matsuzaka, and T. Shimojo. A comparative study of the lipid composition of white, intermediate, red and heart muscle in rats. *Biochim. Biophys. Acta* 619: 167–175, 1980.
197. Okano, G., and T. Shimojo. Utilization of long-chain free fatty acids in white and red muscle of rats. *Biochim. Biophys. Acta* 710: 122–127, 1982.
198. Olsson, A. G., B. Eklund, L. Kaijser, and L. A. Carlson. Extraction of endogenous plasma triglycerides by the working human forearm muscle in the fasting state. *Scand. J. Clin. Lab. Invest.* 35: 231–236, 1975.
199. Orfali, K. A., L. G. D. Fryer, M. J. Holness, and M. C. Sugden. Longterm regulation of pyruvate dehydrogenase kinase by high-fat feeding. Experiments in vivo and in cultured cardiomyocytes. *FEBS Lett.* 336: 501–505, 1993.
200. Oscai, L. B., R. A. Caruso, and C. Wergeles. Lipoprotein lipase hydrolyzes endogenous triacylglycerols in muscle of exercised rats. *J. Appl. Physiol.* 52: 1059–1063, 1982.
201. Oscai, L. B., D. A. Essig, and W. K. Palmer. Lipase regulation of muscle triglyceride hydrolysis. *J. Appl. Physiol.* 69: 1571–1577, 1990.
202. Oscai, L. B., J. Górski, W. C. Miller, and W. K. Palmer. Role of the alkaline TG lipase in regulating intramuscular TG content. *Med. Sci. Sports Exerc.* 20: 539–544, 1988.
203. Osmundsen, H., J. Bremer, and J. I. Pedersen. Metabolic aspects of peroxisomal β-oxidation. *Biochim. Biophys. Acta* 1085: 141–158, 1991.
204. Owen, O. W., and G. A. Reichard. Fuels consumed by man: the interplay between carbohydrates and fatty acids. *Prog. Biochem. Pharmacol.* 6: 177–213, 1971.
205. Pande, S. V., and J. F. Mead. Distribution of long-chain fatty acidactivating enzymes in rat tissues. *Biochim. Biophys. Acta* 152: 636–638, 1968.
206. Paul, P. FFA metabolism of normal dogs during steady-state exercise at different work loads. *J. Appl. Physiol.* 28: 127–132, 1970.
207. Paul, P. Uptake and oxidation of substrates in the intact animal during exercise. In: *Muscle Metabolism During Exercise*, edited by B. Pernow and B. Saltin. New York: Plenum Press, 1971, p. 225–247.
208. Paulussen, R. J. A., M. J. H. Geelen, A. C. Beynen, and J. H. Veerkamp. Immunochemical quantitation of fatty-acid-binding proteins. I. Tissue and intracellular distribution, postnatal development and influence of physiological conditions on rat heart and liver FABP. *Biochim. Biophys. Acta* 1001: 201–209, 1989.
209. Paulussen, R. J. A., H. T. B. Van Moerkerk, and J. H. Veerkamp. Immunochemical quantification of fatty acid-binding proteins. Tissue distribution of liver and heart FABP types in human and porcine tissues. *Int. J. Biochem.* 22: 393–398, 1990.
210. Pearsall, D., and W. K. Palmer. Triacylglycerol metabolism in rat skeletal muscle after exercise. *J. Appl. Physiol.* 68: 2451–2456, 1990.
211. Peeters, R. A., J. M. Ena, and J. H. Veerkamp. Expression in Eschericia coli and characterization of the fatty-acid-binding protein from human muscle. *Biochem. J.* 278: 361–364, 1991.
212. Peeters, R. A., M. A. In 't Groen, and J. H. Veerkamp. The fatty acidbinding protein from human skeletal muscle. *Arch. Biochem. Biophys.* 274: 556–563, 1989.
213. Peeters, R. A., J. H. Veerkamp, and R. A. Demel. Are fatty acid-binding proteins involved in fatty acid transfer? *Biochim. Biophys. Acta* 1002: 8–13, 1989.
214. Peeters, R. A., J. H. Veerkamp, A. G. Van Kessel, T. Kanda, and T. Ono. Cloning of the cDNA encoding human skeletal-muscle fatty-acid-binding protein, its peptide sequence and chromosomal localization. *Biochem. J.* 276: 203–207, 1991.
215. Phinney, S. D., B. R. Bistrian, W. J. Evans, E. Gervino, and G. L. Blackburn. The human metabolic response to chronic ketosis without caloric restriction: preservation of submaximal exercise capability with reduced carbohydrate oxidation. *Metabolism* 32: 769–776, 1983.
216. Powers, S. K., W. Riley, and E. T. Howley. Comparison of fat metabolism between trained men and women during prolonged aerobic work. *Res. Q. Exerc. Sport* 51: 427–431, 1980.
217. Pratt, C. A. Lipoprotein lipase and triglyceride in skeletal and cardiac muscles of rats fed lard or glucose. *Nutr. Res.* 9: 47–55, 1989.
218. Putman, C. T., L. L. Spriet, E. Hultman, M. I. Lindinger, L. C. Lands, R. S. McKelvie, G. Cederblad, N. L. Jones, and G. J. F. Heigenhauser. Pyruvate dehydrogenase activity and acetyl group accumulation during exercise after different diets. *Am. J. Physiol.* 265 (*Endocrinol. Metab.* 28): E752–E760, 1993.
219. Rabin, R. A., and D. O. Allen. Role of protein kinase and contractile force in the regulation of myocardial lipolysis. *Horm. Metab. Res.* 16: 465–467, 1984.
220. Randle, P. J., C. N. Hales, P. B. Garland, and E. A. Newsholme. The glucose fatty-acid cycle. Its role in insulin sensitivity and the metabolic disturbances of diabetes mellitus. *Lancet* 34: 785–789, 1963.
221. Randle, P. J., E. A. Newsholme, and P. B. Garland. Regulation of glucose uptake by muscle. 8. Effects of fatty acids, ketone bodies and pyruvate, and of alloxan-diabetes and starvation, on the uptake and metabolic fate of glucose in rat and diaphragm muscles. *Biochem. J.* 93: 652–665, 1964.
222. Randle, P. J., D. A. Priestman, S. C. Mistry, and A. Halsall. Glucose fatty acid interactions and the regulation of glucose disposal. *J. Cell. Biochem.* 55S: 1–11, 1994.
223. Ravussin, E., C. Bogardus, K. Scheidegger, B. LaGrange, E. D. Horton, and E. S. Horton. Effect of elevated FFA on

carbohydrate and lipid oxidation during prolonged exercise in humans. *J. Appl. Physiol.* 60: 893–900, 1986.
224. Reed, D. R., M. G. Tordoff, and M. I. Friedman. Enhanced acceptance and metabolism of fats by rats fed a high-fat diet. *Am. J. Physiol.* 261 (*Regulatory Integrative Comp. Physiol.* 30): R1084–R1088, 1991.
225. Reimer, F., G. Löffler, G. Henning, and O. H. Wieland. The influence of insulin of glucose and fatty acid metabolism in the isolated perfused rat hind quarter. *Hoppe-Seyler's Z. Physiol. Chem.* 356: 1055–1066, 1975.
226. Reitman, J., K. M. Baldwin, and J. O. Holloszy. Intramuscular triglyceride utilization by red, white, and intermediate skeletal muscle and heart during exhausting exercise. *Proc. Soc. Exp. Biol. Med.* 142: 628–631, 1973.
227. Rennie, M. J., and J. O. Holloszy. Inhibition of glucose uptake and glycogenolysis by availability of oleate in well-oxygenated perfused skeletal muscle. *Biochem. J.* 168: 161–170, 1977.
228. Rennie, M. J., W. W. Winder, and J. O. Holloszy. A sparing effect of increased plasma fatty acids on muscle and liver glycogen content in the exercising rat. *Biochem. J.* 156: 647–655, 1976.
229. Rocchiccioli, F., R. J. A. Wanders, P. Aubourg, C. Vianey-Liaud, L. IJlst, M. Fabre, M. Cartier, and P. F. Bougneres. Deficiency of long-chain 3-hydroxyacyl-CoA dehydrogenase: a cause of lethal myopathy and cardiomyopathy in early childhood. *Pediatr. Res.* 28: 657–662, 1990.
230. Romijn, J. A., S. Klein, E. F. Coyle, L. S. Sidossis, and R. R. Wolfe. Strenuous endurance training increases lipolysis and triglyceride-fatty acid cycling at rest. *J. Appl. Physiol.* 75: 108–113, 1993.
231. Rowell, L. B., E. J. Masoro, and M. J. Spencer. Splanchnic metabolism in exercising man. *J. Appl. Physiol.* 20: 1032–1037, 1965.
232. Saggerson, D., I. Ghadiminejad, and M. Awan. Regulation of mitochondrial carnitine palmitoyltransferase from liver and extrahepatic tissues. *Adv. Enzyme Regul.* 32: 285–306, 1992.
233. Saggerson, E. D., and C. A. Carpenter. Carnitine palmitoyltransferase and carnitine octanoyltransferase activities in liver, kidney cortex, adipocyte, lactating mammary gland, skeletal muscle and heart. *FEBS Lett.* 129: 229–232, 1981.
234. Saltin, B. Physiological adaptation to physical conditioning. Old problems revisited. *Acta Med. Scand. Suppl.* 711: 11–24, 1986.
235. Saltin, B. (1990). Maximal oxygen uptake: Limitation and malleability. In: *International Perspectives in Exercise Physiology*, edited by K. Nazar. Champaign, IL: Human Kinetics Publishing Company, 1990, p. 26–40.
236. Saltin, B., and P.-O. Åstrand. Free fatty acids and exercise. *Am. J. Clin. Nutr.* 57 (Suppl.): 752S–758S, 1993.
237. Saltin, B., and P. D. Gollnick. Skeletal muscle adaptability: significance for metabolism and performance. In: *Handbook of Physiology, Skeletal Muscle, Skeletal Muscle*, edited by L. D. Peachy. Washington, DC: Am. Physiol. Soc., 1983, p. 555–631.
238. Saltin, B., and J. Karlsson. Muscle ATP, CP, and lactate during exercise after physical conditioning. In: *Muscle Metabolism During Exercise*, edited by B. Pernow and B. Saltin. New York, London: Plenum Press, 1971, p. 395–399.
239. Saltin, B., B. Kiens, and G. Savard. A quantitave approach to the evaluation of skeletal muscle substrate utilization in prolonged exercise. In: *Biochemical Aspects of Physical Exercise*, edited by G. Benzi, L. Packer, and N. Siliprandi. Amsterdam, Elsevier Science Publications, 1986, p. 235–244.
240. Schantz, P., J. Henriksson, and E. Jansson. Adaptation of human skeletal muscle to endurance training of long duration. *Clin. Physiol.* 3: 141–151, 1983.
241. Schnitzer, J. E., A. Sung, R. Horvat, and J. Bravo. Preferential interaction of albumin-binding proteins, gp30 and gp18, with conformationally modified albumins. Presence in many cells and tissues with a possible role in catabolism. *J. Biol. Chem.* 34: 24544–24553, 1992.
242. Scholte, H. R. The biochemical basis of mitochondrial diseases. *J. Bioenerg. Biomembr.* 20: 161–191, 1988.
243. Scholte, H. R., F. G. I. Jennekens, and J. J. B. J. Bouvy. Carnitine palmitoyltransferase II deficiency with normal carnitine palmitoyltransferase I in skeletal muscle and leucocytes. *J. Neurol. Sci.* 40: 39–51, 1979.
244. Scholte, H. R., R. Rodrigues Pereira, P. C. De Jonge, I. E. M. Luyt-Houwen, M. H. M. Verduin, and J. D. Ross. Primary carnitine deficiency. *J. Clin. Chem. Clin. Biochem.* 28: 351–357, 1990.
245. Scholte, H. R., J. D. Ross, W. Blom, A. M. C. Boonman, O. P. Van Diggelen, C. L. Hall, J. G. M. Huijmans, I. E. M. Luyt-Houwen, W. J. Kleijer, and J. B. C. De Klerk. Assessment of deficiencies of fatty acyl-CoA dehydrogenases in fibroblasts, muscle and liver. *J. Inherit. Metab. Dis.* 15: 347–352, 1992.
246. Schonfeld, G., and D. M. Kipnis. Glucose-fatty acid interactions in the rat diaphragm in vivo. *Diabetes* 17: 422–426, 1968.
247. Schoonderwoerd, K., S. Broekhoven-Schokker, W. C. Hülsmann, and H. Stam. Properties of phosphatidate phosphohydrolase and diacylglycerol acyltransferase activities in the isolated rat heart. Effect of glucagon, ischaemia and diabetes. *Biochem. J.* 268: 1–6, 1990.
248. Schulz, H. Beta oxidation of fatty acids. *Biochim. Biophys. Acta* 1081: 109–120, 1991.
249. Scow, R. O., E. J. Blanchette-Mackie, and L. C. Smith. Transport of lipid across capillary endothelium. *Federation Proc.* 39: 2610–2617, 1980.
250. Seitz, H. J., H. Bühring, H. Feldmann, and W. Lierse. Modelluntersuchungen über die Bedeutung des interstitiellen Fettgewebes der Muskulatur. *Hoppe-Seyler's Z. Physiol. Chem.* 350: 951–965, 1969.
251. Severson, D. L., and M. Hee-Cheong. Monoacylglycerol lipase activity in cardiac myocytes. *Biochem. Cell. Biol.* 66: 1013–1018, 1988.
252. Simi, B., B. Sempore, M.-H. Mayet, and R. J. Favier. Additive effects of training and high-fat diet on energy metabolism during exercise. *J. Appl. Physiol.* 71: 197–203, 1991.
253. Simonelli, C., and R. P. Eaton. Reduced triglyceride secretion: a metabolic consequence of chronic exercise. *Am. J. Physiol.* 234 (*Endocrinol. Metab. Gastrointest. Physiol.* 3): E221–E227, 1978.
254. Small, C. A., A. J. Garton, and S. J. Yeaman. The presence and role of hormone-sensitive lipase in heart muscle. *Biochem. J.* 258: 67–72, 1989.
255. Snow, D. H., and P. S. Guy. The effect of training and detraining on several enzymes in horse skeletal muscle. *Arch. Int. Physiol. Biochem.* 87: 87–93, 1979.
256. Spriet, L. L., D. J. Dyck, G. Cederblad, and E. Hultman. Effects of fat availability on acetyl-CoA and acetylcarnitine metabolism in rat skeletal muscle. *Am. J. Physiol.* 263 (*Cell Physiol.* 32): C653–C659, 1992.
257. Spriet, L. L., G. J. F. Heigenhauser, and N. L. Jones. Endogenous triacylglycerol utilization by rat skeletal muscle during tetanic stimulation. *J. Appl. Physiol.* 60: 410–415, 1986.

258. Spriet, L. L., D. A. MacLean, D. J. Dyck, E. Hultman, G. Cederblad, and T. E. Graham. Caffeine ingestion and muscle metabolism during prolonged exercise in humans. *Am. J. Physiol.* 262 (*Endocrinol. Metab.* 25): E891–E898, 1992.
259. Spriet, L. L., S. J. Peters, G. J. F. Heigenhauser, and N. L. Jones. Rat skeletal muscle triacylglycerol utilization during exhaustive swimming. *Can. J. Physiol. Pharmacol.* 63: 614–618, 1985.
260. Stam, H., S. Broekhoven-Schokker, and W. C. Hülsmann. Characterization of mono-, di- and triacylglycerol lipase activities in the isolated rat heart. *Biochim. Biophys. Acta* 875: 76–86, 1986.
261. Standl, E., N. Lotz, T. Dexel, H.-U. Janka, and H. J. Kolb. Muscle triglycerides in diabetic subjects. Effect of insulin defiency and exercise. *Diabetologia* 18: 463–469, 1980.
262. Stankiewicz-Choroszucha, B., and J. Górski. Effect of beta-adrenergic blockade on intramuscular triglyceride mobilization during exercise. *Experientia* 34: 357–358, 1978.
263. Stankiewicz-Choroszucha, B., and J. Górski. Effect of decreased availability of substrates on intramuscular triglyceride utilization during exercise. *Eur. J. Appl. Physiol.* 40: 27–35, 1978.
264. Stanley, C. A., D. E. Hale, G. T. Berry, S. Deleeuw, J. Boxer, and J.-P. Bonnefont. Brief report: a deficiency of carnitine-acylcarnitine translocase in the inner mitochondrial membrane. *N. Engl. J. Med.* 327: 19–23, 1990.
265. Staron, R. S., R. S. Hikida, T. F. Murray, F. C. Hagerman, and M. T. Hagerman. Lipid depletion and repletion in skeletal muscle following a marathon. *J. Neurol. Sci.* 94: 29–40, 1989.
266. Storlien, L. H., A. B. Jenkins, D. J. Chisholm, W. S. Pascoe, S. Khouri, and E. W. Kraegen. Influence of dietary fat composition on development of insulin resistance in rats. Relationship to muscle triglyceride and ω-3 fatty acids in muscle phospholipid. *Diabetes* 40: 280–289, 1991.
267. Stremmel, W. Fatty acid uptake by isolated rat heart myocytes represents a carrier-mediated transport process. *J. Clin. Invest.* 81: 844–852, 1988.
268. Strohfeldt, P., and C. Heugel. Characterization of triglyceride lipase activities in rat skeletal muscle. *Biochem. Biophys. Res. Commun.* 121: 87–94, 1984.
269. Sugden, M. C., and M. J. Holness. Interactive regulation of the pyruvate dehydrogenase complex and the carnitine palmitoyltransferase system. *FASEB J.* 8: 54–61, 1994.
270. Sugden, M. C., M. J. Holness, and R. M. Howard. Changes in lipoprotein lipase activities in adipose tissue, heart and skeletal muscle during continuous or interrupted feeding. *Biochem. J.* 292: 113–119, 1993.
271. Tan, M. H., T. Sata, and R. J. Havel. The significance of lipoprotein lipase in rat skeletal muscles. *J. Lipid. Res.* 18: 363–370, 1977.
272. Tarnapolsky, L. J., J. D. MacDougall, S. A. Atkinson, M. A. Tarnapolsky, and J. R. Sutton. Gender differences in substrate for endurance exercise. *J. Appl. Physiol.* 68: 302–308, 1990.
273. Taskinen, M.-R., E. A. Nikkilä, S. Rehunen, and A. Gordin. Effect of acute vigorous exercise on lipoprotein lipase activity of adipose tissue and skeletal muscle in physically active men. *Artery* 6: 471–483, 1980.
274. Taylor, A. W. The effects of different feeding regimens and endurance exercise programs on carbohydrate and lipid metabolisms. *Can. J. Appl. Sports Sci.* 4: 126–130, 1979.
275. Tein, I., C. De Vivo, F. Bierman, P. Pulver, L. J. De Meirleir, L. Cvitanovic-Sojat, R. A. Pagon, E. Bertini, C. Dionisi-Vici, and S. Servidei. Impaired skin fibroblast carnitine uptake in primary systemic carnitine deficiency manifested by childhood carnitine-responsive cardiomyopathy. *Pediatr. Res.* 28: 247–255, 1990.
276. Terjung, R. L. Endocrine response to exercise. *Exerc. Sport Sci. Rev.* 7: 153–180, 1979.
277. Terjung, R. L., L. Budohoski, K. Nazar, A. Korbryn, and H. KaciubaUscilko. Chylomicron triglyceride metabolism in resting and exercising fed dogs. *J. Appl. Physiol.* 52: 815–820, 1982.
278. Terjung, R. L., and H. Kaciuba-Uscilko. Lipid metabolism during exercise: Influence of training. *Diabetes Metab. Rev.* 2: 35–51, 1986.
279. Terjung, R. L., B. G. Mackie, G. A. Dudley, and H. Kaciuba-Uscilko. Influence of exercise on chylomicron triacylglycerol metabolism: plasma turnover and muscle uptake. *Med. Sci. Sports Exerc.* 15: 340–347, 1983.
280. Therriault, D. G., G. A. Beller, J. A. Smoake, and L. H. Hartley. Intramuscular energy sources in dogs during physical work. *J. Lipid. Res.* 14: 54–60, 1973.
281. Thiébaud, D., R. A. DeFronzo, E. Jacot, A. Golay, K. Acheson, E. Maeder, E. Jéquier, and J.-P. Felber. Effect of long chain triglyceride infusion on glucose metabolism in man. *Metabolism* 31: 1128–1136, 1982.
282. Treem, W. R., C. A. Stanley, D. N. Finegold, D. E. Hale, and P. M. Coates. Primary carnitine deficiency due to a failure of carnitine transport in kidney, muscle and fibroblasts. *N. Engl. J. Med.* 319: 1331–1336, 1988.
283. Treem, W. R., C. A. Stanley, D. E. Hale, H. B. Leopold, and J. S. Hyams. Hypoglycemia, hypotonia, and cardiomyopathy: the evolving clinical picture of long-chain acyl-CoA dehydrogenase deficiency. *Pediatrics* 87: 328–333, 1991.
284. Trumble, G. E., M. A. Smith, and W. W. Winder. Evidence of a biotin dependent acetyl-coenzyme A carboxylase in rat muscle. *Life Sci.* 49: 39–43, 1991.
285. Turcotte, L. P., B. Kiens, and E. A. Richter. Saturation kinetics of palmitate uptake in perfused skeletal muscle. *FEBS Lett.* 279: 327–329, 1991.
286. Turcotte, L. P., E. A. Richter, A. K. Srivastava, and J.-L. Chiasson. First evidence for the existence of a fatty acid binding protein in the plasma membrane of skeletal muscle. *Diabetes* 41 (Suppl. 1): 172A, 1992.
287. Vaag, A. A., A. Handberg, P. Skøtt, E. A. Richter, and H. Beck-Nielsen. Glucose-fatty acid cycle operates in humans at the levels of both whole body and skeletal muscle during low and high physiological plasma insulin concentrations. *Eur. J. Endocrinol.* 130: 70–79, 1994.
288. Van Breda, E. (1994). The effect of testosterone on skeletal muscle energy metabolism in diabetic and non-diabetic endurance trained rats. University of Limburg, Maastricht, The Netherlands.
289. Van Breda, E., H. A. Keizer, M. M. Vork, D. A. M. Surtel, Y. F. De Jong, G. J. Van der Vusse, and J. F. C. Glatz. Modulation of fatty-acidbinding protein content of rat heart and skeletal muscle by endurance training and testosterone treatment. *Pflugers Arch.* 421: 274–279, 1992.
290. Van der Horst, D. J., J. M. Van Doorn, P. C. C. M. Passier, M. M. Vork, and J. F. C. Glatz. Role of fatty acid-binding protein in lipid metabolism of insect flight muscle. *Mol. Cell. Biochem.* 123: 145–152, 1993.
291. Van der Vusse, G. J., J. F. C. Glatz, H. C. G. Stam, and R. S. Reneman. Fatty acid homeostasis in the normoxic and ischemic heart. *Physiol. Rev.* 72: 881–940, 1992.
292. Van der Vusse, G. J., and R. S. Reneman. The myocardial non-esterified fatty acid controversy. *J. Mol. Cell. Cardiol.* 16: 677–682, 1984.

293. Van der Vusse, G. J., and T. H. M. Roemen. Gradient of fatty acids from blood plasma to skeletal muscle in dogs. *J. Appl. Physiol.* 78: 1839–1843, 1995.
294. Van Nieuwenhoven, F. A., C. P. H. J. Verstijnen, G. J. J. M. Van Eijs, E. Van Breda, Y. F. De Jong, G. J. Van der Vusse, and J. F. C. Glatz. Fatty acid transfer across the myocardial capillary wall: No evidence for a substantial role of cytoplasmic fatty acid-binding protein. *J. Mol. Cell. Cardiol.* 26: 1635–1647, 1994.
295. Veerkamp, J. H., and R. J. A. Paulussen. Fatty acid-binding proteins of various tissues. In: *Drugs Affecting Lipid Metabolism*, edited by R. Paoletti, Berlin: Springer-Verlag, 1987, p. 98–103.
296. Veerkamp, J. H., T. H. M. S. M. Van Kuppevelt, R. G. H. J. Maatman, and C. F. M. Prinsen. Structural and functional aspects of cytosolic fatty acidbinding proteins. *Prostaglandins Leuko. Essent. Fatty Acids* 49: 887–906, 1993.
297. Veerkamp, J. H., and H. T. B. Van Moerkerk. The fatty acid binding protein content and fatty acid oxidation capacity of rat tissues. In: *New Developments in Fatty Acid Oxidations*. New York: Wiley-Liss, Inc., 1992, p. 205–210.
298. Veerkamp, J. H., and H. T. B. Van Moerkerk. Fatty acid-binding protein and its relation to fatty acid oxidation. *Mol. Cell. Biochem.* 123: 101–106, 1993.
299. Veerkamp, J. H., and J. L. Zevenbergen. Effect of dietary fat on total and peroxisomal fatty acid oxidation in rat tissues. *Biochim. Biophys. Acta* 878: 102–109, 1986.
300. Vork, M. M., J. F. C. Glatz, D. A. M. Surtel, H. J. M. Knubben, and G. J. Van der Vusse. A sandwich enzyme linked immuno-sorbent assay for the determination of rat heart fatty acid-binding protein using the streptavidin-biotin system. Application to tissue and effluent samples from normoxic rat heart perfusion. *Biochim. Biophys. Acta* 1075: 199–205, 1991.
301. Vork, M. M., J. F. C. Glatz, and G. J. Van der Vusse. On the mechanism of long chain fatty acid transport in cardiomyocytes as facilitated by cytoplasmic fatty acid-binding protein. *J. Theor. Biol.* 160: 207–222, 1993.
302. Walker, M., G. R. Fulcher, C. F. Sum, H. Orskov, and K. G. M. M. Alberti. Effect of glycemia and nonesterified fatty acids on forearm glucose uptake in normal humans. *Am. J. Physiol.* 261 (*Endocrinol. Metab.* 24): E304–E311, 1991.
303. Wanders, R. J. A., M. Duran, L. IJlst, J. P. De Jager, A. H. Van Gennip, G. Jakobs, L. Dorland, and F. J. Van Sprang. Sudden infant death and long-chain 3-hydroxyacyl-CoA dehydrogenase. *Lancet* ii: 52–53, 1989.
304. Watanabe, M., T. Ono, and H. Kondo. Immunohistochemical studies on the localisation and ontogeny of heart fatty acid binding protein in the rat. *J. Anat.* 174: 81–95, 1991.
305. Wilson, D. F. Factors affecting the rate and energetics of mitochondrial oxidative phoshorylation. *Med. Sci. Sports Exerc.* 26: 37–43, 1994.
306. Winder, W. W., J. Arogyasami, R. J. Barton, I. M. Elayan, and P. R. Vehrs. Muscle malonyl-CoA decreases during exercise. *J. Appl. Physiol.* 67: 2230–2233, 1989.
307. Winder, W. W., R. W. Braiden, D. C. Cartmill, C. A. Hutber, and J. P. Jones. Effect of adrenodemedullation on decline in muscle malonyl-CoA during exercise. *J. Appl. Physiol.* 74: 2548–2551, 1993.
308. Winder, W. W., R. C. Hickson, J. M. Hagberg, A. A. Ehsani, and J. A. McLane. Training-induced changes in hormonal and metabolic responses to submaximal exercise. *J. Appl. Physiol.* 46: 766–771, 1979.
309. Woeltje, K. F., V. Esser, B. C. Weis, W. F. Cox, J. G. Schroeder, S.-T. Liao, D. W. Foster, and J. D. McGarry. Inter-tissue and inter-species characteristics of the mitochondrial carnitine palmitoyltransferase enzyme system. *J. Biol. Chem.* 265: 10714–10719, 1990.
310. Wolfe, B. M., S. Klein, E. J. Peter, B. F. Schmidt, and R. R. Wolfe. Effect of elevated free fatty acid acids on glucose oxidation in normal humans. *Metabolism* 37: 323–329, 1988.
311. Wolfe, R. R., S. Klein, F. Carraro, and J.-M. Weber. Role of triglyceride-fatty acid cycle in controlling fat metabolism in humans during and after exercise. *Am. J. Physiol.* 258 (*Endocrinol. Metab.* 21): E382–E389, 1990.
312. Yamaguchi, S., Y. Indo, P. M. Coates, T. Hashimoto, and K. Tanaka. Identification of very-long-chain acyl-CoA dehydrogenase deficiency in three patients previously diagnosed with long-chain acyl-CoA dehydrogenase deficiency. *Pediatr. Res.* 34: 111–113, 1993.
313. Yamaguchi, S., T. Orii, K. Maeda, M. Oshima, and T. Hashimoto. A new variant of glutaric aciduria type II: deficiency of β-subunit of electron transfer flavoprotein. *J. Inherit. Metab. Dis.* 13: 783–786, 1990.
314. Yeaman, S. J. Hormone-sensitive lipase—a multipurpose enzyme in lipid metabolism. *Biochim. Biophys. Acta* 1052: 128–132, 1990.
315. Yki-Järvinen, H., I. Puhakainen, and V. A. Koivisto. Effect of free fatty acids on glucose uptake and nonoxidative glycolysis across human forearm tissues in the basal state and during insulin stimulation. *J. Clin. Endocrinol. Metab.* 72: 1268–1277, 1991.
316. Yki-Järvinen, H., I. Puhakainen, C. Saloranta, L. Groop, and M.-R. Taskinen. Demonstration of a novel feedback mechanism between FFA oxidation from intracellular and intravascular sources. *Am. J. Physiol.* 260 (*Endocrinol. Metab.* 23): E680–E689, 1991.
317. Yokota, I., Y. Indo, P. M. Coates, and K. Tanaka. Molecular basis of medium chain acyl-coenzyme A dehydrogenase deficiency. An A to G transition at position 985 that causes a lysine-304 to glutamate substitution in the mature protein is the single prevalent mutation. *J. Clin. Invest.* 86: 1000–1003, 1990.
318. Young, D. R., J. Shapira, R. Forrest, K. R. Adachi, R. Lim, and R. Pelligra. Model for evaluation of fatty acid metabolism for man during prolonged exercise. *J. Appl. Physiol.* 23: 716–725, 1967.
319. Zierler, K. L. Fatty acids as substrates for heart and skeletal muscle. *Circ. Res.* 38: 459–463, 1976.
320. Zierz, S., and A. G. Engel. Regulatory properties of a mutant carnitine palmitoyltransferase in human skeletal muscle. *Eur. J. Biochem.* 149: 207–214, 1985.
321. Zierz, S., and A. G. Engel. Are there two forms of carnitine palmitoyltransferase in muscle? *Neurology* 37: 1785–1790, 1987.
322. Zierz, S., S. Neumann-Schmidt, and F. Jerusalem. Inhibition of carnitine palmitoyltransferase in normal human skeletal muscle and in muscle of patients with carnitine palmitoyltransferase deficiency by long- and shortchain acylcarnitine and acyl-coenzyme A. *Clin. Invest.* 71: 763–769, 1993.
323. Zorzano, A., T. W. Balon, L. J. Brady, P. Rivera, L. P. Garetto, J. C. Young, M. N. Goodman, and N. B. Ruderman. Effects of starvation and exercise on concentrations of citrate, hexose phosphates and glycogen in skeletal muscle and heart. Evidence for selective operation of the glucose-fatty acid cycle. *Biochem. J.* 232: 585–591, 1985.

22. Influence of exercise on protein and amino acid metabolism

MICHAEL J. RENNIE | *Department of Anatomy & Physiology, University of Dundee, Dundee, Scotland*

CHAPTER CONTENTS

THE EFFECTS OF PHYSICAL ACTIVITY on protein and amino acid metabolism of the whole body and of individual tissues and organs seems a natural subject for study within the overall context of physiology. Apart from water and a few salts, muscles after all are mainly made of protein, and since it is a common experience that alterations of physical activity lead to muscle growth or wasting with implied changes in the protein architecture of muscle, it makes sense that these changes would be the result of alterations in protein metabolism. Furthermore, the novice physiologist soon learns that muscles are remarkable in their capacity to use a wide variety of metabolic fuels—not just fatty acids, sugars, and organic acids but also amino acids. The capacity to use amino acids as fuel may seem counterintuitive: Why would muscle burn its own house down? This is a problem that remains to be solved. Lastly, it is probably not exaggerating to say that a whiff of vitalism (and in particular the belief that protein is imbued with some special life force) still lingers around the whole question of contractile activity and protein metabolism. For many professional, and committed amateur, athletes and their trainers, the false idea of the primacy of protein in some hypothetical league of nutrients appears to be unassailable. The study of exercise metabolism is not, however, an activity of interest only to athletes and trainers.

As for other branches of metabolism, the study of the influences of contractile activity on protein metabolism has been illuminating for our understanding of the metabolic control of whole-body fuel and nitrogen metabolism in general (130, 181, 197). In addition, our concepts of the control of the lean body mass (186) have been markedly influenced by studies involving exercise or immobility, and many of the lessons learned have direct application to the rehabilitation of patients who have lost lean body mass through malnutrition, trauma, burns, sepsis, or immobility (79, 209). Furthermore, the study of protein metabolism and physical activity provides evidence of the beneficial effects of exercise in both development and maintenance of lean body mass throughout middle and old age and in the potential for reversing the muscle wasting associated with aging (62, 75, 76).

This chapter has been written as an overview of the most important knowledge of protein and amino acid metabolism during exercise that is relevant to human physiology. The major concepts used to classify and make sense of that knowledge are discussed without necessarily exploring all of the byways. However, there are some pieces of information which do not fit into the broad picture but which are so puzzling or simply entertaining that it would be a pity to leave them out.

GENERAL ASPECTS OF AMINO ACID AND PROTEIN METABOLISM IN MUSCLE

Amino acid metabolism in general is complicated. There are, after all, 20 physiologically important amino acids, and they are involved in a wide array of physiological processes, some common to all and some restricted to particular amino acids. The general processes include (*1*) protein turnover—amino acids being constantly removed from the metabolic pool during the synthesis of a bewildering array of different functional and structural proteins and reappearing in the pool as the result of protein breakdown, and (2) amino acid transport—the influx and efflux of amino acids across the cell membrane (Fig. 22.1). In addition, the composition of the free amino acid pool itself is continually being rearranged as a result of de novo synthesis, interconversion, and irreversible catabolism of particular amino acids (Fig. 22.2). Furthermore, the intermediary metabolism of amino acids, within and beyond muscle, is linked to a very wide variety of metabolic functions. The intracellular functions include maintenance of adenine nucleotide concentrations; de novo synthesis of purine and pyrimidine bases; the transfer of reducing equivalents into mitochondria; anaplerotic maintenance of intermediates in the Krebs cycle; and extramuscular functions that include provision of fuel for cells of the immune system, acid–base regulation, gluconeogenesis, and ureagenesis. Perhaps because muscle is often seen as a tissue the overriding function of which is to transform chemical to mechanical energy, it may surprise some readers to realize that all of the above activities are significantly affected by contractile activity in its various modes.

Amino Acid Transport and the Free Amino Acid Pool

The concentration within the free amino acid pool of various amino acids probably has important modulatory effects on their metabolism and possibly on protein metabolism in general. For example, the catabolism of the branched chain amino acids (BCAA) via transamination and decarboxylation is accelerated as their concentration rises due to the high K_m of the BCAA transaminases relative to their concentrations in intracellular fluid (109, 155). Furthermore, amino acids themselves have modest but significant modulatory effects in stimulating protein anabolism in muscle (12, 13, 276); particular amino acids such as leucine (or its ketoacid metabolites) and glutamine may have specific anabolic effects (28, 171, 173, 257, 288) in promoting protein synthesis and inhibiting protein breakdown.

The overall size of the free amino acid pool of the whole body (273) is the algebraic result of dietary input via the gut, de novo synthesis of amino acids, protein breakdown and withdrawal of amino acids into protein synthesis, and synthesis of nucleotides and neurotransmitters as well as catabolic pathways leading to ammonia and urea. As a result of a substantial amount of work in the past 10 years it is now becoming recognized that, despite previously being almost ignored as control elements, the amino acid transporters are involved not only in contributing to the control of the pool sizes of amino acids in the tissues but also in regulating the concentration of amino acids in the blood and thus contributing to the control of whole-body nitrogen metabolism (44, 200). However, it should not be imagined that amino acid transporters play as substantial a part in the regulation of nitrogen metabolism as do the glucose transporters for carbohydrate metabolism. There are after all seven known transporters for a single sugar (i.e., glucose). One of them, GLUT4, exhibits a range of modulatory behavior in response to stimulation by insulin and contractile activity, such as translocation from endosomal sites to the membrane, which is simply unknown for amino acid transport, although it has been looked for. Nevertheless, there is good evidence from animal work (reviewed in 169) and increasingly from studies using various isotope dilution techniques in people in vivo (17) that for skeletal muscle amino acid metabolism, control of transport is significant, particularly in the regulation of the muscle glutamine pool in its role

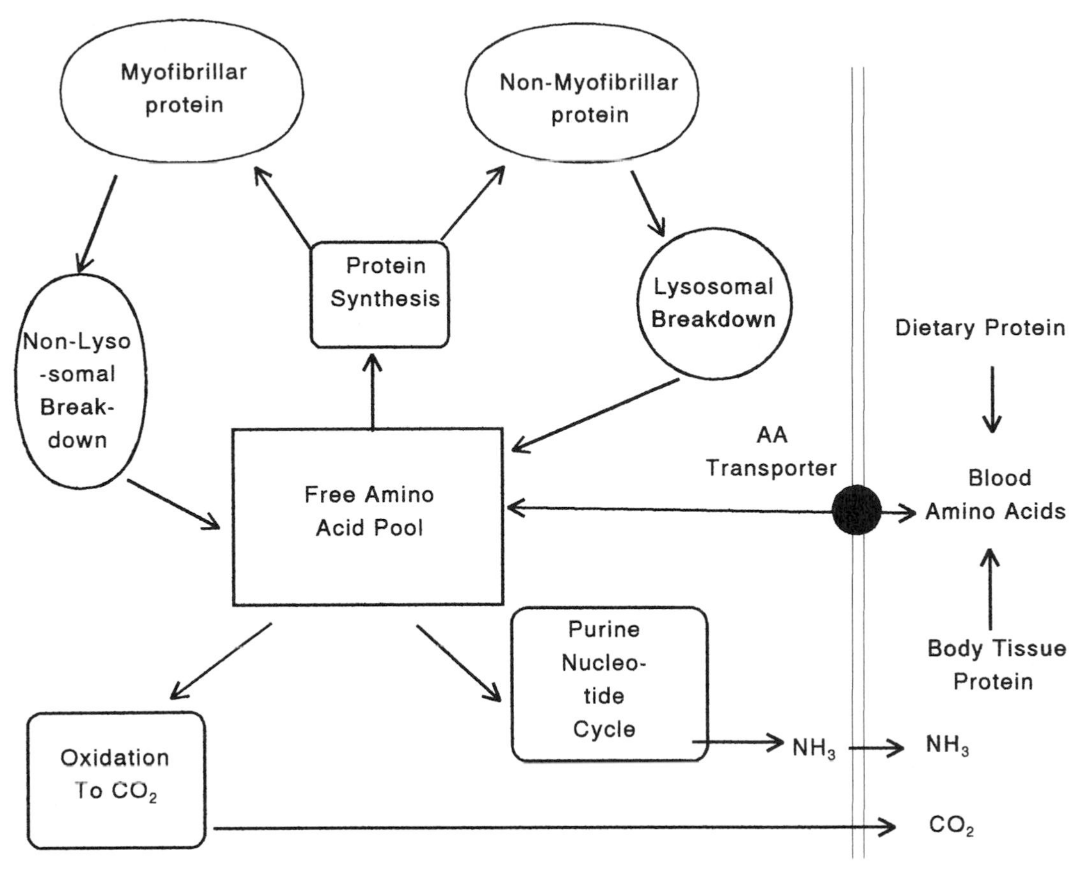

FIG. 22.1. General scheme of protein and amino acid metabolism in skeletal muscle.

as a buffer or short-term store of carbon and nitrogen for the rest of the body. The availability of muscle glutamine for extramuscular metabolism is likely to be important in the control of whole-body acid–base balance (69, 150), hepatic amino acid catabolism (164), and immunocompetence (178). Furthermore, regulation of the blood concentration ratio between the aromatic amino acids (particularly tryptophan) and BCAA may be important in regulating substrate supply for neurotransmitter synthesis in the central nervous system (CNS) (39, 234). An understanding of the characteristics of the transport mechanisms involved in each case is crucial to the critical appraisal of the arguments involved.

Transmembrane transport of amino acids in mammals is the result of the activities of a number of transporter proteins of overlapping specificities (46). For many years these were classified purely on the basis of their substrate specificity, ion dependence, and kinetics; transporters for particular groups of amino acids were identified by single letters indicating the name of a paradigm substrate; for example, System-A for short-chain neutral amino acids (of which alanine was a major substrate) or System-L for the large neutral amino acids (of which leucine was the best example) (see Table 22.1). Although a substantial amount of work has been done in characterizing the overlapping specificities and kinetics (45) using nonmetabolizable amino acids, such as *N*-methylaminoisobutyrate (MeAIB) for System-A or by 2-amino bi-cyclo[2.2.1]heptane-2-carboxylic acid (BCH) for System-L, it has not always been easy unequivocally to identify the mode of transport of a particular amino acid or to predict its transport behavior or that of its close relatives from the kinetic characteristics of a single transporter known to handle it. Now that a somewhat belated start has been made in identifying specific transmembrane-spanning proteins as being responsible for the activity of particular transport systems [e.g., the lysine transporter, System y^+ (149), the cystine transporter x_c^- (129), the taurine transporter (261), and the glutamate transporters (198), etc. (15, 191)], it is likely that, ultimately, we will be able to understand amino acid transport in the tissues in terms of structure and function. However, currently, especially for muscle and liver, such information as is available has had little impact on our understanding of metabolic events.

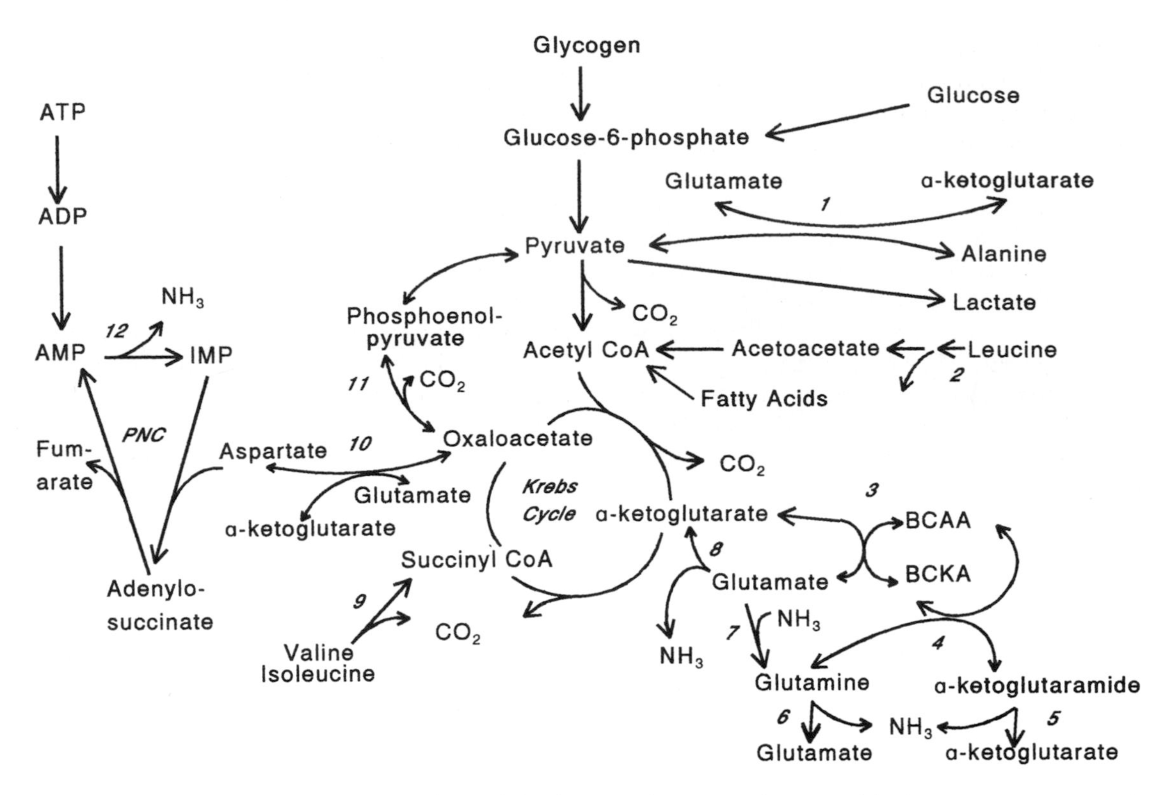

FIG. 22.2 Intermediary metabolism of amino acids in skeletal muscle. Reaction steps referred to are as follows: *1*, alanine aminotransferase; *2*, leucine decarboxylation and catabolism to acetoacetate; *3*, branched chain aminotransferase; *4*, glutamine transaminase; *5*, ω-amidase; *6*, glutaminase; *7*, glutamine synthetase; *8*, glutamate dehydrogenase; *9*, valine and isoleucine catabolism to succinate via BCKA dehydrogenase; *10*, aminotransferase; *11*, phospho*enol*pyruvate carboxykinase; *12*, AMP deaminase.

Amino Acid Transport in Skeletal Muscle and Heart. In muscle there exists a wide variety of amino acid transport modalities (see Table 22.1), and the transport of most amino acids is probably of minor importance in relationship to regulation of metabolism. However, for amino acids of metabolic importance (like alanine, glutamine, and the BCAA) involved with tidal flow of carbon and nitrogen between the viscera and muscle and vice versa, the transporter involved may be of substantial importance. The important candidates are Systems-A, -ASC, -L, and -N. System-A was among the first

TABLE 22.1. *Metabolically Important Amino Acid Transporters in Skeletal Muscle*

System	Substrates	Capacity, V_{max} nmol · min^{-1} · g^{-1}	Affinity, K_m mm	Na-Dependent	Hormone Sensitivity	E_m-Sensitive
A	MeAIB AIB Alanine Methionine	Low (< 100)	High (< 1)	Yes	Insulin (inwards)	Yes
ASC	Alanine Serine Cysteine	Medium (400)	Medium (3)	Yes	No	Yes
N^m	Glutamine Asparagine Histidine 3-Me His	High (1000)	Low (8)	Yes	Insulin (inwards) Corticosteroid (outward)	Yes
L	BCAA Aromatic AA	Very high (3000)	Very low (20)	Yes	No	Yes
X^-_{ac}	Glutamate Aspartate	Low (80)	High (1)	No	No	No

amino acid transport system to be kinetically characterized and to be identified as occurring in muscle (3, 151). It is a high-affinity, low-capacity transporter that is sodium-dependent and stimulated by insulin. It transports small, neutral amino acids, particularly alanine and glycine, although its paradigm, defining substrate is MeAIB, an artificial nonmetabolizable chemical. (It is worth noting that the unmethylated version, AIB, is a substrate for both System-A and System-ASC, and results from its use should be interpreted accordingly.) Since System-A was one of the first amino acid transporters identified in muscle, a substantial amount of interest has focused upon it, especially since alanine is a major muscle metabolite.

However, there must be some doubt as to how important System-A is for muscle alanine metabolism and sarcolemmal transport. A substantial part of the exchange of alanine between blood and muscle appears in fact to occur via Systems-ASC (or possibly its sodium-independent variant, asc) and -L (88, 169), which are unresponsive to insulin in skeletal muscle (Table 22.1). Also, in tissues in which the System-A component is the major alanine transporter [e.g., in cardiomyocytes in culture (99)], insulin stimulation may markedly increase alanine transport. However, in isolated, incubated muscle (211), in perfused rat muscle (124), in rabbit muscle (9), or in the human forearm (22, 232), insulin stimulation of the System-A transporter rarely exceeds 30% (i.e., much less than the doubling commonly seen for glucose transport). Much of the effect may in fact be due either to stimulatory effects on the Na^+/K^+-ATPpase pump (47) (decreasing intracellular Na^+ and thus increasing the electrochemical potential for alanine + Na^+) and in vivo, especially, to stimulation of muscle blood flow by insulin (10).

System-A shows a substantial up-regulation of its activity when alanine concentrations are low (102, 162). The capacity of muscle to up-regulate amino acid transport systems is one shared by heart, liver, and possibly other tissues (101). Its physiological significance is unknown, since in the model circumstances in which the phenomenon is exhibited, low concentrations of the amino acid need to be maintained for hours before up-regulation is observed. The up-regulation appears to be the result of de novo gene transcription and translation, since it is blocked by actinomycin and cycloheximide (102, 162).

System-L is a low-affinity, high-capacity transporter (46, 124) which, in muscle, handles the BCAA and aromatic amino acids but appears not to transport glutamine to any extent (124), unlike System-L in other tissues (234). System-L activity is unaffected by insulin or other hormones (86, 123, 124). It is a sodium-independent system and, since none of the amino acids it transports is charged at physiological pH, it effectively acts as a means of equalizing concentrations of its substrates across the sarcolemmal membrane. However, because alanine can be a System-L substrate (albeit a poor one) this, together with the capacity of the L-transporter to exhibit the phenomenon of transstimulation is likely to explain the slight muscle/blood concentration gradient for the BCAA and aromatic amino acids. Alanine, either generated within muscle or possibly concentrated by means of the System-A transporter, shows a substantial concentration gradient of up to 3:1; since alanine is a substrate for System-L, its outward passage via this system can drive the countertransport of BCAA to reach a distribution ratio between muscle and the extracellular space of about 1.2:1.

The fact that the System-L transporter has such a high K_m relative to the prevailing intracellular and extracellular concentrations (123, 124) means that the relative transmembrane flux will be governed largely by the size of the gradient and, of course, by blood flow to the tissues. Thus, after a meal when blood BCAA concentrations rise as a result of dietary input, there will be a net inward flux of the amino acids that will be sustained by their removal from the free amino acid pool into protein synthesis (58); however, in the postabsorptive state as net protein breakdown rises, the free amino pool of BCAA will increase in size (182), and even though BCAA catabolism will be stimulated, protein synthesis will be inhibited by the lack of insulin, so BCAA leave muscle (57, 201).

System-N^m, the muscle variant (2, 123) of the System-N transporter first discovered in hepatocytes (148), is unusual in being a high-capacity, low-affinity, sodium-dependent transporter with a remarkably narrow range of specificity, taking only glutamine, asparagine, and histidine as major substrates; 3-methylhistidine is probably also a minor substrate for this transporter (124). The transporter has not yet been cloned, but there is a substantial amount of information regarding its substrate specificity, kinetics, and behavior in muscle tissue under various physiological and pathophysiological circumstances (169). The System-N^m transporter appears to play a marked role in normal net delivery of glutamine to the circulation, and its activity is elevated under conditions of acidosis, corticosteroid treatment, trauma, burns, and sepsis; by mechanisms which are not understood but that may involve the elevation of intracellular sodium (219); and possibly by the synthesis of new transporter proteins (251). Newsholme and

Parry-Billings have pointed out, correctly, that the maintenance of the glutamine gradient across skeletal muscle requires an input of energy (190) but have calculated, incorrectly in our view (225), that inward glutamine transport requires 12 kJ/mol. By our calculation the amount of energy required is much less, around 2–3 kJ/mol, and thus the inward transport step cannot be said to be irreversible. Nevertheless, Newsholme and Parry-Billings have used the concept of irreversible inward glutamine transport to construct a hypothesis of glutamine cycling through two transporters, the N^m transporter inward and another unidentified sodium-independent transporter operating in an outward direction. Unfortunately, the only known sodium-independent transporter likely to have a sufficiently large capacity to handle the size of flux of glutamine observed would be System-L, but glutamine efflux from isolated incubated skeletal muscle is not inhibited by System-L substrates (280), suggesting that the putative transporter required by the hypothesis is not System-L (169). Unfortunately, no other candidate springs to mind, and until more evidence can be produced to confirm or deny this interesting hypothesis it must remain simply that.

Like System-A transport, the upregulation of System-N^m in response to low tissue or extracellular glutamine concentration appears (251) to be the result of elevated gene transcription and translation of gene product rather than some posttranslational activation of the transporter; control of up-regulation of glutamine synthetase and System-N^m may be coordinated (251).

Glutamate, from which glutamine is made (see later), is a pivotal intermediary metabolite in many tissues including muscle, but the tissue-blood exchange of this amino acid usually occurs at very low rates in most tissues probably because of the low activity of the transporter in the membrane. In rat (and probably human skeletal muscle), the glutamate transporter x^-_{AG} (169) has a high-affinity and low-capacity and is sodium-independent but H^+ dependent. One of the fascinating aspects of this transporter is that under conditions in which glutamine concentrations fall, the capacity of the skeletal muscle glutamate transporter is elevated and this upregulation follows the general pattern for such adaptation being the result of elevated gene transcription and translation (163).

Cardiac amino acid transport is a somewhat undeveloped area, although there has been a fair amount of work carried out in cardiomyocytes of both fetal chick and rat (77, 100), but only a little work has been carried out on perfused rat heart (258). Most of the normal transport activities appear to be present. In the rat heart there is a high-capacity, low-affinity transporter for glutamine probably similar to that observed in skeletal muscle (S. O. Khogali and M. J. Rennie, unpublished results). However, glutamate transport in the heart appears to occur at a much faster rate than in skeletal muscle, and the cardiac glutamate transporter is likely to be quite unlike that found in skeletal muscle, since it appears to be sodium dependent and membrane potential-dependent (A. Ahmed and M. J. Rennie, unpublished work).

Hepatic, Blood-Brain Barrier, and Small Intestinal Blood-Facing AA Transporters. The relevance of these transporters to amino acid and protein metabolism during exercise depends upon the exercise-induced alterations of the blood amino acid concentrations (see later). The amino acid concentrations within the intracellular water of the liver vary much more widely than do those of other tissues (165, 256)—for obvious reasons (i.e., the large variation with feeding and fasting in the systemic and hepatic portal blood concentrations and in rates of ureagenesis and gluconeogenesis). Although the main hepatic amino acid transporters for alanine and glutamine (Systems-A and -N respectively) are relatively low affinity and high capacity, sodium-dependent transporters (107, 135, 148, 165), features which would all tend to make the entry of their substrates into the liver dependent upon delivery (210), amino acid disposal by the liver usually occurs at a rate faster than transmembrane transport (210). Thus, the rate of inward transport of amino acids is limiting for amino acid–derived gluconeogenesis and ureagenesis and the rate of delivery to the liver of amino acids is crucial (112, 136, 175). The overall hepatic catabolism of the aromatic amino acids is also, to a large extent, limited by the rather small capacity of transmembrane transport; also, the transporter for the aromatic amino acids including tryptophan is capable of being competitively inhibited by BCAA. Thus, any circumstances in which BCAA concentration fluctuates will have a predictable effect upon the net catabolism of the aromatic amino acids and also upon the availability of these amino acids for neurotransmitter synthesis in the brain (234).

The blood-brain barrier transporters conform to the general System-L type (194) and here too the availability of tryptophan for synthesis of serotonin in the brain should, to some extent, depend upon the presence, or not, of competing long-chain amino acids (particularly BCAA) and the extent to which the tryptophan is displaced from albumin by nonesterified fatty acids (48). Little is known about the extent to which amino acid transport across the blood-brain barrier can be modulated by other physiological influences likely to occur during exercise, such as decreased pH and altered substrate and hormone concentrations.

The blood facing membranes of the small intestine contain high-capacity sodium-independent transporters whose function is presumably to transfer absorbed amino acids to the circulation in proportion to the gut cell amino acid concentration (44, 46, 255). These transporters are also likely to be active under circumstances in which small intestinal proteolysis is stimulated; this phenomenon may confer upon the gut the property of being a store of protein-bound amino acid that can be called upon during glucopenia, possibly including long-term exercise.

Regulation of Transmembrane Transport of Amino Acids as a Result of Contractile Activity. There is good evidence from work on isolated incubated and perfused muscle that inward transport of alanine and AIB is acutely stimulated by contractile activity and that the stimulation persists afterwards (84–86, 187, 296). The relatively large effects of contraction with and without insulin seen in rat muscle in vivo (260) are probably exacerbated by capillary recruitment (10), since the effects seen in isolated muscles are usually small, about 30% at most. The effect is most likely to be due to System-A, although surprisingly few studies have been carried out with the specific System-A substrate, MeAIB. The effects are not due to transcription of new genetic information or to synthesis of new proteins, since they are unaffected by inhibitors of these processes (86), but do seem to be dependent upon the presence of a protein in the membrane, since incubation with trypsin inhibits the effect (187). Some, but not all, of the increased activity after contractile activity is due to alterations of the membrane potential or the Na^+/K^+-ATPase (296), and its basis is a mystery. The effect appears to occur via pathways distinct from those by which insulin stimulates system A transport (103).

The physiological significance of stimulation of inward alanine transport is somewhat mysterious, since muscle is a net producer of alanine. Maybe increased System-A transport contributes to the observed increased *efflux* of alanine during contractile activity (66). However, because of the relatively small capacity of System-A [in rat and human skeletal muscle at least (169)], it is unlikely that the transport activity has much influence on the nitrogen balance of muscle during or after exercise. Alanine is made in such large amounts during contractile activity that the muscle alanine content rises (142, 143), suggesting that the transporter is unable to keep up with production rate. It is also difficult to see an important functional role for increased uptake of System-A substrates in the postcontractile phase, since none of the substrates for System-A (with the possible exception of methionine, which can also be transported on System-L) could be regarded as being likely to be limiting for protein synthesis or other metabolic pathways (273, 274). A role for alanine as a possible precursor for postexercise glycogen synthesis in human muscle can probably be ruled out (M. Varnier, G. Lease, and M. J. Rennie, unpublished work).

For other sodium-dependent transporters such as System-N^m, and possibly System-ASC, which have a much higher capacity than System-A in muscle (123, 124), there is no evidence of an acute stimulatory effect on inward transport, although there is some evidence of a small stimulatory effect on outward transport (122). The latter may be because contractile activity is associated with an increase in intracellular sodium and membrane depolarization, both of which would decrease the inward driving force for accumulation of amino acids. Such mechanisms may also be involved in the increased efflux of alanine and glutamine observed during exercise (see later) but the evidence is sparse and indeed, and since alanine and glutamine concentrations within muscle rise during short-term moderate exercise, any stimulation of the transport process is obviously insufficient to deplete the intracellular pools of these amino acids, unlike the stimulation of transport that occurs as a result of corticosteroids, sepsis, or injury (222). However, longer term exercise can reduce muscle glutamine concentrations below normal (217). One hypothesized explanation of the "overtraining syndrome" (196) is that it is associated with chronic depletion of muscle and blood glutamine, which reduces the effectiveness of the immunological defense functions of white cells, and increases the susceptibility of the body to viral and bacterial infection. Whether the decreased blood and muscle glutamine is "chicken" or "egg" in this situation is difficult to judge.

One interesting phenomenon that may be a direct consequence of exercise-induced stimulation of amino acid transport is the acute increase in the efflux of 3-methylhistidine when measured as the arteriovenous (AV) difference across working legs (168). We have shown that 3-methylhistidine is transported via the System-N^m transporter (124), and thus the observed increase in its efflux during acute exercise may be due to increased activity of the transporter. Obviously, changes in 3-methylhistidine pool size as a result of exercise would tend to confound interpretations of altered myofibrillar protein breakdown based upon alterations of 3-methylhistidine production (54, 217).

For sodium-independent amino acid transporters, such as System-L, it is difficult to imagine a mechanism whereby increased muscle activity would alter the transporter activity in either direction (inward or outward) of large neutral amino acids, since changes in membrane potential would have no effect on the driving force for membrane transport. No contraction-related changes of uptake of substrates for System-L have ever been reported (86), and it seems more likely that the major forces driving muscle BCAA transport during exercise are the changes in their transmembrane concentration gradients, which will to some extent depend upon blood flow through working muscle. For example, if, compared to the resting situation, muscle synthesizes more alanine and glutamine and oxidizes more BCAA, the relative gradients between muscle and blood of alanine and glutamine will rise and those of the BCAA fall. The exercise-induced increase in blood flow will exacerbate the transmembrane difference, and thus the flow of alanine and glutamine away from muscle to the viscera and the flow of BCAA to muscle should increase.

The fact that, during exercise, the leg arteriovenous differences of amino acids appear to be little different between normal subjects and patients with chronic hypoxia (168) suggests that in human beings amino acid transport per se is not acutely sensitive to hypoxia itself or metabolic events which result from it.

There have been a limited number of studies in dogs and human beings of exchange across the heart of amino acids at rest (244, 290, 293) and during pacing to increased heart work (290). It seems likely that the normally high cardiac blood flow makes it difficult to observe significant A-V differences of most amino acids, but nevertheless there do appear to be net positive uptakes of glutamate and the BCAA at rest. Because of the increase of blood flow during ventricular pacing, the arterial–coronary sinus concentration differences decrease somewhat, but the flow increase is likely to be so great that the inward flux increases also. By similar arguments, it seems likely that alanine efflux increases with exercise, as it does in skeletal muscle. In patients with coronary artery disease, such changes are small or occur in the opposite direction (290)! Glutamine efflux from the heart is substantial in the postabsorptive state at normal "resting" heart rates, but unfortunately no information is available on possible changes during pacing, though it would be expected to increase.

Predicted Hormonal Effects on Transport of Amino Acids during and after Exercise. Physical activity is associated with increases in the secretion and blood concentrations of glucagon, cortisol, adrenaline, noradrenaline, and growth hormone and with decreases in insulin secretion and blood concentration (105, 220, 221). To what extent these hormonal alterations have direct or indirect effects on muscle amino acid transport is difficult to say for certain, except for glucagon in which all direct effects can probably be ruled out, since there are no glucagon receptors in skeletal muscle, and infusion of glucagon has no direct effect on skeletal muscle in human forearm (202). Indirectly, glucagon may predispose muscle to export alanine and glutamine by its lowering of the blood amino acid concentration secondary to stimulation of the catabolism of these amino acids in the viscera. Corticosteroids and adrenaline both appear to stimulate muscle glutamine efflux acutely (121, 123, 124) and may play a part in its exercise-induced loss. The decrease in blood insulin concentration should diminish insulin-sensitive inward amino acid transport (of alanine and glutamine) during exercise, but growth hormone, the secretion of which rises during exercise, probably has an acute stimulatory effect on System-A transport (153, 226). Since an increased net efflux of both alanine and glutamine are observed (see later), it is impossible to precisely align cause and effect in these cases, but it is likely that hormonal effects are minor. After exercise, there is a normalization of the hormonal concentrations in blood, with a large rebound of insulin that possibly contributes to a net switch towards postexercise anabolism in muscle (see later).

Transport Effects during Exercise in Liver and Brain. In the liver, the fall in insulin and the rise in glucagon availability should stimulate the net influx of amino acids via System-A and System-N. Glucagon acutely stimulates inward amino acid transport in the liver, probably by increasing the activity of the various mechanisms for causing efflux of sodium, hence increasing the sodium gradient and thus stimulating secondary active amino acid transporters. Also, since insulin normally inhibits gluconeogenesis and ureagenesis, the release of such an inhibition would tend to reduce the intrahepatic concentration of amino acids, hence decreasing the gradient against which the transporters needed to work. These changes would be consistent with the increased hepatic catabolism of amino acids, particularly glutamine and alanine, observed as a result of exercise (64, 272).

Tryptophan and Central Fatigue. During long-term exercise, it is likely that catabolism of BCAA in muscle and the increase in whole-body protein breakdown (see later) result in the observed rise in the concentration ratio of aromatic amino acids to BCAA in the blood (28, 50, 108). For tryptophan, of which the major part of the total blood burden is bound to albumin, any exercise-induced rise in nonessential fatty acids is also likely to increase the free tryptophan by displacing the amino acid from it, since both compete for nonspecific binding sites on the protein. The net result will be a rise in the free tryptophan/BCAA ratio, and the blood-brain barrier transport of tryptophan via System-L might be increased as a result with the possibility of a consequent increase in brain synthesis of serotonin, for which tryptophan availability is usually limiting. Increases in brain tryptophan are said to occur under circumstances of depression and fatigue (39), so a mechanism like that outlined above has been hypothesized to underlie the causes of "central fatigue" observed during long-term exercise (20). Evidence for this concept is mixed: it is true that in plasma and in brain of exercising rats concentrations of tryptophan increase, but this occurs without any increase in blood-free BCAA (39). The blood-free tryptophan also rises in cross-country running (21) and even in exercise mild enough not to broach the lactate threshold (71). The serotonin-reuptake inhibitor paroxetine (Prozac, which acts like a serotonin agonist) does reportedly decrease endurance performance when administered to running rats and to men (281), but so far there have been no convincing results of interventions increasing the availability of blood tryptophan per se to cause an increase in fatigue or indeed increasing the availability of BCAA to decrease fatigue. The results of work carried out on the effects of BCAA supplementation on development of fatigue during endurance exercise are equivocal, mainly because the effects seem so small and variable. Use of the Stroop color-and-word tests before and after 30 km of cross-country running produced very small (~5%) changes in two out of three measures of mental alertness; the changes themselves were of the order of the standard errors of the mean values (21). In another series of experiments by the same group on mood profiles conducted before and after exercise, a cross-sectional study of BCAA supplementation produced no significant evidence of a BCAA-associated decrease of fatigue, or indeed any other definite alteration of mood profile (19).

The claimed improvements in physical performance in marathon runners given BCAA were also small and did not reach significance for the whole group (21). However, the authors examined their data and discovered that if the runners were divided according to performance capability, the slower runners in the BCAA group had run marginally faster than the placebo group. No effect was seen for the better runners, possibly, claimed the authors, because these athletes' plasma free fatty acids had not risen as much as in the less fit runners. Unfortunately, no free fatty acid concentrations were measured! Furthermore, recently Wagenmakers and coworkers have demonstrated that the time to exhaustion during bicycle exercise is not altered as a result of increased availability of BCAA during exercise at 70% $\dot{V}O_{2max}$ on a bicycle ergometer (mean time to exhaustion, 122 min) (262).

There is another interesting side to the tryptophan-exercise story. The hypothalamic hormone prolactin increases during exercise in a manner that correlates positively with free tryptophan, both peaking 10 min after 1 hour of bicycle exercise (71). In a similar study carried out by other workers, giving oral BCAA before exercise reduced the exercise-stimulated postexercise increase of prolactin and growth hormone (33).

Outline of the Metabolism of Amino Acids in Muscle in Relation to Exercise

The repertoire of reactions involving amino acids in skeletal muscle is relatively meager compared to that shown by other tissues, particularly the liver, gut, and kidney (Fig. 22.2). The textbooks tell us that only six of the common physiological amino acids can be oxidized in muscle (the BCAA: Ile, Leu, Val, plus Glu, Asp, and Ala). The others, on release from protein breakdown, leave muscle intact (Table 22.2). Nevertheless, during a normal day in the life of an active adult male, it is likely that of all the amino acid oxidized in the body, the muscle accounts for 60% (136). Furthermore, in the postabsorptive state, between meals 60% of the total amino acid leaving muscle is in the form of alanine and glutamine (about half each) despite the fact that together these amino acids constitute only about 10% of muscle protein (64). In the fed state the amount of alanine released stays almost constant, but there is a marked rise in the amount of glutamine released, which then accounts for seven-eighths of the total amino acid leaving muscle (58). These phenomena can be understood in relation to the facts that the BCAA make up a large part (~20%) of muscle (and other first-class) protein and muscle has a virtual monopoly on the enzymes of their catabolism (125, 147). Jungas and colleagues, in a stimulating review (136), suggest that there are advantages to the organism of arranging the metabolic capacities of the

TABLE 22.2. *Muscle Amino Acids: Concentration and Exchange in Postabsorptive State*

Amino Acid	Concentration μmol/liter Intracellular H_2O	A-V Flux nmol · 100 g forearm^{-1} · min^{-1}
Ile	110	− 16
Leu	225	− 20
Val	320	− 18
Met	60	− 9
Phe	85	− 15
Thr	770	− 33
Lys	1110	− 35
Tyr	122	− 13
His	430	− 21
Arg	680	− 20
Ala	2860	−195
Asp	1650	− 1
Asn	420	− 25
Glu	3960	+ 80
Gln	19,970	−200
Gly	1660	− 52
Orn	350	0
Ser	900	+ 9
Tau	17,680	− 17

tissues in this way, a major one being simply that the liver could not both make glucose carbon from prandial amino acids and oxidize them simultaneously, and that the anabolic requirements of the liver would not satisfy the extra adenosine triphosphate (ATP) produced. There are other advantages to having the capabilities for amino acid metabolism partitioned in the way they are: these include the ability of muscle to act as a store of gluconeogenic carbon and fuel for the immune system, as a detoxifier of ammonia produced in intense exercise, and as an active participant in whole-body acid–base balance (277) (against which some of the most acute perturbations are generated by contractile activity).

The branched chain amino transferases are found in different isoenzyme forms in muscle cytoplasm and mitochondria. Most of the cytoplasmic forms are found in pale, less oxidative, more glycolytic muscle and the mitochondrial forms are in greater abundance in redder, more oxidative muscle, with this being the only form found in heart (125). In mitochondria, the branched chain aminotransferase also has a function as a transporter protein, channeling branched chain keto acids (BCKA) directly into mitochondria (126), which allows red-fiber muscle to oxidize BCKA produced elsewhere. The transaminating capacity of human muscle is about 280 μmol · kg^{-1} · min^{-1} (90), so the enzyme capacity is certainly capable of processing sufficient BCAA to account for observed rates of leucine oxidation (see later). The branched transaminase activity in muscle is due to isoenzymes I and III, which show the same substrate specificities for the three BCAA, and the maximal activities using these three substrates is almost identical. The K_m values are 5 mM for valine and 1 mM for both leucine and isoleucine.

As in all cell types, the aminotransferase that is involved in the malate shuttle of reducing equivalents across the mitochondrial membrane, aspartate aminotransferase, is also present in muscle in considerable amounts (128). The other major transaminase is alanine aminotransferase, the distribution of which in muscle parallels enzymes of pyruvate metabolism (184), as might be expected of its physiological role as a virtual extension of carbohydrate metabolism and as a major gluconeogenic substrate.

Skeletal muscle is capable of synthesizing glutamine from glutamate, ATP, and ammonia (not ammonium) via the cytoplasmic glutamine synthase reaction (150, 228). In rat skeletal muscle, the K_m of the enzyme for glutamate is 4 mM (227), suggesting that the rate of the reaction is not dependent upon the availability of glutamate at normal glutamate concentrations (4–8 mM) within muscle. The facts that glutamine production is stimulated even though the steady-state ATP/ADP ratio falls during contractile activity (143) and that the production of ammonia rises (93, 143), probably due to the adenosine deaminase reaction of the purine nucleotide cycle, is evidence in favor of the idea that availability of ammonia, to some extent, controls the rate of production of glutamine. Muscle also contains mitochondrial glutamate dehydrogenase (GDH) (7, 241, 279). The physiological activity of this enzyme in muscle is worthy of discussion, because of its possible relevance to the formation of ammonia (as a substrate for glutamine synthesis at rest and during exercise) and of α-ketoglutarate, which would help to replenish tricarboxylic acid cycle intermediates (termed anaplerosis) drained off (possibly by the decarboxylating malic enzyme or the activity of phosphoenolpyruvate carboxykinase) during exercise (233). Lowenstein and colleagues claim that the activity is too low (7, 167) to be important as part of an anaplerotic mechanism during exercise. On the other hand, Jungas and colleagues suggest (136) that in human muscle the activity of glutamate dehydrogenase (70, 241) is at least 100 times greater than required to account for the rate of glutamine synthesis at rest, so long as sufficient ADP is available. More recently, Wibom and Hultman have reported even greater activities of GDH in human muscle (280). Since more ADP is likely to be available during exercise than at rest, the GDH enzyme may after all be important for anaplerosis, which has implications for the operation of the purine nucleotide cycle and the source of exercise-generated ammonia (see below).

Because GDH is a mitochondrial enzyme which uses NAD/NADH as cofactors, the mass-action ratio of its substrates and products has been used to estimate the redox potential of the mitochondria during exercise (96). Problems about the low activity of the enzyme and whether it is actually at equilibrium both throw some doubt on this approach; certainly under conditions in which leg muscle mitochondria almost certainly do become substantially reduced (i.e., during occlusion of resting muscle or during fatiguing isometric contractions), the mass action ratio did not change (144).

Enzymes of glutaminolysis include a mitochondrial phosphate-dependent kidney type of glutaminase (250); also, in rat muscle at least, there are K- and L-type glutamine transaminases (289) that transaminate keto acids such as phenylpyruvate and ketomethionine to produce phenylalanine and methionine; the other main product is α-ketoglutaramide. There is apparently sufficient ω-amidase in rat and chicken skeletal muscle for the next step, the deamidation of α-ketoglutaramide to ammonia and α-ketoglutamate. The capacities of the glutamine transaminase in human muscle are unknown, but in any case their activity as enzymes of glutamine catabolism depends upon the availability of amino-acceptor molecules, and apart from pyruvate (which is a poor substrate), the concentrations of keto acids in muscle are probably too low (161) to allow the pathway to function physiologically.

The existence of enzymes which synthesize and degrade glutamine within the same compartment might be thought to give rise to cycling of substrates with the sarcoplasm, with the possible implication that such cycling confers sensitivity of control upon the steady-state concentrations of muscle free glutamine concentration and its utilization for other cells and tissues (188, 190). In fact, it appears that this is unlikely for glutamine metabolism, since although glutamine synthetase appears to be exclusively found within muscle cells, when it is attempted to localize glutaminase by immunocytochemical methods it appears to be mainly outside muscle cells, principally in infiltrating white cells, fibroblasts, and capillary cells (N. Willhoft and M. J. Rennie, unpublished results). These findings lessen the likelihood of there being major intracellular substrate cycling between glutamate, glutamine, α-ketoglutarate, and ammonia but does not rule out the possible existence of cycles involving more than one cell type. What the functional correlates of this would be and how they might alter with contractile activity are not easily identified.

Alanine and aspartate can both be synthesized in muscle through reactions catalyzed by their respective aminotransferase enzymes, given a sufficient availability of both glutamate as amino donor and the appropriate keto acid (pyruvate or malate); the aminotransferase reactions are near equilibrium and therefore can be driven in either direction, according to the availability of substrate. The branched-chain aminotransferase enzymes are capable of utilizing isoleucine, valine, and methionine as substrates to produce the respective branched chain keto acid and, by adding an amino group to α-ketoglutarate, glutamate as the other main product.

The BCAA (and methionine) can be catabolized via initial transamination then oxidation of the keto acid within mitochondria by the BCAA dehydrogenase (57, 245). The BCKA dehydrogenase is a multisubunit enzyme that is subject to phosphorylation and dephosphorylation, the latter causing activation (195). Contractile activity stimulates the BCKA dehydrogenase in both rat (140, 270) and human muscle (268), as does the provision of additional BCAA substrate (18). Acidosis also seems to activate the enzyme (174). Such characteristics predispose muscle to a stimulation of BCAA catabolism during exercise, especially under conditions in which net loss of protein (by whatever mechanism) increases the acute availability of substrate. In human muscle, one indication that the capacity of the BCAA dehydrogenase closely matches that of the transaminase is that little if any BCKA escape muscle (57, 58). Indeed, BCKA can be taken up as a fuel by human muscle (41), especially during exercise (215, 217) but, as mentioned above, this is not proof of complete oxidation of the carbon chain of the BCAA. In the rat, muscle transaminase activity is greater than the muscle dehydrogenase activity, and rat muscle exports BCKA to the bloodstream from where they are extracted for complete hepatic catabolism (127, 128). Maximal activity of the branched chain transaminase is about 100 μmol · min^{-1} · kg^{-1} wet weight (90), and that of the fully activated branched chain keto acid dehydrogenase complex is about 25 μmol · min^{-1} · kg^{-1} wet weight (267). These activities are certainly sufficient to account for the observed rates of leucine oxidation observed during exercise.

Interrelationship of BCAA, Alanine, and Glutamine Metabolism

Many studies of muscle amino acid catabolism have utilized keto or amino acids labeled on the carboxyl group (161), and it is often assumed that decarboxylation indicates complete catabolism of the carbon chain. For leucine this is likely to be true, since the distal steps of leucine catabolism produce first acetoacetyl-CoA, then acetyl-CoA, which cannot be converted to α-ketoglutarate or further to oxalacetate. In human muscle, leucine carbon is therefore probably completely oxidized, since little α-ketoisocaproate leaves human muscle at rest or in exercise. However, for valine and isoleucine, oxidation eventually produces succinyl CoA which can be converted to α-ketoglutarate, which may "top-up" the concentration of Krebs cycle intermediates or be further converted to oxalacetate. Oxalacetate may then either be transaminated to aspartate or converted via the malic enzyme or phosphoenolpyruvate carboxykinase to pyruvate; the latter could then be transaminated to alanine.

It is clear that the amino groups of the BCAA undergoing transamination will probably end up in glutamine or alanine in resting muscle [though exactly how much serves to form ammonia in exercising muscle, under different conditions, is an unresolved question (269)]. It is also clear that the carbon from any two of the potentially oxidizable amino acids in muscle (except leucine) can be used to produce α-ketoglutarate and thus glutamate and glutamine (189). However, there is an unresolved controversy about how much of the carbon for alanine comes from the BCAA and how much comes from pyruvate. The problem concerns the extent to which the Krebs cycle intermediates produced from the amino acids (except leucine) are able to be diverted via oxalacetate and the phospho*enol*pyruvate carboxykinase (PEPCK) reactions to form pyruvate. Snell and Newsholme (see 189) for the argument in full) base their case on the observed decrease in alanine production in postabsorptive incubated rat muscle treated with a PEPCK inhibitor, mercaptopicolinate. The argument is bolstered by pointing out that unless carbon from the amino acids does reach pyruvate, the "glucose-alanine cycle," the supposed mechanism by which muscle carbon is turned into glucose in the liver (65), becomes futile; it would then be of little use in starvation or exercise when glucose availability would otherwise diminish. The counterarguments come from Goldberg and Chang, who showed that most of the label from universally ^{14}C-labeled succinate or aspartate or either valine or isoleucine appeared in glutamine (about one-half) or CO_2 (about one-fifth), but only 2% appeared in alanine; furthermore, so long as glycolytic substrates were available, addition of any of the BCAA increased production of alanine (83). This evidence seems robust, especially given the fact that mercaptopicolinate is not a very specific agent in muscle (193), and careful examination of its effects (193) seems to show the veracity of the scheme proposed by Goldberg and Chang.

Recently, Brosnan and Letto (26) and Palmer and co-workers (192) have independently demonstrated that there is incomplete oxidation of the carbon chain of some BCAA both in heart and in skeletal muscle in rats. The branched chain hydroxyacids produced may find their way back into intermediary metabolism (e.g., as gluconeogenic precursors or as precursors of other metabolites), without having to be converted into glutamine or alanine and later metabolism in the gut or kidney (136).

The Purine Nucleotide Cycle in Muscle

A metabolic feature of some importance in skeletal muscle is the purine nucleotide cycle (PNC) [Fig. 22.2); (7, 166, 167)]. In muscle in which myosin ATPase is activated (i.e., hydrolyzing ATP during cross-bridge cycling), the action of the myokinase reaction maintains ATP concentrations at the expense of two molecules of adenosine diphosphate (ADP) but with the formation of adenosine monophosphate (AMP). Since the myokinase reaction would normally come to equilibrium if allowed to, with a loss of effectiveness in resynthesis of ATP, the action of AMP deaminase to produce inosine monophosphate (IMP) and ammonia would shift the equilibrium to the right, helping to maintain the steady-state concentrations of ATP during accelerated cross-bridge cycling. The AMP deaminase reaction is one of three reactions that constitute the PNC, the others being adenylosuccinate synthetase, which transforms IMP to adenylosuccinate (by reacting it with aspartate and GTP), and adenylosuccinate lyase, which releases fumarate from adenylosuccinate to reform AMP. For the purposes of the present discussion, of all the possible beneficial functions outlined by Lowenstein for the PNC (158), the replenishment of citric cycle intermediates via the production of fumarate and the deamination of amino acids prior to oxidative metabolism are of most interest, since there is no doubt that the tricarboxylic acid cycle intermediates can become depleted in long-term exercise (233); they may, of course, actually rise in the short term as a result of the acceleration of oxidative metabolism (7). The pro's and con's of this argument will be presented later.

Although the cycle is a net producer of ammonia, it is not clear whether this is functionally important for the control of metabolism or not. Lowenstein originally suggested that the ammonium ion helped to stimulate phosphofructokinase (166), thus accelerating glycolysis—certainly an appropriate action in the context of muscle activity. Other properties consonant with the idea of a role of the PNC in exercise metabolism are that AMP deaminase is activated by increasing concentrations of free ADP, inorganic phosphate, and protons, and that additionally it can be activated by binding of the enzyme to myosin during contractile activity (229, 230). If the PNC has evolved to subserve the preservation of the adenine nucleotide phosphorylation state during exercise, this fits well with the fiber-type distribution of adenosine deaminase, which is more than twice as abundant in rat fast-twitch white muscle than in slow-twitch oxidative red muscle. Nevertheless, a major increase in metabolic stress to oxidative muscle such as imposition of electrically induced contraction during a low rate of perfusion will cause about as much increase in IMP and ammonia as in more glycolytic fibers (259). The fiber-type distribution of enzymes of the PNC in rat muscle does not support the idea of a beneficial role in anaplerosis for the Krebs cycle, given that the abundance of enzymes in the two pathways would be inversely related in white and red muscle.

Amino Acid Catabolism and Gluconeogenesis from Amino Acids in Liver and Kidney

As pointed out above, the entry of amino acids into the liver is a site of control for disposal of amino acids via oxidation. Another particularly important site of control is carbamoylphosphate synthetase, which is stimulated by ammonia, the source of which is mainly hepatic deamidation of glutamine to glutamate (40, 175). However, the availability of ammonia in the bloodstream effectively exacerbates the stimulation of ureagenesis driven by the availability of amino acid substrate (30), and this has obvious relevance for control of ureagenesis during muscular work in which the systemic concentration of ammonia rises (93, 170, 263). The fates of amino acids after oxidative deamination in liver vary, but a substantial portion of the glucogenic amino acids are converted eventually, via oxalacetate and phosphoenolpyruvate, to glucose (1, 66). The portion not so converted is oxidized or, in the case of the ketogenic amino acids (Phe, Tyr, Leu, Lys, Try, and half of Ile), converted to acetoacetate and 3-hydroxybutarate. Alanine is par excellence a glucogenic amino acid but in liver glutamine is not (136); however, glutamine is a substrate for renal gluconeogenesis, although this is only likely to be important in the postexercise situation, since during exercise production of ammonium ions, plus bicarbonate from glutamine and glutamate, is likely to be more advantageous to the organism in the context of the control of the lactic acidosis produced by contractile activity (277). Glutamine is also processed by the gut to release alanine into the hepatic portal vein (255, 277, 282, 283) effectively providing a mechanism by which muscle protein can be made available for gluconeogenesis even if not via alanine leaving muscle.

Training Effects on the Capacities of Muscle Enzymes of Amino Acid Metabolism

There is little information on this topic. However, it might be expected that for those enzymes of amino acid metabolism found in mitochondria (e.g., mitochondrial aspartate aminotransferase and glutamate dehydrogenase), repeated medium-intensity exercise of the kind that results in increased mitochondrial density (117) would increase their abundance in muscle. There is some evidence of this for glutamate dehydrogenase at least (115, 279), and also for the other enzyme involved in the mitochondrial half of the malate-aspartate shuttle, malate dehydrogenase (132). Muscle aspartate aminotransferase increases with training in horses (104), and alanine aminotranferase also shows training-related increases in the muscles of trained horses (104) and rats (183); the response of the alanine aminotransferase is probably an adaptation to increased efficiency of pyruvate handling (183).

No data seem to exist concerning the possible response of glutamate synthetase to endurance training, but it might be predicted from previous work (251) that depletion of glutamine in muscle and blood by repeated training (196) would act as a stimulus to the production of the enzyme and possibly also to the glutamine transporter. Compensatory hypertrophy, caused by tenotomy of a synergistic muscle, is associated with a stimulation of the capacities of enzymes of glutamine metabolism, both glutamine synthetase and glutaminase (145). However, although the increase in capacity of the synthetic enzyme appears to occur in muscle tissue itself, the increases in the glutaminase seem to occur in accessory, nonmuscle cells (white cells, fibroblasts), which seem to have increased as part of an inflammatory response to the acute increase in strain imposed by the tenotomy. Since nonmuscle cells may account for about half of all cells in a muscle, these results highlight the need to be vigilant and cautious in ascribing whole-tissue changes to muscle cells.

The Effects of Contractile Activity on Ammonia Production and its Relation to the Free Amino Acid Pool

Theoretically, the ultimate function of all metabolic processes showing increases during contractile activity should be the maintenance of the steady-state concentrations of ATP and of the ATP/ADP ratio in muscle. It might therefore be expected that the amino acids and their metabolites showing the most marked changes in concentration would be ones most closely connected to those pathways of fuel metabolism which exhibit the greatest acceleration during contractile activity. On this basis, the alterations observed in muscle alanine (in close connection to glycolysis and BCAA transamination) and muscle glutamine (in close connection to Krebs cycle activity) are readily understandable.

Of course, it should always be borne in mind that any changes in the concentrations of amino acids and their metabolites in the intramuscular compartment, in the extracellular water, and in the blood (both plasma and red cells) will be influenced by the pattern of blood flow through the working tissue and the fluid shifts which occur as a result of osmotic, mechanical, and hydraulic forces.

The processes most closely interlinked with intermediary metabolism of amino acids in muscle are adenine nucleotide metabolism, glycolysis, and mitochondrial oxidative decarboxylation, occurring mainly in the Krebs cycle (Fig. 22.2). It might, a priori, be expected that certain particular changes in amino acid–related metabolism would be greatest for each of these three processes under the following conditions: first, adenine nucleotide catabolism and ammonia generation should be most stimulated during explosive events such as throwing or weight lifting; second, glycolysis-related metabolism and alanine production might show the biggest change during activities which take long enough for glycolysis to be fully activated, such as sprinting; and third, any changes in amino acid metabolism related to oxidative catabolism (e.g., increased utilization of glutamate or BCAA) would be most obvious during longer term activities, such as middle- to long-distance running, cycling, rowing, and so forth. By and large, these expectations are borne out, but a substantial number of surprises and paradoxes remain.

It is well known that exercise in people and in animals raises blood ammonia (8, 263); the rise is disproportionately greater as the work rate increases (Fig. 22.3). At rest, plasma ammonia is about 30

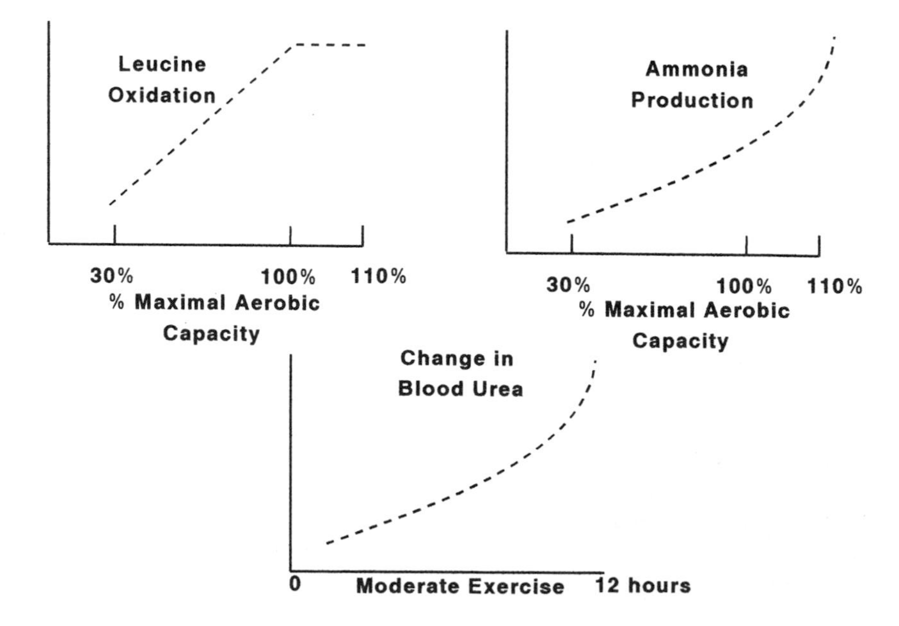

FIG. 22.3 Amino acid catabolism illustrated by CO_2 production from branched chain amino acids, ammonia production, and blood urea concentration. Notice that ammonia production and CO_2 production at high levels of exercise show a different pattern, suggesting that the processes are not necessarily linked at high exercise intensity. Notice also that urea production is only marked after long periods of exercise, presumably when glycogen stores are low.

μmol/liter. The value of whole-blood ammonia is higher (180 μmol/liter) than that of plasma ammonia because of the concentration of ammonium within red cells. In resting muscle it is about 420 μmol/liter in the intramuscular water (i.e., there is a distribution ratio of about 20:1). After exhausting dynamic exercise, muscle ammonia rises 3.75-fold and that in venous blood somewhat more, so that the distribution ratio falls to about half (94); the resting ratio is only reattained after 60 min of rest.

Given a pK_a of NH_4^+ of 9.5, the ammonia concentration in muscle cells is likely to be overwhelmingly in the form of ammonium at physiological pH (7.2); decreasing the value of intracellular pH in going from rest to exhaustion (pH 6.7) is unlikely to make more than a few percent difference in the ratio. Thus, it would be expected that the efflux of ammonia from muscle would be simply concentration dependent. In fact, this is too simplistic; ammonia may diffuse rapidly across membranes in its unprotonated form, but it may also move via potassium channels, with a conductance of about one-tenth of the potassium itself (94). Intramuscular potassium concentrations fall during exercise, which should decrease the competition for ammonia efflux, possibly explaining the lowered distribution ratio for muscle to blood ammonia during exercise.

If functioning completely, the PNC would produce IMP and ammonia from AMP, and would consume aspartate, which in the steady state could be replenished by transamination reactions drawing α-amino nitrogen from the BCAA. How well does this theoretical model fit the observed facts?

There is good evidence that in rat muscle during contractile activity ammonia and IMP are produced (167) and provision of ^{15}N-labeled leucine after contraction results in labeling of AMP (91). However, there is some uncertainty about whether the PNC actually operates in its full form during intense exercise. The evidence comes from studies of contracting rat and human muscle. In electrically stimulated rat muscle (177) inhibition of IMP reamination (by the adenylosuccinate synthetase inhibitor hadacidin) has no effect on production of ammonia via AMP deaminase, although the increase of fumarate and Krebs cycle intermediates is diminished (7). Thus, the contraction-induced production of ammonia is not dependent upon operation of the full cycle. In electrically stimulated rat muscle (177) and in human muscle during short-term intense dynamic exercise, or isometric exercise (at a rate that caused rapid exhaustion), there are stoichiometrically similar increases in muscle ammonia and IMP concentrations (94, 143); also, the size of the total adenine pool falls by an amount which matches (±10%–20%) the rise in IMP. All these effects strongly suggest that the ammonia is produced from deamination of AMP. The fact that use of the adenylosuccinate inhibitor hadacidin during electrical stimulation does not result in a larger than observed increase in IMP argues strongly that the enzymes of the PNC do no operate as a full cycle during contractile activity intense enough to diminish the total adenine nucleotide pool (177). A similar conclusion can be reached by considering that if the enzymes operate as a cycle, then the measured increase in ammonia should exceed the fall in the adenine nucleotide pool, but it does not (94, 143). Afterwards, IMP concentrations fall, but this in itself is not evidence of reamination; however, when hadacidin is used in rat muscle there is no such postcontraction fall, which is consistent with the action of adenylosuccinate synthetase reaminating IMP only after contractile activity (177).

The time course of the changes in the putative activators of AMP deaminase during short-term intense exercise suggests that increases in ADP, AMP, and H^+ were not as great as theoretically required to cause activation of the enzyme (i.e., some other activating process was more important). The binding of the AMP deaminase to myosin may fulfill the requirement (231). Also, the fact that increases in muscle lactate (94) precede the elevation of muscle ammonia disposes of the idea of ammonia as a primary stimulator of glycolysis (166).

If there is no reamination of IMP during contractile activity, there can be no anaplerotic replenishment of Krebs cycle intermediates, but perhaps it might be expected that such changes would only occur during exercise taking place for longer than a few minutes.

When the changes in ammonia production, adenine nucleotides, and amino acids are estimated during and after bicycle exercise at 75% of $\dot{V}O_{2max}$ until exhaustion (170), the diminutions of the nucleotide pool were almost negligible, but there were increases in muscle and plasma ammonia, and even if they were smaller than during more intense exercise, they exceed the change in the adenine pool. However, it appears that the total muscle concentration of aspartate is insufficient to account for all of the ammonia produced. Indeed, far from falling, as might be expected if the PNC were operational, it actually increases during the early part of exercise and shows only minor falls at exhaustion. Perhaps the most damning evidence against the idea of a fully functional PNC comes from a consideration of the muscle and blood glutamate concentrations during bicycling: there were substantial decreases in the muscle glutamate pool (170). Since it is likely that human muscle activity of glutamate dehydrogenase is in fact sufficient to cope with the demands of ammonia production at the rates observed (170, 279), the next question must be, Was the decrease in the muscle glutamate pool sufficient to account for the observed ammonia production rate? The answer is probably in the affirmative, given the size of the experimental errors involved. However, it was not big enough to account for both the rise in ammonia and the observed rise in muscle glutamine and alanine concentrations: for these to be accommodated, BCAA must have been transdeaminated. That there was a general increase in the muscle and plasma concentrations of the aromatic amino acids (which, not being catabolizable in muscle, may be indicators of the state of muscle net amino acid balance) suggests that this was negative (i.e., there was a state of muscle amino acid loss). Nevertheless, blood and muscle BCAA did not rise in parallel with the aromatic amino acids, suggesting that they could easily have been the source of the N for ammonia production.

This interpretation is strengthened by examination of other available data. For example, provision of extra fatty acids during exercise diminished the efflux of noncatabolizable amino acids (lysine, phenylalanine, and tyrosine) from working muscle (95), suggesting a diminution of net protein breakdown [a previously reported effect of fatty acids (11)]. Furthermore, the leg production of ammonia decreased (95). Also, patients with McArdle's disease, who lack myophosphorylase and cannot utilize muscle glycogen during exercise, have a greater than normal exercise-induced activation of branched chain keto acid dehydrogenase; they take up more BCAA from the blood than normal healthy subjects and, most importantly for this argument, they produce more than normal amounts of ammonia (269).

During moderate submaximal exercise, it might be expected that the drain on the adenine nucleotide pool would be small and most of the ammonia produced would come from amino acids, ultimately the BCAA. If so, then the maneuvers which increase the availability of BCAA (such as intravenous infusion or oral ingestion of BCAA, or brief starvation or a high-protein diet) should increase muscle ammonia production. Conversely, consumption of a high-carbohydrate diet (which by stimulating insulin secretion and the availability of blood glucose inhibits both protein breakdown and gluconeogenesis) should diminish ammonia production. By and large, this is indeed what happens (267, 269).

Presumably because muscle is at a much lower pH than the pK_a for ammonium (9.5), ammonia tends to be sequestered in muscle as ammonium during exercise, and the appearance of ammonia in blood lags behind the production in muscle, only reaching a peak some 2–3 min after the end of exercise. In the study by Graham and colleagues (94), 74% of the total ammonia remained in the muscle at the end of exercise, but almost 84% of the total was released from muscle during exercise and by 60 min afterwards, suggesting that none of the ammonia could have been made available for glutamine synthesis, unless ammonia and glutamine production were continuing together even as muscle ammonia fell. Unfortunately, no amino acid measurements were made in this study.

The picture drawn above is consistent with the idea that the higher the rate of ATP turnover, the more the requirement to maintain the steady-state ATP/ADP ratio and thus the greater the need to draw on the activity of the PNC, which appears to be operationally incapable of working in its complete form at high levels of intensity of contraction (>70% $\dot{V}O_{2max}$). Whether it is able to function completely at much lower rates of contraction in human muscle is presently unknown. Certainly, Meyer and Terjung were doubtful that even at low rates of stimulation deamination and reamination occurred simultaneously in perfused rat muscle (177). If no complete operation of the PNC does occur, then the putative advantages attaching to its function disappear and the anaplerotic role in particular could be accomplished by the activity of glutamate dehydrogenase.

In summary, therefore: at high intensities the source of the ammonia that rises exponentially in concentration with intensity of contractile activity, both dynamic and isometric, is likely to be derived from adenine nucleotides. At lower rates of contraction the ammonia probably derives from amino acids, mainly BCAA.

Alterations of Muscle and Blood Amino Acid Concentrations during Exercise

The size of the free pool of amino acids tells us something about the metabolic processes at work in the whole body, but care should be taken not to overinterpret the information available. The body water pool and its distribution between the intracellular and extracellular spaces and the size of the free amino acid pool can vary in complicated ways during exercise under different conditions. This makes interpretation of changes in the free concentrations of amino acids difficult.

The amino acids of most interest in the context of muscle metabolism are those concerned with intermediary metabolism (alanine, glutamate, glutamine,

BCAA, aspartate) and those amino acids which, because they are not metabolized in muscle, may act as indicators of the state of the net nitrogen balance of the tissue (the aromatic amino acids and lysine particularly). Other amino acids of interest are 3-methylhistidine and hydroxyproline, which are formed by posttranslational modifications of actin + myosin and collagen, respectively, and whose appearance in the free pool should theoretically be good indicators of net myofibrillar and collagen breakdown, respectively. For the present purposes, the following discussion will be confined to these amino acids and to various intermediary metabolites such as α-ketoglutarate, pyruvate, and the branched chain keto acids, which relate to intermediary metabolism.

During short-term exercise, blood ammonia, alanine, and glutamine concentrations rise, with very little change in other amino acids [Table 22.3; (8, 114, 142)]. Particularly noteworthy is the fact near that the blood BCAA concentrations do no change. The same pattern is also seen for muscle, except that the increases in ammonia alanine and glutamine are somewhat bigger (114, 142).

In exercise at a rate that can be sustained for an hour or longer, the pattern of responses in muscle and blood appears to be somewhat different to that observed during shorter term exercise. For example (170), whereas during short-term exercise aspartate concentrations generally rise from about 250 μmol/kg of wet muscle to about 400 μmol/kg, after bicycle exercise at 75% of maximum to exhaustion at about 3 h, aspartate concentrations in muscle fall to about 75% of normal. Glutamate concentrations appear to fall early during exercise and to remain at about two-thirds of the normal concentration (i.e., ~ 2.5 mmol/kg) and muscle glutamine concentration shows hardly any change from 14–18 mmol/kg. The concentrations of the sum of the other nonessential amino acids shows an increase of about 20%, whereas the sum of the BCAA shows no significant change (170).

Blood concentrations of most amino acids are steady for up to about 90 min of exercise, but beyond this there appears to be a general tendency for the BCAA to fall by up to 50% (20, 119, 267, 269).

There have been many reports (20, 50, 170) that long-term exercise is associated with increases in the aromatic amino acids and lysine in muscle and blood, suggesting an elevation of muscle protein breakdown. Maclean and co-workers did not notice any effects of exercise to exhaustion on muscle free hydroxyproline concentration in muscle, suggesting no acute increase in collagen breakdown; they did not measure 3-methylhistidine (170). Henriksson and co-workers noticed elevations of tyrosine, phenylalanine, and 3-methylhistidine, but no alteration in muscle BCAA (114).

Bicycling may have effects substantially different from those of running. For example, Décombaz found that immediately after a 100 km run most free amino acid concentrations in the blood of the athletes were reduced by 30%–90% (50). Also, in rats that had run to exhaustion (51), the concentrations of most amino acids fell, with the exception of the BCAA (which show a 20% rise) and the aromatic amino acids (which almost double). This work is particularly interesting, since free amino acid concentrations were measured in muscle and in liver. Both alanine and glutamine concentrations were only 80% of the normal resting value in muscle, whereas aspartate was almost double and tyrosine increased by 50%; concentrations of leucine and isoleucine were also increased by about 20%. However, the most spectacular change occurred in the liver, where most amino acids showed a substantial elevation between 30% and 300%. Glutamate concentration increased by 80% and the BCAA were about twice the preexercise value. Overall, these changes

TABLE 22.3. *Effects of Exercise Mode on Likely Pattern of Changes in Muscle and Blood Amino Acid Concentrations*

	Short-Term (0–30 min) Mild 40%–60% $\dot{V}O_{2max}$		Short-Term Intense (75%–110% $\dot{V}O_{2max}$		Long-Term (60–120 + min) Moderate (60%–75% $\dot{V}O_{2max}$)	
	Muscle	Blood	Muscle	Blood	Muscle	Blood
Alanine	↑ ↑	↑	↑ ↑ ↑	↑ ↑ ↑	↑	↑
Glutamine	↑ ↑	↑ ↑	↑ ↑ ↑	↑ ↑ ↑	↓	↓
Glutamate	=	=	↓	↓	↓	↓
NH_3	↑	↑	↑ ↑ ↑	↑ ↑	↑	↑
BCAA	=	=	=	=	↓	↓ ↓
Tyrosine/Phenylalanine	=	–	=	=	↑ ↑	↑ ↑
Try	?	=	?	?		↑

are suggestive of a very marked increase in hepatic proteolysis.

Production and Consumption of Amino Acids by Muscle during Exercise

During short-term intense dynamic exercise which results in exhaustion in a few minutes, muscle is effectively working as a quasi-isolated preparation, and many of the metabolic changes observed occur without much influence of the circulation. For example, in 5 min of exercise at 100% $\dot{V}O_{2max}$, less than 20% of the ammonia or lactate produced escapes from muscle into the blood (142). Of course, during isometric exercise at or above 30% maximum voluntary contraction (MVC) there will be no exchange with the blood at all (59). It is remarkable that glycolysis and oxidative metabolism are turned on rapidly after the onset of contractile activity, probably before ammonia production from AMP, and thus amino acids present in muscle at the beginning of exercise will be able to interact with the metabolic products of glycolysis and possibly with oxidative processes also.

Exercise is usually carried out in the postabsorptive state, when resting human muscle is an exporter of alanine, glutamine, and BCAA and an importer of glutamate (6, 58). During short-term, high-intensity exercise it seems unlikely that there is any net increase in the uptake of amino acids from the blood (142). Thus, assuming that the alanine aminotransferase reaction is at equilibrium, it could be predicted that production of alanine would be driven by an increased delivery of pyruvate via accelerated glycolysis, given sufficient availability of glutamate. Indeed, there is a large amount of information suggesting that muscle alanine concentrations increase markedly in a fashion that correlates with the increase in glycolytic flux and pyruvate production, and glutamate concentrations fall, even in isometric exercise in which the contribution from the blood will be less (14, 142, 143). It is interesting that the pattern of change in alanine and glutamine production by muscle as a result of exercise is unlike that which occurs simply by presenting muscle with increased amounts of BCAA at rest. Under these circumstances, alanine production hardly changes (58), whereas glutamine production triples. The difference in exercise is that alanine production appears to increase more than glutamine production, presumably as a result of increased activation of glycolysis and the provision of pyruvate to accept α-amino nitrogen.

For example, during 5 min dynamic exercise at 100% $\dot{V}O_{2max}$, conditions under which fatigue occurs in just over 5 min (142), the glycolytic flux (calculated as the sum of muscle accumulation and efflux into the venous blood of pyruvate + lactate + alanine) is about 16 μmol/min from one leg, of which alanine production accounts for only about 5%. The alanine production rate of about 0.45 mmol/kg wet wt muscle per minute was about three times the glutamate consumption (calculated from the size of the fall observed in intramuscular glutamate + leg glutamate uptake) of 0.17 mmol $\cdot$ kg^{-1} $\cdot$ min^{-1}, leaving a shortfall of about 0.28 mmol $\cdot$ kg^{-1} $\cdot$ min^{-1}. Given that the intramuscular free concentration of the BCAA is about 0.7 mmol/kg and that net uptake of BCAA from the blood is undetectable during exercise of this intensity or duration (114), even during exercise of only 5 min duration there would have to be a substantial rise in the delivery of BCAA from protein turnover to supply the required α-amino nitrogen for alanine synthesis, assuming that glutaminolysis is unimportant. As discussed below, protein turnover within muscle probably could not supply this.

In the work by Katz and colleagues (142), no significant change in the glutamine intramuscular pool size (normally about 14–18 mmol/kg) could be detected, which is in line with the previous findings concerning muscle glutamine concentration during isometric contraction; there was a small release of glutamine detected (about 16 μmol $\cdot$ kg^{-1} $\cdot$ min^{-1}), but this would make no discernable impact on the size of the intracellular glutamine pool. If this glutamine were synthesized in muscle rather than simply being subtracted from the intracellular pool it would add to the deficit of glutamate noted above. Even assuming that under the conditions of a high rate of muscle work, the ammonia production can be quantitatively assigned to the deficit in the total adenine nucleotide pool, so that it would not have to be derived from amino acids, it is not easy to quantify the size of the change in the net α-amino nitrogen balance and balance it against the changes in the metabolites accounting for it.

During dynamic exercise at a slightly lower percentage of maximal aerobic capacity—75%–80% of $\dot{V}O_{2max}$—there appears to be no activity of adenosine deaminase, as judged from a lack of a fall in the adenine nucleotide pool (170), and exercise can be sustained for at least an hour. Nevertheless, ammonia production on the order of 14–26 μmol $\cdot$ kg muscle^{-1} $\cdot$ min^{-1}, alanine production 14–40 μmol $\cdot$ kg muscle^{-1} $\cdot$ min^{-1} and glutamine production 20–28 μmoles $\cdot$ kg muscle^{-1} $\cdot$ min^{-1} (59–95). If average figures are taken, then it can be calculated that about

96 μmol · kg^{-1} · min^{-1} of α-amino nitrogen leaves muscle as ammonia + alanine + glutamine and that only 12–24 μmol · kg^{-1} · min^{-1}, are taken up as glutamate (i.e., there is a net loss to muscle of about 72–84 μmol · kg^{-1} · min^{-1}, of α-amino nitrogen. It can be shown that at rest muscle protein breakdown in leg muscle of normal healthy men contributes about 1 μmol · kg^{-1} · min^{-1} (12) (i.e., probably about 2.3 μmol of total BCAA · kg^{-1} · min^{-1}. Even if muscle protein synthesis (which consumes about 1.6 μmol · kg^{-1} · min^{-1} of BCAA in the postabsorptive state) is totally shut down, this would only bring the total availability of BCAA for ammonia, alanine, and glutamine synthesis to 3.9 μmol · kg^{-1} · min^{-1} leaving a substantial shortfall of about 68–80 μmol · kg^{-1} · min^{-1} of BCAA. The shortfall in BCAA does not seem to come from the blood and indeed it is remarkable that most workers in the last 5–10 years have been unable to reproduce the findings of Ahlborg et al. (1) of a marked increase in the uptake the BCAA by working muscle. In this classic study of bicycle exercise at 40% of maximal power output, BCAA flux across the leg was negative at rest, but by 40 min a marked positive balance of the BCAA became established. A study of this sort has not, so far as I am aware, ever been observed in exercise at higher work rates, and unfortunately the experiment itself has not been repeated by other workers.

The results of these conjectures are particularly puzzling because there does seem to be a good match between the measured rates of whole-body oxidation of BCAA and the rates of appearance of α-amino nitrogen from muscle. The problem is best seen by considering the production rates of ammonia, alanine, and glutamine during bicycle exercise at 55% of $\dot{V}O_{2max}$ (59), a type and intensity of exercise for which data are available on leucine oxidation. Eriksson and colleagues found that the total release from alanine, glutamine, and ammonia was about 200 μmol/min for two exercising legs. Now if this is ultimately derived from the BCAA, then these must be transaminated, and since it is likely that in human muscle quantitatively insignificant amounts of keto acids are released, most being completely oxidized (41, 42, 58), the oxidation rate should provide a good estimate of the transamination rate. We have previously shown that during bicycle ergometer exercise leucine oxidation is directly proportionate to the aerobic power (181), and it is possible to calculate from this information and the results of Knapik and co-workers (152) that total leucine oxidation during bicycle hydrometer exercise at 55% $\dot{V}O_{2max}$ would be about 100 μmol/min; if leucine is about 43% of the total BCAA available (as in protein), then the total BCAA oxidation should be about 240 μmol/min. Thus, the transamination rate of BCAA is probably sufficient to account for the α-amino nitrogen lost by muscle during exercise, but the question remains: Where does the BCAA come from? Since the whole-body leucine turnover rate does not change [i.e., leucine appearance from breakdown is not elevated markedly during bicycle ergometer exercise (152)] and muscle protein breakdown in the forearm apparently decreases during exercise (224), the leucine oxidized must come from either a depression in muscle protein synthesis or increased net uptake. However, neither of these processes seems to occur fast enough, and a clear balance sheet for amino acid transamination and oxidation cannot be drawn up.

Even if the primary source for alanine and glutamine in short-term exercise is actually glutamate, which falls about 1.8 mmol/kg, this would only supply the observed rates of efflux for 20–30 min, whereas the rates of efflux cited above can be sustained for up to an hour (95). Thus, either muscle protein breakdown must increase 10- to 20-fold as a result of exercise at above 50% of $\dot{V}O_{2max}$ (which seems very unlikely), or amino acids other than BCAA must contribute substantially to the transaminating pool, or there is in fact a net loss of glutamine from the muscle free pool. The latter is certainly a possibility and could occur either by increased outward transport (due to a rise in intracellular Na^+ and a decrease in membrane potential) or by glutaminolysis via glutaminase, or less likely via glutamine transaminase. Because the glutamine pool is so large, it would be difficult to detect a fall which could completely account for all the observed production of glutamine, at least during the early part of exercise.

Obviously, more work needs to be done in this area before we can claim to understand completely muscle amino acid metabolism in short-term or long-term exercise.

The rates of glutamine production observed during exercise at about 80% $\dot{V}O_{2max}$ (i.e., 24 μmol · kg^{-1} · min^{-1} are certainly within the capacity of glutamate dehydrogenase to supply ammonia for the glutamine synthetase reaction, since GDH activity is on the order of 1 mmol · kg muscle $^{-1}$ · min^{-1} (279). By using values for glutamine synthetase measured in rat muscle (150) and by assuming the K_m for glutamate is about 5 mM in human muscle, then the capacity of glutamine synthetase in muscle can be calculated to be about 100 μmol · kg^{-1} · min^{-1} (i.e., more than enough to accommodate observed rates of glutamine synthesis).

However, exercise at 75% $\dot{V}O_{2max}$ substantially decreases muscle α-ketoglutarate from about 13 to 9 μmol/kg wet weight in 5 min (96). This suggests that the availability of α-ketoglutarate for transamination of BCAA decreases during exercise. Nevertheless, it seems unlikely that, in short-term exercise at least, the α-ketoglutarate availability is limiting, since BCAA oxidation [the extent of which is linearly related to aerobic power output (215)] can continue to increase at work rates beyond 75% of $\dot{V}O_{2max}$ (Fig. 22.3).

Amino Acid Oxidation and Contractile Activity. Many workers have demonstrated that exercise is associated with increased oxidation of leucine (106, 152, 181, 212, 217, 278, 285), but there seems to be no data available for any other BCAA. BCKA dehydrogenase enzymes in both rat and human skeletal muscle are activated during exercise, possibly as a result of increases in ADP concentration (139, 270) or perhaps due to an increase in H^+ concentration. The observed increase in leucine oxidation appears to be in proportion to the aerobic power output up to $\dot{V}O_{2max}$ (215, 278). Since the K_m of the transaminase is sufficiently high (1 mM for leucine and isoleucine and 5 mM for valine), it seems likely that the transaminase would never be saturated under physiological conditions, given that the total muscle BCAA concentration is only 0.6–1.20 mmol/kg. Thus, control of the oxidation of the BCAA resides with the BCKA dehydrogenase. Despite being activated during exercise, it appears that at very high work rates the rate of transamination may exceed the rate of oxidation according to the increase in concentration of the BCKA observed in muscle (67). What is puzzling about these observations is why the branched chain transaminase activity increases more than the dehydrogenase activity, since the concentration of the BCAA does not show a sufficient rise during short-term exercise to explain the marked increase in activity. It may be that the observed increase in the transaminase activity is mainly due to the observed fall in glutamate concentration in muscle during exercise. Since the loss of glutamate is probably driven by an increase in pyruvate accumulation and thus alanine production, it is likely that the transamination of the BCAA is indirectly controlled by the rate of glycolysis, whereas the rate of decarboxylation of the keto acids depends upon the activation state of the dehydrogenase.

The higher than normal rate of leucine oxidation observed during exercise after fasting (152) is probably the result of increased muscle BCAA concentrations commonly observed during fasting as well as an increased activation of the dehydrogenase. Kasperek and co-workers have shown that exercise plus starvation cause a greater increase in rat muscle dehydrogenase activity than exercise alone (140).

Leucine oxidation during exercise can be inhibited by provision of glucose during exercise (218) as expected from knowledge of the interaction between glucose and BCAA oxidation (27) and the effect of insulin in depressing the activation of the enzyme (195). Consumption of a high-protein diet probably increases the capacity for BCAA oxidation in muscle by increasing the capacity of the transaminase and keto acid dehydrogenase (18), and it is not surprising to discover that consumption of a high-protein diet leads to increased rates of leucine oxidation during exercise (214).

Availability of medium-chain triglycerides inhibits leucine oxidation at rest (11) and long-chain fatty acids should do likewise (18). It might therefore be expected that during exercise the maximum rate of BCAA oxidation would be, to some extent, limited by lipolysis and fat oxidation, but so far as I am aware no relevant data exist regarding this question.

Branched Chain Amino Acids as Precursors of Tricarboxylic Acid Intermediates. At the beginning of contractile activity the concentrations of some Krebs cycle intermediates (fumarate, malate) probably increase (7). However, α-ketoglutarate concentration is known to fall during intense exercise (96); this fall is associated with a generalized loss of cycle intermediates (233), but it is not known whether the two are causally linked or if the changes in α-ketoglutarate are mainly cytoplasmic or mitochondrial changes. Either is possible due to transamination in the cytoplasm, or cataplerotic metabolism in the mitochondria. Partial oxidation of valine and isoleucine could provide a source of Krebs cycle intermediates to help maintain their steady-state concentrations and thus ensure continued operations of the cycle to allow full oxidation of fat and carbohydrate. However, in order for BCAA to be oxidized they must first be transaminated, and transamination drains the α-ketoglutarate pool. Wagenmakers has suggested that under conditions in which the provision of anaplerotic precursors from carbohydrate metabolism is diminished (e.g., during long-term exercise when muscle glycogen concentrations fall), BCAA transamination and oxidation may further deplete the pool of Krebs cycle intermediates, thereby diminishing the ability of muscle to oxidize fat and carbohydrate adequately (266, 267). Moreover, in patients with McArdle's disease who cannot replenish TCA cycle intermediates from glycogen metabolism due to a lack of phosphorylase, BCAA supplementation during exercise leads to a decreased exercise performance (269). However, when BCAA supplements were given to healthy subjects in a normal or glycogen-depleted state during exercise to exhaustion on a bicycle ergometer at 70%–75% maximal aerobic power, no diminution of exercise performance could be determined. Thus, it appears that oxidative metabolism is not limited by the drain of α-ketoglutarate.

Effects of Training on Amino Acid Metabolism during Exercise

Exercise increases the capacity of muscle to maintain a constant ATP/ADP ratio partly due to an increase in the mitochondrial content (116). Thus, trained animals and humans are able to exercise at higher absolute power outputs than untrained subjects, and they can rely more on fat metabolism at the given percentage of maximal aerobic capacity. It might be expected therefore that in trained subjects there would be a rather good match between rates of glycolysis and rates of pyruvate oxidation. Lactate production at the same absolute or relative submaximal workload is lower in trained subjects (220). If pyruvate is rapidly and efficiently routed towards mitochondrial oxidation, less of it will accumulate and be available as a substrate for transamination, although the capacity of alanine aminotransferase is reportedly elevated in trained rat and horse muscle (104, 132). Trained athletes and rats have lower plasma concentrations of alanine during exercise than untrained subjects (133, 220), which would be consistent with a decreased production (as argued above) or an increased clearance, presumably in liver. However, Hood and Terjung found, perhaps somewhat surprisingly, that the output of alanine from isolated electrically stimulated rat muscle taken from trained rats shows increased amounts of alanine being released compared to muscles from untrained rats (120). Phenylalanine release did not differ between the two, suggesting that the appearance of amino acids from protein degradation, and thus the input of transaminating substrate, is the same in trained as in untrained muscle. They interpret the available data as indicating that physical training improves all components of the whole metabolic system for maintenance of gluconeogenesis during exercise. Nothing substantial seems to be known about the effects of training on muscle glutamine metabolism. Trained rat muscle has a greater activity of glutamine synthase activity than untrained muscle (63), but Hood and Terjung were unable to find any differences in glutamine output from stimulated isolated incubated rat muscle (120). Theoretically, if trained muscle oxidizes fat and carbohydrate more efficiently, as it seems likely to do, then BCAA oxidation would not be favored so long as the ATP/ADP ratio remained high; thus BCAA transamination should not be accelerated, reducing the input of α-amino nitrogen for alanine, glutamate, and glutamine synthesis, so glutamine production might be lessened. On the other hand, muscle contains a substantial amount of glutamate, and trained muscle has more glutamate dehydrogenase (279), so an elevated production of glutamine is also possible!

The capacity for leucine oxidative decarboxylation is greater in trained muscle than in untrained muscle, simply because of the increased mitochondrial density. When muscle in isolated perfused rat hind leg was electrically stimulated, trained muscle was able to maintain a greater tension and a greater oxygen consumption than untrained muscle and the rate of leucine oxidation was a smaller proportion of the total oxidative flux than for the untrained rats (118). These results are in agreement with the proposition above suggesting that the trained rats preferentially use fuels other than protein, and muscle production of alanine and glutamine should be lower in the trained state.

Interrelationships between Working Muscle and the Viscera during Exercise

The increased flux of alanine and glutamine from working muscle in longer term exercise serves to underpin gluconeogenesis (136) and acid–base regulation (243), with ureagenesis as an obligatory counterpart. The definition of longer term exercise is necessarily elastic, since it must encompass bouts of exercise possibly as short as half an hour up through periods of time appropriate for running marathons or taking part in triathlons and various orienteering and mountain running events which can last for days. Of course, the always heavy and intermittently intense exercise required of mountaineering expeditions may require weeks of effort in hypoxic and dehydrating conditions where food and water are in short supply. Unfortunately, our knowledge of the changes which occur in amino acid and protein metabolism over the full range of such types of physical activity is extremely limited.

The observed increased efflux of ammonia, alanine, and glutamine from muscle, and the increase in the plasma glucagon/insulin ratio should stimulate ureagenesis in liver. Ahlborg and co-workers (1) demonstrated that the fractional hepatic extraction of alanine, threonine, serine, proline, glycine, and methionine almost doubled after 4 h of exercise at 30% $\dot{V}O_{2max}$; unfortunately, glutamine exchange was not measured. The output of alanine via muscle was statistically indistinguishable from the uptake of alanine by the splanchnic region. The total amino acid uptake by the liver accounted for about 18% of the total uptake of gluconeogenic substrates in terms of glucose equivalents, and if glutamine had been measured, it is likely that this figure could have been increased to about 25%. Unfortunately, in these classic experiments, not only were leg and muscle glutamine not measured, but urea production was not measured either.

The work of Felig and Wahren and colleagues (1, 60, 66, 271) on human exercise metabolism has provided valuable information about splanchnic and muscle exchange of amino acids, but no division was possible between gastrointestinal and liver metabolism and no information is currently available about renal metabolism during exercise in people: the major limitation is, of course, the difficulty of placing sampling cannulae in appropriate vessels. Similar constraints do not exist with animal work, and the results of Wasserman and co-workers have provided a unique insight into the hepatic splanchnic exchanges occurring with exercise in dogs (272). As expected, muscle production of glutamine and alanine increased (and thus increased hepatic extraction followed). A remarkable, unexpected observation was that exercise caused the gut to become a net exporter of amino acids to the liver, presumably as a result of increased net protein degradation, and with the benefit of blood glucose maintenance (272).

The idea that the protein of the gastrointestinal tract is a buffer against glucopenia, as well as supplying BCAA to working muscle, is an interesting and potentially important one. Increased net degradation in the viscera has been reported in exercising rats (54), and studies carried out in exercising man by our group 10 years ago suggested that visceral protein breakdown may be a substantial source of substrate during exercise (217).

In exercising dogs (272), hepatic amino acid and ammonia uptake from the portal blood closely matched their delivery from the gut under circumstances in which it is known that hepatic glucose output increases, suggesting increased gluconeogenesis as the fate of the amino acids. However, in these experiments, the output of urea from the liver, although elevated, did not match quantitatively the uptake of amino acids and ammonia from the blood, suggesting that there was some other route of disposal of the α-amino nitrogen. One possibility is that even during exercise hepatic export-protein synthesis (possibly including acute-phase proteins) is stimulated (34). Another possibly important finding is that the fractional extraction of glutamine by the gut and the liver in exercising dogs was increased more than the delivery of glutamine from the periphery. The results suggest the involvement of some hormonal or nervous stimulatory effect on hepatic and gastrointestinal glutamine utilization; the most likely candidate is glucagon, the secretion of which increases during exercise (105) and which is able to stimulate both gastrointestinal and hepatic utilization of glutamine (5).

Much of our current understanding of whole-body amino acid oxidation during exercise is derived from information concerning changes in urea production gauged from changes in urea pool size and excretion rates of urea both in urine and in sweat (55, 159, 207, 216). Even taking into account the difficulties imposed by the fall in renal blood flow during exercise (38), which delays the appearance of urea produced during the exercise period until the postexercise period (216), there appears to be overwhelming evidence that exercise is associated with an increase in urea production and hence by inference an increase in amino acid oxidation (Fig. 22.3). The problem with this interpretation is that when urea turnover is examined by isotopic techniques (35, 286), no increase in urea production could be discerned during exercise. Furthermore, the rate of appearance of ^{15}N in urea after infusion of [^{15}N]leucine is unchanged as a result of exercise, although the rate of transfer of leucine-N to alanine increases by about 150% (286). Wolfe, in considering all these data (284), concludes that *(1)* the oxidative catabolism of leucine is not necessarily a guide to the oxidative catabolism of other essential amino acids such as lysine, and *(2)* urea production is not increased during exercise. However, this conclusion is impossible to square not only with the urea excretion data but with the observations of Wasserman and colleagues who demonstrated that increased hepatic amino acid uptake in the exercising dog was accompanied by increased urea production, although the size of the increase in urea production was less than might have been expected (272). More recently, Wolfe and co-workers, using a new technique in exercising man to partition the amount alanine derived from pyruvate synthesis and protein breakdown (292), have shown that exercise does increase net protein breakdown (i.e., promotes negative tissue nitrogen balance), which must eventually cause elevated urea production.

How are we to reconcile the different pieces of evidence available? It seems clear that exercise is associated with an increase in BCAA transamination and an increase in leucine oxidation and probably also in the complete oxidation of isoleucine and valine (though there is no good evidence on this latter point). Even if the BCAA (which account for 20% of protein) are selectively oxidized, this means that the other 80% of amino acids released by net proteolysis have to be processed somehow by the body, and that means disposal either by urea synthesis or incorporation into protein. Since most proteins contain all amino acids, it is difficult to conceive of the extra non-BCAA amino acids being disposed of by protein synthesis. However, recently Carraro and co-workers have shown that postexercise synthesis of the hepatic export protein fibronectin was significantly increased; there is also a trend towards an increase in albumin synthesis, although this did not reach significance (36). We have recently investigated albumin synthesis after higher rates of exercise than those used by Carraro and colleagues and demonstrated that it increases significantly (J. J. Walker and M. J. Rennie, unpublished results). Since albumin and fibronectin are relatively depleted in BCAA compared to most tissue protein, their postexercise synthesis may be a way of absorbing some of the non-BCAA amino acids released by the increase in net protein breakdown, but this cannot be the entire explanation. What seems most likely is that (for reasons not understood) measurements of urea turnover, and possibly of protein and amino acid turnover during exercise using isotopes are in some way flawed, giving only partially correct answers.

PROTEIN TURNOVER DURING EXERCISE

Most of the information that is currently available concerning changes in rates of protein synthesis and protein breakdown in muscle or other tissues during contractile activity come to us via work in animals (25, 54). These facts should not be a surprise when it is considered that the whole question of the measurement of protein turnover in human beings is currently the subject of vigorous debate (16). The area is bedeviled by the lack of agreement concerning the best methods to use and the interpretation of results obtained with particular types of methods. It is my personal view that for the measurement of tissue protein synthesis, including muscle, the best method remains the primed, constant infusion of tracer amino acids with measurement of tracer incorporation into protein as the index of protein synthesis (247). A method which looks promising is the compartmental analysis technique recently developed by Biolo, Wolfe, and co-workers (17); this method has the advantage that amino acid transport, protein synthesis, and protein breakdown may be measured together. However, the method is somewhat cumbersome inasmuch as besides arterial and venous cannulation it also requires accurate measurements of blood flow by a dye-dilution method, and a muscle biopsy must be taken at steady state in order to measure the enrichment of the muscle-free pool; it is therefore difficult to see it becoming widely applied for the study of exercise or exercise-induced alterations in muscle protein.

Muscle protein breakdown is harder to measure than protein synthesis; methods based on stable or radioactive amino acid tracer dilution between arterial blood and venous blood leaving organs or limbs probably underestimates tissue protein turnover unless the intracellular pool is sampled by biopsy (17). Semiquantitative methods, measuring the efflux from muscle of tyrosine and 3-methylhistidine (neither of which are metabolized in muscle), as indices of breakdown of total muscle protein and myofibrillar protein, respectively, have been applied in A-V balance studies across limbs (213) as well as in incubated (141) and perfused muscle preparations (138). These latter methods are useful in allowing some insight into the breakdown of the two major pools of muscle, but the results they provide need to be carefully interpreted. The tyrosine efflux, unless measured in the presence of a protein synthesis inhibitor, provides an indicator of net balance between synthesis and breakdown, theoretically for all muscle protein. The efflux of 3-methylhistidine is a specific index of actin and myosin breakdown.

That habitual exercise causes adaptations in muscle composition and muscle fiber size, depending upon the type of exercise undertaken, strongly suggests that there are changes in muscle protein synthesis as a result of exercise. Whether there are also alterations in protein breakdown is much harder to decide, because direct methods of measuring protein breakdown are not available, except semiquantitatively as 3-methylhistidine. The evidence for and against such changes will be reviewed below.

Effects of Acute Contractile Activity on Protein Turnover

Protein Synthesis. There is now a substantial amount of evidence available from work on running rats (53, 215), on perfused electrically stimulated rat hindlimb muscle (31, 215), and in human forearm muscle isometrically contracting at low tensions (214): the results of all of these studies (and those by other workers) suggested that there was a fall in the rate of muscle protein synthesis during contractile activity (Table 22.4). However, when the muscle-biopsy, leucine-incorporation method for protein synthesis was applied to the study of human muscle before, during, and after 4 h exercise, Wolfe and colleagues

TABLE 22.4. *Likely Involvement of Tissues in Changes in Protein Metabolism as a Result of Exercise Relative to Preexercise Postabsorptive State*

	Exercise			Recovery Fasted			Recovery Fed		
	Ox	Syn	Bkdn	Ox	Syn	Bkdn	Ox	Syn	Bkdn
Muscle	↑↑	↓	↑	=	↑	↑↑	↑	↑↑↑	↑
Liver	↑	↓↓	↑↑	↑	↑	↑↑	↑↑	↑↑	↑
Gut	=	↓↓	↑↑	=	↓	↑↑	=	↑↑	↑

(37) were unable to discern more than a slight nonsignificant fall in the incorporation of tracer leucine during 40% $\dot{V}O_{2max}$. It may be that the exercise intensity used was insufficient to demonstrate the fall that has been observed by other workers in other preparations and models. There certainly appears to be a fall of some magnitude in whole-body protein synthesis determined either from [^{15}N]glycine end-product methods or by [^{13}C]leucine plasma turnover methods during exercise at 60% $\dot{V}O_{2max}$ (106, 181, 215, 217). The implication is that this fall occurs in muscle, but it could also occur in visceral tissue, which suffers some fall in blood flow and possibly oxygenation as exercise continues.

The mechanism of any fall in muscle protein synthesis is difficult to ascertain. Bylund-Fellenius and colleagues (31) suggested that in electrically stimulated perfused rat hindlimb muscle the fall was due to a decrease in the muscle ATP/ADP ratio, which is plausible, since in acute hypoxia in normal subjects the net protein balance of muscle determined by [^{13}C]leucine exchange becomes more negative (212). A similar relationship has been found in resting muscle, in which hypoxia and ischemia cause a fall in the ratio of creatine phosphate to creatine, and there is a linear relationship between this ratio and the rate of muscle protein synthesis (31, 171).

Protein Breakdown. Acute changes in muscle protein breakdown as a result of increased contractile activity are harder to pin down. Muscle protein breakdown occurs by a variety of different mechanisms involving at least four different subcellular systems such as the lysosome, the ATP-dependent ubiquitin system, an ATP-independent ubiquitin system, and calcium-dependent proteases with high and low affinities for calcium (see 146 for review). It now seems reasonably clear that the lysosomal systems are physiologically important only for turnover of nonmyofibrillar protein and that the calcium-dependent systems are probably involved only in end-stage degradation, possibly as a result of massive muscle damage or remodeling (Fig. 22.1; Tables 22.4 and 22.5). The myofibrillar apparatus is probably degraded by a nonlysosomal pathway, most likely a ubiquitin-dependent pathway. The lysosomal mechanisms are insulin sensitive and also sensitive to prevailing concentrations of amino acids, especially leucine; it may therefore be predicted that as the anabolic environment of muscle is diminished during exercise by falls in blood insulin concentration and in the intramuscular and blood amino acid concentrations, protein breakdown by the lysosomal pathways would be accelerated. There is, however, no good evidence that muscle lysosomal enzyme activities increase acutely during short-term contractile activity sufficient to cause a stimulation of mitochondrial adaptation (242). There certainly is a wealth of evidence that after exercise, especially during a chronic exercise training program, lysosomal enzyme activity rises (264, 265), suggesting that a postexercise adaptation occurs. Nevertheless, there is evidence that acute exercise is accompanied by an increase in the muscle concentration and release of those amino acids which are not subject to catabolism in muscle such as phenylalanine, tyrosine, and lysine (141, 146); furthermore, in the isolated perfused rat hindlimb, the increased exercise-induced, postexercise tyrosine efflux can be only partially and not completely diminished by the application of the lysosomal

TABLE 22.5. *Likely Pattern of Changes in Protein Synthesis and Breakdown in Myofibrillar and Nonmyofibrillar Protein as a Result of Immobilization, Moderate and Severe Exercise, and during Recovery*

	Immobilization		Moderate Aerobic Exercise		Strenous Power Exercise		Postexercise	
	Syn	Bkdn	Syn	Bkdn	Syn	Bkdn	Syn	Bkdn
Myofibrillar	↓↓	↓	↓	=	↓	=	↑↑	=
Nonmyofibrillar	↓	↓	↓	↑↑	↓	=	↑↑	↑

protease inhibitor chloroquine (138, 141), suggesting that nonlysosomal pathways of proteolysis are activated. However, the efflux of 3-methylhistidine from rat hindlimb muscle is largely unaffected by preceding exercise, whether mainly concentric or with a substantial eccentric component, suggesting that myofibrillar protein breakdown is not accelerated by preceding exercise. It is worth noting that although the nonmyofibrillar soluble protein pool of muscle constitutes only about 50% of the mass of the myofibrillar pool, it has an intrinsically higher rate of turnover (146, 179), and so an elevation of the rate of breakdown of the soluble proteins may make a substantial contribution to alanine and glutamine production by muscle during acute exercise.

The question of an alteration (usually assumed to be an increase) of the degradation rate of myofibrillar protein has been a vexed one for some years (54, 197). Virtually the only way in which to approach this problem has been to measure the efflux from muscle of 3-methylhistidine, which is produced by the posttranslational modification of histidine residues in actin and myosin and which cannot be reincorporated into protein; 3-methylhistidine is excreted in urine unchanged in humans, but in rodents it may be acetylated (294). There is a great amount of disagreement in the literature concerning postexercise urinary 3-methylhistidine production, but current authors reviewing the literature tend to agree that, as originally suggested, there is no exercise-associated increase (24, 56, 197). When the topic was first of interest it was impossible to measure 3-methylhistidine at low concentrations (e.g., in blood or incubation media due to lack of sensitivity of classical amino acid analyzers). However as methods improved, particularly with the adoption of reverse phase high-performance liquid chromatography (HPLC) with fluorescent detection, we can have increasing confidence in the results using efflux of 3-methylhistidine into the plasma or perfusion or incubation media, and the method has gained widespread use (89, 110, 141). Obviously, application of such methods makes it easier to determine whether the amino acid is coming directly from muscle, and a substantial amount of information on this point is now available.

In my view, the balance of evidence now appears to suggest that myofibrillar protein breakdown is *not* elevated during acute aerobic exercise and probably not elevated acutely as a result of strength-training exercise [Table 22.5; (197, 199, 206)]. The intramuscular concentration of 3-methylhistidine may actually fall as a result of moderate aerobic exercise (217), and this fall may be due either to a decrease in breakdown or a decrease in the intracellular pool of the amino acid due to an increased outward transport, as has been observed when A-V differences were measured during moderate exercise (168). There is quite a body of literature suggesting that in rats and people there is an increased postexercise excretion of 3-methylhistidine. Unfortunately, a considerable body of evidence (197) suggests no such increase! One of the possible explanations for these contradictions is that if renal plasma flow falls during exercise, as it usually does at intensities above about 50% $\dot{V}O_{2max}$ (38), clearance of low-molecular-weight substances will fall and the plasma pool will expand during exercise. Thus, apparently (falsely) increased excretion will occur after exercise. In any case, such an increase in 3-methylhistidine production does not necessarily signify that muscle protein breakdown has been elevated; some years ago Joe Millward and I drew attention to the possibility that nonmuscular sources of 3-methylhistidine, principally smooth muscle actin which had an inherently fast turnover rate, could contribute to whole-body production (i.e., excretion) of 3-methylhistidine and cause errors to be made in the estimate of its production and hence of the fractional turnover rate of muscle (223). Although in certain conditions (e.g., post-trauma, sepsis, starvation) in hospital patients these worries have probably turned out to be less important than we thought they might have been (246), there is still cause for concern that postexercise increases of 3-methylhistidine excretion do not necessarily represent elevations of muscle protein breakdown. The problem can be neatly illustrated by the work of Kasperek and co-workers (52, 55), who have, over the years, produced a substantial amount of evidence for increased 3-methylhistidine production by running rats in the postexercise period, suggesting that myofibrillar protein breakdown was elevated. However, in studies of isolated incubated muscle (141) and of perfused muscle taken from rats previously run on a treadmill (138), they were unable to detect any increases in 3-methylhistidine production despite the substantial elevation in muscle tyrosine production. Inhibitors of lysosomal proteolysis, as mentioned above, inhibited tyrosine release but had no effect on methylhistidine release. This argues very strongly that the rate of myofibrillar protein breakdown is not elevated as a result of exercise.

Effects of Eccentric and Concentric Exercise on Muscle Protein Turnover. The whole question of whether contractile activity in the concentric or eccentric mode is more efficient at stimulating adaptation or hypertrophy of muscle is difficult to sort out. Jones and Rutherford have shown convincingly that there is no difference in the extent of changes in muscle fiber size in groups of subjects who undertook isometric, concentric, or eccentric exercise for strength training (134). These results are not what would have been predicted by Evans and co-workers (61), who believe that muscle hypertrophy depends upon some element of concentric exercise.

One of the difficulties that bedevils the subject is the relatively slow rate of muscle protein turnover and therefore the inordinate length of time required for changes in muscle protein synthesis to manifest themselves as measurable changes in the muscle or lean body mass. Since animals have faster rates of muscle protein turnover, it might be assumed that work using animal models would provide more clear-cut results. However, when Wong and Booth carried out a series of pertinent studies, the results were not straightforward. These workers examined protein synthesis and related indices as a result of acute and chronic eccentric or concentric contractile activity induced by electrical stimulation of leg muscles in ether-anesthetized rats (213, 287). The gastrocnemius muscle was stimulated to contract concentrically and the anterior tibialis to contract eccentrically. Different patterns of electrical stimulation, effectively modeling high-repetition, low-intensity exercise and high-intensity, low-repetition exercise, were used. Muscle protein synthesis was measured at 17 or 34 h after a single bout of acute exercise and total muscle mRNA, ribosomal RNA, and amounts of RNA for α-actin and cytochrome *c* measured before and after 12 weeks of chronic exercise. The results were something of a puzzle. To their surprise they found that concentric exercise in this model caused no muscle hypertrophy, even though acute concentric exercise stimulated muscle protein synthesis. Also, the extent of the changes in protein synthesis as a result of the acute concentric exercise bout were about equal, irrespective of the different patterns of contractile activity. There were no increases in muscle protein concentration, but at the end of the 12 weeks of chronic concentric exercise the total amounts of RNA and DNA in the muscle appeared to be increased, although specific α-actin and cytochrome *c* mRNA did not change. These results were particularly surprising, since Wong and Booth had previously shown that their model *did* produce gastrocnemius muscle hypertrophy. However, eccentric contraction of the anterior tibialis did induce muscle hypertrophy and the extent of the increase was almost as great for low-frequency, high-resistance exercise (+30%) as for high-frequency, low-resistance exercise (+45%) lasting eight times longer. Also, no specific increases in specific mRNA amounts could be detected. An attempt was made to explain their puzzling findings by suggesting that the differences in response may have been due to the greater specific tension imposed on the tibialis anterior (0.6 g) than on the gastrocnemius (1.6 g). The results suggest that the increases in protein synthesis observed were greater than could be explained by alterations in either messenger or ribosomal RNA, and Wong and Booth suggest that in their model the increases occurred as a result of posttranscriptional or translational mechanisms.

A major worry in the interpretation of all of these results is the extent to which the alterations in RNA and protein turnover were due to increases in connective tissue turnover or in inflammatory cell protein turnover. Wong and Booth point out, however, that there were 54%–65% increases in rates of synthesis of protein, which their extraction procedure suggested should be myofibrillar, whereas the myofibrillar protein content of nonmuscle cells is virtually nil. Whatever else these studies show, they demonstrate that large increases in muscle protein synthesis can occur after acute eccentric exercise without apparently much change in transcription; this is what might have been expected from the large rapid increases observed as a result of human resistance exercise (see below). However, unfortunately, the results appear to me not to unequivocally answer the question of whether eccentric or concentric exercise is the more powerful in producing hypertrophy or alterations in muscle protein turnover.

Unfortunately, no measurements of human muscle protein synthesis using amino acid tracers and the biopsy technique have been carried out during eccentric exercise, although they must surely come. Reichson and co-workers examined the amounts of muscle proteins relative to myofibrillar protein in biopsy samples taken from subjects 2 days after a bout of eccentric exercise using the biceps brachii (208). They found no gross changes in total protein or myofibrillar protein, but they did notice that there were large (1.5-fold) increases in three minor proteins which together accounted for only 14% of total protein. They suggested that two of these proteins may have been heat shock proteins and the third ubiquitin, the molecule that attaches to proteins destined for breakdown via the ubiquitin-dependent pathway (146), which may be responsible for myofibrillar degradation.

Eccentric Contractile Activity and Protein Breakdown. Eccentric exercise has been identified as a circumstance in which muscle proteolysis might be likely to become increased (68, 138, 249). This is because eccentric exercise is a mode of contractile activity in which muscle is activated to contract as it is being stretched, which leads to muscle damage, as indicated by the histochemical appearance of muscle with derangement of the muscle architecture (i.e., with disruption of T-tubular and sarcolemmal-tubular structures and tearing of intersarcomere Z disks and of actin-α actinin connections); there is also a substantial increase in the efflux from muscle of soluble enzymes. The evidence from the studies of isolated muscles of rats which had been previously made to run downhill (i.e., involving more eccentric contraction than running on the flat) suggests that there was no acute increase in myofibrillar degradation as a result of this activity, although nonmyofibrillar protein degradation was increased (138).

However, it may be that there are important longer term changes which are not picked up by these techniques. In a well-designed study by Evans and co-workers, young and old men were subjected to bouts of high-intensity eccentric cycling exercise (attempting to cycle backwards against an electrically driven bicycle ergometer) (68). In this study there appeared to be a marked rise in whole-body 3-methylhistidine production (measured in urine)—but only after 10 days following exercise! In these experiments the subjects ate the same non–meat containing food throughout the entire period of the study and the rises of 3-methylhistidine production appeared to be marked and significant. However, they did not occur in the immediate postexercise phase and are most likely to have represented proteolysis-dependent remodeling of muscle in response to muscle damage and possibly to cytokine-related events (32).

Postexercise Alterations in Muscle Protein Synthesis

In the 1970s Holloszy and Booth provided a substantial amount of evidence (116) that exercise of a type associated with increases in mitochondrial volume (but no hypertrophy of muscle fibers) increases the rate of synthesis of cytochrome *c* and of δ-aminolevulinate synthase. When hypertrophy can be induced in a variety of different experimental models used in animals, such as tenotomy of synergistic muscles or forced jumping exercise, or increased muscle stretch through limb loading [e.g., in chickens forced to carry weights on their wings (157)], an increase of muscle fiber size does occur, and this increase is accompanied by marked increases in muscle protein synthesis, including collagen synthesis (84, 157, 179). The large increases in synthesis are also accompanied by large but somewhat smaller increases in protein breakdown. The possibility exists that these increases in breakdown are required for remodeling of muscle and that there is, therefore, some inevitable wastage during hypertrophy (180).

As explained above, it appears that in human beings whole-body and muscle protein synthesis are depressed during exercise but show a recovery or rebound in the postexercise period (34, 37, 181, 217); skeletal muscle can be shown to contribute to this recovery by means of various tracer-based techniques including tracer exchange and incorporation methods (Tables 22.4 and 22.5). Isometric forearm exercise increases muscle anabolism in the postexercise period (224), and 4 h of treadmill exercise at 40% $\dot{V}O_{2max}$ also results in a modest increase in incorporation of [^{13}C]leucine into muscle protein afterwards (37).

The effect of intense aerobic exercise on the postexercise metabolism of nonworking muscle has been examined by Devlin and co-workers (49). Their principal findings were that the anabolic effect of exercise in the postexercise period is not generalized to include all muscle whether previously working or not, but probably only occurs in previously working muscle; furthermore, the increased leucine oxidation associated with exercise persists for some time after exercise, when muscle is at rest, presumably implicating sites other than nonworking muscle, possibly liver.

A single bout of multiple repetitions of weight lifting can be shown to cause a marked increase in incorporation into muscle protein within 4 h of the end of the exercise, and this increase is sustained for at least 24 h (43). In men or women carrying out a program of training using resistance exercise, muscle protein synthesis can be stimulated by 50%–60% over a period of 2 weeks (291), and the stimulation is seen irrespective of age or gender. In fact, the relative increase is appreciably greater in elderly men because, in them, muscle protein synthesis in the basal state is diminished compared to that in younger men.

In all of these situations the observed increases in the rate of muscle protein synthesis are more than the increases in the rate of accumulation of muscle mass, suggesting that muscle protein breakdown must have also been elevated. Obviously, this conclusion is difficult to accommodate within the framework of other results which generally show no change in myofibrillar protein breakdown turnover in the postexercise period. One possibility is that most of the observed increase in muscle protein synthesis in people is of nonmyofibrillar protein, but the wealth of animal data cited above makes this hard to accept. Unfortunately, the crucial experiments have not been done.

Effects of Habitual Exercise on Whole-Body Protein Turnover

Whole-body protein turnover is hardly affected by periods of competitive short-term intense exercise such as those carried out by a weight lifter during training (253). Furthermore, whole-body protein turnover per kilogram of lean body mass is not affected in subjects accustomed to regular resistance exercise, although in habitual middle- to long-distance runners there may be a slight increase (62, 176). Separating the effects of the last bout of exercise from an underlying trend towards increased protein turnover is difficult, but there must be a suspicion that this is a contributory factor. Habitual moderate exercise appears to increase the efficiency of protein utilization. A very careful series of studies by Butterfield and Calloway in young, healthy subjects showed this in a convincing fashion (29). In studies carried out in intravenously fed young men, daily aerobic bicycle exercise was associated with a better balance of amino acid across leg tissue; 3-methylhistidine efflux from the leg under resting conditions was decreased compared to that observed in sedentary subjects, suggesting that steady-state myofibrillar protein breakdown was diminished under these circumstances (4).

Effects of Immobilization and Disuse

It is well known from work in animals, from the study of hospital patients, and from astronauts that disuse, immobilization, and a low-gravity environment result in the wasting of muscle (23). In immobilization induced by plaster casting after injury in people, both fiber types waste, contributing equally to loss of cross-sectional area (78, 236) and thus to loss of strength, but mitochondrial enzymes appear to be lost preferentially compared to cytoplasmic enzymes (111). The loss of muscle protein may occur through a variety of mechanisms, the most obvious being a depression of protein synthesis, with either no change, a rise, or a smaller fall in protein breakdown (Table 22.5). Watson and colleagues found that gene translational activity (i.e., protein synthesis) for muscle actin fell rapidly (by 66%) within 6 h of immobilization in gastrocnemius of hindlimb-immobilized rats, whereas the abundance of actin mRNA in the muscle did not fall until after 72 h; by 6 days afterwards the mRNA had fallen by about 50% (275). The results confirmed earlier work of the same group suggesting that 6 h of immobilization was enough to inhibit synthesis of mixed muscle proteins and cytochrome *c*. Thus, modulation of gene transcription appears not to be particularly important for either the up-regulation or the down-regulation of muscle mass, with most of the control residing in regulation of translation and possibly elongation. In the work by Watson et al., the muscle size certainly did not fall appreciably by 6 h, suggesting that protein breakdown must have fallen. Nevertheless, in a different model of immobilization, the tail-cast suspension method, Jaspers and Tischler found that when measured in vitro after 6 days, not only was protein synthesis depressed but protein breakdown was elevated (131). The authors make the point that the results should be seen as only qualitative, since muscles studied in vitro are always in negative nitrogen balance, which may distort the extent of the changes observed.

We have investigated the effects on muscle protein synthesis of limb immobilization during plaster casting used therapeutically after fracture of the tibia (78). In our subjects, in whom the rates of muscle wasting and muscle protein synthesis in the casted leg with 7 weeks of immobilization were compared with the rates of muscle protein synthesis in the uncasted leg, there was evidence that muscle protein synthesis fell dramatically as a result of casting. This fall in muscle protein synthesis appears to be associated with a fall in muscle protein breakdown, since the loss of muscle mass was less than might have been expected from the extent of the fall in muscle protein synthesis. The fall in muscle protein synthesis appeared to be associated with a fall in the muscle protein synthetic rate per unit of RNA (i.e., to represent a diminution of translational activity). The diminution of muscle protein turnover by immobilization appeared to be prevented or reversed by mild electrical stimulation of the muscle for only 1 h/day (81, 82).

An opportunity to study the effects of immobilization and chronic stretch is presented by the study of protein synthesis in spinal muscle in adolescent children with scoliosis; on only one side of the spine is the muscle stretched, and the contralateral muscle is flaccid as a result of the spinal curvature (80). Our evidence of the incorporation of tracer [^{13}C]leucine into muscle suggests that muscle stretch is associated with chronically increased muscle protein synthesis; also, the incorporation of tracer into the flaccid muscle was diminished.

Collagen Turnover in Muscle

The extracellular matrix of connective tissue in muscle is an important mechanical element supporting individual muscle fibers; it is particularly important in muscles in which the fibril arrangement forming connections to the tendons to which muscle force is transmitted is not axial but pennate (92). Most of the collagen in skeletal muscle occurs in the epimysial sheath which supports whole muscles; the perimysial and endomysial collagen support fiber bundles and individual fibers, respectively. The collagen is synthesized not in muscle cells but in fibroblasts, which are found scattered within the tissue and which may proliferate, migrate, or necrose according to their circumstances. The amount of hydroxyproline, and therefore the amount of collagen, associated with slow-twitch fibers is greater than that associated with fast-twitch fibers (154). Even within a single muscle there appears to be more collagenous material associated with the slow-twitch than with the fast-twitch fibers, both at the level of the perimysium and endomysium. This pattern was not affected by endurance training (154). The authors point out that slow-twitch muscle is less elastic than fast-twitch muscle, which may be related to a higher proportion of stiffer collagen types (e.g., more type IV than types I and III) in the slow-twitch muscle.

Given the importance of collagen to skeletal muscle function, it is surprising that we know so little about what controls the steady-state mass of muscle collagen, or the possible effects of altered contractile activity. It ought to be possible to estimate collagen turnover in muscles of limbs from A-V differences of hydroxyproline, the posttranslationally modified derivative of proline found exclusively in collagen. Unfortunately, most workers do not report hydroxyproline blood concentrations. Where they have been reported (95) the A-V difference is, however, very small and the standard errors of flux measurements large; nevertheless, there seems to be a doubling of hydroxyproline output at the end of 1 h of one-legged knee-extensor exercise at 80% of maximal, suggesting that the collagen breakdown is acutely increased by exercise. However, Maclean and colleagues were able to determine no effect of exhausting exercise on muscle free hydroxyproline (170). Unfortunately, there appear to be no data available for the effects of exercise on urinary excretion of hydroxyproline.

Much of what is known comes from the work of a single group of Finnish workers. Vihko and colleagues have shown that acute exhausting exercise markedly increases the activities of enzymes of collagen turnover (185, 264, 265). These workers examined the effect of a 9 h bout of running on muscle concentrations of hydroxyproline, reticulin, and collagen types III, IV, and V, as well as the activities of propyl 4-hydroxylase and β-glucuronidase. Two days after the exercise bout, the activities of the collagen synthetic enzymes were increased, with the largest increases being seen in red rather than in white muscle; about 20 days after exercise, the enzyme activities had returned to normal. The hydroxyproline content and collagen contents of muscle were increased for up to 20 days after the single bout of exercise. These changes were much less in the muscles of trained animals in which the hydroxyproline concentrations and propyl 4-hydroxylase (PH) activity were no different from those in control mice, suggesting that accustomed exercise protected against the damage. The authors interpreted their results as suggesting that the single acute bout of exercise caused muscle fiber overload, and consequent necrosis, with the subsequent changes in collagen and associated enzymes being part of the repair process rather than a simple physiological adaptation. It may be that the changes in markers of collagen metabolism are greater in soleus than gastrocnemius or plantaris because of the strict order of recruitment of rodent muscle fibers (in the order of slow red, fast red, white), which would have possibly caused greatest exercise-induced damage in the slow red soleus, or simply that there is more collagen in the slow-twitch muscle.

The same group used a different intervention to alter the amount of collagen in studies of collagen synthesis during hypertrophy and atrophy of rat skeletal muscle (238). They measured synthetic and proteolytic enzymes of collagen metabolism in muscles which have been immobilized in the lengthened or shortened position, which results in hypertrophy and atrophy, respectively. Somewhat surprisingly, there were no increases in the activities of PH and galactosylhydroxylysyl glucosyltransferase (GGT) in the lengthened plantar flexors, whereas there was substantial decrease (by up to 50%) in the PH activity of immobilized, flaccid gastrocnemius and soleus. The collagen proteolytic activities of the shortened muscles were also substantially elevated, but there were no such increases observed in the stretched muscles. In a further study, the same authors examined the effect of electrical stimulation on the extent of the disuse atrophy alterations of enzymes of collagen synthesis and of hydroxyproline content in rat tibialis anterior, gastrocnemius, and soleus muscles (239). Once again, they found that the synthetic activities decreased by about 50% within a week and fell to 75% below normal after 3 weeks for PH; GGT activities also fell, but by a smaller amount. The most pronounced decreases were observed in soleus muscles, with the paler gastrocnemius and tibialis anterior muscles being affected less. Hydroxyproline content showed a surprising increase during the first week of immobilization, but by 3 weeks the total content was reduced markedly. Electrical stimulation of the sciatic nerve partially prevented the tissue atrophy as well as the decreases in the enzyme activities and hydroxyproline content in the tibialis anterior, but not in the gastrocnemius or soleus muscles.

The denervation of muscles causes surprising, counterintuitive changes in the activity of the collagen synthetic enzymes PH and GGT and also in total muscle hydroxyproline concentrations (237). There were substantial increases (up to 215%) in PH activity in the denervated gastrocnemius, with GGT activity increasing less; a marked elevation in muscle hydroxyproline concentration was also noted. Whether the denervated muscles were immobilized in the lengthened or shortened position made no difference to the responses of the enzymes and hydroxyproline. When the tendons of the same muscles were examined, the specific activities of the synthetic enzymes was unaffected in tendons of muscles immobilized in the lengthened position, but fell dramatically in tendons of muscles immobilized in the shortened position. The changes in the specific activities of the collagen synthetic enzymes at a time when total muscle protein content is decreasing as a result of denervation atrophy suggests that the increases in collagen concentrations observed in this condition are not simply the result of a concentration effect due to the disappearance of noncollagen protein.

Other work from the same group (137) has shown that during remobilization after 7 days of casting immobilization, the activities of PH and GGT and the concentration of hydroxyproline increase rapidly. GGT activity actually overshoots the control value at 3 days, before coming back to the control value after 2 weeks. A single bout of treadmill running for 3–12 h causes dramatic increase in PH activity in soleus and tibialis anterior muscles of previously immobilized limbs. However, exercise did not cause elevation in the activities of either PH or GGT in the previously slack Achilles tendons. Such a result is surprising, since Achilles tendon immobilization caused a decrease in PH and GGT activities. It may be that the single bout of exercise that is able to stimulate muscle collagen synthesis is insufficiently powerful to stimulate tendon synthesis. This inference is supported by the results of an investigation of the effects of a week of treadmill running on the tendons of flexor digitorum longus muscles from young mice (178). Within 1 week of beginning training there was an increase in the mean diameter number and cross-sectional area of tendon collagen fibrils. By 10 weeks, the number of collagen fibrils had increased but there had been a fall in the mean diameter, suggesting that the fibrillar packing density was greater in the tendons of the trained rather than the untrained animals.

The only extant description of skeletal muscle collagen turnover per se using isotope tracer methods has been provided by Laurent and co-workers (156), who studied the changes consequent upon stretch-induced hypertrophy of the anterior and posterior latissimus dorsi muscles (ALD and PLD) in chickens. They measured the hydroxyproline/proline ratios and the incorporation of [^{14}C]proline in the collagen of the muscles over 58 days. In the ALD muscle, collagen content almost doubled over the period, whereas noncollagen protein content increased by 140%. Collagen synthesis increased dramatically up to 7 days (at which time it had increased about eightfold), but then the rates of synthesis fell even though collagen content continued to increase, albeit more slowly. The turnover rate of noncollagen muscle proteins in red PLD muscle was two to three times faster that in the white PLD muscle, but the rates of collagen synthesis were identical in each. The authors point out that there is no reason, a priori, to expect that the metabolism of fibroblasts producing the additional collagen should vary quantitatively between muscle types. The authors compared the change in collagen synthesis rate with actual rate of accumulation of collagen and concluded that 50%–70% of all newly synthesized collagen was wasted (156) during the hypertrophy.

Presumably, alterations in physical activity and in the type of physical activity must have effects on collagen metabolism in bone, since it is likely that weight-bearing exercise and resistance exercise optimize accretion and maintenance of skeletal bone mass (248). Nevertheless, nothing seems to be known about the effects of exercise on bone collagen turnover, an area of obvious interest given the relevance to osteoporosis in middle and old age. Studies have been carried out on the effects of running exercise on the amount of collagen and proteoglycans in the intervertebral disk of young dogs (240). Fifteen weeks of 20 km/day running exercise caused an increase of about 35% in the collagen content of the annulus fibrosus, the outer ring of the disk. The total amount of proteoglycans did not increase, so that the annulus fibrosus became relatively depleted of them. Since the collagen content of connective tissues is related to tensile strength and the proteoglycan content to the resilience of tissues, it appears that the disks from the trained animals were likely to have increased tensile strength and decreased viscoelasticity. The changes observed were unlike those expected from aging and degeneration which normally results in the accumulation of chondroitin-6-sulphate, which did not occur. The authors concluded that the changes observed were a specific adaptation to the running exercise.

Physical Activity and Protein Requirements

It is relatively easy to identify two separate mechanisms by which people might increase their protein requirements as a result of physical activity. Obviously, an increase in the obligatory oxidation of amino acids as the result of exercise carried out on a habitual basis could theoretically elevate protein requirements, and if the BCAA are disproportionately represented among those amino acids oxidized, this might increase the requirement for first-class protein. Second, acute adaptation or sustained growth of elements of the muscle architecture would certainly increase the requirements for protein to allow restructuring or addition of new muscle protein. So much can be agreed on by everyone with a scientific interest in the area. However, controversy exists concerning *(1)* the extent of any increases in the requirements for dietary protein and *(2)* whether these increased requirements would mean an alteration in the protein/energy density of the diet.

Let us deal first with the consequences of increases in lean body mass, since the issues are reasonably straightforward. It makes sense that anybody who undertakes a program of regular resistance exercise such as weight lifting will increase total energy requirements, but it appears from the work by Tarnopolsky that there is little, if any, acute increase in whole-body protein turnover or amino acid oxidation as the result of a typical bout of weight training (253). Thus, the increases in lean body mass, principally muscle and possibly bone mass, associated with muscle hypertrophy are likely to represent the only important extra requirement for dietary protein. Millward and co-workers have demonstrated that the linear relationship between lean body mass and height (73, 74) is shifted upwards for body builders and rowers compared to normal control subjects of both sexes (204). Even if it is assumed that the extra lean body mass at a given height in the athletes is the result of a relatively rapid accretion, say over 3 years, the accretion rate is equivalent to about 20–30 mg of protein $\cdot$ kg^{-1} $\cdot$ day^{-1}. This is obviously a very small amount of protein in terms of normal protein requirements, being less than 5% of the recommended daily allowances (RDA) in the United States and of the dietary reference value of the Department of Health in the United Kingdom. Forbes has suggested that, by the use of anabolic steroids, substantially faster rates of gain of mean body mass can be achieved, up to about 0.3 g protein $\cdot$ kg^{-1} $\cdot$ day^{-1} over a period of 6 weeks (72, 98). If the population of the United Kingdom can be regarded as representative of populations elsewhere in the developed world, then the mean protein intake of an adult male is 1.12 g $\cdot$ kg^{-1} $\cdot$ day^{-1} (97). Since, as indicated by Quevedo et al. (204), body builders have a daily energy expenditure of about twice their resting metabolic rate, they would require a 42% increase in energy intake for balance, but at a protein/energy density of 140 kJ/MJ (a reasonable value for most Western foodstuffs) this would supply an extra 460 mg of protein $\cdot$ kg^{-1} $\cdot$ day^{-1} (i.e., 1.5 times as much protein as would be required by the maximal rate of accretion for steroid-induced weight gain!). There is no evidence that maintenance of extra lean body mass is more expensive per kilogram in terms of energy or protein requirements than normal lean body mass and therefore no extra requirements of dietary protein are likely to be engendered by increasing lean body mass.

The second possible mechanism whereby protein requirements might be increased is the elevated amino acid oxidation associated with exercise. A number of workers have suggested that this extra amino acid oxidation is sufficiently large to impose an additional protein requirement. There is a large body of evidence suggesting that exercise is associated with amino acid catabolism (152, 160, 235, 285), although we should acknowledge that our understanding of the exercise-induced increase in amino acid oxidation is far from perfect. For example, we do not know to what extent oxidation of the BCAA is actually complete, or whether amino acids which are liberated from protein but not catabolized during increased physical activity have a greater propensity to be incorporated into hepatic export protein. Both hypothetical phenomena might explain the apparent discrepancy between increased protein breakdown and amino acid catabolism in the face of little increase in whole-body urea turnover. Nevertheless there is, primae facie, the possibility of an extra requirement. Does the evidence support such a need?

As mentioned earlier, the studies of Butterfield and Calloway (29), which involved measurement over five successive 16 day balance periods during which energy intake/expenditure and nitrogen balance were carefully monitored, demonstrate that nitrogen balance is actually improved by physical activity and that the extent of the improvement increases if energy intake is increased. In other words, physical activity optimizes dietary protein utilization. Also, the careful and elegant studies of Gonzea et al. (87) 20 years ago suggest that stepwise increase in physical activity in young healthy but untrained individuals resulted in only a transient decrease in nitrogen balance; within 10 days zero nitrogen balance was restored on an intake of 1 g protein · kg body weight^{-1} · day^{-1}.

Nevertheless, there are reports of measurements of nitrogen balance in athletes suggesting that athletes undertaking high levels of physical activity have increased protein requirements (176, 252, 254). Meredith and co-workers examined nitrogen balance in young and middle-aged runners in whom nitrogen balance was assessed at three rates of dietary protein intake. Both the young and the middle-aged runners achieved nitrogen balance at a value of about 0.94 g protein · kg^{-1} · day^{-1}, which is nearly 20% above the current U.S. recommended dietary allowance. Unfortunately, in this study no sedentary controls were studied, and it is not at all clear whether the protein intake for zero balance in the runners was actually elevated compared to age- and lean body mass–matched sedentary members of the population. In the studies by Tarnopolski, nitrogen balance was measured in three groups of subjects: sedentary subjects, athletes undergoing strength training, and runners (252). Nitrogen balance was measured at the normal habitual dietary intake and at one other higher level. Extrapolation of the relationship between N excretion and protein utilization to zero balance indicated that the protein requirements for the control subjects, the strength training athletes, and the runners would be 0.73, 0.82, and 1.37 g · kg^{-1} · day^{-1}, respectively. This study was substantially less stringent in design than that carried out by Meredith and colleagues; there was no attempt at randomly ordering the treatment, no truly low-protein diet was examined, and no individuals in fact ever experienced negative nitrogen balance. The results suggest that the endurance athletes required 67% more protein than the recommended dietary allowance to achieve balance, but they also apparently sustained very large positive balances such that the increases of lean body mass would also have been large and easily measurable and equivalent to about 500 g of lean tissue per day, which is simply not biologically feasible.

In fact, as pointed out elsewhere (214) nitrogen balance studies of this kind are easily open to misinterpretation for a variety of reasons. One of these concerns the adaptation of amino acid catabolic enzymes, which can take a week to increase in response to a high dietary protein intake. Thus, the lack of adaptation of the catabolic enzymes can result in an apparently increased positive nitrogen balance for a short period. Furthermore, going from a high-protein diet to a low-protein diet takes some time for the capacity of the catabolic enzymes to fall to an appropriately low level, so that excessive losses of nitrogen are seen during the change to a lower intake. What this means is that the slope of a regression line between nitrogen balance and dietary intake will be steeper than it ought to be, ideally, if the data have been collected without due regard to the substantial periods of time required for adaptation. The evidence for shifts in the amplitude of anabolic gains and catabolic losses with dietary protein intake has been reviewed in detail by Millward and co-workers elsewhere (203, 205).

The physiological mechanisms underlying the adaptations mean that once individuals begin consuming high-protein diets, they are effectively trapped into continuation of this level of dietary protein intake if they are to maintain their lean body mass because to move to a lower level of intake would risk losing body protein in the period before adaptation occurs (see 205). However, consuming a high intake of protein confers little advantage in terms of increased storage of protein at rest, during physical activity, or afterwards, since the adaptations that occur in amino acid oxidation are exacerbated during exercise (214).

It seems, therefore, that there is no case to be made for supplementing diets to achieve a higher protein/energy density of intakes. Such a conclusion may come as bad news to companies selling dietary protein or amino acid supplements, but it is nevertheless likely to be the case. There may also be substantial disadvantages to increased dietary protein intake that have nothing to do with muscle protein turnover. Increased protein consumption is usually associated with increased nucleic acid intake and hence increased phosphate intake. It has been hypothesized that the increased production of so-called fixed acids (i.e., phosphoric acid, sulphuric acid) associated with increased protein intake may alter renal calcium reabsorption and that increased phosphate loads also increased calcium loss. In both male and female distance runners, weakening of the bone matrix is a serious problem, especially so in women who suffer amenorrhoea as a result of exercise. So far as I am aware no studies have been carried out to specifically investigate this problem, but it may well be important and theoretically, at least, there is a case for maintaining protein intake at about the RDA.

Outstanding Questions

There are a number of obvious questions which ought to be capable of resolution relatively easily. These include whether or not the BCAA are completely catabolized, which ought to be addressable by the use of BCAA labeled in positions other than the carboxyl group. Also, it would be reassuring to be able to pin down exactly where the BCAA for muscle transamination originate from. There is the question of differential rates of protein synthesis of individual muscle proteins, which again ought to be soluble using modern methods of protein isolation and estimates of labeling at low levels. There are the questions of the relationship between protein breakdown and contractile activity and which groups of protein (even which tissues!) are particularly susceptible. These questions ought to be soluble via the application of new techniques of mass isotopomer distribution analysis (113) applied to particular proteins of the myofibrillar and sarcoplasmic pools. The whole problem of the control of amino acid and protein metabolism as a result of physical exercise remains a fascinating one, and the area ought to be susceptible to approaches that combine the best of molecular biology with the best of modern integrative physiological chemistry. The next 20 years is likely to be particularly fruitful from this point of view.

REFERENCES

1. Ahlborg, G., P. Felig, L. Hagenfeldt, R. Hendler, and J. Wahren. Substrate turnover during prolonged exercise in man. *J. Clin. Invest.* 53: 1080–1090, 1974.
2. Ahmed, A., D. L. Maxwell, P. M. Taylor, and M. J. Rennie. Glutamine transport in human skeletal muscle. *Am. J. Physiol.* 264: 993–1000, 1993.
3. Akedo, H., and H. N. Christensen. Nature of insulin action on amino acid uptake by isolated diaphragm. *J. Biol. Chem.* 237: 118–127, 1962.
4. Albert, J. D., D. E. Matthews, A. Legaspi, K. J. Tracey, M. Jeevanandam, M. F. Brennan, and S. F. Lowry. Exercise-mediated peripheral tissue and whole-body amino acid metabolism during intravenous feeding in normal man. *Clin. Sci.* 77: 113–120, 1977.
5. Almdal, T. P., and H. Vilstrup. Exogenous hyperglucagonaemia in insulin controlled diabetic rats increases urea excretion and nitrogen loss from organs. *Diabetologia* 31: 836–841, 1988.
6. Aoki, T. T., M. F. Brennan, W. A. Muller, F. D. Moore, and G. F. Cahill. Effect of insulin on muscle glutamate uptake. *J. Clin. Invest.* 51: 2889–2894, 1972.
7. Aragón, J., and J. M. Lowenstein. The purine-nucleotide cycle. Comparison of the levels of citric acid cycle intermediates with the operation of the purine nucleotide cycle in rat skeletal muscle during exercise and recovery from exercise. *Eur. J. Biochem.* 110: 371–377, 1980.
8. Babij, P., S. M. Matthews, and M. J. Rennie. Changes in blood ammonia, lactate and amino acids in relation to workload during bicycle ergometer exercise in man. *Eur. J. Appl. Physiol.* 50: 405–411, 1983.
9. Bading, J. R., M. T. Corbally, J. D. Fissekis, G. R. DiResta, and M. F. Brennan. Effects of starvation on [^{11}C]-2-aminoisobutyrate transport in skeletal muscle. *J. Nucl. Med.* 28: 650, 1987.
10. Baron, A. D. Cardiovascular actions of insulin in humans. Implications for insulin sensitivity and vascular tone. In: *Insulin Resistance and Disease*, edited by E. Ferranini. London: Baillière Tindall, 1993, p. 961–988.
11. Beaufrere, B., P. Tessari, M. . Cattalini, J. Miles, and M. W. Haymond. Apparent decreased oxidation and turnover of leucine during infusion of medium-chain triglycerides. *Am. J. Physiol.* 249: 175–182, 1985.
12. Bennet, W. M., A. A. Connacher, C. M. Scrimgeour, and M. J. Rennie. The effect of amino acid infusion on leg protein turnover assessed by L-[^{15}N]phenylalanine and L-[^{13}C]leucine exchange. *Eur. J. Clin. Invest.* 20: 37–46, 1990.
13. Bennet, W. M., A. A. Connacher, C. M. Scrimgeour, K. Smith, and M. J. Rennie. Increase in anterior tibialis muscle protein synthesis in healthy man during mixed amino acid infusion: studies of incorporation of 1-[13C]leucine. *Clin. Sci.* 76: 447–454, 1989.
14. Bergstrom, J., P. Fürst, and E. Hultman. Free amino acids in muscle tissue and plasma during exercise in man. *Clin. Physiol.* 5: 155–160, 1985.
15. Bertran, J., A. Werner, G. Stange, D. Markovic, J. Biber, X. Testar, A. Zorzano, M. Palacin, and H. Murer. Expression of Na$^+$-independent amino acid transport in *Xenopus laevis* oocytes by injection of rabbit kidney cortex mRNA. *Biochem. J.* 281: 717–723, 1992.
16. Bier, D. M. Intrinsically difficult problems: the kinetics of body proteins and amino acid in man. *Diabetes Metab. Rev.* 5: 111–132, 1989.
17. Biolo, G., D. Chinkes, X. J. Zhang, and R. R. Wolfe. A new model to determine in vivo the relationship between amino acid transmembrane transport and protein kinetics in muscle. *J. Parenter. Enteg. Nutr.* 16: 305–315, 1992.
18. Block, K. P., R. P. Aftring, W. B. Mehard, and M. G. Buse. Modulation of rat skeletal muscle branched-chain α-keto acid dehydrogenase in vivo. Effects of dietary protein and meal consumption. *J. Clin. Invest.* 79: 1349–1358, 1987.
19. Blomstrand, E. Branched-chain amino acids and neurotransmission in intense efforts. In: *Branched-Chain Amino Acids: Biochemistry, Physiopathology and Clinical Science*, edited by P. Schauder, J. Wahren, R. Paoletti, R. Bernardi, and M. Rinetti. New York: Raven Press, 1992, p. 31–41.
20. Blomstrand, E., F. Celsing, and E. A. Newsholme. Changes in plasma concentrations of aromatic and branched-chain amino acids during sustained exercise in man and their possible role in fatigue. *Acta Physiol. Scand.* 133: 115–121, 1988.
21. Blomstrand, E., P. Hassmén, B. Ekblom, and E. A. Newsholme. Administration of branched-chain amino acids during sustained exercise—effects on performance and on plasma concentration of some amino acids. *Eur. J. Appl. Physiol.* 63: 83–88, 1991.
22. Bonadonna, R. C., M. P. Saccomani, C. Cobelli, and R. A. DeFronzo. Effect of insulin on system A amino acid transport in human skeletal muscle. *J. Clin. Invest.* 91: 514–521, 1993.
23. Booth, F. W., and P. D. Gollnick. Effects of disuse on the structure and function of skeletal muscle. *Med. Sci. Sports Exerc.* 15: 415–420, 1983.
24. Booth, F. W., and P. A. Watson. Control of adaptations in protein levels in response to exercise (review). *Federation Proc.* 44: 2293–2300, 1985.
25. Brooks, G. A. Amino acid and protein metabolism during exercise and recovery. *Med. Sci. Sports Exerc.* 19: 5150–5156, 1987.

26. Brosnan, M. E., and J. Letto. Interorgan metabolism of valine. *Amino Acids* 1: 29–35, 1991.
27. Buse, M. G., F. J. Biggers, K. H. Friderici, and J. F. Buse. Oxidation of branched chain amino acids by isolated hearts and diaphragms of the heart: The effect of fatty acids, glucose, and pyruvate respiration. *J. Biol. Chem.* 247: 8085–8096, 1972.
28. Buse, M. G., and S. S. Reid. Leucine: a possible regulator of protein turnover in muscle. *J. Clin. Invest.* 56: 1250–1261, 1975.
29. Butterfield, G. E., and D. H. Calloway. Physical activity improves protein utilization in young men. *Br. J. Nutr.* 51: 171–184, 1984.
30. Buttrose, M. E., D. McKellar, and T. E. Welbourne. Gut-liver interaction in glutamine homeostasis: portal ammonia role in uptake and metabolism. *Am. J. Physiol.* 252 (*Endocrinol. Metab.* 15): E746–E750, 1987.
31. Bylund-Fellenius, A.-C., K. M. Ojamaa, K. E. Flaim, J. B. Li, S. J. Wassner, and L. S. Jefferson. Protein synthesis versus energy state in contracting muscle of perfused rat hindlimb. *Am. J. Physiol.* 246 (*Endocrinol. Metab.* 9): E297–E305, 1984.
32. Cannon, J. G., R. A. Fielding, M. A. Fiatarone, S. F. Orencole, C. Dinarello, and W. J. Evans. Increased interleukin 1 beta in human skeletal muscle after exercise. *Am. J. Physiol.* 257 (*Regulatory Integrative Comp. Physiol.* 20): R451–R455, 1989.
33. Carli, G., M. Bonifazi, L. Lodi, C. Lupo, G. Martelli, and A. Viti. Changes in the exercise-induced hormone response to branched chain amino acid administration. *Eur. J. Appl. Physiol.* 64: 272–277, 1992.
34. Carraro, F., W. H. Hartl, C. A. Stuart, D. K. Layman, F. Jahoor, and R. R. Wolfe. Whole body and plasma protein synthesis in exercise and recovery in human subjects. *Am. J. Physiol.* 258 (*Endocrinol. Metab.* 21): E821–E831, 1990.
35. Carraro, F., T. D. Kimbrough, and R. R. Wolfe. Urea kinetics in humans at two levels of exercise intensity. *J. Appl. Physiol.* 75: 1180–1185, 1993.
36. Carraro, F., J. Rosenblatt, and R. R. Wolfe. Isotopic determination of fibronectin synthesis in humans. *Metabolism* 40: 553–561, 1991.
37. Carraro, F., C. A. Stuart, W. H. Hartl, J. Rosenblatt, and R. R. Wolfe. Effect of exercise and recovery on muscle protein synthesis in human subjects. *Am. J. Physiol.* 259 (*Endocrinol. Metab.* 22): E470–E476, 1990.
38. Castenfors, J. Renal function during exercise. *Acta Physiol. Scand.* 70 (Suppl. 293): 1–40, 1967.
39. Chaouloff, F., G. A. Kennett, B. Serrurrier, D. Merino, and G. Curzon. Amino acid analysis demonstrates that increased plasma free tryptophan causes the increase of brain tryptophan during exercise in the rat. *J. Neurochem.* 46: 1647–1650, 1986.
40. Cheek, D. B. Muscle cell growth in normal children. In: *Human Growth*, edited by D. B. Cheek. Philadelphia: Lea & Febiger, 1968, p. 337–351.
41. Cheng, K. N., F. Dworzak, G. C. Ford, M. J. Rennie, and D. Halliday. Direct determination of leucine metabolism and protein breakdown in humans using L-[^{13}C,^{15}N]leucine and the forearm model. *Eur. J. Clin. Invest.* 15: 349–354, 1986.
42. Cheng, K. N., P. J. Pacy, F. Dworzak, G. C. Ford, and D. Halliday. Influence of fasting on leucine and muscle protein metabolism across the human forearm determined using L-[1-^{13}C,^{15}N]leucine as the tracer. *Clin. Sci.* 73: 241–246, 1987.
43. Chesley, A., J. D. MacDougall, M. A. Tarnopolsky, S. A. Atkinson, and K. Smith. Changes in human muscle protein synthesis following resistance exercise. *J. Appl. Physiol.* 73: 1383–1388, 1992.
44. Christensen, H. N. Interorgan amino acid nutrition. *Physiol. Rev.* 62: 1193–1233, 1982.
45. Christensen, H. N. On the strategy of kinetic discrimination of amino acid transport systems. *J. Mol. Biol.* 84: 97–103, 1985.
46. Christensen, H. N., and M. S. Kilberg. Amino acid transport across the plasma membrane: role of regulation of interorgan flows. In: *Amino Acid Transport in Animal Cells*, edited by D. L. Yudilevich and C. A. R. Boyd. Manchester: Manchester University Press, 1987, p. 10–46
47. Clausen, T., and P. G. Kohn. The effect of insulin on the transport of sodium and potassium in rat soleus muscle. *J. Physiol. (Lond.)* 265: 19–42, 1977.
48. Curzon, G., J. Friedel, and P. J. Knott. The effect of fatty acids on the binding of tryptophan to plasma protein. *Nature* 242: 198–200, 1973.
49. Devlin, J. T., I. Brodsky, A. Scrimgeour, S. Fuller, and D. M. Bier. Amino acid metabolism after intense exercise. *Am. J. Physiol.* 258 (*Endocrinol. Metab.* 21): E249–E255, 1990.
50. Décombaz, J., P. Reinhardt, K. Anantharaman, G. van Glutz, and J. R. Poortmans. Biochemical changes in a 100km run: free amino acids, urea and creatinine. *Eur. J. Appl. Physiol.* 41: 61–72, 1979.
51. Dohm, G. L., G. R. Beecher, R. Q. Warren, and R. T. Williams. The influence of exercise on free amino acid concentrations in rat tissues. *J. Appl. Physiol.* 50: 41–44, 1982.
52. Dohm, G. L., G. J. Kasperek, E. B. Tapscott, and G. R. Beecher. Effect of exercise on synthesis and degradation of muscle protein. *Biochem. J.* 188: 255–262, 1980.
53. Dohm, G. L., E. B. Tapscott, H. A. Barakat, and G. J. Kasperek. Measurement of in vivo protein synthesis in rats during an exercise bout. *Biochem. Med.* 27: 367–373, 1982.
54. Dohm, G. L., E. B. Tapscott, and G. J. Kasperek. Protein degradation during endurance exercise and recovery. *Med. Sci. Sports Exerc.* 19: 5166–5172, 1987.
55. Dohm, G. L., R. T. Williams, G. J. Kasperek, and A. M. van Rij. Increased excretion of urea and N^{τ}-methylhistidine by rats and humans after a bout of exercise. *J. Appl. Physiol.* 52: 27–33, 1982.
56. Elia, M., A. Carter, S. Bacon, C. G. Winearls, and R. Smith. Clinical usefulness of urinary 3-methylhistidine excretion in indicating muscle protein breakdown. *BMJ* 282: 351–354, 1981.
57. Elia, M., and G. Livesey. Branched chain amino acid and oxo acid metabolism in human and rat muscle. In: *Metabolism and Clinical Implications of Branched Chain Amino and Ketoacids*, edited by M. Walser and J. R. Williamson. New York, Amsterdam, and Oxford: Elsevier/North Holland, 1981, p. 257–262.
58. Elia, M., and G. Livesey. Effects of ingested steak and infused leucine on forelimb metabolism in man and the fate of the carbon skeletons and amino groups of branched-chain amino acids. *Clin. Sci.* 64: 517–526, 1983.
59. Eriksson, L. S., S. Broberg, O. Björkman, and J. Wahren. Ammonia metabolism during exercise in man. *Clin. Physiol.* 5: 325–336, 1985.
60. Eriksson, L. S., L. Hagenfeldt, P. Felig, and J. Wahren. Leucine uptake by splanchnic and leg tissues in man: relative independence of insulin levels. *Clin. Sci.* 65: 491–498, 1983.

61. Evans, W. J. Exercise and muscle metabolism in the elderly. In: *Nutrition and Aging*, edited by M. L. Hutchinson and H. N. Munro. San Diego, CA: Academic Press, 1986, p. 170–191.
62. Evans, W. J., and C. N. Meredith. Exercise and nutrition in the elderly. In: *Nutrition, Ageing and the Elderly*, edited by H. N. Munro and D. E. Danford. New York and London: Plenum Press, 1989, p. 89–125.
63. Falduto, M. J., R. C. Hickson, and A. P. Young. Antagonism by glucocorticoids and exercise on expression of glutamine synthetase in skeletal muscle. *FASEB J.* 3: 2623–2628, 1989.
64. Felig, P. Amino acid metabolism in man. *Annu. Rev. Biochem.* 44: 933–955, 1975.
65. Felig, P., T. Pozefsky, C. Marliss, and G. F. Cahill. Alanine: key role in gluconeogenesis. *Science* 167: 1003–1004, 1970.
66. Felig, P., and J. Wahren. Amino acid metabolism in exercising man. *J. Clin. Invest.* 50: 2703–2709, 1971.
67. Fielding, R. A., W. J. Evans, V. A. Hughes, L. L. Moldawer, and B. R. Bistrian. The effects of high intensity exercise on muscle and plasma levels of alpha-ketoisocaproic acid. *Eur. J. Appl. Physiol.* 55: 482–485, 1986.
68. Fielding, R. A., C. N. Meredith, K. P. O'Reilly, W. R. Frontera, J. G. Cannon, and W. J. Evans. Enhanced protein breakdown after eccentric exercise in young and older men. *J. Appl. Physiol.* 71: 674–679, 1991.
69. Fine, A., F. I. Bennett, and G. A. O. Alleyne. Effects of acute acid-base alterations of glutamine metabolism and renal ammoniagenesis in the dog. *Clin. Sci. Mol. Med.* 54: 503–508, 1978.
70. Finocchiaro, G., F. Taroni, and S. Di Donato. Glutamate dehydrogenase in olivopontocerebellar atrophies: leukocytes, fibroblasts, and muscle mitochondria. *Neurology* 36: 550–553, 1986.
71. Fischer, H. G., W. Hollmann, and K. De Meirleir. Exercise changes in plasma tryptophan fractions and relationship with prolactin. *Int. J. Sports Med.* 12: 487–489, 1991.
72. Forbes, G. B. The effect of anabolic steroids on lean body mass: the dose response curve. *Metabolism* 34: 571–573, 1985.
73. Forbes, G. B. Body composition as affected by physical activity and nutrition. *Federation Proc.* 44: 343–347, 1985.
74. Forbes, G. B. *Human Body Composition: Growth, Aging, Nutrition and Activity*. New York: Springer-Verlag, 1987, p. 171.
75. Frontera, W. R., C. N. Meredith, K. P. O'Reilly, and W. J. Evans. Strength training and determinants of $\dot{V}O_{2max}$ in older men. *J. Appl. Physiol.* 68: 329–333, 1990.
76. Frontera, W. R., C. N. Meredith, K. P. O'Reilly, H. G. Knuttgen, and W. J. Evans. Strength conditioning in older men: skeletal muscle hypertrophy and improved function. *J. Appl. Physiol.* 64: 1038–1044, 1988.
77. Gazzola, G. C., R. Franchi, V. Saibene, P. Ronchi, and G. G. Guidotti. *Biochim. Biophys. Acta* 266: 407–421, 1972.
78. Gibson, J. N. A., D. Halliday, W. L. Morrison, P. J. Stoward, G. A. Hornsby, P. W. Watt, G. Murdoch, and M. J. Rennie. Decrease in human quadriceps muscle protein turnover consequent on leg immobilization. *Clin. Sci.* 72: 503–509, 1987.
79. Gibson, J. N. A., D. Halliday, P. W. Watt, P. J. Stoward, W. L. Morrison, and M. J. Rennie. Decrease in human quadriceps muscle protein turnover consequent upon leg immobilisation. *Clin. Sci.* 72: 503–509, 1987.
80. Gibson, J. N. A., M. J. McMaster, C. M. Scrimgeour, P. J. Stoward, and M. J. Rennie. Rates of muscle protein synthesis in paraspinal muscles: lateral disparity in children with idiopathic scoliosis. *Clin. Sci.* 75: 79–83, 1988.
81. Gibson, J. N. A., W. L. Morrison, C. M. Scrimgeour, K. M. Smith, P. J. Stoward, and M. J. Rennie. Effects of therapeutic percutaneous electrical stimulation of atrophic human quadriceps on muscle composition protein synthesis and contractile properties. *Eur. J. Clin. Invest.* 19: 206–212, 1989.
82. Gibson, J. N. A., K. Smith, and M. J. Rennie. Prevention of disuse muscular atrophy by means of electrical stimulation: maintenance of protein synthesis. *Lancet* ii: 767–770, 1988.
83. Goldberg, A. L., and T. W. Chang. Regulation and significance of amino acid metabolism in skeletal muscle. *Federation Proc.* 37: 2301–2307, 1978.
84. Goldberg, A. L., J. D. Etlinger, D. F. Goldspink, and C. Jablecki. Mechanism of work-induced hypertrophy of skeletal muscle. *Med. Sci. Sports* 7: 248–261, 1975.
85. Goldberg, A. L., and H. M. Goodman. Amino acid transport during work-induced growth of skeletal muscle. *Am. J. Physiol.* 216: 1111–1115, 1969.
86. Goldberg, A. L., C. Jablecki, and J. B. Li. Effects of use and disuse on amino acid transport and protein turnover in muscle. *Ann. N. Y. Acad. Sci.* 228: 190–201, 1974.
87. Gontzea, I., P. Sutzescu, and S. Dumitrache. The influence of adaptation to physical effort on nitrogen balance in man. *Nutr. Rep. Int.* 22: 231–236, 1975.
88. Goodman, M. N. Acute alterations in sodium flux in vitro lead to decreased myofibrillar protein breakdown in rat skeletal muscle. *Biochem. J.* 247: 151–156, 1987.
89. Goodman, M. N. Myofibrillar protein breakdown in skeletal muscle is diminished in rats with chronic streptozocin-induced diabetes. *Diabetes* 36: 100–105, 1987.
90. Goro, M., H. Shinno, and A. Ichihara. Isozyme patterns of branched-chain amino transaminase in human tissues and tumors. *Gann* 68: 663–667, 1977.
91. Gorski, J., D. A. Hood, O. M. Brown, and R. L. Terjung. Incorporation of 15N-leucine amine into ATP of fast-twitch muscle following stimulation. *Biochem. Biophys. Res. Commun.* 128: 1254–1260, 1985.
92. Gould, R. P. Collagen. In: *The Structure and Function of Muscle*, edited by G. J. Bourne. New York: Academic Press, 1973, p. 186–243.
93. Graham, T., J. Bangsbo, and B. Saltin. Skeletal muscle ammonia production and repeated, intense exercise in humans. *Can. J. Physiol. Pharmacol.* 71: 484–490, 1993.
94. Graham, T. E., J. Bangsbo, P. D. Gollnick, C. Juel, and B. Saltin. Ammonia metabolism during intense dynamic exercise and recovery in humans. *Am. J. Physiol.* 259: 170–176, 1990.
95. Graham, T. E., B. Kiens, M. Hargreaves, and E. A. Richter. Influence of fatty acids on ammonia and amino acid flux from active human muscle. *Am. J. Physiol.* 261 (*Endocrinol. Metab.* 24): E168–E176, 1991.
96. Graham, T. E., and B. Saltin. Estimation of the mitochondrial redox state in human skeletal muscle during exercise. *J. Appl. Physiol.* 66: 561–566, 1989.
97. Gregory, J., K. Foster, H. Tyler, and M. Wiseman. *The Dietary and Nutritional Survey of British Adults*. London: H.M. Stationery Office, 1990.
98. Griggs, R. C., W. Kingston, R. F. Jozefowicz, B. E. Herr, G. Forbes, and D. Halliday. Effect of testosterone on muscle mass and muscle protein synthesis. *J. Appl. Physiol.* 266 (*Endocrinol. Metab.* 29): E498–E503, 1989.

99. Guidotti, G. G., A. F. Borghetti, and G. C. Gazzola. The regulation of amino acid transport in animal cells. *Biochim. Biophys. Acta* 515: 329–366, 1978.
100. Guidotti, G. G., R. Franchi-Gazzola, G. C. Gazzola, and P. Ronchi. Regulation of amino acid transport in chick embryo heart cells. IV. Site and mechanisms of insulin action. *Biochim. Biophys. Acta* 356: 219–230, 1974.
101. Guidotti, G. G., G. C. Gazzola, A. M. Borghetti, and R. Franchi-Gazzola. Adaptive regulation of amino acid transport across the cell membrane in avian and mammalian tissues. *Biochim. Biophys. Acta* 406: 264–279, 1991.
102. Gulve, E. A., G. D. Cartee, J. H. Youn, and J. O. Holloszy. Prolonged incubation of skeletal muscle increases system A amino acid transport. *Am. J. Physiol.* 260 (*Cell Physiol.* 29): C88–C95, 1991.
103. Gumà, A., M. Camps, M. Palacin, X. Testar, and A. Zorzano. Protein kinase C activators selectively inhibit insulin-stimulated system A transport activity in skeletal muscle at a post-receptor level. *Biochem. J.* 268: 633–639, 1990.
104. Guy, P. S., and D. H. Snow. The effect of training and detraining on muscle composition in the horse. *J. Physiol. (Lond.)* 269: 33–51, 1977.
105. Gyntelberg, F., M. J. Rennie, R. C. Hickson, and J. O. Holloszy. Effect of training on the response of plasma glycagon to exercise. *J. Appl. Physiol.* 43: 302–305, 1977.
106. Hagg, S. A., E. L. Morse, and S. A. Adibi. Effect of exercise on rates of oxidation, turnover and plasma clearance of leucine in human subjects. *Am. J. Physiol.* 242 (*Endocrinol. Metab.* 11): E407–E410, 1985.
107. Handlogten, M. E., M. S. Kilberg, and H. N. Christensen. Incomplete correspondence between repressive and substrate action by amino acids on transport systems A and N in monolayered rat hepatocytes. *J. Biol. Chem.* 257: 345–348, 1982.
108. Haralambie, G. and A. Berg. Serum urea and amino nitrogen changes with exercise duration. *Eur. J. Appl. Physiol.* 36: 39–48, 1976.
109. Harper, A. E. Some recent developments in the study of amino acid metabolism. *Proc. Nutr. Soc.* 42: 437–449, 1983.
110. Hasselgren, P.-O., M. Hall-Ångeras, U. Ångeras, D. Benson, J. H. James, and J. E. Fischer. Regulation of total and myofibrillar protein breakdown in rat extensor digitorum longus and soleus muscle incubated flaccid or at resting length. *Biochem. J.* 267: 37–44, 1990.
111. Häggmark, T. A study of morphologic and enzymatic properties of the skeletal muscles after injuries and immobilization in man. Ph.D. Thesis: Karolinska Institute, Stockholm, 1978.
112. Häussinger, D., S. Kaiser, T. Stehle, and W. Gerok. Structural and functional organization of hepatic ammonia metabolism: pathophysiological consequences. In: *Advances in Ammonia Metabolism and Hepatic Encephalopathy*, edited by P. B. Soeters, J. H. P. Wilson, A. J. Meijer, and E. Holm. Amsterdam: Elsevier Scientific Publishers B.V. (Biomedical Division), 1988, p. 26–36.
113. Hellerstein, M. K., and R. A. Neese. Mass isotopomer distribution analysis: a technique for measuring biosynthesis and turnover of polymers. *Am. J. Physiol.* 263 (*Endocrinol. Metab.* 32): E988–E1001, 1992.
114. Henriksson, J. Effect of exercise on amino acid concentrations in skeletal muscle and plasma. *J. Exp. Biol.* 160: 149–165, 1991.
115. Henriksson, J., M. M.-Y. Chi, C. S. Hintz, D. A. Young, K. Kaiser, S. Salmons, and O. H. Lowry. Chronic stimulation of mammalian muscle: changes in enzymes of six metabolic pathways. *Am. J. Physiol.* 251: 614–632, 1986.
116. Holloszy, J. O., and F. W. Booth. Biochemical adaptations to endurance exercise in muscle. *Annu. Rev. Physiol.* 38: 273–291, 1976.
117. Holloszy, J. O., L. B. Oscai, I. J. Don, and P. A. Mole. Mitochondrial citric acid cycle and related enzymes: adaptive response to exercise. *Biochem. Biophys. Res. Commun.* 40: 1368–1373, 1970.
118. Hood, D. A., and R. L. Terjung. Effect of endurance training on leucine metabolism in perfused rat skeletal muscle. *Am. J. Physiol.* 253 (*Endocrinol. Metab.* 16): E648–656, 1987.
119. Hood, D. A., and R. L. Terjung. Amino acid metabolism during exercise and following endurance training. *Sports Med.* 9: 23–35, 1990.
120. Hood, D. A., and R. L. Terjung. Endurance training alters alanine and glutamine release from muscle during contractions. *FEBS Lett.* 340: 287–290, 1994.
121. Hundal, H. S., P. Babij, P. M. Taylor, P. W. Watt, and M. J. Rennie. Effects of corticosteroid on the transport and metabolism of glutamine in rat skeletal muscle. *Biochim. Biophys. Acta* 1092: 376–383, 1991.
122. Hundal, H. S., and M. J. Rennie. Effects of electrical stimulation on perfused rat skeletal muscle glutamine transport. *J. Physiol. (Lond.)* 392: 28P, 1987 (Abstract).
123. Hundal, H. S., M. J. Rennie, and P. W. Watt. Characteristics of L-glutamine transport in perfused rat skeletal muscle. *J. Physiol. (Lond.)* 393: 283–305, 1987.
124. Hundal, H. S., M. J. Rennie, and P. W. Watt. Characteristics of acidic, basic and neutral amino acid transport in perfused rat hindlimb. *J. Physiol. (Lond.)* 408: 93–114, 1989.
125. Hutson, S. M. Subcellular distribution of branched-chain aminotransferase activity in rat tissues. *J. Nutr.* 118: 1475–1481, 1988.
126. Hutson, S. M., and T. R. Hall. Identification of the mitochondrial branched chain aminotransferase as a branched chain alpha-keto acid transport protein. *J. Biol. Chem.* 268: 3084–3091, 1993.
127. Hutson, S. M., and A. E. Harper. Blood and tissue branched-chain amino and α-keto acid concentrations: effect of diet, starvation and disease. *Am. J. Clin. Nutr.* 34: 173–183, 1981.
128. Hutson, S. M., C. Zapalowski, T. C. Cree, and A. E. Harper. Regulation of leucine and α-ketoisocaproic acid metabolism in skeletal muscle. Effects of starvation and insulin. *J. Biol. Chem.* 255: 2418–2426, 1980.
129. Ishii, T., K. Nakayama, H. Sato, K. Miura, M. Yamada, K. Yamada, Y. Sugita, and S. Bannai. Expression of mouse macrophage cystine transporter in Xenopus laevis oocytes. *Arch. Biochem. Biophys.* 289: 71–75, 1991.
130. Jahoor, F., and R. R. Wolfe. Re-assessment of the primed-constant infusion tracer technique as a tool for the measurement of urea production in humans. *Am. J. Physiol.* 252 (*Endocrinol. Metab.* 15): E557–E564, 1987.
131. Jaspers, S. R., and M. E. Tischler. Atrophy and growth failure of rat hindlimb muscles in tail-cast suspension. *J. Appl. Physiol.* 57: 1472–1479, 1984.
132. Ji, L. L., D. L. Lennon, R. G. Kochan, F. J. Nagle, and H. A. Lardy. Enzymatic adaptation to physical training under beta-blockade in the rat. Evidence of a beta 2-adrenergic mechanism in skeletal muscle. *J. Clin. Invest.* 78: 771–778, 1986.
133. Ji, L. L., R. H. Miller, F. J. Nagle, H. A. Lardy, and F. W. Stratman. Amino acid metabolism during exercise in

trained rats: the potential role of carnitine in the metabolic fate of the branched chain amino acids. *Metabolism* 8: 748–752, 1987.

134. Jones, D. A., and O. M. Rutherford. Human muscle strength training: the effects of three different regimes and the nature of the resultant changes. *J. Physiol. (Lond.)* 391: 1–11, 1987.
135. Joseph, S. K., N. M. Bradford, and J. D. McGivan. Characteristics of the transport of alanine, serine and glutamine across the plasma membrane of isolated liver cells. *Biochem. J.* 176: 827–836, 1978.
136. Jungas, R. L., M. L. Halperin, and J. T. Brosnan. Quantitative analysis of amino acid oxidation and related gluconeogenesis in humans. *Physiol. Rev.* 72: 419–448, 1992.
137. Karpakka, J., K. Väänänen, P. Virtanen, J. Savolainen, S. Orava, and T. E. S. Takala. The effects of remobilization and exercise on collagen biosynthesis in rat tendon. *Acta Physiol. Scand.* 139: 139–145, 1990.
138. Kasperek, G. J., G. R. Conway, D. S. Krayeski, and J. J. Lohne. A reexamination of the effect of exercise on rate of muscle protein degradation. *Am. J. Physiol.* 263 (*Endocrinol. Metab.* 26): E1144–E1150, 1992.
139. Kasperek, G. J., G. L. Dohm, and R. D. Snider. Activation of branched chain keto acid dehydrogenase by exercise. *Am. J. Physiol.* 248 (*Regulatory Integrative Comp. Physiol.* 17): R166–R171, 1985.
140. Kasperek, G. J., and R. D. Snider. Effect of exercise intensity and starvation on activation of branched-chain keto acid dehydrogenase by exercise. *Am. J. Physiol.* 252 (*Endocrinol. Metab.* 15): E22–E37, 1987.
141. Kasperek, G. J., and R. D. Snider. Total and myofibrillar protein degradation in isolated soleus muscles after exercise. *Am. J. Physiol.* 257 (*Endocrinol. Metab.* 20): E1–E5, 1989.
142. Katz, A., S. Broberg, K. Sahlin, and J. Wahren. Muscle ammonia and amino acid metabolism during dynamic exercise in man. *Clin. Physiol.* 6: 365–379, 1986.
143. Katz, A., K. Sahlin, and J. Henriksson. Muscle ammonia metabolism during isometric contraction in humans. *Am. J. Physiol.* 250 (*Cell Physiol.* 19): C834–C840, 1986.
144. Katz, A., M. K. Spencer, and K. Sahlin. Failure of glutamate dehydrogenase system to predict oxygenation state of human skeletal muscle. *Am. J. Physiol.* 259 (*Cell Physiol.* 28): C26–C28, 1990.
145. Kelso, T. B., C. R. Shear, and S. R. Max. Enzymes of glutamine metabolism in inflammation associated with skeletal muscle hypertrophy. *Am. J. Physiol.* 257 (*Endocrinol. Metab.* 20): E885–E894, 1989.
146. Kettelhut, I. C., S. S. Wing, and A. L. Goldberg. Endocrine regulation of protein breakdown in skeletal muscle. *Diabetes Metab. Rev.* 4: 751–772, 1988.
147. Khatra, B. S., R. K. Chawla, C. W. Sewell, and D. Rudman. Distribution of branched-chain α-keto acid dehydrogenases in primate tissues. *J. Clin. Invest.* 59: 558–564, 1977.
148. Kilberg, M. S., M. E. Handlogten, and H. N. Christensen. Characteristics of an amino acid transport system in rat liver for glutamine, asparagine, histidine and closely related analogs. *J. Biol. Chem.* 255: 4011–4019, 1980.
149. Kim, J. W., E. I. Closs, L. M. Albritton, and J. M. Cunningham. Transport of cationic amino acids by the mouse ecotropic retrovirus receptor. *Nature* 352: 725–728, 1991.
150. King, P. A., L. Goldstein, and E. A. Newsholme. Glutamine synthetase activity of muscle in acidosis. *Biochem. J.* 216: 523–525, 1983.
151. Kipnis, D. M., and M. W. Noall. Stimulation of amino acid transport by insulin in the isolated rat diaphragm. *Biochim. Biophys. Acta* 228: 226–227, 1958.
152. Knapik, J., C. Meredith, B. Jones, R. Fielding, V. R. Young, and W. Evans. Leucine metabolism during fasting and exercise. *J. Appl. Physiol.* 70: 43–47, 1991.
153. Kostyo, J. L. Rapid effects of growth hormone on amino acid transport and protein synthesis. *Ann. N. Y. Acad. Sci.* 148: 389–407, 1968.
154. Kovanen, V., H. Suominen, and E. Heikkinen. Collagen of slow twitch and fast twitch muscle fibre types in different types of rat skeletal muscle. *Eur. J. Appl. Physiol.* 52: 235–242, 1984.
155. Krebs, H. A. Regulation of fuel supply in animals. *Adv. Enzyme Regul.* 10: 406–413, 1972.
156. Laurent, G. J., M. P. Sparrow, P. C. Bates, and D. J. Millward. Collagen content and turnover in cardiac and skeletal muscles of the adult fowl and the changes during stretch-induced growth. *Biochem. J.* 176: 419–427, 1978.
157. Laurent, G. J., M. P. Sparrow, and D. J. Millward. Turnover of muscle protein in the fowl. Changes in rates of protein synthesis and breakdown during hypertrophy of the anterior and posterior latissimus dorsi muscles. *Biochem. J.* 176: 407–417, 1978.
158. Leighton, B., R. Curi, A. Hussein, and E. A. Newsholme. Maximum activities of some key enzymes of glycolysis, glutaminolysis, Krebs cycle and fatty acid utilization in bovine pulmonary endothelial cells. *FEBS Lett.* 225: 93–96, 1987.
159. Lemon, P. W., and J. P. Mullin. Effect of initial muscle glycogen levels on protein catabolism during exercise. *J. Appl. Physiol.* 48: 624–629, 1980.
160. Lemon, P. W. R., F. J. Nagle, J. P. Mullin, and N. J. Benevenga. In vivo leucine oxidation at rest and during two intensities of exercise. *J. Appl. Physiol.* 53: 947–954, 1982.
161. Livesey, G., and P. Lund. Enzymic determination of branched-chain amino acids and 2-oxoacids in rat tissues. *Biochem. J.* 188: 705–713, 1980.
162. Logan, W. J., A. Klip, and E. Gagalang. Regulation of amino acid transport into L6 muscle cells: I. Stimulation of transport System A by amino acid deprivation. *J. Cell. Physiol.* 112: 229–236, 1982.
163. Low, S. Y., M. J. Rennie, and P. M. Taylor. Sodium-dependent glutamate transport in cultured rat myotubes increases after glutamine deprivation. *FASEB J.* 8: 127–131, 1994.
164. Low, S. Y., M. Salter, R. G. Knowles, C. I. Pogson, and M. J. Rennie. A quantitative analysis of the control of glutamine catabolism in rat liver cells: use of selective inhibitors. *Biochem. J.* 295: 617–624, 1993.
165. Low, S. Y., P. M. Taylor, H. S. Hundal, C. I. Pogson, and M. J. Rennie. Transport of L-glutamine and L-glutamate across sinusoidal membranes of rat liver. Effects of starvation, diabetes and corticosteroid treatment. *Biochem. J.* 284: 333–340, 1992.
166. Lowenstein, J. M. Ammonia production in muscle and other tissues: the purine nucleotide cycle. *Physiol. Rev.* 52: 382–414, 1972.
167. Lowenstein, J. M. and M. N. Goodman. The purine nucleotide cycle in skeletal muscle. *Federation Proc.* 37: 2308–2312, 1978.
168. Lundgren, F., H. Sachrisson, P. Emery, A.-C. Bylund-Fellenius, A. Elander, K. Bennegård, T. Scherstén, and K. Lundholm. Leg exchange of amino acids during exercise in patients with arterial insufficiency. *Clin. Physiol.* 8: 227–241, 1988.
169. Mackenzie, B., A. Ahmed, and M. J. Rennie. Muscle amino acid metabolism and transport. In: *Mammalian Amino*

Acid Transport: Mechanism and Control, edited by M. S. Kilberg and D. Häussinger. New York: Plenum Publishing, 1992.

170. MacLean, D. A., L. L. Spriet, E. Hultman, and T. E. Graham. Plasma and muscle amino acid and ammonia responses during prolonged exercise in humans. *J. Appl. Physiol.* 70: 2095–2103, 1991.
171. MacLennan, P. A., R. A. Brown, and M. J. Rennie. A positive relationship between protein synthetic rate and intracellular glutamine concentration in perfused rat skeletal muscle. *FEBS Lett.* 215: 187–191, 1987.
172. MacLennan, P. A., and M. J. Rennie. Effects of ischaemia, blood loss and reperfusion on rat skeletal muscle protein synthesis *in vivo*. *Biochem. J.* 260: 195–200, 1989.
173. MacLennan, P. A., K. Smith, B. Weryk, P. W. Watt, and M. J. Rennie. Inhibition of protein breakdown by glutamine in perfused rat skeletal muscle. *FEBS Lett.* 237: 133–136, 1988.
174. May, R. C., Y. Hara, R. A. Kelly, K. P. Block, M. G. Buse, and W. E. Mitch. Branched-chain amino acid metabolism in rat muscle: abnormal regulation in acidosis. *Am. J. Physiol.* 252 (*Endocrinol. Metab.* 15): E712–E718, 1987.
175. Meijer, A. J., C. Lof, I. C. Ramos, and A. J. Verhoeven. Control of ureagenesis. *Eur. J. Biochem.* 148: 189–196, 1985.
176. Meredith, C. N., M. J. Zackin, W. R. Frontera, and W. J. Evans. Dietary protein requirements and body protein metabolism in endurance-trained men. *J. Appl. Physiol.* 66: 2850–2856, 1989.
177. Meyer, R. A., and R. L. Terjung. AMP deamination and IMP reamination in working skeletal muscle. *Am. J. Physiol.* 237: 111–118, 1979.
178. Michna, H., and G. Hartmann. Adaptation of tendon collagen to exercise. *Int. Orthopaed.* 13: 161–163, 1989.
179. Millward, D. J. Protein turnover in cardiac and skeletal muscle during normal growth and hypertrophy. In: *Degradative Processes in Skeletal and Cardiac Muscle*, edited by K. Wildenthal. New York: Elsevier-North Holland, 1980, p. 161–200.
180. Millward, D. J., P. C. Bates, J. G. Brown, S. R. Rosochacki, and M. J. Rennie. Protein degradation and the regulation of protein balance in muscle. In: *Protein Degradation in Health and Disease*, edited by D. Evered and J. Whelan. Amsterdam, Excerpta Medica, 1980, p. 307–329.
181. Millward, D. J., C. T. M. Davies, D. Halliday, S. L. Wolman, D. E. Matthews, and M. J. Rennie. Effect of exercise on protein metabolism in humans as explored with stable isotopes. *Federation Proc.* 41: 2686–2691, 1982.
182. Millward, D. J. and J. C. Waterlow. Effect of nutrition on protein turnover in skeletal muscle. *Federation Proc.* 37: 2283–2290, 1978.
183. Mole, P. A., K. M. Baldwin, R. L. Terjung, and J. O. Holloszy. Enzymatic pathways of pyruvate metabolism in skeletal muscle: adaptations to exercise. *Am. J. Physiol.* 224: 50–54, 1973.
184. Mole, P. A., L. B. Oscai, and J. O. Holloszy. Adaptation of muscle to exercise. Increase in levels of palmityl Coa synthetase, carnitine palmityltransferase, and palmityl Coa dehydrogenase, and in the capacity to oxidize fatty acids. *J. Clin. Invest.* 50: 2323–2330, 1971.
185. Myllyla, R., A. Salminen, L. Peltonen, T. E. Takala, and V. Vihko. Collagen metabolism of mouse skeletal muscle during the repair of exercise injuries. *Pflugers Arch.* 407: 64–70, 1986.
186. Nair, K. S., D. Halliday, D. E. Matthews, and S. L. Welle. Hyperglucagonemia during insulin deficiency accelerates protein catabolism. *Am. J. Physiol.* 253 (*Endocrinol. Metab.* 16): E208–E213, 1987.
187. Narahara, H. T., and J. O. Holloszy. The actions of insulin, trypsin and electrical stimulation on amino acid transport in muscle. *J. Biol. Chem.* 249: 5435–5443, 1974.
188. Newsholme, E. A., and B. Crabtree. Flux-generating and regulatory steps in metabolic control. *Trends Biochem. Sci.* 00: 53–56, 1981.
189. Newsholme, E. A., and A. R. Leach. *Biochemistry for the Medical Sciences*. Chichester: John Wiley & Sons, 1983.
190. Newsholme, E. A., and M. Parry-Billings. Properties of glutamine release from muscle and its importance for the immune system. *J. Parenter. Enter. Nutr.* 14: 63S–67S, 1990.
191. Palacin, M., A. Werner, J. Dittmer, H. Murer, and J. Biber. Expression of rat liver Na^+/L-alanine co-transport in *Xenopus laevis* oocytes. *Biochem. J.* 270: 189–195, 1990.
192. Palmer, T. N., M. A. Caldecourt, K. Snell, and M. C. Sugden. Alanine and inter-organ relationships in branched-chain amino and 2-oxo acid metabolism. *Biosci. Rep.* 5: 1015–1033, 1985.
193. Palmer, T. N., M. A. Caldecourt, J. P. Warner, and M. C. Sugden. The role of phosphenolpyruvate carboxykinase in muscle alanine synthesis. *Biochem. J.* 224: 971–976, 1984.
194. Pardridge, W. M. Tryptophan transport through the blood-brain barrier: in vivo measurement of free and albumin bound amino acid. *Life Sci.* 25: 1519–1528, 1979.
195. Parker, P. J., and P. J. Randle. Active and inactive forms of branched-chain 2-oxoacid dehydrogenase complex in rat heart and skeletal muscle. *Biomed. Press* 112: 186–190, 1980.
196. Parry-Billings, M., R. Budgett, Y. Koutedakis, E. Blomstrand, S. Brooks, D. Williams, P. C. Calder, S. Pilling, R. Baigrie, and E. A. Newsholme. Plasma amino acid concentrations in the overtraining syndrome: possible effects on the immune system. *Med. Sci. Sports Exerc.* 24: 1353–1358, 1992.
197. Paul, G. L. Dietary protein requirements of physically active individuals. *Sports Med.* 8: 154–176, 1989.
198. Pines, G., N. C. Danbolt, M. Bjoras, Y. Zhang, A. Bendahan, L. Eide, H. Koepsell, J. Storm-Mathisen, E. Seeberg, and B. I. Kanner. Cloning and expression of a rat brain L-glutamate transporter. *Nature* 360: 464–467, 1992.
199. Plante, P. D., and M. E. Houston. Effects of concentric and eccentric exercise on protein catabolism in man. *Int. J. Sports Med.* 5: 174–178, 1984.
200. Pogson, C. I., S. Y. Low, R. G. Knowles, M. Salter, and M. J. Rennie. Application of metabolic control theory to amino acid metabolism in liver. In: *Regulation of Hepatic Function: Alfred Benzon Symposium 30*, edited by N. Grunnet and B. Quistorff. Copenhagen: Munksgaard, 1990, p. 262–272.
201. Pozefsky, T., P. Felig, J. D. Tobin, J. S. Soeldner, and G. F. Cahill. Amino acid balance across tissues of the forearm in postabsorptive man. Effects of insulin at two dose levels. *J. Clin. Invest.* 48: 2273–2282, 1969.
202. Pozefsky, T., R. G. Tancredi, R. T. Moxley, J. Dupre, and J. D. Tobin. Metabolism of forearm tissues in man. Studies with glucagon. *Diabetes* 25: 128–134, 1976.
203. Price, G. M., D. Halliday, P. J. Pacy, R. M. Quevedo, and D. J. Millward. Nitrogen homeostasis in man: 1. Influence of protein intake on the amplitude of diurnal cycling of body nitrogen. *Clin. Sci.* 86: 91–102, 1994.
204. Quevedo, R. M., M. Cox, W. A. Coward, D. Jones, P. Pacy, I. Smeaton, D. Thorpe, and D. J. Millward. Energy intake and expenditure in body builders. *Proc. Nutr. Soc.* 50: 238A, 1991.

205. Quevedo, R. M., G. M. Price, D. Halliday, P. J. Pacy, and D. J. Millward. Nitrogen homeostasis in man: 3. Diurnal changes in nitrogen excretion, leucine oxidation and whole body leucine kinetics during a reduction from a high to a moderate protein intake. *Clin. Sci.* 86: 185–193, 1994.
206. Radha, E., and S. P. Bessman. Effect of exercise on protein degradation: 3-methylhistidine and creatinine excretion. *Biochem. Med.* 29: 96–100, 1983.
207. Refsum, H. W., and S. B. Strömme. Urea and creatinine production and excretion in urine during and after prolonged heavy exercise. *J. Lab. Clin. Invest.* 33: 247–254, 1974.
208. Reichsman, F., S. P. Scordilis, P. M. Clarkson, and W. J. Evans. Muscle protein changes following eccentric exercise in humans. *Eur. J. Appl. Physiol.* 62: 245–250, 1991.
209. Rennie, M. J. Muscle protein turnover and the wasting due to injury and disease. *Br. Med. Bull.* 41: 257–264, 1985.
210. Rennie, M. J., A. Ahmed, S. Y. Low, H. S. Hundal, P. W. Watt, P. A. Lennan, and C. J. Egan. Transport of amino acids in muscle, gut and liver: relevance to metabolic control. *Biochem. Soc. Trans.* 18: 1140–1141, 1991.
211. Rennie, M. J., A. Ahmed, G. W. A. Thompson, K. Smith, W. M. Bennet, and P. W. Watt. Effects of insulin on amino acid transport and protein synthesis in skeletal muscle. In: *Protein Metabolism in Diabetes Mellitus*, edited by K. S. Nair. London: Smith-Gordon, 1992, p. 173–180.
212. Rennie, M. J., P. Babij, J. R. Sutton, W. W. Tonkins, W. W. Read, C. Ford, and D. Halliday. Effects of acute hypoxia on forearm leucine metabolism. *Prog. Clin. Biol. Res.* 136: 317–323, 1983.
213. Rennie, M. J., C. Bennegård, E. Edén, P. W. Emery, and K. Lundholm. Urinary excretion and efflux from the leg of 3-methylhistidine before and after major surgical operation. *Metabolism* 33: 250–256, 1984.
214. Rennie, M. J., J. L. Bowtell, and D. J. Millward. Physical activity and protein metabolism. In: *Physical Activity, Fitness and Health. International Consensus Statements*, edited by C. Bouchard, R. J. Shepherd, and T. Stephens. Champaign, IL: Human Kinetics Publishers, 1994.
215. Rennie, M. J., R. H. T. Edwards, C. T. M. Davies, S. Krywawych, D. Halliday, J. C. Waterlow, and D. J. Millward. Protein and amino acid turnover during and after exercise. *Biochem. Soc. Trans.* 8: 499–501, 1980.
216. Rennie, M. J., R. H. T. Edwards, D. Halliday, D. E. Matthews, S. L. Wolman, and D. J. Millward. Muscle protein synthesis measured by stable isotope techniques in man: the effects of feeding and fasting. *Clin. Sci.* 63: 519–523, 1982.
217. Rennie, M. J., R. H. T. Edwards, S. Krywawych, C. T. M. Davies, D. Halliday, J. C. Waterlow, and D. J. Millward. Effect of exercise on protein turnover in man. *Clin. Sci.* 61: 627–639, 1981.
218. Rennie, M. J., D. Halliday, C. T. M. Davies, R. H. T. Edwards, S. Krywawych, D. J. Millward, and D. E. Matthews. Exercise induced increase in leucine oxidation in man and the effect of glucose. In: *Metabolism and Clinical Implications of Branched Chain Amino and Keto Acids*, edited by M. Walser and J. R. Williamson. New York: Elsevier-North Holland, 1981, p. 361–366.
219. Rennie, M. J., H. S. Hundal, P. Babij, P. A. MacLennan, P. W. Watt, M. M. Jepson, and D. J. Millward. Characteristics of a glutamine carrier in skeletal muscle have important consequences for nitrogen loss in injury, infection, and chronic disease. *Lancet* ii: 1008–1012, 1986.
220. Rennie, M. J., S. M. Jennett, and R. H. Johnson. The metabolic effects of strenous exercise: a comparison between untrained subjects and racing cyclists. *Q. J. Exp. Physiol.* 59: 201–212, 1974.
221. Rennie, M. J., and R. H. Johnson. Alteration of metabolic and hormonal responses to exercise by physical training. *Eur. J. Appl. Physiol.* 33: 215–226, 1974.
222. Rennie, M. J., P. A. MacLennan, H. S. Hundal, B. Weryk, K. Smith, P. M. Taylor, and C. Egan. Skeletal muscle glutamine transport, intramuscular glutamine concentration, and muscle-protein turnover. *Metabolism* 38: 47–51, 1989.
223. Rennie, M. J., and D. J. Millward. 3-Methylhistidine excretion and the urinary 3-methylhistidine/creatinine ratio are poor indicators of skeletal muscle protein breakdown. *Clin. Sci.* 65: 217–225, 1983.
224. Rennie, M. J., N. M. Willhoft, A. Ahmed, P. W. Watt, P. M. Taylor, and H. S. Hundal. Amino acid and protein metabolism during exercise. In: *Diabetes Mellitus and Exercise*, edited by J. Devlin, E. S. Horton, and M. Vranic. London: Smith-Gordon, 1993, p. 139–150.
225. Rennie, M. J., N. M. Willhoft, and P. M. Taylor. Glutamine transport and metabolism in mammalian skeletal muscle. *Biochem. J.* 285: 339–344, 1992.
226. Riggs, T. R., and L. M. Walker. Growth hormone stimulation of amino acid transport into rat tissues *in vivo*. *J. Biol. Chem.* 235: 3603–3607, 1960.
227. Rowe, W. B. Glutamine synthetase from muscle. *Methods Enzymol.* 113: 199–212, 1985.
228. Ruderman, N. B., and P. Lund. Amino acid metabolism in skeletal muscle: regulation of glutamine and alanine release in the perfused rat hindquarter. *Isr. J. Med. Sci.* 8: 295–302, 1972.
229. Rundell, K. W., P. C. Tullson, and R. L. Terjung. AMP deaminase binding in contracting rat skeletal muscle. *Am. J. Physiol.* 263 (*Cell Physiol.* 32): C287–C293, 1992.
230. Rundell, K. W., P. C. Tullson, and R. L. Terjung. Altered kinetics of AMP deaminase by myosin binding. *Am. J. Physiol.* 263 (*Cell Physiol.* 32): C294–C299, 1992.
231. Rundell, K. W., P. C. Tullson, and R. L. Terjung. AMP deaminase binding in rat skeletal muscle after high-intensity running. *J. Appl. Physiol.* 74: 2004–2006, 1993.
232. Saccomani, M. P., C. Cobelli, R. A. De Fronzo, and R. C. Bonadonna. Effect of insulin on aminoacid trans-membrane transport and metabolism in human skeletal muscle assessed by a compartmental-model. *San Raffaele Proc. Milan* 1: 32P, 1990.
233. Sahlin, K., A. Katz, and S. Broberg. Tricarboxylic acid cycle intermediates in human muscle during prolonged exercise. *Am. J. Physiol.* 259 (*Cell Physiol.* 28): C834–C841, 1990.
234. Salter, M., R. G. Knowles, and C. I. Pogson. Quantification of the importance of individual steps in the control of aromatic amino acid metabolism. *Biochem. J.* 234: 635–647, 1986.
235. Saltin, B., J. Henriksson, E. Nygaard, and P. Andersen. Fiber types and metabolic potentials of skeletal muscles in sedentary man and endurance runners. *Ann. N. Y. Acad. Sci.* 301: 3–29, 1977.
236. Sargeant, A. J., A. Young, C. T. M. Davies, C. Maunder, and R. H. T. Edwards. Functional and structural changes following disuse of human muscle. *Clin. Sci.* 52: 342, 1977.
237. Savolainen, J., V. Myllyla, R. Myllyla, V. Vihko, K. Vaananen, and T. E. Takala. Effects of denervation and immobilization on collagen synthesis in rat skeletal muscle and tendon. *Am. J. Physiol.* 254 (*Regulatory Integrative Comp. Physiol.* 23): R897–R902, 1988.
238. Savolainen, J., K. Vaananen, J. Puranen, T. E. Takala, J. Komulainen, and V. Vihko. Collagen synthesis and proteo-

lytic activities in rat skeletal muscles: effect of cast-immobilization in the lengthened and shortened positions. *Arch. Phys. Med. Rehabil.* 69: 964–969, 1988.

239. Savolainen, J., K. Vaananen, V. Vihko, J. Puranen, and T. E. Takala. Effect of immobilization on collagen synthesis in rat skeletal muscles. *Am. J. Physiol.* 252 (*Regulatory Integrative Comp. Physiol.* 21): R883–R888, 1987.
240. Säämänen, A.-M., K. Puustjärvi, K. Ilves, and M. Tammi. Effect of running exercise on proteoglycans and collagen content in the intervetebral disc of young dogs. *Int. J. Sports Med.* 14: 48–51, 1993.
241. Scholte, H. R., and H. F. Busch. Early changes of muscle mitochondria in Duchenne dystrophy. Partition and activity of mitochondrial enzymes in fractionated muscle of unaffected boys and adults and patients. *J. Neurol. Sci.* 45: 217–234, 1980.
242. Schott, L. H., and R. L. Terjung. The influence of exercise on muscle lysosomal enzymes. *Eur. J. Appl. Physiol.* 42: 175–182, 1979.
243. Schröck, H., C. J. Cha, and L. Goldstein. Glutamine release from hind limb and uptake by kidney in the acutely acidotic rat. *Biochem. J.* 188: 557–560, 1980.
244. Schwartz, R. G., E. J. Barrett, C. K. Francis, R. Jacob, and B. L. Zaret. Regulation of myocardial amino acid balance in the conscious dog. *J. Clin. Invest.* 75: 1204–1211, 1985.
245. Scislowski, P. W. D., B. M. Hokland, W. I. A. Davis-van Thienen, J. Bremer, and E. J. Davis. Methionine metabolism by rat muscle and other tissues. *Biochem. J.* 247: 35–40, 1987.
246. Sjölin, J., H. Stjernström, S. Henneberg, E. Andersson, J. Martensson, G. Griman, and J. Larsson. Splanchnic and peripheral release of 3-methylhistidine in relation to its urinary excretion in human infection. *Metabolism* 38: 23–29, 1989.
247. Smith, K., J. M. Barua, C. M. Scrimgeour, and M. J. Rennie. Flooding with L-[1-^{13}C]leucine stimulates human muscle protein incorporation of continuously infused L-[1-^{13}C]valine. *Am. J. Physiol.* 262 (*Endocrinol. Metab.* 25): E372–E376, 1992.
248. Snow-Harter, C., and R. Marcus. Exercise, bone mineral density and osteoporosis. In: *Exercise and Sports Science Reviews*, edited by J. O. Holloszy. Baltimore: Williams & Wilkins, 1991, p. 351–388.
249. Stauber, W. T., P. M. Clarkson, V. K. Fritz, and W. J. Evans. Extracellular matrix disruption and pain after eccentric muscle action. *J. Appl. Physiol.* 69: 868–874, 1990.
250. Swierczynski, J., Z. Bereznowski, and W. Makarewicz. Phosphate-dependent glutaminase of rat skeletal muscle. Some properties and possible role in glutamine metabolism. *Biochim. Biophys. Acta* 1157: 55–62, 1993.
251. Tadros, L. B., N. M. Willhoft, P. M. Taylor, and M. J. Rennie. Effects of glutamine deprivation on glutamine transport and synthesis in primary tissue culture of rat skeletal muscle. *Am. J. Physiol.* 265: 935–942, 1993.
252. Tarnopolsky, M. A., S. A. Atkinson, J. D. MacDougall, A. Chesley, S. Phillips, and H. P. Schwarcz. Evaluation of protein requirements for trained strength athletes. *J. Appl. Physiol.* 73: 1986–1995, 1992.
253. Tarnopolsky, M. A., S. A. Atkinson, J. D. MacDougall, B. B. Senor, P. W. R. Lemon, and H. Schwarcz. Whole body leucine metabolism during and after resistance exercise in fed humans. *Med. Sci. Sports Exerc.* 23: 326–333, 1991.
254. Tarnopolsky, M. A., J. D. MacDougall, and S. A. Atkinson. Influence of protein intake and training status on nitrogen balance and lean body mass. *J. Appl. Physiol.* 64: 187–193, 1988.
255. Taylor, P. M., C. J. Egan, and M. J. Rennie. Transport of glutamine across blood-facing membranes of perfused rat jejunum. *Am. J. Physiol.* 256 (*Endocrinol. Metab.* 19): E550–E558, 1989.
256. Taylor, P. M., and M. J. Rennie. Amino acid fluxes across sinusoidal membranes of perfused rat liver: relationship with portal ammonia concentrations. In: *Advances in Ammonia Metabolism and Hepatic Encephalopathy*, edited by P. B. Soeters, J. H. P. Wilson, A. J. Meijer, and E. Holm. Amsterdam: Elsevier (Biomedical Division), 1988, p. 45–52.
257. Tischler, M. E., M. Desautels, and A. L. Goldberg. Does leucine, leucyl-tRNA, or some metabolite of leucine regulate protein synthesis and degradation in skeletal and cardiac muscle? *J. Biol. Chem.* 257: 1613–1621, 1982.
258. Tovar, A. R., J. K. Tews, N. Torres, D. C. Madsen, and A. E. Harper. Competition for transport of amino acids into rat heart: effect of competitors on protein synthesis and degradation. *Metabolism* 41: 925–933, 1992.
259. Tullson, P. C., and R. L. Terjung. Adenine nucleotide metabolism in contracting skeletal muscle. *Exerc. Sport Sci. Rev.* 19: 507–537, 1991.
260. Turinsky, J. Glucose and amino acid uptake by exercising muscles *in vivo* effect of insulin, fiber population and denervation. *Endocrinology* 121: 528–535, 1987.
261. Uchida, S., H. M. Kwon, A. S. Preston, and J. S. Handler. Expression of Madin-Derby canine kidney cell Na^+- and Cl^--dependent taurine transporter in *Xenopus laevis* oocytes. *J. Biol. Chem.* 266: 9605–9609, 1991.
262. Van Hall, G., J. S. H. Raaymakers, W. H. M. Saris, and A. J. M. Wagenmakers. Effect of branched-chain amino acid supplementation on performance during prolonged exercise. *J. Physiol.* 479: 51P, 1994.
263. Vanuxem, D., S. Delpierre, A. Barlatier, and P. Vanuxem. Changes in blood ammonia induced by a maximum effort in trained and untrained subjects. *Arch. Int. Physiol. Biochim. Biophys.* 101: 405–409, 1993.
264. Vihko, V., A. Salminen, and J. Rantamaki. Acid hydrolase activity in red and white skeletal muscle of mice during a two-week period following exhausting exercise. *Pflugers Arch.* 378: 99–106, 1978.
265. Vihko, V., A. Salminen, and J. Rantamaki. Oxidative and lysosomal capacity in skeletal muscle of mice after endurance training of different intensities. *Acta. Physiol. Scand.* 104: 74–81, 1978.
266. Wagenmakers, A. J. Amino acid metabolism, muscular fatigue and muscle wasting. speculations on adaptations at high altitude (review). *Int. J. Sports Med.* 13(Suppl. 1): S110–S113, 1992.
267. Wagenmakers, A. J. M., E. J. Beckers, F. Brouns, H. Kuipers, P. B. Soeters, G. J. van der Vusse, and W. H. M. Saris. Carbohydrate supplementation, glycogen depletion and amino acid metabolism during exercise. *Am. J. Physiol.* 260 (*Endocrinol. Metab.* 23): E883–E890, 1991.
268. Wagenmakers, A. J. M., J. H. Brookes, J. H. Coakley, T. Reilly, and R. H. T. Edwards. Exercise-induced activation of the branched-chain 2-oxo acid dehydrogenase in human muscle. *Eur. J. Appl. Physiol.* 59: 159–167, 1989.
269. Wagenmakers, A. J. M., J. H. Coakley, and R. H. T. Edwards. Metabolism of branched-chain amino acids and ammonia during exercise: clues from McArdle's disease. *Int. J. Sports Med* 11: S101–S113, 1990.
270. Wagenmakers, A. J. M., J. T. G. Schepens, and J. H. Veerkamp. Effect of starvation and exercise on actual and total activity of the branched chain 2-oxo acid dehydrogenase

complex in rat skeletal tissues. *Biochem. J.* 223: 815–821, 1984.
271. Wahren, J., P. Felig, and L. Hagenfeldt. Effect of protein ingestion on splanchnic and leg metabolism in normal man and in patients with diabetes mellitus. *J. Clin. Invest.* 57: 987–999, 1976.
272. Wasserman, D. H., R. J. Geer, P. E. Williams, T. Becker, D. B. Lacy, and N. N. Abumrad. Interaction of gut and liver in nitrogen metabolism during exercise. *Metabolism* 40: 307–314, 1991.
273. Waterlow, J. C., and E. B. Fern. Free amino acid pools and their regulation. In: *Nitrogen Metabolism in Man.* Chichester, England: Applied Science Publishers, 1981, p. 1–16.
274. Waterlow, J. C., P. J. Garlick, and D. J. Millward. *Protein Turnover in Mammalian Tissues and in the Whole Body.* Amsterdam: Elsevier-North Holland, 1978.
275. Watson, P. A., J. P. Stein, and F. W. Booth. Changes in actin synthesis and α-actin-mRNA content in rat muscle during immobilization. *Am. J. Physiol.* 247: 39–44, 1984.
276. Watt, P. W., M. E. Corbett, and M. J. Rennie. Stimulation of protein synthesis in pig skeletal muscle by infusion of amino acids during constant insulin availability. *Am. J. Physiol.* 263: 453–460, 1992.
277. Welbourne, T. C. Interorgan glutamine flow in metabolic acidosis. *Am. J. Physiol.* 253 (*Renal Fluid Electrolyte Physiol.* 22): F1069–F1076, 1987.
278. White, T. P., and G. A. Brooks. [U-^{14}C]glucose, -alanine, and -leucine oxidation in rats at rest and two intensities of running. *Am. J. Physiol.* 240: 155–165, 1981.
279. Wibom, R., and E. Hultman. ATP production rate in mitochondria isolated from microsamples of human muscle. *Am. J. Physiol.* 259 (*Endocrinol. Metab.* 22): E204–E209, 1990.
280. Willhoft, N. M., and M. J. Rennie. Characteristics of L-glutamine efflux from incubated rat soleus muscle. *J. Physiol. (Lond.)* 446: 10P, 1992.
281. Wilson, W. M., and R. J. Maughan. Evidence for a possible role of 5-hydroxytrypamine in the genesis of fatigue in man: administration of paroxetine, a 5-HT re-uptake inhibitor, reduces the capacity to perform prolonged exercise. *Exp. Physiol.* 77: 921–924, 1992.
282. Windmueller, H. G., and A. E. Spaeth. Uptake and metabolism of plasma glutamine by the small intestine. *J. Biol. Chem.* 249: 5070–5079, 1974.
283. Windmueller, H. G., and A. E. Spaeth. Identification of ketone bodies and glutamine as the major respiratory fuels in vivo for post-absorptive rat small intestine. *J. Biol. Chem.* 253: 69–76, 1978.
284. Wolfe, R. R. Does exercise stimulate protein breakdown in humans?: isotopic approaches to the problem. *Med. Sci. Sports Exerc.* 19: 172–178, 1987.
285. Wolfe, R. R., R. D. Goodenough, M. H. Wolfe, F. T. Royle, and E. R. Nadel. Isotopic analysis of leucine and urea metabolism in exercising humans. *J. Appl. Physiol.* 52: 458–466, 1982.
286. Wolfe, R. R., M. H. Wolfe, E. R. Nadel, and J. H. F. Shaw. Isotopic determination of amino acid-urea interactions in exercise in humans. *J. Appl. Physiol.* 56: 221–229, 1984.
287. Wong, T. S., and F. W. Booth. Protein metabolism in rat gastrocnemius muscle after stimulated chronic concentric exercise. *J. Appl. Physiol.* 69: 1709–1717, 1990.
288. Wu, G., and J. R. Thompson. The effect of glutamine on protein turnover in chick skeletal muscle *in vitro*. *Biochem. J.* 265: 593–598, 1990.
289. Wu, G., J. R. Thompson, and V. E. Baracos. Glutamine metabolism in skeletal muscles from the broiler chick (*Gallus domesticus*) and the laboratory rat (*Rattus norvegicus*). *Biochem. J.* 274: 769–774, 1991.
290. Yamada, Y., T. Ishihara, M. Fujiwara, S. Tamoto, I. Seki, and N. Ohsawa. Effects of exercise and pacing loads on myocardial amino acid balance in patients with normal and stenotic coronary arteries, with special reference to branched chain amino acids. *Jpn. Circ. J.* 57: 272–282, 1993.
291. Yarasheski, K. E., J. J. Zachwieja, and D. M. Bier. Acute effects of resistance exercise on muscle protein synthesis rate in young and elderly men and women. *Am. J. Physiol.* 265 (*Endocrinol. Metab.* 23): E210–E214, 1993.
292. Yki Jarvinen, H., K. Sahlin, J. M. Ren, and V. A. Koivisto. Localization of rate-limiting defect for glucose disposal in skeletal muscle of insulin-resistant type I diabetic patients. *Diabetes* 39: 157–167, 1990.
293. Young, L. H., P. H. McNulty, C. Morgan, L. I. Deckelbaum, B. L. Zaret, and E. J. Barrett. Myocardial protein turnover in patients with coronary artery disease. Effect of branched chain amino acid infusion. *J. Clin. Invest.* 87: 554–560, 1991.
294. Young, V. R., and H. N. Munro. N^{τ}-Methylhistidine (3-methylhistidine) and muscle protein turnover: an overview. *Federation Proc.* 37: 2291–2300, 1978.
295. Zorzano, A., T. W. Balon, L. P. Garetto, M. N. Goodman, and N. B. Ruderman. Muscle α-aminoisobutyric acid transport after exercise: enhanced stimulation by insulin. *Am. J. Physiol.* 248 (*Endocrinol. Metab.* 11): E546–E552, 1985.

23. Regulation of extramuscular fuel sources during exercise

DAVID H. WASSERMAN
ALAN D. CHERRINGTON | *Department of Molecular Physiology and Biophysics, Vanderbilt University School of Medicine, Nashville, Tennessee*

CHAPTER CONTENTS

INTRAMUSCULAR FUEL STORES ARE LIMITED IN QUANTITY and cannot, in and of themselves, provide adequate energy for sustained exercise. Potential energy is, contained outside the working muscle in quantities that are sufficient for exercise of extended duration. Extramuscular fuel sources are present as fats in adipose tissue and carbohydrates in liver. Fat stores, even in lean individuals, are effectively limitless. Hepatic carbohydrate stores, on the other hand, are finite and may deplete during prolonged exercise. Fortunately, the availability of blood glucose for the working muscle can be sustained, to a large extent, by hepatic gluconeogenesis and the ingestion of carbohydrate-based fuels. Although the amount of protein in the body is vast, excessive proteolysis may compromise cell function, and amino acids therefore are used only sparingly as a fuel. The mechanisms involved in the exercise-induced increase in fuel utilization have become better defined in recent years. It is apparent that although the different extramuscular fuels are mobilized from anatomically distinct sites and are regulated by diverse mechanisms, the processes involved are coordinated both quantitatively and temporally to meet the metabolic needs of the working muscle. This is the case regardless of whether the working muscle is engaged in a high-intensity sport or a prolonged task. The aim of this chapter is to characterize the role of extramuscular fuel sources and describe the means by which the endocrine and autonomic nervous systems regulate the mobilization of these fuels. In addition to the role and regulation of endogenous fuel supplies, the effectiveness with which exogenous (ingested) fuels are made available to the working muscle and the circumstances in which fuel ingestion may be important will be described.

FUEL REQUIREMENTS OF THE WORKING MUSCLE

Patterns of fuel utilization during exercise have been comprehensively described in studies using pulmonary gas exchange, tissue biopsy, arteriovenous difference, isotopic, and nuclear magnetic resonance techniques, and this information is now a fundamental component of our understanding of intermediary metabolism. It is well documented that the increased energy demand of muscular work in the postabsorptive state necessitates an accelerated flow of carbohydrate and fat from their storage sites to the energy-transducing machinery in the working muscle. To a lesser extent, amino acids may be used as fuel, particularly when the availability of other substrates is limited. The precise contribution of each of these substrates to the metabolic demand of the working muscle will depend on a number of different variables relating to subject characteristics (e.g., fitness, nutritional state, specific health deficits) and exercise conditions (e.g., high altitude, temperature extremes). The most important determinants of the type and amount of fuel utilized are the duration and intensity of exercise. The impact of these two primary exercise parameters in postabsorptive states is discussed below.

Effect of Exercise Duration

During the transition from rest to moderate-intensity exercise, the muscle shifts from using primarily circulating nonesterified fatty acids (NEFAs) to using a blend of NEFAs, extramuscular glucose, and muscle glycogen (6, 20, 292). During the early stages of exercise, muscle glycogen is an important source of energy, with significant contributions also derived from circulating glucose and NEFAs. With increasing exercise duration the uptake of circulating glucose by the working muscle of overnight-fasted humans increases gradually for approximately the first 60–120 min of moderate-intensity exercise, after which it declines slowly (6). During exercise of moderate duration (approximately <60 min) hepatic glucose output is reasonably well matched to the increment in glucose uptake by the working muscles and glucose homeostasis is maintained (6, 306). With prolonged exercise, hepatic glucose output becomes slightly less than glucose utilization and blood glucose levels fall gradually. In contrast, the contribution of circulating NEFAs increases progressively with prolonged exercise (6, 331). It can be estimated, assuming that all the NEFAs extracted by the working limb are completely oxidized, that this fuel satisfies ~30% of the energy requirement of the working limb after 40 min of moderate exercise (40% $V_{O_{2max}}$) and greater than 60% after 4 h in overnight-fasted untrained subjects (6). The transition to a greater utilization of circulating NEFAs during prolonged exercise is important, since it curtails the rate at which glycogen stores are depleted. Fats are the preferable fuel for long-term exercise, since differences in the degree of saturation between fatty acids and glucose predict that more than twice as much energy is derived from 1 g of fat than from 1 g of carbohydrate. As a result, fatty acids are the most economical fuel for long-duration exercise from the standpoint of both its storage and metabolism. The importance of the economical storage of fats is readily evident in nature by the massive fat deposition that occurs in migratory birds prior to spring and fall migration or in the muscle of salmon prior to the spawning migration. Although branched chain amino acids (BCAAs) released from the splanchnic bed can be oxidized by the working muscle (84, 239, 330), it is unlikely that this fuel can satisfy more than a small fraction of the energy requirement (<10%) even during prolonged exercise in excess of 2 h (231). Protein breakdown may play a more important role in supplying amino acids for gluconeogenesis (84, 312) and/or protein synthesis within the liver (42). Formation of amino acids, de novo, may be important in nitrogen transport. Although amino acids utilized in this way are not a direct energy source, it is necessary for high metabolic rates to be sustained.

Effect of Exercise Intensity

With increasing exercise intensity the balance of substrate usage shifts to a greater oxidation of carbohydrates (120, 154, 292). This is due both to an increase in muscle glycogenolysis and muscle glucose uptake from the blood. The relationship between carbohydrate metabolism and work rate is not linear but increases disproportionately at higher work rates [Fig. 23.1; (57, 58, 120, 154, 292)]. The work rate beyond which muscle glycogen and glucose metabolism increases disproportionately has been proposed to correspond to the lactate threshold (57). One advantage of carbohydrates at high work intensities is that they can be metabolized in the cytosol by the glycolytic pathway which, due to the high activities of the enzymes that comprise this pathway, can produce adenosine triphosphate (ATP) rapidly. A second advantage is that, for complete oxidation, glucose requires less oxygen (O_2) compared to fats per carbon atom. Consequently, conditions during which O_2 availability may be limiting such as during heavy exercise (161, 292) or exercise with anemia (105, 308), while breathing a hypoxic gas mixture (58, 162) or while breathing at high altitude result in a greater utilization of glucose, since it is the most efficient fuel metabolically (33). In contrast to the high rate of carbohydrate metabolism during high-intensity exercise, the utilization of NEFAs by the working muscle is reduced (151). Although the ca-

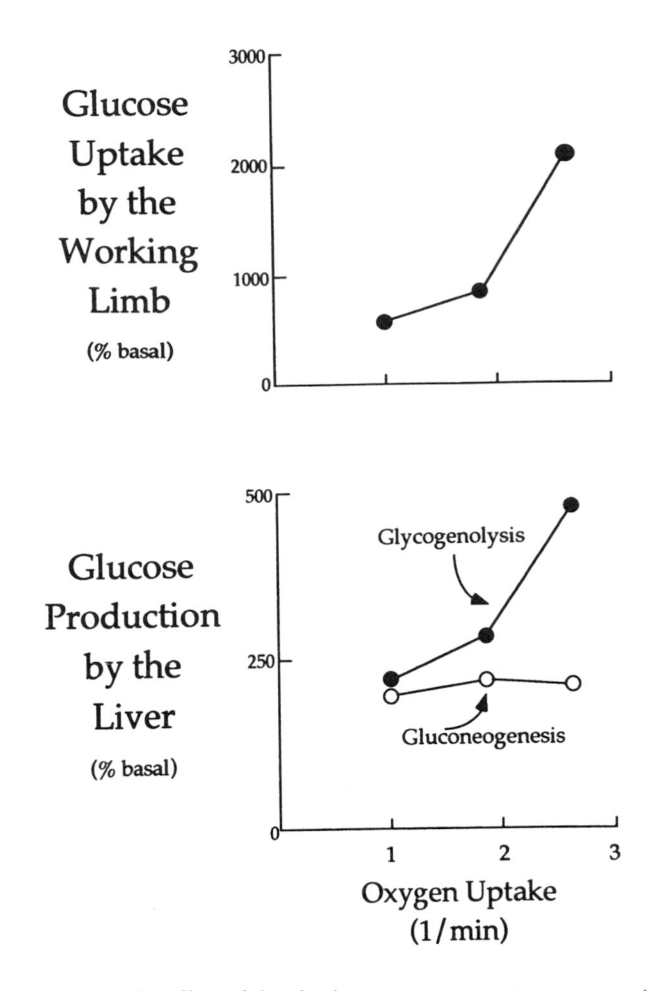

FIG. 23.1. The effect of the absolute exercise intensity (expressed as O_2 uptake) on limb glucose uptake *(A)* and hepatic glycogenolysis and gluconeogenesis *(B)* in untrained subjects. The increase in limb glucose uptake and hepatic glucose production per increase in work intensity is greater at higher work rates. The increase in hepatic glucose production is due strictly to an increase in hepatic glycogenolysis (see HEPATIC GLUCOSE PRODUCTION). All measurements were made at 40 min of exercise. [Modified from the data of Wahren et al. (292).]

pacity for BCAA oxidation is increased at higher work rates (127, 316), it is still unlikely that this substrate contributes significantly to energy production.

EXERCISE RESPONSES OF HORMONES AND NERVES INVOLVED IN ACUTE METABOLIC REGULATION

The importance of the endocrine system in metabolic regulation was recognized beginning almost immediately after the concept of a hormone as a bloodborne messenger was introduced. Since that time, the metabolic role of the endocrine system has been studied extensively. The development of sensitive hormone assays over the last 30 years has been instrumental in describing the endocrine response to muscular work (92). Measurements of increased circulating norepinephrine levels (52, 92) and direct measurements of nerve activity (286) indicate that sympathetic activity is also affected by exercise (See Part II of this *Handbook* for details of the regulation of sympathetic nerve activity). These hormonal and neural responses are generally more pronounced with increased exercise duration and intensity. Other factors such as age, nutritional status, and fitness level are also important in determining the responses of the endocrine and nervous systems to exercise. Exercise in the postabsorptive state is characterized by a fall in arterial insulin; an increase or no change in arterial glucagon; and increases in arterial catecholamine, growth hormone, thyroid hormone, adrenocorticotrophic hormone (ACTH), β-endorphin, gastrointestinal hormones, renin, and gonadal hormone levels, among others (for review, see 92). An important characteristic of the endocrine response to exercise is that it can synergize with other hormonal stimuli. Specifically, the catecholamines, glucagon, and cortisol are generally stimulated synergistically by exercise in the presence of hypoglycemia (9, 272, 303, 307) or hypoxia (58, 105, 308). The absorption of nutrients in the gastrointestinal tract can also alter many of the hormonal responses to exercise (3). The precise effects will depend on meal size, content, and timing with respect to exercise.

Despite the extensive documentation of the arterial hormone responses to exercise, two major features are not well established. First of all, arterial or peripheral plasma measurements do not always reflect the concentrations that are present at the site of action. This is particularly important when trying to assess the pancreatic hormone levels at the liver, since portal vein glucagon and insulin levels are different from arterial levels (302, 304), and when attempting to estimate norepinephrine levels at the synaptic clefts of potential target organs (52). The second component of the endocrine and autonomic nervous responses to exercise that has not been comprehensively defined is the signal or signals that initiate these responses. It has been postulated and there is evidence to support the concept that subtle changes in glycemia (18, 146, 147), neural or chemical feedback originating from the working muscle (18, 146, 147) neural feedback from the liver (176, 182), and/or feedforward mechanisms originating in the hypothalamus (170, 289, 290) may be involved. These putative mechanisms are illustrated in Figure 23.2.

It has been proposed that some of the changes in hormone levels are due to a decrease in blood flow to the clearing organ (277). In the presence of either

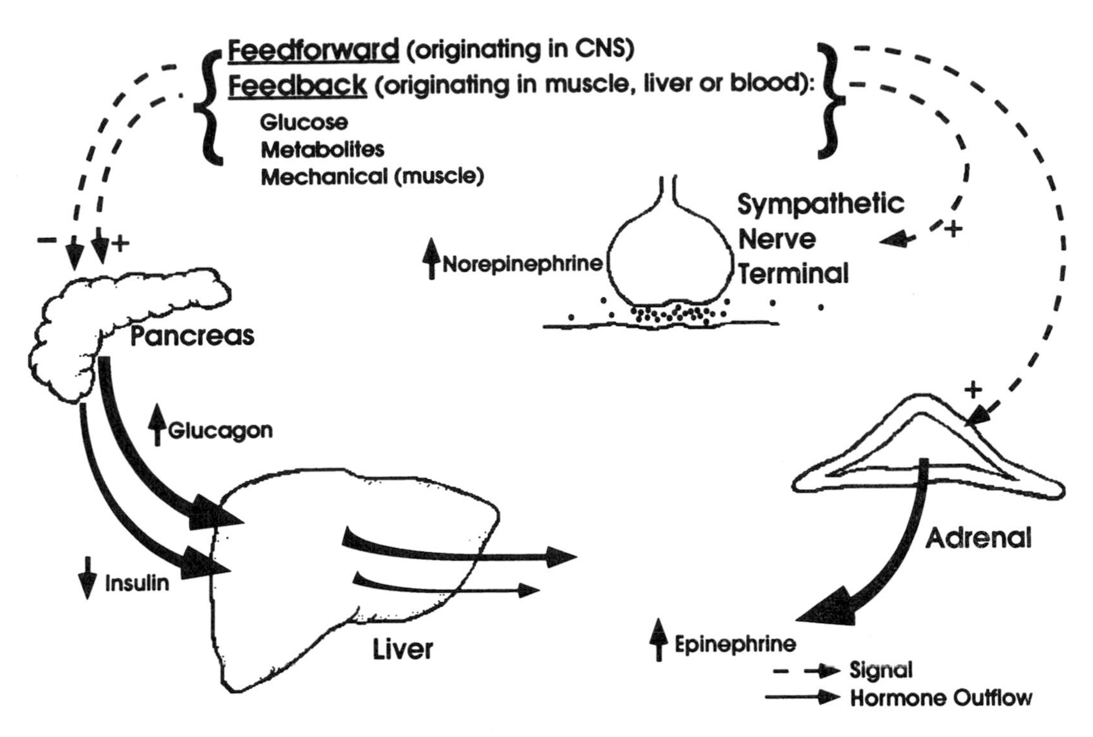

FIG. 23.2. Mechanisms that have been proposed to control the secretion of hormones involved in acute metabolic regulation and the activity of sympathetic nerves during exercise. Glucagon and insulin are secreted from the pancreas into the portal vein after which a percentage is extracted by the liver before reaching the systemic circulation. Sympathetic nerve activity is increased to specific target organs where norepinephrine is released into the synaptic cleft. Norepinephrine levels in the blood represent mainly that which escapes reuptake and spills over from the synaptic cleft.

pharmacological suppression of endogenous insulin secretion (122, 310, 332) or the elimination of endogenous epinephrine (210) by adrenalectomy, constant venous infusions from rest through exercise of the deficient endogenous hormone results in constant levels. This suggests that the clearances of these hormones do not change appreciably during exercise and the mechanism by which their levels are affected is via changes in secretion. Regulation of glucagon clearance is more complex. As addressed in a later section, evidence exists that the efficiency of hepatic glucagon removal may be increased by exercise.

Specific hormone responses are discussed below. Only the hormones that are likely to be involved in the acute regulation of extramuscular fuel metabolism will be discussed. Hormones such as growth hormone and the gonadal hormones are not likely to participate in the acute metabolic response to exercise, but may contribute to the long-term metabolic adaptations. The role of the endocrine system in an adaptive capacity is discussed elsewhere in this *Handbook*.

Insulin Response

The pancreas and the liver are anatomically in series, with the portal vein the conduit between these two organs. Flow through the portal vein comprises the majority (~80%) of the total hepatic blood flow, with arterial flow supplying the balance (104). Since the liver extracts ~50% of the insulin with which it is presented, arterial levels will be less than those at the liver (246). For this reason changes in insulin secretion will lead to smaller changes in arterial insulin levels (304). The reduction in insulin levels with exercise is due to a decrease in β-cell secretion, as evidenced by a fall in C-peptide levels (51, 121, 178, 267, 326), decreased net insulin release from extrahepatic splanchnic tissue (pancreas inclusive) (304), and an increase in plasma insulin-specific activity during isotopic insulin infusion (90). The magnitude of the fall in insulin levels is directly related to work duration. A fall in plasma insulin levels of ~50% is present after 2 h of moderate exercise in postabsorptive subjects (92). The fall in insulin will also increase with more intense exercise, provided that an increase in the blood glucose level does not occur (92). An increase in blood glucose of ~10–20 mg/dl commonly occurs during high-intensity exercise and may attenuate the fall in insulin and perhaps even increase the levels of this hormone slightly (36, 193, 266).

Neural input to the pancreas has been proposed to comprise a component of the effector system that regulates the pancreatic hormone response to exercise. Stimulation of α-adrenergic receptors suppress pancreatic β-cell insulin release (232, 255) and may be directly responsible for the exercise-induced decrease in insulin secretion. This is supported by the demonstration that α-adrenergic blockade prevents the fall in insulin in exercising humans (93, 267). The fall in insulin is retained in human subjects who are adrenalectomized for treatment of pheochromocytoma, again suggesting that the sympathetic nerves mediate this hormonal change (125, 145). The importance of sympathetic nerves is further supported by the demonstration that insulin levels in long-term islet cell autografted dogs are actually increased by exercise (233).

Arterial and portal vein plasma insulin levels are very sensitively regulated by the circulating glucose, level, particularly during exercise (18). It is possible that a decrease in insulin secretion during exercise is a result of small decrements in glycemia (<5 mg/dl) acting on the β-cell either directly or via the sympathetic nervous system. This is supported by the observation cited above that the fall in insulin level may be attenuated or even increased by high-intensity exercise that results in an increase in circulating glucose (36, 193). Glucose sensors exist at the liver, and evidence exists that this site may be important in monitoring blood glucose during exercise (176). A basis for an important role of portal vein/hepatic sensing mechanisms was suggested by the demonstration that hepatic vagotomy attenuates the exercise-induced reduction in insulin and increase in glucagon in the rat (182). Furthermore, a role of portal vein/hepatic glucose sensors is suggested from a study in the dog in which an intraportal glucose infusion of ~2.3 $mg \cdot kg^{-1} \cdot min^{-1}$ results in an *increase* in insulin of about twofold at 60 min of moderate-intensity exercise compared to exercise with an equivalent peripheral vein infusion (176). This study illustrates the potential importance of the portal vein glucose concentration to insulin levels during exercise. A possible role for afferent nerves in mediating this response contrasts, however, with the observation that complete surgical denervation of the liver does not affect the responses of the pancreatic hormones or hepatic glucose production to exercise (167, 271, 311). It is possible that other mechanisms adapt and become important following total hepatic denervation or that the removal of sympathetic nerves compensates for the absence of parasympathetic nerves.

Glucagon Response

Perfusing the liver with pancreatic venous drainage is efficient for glucoregulation, since it permits glucagon to have rapid and potent effects at the liver without the need for excessive glucagon secretion and high arterial levels. This is an efficient arrangement physiologically but adds a degree of difficulty to the assessment of changes in glucagon secretion experimentally. This is because arterial and peripheral venous blood vessels are the only readily accessible sampling sites in conscious human subjects and, as noted earlier, changes in glucagon levels at the liver are not necessarily reflected by those in the systemic circulation, particularly under non–steady-state conditions (230, 268, 302). Increases in arterial and peripheral venous glucagon levels are often small (19, 97, 121, 124) or undetectable (171, 267, 272, 332) in humans after short or moderate duration exercise (less than ~45 min). A decrease in peripheral glucagon levels may even occur during brief bouts of high-intensity exercise (95, 97). Exercise longer than 60 min in duration generally results in an unequivocal increase (5, 19, 92). Studies in dogs with indwelling arterial and portal vein catheters show that arterial glucagon levels greatly underestimate the levels to which the liver is exposed during moderate-intensity exercise (302). The portal vein/arterial glucagon gradient was 15 pg/ml at rest in these studies but was extended to 130 pg/ml during exercise. The widened arterial/portal vein gradient was due primarily to a fivefold increase in net glucagon release from the extrahepatic splanchnic tissue. This increase is consistent with investigations in exercising dogs (309, 310) and humans (122) in which glucagon and insulin secretion rates were suppressed with somatostatin and these hormones were replaced at rates designed to recreate the hepatic response present under these conditions. These studies showed that increases in the glucagon infusion rate of five- and fourfold, respectively, were required. Thus, the measured increase in immunoreactive glucagon release from extrahepatic splanchnic tissue is indistinguishable from the increments in the glucagon infusion rate required to recreate the normal metabolic response of the liver during moderate-intensity exercise. The reason that increases in glucagon release do not translate into proportional increases in arterial levels may be due to an increased hepatic extraction of glucagon by the liver (302). The dissociation of arterial and portal vein glucagon levels observed in the dog emphasizes the need for caution when extrapolating arterial levels to the potential for glucagon action at the liver.

Although extrapancreatic sites in the gastrointestinal tract synthesize and release immunoreactive glucagon, any increase in glucagon during exercise is probably derived from the pancreatic α-cell, since extrapancreatic sources of immunoreactive glucagon are largely unaffected by acute stimuli that regulate the pancreas (185). This is exemplified by the fact that the depancreatized dog, which has normal circulating glucagon levels at rest, does not have increased glucagon during exercise (291, 297).

The importance of the increase in immunoreactive glucagon at the liver is determined by the fraction that is the biologically active 3500 dalton (D) component. In this regard, the larger molecular weight immunoreactive glucagon, which is not biologically active, is not as readily affected by acute stimuli such as exercise (137), epinephrine (185), and changes in glucose availability (183, 282) as the 3500 D molecule. Therefore, any increase in immunoreactive glucagon observed in the plasma with exercise is probably due to an increase in 3500 D glucagon.

As is the case with the exercise-induced fall in insulin, an exercise-induced increase in glucagon is, at least in part, due to adrenergic stimulation (92). In addition, during prolonged exercise, a fall in circulating glucose is probably an important stimulus (94, 98). There are several lines of evidence that support the possibility that adrenergic drive stimulates glucagon release during exercise. First, both α- and/or β-adrenergic stimulation can stimulate glucagon release from pancreatic α-cells (255). Second, adrenergic blockade attenuates the increment in arterial glucagon during exercise in animal models (114, 188). Finally, splanchnic nerve section reduces the glucagon response to exercise in the dog (101). The view that glucose is an important determinant of the glucagon response to exercise is supported by the demonstration that the rise in glucagon is abolished when glucose is ingested prior to (4) or during (3, 189) exercise and results in an increase in blood glucose. In contrast to these findings in humans, a recent study conducted in the dog showed that glucagon rose normally during exercise even when glucose was infused at a rate designed to mimic the increase in glucose utilization (18). The lack of an effect of the glucose infusion may have been due to the very small changes in glucose that were present (<5 mg/dl greater than normal exercise levels) or, possibly, due to the presence of a species difference. Regardless, the results of this study suggest that an increase in glucagon during exercise in the dog does not require feedback from circulating glucose. It has been proposed that the initial signal for the exercise-induced rise in glucagon originates in the portal circulation or at the liver, since hepatic vagotomy blunts the response in rats (182). As is the case with the insulin response, surgical denervation of the liver that removes afferent as well as efferent nerves does not affect the glucagon response.

Catecholamine Responses

Epinephrine secretion from the adrenal medulla increases with exercise, resulting in elevated circulating levels of this hormone (92). The magnitude of this increase is directly related to the duration and intensity of exercise. In one study, for example, epinephrine had risen by about twofold after 30 min of moderate-intensity exercise (60% of the maximum O_2 uptake) and by about tenfold after 3 h (5). The relationship between exercise intensity and epinephrine response is such that increments in work rate above ~50% of the maximum O_2 uptake (roughly above the lactate threshold) are far greater than similar increments constrained to be below this work rate (97). During exhaustive exercise at 100% of the subject's maximum O_2 uptake, epinephrine can increase by as much as 10- to 20-fold in less than 15 min (193).

Norepinephrine is also released from the adrenal medulla (80). More importantly, norepinephrine is released from sympathetic nerve endings, resulting in very high levels in sympathetic synaptic clefts (80). Exercise is a well recognized means of increasing sympathetic nerve activity (92, 286). Existing evidence supports the contention that sympathetic nerve activity is increased to the two major extramuscular fuel depots, liver (321) and adipose tissue (261). As is the case with the response of epinephrine to exercise, the norepinephrine response is also directly related to exercise duration and intensity (92). The response of norepinephrine is different from the epinephrine response in two ways. The norepinephrine response occurs both more rapidly during constant-load exercise (94, 312) and more markedly at low work rates (97). Studies using ^{3}H-norepinephrine have shown that the increase in circulating norepinephrine during low-intensity exercise is due to an increased release, as norepinephrine clearance is unaffected (184). A reduction in norepinephrine clearance may make a small contribution to the increase in norepinephrine levels with high-intensity exercise (184). The signal for the increase in adrenergic drive during exercise has not been fully established. It has been shown that an intraportal glucose infusion that has no effect on arterial glucose attenuates the exercise-induced increase in norepinephrine, suggesting that the response is due to a metabolic signal initiated in the portal venous circulation or at the liver (176). These findings are supported by the demonstration that preventing the fall in blood glucose during prolonged exercise attenuates the increase in epinephrine (94) and is consistent with the observation that a prolonged fast accentuates the rise in catecholamines with exercise (95).

EXTRAMUSCULAR FUEL SOURCES

There are two primary extramuscular fuel depots in postabsorptive humans. These are the adipose tissue and liver. Adipose tissue stores pure triglyceride to such a great extent that it can comprise greater than 80% of the adipocyte volume. In response to lipoytic agents, NEFAs are released from adipose tissue, bound to albumin, and made available to other tissues. The liver stores glycogen in high concentrations and contains the enzymatic machinery necessary to mobilize it as glucose. The liver also has a high capacity for gluconeogenesis and, by this mechanism, provides a second source of glucose for the cells of the body. Physical exercise can lead to the stimulation of fuel mobilization from each of these depots. Although both fuel stores are essential for sustained muscular work, the bases for their essentiality are clearly different. Adipose tissue is important by virtue of its size. Contained in the cells of this tissue are greater than 95% of the body's fuel stores (discounting the contribution of endogenous protein). The liver, on the other hand, has two important metabolic roles. First, the liver is the only net source of glucose in the body. This, of course, is important because glucose is the obligate fuel for the central nervous system (CNS) as well as certain other tissues. Furthermore, a requisite rate of glycolysis is necessary in skeletal muscle and other tissues to provide metabolic intermediates for β-oxidation of fatty acids. The second important function of the liver in fuel metabolism is its ability to scavenge metabolic by-products and metabolize them or recycle the component atoms. The rate at which glucose is released by the liver and NEFAs are released by adipose tissue during muscular work will depend on a number of factors (health, nutritional state, body composition), the most important of which are the exercise intensity and duration.

Because of the sizeable fat stores contained within adipose tissue, the supply of NEFAs for the working muscle is, for all intents and purposes, limitless. In marked contrast, prolonged exercise may lead to hepatic glycogen depletion and reduce the ability of the liver to supply glucose, which may lead to hypoglycemia and result in exhaustion. Hepatic glycogen depletion and the associated deficits can be circumvented by carbohydrate ingestion. This, in effect, makes the gastrointestinal tract an important third source of fuel for the working muscle.

Two other extramuscular processes may have roles in substrate metabolism in postabsorptive individuals. First, the liver, besides supplying glucose, produces the vast majority of lipoprotein and, as a consequence, is the chief source of circulating triglyceride. Second, tissues of the splanchnic bed are characterized by the highest protein turnover rates in the body and contain a labile protein pool that can be mobilized during exercise. Amino acid metabolism can only account for a small percentage of the O_2 uptake of the working limb and it does so most notably when exercise duration is protracted. The importance of splanchnic amino acid metabolism probably rests with its capacity to increase the supply of substrates for liver gluconeogenesis and/or protein synthesis or with its role in nitrogen metabolism.

NEFA MOBILIZATION FROM ADIPOSE TISSUE

Basic Mechanisms that Influence NEFA Availability

NEFA mobilization from adipose tissue is determined by the activities of two opposing nonequilibrium reactions (31, 219). These two reactions form a substrate cycle, the rate of which depends on the rate that triglycerides are hydrolyzed to glycerol and NEFAs (lipolysis) and the rate of at which NEFAs are reesterified to glycerol 3-phosphate with the formation of triglycerides (reesterification). Substrate cycling is a means of causing large changes in substrate flux without extreme activation or inactivation of any one reaction (220). The function of this substrate cycle during exercise is to amplify the rate that NEFAs are mobilized from adipose tissue. Triglyceride-NEFA substrate cycles are illustrated schematically in Figure 23.3. In response to exercise both limbs of the substrate cycle, lipolysis and reesterification, are modified in such a way as to increase the flux of NEFAs into the blood. The stimulation of lipolysis, however, is considerably more important. The intracellular events that lead to an increase in lipolysis begin with the formation of cyclic adenosine monophosphate (cAMP) (245). cAMP, in turn, activates a protein kinase that phosphorylates, thereby activating, hormone-sensitive lipase (131, 132). Hormone-sensitive lipase catalyzes the hydrolysis of triglycerides to three molecules of NEFAs and one of glycerol (285). This reaction is rate limiting and, therefore, of major importance in lipolysis (275). These reactions are stimulated by catecholamines (245) and inhibited by insulin (275) after interaction with their respective cell surface receptors.

Reesterification requires the activation of NEFA to acyl-CoA by the enzyme acyl CoA synthetase and the presence of glycerol 3-phosphate (31, 216). One aspect of the latter requirement is particularly notable. The adipocyte lacks the enzyme glycerokinase and, as a result, cannot utilize glycerol released in

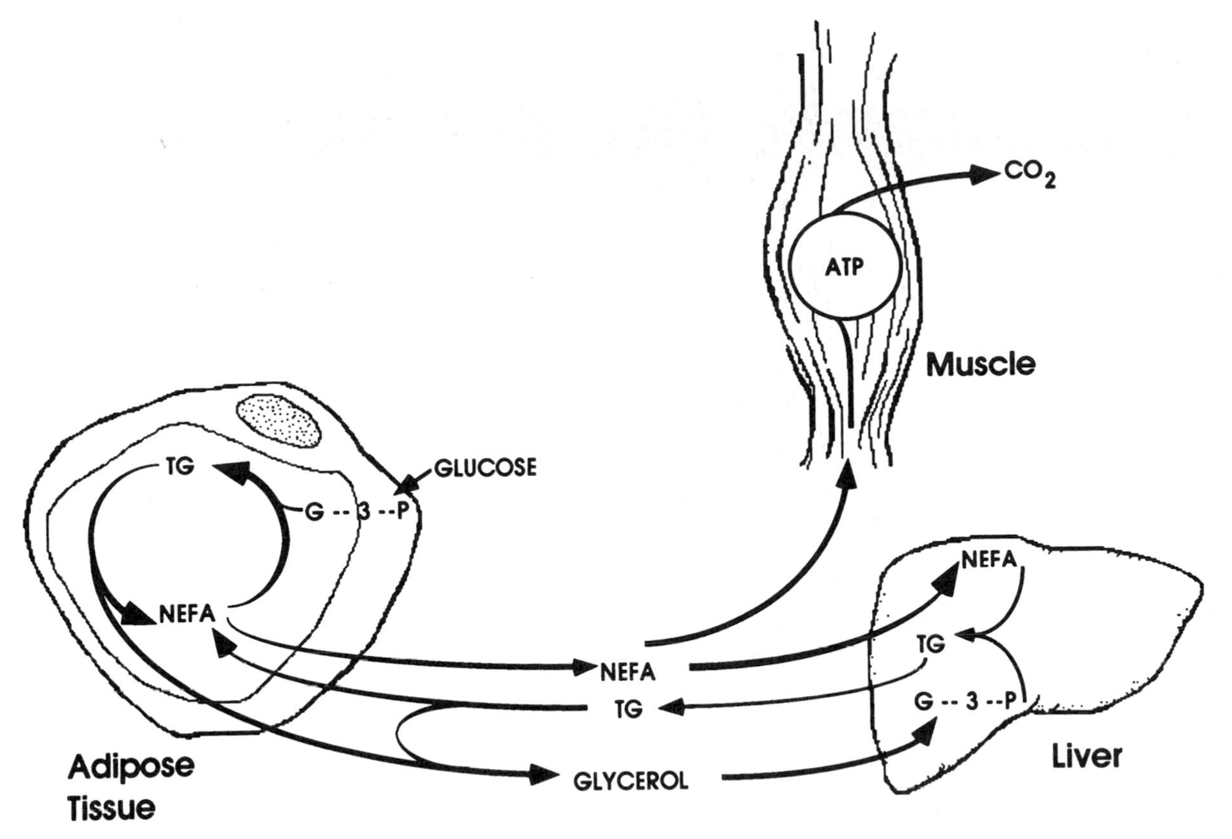

FIG. 23.3. Pathways involved in the regulation of NEFA mobilization and availability to working muscle. Substrate cycling occurs due to concurrent lipolysis in adipocytes and re-esterification in liver (see HEPATIC FAT METABOLISM: OXIDATION AND TRIGLYCERIDE SYNTHESIS) and adipocytes. These cycles increase the sensitivity of NEFA fluxes to regulatory factors. TG refers to triglycerides. [Adapted from Wolfe and George (329).]

lipolysis (262). Consequently, glycerol 3-phosphate must be derived from the glycolytic metabolism of glucose. The availability of glycerol 3-phosphate is limiting for reesterification (31). Any factor, such as insulin, that stimulates glycolysis in the adipocyte may enhance reesterification (31). Triglycerides are formed from acyl-CoA and glycerol 3-phosphate in acyltransferase reactions (216). Studies using stable isotope methodology have estimated that NEFA reesterification in the adipocyte is 20% and 12% of the lipolytic rate in humans at rest and during prolonged exercise, respectively (331). As a result of this reduction, more NEFAs leave the cell and are available for metabolism in the working muscle.

Regulatory Factors

Lipolytic rate and NEFA mobilization, as determined by the increase in blood glycerol levels and isotopic techniques, increase with the onset of moderate-intensity exercise (331). Arterial NEFA levels, however, increase gradually (153, 305, 331). The slower time course for the rise in plasma NEFA levels reflects an increase in the clearance of this fuel, presumably by the working muscle, since the percentage of NEFAs that are reesterified is actually reduced (331). As mentioned above, the two main regulators of lipolysis are the stimulatory effects of catecholamines and the inhibitory effects of insulin. It is, in fact, the β-adrenergic effects of the catecholamines (8, 133, 295) and the fall in insulin (305) that are important during muscular work. Circulating NEFA levels are diminished during exercise by β-adrenergic blockade (124, 133, 267). A parallel reduction in tracer-determined glycerol appearance indicates that this is due to a suppression of lipolytic activity (133). The exercise-induced increase in NEFA levels is retained in adrenalectomized (or adrenodemedullated) animals (210, 261, 325) and humans (125), suggesting that norepinephrine released from the sympathetic nerves is the important lipolytic stimulus. The mechanism by which catecholamines stimulate lipolysis is related not only to an increase in sympathetic nerve activity but also to an increased efficacy of β-adrenergic stimulation (295). Adipocytes taken from human subjects following exercise have an increased lipolytic responsiveness to catecholamines that is mediated through β-adrenergic mechanisms (295). This effect occurs without an increase in the binding of the β-receptor–specific catecholamine, ^{125}I-cyanopindolol, suggesting that a step distal to ligand binding is expected. Prevention of the exercise-induced fall in insulin with an exogenous infusion of the hormone also attenuates the increase in arterial NEFA levels (122, 305). Since this is accompanied by a diminished increase in circulating glycerol levels, it is likely that the fall in insulin increases NEFA levels, at least in part, by stimulating lipolysis (305). Nevertheless, the possibility of a decrease in reesterification resulting from the exercise-induced fall in insulin cannot be excluded. The ability of small changes in insulin to affect NEFA availability during exercise may be facilitated by an increase in insulin action at the adipocyte (15, 174, 299). An experiment in human subjects demonstrated that moderate-intensity exercise results in a twofold increase in the absolute magnitude of insulin-induced suppression of plasma NEFA levels (299).

In contrast to the importance of NEFA mobilization from adipose tissue during moderate-intensity exercise, its role during high-intensity exercise is considerably less. Despite the increased adrenergic drive that is present during high-intensity work, the arterial NEFA levels and the rate of NEFA appearance into the blood decrease (151). The contributions of a diminished lipolytic response and increased rate of reesterification to the diminished increase in NEFA mobilization have not been examined (151, 292). It is notable, in this regard, that blood glycerol levels may still rise during heavy exercise. One explanation for this apparent discrepancy is that the increased blood glycerol levels are due to release from triglycerides within the working muscle and the NEFA, that are liberated in the process are oxidized locally, within the muscle.

There are several regulatory factors that could explain the diminished capacity for NEFA mobilization in the presence of strong adrenergic drive. One such mechanism may relate to the marked increase in lactate that occurs under these conditions. High lactate levels inhibit lipase activation in vitro (23) and in vivo (28, 136) and it appears that during high-intensity exercise inhibitory concentrations are attained. High lactate levels may also decrease NEFA levels by increasing the reesterification rate (136). Circulating glucose levels may increase during heavy exercise (193) and thereby stimulate reesterification and decrease NEFA release from adipose tissue. If the increase in glucose prevents the exercise-induced fall in insulin, it may also work to inhibit NEFA mobilization through the actions of this hormone (305). It has also been postulated that a reduction in adipose tissue blood flow may contribute to the reduction in circulating NEFA levels during exercise (249).

Lipolysis is not regulated homogenously in all human adipose tissue. Adipose tissue in the femoral and gluteal regions, for example, is less lipolytically active than abdominal subcutaneous adipose tissue (8, 160, 269). Intra-abdominal depots seem particularly sensitive to lipolytic stimuli (223) and are relatively insensitive to insulin (26). This is consistent with the demonstration that the exercise-induced release of glycerol from abdominal fat depots is about two- to threefold greater than release from gluteal fat depots in humans as determined by a microdialysis technique (8). There also appears to be a significant gender difference in the lipolytic response to exercise. This is evident by the twofold greater release of glycerol from abdominal adipose tissue of women compared to men (8). The ability to mobilize NEFAs during exercise may also be affected by the presence of obesity. For example, women characterized by upper body obesity have a 50% reduction in the exercise-induced increase in NEFA availability in comparison to women with lower body obesity (153). This may reflect an impairment in catecholamine-stimulated NEFA mobilization of intra-abdominal fat stores (148).

HEPATIC GLUCOSE PRODUCTION

Exercise Response

The sum of exercise-induced increments in hepatic glycogenolysis and gluconeogenesis closely approximates the increased rate of muscle glucose utilization and, as a result, arterial glucose is maintained within narrow limits. The importance of this coupling process is illustrated by the precipitous fall in circulating glucose that would result if hepatic glucose production did not increase in synchrony with glucose utilization. Glucose utilization may rise by 3 $mg \cdot kg^{-1} \cdot min^{-1}$ in response to just moderate-intensity exercise. If the liver did not respond to the exercise stimulus, blood glucose levels would decrease at a rate of ~1.5 mg/dl every minute and overt hypoglycemia would be present in just 30 min.

Hepatic glycogenolysis is determined by the degree of activation of the enzyme, phosphorylase *a* (118). Activation occurs due to the phosphorylation of the inactive enzyme, phosphorylase *b* (328), and is stimulated by at least two basic cascade systems. A number of effectors (glucagon, β-adrenergic stimulation, vasoactive intestinal polypeptide, secretin) act by stimulation of adenylate cyclase and the formation of cAMP (118). These activate cAMP-dependent protein kinase and ultimately result in an increase in phosphorylase *a* (82). The second cascade system is initiated by α-adrenergic stimulation and involves an increase in the concentration of cytosolic Ca^{2+} ions (118). In contrast to hepatic glycogenolysis in which stimulation is brought about by an increase in phosphorylase *a* activity within the liver, the means by which gluconeogenesis is stimulated involves diverse mechanisms. Gluconeogenesis is regulated by mechanisms that influence gluconeogenic precursor delivery to, extraction by, and efficiency of conversion to glucose within the liver [Figure 23.4; (47)]. Exercise stimulates all three of these processes. Accelerated rates of protein breakdown, lipolysis, and glycolysis increase amino acid, glycerol, lactate, and pyruvate production and may enhance their hepatic availability. The hepatic fractional extraction of gluconeogenic amino acids is increased in response to exercise, indicating that amino acid transport systems are stimulated (84, 300, 312). Hepatic alanine extraction increases gradually with exercise (84, 312), whereas the extraction of glutamine increases promptly (300). Alanine and glutamine are transported across the liver plasma membrane by the A- and N-transport systems, respectively (47). The relatively different time course for the increase in net fractional extraction of these amino acids may reflect differential regulation of these transport systems by exercise. Evidence that intrahepatic gluconeogenic mechanisms are stimulated during exercise is twofold. First, gluconeogenic enzyme activities [e.g., phospho*enol*pyruvate carboxykinase (PEPCK), fructose-1,6-bisphosphatase, glucose 6-phosphatase] are elevated (73, 74, 130), whereas the activity of the glycolytic enzyme, phosphofructokinase, is diminished by exercise (73). Second, the intrahepatic gluconeogenic efficiency, as determined by the fraction of ^{14}C-alanine consumed by the liver that is channeled into ^{14}C-glucose, is increased (312). The mechanism for the increase in intrahepatic gluconeogenic efficiency may be due, at

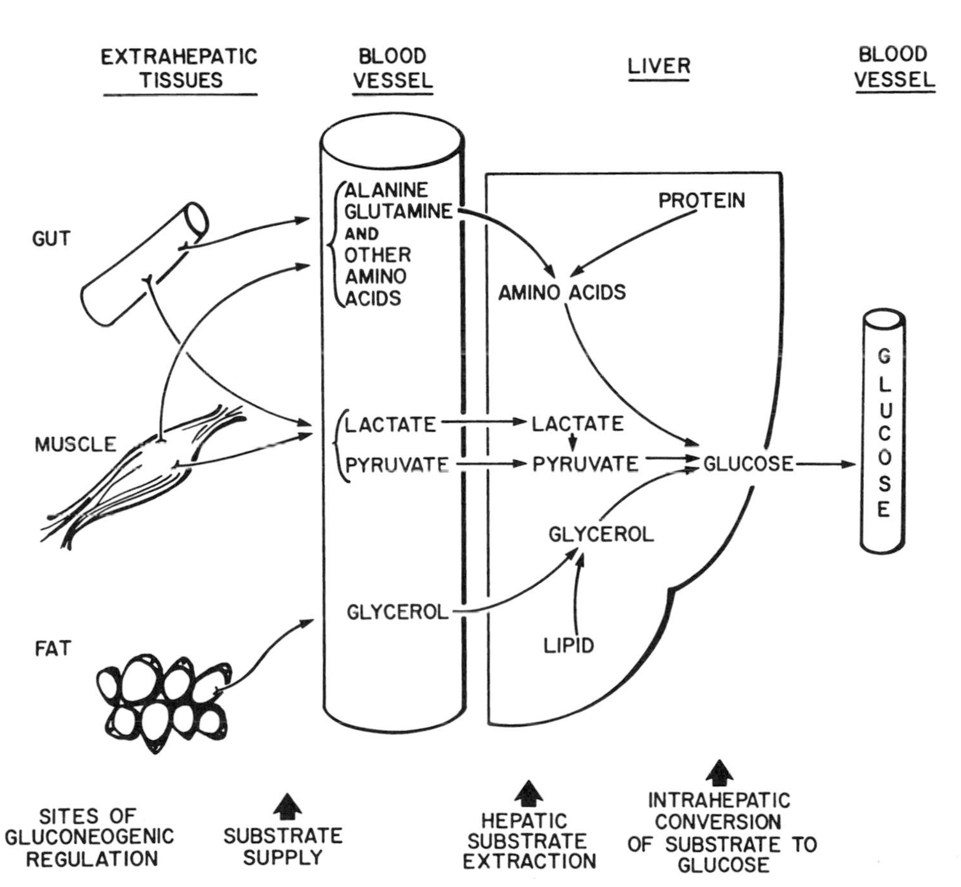

FIG. 23.4. Gluconeogenic regulation during exercise. Gluconeogenesis is increased during exercise as accelerated rates of protein degradation, lipolysis, and glycolysis lead to increased rates of amino acid, glycerol, lactate, and pyruvate production and subsequent delivery to the liver. The hepatic extraction of gluconeogenic precursors is enhanced by exercise, as is the efficiency of intrahepatic conversion of precursors into glucose. The importance of each of these regulatory sites is determined by the intensity and duration of exercise and the absorptive state of the subject. [Modified from Cherrington (47).]

least in part, to increases in the transcription of genes that encode key gluconeogenic enzymes. Exercise in mice results in an increase in PEPCK gene transcription and leads to a threefold rise in liver PEPCK mRNA after just 30 min (91). The mechanism for the increase in PEPCK gene transcription may be related to the parallel increases in the transcription of the genes for the nuclear proteins, CCAAT/enhancer-binding protein β and C-jun, both of which stimulate this process (91).

One site of regulation that is common to hepatic glycogenolysis and gluconeogenesis is the substrate cycle that is regulated by glucokinase and glucose 6-phosphatase activity and interconverts glucose to glucose 6-phosphate within the liver (220). As discussed previously, the existence of a substrate cycle may amplify flux through a pathway. A study that used stable isotope methodology in exercising humans showed that the rate of substrate cycling between glucose and glucose 6-phosphate remains a constant fraction of the total glucose flux during rest and exercise (313). This suggests that, whereas glucose production can respond extremely quickly to large increases in energy requirement, substrate cycling does not have an important role in amplifying the response.

The relative contributions of hepatic glycogenolysis and gluconeogenesis are determined by the duration and intensity of exercise and the absorptive state of the subject. In overnight-fasted humans and dogs (both of whom have substantial liver glycogen stores), the initial increment in hepatic glucose production that occurs with exercise is due almost entirely to an increase in glycogenolysis (292, 312). The magnitude of the early increase in hepatic glycogenolysis in the dog is evident by the large glycolytic flux that may result in hepatic lactate output, particularly during the transition from rest to exercise (306). Wahren and colleagues concluded, by summing the splanchnic lactate, pyruvate, glycerol, and amino acid uptakes, that gluconeogenesis does not contribute significantly to the increase in splanchnic glucose output evident at 40 min of light, moderate, or heavy exercise in overnight-fasted humans even if the liver channels all of the gluconeogenic precursor carbons into glucose (292). Measurements of splanchnic balance in the exercising dog yield results similar to those obtained in humans (300, 312). The ability to measure net hepatic (rather than splanchnic) balance in the dog, coupled with isotopic methods, has allowed more accurate estimates of the exercise-induced increase in gluconeogenesis. If the hepatic uptakes of all gluconeogenic precursors are summed it is apparent that gluconeogenesis may contribute at the most 15% to the increment in glucose production at 30 min of exercise in the overnight-fasted dog (300, 312). Based on the proportion of ^{14}C-alanine extracted by the liver and converted to ^{14}C-glucose, a minimum estimate of the intrahepatic efficiency with which extracted precursors are converted to glucose can be obtained. Isotope dilution in the oxaloacetate pool, which is common to gluconeogenic and oxidative processes, prevents precise determination of gluconeogenic efficiency using this method. Results obtained by using this isotopic technique indicate that a minimum of one-third of the precursors extracted by the liver are channeled into glucose after 30 min of exercise (312). Thus, minimum (total hepatic precursor uptake $\times$ intrahepatic gluconeogenic efficiency) and maximum (total hepatic precursor uptake) estimates of gluconeogenesis indicate that between 5% and 15% of the increment in hepatic glucose production is due to this pathway at this interval. Gluconeogenesis becomes increasingly more important with more prolonged exercise as hepatic glycogen stores decrease, comprising 18%–22% of the increase in glucose production after 150 min of moderate exercise in the overnight-fasted dog (300, 312). The greater gluconeogenic rate is due, in part, to increases in hepatic gluconeogenic precursor delivery and fractional extraction. Moreover, the intrahepatic gluconeogenic efficiency is nearly maximal, rising by about threefold. Almost all the glucose produced gluconeogenically by the liver over a 150 min exercise period in the dog is released, as less than 2% of the label from ^{14}C-alanine that was incorporated into ^{14}C-glucose is detectable in glycogen (312). When the exercise duration is extended to 4 h in overnight-fasted human subjects, it can be calculated using splanchnic balances that gluconeogenesis comprises 45% of the total glucose output if it is assumed that the liver is 100% efficient at channeling precursor into glucose (6). In the postexercise state, gluconeogenesis remains high, as the increases in gluconeogenic precursor uptake (5, 312) and intrahepatic gluconeogenic efficiency (312) persist. The gluconeogenic response during 150 min of exercise and 90 min of exercise recovery, as compiled from studies in the dog (300, 312), is presented schematically in Figure 23.5.

The increase in gluconeogenesis observed with prolonged exercise plays a key role in delaying the depletion of liver and muscle glycogen by transforming the energy provided by hepatic fat oxidation to the conversion of amino acids, glycerol, pyruvate, and lactate to glucose. This is exemplified by the more rapid depletion of liver and muscle glycogen and a reduced endurance time when gluconeogenesis is inhibited with mercaptopicolinic acid in rats (150,

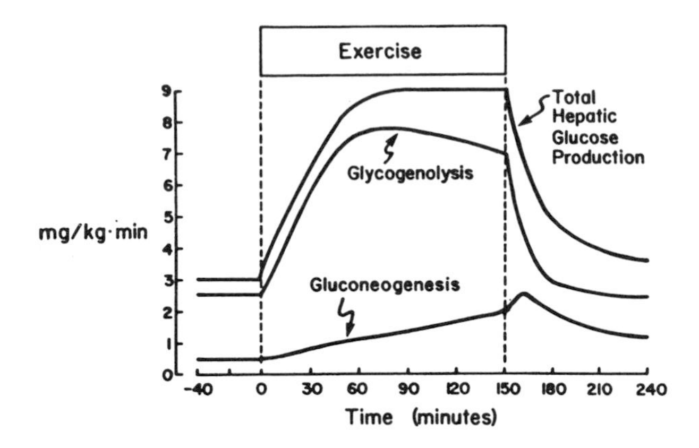

FIG. 23.5. Schematic representation of the minimal glycogenolytic and maximal gluconeogenic contributions to total glucose production during rest, exercise, and recovery. These responses are based on studies in the overnight-fasted dog (300, 312). [From Wasserman and Cherrington (298).]

281). The importance of gluconeogenesis during prolonged exercise in humans is illustrated by the ~30% reduction in splanchnic glucose output that occurs after 3 h of exercise in the presence of an ethanol infusion that inhibits splanchnic gluconeogenic substrate uptake by ~50% (152).

The importance of exercise intensity as a determinant of glucose flux is illustrated by the increased hepatic glucose output that occurs with more strenuous work (57, 292). As shown in Figure 23.1, the increase in hepatic glucose production per increase in work intensity is greater at higher work rates (57). Furthermore, exercise in anemic subjects (105, 308) or in subjects breathing air with a reduced fraction of inspired O_2 (58) stimulates glucose fluxes relative to controls even when the energy requirement is not different. The added increment in glucose production that occurs with heavy exercise is due generally to an increased rate of hepatic glycogenolysis (292). Nevertheless, measurements of splanchnic gluconeogenic precursor uptake indicate that if heavy exercise can be sustained, gluconeogenesis will likely become important more rapidly because the finite glycogen stores will deplete at a faster rate and hormonal signals will be greater (5, 6).

Regulation by the Endocrine Pancreas

The role of glucagon in the regulation of hepatic glucose production during exercise was initially assessed by examining the effects of suppressing this hormone below basal levels using somatostatin. Studies in the dog demonstrated that glucagon suppression results in a reduction in hepatic glucose production and a fall in circulating glucose that is normalized by glucagon replacement (137). This finding is in agreement with studies conducted in exercising sheep that showed that a somatostatin-induced attenuation of the normal rise in glucagon results in a smaller rise in glucose production and a relative reduction in glucose levels (30). The results obtained with somatostatin-induced glucagon suppression were further substantiated by the observation that rats treated with glucagon antibodies exhibit a reduction in exercise-stimulated hepatic glycogen breakdown (242). Although these studies demonstrated that the presence of glucagon is necessary for normal glucoregulation during exercise, compensatory changes elicited in response to a reduction in glycemia prevented the determination of a quantitative role for the hormone. Subsequent studies in the dog established the physiological role of glucagon during exercise, as well as the role of counterregulation, which occurs in its absence (307). These studies demonstrated, by suppressing glucagon with somatostatin and preventing counterregulation by clamping glucose, that this hormone is necessary for over 60% of the total glucose production during exercise. This percentage is similar to that observed under resting conditions in dogs (50) and humans (186); however, because hepatic glucose production is so much greater during exercise, the absolute role of glucagon is greater. Furthermore, it was determined that counterregulatory mechanisms that occurred when glucose was allowed to fall could compensate for ~40% of the deficit in hepatic glucose production created by glucagon deficiency.

Although the studies cited above demonstrate that glucagon is important in regulating glucose production during exercise, they do not differentiate between the role of basal glucagon and the added glucagon that is released. The role of the increase in glucagon and the fall in insulin has been examined in exercising humans by infusing somatostatin to suppress endogenous insulin and glucagon release and then by replacing these hormones via a peripheral vein at rates designed to recreate normal basal arterial levels during rest and throughout exercise (122, 166, 332). This approach prevents exercise-induced changes in peripheral glucagon and insulin. Under these conditions the increase in hepatic glucose production is attenuated and plasma glucose falls by ~25–50 mg/dl within 60 min of moderate-intensity exercise despite a large compensatory increase in the catecholamines (122, 166, 332). The conclusion from these studies was that changes in glucagon and/or insulin are essential to the maintenance of glucose homeostasis during exercise. Subsequently, the pancreatic clamp technique was used to study the role of the exercise-induced changes in glucagon and insulin independently in humans. Selective deletion of either the exercise-induced fall in insulin or rise in glucagon led to a 30 mg/dl fall in plasma glucose within 60 min (122). This approach may have overestimated the essential nature of the roles of glucagon and insulin, since the use of somatostatin may have prevented compensatory changes in glucagon and insulin when the fall in insulin and rise in glucagon, respectively, were eliminated.

The experiments described above show the important role of changes in glucagon and insulin to the increment in hepatic glucose production during moderate-intensity exercise. They did not, however, define the precise role for these hormones, since once again hypoglycemia ensued. Studies during treadmill exercise in the dog determined the role of these hormone changes in the presence of euglycemia (304, 310). Furthermore, arteriovenous differences and isotopic techniques were combined in the dog model to determine hepatic glycogenolysis and gluconeogenesis, differentially. An additional advantage in using the dog to investigate the role of glucagon and insulin is that these hormones can be replaced at their physiological entry site, the portal vein, thus preserving their normal portal/peripheral gradient. To selectively determine the role of the exercise-induced increment in glucagon, somatostatin was infused to suppress endogenous pancreatic hormone release and glucagon was replaced at a basal rate during rest and was either maintained at resting values or increased to simulate the normal response during exercise (310). Insulin was replaced intraportally at basal rates at rest and with the normal fall in this hormone simulated during exercise. Circulating glucose levels were clamped to prevent the confounding effects of hypoglycemic counterregulation. These studies showed that just as the *total* glucagon level controls ~60% of the *total* rate of hepatic glucose production during exercise (307), the *exercise-induced increment* in glucagon controls ~60% of the *exercise-induced increment* in glucose production. Furthermore, it was determined that the rise in glucagon is necessary for the full increment in both hepatic glycogenolysis and gluconeogenesis (determined by the rate of conversion of ^{14}C-alanine to ^{14}C-glucose). This stimulatory effect of glucagon on gluconeogenesis was due to an accelerated rate of gluconeogenic precursor extraction by the liver and enhanced channeling of precursor to glucose within the liver (Fig. 23.6).

The role of the fall in the insulin level was elucidated by infusing insulin intraportally at a rate designed to prevent the decrease in this hormone during treadmill exercise in the dog (304). Glucose levels were clamped throughout the exercise period. In the absence of the fall in insulin, the exercise-induced rise in glucagon was attenuated and the increases in both hepatic glycogenolysis and gluconeogenesis were impaired. When the normal exercise-induced glucagon levels were restored with an intraportal infusion of the hormone, the full role of the fall in insulin was manifest. Under this condition, the fall in insulin controlled 55% of the increase in hepatic glucose production. This stimulatory effect was almost entirely related to hepatic glycogenolysis, as the change in insulin had only a small effect on the intrahepatic gluconeogenic efficiency. When the fall in insulin was prevented and glucose levels were not clamped, severe hypoglycemia was prevented by the increase in the counterregulatory hormones, which stimulated hepatic glycogenolysis and gluconeogenesis (303). The compensatory increase in gluconeogenesis was due to effects on hepatic gluconeogenic precursor delivery and extraction, as well as an increase in intrahepatic gluconeogenic efficiency. The advantage to preventing the fall in insulin using this approach, in which somatostatin was not used, is that counterregulation due to the compensatory glucagon response is intact. It is likely that glucagon is an important component of the counterregulatory response, since the effects on hepatic gluconeogenic precursor extraction and efficiency are both hallmark effects of glucagon. Second, if the glucagon response is prevented under similar conditions in humans, the fall in glucose is approximately threefold more rapid. Thus, whereas the fall in insulin has an important physiological role at the liver, effective counterregulation partially compensates for the absence of the exercise-induced decrease in this hormone and the fall in glucose is minimized.

The discussion above reflects the importance of changes in glucagon and insulin in accounting for virtually the entire increment in hepatic glycogenolysis and gluconeogenesis during moderate-intensity exercise. Whereas changes in glucagon and insulin are individually very important, several lines of evidence indicate that it is the interaction of these changes that is most critical (298). First, although changes in glucagon and insulin are both well correlated to the increase in hepatic glucose production, the ratio between glucagon and insulin exhibits the strongest correlation to this variable (134, 307). Second, the increment in glucagon controls about fourfold more of the increment in glucose production when insulin is allowed to fall compared to when it is maintained at basal levels (304, 310). Hence, during exercise, as is the case at rest (49), a fall in insulin sensitizes the liver to the effects of glucagon. Third, in the absence of biologically active glucagon,

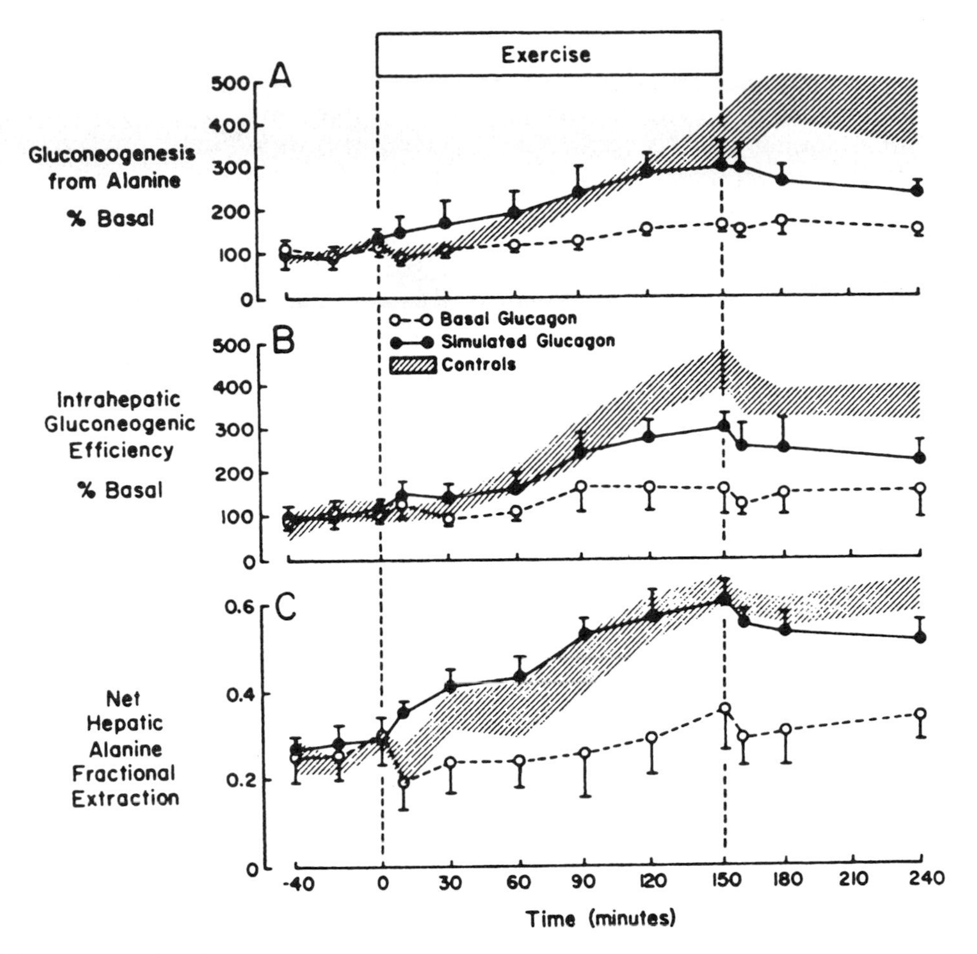

FIG. 23.6. Role of the exercise-induced increase in glucagon in gluconeogenic regulation. Effect of exercise alone *(shaded area)*, exercise with somatostatin + simulated glucagon and insulin *(solid line)* and somatostatin + basal glucagon and simulated insulin *(dashed line)* on *(A)* gluconeogenic conversion from alanine; *(B)* intrahepatic gluconeogenic efficiency from alanine; and *(C)* hepatic fractional alanine extraction. The exercise-induced increment in glucagon increases gluconeogenesis by stimulating the gluconeogenic precursor extraction by the liver and channeling into glucose within the liver. Data are mean ± SE. [Modified from Wasserman et al. (310).]

the exercise-induced fall in insulin does not stimulate hepatic glucose production (338). This suggests that the fall in insulin acts by potentiating the actions of glucagon. Finally, the roles of the increase in glucagon and the fall in insulin determined individually sum to control over 100% of the total increment in glucose production (304, 310). This implies that an overlap in the mechanisms of action of these hormones exists.

Role of Epinephrine

Epinephrine can stimulate hepatic glucose production independent of changes in the pancreatic hormones (48, 253). The majority of the literature indicates, however, that epinephrine is not an important determinant of the increase in hepatic glucose production, at least during moderate-intensity exercise of less than 90 min duration (reviewed in 298). While adrenodemedullation in the rat has been shown to reduce hepatic glycogenolysis (241) and tracer-determined glucose production (271) during exercise in some studies, most studies in this model indicate that the absence of epinephrine has no effect on the liver (7, 40, 103, 191, 324, 325). The results of studies in adrenalectomized rats have been difficult to interpret in terms of establishing a direct physiological role for epinephrine, since these animals generally have elevated arterial insulin levels (7, 40, 241, 242, 271, 324), whereas the increase in arterial glucagon can be augmented (7, 324), reduced (191, 241), or normal (40, 271). Furthermore, it is also possible that an augmented sympathetic drive may compensate for a deficiency of epinephrine. Nevertheless, human subjects adrenalectomized for treatment of Cushing's disease or bilateral pheochromocytoma have a normal increase in glucose production during 60 min of moderate-intensity exercise even when the pancreatic hormone changes are similar to those in normal controls (125). Similarly, glucose production was the same for the first 120 min of muscular work in adrenalectomized dogs receiving basal and exercise-simulated epinephrine replacement (210). The rise in epinephrine, however, controlled a significant proportion of the increase in glucose output from 120–150 min of exercise. This stimulatory effect of epinephrine occurred even though the glucagon and insulin responses were normal. Since epinephrine stimulates glucose production only after prolonged exercise when gluconeogenesis is accelerated and it coincides with a diminished arterial lactate response, one can speculate that the effect of epinephrine is to facilitate gluconeogenic substrate mobilization from peripheral sites. This hypothesis is supported by the increased importance of epinephrine to glucoregulation in fasted rats, which are far more reliant on gluconeogenesis (324). It may be that epinephrine may have to reach a critically high level, such as it does with prolonged or heavy exercise (92), to play a role in the regulation of glucose production.

Role of Sympathetic Nerve Activity and Norepinephrine

Hepatic nerves have been proposed to have an important function in the stimulation of hepatic glucose production during exercise based on two premises. First, an increase in phosphorylase *a* activity (113, 265) and hepatic glycogenolysis (99, 113, 181) occur with direct stimulation of the nerves to the liver, presumably caused by α- and β-adrenergic receptor activation. Second, the exercise-induced increase in hepatic glucose production is more rapid than changes in arterial glucagon, insulin, and epinephrine levels (92) [although portal vein glucagon may rise more rapidly (302)] . The first observation establishes the potential of hepatic nerves to control hepatic glucose production, while the second implies that a factor other than arterial glucoregulatory hormone levels may be important during exercise. Despite the circumstantial evidence that seems to implicate the sympathetic nerves, no role during exercise has been demonstrated. Combined α- and β-adrenergic blockade does not impair the increase in hepatic glucose production during muscular work in humans (124, 192, 267), implying that sympathetic drive is unimportant to this process. In one recent study sympathetic nerve activity to the liver and adrenal medulla were blocked with local anesthesia of the celiac ganglion prior to exercise and the pancreatic hormone responses were controlled using somatostatin with insulin and glucagon replacement (166). Hepatic glucose production increased in a fashion similar to controls despite the presumed absence of sympathetic nerve activity to the liver and adrenal medulla. In further support of the absence of a role of hepatic innervation is the demonstration that liver-transplanted human subjects have a normal increase in glucose production during exercise (167). Animal studies also indicate that hepatic innervation does not play an important role during exercise. A general sympathectomy with 6-OH dopamine does not reduce hepatic glycogen breakdown during exercise in rats (242, 261) and surgical hepatic denervation does not diminish the increment in hepatic glucose production in the rat (271) or the dog (311). Furthermore, the exercise-induced increases in hepatic glycogenolysis and gluconeogenesis in the dog do not depend on hepatic innervation (311). In the hepatic-denervated dog model, arterial glucagon and insulin respond normally to exercise, but epinephrine tends to be elevated. It is possible, therefore, that epinephrine may have a small compensatory role, thereby masking a physiological effect of the hepatic nerves. Clearly, however, hepatic nerves are not essential to the increase in glucose production or in maintaining glucose homeostasis during moderate-intensity exercise.

From what is known about hepatic parasympathetic nerve function, it seems unlikely that efferents from these autonomic nerves are important during instances, such as exercise, which are characterized by high rates of hepatic glucose output (180). Nevertheless, parasympathetic afferent nerves transmit information regarding hemodynamic, thermoregulatory, and nutritional variables to the central nervous system (258). As discussed earlier it has been postulated that these nerves may be important in transmitting information to the brain during exercise and other conditions.

Role of Cortisol

Although the acute effects of glucocorticoids are usually considered minimal (102), they may play a role in the exercise-induced increase in gluconeogenesis. In transgenic mice carrying a gene consisting of the PEPCK promotor linked to a reporter gene for bovine growth hormone (bGH), the level of hepatic bGH mRNA increased by nearly fivefold in response to exercise (91). However, transgenic mice with a deletion in the PEPCK gene glucocorticoid regulatory element did not. This observation was supported by the finding that the exercise-induced increase in PEPCK mRNA is markedly attenuated in adrenalectomized mice and dexamethasone corrects the impairment (91). The importance of this interesting finding is not altogether clear, since adrenalectomized rats deprived of cortisol have similar liver glycogen and blood glucose levels after exhaustive exercise as adrenalectomized corticosterone-replaced controls (260).

Figure 23.7 summarizes studies in the dog (210, 304, 310) that illustrate the role of the endocrine system in regulating the increase in hepatic glucose production during moderate-intensity exercise.

Regulation during High-Intensity Exercise

The majority of work in the regulation of hepatic function during exercise has addressed mechanisms that are operative at moderate intensities (~50% maximum oxygen uptake). The discussion above reflects this emphasis. The main identifiable difference in glucoregulation during high-intensity exercise (above ~75% maximum oxygen uptake) is that the increase in hepatic glucose production no longer matches but in fact exceeds the rise in glucose utilization. This results in an increase in arterial glucose levels that may extend into the postexercise state (36, 161, 193, 292). The postulate that the increase in catecholamines, and not changes in glucagon and insulin, is important for the increase in hepatic glycogenolysis during high-intensity exercise is based on several lines of evidence. First, during high-intensity exercise, catecholamines may increase by tenfold, while arterial glucagon levels may increase, remain the same, or even decrease (92). Second, circulating glucose levels generally increase with heavy exercise, and this may prevent the fall or even lead to an increase in insulin levels (92, 193). This is significant, since insulin suppresses glucagon's stimulatory effect on R_a, but has considerably less effect on catecholamine action (70, 252). Finally, adrenalectomized rats were shown to have a decreased net liver glycogen breakdown during high-intensity exercise, but generally not during exercise of lesser intensities (191). The glucagon response to high-intensity exercise was attenuated in these studies and may have led to the impairment in liver glycogen breakdown (191). Whereas the evidence cited above is consistent with the possibility that catecholamines may be important during heavy exercise, studies in human subjects have been negative. In one study, attenuation of the sympathetic nerve activity to the liver and adrenal medulla by anesthetic blockade of the celiac ganglion did not alter hepatic glucose production during high-intensity exercise (~75% maximum oxygen uptake) (166). A second study showed that liver transplant patients have a normal hepatic glucose production response to high-intensity exercise (~82% maximum oxygen uptake) (167). When β-adrenergic blockade was employed in healthy subjects exercising at 100% maximum oxygen uptake (266), hepatic glucose production was actually increased. Again, these studies emphasize the apparent absence of a role for the catecholamines in hepatic glucoregulation during high-intensity exercise.

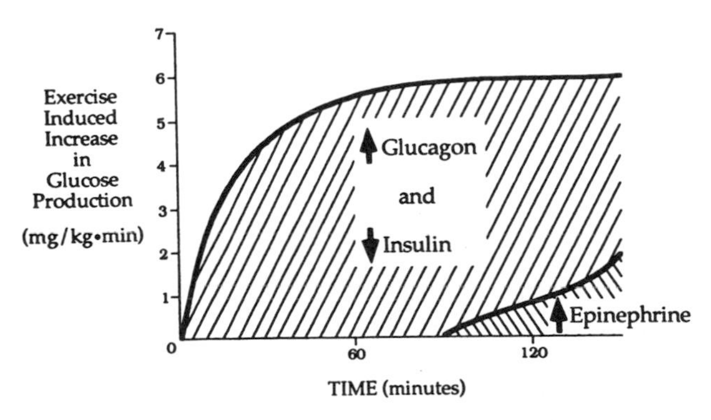

FIG. 23.7. Schematic representation of the rise in glucose production during moderate-intensity exercise and the impact of the fall in insulin and rise in glucagon and the role of the increase in epinephrine on this response. [Modified from Wasserman and Cherrington (298).]

HEPATIC FAT METABOLISM: OXIDATION AND TRIGLYCERIDE SYNTHESIS

From the standpoint of fuel metabolism, there are two avenues for hepatic fat metabolism that are of note. These are fatty acid oxidation and incorporation into triglycerides. The pathways involved are most frequently assessed by the dynamics of circulating ketone bodies and lipoproteins, respectively. In postabsorptive, healthy individuals neither fate provides appreciable amounts of fuel to the working muscle directly. As will be explained, the regulation of hepatic fatty acid oxidation and triglyceride synthesis can, nevertheless, have important effects on muscle fuel metabolism by indirect mechanisms.

Regulation of Ketogenesis

Ketone bodies (acetoacetate, acetone, and β-hydroxybutyrate) are produced in the liver by a process that can be conveniently divided into two sections (201). The first is the β-oxidation sequence that involves the generation of acetyl-CoA from long-chain fatty acids. The second is the synthesis of acetoacetate from two acetyl-CoA molecules. Acetoacetate either remains as such, is decarboxylated to acetone, or is reduced to β-hydroxybutyrate. Regulation of ketogenesis can be exerted through effects on the mobilization of NEFAs from adipose tissue and delivery to the liver, the extraction of NEFAs by the liver, and the conversion of NEFAs to ketone bodies within the liver (294). Ketogenesis is increased with prolonged exercise due to the stimulation of each of these processes (293, 294). The rate at which ketone bodies are released by the liver is quantitatively unimportant as a fuel for the working muscle in healthy humans. The significance of hepatic ketogenesis rests with the fact that it is a reflection of the energy state of the liver. It is a marker of fat oxidation, a key pathway in providing energy to fuel gluconeogenesis (201). In this regard, acute and chronic circumstances that require accelerated gluconeogenic rates are characterized by high rates of ketogenesis (201). It has been shown that inhibiting fat oxidation pharmacologically reduces basal glycemia and hepatic glycogen (337), as well as the exercise-induced increase in glucose production (334) in animal models of diabetes that are heavily reliant on gluconeogenesis. In addition, increasing NEFA availability in the exercising rat spares liver glycogen, perhaps by increasing the capacity for gluconeogenesis (240). It is important to recognize that, besides direct effects on the liver, increased NEFA availability and oxidation may indirectly preserve liver glycogen and reduce total hepatic glucose production by reducing the need for glucose in muscle.

Although it is known from in vitro studies that many hormonal and neural effectors may impact on ketogenesis (201), very few studies have assessed the role of these potential controllers during muscular work. Regardless, any hormone or neurotransmitter that regulates NEFA mobilization (described previously), hepatic NEFA extraction, or intrahepatic fat oxidation may play a role in the regulation of ketogenesis during exercise. Hepatic NEFA delivery and ketone body output are closely correlated during rest and exercise (259). Moreover, when circulating NEFA levels are elevated chronically, as may occur with starvation (85), diabetes (259, 293, 294), or in response to peripheral fat infusion (163, 208), ketogenesis is stimulated. Any factor that provides, therefore, a sufficient stimulus to NEFA mobilization such as the fall in insulin (305) and the β-adrenergic effects of the catecholamines (124) may stimulate ketogenesis.

Mobilization of intrahepatic fat stores during exercise could also provide NEFAs for oxidation within the liver as well as glycerol for gluconeogenesis. The release of oleic acid from the splanchnic bed, as determined with ^{14}C-oleic acid, rises by approximately threefold at 60 min of exercise in humans even though net uptakes of oleic acid and total NEFAs are present with exercise (294). The precise source of the oleic acid within the splanchnic bed is probably mesenteric and omental adipose tissue, as experiments in the dog show that net gut NEFA output increases, while the liver exhibits net uptake (305). It seems likely, therefore, that extrahepatic tissues is the main site of the exercise-induced increase in splanchnic oleic acid production.

Hepatic NEFA uptake is primarily determined by the hepatic NEFA delivery rate. Studies in normal and diabetic subjects show that hepatic NEFA load and uptake are strongly correlated during rest and exercise (259, 294). Wahren and colleagues demonstrated that splanchnic oleic acid load and uptake are characterized by a correlation coefficient in excess of 0.94 during both rest and at 60 min of muscular work in insulin-dependent diabetics and healthy controls (294). The slope of this relationship rises with exercise, reflecting an increase in splanchnic fractional oleic acid extraction (294). This suggests that although hepatic NEFA delivery is important to hepatic NEFA uptake, exercise exerts an independent effect. When the exercise-induced fall in insulin is prevented in the dog with an intraportal infusion of the hormone, the small exercise-induced rise in hepatic fractional NEFA extraction does not occur (305). Therefore, the fall in insulin enhances ketogenesis not only by enhancing NEFA mobilization but also by increasing hepatic fractional NEFA extraction. It is unknown whether the effect on NEFA extraction is due to a direct transport effect or whether it is due to a primary increase in intrahepatic fat oxidation that may effectively "pull" NEFAs into the cell.

The splanchnic ketone body output divided by the splanchnic NEFA uptake has been used to provide an index of intrahepatic ketogenic efficiency in human subjects. This variable increases from 20% at rest to 40% after 60 min of moderate-intensity exercise in healthy subjects, indicating that a greater proportion of NEFA carbons is channeled into ketones (294). In insulin-dependent diabetics in poor control the intrahepatic ketogenic efficiency is elevated to 61% at rest and increases to essentially 100% after 60 min of exercise (294). Further evidence that intrahepatic changes facilitate fat oxidation during exercise is illustrated by the increased capacity to oxidize 1-^{14}C-palmitate (13) and the greater respiratory capacity (278) of livers from exercised rats. Experiments in the dog suggest that the rise in glucagon during prolonged exercise is the stimulus for the increase in ketogenic efficiency. When the exercise-induced rise in glucagon is eliminated using somatostatin with glucagon and insulin replaced in the portal vein to desired rates it can be demonstrated that the increment in this hormone controls ~90% and 20% of the increments in net hepatic β-hydroxybutyrate and acetoacetate output, respectively, between 90 and 150 min of exercise (309). The rise in glucagon exerts its effects on ketogenesis solely through intrahepatic mechanisms, as hepatic NEFA delivery and extraction are the same regardless of whether the hormone is increased. This finding is consistent with the observation that elevated glucagon levels increase ketone body production in resting humans provided that insulin levels are reduced and NEFA levels are elevated (208), such as they are during exercise. It is also in agreement with the close correlation between splanchnic ketone body output and hepatic vein glucagon levels in humans (259) and the demonstration that glucagon can enhance the activity of the key ketogenic enzyme, carnitine acyltransferase, in the rat (201).

Triglyceride Synthesis

In an earlier segment of this chapter, substrate cycling between triglycerides and NEFA in the adipocyte was discussed. Substrate cycling also occurs at the organ level as NEFA, mobilized from adipose tissue are released, transported to and extracted by the liver, synthesized into triglyceride, and incorporated into lipoprotein. The fatty acids from these triglycerides will be hydrolyzed and metabolized in various tissues. If these fatty acids form triglyceride in adipose tissue, a substrate cycle will exist. During exercise, modification of this interorgan substrate cycle may be significant in amplifying the rate that NEFAs are made available to the working muscle. Stable isotope methodology was used to determine that ~60% of the NEFA released from adipose tissue is reesterified by the liver in resting humans, while only ~20%–25% is reesterified during exercise (331). These data show that fat oxidation attributable to a reduction in reesterification is ~40%–50% of the total fat oxidation rate during exercise. This reduction is, in large part, probably a result of hemodynamic shifts leading to a reduction in blood flow to the liver and an increase in that to the skeletal muscle. For reasons summarized previously (280), it is unlikely that triglyceride release by the liver is a significant source of fuel for the working muscle in postabsorptive subjects (supplying <10% of the total energy cost). The half-life of very-low-density lipoprotein (VLDL), the main circulating form of triglyceride in the postabsorptive state, is on the order of hours and the circulating concentration is not sufficiently high to compensate for this low clearance (279). Exercise appears to have a stimulatory effect on the utilization of circulating triglycerides, as the levels of this substrate are reduced in response to muscular work (41). Hepatic triglyceride synthesis is apparently not greatly affected by exercise, as changes in endogenously labeled trigyceride-specific activity (336) and hepatic balance (251) do not change markedly. After consuming a meal containing fat, the main source of circulating triglyceride is chylomicrons formed in the intestine. Chylomicrons have a considerably higher turnover rate than VLDL and may obtain levels that permit them to be a significant fuel for working muscle (279). In the dog, ~25% of the circulating chylomicron triglyceride pool turns over every minute at rest, while during exercise this turnover rate increases slightly to ~33% (279).

SPLANCHNIC BED AMINO ACID METABOLISM

Because of the central role of amino acids in a variety of biochemical processes, their metabolism is of great significance during exercise. In addition to being constituents of protein, amino acids may actually serve a regulatory role in controlling the balance of protein synthesis and breakdown (1,200). Moreover, amino acids perform functions essential to nitrogen metabolism, are substrates for gluconeogenesis and oxidation, and are involved in acid–base regulation (1). Their relative importance to various pathways is specific to the amino acid. Despite the essential role of amino acids to the structure and function of the cell, organ, and body as a whole, major gaps in the understanding of their role and regulation still exist. In a fundamental sense it is known that amino acid metabolism, like the metabolism of other substrates, is regulated by nutritional status, the hormonal and metabolic environment of the body, and the degree of nervous activity (1). Exercise can lead to changes in all of these factors. The splanchnic bed has at least two important functions during a condition that is characterized by high metabolic demand, such as exercise. First, the tissues of the gastrointestinal tract exhibit the highest protein turnover rates in the body and are extremely sensitive to proteolytic stimuli. Therefore, one function is to mobilize amino acids as substrates for liver and muscle. Second, under conditions of increased metabolic demand the production and interorgan flux of nitrogenous compounds (glutamine, alanine, NH_3) are often increased. The tissues of the splanchnic bed, particularly the liver, are primary sites for nitrogen metabolism and are important in this capacity during sufficiently demanding exercise.

Protein Breakdown

Studies utilizing isotopes of the essential amino acid leucine generally show that the total rate of leucine flux is minimally affected by moderate exercise (42, 45, 108, 119, 239), but that there is a shift in the route of leucine utilization, such that more of the amino acid is oxidized and less is involved in protein synthesis (108, 119, 239, 316, 330, 333). This results in an overall increase in protein catabolism. In contrast to the studies using isotopic leucine, a study using a dual stable isotope method in humans showed that there is an increase in the rate of appearance of alanine formed from proteolysis during 2 h of moderate exercise (44). Regardless of the mechanism (i.e., increased proteolysis and/or decreased protein synthesis), net protein catabolism and, as a result, amino acid availability is increased by exercise. Most of the emphasis has been placed on the skeletal muscle as an important site of protein catabolism. Evidence as to the importance of exercise-induced skeletal muscle protein catabolism is equivocal. 3-Methylhistidine is abundant in myofibrillar protein, and plasma and urine levels are used as an index of myofibrillar protein catabolism. Exercise has been shown to decrease (72, 239), increase (72), or not change (37, 68) the 3-methylhistidine production rate in humans. This discrepancy is apparently due to a biphasic response of 3-methylhistidine so that samples taken during or immediately after exercise show a decrease in the levels of this free amino acid, while with more prolonged recovery a rise is present (72). Since 3-methylhistidine is not elevated until recovery from exercise, any protein breakdown during the work period must be a result of nonmyofibrillar protein degradation. Total protein breakdown from muscle of exercised rats has been generally shown to increase with contraction (76, 155, 159). This finding, however, has not been completely uniform (12). It was calculated, using the enrichments of α-ketoisocaproic acid and leucine during a ^{13}C-leucine infusion in exercising humans, that 50% of the leucine oxidized during exercise was derived from plasma and 50% was derived from within the cell (333). If one assumes that leucine is oxidized mainly within the working muscle (see below), a corollary must be that substantial muscle protein catabolism is occurring. It is important to note that the efflux of nitrogenous compounds from working muscle does not represent the amino acid content of muscle protein, but occurs mostly in the form of alanine, glutamine, and free NH_3 (84). This indicates that either the amino acids released from skeletal muscle protein undergo transamination (or deamination) or that a source of nitrogenous compounds in skeletal muscle other than protein may predominate during exercise [e.g., nucleotides (206)].

Although less attention has been focused on the role of protein catabolism in the splanchnic bed, experiments in humans have shown that BCAAs (leucine, isoleucine, valine) are released from these tissues and that the rate of release is elevated during exercise (6, 79, 84). The original presumption was that the source of these amino acids was the liver. This premise was supported by studies in the rat that showed prolonged exercise (>2 h) resulted in a 10%–15% fall in hepatic protein content (156). This decrease was associated with morphologic changes in lysosomes and an increase in the activity of free lysosomal enzymes, indicating that this reduction was due to an accelerated proteolytic rate (157). Data from experiments in the dog suggest that extrahepatic splanchnic tissues (primarily gastrointestinal tract) are, in fact, the primary source of the amino acids released by the splanchnic bed (300, 317). Since the essential amino acid leucine is amongst those released by the gut, it would seem that an increase in proteolysis and/or a decrease in protein synthesis must be involved (317). In contrast to the fall in hepatic protein content seen after treadmill exercise in the rat, studies in the dog give no indication that net hepatic protein catabolism is increased. The differences between results obtained in the dog and rat models may be due to the means of estimating protein catabolism (biopsy vs. arteriovenous and isotope), a species difference, or the intensity and duration of exercise used. A significant decrease in hepatic protein content was not present until 2 h of exercise in the rat (156), whereas the dogs in the experiments in which leucine enrichment was measured across the liver were exercised for only 90 min. Interestingly, most of the amino acids released by the gut are consumed by the liver and only a small portion appear in the systemic circulation (300). A corollary to the finding that amino acids are released by the gut is that previous studies in humans, in which only splanchnic balance was measured, greatly underestimated the rate that amino acids were consumed by the liver. An important role for the gut during exercise is consistent with the demonstration that the gastrointestinal tract is responsible for almost the entire increase in protein catabolism during another metabolic stress, insulin-induced hypoglycemia (128). Furthermore, it is consistent with studies in cattle (187) and rats (202) that show that tissues of the gastrointestinal tract have the highest protein turnover rate in the body. Thus, it appears that the gut contains a labile pool of amino acids that is mobilized during exercise. The signal (e.g., hormonal, neural, metabolic) that triggers this effect is unclear.

Amino Acids as a Carbon Source for Gluconeogenesis and Oxidation

Once they are made available, amino acids can be metabolized by several different routes, and their metabolism can serve several functions. The amino acids glutamine, glutamate, alanine, threonine, serine, and glycine can also be important gluconeogenic substrates (47). After an overnight fast, alanine (84, 312) and glutamine (300) appear to be the most quantitatively important during exercise. The release of alanine and glutamine from the working limb increases with exercise intensity (79) and duration (301), thereby providing more gluconeogenic substrate to the liver. Certainly, the rate of amino acid delivery from the gut, muscle, and other tissues must be considered an important determinant of hepatic amino acid uptake. Nevertheless, the increased hepatic uptake of amino acids can occur in the absence of an increase in hepatic delivery as the fractional extraction of amino acids is increased (84, 300, 312). This reflects regulation directly at the liver. The regulation of hepatic alanine extraction and intrahepatic conversion into glucose was discussed in a previous section. To reiterate briefly, the increase in gluconeogenesis from alanine is due to an increase in the fractional extraction of the amino acid by the liver and enzymatic conversion to glucose within the liver (312). The exercise-induced increase in glucagon is the primary stimulus for these processes (310). The net uptake of glutamine by the liver also increases (300). Studies conducted in the perfused rat liver (115) and in the resting conscious dog (100) suggest that glucagon may, as it does in the control of hepatic alanine metabolism, have important effects on hepatic glutamine metabolism. If hepatic proteolysis is appreciable, this process could also provide carbons for gluconeogenesis (212). Estimates of the gluconeogenic amino acid uptake by the liver are, nevertheless, approximately equal to the urea nitrogen released by the liver during 150 min of exercise in the dog, suggesting that there is no other major source of amino acids for this pathway (298).

Glutamine (1) and the BCAAs (200) are readily oxidized in the gastrointestinal tract and skeletal muscle, respectively. Net gut glutamine uptake increases transiently during exercise in the dog (300). Moreover, leucine oxidation by the perfused rat hindlimb is increased when the muscles are stimulated to contract, and this increase is directly related to the duration and intensity of contraction (127). The observation that leucine oxidation is increased with exercise is supported by the increased activity of the enzyme that catalyzes the transamination of BCAAs in muscle, branched chain keto acid dehydrogenase (127, 158). Despite these changes in the working muscle it is unlikely that the added BCAAs made available by protein catabolism during exercise contribute markedly to the metabolic requirement.

Uptake of Nitrogenous Compounds by the Splanchnic Bed

Because exercise increases the rates of amino acid oxidation and adenosine monophosphate deamination (206) in the muscle and gluconeogenesis within the liver, NH_3 formation is accelerated. As a result, NH_3 metabolism must also be increased. NH_3 leaves the working muscle and enters the circulation carried by glutamine, alanine, or as free NH_3. The muscle efflux rate of these nitrogenous compounds increases with exercise intensity (79) and duration (301). Since gluconeogenesis increases gradually with exercise, it is likely that the formation of NH_3 from this pathway increases with a similar time course (6, 312).

Regardless of the site of NH_3 formation and the pathways involved, the liver represents an important site for the metabolism of this compound. The efficiency of the liver in nitrogen removal during exercise is apparent from the fact that in the presence of a twofold increase in gut protein catabolism, only BCAA escape from the splanchnic bed is increased. The net hepatic uptake of NH_3 and total α-amino-nitrogens is equal to or greater than their respective release by the gut. Due to its high circulating level and the fact that it carries amine and amide groups, glutamine is an extremely important nitrogen carrier. During exercise in the immediate postabsorptive state, it appears to be the most important quantitatively (79, 300). Most of the glutamine extracted by the splanchnic bed is metabolized in the gut in the basal state (1, 273, 300). Exercise results in an increased net gut uptake of glutamine (300). Net hepatic glutamine uptake increases to a greater extent, however, and as a result the transition from rest to exercise leads to a shift from mainly gut to liver glutamine utilization (300). In addition, some of the glutamine carbons extracted by the gut are liberated as glutamate and a portion of the nitrogens are released as free NH_3 or participate in the transamination of keto acids (300). Remarkably, glutamate, NH_3, and alanine (gut and hepatic balances of other nitrogenous compounds have not been assessed during exercise) are consumed by the liver at nearly the same rate that they are liberated from the gut (300). Gut glutamine metabolism serves to facilitate nitrogen metabolism at the liver. The close coupling of the hepatic deliveries of various nitrogenous compounds via the portal vein to their respective hepatic uptakes implies that some feature of the increase in portal vein level or delivery is of significance. The efficient role of the liver in nitrogen metabolism is consistent with the experimental observation that none of an intraportal infusion of NH_3 escapes the splanchnic bed (35, 46).

Glutamine metabolism within the liver is complex, as the amino acid is produced and consumed simultaneously by this organ. The pathway that predominates is determined by the relative activities of the synthetic enzyme, glutamine synthetase, and the degrading enzyme, glutaminase (203). The simultaneous activation of pathways for formation and degradation of glutamine results in an energy-consuming cycle, but makes the regulation of hepatic glutamine metabolism far more sensitive (115, 203). As indicated above, hepatic glutamine uptake predominates during exercise. The means by which this occurs has not been studied. Note, however, that the exercise-induced increase in hepatic glutamine uptake does not require an increase in load (i.e., occurs as a result of an increase in fractional extraction). Several factors are known to affect hepatic glutamine balance in the resting state and may be important during exercise. Glucagon is a potent stimulator of glutamine metabolism due to both stimulation of glutaminase and inhibition of glutamine synthetase (115). NH_3 stimulates glutamine cycling and may sensitize the liver to other regulatory factors. Perfusion of a rat liver with glucagon in the presence of elevated NH_4Cl causes a twofold greater increase in glutamine utilization than when the liver is perfused with glucagon alone (115). In addition to NH_3 and glucagon, pH can also regulate glutamine metabolism (1, 314). Since exercise can increase the rate of hepatic ammonia delivery, raise glucagon levels, and change pH, these may all be factors that potentially control glutamine metabolism during muscular work.

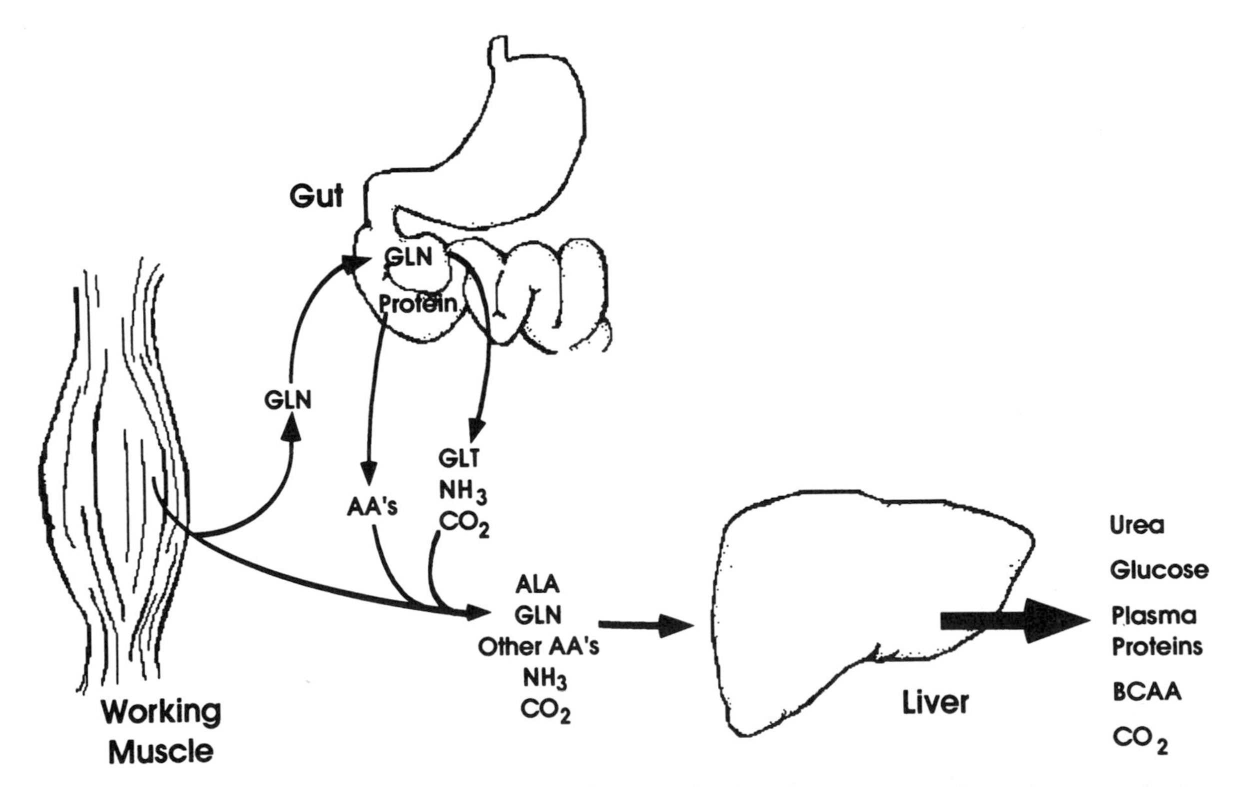

FIG. 23.8. Proposed pathways for amino acid metabolism in the splanchnic bed. Amino acids, primarily alanine and glutamine, are released by working muscle. Glutamine (GLN) is deaminated in the gastrointestinal tract forming glutamate (GLT), which is released or oxidized. Amino acids are released from the gastrointestinal tract as a result of proteolysis. The liver takes up amino acids where they are converted into glucose, oxidized, or incorporated into protein. Only the branched chain amino acids (leucine, isoleucine, valine) are consistently released from the splanchnic bed in a net sense. Nitrogen released during metabolism of amino acids may be converted to urea.

Fate of Nitrogenous Compounds in the Liver

The fate of the nitrogenous compounds once they are consumed by the liver during exercise has not been clearly defined. In the exercising dog, net hepatic urea output increases (300), whereas in the exercising human the body urea pool has been reported to expand (239) and urea can be detected in the sweat and urine (109, 236). On the other hand, an increase in ureagenesis is undetectable by use of stable isotopes (43, 333) even at high work intensities (43). Keep in mind that the increase in hepatic urea output present during exercise in the dog cannot nearly account for the uptake of nitrogenous compounds by the liver (300). It can be estimated by summing the hepatic uptakes of α-amino nitrogen, ammonia, and the glutamine amide group that nitrogen uptake by the liver exceeds the rate at which nitrogen exits the liver via urea by twofold. The fate of the rest of the nitrogen that is extracted by the liver remains to be assessed. It has been proposed that hepatic uptake of nitrogenous compounds during exercise may be important for the accelerated formation of plasma proteins by the liver (42). In this regard, the fractional synthetic rates of fibronectin and fibrinogen are increased at 4 h of exercise and after recovery from 4 h of exercise, respectively, in humans (42). A previous study in the dog has shown that all the leucine used in fibronectin synthesis comes from the portal vein (17). This would seem to imply that there is a distinct advantage to the exercise-induced increase in gut protein catabolism and consequent amino acid efflux, insofar as the synthesis of this plasma protein is concerned.

From the preceding it is evident that amino acid metabolism is an integral part of the exercise response. Muscular work stimulates protein catabolism, resulting in the mobilization of amino acids. This provides a small source of oxidative fuel and important substrates for gluconeogenesis, but necessitates that the nitrogen formed as the amino acids are metabolized be disposed of. The liver has at least two primary functions in the increased amino acid metabolism during exercise. These are the channeling of carbon compounds for use in gluconeogenesis and the metabolism of nitrogen produced in extrahepatic (and possibly hepatic) tissues. A third function may be to provide amino acids for incorporation into proteins within the liver. Despite the important role of exercise-induced changes in amino acid metabolism, the response remains to be described fully and the factors involved in its regulation continue to be largely unknown. Figure 23.8 summarizes the postulated roles of the splanchnic bed in amino acid metabolism during exercise.

GASTROINTESTINAL TRACT AS A SOURCE OF GLUCOSE: EFFECT OF CARBOHYDRATE INGESTION

Importance

Endogenous carbohydrate stores are finite, and in the postabsorptive state their depletion represents one factor that may be limiting for prolonged exercise. The limitations posed by the exhaustible carbohydrate stores of the body can be circumvented by carbohydrate ingestion and subsequent gastrointestinal absorption. The important role carbohydrate ingestion can play in exercise tolerance was demonstrated by Dill and colleagues in 1932, when they showed that intermittent glucose feeding (20 g every hour) increased endurance time in the exercising dog by over threefold (71). Moreover, these investigators showed that ingestion of 40 g of glucose allowed a dog exhausted by over 4 h of exercise to run for an added 90 min. In the 60 years since these experiments were conducted, numerous studies have demonstrated the potential importance of glucose ingestion in exercising humans. The mechanism by which carbohydrate ingestion delays fatigue is related to an increased availability of glucose to the working muscle (55). The ability of carbohydrate ingestion to prevent neuroglucopenia is probably not of primary importance in delaying fatigue, since severe hypoglycemia is not necessarily present at exhaustion from prolonged exercise (53, 54).

Carbohydrate ingestion may also delay glycogen depletion by preventing the counterregulatory response that occurs as circulating glucose availability falls. The development of just moderate hypoglycemia may contribute to glycogen depletion by accentuating the exercise-induced increases in glucagon and catecholamines. These counterregulatory hormone changes are highly sensitized by exercise, as marked responses occur with small changes in blood glucose (9, 272, 303, 307). These hormonal changes, in turn, accelerate glycogen breakdown. What, in effect, may occur is a self-propagating cycle triggered during prolonged exercise by diminished glycogen stores, resulting in a reduction in glycemia. This, then, elicits a counterregulatory response which, in turn, further accelerates glycogen depletion. This cycle can be broken by supplementation of endogenous carbohydrate stores with ingested glucose. The effectiveness with which carbohydrate feeding maintains glucose availability to the working muscle will depend on the amount and form of ingested glucose.

Moreover, the timing of glucose ingestion with respect to exercise will be a key determinant of how it affects metabolism. Finally, exercise factors related to duration and intensity will to a large extent determine the contribution of ingested glucose to exercise metabolism.

Determinants of the Metabolic Availability of Ingested Carbohydrates

The effectiveness with which ingested glucose enters the blood and is, thereby, made available to the tissues of the body is dependent on the transit time through the gastrointestinal tract and absorption by the gastrointestinal tract. Gastric emptying is a key factor in determining transit time (63). Several factors influence this variable, including volume (222), osmolality (144, 190), temperature (222), energy content (29), and acidity (222). In addition, a number of specific nutrients affect gastric emptying (129, 190). The volume of the solution in the stomach has the most powerful direct relationship to gastric emptying. The most potent inhibitor of gastric emptying of ingested carbohydrate is the amount of carbohydrate in the solution itself (222). Even though the total volume of fluid emptied from the stomach is reduced with high-carbohydrate solution, the rate that carbohydrate is delivered to the small intestine will usually be sustained by the higher carbohydrate concentration. The results of initial studies addressing the effects of exercise on gastric emptying suggest that low- and high-intensity exercise stimulate and inhibit it, respectively (39, 117). More recent work yielded conflicting results, showing that exercise at 70% of maximum oxygen uptake may increase (218), decrease (83, 224), or not alter (62, 63, 224) gastric emptying. At exercise intensities above 70% maximum oxygen uptake, a decrease in gastric emptying has been consistently demonstrated (87, 218, 237, 270). Reasons for the discrepancies at the lower work rates may pertain to differences in the methods used to measure gastric emptying and study design. If exercise is accompanied by dehydration, gastric emptying is likely to be reduced. Furthermore, certain hormones and neurotransmitters that accompany anxiety, such as those that may occur during serious competition, may impair gastric emptying (106, 110).

Motility of the small intestine is a second determinant of gastrointestinal transit time. Gastric emptying will be facilitated by a high ratio of gastric/duodenum contractile activity. This, in effect, creates a better pressure gradient for the bulk transport of solution from stomach to small intestine. Not only does low small intestine contractile activity improve the movement of a solution from stomach to small intestine, but it also increases the transit time within the small intestine. Since the small intestine is the predominant site of nutrient absorption, any factor that increases the transit time in this section of the gastrointestinal tract may potentially enhance nutrient availability to the tissues of the body. A high level of small intestine contractile activity will cause the reverse effects on gastric emptying (i.e., a decrease). Experiments generally show that in the small intestine, transit time is increased by exercise (81, 205, 213, 214) provided that work intensity is sufficiently high (38). In contrast to the increase in transit time through the small intestine, transit time through the colon is decreased. Most of the transit time throughout the gastrointestinal tract is spent in the colon. As a result, the net whole gut transit time may reflect the decreased transit time in the colon (59). Nevertheless, since the vast majority of sugar absorption occurs in the small intestine, the increased transit time along this segment should facilitate the availability of ingested glucose in the blood.

The direct influence of exercise on intestinal absorption has not been studied extensively. In one early investigation it was shown that exercise at 71% of the maximum oxygen uptake for 1 h had no effect on jejunal or ileum absorption of water or glucose using a jejunal perfusion technique (87). In a more recent study in humans, moderate-intensity cycling (~45% maximum oxygen uptake) led to a reduction in water and electrolyte absorption as determined using jejunal perfusion (14). This finding is consistent with other work that showed that the vascular appearance of ingested deuterium oxide was reduced by high-intensity exercise (199). Studies in the dog have shown that an impaired absorption rate may occur as a result of a decrease in blood flow to the tissues of the small intestine (284, 318). Exercise reduces splanchnic blood flow in humans by as much as 70% during high-intensity exercise (250). This hemodynamic change may, therefore, impair the absorption of ingested glucose.

The metabolic availability of ingested carbohydrates has been assessed in numerous studies by spiking the oral load with sugar labeled with isotopic carbon and measuring the appearance of the isotope in expired carbon dioxide (CO_2). Initial studies were done using ^{14}C-glucose to trace the oxidation rate of ingested glucose (60, 283). It was shown in one study that although ~60% of the circulating glucose during 60 min of moderate exercise was derived from ingested glucose, the appearance of $^{14}CO_2$ in the breath was low and the contribution of ingested glucose to total carbohydrate oxidation was calculated to equal only 5% (60). The conclusion from this study was that ingested glucose was of little importance for metabolism of the working muscle. The recovery of $^{14}CO_2$, however, was probably underestimated due to technical problems that arise from the extensive interval required for the $H^{14}CO_3$ to equilibrate with the endogenous HCO_3 stores. In subsequent years the metabolic availability of ingested glucose was measured using ^{13}C-labeled sugars. Use of this label, on the other hand, has given rise to large overestimates due to the presence of naturally occurring ^{13}C-label. Since the ^{13}C enrichment of glucose is greater than fats, an increased contribution of carbohydrate to total oxidation will result in an increase in $^{13}CO_2$ production. Since oxidation of ingested ^{13}C-labeled sugars cannot be distinguished from oxidation of endogenous stores, an overestimate of the oxidation of ingested ^{13}C-labeled sugar occurs when the metabolic contribution of endogenous carbohydrate is increased. Early work that did not consider the contribution of endogenous carbohydrates may have overestimated the rate of ingested carbohydrate oxidation by as much as 75% (226). The precise metabolic availability of ingested carbohydrate will depend on many factors related to the composition and quantity of the substrate load. In addition, exercise parameters (i.e., work intensity, duration, modality) will also be important determinants of how readily ingested glucose will be made available. As a consequence, it is difficult to ascribe an exact efficiency for metabolism of ingested glucose. In any case, a reasonable estimate might be that ~40% of a 50 g oral glucose load, ingested at the start of moderate-intensity exercise, is metabolized during the first hour (2).

During very light rates of exercise there is probably very little difficulty in deliverying adequate amounts of ingested glucose to the working muscle. As exercise intensity increases and glucose oxidation by the working muscle increases it may no longer be possible to absorb adequate amounts of ingested glucose from the gastrointestinal tract. As a result the limitation for the oxidation of ingested glucose may shift with increasing work rate so that the low muscle demand limits glucose oxidation at light work rates, whereas absorption from the gastrointestinal tract limits it at high work rates. One study showed that as exercise intensity increased from 22% to 51% of the maximum oxygen uptake the oxidation of ingested glucose (100 g) increased proportionally (227). With further increases in work rate, total carbohydrate oxidation continued to rise; the oxidation of ingested glucose, however, increased no further. This suggested that the rate that glucose is made available from the gastrointestinal tract has become limiting.

One approach for increasing the amount of carbohydrate that enters the blood from the gut is simply to increase the mass of ingested glucose. While this is an effective approach in increasing the absolute mass of glucose that is metabolically available, the fraction of the ingested glucose that is made available for metabolism is actually decreased. For example, in one study an increase in ingested glucose of 58 g to 220 g prior to exercise increased the amount of glucose that was oxidized from 32 g to only 42 g. With the lower mass of ingested glucose 55% was oxidized, compared to 19% when the greater mass was ingested (238). This is consistent with findings from other studies (2, 225). One reason for the decreased percentage of metabolized glucose with larger glucose loads is that more glucose remains in the gastrointestinal tract (238). In any case, the decreased percentage of ingested glucose that is oxidized when larger quantities of glucose are consumed orally suggests one or more steps involved in the intestinal absorption of glucose or delivery of glucose to the working muscle has become saturated. This saturation can be circumvented and more carbohydrate can be metabolically available by using different sugar types. A greater percentage of ingested sugar is oxidized during exercise if 50 g of glucose and 50 g of fructose are ingested than if 100 g of either sugar alone is consumed (2). The approach of using multiple feedings distributed over the duration of the work period instead of a single ingestion of an equal amount of glucose does not, in general, facilitate the oxidation of ingested glucose (116). This may be due to the normally slow absorption profile of ingested sugar, as peak rates do not occur with a single ingestion of sugar until well into the second hour of prolonged exercise (143, 144, 179, 228, 229). Therefore, the benefits of subsequent ingestions may not be evident within the context of even prolonged exercise. The exact time at which carbohydrates are ingested during exercise does not seem to be of major importance in sustaining work performance, provided that signs of fatigue are not already present (55). Glucose ingestion, from the onset of muscular work at 70%–75% maximum oxygen uptake until exhaustion (64) or glucose ingestion beginning 30 min prior to the anticipation of fatigue at the same work rate (54) both delay fatigue by ~50 min. Ingestion of glucose is somewhat less effective in restoring work capacity in an individual once fatigue has been established (53). Carbohydrate ingestion may result in a paradoxical decrease in plasma glucose that is counterproductive for work performance if it precedes exercise by an interval (~45 min) that causes the onset of exercise to coincide with peak insulin levels (61, 88, 173).

The form of the ingested sugar may be important to its ultimate metabolic availability. It probably makes very little difference whether the carbohydrate is in a solid or liquid form as long as the sugars themselves are the same (55). If, however, an insoluble sugar (e.g., amylopectin) is ingested, the rate at which glucose is made available to the working muscle will be reduced compared to the same quantity of a soluble sugar (107, 256). Ingestion of glucose polymers has been frequently employed during exercise (89, 138, 217, 224, 270, 315). The basis for consuming this form of sugar is that the osmolarity of the ingested solution will be reduced, thereby decreasing the movement of water and electrolytes into the gastrointestinal tract. It was also thought that the higher osmolarity would facilitate gastric emptying. This does not appear to be case (55, 116). Once in the small intestine, the glucose polymers are rapidly hydrolyzed to free glucose and absorbed in this form. Therefore, upon absorption from the gastrointestinal tract, they are metabolized with the same efficiency as that of ingested glucose. Sucrose ingestion has been used as a source of substrate during exercise with effectiveness similar to that of ingested glucose (16, 215). This is not surprising since, again, the hydrolysis of this sugar leads to the entry of glucose into the circulation.

Effect of Carbohydrate Ingestion on Endogenous Substrates

Carbohydrate ingestion is accompanied by hormonal and metabolic changes that will impact on the fuel supply to the working muscle. Carbohydrate ingestion slows the rate of fall of circulating glucose that generally occurs with prolonged exercise or leads to an overt increase in circulating glucose (55). At least two important endocrine changes accompany the increase in glucose availability. The exercise-induced fall in insulin and rise in glucagon are attenuated or eliminated altogether (3). The absence of the fall in insulin will suppress both the mobilization of NEFA from adipose tissue and glucose from the liver (122, 304), while a reduction in glucagon will reduce the latter (122, 310). Insulin will, of course, stimulate glucose transport at the working muscle, a process that may also be increased by a reduction in NEFA levels (21, 234). Although insulin acts to suppress net muscle glycogen breakdown (67), multiple signals are present in the working muscle and the antiglycogenolytic effects of insulin more often than not are counterbalanced by these. The effects of carbohydrate ingestion on muscle glycogen breakdown during exercise have yielded conflicting results. An attenuation (22, 78, 112, 335) and no effect (64, 86, 111, 172, 209, 221) have been observed when exercise is accompanied by glucose ingestion. These variable results may be due to differences in exercise intensity and duration or to other technical differences. In addition, it is possible that the decreased availability of circulating NEFA under these conditions may require continued utilization of muscle glycogen which, in some cases, may offset the effects of insulin and glucose on muscle glycogen breakdown.

The insulin response to fructose is markedly reduced compared to the response to glucose (172, 173). For this reason fructose ingestion has been used as a fuel during exercise with the expectation that it would prevent an increase in insulin and minimize the antilipolytic effect of the hormone. Despite the diminished insulin response, fructose ingestion does not, however, normally seem to improve exercise performance (22, 215) or slow muscle glycogen depletion (172). The inability of fructose to lead to a more favorable response to exercise is consistent with a slower rate of oxidation of ingested fructose compared to ingested glucose over the course of prolonged exercise (195, 196). This reduced oxidation rate is most likely due to a slower absorption rate from the gastrointestinal tract and also to the fact that fructose must be converted to glucose via hepatic gluconeogenesis in order to be metabolized in the working muscle. It is noteworthy that when subjects are exercised after a prolonged fast that stimulates gluconeogenic processes, the oxidation rate of ingested fructose becomes similar to that of an equal quantity of glucose (69, 197).

Because of the difficulties in studying liver metabolism directly in humans and the complexities in using tracer methods in the presence of glucose absorption, very little direct information as to the effects of carbohydrate ingestion on hepatic glucose production are available. The data that are available, however, are all uniform in suggesting that exogenous glucose reduces the demands on the liver. Glucose infusion reduces liver glycogen breakdown and hepatic glucose production during low- and moderate-intensity exercise in humans (146, 147) and animal models (18, 135, 320). Furthermore, glucose ingestion inhibits the uptake of gluconeogenic precursors by the splanchnic bed during prolonged low-intensity exercise (3). It has been demonstrated that ingested glucose can comprise nearly 70% of the circulating glucose pool during moderate-intensity exercise (60, 283). The potent effect of glucose infusion and carbohydrate ingestion at the liver is probably mediated, in large part, by a highly sensitive pancreatic hormone response (18).

TRAINING-INDUCED ADAPTATIONS IN EXTRAMUSCULAR FUEL MOBILIZATION

The result of the adaptations to repeated bouts of exercise is an improved capacity to perform subsequent bouts. Training-induced adaptations provide insight into the mechanisms that the body perceives to be limiting for work performance. During very-high-intensity exercise that can be maintained for only short intervals, the availability of extramuscular fuels is not limiting. One would predict, therefore, that adaptations in the processes responsible for the provision of these fuels are minimal. Instead, it is more likely that under these conditions the important metabolic adaptations occur within the muscle itself. The adaptations to regular bouts of prolonged exercise, on the other hand, reflect the importance of extramuscular fuels during work of this type. Functional changes in the efficiency with which these substrates are stored, mobilized, delivered, and utilized all come about in response to regular exercise of this type. The result of participation in chronic endurance-type exercise is an increased ability to preserve glucose homeostasis and maintain tissue glycogen stores during prolonged exercise. The primary mechanisms by which this is accomplished occurs through adaptations in the endocrine system and within adipose tissue and liver. The following discussion addresses the nature of these adaptations.

Endocrine Adaptations to Physical Training

The greater metabolic efficiency of the trained organism is evident by the reduced hormone response to exercise that is required at any absolute work intensity (92). The exercise-induced increases in glucagon, norepinephrine, and epinephrine and the exercise-induced reduction in circulating insulin are all blunted with endurance training (92). These adaptations occur rapidly and are essentially complete within ~2 weeks (204, 322, 323). The mechanisms behind these blunted responses are unknown. It is possible that an attenuation of the catecholamine response is a common denominator. Catecholamines can increase glucagon and reduce circulating insulin levels. For this reason one may speculate that the reduced catecholamine response could be the cause of these other endocrine changes. It is also possible that a blunted endocrine response to prolonged exercise may occur via an improved capacity to maintain glucose homeostasis. It is noteworthy that despite the reduced counterregulatory hormone responses to exercise at the same intensity of work, the increase in epinephrine in response to various stimuli, such as hypoglycemia (169), glucagon (168), and hypoxia (168), is actually increased in the trained state.

The adaptation of the pancreatic β-cell to exercise training has been the most widely assessed of the endocrine organs. Basal (24) and glucose-stimulated (141, 207, 247) insulin levels are both reduced in response to regular exercise. Although the reduction in glucose-stimulated insulin levels appears to be greater than that which can be explained by the effects of a single bout of prior exercise (141), studies in humans suggest that the effect of training on plasma insulin levels is short lived in relation to other adaptations (165). Insulin release into the circulation of trained rats as assessed using ^{125}I-insulin is reduced in the fasted state (327). Furthermore, glucose-stimulated insulin release from pancreatic islets isolated from trained rats is lower than that observed in sedentary controls (96, 235). These experiments demonstrate that the lower basal and glucose-stimulated insulin levels after training are primarily the result of a decreased insulin secretion rate. Evidence also exists that insulin clearance is elevated and may make a small contribution to the lower insulin levels in trained humans (326) and rats (327). In support of a direct effect on the pancreas is the demonstration that exercise training, or an associated weight loss, reverses the β-cell damage and fibrosis associated with aging in sedentary rats (235). Training results in decreases in the mRNA for proinsulin and glucokinase in the pancreas (175). This suggests that there are at least two potential cellular mechanisms for the decreased insulin secretion. First, the existence of a reduction in proinsulin mRNA suggests that the synthesis of insulin is reduced. Second, it has been hypothesized that the reaction catalyzed by glucokinase (i.e., the phosphorylation of glucose) serves as the glucose sensor in the pancreas (198). Since glucokinase mRNA is reduced it is possible that glucokinase activity is reduced, thereby explaining the decreased sensitivity of the β-cell to glucose. The events that trigger these effects at the cell may be related to some event relating to catecholamine action, since either phentolamine (177) or adrenalectomy (243) can prevent the effect of exercise training on insulin secretion.

Adaptations of Extramuscular Fuel Sources to Physical Training

An extension of the effects of training on the endocrine and sympathetic nervous systems is that the metabolic fuel depots that are so closely regulated by them must adapt as well. The adipocyte of the trained organism has an increased ability to mobilize and store NEFAs. This allows for improved fuel provisions to the muscle during exercise despite reduced sympathetic nerve activity (at a given absolute work rate) and better replenishment of triglyceride stores afterwards despite reduced pancreatic insulin secretion during feeding. The increase in the capacity of these pathways is illustrated by the increased basal glycerol and palmitate flux rates and the greater rate of triglyceride–fatty acid cycling in highly trained human subjects (248). The increased ability to mobilize NEFAs occurs as a result of an increased adipocyte sensitivity to the catecholamines (11, 34, 66, 139, 194, 319) and is mediated by an increased formation (139, 319) and/or improved effectiveness of cAMP (139). This sensitization to the catecholamines can occur in the absence of an increase in β-receptor number or agonist-binding affinity on the plasma membrane of isolated adipocytes (34, 319). It has been proposed instead to involve an increase in the coupling of the plasma membrane receptor to adenylate cyclase due to a modification of the G protein that links them (319). This hypothesis was supported by the demonstration that guanine nucleotides were more potent in stimulating adenylate cyclase in adipocyte plasma membranes isolated from trained as compared to sedentary rats (140). Despite evidence that catecholamine-stimulated adenylate cyclase activity is increased in adipocytes isolated from trained rats, phosphodiesterase activity is also increased, leading to an overall reduction in cAMP levels (10, 164). This would seem to indicate that a step distal to the formation of cAMP causes the increased lipolytic rate. This concept is supported by the demonstration that dibutyryl cAMP-stimulated (34, 244) and cAMP-stimulated (139) lipolysis in normal and permeabilized adipocytes, respectively, is increased in the trained state. Nevertheless, neither the activity of cAMP protein kinase (264) nor hormone-sensitive lipase (263) has been shown to be increased.

The rate-limiting process for triglyceride formation is the provision of glycerol 3-phosphate. As a result, the increased capacity to store triglyceride in the trained state must involve adaptations in the ability of the fat cell to metabolize glucose, the carbon source of this compound. Consistent with this is the demonstration that exercise training increases the glucose transporter number in adipocytes (123, 288). Both basal glucose transport and metabolism were reported to increase (296) and to be unchanged (287) in adipocytes isolated from trained rats. There is an unequivocal increase in adipocyte insulin-stimulated glucose transport (65, 287, 296), oxidation (65, 287, 296), and incorporation into lipid (65, 142, 257, 287, 296) in the trained state. Exercise training results in a reduction in adipocyte size (11, 34, 65, 287) which, in turn, is an independent determinant of insulin sensitivity (254). The reduced size of the adipocyte is probably a major reason for the increased capacity to transport and metabolize glucose. Nevertheless, training appears to increase glucose transport and metabolism by other mechanisms as well, since adaptations can occur in the absence of a reduction in adipocyte cell size (296). In addition to the effects on adipocyte glucose metabolism, adipose tissue mitochondrial enzyme activity is increased in the trained state (274). This may be important in supplying the ATP that is necessary for the formation of glycerol 3-phosphate.

Prolonged exercise places considerable demands on the glucoregulatory system. It is not surprising, therefore, that there are adjustments in hepatic function that occur after endurance-type training. These adaptations improve the ability of an organism to maintain glucose homeostasis in response to exercise (32, 77, 204). Training increases the capacity for hepatic gluconeogenesis (77, 276), a pathway critical in counteracting hypoglycemia during long-duration exercise. This is evident from studies that show that maximal rates of gluconeogenesis from lactate are increased in perfused rat livers from trained rats (276) and further supported by the demonstration that exercise-stimulated gluconeogenesis from various precursors is increased in hepatocytes isolated from trained rats (25). The intrahepatic mechanism for this increase in gluconeogenic capacity is unclear. The activity of the key gluconeogenic enzyme phosphoenolpyruvate carboxykinase is not elevated in the basal state, but may increase more in response to exercise in the trained state (130). In addition, a reduction in hepatic phosphodiesterase activity has been reported to occur in response to endurance training (75). This adaptation may increase the responsiveness of the gluconeogenic pathway to hormones and thereby enhance the exercise response. Hepatic fuel oxidation is necessary to supply energy for gluconeogenesis. In this regard, it is notable that endurance training leads to an increase in the oxidative capacity of the liver (149, 276). Although the stimulus for these changes in hepatic function have not been studied extensively, the increase in hepatic oxidative capacity seems to be mediated by β-adrenergic stimulation (149).

The ability to maintain glucose homeostasis during exercise is facilitated by a decreased glucose demand at any given submaximal work rate after endurance training (126). Studies in trained human subjects show that hepatic glucose production is reduced in accordance with the lower requirement (56, 204). The mechanism for this reduction may relate to the concurrent attenuation in counterregulatory hormone responses (204) or an altered hormonal responsiveness of the liver (75, 204). Just 10 days of endurance training reduced the response of hepatic glucose production to 2 h of exercise by a mean of 25% in human subjects [Fig. 23.9; (204)]. After 12 weeks of training the increase in hepatic glucose production was reduced by over 40% of pretraining values. Trained, long-term–fasted rats have a greater increase in response to submaximal exercise than their sedentary counterparts (77). This discrepancy with results obtained in humans may reflect the glycogen-depleted state and a greater reliance on the gluconeogenic pathway which, as noted above, may have a greater capacity after training. Studies in the rat also show that training-induced adaptations may actually increase the capacity for hepatic glucose production so that higher rates can be achieved in response to high-intensity exercise (32).

There is little evidence that hepatic glucose uptake or glycogen storage is improved after training. Glucose uptake by the perfused livers of trained rats is no greater than that of sedentary controls in the presence or absence of insulin (211). Furthermore, glycogen deposition assessed following hyperinsulinemic glucose clamps is not increased by training in rats (142). This is consistent with the finding that insulin binding to the liver of trained rats is not increased (27).

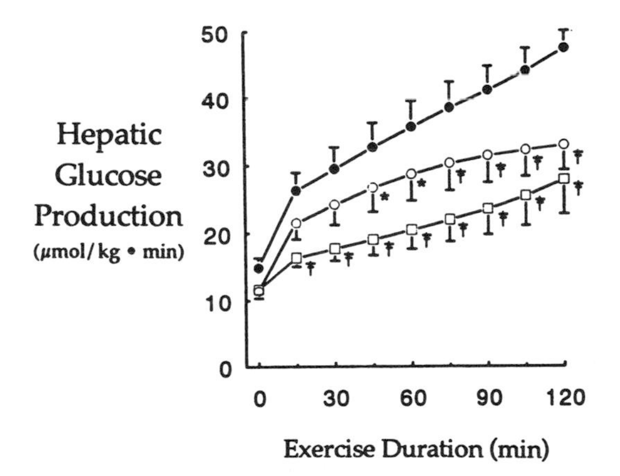

FIG. 23.9. Rate of appearance of plasma glucose at rest and during exercise before *(closed circles)* and after 10 days *(open circles)* and 12 weeks *(open squares)* of endurance training. Subjects were exercised at 60% of their pretraining maximum oxygen uptakes. Significantly different than before training ($P<0.05$). ‡Significantly different than before training ($P<0.001$). [Modified from Mendenhall et al. (204).]

SUMMARY

The increased metabolic demands of muscular work require an increase in fuel metabolism. For the greater energy needs to be sustained, fuels present outside the muscle must be mobilized, delivered, and consumed by the muscle. In healthy, postabsorptive individuals, adipose tissue lipolysis and hepatic glycogenolysis and gluconeogenesis are the critical pathways for fuel mobilization. The precise contribution from each pathway is not arbitrary, but is based on a number of variables, most importantly the exercise duration and intensity. The importance of NEFAs from adipose tissue increases with exercise duration, while the role of glucose derived from the liver is greater at higher work intensities. The mobilization of these substrates is regulated by a complex hormonal and neural response that is not entirely understood. During moderate-intensity exercise, the increment in NEFA mobilization is primarily due to accelerated lipolysis resulting from increased adrenergic drive to adipose tissue and reduced pancreatic insulin secretion (Figure 23.10). Hepatic glucose production is controlled by an increase in glucagon secretion from the pancreas and a decrease in insulin secretion (Fig. 23.10). The hepatic response can be considered in terms of effects on glycogenolysis and gluconeogenesis. Hepatic glycogenolysis is stimulated by changes in both glucagon and insulin secretion, while gluconeogenesis is regulated by the increase in glucagon. The increase in gluconeogenesis is reliant on the mobilization of precursors generated by lipolysis, glycolysis, and proteolysis in extrahepatic tissues. While much has been learned in recent years regarding these processes, there is particular uncertainty regarding two features of the regulation of extramuscular sources of fuel. First, the factors that determine the hormonal and neural responses that are so important to these processes are not well defined. Second, it is unclear whether the same regulators that are important during moderate-intensity exercise are equally as important during heavy exercise.

Most of the research conducted in the area of regulation of fuel metabolism during exercise has focused on understanding the postabsorptive state. Exercise, however, is frequently undertaken while gastrointestinal fuel absorption is present. Metabolic substrates absorbed from the intestine can be an abundant and readily available fuel source. This may be an important vehicle for supplying carbohydrate to the working muscle, since the endogenous stores of this substrate are limited in quantity. The effect of ingested sugars is complex, as increased intestinal absorption will attenuate many of the hormonal

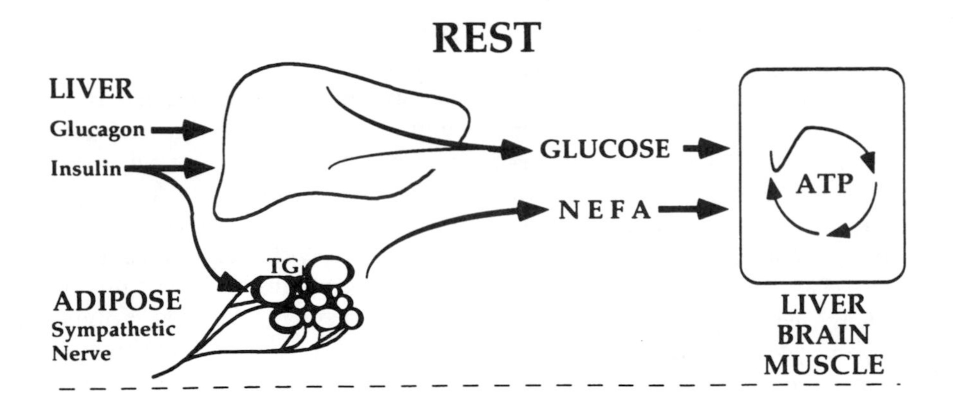

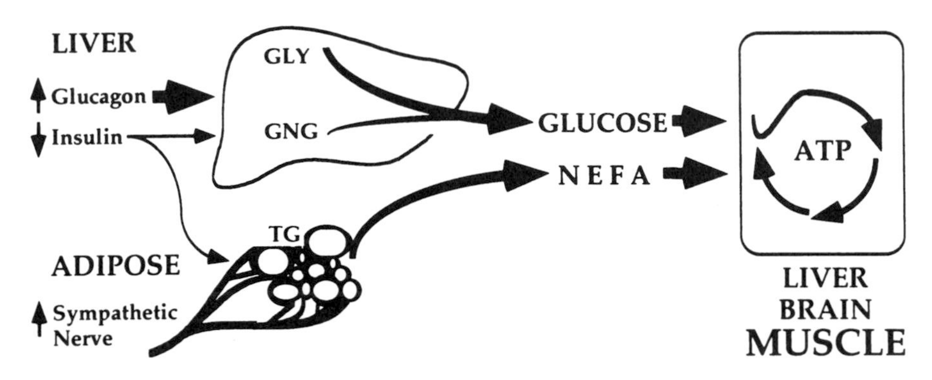

FIG. 23.10. Summary of hormones and nerves involved in the regulation of glucose from the liver and NEFA from adipose tissue during moderate-intensity exercise.

changes that occur with exercise and inhibit the mobilization of NEFA from adipose tissue and glucose from the liver. Nevertheless, carbohydrate ingestion can be effectively used during prolonged exercise to preserve glucose homeostasis and sustain glucose delivery to the muscle and, as a consequence, increase endurance time.

The adaptations that occur with endurance training improve the capacity to mobilize NEFAs and preserve glucose homeostasis. The ability to perform prolonged exercise is improved, probably in large part, due to these adaptations. These metabolic effects are accompanied by a reduced endocrine response and adaptations within the adipocyte and hepatocyte. In adipose tissue, the ability to both mobilize and store NEFAs is increased by training. At the liver the effects of training are less clear. The improved ability to mobilize NEFAs appears to decrease the reliance of muscle on glucose; as a result, hepatic glucose production is reduced. In addition, the ability to maintain glucose homeostasis may be aided by an increased gluconeogenic capacity.

The mechanisms by which fuels are delivered to the working muscle involve the integration of processes in diverse organ systems. The responses of these different organs are coordinated to best meet the metabolic needs of the muscle. The close relationship between the improved capacity to provide fuels to the working muscle and endurance emphasizes the importance of these processes. Future research will be important in further defining the means by which these processes are regulated at the cellular and organ levels. Because exercise, and specifically fuel mobilization, involves the integration of many distinct processes, continued investigation of the response at the level of the whole organism remains essential.

REFERENCES

1. Abumrad, N. N., P. E. Williams, M. Frexes-Steed, R. Geer, P. Flakoll, E. Cersosimo, L. L. Brown, I. Melki, N. Bulus, H. Hourani, M. Hubbard, and F. Ghishan. Inter-organ metabolism of amino acids in vivo. *Diabetes Metab. Rev.* 5: 213–226, 1989.
2. Adopo, E., F. Peronnet, D. Masicotte, G. R. Brisson, and C. Hillaire-Marcel. Respective of oxidation of exogenous glucose and fructose given in the same drink during exercise. *J. Appl. Physiol.* 76: 1014–1019, 1994.
3. Ahlborg, G., and P. Felig. Influence of glucose ingestion on fuel-hormone response during prolonged exercise. *J. Appl. Physiol.* 41: 683–688, 1976.

4. Ahlborg, G., and P. Felig. Substrate utilization during prolonged exercise preceded by ingestion of glucose. *Am. J. Physiol.* 233 (*Endocrinol. Metab. Gastrointest. Physiol.* 2): E188–E194, 1977.
5. Ahlborg, G., and P. Felig. Lactate and glucose exchange across the forearm, legs, and splanchnic bed during after prolonged leg exercise. *J. Clin. Invest.* 69: 45–54, 1982.
6. Ahlborg, G., P. Felig, L. Hagenfeldt, R. Hendler, and J. Wahren. Substrate turnover during prolonged exercise in man. *J. Clin. Invest.* 53: 1080–1090, 1974.
7. Arnall, D. A., J. C. Marker, R. K. Conlee, and W. W. Winder. Effect of infusing epinephrine on liver and muscle glycogenolysis during exercise. *Am. J. Physiol.* 250 (*Endocrinol. Metab.* 13): E641–E649, 1986.
8. Arner, P., E. Kriegholm, P. Engfeldt, and J. Bolinder. Adrenergic regulation of lipolysis in situ at rest and during exercise. *J. Clin. Invest.* 85: 893–898, 1990.
9. Arogyasami, J., T. L. Sellers, J. P. Jones, C. Duan, and W. W. Winder. Insulin-induced hypoglycemia in fed and fasted exercising rats. *J. Appl. Physiol.* 72: 1992–1998, 1989.
10. Askew, E. W., A. L. Hecker, V. G. Coppes, and F. B. Stifel. Cyclic AMP metabolism in adipose tissue of exercise-trained rats. *J. Lipid. Res.* 19: 729–736, 1978.
11. Askew, E. W., R. L. Huston, C. G. Plopper, and A. L. Hecker. Adipose tissue cellularity and lipolysis: response to exercise and cortisol treatment. *J. Clin. Invest.* 56: 521–529, 1975.
12. Balon, T. W., A. Zorzano, J. L. Treadway, M. N. Goodman, and N. B. Ruderman. Effect of insulin on protein synthesis and degradation in skeletal muscle after exercise. *Am. J. Physiol.* 258 (*Endocrinol. Metab.* 21): E92–E97, 1990.
13. Barakat, H. A., G. J. Kasperek, and G. L. Dohm. Progressive changes in fatty acid metabolism in rat liver and muscle during exercise. *Biochem. Med.* 29: 298–306, 1983.
14. Barclay, G. R., and L. A. Turnberg. Effect of moderate exercise on salt and water transport in the human jejunum. *Gut* 29: 816–820, 1988.
15. Begum, N., R. L. Terjung, H. M. Tepperman, and J. Tepperman. Effect of acute exercise on insulin generation of pyruvate dehydrogenase activator by rat liver and rat adipocyte plasma membranes. *Diabetes* 35: 785–790, 1986.
16. Benade, A. J. S., C. H. Wyndham, C. R. Jansen, G. G. Rogers, and E. J. P. Debruin. Plasma insulin and carbohydrate metabolism after sucrose ingestion during rest and prolonged exercise. *Pflugers Arch.* 342: 207–218, 1973.
17. Bennet, W. M., and M. W. Haymond. Plasma pool source for fibrinogen synthesis in postabsorptive conscious dogs. *Am. J. Physiol.* 260 (*Endocrinol. Metab.* 23): E581–E587, 1991.
18. Berger, C. M., P. J. Sharis, D. P. Bracy, D. B. Lacy, and D. H. Wasserman. Sensitivity of the exercise-induced increments in hepatic glycogenolysis and gluconeogenesis to glucose supply and demand. *Am. J. Physiol.* 267 (*Endocrinol. Metab.* 30): E411–E421, 1994.
19. Berger, M., P. Berchtold, H. J. Kuppers, H. Drost, H. K. Kley, W. A. Muller, W. Wiegelmann, H. Zimmerman-Telschow, F. A. Gries, H. L. Kruskemper, and H. Zimmerman. Metabolic and hormonal effects of muscular exercise in juvenile type diabetics. *Diabetologia* 13: 355–365, 1977.
20. Bergstrom, J., L. Hermansen, E. Hultman, and B. Saltin. Diet, muscle glycogen and physical performance. *Acta Physiol. Scand.* 71: 140–150, 1967.
21. Bjorkman, O., P. Miles, D. H. Wasserman, L. Lickley, and M. Vranic. Muscle glucose uptake during exercise in total insulin deficiency: No effect of beta-adrenergic blockade. *J. Clin. Invest.* 81: 1759–1767, 1988.
22. Bjorkman, O., K. Sahlin, L. Hagenfeldt, and J. Wahren. Influence of glucose and fructose ingestion on the capacity for long-term exercise in well-trained men. *Clin. Physiol.* 4: 483–494, 1984.
23. Bjorntorp, P. The effect of lactic acid on adipose tissue metabolism in vitro. *Acta Med. Scand.* 178: 253–258, 1965.
24. Bjorntorp, P., K. Dejounge, L. Sjostrom, and L. Sullivan. The effect of physical training on insulin production in obesity. *Metabolism* 19: 631–638, 1970.
25. Bobyleva-Guarriero, V., and H. Lardy. The effect of different types of physical exercise on glucose and citrulline synthesis in isolated rat liver parenchymal cells. *FEBS Lett.* 194: 56–59, 1986.
26. Bolinder, J., L. Kager, J. Ostman, and P. Arner. Differences at the receptor and post-receptor levels between human omental and subcutaneous adipose tissue in the action of insulin on lipolysis. *Diabetes* 32: 117–129, 1983.
27. Bonen, A., P. A. Clune, and M. H. Tan. Chronic exercise increases insulin binding in muscles but not liver. *Am. J. Physiol.* 251 (*Endocrinol. Metab.* 14): E196–E203, 1986.
28. Boyd, A. E., S. R. Giamber, M. Mager, and H. E. Lebovitz. Lactate inhibition of lipolysis in exercising man. *Metabolism* 23: 531–542, 1974.
29. Brenner, W., T. R. Hendrix, and P. R. McHugh. Regulation of the gastric emptying of glucose. *Gastroenterology* 85: 76–82, 1983.
30. Brockman, R. P. Effect of somatostatin on plasma glucagon and insulin, and glucose turnover in exercising sheep. *J. Appl. Physiol.* 47: 273–278, 1979.
31. Brooks, B., J. R. S. Arch, and E. A. Newsholme. Effects of hormones on the rate of the triacylglycerol/fatty acid substrate cycle in adipocytes and and epididymal fat pads. *FEBS Lett.* 146: 327–330, 1982.
32. Brooks, G. A., and C. M. Donovan. Effect of endurance training on glucose kinetics during exercise. *Am. J. Physiol.* 244 (*Endocrinol. Metab.* 7): E505–E512, 1983.
33. Brooks, G. A., E. E. Wolfel, B. M. Groves, P. R. Bender, G. E. Butterfield, A. Cymerman, R. S. Mazzeo, J. R. Sutton, R. R. Wolfe, and J. T. Reeves. Muscle accounts for glucose disposal but not blood lactate appearance during exercise after acclimatization to 4,300 m. *J. Appl. Physiol.* 72: 2435–2445, 1992.
34. Bukowiecki, L., J. Lupien, N. Follea, D. Paradis, D. Richard, and J. Leblanc. Mechanism of enhanced lipolysis in adipose tissue of exercise-trained rat. *Am. J. Physiol.* 239 (*Endocrinol. Metab.* 2): E422–E429, 1980.
35. Buttrose, M., D. McKellar, and T. C. Welbourne. Gut-liver interaction in glutamine homeostasis: portal ammonia role in uptake and metabolism. *Am. J. Physiol.* 252 (*Endocrinol. Metab.* 15): E746–E750, 1987.
36. Calles, J., J. J. Cunningham, L. Nelson, N. Brown, E. Nadel, R. S. Sherwin, and P. Felig. Glucose turnover during recovery from intensive exercise. *Diabetes* 32: 734–738, 1983.
37. Calles-Escandon, J., J. J. Cunningham, P. Snyder, R. Jacob, G. Huszar, J. Loke, and P. Felig. Influence of exercise on urea, creatinine, and 3-methylhistidine excretion in normal human subjects. *Am. J. Physiol.* 246 (*Endocrinol. Metab.* 15): E334–E339, 1984.
38. Cammack, J., N. W. Read, P. A. Cann, B. Greenwood, and A. M. Holgate. Effect of prolonged exercise on the pasage of a solid meal through the stomach and small intestine. *Gut* 23: 957–961, 1982.

39. Campbell, J. M. H., G. O. Mitchell, and A. T. W. Powell. The influence of exercise on digestion. *Guy's Hosp. Rep.* 78: 279–293, 1928.
40. Carlson, K. I., J. C. Marker, D. A. Arnall, M. L. Terry, H. T. Yang, L. G. Lindsay, M. E. Bracken, and W. W. Winder. Epinephrine is unessential for stimulation of liver glycogenolysis during exercise. *J. Appl. Physiol.* 58: 544–548, 1985.
41. Carlson, L. A., and F. Mossfeldt. Acute effects of prolonged, heavy exercise on the concentration of plasma lipids and lipoproteins in man. *Acta Physiol. Scand.* 62: 51–59, 1964.
42. Carraro, F., W. H. Hartl, C. A. Stuart, D. K. Layman, F. Jahoor, and R. R. Wolfe. Whole body and plasma protein synthesis in exercise and recovery in human subjects. *Am. J. Physiol.* 258 (*Endocrinol. Metab.* 21): E821–E831, 1990.
43. Carraro, F., T. D. Kimbrough, and R. R. Wolfe. Urea kinetics in humans at two levels of exercise intensity. *J. Appl. Physiol.* 75: 1180–1185, 1993.
44. Carraro, F., A. Naldini, J. M. Weber, and R. R. Wolfe. Alanine kinetics in humans during low-intensity exercise. *Med. Sci. Sports Exerc.* 26: 348–353, 1994.
45. Carraro, F., C. A. Stuart, W. H. Hartl, J. Rosenblatt, and R. R. Wolfe. Effect of exercise and recovery on muscle protein synthesis in human subjects. *Am. J. Physiol.* 259 (*Endocrinol. Metab.* 22): E470–E476, 1990.
46. Cersosimo, E., P. E. Williams, R. J. Geer, T. Lairmore, F. Ghishan, and N. N. Abumrad. Importance of ammonium ions in regulating hepatic glutamine synthesis during fasting. *Am. J. Physiol.* 257 (*Endocrinol. Metab.* 20): E514–E519, 1989.
47. Cherrington, A. D. Gluconeogenesis: its regulation by glucagon and insulin. In: *Diabetes Mellitus*, edited by M. Brownlee. New York: Garland, 1981.
48. Cherrington, A. D., H. Fuchs, R. W. Stevenson, P. E. Williams, K. G. M. M. Alberti, and K. E. Steiner. Effect of epinephrine on glycogenolysis and gluconeogenesis in conscious overnight-fasted dogs. *Am. J. Physiol.* 247 (*Endocrinol. Metab.* 10): E137–E144, 1984.
49. Cherrington, A. D., W. W. Lacy, and J. L. Chiasson. Effect of glucagon on glucose production during insulin deficiency in the dog. *J. Clin. Invest.* 62: 664–677, 1978.
50. Cherrington, A. D., J. E. Liljenquist, G. I. Shulman, P. E. Williams, and W. W. Lacy. Importance of hypoglycemia-induced glucose production during isolated glucagon deficiency. *Am. J. Physiol.* 236 (*Endocrinol. Metab. Gastrointest. Physiol.* 5): E263–E271, 1979.
51. Chisholm, D. J., A. B. Jenkins, D. E. James, and E. W. Kraegan. The effect of hyperinsulinemia on glucose homeostasis during moderate exercise in man. *Diabetes* 31: 603–608, 1982.
52. Christensen, N. J., and H. Galbo. Sympathetic nerve activity during exercise. *Annu. Rev. Physiol.* 45: 139–153, 1983.
53. Coggan, A. R., and E. F. Coyle. Reversal of fatigue during prolonged exercise by carbohydrate infusion or ingestion. *J. Appl. Physiol.* 63: 2388–2395, 1987.
54. Coggan, A. R., and E. F. Coyle. Metabolism and performance following carbohydrate ingestion late in exercise. *Med. Sci. Sports Exerc.* 21: 59–65, 1989.
55. Coggan, A. R., and E. F. Coyle. Carbohyrate ingestion during prolonged exercise: effects on metabolism and performance. *Exerc. Sports Sci. Rev.* 19: 1–40, 1991.
56. Coggan, A. R., W. M. Kohrt, R. J. Spina, D. M. Bier, and J. O. Holloszy. Endurance training decreases plasma glucose turnover and oxidation during moderate intensity exercise in men. *J. Appl. Physiol.* 68: 990–996, 1990.
57. Cooper, D. M., T. J. Barstow, A. Bergner, and W. P. Lee. Blood glucose turnover during high- and low-intensity exercise. *Am. J. Physiol.* 257 (*Endocrinol. Metab.* 20): E405–E412, 1989.
58. Cooper, D. M., D. H. Wasserman, M. Vranic, and K. Wasserman. Glucose turnover in response to exercise during high- and low-FiO2 breathing in humans. *Am. J. Physiol.* 14 (*Endocrinol. Metab.* 14): E209–E214, 1986.
59. Cordain, L., R. W. Latin, and J. J. Behnke. The effects of an aerobic running programme on bowel transit time. *J. Sports Med.* 26: 101–104, 1986.
60. Costill, D. L., A. Bennett, G. Branam, and D. Eddy. Glucose ingestion at rest and during prolonged exercise. *J. Appl. Physiol.* 34: 764–769, 1973.
61. Costill, D. L., E. Coyle, G. P. Dalsky, W. Evans, W. Fink, and D. Hoopes. Effects of elevated plasma FFA and insulin on muscle glycogen usage during exercise. *J. Appl. Physiol.* 43: 695–699, 1977.
62. Costill, D. L., W. F. Kammer, and A. Fisher. Fluid ingestion during distance running. *Arch. Environ. Health* 21: 520–525, 1970.
63. Costill, D. L., and B. Saltin. Factors limiting gastric emptying. *J. Appl. Physiol.* 37: 679–683, 1974.
64. Coyle, E. F., A. R. Coggin, M. K. Hemmert, and J. L. Ivy. Muscle glycogen utilization during prolonged strenuous exercise when fed carbohydrate. *J. Appl. Physiol.* 61: 165–172, 1986.
65. Craig, B. W., G. T. Hammons, S. M. Garthwaite, L. Jarett, and J. O. Holloszy. Adaptation of fat cells to exercise: response of glucose uptake and oxidation to insulin. *J. Appl. Physiol.* 51: 1500–1506, 1981.
66. Crampes, F., M. Beauville, D. Riviere, and M. Garrigues. Effect of physical training in humans on the response of isolated fat cells to epinephrine. *J. Appl. Physiol.* 61: 25–29, 1986.
67. Danforth, W. H. Glycogen synthetase activity in skeletal muscle: interconversion of two forms and control of glycogen synthesis. *J. Biol. Chem.* 2: 588–593, 1965.
68. Decombaz, J., P. Reinhardt, K. Anantharaman, G. V. Glutz, and J. R. Poortsman. Biochemical changes in a 100 km run: free amino acids, urea, and creatinine. *Eur. J. Appl. Physiol.* 41: 61–72, 1979.
69. Decombaz, J., D. Sartori, M. J. Arnaud, A. L. Thelin, P. Schurch, and H. Howald. Oxidation of metabolic effects of glucose ingested before exercise. *Int. J. Sports Med.* 6: 282–286, 1985.
70. Deibert, D. C., and R. A. Defronzo. Epinephrine-induced insulin resistance in man. *J. Clin. Invest.* 65: 717–721, 1980.
71. Dill, D. B., H. T. Edwards, and J. H. Talbott. Studies in muscular activity. VII. Factors limiting the capacity to work. *J. Physiol.* 77: 49–62, 1932.
72. Dohm, G. L., R. G. Israel, R. L. Breedlove, R. T. Williams, and E. W. Askew. Biphasic changes in 3-methylhistidine excretion in humans after exercise. *Am. J. Physiol.* 248 (*Endocrinol. Metab.* 11): E588–E592, 1985.
73. Dohm, G. L., G. J. Kasperek, and H. A. Barakat. Time course of changes in gluconeogenic enzyme activities during exercise and recovery. *Am. J. Physiol.* 249 (*Endocrinol. Metab.* 12): E6–E11, 1985.
74. Dohm, G. L., and E. A. Newsholme. Metabolic control of hepatic gluconeogenesis during exercise. *Biochem. J.* 212: 633–639, 1983.

75. Dohm, G. L., S. N. Pennington, and H. Barakat. Effect of exercise training on adenylyl cyclase and phosphodiesterase in skeletal muscle, heart, and liver. *Biochem. Med.* 16: 138–142, 1976.
76. Dohm, G. R., G. J. Kasperek, E. B. Tapscott, and G. R. Beecher. Effect of exercise on synthesis and degradation of muscle protein. *Biochem. J.* 188: 255–262, 1985.
77. Donovan, C. M., and K. D. Sumida. Training improves glucose homeostasis in rats during exercise via glucose production. *Am. J. Physiol.* 258 (*Regulatory Integrative Comp. Physiol.* 27): R770–R776, 1990.
78. Erikson, M. A., R. J. Schwarzkopf, and R. D. McKenzie. Effects of caffeine, fructose, and glucose ingestion on muscle glycogen utilization during exercise. *Med. Sci. Sports Exerc.* 19: 579–583, 1987.
79. Eriksson, L. S., S. Broberg, O. Bjorkman, and J. Wahren. Ammonia metabolism during exercise in man. *Clin. Physiol.* 5: 325–336, 1985.
80. Euler, U. S. V. *Adrenal Medullary Secretion and its Neural Control.* New York: Academic Press, 1967.
81. Evans, D. F., G. E. Foster, and J. D. Hardcastle. Does exercise affect small bowel motility in man? *Gut* 24: A1012, 1989.
82. Exton, J. H., and S. C. Harper. Role of cyclic-AMP in the actions of the catecholamines in hepatic carbohydrate metabolism. *Adv. Cyclic Nucleotide Res.* 5: 519–532, 1975.
83. Feldman, M., and J. V. Nixon. Effect of exercise on postprandial gastic secretion and emptying in humans. *J. Appl. Physiol.* 53: 851–854, 1982.
84. Felig, P., and J. Wahren. Amino acid metabolism in exercising man. *J. Clin. Invest.* 50: 2703–2711, 1971.
85. Fery, F., and E. O. Balasse. Response of ketone body metabolism to exercise during transition from post-absorptive to fasted state. *Am. J. Physiol.* 250 (*Endocrinol. Metab.* 13): E495–E501, 1986.
86. Fielding, R. A., D. L. Costill, W. J. Fink, D. S. King, M. Hargreaves, and J. E. Kovaleski. Effect of carbohydrate feeding frequency and dosage on muscle glycogen use during exercise. *Med. Sci. Sports Exerc.* 17: 472–476, 1985.
87. Fordtran, J. S., and B. Saltin. Gastric emptying and intestinal absorption during prolonged severe exercise. *J. Appl. Physiol.* 23: 555–559, 1967.
88. Foster, C., D. L. Costill, and W. J. Fink. Effects of pre-exercise feedings on endurance performance. *Med. Sci. Sports Exerc.* 11: 1–5, 1979.
89. Foster, C., D. L. Costill, and W. J. Fink. Gastric emptying characteristics of glucose and glucose polymer solution. *Med. Sci. Sports Exerc.* 51: 299–305, 1980.
90. Franckson, J. R. M., R. Vanroux, R. Leclercq, H. Brunengraber, and H. A. Ooms. Labelled insulin catabolism and pancreatic responsiveness during long-term exercise in man. *Horm. Metab. Res.* 3: 366–373, 1979.
91. Friedman, J. E. Role of glucocorticoids in activation of hepatic PEPCK gene transcription during exercise. *Am. J. Physiol.* 266 (*Endocrinol. Metab.* 29): E560–E566, 1994.
92. Galbo, H. *Hormonal Adaptations to Exercise.* New York: Thieme-Stratton, Inc., 1983.
93. Galbo, H., N. J. Christensen, and J. J. Holst. Catecholamines and pancreatic hormones during autonomic blockade in exercising man. *Acta Physiol. Scand.* 101: 428–437, 1977.
94. Galbo, H., N. J. Christensen, and J. J. Holst. Glucose-induced decrease in glucagon and epinephrine responses to exercise in man. *J. Appl. Physiol.* 42: 525–530, 1977.
95. Galbo, H., N. J. Christensen, K. J. Mikines, B. Sonne, J. Hilsted, C. Hagen, and J. Fahrenkrug. The effect of fasting on the hormonal response to graded exercise. *J. Clin. Endocrinol. Metab.* 52: 1106–1112, 1981.
96. Galbo, H., C. J. Hedeskov, K. Capito, and J. Vinten. The effect of physical training on insulin secretion of rat pancreatic islets. *Acta Physiol. Scand.* 111: 75–79, 1981.
97. Galbo, H., J. J. Holst, and N. J. Christensen. Glucagon and plasma catecholamine responses to graded and prolonged exercise in man. *J. Appl. Physiol.* 38: 70–76, 1975.
98. Galbo, H., J. J. Holst, and N. J. Christensen. The effect of different diets and of insulin on the hormonal response to prolonged exercise in man. *Acta Physiol. Scand.* 107: 19–32, 1979.
99. Garceau, D., N. Yamaguchi, R. Goyer, and F. Guitard. Correlation between endogenous noradrenaline and glucose released from the liver upon hepatic sympathetic nerve stimulation in anesthetized dogs. *Can. J. Physiol. Pharmacol.* 62: 1086–1091, 1984.
100. Geer, R. J., P. E. Williams, T. Lairmore, and N. N. Abumrad. Glucagon: an important stimulator of gut and hepatic glutamine metabolism. *Surg. Forum* 38: 27–29, 1987.
101. Girardier, L., J. Seydoux, M. Berger, and A. Veicsteinas. Selective pancreatic nerve section. An investigation of neural control of glucagon release in the conscious unrestrained dog. *J. Physiol. (Paris)* 74: 731–735, 1978.
102. Goldstein, R. E., G. W. Reed, D. H. Wasserman, P. E. Williams, D. B. Lacy, R. Buckspan, N. N. Abumrad, and A. D. Cherrington. The effects of acute elevations in plasma cortisol on alanine metabolism in the conscious dog. *Metabolism* 41: 1295–1303, 1992.
103. Gollnick, P. D., R. G. Soule, A. W. Taylor, C. Williams, and C. D. Ianuzzo. Exercise-induced glycogenolysis and lipolysis in the rat: hormonal influences. *Am. J. Physiol.* 219: 729–733, 1970.
104. Greenway, C. V., and R. D. Stark. Hepatic vascular bed. *Physiol. Rev.* 51: 23–65, 1971.
105. Gregg, S. G., M. Kern, and G. A. Brooks. Acute anemia results in an increased glucose dependence during sustained exercise. *J. Appl. Physiol.* 66: 1874–1880, 1989.
106. Gue, M., T. Peeters, I. Depoortere, G. Vantrappen, and L. Bueno. Stress induced changes in gastric emptying motilitly and plasma gut hormone levels in dogs. *Gastroenterology* 97: 1101–1107, 1989.
107. Guezennec, C. Y., P. Satapin, F. Duforez, D. Merino, F. Peronnet, and J. Koziet. Oxidation of corn starch, glucose, and fructose ingested before exercise. *Med. Sci. Sports Exerc.* 21: 45–50, 1989.
108. Hagg, S. A., E. L. Morse, and S. A. Adibi. Effect of exercise on rates of oxidation, turnover, and plasma clearance of leucine in human subjects. *Am. J. Physiol.* 242 (*Endocrinol. Metab.* 5): E407–E410, 1982.
109. Haralambie, G., and L. Senser. Metabolic changes in man during long-distance swimming. *Eur. J. Appl. Physiol.* 43: 115–125, 1980.
110. Harber, V. J., and J. R. Sutton. Endorphins and exercise. *Sports Med.* 1: 154–174, 1984.
111. Hargreaves, M., and C. A. Briggs. Effect of carbohydrate ingestion on exercise metabolism. *J. Appl. Physiol.* 65: 1553–1555, 1988.
112. Hargreaves, M., D. Costill, A. Coggan, W. J. Fink, and D. Nishibata. Effect of carbohydrate feeding on muscle glycogen utilization and exercise performance. *Med. Sci. Sports Exerc.* 16: 219–222, 1984.
113. Hartmann, H., K. Beckh, and K. Jungermann. Direct control of glycogen metabolism in the perfused rat liver by the sympathetic innervation. *Eur. J. Biochem.* 123: 521–526, 1982.

114. Harvey, W. D., G. R. Faloona, and R. H. Unger. The effect of adrenergic blockade on exercise-induced hyperglucagonemia. *Endocrinology* 94: 1254–1258, 1974.
115. Haussinger, D., W. Gerok, and H. Sies. Regulation of flux through glutaminase and glutamine synthetase in isolated perfused rat liver. *Biochim. Biophys. Acta* 755: 272–278, 1983.
116. Hawley, J. A., S. C. Dennis, and T. D. Noakes. Oxidation of carbohydrate ingested during prolonged endurance exercise. *Sports Med.* 14: 27–42, 1992.
117. Hellebrandt, F. A., and R. H. Tepper. Studies on the influence of exercise on the digestive work of the stomach. II. Its effect on emptying time. *Am. J. Physiol.* 107: 355–363, 1934.
118. Hems, D. A., and P. D. Whitton. Control of hepatic glycogenolysis. *Physiol. Rev.* 60: 1–50, 1980.
119. Henderson, S. A., A. L. Black, and G. A. Brooks. Leucine turnover and oxidation in trained rats during exercise. *Am. J. Physiol.* 249 (*Endocrinol. Metab.* 12): E137–E144, 1985.
120. Hermansen, L., E. Hultman, and B. Saltin. Muscle glycogen during prolonged severe exercise. *Acta Physiol. Scand.* 71: 129–139, 1967.
121. Hilsted, J., H. Galbo, B. Sonne, T. Schwartz, J. Fahrenkrug, O. B. S. D. Muckadell, K. B. Lauritsen, and B. Tronier. Gastroenteropancreatic hormonal changes during exercise. *Am. J. Physiol.* 239 (*Gastrointest. Liver Physiol.* 2): G136–G140, 1980.
122. Hirsh, I. B., J. C. Marker, L. J. Smith, R. Spina, C. A. Parvin, J. O. Holloszy, and P. E. Cryer. Insulin and glucagon in the prevention of hypoglycemia during exercise in humans. *Am. J. Physiol.* 260 (*Endocrinol. Metab.* 23): E695–E704, 1991.
123. Hirshman, M. F., L. J. Wardzala, L. J. Goodyear, S. P. Fuller, E. D. Horton, and E. S. Horton. Exercise training increases the number of glucose transporters in rat adipose cells. *Am. J. Physiol.* 257 (*Endocrinol. Metab.* 20): E520–E530, 1989.
124. Hoelzer, D. R., G. P. Dalsky, W. E. Clutter, S. D. Shah, J. O. Holloszy, and P. E. Cryer. Glucoregulation during exercise: hypoglycemia is prevented by redundant glucoregulatory systems, sympathochromaffin activation, and changes in islet hormone secretion. *J. Clin. Invest.* 77: 212–221, 1986.
125. Hoelzer, D. R., G. P. Dalsky, N. S. Schwartz, W. E. Clutter, S. D. Shah, J. O. Holloszy, and P. E. Cryer. Epinephrine is not critical to prevention of hypoglycemia during exercise in humans. *Am. J. Physiol.* 251 (*Endocrinol. Metab.* 14): E104–E110, 1986.
126. Holloszy, J. O., and E. Coyle. Adaptations of skeletal muscle to endurance exercise and their metabolic consequences. *J. Appl. Physiol.* 56: 831–838, 1984.
127. Hood, D. A., and R. L. Terjung. Leucine metabolism in perfused rat skeletal muscle during contractions. *Am. J. Physiol.* 253 (*Endocrinol. Metab.* 16): E636–E647, 1987.
128. Hourani, H., P. E. Williams, J. A. Morris, M. E. May, and N. N. Abumrad. Effect of insulin-induced hypoglycemia on protein metabolism in vivo. *Am. J. Physiol.* 259 (*Endocrinol. Metab.* 22): E342–E350, 1990.
129. Hunt, J. N., J. L. Smith, and C. L. Jiang. Effect of meal volume and energy density on the gastric emptying of carbohydrates. *Gastroenterology* 89: 1326–1330, 1985.
130. Huston, R. L., P. C. Weiser, G. L. Dohm, E. W. Askew, and J. B. Boyd. Effect of training, exercise, and diet on muscle glycogenolysis and liver gluconeogenesis. *Life Sci.* 17: 369–376, 1975.
131. Huttunen, J. K., and D. Steinberg. Activation and phosphorylation of purified adipose tissue hormonse-sensitive lipase by cyclic AMP-dependent protein kinase. *Biochim. Biophys. Acta* 239: 411–427, 1971.
132. Huttunen, J. K., D. Steinberg, and S. E. Mayer. ATP-dependent and cyclic AMP-dependent activation of rat adipose tissue lipase by protein kinase from rabbit skeletal muscle. *Proc. Natl. Acad. Sci. U. S. A.* 67: 290–295, 1970.
133. Issekutz, B. Role of beta-adrenergic receptors in mobilization of energy sources in exercising dogs. *J. Appl. Physiol.* 44: 869–876, 1978.
134. Issekutz, B. The role of hypoinsulinemia in exercise metabolism. *Diabetes* 29: 629–635, 1980.
135. Issekutz, B. Effects of glucose infusion on hepatic and muscle glycogenolysis in exercising dogs. *Am. J. Physiol.* 240 (*Endocrinol. Metab.* 3): E451–E457, 1981.
136. Issekutz, B., W. A. S. Shaw, and T. B. Issekutz. Effect of lactate on FFA and glycerol turnover in resting and exercising dogs. *J. Appl. Physiol.* 39: 349–353, 1975.
137. Issekutz, B., and M. Vranic. Significance of glucagon in the control of glucose production during exercise. *Am. J. Physiol.* 238 (*Endocrinol. Metab.* 1): E13–E20, 1980.
138. Ivy, J. L., W. Miller, V. Dover, L. J. Goodyear, W. M. Sherman, S. Farrell, and H. Williams. Endurance improved by ingestion of a glucose polymer supplement. *Med. Sci. Sports Exerc.* 15: 466–471, 1983.
139. Izawa, T., T. Komabayashi, T. Mochizuki, K. Suda, and M. Tsuboi. Enhanced coupling of adenylate cyclase to lipolysis in permeabilized adipocytes from trained rats. *J. Appl. Physiol.* 71: 23–29, 1991.
140. Izawa, T., T. Komabayashi, M. Tsuboi, E. Koshimizu, and K. Suda. Augmentation of catecholamine-stimulated [3H] GDP release in adipocyte membranes from exercise-trained rats. *Jpn. J. Physiol.* 36: 1039–1045, 1986.
141. James, D. E., K. M. Burleigh, E. W. Kraegen, and D. J. Chisholm. Effect of acute exercise and prolonged training on insulin response to intravenous glucose in vivo in rat. *J. Appl. Physiol.* 55: 1660–1664, 1983.
142. James, D. E., E. W. Kraegen, and D. J. Chisholm. Effect of exercise training on in vivo insulin action in individual tissues of the rat. *J. Clin. Invest.* 76: 657–666, 1985.
143. Jandrain, B. J., G. Krzentowski, F. Pirnay, F. Morosa, A. J. Scheen, and P. J. Lefebvre. Metabolic availability of glucose ingested 3 h before prolonged exercise in humans. *Eur. J. Appl. Physiol.* 56: 1314–1319, 1984.
144. Jandrain, B. J., F. Pirnay, M. Lacroix, F. Morosa, A. J. Sheen, and P. J. Lefebvre. Effect of osmolality on availability of glucose ingested during prolonged exercise in humans. *J. Appl. Physiol.* 67: 76–92, 1989.
145. Jarhult, J., and J. J. Holst. The role of the adrenergic innervation to the pancreatic islets in the control of insulin release during exercise in man. *Pflugers Arch.* 383: 41–45, 1979.
146. Jenkins, A. B., D. J. Chisholm, K. Y. Ho, and E. W. Kraegen. Exercise induced hepatic glucose output is precisely sensitive to the rate of systemic glucose supply. *Metabolism* 34: 431–434, 1985.
147. Jenkins, A. B., S. M. Furler, D. J. Chisholm, and E. W. Kraegen. Regulation of hepatic glucose output during exercise by circulating glucose and insulin in humans. *Am. J. Physiol.* 250 (*Regulatory Integrative Comp. Physiol.* 19): R411–R417, 1986.
148. Jensen, M. D., M. W. Haymond, R. A. Rizza, P. E. Cryer, and J. M. Miles. Influence of body fat distribution on free fatty acid metabolism in obesity. *J. Clin. Invest.* 83: 1168–1173, 1989.

149. Ji, L. L., D. F. Lennon, R. G. Kochan, F. J. Nagle, and H. A. Lardy. Enzymatic adaptation to physical training under β-blockade in the rat. Evidence of a β2-adrenergic mechanism in skeletal muscle. *J. Clin. Invest.* 78: 771–778, 1986.
150. John-Adler, H. B., R. M. McAllister, and R. L. Terjung. Reduced running endurance in gluconeogenesis-inhibited rats. *Am. J. Physiol.* 251 (*Regulatory Integrative Comp. Physiol.* 14): R137–R142, 1986.
151. Jones, N. L., G. J. F. Heigenhauser, A. Kuksis, C. G. Matsos, J. R. Sutton, and C. J. Toews. Fat metabolism during heavy exercise. *Clin. Sci.* 59: 469–478, 1980.
152. Juhlin-Dannfeldt, A., G. Ahlborg, L. Hagenfeldt, L. Jorfeldt, and P. Felig. Influence of ethanol on splanchnic and skeletal muscle substrate turnover during prolonged exercise in man. *Am. J. Physiol.* 233 (*Endocrinol. Metab. Gastrointest. Physiol.* 2): E195–E202, 1977.
153. Kanaley, J. A., P. E. Cryer, and M. D. Jensen. Fatty acid kinetic responses to exercise. Effects of obesity, body fat distribution, and energy-restricted diet. *J. Clin. Invest.* 92: 255–261, 1993.
154. Karlsson, J., and B. Saltin. Lactate, ATP, and CP in working muscles during exhaustive exercise in man. *J. Appl. Physiol.* 29: 598–602, 1970.
155. Kasperek, G. J., G. R. Conway, D. S. Krayeski, and J. J. Lohne. A re-examination of the effect of exercise on rate of muscle protein degradation. *Am. J. Physiol.* 263 (*Endocrinol. Metab.* 26): E1144–E1150, 1992.
156. Kasperek, G. J., G. L. Dohm, H. A. Barakat, P. H. Strausbauch, D. W. Barnes, and R. D. Snider. The role of lysosomes in exercise-induced hepatic protein loss. *Biochem. J.* 202: 281–288, 1982.
157. Kasperek, G. J., G. L. Dohm, E. B. Tapscott, and T. Powell. Effect of exercise on liver protein loss and lysosomal enzyme levels in fed and fasted rats. *Proc. Soc. Exp. Biol. Med.* 164: 430–434, 1980.
158. Kasperek, G. J., and R. D. Snider. Effect of exercise intensity and starvation on activation of branched-chain keto acid dehydrogenase by exercise. *Am. J. Physiol.* 253 (*Endocrinol. Metab.* 16): E33–E37, 1987.
159. Kasperek, G. J., and R. D. Snider. Total and myofibrillar protein degradation in isolated soleus muscle after exercise. *Am. J. Physiol.* 257 (*Endocrinol. Metab.* 20): E1–E5, 1989.
160. Kather, H., F. Schroeder, B. Simon, and G. Schlierf. Human fat cell adenylate cyclase: Regional differences in hormone sensitivity. *Eur. J. Clin. Invest.* 7: 595–597, 1977.
161. Katz, A., S. Broberg, K. Sahlin, and J. Wahren. Leg glucose uptake during maximal dynamic exercise in humans. *Am. J. Physiol.* 251 (*Endocrinol. Metab.* 14): E65–E70, 1986.
162. Katz, A., and K. Sahlin. Effect of hypoxia on glucose metabolism in human skeletal muscle during exercise. *Acta Physiol. Scand.* 136: 377–382, 1989.
163. Keller, U., P. P. G. Gerber, and W. Stauffacher. Fatty acid-independent inhibition of hepatic ketone body production in humans. *Am. J. Physiol.* 254 (*Endocrinol. Metab.* 17): E694–E699, 1988.
164. Kenno, K. A., J. L. Durstine, and R. E. Shepherd. Distribution of cyclic AMP phosphodiesterase in adipose tissue from trained rats. *J. Appl. Physiol.* 56: 845–848, 1986.
165. King, D. S., G. P. Dalsky, W. E. Clutter, D. A. Young, M. A. Staten, P. E. Cryer, and J. O. Holloszy. Effects of lack of exercise on insulin secretion and action in trained subjects. *Am. J. Physiol.* 254 (*Endocrinol. Metab.* 17): E537–E542, 1988.
166. Kjaer, M., K. Engfred, A. Fernandez, N. Secher, and H. Galbo. Regulation of hepatic glucose production during exercise in humans: role of sympathoadrenergic activity. *Am. J. Physiol.* 265 (*Endocrinol. Metab.* 28): E275–E283, 1993.
167. Kjaer, M., K. Engfred, H. Galbo, B. Sonne, K. Rasmussen, and S. Keiding. Hepatic glucose production during exercise in liver-transplanted subjects (Abstract). *Scand. J. Gastroenterol.* 26 (Suppl.): 46A, 1991.
168. Kjaer, M., and H. Galbo. Effect of physical training on the capacity to secrete epinephrine. *J. Appl. Physiol.* 64: 11–16, 1988.
169. Kjaer, M., K. J. Mikines, N. J. Christensen, B. Tronier, J. Vinten, B. Sonne, E. A. Richter, and H. Galbo. Glucose turnover and hormonal changes during insulin-induced hypoglycemia in trained men. *J. Appl. Physiol.* 57: 21–27, 1984.
170. Kjaer, M., N. H. Secher, F. W. Bach, and H. Galbo. Role of motor center activity for hormonal changes and substrate mobilization in humans. *Am. J. Physiol.* 253 (*Regulatory Integrative Comp. Physiol.* 22): R687–R695, 1987.
171. Kjaer, M., N. H. Secher, F. W. Bach, S. Sheikh, and H. Galbo. Hormonal and metabolic responses to exercise in humans: effect of sensory nervous blockade. *Am. J. Physiol.* 257 (*Endocrinol. Metab.* 20): E95–E101, 1989.
172. Koivisto, V. A., M. Harkonen, S. Karonen, P. H. Groop, R. Elovaino, E. Ferrannini, L. Sacca, and R. A. Defronzo. Glycogen depletion during prolonged exercise: influence of glucose fructose, or placebo. *J. Appl. Physiol.* 58: 731–737, 1985.
173. Koivisto, V. A., S. Karonen, and E. A. Nikkila. Carbohydrate ingestion before exercise: comparison of glucose, fructose, and sweet placebo. *J. Appl. Physiol.* 51: 783–787, 1981.
174. Koivisto, V. A., and H. Yki-Jarvinen. Effect of exercise on insulin binding and glucose transport in adipocytes of normal humans. *J. Appl. Physiol.* 63: 1319–1323, 1987.
175. Koranyi, L. I., R. E. Bourey, C. A. Slentz, and J. O. Holloszy. Coordinate reduction of rat pancreatic islet glucokinase and proinsulin mRNA by exercise training. *Diabetes* 40: 401–404, 1991.
176. Kozlowski, S., K. Nazar, Z. Brzezinska, D. Stephens, H. Kaciuba-Uscitko, and A. Kobryn. Mechanism of sympathetic activation during prolonged physical exercise in dogs. *Pflugers Arch.* 399: 63–67, 1983.
177. Krotkiewski, M., and J. Groski. Effect of muscular exercise on plasma C-peptide and insulin in obese non-diabetics and diabetics, type II. *Clin. Physiol.* 6: 499–506, 1986.
178. Krzentowski, G., F. Pirnay, N. Pallikarakis, A. S. Luyckx, M. Lacroix, F. Mosora, and P. J. Lelfebvre. Glucose utilization during exercise in normal and diabetic subjects. The role of insulin. *Diabetes* 30: 983–989, 1981.
179. Krzentowski, G. B., B. Jandrain, F. Pirnay, F. Morosa, A. S. Lacroix, and P. Lefebvre. Availability of glucose given orally during exercise. *J. Appl. Physiol.* 56: 315–320, 1984.
180. Lautt, W. Afferent and efferent neural roles in liver function. *Prog. Neurobiol.* 21: 323–348, 1983.
181. Lautt, W. W., and C. Wong. Hepatic glucose balance in response to direct stimulation of sympathetic nerves in the intact liver of cats. *Can. J. Physiol. Pharmacol.* 56: 1022–1028, 1978.
182. Lavoie, J. M., S. Cardin, and B. Doiron. Influence of hepatic vagus nerve on pancreatic hormone secretion. *Am. J. Physiol.* 257 (*Endocrinol. Metab.* 20): E855–E859, 1989.

183. Leclerq-Meyer, V., J. Marchand, and R. Leclerq. Studies on the molecular forms of glucagon immunoreactivity (GLI) released by the in vitro perfused pancreas. *Diabetologia* 19: 294–300, 1980.
184. Leuenberger, U., L. Sinoway, S. Gubin, L. Gaul, D. Davis, and R. Zelis. Effects of exercise intensity and duration on norepinephrine spillover and clearance in humans. *Am. J. Physiol.* 75: 668–674, 1993.
185. Lickley, H. L. A., F. W. Kemmer, D. E. Gray, N. Kovacevic, T. W. Hatton, G. Perez, and M. Vranic. Chromatographic pattern of extrapancreatic glucagon and glucagon-like immunoreactivity before and during stimulation by epinephrine, and participation of glucagon in epinephrine-induced hepatic glucose overproduction. *Surgery* 90: 186–194, 1981.
186. Liljenquist, J. E., G. L. Mueller, A. D. Cherrington, U. Keller, J. L. Chiasson, J. M. Perry, W. W. Lacy, and D. Rabinowitz. Evidence for an important role of glucagon in the regulation of hepatic glucose production in normal man. *J. Clin. Invest.* 59: 369–374, 1977.
187. Lobley, G. E., V. Milne, J. M. Lovie, P. J. Reeds, and K. Pennie. Whole body and tissue protein synthesis in cattle. *Br. J. Nutr.* 43: 491–502, 1980.
188. Luyckx, A. S., and P. J. Lefebvre. Mechanisms involved in the exercise-induced increase in glucagon secretion in rats. *Diabetes* 23: 81–93, 1974.
189. Luyckx, A. S., F. Pirnay, and P. J. Lefebvre. Effect of glucose on plasma glucagon and free fatty acids during prolonged exercise. *Eur. J. Appl. Physiol.* 39: 53–61, 1978.
190. Macleod, J. J. R., H. E. Magee, and C. B. Purves. Selective absorption of carbohydrates. *J. Physiol. (Lond.)* 70: 404–413, 1930.
191. Marker, J. C., D. A. Arnall, R. K. Conlee, and W. W. Winder. Effect of adrenodemedullation on metabolic responses to high-intensity exercise. *Am. J. Physiol.* 251 (*Regulatory Integrative Comp. Physiol.* 20): R552–R559, 1986.
192. Marker, J. C., I. B. Hirsh, L. J. Smith, C. A. Parvin, J. O. Holloszy, and P. E. Cryer. Catecholamines in prevention of hypoglycemia during exercise in humans. *Am. J. Physiol.* 260 (*Endocrinol. Metab.* 23): E705–E712, 1991.
193. Marliss, E. B., E. Simantirakis, C. Purdon, R. Gougeon, C. J. Field, J. B. Halter, and M. Vranic. Glucoregulatory and hormonal responses to repeated bouts of intense exercise in normal male subjects. *J. Appl. Physiol.* 71: 924–933, 1991.
194. Martin, W. H., E. F. Coyle, M. Joyner, D. Santesusanio, A. A. Ehsani, and J. O. Holloszy. Effect of stopping exercise training on epinephrine-stimulated lipolysis in humans. *J. Appl. Physiol.* 56: 845–848, 1984.
195. Massicotte, D., F. Peronnet, C. Allah, C. Hillaire-Marcel, M. Ledoux, and G. Brisson. Metabolic response of to [13C]-glucose and [13C]-fructose ingestion during exercise. *J. Appl. Physiol.* 61: 1180–1184, 1986.
196. Massicotte, D., F. Peronnet, G. Brisson, K. Bakkouch, and C. Hillaire-Marcel. Oxidation of glucose polymer during exercise: comparison with glucose or fructose. *J. Appl. Physiol.* 66: 179–183, 1989.
197. Massicotte, D., F. Peronnet, G. Brisson, L. Boivin, and C. Hillaire-Marcel. Oxidation of exogenous carbohydrate during prolonged exercise in fed and fasted conditions. *Int. J. Sports Med.* 11: 253–258, 1990.
198. Matchinsky, F. M. Glucokinase as glucose sensor and metabolic signal generator in pancreatic B-cells and hepatocytes. *Diabetes* 39: 647–652, 1990.
199. Maughan, R. J., J. B. Leiper, and A. McGaw. Effects of exercise intensity on absorption of ingested fluids in man. *Exp. Physiol.* 75: 419–421, 1990.
200. May, M. E., and M. G. Buse. Effects of branched chain amino acids on protein turnover. *Diabetes Metab. Rev.* 5: 227–245, 1989.
201. McGarry, J. D., and D. W. Foster. Regulation of hepatic fatty acid oxidation and ketone body production. *Annu. Rev. Biochem.* 49: 395–420, 1980.
202. McNurlan, M. A., and P. J. Garlick. Contribution of liver and gastrointestinal tract to whole-body protein synthesis in the rat. *Biochem. J.* 186: 381–383, 1980.
203. Meister, A. Enzymology of glutamine metabolism. In: *Glutamine Metabolism in Mammalian Tissues*, edited by D. Haussinger and H. Sies, New York: Springer-Verlag, 1984.
204. Mendenhall, L. A., S. C. Swanson, D. L. Habash, and A. R. Coggan. Ten days of exercise training reduces glucose production and utilization during moderate-intensity exercise. *Am. J. Physiol.* 266 (*Endocrinol. Metab.* 29): E136–E143, 1994.
205. Meshkinpour, H., C. Kemp, and R. Fairster. The effect of aerobic exercise on mouth to cecum transit time. *Gastroenterology* 96: 938–941, 1989.
206. Meyer, R. A., and R. L. Terjung. Differences in ammonia and adenylate metabolism in contracting fast and slow muscle. *Am. J. Physiol.* 237 (*Cell Physiol.* 6): C111–C118, 1979.
207. Mikines, K. J., B. Sonne, P. A. Farrell, B. Tronier, and H. Galbo. Effect of training on the dose-response relationship for insulin action in men. *J. Appl. Physiol.* 66: 695–703, 1989.
208. Miles, J. M., M. W. Haymond, S. L. Nissen, and J. E. Gerich. Effects of free fatty acid availability, glucagon excess, and insulin deficiency on ketone body production in postabsorptive man. *J. Clin. Invest.* 71: 1554–1561, 1983.
209. Mitchell, J. B., D. L. Costill, J. A. Houmard, W. J. Fink, R. A. Robergs, and J. A. Davis. Influence of carbohydrate dosage on exercise performance and glycogen metabolism. *J. Appl. Physiol.* 67: 1843–1849, 1989.
210. Moates, J. M., D. B. Lacy, A. D. Cherrington, R. E. Goldstein, and D. H. Wasserman. The metabolic role of the exercise-induced increment in epinephrine. *Am. J. Physiol.* 255 (*Endocrinol. Metab.* 18): E428–E436, 1988.
211. Mondon, C. E., C. B. Dolkas, and G. M. Reaven. Site of enhanced insulin sensitivity in exercise-trained rats at rest. *Am. J. Physiol.* 239 (*Endocrinol. Metab.* 2): E169–E177, 1980.
212. Mortimore, G. E., A. R. Poso, and B. R. Lardeux. Mechanism and regulation of protein degradation in liver. *Diabetes Metab. Rev.* 5: 49–70, 1989.
213. Moses, F. M., C. Ryan, J. Debolt, and B. Smoak. Oral cecal transit time during a 2 h run with ingestion of water of glucose polymer. *Am. J. Gastroenterol.* 83: 1055–1061, 1988.
214. Moses, F. M., A. Singh, V. V. Nueva, B. Kelsey, and B. Smoak. Lactate absorption and transit during prolonged exercise. *Am. J. Gastroenterol.* 84: 1192–1201, 1989.
215. Murray, R., G. L. Paul, J. G. Siefert, D. E. Eddy, and G. L. Halaby. The effects of of glucose, fructose, and sucrose ingestion during exercise. *Med. Sci. Sports Exerc.* 21: 275–282, 1989.
216. Murray, R. K., D. K. Granner, P. A. Mayes, and V. W. Rodwell. *Harper's Biochemistry*. Englewood Cliffs, NJ: Prentice Hall, 1990.
217. Neufer, P. D., D. L. Costill, W. J. Fink, J. P. Kirwin, R. A. Fielding, and M. G. Flynn. Effects of exercise and carbo-

hydrate composition on gastric emptying. *Med. Sci. Sports Exerc.* 18: 658–662, 1986.

218. Neufer, P. D., A. J. Young, and M. N. Sawka. Gastric emptying during exercise: effects of heat stress and hypohydration. *J. Appl. Physiol.* 58: 433–439, 1989.
219. Newsholme, E. A. A possible metabolic basis for the control of body weight. *N. Engl. J. Med.* 302: 400–405, 1980.
220. Newsholme, E. A., and B. Crabtree. Substrate cyclesin metabolic regulation and in heat generation. *Biochem. Soc. Symp.* 41: 61–109, 1976.
221. Noakes, T. D., E. V. Lambert, M. I. Lambert, P. S. McArthur, K. H. Myburgh, and A. J. S. Benade. Carbohydrate ingestion and muscle glycogen depletion during marathon and ultramarathon racing. *Eur. J. Appl. Physiol.* 57: 482–489, 1988.
222. Noakes, T. D., N. J. Reher, and R. J. Maughan. The importance of emptying volume in regulating gastric emptying. *Med. Sci. Sports Exerc.* 23: 307–313, 1991.
223. Ostman, J., P. Arner, P. Engfeldt, and L. Kager. Regional differences in the control of lipolysis in human adipose tissue. *Metabolism* 28: 1198–1203, 1979.
224. Owen, M. D., K. C. Kregel, P. T. Wall, and C. V. Gisolfi. Effects of ingesting carbohydrate beverages during exercise in the heat. *Med. Sci. Sports Exerc.* 18: 568–575, 1986.
225. Pallikarakis, N., B. Jandrain, F. Pirnay, F. Mosora, M. Lacroix, A. S. Luycks, and P. J. Lefebvre. Remarkable metabolic availability of oral glucose during long-duration exercise in humans. *J. Appl. Physiol.* 60: 1035–1042, 1986.
226. Peronnet, F., D. Massicotte, G. Brisson, and C. Hillaire-Marcel. Use of 13C substrates for metabolic studies in exercise: methodological considerations. *J. Appl. Physiol.* 69: 1047–1052, 1990.
227. Pirnay, F., J. M. Crielaard, N. Pallikarakis, M. Lacroix, F. Mosora, A. Luyckx, and P. J. Lefebvre. Fate of exogenous glucose during exercise of different intensities in humans. *J. Appl. Physiol.* 43: 258–261, 1982.
228. Pirnay, F., M. Lacroix, F. Mosora, A. Luyckx, and P. Lefebvre. Effect of glucose ingestion on energy substrate utilization during prolonged exercise in man. *Eur. J. Appl. Physiol.* 36: 247–254, 1977.
229. Pirnay, F., M. Lacroix, F. Mosora, A. Luyckx, and P. J. Lefebvre.. Glucose oxidation during prolonged exercise evaluated with naturally labelled 13C glucose. *J. Appl. Physiol.* 43: 258–261, 1977.
230. Polonsky, K., J. Jaspan, W. Pugh, J. Dhorajiwala, M. Abraham, P. Blix, and A. R. Moosa. Insulin and glucagon breakthrough of somatostatin suppression. Importance of portal vein hormone measurements. *Diabetes* 30: 664–669, 1981.
231. Poortmans, J. R. Protein turnover and amino acid oxidation during and after exercise. *Med. Sports Sci.* 17: 130–147, 1984.
232. Porte, D., A. L. Graber, T. Kuzuya, and R. H. Williams. The effects of epinephrine on IRI levels in man. *J. Clin. Invest.* 45: 228–236, 1966.
233. Portis, A. J., G. L. Warnock, D. T. Finegood, A. N. Belcastro, and R. V. Rajotte. Glucoregulatory response to moderate exercise in long-term islet cell autografted dogs. *Can. J. Physiol. Pharmacol.* 68: 1308–1312, 1990.
234. Randle, P. J., P. B. Garland, C. N. Hales, and E. A. Newsholme. The glucose-fatty acid cycle its role in insulin sensitivity and the metabolic disturbances of diabetes mellitus. *Lancet* i: 785–789, 1963.
235. Reaven, E. P., and G. M. Reaven. Structure and function changes in the endocrine pancreas of aging rats with reference to the modulating effects of exercise and caloric restriction. *J. Clin. Invest.* 68: 75–84, 1981.
236. Refsum, H. E., R. Gjessing, and S. B. Stromme. Changes in plasma amino acid distribution and urine amino acid excretion during prolonged heavy exercise. *Scand. J. Clin. Lab. Invest.* 39: 407–413, 1979.
237. Rehrer, N. J., E. Beckers, F. Brouns, W. H. M. Saris, and F. T. Hoor. Effects of dehydration on gastric emptying and gastrointestinal distress while running. *Med. Sci. Sports Exerc.* 22: 790–795, 1990.
238. Rehrer, N. J., A. J. M. Wagenmakers, E. J. Beckers, D. Halliday, J. B. Leiper, F. Brouns, R. J. Maughan, K. Westerterp, and W. H. M. Saris. Gastric emptying, absorption, and carbohydrate oxidation during prolonged exercise. *J. Appl. Physiol.* 72: 468–475, 1992.
239. Rennie, M. J., R. H. T. Edwards, S. Krywawyck, C. T. M. Davies, D. Halliday, J. C. Waterlow, and D. J. Millward. Effect of exercise on protein turnover in man. *Clin. Sci.* 61: 627–639, 1981.
240. Rennie, M. J., W. W. Winder, and J. O. Holloszy. A sparing effect of increased plasma fatty acids on muscle and liver glycogen content in the exercising rat. *Biochem. J.* 156: 647–655, 1976.
241. Richter, E. A., H. Galbo, and N. J. Christensen. Control of exercise-induced muscular glycogenolysis by adrenal medullary hormones in rats. *J. Appl. Physiol.* 50: 21–26, 1981.
242. Richter, E. A., H. Galbo, J. J. Holst, and B. Sonne. Significance of glucagon for insulin secretion and hepatic glycogenolysis during exercise in rats. *Horm. Metab. Res.* 13: 323–326, 1981.
243. Richter, E. A., H. Galbo, B. Sonne, J. J. Holst, and N. J. Christensen. Adrenal medullary control of muscular and hepatic glycogenolysis and of pancreatic hormonal secretion in exercising rats. *Acta Physiol. Scand.* 108: 1980, 1980.
244. Riviere, D., F. Crampes, M. Beauville, and M. Garrigues. Lipolytic response of fat cells to catecholamines in sedentary and exercise-trained women. *J. Appl. Physiol.* 66: 330–335, 1989.
245. Rizack, M. A. Activation of an epinephrine-sensitive lipolytic activity from adipose tissue by adenosine 3′, 5′ phosphate. *J. Biol. Chem.* 239: 392–395, 1964.
246. Rodjkmark, S., G. Bloom, M. C. Y. Chou, and J. B. Field. Hepatic extraction of exogenous insulin and glucagon in the dog. *Endocrinology* 102: 806–813, 1978.
247. Rodnick, K. J., W. L. Haskell, A. L. M. Swislocki, J. E. Foley, and G. M. Reaven. Improved insulin action in muscle, liver, and adipose tissue in physically trained human subjects. *Am. J. Physiol.* 253 (*Endocrinol. Metab.* 16): E489–E495, 1987.
248. Romijn, J. A., S. Klein, E. F. Coyle, L. S. Sidossis, and R. R. Wolfe. Strenuous endurance training increases lipolysis and triglyceride-fatty acid cycling at rest. *J. Appl. Physiol.* 75: 108–113, 1993.
249. Rosell, S., and E. Belfrage. Blood circulation in adipose tissue. *Physiol. Rev.* 59: 1078–1104, 1979.
250. Rowell, L. B., J. R. Blackmon, and R. A. Bruce. Indocyanine green clearance and estimated blood flow during mild to maximal exercise in upright man. *J. Clin. Invest.* 43: 1677–1690, 1964.
251. Rowell, L. B., E. J. Masoro, and M. J. Spenser. Splanchnic metabolism in exercising man. *J. Appl. Physiol.* 20: 1032–1037, 1965.
252. Sacca, L., N. Eigler, P. E. Cryer, and R. S. Sherwin. Insulin antagonistic effects of epinephrine and glucagon in the dog. *Am. J. Physiol.* 237 (*Endocrinol. Metab. Gastrointest. Physiol.* 6): E487–E492, 1979.

253. Sacca, L. C., C. Vigorito, M. Cicala, G. Corso, and R. S. Sherwin. Role of gluconeogenesis in epinephrine-stimulated hepatic glucose production in humans. *Am. J. Physiol.* 245 (*Endocrinol. Metab.* 8): E294–E302, 1983.
254. Salans, L. B., and J. W. Doherty. The effect of insulin upon glucose metabolism by adipose cells of different size. *J. Clin. Invest.* 50: 1399–1410, 1971.
255. Samols, E., and G. C. Weir. Adrenergic modulation of pancreatic A, B, and D cells. *J. Clin. Invest.* 63: 230–238, 1979.
256. Saris, W. H. M., B. H. Goodpaster, A. E. Jeukendrup, F. Brouns, D. Halliday, and A. J. M. Wagenmakers. Exogenous carbohydrate oxidation from different carbohydrate sources during exercise. *J. Appl. Physiol.* 75: 2168–2172, 1993.
257. Savard, R., J. P. Despres, M. Marcotte, and C. Bouchard. Endurance training and glucose conversion into triglycerides in human fat cells. *J. Appl. Physiol.* 58: 230–235, 1985.
258. Sawchenko, P. E., and M. I. Friedman. Sensory functions of the liver-a review. *Am. J. Physiol.* 236 (*Regulatory Integrative Comp. Physiol.* 5): R5–R20, 1979.
259. Seftoft, L., J. Trap-Jensen, J. Lyngsoe, J. P. Clausen, J. J. Holst, S. L. Nielsen, J. F. Rehfeld, and O. S. D. Muckadell. Regulation of gluconeogenesis and ketogenesis during rest and exercise in diabetic subjects and normal men. *Clin. Sci. Mol. Med.* 53: 411–418, 1977.
260. Sellers, T. L., A. W. Jaussi, H. T. Yang, R. W. Heninger, and W. W. Winder. Effect of the exercise-induced increase in glucocorticoids on endurance in the rat. *J. Appl. Physiol.* 65: 173–178, 1988.
261. Sembrowich, W. L., C. D. Ianuzzo, C. W. Saubert, R. E. Shepherd, and P. D. Gollnick. Substrate mobilization during prolonged exercise in 6-hydroxydopamine treated rats. *Pflugers Arch.* 349: 57–62, 1974.
262. Shapiro, B., I. Chowers, and G. Rose. Fatty acid uptake and esterification in adipose tissue. *Biochim. Biophys. Acta* 23: 115–120, 1957.
263. Shepherd, R. E., E. G. Noble, G. A. Klug, and P. D. Gollnick. Lipolysis and cAMP accumulation in adipocytes in response to physical training. *J. Appl. Physiol.* 50: 143–148, 1981.
264. Shepherd, R. E., W. L. Sembrowich, H. E. Green, and P. D. Gollnick. Effect of physical training on control mechanisms of lipolysis in rat fat cell ghosts. *J. Appl. Physiol.* 42: 884–888, 1977.
265. Shimazu, T., and M. Usami. Further studies on the mechanism of phosphorylase activation in rabbit liver in response to splanchnic nerve stimulation. *J. Physiol. (Lond.)* 329: 231–242, 1982.
266. Sigal, R. J., C. Purdon, D. Bilinski, M. Vranic, J. B. Halter, and E. B. Marliss. Glucoregulation during and after intense exercise: effects of beta-blockade. *J. Clin. Endocrinol. Metab.* 78: 359–366, 1994.
267. Simonson, D. C., V. A. Koivisto, R. S. Sherwin, E. Ferrannini, R. Hendler, and R. A. Defronzo. Adrenergic blockade alters glucose kinetics during exercise in insulin-dependent diabetics. *J. Clin. Invest.* 73: 1648–1658, 1984.
268. Sirek, A., M. Vranic, O. V. Sirek, M. Vigas, and Z. Policova. Effect of growth hormone on acute glucagon and insulin release. *Am. J. Physiol.* 237 (*Endocrinol. Metab. Gastrointest. Physiol.* 6): E107–E112, 1979.
269. Smith, U., J. Hammarsten, P. Bjorntorp, and J. Kral. Regional differences and effect of weight reduction on human fat cell metabolism. *Eur. J. Clin. Invest.* 9: 327–333, 1979.
270. Sole, C. C., and T. D. Noakes. Faster gastric emptying for glucose-polymer and fructose solutions than for glucose in humans. *Eur. J. Appl. Physiol.* 58: 605–612, 1989.
271. Sonne, B., K. J. Mikines, E. A. Richter, N. J. Christensen, and H. Galbo. Role of liver nerves and adrenal medulla in glucose turnover of running rats. *J. Appl. Physiol.* 59: 1650–1656, 1985.
272. Sotsky, M., S. Shilo, and H. Shamoon. Regulation of counterregulatory hormone secretion in man during exercise and hypoglycemia. *J. Clin. Endocrinol. Metab.* 68: 9–16, 1989.
273. Souba, W. W., R. J. Smith, and D. W. Wilmore. Glutamine metabolism by the intestinal tract. *J. Parenter. Enter. Nutr.* 9: 608–617, 1985.
274. Stallknecht, B., J. Vinten, T. Ploug, and H. Galbo. Increased activities of mitochondrial enzymes in white adipose tissue in trained rats. *Am. J. Physiol.* 261 (*Endocrinol. Metab.* 24): E410–E414, 1991.
275. Stralfors, P., H. Olsson, and P. Belfrage. Hormone sensitive lipase. *Enzymes* 18: 147–177, 1987.
276. Sumida, K. D., J. H. Urdiales, and C. M. Donovan. Enhanced gluconeogenesis from lactate in perfused livers after endurance training. *J. Appl. Physiol.* 74: 782–787, 1993.
277. Sutton, J. R. Hormonal and metabolic responses to exercise in subjects of high and low work capacities. *Med. Sci. Sports Exerc.* 10: 1–6, 1978.
278. Tate, C. A., P. E. Wolkowicz, and J. McMillin-Wood. Exercise-induced alterations of hepatic mitochondrial function. *Biochem. J.* 208: 695–701, 1982.
279. Terjung, R. L., L. Budohoski, K. Nazar, A. Kobryn, and H. Kaciuba-Uscilko. Chylomicron triglyceride metabolism in resting and exercising dogs. *J. Appl. Physiol.* 52: 815–820, 1982.
280. Terjung, R. L., and H. Kaciuba-Uscilko. Lipid metabolism during exercise: influence of training. *Diabetes Metab. Rev.* 2: 35–51, 1986.
281. Turcotte, L. P., A. S. Rovner, R. R. Roark, and G. A. Brooks. Glucose kinetics in gluconeogenesis-inhibited rats during rest and exercise. *Am. J. Physiol.* 258 (*Endocrinol. Metab.* 21): E203–E211, 1990.
282. Valverde, I., M. Ghiglione, R. Matesanz, and S. Casado. Chromatographic pattern of gut glucagon-like immunoreactivity (GLI) in plasma before and during glucose absorption. *Horm. Metab. Res.* 11: 343–346, 1979.
283. Vanhandel, P. J., W. J. Fink, G. Branam, and D. Costill. Fate of 14C gluocse ingested during prolonged exercise. *Int. J. Sports Med.* 1: 127–131, 1980.
284. Varro, G. E., J. A. Harris, and J. E. Geenen. Effect of decreased local circulation on the absorptive capacity of a small intestine loop in the dog. *Am. J. Dig. Dis.* 10: 170–177, 1965.
285. Vaughan, M., and D. Steinberg. Effect of hormones on lipolysis and re-esterification of free fatty acids during incubation of adipose tissue in vitro. *J. Lipid Res.* 4: 193–199, 1963.
286. Victor, R. G., D. R. Seals, and A. L. Mark. Differential control of heart rate and sympathetic nerve activity during dynamic exercise. Insight from intraneural recordings in humans. *J. Clin. Invest.* 79: 508–516, 1987.
287. Vinten, J., and H. Galbo. Effect of physical training on transport and metabolism of glucose in adipocytes. *Am. J. Physiol.* 244 (*Endocrinol. Metab.* 7): E129–E134, 1983.
288. Vinten, J., and H. Galbo. Effect of physical training on transport and metabolism of glucose in adipocytes. *Biochim. Biophys. Acta* 841: 223–227, 1985.

289. Vissing, J., G. A. Iwamoto, K. J. Rybicki, H. Galbo, and J. H. Mitchell. Mobilization of glucoregulatory hormones and glucose by hypothalamic locomotor centers. *Am. J. Physiol.* 257 (*Endocrinol. Metab.* 20): E722–E728, 1989.
290. Vissing, J., J. L. Wallace, A. J. W. Scheurink, H. Galbo, and A. B. Steffens. Ventromedial hypothalamic regulation of hormonal and metabolic responses to exercise. *Am. J. Physiol.* 256 (*Regulatory Integrative Comp. Physiol.* 25): R1019–R1026, 1989.
291. Vranic, M., R. Kawamori, S. PEK, N. Kovacevic, and G. Wrenshall. The essentiality of insulin and the role of glucagon in regulating glucose utilization and production during strenuous exercise in dogs. *J. Clin. Invest.* 57: 245–255, 1976.
292. Wahren, J., P. Felig, G. Ahlborg, and L. Jorfeldt. Glucose metabolism during leg exercise in man. *J. Clin. Invest.* 50: 2715–2725, 1971.
293. Wahren, J., L. Hagenfeldt, and P. Felig. Splanchnic and leg exchange of glucose, amino acids, and free fatty acids during exercise in diabetes mellitus. *J. Clin. Invest.* 55: 1303–1314, 1975.
294. Wahren, J., Y. Sato, J. Ostman, L. Hagenfeldt, and P. Felig. Turnover and splanchnic metabolism of free fatty acids and ketones in insulin-dependent diabetics during exercise. *J. Clin. Invest.* 73: 1367–1376, 1984.
295. Wahrenberg, H., P. Engfeldt, J. Bolinder, and P. Arner. Acute adaptation in adrenergic control of lipolysis during physical exercise in humans. *Am. J. Physiol.* 253 (*Endocrinol. Metab.* 16): E383–E390, 1987.
296. Wardzala, L. J., M. Crettaz, E. D. Horton, B. Jeanrenaud, and E. S. Horton. Physical training of lean and genetically obese Zucker rats: effect of fat cell metabolism. *Am. J. Physiol.* 243 (*Endocrinol. Metab.* 6): E418–E426, 1982.
297. Wasserman, D. H., J. L. Bupp, J. L. Johnson, D. Bracy, and D. B. Lacy. Glucoregulation during rest and exercise in depancreatized dogs: role of the acute presence of insulin. *Am. J. Physiol.* 262 (*Endocrinol. Metab.* 25): E574–E582, 1992.
298. Wasserman, D. H., and A. D. Cherrington. Hepatic fuel metabolism during exercise: role and regulation. *Am. J. Physiol.* 260 (*Endocrinol. Metab.* 23): E811–E824, 1991.
299. Wasserman, D. H., R. J. Geer, D. E. Rice, D. Bracy, P. J. Flakoll, L. L. Brown, J. O. Hill, and N. N. Abumrad. Interaction of exercise and insulin action in man. *Am. J. Physiol.* 260 (*Endocrinol. Metab.* 23): E37–E45, 1991.
300. Wasserman, D. H., R. J. Geer, P. E. Williams, D. B. Lacy, and N. N. Abumrad. Interaction of gut and liver in nitrogen metabolism during exercise. *Metabolism* 40: 307–314, 1991.
301. Wasserman, D. H., D. B. Lacy, D. Bracy, and P. E. Williams. Metabolic regulation in peripheral tissues and transition to increased gluconeogenic mode during prolonged exercise. *Am. J. Physiol.* 263 (*Endocrinol. Metab.* 26): E345–E354, 1992.
302. Wasserman, D. H., D. B. Lacy, and D. P. Bracy. Relationship between arterial and portal vein immunoreactive glucagon during exercise. *J. Appl. Physiol.* 75: 724–729, 1993.
303. Wasserman, D. H., D. B. Lacy, C. A. Colburn, D. P. Bracy, and A. D. Cherrington. Efficiency of compensation for the absence of the fall in insulin during exercise. *Am. J. Physiol.* 261 (*Endocrinol. Metab.* 24): E587–E597, 1991.
304. Wasserman, D. H., D. B. Lacy, R. E. Goldstein, P. E. Williams, and A. D. Cherrington. Exercise-induced fall in insulin and hepatic carbohydrate metabolism during exercise. *Am. J. Physiol.* 256 (*Endocrinol. Metab.* 19): E500–E508, 1989.
305. Wasserman, D. H., D. B. Lacy, R. E. Goldstein, P. E. Williams, and A. D. Cherrington. Exercise-induced fall in insulin and the increase in fat metabolism during prolonged exercise. *Diabetes* 38: 484–490, 1989.
306. Wasserman, D. H., D. B. Lacy, D. R. Green, P. E. Williams, and A. D. Cherrington. Dynamics of hepatic lactate and glucose balances during prolonged exercise and recovery. *J. Appl. Physiol.* 63: 2411–2417, 1987.
307. Wasserman, D. H., H. L. A. Lickley, and M. Vranic. Interactions between glucagon and other counterregulatory hormones during normoglycemic and hypoglycemic exercise in dogs. *J. Clin. Invest.* 74: 1404–1413, 1984.
308. Wasserman, D. H., H. L. A. Lickley, and M. Vranic. Effect of hematocrit reduction on hormonal and metabolic responses to exercise. *J. Appl. Physiol.* 58: 1257–1262, 1985.
309. Wasserman, D. H., J. S. Spalding, D. P. Bracy, D. B. Lacy, and A. D. Cherrington. Exercise-induced rise in glucagon and the increase in ketogenesis during prolonged muscular work. *Diabetes* 38: 799–807, 1989.
310. Wasserman, D. H., J. S. Spalding, D. B. Lacy, C. A. Colburn, R. E. Goldstein, and A. D. Cherrington. Glucagon is a primary controller of the increments in hepatic glycogenolysis and gluconeogenesis during exercise. *Am. J. Physiol.* 257 (*Endocrinol. Metab.* 20): E108–E117, 1989.
311. Wasserman, D. H., P. E. Williams, D. B. Lacy, D. Bracy, and A. D. Cherrington. Hepatic nerves are not essential to the increase in hepatic glucose production during muscular work. *Am. J. Physiol.* 259 (*Endocrinol. Metab.* 22): E195–E203, 1990.
312. Wasserman, D. H., P. E. Williams, D. B. Lacy, D. R. Green, and A. D. Cherrington. Importance of intrahepatic mechanisms to gluconeogenesis from alanine during prolonged exercise and recovery. *Am. J. Physiol.* 254 (*Endocrinol. Metab.* 17): E518–E525, 1988.
313. Weber, J. M., S. Klein, and R. R. Wolfe. Role of the glucose cycle in control of net glucose flux in exercising humans. *J. Appl. Physiol.* 68: 1815–1819, 1990.
314. Welbourne, T. C. Interorgan glutamine flow in metabolic acidosis. *Am. J. Physiol.* 253 (*Endocrinol. Metab.* 16): E1069–E1076, 1987.
315. Wheeler, K. B., and J. G. Banwell. Intestinal water and electrolyte flux of glucose polymer electrolyte solutions. *Med. Sci. Sports Exerc.* 18: 436–439, 1986.
316. White, T. P., and G. A. Brooks. [u-14c]-glucose, -alanine, and -leucine oxidation in rats at rest and two intensities of running. *Am. J. Physiol.* 240 (*Endocrinol. Metab.* 3): E155–E165, 1981.
317. Williams, B. D., R. R. Wolfe, D. P. Bracy, and D. H. Wasserman. Gut proteolysis contributes essential amino acids during exercise. *Med. Sci. Sports Exerc.* 24: 1062, 1992.
318. Williams, J. H., M. Mager, and E. D. Jacobson. Relationship of mesenteric blood flow to intestinal absorption of carbohdyrates. *J. Lab. Clin. Med.* 63: 853–862, 1964.
319. Williams, R. S., and T. Bishop. Enhanced receptor-cyclase coupling and augmented catecholamine-stimulated lipolysis in exercising rats. *Am. J. Physiol.* 243 (*Endocrinol. Metab.* 6): E345–E351, 1982.
320. Winder, W. W., J. Arogyasami, H. T. Yang, K. G. Thompson, L. A. Nelson, K. P. Kelly, and D. H. Han. Effects of glucose infusion in exercising rats. *J. Appl. Physiol.* 64: 2300–2305, 1988.
321. Winder, W. W., M. A. Beattie, C. Piquette, and R. T. Holman. Decrease in liver norepinephrine in response to ex-

ercise and hypoglycemia. *Am. J. Physiol.* 244 (*Regulatory Integrative Comp. Physiol.* 13): R147–R152, 1983.
322. Winder, W. W., J. M. Hagberg, R. C. Hickson, A. A. Ehsani, and J. O. Holloszy. Time course of sympathoadrenal adaptation to endurance training in man. *J. Appl. Physiol.* 45: 370–374, 1978.
323. Winder, W. W., R. C. Hickson, J. M. Hagberg, A. A. Ehsani, and J. McLane. Training-induced changes in the hormonal and metabolic response to submaximal exercise. *J. Appl. Physiol.* 46: 766–771, 1979.
324. Winder, W. W., M. L. Terry, and V. M. Mitchell. Role of plasma epinephrine in fasted exercising rats. *Am. J. Physiol.* 248 (*Regulatory Integrative Comp. Physiol.* 17): R302–R307, 1985.
325. Winder, W. W., H. T. Yang, A. W. Jaussi, and C. R. Hopkins. Epinephrine, glucose, and lactate infusion in exercising adrenomedullated rats. *J. Appl. Physiol.* 62: 1442–1447, 1987.
326. Wirth, A., C. Diehm, H. Mayer, H. Morl, I. Vogel, P. Bjorntorp, and G. Schlierf. Plasma C-peptide and insulin in trained and untrained subjects. *J. Appl. Physiol.* 50: 71–77, 1981.
327. Wirth, A., G. Holm, B. Nilsson, U. Smith, and P. Bjorntorp. Insulin kinetics and insulin binding in physically trained and food-restricted rats. *Am. J. Physiol.* 238 (*Endocrinol. Metab.* 1): E108–E115, 1980.
328. Wolf, P. D., E. H. Fischer, and E. G. Krebs. Amino acid sequence of the phosphorylated site in rabbit liver glycogen phosphorylase. *Biochemistry* 9: 1923–1929, 1970.
329. Wolfe, R. R., and S. George. Stable isotope methods for studying metabolism. *Exerc. Sports Sci. Rev.* 21: 3–23, 1993.
330. Wolfe, R. R., R. D. Goodenough, M. H. Wolfe, G. T. Royle, and E. R. Nadel. Isotopic analysis of leucine and urea metabolism in exercising humans. *J. Appl. Physiol.* 52: 458–466, 1982.
331. Wolfe, R. R., S. Klein, F. Carraro, and J. M. Weber. Role of triglyceride-fatty acid cycle in controlling fat metabolism in humans during and after exercise. *Am. J. Physiol.* 258 (*Endocrinol. Metab.* 21): E382–E389, 1990.
332. Wolfe, R. R., E. R. Nadel, J. H. F. Shaw, L. A. Stephenson, and M. Wolfe. Role of changes in insulin and glucagon in glucose homeostasis in exercise. *J. Clin. Invest.* 77: 900–907, 1986.
333. Wolfe, R. R., M. H. Wolfe, E. R. Nadel, and J. H. F. Shaw. Isotopic determination of amino acid urea interactions in exercise in humans. *J. Appl. Physiol.* 56: 221–229, 1984.
334. Yamatani, K., Z. Shi, A. Giacca, R. Gupta, S. Fisher, H. L. A. Lickley, and M. Vranic. Role of FFA-glucose cycle in glucoregulation during exercise in total absence of insulin. *Am. J. Physiol.* 263 (*Endocrinol. Metab.* 32): E646–E653, 1992.
335. Yaspelkis, B. B., J. G. Patterson, P. A. Anderla, Z. Ding, and J. L. Ivy. Carbohydrate supplementation spares muscle glycogen during variable-intensity exercise. *J. Appl. Physiol.* 75: 1477–1485, 1993.
336. Young, D. R., J. Shapira, R. Forrest, R. R. Adachi, R. Lim, and R. Pelligra. Model for evaluation of fatty acid metabolism in man during prolonged exercise. *J. Appl. Physiol.* 23: 716–725, 1967.
337. Young, J. C., J. L. Treadway, E. I. Fader, and R. Caslin. Effects of oral hypoglycemic agent methylpalmoxirate on exercise capacity of streptozotocin diabetic rats. *Diabetes* 35: 744–748, 1986.
338. Zinker, B. A., T. Mohr, P. Kelly, K. Namdaran, D. P. Bracy, and D. H. Wasserman. Exercise-induced fall in insulin: mechanism of action at the liver and effect on skeletal muscle glucose metabolism. *Am. J. Physiol.* 266 (*Endocrinol. Metab.* 29): E683–689, 1994.

24. Muscle plasticity: energy demand and supply processes

FRANK W. BOOTH | *Department of Integrative Biology, University of Texas Medical School, Houston, Texas*

KENNETH M. BALDWIN | *Department of Physiology and Biophysics, University of California at Irvine, Irvine, California*

CHAPTER CONTENTS

ALL LIVING ORGANISMS possess the inherent capacity to alter the structural and functional properties of their organ systems in accordance with the environmental conditions imposed on a particular system. The goal of this chapter is to review the state of knowledge concerning the plasticity of striated muscle; that is, the ability of muscle cells to alter the amount and composition of their subcellular components (such as contractile machinery, mitochondrial and glycogenolytic enzyme levels, calcium-cycling properties) in response to a variety of chronic perturbations including, but not limited to, altered states of neural activity, mechanical stress and physical activity, hormonal manipulation, and pharmacological intervention. The topics to be covered include: *(1)* fundamental concepts relevant to muscle plasticity, *(2)* the organization of striated muscle cells into functional units based on common patterns of protein expression, *(3)* organelle plasticity in response to various experimental paradigms, and *(4)* the regulatory factors (mechanisms) involved in the adaptive process. Since insufficient space is available to cover all aspects of those proteins thought to be involved in the adaptative process in response to the various activity patterns, the reader is referred to several other excellent reviews of this general topic (10, 99, 138, 255, 278, 298, 317).

GOALS AND FUNDAMENTAL CONCEPTS

The Concept of Plasticity

In this chapter muscle plasticity is defined as the ability of a given muscle cell to alter (*1*) the quantity (amount) of and/or (2) the type of protein (i.e., phenotype or isoform) comprising its different subcellular components in response to any type of stimulus that disrupts its normal homeostasis. For example, a given muscle fiber may respond to chronic increases in mechanical stress (physical activity) by increasing its cross-sectional area so that all of the subcellular components remain in normal proportion to one another and the same specific protein phenotypes are maintained in normal expression. In this case the muscle expands its protein mass and mechanical strength without qualitatively changing any other inherent functional property such as endurance and/or contractile speed. On the other hand, a given fiber may respond to the same perturbation by both increasing its mass and altering the type of myosin heavy chain (MHC) isoform that it expresses in the myofilaments. In this situation, while the muscle becomes both larger and stronger, due to the increase in contractile protein accumulation, its intrinsic contractile properties also become transformed due to the altered myosin phenotype that is expressed. Thus, the muscle's plasticity potential may involve (*1*) a change in the amount of protein, (*2*) the type of protein isoform it expresses, and (*3*) a combination of the two. However, the functional consequences of such a transformation will depend on which component(s) of the cell is altered in terms of the quantity and quality of protein expression.

The Concept of Protein Isoforms

From the above discussion, one begins to see that a significant factor dictating a muscle fiber's adaptational capacity is related to its genetic capability of expressing different isoforms (molecular species) of a given protein. By definition, isoforms of a particular protein are molecules with slight variations in amino acid composition, thereby altering either the structural, functional, and/or enzymatic properties of that protein. Isoform species have been identified for a large number of muscle proteins involved in processes governing ion transport, contraction and relaxation, and energy metabolism. In the different sections of this chapter, emphasis will be given to the effects of physical activity and altered hormonal state on the pattern of protein isoform expression in both skeletal and cardiac muscle.

The Concept of Protein Turnover

The continuous turnover of proteins permits muscle plasticity (110). The ability of muscle to adapt to a chronic change in its contractile activity (in Darwinian terms, its environment) would be eliminated if its proteins were inert (i.e., they did not turn over). For example, in the switching of protein isoforms, one isoform must be decreased. Thus, protein turnover is one of two determinants of muscle plasticity. The other determinant of plasticity is protein synthesis rate, which will be discussed later.

The time required to alter muscle plasticity is solely a function of the protein half-life, (294). Thus, proteins that turn over rapidly can reach a new steady-state level faster than those that turn over slowly during adaptation to exercise. Proteins turning over rapidly must also have high rates of protein synthesis. Goldberg (110) has remarked that short half-lives may have evolved in order that certain crucial enzymes can fluctuate rapidly with changing physiological conditions. This could provide an enhanced survival, or a more rapid adaptability to exercise training.

ORGANIZATION OF MUSCLE CELLS INTO FUNCTIONAL UNITS BASED ON PATTERNS OF PROTEIN EXPRESSION

The purpose of this section is to provide a brief review of the functional processes of skeletal muscle.

Cellular Processes Involved in Contraction and Relaxation: Role of Cross-Bridge and Calcium Cycling Isoforms

For over 100 years, it has been widely appreciated that muscles (including single fibers) can be categorized into distinct types, based on both their gross appearance (red vs. white) and their contractile speed (fast vs. slow) (121, 278). Furthermore, it is widely accepted that the functional unit of a muscle is the "motor unit," consisting of a motoneuron innervating a collection of fibers (ranging from 100–1000) of relatively similar mechanical, biochemical, and metabolic properties (121). Studies performed on individual motor units, corresponding to the simplified scheme identified above, clearly suggest that those units capable of developing force and shortening rapidly also have rapid relaxation properties (121, 254, 255, 278). Furthermore, additional studies have shown that the maximal shortening velocity of skeletal muscle is related to the specific activity of its myosin adenosine triphosphatase (ATPase), which is thought to control the cycling kinetics of the cross-bridge machinery (45, 228, 261). On the other hand, both the time course of muscle force generation and of relaxation appear to be correlated with the kinetic properties of calcium transport processes [defined herein as the coupled process of releasing and sequestering calcium ions across the sarcoplasmic reticulum (SR) network] (255, 289). Thus, muscle fibers function in highly organized motor units, consisting largely of distinct protein isoforms possessing different kinetic properties for cycling the cross-bridges that are formed during contractile activity and for cycling the calcium that must be processed for both the activation of and relaxation of the contractile machinery. The inherent properties governing contraction and relaxation processes need to be precisely regulated; otherwise, it would be impossible to coordinate the cyclic behavior of limb movement in performing the complex motor activities involved in routine locomotion (278, 346). The above discussion has focused on a simple functional example of fast and slow. However, with the refinement of modern immunological (16, 68, 293), biochemical (99, 228, 336), and mechanical analytical technologies (45, 46, 204, 228, 261), it is now apparent that the simple fast-slow contractile scheme needs to be modified appreciably into a more complex scheme representing a continuum of mechanical and metabolic properties as discussed below (see Table 24.1). This is necessary in order to account for the spectrum of mechanical/energetic gradations that are now recognized for muscle function, due, in part, to the many isoforms of MHC (16, 68, 184, 204, 293) and calcium cycling proteins (11, 175, 255, 289, 370) that are known to be expressed in mammalian muscle. Therefore, fundamental questions arise as to whether there is always precise coupled regulation of expression of the protein isoforms governing both cross-bridge and calcium cycling processes, and whether these interrelated systems are always altered in parallel with one another in response to interventions inducing transformations in either system.

Cellular Processes Involving Oxidative Metabolism

Muscle processes involved in oxidative metabolism can be conceptualized as the flow of oxygen and substrates from the blood to mitochondria. The delivery of oxygen and substrates is dependent on cap-

TABLE 24.1. *Organization of Muscle Fibers into Functional Units of Common Metabolic and Biochemical Properties and their Primary Adaptive Change*

Properties	Unit Types			
	I	IIa	IIx	IIb
Predominant MHC type	I (IIa, IIx)	IIa (I, IIx)	IIx (IIa, IIb)	IIb (IIx)
Contractile speed	Slow (↑)	Fast (↓)	Fast (↑)	Fast (↓)
Myofibril ATPase	Low (↑)	Mod. high (↓)	High (↑)	High (↓)
SR Ca^{2+}-ATPase	Low (↑)	Mod. high (↓)	High	High (↓)
Glycolytic Enzymes	Low (↑)	Mod. high (↓)	High (?)	High (↓)
ATP buffering enzyme	Low (↑)	Mod. high (↓)	Mod. high	High (↓)
High-energy phosphate levels	Low (↑)	Mod. (↓)	—	High
Oxidative enzymes	Mod. high (↑)	High (↑)	Mod. high (↑)	Low (↑)
Blood flow	Mod. high	High	—	Low (↑)
Fatigability	Low (↓)	Mod. (↓)	Mod. high (↓)	High (↓)

The myosin heavy chains listed in parentheses reflect which isoform the primary myosin heavy chain is transformed into during adaptations in response to either increases or decreases in mechanical activity. The arrows listed in parenthesis reflects either increases or decreases in the relative expression of a given property or enzyme system in response to increases or decreases in mechanical activity imposed on that specific motor unit. For example, the adapative response typically seen in slow, type I units represents an upregulation of properties typically seen in faster motor units and vice versa.

illary number per unit of volume, capillary length, and blood flow through these capillaries. The transfer of oxygen and substrates from blood to mitochondria can be understood by considering the proteins facilitating their transfer. For example, oxygen requires myoglobin to facilitate its transfer through the sarcoplasm. Other proteins involved in transport processes (GLUT1 and GLUT4 protein, lipoprotein lipase, albumin, fatty acid–binding proteins, carnitine palmitoyltransferases I and II) increase with endurance types of training, as shown in Table 24.2.

Increases in 11–12 of the 14 proteins/structures involved in transferring oxygen/substrates into adenosine triphosphate (ATP) in muscle are shown in Table 24.2. The two not increasing are submaximal blood flow per unit of muscle mass and glycolytic enzyme levels. The remainder of this paragraph will speculate on why these two transfer functions are not increased by endurance types of training. Blood flow does not increase, and may decrease, per unit of muscle mass when major muscle groups are recruited during exercise at a given submaximal work intensity after training. However, blood flow is redistributed within a muscle as a result of endurance training. In trained rats there is a higher blood flow in muscular regions composed of type IIa fibers (13). Glycolytic enzymes and mRNAs decrease in fast muscles with endurance types of training. A benefit of this decrease could be surmised to be a sparing of carbohydrate, as endurance-trained muscle has a greater capacity to oxidize fatty acids. The reason for the species difference in myoglobin protein gene expression with endurance types of training is not understood (i.e., why endurance training increases myoglobin concentration in rodents, but not in human beings). As a general rule, changes in rodent and mammalian protein quantities in skeletal muscle are in similar directions as a result of endurance training.

Differences in transporting processes found between wild and domesticated animals are in the same directions as those occurring with endurance training. The hypothesis of functional coadaptation between oxygen and metabolic fuel supply systems in migratory and sedentary animals was used by Weber to predict that the capacity of key enzymes, transmembrane transporter proteins, glucose precursor supply, and soluble fatty acid transport proteins must all be geared to support higher maximal glucose, fatty acid, and oxygen fluxes in wild, more aerobic animals than in their sedentary counterparts for a given species (351).

Hoppeler and Billeter (152) conclude that the rate-limiting factor for the continuation of mild aerobic work is the supply of oxygen and substrates from the circulation to the muscle fiber. They contend that

TABLE 24.2. *Most Processes Involved in Transfer of Oxygen and Substrates Increase in Response to Endurance Types of Training*

Item Transferred	Protein/Structure Involved in Transfer	Directional Change to Endurance Types of Training	References
Blood	Capillary density	↑	See 287 for references
	Mean capillary transit time (at a given $\dot{Q}$)	↑,	286
	Blood flow through muscle		
	Same submaximal work intensity	→	See 56, 205 for references
	Maximal work	↑	205
Oxygen	Arterial–venous O_2 difference		276
	Small mass of exercising muscle	→	
	Large mass of exercising muscle	↑	
	Myoglobin		
	Animals	↑	252
	Human beings	→	169
	Krebs cycle enzyme activities	↑	147
	Electron transport chain activities	↑	25, 66, 143
Glucose	GLUT4	↑	105, 257, 272
	Glycolytic enzyme activities		
	1–2 h exercise per day	↓ type IIa	24
		↑ type I	24
	8–24 h continuous stimulation per day	↓	361
Fatty acids	Lipoprotein lipase	↑	
	Albumin	↑	131
	Fatty acid–binding protein	↑	177
	Carnitine palmitoyltransferase	↑	236
	Capacity to oxidize fatty acids	↑	236

transport is the primary limitation to work. Myofibrils must be provided with newly synthesized ATP to fuel myosin ATPase for contraction in the exercising muscle. An overview of these processes is shown in Figure 24.1. Adaptations of these processes will be discussed in a later section.

From information such as the above, others have suggested that one strategy of skeletal muscle adaptation to endurance training is to increase almost all components of the systems involved in the transfer of oxygen and substrates from blood to their conversion to ATP. Weibel et al. (353) tested the hypothesis that the quantitative design of a system matches its functional parameters, termed "symmorphorosis". They concluded: (*1*) that the amount of mitochondria expression is directly proportional to $\dot{V}O_{2max}$, which determines maximal oxidative capacity; (*2*) that the quantity of capillaries and the concentration of O_2-carrying erythrocytes in capillary blood contribute equally to establishing oxygen supply; and (*3*) that stroke volume and hematocrit match $\dot{V}O_{2max}$ (353). Weibel et al. (353) did not find that pulmonary diffusing capacity was proportional to $\dot{V}O_{2max}$, either singularly or in combination with other factors. Weibel et al. (353) concluded that structural design is matched to functional demand for all systems, except the pulmonary, that are involved in the supply of oxygen and substrate to muscle mitochondria.

Others have examined the relationship between structure and function. For example, (*1*) a correlation of 0.75 between cytochrome oxidase activity in the vastus lateralis muscle of young men and their $\dot{V}O_{2max}$ was reported by Booth and Narahara in 1974 (33); (*2*) aerobic enzyme activities of muscle tissue are linearly dependent on the absolute volume of mitochondria it contains (296); and (*3*) a significant correlation exists between mitochondrial volume density (cm^2) and capillary length density (km) (152, 153); and (*4*) a ratio of 1:200 exists between the surface area of the capillary wall and that of the inner mitochondrial membrane (152).

Cellular Processes Involving Anaerobic Metabolism and High-Energy Phosphate Buffering

During relatively short-term exercise of very high intensity, in which the rate of ATP synthesis derived

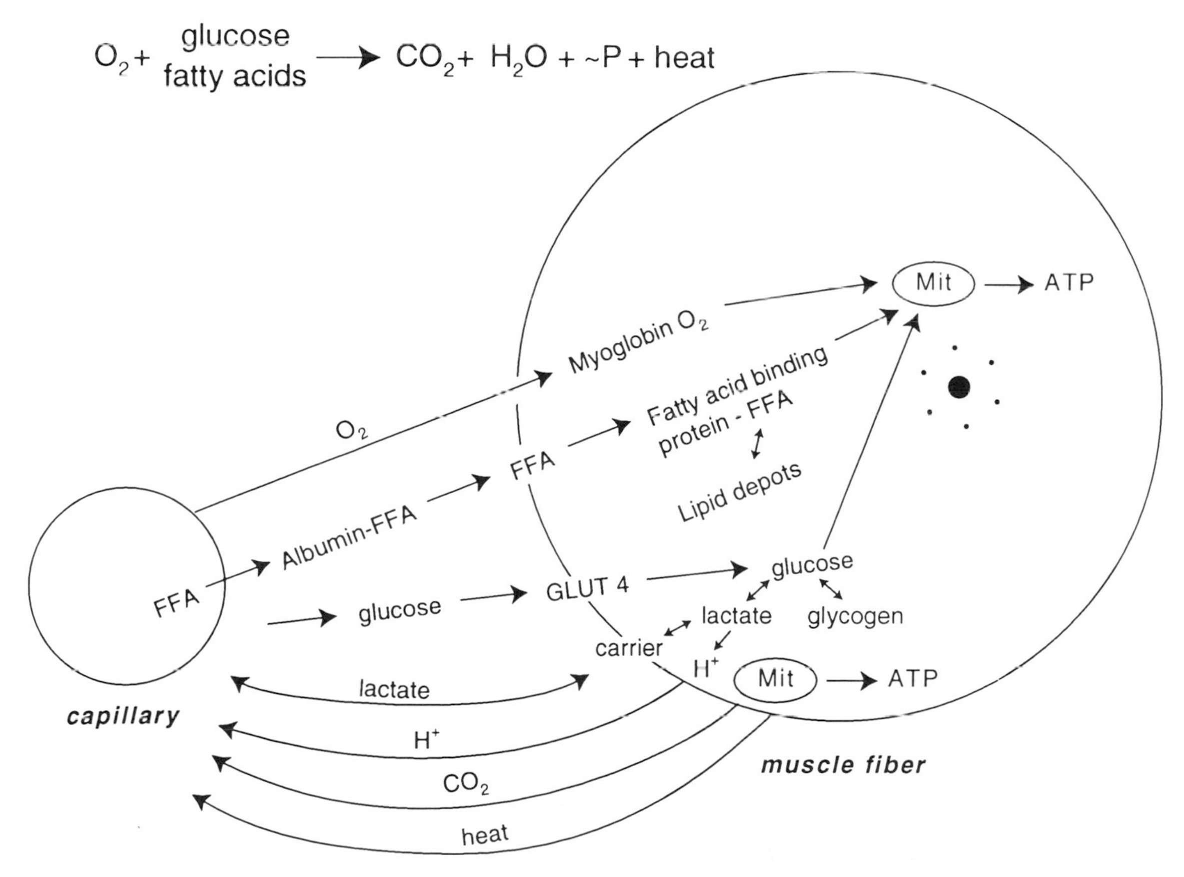

FIG. 24.1. Diagram of intermediary steps involved in the transfer of substrates to and from skeletal muscle. Mit, mitochondria; FFA, free fatty acids; GLUT 4 is glucose transport protein 4. [Adapted from a review by Hoppeler and Billeter (152).]

from oxidative processes is unlikely capable of matching the rate of energy expenditure occurring in the contractile and SR component, the muscle cell becomes highly dependent on energy-transforming processes linked to two separate but interrelated pathways involving ATP synthesis independent of oxidative metabolic pathways. The first system involves high-energy phosphate transformations involving the coupling of the creatine kinase, the adenylate kinase, and the adenylate deaminase enzyme systems [see Fig. 24.2; 99, 35]. These enzymes are linked to the buffering of ATP at the expense of lowering the cellular levels of phosphocreatine while elevating the levels of creatine, and of free adenosine diphosphate (ADP), adenosine monophosphate (AMP), and inosine monophosphate (IMP) (335). These coupled reactions ensure that the ATP levels remain in proximity to resting levels, while the change in both the level of substrates and products in these reactions contribute to the modulation of other metabolic processes governing intracellular substrate mobilization.

The second pathway of importance in regulating ATP levels independent of oxidative processes involves the mobilization of endogenous glycogen through the glycolytic pathway to pyruvate and/or lactic acid, whereby 3 moles of ATP are generated per mole of glucose equivalent utilized (99). It is interesting that in those motor units expressing both the fast myosin isoforms and fast calcium pump isoforms—that is, the so-called type IIa and IIb (and likely the IIx) motor units—these same motor units maintain a three to fivefold greater level of the glycogenolytic enzymes as well as the above-described enzymes involved in ATP buffering as compared to the type I (slow) motor unit, which inherently expresses the slow isoforms governing cross-bridge and calcium cycling (24, 99). Furthermore, the steady, state levels of high energy phosphates at rest are greater in the fast(er) motor units (99). These observations suggest that in addition to the coregulation of protein systems involved in contraction-relaxation processes, there appears to be a coupled regulation of these contractile enzyme systems to those enzyme systems involved in the anaerobic generation of ATP (see Fig. 24.2). On the other hand, the level of mitochondria maintained in a given muscle fiber appears to be independently regulated relative to either the type of contractile machinery or the level of anaerobic enzymatic activity that is expressed in the muscle fiber, because fibers expressing either the fast IIa or slow (type I) MHCs (and other related contractile isoforms) inherently express a high level of mitochondria. On the other hand, there is a large discrepancy in mitochondrial levels among fibers expressing the fast MHC isoforms (20, 142, 298). Furthermore, as discussed below, the level of mitochondria can be altered in skeletal muscle independently of any altered expression in contractile protein isoforms. Therefore, from a regulation standpoint it is of interest to determine which components of the cell display adaptive plasticity in response to the various activity/hormonal/pharmacological paradigms imposed on the muscle.

Interrelationships in Cellular Processes

Blood Flow and Oxidative Metabolism. The reader is referred to a recent review on the distribution of blood flow within and among skeletal muscles in conscious animals during locomotory exercise for a more detailed account (12). In brief, once a muscle fiber type is recruited, blood flow increases proportionally with increases in the speed of treadmill run-

$$\text{ATP} \xrightarrow{\text{Actomyosin ATPase}} \text{ADP} + \text{P}_i + \text{Free Energy}$$

$$\text{ADP} + \text{P}_{Cr} \xrightarrow{\text{Creatine Kinase}} \text{ATP} + \text{Creatine}$$

$$\text{ADP} + \text{ADP} \xrightarrow{\text{Adenylate Kinase}} \text{ATP} + \text{AMP}$$

$$\text{AMP} + \text{H}_2\text{0} \xrightarrow{\text{AMP Deaminase}} \text{IMP} + \text{NH}_3$$

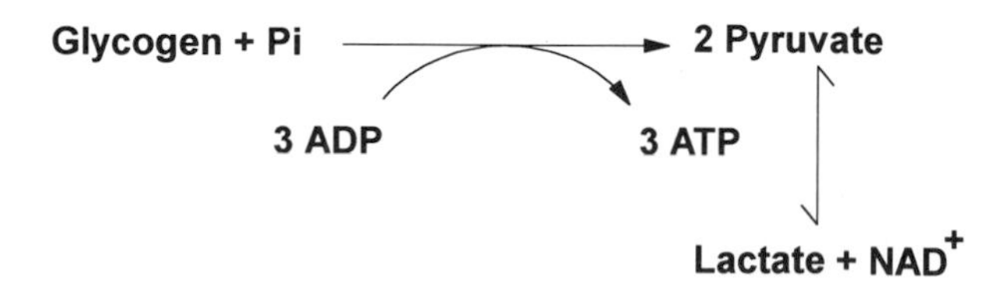

FIG. 24.2. Enzymatic reactions designed to buffer ATP turnover independent of aerobic metabolic processes.

ning by the animal until reaching a peak flow either below, or at, $\dot{V}O_{2max}$. Thus, a close matching of blood flow to the percentage of activated muscle fibers has been shown.

Are there vascular adaptations in muscle that benefit endurance performance? The answer to this question depends on the mass of muscle exercising and whether one refers to submaximal or maximal exercise. During intense exercise with a small or large muscle mass, an increase in maximal vascular conductance in trained muscle (205) could benefit endurance via an increase in peak muscle flow. However, during maximal exercise with a large mass, blood flow to muscle is limited by the pumping capacity of the heart and by any further rise in muscle blood flow being prevented by the fall in vascular conductance needed to maintain arterial blood pressure (275, 277, 288). Therefore, any increases in peak muscle blood flow observed during maximal exercise after training are concluded to be a result of an increased cardiac output along with a compensatory rise in muscle vascular conductance produced by less sympathetic vasoconstriction. A well-documented adaptation that is listed in Table 24.2 is an increase in capillary density.

Endurance types of training increase the potential for maximal blood flow per unit of trained skeletal muscle during aerobic exercise. Capillary density per unit of volume of muscle increases after either endurance training (287) or chronic stimulation (40). Functional importances of increased capillary density with endurance training seem to be for improved O_2 diffusion by having more capillaries per muscle fiber, more capillaries per square millimeter of tissue, and less muscle tissue supplied by each capillary (179). Endurance types of training increase both aerobic enzyme activity of trained muscle and steady-state blood flow to muscle at the maximal work intensity after training, as compared to pretraining. The increase in muscle blood flow as $\dot{V}O_{2max}$ increases with training without any effect on arterial blood pressure is because cardiac output and muscle vascular conductance rise in the same relative proportions (276).

During the adaptation to chronic electrical stimulation, Simoneau et al. (307) present data showing that the increase in resistance to fatigue observed in chronically low-frequency–stimulated muscle does not have exactly the same time course of adaptation as the increase in citrate synthase activity. They suggest that the increased resistance to fatigue in chronic stimulation may not entirely be determined by elevations in the capacity of the citric acid cycle and other related metabolic pathways of aerobic metabolism (307).

The critical question of what factors induce angiogenesis in skeletal or heart muscles has yet to be answered (156). Hudlicka et al. (156) indicate that chronic increases in muscle contraction increase capillary red blood cell flow and shear stress, as well as increasing capillary wall tension. They speculate that these changes are likely to disturb the luminal side of the capillary endothelial cells and consequently release bound proteases that would damage the basement membrane, which would release basic fibroblast growth factor (FGF). Morrow et al. (241) reported that chronic stimulation doubled the acidic and basic FGF in muscle. They speculate that increased FGF could induce vascular growth and satellite cell proliferation (241). Henriksson (133) indicates that a lack of information exists concerning to what extent neoformation is dependent on training intensity and duration.

ORGANELLE PLASTICITY IN RESPONSE TO INTERVENTIONS

The goal of this section is to delineate some of the adaptations in skeletal muscle that occur in response to a variety of models that have been developed to study muscle plasticity.

Contractile Machinery

Myosin Heavy Chains. Adult mammalian skeletal muscle fibers express at least four specific types of MHC: slow type I, fast IIa, fast IIx (also designated as IId), and fast IIb. These MHCs have been identified at the protein level on the basis of their mobility under denaturing gel electrophoresis (43, 319), and the pattern of their reactivity to a battery of monoclonal antibodies specific to the MHCs (16, 68, 204, 293). The type I MHC is known to have low ATPase activity, and it predominates in muscle fibers (motor units) used extensively for antigravity function and locomotion (280). In most species, including humans, this isoform is most abundantly expressed in the soleus and vastus intermedius muscles. Also, it is expressed extensively in the deep, "red" region of most mammalian muscles used extensively in locomotion (279). In contrast, the faster isoforms are expressed abundantly in muscles of all the extremities (5, 292, 310). Motor units that are used almost exclusively for short-duration, high-power output activity, such as sprinting and power weight lifting, express chiefly the IIb and IIx MHCs (5, 6); whereas, fast motor units used for more endurance types of activity (i.e., the deep red regions of most mammalian muscles) appear to abundantly express the IIa MHC isoform (125). Estimates of myofibril/myosin ATPase activity among the three fast isoforms suggest the IIb MHC has the highest specific activity followed by the IIx and IIa isoforms (45, 46). Consequently, there appears to be both functional and energetic correlates to the pattern of expression of these MHC phenotypes in the musculature. However, there is not yet a clear-cut differentiation of mechanical properties in fibers expressing the IIa vs. IIx isoform (204). In the heart, two MHC isoforms have been identified. One isoform is the same protein product as the slow type I MHC gene identified in slow-twitch skeletal muscle, and it has been designated as the low ATPase, β-MHC (75, 161, 318). The other isoform, designated as α, has relatively high ATPase activity. Like skeletal muscle, these two isoforms are highly plastic in that their relative expression in cardiac tissue is dependent on the animal species (the β-MHC predominates in larger mammals and vice versa), the hormonal status of the animal, and the mechanical loading state imposed on the heart (discussed later).

Myosin Light Chains. In each native myosin molecule, two pairs of light chains, ranging in molecular weight from 16–30 kDa, have been identified (255). One pair of the myosin light chains (MLCs) has been designated as the alkali or essential light chain (255); whereas, the other pair is designated as the phosphorylatable (P or DTNB, or regulatory) light chain (255). Collectively, it is thought that the role of these light chains is to modulate the force generation (P light chain) and ATPase activity (alkali light chain) of myosin in the context of its interaction with actin during contraction (228, 255). Isoform-specific essential and regulatory light chains have been identified for fast-twitch, slow-twitch, and cardiac muscle, giving rise to a large number of possible native myosin protein isoforms depending on the post-translational processing of both the MHCs and the MLCs (255). Although the evidence suggests a high level of plasticity of expression of these MLCs, (which may parallel that seen for the MHCs as discussed below), a comprehensive review of MLC plasticity is beyond the scope of this chapter (for excellent reviews see 228, 255). A comprehensive update of directional changes in MLC mRNAs with different exercise models is given in Table 24.4 later in chapter.

MHC Plasticity

Effects of loading state. Exposure of rodents to microgravity and to ground-based models (hindlimb suspension and limb immobilization) of muscle unloading induce alterations in both fiber mass and MHC phenotype in the unloaded skeletal muscles (19, 47, 71, 126, 173, 222, 247, 323). Available evidence suggests that a subpopulation of fibers, normally expressing predominantly either the type I or IIa MHC, undergo both atrophy (5, 43, 173, 247) and a transformation whereby the IIx and IIb MHCs are up-regulated in expression at both the protein and mRNA level (5, 43, 126). These transforming fibers appear largely as hybrids in which both the slow(er) and faster MHCs are coexpressed (43, 173, 247). It remains to be seen whether a complete change in phenotype occurs in these transforming fibers.

A significant pool of slow fibers in the soleus muscle appears to be unaffected by unloading (43, 173). As we discuss later in the chapter, these soleus fibers may represent a developmentally regulated, non-adapting pool of fibers that do not possess the genetic capability of expressing the faster MHCs. In contrast to the pattern of response seen for the antigravity muscles, fast muscles, used chiefly for locomotor and burst activity, demonstrate lesser degrees of both atrophy (5, 19, 71, 173) and capability for MHC transformation in response to unloading (5, 19, 71, 173).

At the other end of the spectrum, if weight-bearing stress is chronically imposed on a fast muscle, by eliminating its synergists, a significant pool of fibers, located chiefly in the inner core of the overloaded muscle, will both hypertrophy and up-regulate expression of the type I MHC (22, 74, 158, 159, 279, 313, 319, 334). However, fibers in the superficial regions of the muscle appear to be less adaptable in terms of MHC expression. While these fibers, chiefly expressing the IIb MHC, also hypertrophy, they alter phenotype by up-regulating expression of the IIx and/or IIa MHCs (22, 44). These types of adaptation suggest that there may be a limit to the MHC phenotype(s) that can be expressed in different types of fiber as a result of their embryonic/neonatal developmental history. In the context of the these changes seen in skeletal muscle, it is interesting that in the rat heart, which normally expresses the fast (α) type of cardiac MHC, chronic functional overload (i.e., increases in blood pressure) in addition to inducing fiber hypertrophy, induces the up-regulation of the slow, β-MHC in proportion to the level of afterload imposed on the heart (161). This response is consistent with the hypothesis that in muscle cells that are not normally accustomed to slow cross-bridge cycling kinetics, the up-regulation of slower isoforms is an inherent adaptation to better accommodate the cell to handle the increased load. These types of adaptive processes are further exemplified in the continuous stretch model involving avian wing muscle. Results from this model further suggest that fiber enlargement induced by mechanical stress transforms the MHC phenotype, indicative of slower MHC expression in selected pools of fibers (10). However, unlike the mammalian overload model, increases in fiber length are routinely observed in that more sarcomeres are being added in response to the stretch (10, 326). Consequently, when continuous stress is imposed on muscle cells, the adaptation increases the quantity of contractile protein in order to compensate for the elevation in mechanical stress. In addition, there is some level of alteration in the contractile protein phenotype favoring increased expression of slower MHC isoforms in order to enable a limited subset of the total fiber pool to sustain the mechanical stress more economically.

Resistance training using animals. Several approaches have been used to induce intermittent heavy resistance stress on the musculature of animals. For example, rodents have been forced to climb vertical inclines carrying varying amounts of weight (up to 150% of body weight) several times per day over a period of weeks (376). The adaptation has modestly increased muscle mass (376) and altered fiber types, indicative of a greater fast glycolytic cross-sectional area (376). However, the chief drawback of this particular model is that it is impossible to ascertain how the increase in load-bearing activity is distributed across the musculature of interest. To overcome this problem, others (47, 72, 367, 368) have developed an animal model in order to simulate heavy resistance training programs routinely used to induce hypertrophy in human skeletal muscle. The key feature of this model is the implantation of electrodes into the muscle to be trained by electrically activating it to perform heavy resistance training paradigms against a computer-controlled ergometer so that precise loading conditions and velocities of contraction can be controlled (46, 72). Caiozzo et al. (46) used a variety of high-resistance (90% maximal force) programs of either the concentric or eccentric type, spanning 6–8 weeks, and they observed modest increases in muscle mass (14%–18%) (46). This enlargement accompanied a decrease in the relative expression of IIb MHC and a concomitant increase in the relative content of IIa/IIx MHCs in regions of muscle typically expressing chiefly the IIb isoform (46). Others found that these programs induced greater increases in protein synthesis in the trained muscles after as little as a single training session (367, 368). Interestingly, in this model, expression of the slow type I MHC with these training paradigms appears not to be increased. However, Diffee et al. (72) found isometric training programs to be successful in partially preventing the down-regulation of type I MHC expression that occurs in antigravity muscles such as the soleus in response to continuous hindlimb unloading. Changes in MHC mRNA have been observed in compensatory hypertrophy (See Table 24.4 later in chapter). Collectively, these findings suggest that the plasticity of MHC expression in response to resistance training may be dependent on both the amount and type of mechanical stress imposed on the muscle.

Several investigators have used a chronic heavy resistance training model involving the voluntary training of the forearm musculature of cats (10, 118, 229, 326). With this particular model, the results suggest that variable increases in both muscle fiber mass (11%) and total fiber number (9%) can be induced following prolonged training (100–150 weeks) without any appreciable change in the pattern of fiber-type expression (118, 229). However, with this model, the voluntary induced mechanical activity of the cats is quite variable, with some animals demonstrating ballistic types of contractions, whereas others employ slower deliberate activity (75, 229). Also, most of the force developed against the load was from muscles other than the forearm. These contrasting patterns of mechanical activity make it difficult to link specific mechanical factors to the adaptational processes.

Human models of resistance training. In human studies, it is well established that heavy resistance training over approximately 6 months increases both strength and muscle fiber enlargement in the range of 12%–25% (6, 81, 217, 310, 326). Furthermore, these longitudinal training programs appear not to change in the relative proportion of fast vs. slow fibers (310, 326). However, athletes who have trained for years have larger muscle fibers than those who have trained for relatively short periods (117, 326). Interestingly, only recently have attempts been made to partition out the contribution of specific contractile variables in the adaptive process. These recent studies suggest that the eccentric component of most training programs may be a pivotal factor for inducing increases in strength and fiber size (81). Furthermore, examination of myosin phenotype by histochemical (310) and electrophoretic techniques (6) suggests that resistance training induces transformations in fiber typing and MHC expression among the fast types of fibers without much change in the relative expression of slow fibers (6, 310). These adaptations involve an apparent down-regulation of the IIb MHC with concomitant up-regulation of the IIa MHC in both male and female subjects (310).

Thus, these findings on human subjects resemble the adaptive process (as discussed above) seen in rodent skeletal muscle electrically activated to perform heavy resistance contractions (46).

Endurance exercise. Vertical population studies comparing individuals who have trained for endurance over months to years with more sedentary populations suggest that the former athletes have a greater proportion of slow-twitch fibers in their trained musculature than do their nontrained counterparts (23, 125, 216, 255, 292). Similar responses have been observed in rats who have exercised on the treadmill for long periods of time (23, 102, 125). On the other hand, longitudinal studies involving humans examined in both the trained and nontrained state suggest that the changes in myosin phenotype are more subtle, likely involving transformations either among the faster MHCs or the formation of fiber types bridging the fast vs. slow types (255, 292). Similar studies in the endurance-trained rodent reveal that native myosin isoforms, largely comprised of the type IIa MHC, are up-regulated in regions of hindlimb muscle used extensively in running (101, 102, 125). Collectively, these observations suggest that low-force, high-frequency activity patterns in the rat are capable of inducing transformations in MHC phenotype to the "slower" isoforms seen in the trained musculature. This response is qualitatively similar to that seen with the model of chronic electrical stimulation as discussed below.

Chronic electrical stimulation. Continuous chronic electrical stimulation (generally of low frequency; 10–20 Hz) of rodent fast-twitch and slow-twitch muscle exerts a major impact on MHC phenotype (16, 184, 186, 254, 255). In general, after a sufficient period of stimulation (20–30 days), there is nearly complete repression of IIb MHC expression coupled with increased levels of both the IIx (transiently) and IIa MHCs in both the tibialis anterior and extensor digitorum muscles of rodents (16, 186, 255). Unlike rabbit muscle, in which chronic electrical stimulation increases type I MHC expression across the fiber pool (254, 255), rodent muscle responds with relatively little up-regulation in type I MHC in stimulated muscles (184, 186, 255). However, recent observations (223) indicate that prolonged continuous stimulation at 10–20 Hz can significantly up-regulate the expression of type I MHC in rodent fast muscle. These findings suggest lower responsiveness in the transforming capacity to express type I MHC, particularly in the ankle flexor muscles (which generally are not involved in weight-bearing activity). In other investigations, repetitive high-frequency (150 Hz), short-duration (0.16) bursts of activation of rodent soleus muscle down-regulated type I MHC expression (16). Interestingly, this transformation in MHC expression closely resembles the pattern reported above when soleus muscles are subjected to chronic periods of non–weight-bearing activity (5, 71). As an aside, it has been reported that chronic electrical stimulation of the ankle flexor muscles causes their atrophy (255). This suggests that this model may not provide a true physiological stimulus for the normal regulation of MHC adaptation . For example, hypertrophy is the physiological end result when the muscle is electrically stimulated to contract under controlled loading conditions requiring high force production (47, 72). Consequently, the relative loading state imposed on a muscle appears to be an important variable that can dictate the degree and type of adaptation induced in MHC phenotype among the different fiber types.

Thyroid state

HYPOTHYROIDISM. Depending on the type of muscle, hypothyroidism [a reduction in circulating thyroid hormone (T_3)] and muscle overload both alter MHC phenotype in a similar manner, but the magnitude is less in the former. In the soleus muscle of rodents, hypothyroidism induces all of the IIa fibers, which normally make up 15%–20% of the fiber pool, to express only the type I MHC (46, 48). Since functional overload appears to cause the same response in the soleus (160, 279), these interventions represent the only type of stimuli that we think are capable of inducing expression of only one type of MHC (i.e., type I) in a particular muscle.

In another slow muscle such as the vastus intermedius, a similar response to hypothyroidism occurs, but not all the IIa and IIx fibers shift to type I fibers (46, 48). In faster muscles such as the plantaris and the red medial gastrocnemius, the same general pattern of response occurs as seen in the vastus intermedius, but the degree of change is small (4%–7%) (46). Regions of adult muscle chiefly expressing the IIb fibers are largely unresponsive to hypothyroidism. These findings suggest that there is a relatively small core of fibers within slow muscles, and likely within the red region of fast muscles (likely IIa and/or IIx fibers), that revert to expressing the type I MHC in the absence of sufficient levels of circulating thyroid hormone.

HYPERTHYROIDISM. In contrast, hindlimb muscle responds to a hyperthyroid state (increased levels of circulating T_3) remarkably similar in pattern to that seen for chronic states of unloading (45). The key observations are as follows: (*1*) in the soleus, there is up-regulation of IIa (and possibly IIx) in approximately 30%–40% of the fibers, with the remaining type I fibers being unresponsive (45); (2) a prolonged state of hyperthyroidism (20 weeks) does not induce type IIb expression in the soleus (45, 48); and (3) in the vastus intermedius and red medial gastrocnemius, and plantaris muscles, there is a decrease in type I, IIa, and IIx MHC expression and an increase in type IIb MHC expression, but these transformations are relatively small (12%–20%) (319). Like skeletal muscle, heart muscle is highly sensitive to thyroid hormone. For example, in the rat, hypothyroidism induces concomitant up-regulation of the slow, β-myosin gene and down-regulation of the fast, α-MHC gene and vice versa (75). Generally, the shifts in MHC expression in response to thyroid state are mirrored by changes in the relative content of mRNA for the various MHCs, suggesting that the myosin genes are regulated by thyroid hormone via pretranslational (transcriptional and/or mRNA stability) processes (73, 319).

Interaction of thyroid state and weight bearing activity on MHC phenotype. As indicated above, both hyperthyroidism and functional overload produce opposite effects on MHC expression. Thus, when these two interventions compete, the hyperthyroid state can blunt the overload-induced increase in type I MHC in both slow and fast muscles (160, 319). However, the hyperthyroid state could not completely prevent the altered expression of the three fast MHCs in response to functional overload (319). Similar patterns of adaptive response accompanied chronic electrical stimulation of skeletal muscle in conjunction with hyperthyroidism (i.e., the hyperthyroid state is partially effective in blunting the isomyosin shifts associated with chronic low-frequency stimulation) (186). This latter response suggests that some fibers are sensitive to increased loading states and chronic electrically induced activity independently of thyroid state. On the other hand, when the intervention of hypothyroidism was interacted with hindlimb unloading, the former was completely effective in preventing the unloading-induced increases in fast MHC expression that occurred in both the soleus and VI muscles (73). As observed for the thyroid studies, the level of regulation of these adaptations appears to be at the pretranslational level (73).

Sarcoplasmic Reticulum. The SR, including the T-tubular network, is the subcellular component involved chiefly in calcium cycling (255, 289). Recent findings suggest that a protein complex, designated as the dihydropyridine receptor (DHP), is a regulatory protein involved in triggering the calcium release from the SR (175, 269). The DHP receptor is located in the T tubules and acts as a voltage sensor, coupling the depolarization of the T-tubular membrane to the SR for release of calcium via calcium-specific channels to the myofilaments. The DHP receptor is a complex protein containing four specific subunits (α_1, α_2, β, and γ). The α_1-subunit is known to confer DHP-binding and voltage-sensing properties (269). Skeletal muscle isoform specific α_1-subunits have been identified (269), and the mRNA abundance for the DHP receptor is markedly different in fast vs. slow skeletal muscles (i.e., greater in fast-twitch vs. slow-twitch muscles) (269). These differences are in keeping with the notion that fast-twitch muscles have a greater abundance of DPH receptors and hence generate faster kinetics in the release of calcium to activate the contractile machinery.

A second key protein in the modulation of calcium cycling is the SR calcium-ATPase pump that actively transports calcium into the SR to lower the free calcium in the myoplasm (255, 289, 291, 308, 370). Two isoforms of calcium pump protein exist in adult skeletal muscle, a slow and a fast isoform that are differentially expressed in fast- and slow-twitch skeletal muscle (255, 370). Although the specific functional difference of these two isoforms is not well defined (370), the relative density of expression of each isoform in their respective fast and slow muscles appears to be associated with the differences in the relaxation kinetics in two muscle types (255).

In addition to these primary proteins that regulate calcium cycling, three additional proteins have been identified in skeletal muscle, and these may exert modulatory roles in calcium transport. The first is phospholamban, a phosphorylatable protein that appears to be associated with the calcium ATPase pump of cardiac and slow skeletal muscle, but not fast-twitch skeletal muscle (209). This protein is thought to modulate the calcium transport process in slow skeletal muscle. The second protein is calsequestrin, a calcium-binding protein found in the SR. While cardiac- and skeletal-specific isoforms have been identified (254, 255), both fast- and slow-twitch skeletal muscles appear to express the skeletal type. Consequently, it appears that the two types of muscle are differentiated by the amount of calsequestrin expressed (i.e., greater content being expressed in the fast type). These observations have suggested that this protein acts as a sink to bind calcium as it is transported into the reticulum. A third protein, parvalbumin, has been identified in fast but not in slow skeletal muscle (255). This low-molecular-weight protein is thought to act as a buffer for calcium and magnesium in the cytosol and may be essential in the early phase of relaxation by binding calcium as it is released from troponin (255).

Sarcoplasmic Reticulum Plasticity

Effects of loading state. Chronic muscle overload caused by surgical removal of synergists reduces slightly (10%–15%) the kinetic properties of rodent slow-twitch and fast-twitch skeletal muscle relaxation in response to an isometric contraction (21, 279, 280). These studies employ indices such as the time to peak tension and the one-half relaxation time as the chief functional markers during the time course of an isometric contraction. The small changes correlate well with kinetics of calcium uptake measured on isolated preparations of sarcoplasmic reticulum, corresponding to the early phases of the reaction process (i.e., the first minute) (21). These observations suggest that there is relatively little alteration in either the density or type of calcium pump isoform being expressed in the SR network for both calcium delivery and sequestration in the overloaded muscles (21, 279). These small changes in calcium cycling properties are not as striking as the changes observed in both MHC phenotype and force–velocity properties for the same overloaded muscles (21, 279). These observations suggest that there is some degree of dissociation in the regulation of calcium cycling vs. that of cross-bridge cycling in the affected fibers (280). The functional significance of this adaptive process remains to be elucidated.

On the other hand, when slow-twitch muscles such as the soleus are chronically unloaded there is evidence, based on contractile (71), SR DHP receptor (175), SR calcium ATPase kinetic (255), and SR calcium ATPase pump isoform (87) (see Table 24.1) data, to indicate that the calcium cycling properties are enhanced in the unloaded muscles. Under these conditions of altered activity, the changes seen in calcium cycling properties are in line with the degree of MHC transformation and hence the speeding of the intrinsic shortening velocity of the muscle (295). Similar directional changes are seen in unloaded fast-twitch muscles (71), but their magnitude is considerably less than that seen in the antigravity muscles. A summary of changes in mRNAs for calcium handling proteins is given in Table 24.4 later in chapter.

Chronic electrical stimulation. When fast-twitch muscles are chronically stimulated at low frequency, there is a rapid slowing in the relaxation properties of the muscle. This occurs in a few days rather than in weeks (190, 209, 254, 255). The slowing in relaxation properties is correlated with reductions in the calcium pump ATPase activity (209, 254, 255) with a reduction in the expression of parvalbumin (190, 254, 255), as well as with changes in the type of calcium pump that is expressed in the affected muscle (255). Changes in the mRNAs of calcium handling proteins during chronic stimulation are summarized in Table 24.4 later in chapter. However, the changes in calcium pump isoform is a late manifestation of the adaptation process (209). Importantly, the changes in calcium cycling properties appear to precede the down-regulation of the fast MHC isoforms (254, 255). Thus, depending on its time frame, chronic electrical stimulation may serve as a useful model for uncoupling the role of the SR from that of the myosin isoforms in the regulation of the cyclic mechanical behavior of skeletal muscle. This experimental manipulation may enable one to model the kinetics of cross-bridge cycling and relaxation processes in performing cyclic movement activities such as running and other modes of locomotion.

Thyroid state. Chronic elevation of thyroid hormone exerts a profound affect indicative of faster kinetics in the contraction time and SR calcium-sequestering properties of slow skeletal muscle (45, 101, 255, 291). These changes are manifest in greater calcium pump ATPase both per gram of tissue and per unit of SR protein. This indicates that both quantitative and qualitative changes are occurring in this machinery (11, 291, 308). Hypothyroidism produces the opposite affects (46, 48). Thus, the SR is similar to the contractile apparatus in that it is keenly sensitive to both mechanical activity and to thyroid hormone in the regulation of its plasticity. Accordingly, a fundamental question is whether activity-related changes in the plasticity of the contractile and SR systems are mediated through changes in the muscle's responsiveness to thyroid hormone.

Mitochondria and Substrate Provision (Oxidative Processes)

Aerobic types of exercise increase the density of mitochondria in endurance-trained skeletal muscles (25, 66, 143), whereas resistance training does not alter mitochondrial density (144; for reviews, see 34, 144, 146 and also Fig. 24.3). After endurance training, exercise at a given submaximal $\dot{V}O_2$ elicits smaller increases in muscle and blood lactate concentrations, a slower utilization rate of carbohydrate, and an increased reliance on fat oxidation as an energy source occur (see Chapters 19, 20, 21, and 23). These changes are associated with increased mitochondrial density in the trained skeletal muscle. Holloszy and Coyle (146) suggest that it seems probable that these interrelated metabolic adaptations to endurance training are largely responsible for the increased endurance in the trained state. Chapters 21

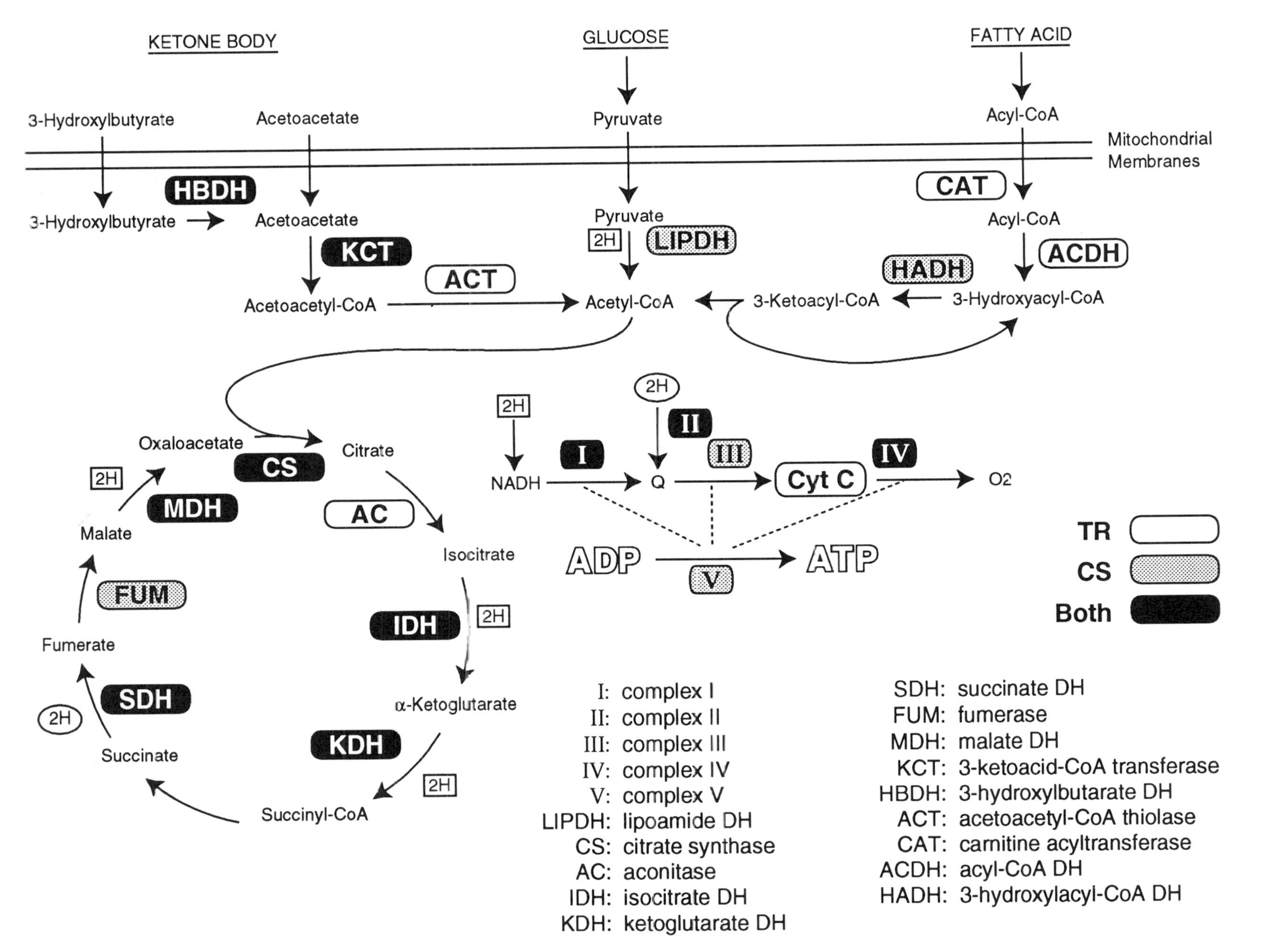

FIG. 24.3. Adaptive increases in mitochondrial enzymes to either treadmill running or chronic electrical stimulation. (Contributed by Zhen Yan.)

and 23 provide excellent reviews on fatty acid metabolism.

Green et al. (124) observed that metabolic adaptations, such as muscle glycogen sparing and lower levels of muscle lactate, occur prior to increases in muscle mitochondrial volume in humans during moderate endurance training. After 5–7 days of this training, neither citrate synthase nor succinate dehydrogenase activities changed. The two authors (124) suggested that other adaptations early in training may promote enhancement of metabolic adaptations.

In rats trained by running 2 h/pday, the capacity of isolated mitochondria to oxidize both pyruvate and malate (143) and also palmitic acid (236) doubled when data were expressed per gram of muscle wet weight basis. mRNAs for mitochondrial enzymes do not always increase in skeletal muscles from rats who have undergone treadmill run training (see Table 24.4 later in chapter).

Glycogenolytic Activity and Glucose Transport for Anaerobic Processes

The capacity to mobilize endogenous glycogen is influenced by the absolute level of glycogenolytic enzymes expressed in the muscle fibers, and by the rate of ATP turnover during sustained contractile activity, which in turn alters the level of metabolites and other allosteric factors involved in regulating the flux through this pathway. Chronic physical activity (functional overload) and hormonal manipulation such as hypothyroidism (i.e., paradigms that result in down-regulation of contractile/relaxation processes indicative of a slower phenotype, and vice versa) are generally associated with a decrease in the relative level of expression of key glycogenolytic enzymes such as phosphorylase, phosphofructokinase, and lactic dehydrogenase (21, 23, 24, 99). Although these enzyme alterations should theoretically lower the maximal flux rate through the glycogenolytic pathway when it is fully activated, the actual rate of glycogen mobilization increases during sustained contractile activity (i.e., nonburst activity). Its mobilization is under the control of metabolic processes that are activated by changes in the operational level of ATP turnover (ATP synthesis to ATP degradation). For example, at submaximal rates of energy turnover, the actual rate of glycogenolysis is dependent on both the production and/or reduction of key metabolites involved in energy metabolism (e.g., citrate, free creatine, ATP, ADP) that collectively regulate the flux through key enzymatic steps in the glycogenolytic pathway (i.e., phosphofructokinase). Consequently, while there may be an activity-induced reduction in the level of the glycogenolytic enzymes expressed in skeletal muscle, the operational level of the glycogen mobilization pathway is dependent on the other factors controlling this complex process. Therefore, the extent that glycogen contributes to the overall energy balance in a particular type of muscle fiber during any given bout of exercise following physical training likely involves the integration of several factors including altered enzyme expression (both oxidative and glycogenolytic/glycolytic), altered hormonal status (chiefly insulin, catecholamines, and glucagon), and the availability of alternative substrates such as glucose and free fatty acids. Since these factors also are collectively altered during physical conditioning (188, 317), the overall metabolic profile during any given bout of exercise performed as a result chronic physical activity is a reflection of altered exogenous substrate mobilization, enzymatic capacity in the muscle, and the metabolic regulation taking place both in the muscle and in the organism.

Glucose Transport/Flux Processes. Uptake of glucose from plasma by muscle is important both during and after exercise (145). Muscle oxidizes both plasma glucose and glycogen during exercise. After exercise, depleted glycogen is replaced with the glucose from the plasma. The rate-limiting step for glucose use by muscle is glucose transport (204, 262). Glucose uptake across the sarcolemma into skeletal muscle occurs by facilitated diffusion with glucose transporters. Skeletal muscle expresses two isoforms, GLUT1 and GLUT4, of the glucose transporter family (53, 167). A comprehensive review of the glucose transporter family appeared recently (123). There appears to be a close correlation between the maximal capacity of muscles to transport glucose and their GLUT4 protein content (131, 167, 178). The values for GLUT4 protein content and 2-deoxyglucose uptake were related to the type of muscle fiber, with the relative rates being (92% type IIa) > (84% type I) > (a mixture of 57% type IIa and 40% type IIb) > (65% type IIb) (131). This relationship more closely correlates to oxidative capacity than to fiber type in skeletal muscle.

Both acute exercise and chronic exercise training increase the sensitivity of glucose uptake for a given insulin concentration across the sarcolemma. These affects appear to be through changes in GLUT4. A single acute bout of contractile activity causes a translocation of GLUT4 transporters from an intracellular storage site to the sarcolemma (78, 107, 139, 181, 311) without reducing the quantity of GLUT4 in the insulin-sensitive intracellular pool

(78, 79). These investigators suggest that there exists either a distinct exercise-sensitive intracellular pool of GLUT4, or that masked GLUT4 in the sarcolemma is unmasked by the initial bout of contractile activity (78, 79). Both the increase in glucose transport (256, 345) and the increase in the number and activity of GLUT4 in the sarcolemma (119) during acute exercise does not require the presence of insulin. Physical training improves glucose tolerance and insulin sensitivity of skeletal muscle glucose metabolism (28, 166, 237, 257, 273). Chronic aerobic training is associated with an increase in the quantity of GLUT4 protein in muscle (271). Changes in GLUT4 mRNA are summarized in Table 24.4 later in chapter.

Transgenic mice overexpressing GLUT1 glucose transporter, with no alteration in GLUT4 concentrations, had a 4.5-fold increase in basal 2-deoxyglucose uptake into the epitrochlearis muscle that was associated with an 18% and 30% decrease in blood glucose in the fed and fasted states, respectively (221). Since exercise does not alter GLUT1 concentration in skeletal muscle, the action of GLUT1 does not explain the increased insulin sensitivity of muscle after exercise.

The functional importance of glucose uptake by contracting skeletal muscle is well established. Depletion of muscle glycogen is associated with an inability to continue physical work at the same intensity (135). Uptake of glucose from the blood during exercise allows work to continue past the normal time point of exhaustion as compared to when no exogenous glucose was supplied (55, 116). Production of hyperglycemia during 2 h of cycling at 73% of maximal oxygen consumption, did not alter the usage of muscle glycogen in eight men (62). Others have found decreased glycogen utilization if blood glucose is maintained during exercise (see 62 for refences). Coyle et al. (62) suggest that the differences between these studies is due to the training status of the subjects. The prolongation of exercise time by glucose infusion is likely mediated through the maintenance of blood glucose. Brain and nervous tissue do not oxidize fatty acids. When hypoglycemia occurs during exercise, nerve transmission of action potentials is likely diminished, which leads to an inability to continue work at the same intensity. Endurance training also alters the pretranslational regulation of proteins involved in glucose flux in skeletal muscle (see Table 24.4 later in chapter).

Fatty Acid Transfer and Oxidation

Fatty acids have low solubility in water and must be bound for transport, either through the circulatory system or through the interstitial and intracellular compartments. Albumin and fatty acid–binding protein (FABP) function to transfer fatty acids from the vascular compartment to the outer membrane of the mitochondria. Albumin concentration of striated muscle parallels its mitochondrial density, having the rank order: heart > soleus > tibialis anterior muscle (128). Albumin is in the extravascular component of the interstitial space (128), including the T tubules (381), of skeletal muscle and may function in the transfer of fatty acids from the vascular to intracellular compartment of muscle. Chronic stimulation of the tibialis anterior muscle results in five- to sixfold increases in chloride space (134) and albumin concentration in muscle (128). Heilig and Pette (130) conclude that the increase in albumin is due to an enhanced transcapillary filtration in response to the drastic increase in contractile activity. Heilig and Pette (130) suggest that albumin could play a role in enhancing the transfer of fatty acids from capillaries to muscle fibers during the period of increased substrate demand of the contracting muscle in chronic stimulation.

Although isoforms of FABP exist, the same isoform is present in heart and skeletal muscles (231). In the heart, FABP comprises 5% of the cytosolic mass and 25%–35% of the number of soluble proteins (108). The concentration of FABP is correlated with mitochondrial density in various types of striated muscle. Both FABP and cytochrome-*c* oxidase activity have the rank order: heart > soleus > extensor digitorum longus muscles (339). The concentration of FABP and intracellular lipase activity are also correlated by fiber type; both having the rank order: soleus > red vastus > white vastus (36, 231). However, this correlation breaks down when FABP and the capacity for fatty acid oxidation are related; they are inverted in a comparison of two types. Whereas slow red muscle has a higher FABP than fast red, the opposite directionality exists for fatty acid oxidation in rat skeletal muscle (231). The functions of FABP are circumstantial according to a review by Glatz and van der Vusse (108). They suggest that FABP may facilitate transcytosolic movement of poorly soluble fatty acyl-CoAs from their sites of entry or synthesis to their sites of esterification or oxidation (108).

FABP concentration increases 250% in the 21 day stimulated tibialis anterior muscle of rabbits (177). In contrast, endurance training had little affect on skeletal muscle FABP. After 9 weeks of treadmill running (completing 30 m/min during the final 3 weeks of training 5 days/week), FABP concentration remained unchanged in the trained soleus muscle, which showed a 14% increase in cytochrome-*c* oxidase activity (339). The lack of an affect on FABP is due possibly to the relatively low increase in cytochrome-*c* oxidase activity, implying a lack of an aerobic training effect. Hearts in the same trained rats had a 29% higher FABP. After 28 days of chronic stimulation of the rabbit tibialis anterior muscle, a 200% increase occurred in selected enzymes of fatty acid oxidation (3-hydoxyyacyl-CoA dehydrogenase, 3-ketoacyl-CoA thiolase, and carnitine:palmitoyl-CoA transferase activities), which paralleled increases in the activities of components of the citric acid cycle and the respiratory chain (260). A 100% increase in the activities of carnitine palmitoyltransferase, palmitoyl CoA dehydrogenase, and mitochondrial ATP-dependent palmitoyl CoA synthetase per gram of wet weight occurred in the gastrocnemius and quadriceps muscles after a 12 week running program that was progressively increased to 2 h of running per day (236). These increases in fat-oxidizing enzymes also paralleled increases in respiratory activity in skeletal muscle of rats who were running 2 h/day on motorized treadmills (147). Carnitine palmitoyltransferase mRNA increases in skeletal muscle of treadmill-trained rats (see Table 24.4 later in chapter). FABP is markedly depressed in the adductor longus muscle of rats after 14 days of spaceflight (267). This muscle switches from 90% to 65% slow fibers after 14 days of spaceflight (267).

Fiber-Type Plasticity

The plasticity of the contractile/relaxation machinery in the majority of the interventions discussed above suggests that only a selective subpopulation of fibers representing any given fiber type (I, IIa, IIx, IIb) adapt to a particular type of stimulus (48, 173, 174, 247). For example, approximately 90% of the soleus muscle fibers are comprised of type I (slow-oxidative), with the remainder of the fibers expressing the IIa MHC (fast-oxidative glycolytic fibers). During either hindlimb suspension or treatment with T_3, a large number of the type I fibers (35%–40%) are transformed to express type IIa and/or IIx MHC; they also appear to possess a high oxidative profile (48, 142, 173, 174, 222). Thus, following these interventions almost one-half of the fiber pool in the soleus muscle becomes type IIa/IIx and the other half remains as type I (48, 142). This raises a fundamental question: What causes the selective plasticity of the fiber-type pool(s) in a given muscle in response to any given intervention? It is speculated that the specificity of fiber-type adaptation lies in the developmental history of the fibers making up the limb musculature as outlined below in the case of rat muscle.

Embryonic development of the rat occurs over approximately 21–22 days (59, 60) during which skeletal muscle develops in two specific stages. The first stage is between days 15 and 20 and involves the transformation of primary myotubes into distinct fibers. The second stage occurs primarily during days 20 and 21 (and likely continues into the neonatal stage. This latter embryonic stage involves secondary myotube fusion into distinct fibers. Both the primary and secondary myotube transformation processes have unique features, that undoubtedly affect both (*1*) the pattern of MHC and other contractile protein expression that evolves in the adult musculature and (*2*) the degree of fiber-type diversity and plasticity that occurs in response to mechanical/hormonal intervention in both the neonatal and adult states.

One clue concerning the development of muscle may lie in the type of MHC (and other protein isoforms) that is programmed into the muscle fiber (59, 60). For example, one type of primary myotube is characterized by its expression first of embryonic myosin followed later by its gradual expression of slow (type I) MHC, the latter of which is retained in the maturing fiber (59, 60). These myotubes are generally abundant in the center (core) of all limb muscles and, in particular, they dominate the anatomical region serving as the precursor anatomy for the soleus muscle (59, 60). A second primary subset has been identified, which evolves as described above, but in this particular subset the slow myosin is replaced gradually with neonatal myosin. Neonatal myosin is thought to be a precursor of the fast myosin isoforms that are eventually expressed in the fibers following birth (59, 60). Thus, it is important to note that one of the primary myotube subsets is programmed to express both slow and neonatal (fast) isoforms, whereas the other expresses only the slow isoform. This has led to the postulate that this latter subset represents a slow type of MHC fiber (i.e., a primary slow fiber) that may not be capable of being transformed into a faster phenotype due to its unique lineage of not expressing neonatal myosin (59, 60, 312).

The developmental process is further complicated by an additional process involving secondary myotube development, which occurs just prior to birth. One type of secondary myotube has been identified that emerges initially expressing both embryonic and neonatal MHC. These developing fibers fill in around the primary (i.e., chiefly the slow fibers described above), eventually making up the more superficial regions of certain muscles such as the plantaris, medial and lateral gastrocnemius, and so forth

(59, 60). In the adult animal, these superficial regions consist primarily of the motor units expressing chiefly the IIb and IIx MHCs. Furthermore, an additional type of secondary myotube has been identified (although small in relative number) that evolves as just described (i.e., first expressing both embryonic and neonatal MHC); however, the latter two MHCs are replaced with slow MHC. This subset appears to be localized in deep regions of the dorsal antigravity and locomotor muscles. Note that the majority of the secondary developing fibers are not programmed to express slow myosin in the embryonic state. This could have important bearing on the degree of plasticity that enables adult fast fibers to be transformed into slower contracting fibers during interventions involving chronic functional overload and resistance training in the adult stages of life. Thus, the developmental history of the fibers comprising both antigravity and locomotor muscles may largely determine both the type and degree of plasticity that occurs in the various fiber pools in response to various activity patterns.

Furthermore, new evidence suggests that certain pools within a given fiber type have an inherent capacity to transform phenotype with or without the presence of "activity/neural" factors. For example, when the spinal cord of a cat at any age is transected, the muscles in the lower extremity are rendered almost totally inactive (142, 281). In antigravity muscles such as the soleus, its slow-twitch fibers (which are almost exclusively expressed in this type of muscle in the cat), undergo modest reductions in size, accompanied by transformations in myosin phenotype (slow to fast MHC transformations), increases in glycogenolytic enzyme activity, and increases in oxidative enzyme activity indicating that the fibers are transforming into a phenotype consistent with that typically expressed in the high oxidative–fast glycolytic fiber type (142). Since endurance training causes up-regulation of fast oxidative fibers in several species (255, 298), including trained humans (298), it appears that factors related and unrelated to activity are involved in regulating gene expression in certain types of fibers that have the plasticity characteristics to be transformed in response to various stimuli. This raises a fundamental question: What are the underlying factors in the regulation of muscle plasticity?

REGULATORY FACTORS

We have presented considerable evidence demonstrating that altered levels of mechanical activity can lead to adaptations in the subcellular systems that regulate contraction/relaxation processes as well as processes that involve both anaerobic and oxidative energy transformations. Furthermore, certain hormonal (and metabolic) states and activity paradigms induce similar adaptations in phenotype in the musculature of humans and nonhuman species. For example, both a hyperthyroid state and chronic muscle unloading (e.g., by hindlimb suspension and space flight) appear to induce slow to fast phenotype transformations (43, 45, 48, 222). Conversely, hypothyroidism and chronic increases in functional stress induce the opposite types of transformations (18, 46, 48, 279, 280). Similarly, chronic states of creatine phosphate depletions (i.e., feeding animals β-guanidinopropionic acid (BPGA) induce adaptations remarkably similar to those seen during endurance training (5). Other findings suggest that chronic treatment of animals with either catecholamine derivatives (clenbuterol) (328, 380) or other compounds that have insulin-like effects (i.e., that increase either the uptake, flux, and/or utilization of exogenous glucose as a source of energy), enhance tissue mass both in selected skeletal muscles and in the heart, depending on which type of tissue is targeted. Collectively, these findings suggest that mechanical activity, certain hormones, and metabolic states may be generating the same subcellular signals and/or targeting similar cellular messenger systems and that these eventually regulate gene expression in the affected fibers. The purpose of the next section is to consider some of the cellular and molecular events that have been identified as controlling the plasticity of skeletal muscle.

External to the Muscle

Ligands. Factors that reach the external side of the sarcolemma, either from the circulation or by autocrine or paracrine secretion, bind to receptors on either the sarcolemma (proteins, peptides) or the cytoplasm (steroids). The interaction between muscle activity and hormone action has long been appreciated. More active muscles have less muscle atrophy after cortisone administration than do less active muscles in rats (111). The combination of human growth hormone (HGH), insulin-like growth factor I (IGF-I), and ladder climbing exercise prevented atrophy of soleus muscles of hypophysectomized rats during a 10 day period of hindlimb unloading. Conversely, neither HGH alone, nor IGF-I alone, nor ladder climbing alone prevented the atrophy (122), suggesting that an interaction among these factors must occur beyond the receptor. IGF-I and IGF-II mRNAs increase in compensatory hypertrophied muscle (see Table 24.4 later in chapter).

Basal Lamina. Expression of the adult ε-subunit of the nicotinic receptor gene is not responsive to electrical activity, but appears to be regulated, in part, by the basal lamina in noninnervated, regenerating muscle (114). The adult basal lamina suppresses the expression of extrajunctional adult ε-subunits while inducing ε-subunit expression at the end-plate. However, the chemical factors in the basal lamina responsible for inducing adult nicotinic receptor gene expression are unknown (114).

Yamada et al. (371) speculate that satellite cell activation occurring during muscle fiber regeneration and work-induced hypertrophy involves a release of FGF and/or satellite cells from the heparin component of the basal lamina. One possible mechanism that Yamada et al. (371) suggest for a release of FGF and satellite cells is the partial digestion of basement membranes by invading lymphocytes during the post-exercise inflammatory response produced by damage during the exercise.

Oxygen/Hypoxia. Sundberg (315) reported that after 4 weeks of training, skeletal muscle of ischemic-trained legs had greater citrate synthase activity and capillaries per muscle fiber, and lower type IIb proportion, than the contralateral nonischemically trained leg. He wrote: "It can be concluded that intermittent reduction of oxygen availability during exercise, brought about by reduced blood flow or arterial hypoxia, is a very strong candidate as a direct or indirect stimulus for the greater adaptive effect observed with ischemic training." Evidence exists that alterations in oxygen levels can regulate new levels of gene expression.

Regulatory regions that sense oxygen levels in a small number of genes that are not expressed to skeletal muscle have been found with molecular biological techniques. The question is then raised whether regulatory elements that sense oxygen levels are present in genes that are expressed in skeletal muscle and, if so, whether these oxygen-sensing regulatory regions are functional transformers to adaptations to endurance training.

Much of the early molecular research on "low oxygen-sensing" gene elements has centered on erythropoiesis. (Molecular biology publications have termed gene regulatory regions that sense low oxygen as "hypoxic-sensing elements of genes.") At present, the quantitative usage of the term "hypoxic" may differ in molecular biology and physiology. Low oxygen increases erythropoietin transcription and mRNA concentration (171). Both a hypoxic responsive enhancer [in the 3′ flanking region of the human and mouse erythropoietin gene (27)] and a nuclear protein (HIF-1) that binds to the hypoxic responsive enhancer (found in nuclear extracts of Hep3B cells) have been found. HIF-1 binds specifically to a 50-nucleotide enhancer of the erythropoietin gene (299). Furthermore, Beck et al. (27) identified three different areas within a 29 bp segment (designated as the hypoxic-response enhancer) in the 3′ flanking region of the mouse and human erythropoietin gene that is necessary for its full transcriptional activity. Both cycloheximide and Anisomycin block induction of the nuclear binding protein, HIF-1. Therefore, de novo synthesis of the HIF-1 occurs in response to low oxygen (27, 299).

Many mammalian cell types, including C_2C_{12} myoblasts (352), alter their gene expression in response to low oxygen partial pressure. HIF-1 DNA binding activity, determined by electrophoretic-mobility-shift assay, is present in nuclear extracts with low oxygen, but not from high oxygen, tissue-culture cell lines (including the following types of cells: liver, fibroblasts, ovary, kidney, cervical, and muscle) (347). Wang and Semmenza (347) conclude that it appears that many cell types can sense oxygen tension and respond to low oxygen partial pressure by changes in gene expression. Likewise, Beck et al. (27) found that a 120-kDa protein, which binds to the hypoxic-response enhancer of the erythropoietin gene, was present in low oxygen but was not present in high oxygen partial pressure nuclear extracts from both erthryopoietin-producing and non–erythropoietin-producing cells (such as fibroblasts, epithelial, mesangial, endothelial cell lines). They suggested that the hypoxic-inducible nuclear protein could be involved in a more generalized mechanism of cellular response to low oxygen partial pressure, since it was induced in cells not producing erythropoietin (27). Genes in endothelial cells respond to low oxygen partial pressure. Low oxygen partial pressure induces endothelial growth factor mRNA expression in brain tumor cells (306), heart (201), and umbilical vein endothelial cells (195). They interpreted that vascular endothelial factor induced by low oxygen partial pressure may mediate hypoxia-induced angiogenesis (201, 306). Low oxygen partial pressure also induces interleukin-1α activity (305) and platelet-derived growth factor-B chain mRNA in endothelial cells (194). In addition to the aforementioned erythropoietin gene, platelet-derived growth factor B chain, endothelin, interleukin-1α, ornithine decarboxylase, vascular endothelial growth factor, *jun*, and *fos* are up-regulated in response to low oxygen partial pressure. Goldberg et al. (112) have suggested a model whereby a heme protein is the oxygen sensor in the regulation of erythropoietin production. They propose that when oxygen tension is sufficiently low, this heme protein is in the deoxy conformation and it triggers increased expression of the erythropoietin gene. On the other hand, they suggest that when oxygen tension is sufficiently high, the heme protein is in its inactive oxy conformation and does not stimulate erythropoietin production. Cowan et al. (61) identified two oxygen responsive *cis*-acting elements (ORE1 and ORE2) in the 5′-flanking region of the human glutathione peroxidase gene. These two elements bound different proteins. When each ORE is placed upstream of a reporter gene and either construct is transfected into the culture medium surrounding human ventricular myocytes, expression of the reporter gene is higher for those incubated with an oxygen tension of 150 mm Hg as compared to cells growing in 40 mm Hy oxygen.

High-Energy Phosphates. β-Guanidinopropionic acid (β-GPA), when fed to animals, results in low levels of phosphocreatine and ATP in their skeletal muscle (97, 98). Initially this treatment was used to study fatigue patterns of muscles. The tibialis anterior muscle from rats fed β-GPA (chronic depletion of high-energy phosphates) failed to exhibit the staircase phenomena and developed 25% less tension than control muscles during hypoxic isometric contractions (97).

Later it was found that β-GPA feeding results in alterations in activities of metabolic enzyme in skeletal muscle. Shoubridge et al. (304) observed that 6-phosphofructokinase and creatine kinase activities decrease in parallel in skeletal muscles of rats fed β-GPA. An increase in mitochondrial enzymes in some, but not all, skeletal muscles of rats fed β-GPA was also noted (203, 304). Cytochrome *c* mRNA is increased in some, but not all, skeletal muscles in rats fed β-GPA (203). A later study reports that GLUT4 mRNA, GLUT4 protein, citrate synthase activity, cytochrome *c* protein, and hexokinase activity all increase by similar percentages in skeletal muscles of rats fed β-GPA (263). Ren et al. (263) interpret these observations to support the hypothesis that the levels of mitochondrial enzymes, hexokinase, and GLUT4 are coregulated in striated muscles. They further suggest that a decrease in the quantity of high-energy phosphate is involved in inducing the adaptive increase in the capacity for aerobic metabolism (i.e., increase in mitochondria, hexokinase, and GLUT4) (263). Shoubridge et al. (304) had earlier suggested that directional changes in muscle proteins of skeletal muscle are similar in β-GPA feeding and in endurance type of physical training (Table 24.3). A change in the energy state of the muscle has been proposed to be the trigger for the adaptive increase in aerobic potential that occurs in skeletal muscle of patients with peripheral vascular insufficiency (149) and in rats fed β-GPA (304).

Another consequence of the β-GPA feeding is a conversion of MHC protein isoforms from faster to slower isomyosins. For example, the percentage of slow MHC chain increased from 37% to 68% in the soleus muscle of mice fed β-GPA (235). A shift from fast native myosin 1 isoform to native isoform 3 also occurred in the extensor digitorum longus muscle of β-GPA–fed mice. Interestingly, parvalbumin is also de novo expressed in the extensor digitorum longus muscle of β-GPA–fed rats. Moerland et al. (235) suggest that the simultaneous adaptations in myosin isoforms and oxidative capacity with β-GPA feeding function to enhance the capacity for sustained performance.

Increased expression of GLUT4 in skeletal muscles of rats fed β-GPA was associated with a doubling of glycogen concentrations in these muscles (263, 304). Furthermore, the GLUT4 protein concentration increased in parallel with the increase in maximal insulin-stimulated glucose uptake in the epitrochlearis muscle of rats fed β-GPA (263). Ren et al. (263) interpret these findings to mean that when the signaling pathways for GLUT4 translocation and activation are intact, it is the concentration of GLUT4 protein that determines the maximal transport activity in striated muscle.

Internal to Muscle

Mechanical and Load-Bearing States. Both the specific type and quantity of mechanical activity im-

TABLE 24.3. *Directional Changes in Muscle Plasticity During β-GPA Feeding or Endurance Training*

Muscle Protein	β-GPA Feeding	Endurance Training
Mitochondria concentration	↑	↑
Hexokinase activity	↑	↑
GLUT4 concentration	↑	↑
Glycogen concentration	↑	↑
Increased myosin heavy chain I	↑	↑
Diameter of type IIb fibers	↓	↓

posed on muscle systems may play a pivotal role in determining the type of contractile system and metabolic apparatus that is expressed within those adaptable fibers. Intermittent, high-frequency activity of relatively low force output (i.e., as occurring during running, cycling, swimming, and so forth) initiates a high energy turnover rate along with adaptations in the metabolic apparatus without marked changes in the contractile system of the affected muscle (292). On the other hand, mechanical activity patterns that impact heavily on the muscle's chronic force requirements (i.e., either overload or exposure to microgravity) appear to impact on the type and amount of contractile system expressed in the affected fibers, with lesser impact on the metabolic pathways associated with oxidative metabolism (278). Furthermore, activity requiring periodic high force output, such as during heavy resistance training, appears to impact on muscle mass, with only limited transformations in either the phenotype of the contractile machinery or oxidative metabolic apparatus (22, 217). However, in these latter paradigms, the contractile apparatus may be expanded, such that the mitochondrial system is diluted by the pattern of protein accumulation (217), thereby resulting in a lower oxidative capacity in the affected fibers.

In each of the above-described paradigms, the adaptive process may be fundamentally linked to the type of contractile machinery that is being programmed into the muscle. For example, any functional state that induces high levels of cross-bridge cycling, and hence high rates of ATP turnover, may serve as a signal to up-regulate the number of mitochondria in the affected fibers. However, the manner in which the cross-bridges are cycled during any given contraction pattern could potentially dictate the type of MHC and SR calcium pump system that is most appropriate or efficient for supporting that type of activity. For example, models that require more continuous isometric contractile responses may be more useful for ground-supported activities that are opposed by gravity. Consequently, in the absence of gravity, those muscles expressing slow contractile apparatus down-regulate the expression of the slow machinery. This is efficient because muscle no longer derives advantage from expressing a slow motor system when its usefulness is reduced. In this context, isometric training programs may be more effective than isovelocity training paradigms in conserving both slow muscle mass and slow MHC expression in chronically unloaded skeletal muscle (70, 74). Bear in mind that the usage of slow antigravity muscles (i.e., standing) is largely isometric. Conversely, activities that require dynamic high power output activity may require a faster type of contractile machinery if the muscle is to become more effective in performing high power output activity whereby the expression of rapid cross-bridge and calcium cycling kinetic properties would enable the muscle to generate more velocity for any given submaximal resistance encountered.

The magnitude of the force generated in the muscle fiber (i.e., the number of cross-bridges that need to be interacted in the power stroke of contraction) may dictate the size of the fibers in both antigravity and locomotor muscles. This is illustrated by the fact that in the antigravity muscles of rodents such as the soleus, the type I (slow) fibers are significantly larger than the type II fibers under normal conditions (247). In contrast, in the fast locomotor muscles such as the gastrocnemius/plantaris the opposite is true; type IIb fibers are the largest and the type I fibers are the smallest (173). The type IIa fibers are of similar size in both fast and slow muscle (173, 247). Also, both fast and slow fibers can undergo either enlargement (seen more so in fast fibers) or atrophy (seen more so in slow fibers) depending on the muscle and the type of altered activity imposed. This suggests that all fibers in load-bearing muscles are sensitive to the activity state chronically imposed on them. If so, it is logical to ask what specific mechanical factor(s) associated with the activity pattern of the animal is critical in maintaining the mass of the fibers across the musculature supporting weight-bearing activities. It is possible that the force requirement imposed on the muscle fiber, rather than how the muscle fiber is programmed to contract (i.e., isometrically, concentrically, eccentrically), is that which primarily determines muscle size. Requirements for force generation are entirely different during isometric contractions as opposed to dynamic exercise such as sprinting. Since fast IIb (and likely IIx) motor units develop the force required during high burst activity (346), the mechanical factors associated with such activities may be pivotal in maintaining the size of the type II fibers. The concepts presented in this section are all somewhat speculative in nature. Future research should examine the relationship of specific mechanical factors to the adaptive responses of the muscle. It is also necessary to ascertain the fundamental links of the putative mechanical signals to subcellular events resulting in the accumulation of protein in muscle fibers.

Regulation of Gene Expression

Protein synthesis and degradation. The level of a protein is determined by the magnitude of the rates of its synthesis and degradation. Exercise usually alters both rates for mixed proteins in skeletal muscle (see 35, 77, 115 for detailed reviews). Chronic increases or decreases in contractile activity increase protein degradation rates in skeletal muscle (see 34, 35 for reviews). For example, cytochrome *c* degradation rate increases in aerobically trained skeletal muscle as its concentration rises (32). Usage seems to be associated with faster protein turnover (109). Increases in contractile activity are associated with increases in protein synthesis rates of mixed proteins in skeletal muscle, while decreased contractile activity is related to decreased protein synthesis (see 34, 35, 77, 115 for reviews).

During periods of enlargement of protein content, an apparent overshoot in necessary increase in protein synthesis, which is needed to produce a given growth of skeletal muscle, occurs. For example, a 129% increase was found 24 h after a bout of heavy resistance exercise in men (218). Biceps muscle protein synthesis rates were increased 50% and 109% 4 h and 24 h later, respectively, after repeated repetitions of forceful dynamic contractions of the biceps at 80% of maximal force (54). Both the prolonged time of increased protein synthesis after exercise and the magnitude of its relative increase were surprising. These observations on humans confirmed earlier analogous findings in other species. Rates of either mixed or myofibrillar protein synthesis were increased 32%–45% 12–17 h after either 24 or 192 eccentric contractions; these rates remained elevated 41%–65% at 36–41 h afterwards (368). The protracted period increase in muscle protein synthesis rate after a single bout of resistance exercise implies that the unknown mechanisms that regulate this synthesis are imprinted for long periods after the exercise bout. In addition, the magnitude of the increases in protein synthesis greatly exceeds the rate of muscle enlargement. Since muscle growth is only 1%–3% per week across species during programs of resistance training, increases in the rates of protein synthesis of 25%–129% for at least 1 day after the exercise bout far exceed that required to account for the final increase in muscle mass. This observation implies that much of the increase in protein synthesis could be "wasted" (i.e., degraded before the newly synthesized protein is assembled). The "wastage" concept has been described earlier by Millward (232). He estimated that 80% of the increase in mixed muscle protein synthesis is wasted when the chicken anterior latissimus dorsi muscle enlarges by 140% during overload-induced hypertrophy, which involves the chronic attachment of a load to one wing.

In young men, resistance training with and without administration of recombinant growth hormone evoked similar increments in muscle size, strength, and muscle protein synthesis. The investigators concluded that the growth hormone did not enhance muscle anabolism and function (377).

Denatured or misfolded proteins, as well as proteins containing oxidized or otherwise abnormal amino acids, are recognized and degraded by ubiquitin-dependent proteolytic systems. Ubiquitination of proteins has been implicated in a variety of processes such as the heat shock response, among other functions (136). Riley et al. (268) found increased ubiquitination of disrupted myofibrils in degrading myofilaments in the atrophying soleus muscle of rats after 12.5 days of spaceflight. Ubiquitin is twice as high in slow- as in fast-twitch skeletal muscle (266).

mRNA. Contractile activity modulates mRNA concentration. As a general rule, the directional change of a given mRNA is the same as the directional change of the protein during its adaptation to a new steady level in response to an inherent change in contractile activity. Table 24.4 lists the changes in various mRNA species occurring as a result of a change in the inherent level of contractile activity in innervated skeletal muscle. Purposes of Table 24.4 are to provide a single-source reference of those mRNAs that have been measured in exercise models that we were able to locate in 1994 and to show the magnitude of this information.

Protein translation. The synthesis of new proteins occurs on polyribosomes. The rate of synthesis could be modulated by the quantity of mRNA, rRNA, aminoacylated tRNAs, factors initiating translation of new protein on polyribosomes, factors determining rates of elongation (i.e., rates that amino acids are added to growing protein), and factors regulating termination of protein synthesis. Some of these six regulatory processes involved in protein synthesis are modulated by changes in contractile activity (i.e., mRNA and rRNA).

A decrease in the rate of translation of mRNAs has been inferred based on comparisons of the time course of change in mRNA and protein synthesis rates in earlier studies. These experiments found changes in the rate of protein synthesis without a concurrent alteration in the quantity of mRNA for the protein whose synthesis is measured. Some examples are as follows. Synthesis rates for both actin and cytochrome c protein decrease in skeletal muscle in the first 6 h of limb immobilization. During the same period, the quantity of either skeletal α-actin mRNA or cytochrome *c* mRNA did not change (see Table 24.4). The conclusion was that translation of the skeletal α-actin mRNA and cytochrome *c* mRNA had decreased.

TABLE 24.4. *Response of mRNAs to Altered Contractile Activity*

Skeletal Muscle mRNA	Directional Change	Time of Measurement	Contractile Activity Model	Muscle	Species	References
α-Actin, skeletal	↓	7 days	Limb immobilization	Gastrocnemius	Rat	348
	↓	7 days	Non-weight bearing	Soleus	Rat	17
	↓	1–7 days	Non-weight bearing	Soleus, gastrocnemius	Rat	154
	↑	14 days	Treadmill running	Plantaris, red	Rat	238
	↑	10 weeks	Resistance training	Tibialis anterior	Rat	368
	↑	10 weeks	Resistance training	Gastrocnemius	Rat	367
	↓	14 days	Spaceflight	Vastus intermedius	Rat	323
	↓	10–21 days	Chronic stimulation	Tibialis anterior	Rabbit	128, 147
β-Actin, cytoskeletal	↑	2 days–7 weeks	Compensatory overload	Plantaris	Mouse	333
Acyl CoA synthetase	→	7 days	Treadmill running	Gastrocnemius	Rat	303
Aldolase A	↓	21 days	Chronic stimulation	Tibialis anterior	Rabbit	297, 361
5-Aminolevulinate synthase	→	1–28 days	Treadmill running	Plantaris	Rat	329
	↑	7 days	Compensatory hypertrophy	Patagialis	Chicken	91
F_1ATPase, β-subunit	↑	9–21 days	Chronic stimulation	Tibialis anterior	Rabbit	197, 361
Ca^{2+}-ATPase, fast SR	↑	1–28 days	Non-weight bearing	Soleus	Rat	295
Ca^{2+}-ATPase, fast Sr	↓	52–117 days	Chronic stimulation	EDL	Rabbit	209
Ca^{2+}-ATPase, slow SR	→/↑	1–28 days	Non-weight bearing	Soleus	Rat	295
Ca^{2+}-ATPase, slow SR	↑	52–117 days	Chronic stimulation	EDL	Rabbit	209
Ca^{2+}-ATPase, mixed SR	↓	30–50 days	Chronic stimulation	EDL	Rabbit	210
Carbonic anhydrase	→	0–56 days	Chronic stimulation	Tibialis anterior	Rat	170
Carnitine palmitoyltransferase	↑	2 weeks	Treadmill running	Plantaris	Rat	375
	↑	9 days	Chronic stimulation	Tibialis anterior	Rat	373
Citrate synthase	↑	8–50 days	Chronic stimulation	EDL	Rabbit	297
	↑	3 days	Chronic stimulation	Tibialis anterior	Rabbit	9
Creatine kinase, muscle	↓	2 days–6 weeks	Compensatory overload	Plantaris	Mouse	332
αβ-Crystalline	↓	36 h–1 week	Non-weight bearing	Soleus	Rat	15
Cytochrome *b*	↑	9–21 days	Chronic stimulation	Tibialis anterior	Rabbit	361
Cytochrome *c*	↓	7 days	Limb immobilization	Red quadriceps	Rat	239
	↓	7 days	Non-weight bearing	Soleus	Rat	17
	↑	14 days	Treadmill running	Plantaris, red quadriceps	Rat	238
	↑	10 weeks	Resistance training	Tibialis anterior	Rat	368
	↑	10 weeks	Resistance training	Gastrocnemius	Rat	367
	↓	14 days	Spaceflight	Vastus intermedius	Rat	323
	↑	9 days	Chronic stimulation	Tibialis anterior	Rat	374
Cytochrome oxidase						
Subunits III and IV	→	1–28 days	Treadmill running	Plantaris	Rat	329
Subunit III	↑	7–35 days	Chronic stimulation	Tibialis anterior	Rat	150, 151
Subunit VIc	↑	7–35 days	Chronic stimulation	Tibialis anterior	Rat	150, 151
Subunit VIc	↑	21 days	Chronic stimulation	Tibialis anterior	Rabbit	361
Dihydropyridine receptor	↑	1–28 days	Non-weight bearing	Soleus	Rat	175
c-*fos*	→	12 h	Compensatory overload	Plantaris	Rat	359
	↑	1 h	Compensatory overload	Plantaris	Mouse	333
GLUT4	↑	10 weeks	Swimming	Fast red	Rat	257
	↑	3 weeks	Voluntary wheel running	Plantaris, quadriceps	Rat	344
	→	0 h	After cycling	Vastus lateralis	Human	191
	↓	0 h	After cycling	Vastus lateralis	Human type 1 diabetic	191
	→	7 days	Treadmill running	Gastrocnemius	Rat	303
Glutamine synthetase	↓	12–16 weeks	Endurance run training	Fast red	Rat	93
	↓	30 days	Compensatory hypertrophy	Plantaris	Rat	95
	↓	11 days	Treadmill running	Fast red	Rat	94
Glyceraldehyde phosphate dehydrogenase	→	0–35 days	Chronic stimulation	Tibialis anterior	Rat	151
α-glycerol phosphate dehydrogenase	↓	2 days–6 weeks	Compensatory overload	Plantaris	Mouse	333

TABLE 24.4. *Continued*

Skeletal Muscle mRNA	Directional Change	Time of Measurement	Contractile Activity Model	Muscle	Species	References
Glyceraldehyde-3-phosphate dehydrogenase	↓	2 days–6 weeks	Compensatory overload	Plantaris	Mouse	332
Glycogen synthase	↑	36 h post-exercise	Long-distance runners	Vastus lateralis	Human	340
Hexokinase II	↑	0–3 h post-exercise	30 min treadmill run	Soleus, gastrocnemius White vastus	Rat	246
hsp70	↑	0–1 h	After treadmill run	Many hindlimb	Rat	285
IGF-I	↑	2–8 days	Compensatory hypertrophy	Soleus, plantaris	Rat	70
IGF-II	↑	4–8 days	Compensatory hypertrophy	Soleus, plantaris	Rat	70
c-*jun*	↑	45 min–1 h	Chronic stimulation	Gastrocnemius	Mice	2
JunB	Slight ↑		Chronic stimulation	Gastrocnemius	Mice	2
Lactate dehydrogenase						
Heart subunit	↑	6–50 days	Chronic stimulation	EDL	Rabbit	297
Muscle subunit	↓	6–50 days	Chronic stimulation	EDL	Rabbit	297
Lipoprotein lipase	↑	0 h	After acute swimming	Red and white vastus lateralis,	Rat	202
	→	7 days	Treadmill running	Gastrocnemius	Rat	303
MLC, 1 fast	↑	35 days	Compensatory hypertrophy	Plantaris	Rat	31
	↓	91–117 days	Chronic stimulation	EDL	Rabbit	182
MLC, 1 fast	↑	14–42 days	Chronic stimulation	Tibialis anterior	Rat	188, 186
MLC, 1 fast	↑	9 days	Spaceflight	Soleus, EDL	Rat	88
MLC, 2 fast	↑	35 days	Compensatory hypertrophy	Plantaris	Rat	31
MLC, 2 fast	↓	7–117 days	Chronic stimulation	EDL	Rabbit	182
MLC, 2 fast	→	0–42 days	Chronic stimulation	Tibialis anterior	Rat	185, 186
MLC, 2 fast	↑	9 days	Spaceflight	Soleus, EDL	Rat	88
MLC, 3 fast	↓	7–117 days	Chronic stimulation	EDL	Rabbit	182
MLC, 3 fast	↓	14–42 days	Chronic stimulation	Tibialis anterior	Rat	185, 186
MLC, 1 slow	↑	35 days	Compensatory hypertrophy	Plantaris	Rat	31
MLC, 1 slow	↑	70–117 days	Chronic stimulation	EDL	Rabbit	182
MLC, 1 slow	↑	28–42 days	Chronic stimulation	Tibialis anterior	Rat	185
MLC, 1 slow	→	35 day	Chronic stimulation	Tibialis anterior	Rat	186
MLC, 1 slow	↓	9 days	Spaceflight	Soleus, EDL	Rat	88
MLC, 1 slow	↑	3–9 weeks	Overload	Plantaris	Mouse	354
MLC, 2 slow	↑	7–117 days	Chronic stimulation	EDL	Rabbit	182
MLC, 2 slow	→	0–42 days	Chronic stimulation	Tibialis anterior	Rat	185
MLC, 2 slow	↑	35 day	Chronic stimulation	Tibialis anterior	Rat	186
MLC, 2 slow	↓	9 days	Spaceflight	Soleus, EDL	Rat	88
MLC, 2 slow	↑	3 weeks	Compensatory overload	Plantaris	Mouse	354
MHC, embryonic	↑	2 weeks	Continuous stretch	Patagialis	Chicken	89
MHC, slow/I	↑	4–11 weeks	Compensatory hypertrophy	Plantaris	Rat	253
MHC, slow/I	→	7 days	Non-weight bearing	Soleus	Rat	321
MHC, slow/I	↑	21–117 days	Chronic stimulation	EDL	Rabbit	182
MHC, slow/I	→	0–56 days	Chronic stimulation	Tibialis anterior	Rat	170, 186
MHC, slow/I	↑	4–6 days	Continuous stretch	Tibialis anterior	Rabbit	76
MHC, slow/I	↓	14 days	Non-weight bearing	Soleus, plantaris	Rat	73
MHC, slow/I	↑	9 days	Spaceflight	Soleus, EDL	Rat	88
MHC, slow/I	↑	3–9 weeks	Overload	Plantaris	Mouse	354
MHC, fast IIa	↑	4–11 weeks	Compensatory hypertrophy	Plantaris	Rat	253
MHC, fast IIa	↓	35–117 days	Chronic stimulation	EDL	Rabbit	182
MHC, fast IIa	↑	4–35 days	Chronic stimulation	Tibialis anterior	Rat	183, 186
MHC, fast IIa	↓	14 days	Non-weight bearing	Soleus, vastus lateralis	Rat	75
MHC, fast IIa	→	9 days	Spaceflight	EDL	Rat	88
MHC, fast IIa	↓	9 days	Spaceflight	Soleus	Rat	88
MHC, fast IIb	↓	4–11 weeks	Compensatory hypertrophy	Plantaris	Rat	253
MHC, fast IIb	↓	4–35 days	Chronic stimulation	Tibialis anterior	Rat	183, 186

Table continues

TABLE 24.4. *Continued*

Skeletal Muscle mRNA	Directional Change	Time of Measurement	Contractile Activity Model	Muscle	Species	References
MHC, fast IIb	↑	21 h	Recovery from 15 days of chronic stimulation	Tibialis anterior	Rat	183
MHC, fast IIb	↑	14 days	Non-weight bearing	Soleus, plantaris, Vastus lateralis	Rat	73
MHC, fast IIb	↑	9 days	Spaceflight	Soleus, EDL	Rat	88
MHC, fast IId	↑	35 days	Chronic stimulation	Tibialis anterior	Rat	186
MHC, fast IId/x	↑	9 days	Spaceflight	Soleus	Rat	88
MRF4	↑	2 h	Stretch and stimulation	Tibialis anterior	Rat	165
c-*myc*	↑	3–24 h	Compensatory overload	Soleus	Rat	359
	↑	12–24 h	Compensatory overload	Plantaris	Rat	359
	↑	0.5–24 h	Chronic stretch	Tibialis anterior	Chicken	87
	↑	3 h	Compensatory overload	Plantaris	Mouse	333
Myf-5	↑	2 h	Stretch and stimulation	Tibialis anterior	Rat	165
Myogenin	↑	9 days	Spaceflight	Soleus	Rat	88
Myogenin	→	2 h	Stretch and stimulation	Tibialis anterior	Rat	165
Myoglobin	↑	21 days	Chronic stimulation	Tibialis anterior	Rabbit	197, 337
nur77	→		Chronic stimulation	Gastrocnemius	Mice	2
Parvalbumin	↓	4–50 days	Chronic stimulation	EDL	Rabbit	210
Phospholamban	↑	35–90 days	Chronic stimulation	EDL	Rabbit	209
Phosphofructokinase	→	36 h post-exercise	Long-distance runners	Vastus lateralis	Human	340
*qmf*1 (avian myoD)	↑	0.5–6 h	Chronic stretch	Tibialis anterior	Chicken	87
α-Tropomyosin, fast	↑	9 days	Spaceflight	Soleus, EDL	Rat	88
α-Tropomyosin, slow	↓	9 days	Spaceflight	Soleus, EDL	Rat	88
β-Tropomyosin/ α-Tropomyosin	↑	35 days	Compensatory hypertrophy	Plantaris	Rat	31
Troponin C, fast	↓	8–91 days	Chronic stimulation	Tibialis anterior EDL	Rabbit	129, 211
Troponin C, fast	↑	9 days	Spaceflight	Soleus	Rat	88
Troponin C, fast	↓	9 days	Spaceflight	EDL	Rat	88
Troponin C, skeletal	↓	1–9 weeks	Overload	Plantaris	Mouse	354
Troponin C, slow	↑	14–117 days	Chronic stimulation	EDL	Rabbit	129
Troponin C, slow	↑	9 days	Spaceflight	Soleus	Rat	88
Troponin C, slow	↑	1–9 weeks	Overload	Soleus, plantaris	Mouse	354
Troponin I, fast	↑	9 days	Spaceflight	Soleus, EDL	Rat	88
Troponin I, slow	↓	9 days	Spaceflight	Soleus	Rat	88
Troponin I, slow	↑	11–60 days	Chronic stimulation	Tibialis anterior	Rabbit	211
Troponin T, fast	↓	7–91 days	Chronic stimulation	EDL	Rabbit	128, 129
Troponin T, fast	↑	9 days	Spaceflight	Soleus, EDL	Rat	88
Troponin T, slow	↑	9 days	Spaceflight	Soleus	Rat	88
zif268	↑	30 min-4 h	Chronic stimulation	Gastrocnemius	Mice	2

In a more direct measurement of translation, polyribosomes were isolated from the soleus muscle in the 18th hour of non-weight bearing and fractionated according to size (199). Skeletal α-actin mRNA and 18S rRNA were shifted to larger masses of polysomes at the 18th hour of non-weight bearing (199). Ku and Thomason (199) suggest that additional ribosomes were attached to each mRNA during the first 18 hours of non-weight bearing by the soleus muscles. They also noted that additional rRNA was mobilized into the polysome pool, suggesting to them that the initiation of protein synthesis was not rate limiting during the 18th hour of limb immobilization (199). Rather, they explain their results as a slowing of nascent polypeptide chain elongation (i.e., a "traffic jam" of ribosomes exists on each mRNA). The decreased elongation is the reason for the fall in protein translation. The signals from non–weight-bearing muscle that induce the decrease in protein elongation are unknown.

Heat shock proteins. Heat shock proteins (hsp) are those whose synthesis is increased by a stress factor, such as an elevated temperature (63). Later it was observed that several other metabolic insults increased the expression of the so-called hsp. In order to characterize the broader reaction of hsp to homeostatic disruptions, they are also called "stress proteins" (357). The following factors, in addition to heat, have been identified as inducers of stress protein formation in cells or cell cultures: hypoxia, glucose deprivation, calcium ionophores, glucose or amino acid analogues, ethanol, sodium arsenite, 2-mercaptoethanol, cadmium, and 2,4-nitrophenol [see Locke et al. (218) for references].

Heat shock proteins function as molecular chaperons because they are directly involved in the biogenesis of proteins from the time of synthesis as nascent chains until the assembly of multimeric complexes (63). In a recent review, Craig et al. (63) proposed that molecular chaperons bind transiently and noncovalently to nascent polypeptides and to unfolded or unassembled proteins. These authors maintain that this binding with a chaperon aids protein biogenesis in two general ways: First, it blocks nonproductive protein–protein interactions; and second, it mediates the folding of proteins to their native state by sequestering folding intermediates, allowing the concerted folding by domains and assembly of oligomers. Thomason suggests that heat shock cognate proteins could mediate the increased elongation rate of nascent polypeptides during muscle atrophy.

In the justification for their hypothesis that exercise might increase stress proteins, Locke et al. (213) suggest that homeostatic disruptions within the muscle during exercise (e.g., elevated temperature, glycogen depletion, pH alteration, increased lactate), and changes in intracellular calcium could provide signals to induce hsp synthesis. In testing their hypothesis, Locke et al. (213) reported that synthesis of proteins of ~65, 72, 90, and 100 kDa in lymphocytes, spleen cells, and soleus muscle was enhanced after rats ran to exhaustion. Since the molecular weights and isoelectric points of these proteins correspond to hsp synthesized by spleen cells exposed to temperatures that cause heat shock, Locke et al. (213) suggested that exhaustive exercise is a sufficient stimulus to induce or enhance the synthesis of hsp in peripheral lymphocytes, spleen cells, and the soleus muscle. In later studies, an increase in hsp72 protein was found in muscle either experiencing overload-induced hypertrophy in the rat (180) or stretch-overload–induced hypertrophy in the chicken (180). In addition, it has been reported that more hsp72 is found in type I than type II muscle, which supports a role of contractile activity in its regulation (214). Treadmill running increases hsp70 mRNA, while unloading decreases $\alpha\beta$-crystalline mRNA (see Table 24.3).

Assembly of mitochondria. Neupert and Pfanner (245) have reviewed the role of hsp's in mitochondrial biogenesis. They conclude that molecular chaperons (hsp70 and hsp60) are essential components of the machinery facilitating the import and eventual assembly of nuclear-encoded proteins into mitochondrial membranes. Various hsp members contribute to the assembly of mitochondrial proteins. For example, cytosolic hsp70 maintains precursors in a translocation-competent state, facilitating import across the outer and inner mitochondrial membranes, probably by assisting the unfolding of proteins in the cytosol. Mitochondrial hsp60, located in the matrix of mitochondria, facilitates folding and assembly of imported polypeptide chains into mitochondrial membranes (245). Hsp70 mRNA was elevated immediately after rats ran to exhaustion, and remained elevated for up to 6 h after exercise in the plantaris, extensor digitorium longus, heart, and soleus muscles (see Table 24.4). Salo et al. (285) speculate that hsp70 could provide a vital link in the mechanism of exercise-induced mitochondrial biogenesis. This is a reasonable hypothesis. However, an increase in hsp70 mRNA in and of itself is not sufficient to increase mitochondrial biogenesis. Hsp70 increased in the extensor digitorum longus muscle, a muscle in which increases in mitochondria do not occur during running by the rat.

Essig et al. (90) recently found that heme oxygenase-1 mRNA increased 32-fold 1.5 h after an acute 3 h stimulation at 10 Hz. Heme oxygenase-1 is an inducible stress protein that degrades free heme. As such, heme oxygenase is not only a stress protein, but it plays an antioxidant role by degrading heme. Iron, a component of heme, can convert superoxide (O_2^-) and hydrogen peroxide (H_2O_2) to the hydroxyl radical (OH^-), which is one of the most reactive oxygen free radicals. In 1979, Holloszy and Winder (148), noted that 5′-aminolevulinate synthase activity was increased 18 h after a single bout of exercise. [The reader is referred to Town and Essig (329) for a further discussion of details.]

*Nuclear domains.** The concept of a nuclear control domain is defined as the volume of cytoplasm controlled by a single nucleus (127). Two major classes of proteins—structural and metabolic—account for much of the protein synthesis required from a myonucleus in a resting muscle cell. Small cytoplasmic volumes per myonucleus seem to be related to both slow myosin isoform and high oxidative levels (330). The slow myosin isoform predominates in muscle with a more rapid turnover of contractile proteins, which requires more nuclear activity, and thus slow muscles have smaller cytoplasmic volumes per myonucleus than do fast muscles (see 330 for references). Eisenberg et al. (86) and Tseng et al. (330) found that fibers with high oxidative capacities had smaller cytoplasmic volumes per myonucleus. Tseng et al. (330) reported that slow and fast fibers of the soleus muscle, as well as slow fibers of the plantaris muscle of rats, had high succinate dehydrogenase (SDH) activities and low

*Section coauthored with Brian S. Tseng.

cytoplasmic volume/myonucleus ratios. In contrast, fast fibers of the rat plantaris muscle had less SDH activity and high cytoplasmic volume/myonucleus ratios (330).

Edgerton and Roy (82) suggest that the cytoplasmic/myonucleus ratio is a function of the myosin type and the amount and/or rate of protein synthesis and degradation. Tseng et al. (330) extend this suggestion by proposing that the maximal volume of cytoplasm that a given myonucleus can control is limited by the capacity of a myonucleus to support protein turnover rates as well as increased synthesis of perturbed protein classes (e.g., structural or oxidative). Tseng suggests that since intense training increases protein synthesis to rates that exceed basal requirements, a given myonucleus can reallocate its activity to support maximally increased rates of synthesis for either structural or oxidative proteins, but not maximally for both simultaneously. Tseng offered the following hypothesis: within a window of adaptive potential, a muscle cell has a significant ability to alter its size and phenotype, but if challenged to extreme limits for either increasing its size (cross-sectional area) in strength training or oxidative potential (mitochondrial content) in endurance training, the muscle cell must make a trade-off decision either to give up oxidative capacity for maximal size or relinquish size for maximal oxidative capacity, but not both (designated as the nuclear domain limitation hypothesis). Nuclear domains appear to play a critical role in establishing these limitations, and likewise the limited satellite cell population may also be important.

Tseng suggests that the nuclear domain limitation hypothesis could largely explain why the world-class decathlete doesn't achieve top power (e.g., javelin, shot put, sprint, long jump) or endurance (running 1500 m) equivalent to that achieved by top athletes trained in only one of these events. Several recent reports support the nuclear domain limitation hypothesis (85, 137, 196, 361). Williams et al. (361) have maximized mitochondrial synthesis by chronic electrical stimulation of skeletal muscle for 24h/day. After 3 weeks of chronic stimulation, mitochondria increased 400% (361), while whole muscle (361) and muscle fiber diameter (284) atrophied 25%. This finding demonstrates that the muscle made a trade-off decision to give up size for maximal oxidative capacity. Kraemer et al. (196) found that the cross-sectional area of type I and IIC muscle fibers increased significantly with high-intensity strength training; this area decreased significantly with high-intensity endurance training; and finally it was unchanged in a group of subjects who had combined both high-intensity strength and endurance training. Thus, myonuclei were unable to direct an increase in the cross-sectional area of type I and IIC muscle fibers when confronted with both strength and endurance training stimuli. To further test the nuclear domain limitation hypothesis requires the measurements of oxidative capacities in combined strength and endurance training.

Three other tissues show this limitation of maximizing both structure and mitochondria within their cells. Larger motoneurons are generally limited to only low SDH activities, while smaller motoneurons can have either high or low SDH activities (52). Aaraether et al. (1) showed that feeding ethionine reduced the volume of liver cells while increasing the volume fraction of the liver cell that is composed of mitochondria and nuclei. Swimming by rats increases the width of the cardiac muscle fibers by 30%, while there was no change in the volume percentage of mitochondria in cardiac muscle cells (106).

Cell Signalling. A schematic overview of the signal transduction pathway from ligand binding to a cell receptor to binding of the signal to a DNA element on a gene is given in Figure 24.4 (157). We speculate that signals from altered contractile activity can enter this signaling pathway at any point from the ligand to the second messenger. For example, insulin-like growth factor can have an autocrine effect on its muscle fiber. Contractile responses could alter [cAMP], a second messenger. The effect, or potential effect, of exercise on selected examples of each component of the signaling pathway is given.

Sadoshima et al. (283) have suggested that the simultaneous activation of multiple second-messenger systems by imposed stretch of cultured cardiomyocytes is remarkably similar to intracellular signaling initiated by growth factors. Stretching of cultured cardiac myocytes activates multiple signaling pathways [i.e., phospholipases C, D, and A_2; protein kinase C; tyrosine kinases; $p21^{ras}$; mitogen-activated protein kinases; and 90 kDa S6 kinase (282, 372).

Receptor.

THYROID HORMONE RECEPTORS. In view of the role that thyroid hormone plays in the regulation of muscle plasticity, it is important to examine the properties of this regulatory factor. Current evidence indicates that T_3 largely exerts its effects by first interacting with receptor complexes in the nucleus of the cell. Thyroid hormone receptors are protein products of the c-*erb*-A protooncogene superfamily, which encode for a family of receptors that also include steroid hormones, vitamin D, and retinoic acid receptors (140, 141, 192, 207, 208, 242, 324, 355). Each member of the superfamily has a conserved

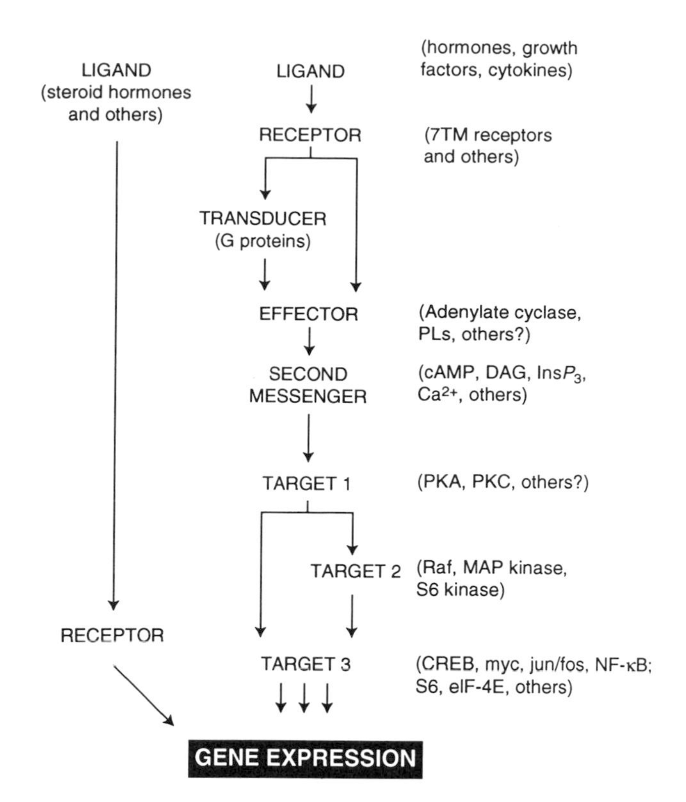

FIG. 24.4. Schematic overview of signal transduction pathways. TM, transmembrane; PL, phospholipases; DAG, diacylglycerol; $InsP_3$, inositol 1,4,5-triphosphate; PKA, protein kinase A; PKC, protein kinase C; MAP kinase, mitogen-activated protein kinase. [Reprinted with permission from the publisher from Hug and Sarre (157).]

DNA-binding domain and a separate carboxyl terminal ligand (hormone)–binding domain (208). Chromosomal and hybridization studies have revealed the existence of two distinct but similar T_3 receptor genes designated as c-*erb*-A α and c-*erb*-A β, which are located on chromosome 17 and chromosome 3, respectively (140, 207, 208). The α gene encodes multiple mRNA species, generated by alternative splicing of its transcripts that give rise to at least two products: T_3-receptor α-$_1$ and T_3-receptor α_2 (140, 228, 234). TR-α_1 has in vitro receptor binding properties of the TR receptor, whereas TR-α_2 does not bind T_3. Rather, TR-α_2 binds to DNA segments designated as the thyroid responsive element (TRE), and it is thus thought to serve as a negative regulator to thyroid hormone action (234). The c-*erb*-A β gene encodes at least two mRNA species that give rise to two distinct proteins, β_1 and β_2. α_1 is expressed in all thyroid-responsive tissue, whereas β_2 is expressed only in pituitary tissue (140). Both β_1 and β_2 are high-affinity T_3 receptors. Available evidence further suggests that TR expression can be regulated at a pretranslational level (207). Thus, it is of interest to understand the physiological factors associated with both TR mRNA and protein regulation in the various models of muscle plasticity.

The subcellular action of thyroid hormone–thyroid receptor interaction is thought to be mediated via their combined interaction with DNA sequences located in the promotor (regulatory) regions of thyroid-responsive genes designated as the TRE (103, 104, 219, 274, 325). Depending on the particular gene, the TRE can be designated as either positive or negative, according to whether thyroid hormone either up-regulates or down-regulates the transcriptional activity of the gene. In addition, nuclear protein factors, designated as thyroid receptor auxiliary proteins (TRAPs), have been identified (378), which bind to TRs and form heterodimer complexes with the TRE to enhance transcriptional activity of the T_3-TR (378). Therefore, this complex of proteins in combination with the availability of T_3 can exert significant impact on those genes under the transcriptional control of thyroid hormone. Interestingly, the MHC gene family is an important muscle protein constituent that is now thought to be under the control of T_3 in both an MHC isoform and tissue-specific fashion, as discussed below.

β-ADRENERGIC RECEPTOR. Three types of studies suggest that changes in the β-adrenergic system are involved in oxidative adaptations to endurance training (see 258). First, the density of β-adrenergic receptors in muscles is greatest in those undergoing the most contractile activity (360). Furthermore, β-adrenergic receptor density was correlated positively with the oxidative capacity in skeletal muscle (360). Second, effective β-adrenergic blockade inhibits some but not all oxidative changes (172). Third, administration of β-adrenergic agonists to humans during continuous bedrest maintains or increases the activities of citrate synthase and succinate dehydrogenase in skeletal muscle (314). Kraus et al. (197) supported the conclusion that contractile activity alone, in the absence of β-adrenergic activation, is a stimulus sufficient to evoke increased expression of genes that encode proteins of oxidative metabolism. They were able to remove the influence of the β-adrenergic receptors by the administration of propranolol to animals undergoing chronic stimulation. They postulated that cyclic adenosine monophosphate (cAMP) stimulates the expression of nuclear genes encoding mitochondrial proteins (197). This suggests that increased contractile activity enhances cAMP by β-adrenergic–independent pathway.

Immediately after a single bout of low-intensity treadmill running, about 35% of β-adrenergic receptors in the rat heart were transferred from a presumably intracellular site (light vesicles) to functional membrane fractions (sarcolemmal membranes)

(163). This suggests that as with protein kinase C and GLUT4, exercise modulates intracellular trafficking. Based on the overexpression of β_2-adrenergic receptors in hearts of transgenic mice increasing left ventricular function in vivo (230), we speculate that an addition of β-adrenergic receptors to the sarcolemma during exercise could foster further increase myocardial contractility during the exercise.

Transducer (G proteins). Kraus et al. (198) found no changes in $G_{s\alpha}$ protein in skeletal muscle chronically stimulated for 21 days. In the rat, treadmill training reduces the quantity of $G_{i\alpha}$ protein in the heart (30), but in hamster heart this training reduces G_s activity in normal hearts, but improves the functional abnormality of G_s protein in cardiomyopathetic BIO 53.58 hearts (327).

Low-molecular-weight GTP-binding proteins. Ten minutes of contraction significantly increased the plasma membrane content of GTP-binding proteins (63%) and GLUT4 protein (68%) in muscles of the perfused hindlimb (92). Insulin had a similar effect. Etgen et al. (92) suggest that there may be an involvement of GTP-binding proteins in the regulation of GLUT4 protein translocation by both contractile activity and insulin. It has been suggested that GTP-binding proteins are involved in various aspects of vesicular trafficking, including endocytosis and exocytosis.

Effector. Endurance training increased basal adenylate cyclase activity approximately 2.5-fold in the red vastus muscle of rats (42). In the same rats, non–receptor-mediated adenylate cyclase activity was stimulated two-fold by either NaF or forskolin in the trained red vastus and white vastus muscles (42). An acute bout of exercise did not alter adenylate cyclase activity (42). Chronic increases in contractile activity increase adenylate cyclase activity (198).

Adenylate cyclase activity is increased following the swelling of S49 mouse lymphoma cells in hypotonic medium through a mechanism independent of the G-proteins that are involved in hormonal regulation of the enzyme (349). Watson (350) proposes that stretch increases the catalytic activity of adenylate cyclase by mechanical deformation of the protein. He suggests that tactile forces or tension in the extracellular matrix would be communicated across the sarcolemma through the cell-surface receptors for extracellular proteins. The forces would be transmitted through the cytoskeletal filaments, which are attached to adenylate cyclase. Thus, the secondary/tertiary structure of adenylate cyclase will be altered by the force transmitted through its attached cytoskeletal components. Watson (350) predicts that conformational changes in the cytoplasmic domain in response to alteration in the free energy of the cyclase molecule would result in an increase in its catalytic activity.

Second messengers.

CYCLIC ADENOSINE MONOPHOSPHATE. Increases in [cAMP] have been found in exercising skeletal muscle. Kraus et al. (197) observed a similar time course for the increases in [cAMP], β-adrenergic receptor density, mitochondrial enzyme activities, mitochondrial RNA, β-F_1ATPase mRNA, and myoglobin mRNA during the continuous chronic stimulation of the tibialis anterior muscle of rabbits. As mentioned above, these changes occurred in the presence of propranolol, thereby leading them to conclude that increased mitochondria expression during chronic stimulation does not require the concomitant stimulation of β-adrenergic receptors (197). Kraus et al. (197) hypothesized that while these correlations do not establish a direct causal relationship between cAMP and gene expression in skeletal muscle, the data do provide a rationale for specific, experimentally testable hypotheses concerning the role of cAMP in the adaptive increase in mitochondria in chronically stimulated skeletal muscle.

However, other findings suggest that any increased transcription of nuclear genes for mitochondrial proteins would require more than a single inducer, such as cAMP. The findings supporting this suggestion are as follows. Cytochrome *c* mRNA, but not cytochrome oxidase IV mRNA, is induced by cAMP through a mechanism involving transcriptional activation (120). Gopalakrishnan and Scarpulla (120) suggest that this differential regulation of cytochrome *c* and cytochrome oxidase mRNAs in response to altered cAMP levels argues against the notion that respiratory chain genes are uniformly regulated under all physiological conditions. This observation confirms a previous study (342), showing that the administration of thyroid hormone to hypothyroid rats increased cytochrome *c* mRNA, but not cytochrome oxidase subunit IV mRNA. Thus, only one of two mRNAs for nuclear-encoded mitochondrial proteins responded to thyroid hormone. They concluded that the cellular mechanisms by which demands for cellular energy are met may not be satisfactorily explained by a single universal regulator of nuclear genes for mitochondrial proteins (342).

Kraus et al. (197) found that the activity-induced down-regulation of aldolase A gene expression is blunted by propranolol, despite the failure of this drug to inhibit activity-induced elevations of cAMP. They indicate that since propranolol suppresses both lipolysis in adipocytes and the supply of free fatty acids to the muscle, the signal producing the decreased glycolytic enzyme activities is the reduction in free fatty acid oxidation in the contracting muscle. [cAMP] does not appear to be the signal inducing the down-regulation of glycolytic enzyme activity.

Increases in [cAMP] and protein kinase A activities have been suggested to be a second messenger in the changes in muscle gene expression induced by denervation. These changes occur in denervated, and not in innervated, adult muscles and in noncontracting muscle cells in culture (50). The addition of cAMP to rat primary muscle cells during the electrical stimulation of these cultured cells prevented much of the down-regulation of MyoD, myogenin, nicotinic receptor subunit, and tetrodotoxin-sensitive sodium channel mRNAs that occurs with electrical stimulation in the absence of cAMP (50). It has also been reported that cAMP up-regulates nicotinic receptor protein synthesis in primary chicken muscle cells in culture (29). Chahine et al. (50) propose the following model for the chemical link from electrical activity in the sarcolemma to down-regulation of the family of electrically sensitive genes (50). In the process of excitation-contraction coupling, calcium is released from the sarcoplasmic reticulum, raising intracellular Ca^{2+} levels; and via interaction with calmodulin, Ca^{2+} stimulates cAMP phosphodiesterase activity. Thus, activation of this enzyme maintains a low level of cAMP, and therefore a low level of protein kinase A activity in the innervated adult skeletal muscle. The mechanisms by which the altered cAMP levels are transduced to the genome are unknown (50). However, gene regions with electrically responsive elements have been identified. The first 850 bp upstream to the start of transcription of the chicken α-subunit gene is responsible for its down-regulation during innervation in transgenic mice (226). The region between -677 and -550 bp of the δ-subunit of the rat nicotinic receptor gene suppresses its expression during electrical stimulation of primary rat muscle cells in culture (51). Thus, regions of promoters containing the gene element that is responsible for the down-regulation of two members of the family of genes responding to electrical activity/innervation have been reported.

CA^{2+}. Chronic blockage of sodium channels with tetrodotoxin increases the number of tetrodotoxin-sensitive sodium channels in primary muscle cells in culture (39, 300). Increased cytoplasmic Ca^{2+} produced by the Ca^{2+} ionophore A23187, independent of electrical activity, reduces the density of sarcolemmal tetrodotoxin-sensitive sodium channels in cultured rat muscle cells (300). Sherman and Catterall (300) and Brodie et al. (39) conclude that electrical and mechanical activity of cultured myotubes regulate de novo synthesis of sodium channels through alterations in the level of cytosolic Ca^{2+}. It is likely that Ca^{2+} could play a role in the signal transduction of other genes during alterations in contractile activity.

Target 1. Alterations in activities of protein kinase A or C could be intermediates between second messengers and changes in gene transcription. Protein kinase C translocation and activation during muscle contraction has been suggested to play a regulatory role during contraction, possibly in the activation of glucose transport (57, 265). Henriksen et al. (132) suggest that exercise increases cytoplasmic Ca^{2+}, which would in turn increase protein kinase C activity, thereby activating glucose transport in skeletal muscle. Electrical stimulation increases the activity of protein kinase C in the nucleus by over two orders of magnitude within 10 min (155). The activity-triggered gene inactivation of the transcription of genes encoding different subunits of the acetylcholine receptor is blocked by staurosporine, a protein kinase C inhibitor, or by depletion of protein kinase C with chronic pretreatment of the muscle with phorbol esters (155).

Target 2. Little information is available as to how either running or resistance exercise of animals alters Raf, MAP kinase, or S6 kinase.

Target 3: nuclear binding proteins.

SKI. The viral-*ski* oncogene is a truncated form of the cellular form of *ski* (212). The *ski* oncogene has been shown to stimulate proliferation as well as the transformation and differentiation to myoblasts from quail fibroblastoid embryo cells in culture (58). The *ski* oncogene also produces increased muscle mass in transgenic mice by selective hypertrophy of type IIb and likely IIx fibers (36), but the hypertrophied fibers have low specific tensions.

MYOD FAMILY. The *MyoD* family consists of the four related nuclear binding proteins: *MyoD* (67), myogenin (83, 369), *Myf-5* (38) and *mrf4/herculin/myf-6* (37, 233, 264). This gene family produces proteins that are members of the basic-helix-loop-helix family of transcription factors that form heterodimers and bind in vitro to the consensus "E-box" recognition sites (243). Three lines of evidence support a role for the MyoD family of regulators in skeletal muscle myogenesis (251); they are: (*1*) All four MyoD family members can recruit cultured nonmuscle cells to be a skeletal muscle phenotype (249, 356), (*2*) E-box sequences exist on numerous muscle-specific genes (249, 356), and (*3*) the appearance of the MyoD family of proteins occurs prior to overt differentiation into muscle during development (249, 290). Although the upregulation of MyoD and myogenin are described for denervation, the role of the MyoD family in adaptations to exercise in adult skeletal muscle is not well described. Changes in MyoD family mRNAs are given in Table 24.4.

C-MYC. c-*myc* mRNA concentration increases from 3–24 h and 12–24 h after the initiation of compensatory hypertrophy in the soleus and plantaris muscles, respectively (359). However, no significant change in c-*myc* mRNA was noted in either muscle 48 h after starting their hypertrophy. These time course data imply that the functional consequence of the increase in c-*myc* is within the first day of hypertrophy even though most of the muscle growth occurs after the first day of hypertrophy. Administration of clenbuterol also increased c-*myc* mRNA concentration within 24 h of injection, but no other time points were examined (359).

Overexpression of Myc protein not only promotes cellular proliferation, but also increases the rate of programmed cell death (193). The role of c-*myc* in muscle has been reviewed by Meichle et al. (225). c-*myc* expression decreases in parallel with the differentiation of muscle cells. Indeed, overexpression of c-*myc* protein interferes with muscle cell differentiation (225), likely by a sustained proliferative stimulus provided by c-*myc*. A potential mechanism according to Meichle et al. (225) is that myc expression may block the ability of MyoD to induce myogenin, which is an essential myogenic factor required to induce differentiation of cultured muscle cells.

MRNAS FOR NUCLEAR BINDING PROTEINS. These are included in Table 24.4.

OXYGEN FREE RADICALS. During reduction of molecular oxygen to water in cellular respiration, partially reduced oxygen species are produced that are very reactive with protein, lipids, and DNA, producing deleterious effects/damage on cells (e.g., cross-linking of proteins, peroxidation of lipids, and cross-linking of DNA) (168). Since the reduction of molecular oxygen to water in the electron transport chain increases in contracting muscle, more oxygen species free radicals are formed during exercise. In 1982, Davies et al. (67) reported a two- to three-fold increase in the concentrations of free radical in both muscle and liver following exercise to exhaustion in rats. They also observed an increased rate of basal respiration after exhaustive exercise in rats. They interpreted this to mean that the integrity of the sarcoplasmic reticulum and endoplasmic reticulum in muscle and liver was impaired by the exercise. Lipid peroxidation was also increased in these exhausted animals. Vitamin E–deficient rats had a 40% decrease in the running time to exhaustion, but no change in $\dot{V}O_{2max}$, respiratory exchange ratio, and maximal workload at $\dot{V}O_{2max}$. Davies et al. (67) suggested that the decreased endurance time in the vitamin E–deficient rats is precipitated by peroxidative damage to mitochondria. Finally, they conclude that exercise-induced free radicals may cause limited damage to mitochondrial membranes which, in a chronic training situation, may be the initiating stimulus to mitochondrial biogenesis.

The reader is referred to reviews (7, 69, 250, 309, 363) of the numerous papers in this area. The majority of the evidence supports the conclusion that endurance training increases antioxidant enzymes [glutathione peroxidase (GPX), mitochondrial GPX, glutathione reductase, and superoxide dismutase (SOD)] in skeletal muscle. Powers et al. (259) have recently shown that high-intensity exercise training is generally necessary for up-regulation of SOD and GPX activities in rat skeletal muscle and that the magnitude of the increase in oxidative enzymes do not parallel the exercise-induced increases in oxidative enzymes. Furthermore, the authors reported fiber-type differences in the response of antioxidant enzymes to treadmill training. The functional significance as well as the underlying mechanisms responsible for the training-induced up-regulation of skeletal muscle antioxidant enzymes remains to be elucidated.

GENE EXPRESSION. Gene expression is defined as a steady-state alteration in the content (amount per muscle) of a given protein. Actin and myosin gene expression are increased in hypertrophied muscle, but are decreased in muscle atrophy. There are multiple sites for the regulation of gene expression, as illustrated in Figure 24.5.

Observations to date lead to the conclusion that alterations in contractile activity produce changes at many sites in the regulatory cascade for gene expression (Figure 24.5). Three different experimental approaches support this conclusion, and they are described briefly in the next section.

The first experimental approach is to directly measure protein synthesis and RNA, from which deductions are made about changes in regulatory sites of gene expression. For example, increases in the categories of pretranslational, translational, and posttranslational regulation were noted by Laurent et al. (206) in the stretch-overload model of muscle hypertrophy. An increase in the fractional rate of protein synthesis (i.e., an increase in translational regulation) was directly measured in the chicken anterior latissimus dorsi muscle that was undergoing chronic stretch-overload. From the greater percentage increase in protein synthesis as compared to muscle protein, they deduced that rates of protein degradation must have also increased (i.e., an alteration in posttranslational control). They also noted

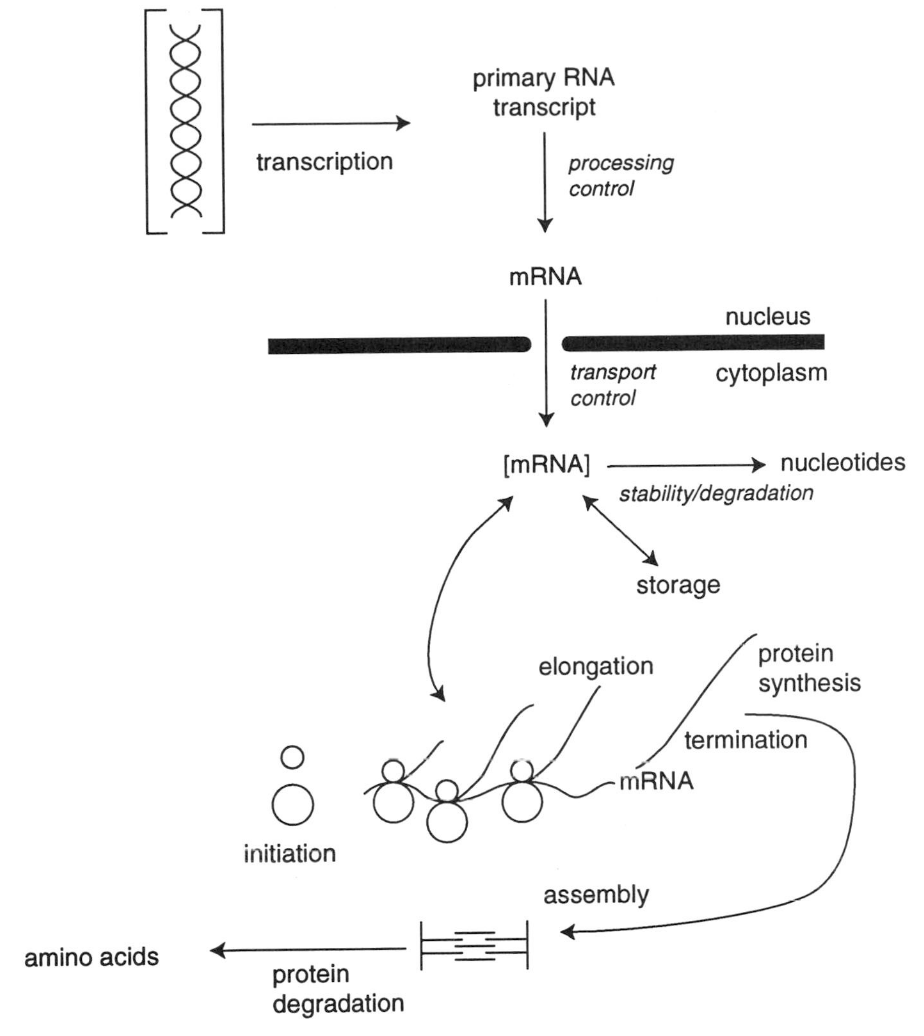

FIG. 24.5. Multiple steps in the pathway of gene expression are modulated by changes in the inherent contractile activity.

that RNA content increased, (i.e., an alteration in pretranslational control). The initial increase in protein synthesis after the first day of stretch-overload was mediated by an increase in the efficiency of translation (i.e., the grams of protein synthesized per gram of RNA increased during the first treatment day). Thereafter, the capacity for translation increased (i.e., the increases in protein synthesis and [RNA] were proportional). Thus, the report of Laurent et al. (206) suggested that adaptations to stretch-overload occurred at pretranslational, translational, and posttranslational sites.

A second experimental approach used direct measurements of protein synthesis and mRNA. This approach found that rates of synthesis for a specific protein did not always change with the same percentage as was the percentage change of its mRNA. The mRNAs for actin, cytochrome *c*, and β-MHC were used for these studies. For actin, the model of producing muscle atrophy in rats by hindlimb immobilization or recovery of muscle from atrophy was employed. Whereas actin protein synthesis decreased in a fast-twitch muscle during the first 6 h of limb immobilization, a procedure leading to muscle atrophy, the amount of skeletal α-actin mRNA per unit of RNA did not change in this muscle for the first 3 days of limb immobilization (348). Watson et al. (348) concluded that an alteration in translation must account for the early decline in actin protein synthesis. Thus, changes in translation of the skeletal α-actin mRNA play a more predominant early role, but changes in pretranslational regulation of the skeletal α-actin mRNA occur somewhat later. This sequence of regulation was reversed during regrowth from atrophy. Rates of actin protein synthesis and the percentage of α-actin mRNA per unit of

RNA increase in parallel during first 2 days of recovery from a 7 days of limb immobilization (240). These data suggest both a pretranslational and translational regulation during the first few days of regrowth. However, the further increase in actin protein synthesis in the third to fourth day after removing the plaster cast was not associated with as large of a percentage increase in skeletal α-actin mRNA per unit of RNA as was the percentage increase in actin protein synthesis rate. These data can be interpreted to mean that translational processes are being up-regulated more than pretranslational processes as recovery progresses in the third to fourth day. Since muscle mass was unchanged during the first 4 days of recovery, the increase in actin protein synthesis was likely without a concurrent accretion of protein, which suggests a posttranslational regulation (i.e., either the new actin is not assembled, but is degraded, or that the newly synthesized actin is assembled, but other actin is degraded as protein turnover is increased in muscle regrowing from atrophy).

A similar study was performed with cytochrome *c* in which its protein synthesis rate decreased 27% in type II muscle during the first 6 h of hindlimb immobilization in rats while cytochrome *c* mRNA was unchanged (239). By the seventh day of limb immobilization, cytochrome *c* mRNA had decreased 40%. Thus, an early decrease in cytochrome *c* translation was followed by a decrease in its pretranslational regulation. During recovery from 7 days of limb immobilization, cytochrome *c* protein synthesis rate and mRNA both doubled from their atrophied level by the fourth day of recovery (239). Thus, both pretranslational control and translational regulation of cytochrome *c* are inferred to be up-regulated as the muscle underwent the first 4 days of recovery from a 7 day period of atrophy.

Another study related myofibrillar protein synthesis rates to two myofibrillar mRNAs. At the seventh day of non-weight bearing by the rat soleus muscle, myofibrillar protein synthesis is decreased 59% (321). On the other hand, only one of the two measured myofibrillar mRNAs decreased at this time. Skeletal α-actin mRNA decreases, but β-MHC mRNA is unchanged on the seventh day of soleus muscle atrophy during non-weight bearing (321). These results suggest that pretranslational regulation could differ between the two major myofibrillar proteins during non–weight-bearing atrophy of the type I muscle. Furthermore, the results suggest a decrease in β-MHC mRNA translation during non–weight-bearing atrophy of the rat soleus muscle.

A 41%–65% increase in myofibrillar protein synthesis rates, without any change in skeletal α-actin mRNA content occurred in the 12–41 h period after 192 eccentric contractions (368). These data indicate an acute translational regulation in response to eccentric contraction. However, after 10 weeks of resistance training consisting of twice-weekly bouts of 192 eccentric contractions, skeletal α-actin mRNA had increased 34%–67% when calculated per whole muscle (368).

A third experimental approach examined the relative changes in pretranslational and posttranscriptional regulation by measuring transcription rate for an mRNA by nuclear run-on and the quantity of that mRNA by northern blots. Transcription run-on analysis provides a reasonably accurate measure of the transcription rate of any given gene of interest at the time of sacrifice. The results of this experiment are given in Table 24.5.

These data were interpreted by Neufer and Dohm (244) to indicate that the early increase in GLUT4 protein content in endurance-trained skeletal muscle predominately involves translational and/or post-

TABLE 24.5. *Response of Red Hindlimb Skeletal Muscle to 1 Week of 80 Min Daily Duration Running on a Treadmill by Rats**

Item	Transcriptional Run-on	mRNA from Northern Blot	Protein from Western Blot
GLUT4	↑ 3 h postexercise → 30 min and 24 h postexercise	NS	↑ 76%
Citrate synthase	↑ 3 and 24 h postexercise	NS	↑ 30%
GLUT1	→		
Cytochrome *c*	→		
βC/EBP	→		

*Data taken from Neufer and Dohm (244).

translational mechanisms. They further propose that the increase in GLUT4 mRNA evident with extended periods of training is generated from the summing of small increases with repeated postexercise transient increases in GLUT4 gene transcription. Thus, in the trained steady-state level, GLUT4 mRNA increases due to pretranscriptional regulation, in part due to increased transcription.

Another discordancy between percentage changes in mRNA and protein quantities is found in the study of Vestergaard et al. (340). They noted a 40% increase in glycogen synthase mRNA, a 34% increase in glycogen synthase activity in the presence of its allosteric activator, glucose 6-phosphate, and no change in immunoreactive glycogen synthase. These findings suggest an increased pretranslational regulation (i.e., the increase in mRNA) and either a decreased translational regulation or an altered posttranslational regulation (i.e., a decreased assembly or increased protein degradation) (340). Vestergaard et al. (340) also observed a 15% reduction in phosphofructokinase activity, a 20% decrease in immunoreactive phosphofructokinase, and no change in phosphofructokinase mRNA. A 20% decline in mRNA may not have been detectable, so it is not possible to interpret fully these data.

These three experimental approaches demonstrate that changes in gene expression in skeletal muscle adapting to alterations in contractile activity invoke altered regulation at multiple sites, including pretranslational, translational, and posttranslational. A complex combination of synergistic signaling pathways could be involved in the regulation of gene expression. Regulation of gene expression could also be via a sole signaling pathway interacting at multiple sites. The challenge of future research is to unravel these possibilities.

TRANSCRIPTIONAL AND PRETRANSLATIONAL CONTROL OF MHC GENE PLASTICITY. Experiments conducted to date clearly suggest that under steady-state conditions, the level of mRNA for a given MHC largely parallels the relative level of expression of that MHC (73, 126, 164, 302, 318, 319). This general pattern appears to apply to conditions of adaptation involving functional overload (319), muscle unloading involving both ground base and spaceflight experiments (73, 126), and perturbations designed to chronically reduce phosphocreatine levels in skeletal muscle (235). Since there is alteration in both mRNA and protein content for the MHCs undergoing the adaptive transformation, it appears that the MHC gene family is chiefly regulated at the pretranslational level. However, this may not be the case during the early stages of the adaptation process. For example, there is evidence that during the initial stages of muscle unloading, there are reductions in expression of slow MHC without evidence of a reduction in mRNA levels (321), suggesting that posttranslational events can also impact on MHC plasticity.

At the present time there is a scarcity of information concerning the regulation of fast MHC gene expression. Nevertheless, there has been some preliminary characterization of the IIb MHC promotor in the mouse (320). The findings suggest that there are both positive and negative regulatory sequences, and one of the positive sequences contains a motif that binds the MyoD family of nuclear proteins (320).

On the other hand, there is some definitive information available concerning transcriptional control of the slow MHC. Investigations of control of the slow MHC gene have largely focused on cardiac muscle, which expresses two MHC genes, one encoding for the α (cardiac specific fast) and the other for the β (type I or slow), MHC, respectively (104, 105, 274, 302). These α- and β-MHCs form native myosins (the fast V1 and the slow V3), which are responsible for the intrinsic functional properties of the cardiac cell. The contractile properties of the V1 and V3 isoforms are analogous to the fast and slow contractile properties demonstrated in skeletal muscle fiber types (8). Available information suggests that there is a TRE upstream of the promoter region of both the α- and β-MHC genes that binds T_3-TR complexes, and the interaction of the T_3-TR-TRE exerts positive transcriptional control on the α gene and negative control on the β-MHC gene (104, 105). Additional studies have also reported the existence of different T_3 isoforms (designated as α_1, α_2, and β_1; see above) as well as TRAPs that have been implicated in the differential control of genes containing the TRE (378). These findings suggest that both the type and level of TRs maintained in the cell, as well as the level of TRAP protein, may play an important role in the regulation of MHC expression in different type of muscle. Consistent with this notion, it has recently been reported that exogenous T_3 treatment induces reduced expression of type I MHC coupled with a concomitant increase in expression of type IIa and IIx MHC in slow, soleus muscle (319). However, in fast muscle hyperthyroidism causes reduced expression of type I, IIa, and IIx MHC expression with a concomitant increase in IIb MHC expression (319). These collective observations suggest that all the adult MHC genes may be under some control of T_3, but the nature of this control is tissue specific, because it appears that the IIa and IIx MHCs are up-regulated by T_3 in slow muscle and down-regulated by T_3 in fast skeletal muscle. Furthermore, the unique impact of T_3 on slow MHC expression can be seen when mechanical interventions inducing altered expression of type I MHC expression are performed in conjunction with altered thyroid state. Under these conditions, it appears that thyroid state can blunt the mechanical signal inducing type I MHC transformation (319). These findings suggest that thyroid state may be a pivotal regulatory component on the plasticity of the slow MHC gene in both cardiac and skeletal muscle fibers.

Recently, another nuclear factor has been identified in rodent cardiac cells that has been shown to bind to an enhancer segment in the β (type I) gene. This so-called β-f1 protein is necessary for optimal transcription of the β-MHC gene, and it can be expressed in skeletal muscle (104, 302, 325). Based on these observations, it is possible that cell expressing the β or type I MHC require the presence of the β-f1 factor for optimal transcription of the gene. Thus, it will be of interest in the future to determine the role of TRs, TRAPs, and other factors (β-f1), in the context of slow MHC plasticity in response to altered physical activity. Furthermore, it is essential that future research focus on understanding the factors that regulate promotor activity in the various fast MHC genes.

ELECTRICALLY SENSITIVE GENES. Early findings indicated that denervated skeletal muscles had an increased sensitivity to acetylcholine sensitivity by an up-regulation of extrajunctional acetylcholine receptors. Direct electrical stimulation of denervated skeletal muscles reversed the increased acetylcholine sensitivity (80, 215). These findings suggested that acetylcholine receptors could be regulated by depolarization of the sarcolemma. A family of genes is regulated by the electrical activity (i.e., depolarization) of the sarcolemma and are summarized in Table 24.6. The electrical signal from a single motoneuron is amplified 120,000 times. Tseng et al. (330) calculate that there are 120,000 myonuclei under the influence of electrical signals produced by a single motor nerve in the rat soleus and plantaris muscles (330).

However, not all muscle genes are regulated by electrical activity (Table 24.7).

Two experimental models have been employed to test for electrically responsive genes. In one model, stimulating electrodes are immersed in the culture medium and the muscles are stimulated chronically for 3–7 days with 100 Hz trains, 1 s duration, applied once every 100 s (51). In the second model, muscles are denervated, so that muscles do not generate action potentials in the sarcolemma from neural input.

Merlie et al. (227) showed electrically responsive regions of two genes in transgenic mice. An 111 bp and a 335 bp region from the promoters of the acetylcholine α-subunit and myogenin genes, respectively, conferred activity-dependent regulation to a linked reporter gene in transgenic mice. Binding sites for myogenic helix-loop-helix proteins were present in both the acetylcholine α-subunit and myogenin promoters. They suggest that the presence of these E-boxes is consistent with the hypothesis that myogenic regulators serve as nuclear targets for the signaling cascade through which motor innervation leads to changes in the transcription of "electrically sensitive" genes in skeletal muscle (227). A model (249) for the pathway from membrane depolarization to the inhibition of transcription of the acetylcholine α-subunit shows that free Ca^{2+} increases in the cytoplasm by the process of excitation-contraction coupling and activates protein kinase C, which phosphorylates myogenin, abolishing its ability to bind to the DNA sequence containing the E-box of the promoter DNA for the acetylcholine α-subunit. Thus, the acetylcholine α-subunit is not transcribed. This model would explain why extrajunctional receptors for acetylcholine do not appear in innervated skeletal muscles.

The δ-subunit of the nicotinic acetylcholine receptor is only transcribed for extrajunctional receptors when electrical activity is absent. When primary rat muscle cells in culture were stimulated via electrodes, DNA elements conferring suppression of the δ-subunit promoter of the nicotinic acetylcholine base pair region (-677 to -550 bp) were located (50). This sequence contains the consensus sequence for the E-box (CAACTG).

Animal Models to Study Gene Expression

Transgenic. Transgenic mice were employed to determine transcriptional regulation of the MM-creatine kinase (MCK) isozyme during mechanical overload hypertrophy. Tsika et al. (333) observed a 2.6-fold repression in MCK activity, a 3.6-fold repression in MCK mRNA, and a 5-fold repression in chloramphenicol acetyltransferase activity driven from a -3300 bp MCK promoter in 2 day hypertrophied muscle. They concluded that regulatory elements upstream of previously identified muscle-specific and differentiation-specific elements contribute to the transcriptional regression. β-MHC transgenes are induced ten-fold after 6–8 weeks of work overload. Both muscle and human β-MHC genes require only 600 bp of their 5′ promoter (270).

Transgenic mice overexpressing glucose transporter protein, GLUT1, in skeletal muscle have a

TABLE 24.6. *Genes Responsive to Electrical Activity or Electrical Activity and cAMP in Either Cultured Muscle Cells or in Denervated Muscles*

Gene	Denervation or No Electrical Activity	Electrical Stimulation of Denervated Muscle or of Muscle Cells in Culture	Application of cAMP to Stimulated Muscle Cells in Culture	References
MyoD	↑	↓	↑	50, 84
Myogenin	↑	↓	↑	50, 84
Nicotinic acetylcholine receptor				
α-Subunit	↑	↓	↑	51, 113, 189
β-Subunit	↑	↓	↑	50, 113
γ-Subunit	↑	↓	↑	50, 113
δ-Subunit	↑	↓	↑	50, 113
Tetrodotoxin-insensitive sodium channel	↑	↓	↑	50, 300, 301

ten-fold increase in muscle glycogen concentration that is not due either to an increase in muscle glycogen synthase activity or to a decrease in muscle glycogen phosphorylase activity (262). Glucose transport activity is seven-fold higher in mice overexpressing GLUT1 than in control animals. Since a four-fold increase in muscle free glucose occurred in the transgenic mouse muscle, with no significant change in hexokinase activity, Ren et al. (262) conclude that glucose transport is the rate-limiting step for muscle glucose disposal in normal, resting mice. These data illustrate one usage of transgenic animals (i.e., overexpression of a protein to delineate function).

Homologous recombination: null mutations of muscle genes. Null mutations involve a procedure that removes a part of a gene in the germ line of mice. As a result the mRNA and protein are not present in animals with the missing gene. Null mutations are the laboratory equivalent of the clinical disease of Duchenne muscular dystrophy, in which a part of a gene is missing. Other terms synonymous with "null mutation" are "knockout" mice and "homologous recombination."

An example of the usage in null mutation with application to exercise sciences is the production of a line of mice deficient in exon 2 of M-creatine kinase. M-creatine kinase (M-CK) null alleles were generated by gene targeting in the 129SvE-derived ES cell line AB-1 (224, 338). These mice had no M-CK mRNA or M-CK protein subunits in either their heart or skeletal muscles. Functions of M-CK enzyme activity were determined by work tests in the absence of the enzyme. Absence of M-CK was associated with a loss of "burst" work capacity, and an enhancement of endurance capacity (338). A more rapid decline in twitch force occurred in M-CK–null mice during 5 Hz stimulation. Nevertheless, M-CK mice had an increased intermyofibrillar mitochondrial network developed in type II, but not type I, fibers. Cytochrome oxidase and citrate synthase activities were 50%–80% higher in whole-muscle preparations. This is striking because the absence of one enzyme that functions in the transfer of high-energy phosphate was sufficient to induce an increase in mitochondrial density. M-CK–null mice had 60% more glycogen in gastrocnemius-plantaris-soleus muscles than wild-type mice. Although glycogen depletion was more rapid in these muscles during 5 Hz stimulation, muscle lactates were similar. Surprisingly, creatine phosphate concentrations decreased normally during muscle exercise in M-CK–null mice. Van Deursen et al. (338) interpret this finding to suggest that M-CK–mediated conversion is not the only route for phosphocreatine conversion in contracting muscle. Thus, the null mouse model can provide many new, unexpected findings, hinting at additional future experiments.

Another interesting comparison is that some of the mitochondrial adaptations occurring in skeletal muscle are similar in the M-CK–null mouse and in rats being fed β-GPA. One interpretation is that the transportation of energy in the muscle fiber could be sensed in some manner and the rate of flux could induce a signal for adaptive increases in mitochondria.

Direct plasmid injection. Skeletal muscles of rodents have been reported to take up directly injected plasmid DNA and to express reporter genes from

TABLE 24.7. *Genes Not Responsive to Electrical Activity in Cultured Muscle Cells*

Gene	Reference
α-Actin mRNA	189
Adult-type ε-subunit of nicotinic acetylcholine receptor	50
Creatine kinase	50

viral- and muscle-specific regulatory sequences (3, 64, 220, 336, 341, 358, 364–366). Direct injections of plasmids into the heart results in a higher level of expression of reporter genes than in skeletal muscle (187, 341, 343). Others have demonstrated the uptake and expression of plasmids containing promoter-reporter genes in the heart (4, 248).

Variability is one of the major limitations of analysis of reporter genes directed by promoters after the direct injection of plasmids containing these constructs into skeletal muscles. Methods reported to minimize this variability are: (*1*) use of single batches of plasmid DNA (220); (*2*) intramuscular injection of plasmid in saline (366), rather than water (220); (*3*) preinjection of muscles with a relatively large volume of hypertonic sucrose (64); and (*4*) injection of the plasmid in relatively large, rather than small, volumes (64). Optimization of reporter expression is suggested to occur if 3- to 4-week-old male rats, rather than if older male or female rats are employed (358), and if closed circular, instead of linearized, plasmid (220) is used. In order to correct for variability of injection (both DNA uptake and expression), a second plasmid containing a viral promoter directing the expression of a second reporter gene should be co-injected with the plasmid containing the muscle-specific promoter directing the first reporter gene. A high degree of correlation between expression of two injected plasmids supports the validity of normalizing the activity of reporter directed by the muscle-specific promoter to the activity of the second reporter directed by the prokaryotic promoter (343, 373). Recently, Booth has observed treatment effects on the CAT reporter gene. For example, chronic stimulation and stretch overload increased CAT reporter gene while limb immobilization decreased its expression in skeletal muscle after CAT reporter gene injection into skeletal muscle. It is not known whether the responses of the reporter gene are attributable to the sequences in the viral promoter that directs the gene expression or to the post-transcriptional processes of the reporter gene RNA and protein. This information raises an important consideration in interpreting results. In any case, proper control should be included during experimental design to monitor treatment effects on reporter genes.

The expression of the reporter gene directed by the −613 α-MHC promoter, after its injection into rat heart with a second plasmid for normalization of injection efficiency, was responsive to the thyroid state of the animal (187). The ratio of the mean luciferase activity divided by chloramphenicol (CAT) activity in the hearts of hypothyroid rats treated with T_3 is approximately three times greater than that of the hypothyroid animals not treated with T_3, and is two times greater than that of euthyroid controls (187). Kitsis et al. (187) conclude expression of injected genes can be targeted to specific cell types in vivo and can be modulated by the hormonal status of the animal.

Vincent et al. (341) directly injected plasmids containing various lengths of the promoter of the M isozyme of creatine kinase (MCK) into the heart and skeletal muscles of rats to determine regulatory sequences of this gene in the animal. They found that the overall expression of the −650 MCK 5′-flanking region is much higher in heart than in skeletal muscle. Deletion constructs showed that the MCK gene is controlled by different regulatory programs in adult cardiac and skeletal muscle. Vincent et al. (341) observed that deletion of the enhancer region of the MCK gene significantly decreased MCK promoter expression in skeletal muscle, but that this deletion had no detectable effect on expression in the heart. Additional deletions uncovered a serum response element (SRE) (i.e., CArG sequence) motif at sequence −179 in the MCK promoter that is essential for cardiac-specific expression.

Von Harsdorf et al. (343) injected into dog heart constructs containing serial deletions of the 5′-flanking region of the β-MHC gene, which was contained in a closed circular plasmid. The −667 rat β-MHC construct is more active in the heart than in skeletal muscle. Von Harsdorf et al. (343) suggest that this could reflect the existence of a positive regulatory element between nucleotide positions −667 and −354, which is recognized specifically in cardiocytes and acts cooperatively with other positive regulatory elements, likely between −215 and −186 bp from the transcription start site. They conclude that the method of direct injection of plasmids into the heart of dogs is a model that can be used to map promoter regions and identify important regulatory sequences in living animals.

Yan and Booth (373) observed that chronic electrical stimulation caused a six-fold higher expression of the reporter gene, chloramphenicol acetyltransferase activity, directed by either the −726 or −146 bp promoters of the rat somatic cytochrome *c* gene after their injection into the tibialis anterior muscle of rats (362). These data indicate that the region between −726 and −146 does not contain the sequence element(s) necessary to cause the increase in the promoter activity of the cytochrome *c* promoter in response to chronic stimulation in intact rats. The data further suggest that the 3′ untranslated region of the rat somatic cytochrome *c* gene is the region of the gene responding to chronic stimulation.

Carson et al. (49) have used the model of stretch overload (i.e., weighting the wing of a chicken) to identify which regulatory sequences of the skeletal α-actin are important during hypertrophy in living animals. Six days after placing 10% of the bird's body weight on its left wing, the anterior latissimus dorsi (ALD) muscle enlarges 110% and has a 209% increase in the luciferase/CAT ratio activity from the −2090 α-actin promoter directing luciferase expression. The −424, −202, and −99 deletion constructs of the skeletal α-actin promoter all have a significantly higher luciferase/CAT ratio in the hypertrophied ALD muscle (229%, 125%, and 225%, respectively) (49). The −77 actin-luciferase construct did not show a significant difference in the luciferase/CAT ration the ALD muscle between stretch and control wings. These data not only show that the promoter activity of the skeletal α-actin gene is upregulated during stretch-overload–induced hypertrophy, but that the serum response element 1 −91 to −81) is a stretch-hypertrophy response element in the chicken skeletal α-actin promoter.

CLINICAL SIGNIFICANCE OF MUSCLE PLASTICITY

A few brief examples of the clinical application of muscle plasticity research are given here. Skeletal muscle mass peaks about age 25 years, and then atrophies (see 331 for references). Resistance training has been shown to compensate for loss of muscle, delaying frailty and the loss of independence of living (see 41 for references). Old muscle is plastic and retains some of its ability to enlarge during resistance training (see 96 for references). Insulin resistance of skeletal muscle may be the underlying factor for the development of obesity, non–insulin-dependent diabetes mellitus, hypertension, hyperlipidemia, and reduced high-density lipoprotein (see 26 for references). A single bout of contractile activity reverses insulin resistance (see 162 for references). Muscle plasticity research has given us insight into these clinical processes.

SUMMARY

A Greek living in the sixth century B.C. is reputed to have been the first to practice progressive resistance training (14). Thus, awareness of skeletal muscle plasticity is old. However, it was not until the second half of the twentieth century that detailed reports of adaptative changes in contractile properties, morphology, biochemistry, cellular, and molecular biology of skeletal muscle during alterations in the use of skeletal muscle have appeared. For example, resistance training decreases the Ca^{2+} concentration needed to elicit 50% of maximal tension (176), decreases MHC IIb gene expression, and increases contractile proteins in parallel, which permits greater absolute loads to be moved. Serum response element 1 of the skeletal α-actin promoter is a member of a mechanotransduction pathway for enhancing actin gene transcription, which enlarges muscle. In a second example, endurance training increases the maximal velocity of contraction, the percentage volume occupied by mitochondria, the capacity to oxidize substrates, and MHC type I in skeletal muscle. Furthermore, endurance training increases and decreases the V_{max} of individual slow and fast fibers, respectively (100). All these changes contribute to an improved endurance performance. The pathway from aerobic exercise that signals mitochondria to increase is not known, but an initial clue may ensue from the identification that the 3′-end of the rat somatic cytochrome *c* gene is a regulator of its mRNA level in response to aerobic activity. This review has indicated many other changes. Indeed, it is difficult to name much that does not change in skeletal muscle as it adapts to a new level of use. Because so many things change in exercising skeletal muscle, it will be difficult to establish cause-and-effect relationships of signaling pathways. The cellular and molecular regulations of muscle plasticity are just beginning to be investigated. Early data indicate that very complex cellular and molecular regulations underlie the response of muscle proteins to changes in contractile activity in the living animal. The difficulty of this task is amplified by the integrative nature of muscle plasticity. Gene expression in exercising muscle is modulated by many different kinds of clues: nerves, cytokines (often of immune origin), autocrine and paracrine substances (local growth factors), hormones, temperature (heat shock proteins), circulatory changes (alterations in blood flow change supply of factors to muscle), fluid shifts within muscle that alter the concentration of factors, and so forth. Because of the complicated integration of multiple factors, what can be measured in human beings is often limited, which necessitates animal models that have their own limitations. Many facets of gene expression (pretranslational, translational, and posttranslational regulation) are involved. These events often occur in different time frames. Thus, delineating signaling pathways from the exercise signal to the change in gene expression will be a difficult and lengthy research endeavor.

We thank Ms. Leslie Sanders for editing and word processing assistance. This work was supported by U.S. Public Health Service grants NIH AR19393 (FWB), NIH AR30346 (KMB), NIH HL38819 (KMB), and NASA NAG2-555 (KMB), and NASA NAGW3908 (FWB).

REFERENCES

1. Aarsaether, N., A. Aarsland, H. Kryvi, A. Nilsson, A. Svardal, P. M. Ueland and R. K. Berge. Changes in perioxisomes and mitochondria in liver of ethionine exposed rats: a biochemical and morphological investigation. *Carcinogenesis* 10: 987–994, 1989.
2. Abu-Shakra, S. R., A. J. Cole, and D. B. Drachman. Nerve stimulation and denervation induce differential patterns of immediate early gene mRNA expression in skeletal muscle. *Mol. Brain Res.* 18: 216–220, 1993.
3. Acsadi, G., G. Dickson, D. R. Love, A. Jani, F. S. Walsh, A. Gurusinghe, J. A. Wolff, and K. E. Davies. Human dystrophin expression in mdx mice after intramuscluar injection of DNA constructs. *Nature* 352: 815–818, 1991.
4. Acsadi, G., S. Jiao, A. Jani, D. Duke, P. Williams, W. Chong, and J. A. Wolff. Direct gene transfer and expression into rat heart in vivo. *New Biol.* 3: 71–81, 1991.
5. Adams, G. R., F. Haddad, and K. M. Baldwin. Interaction of chronic creative depletion and hindlimb non-weight bearing activity: effects on postural and locomotor muscles. *J. Appl. Physiol.* 77: 1198–1205, 1994.
6. Adams, G. R., B. M. Hather, K. M. Baldwin, and G. A. Dudley. Skeletal muscle myosin heavy chain composition and resistance training. *J. Appl. Physiol.* 74: 911–915, 1993.
7. Alessio, H. M. Exercise-induced oxidative stress. *Med. Sci. Sports Exerc.* 25: 218–224, 1993.
8. Alpert, N. R., and L. A. Mullieri. Functional consequences of altered cardiac myosin isoenzymes. *Med. Sci. Sports Exerc.* 18: 309–313, 1986.
9. Annex, B. H., W. E. Kraus, G. L. Dohm, and R. S. Williams. Mitochondrial biogenesis in striated muscles: rapid induction of citrate synthase mRNA by nerve stimulation. *Am. J. Physiol.* 260 (*Cell Physiol.* 29): C266–C270, 1991.
10. Antonio, J., and W. J. Gonyea. Skeletal muscle hyperplasia. *Med. Sci. Sports Exerc.* 25: 1333–1345, 1993.
11. Arai, M., K. Otsu, D. H. MacLennan, and M. Periasamy. Regulation of sarcoplasmic reticulum gene expression during cardiac and skeletal muscle development. *Am. J. Physiol.* 262 (*Cell Physiol.* 31): C614–C620, 1992.
12. Armstrong, R. B. Distribution of blood flow in the muscles of conscious animals during exercise. *Am. J. Cardiol.* 62: 9E-14E, 1988.
13. Armstrong, R. B., and M. H. Laughlin. Exercise blood flow patterns within and among rat muscles after training. *Am. J. Physiol.* 246 (*Heart Circ. Physiol.* 15): H59–H68, 1984.
14. Atha, J. Strengthening skeletal muscle. *Exerc. Sport Sci. Rev.* 9: 1–73, 1981.
15. Atomi, Y., S. Yamada, and T. Nishida. Early changes of αB-crystallin in rat skeletal muscle to mechanical tension and denervation. *Biochem. Biophys. Res. Commun.* 181: 1323–1330, 1991.
16. Ausoni, S., L. Gorza, S. Schiaffino, K. Gundersen, and T. Lomo. Expression of myosin heavy chain isoforms in stimulated fast and slow rat muscles. *J. Neurosci.* 10: 153–160, 1990.
17. Babij, P., and F. W. Booth. α-Actin and cytochrome *c* mRNAs in atrophied adult rat skeletal muscle. *Am. J. Physiol.* 254 (*Cell Physiol.* 23): C651–C656, 1988.
18. Baldwin, K. M., W. G. Cheadle, O. M. Martinez, and D. A. Cooke. Effect of functional overload on enzyme levels in different types of skeletal muscle. *J. Appl. Physiol.* 42: 312–317, 1977.
19. Baldwin, K. M., R. E. Herrick, and E. Ilyina-Kakeuva, and U. S. Oganov. Effects of zero gravity of myofibril content and isomyosin distribution in rodent skeletal muscle. *FASEB J.* 4: 79–83, 1990.
20. Baldwin, K. M., R. R. Roy, R. D. Sacks, C. Blanco, and V. R. Edgerton. Relative independence of metabolic enzymes and neuromuscular activity. *J. Appl. Physiol. Respir. Environ. Exerc. Physiol.* 56: 1602–1607, 1984.
21. Baldwin, K. M., V. Valdez, R. E. Herrick, A. M. MacIntosh, and R. R. Roy. Biochemical properties of overloaded fast-twitch skeletal muscle. *J. Appl. Physiol. Respir. Environ. Exerc. Physiol.* 52: 467–472, 1982.
22. Baldwin, K. M., V. Valdez, L. F. Schrader, and R. E. Herrick. Effect of functional overload on substrate oxidation capacity of skeletal muscle. *J. Appl. Physiol.* 50: 1272–1276, 1981.
23. Baldwin, K. M., W. W. Winder, and J. O. Holloszy. Adaptation of actomyosin ATPase in different types of muscle to endurance exercise. *Am. J. Physiol.* 229: 422–426, 1975.
24. Baldwin, K. M., W. W. Winder, R. L. Terjung, and J. O. Holloszy. Glycolytic enzymes in different types of skeletal muscle. *Am. J. Physiol.* 225: 962–966, 1973.
25. Barnard, R. J., and J. B. Peter. Effect of exercise on skeletal muscle. III. Cytochrome changes. *J. Appl. Physiol.* 31: 904–908, 1971.
26. Barnard, R. J. and S. J. Wen. Exercise and diet in the prevention and control of the metabolic syndrome. *Sports Med.* 18: 218–228, 1994.
27. Beck, I., R. Weinmann, and J. Caro. Characterization of hypoxia-responsive enhancer in the human erythropoietin gene shows presence of hypoxia-inducible 120-Kd nuclear DNA-binding protein in erythropoietin-producing and nonproducing cells. *Blood* 82: 704–711, 1993.
28. Berger, M., F. W. Kemmer, K. Becker, L. Herberg, M. Schwenen, A. Gjinavci, and P. Berchtold. Effect of physical training on glucose tolerance and on glucose metabolism of skeletal muscle in anaesthetized normal rats. *Diabetologia* 16: 179–184, 1979.
29. Betz, H., and J.-P. Changeux. Regulation of muscle acetylcholine receptor synthesis in vitro by cyclic nucleotide derivatives. *Nature* 278: 749–752, 1979.
30. Bohm, M., H. Dorner, P. Htun, H. Lensche, D. Platt, and E. Erdmann. Effects of exercise on myocardial adenylate cyclase and G_i alpha expression in senescence. *Am. J. Physiol.* 264 (*Heart Circ. Physiol.* 33): H805–H814, 1993.
31. Boissonneault, G., J. Gagnon, M. A. Ho-Kim, and R. R. Tremblay. Lack of effect of anabolic steroids on specific mRNAs of skeletal muscle undergoing compensatory hypertrophy. *Mol. Cell. Endocrinol.* 51: 19–24, 1987.
32. Booth, F. W. Cytochrome c protein synthesis rate in rat skeletal muscle. *J. Appl. Physiol.* 71: 1225–1230, 1991.
33. Booth, F. W., and K. A. Narahara. Vastus lateralis cytochrome oxidase activity and its relationship to maximal oxygen consumption in man. *Pflugers Arch.* 349: 319–324, 1974.
34. Booth, F. W., and D. B. Thomason. Molecular and cellular adaptation of muscle in response to exercise: perspectives of various models. *Physiol. Rev.* 71: 541–585, 1991.
35. Booth, F. W., and P. A. Watson. Control of adaptations in protein levels in response to exercise. *Federation Proc.* 44: 2293–2300, 1985.

36. Borensztajn, J., M. S. Rone, S. P. Babirak, J. A. McGarr, and L. B. Oscai. Effect of exercise on lipoprotein lipase activity in rat heart and skeletal muscle. *Am. J. Physiol.* 229: 394–397, 1975.
37. Braun, T., E. Bober, B. Winter, N. Rosenthal, and H. H. Arnold. Myf-6, a new member of the human gene family of myogenic determination factors: evidence for a gene cluster on chromosome 12. *EMBO J.* 9: 821–831, 1990.
38. Braun, T., G. Buschhausen-Denker, G. Bober, E. Tannich, and H. H. Arnold. A novel human muscle factor related to but distinct from MyoD1 induces myogenic conversion in 10T1/2 fibroblasts. *EMBO J.* 8: 701–709, 1989.
39. Brodie, C., M. Brody, and S. R. Simpson. Characterization of the relation between sodium channels and electrical activity in cultured rat skeletal myotubes: regulatory aspects. *Brain Res.* 488: 186–194, 1989.
40. Brown, M. D., M. A. Cotter, O. Hudlicka, and G. Vrbova. The effects of different patterns of muscle activity on capillary density, mechanical properties and structure of slow and fast rabbit muscles. *Pflugers Arch.* 361: 241–250, 1976.
41. Buchner, D. M., and E. H. Wagner. Preventing frail health. *Clin. Geriatr. Med.* 8: 1–17, 1992.
42. Buckenmeyer, P. J., A. H. Goldfarb, J. S. Partilla, M. A. Pineyro, and E. M. Dax. Endurance training, not acute exercise, differentially alters beta receptors and cyclase in skeletal muscle fiber types. *Am. J. Physiol.* 258 (*Endocrinol. Metab.* 21): E71–E77, 1990.
43. Caiozzo, V. J., M. J. Baker, R. E. Herrick, M. Tao, and K. M. Baldwin. Effect of spaceflight on skeletal muscle: mechanical properties and myosin isoform content of a slow antigravity muscle. *J. Appl. Physiol.* 76: 1764–1773, 1994.
44. Caiozzo, V. J., F. Haddad, M. J. Baker, and K. M. Baldwin. The influence of mechanical loading on myosin heavy chain protein and mRNA expression. *J. Appl. Physiol.* (in press).
45. Caiozzo, V. J., R. E. Herrick, and K. M. Baldwin. The influence of hyperthyroidism on the maximal shortening velocity and myosin isoform distribution in slow and fast skeletal muscle. *Am. J. Physiol.* 261 (*Cell Physiol.* 30): C285–C295, 1991.
46. Caiozzo, V. J., R. E. Herrick, and K. M. Baldwin. Response of slow and fast skeletal muscle to hypothyroidism; maximal shortening velocity and myosin isoforms. *Am. J. Physiol.* 263 (*Cell Physiol.* 32): C86–C94, 1992.
47. Caiozzo, V. J., E. Ma, S. A. McCue, R. E. Herrick, and K. M. Baldwin. A new animal model for modulating myosin isoform expression by mechanical activity. *J. Appl. Physiol.* 73: 1432–1440, 1992.
48. Caiozzo, V. J., S. Swoap, M. Tao, R. Vandergriff, D. B. Menzel, and K. M. Baldwin. Quantitative single fiber analysis of type IIA myosin heavy chain distribution in hyper and hypothyroid soleus. *Am. J. Physiol.* 265 (*Cell Physiol.* 34): C842–C849, 1993.
49. Carson, J. A., Z. Yan, R. J. Schwartz, F. W. Booth, and C. S. Stump. Regulation of skeletal α-actin promotor in young chickens during hypertrophy caused by stretch overload. *Am. J. Physiol.* 268 (*Cell Physiol.* 37): C918–C929, 1995.
50. Chahine, K. G., E. Baracchini, and D. Goldman. Coupling muscle electrical activity to gene expression via a cAMP-dependent second messenger system. *J. Biol. Chem.* 268: 2893–2898, 1993.
51. Chahine, K. G., W. Walke, and D. Goldman. A 102 base pair sequence of the nicotinic acetylcholine receptor delta-subunit gene confers regulation by muscle electrical activity. *Development* 115: 213–219, 1992.
52. Chalmers, G. R., R. R. Roy, and V. R. Edgerton. Adaptability of the oxidative capacity of motoneurons. *Brain Res.* 570: 1–10, 1992.
53. Charron, M. J., F. C. Brosius, S. L. Alper, and H. F. Lodish. A glucose transport protein expressed predominately in insulin-responsive tissues. *Proc. Natl. Acad. Sci. U. S. A.* 86: 2535–2539, 1989.
54. Chesley, A., J. D. MacDougall, M. A. Tarnopolsky, S. A. Atkinson, and K. Smith. Changes in human muscle protein synthesis after resistance exercise. *J. Appl. Physiol.* 73: 1383–1388, 1992.
55. Christensen, E. H., and O. Hansen. Arbeitsfahigkeit und ehrnahrung. *Scand. Arch. Physiol.* 81: 160–175, 1939.
56. Clausen, J. P. Effect of physical training on cardiovascular adjustments to exercise in man. *Physiol. Rev.* 57: 779–815, 1977.
57. Cleland, P. J., G. J. Appleby, S. Rattigan, and M. G. Clark. Exercise-induced translocation of protein kinase C and production of diacylglycerol and phosphatic acid in rat skeletal muscle in vivo. *J. Biol. Chem.* 264: 17704–17711, 1989.
58. Colmenares, C., and E. Stavnezer. The *ski* oncogene induces muscle differentiation in quail embryo cells. *Cell* 59: 293–303, 1989.
59. Condon, K., L. Siberstein, H. M. Blau, and W. J. Thompson. Development of muscle fiber types in prenatal rat hindlimb. *Dev. Biol.* 138: 256–274, 1990.
60. Condon, K., L. Silberstein, H. M. Blau, and W. J. Thompson. Differentiation of fiber-types in aneural musculature of prenatal rat hindlimb. *Dev. Biol.* 138: 275–295, 1990.
61. Cowan, D. B., R. D. Weisel, W. G. Williams, and D. A. G. Mickle. Identification of oxygen responsive elements in the 5′-flanking region of the human glutathione peroxidase gene. *J. Biol. Chem.* 268: 26904–26910, 1993.
62. Coyle, E. F., M. T. Hamilton, J. G. Alonso, S. J. Montain, and J. L. Ivy. Carbohydrate metabolism during intense exercise when hyperglycemic. *J. Appl. Physiol.* 70: 834–840, 1991.
63. Craig, E. A., B. D. Gambill, and R. J. Nelson. Heat shock proteins: molecular chaperones of protein biogenesis. *Microbiol. Rev.* 57: 402–414, 1993.
64. Davies, H. L., R. G. Whalen, and B. A. Demeneix. Direct gene transfer into skeletal muscle in vivo: factors affecting efficiency of transfer and stabilty of expression. *Hum. Gene Ther.* 4: 151–159, 1993.
65. Davies, K. J. A., L. Packer, and G. A. Brooks. Biochemical adaptation of mitochondria, muscle, and whole animal respiration to endurance training. *Arch. Biochem. Biophys.* 209: 539–554, 1981.
66. Davies, K. J. A., A. T. Quintanilda, G. A. Brooks, and L. Packer. Free radicals and tissue damage produced by exercise. *Biochem. Biophys. Res. Commun.* 107: 1198–1205, 1982.
67. Davis, R. L., H. Weintaub, and A. B. Lasser. Expression of a single transfected cDNA converts fibroblasts to myoblasts. *Cell* 51: 987–1000, 1987.
68. Denardi, C., S. Ausoni, P. Moretti, L. Gorza, M. Velleca, M. Buckingham, and S. Schiaffino. Type 2X-myosin heavy chain is coded by a muscle fiber-type-specific and developmentally regulated gene. *J. Cell Biol.* 123: 823–835, 1993.
69. deQuiroga, G. B. Brown fat thermogenesis and exercise: two examples of physiological oxidative stress? *Free Rad. Biol. Med.* 13: 325–340, 1992.
70. DeVol, D. L., P. Rotwein, J. L. Sadow, J. Novakoski, and P. J. Bechtel. Activation of insulin-like growth factor gene expression during work-induced skeletal muscle growth.

Am. J. Physiol. 259 (*Endocrinol. Metab.* 22): E89–E95, 1990.
71. Diffee, G. M., V. J. Caiozzo, R. E. Herrick, and K. M. Baldwin. Contractile and biochemical properties of rat soleus and plantaris following hindlimb suspension. *Am. J. Physiol.* 260 (*Cell Physiol.* 29): C528–C534, 1991.
72. Diffee, G. M., V. J. Caiozzo, S. A. McCue, R. E. Herrick, and K. M. Baldwin. Activity-induced regulation of myosin isoform distribution: comparison of two contractile activity programs. *J. Appl. Physiol.* 74: 2509–2516, 1993.
73. Diffee, G. M., F. Haddad, R. E. Herrick, and K. M. Baldwin. Control of myosin heavy chain expression: interaction of hypothyroidism and hindlimb suspension. *Am. J. Physiol.* 261 (*Cell Physiol.* 30): C1099–C1106, 1991.
74. Diffee, G. M., S. McCue, A. LaRossa, R. E. Herrick, and K. M. Baldwin. Interaction of various activity models in the regulation of myosin heavy chain isoform expression. *J. Appl. Physiol.* 74: 2517–2522, 1993.
75. Dillman, W. H. Diabetes mellitus and hypothyroidism induce changes in myosin isoenzyme distribution in the rat heart—do alterations in fuel flux mediate these changes? *Adv. Exp. Med. Biol.* 194: 469–479, 1986.
76. Dix, D. J., and B. R. Eisenberg. Myosin mRNA accumulation and myofibrillogenesis at the myotendinous junction of stretched muscle fibers. *J. Cell Biol.* 111: 1885–1894, 1990.
77. Dohm, G. L., E. B. Tapscott, and G. J. Kasperek. Protein degradation during endurance exercise and recovery. *Med. Sci. Sports Exerc.* 19: S166–S171, 1987.
78. Douen, A. G., T. Ramlal, A. Klip, D. A. Young, G. D. Cartee, and J. O. Holloszy. Exercise-induced increase in glucose transporters in plasma membranes of rat skeletal muscle. *Endocrinology* 124: 449–454, 1989.
79. Douen, A. G., T. Ramlal, S. Rastogi, P. J. Bilan, G. D. Cartee, M. Vranic, J. O. Holloszy, and A. Klip. Exercise induces recruitment of the "insulin-responsive glucose transporter." *J. Biol. Chem.* 265: 13427–13430, 1990.
80. Drachman, D. B., and F. Witzke. Trophic regulation of acetylcholine sensitivity of muscle: effect of electrical stimulation. *Science* 176: 514–516, 1972.
81. Dudley, G. A., P. A. Tesch, B. J. Miller, and P. Buchannan. Importance of eccentric actions in performance adaptations to resistance training. *Aviat. Space Environ. Med.* 62: 543–550, 1991.
82. Edgerton, V.R., and R.R. Roy. Regulation of skeletal muscle fiber size, shape and function. *J. Biomech.* 24 (Suppl. 1): 123–133, 1991.
83. Edmondson, D. G., and E. N. Olson. A gene with homology to the *myc* similarity region of MyoD1 is expressed during myogenesis and is sufficient to activiate the muscle differentiation program. *Genes Dev.* 3: 628–640, 1989.
84. Eftimie, E., H. R. Brenner, and A. Buonanno. Myogenin and MyoD join a family of skeletal muscle genes regulated by electrical activity. *Proc. Natl. Acad. Sci. U. S. A.* 88: 1349–1353, 1991.
85. Eisenberg, B. R., J. M. C. Brown, and S. Salmons. Restoration of fast muscle characteristics following cessation of chronic stimulation. *Cell Tiss. Res.* 238: 221–130, 1984.
86. Eisenberg, B. R., J. M. Kennedy, M. P. Wenderoth, and D. J. Dix. Satellite cells, isomyosin switching and muscle growth. In: *Cellular and Molecular Biology of Muscle Development*. New York: Alan R. Liss, 1989, p. 451–460.
87. Eppley, Z. A., J. Kim, and B. Russell. A myogenic regulatory gene, *qmf*1, is expressed by adult myonuclei after injury. *Am. J. Physiol.* 265 (*Cell Physiol.* 34): C397–C405, 1993.
88. Esser, K. A., and E. C. Hardeman. Changes in contractile protein mRNA accumulation in response to spaceflight. *Am. J. Physiol.* 268 (*Cell Physiol.* 37): C466–C471, 1995.
89. Essig, D. A., D. L. DeVol, P. J. Betchel, and T. J. Trannel. Expression of embryonic myosin heavy chain mRNA in stretched adult chicken skeletal muscle. *Am. J. Physiol.* 260 (*Cell Physiol.* 29): C1325–C1331, 1991.
90. Essig, D. A., D. A. Jackson, and D. R. Borger. A heme oxygenase mRNA is induced in skeletal muscle following 3 hours of nerve stimulation. *Med. Sci. Sports Exerc.* 26: 594, 1994.
91. Essig, D. A., J. M. Kennedy, and L. A. McNabney. Regulation of 5′-aminolevulinate synthase activity in overloaded skeletal muscle. *Am. J. Physiol.* 259 (*Cell Physiol.* 28): C310–C314, 1990.
92. Etgen, G. T., A. R. Memon, G. A. Thompson, Jr., and J. L. Ivy. Insulin- and contraction-stimulated translocation of GTP-binding proteins and GLUT4 protein in skeletal muscle. *J. Biol. Chem.* 268: 20164–20169, 1993.
93. Falduto, M. T., A. P. Young, and R. C. Hickson. Exercise inhibits glucocorticoid-induced glutamine synthatase expression in red skeletal muscles. *Am. J. Physiol.* 262 (*Cell Physiol.* 31): C214–C220, 1992.
94. Falduto, M. T., A. P. Young, and R. C. Hickson. Exercise interrupts ongoing glucocorticoid-induced muscle atrophy and gultamine synthetase induction. *Am. J. Physiol.* 263 (*Endocrinol. Metab.* 26): E1157–E1163, 1992.
95. Falduto, M. T., A. P. Young, G. Smyrniotis, and R. C. Hickson. Reduction of glutamine synthetase mRNA in hypertrophied skeletal muscle. *Am. J. Physiol.* 262 (*Regulatory Integrative Comp. Physiol.* 31): R1131–R1136, 1992.
96. Fiatarone, M. A., E. F. O'Neill, N. D. Ryan, K. M. Clements, G. R. Solares, M. E. Nelson, S. B. Roberts, J. J. Lipsitz, and W. J. Evans. Exercise training and nutritional supplements for physical frailty in very elderly people. *N. Engl. J. Med.* 330: 1769–1775, 1994.
97. Fitch, C. D., M. Jellinek, R. H. Fitts, K. M. Baldwin, and J. O. Holloszy. Phosphorylated β-guanidinopropionate as a substitute for phosphocreatine in rat muscle. *Am. J. Physiol.* 228: 1123–1125, 1975.
98. Fitch, C. D., M. Jellinek, and E. J. Mueller. Experimental depletion of creatine and phosphocreatine from skeletal muscle. *J. Biol. Chem.* 249: 1060–1063, 1974.
99. Fitts, R. H. Substrate supply and energy metabolism during brief high intensity exercise: importance in limiting performance. In: *Perspectives in Exercise Science and Sports Medicine*, edited by D. R. Lamb and C. V. Gisolfi. Indianapolis: Benchmark, 1992, p. 53–107.
100. Fitts, R. H., D. L. Costill, and P. R. Gardetto. Effect of swim training on human muscle fiber function. *J. Appl. Physiol.* 66: 465–475, 1989.
101. Fitts, R. H., W. W. Winder, M. H. Brooke, K. K. Kaiser, and J. O. Holloszy. Contractile, biochemical, and histochemical properties of thyrotoxic rat soleus muscle. *Am. J. Physiol.* 238 (*Cell Physiol.* 7): C15-C20, 1980.
102. Fitzsimons, D. P., G. M. Diffee, R. E. Herrick, and K. M. Baldwin. Effect of endurance exercise on isomyosin patterns in fast- and slow-twitch skeletal muscle. *J. Appl. Physiol.* 68: 1950–1955, 1990.
103. Flink, I. L., J. G. Edwards, J. J. Bahl, C. C. Liaw, M. Sole, and E. Mortin. Characterization of a strong positive cis element of the human beta-myosin heavy chain gene in fetal rat heart cells. *J. Biol. Chem.* 267: 9917–9924, 1992.
104. Flink, I. L., and E. Mortin. Interaction of thyroid hormone receptors with strong and weak cis acting elements in hu-

man alpha-myosin heavy chain gene promotor. *J. Biol. Chem.* 265: 11233–11237, 1990.
105. Freidman, J. E., W. M. Sherman, M. J. Reed, C. W. Elton, and G. L. Dohm. Exercise training increases glucose transporter protein GLUT-4 in skeletal muscle of obese Zucker (fa/fa) rats. *FEBS Lett.* 268: 13–16, 1990.
106. Frenzel, H., B. Schwartzkopff, W. Holtermann, H. G. Schurch, A. Novi, and W. Hort. Regression of cardiac hypertrophy: morphometric and biochemical studies in rat heart after swimming training. *J. Mol. Cell. Cardiol.* 20: 737–751, 1988.
107. Fushiki, T., J. A. Wells, E. B. Tapscott, and G. L. Dohm. Changes in glucose transporters in muscle in response to exercise. *Am. J. Physiol.* 256 (*Endocrinol. Metab.* 19): E580–E587, 1989.
108. Glatz, J. F. C., and G. J. ver der Vusse. Intracellular transport of lipids. *Mol. Cell. Biochem.* 88: 37–44, 1989.
109. Goldberg, A. L. Protein synthesis in tonic and phasic skeletal muscles. *Nature* 216: 1219–1220, 1967.
110. Goldberg, A. L., and J. F. Dice. Intracellular protein degradation in mammalian and bacterial cells. *Annu. Rev. Physiol.* 43: 835–869, 1974.
111. Goldberg, A. L., and H. M. Goodman. Relationship between cortisone and muscle work in determining muscle size. *J. Physiol. (Lond.)* 200: 667–675, 1969.
112. Goldberg, M. A., S. P. Dunning, and H. F. Bunn. Regulation of the erythropoietin gene: evidence that the oxygen sensor is a heme protein. *Science* 242: 1412–1415, 1988.
113. Goldman, D., H. R. Brenner, and S. Heineman. Acetylcholine receptor α-, β-, γ-, and δ-subunit mRNA levels are regulated by muscle activity. *Neuron* 1: 329–333, 1988.
114. Goldman, D., B. M. Carlson, and J. Staple. Induction of adult-type nicotinic acetylcholine receptor gene expression in noninnervated regenerating muscle. *Neuron* 7: 649–658, 1991.
115. Goldspink, D. F. Exercise-related changes in protein turnover in mammalian striated muscle. *J. Exp. Biol.* 160: 127–148, 1991.
116. Gollnick, P. D. Energy metabolism and prolonged exercise. In: *Perspectives in Exercise Science and Sports in Medicine. Prolonged Exercise*, edited by D. R. Lamb and R. Murray. Indianapolis: Benchmark, 1988, p. 1–37.
117. Gollnick, P. D., R. B. Armstrong, C. W. Saubert, K. Piehl, and B. Saltin. Enzyme activity and fiber composition in skeletal muscle of untrained and trained men. *J. Appl. Physiol.* 33: 312–319, 1972.
118. Gonyea, W. J., D. G. Sale, F. B. Gonyea, and A. Mikesky. Exercise induced increases in muscle fiber number. *Eur. J. Physiol.* 55: 137–141, 1986.
119. Goodyear, L. J., P. A. King, M. F. Hirshman, C. M. Thompson, E. D. Horton, and E. S. Horton. Contractile activity increases plasma membrane glucose transporters in absence of insulin. *Am. J. Physiol.* 258 (*Endocrinol. Metab.* 21): E667–E672, 1990.
120. Gopalakrishnan, L., and R. C. Scarpulla. Differential regulation of respiratory subunits by a CREB-dependent signal transduction pathway. *J. Biol. Chem.* 269: 105–113, 1994.
121. Gordon, T., and M. Pattullo. Plasticity of muscle fiber and motor unit types. *Exerc. Sports Sci. Rev.* 21: 331–362, 1993.
122. Gosselink, K. L., R. E. Grindeland, R. R. Roy, V. R. Muukku, R. J. Talmadge, V. R. Edgerton, and J. K. Linderman. Effects of growth hormone and insulin-like growth factor-I with or without exercise on hypophysectomized hindlimb suspended rats. *Am. J. Physiol.* 267 (*Regulator Integrative Comp. Physiol.* 38): R365–R371, 1994.
123. Gould, G. W., and G. D. Holman. The glucose transporter family: structure, function and tissue-specific expression. *Biochem. J.* 295: 329–341, 1993.
124. Green, H. J., H. Helyar, M. Ball-Burnett, N. Kowalchuk, S. Symon, and B. Farrance. Metabolic adaptations to training precede changes in muscle mitochondrial capacity. *J. Appl. Physiol.* 72: 484–491, 1992.
125. Green, H. J., G. A. Klug, H. Reichman, U. Seedorf, W. Wiehrer, and D. Pette. Exercise-induced fiber-type transitions with regard to myosin, parvalbumin, and sarcoplasmic reticulum in muscles of the rat. *Pflugers Arch.* 400: 432–438, 1984.
126. Haddad, F., R. E. Herrick, G. R. Adams, and K. M. Baldwin. Myosin heavy chain expression in rodent skeletal muscle: Effects of exposure to zero gravity. *J. Appl. Physiol.* 75: 2471–2477, 1993.
127. Hall, Z. W., and E. Ralston. Nuclear domains in muscle cells. *Cell* 59: 771–772, 1989.
128. Hartner, K. T., B. J. Kirschbaum, and D. Pette. The multiplicity of troponin T isoforms. Distribution on normal rabbit muscles and effects of chronic stimulation. *Eur. J. Biochem.* 179: 31–38, 1989.
129. Hartner, K. T., and D. Pette. Fast and slow isoforms of troponin I and troponin C. Distribution in normal rabbit muscles and effects of chronic stimulation. *Eur. J. Biochem.* 188: 261–267, 1990.
130. Heilig, A., and D. Pette. Albumin in rabbit skeletal muscle. Origin, distribution and regulation by contractile activity. *Eur. J. Biochem.* 171: 503–508, 1988.
131. Henriksen, E. J., R. E. Bourey, K. J. Rodnick, L. Koranyi, M. A. Permutt, and J. O. Holloszy. Glucose transporter protein content and glucose transport capacity in rat skeletal muscles. *Am. J. Physiol.* 259 (*Endocrinol. Metab.* 22): E593–E598, 1990.
132. Henriksen, E. J., K. J. Rodnick, and J. O. Holloszy. Activation of glucose transport in skeletal muscle by phospholipase C and phorbol ester. Evaluation of the regulatory roles of protein kinase C and calcium. *J. Biol. Chem.* 264: 21536–21543, 1989.
133. Henriksson, J. Effects of physical training on the metabolism of skeletal muscle. *Diabetes Care* 15 (Suppl. 4): 1701–1711, 1992.
134. Henriksson, J., M. M.-Y. Chi, C. S. Hintz, D. A. Young, K. K. Kaiser, S. Salmons, and O. H. Lowry. Chronic stimulation of mammalian muscle: changes in enzymes of six metabolic pathways. *Am. J. Physiol.* 251 (*Cell Physiol.* 20): C614–C632, 1986.
135. Hermansen, L., E. Hultman, and B. Saltin. Muscle glycogen during prolonged exercise. *Acta Physiol. Scand.* 71: 129–139, 1967.
136. Hershko, A., and A. Ciechanover. The ubiquitin system for protein degradation. *Annu. Rev. Biochem.* 61: 761–807, 1992.
137. Hickson, R. C. Interference of strength development by simultaneously training for strength and endurance. *Eur. J. Appl. Physiol.* 45: 255–263, 1980.
138. Hickson, R. C., and J. R. Marone. Exercise and inhibition of glucocorticoid induced muscle atrophy. *Exerc. Sport Sci. Rev.* 21: 135–167, 1993.
139. Hirshman, M. F., H. Wallberg-Henriksson, L. J. Wardzala, E. D. Horton, and E. S. Horton. Acute exercise increases the number of plasma membrane glucose transporters in rat skeletal muscle. *FEBS Lett.* 238: 235–239, 1988.
140. Hodin, R. A., M. A. Lazar, W. W. Chin. Differential and tissue-specific regulation of the multiple rat c-erbA messen-

ger RNA species by thyroid hormone. *J. Clin. Invest.* 85: 101–105, 1990.
141. Hodin, R. A., M. A. Lazar, B. I. Wintman, D. S. Darling, R. J. Koenig, P. R. Larsen, D. D. Moore, W. W. Chin. Identification of a thyroid hormone receptor that is pituitary-specific. *Science* 244: 76–79, 1989.
142. Hoffman, S. J., R. R. Roy, C. E. Blanco, and V. R. Edgerton. Enzyme profiles of single muscle fibers never exposed to neuromuscular activity. *J. Appl. Physiol.* 69: 1150–1158, 1990.
143. Holloszy, J. O. Biochemical adaptations in muscle: effects of exercise on mitochondrial oxygen uptake and respiratory enzyme activity in skeletal muscle. *J. Biol. Chem.* 242: 2278–2282, 1967.
144. Holloszy, J. O., and F. W. Booth. Biochemical adaptations to endurance exercise in muscle. *Annu. Rev. Biochem.* 38: 273–291, 1976.
145. Holloszy, J. O., S. H. Constable, and D. A. Young. Activation of glucose transport in muscle by exercise. *Diabetes Metab. Rev.* 1: 409–423, 1986.
146. Holloszy, J. O., and E. F. Coyle. Adaptations of skeletal muscle to endurance exercise and their metabolic consequences. *J. Appl. Physiol.* 56: 831–838, 1984.
147. Holloszy, J. O., L. B. Oscai, I. J. Don, and P. A. Mole. Mitochondrial citric acid cycle and related enzymes: adaptive response to exercise. *Biochem. Biophys. Res. Commun.* 40: 1368–1373, 1970.
148. Holloszy, J. O., and W. W. Winder. Induction of δ-aminolevulinic acid synthetase in muscle by exercise or thyroxine. *Am. J. Physiol.* 236 (*Regulatory Integrative Conp. Physiol.* 5): R180–R14, 1979.
149. Holm, J., P. Bjorntorp, and T. Schersten. Metabolic activity in rat skeletal muscle. *Eur. J. Clin. Invest.* 3: 279–283, 1973.
150. Hood, D. A., J. A. Simoneau, A. M. Kelly, and D. Pette. Effect of thyroid status on the expression of metabolic enzymes during chronic stimulation. *Am. J. Physiol.* 263 (*Cell Physiol.* 32): C788–C793, 1992.
151. Hood, D. A., R. Zak, and D. Pette. Chronic stimulation of rat skeletal muscle induces coordinate increases in mitochondrial and nuclear mRNAs of cytochrome-c-oxidase subunits. *Eur. J. Biochem.* 179: 275–280, 1989.
152. Hoppeler, H., and R. Billeter. Conditions for oxygen and substrate transport in muscles of exercising mammals. *J. Exp. Biol.* 160: 263–283, 1991.
153. Hoppeler, H., and S. R. Kayar. Capillary and oxidative capacity of muscles. *News Physiol. Sci.* 3: 113–116, 1988.
154. Howard, G., J. M. Steffen, and T. E. Geoghegan. Transcriptional regulation of decreased protein synthesis during skeletal muscle unloading. *J. Appl. Physiol.* 66: 1093–1098, 1989.
155. Huang, C. F., J. Tong, and J. Schmidt. Protein kinase C couples membrane excitation to acetylcholine receptor gene inactivation in chick skeletal muscle. *Neuron* 9: 671–678, 1992.
156. Hudlicka, O., M. Brown, and S. Egginton. Angiogenesis in skeletal and cardiac muscle. *Physiol. Rev.* 72: 369–417, 1992.
157. Hug, H., and T. F. Sarre. Protein kinase isoenzymes: divergence in signal transduction? *Biochem. J.* 291: 329–343, 1993.
158. Ianuzzo, C. D., and V. Chen. Metabolic character of hypertrophied rat muscle. *J. Appl. Physiol.* 46: 738–742, 1979.
159. Ianuzzo, C. D., N. Hamilton, and B. Li. Competitive control of myosin expression: hypertrophy and hyperthyroidism. *J. Appl. Physiol.* 70: 2328–2330, 1991.
160. Ianuzzo, C. D., N. Hamilton, P. J. O'Brien, C. Desrosiers, and R. Chur. Biochemical transformations of canine skeletal muscle for use in cardiac-assist devices. *J. Appl. Physiol.* 68: 1481–1485, 1990.
161. Imamura, S., R. Matsuoka, E. Hiratsuka, M. Kimura, T. Nakanishi, T. Nishikawa, Y. Furutani, and A. Takao. Adaptational changes of MHC gene expression and isozyme transition in cardiac overloading. *Am. J. Physiol.* 260 (*Heart Circ. Physiol.* 29): H73–H79, 1991.
162. Ivy, J. L. The insulin-like effect of muscle contraction. *Exerc. Sport Sci. Rev.* 15: 29–51, 1987.
163. Izawa, T., T. Komabayashi, K. Suda, Y. Kunisada, S. Shinoda, and M. Tsuboi. An acute exercise-induced translocation of beta-adrenergic receptors in rat myocardium. *J. Biochem. (Tokyo)* 105: 110–113, 1989.
164. Izumo, S., B. Nadal-Ginard, and V. Mahdavi. All members of the MHC multigene family respond to thyroid hormone in a highly tissue specific fashion. *Science* 231: 597–600, 1986.
165. Jacobs-El, J., M.-Y. Zhou, and B. Russell. MRF4, myf4 and myogenin mRNAs in the adaptive responses of mature rat muscle. *Am. J. Physiol.* 268 (*Cell Physiol.* 37): C1045–C1052, 1995.
166. James, D. E., E. W. Kraegen, and D. J. Chisholm. Effects of exercise training on in vivo insulin action in individual tissues of the rat. *J. Clin. Invest.* 76: 657–666, 1985.
167. James, D. E., M. Strube, and M. Mueckler. Molecular cloning and characterization of an insulin-regulatable glucose transporter. *Nature* 338: 83–87, 1989.
168. Janssen, Y. M. W., B. Van Houten, P. J. A. Borm, and B. T. Mossman. Biology of disease. Cell and tissue responses to oxidative damage. *Lab. Invest.* 69: 261–274, 1993.
169. Jansson, E., C. Sylven, and E. Nordevang. Myoglobin in the quadriceps femoris muscle of competitive cyclists and untrained men. *Acta Physiol. Scand.* 114: 627–629, 1982.
170. Jeffery, S., C. D. Kelly, N. Carter, M. Kaufmann, A. Termin, and D. Pette. Chronic stimulation-induced effects point to a coordinated expression of carbonic anhydrase III and slow myosin heavy chain in skeletal muscle. *FEBS Lett.* 262: 225–227, 1990.
171. Jelkmann, W. Erythropoietin: structure, control of production and function. *Physiol. Rev.* 72: 449–489, 1992.
172. Ji, L. L., D. L. F. Lennon, R. G. Kochan, F. J. Nagle, and H. A. Lardy. Enzymatic adaptation to physical training under β-blockade in the rat. Evidence of a β_2-adrenergic mechanism in skeletal muscle. *J. Clin. Invest.* 78: 771–778, 1986.
173. Jiang, B., Y. Ohira, R. R. Roy, Q. Nguyen, E. Ilyina-Kakueva, V. Oganov, and V. R. Edgerton. Adaptation of fibers in fast twitch muscle of rats to space flight and hindlimb suspension. *J. Appl. Physiol.* 73 (Suppl.): 585–655, 1992.
174. Jiang, B., R. R. Roy, and V. R. Edgerton. Enzymatic plasticity of medial gastroenemius fibers in the adult chronic spinal cat. *Am. J. Physiol.* 259 (*Cell Physiol.* 28): C507–C514, 1990.
175. Kandarian, S., S. O'Brien, K. Thomas, L. Schulte, and J. Navarro. Regulation of skeletal muscle dihydropyridine recptor gene expression by biomechanical unloading. *J. Appl. Physiol.* 72: 2510–2514, 1992.
176. Kandarian, S. C., and J. H. Williams. Contractile properties of skinned fibers from hypertrophied skeletal muscle. *Med. Sci. Sports Exerc.* 25: 999–1004, 1993.

177. Kaufmann, M., J.-A. Simoneau, J. H. Veerkamp, and D. Pette. Electrostimulation-induced increases in fatty acid-binding protein and myoglobin in rat fast-twitch muscle and comparison with tissue levels in heart. *FEBS Lett.* 245: 181–184, 1989.
178. Kern, M., J. A. Wells, J. M. Stephens, C. W. Elton, J. E. Friedman, E. B. Tapscott, P. H. Pekala, and G. L. Dohm. Insulin responsiveness in skeletal muscle is determined by glucose transporter (GLUT4) protein level. *Biochem. J.* 270: 397–400, 1990.
179. Keyser, B., H. Hoppeler, H. Clausen, and P. Cerretelli. Muscle structure and performance capacity of Himalayan Sherpas. *J. Appl. Physiol.* 70: 1938–1942, 1991.
180. Kilgore, J. L., B. F. Timson, D. K. Saunders, R. R. Kraemer, R. D. Klemm, and C. R. Ross. Stress protein induction in skeletal muscle: comparison of laboratory models to naturally occurring hypertrophy. *J. Appl. Physiol.* 76: 598–601, 1994.
181. King, P. A., M. F. Hirshman, E. D. Horton, and E. S. Horton. Glucose transport in skeletal muscle vesicles from control and exercised rats. *Am. J. Physiol.* 257 (*Cell Physiol.* 26): C1128–C1134, 1989.
182. Kirschbaum, B. J., A. Heilig, K. T. Hartner, and D. Pette. Electrostimulation-induced fast-to-slow transitions of myosin light and heavy chains in rabbit fast-twitch muscle at the mRNA level. *FEBS Lett.* 243: 123–126, 1989.
183. Kirschbaum, B. J., S. Schneider, S. Izumo, V. Mahdavi, B. Nadal-Ginard, and D. Pette. Rapid and reversible changes in myosin heavy chain expression in response to increased neuromuscular activity of rat fast-twitch muscle. *FEBS Lett.* 268: 75–78, 1990.
184. Kirschbaum, B. J., J. A. Simoneau, P. J. R. Barton, M. E. Buckingham, and D. Pette. Chronic stimulation-induced changes of myosin light chains at the mRNA level and protein levels in rat fast-twitch muscle. *Eur. J. Biochem.* 179: 23–29, 1989.
185. Kirschbaum, B. J., J. A. Simoneau, A. Bar, P. J. Barton, M. E. Buckingham, and D. Pette. Chronic stimulation-induced changes of myosin light chains at the mRNA and protein levels in rat fast-twitch muscle. *Eur. J. Biochem.* 179: 23–29, 1989.
186. Kirschbaum, B. J., H. B. Kucher, A. Termin, A. M. Kelley, and D. Pette. Antagonistic effects of chronic low frequency stimulation and thyroid hormone on myosin expression in rat fast-twitch muscle. *J. Biol. Chem.* 265: 13974–13980, 1990
187. Kitsis, R. N., P. M. Buttrick, E. M. McNally, M. L. Kaplan, and L. A. Leinwand. Hormonal modulation of a gene injected into rat heart in vivo. *Proc. Natl. Acad. Sci. U. S. A.* 88: 4138–4142, 1991.
188. Kjaer, M. Exercise effects on adrenergic regulation of energy metabolism. *Perspect. Exerc. Sci. Sports Med.* 5: 345–381, 1992.
189. Klarsfeld, A., and J.-P. Changeux. Activity regulates the levels of acetylcholine receptor α-subunit mRNA in cultured chicken myotubes. *Proc. Natl. Acad. Sci. U. S. A.* 82: 4558–4562, 1985.
190. Klug, G., H. Reichman, and D. Pette. Rapid reduction in parvalbumin concentration during chronic stimulation of rabbit fast-twitch muscle. *FEBS Lett.* 152: 180–182, 1983.
191. Koivisto, V. A., R. E. Bourey, H. Vuorinen-Markkola, and L. Koranyi. Exercise reduces muscle glucose transport protein (GLUT-4) mRNA in type 1 diabetic patients. *J. Appl. Physiol.* 74: 1755–1760, 1993.
192. Kornig, R. J., R. L. Warne, G. A. Brent, J. W. Harney, P. R. Larsen, and D. D. Moore. Isolation of a cDNA clone encoding a biologically active thyroid hormone receptor. *Proc. Natl. Acad. Sci. U. S. A.* 85: 5031–5035, 1988.
193. Koskinen, P. J., and K. Alitalo. Role of myc amplification and overexpression in cell growth, differentiation and death. *Semin. Cancer Biol.* 4: 3–12, 1993.
194. Kourembanas, S., R. L. Hannan, and D. V. Faller. Oxygen tension regulates the expression of the platelet-derived growth factor-B chain gene in human endothelial cells. *J. Clin. Invest.* 86: 670–674, 1990.
195. Kourembanas, S., P. A. Marsden, L. P. McQuillan, and D. V. Faller. Hypoxia induces endothelin gene expression and secretion in cultured human endothelium. *J. Clin. Invest.* 88: 1054–1057, 1991.
196. Kraemer, W. J., J. F. Patton, S. E. Gordon, E. A. Harman, M. R. Deschenes, K. Reynolds, R. U. Newton, N. T. Triplett, and J. E. Dziados. Compatibility of high intensity strength and endurance training on hormonal and skeletal muscle adaptations. *J. Appl. Physiol.* 78: 976–989, 1995.
197. Kraus, W. E., T. S. Bernard, and R. S. Williams. Interactions between sustained contractile activity and β-adrenergic receptors in regulation of gene expression in skeletal muscles. *J. Appl. Physiol.* 256 (*Cell Physiol.* 25): C506–C514, 1989.
198. Kraus, W. E., J. P. Longabaugh, and S. B. Liggett. Electrical pacing induces adenylyl cyclase in skeletal muscle independent of the β-adrenergic receptor. *Am. J. Physiol.* 263 (*Endocrinol. Metab.* 26): E226–E230, 1992.
199. Ku, Z., and D. B. Thomason. Soleus muscle nascent polypeptide chain elongation slows protein synthesis rate during non-weightbearing. *Am. J. Physiol.* (in press).
200. Kubo, K., and J. E. Foley. Rate-limiting steps for insulin-mediated glucose uptake into perfused rat hindlimb. *Am. J. Physiol.* 250 (*Endocrinol. Metab.* 13): E100–E102, 1986.
201. Ladoux, A., and C. Frelin. Hypoxia is a strong inducer of vascular endothelial growth factor mRNA expression in the heart. *Biochem. Biophys. Res. Commun.* 195: 1005–1010, 1993.
202. Ladu, M. J., H. Kapsas, and W. K. Palmer. Regulation of lipoprotein lipase in muscle and adipose tissue during exercise. *J. Appl. Physiol.* 71: 404–409, 1991.
203. Lai, M. M., and F. W. Booth. Cytochrome c mRNA and β-actin mRNA in muscles of rats fed β-GPA. *J. Appl. Physiol.* 69: 843–848, 1990.
204. Larson, L., L. Edstrom, B. Lindergren, L. Gorza, and S. Schiaffino. MHC composition and enzyme-histochemical and physiological properties of a novel fast-twitch motor unit type. *Am. J. Physiol.* 261 (*Cell Physiol.* 30): C93–C101, 1991.
205. Laughlin, M. H., and R. B. Armstrong. Muscle blood flow during locomotory exercise. *Exerc. Sports Sci. Rev.* 13: 95–136, 1985.
206. Laurent, G. J., M. P. Sparrow, P. C. Bates, and D. J. Millward. Turnover of muscle protein in the fowl. Changes in rates of protein synthesis and breakdown during hypertrophy of the anterior and posterior latissimus dorsi muscles. *Biochem. J.* 176: 407–417, 1978.
207. Lazar, M. A., R. A. Hodin, and W. W. Chin. Human carboxyl-terminal variant of alpha-type c-erbA inhibits transactivation by thyroid hormone receptors without binding thyroid hormone. *Proc. Natl. Acad. Sci. U. S. A.* 86: 7771–7774, 1989.
208. Lazar, M. A., R. A. Hodin, D. S. Darling, and W. W. Chin. A novel member of the thyroid/steroid hormone receptor family is encoded by the opposite strand of the rat c-erbA

alpha transcriptional unit. *Mol. Cell. Biol.* 9: 1128–1136, 1989.

209. Leberer, E., K. T. Hartner, C. Brande, J. Fujii, M. Tada, D. MacLennan, and D. Pette. Slow/cardiac sarcoplasmic reticulum calcium ATPase and phospholamban mRNAs are expressed in chronically stimulated rabbit fast-twitch muscle. *Eur. J. Biochem.* 185: 51–54, 1989.
210. Leberer, E., U. Seedorf, and D. Pette. Neural contol of gene expression in skeletal muscle. Calcium-sequestering proteins in developing and chronically stimulated rabbit skeletal muscles. *Biochem. J.* 239: 195–300, 1986.
211. Leeuw, T., and D. Pette. Coordinate changes in the expression of troponin subunit and myosin heavy-chain isoforms during fast-to-slow transition of low-frequency-stimulated rabbit muscle. *Eur. J. Biochem.* 213: 1039–1046, 1993.
212. Li, Y., C. Magarian, J. K. Teumer, and E. Stavnezer. Unique sequence, *ski*, in Sloan-Kettering avian retroviruses with properties of a new cell-derived oncogene. *J. Virol.* 57: 1065–1072, 1986.
213. Locke, M., E. G. Noble, and B. G. Atkinson. Exercising mammals synthesize stress proteins. *Am. J. Physiol.* 258 (*Cell Physiol.* 27): C723–C729, 1990.
214. Locke, M., E. G. Noble, and B. G. Atkinson. Inducible isoform of HSP70 is constitutively expressed in a muscle fiber type specific pattern. *Am. J. Physiol.* 261 (*Cell Physiol.* 30): C774–C779, 1991.
215. Lomo, T., and J. Rosenthal. Control of ACh sensitivity by muscle activity in the rat. *J. Physiol. (Lond.)* 221: 493–513, 1972.
216. Luginbuhl, A. J., G. A. Dudley, and R. S. Staron. Fiber type changes in rat skeletal muscle after intense interval training. *Histochemistry* 81: 55–58, 1984.
217. MacDougall, J. D., D. G. Sale, J. R. Moroz, G. C. B. Elder, J. R. Sutton, and H. Howald. Mitochondrial volume density in human skeletal muscle following heavy resistance training. *Med. Sci. Sports Exerc.* 11: 164–166, 1979.
218. MacDougall, J. D., M. A. Tarnopoolsky, A. Chesley, and S. A. Atkinson. Changes in muscle protein synthesis following heavy exercise in humans: a pilot study. *Acta Physiol. Scand.* 146: 403–404, 1992.
219. Mahdavi, V., S. Izumo, and B. Nadal-Ginard. Development and hormonal regulation of sarcomeric myosin heavy chain gene family. *Circ. Res.* 60: 804–814, 1987.
220. Manthorpe, M., F. Cornefert-Jensen, J. Hartkka, J. Felgner, A. Rundell, M. Margalith, and V. Dwarki. Gene therapy by intramuscular injection of plasmid DNA: studies on firefly luciferase gene expression in mice. *Hum. Gene Ther.* 4: 419–431, 1993.
221. Marshall, B. W., J.-M. Ren, D. W. Johnson, E. M. Gibbs, J. S. Lillquist, W. C. Soeller, J. O. Holloszy, and M. Mueckler. Germline manipulation of glucose homeostasis via alteration of glucose transporter levels in skeletal muscle. *J. Biol. Chem.* 268: 18442–18445, 1993.
222. Martin, T. P., V. R. Edgerton, and R. E. Grindeland. Influence of spaceflight on rat skeletal muscle. *J. Appl. Physiol.* 65: 2318–2325, 1988.
223. Mayne, C. N., T. Morkrush, C. Jarvis, J. J. Gilroy, and S. Salmons. Stimulation induced expression of slow muscle myosin in a fast muscle of the rat. *FEBS Lett.* 327: 297–300, 1993.
224. McMahon, A. P., and A. Bradley. The *nt-1 (int-1)* proto-oncogene is required for development of a large region of the mouse brain. *Cell* 62: 1073–1085, 1990.
225. Meichle, A., A. Philipp, and M. Eilers. The functions of Myc proteins. *Biochim. Biophys. Acta* 1114: 129–146, 1992.
226. Merlie, J. P., and J. M. Kornhauser. Neural regulation of gene expression by an acetylcholine receptor promoter in muscle of transgenic mice. *Neuron* 2: 1295–1300, 1989.
227. Merlie, J. P., J. Mudd, T. S. Cheng, and E. N. Olsen. Myogenin and acetylcholine receptor α gene promoters mediate transcriptional regulation in response to motor innervation. *J. Biol. Chem.* 269: 2461–2467, 1994.
228. Metzger, J. M. Mechanism of chemomechanical coupling in skeletal muscle during work. In: *Perspectives in Exercise Science and Sports Medicine*, edited by D. R. Lamb and C. V. Gisolfi. Indianapolis: Benchmark, 1992, p. 1–52.
229. Mikesky, A. E., W. Mathews, C. J. Giddings, and W. S. Gonyea. Muscle enlargement and exercise performance in the cat. *J. Appl. Sport Sci. Res.* 3: 85–92, 1989.
230. Milano, C. A., L. F. Allen, H. A. Rockman, P. C. Dolber, T. R. McMinn, K. R. Chien, T. D. Johnson, R. A. Bond, and R. J. Lefkowitz. Enhanced myocardial function in transgenic mice overexpressing the beta 2-adrenergic receptor. *Science* 264: 582–586, 1994.
231. Miller, W. C., R. C. Hickson, and N. B. Bass. Fatty acid binding protein in the three types of rat skeletal muscle. *Proc. Soc. Exp. Biol. Med.* 189: 183–188, 1988.
232. Millward, D. J. Protein turnover in cardiac and skeletal muscle during normal growth and hypertrophy. In: *Degradative Processes in Heart and Skeletal Muscle*, edited by K. Wildenthal. Amersterdam: Elsevier/North Holland, 1980, p. 161–199.
233. Miner, J. H., and B. Wold. Herculin, a fourth member of the *MyoD* family of myogenic regulatory genes. *Proc. Natl. Acad. Sci. U. S. A.* 87: 1089–1093, 1990.
234. Mitsuhashi, T., G. E. Tennyson, and V. M. Nikodem. Alternative splicing generates messages encoding rat c-erbA proteins that do not bind thyroid hormone. *Proc. Natl. Acad. Sci. U. S. A.* 85: 5804–5808, 1988.
235. Moerland, T. S., N. G. Wolfe, and M. J. Kushmerick. Administration of a creatine analogue induces isomyosin transitions in muscle. *Am. J. Physiol.* 257 (*Cell Physiol.* 26): C810–C816, 1989.
236. Mole, P. A., L. B. Oscai, and J. O. Holloszy. Adaptation to exercise: increase in levels of palmityl CoA synthetase, carnitine palmityltransferase, and palmityl CoA dehydrogenase, and in the capacity to oxidase fatty acids. *J. Clin. Invest.* 50: 2323–2330, 1971.
237. Mondon, C. E., C. B. Dolkas, and G. M. Reaven. Site of enhanced insulin sensitivity in exercise-trained rats at rest. *Am. J. Physiol.* 239 (*Endocrinol. Metab.* 2): E169–E177, 1980.
238. Morrison, P. R., R. B. Biggs, and F. W. Booth. Daily running for 2 wk and mRNAs for cytochrome c and α-actin mRNA. *Am. J. Physiol.* 257 (*Cell Physiol.* 26): C936–C939, 1989.
239. Morrison, P. R., J. A. Montgomery, T. S. Wong, and F. W. Booth. Cytochrome c protein-synthesis rates and mRNA contents during atrophy and recovery in skeletal muscle. *Biochem. J.* 241: 257–263, 1987.
240. Morrison, P. R., G. W. Muller, and F. W. Booth. Actin synthesis rate and mRNA level increase during early recovery of atrophied muscle. *Am. J. Physiol.* 253 (*Cell Physiol.* 22): C205–C209, 1987.
241. Morrow, N. G., W. E. Kraus, J. W. Moore, R. S. Williams, and J. L. Swain. Increased expression of fibroblast growth factors in a rabbit muscle model of exercise conditioning. *J. Clin. Invest.* 85: 1816–1820, 1990.
242. Murray, M. B., N. D. Zilz, N. L. McCreary, M. J. MacDonald, and H. C. Towle. Isolation and characterization

of rat cDNA clones for two distinct thyroid hormone receptors. *J. Biol. Chem.* 263: 12770–12777, 1988.
243. Murre, C., P. Schonleber McCaw, H. Vaessin, M. Caudy, L. Y. Jan, Y. N. Jan, C. V. Buskin, S. D. Hauschka, A. B. Lasser, H. Weintaub, and D. Baltimore. Interactions between heterologous helix-loop-helix proteins generate complexes that bind specifically to a common DNA sequence. *Cell* 58: 537–544, 1989.
244. Neufer, P. D., and G. L. Dohm. Exercise induces a transient increase in transcription of the GLUT-4 gene in skeletal muscle. *Am. J. Physiol.* 265 (*Cell Physiol.* 34): C1597–C1603, 1993.
245. Neupert, W., and N. Pfanner. Roles of molecular chaperones in protein targeting to mitochondria. *Philos. Trans. R. Soc. Lond. Biol.* 339: 355–361, 1993.
246. O'Doherty, R. M., D. P. Bracy, H. Osawa, D. H. Wasserman, and D. K. Granner. Rat skeletal muscle hexokinase II mRNA and activity are increased by a single bout of exercise. *Am. J. Physiol.* 266 (*Endocrinol. Metab.* 29): E171–E178, 1994.
247. Ohira, Y., B. Jiang, R. R. Roy, V. Oganov, E. Ilyina-Kakueva, J. F. Marine, and V. R. Edgerton. Rat soleus muscle fiber responses to 14 days of spaceflight and hindlimb suspension. *J. Appl. Physiol.* 73 (Suppl.): 515–575, 1992.
248. Ojamaa, K., and I. Klein. Thyroid hormone regulation of alpha-myosin heavy chain promoter activity assessed by in vivo DNA transfer in rat heart. *Biochem. Biophys. Res. Commun.* 179: 1269–1275, 1991.
249. Olson, E. N. MyoD family: a paradigm for development? *Genes Dev.* 4: 2104–2111, 1990.
250. Packer, L. Protective role of vitamin E in biological systems. *Am. J. Clin. Nutr.* 53: 1050S 1055S, 1991.
251. Patapoutian, A., J. H. Miner, G. E. Lyons, and B. Wold. Isolated sequences from the linked *Myf-5* and *MRF4* genes drive distinct patterns of muscle-specific expression intransgenic mice. *Development* 118: 61–68, 1993.
252. Pattengale, P. K., and J. O. Holloszy. Augmentation of skeletal muscle myoglobin by a program of treadmill running. *Am. J. Physiol.* 213: 783–785, 1967.
253. Periasamy, M., P. Gregory, B. J. Martin, and W. S. Stirewalt. Regulation of myosin heavy chain gene expression during skeletal-muscle hypertrophy. *Biochem. J.* 257: 691–698, 1989.
254. Pette, D. Activity induced fast to slow transitions in mammalian muscle. *Med. Sci. Sports Exerc.* 16: 517–528, 1984.
255. Pette, D., and R. S. Staron. Cellular and molecular diversities of mammalian muscle fibers. *Rev. Physiol. Biochem. Pharmacol.* 116: 1–76, 1990.
256. Ploug, T., H. Galbo, and E. A. Richter. Increased muscle glucose uptake during contractions: no need for insulin. *Am. J. Physiol.* 247 (*Endocrinol. Metab.* 10): E726–E731, 1984.
257. Ploug, T., B. M. Stallknecht, O. Petersen, B. B. Kahn, T. Ohkuwa, J. Vinten, and H. Galbo. Effect of endurance training on glucose transport capacity and glucose transporter expression in rat skeletal muscle. *Am. J. Physiol.* 259 (*Endocrinol. Metab.* 22): E778–E786, 1990.
258. Plourde, G., S. Rousseau-Migneron, and A. Nadeau. Effect of endurance training on β-adrenergic system in three different skeletal muscles. *J. Appl. Physiol.* 74: 1641–1646, 1993.
259. Powers, S. K., D. Criswell, J. Lawler, L. L. Ji, D. Martin, R. A. Herb, and G. Dudley. Influence of exercise and fiber type on antioxidant enzyme activity in rat skeletal muscle. *Am. J. Physiol.* 266 (*Regulatory Integrative Comp. Physiol.* 35): R375–R380, 1994.
260. Reichmann, H., R. Wast, J.-A. Simineau, and D. Pette. Enzyme activities of fatty acid oxidation and the respiratory chain in chronically stimulated fast-twitch muscle of the rabbit. *Pflugers Arch.* 418: 572–574, 1991.
261. Reiser, P. J., R. L. Moss, G. G. Giulian, and M. L. Greaser. Shortening velocity in single fibers from adult rabbit soleus muscle is correlated with myosin heavy chain composition. *J. Biol. Chem.* 260: 9077–9080, 1985.
262. Ren, J.-M., B. A. Marshall, E. A. Gulve, J. Gao, D. W. Johnson, J. O. Holloszy, and M. Mueckler. Evidence from transgenic mice that glucose transport is rate-limiting for glycogen deposition and glycolysis in skeletal muscle. *J. Biol. Chem.* 268: 16113–16115, 1993.
263. Ren, J.-M., C. F. Semenkovich, and J. O. Holloszy. Adaptation of muscle to creatine depletion: effect on GLUT4 glucose transporter expression. *Am. J. Physiol.* 264 (*Cell Physiol.* 33): C146–C150, 1993.
264. Rhodes, S. J., and S. F. Konieczny. Identification of MRF4: a new member of the muscle regulatory factor gene family. *Genes Dev.* 3: 2050–2061, 1989.
265. Richter, E. A., P. J. Cleland, S. Rattigan, and M. G. Clark. Contraction-associated translocation of protein kinase C in rat skeletal muscle. *FEBS Lett.* 217: 232–236, 1987.
266. Riley, D. A., J. L.W . Bain, S. Ellis, and A. L. Haas. Quantitation and immunocytochemical localization of ubiquitin conjugates within rat red and white skeletal muscles. *J. Histochem. Cytochem.* 36: 621–632, 1988.
267. Riley, D. A., S. Ellis, C. S. Giometti, J. F. Y Hoh, E. I. Ilyina-Kakueka, V. S. Organov, G. R. Slocum, L. W. Bain, and F. R. Sedlak. Muscle sarcomere lesions and thrombosis after spaceflight and suspension unloading. *J. Appl. Physiol.* 73: 33S-43S, 1992.
268. Riley, D. A., E. I. Ilyina-Kakueva, S. Ellis, J.L.W. Bain, G. R. Slocum, and F. R. Sedlar. Skeletal muscle fiber, nerve, and blood vessel breakdown in space-flown rats. *FASEB J.* 4: 84–91, 1990.
269. Rios, E., and G. Pizarro. Voltage sensor of excitation-contraction coupling in skeletal muscle. *Physiol. Rev.* 71: 849–908, 1991.
270. Rindt, H., J. Gulick, S. Knotts, J. Neumann, and J. Robbins. *In vivo* analysis of the murine beta-myosin heavy chain gene promoter. *J. Biol. Chem.* 268: 5332–5338, 1993.
271. Rodnick, K. J., E. J. Henriksen, D. E. James, and J. O. Holloszy. Exercise training, glucose transporters, and glucose transport in rat skeletal muscles. *Am. J. Physiol.* 262 (*Cell Physiol.* 31): C9–C14, 1992.
272. Rodnick, K. J., J. O. Holloszy, C. E. Mondon, and D. E. James. Effects of training on insulin-regulatable glucose-transporter protein levels in rat skeletal muscle. *Diabetes* 39: 1425–1429, 1990.
273. Rodnick, K. J., G. M. Reaven, S. Azhar, M. H. Goodman, and C. E. Mondon. Effects of insulin on carbohydrate and protein metabolism in voluntary running rats. *Am. J. Physiol.* 259 (*Endocrinol Metab.* 22): E706-E714, 1990.
274. Rottman, J. N., W. R. Thompson, B. Nadal-Ginard, and V. Mahdavi. Myosin heavy chain gene expression: interplay of cis and trans factors determines hormonal and tissue specificity. In: *Dynamic State of Muscle Fibers*, edited by D. Pette. New York: Walter de Gruyter and Co., 1990, p. 3–16.
275. Rowell, L. B. Muscle blood flow in humans: how high can it go? *Med. Sci. Sports Exerc.* 20: S97–S103, 1988.
276. Rowell, L. B. *Human Cardiovascular Control*. New York: Oxford University Press, 1993.
277. Rowell, L. B., B. Saltin, B. Kiens, and N. J. Christensen. Is peak quadriceps blood flow in humans even higher during

exercise with hypoxemia? *Am. J. Physiol.* 251 (*Heart Circ. Physiol.* 20): H1038–H1044, 1986.
278. Roy, R. R., K. M. Baldwin, and V. R. Edgerton. The plasticity of skeletal muscle: effects of neuromuscular activity. *Exerc. Sports Sci. Rev.* 19: 269–312, 1991.
279. Roy, R. R., K. M. Baldwin, T. P. Martin, S. P. Cimarusti, and V. R. Edgerton. Biochemical and physiological changes in overloaded rat fast-and-slow-twitch ankle extensors. *J. Appl. Physiol.* 59: 639–640, 1985.
280. Roy, R. R., I. D. Meadows, K. M. Baldwin, and V. R. Edgerton. Functional significance of compensatory overloaded rat fast muscle. *J. Appl. Physiol.* 52: 473–478, 1982.
281. Roy, R. R., R. D. Sacks, K. M. Baldwin, M. Short, and V. R. Edgerton. Interrelationships of contraction time, Vmax and myosin ATPase after spinal transection. *J. Appl. Physiol.* 56: 1594–1601, 1984.
282. Sadoshima, J., and S. Izumo. Mechanical stretch rapidly activates multiple signal transduction pathways in cardiac myocytes: potential involvement of an autocrine/paracrine mechanism. *EMBO J.* 12: 1681–1692, 1993.
283. Sadoshima, J., Y. Xu, H. S. Slayter, and S. Izumo. Autocrine release of angiotensin II mediates stretch-induced hypertrophy of cardiac myocytes in vitro. *Cell* 75: 977–984, 1993.
284. Salmons, S., and J. Henriksson. Tha adaptive response of skeletal muscle to increased use. *Muscle Nerve* 4: 94–105, 1981.
285. Salo, D. C., C. M. Donovan, and K. J. A. Davies. HSP70 and other possible heat shock or oxidative stress proteins are induced in skeletal muscle, heart, and liver during exercise. *Free Rad. Biol. Med.* 11: 239–246, 1991.
286. Saltin, B. Hemodynamic adaptations to exercise. *Am. J. Cardiol.* 55: 42D–47D, 1985.
287. Saltin, B., and P. D. Gollnick. Skeletal muscle adaptability: significance for metabolism and performance. In: *Handbook of Physiology, Skeletal Muscle, Skeletal Muscle*, edited by L. D. Peachey. Bethesda, MD: Am. Physiol. Soc., 1985, p. 555–631.
288. Saltin, B. Capacity of blood flow delivery to exercising skeletal muscle in humans. *Am J. Cardiol.* 62: 30E–35E, 1988.
289. Salviati, G., R. Betto, D. Danieli-Betto, and M. Zeviani. Myofibrillar-protein isoforms and sarcoplasmic reticulum calcium transport activity of single human muscle fibers. *Biochem. J.* 224: 215–225, 1983.
290. Sassoon, D., G. Lyons, W. E. Wright, V. Lin, A. Lasser, H. Weintaub, and M. Buckingham. Expression of two myogenic regulatory factors myogenin and MyoD1 during mouse embryogenesis. *Nature* 341: 303–307, 1989.
291. Sayer, M. R., K. K. Rohrer, and W. W. Dillman. Thyroid hormone response of slow and fast-sarcoplasmic reticulum calcium ATPase in RNA in striated muscle. *Mol. Cell. Endocrinol.* 87: 87–93, 1992.
292. Schantz, P., R. Billeter, J. Henriksson, and E. Jansson. Training induced increase in myfibrillar ATPase intermediate fibers in human skeletal muscle. *Muscle Nerve* 5: 628–636, 1982.
293. Schiaffino, S., L. Gorza, S. Sartore, L. Saggin, S. Ausoni, M. Vianello, K. Gundersen, and T. Lomo. Three myosin heavy chains isoforms in type 2 skeletal muscle fibers. *J. Muscle Res. Cell Motil.* 10: 197–205, 1989.
294. Schimke, R. E. Regulation of protein degradation in mammalian tissues. In: *Mammalian Protein Metabolism*, Vol. IV, edited by H. N. Munro. New York: Academic Press, 1970, p. 177–228.
295. Schulte, L. M., J. Navarro, and S. C. Kandarian. Regulation of sarcoplasinic reticulum calcium pump gene expression by hindlimb unweighting. *Am. J. Physiol.* 264 (*Cell Physiol.* 33): C1308–C1315, 1993.
296. Schwerzmann, K., H. Hoppeler, S. R. Kayar, and E. R. Weibel. Oxidative capacity of muscle and mitochondria: correlation of physiological, biochemical, and morphometric characteristics. *Proc. Natl. Acad. Sci. U. S. A.* 86: 1583–1587, 1989.
297. Seedorf, U., E. Leberer, B. J. Kirschbaum, and D. Pette. Neural control of gene expression in skeletal muscle. Effects of chronic stimulation on lactate dehydrogenase isoenzymes and citrate synthase. *Biochem J.* 239: 115–120, 1986.
298. Segal, S. S. Convection, diffusion and mitochondrial utilization of oxygen during exercise. *Perspect. Exerc. Sci. Sports Med.* 5: 269–344, 1992.
299. Semenza, G. L., and G. L. Wang. A nuclear factor induced by hypoxia via de novo protein synthesis binds to the human erythropoietin gene enhancer at a site required for transcriptional activation. *Mol. Cell. Biol.* 12: 5447–5454, 1992.
300. Sherman, S. J., and W. A. Catterall. Electrical activity and cytosolic calcium regulate levels of tetrodotoxin-sensitive sodium channels in cultured rat muscle cells. *Proc. Natl. Acad. Sci. U. S. A.* 81: 262–266, 1984.
301. Sherman, S. J., J. Chriva, and W. A. Catterall. Cyclic adenosine 3′:5′-monophosphate and cytosolic calcium exert opposing effects on biosynthesis of tetrodotoxin-sensitive sodium channels in rat muscle cells. *J. Neurosci.* 5: 1570–1576, 1985.
302. Shimizu, N., E. Dizon, and R. Zak. Both muscle specific and ubiquitous nuclear factors are required for muscle specific expression of myosin heavy chain beta-gene in cultured cells. *Mol. Cell. Biol.* 12: 619–630, 1992.
303. Shimomura, I., K. Tokunaga, K. Kotani, Y. Keno, M. Yanase-Fujiwara, K. Kanosue, S. Jiao, T. Funahashi, T. Kobatake, T. Yamamoto, and Y. Matsuzawa. Marked reduction of acyl CoA synthetase activity and mRNA in intra-abdominal visceral fat by physical exercise. *Am. J. Physiol.* 265 (*Endocrinol. Metab.* 28): E44–E50, 1993.
304. Shoubridge, E. A., A. J. Collins, D. J. Hayes, and G. K. Radda. Biochemical adaptation in the skeletal muscle of rats depleted of creatine with the substrate analogue β-guanidinopropionic acid. *Biochem. J.* 232: 125–131, 1985.
305. Shreeniwas, R., S. Koga, M. Karaurum, D. Pinsky, E. Kaiser, J. Brett, B. A. Wolitzky, C. Norton, J. Piocinski, D. K. Burns, A. Goldstein, and D. Stern. Hypoxia-mediated induction of endothelial cell interleukin-1α. *J. Clin. Invest.* 90: 2333–2339, 1992.
306. Shweiki, D., A. Itin, D. Soffer, and E. Keshet. Vascular endothelial growth factor induced by hypoxia may mediate hypoxia-initiated angiogenesis. *Nature* 359: 843–845, 1992.
307. Simoneau, J.-A., M. Kaufmann, and D. Pette. Asynchronous increases in oxidative capacity and resistance to fatigue of electrostimulated muscles of rat and rabbit. *J. Physiol. (Lond.)* 460: 573–580, 1993.
308. Simonides, W. S., G. C. van der Linden, and C. van Hardeveld. Thyroid hormone differentially affects mRNA levels of calcium ATPase isozymes of sarcoplasmic reticulum in fast and slow skeletal muscles. *FEBS Lett.* 278: 73–76, 1990.
309. Sjodin, B., Y. H. Westing, and F. S. Apple. Biochemical mechanisms for oxygen free radical formation during exercise. *Sports Med.* 10: 236–254, 1990.
310. Staron, R. S., M. J. Leonardi, D. L. Karapondo, E. S. Molicky, J. E. Folkel, F. C. Hagerman, and R. S. Hikida.

Strength and skeletal muscle adaptations in heavy-resistance-trained women after detraining and retraining. *J. Appl. Physiol.* 70: 631–640, 1991.

311. Sternlicht, E., R. J. Barnard, and G. K. Grimditch. Exercise and insulin stimulate skeletal muscle glucose transport through different mechanisms. *Am. J. Physiol.* (*Endocrinol. Metab.* 19) 256: E227–E230, 1989.
312. Stockdale, F. E., and J. B. Miller. The cellular basis of myosin heavy chain isoform expression during development of avian skeletal muscles. *Dev. Biol.* 123: 1–9, 1987.
313. Sugiura, T., H. Miyata, Y. Kawai, H. Matoba, and N. Murakami. Changes in myosin heavy chain isoform expression of overloaded rat skeletal muscle. *Int. J. Biochem.* 25: 1609–1613, 1993.
314. Sullivan, M. J., P. F. Binkley, D. V. Unverferth, J.-H. Ren, H. Boudoulas, T. M. Bashore, A. J. Merola, and C. V. Leier. Prevention of bedrest-induced physical deconditioning by daily dobutamine infusions. *J. Clin. Invest.* 76: 1632–1642, 1985.
315. Sundberg, C. J. Exercise and training during graded leg ischemia in healthy man. *Acta Physiol. Scand.* 150 (Suppl.): 615, 1994
316. Sutrave, P., A. M. Kelly, and S. H. Hughes. *ski* can cause selective growth of skeletal muscle in transgenic mice. *Genes Dev.* 4: 1462–1472, 1990.
317. Sutton, J. R., and P. Farell. Endocrine responses to prolonged exercise. In: *Perspectives in Exercise Science and Sports Medicine*, edited by D. R. Lamb and R. Murray. Indianapolis: Benchmark, 1988, p. 153–212.
318. Swoap, S. J., F. Haddad, P. Bodell, and K. M. Baldwin. Effect of chronic energy deprivation on cardiac thyroid receptor and myosin isoform expression. *Am. J. Physiol.* 266 (*Endocrinol. Metab.* 29): E254–E260, 1994.
319. Swoap, S. J., F. Haddad, V. J. Caiozzo, R. E. Herrick, S. A. McCue, and K. M. Baldwin. Interaction of thyroid hormone and functional overload on skeletal muscle isomyosin expression. *J. Appl. Physiol.* 77: 621–629, 1994.
320. Takeda, S., D. L. North, M. M. Labich, S. D. Russell, and R. G. Whalen. A possible regulatory role for conserved promotor motifs in an adult-specific muscle myosin gene from mouse. *J. Biol. Chem.* 267: 16957–16967, 1992.
321. Thomason, D. B., R. B. Biggs, and F. W. Booth. Protein metabolism and β-myosin heavy-chain mRNA in unweighted soleus muscle. *Am. J. Physiol.* 257 (*Regulatory Integrative Comp. Physiol.* 26): R300–R305, 1989.
322. Thomason, D. B., R. E. Herrick, D. Surdyka, and K. M. Baldwin. Alteration of soleus muscle contractile proteins during hindlimb suspension and subsequent recovery. *J. Appl. Physiol.* 63: 130–137, 1987.
323. Thomason, D. B., P. R. Morrison, V. Oganov, E. Ilyina-Kakueka, F. W. Booth, and K. M. Baldwin. Altered actin and myosin expression in muscle during exposure to microgravity. *J. Appl. Physiol.* 73(Suppl.): 90S–93S, 1992.
324. Thompson, C. C., C. Weinberger, R. Lebo, and R. M. Evans. Identification of a novel thyroid hormone receptor expressed in the mammalian central nervous system. *Science* 237: 1610–1614, 1987.
325. Thompson, W. R., B. Nadal-Ginard, and V. Mahdevi. A myo D-1 independent muscle specific enhancer controls the expression of the beta myosin heavy chain gene in skeletal muscle and cardiac muscles. *J. Biol. Chem.* 266: 22678–22688, 1991.
326. Timson, B. F. Evaluation of animal models for the study of exercise-induced muscle enlargement. *J. Appl. Physiol.* 69: 1935–1945, 1990.
327. Tomita, T., T. Murakami, T. Iwase, K. Nagai, J. Fujita, and S. Sasayamma. Chronic dynamic exercise improves a functional abnormality of the G stimulatory protein in cardiomyopathetic BIO 53.58 Syrian hamsters. *Circulation* 89: 836–845, 1994.
328. Torgan, C. E., J. T. Brozinick, E. A. Banks, M. Y. Cortez, R. E. Wilcox, and J. L. Ivy. Exercise training and clenbuterol reduced insulin resistance of obese Zucker rats. *Am. J. Physiol.* 264 (*Endocrinol. Metab.* 27): E373–E379, 1993.
329. Town, G. P., and D. A. Essig. Cytochrome oxidase in muscle of endurance-trained rats: subunit mRNA contents and heme synthesis. *J. Appl. Physiol.* 74: 192–196, 1993.
330. Tseng, B. S., C. E. Kasper, and V. R. Edgerton. Cytoplasmic-to-myonucleus ratios and succinate dehydrogenase activities in adult rat slow and fast muscle fibers. *Cell Tiss. Res.* 247: 39–49, 1994.
331. Tseng, B. S., D. R. Marsh, M. T. Hamilton, and F. W. Booth. Strength and aerobic training attenuates muscle wasting and improves resistance to the development of disability with aging. *J. Gerontol.* (in press, 1995).
332. Tsika, R. W., S. D. Hauschka, and L. Gao. M-creatine kinase gene in mechanically overloaded skeletal muscle of transgenic mice. *Am. J. Physiol.* 269 (*Cell Physiol.* 38): C665–C674, 1995.
333. Tsika, R. W., and L. Y. Gao. Metabolic and contractile protein adaptations in response to increased mechanical loading. In: *Biochemistry of Exercise*. Champaign, IL: Human Kinetics.
334. Tsika, R. W., R. E. Herrick, and K. M. Baldwin. Time-course adaptations in rat skeletal muscle isomyosins during compensatory growth regression. *J. Appl. Physiol.* 63: 2111–2120, 1987.
335. Tullson, P. C., and R. L. Terjung. Adenine nucleotide metabolism in contracting muscle. *Exerc. Sports Sci. Rev.* 19: 507–538, 1991.
336. Ulmer, J. B., J. J. Donnelly, S. E. Parker, G. H. Rhodes, P. L. Feigner, V. J. Dwarki, S. H. Gromkowski, R. R. Deck, C. M. DeWitt, A. Friedman, L. A. Hawe, K. R. Leander, D. Martinez, H. C. Perry, J. W. Shiver, D. L. Montgomery, and M. A. Liu. Heterologous protection against influenza by injection of DNA encoding a viral protein. *Science* 259: 1745–1749, 1993.
337. Underwood, L. E., and R. S. Williams. Pretranslational regulation of myoglobin gene expression. *Am. J. Physiol.* 252 (*Cell Physiol.* 21): C450–C453, 1987.
338. van Deursen, J., A. Heerschap, F. Oerlemans, W. Ruitenbeek, P. Jap, H. terLaak, and B. Wieringa. Skeletal muscles of mice deficient in muscle creatine kinase lack burst activity. *Cell* 74: 621–631, 1993.
339. van Breda, E., H. A. Keizer, M. M. Vork, D. A. M. Surtel, Y. F. de Jong, G. J. van der Vusse, and J. F. C. Glatz. Modulation of fatty-acid-binding protein content of rat heart and skeletal muscle by endurance training and testosterone treatment. *Pflugers Arch.* 421: 274–279, 1992.
340. Vestergaard, H., P. Andersen, S. Lund, O. Schitz, S. Junker, and O. Pederson. Pre- and posttranslational upregulation of muscle-specific glycogen synthase in athletes. *Am. J. Physiol.* 266 (*Endocrinol. Metab.* 29): E92–E101, 1994.
341. Vincent, C. K., A. Gualberto, C. V. Patel, and K. Walsh. Different regulatory sequences control creatine kinase-M gene expression in directly injected skeletal and cardiac muscle. *Mol. Cell. Biol.* 13: 1264–1272, 1993.
342. Virbasius, J. V., and R. C. Scarpulla. The cytochrome c oxidase subunit IV gene family: tissue-specific and hor-

monal differences in subunit IV and cytochrome c mRNA expression. *Nucleic Acids Res.* 18: 6581–8586, 1990.

343. von Harsdorf, R., R. J. Schott, Y.-T. Shen, S. F. Vatner, V. Mahdavi, and B. Nadal-Ginard. Gene injection into canine myocardium as a useful model for studying gene expression in the heart of large mammals. *Circ. Res.* 72: 688–695, 1993.
344. Wake, S. A., J. A. Sowden, L. H. Storlien, D. E. James, P. W. Clark, J. Shine, D. J. Chisholm, and E. W. Kraegen. Effects of exercise training and dietary manipulation on insulin-regulatable glucose-transporter mRNA in rat muscle. *Diabetes* 40: 275–279, 1991.
345. Wallberg-Henriksson, H., and J. O. Holloszy. Contractile activity increases glucose uptake by muscle in severely diabetic rats. *J. Appl. Physiol.* 57: 1045–1049, 1984.
346. Walmsley, B., J. A. Hodgson, and R. E. Burke. Forces produced by medical gastrocnemius and moving cats. *J. Neurophysiol.* 41: 1203–1215, 1978.
347. Wang, G. L., and G. L. Semenza. General involvement of hypoxia-inducible factor 1 in transcriptional response to hypoxia. *Proc. Natl. Acad. Sci. U. S. A.* 90: 4304–4308, 1993.
348. Watson, P. A., J. P. Stein, and F. W. Booth. Changes in actin synthesis and α-actin-mRNA content in rat muscle during immobilization. *Am. J. Physiol.* 247 (*Cell Physiol.* 16): C39–C44, 1984.
349. Watson, P. A. Accumulation of cAMP and calcium in S49 mouse lymphoma cells following hyposmotic swelling. *J. Biol. Chem.* 264: 14735–14740, 1989.
350. Watson, P. A. Function follows form: generation of intracellular signals by cell deformation. *FASEB J.* 5: 2013–2019, 1991.
351. Weber, J.-M. Pathways for oxidative fuel provision to working muscles: ecological consequences of maximal supply limitations. *Experimentia* 48: 557–564, 1992.
352. Webster, K. A. Regulation of glycolytic enzyme RNA transcriptional rates by oxygen availability in skeletal muscle cells. *Mol. Cell. Biochem.* 77: 19–28, 1987.
353. Weibel, E. R., C. R. Taylor, and H. Hoppler. The concept of symmorphosis: a testable hypothesis of structure-function relationship. *Proc. Natl. Acad. Sci. U. S. A.* 88: 10357–10361, 1991.
354. Wiedenman, J. L., I. Rivera-Rivera, D. Vyas, G. Tsika, L. Gao, K. Sheriff-Carter, L. T. Kwan, and R. W. Tsika. Induction of β-myosin heavy chain and slow myosin light chain transgenes in mechanically overloaded fast-twitch muscle of transgenic mice. *Am. J. Physiol.* (*Cell Physiol*) (in press).
355. Weinberger, C., C. C. Thompson, E. S. Ong, R. Lebo, D. J. Gruol, and R. M. Evans. The c-erb-A gene encodes a thyroid hormone receptor. *Nature* 324: 641–646, 1986.
356. Weintaub, H., R. Davis, S. Tapscott, M. Thayer, M. Krause, R. Benezra, T. K. Blackwell, T. Turner, D. Rupp, R. Rupp, S. Hollenberg, Y. Zhuang, and A. Lasser. The *myoD* gene family: nodal point during specification of the muscle cell lineage. *Science* 251: 761–766, 1991.
357. Welch, W. J. Heat shock proteins functioning as molecular chaperones: their roles in normal and stressed cells. *Philos. Trans. R. Soc. Lond. Biol.* 339: 327–333, 1993.
358. Wells, D. J., and G. Goldspink. Age and sex influence of plasmid DNA directly injected into mouse skeletal muscle. *FEBS Lett.* 306: 203–205, 1992.
359. Whitelaw, P. A., and J. E. Hesketh. Expression of c-*myc* and c-*fos* in rat skeletal muscle. Evidence for increased levels of c-*myc* mRNA during hypertrophy. *Biochem. J.* 281: 143–147, 1992.
360. Williams, R. S., M. G. Caron, and K. Daniel. Skeletal muscle β-adrenegic receptors: variations due to fiber type and training. *Am. J. Physiol.* 246 (*Endocrinol. Metab.* 9): E160–E167, 1984.
361. Williams, R. S., M. Garcia-Moll, J. Mellor, S. Salmons, and W. Harlan. Adaptations of skeletal muscle to increased contractile activity. *J. Biol. Chem.* 262: 2764–2767, 1987.
362. Winder, W. W., K. M. Baldwin, and J. O. Holloszy. Enzymes involved in ketone utilization in different types of muscle: adaptation to exercise. *Eur. J. Biochem.* 47: 461–467, 1974.
363. Witt, E. H., A. Z. Reznick, C. A. Viguie, P. Starke-Reed, and L. Packer. Exercise, oxidative damage and effects of antioxidant manipulation. *Am. J. Nutr.* 122: 766–773, 1992.
364. Wolff, J. A., M. E. Dowty, S. Jiao, G. Repetto, R. K. Berg, J. T. Ludtke, and P. Williams. Expression of naked plasmids by cultured myotubes and entry of plasmids into T tubules and caveolae of mammalian skeletal muscle. *J. Cell Sci.* 103: 1249–1259, 1992.
365. Wolff, J. A., R. W. Malone, P. Williams, W. Chong, G. Acsadi, A. Jani, and P. L. Feigner. Direct gene transfer into mouse muscle in vivo. *Science* 247: 1465–1468, 1990.
366. Wolff, J. A., P. Williams, G. Acsadi, S. Jiao, A. Jani, and W. Chong. Conditions affecting direct gene transfer into rodent muscle in vivo. *Biotechniques* 11: 474–485, 1991.
367. Wong, T. S., and F. W. Booth. Protein metabolism in rat gastrocnemius muscle after stimulated chronic concentric exercise. *J. Appl. Physiol.* 69: 1709–1717, 1990.
368. Wong, T. S., and F. W. Booth. Protein metabolism in rat tibialis anterior muscle after stimulated chronic eccentric exercise. *J. Appl. Physiol.* 69: 1718–1724, 1990.
369. Wright, W. E., D. A. Sassoon, and V. K. Lin. Myogenin, a factor regulating myogenesis, has a domain homologous to MyoD1. *Cell* 56: 607–617, 1989.
370. Wu, K. D., and J. Lytton. Molecular cloning and quantitation of sarcoplasmic reticulum Ca^{2+} ATPase isoforms in rat muscles. *Am. J. Physiol.* 264 (*Cell Physiol.* 33): C333–C341, 1993.
371. Yamada, S., N. Buffinger, J. DiMario, and R. C. Strohman. Fibroblast growth factor is stored in fiber extracellular matrix and plays a role in regulating muscle hypertrophy. *Med. Sci. Sports Exerc.* 21: S173–S180, 1989.
372. Yamazaki, T., K. Tobe, E. Hoh, K. Maemura, T. Kaida, I. Komuro, H. Tanemoto, T. Kadowaki, R. Nagai, and Y. Yazaki. Mechanical loading activates mitogen-activated protein kinase and S6 peptide kinase in cultured rat cardiac myocytes. *J. Biol. Chem.* 268: 12069–12076, 1993.
373. Yan, Z., and F. W. Booth. Potential role of the 3′-untranslated region in cytochrome c gene expression in slow red and fast white skeletal muscle (in press).
374. Yan, Z., Y. Dang, S. Salmons, and F. W. Booth. Skeletal muscle contractile activity increases cytochrome c gene expression: a potential role of decreased RNA-protein interaction in the 3′ untranslated region.
375. Yan, Z., S. Salmons, J. Jarvis, and F. W. Booth. Increased carnitinc palmitoyltransferase mRNA after increased contractile activity. *Am. J. Physiol.* 1995.
376. Yarasheski, K. E., V. Aroniadou, and P. W. R. Lemon. Effect of heavy resistance training on skeletal muscle hypertrophy in rats (Abstract). *Med. Sci. Sports Exerc.* 19: 515, 1987.
377. Yarasheski, K. E., J. A. Campbell, K. Smith, M. J. Rennie, J. O. Holloszy, and D. M. Bier. Effect of growth hormone and resistance exercise on muscle growth in young men. *Am. J. Physiol.* 262 (*Endocrinol. Metab.* 25): E26–E267, 1992.

378. Yen, P. M., D. S. Darling, R. L. Cortez, M. Forgione, P. U. Umeda, and W. W. Chin. T3 decreases binding to DNA by receptor homodymers, but not receptor-auxiliary protein heterodimers. *J. Biol. Chem.* 267: 3565–3568, 1992.
379. Yokota, S. Immunoelectron microscopic localization of albumin in smooth and striated muscle tissues of rat. *Histochemistry* 74: 379–386, 1982.
380. Zemen, R. J., R. Ludeman, T. G. Easton, and J. D. Etlinger. Slow to fast alterations in skeletal muscle fibers caused by clenbuterol, a beta 2-receptor agonist. *Am. J. Physiol.* 254 (*Endocrinol. Metab.* 17): E726–E732, 1988.

25. Regulation of gene expression in skeletal muscle by contractile activity

R. SANDERS WILLIAMS
P. DARRELL NEUFER | *Departments of Internal Medicine and Biochemistry, University of Texas Southwestern Medical Center, Dallas, Texas*

CHAPTER CONTENTS

SKELETAL MUSCLES OF ADULT MAMMALIAN SPECIES, including humans, exhibit a remarkable capacity for stable, long-term adaptation to changing work demands. The processes by which these adaptations occur are distinct from the immediate or short-term physiological responses that provide substrates for muscle work and modulate contractile force during an acute bout of exercise. Most importantly, these long-term responses require changes in gene expression, mediated by changes in the rate of transcription of specific genes and in the rate of synthesis of specific proteins.

Depending on the nature of the inducing stimulus, the adaptive response can take the form of hypertrophy, in which myofibers increase in size but otherwise retain their initial ultrastructural and biochemical properties, or of remodeling without hypertrophy, in which myofibers do not enlarge but acquire markedly different enzymatic and structural characteristics, often accompanied by changes in the microvasculature.

In another volume of this *Handbook*, Saltin and Gollnick (138) summarized the relationships between anatomic and biochemical properties of myofibers and physiological performance, and described in lucid detail many of the changes in these characteristics that are modulated by physical activity. Our chapter brings a different perspective to this subject by focusing explicitly on mechanisms of gene regulation that underlie the striking morphological and biochemical adaptability of skeletal muscle, with specific attention to the following questions: What genes are regulated by contractile activity in skeletal muscle? At what step(s) of gene expression does this regulation take place? In biochemical and molecular terms, how do myocytes sense changing work demands and transduce this information to the relevant genes?

We will begin with some theoretical considerations to provide a structure for subsequent discussions of experimental results. Then we will describe model systems that have been useful in approaching these questions, and will review data on specific genes for which regulatory mechanisms have been examined. Finally, we will review current evidence for specific signal transduction pathways that may link changes in contractile activity to gene expression in skeletal muscles. This remains an emerging, rather than a mature, field of scientific inquiry, so that satisfying and complete answers to the most fundamental questions are unavailable at this time. While we have attempted to provide a thorough and up-to-date summary of current knowledge in this area, we also hope to identify fertile areas for future research.

Several general points merit special attention at the outset. As mentioned above, adaptive responses of skeletal muscle to changing work demands can be divided into two general categories: hypertrophic growth and muscle remodeling. Hypertrophic growth is stimulated by short bursts of muscle activity against high resistance or by prolonged stretch beyond normal resting length. Myofiber hypertrophy is characterized by a generally coordinated increase in abundance, per cell, of most protein constituents of the muscle fibers. Much of what we know of specific mechanisms that lead to hypertrophic growth is derived from studies of cardiac muscle, as opposed to skeletal muscle, but some features of the process appear to be common to both tissues. The hypertrophic process includes, to a limited degree, selective activation of specific genes, in a transient manner in the period immediately following the onset of work overload, and in a sustained manner as the hypertrophic process proceeds and reaches equilibrium. The major events, however, that underlie muscle hypertrophy involve a general and nonspecific augmentation of protein synthesis within the cells. The major physiological consequence of this response is to produce a muscle with a greater capacity for peak force generation.

Remodeling of skeletal muscles, without hypertrophy, is induced by extended periods of tonic contractile activity either sustained continuously or repeated on a regular basis over the course of several weeks. Myofibers do not enlarge, but undergo a striking reorganization, with selective activation or repression of many genes. Mitochondria proliferate and occupy a larger fractional volume within the myofibers. Profiles of expression of many enzymes, cytosolic proteins, and membrane receptors are regulated, and switching among different isoforms of myofibrillar proteins may occur. From a physiological standpoint, this form of adaptation (commonly termed the endurance training response) produces a muscle that is resistant to fatigue during extended periods of repetitive contractions. This latter form of muscle plasticity will be the predominant subject of this review.

Adult skeletal muscles are comprised of a diversity of cell types that can participate in remodeling phenomena. These include mature myofibers of differing subtypes; myogenic satellite cells that can be mobilized in response to muscle injury; motor, sensory, and autonomic neurons; capillary endothelial cells and cellular constituents of larger blood vessels; and fibroblasts. This complexity is germane to the mechanisms that lead to regulation of genes within muscle fibers, in that locally acting paracrine factors released from one cell type may influence gene expression in adjacent cells. Some communication of this type must, for example, be at play in the process that matches increases in capillary density to remodeling effects on muscle fibers that alter the fractional volume of mitochondria in response to endurance training. As we consider experimental models that have been employed to investigate mechanisms of gene regulation in myocytes, it is apparent that cell culture systems consisting only of myotubes may fail to recapitulate important features acting within the more complex environment of the intact muscle.

A third issue that demands attention in studies of gene regulation by contractile activity in skeletal muscle is the complexity and pleiotropic nature of the physical and metabolic stimuli presented to muscle fibers during contractions (Fig. 25.1). Acetylcholine released from motor nerve terminals leads to contraction of the entire fiber, but may induce certain effects that are limited to subcellular domains adjacent to the motor end-plate. Other signaling molecules of neural origin bind cell surface receptors on myofibers and trigger intracellular events that may be linked to changes in gene expression. Contracting myofibers experience mechanical stresses that perturb the sarcolemma and extracellular matrix, as well as exerting tension on the cytoskeleton and organelles. Depending on the duration and intensity of contractions, the cytoplasmic or organellar concentrations of ions and metabolites are altered. Any one of these many changes may, in principle, activate a signaling pathway that ultimately impinges on a single gene or a set of genes.

THEORETICAL AND KINETIC CONSIDERATIONS

The temporal aspects of gene regulation by contractile activity in skeletal muscles make elucidation of the underlying mechanisms a unique and challenging problem. An endurance training regimen of only 30 min of exercise three times weekly is sufficient, after several weeks, to promote easily measurable changes in peak catalytic capacity of enzymes of intermediary metabolism, reflecting induction of genes encoding these proteins. Thus, the physiological stimulus of exercise, delivered only sporadically for brief durations, is capable of producing a significant and long-lived response, but only as a cumulative effect

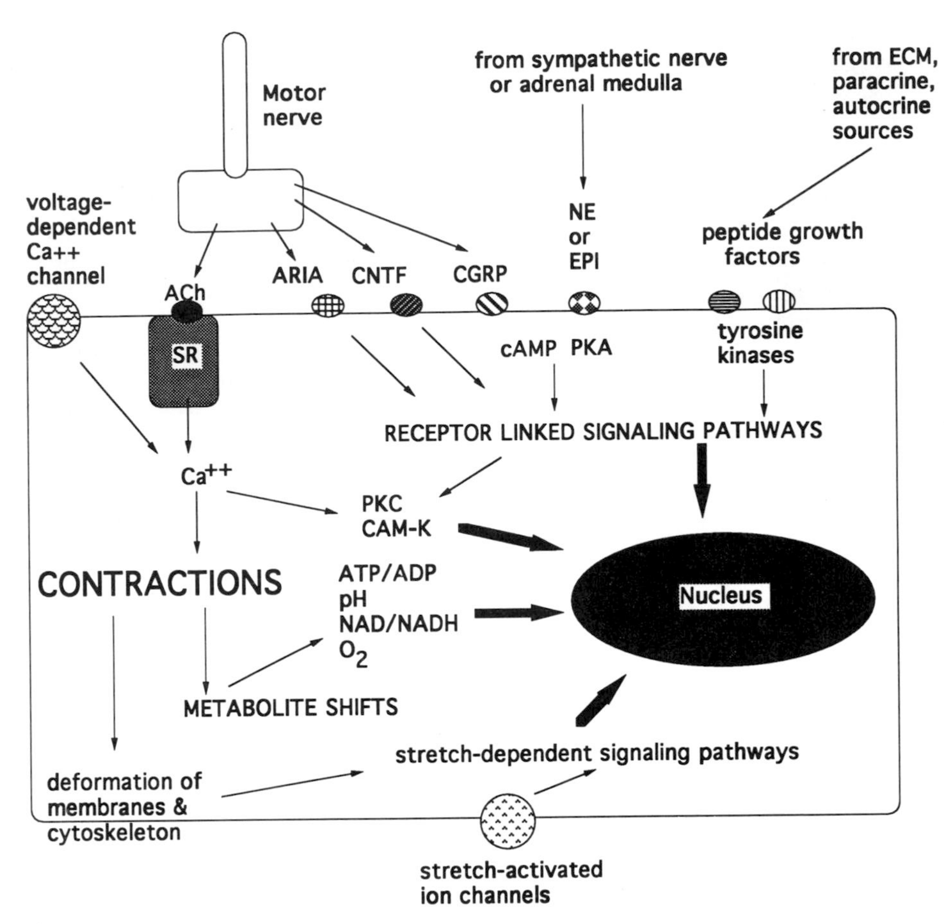

FIG. 25.1. Control of gene expression: potential messengers generated within contracting skeletal myofibers. Acetylcholine (ACh) released from the motor nerve binds its receptor and triggers membrane depolarization, release of calcium (Ca^{2+}) from sarcoplasmic reticulum (SR) stores, and myofiber contractions. Mechanical stresses and metabolic events resulting from contractile activity generate other potential intracellular messengers. Additional extracellular messengers released by the motor nerve or arising from other sources initiate receptor linked signaling pathways. ARIA, acetylcholine receptor inducing activity; CNTF, ciliary neurotrophic factor; CGRP, calcitonin gene-related peptide; NE, norepinephrine; EPI, epinephrine; ECM, extracellular matrix; cAMP, cyclic adenosine monophosphate; PKA, protein kinase A; PKC, protein kinase C; CAM-K, calcium/calmodulin kinase.

of repeated administration of the stimulus. Even if the primary inciting stimulus is delivered at a very intense level on a continuous basis, a condition that can be achieved with electrical pacing of the motor nerve, a latency period of several days separates the initiation of the stimulus from both the onset and the apogee of responses demonstrated by most of the specific genes that have been analyzed.

The signaling mechanisms generated by contractile activity that can modulate expression of specific genes will be governed by certain kinetic principles. Genetic information flows from DNA to RNA to protein (Fig. 25.2), and the abundance of any gene product under steady-state conditions represents a balance between the rate of synthesis (translation of mRNA) and rate of degradation of that protein. The synthesis rate of a given protein is, in part, determined by the concentration of its corresponding mRNA which, in turn, is a function of that mRNA's rate of synthesis (transcription) and rate of degradation. Thus, expression of a given gene represents the integration of a series of synthetic and degradative processes, the overall rates of which will be controlled by the kinetics of the rate limiting steps. Clearly, the rate-limiting step for the synthesis of many proteins resides at the level of transcription. However, expression of other genes may be regulated at different steps to modulate the final concentration of biologically active product. In addition, regulation may shift from one step to another in response to various stimuli. How these regulatory shifts may impact on the overall kinetics of gene ex-

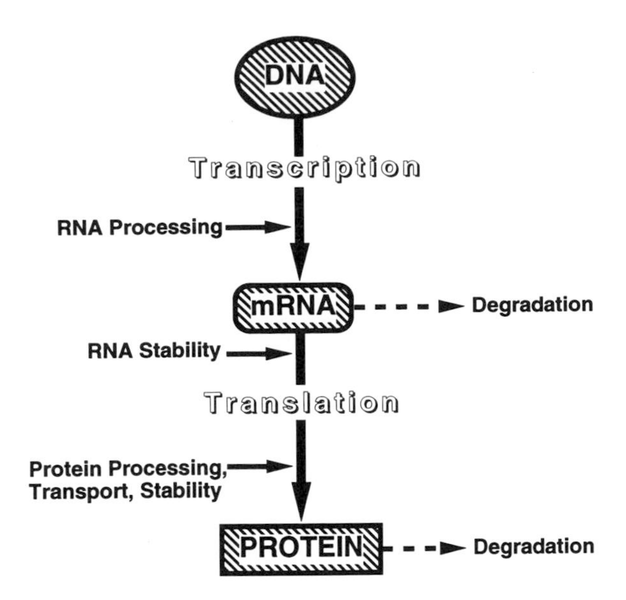

FIG. 25.2. Steps at which gene expression may be controlled.

pression is considered below, with special attention to the response of skeletal muscle to alterations in the chronic level of contractile activity.

Progressive changes in the expression of myofibrillar, Ca^{2+}-sequestering, and mitochondrial proteins induced by exercise training or chronic nerve stimulation have been well characterized (17, 122). Although relatively few studies have focused on changes in protein synthesis with increased contractile activity (9, 15, 16, 84, 155), several lines of evidence suggest that the increase in selected muscle proteins is generated primarily through specific increases in protein synthesis rather than through stabilization of existing proteins. In vivo labeling of nascent polypeptides within skeletal muscle with ^{35}Smethionine reveals enhanced incorporation of label into hexokinase II within hours and into myosin heavy chain (MHC) IIa and IId within 2 days after the onset of continuous nerve stimulation (66, 155). Endurance training also elicits an increase in cytochrome *c* protein synthesis in the red quadriceps muscle of rats within 5 days (15). It should be noted, however, that other models of altered activity of skeletal muscle, particularly those involving sudden reductions in contractile activity by immobilization, unweighting, or denervation, elicit changes in protein expression by altering protein stability (16, 160). The remaining discussion, however, will be limited to theoretical considerations of models of increased contractile activity.

An increase in protein synthesis may be stimulated by a concomitant increase in mRNA and/or by an increase in translational efficiency. Generally, activity-induced modulation of skeletal muscle proteins are preceded by specific changes in corresponding mRNAs (121, 122) and, thus, provide a probable mechanism for eliciting an increase in protein synthesis. As mentioned previously, the steady-state level of a given mRNA is a function of both its rate of synthesis and its rate of degradation, implying that the rate of change in response to a cellular stimulus is dependent on the dynamics of mRNA turnover. This principle is illustrated in Figure 25.3A in which mRNA concentration (mRNA) in response to a stimulus is plotted vs. time. In this example, mRNA degradation is a first-order process (i.e., = kS, where k = degradation rate constant and S = substrate concentration) and unaffected by the stimulus.

Under basal conditions, mRNA is in steady state, reflecting a balance between synthesis and degradation. Introduction of the stimulus elicits an increase in mRNA synthesis that is tempered by an increase in degradation (due to an increase in S, i.e., mRNA). Thus, the resulting rate of increase in mRNA is dependent on the half-life of the message and follows a Michaelis-Menton relationship. In other words, only 50% of the adaptation is realized during the first half-life (12 h in this example) after initiation of the stimulus, and 5 half-lives (2.5 days) are required before ~97% of the new steady-state level is achieved. By the same token, 50% of the adaptive increase in mRNA is lost during the first half-life after the stimulus is removed. The duration for both situations will be longer with more stable messages or may be considerably shorter with mRNAs possessing shorter half-lives (i.e., early-response genes). For example, continuous contractile activity induced by chronic stimulation of the motor nerve elicits marked increases (greater than tenfold) in mRNAs encoding early response genes within hours (106), and in MRP-RNA within 1 day (119), while the induction of other genes requires much longer periods of nerve stimulation (Fig. 25.4) (121, 122). Such differences in the time course of the response of individual genes to contractile activity may be attributable to the half-life of each specific transcript, or to a requirement for intermediate steps in the activation of relevant transcription factors. In either case, the rate of change in mRNA level will be determined by the kinetic properties of each individual message.

The example in Figure 25.3A illustrates the scenario for the rate of increase of a given message in response to a constant stimulus. However, exercise training is typically performed for an hour or more on a daily basis and, thus, represents only an intermittent stimulus. Although both forms of increased contractile activity elicit similar qualitative changes, exercise training requires several weeks to generate

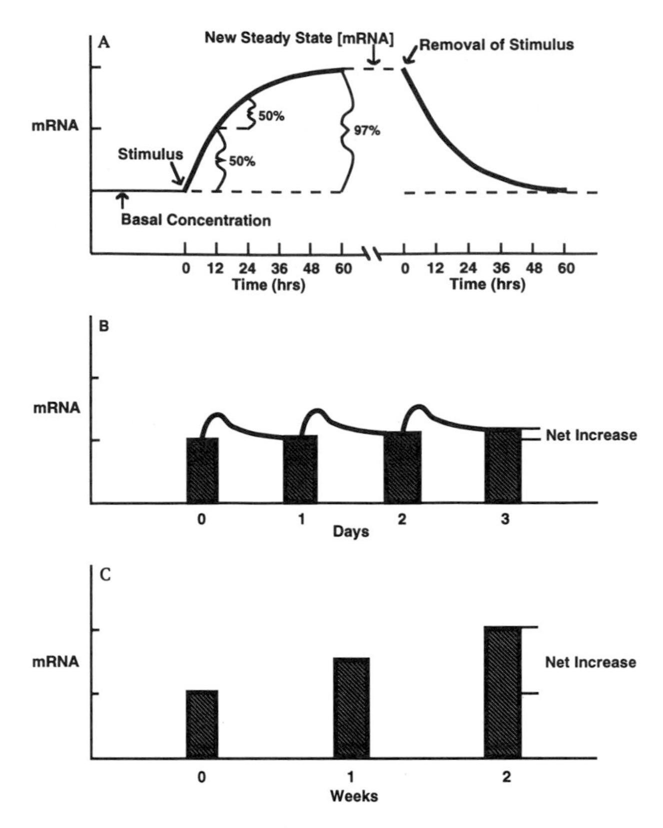

FIG. 25.3. Kinetic features of the regulation of mRNA abundance by a constant or intermittent stimulus. *A*, The effect of a continuous stimulus (e.g., chronic motor nerve stimulation) on abundance of a specific mRNA is plotted as a function of time. Assumptions in this model include: the induction mechanism is triggered immediately when the stimulus is applied; the mRNA half life is 12 h; and mRNA degradation is a first-order process in which the degradation rate constant is unaffected by the stimulus. It is notable that 5 half-lives (2.5 days) are required before ~97% of the new steady-state level is achieved, and 50% of the adaptive increase in [mRNA] is lost during the first half-life after the stimulus is removed. The time required to reach steady state following initiation or withdrawal of the stimulus will be longer with more stable messages and shorter with mRNAs that degrade rapidly (e.g., early response gene products). *B* and *C*, The predicted response to an intermittent stimulus (e.g., treadmill running) delivered for only a fraction of each day. The same assumptions as in *A* apply. Much of the increase evoked by each stimulus period is lost prior to the next stimulus, and changes in mRNA abundance accrue more slowly than with continuous application of the stimulus.

the same adaptive response elicited by only a few days of continuous nerve stimulation. Obviously, the kinetics of each response may differ according to the duration and intensity of the stimulus delivered to the muscle. The time course of the response to an intermittent stimulus is depicted in Figure 25.3B in which mRNA concentration is plotted as a function of consecutive days of training. At time zero, mRNA is at steady-state level, reflecting equal rates of synthesis and degradation. On day 1, exercise triggers a stimulus to induce an increase in synthesis of the selected mRNA. The stimulus, however, is transient and the response abates during the ensuing recovery period. Using the example of an mRNA with a half-life of 12 h and assuming that mRNA degradation is a first-order process, the rate of degradation of the same message is also accelerated during the recovery period due to the small increase in concentration. Thus, the concentration of the selected mRNA rapidly declines toward the preexercise steady-state level, similar to that depicted in Figure 25.3A, until the next exercise bout triggers another period of increased synthesis. Since the recovery period has proceeded through approximately 1.5 half-lives, nearly 65% of the exercise-induced increase in mRNA concentration is lost at the time of the next exercise bout. However, this means that 35% of the increase remains at day 2, resulting in a small net elevation in concentration of the selected mRNA. Each consecutive day of exercise training results in similar fluctuations, eventually culminating in a detectable training-induced increase in mRNA concentration relative to the untrained state (Fig. 25.3C).

Direct evidence for regulation of gene expression during recovery from exercise has recently been demonstrated for the GLUT4 glucose transporter gene (113). Run-on analysis of nuclei isolated from red skeletal muscle of rats after 1 week of training revealed a 1.8-fold increase in GLUT4 gene transcription 3 h after the final exercise bout that was not present either 30 min or 24 h after exercise. A similar transient regulation of gene expression has also been reported for hexokinase II mRNA after a single bout of exercise in untrained rats. Ribonuclease I (RNase) protection analysis revealed an increase in Hexokinase II mRNA immediately after exercise, a further elevation after 3 h of recovery, and a return to basal 24 h after exercise (117). Finally, mRNA encoding δ-aminolevulinate synthase (ALAS), the rate-limiting enzyme for biosynthesis of heme, has also been reported to be elevated in rabbit tibialis anterior muscle after 18 and 48 h of recovery from 7 days of electrical stimulation [3 h/day (153)]. These findings collectively support the concept that cumulative effects of transient changes in gene expression determine the time course of adaptive responses to intermittent periods of increased contractile activity.

There are a few final points to keep in mind concerning the examples presented in Figure 25.3. First, the absolute increase in any mRNA (i.e., the new steady-state level) will vary depending on the intensity of the stimulus. The time required to achieve the new steady-state concentration will, however, be the same as long as the stimulus does not influence the

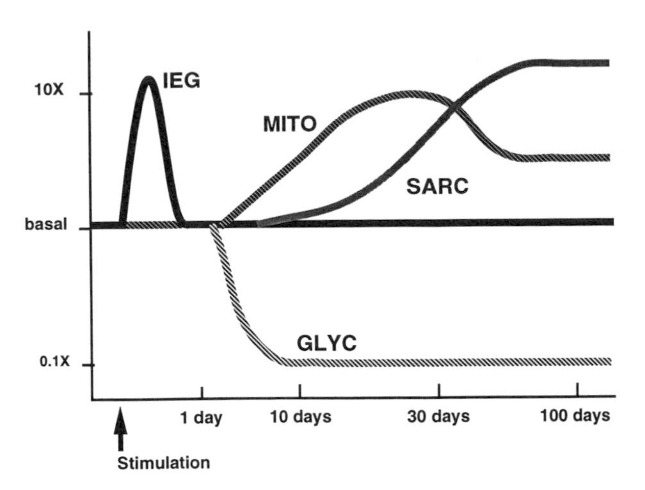

FIG. 25.4. Empirical time course of changes in mRNA abundance evoked by continuous motor nerve stimulation of rabbit tibialis anterior skeletal muscles. Changes in mRNA concentrations (per fiber) are plotted schematically as a function of time following the onset of the stimulus (nonlinear scale). A large but transient induction of immediate early gene (IEG) expression occurs within the first day. Expression of several glycolytic enzymes (GLYC) achieves a new (lower) steady state within the first 5 days. Genes encoding slow isoforms of sarcomeric (SARC) proteins are up-regulated to a new and higher steady state with a somewhat slower time course. Genes encoding mitochondrial (MITO) proteins exhibit a more complex pattern: a period of induction to markedly elevated mRNA concentrations, a plateau phase, and then a decline to a steady state that is above basal levels but below the apogee reached from 3–6 weeks after the onset of nerve stimulation. This figure is based on results from several laboratories, as referenced in the text and tables, with summary data presented in semiquantitative and schematic form only.

degradation rate constant (i.e., mRNA stability). Second, the time at which mRNA concentration is determined in response to a training stimulus is critical. Waiting 24–48 h to measure the "true training effect" will likely underestimate the training-induced increase in mRNAs of average stability. Hypotheses concerning the identity of specific signal molecules and pathways that link contractile activity and gene expression (Fig. 25.1) must accommodate these kinetic considerations, as well as each of the peculiar features of the response of skeletal muscle to changes in work demand that we delineated earlier.

EXPERIMENTAL SYSTEMS AND MODELS FOR STUDY OF GENE REGULATION BY CONTRACTILE ACTIVITY

Both human investigations and a variety of animal models, each with its attendant advantages and shortcomings, have been used to study this problem.

Human Investigations

A rich literature provides details of relationships between work activity and exercise performance in healthy human subjects of varying ages, and in selected populations of patients afflicted with specific diseases (68, 95). The development of methods for muscle biopsy and for noninvasive assessement of muscle metabolism by nuclear magnetic resonance (NMR) spectroscopy and imaging (139) greatly expanded the range of information that could be derived from human studies. Such data are sufficient to conclude that the fundamental adaptations of skeletal muscles to changing work demands are similar in humans and in other mammalian species. We assume, therefore, that exploration of the mechanisms responsible for gene regulation by contractile activity pursued in more tractable animal models will produce information that is pertinent to Homo sapiens.

Animal Studies

Laboratory rodents and other mammalian species can be subjected to treadmill running or swimming so as to generate an endurance training effect in the limb musculature (17, 67). Likewise, load-induced hypertrophy of skeletal muscles in intact mammals or birds can be produced by ablation of antagonist muscles or by other maneuvers to create chronic muscle stretch (48, 131). Atrophy and remodeling phenomena resulting from muscle disuse can be produced in laboratory rodents by tail/hindlimb suspension or immobilization of specific muscle groups in plaster casts (48, 131). Such models have been used widely, and collectively provide an important and extensive body of descriptive data concerning the adaptive responses to each of these forms of disuse or work overload. In addition, valuable insights also may be gleaned from other models of altered gene expression in skeletal muscle, such as temperature acclimation in the striped bass, a species that experiences profound changes in muscle mitochondrial density and oxidative capacity in response to shifts in ambient water temperature (38, 50, 130). The readers are referred Table 25.1 and the indicated references for comprehensive reviews of these models.

A related but different approach to induce remodeling of skeletal muscle is based on manipulation of the motor nerve. Denervation produces a form of disuse atrophy that includes frank degeneration of myofibers, but is accompanied by distinctive changes in gene expression (53, 131). Other manipulations of motor nerves also have provided important insights. A seminal observation in this field came from

TABLE 25.1. *Model Systems Used to Study Gene Expression*

Model	Signal	Physiological Response	References
Intact animals (humans, rats, mice, rabbits, dogs, cats, fish)			
Treadmill running and swimming	Contractile, metabolic, hormonal	↑ Oxidative capacity ↑ Angiogenesis ↑ Gluc. transport capacity ↓ Glycolytic capacity Fast→slow twitch	17, 67 138 122
Motor nerve stimulation	↑ Neural/electrical activity Chronic use	Atrophy Angiogenesis Sarcomeric and Ca^{2+}-Sequestering proteins Fast→slow isoforms ↓ Glycolytic capacity	122 121
Stretch	Mechanical	Hypertrophy Sarcomeric proteins Fast→slow isoforms	48 49
Surgical ablation or tenotomy	Compensatory overload	Hypertrophy Sarcomeric proteins Fast→slow isoforms	16, 131
Immobilization	Disuse	Atrophy Sarcomeric proteins Slow→fast isoforms	16, 131
Hindlimb suspension	Reduced load	Atrophy Sarcomeric and Ca^{2+}-Sequestering proteins Slow→fast isoforms ↑ Glucose transport capacity	16, 131 141 62 53
Cold water acclimation of striped bass	25°C→5°C	↑ Oxidative capacity	38
Denervation	Neural/electrical activity Disuse	Atrophy Sarcomeric proteins Slow→fast isoforms ↓ Oxidative capacity ↓ Glucose transport capacity	17, 131 171 171 62, 103
Hypoxia/ischemia	↓P_{O_2}	↑ Heat shock proteins	11, 12
Pharmacological manipulations			
β-GPA	↓ CrP and ATP	↑ Oxidative capacity	108
hyperthyroidism	↑ T_3	↑ Oxidative capacity	72
hypothyroidism	↓ T_3	↓ Oxidative capacity	72
Muscle cell culture			
Direct stimulation	↑ Electrical activity ↑ Contractile activity	↓ AChR expression Sarcomeric proteins Fast→slow isoforms	118 35
Nerve/muscle co-culture	↑ Neural/electrical activity	↓ AChR expression ↑ Fast myosin isoform	136 36
Stretch	Mechanical	Muscle growth	163
Pharmacological manipulations			
Tetrodotoxin	↓ Contractile activity	↑ AChR expression	93
cAMP	↑ Protein kinase activity	↑ Oxidative capacity	45, 94

studies in which the motor nerves innervating predominantly slow-twitch and fast-twitch fibers were crossed (19). The result of such cross-innervation, after several weeks, was a complete reversal of the phenotypic characteristics of each muscle: the formerly slow-twitch muscle became fast and vice versa. Several studies have confirmed these findings and collectively support the hypothesis that fiber composition is determined by neural input (53). Additional understanding of this property of muscle fibers has been based on the finding that continuous electrical pacing of the motor nerve supplying a predominantly fast-twitch muscle also induces a fast-to-slow transformation (122). Thus, the pattern of neural firing is a powerful determinant of muscle phenotype.

A rabbit model developed by Salmons and Vrbova (137) that involves electrical pacing of the common peroneal nerve innervating the tibialis anterior and extensor digitorum longus muscle of the hindlimb has provided a particularly powerful experimental system. In the native state, these muscles of the adult rabbit are almost entirely comprised of fast-twitch, glycolytic fibers. Within a few days following the onset of nerve pacing, however, expression of glycolytic enzymes and parvalbumin is reduced, while expression of mitochondrial enzymes and myoglobin is markedly enhanced (122). This conversion of the metabolic profile of the fibers is followed by a virtually complete transformation of contractile protein isoforms from fast to slow, and a striking angiogenic response. The transformation process requires 3–5 weeks of continuous nerve stimulation to become complete, and is reversible upon cessation of the stimulus. In addition, and in contrast to exercise training models, muscles electrically stimulated via the motor nerve pass through a phase in which they transiently acquire properties not observed in native skeletal muscles, notably a proliferation of mitochondria approaching that present in cardiac myocytes. After the fibers pass through this transition phase (7–9 weeks), they reach an equilibrium in which the muscle phenotype closely resembles that of native slow oxidative skeletal muscle fibers. The time course of some of these events is illustrated schematically in Figure 25.4.

Endurance training models are advantageous in that they faithfully model forms of work overload in which humans commonly engage. Gene switching events induced by endurance training may require, however, many weeks to become measurable, and the magnitude of some of the pertinent responses, though clearly of physiological significance, is small relative to the precision of many of the biochemical methods that are required for studies of gene regulation. Furthermore, animals often differ in their willingness and ability to complete long and demanding training protocols, and thereby exacerbate variability of measurements. Denervation triggers many striking changes in gene expression events within the muscle, but represents a pathological rather than a physiological state.

Electrical pacing of the motor nerve also provides a potent stimulus to changes in gene expression, and presents several distinct advantages for exploration of the underlying mechanisms. Unlike most endurance training protocols, this model permits comparison of the stimulated muscle to the unstimulated contralateral muscle of the same animal, thereby minimizing intersubject variability. Most of the known effects of nerve stimulation are directionally similar to changes induced by endurance training, but occur more rapidly and are of much greater magnitude. In the model that involves stimulation of the common peroneal nerve of adult rabbits, the muscles innervated by this nerve are sufficiently large (>2 g) to provide ample material for biochemical analyses.

On the other hand, this approach has certain limitations. Muscles of small laboratory rodents are rich in respiratory enzymes in the native state, and changes that result from nerve stimulation are less dramatic than in the rabbit or dog. Some investigators who have studied the rabbit model report accumulation of inflammatory cells, as well as fiber degeneration and regeneration, in chronically stimulated muscles. For unclear reasons, these types of changes seem to occur more commonly with intermittent, as opposed to continuous, nerve stimulation. It is immanently clear, however, that successful application of this model demands exquisite care to avoid injury to the motor nerve during implantation of pacing electrodes. Nerve injury, if present, will result in a mixed picture of degenerating myofibers and healthy fibers undergoing stimulation-induced transformation, and seriously confound results. Finally, while it is likely that pathways linking changes in contractile activity to modulation of specific genes are shared among the response to both endurance training and nerve stimulation, the latter intervention is extreme, by comparison to any stresses that would be experienced by mammalian skeletal muscles in nature. It is conceivable, therefore, that nerve pacing may reveal pathways of gene regulation that, irrespective of their heuristic value, are not evoked during normal environmental conditions.

In this section we have seen how several different experimental models are available for the study of muscle adaptation to changing work demands within intact animals. Most of these models are now well characterized in terms of descriptive morphological and biochemical data that define the time course of specific adaptive responses. As we shall discuss systematically later under MESSENGERS AND SIGNAL TRANSDUCTION PATHWAYS, in many cases such analyses have been extended to include measurements of mRNA transcribed from specific genes. This field has become ripe for investigators to move beyond description and cataloguing to the exploration of underlying mechanisms of gene regulation. This has included exploration of the effects of hypoxia/ischemia on the expression of heat shock proteins as well as various pharmacological/hormonal manipulations designed to investigate the signaling mechanisms that may be involved in modulating gene expression in skeletal muscle. Mechanistic studies of genetic control systems are, however, most productively pursued when appropriate cell culture models are available, and, in the following section, we will discuss attempts to utilize cultured cell systems for studies of physiological modulation of gene expression in skeletal myotubes. However, emerging techniques of somatic cell gene transfer to intact muscles of laboratory animals, as well as more established technology for generation of germline transgenic mice, are currently being brought to bear on this problem and provide potentially exciting and new opportunities for progress using intact animal models.

Studies in Cell Culture

Skeletal myoblasts can be isolated from mammalian or avian embryos, or as satellite cells from adult muscles, and propagated in primary culture as undifferentiated myoblasts. Several clonal derivatives of rodent myoblasts (rat L6, mouse C2C12 or sol8) also are widely available. When grown to confluency in media relatively depleted of growth factors, adherent skeletal myoblasts will differentiate over a matter of days into large multinucleated myotubes that develop cross-striations and contract spontaneously. The relative ease with which this process can be manipulated has given a substantial boost to studies of genetic mechanisms that regulate commitment and differentiation with the skeletal muscle lineage.

To a more limited degree, skeletal myotubes in culture have permitted observations concerning gene regulation by contractile activity. Such models have been applied most productively to studies of subunits of the acetylcholine receptor. While the rate of spontaneous contractions of myotubes in culture is variable, pharmacologic blockage of sarcolemmal sodium channels with tetrodotoxin will result in complete cessation of contractions, and a concomitant increase in abundance of mRNA-encoding subunits of the acetylcholine receptor in primary cultures of myotubes (23, 34, 118). More complicated events with respect to acetylcholine receptors have been modeled by co-culture of skeletal myotubes with neurons derived from spinal cord explants. Innervation of muscle fibers results not only in a decrease in acetylcholine receptor subunit expression but leads to clustering of receptor proteins in the region of the nascent motor end-plate. Once the motor end-plate is formed, activity of the nerve exerts preferential effects on nuclei that are anchored beneath this structure, as compared to more freely mobile nuclei with the fibers that are unassociated with end-plate regions (93).

Other investigators have attempted to modulate the rate of contraction of myotubes in culture by means of electrical stimulation (23, 35, 118). Although some initial applications of this approach seemed promising, there are significant technical as well as biological limitations of this technique. From a technical standpoint, myotube contractions may be sufficiently forceful to disrupt contacts between the cell and the substratum used to coat the culture dish, and cells are lost into the medium. It is difficult, therefore, to maintain vigorously contracting cells for periods of time that may be necessary to model gene-switching events that have a long latency period (see earlier under THEORETICAL AND KINETIC CONSIDERATIONS). From a biological perspective, the artificial environment of cell culture precludes acquisition of traits manifested by mature myofibers in situ. Cultured myotubes are removed from the important influences of the motor nerve, as well as from less well-defined paracrine effects of factors released from endothelial cells or other cellular constituents of the intact muscle. Cells in culture generally are isolated from mechanical stresses experienced by myofibers in situ. Special procedures, such as nerve-muscle co-culture or growth of cells on flexible supports, have allowed investigators to circumvent some of these limitations (163). These efforts, despite their ingenuity, have not yet resulted in the development of a cell culture method in which features of the endurance training response can be modeled faithfully.

WHAT GENES ARE REGULATED BY CONTRACTILE ACTIVITY?

Table 25.2 provides a compendium of specific genes, the protein and/or mRNA products of which have been shown to be regulated in skeletal muscle by contractile activity. Such genes encode proteins of diverse functions: secreted peptide growth factors; nuclear transcription factors including protooncogene products; sarcolemmal surface receptors and transporters; enzymes of the glycolytic pathway, the tricarboxylic acid cycle, and the electron transport chain; many constituents of the contractile apparatus, including both thin and thick filament components; and accessory proteins of respiration (myoglobin) and calcium binding proteins (parvalbumin). The abundance of both large (ribosomal RNA subunits) and small (MRP-RNA) RNA products of nuclear genes is subject to similar control. Finally, expression

TABLE 25.2. *Genes Regulated by Contractile Activity in Skeletal Muscle*

Gene	Model	Protein	mRNA	References
Secreted peptide growth factors				
Heparin-binding mitogen activity	CS	↑		111
Fibroblast growth factors	CS	↑		111
Surface receptors, enzymes, and transporters				
N-Cadherin	EX	↓		56
	DN	↑		
Acetylcholine receptor	DN (ES)	↑	↑	44
Ciliary neurotrophic factor receptor	DN	↑		60
β-Adrenergic receptor	CS,EX	↑	↑	18, 89, 174
Adenylate cyclase	CS	↑		90
Insulin-responsive glucose transporter protein (GLUT4)	CS, EX, HS	↑	↑	39, 62, 87, 114, 146
	DN (ES)	↓	↓	62, 103
Cytosolic transport proteins				
Myoglobin	CS	↑	↑	82, 161
Fatty acid–binding protein	CS, EX	↑	↑	21, 82
Ca^{2+}-sequestering proteins				
Parvalbumin	CS	↑	↑	122
SR Ca^{2+}-ATPase				
Fast→slow isoform	CS	↑	↑	122
Slow→fast isoform	HS	↑	↑	141
Sarcomeric proteins				
Myosin heavy chains:				
HCIIb→HCIId→HCIIa→HCI (fast glycolytic→slow oxidative)	CS, FO ST, EX	↑	↑	48, 121, 131
HCI→HCIIa→HCIId→HCIIb (slow oxidative→fast glycolytic)	IM, HS DN	↓	↓	17, 131
Myosin light chains				
Fast→slow isoforms	CS, FO	↑	↑	122, 131
Troponin subunits TnT, TnI, TnC				
Fast→slow isoforms	CS	↑	↑	122
Glycogen metabolism enzymes				
Phosphorylase	CS	↓		63
Phosphoglucomutase	CS	↓		
Glycogen synthase	CS	nc		
Glycolytic enzymes				
Hexokinase II	CS, EX	↑	↑	66, 117, 167
PFK, Ald, GAPDH, PK, LDH	CS, EX	↓	↓	126
TCA cycle enzymes				
Citrate synthase	CS, EX	↑	↑	4, 89, 110
IDH, KDH, SDH, FUM, MDH	CS	↑		126, 152
Respiratory chain enzymes				
Nuclear encoded				
Cytochrome *c*	EX	↑	↑	15, 110, 126, 152
NADH:cytochrome-*c* oxidoreductase	CS	↑		126
Succinate:cytochrome-*c* oxidoreductase	CS	↑		
Cytochrome oxidase subunit VIC	CS	↑		71, 89, 175
			↑	71, 89, 175
β-F_1-ATPase	CS		↑	89, 175
Mitochondrial encoded				
Cytochrome oxidase, subunit III	CS		↑	73, 89, 126, 175
Cytochrome *b*	CS		↑	175, 176
Mitochondrial membrane phospholipid				
Cardiolipin	DN	↓		171
	CS	↑		152
Fatty acid metabolism enzymes				
CAT, HADH, THIOL	CS	↑		63, 127
Amino acid metabolism enzymes				
Amino acid aminotransferases	CS	↑		63
Glutamine synthetase	DN (GLC)	↑	↑	41
Heme biosynthesis				
Aminolevulinate synthase	CS, EX	↑	nc	153, 158
Transcription factors				
Early response genes				
c-fos, *c-jun*, *egr*-1	CS, EX, FO	↑	↑	106, 170
Myogenic basic helix-loop-helix factors				
MyoD, myogenin	DN (ES)	↑	↑	37, 178

CS, chronic stimulation; EX, exercise training; DN, denervation; DN (ES), denervation + direct electrical stimulation; HS, hindlimb suspension; FO, functional overload elicited by surgical ablation or tenotomy; ST, stretch; IM, immobilization.

of genes encoded within mitochondrial DNA, including both ribosomal RNA and protein-coding genes, is modulated in skeletal myofibers by sustained changes in work demands.

Sarcomeric Proteins

Contractile protein isoforms can be regulated by physiological conditions that promote hypertrophy or atrophy, and in the remodeling response to sustained contractile activity. Hypertrophy induced by functional overload or mechanical stretch generally favors a fast-to-slow fiber-type transition that is associated with corresponding shifts in myosin heavy chain isoform expression (48, 53, 131). In contrast, atrophy of skeletal muscle induced by hindlimb suspension or immobilization elicits a slow-to-fast transition in MHC isoform expression (16, 48, 53, 131). Although the data are incomplete, transitions of MHC isoforms generally are accompained by coordinate changes in isoforms of myosin light chains (131). Motor nerve stimulation in the rabbit model promotes virtually a complete replacement of fast myosin heavy and light chains with their slow muscle counterparts, and a comparable transformation of thin filament components (121, 122). Elevated concentrations of mRNAs encoding slow myosin light chain isoforms are observed within 1 week of the onset of nerve stimulation, while replacement of thick filament proteins requires several weeks to become complete, probably due to their long half-lives. Endurance training protocols also stimulate expression of slow muscle isoforms of contractile proteins, but in a less dramatic manner than continuous nerve stimulation (17).

Enzymes of Glycolysis

Reduced expression of glycolytic enzymes is an early and prominent feature of the response to continuous nerve stimulation (89, 175), and has been observed in muscles from treadmill trained animals as well (8). Curiously, hexokinase II enzyme activity is induced up to 14-fold by chronic contractions (66, 87, 167, 169), in distinct contrast to other enzymes of the Embden-Meyerhof pathway, which are suppressed by fourfold or more (89, 175). Chronic nerve stimulation (39, 87) and exercise training (114, 129, 146) also enhance expression of the insulin-responsive glucose transporter (GLUT4) protein. Although these findings have led to speculation that expression of the GLUT4 and hexokinase II genes may be regulated coordinately with the expression of genes encoding oxidative enzymes (129), the complete loss of contractile activity resulting from denervation alters the expression of these two genes in a divergent manner; hexokinase II activity is increased (169) while GLUT4 expression is reduced (62, 103). The functional implications of these seemingly paradoxical responses to changes in contractile activity are unclear, but perhaps are related to mitochondrial binding of hexokinase II (168).

Mitochondrial Proteins

Perhaps the most distinctive hallmark of the endurance training response is the increased specific activity of mitochondrial enzymes of the Krebs cycle, the electron transport chain, and heme biosynthesis (17, 67). This form of adaptation is so consistent and easily evoked that simple colorimetric assays of mitochondrial enzyme activity are frequently used as internal controls in physiological studies to verify that training effects have occurred. Directionally similar but quantitatively more striking changes result from chronic motor nerve stimulation (122). In either case, induction of mitochondrial enzymes is roughly proportional to the increase in mitochondrial mass observed in ultrastructural studies, and generally proportionate increases in members of functional groups of enzymes [e.g., tricarboxylic acid (TCA) cycle] and in polypeptide components of multisubunit enzymes (e.g., cytochrome-*c* oxidase) are observed. During hypertrophic growth of skeletal muscle, expression of genes encoding mitochondrial enzymes is not induced, such that the fractional volume of mitochondria and specific activities of mitochondrial enzymes either remain constant or are diminished.

An intriguing feature of the stimulation of mitochondrial biogenesis that ensues when skeletal myofibers are tonically active is the participation of the mitochondrial genome in this process. Several mitochondrial enzyme complexes require components produced uniquely as products of mitochondrial DNA. For example, the cytochrome oxidase holoenzyme requires for activity three polypeptide subunits that are encoded only within mitochondrial DNA, in addition to ten subunits derived as products of nuclear genes. To maintain stoichiometry among these subunits under conditions in which the number of functional enzyme units is varying by as much as an order of magnitude, mechanisms must be present to coordinate expression of the relevant genes within the nuclear and mitochondrial compartments. Current evidence suggests that expression of both rRNA and protein coding genes within mitochondrial DNA is increased by tonic contractile activity.

Transcription Factors

The induction of genes encoding transcription factors by contractile activity in skeletal muscle is of special interest, since these gene products may control expression of downstream genes that define muscle phenotype (i.e., myosin isoforms or myoglobin). Recent studies have noted acute induction of immediate early genes encoding transcription factors by changes in neural input and contractile activity in myofibers. Immediate early genes were identified originally on the basis of their rapid and striking induction in culture by mitotic growth factors following serum starvation. These include the protooncogene products Fos and Jun that form heterodimers and comprise the transcription factor AP-1, as well as the zinc finger proteins *egr-1* (*zif268*), which also bind DNA and function as transcriptional activators.

Induction of c-*fos* and c-*myc* in hearts of intact animals occurs as an early response to presure overload (6, 78), and similar effects are evoked by stretching neonatal cardiac myocytes in culture (6, 85, 86). These findings have led to the suggestion that changes in the expression of c-*fos* and c-*myc* may be part of a cascade of events leading to cardiac cell hypertrophy (78). Interestingly, functional overload of the soleus muscle induced by tenotomy also elicits a rapid (3 h) and marked (eightfold) increase in c-*myc* mRNA but fails to produce any alteration in c-*fos* (170).

Alterations in neural activity also affect immediate early gene expression in skeletal myofibers. Stimulation of the nerve innervating the gastrocnemius muscle of mice increases levels of c-*jun* and *egr*-1 mRNA, while denervation results in a marked increase in both c-*jun* and c-*fos* expression (2, 13) without changes in expression of *egr*-1 (2). Motor nerve stimulation in the rabbit model leads to a complex pattern of expression of immediate early genes: an acute but transient induction of c-*fos* mRNA and protein occurs within the first 12 h that is followed by a second and sustained wave of increased c-Fos protein abundance that begins within 7 days and persists for at least 21 days. Other immediate early genes, such as *egr*-1 and c-*jun*, respond in a similar manner while a related *jun* isoform (*jun-D*) is not induced. Increased presense of c-Fos protein is observed within nuclei of both myofibers and capillary endothelial cells, suggesting a role for proteins of this class in gene activation events within postmitotic myocytes as well as in proliferating microvascular cells (106).

Myogenic basic-helix-loop helix (bHLH) transcription factors, which exert essential functions during differentiation of skeletal myotubes, also are regulated in adult muscles in response to denervation or nerve stimulation. In denervated muscle, myogenin mRNA rapidly accumulates between 8 and 16 h, while MyoD transcipt levels increase between 16 and 24 h after denervation (37). Denervation-induced increases in myogenin and MyoD mRNAs have been reported to be in excess of 40- and 15-fold, respectively, relative to innervated muscle (37, 178). It has recently been proposed that denervation also may lead to increased functional activity of myogenin and products of other myogenic determination genes of the bHLH class on the basis of changes in phosphorylation of a critical threonine residue within the basic domain of these proteins. It is proposed that membrane depolarizations of innervated muscle fibers lead to activation of protein kinase C, which phosphorylates myogenin at this site and inhibits DNA-binding activity. Denervation may remove this tonic suppressive effect on the function of myogenic bHLH proteins and augment transcriptional activity of certain promoters (such as acetylcholine receptor subunits) that are dependent upon binding of these factors

A recently identified member of the winged helix or *fkh*/HNF-3 family of transcription factors, termed myocyte nuclear factor (MNF), binds an essential transcriptional control element within an upstream enhancer of the human myoglobin gene. As assessed by immunoblot analysis, the abundance of MNF protein is up-regulated markedly (five- to tenfold) in rabbit skeletal muscles subjected to chronic motor nerve stimulation, in parallel to changes in myoglobin gene expression (10).

Growth Factors and Receptors

Heparin-binding mitogenic activity and immunoreactive fibroblast growth factors are increased in rabbit skeletal muscles subjected to motor nerve stimulation in parallel to remodeling events within myofibers and the angiogenic response that leads to capillary proliferation (111).

Innervation and denervation promote striking changes in expression of subunits of the nicotinic acetylcholine receptor of the motor end-plate. The formation of the neuromuscular junction during development results in a conversion of the nicotinic acetylcholine receptor subunit composition from the embryonic ($\alpha_2\beta\gamma\delta$) to the adult ($\alpha_2\beta\epsilon\delta$) form, an overall repression of nicotinic acetylcholine receptor gene expression, and a redistribution of the protein from throughout the surface of the embryonic myotube to the motor end plate. This switch from embryonic to adult isofoms and repression of extrasynaptic nicotinic acetylcholine receptor gene expression during development has been attributed to the onset of electrical activity and/or neurotrophic factors within the muscle fiber (55, 93). Conversely, as noted previously, denervation of adult skeletal muscle evokes a marked increase in the level of mRNAs encoding for several of the subunits (including the embryonic γ-subunit) of the nicotinic acetylcholine receptor throughout the myofiber, an effect that is suppressed by direct electrical stimulation of the denervated muscle (44, 47).

In addition to the prominent effects of neural activity that control acetylcholine receptors, many other cell surface receptors for growth factors and hormones are modulated by neural input and contractile activity. Denervation leads to overexpression of polypeptide components of the receptor for ciliary neurotrophic factor, a trophic peptide released from motor nerves that appears to have a role in maintaining muscle mass (60). Chronic motor nerve stimulation or endurance training up-regulate β_2 adrenergic receptors (18, 89, 174) as well as peak catecholamine-responsive adenylate cyclase activity (90).

MECHANISMS OF GENE REGULATION

Definitions

In this review we employ the term "gene expression" to indicate the abundance of a product of a specific gene within a given cell. The gene product may be mRNA or protein, depending on the context of the discussion. Using this broad definition, gene expression can be controlled at any of several discrete steps in the synthesis of proteins (Fig. 25.2). Changes in steady-state levels of a specific mRNA induced by a given stimulus most commonly reflect variations in the rate of transcription of the gene encoding that mRNA, but can result from differences in RNA processing (excision of introns or polyadenylation) or in stability of mature mRNA molecules. Expression of some genes expressed in skeletal myofibers are known to be regulated at these posttranscriptional stages. Regulation at any one of these steps is termed "pretranslational." We refer to control mechanisms that alter rates of protein synthesis at constant concentrations of mRNA as "translational" regulation. Finally, the abundance of a specific polypeptide within the cell may be regulated by variations in protein stability, even in the absence of changes in mRNA abundance or in rates of protein synthesis. This form of control is termed "posttranslational."

Transcription

As shown in Table 25.2, the abundance of many mRNA species is regulated by contractile activity in skeletal muscle. It is reasonable to assume that, in most cases, variations in steady-state concentrations of a specific message result from modulation of the rate of transcription of the gene. Direct evidence for transcriptional regulation in response to increased contractile activity is available from recent work on the GLUT4 gene in exercise-trained rats (113) and from studies of denervation-induced up-regulation of acetylcholine receptor subunits (159).

A large and detailed body of information recently has become available concerning transcriptional control during muscle differentiation, and this work provides a framework for future studies of regulation of transcription by contractile work. Transcriptional control regions within many muscle-specific genes have been mapped to high resolution, and members of several families of transcription factors are involved in early or late stages of gene regulation in the developing myofiber. These include the myogenic bHLH proteins (myogenin, MyoD, MRF4, and myf5), MADS-box proteins (MEF-2 and SRF), homeobox proteins (Mhox), winged helix factors (MNF), and others (TEF1). In addition, promoter or enhancer elements that control transcription of nuclear genes encoding mitochodrial proteins have been defined. Only limited data currently implicate any of these elements and their cognate binding proteins in the control of gene transcription by contractile activity in skeletal muscles. In principle, however, it is likely that events illustrated in Figure 25.5 are important in this process. Substantial progress in this area is expected, due to recent advances in gene transfer technologies that make it feasible to conduct detailed promoter analyses in muscles of intact animals.

Myogenic bHLH proteins have been studied in elegant detail, and a variety of mechanisms have been shown to regulate their activity, including phosphorylation by protein kinase A (177), phosphorylation of a specific threonine in the basic domain by protein kinase C (99), competition for cofactors (with Id for E-proteins [115, 154]), and other protein–protein interactions that either enhance or inhibit function of the myogenic factors (98). The abundance of myogenic bHLH proteins is up-regulated by denerva-

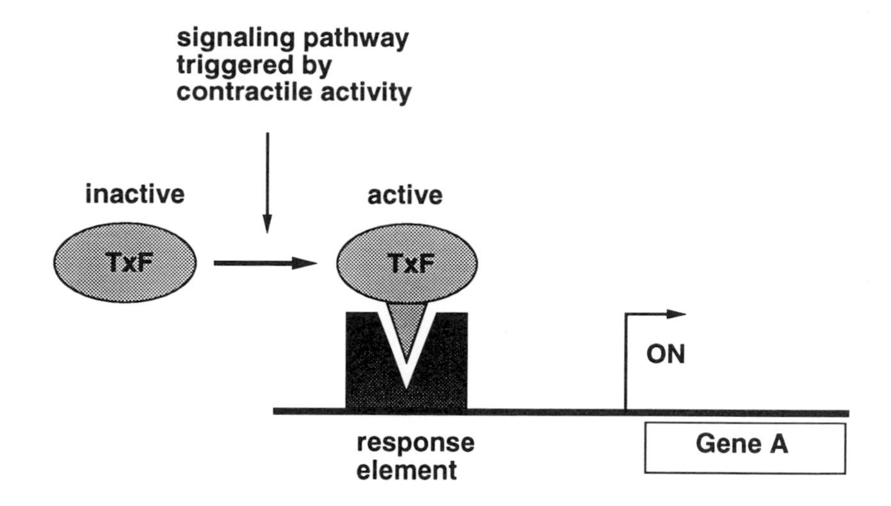

FIG. 25.5. Control of transcription factor activity by signals arising within contracting skeletal myofibers. At the first step in a cascade of gene regulatory events, a preexisting pool of a specific transcription factor (TxF) is present within the cell but is functionally inactive in resting muscles. Nerve stimulation and contractile activity trigger a signaling pathway, the culmination of which is the activation of TxF such that it can bind its cognate response element and induce transcription of a target gene (Gene A). The activation of TxF may be based on translocation from the cytoplasm to the nucleus; unmasking of a DNA binding domain (with or without release from an inhibitory factor); or unmasking of a previously nonfunctional *trans*-activation domain. In this scenario, Gene A itself encodes a transcription factor, the synthesis of which subsequently regulates downstream genes (Gene B and Gene C). Examples of genetic control mechanisms that function in this manner are described in the text.

tion (37, 178), a response that is completely prevented by direct electrostimulation of the denervated muscle (37). Recent gene transfer experiments provide additional evidence supporting a direct role for the myogenic bHLH proteins in regulating the transcription of activity-dependent genes in denervated muscle (14, 105). An 842 bp upstream segment from the acetylcholine receptor α_1-subunit gene was linked to a luciferase reporter gene, packaged into recombinant adenoviral particles and injected in skeletal muscle of adult chickens (14). Denervation led to a tenfold up-regulation of luciferase activity. Point mutations within more proximal of two E-box (CCnnTG) motifs within this segment abolished the response to denervation, suggesting a requirement for bHLH proteins (which bind selectively to E-box sequences) in this response. In support of this concept, Merlie et al. (105) have recently found that a 355 bp region of the myogenin promoter is sufficient to confer up-regulation of reporter gene activity in denervated skeletal muscle of transgenic mice. The presence of E-box sequences within the bHLH myogenin promotor (autoregulatory site) is consistent with the idea that the myogenic bHLH proteins may serve as targets for signaling cascades triggered by changes in neural activity. Indeed, myogenin, which is normally phosphorylated in contracting chick myotubes grown in culture, becomes dephosphorylated when contractile activity is blocked by tetrodoxin treatment (104), a model that mimics denervation of adult skeletal muscle. Dephosphorylation of myogenin coincides with increased binding to E box sequences within the acetylcholine receptor α_1-subunit promotor and with enhanced myogenin-mediated transcriptional activity (104, 181). Moreover, direct electrostimulation reverses the response to denervation by triggering a protein kinase C–mediated inactivation of myogenin and, thus, suppression of nicotinic acetylcholine receptor gene expression (76).

Transcription factors that bind elements common to promotor regions of nuclear-encoded mitochondrial proteins are not as well characterized. Two transcriptional activators, termed nuclear respiratory factor 1 and 2 (NRF1 and NRF2), bind motifs within the cytochrome *c* promoter, as well as upstream regions of genes encoding the nonmitochondrial proteins EIF-2a and hepatic tyrosine aminotransferase (24). These two latter proteins are involved in the rate-limiting steps of their respective pathways; namely, the initiation of translation, an energy-demanding process, and the degradation of tyrosine, an amino acid released from muscle during exercise. As suggested by Chau et al. (24), NRF1 may, therefore, represent an important regulatory mechanism for coordinating the expression of genes involved not only in mitochondrial function but also in other facets of intracellular metabolism that affect overall energy balance.

Recognition sites for NRF2 are found in the 5′-regulatory regions of genes encoding cytochrome c oxidase subunit Vb, β-F_1ATPase, and mitochondrial transcription factor A (mtTFA) (158). The mtTFA gene product binds to both the heavy and light strand promotors of the mitochondrial D-loop region and is believed to be the principal activator of mitochondrial DNA transcription (28). A recognition site for NRF1 is present within the 5′-regulatory region of the gene encoding the RNA subunit of MRP, a mitochondrial endoribonuclease believed to be responsible for generating RNA primers for mitochondrial DNA replication (see later under SPECIAL PATHWAYS FOR CONTROL OF MITOCHONDRIAL GENES). Thus, NRF1 and NRF2 may serve to coordinate expression of both nuclear and mitochondrial-encoded genes during mitochondrial biogenesis (164).

Unique overlapping sequence elements common to the β-F_1ATPase and ANT1 genes have been termed the OXBOX and REBOX motifs (26, 57, 97). The OXBOX is a positive-response element that enhances transcription upon association with a muscle-specific protein factor (96). It is overlapped by a negative response element (REBOX) that binds a ubiquitously expressed, redox-state sensitive nuclear factor (see later under Redox Potential) (26). OXBOX and REBOX specific binding is also present in a conserved OXBOX/REBOX containing sequence within the D-loop region of human mitochondrial DNA (57). Thus, the OXBOX/REBOX region may also be involved in coordinating the expression of nuclear-encoded mitochondrial oxidative phosphorylation genes in response to environmental signals.

RNA Processing, Targeting, and Stability

While there is no current evidence identifying changes in RNA processing, targeting, or stability that result from contractile activity in skeletal muscle, several control mechanisms involving RNA-protein interactions delineated in other cell systems may ultimately prove pertinent to this subject. Proteins that function to protect mRNA from degradation by RNA-protein interaction have been well documented, and recognition sites have been mapped to 5′- and 3′-untranslated regions of various transcripts (79). One such recently described RNA-binding protein, termed COLBP, binds to the 3′-untranslated region of several nuclear-encoded cytochrome-*c* oxidase subunit transcripts (124). Binding activity of COLBP is increased in human Hep G2 liver cells treated with the mitochondrial protein synthesis inhibitor thiamphenicol and is concurrent with thiamphenicol-induced cytochrome-*c* oxidase mRNA protection (25). Interestingly, stability of mRNAs not destined for the mitochondria (e.g., β-actin) are unaffected by the inhibitor (25). Although the mechanism regulating COLBP binding activity has not been established, disruptions in intracellular phosphorylation potential (ATP/ADP ratios) and/or redox state (NADH/NAD) represent possible signaling events, as both would be expected to be compromised in respiratory-deficient cells.

Translational and Posttranslational Control

Translational control also may be important in muscle remodeling in response to chronic motor nerve stimulation. In the rabbit model, ribosomal RNA per unit muscle mass is increased, suggesting increased translational capacity, despite the decline in muscle mass that is characteristic of this model. The abundance of several proteins (cytochrome *c*, δ-aminoluvinate synthase, GLUT4, and citrate synthase) is increased early in the response to exercise training or nerve stimulation in the absence of corresponding changes in mRNA (15, 113, 158). Protein levels may be increased due to enhanced translational efficiency, although direct evidence for an exercise-mediated increase in fractional rates of protein synthesis has yet to be demonstrated (17). Protein stability also may be enhanced by exercise. As discussed earlier under THEORETICAL AND KINETIC CONSIDERATIONS, this latter mechanism may be most pertinent to proteins with relatively short half-lives, such as δ-aminoluvinate synthase (69, 153). For example, hexokinase II enzyme activity increases during recovery (24 h) from chronic stimulation (24 h) despite rapid and concurrent declines in hexokinase II mRNA and ^{35}S methionine incorportation into hexokinase II protein (66). Finally, it is important to recall some of the other kinetic principles raised earlier under THEORETICAL AND KINETIC CONSIDERATIONS. The half-life of a given protein is typically much longer than the half-life of its corresponding mRNA. As such, wide daily fluctations in mRNA may give rise to an apparent stable rate of increase in protein synthesis that is mediated by transcriptional rather than translational control mechanisms (Fig. 25.2). Rigorous tests of these possibilities await development of more sensitive techniques for determining mRNA levels and fractional protein synthesis rates in intact muscles.

MESSENGERS AND SIGNAL TRANSDUCTION PATHWAYS

The concept of primary messengers arising within contracting muscles was presented at the beginning of this chapter, and potential signaling molecules and pathways are illustrated in Figure 25.1. Primary messengers trigger secondary events, examples of which are depicted in Figure 25.6, initiating a cascade (Fig. 25.7) that ultimately alters the morphological, biochemical, and physiological characteristics of the muscle. The focus of this section is on efforts to identify the primary messengers, and the components of signaling pathways that culminate in the gene switching events described earlier under WHAT GENES ARE REGULATED BY CONTRACTILE ACTIVITY? In compiling the following list of candidates, we have considered two major criteria: the concentration of the putative effector must be altered by contractile activity in skeletal muscles; and the putative effector and/or signaling pathway must be known to regulate gene expression, if not in contracting skeletal muscle, than at least in other well-defined biological systems.

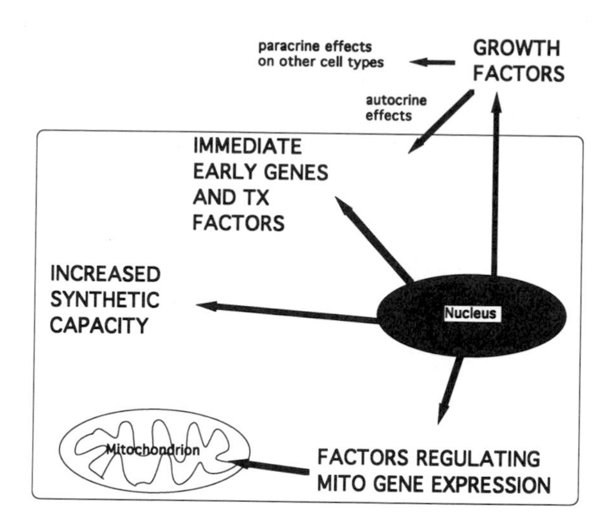

FIG. 25.6. Putative secondary events in the control of gene expression by contractile activity in skeletal muscles. Primary messengers illustrated in Figure 25.1 evoke secondary responses that function as intermediate steps in the response to work overload. Such secondary events are likely to include the elaboration by the myofiber of peptide growth factors (e.g., IGF-1); the induction of immediate early genes and other transcription factors; the increased synthesis of ribosomal RNA and proteins that alter the protein synthetic capacity of the cell; and the production of nuclear gene products that modulate replication or transcription of mitochondrial DNA, or that regulate translation, assembly, or stability of mitochondrial proteins.

Calcium

Alterations in intracellular Ca^{2+} concentration mediate activation/repression of a number of signaling pathways that elicit diverse cellular responses. Calcium ion activates several protein kinases including dedicated protein kinases such as myosin light chain kinase and phosphorylase kinase as well as the multifunctional protein kinase C, protein kinase A, and the Ca^{2+}/calmodulin-dependent protein kinases. In addition, cytosolic Ca^{2+} stimulates glucose transport (61), protein phosphatase 2B activity (29), and the DNA binding and/or transactivation function of several transcription factors (30, 100, 144, 165).

Direct measurement of intracellular Ca^{2+} indicates that total Ca^{2+} concentration is increased nearly sevenfold as early as 1 day after the onset of continuous motor nerve stimulation (147). However, this increase in free Ca^{2+} is no longer evident after 2 weeks of stimulation (147). The transient nature of this elevation could be construed as evidence against free Ca^{2+} as a primary stimulus for the adaptive process (121). However, secondary events triggered by Ca^{2+} may persist beyond the period in which total cellular calcium ion is elevated, or subcellular compartmentalization of Ca^{2+} pools important for regulatory

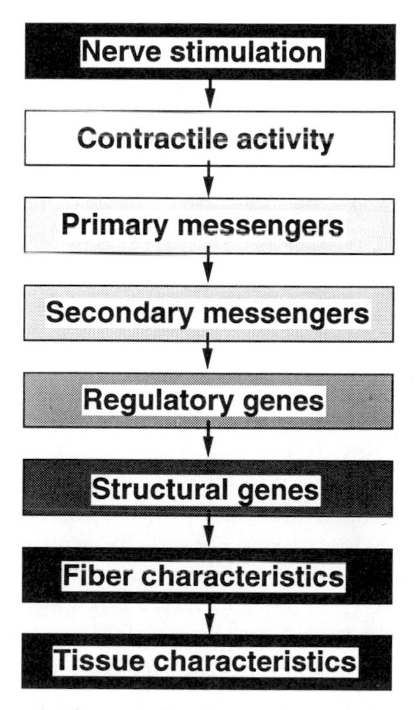

FIG. 25.7. Steps in the cascade of events by which motor nerve activity leads to physiologically relevant alterations of skeletal muscles.

events may persist after the initial phase of calcium increase has abated. For example, down regulation of nicotinic acetylcholine receptor expression during muscle development or in response to electrostimulation of denervated muscle (see earlier under Growth Factors and Receptors and under Transcription) arises from influx of extracellular Ca^{2+} through L-type Ca^{2+} channels (75). Interestingly, release of Ca^{2+} from intracellular sarcoplasmic reticulum stores does not down regulate expression of the receptor, suggesting that influx of extracellular Ca^{2+} triggers activation of a signaling pathway near the point of entry into the cell (75)

The biochemical responses to chronic stimulation of fast-twitch glycolytic muscle include marked and rapid decreases in sarcoplasmic reticulum Ca^{2+}-ATPase activity and in the expression of the Ca^{2+} sequestering protein parvalbumin (122). This early reduction in Ca^{2+}-sequestering capacity may influence free Ca^{2+} concentrations and amplify signaling events initiated by Ca^{2+} that act later in the adaptive process. Similar to chronic stimulation, sarcoplasmic reticulum Ca^{2+}-ATPase activity is depressed for ~30 min following an acute bout of exercise (20, 51). Detailed studies of the sarcoplasmic reticulum Ca^{2+}-ATPase protein indicate that the stimulation-induced decline in enzyme activity results from allosteric modification of the active site rather than a specific decrease in protein content (101). Thus, impairment in the sarcoplasmic reticulum Ca^{2+}-ATPase activity could result in a transient increase in free Ca^{2+} during recovery from exercise. Whether such an increase in Ca^{2+} concentration, if present, participates in the signaling pathways that ultimately lead to the gene regulatory events occurring during recovery from exercise, as discussed earlier under THEORETICAL AND KINETIC CONSIDERATIONS, remains to be determined.

Hydrogen Ion

The accelerated glycolysis associated with muscle contractions leads to generation of lactate and a fall in intracellular pH. Such intracellular acidosis is exacerbated by hypoxia or ischemia, but occurs even in well-perfused muscles, particularly in type IIb fibers during high work rates. The importance of rising hydrogen ion concentration as a stimulus to changes in gene expression in skeletal muscles is currently undefined. It is clear, however, that pathways for gene regulation as a function of pH are present in other mammalian cells. Renal tubular epithelial cells respond to intracellular acidosis by increasing transcription of Na/H antiporter genes via a multistep pathway that includes activation of protein kinase C and tyrosine kinases, as well as induction of immediate early gene transcription (74, 107). Acidosis also may play a role in transcriptional activation of genes encoding heat shock proteins (112).

Energy Charge/Phosphorylation Potential

Muscles stimulated electrically via the motor nerve display a marked reduction in phosphorylation potential of the adenylate system ($ATP/ADP_{free} \times P_{inorganic}$) within 15 min after the initiation of nerve stimulation (54, 70), a condition that persists through 50 days of continuous contractile activity (54). The decreased $ATP/ADP_{free} \times P_{inorganic}$ ratio is due to a persistent reduction in ATP concentration as well as to an increase in both ADP_{free} and $P_{inorganic}$ (54). Phosphorylation potential is also reduced by chronic feeding of the creatine analogue β-guanidinopropionic acid (β-GPA), a drug that competively inhibits creatine uptake in muscle but is a poor substrate for the creatine kinase reaction (43). The resulting β-GPA–induced fall in intracellular PCr and ATP triggers increases in mitochondrial density and gene expression qualitatively similar to the adaptive changes associated with increased contractile activity (91, 108, 128). In addition, elimination of the muscle creatine kinase isozyme through introduction of a null mutation into the germline of mice has recently been shown to result in a twofold increase in the expression of mitochondrial enzymes and total mitochondrial volume (162). Similar to β-GPA feedings, knockout of the muscle creatine kinase isozyme decreased the resting muscle ATP/ADP ratio (162).

These data suggest that changes in energy charge or phosphorylation potential may initiate changes in gene expression in skeletal muscles, although the secondary events that transduce the signal to the responsive genes have not been identified. One possibile mechanism is that a decrease in intracellular phosphorylation potential directly disrupts the phosphorylation state, and thus activity, of key regulatory proteins. In other words, reductions in ATP generated by increased metabolic demand and/or decreased metabolic capacity may limit energy phosphate exchange throughout the cell, resulting in a shift in the ratio of phosphorylated to unphosphorylated (active vs. inactive) forms of key transcription factors and/or signaling proteins.

A second possibility is that a reduction in phosphorylation potential elicits a secondary signaling event that is, in turn, responsible for activating and coordinating the adaptive changes in gene expression. A potential link of this type has recently been made with respect to ATP/ADP ratios, sarcoplasmic reticulum-bound creatine kinase, and regulation of the sarcoplasmic reticulum Ca^{2+} -ATPase enzyme activity. Creatine kinase bound to the sarcoplasmic reticulum catalyzes the local regeneration of ATP, which is used preferentially by the sarcoplasmic reticulum Ca^{2+}-ATPase for Ca^{2+} uptake. However, accumulation of ADP inhibits Ca^{2+}-ATPase activity, an effect that becomes more pronounced as free Ca^{2+} increases (88). Thus, a reduction in phosphorylation potential (increased ADP), generated by contractile activity or altered creatine phosphate transfer capacity, could elicit an increase in free intracellular Ca^{2+}, which may then serve as a secondary messenger by activating downstream signaling events regulating gene expression. This hypothetical mechanism emphasizes the point that multiple and interrelated intracellular signals may participate in the cascade of events leading to the activity-induced modulation of gene expression in skeletal muscle.

Redox Potential

Low-intensity exercise as well as continuous low-frequency stimulation decrease the NADH/NAD ratio in skeletal muscle (54, 135). During chronic stimulation, however, the change in redox state is transient and returns to resting state after 3 days (54). The possibility that alterations in redox state may alter gene expression in skeletal muscle has not been addressed directly, but cellular redox potential clearly is a potent stimulus to gene regulation in other cell types.

The oxidation/reduction status of specific transcription factors was first described in prokaryotes, where the transcriptional regulatory protein OxyR changes DNA-binding specificity according to redox conditions (148). In eukaryotes, evidence for redox-based transcriptional regulation is based on studies of DNA binding in vitro of selected transcription factors. Redox-sensitive DNA binding proteins include Fos and Jun, components of the AP1 transcription factor (1); nuclear factor kB (NFkB), a pleiotropic cellular transcription factor (140, 156); EGR-1, the early growth response factor (77); USF[43], a component of the Pol I transactivator USF (123); and the glucocorticoid and progesterone receptors (120, 145). Redox changes have also been shown to regulate the binding activity of the iron-responsive element–binding protein (IRE-BP) on untranslated portions of ferritin and transferin receptor mRNA (65).

The redox-sensitive proteins identified thus far display a marked but reversible decrease in DNA binding in the oxidized state. In the unbound state, oxidizing conditions are thought to result in the specific formation of both intra- and intermolecular disulfide bonds, or to elicit reversible oxidation of sulfydryl groups (RSH) to sulfenic acid (RSOH) (1, 102, 123). Cysteine residues flanked by one or two basic amino acids represent a highly conserved motif in redox-sensitive proteins (83). It is thought that the microenvironment around these cysteine residues may influence the oxidation constant (K_{ox}) of the sulfydryl groups, allowing the residue to adopt the oxidized form under the normally reducing environment of the cell (179). In the case of Fos and Jun, oxidation of a single cysteine residue in each protein inhibits DNA binding (resting cell), while reduction to the free sulfydryl state promotes protein-DNA interaction (1). A nuclear protein that facilitates in vitro binding of AP-1 sites under oxidizing conditions, termed Ref-1, has recently been identified (179), and presumably acts through reduction of the critical cysteine residues within Fos and Jun. The ability of Ref-1 to activate Fos-Jun DNA binding activity is itself sensitive to oxidative stress, but can be restored by treatment with thioredoxin (179). Ref-1 may, therefore, represent an intracellular redox-sensing protein that reversibly modulates the redox state and DNA-binding activity of redox-sensitive transcription factors which, in turn, regulate the expression of specific redox-sensitive genes (58, 123, 180).

In addition to these direct effects on transcription factors, redox state may also affect other messenger signaling pathways. For example, with respect to Ca^{2+} homeostasis, the sarcoplasmic reticulum Ca^{2+}-ATPase protein contains several reversible disulfide bonds that are critical for full activity of the enzyme (88).

Oxygen Tension

A number of genes are known to be regulated by hypoxia in mammalian cells. In some cases, the response seems to be triggered directly by changes in oxygen tension, while the response of other genes is attributable to metabolic sequelae of hypoxia, rather than to a direct oxygen-sensing mechanism.

Oxygen-dependent modulation of erythropoietin (EPO) gene expression has been studied intensively in recent years, and several components of the mechanism have been defined. A region 3′ to the transcribed portion of the human EPO gene can confer oxygen-regulated transcription to heterologous core promoters and has been termed an oxygen-response element (ORE) (125, 143). This ORE binds specifically to a nuclear protein factor (hypoxia-inducible factor [HIF-1]) that cannot be detected in normoxic cells, but is evident in hypoxic cells (143, 166). Hypoxic induction of this DNA-binding activity requires new RNA and protein synthesis, suggesting that HIF-1 itself is not the oxygen sensor, but is downstream in a multistep process triggered by hypoxia. HIF-1 is induced by cobalt, repressed by carbon monoxide, and unaffected by inhibitors of the electron transport chain, findings all consistent with a direct oxygen-sensing mechanism. These features suggest a functional analogy to the well-defined two-component pathway (FixL/FixJ) for oxygen-dependent regulation of genes required for nitrogen fixation by *Rhizobium meliloti* (3, 46, 109), the bacterium present in root nodules of legume plants. Importantly, HIF-1 is inducible by hypoxia in many cell types, including skeletal and cardiac muscle, that do not express EPO, implying that other downstream genes are regulated by HIF-1. In support of this hypothesis, stimulation of HIF-1 activity in HeLa cells has recently been shown to activate transcription of several genes encoding glycolytic enzymes, providing evidence that HIF-1 may play a more general regulatory role in mediating the adaptive responses to hypoxia (142).

Myogenic cells in culture exposed to hypoxia activate transcription of heat shock protein 70 (hsp70) through mechanisms that involve unmasking the DNA binding activity of a preexistent pool of heat shock transcription factors within the cell (12). Unlike the hypoxic activation of EPO gene expression, however, the effects of oxygen deprivation on transcription of the hsp70 gene appear to be mediated by metabolic sequelae of hypoxia, rather than by diminished oxygen tension per se, since inhibitors of mitochondrial respiration promote identical effects (11).

A number of other genes are induced by hypoxia (59, 81, 173), at least in some cell types. Expression of several glycolytic enzymes, as well as endothelin-1 and vascular endothelial cell growth factor (VEGF), is up-regulated under hypoxic conditions in vascular endothelial cells, and the tyrosine hydroxylyase gene is under exquisite hypoxic control in carotid body cells. Since some of the metabolic sequelae of tonic contractions are similar to those evoked by hypoxia, it is plausible that oxygen-dependent gene regulatory pathways participate in the adaptive responses to contractile activity in skeletal muscle. Moreover, some reports suggest that responses to endurance training are modified by systemic hypoxemia or by local ischemia produced by vascular occlusive disease (116, 150). Competitive athletes may train purposefully at high altitude because of presumed enhancing effects on performance, but the efficacy of this strategy remains controversial. Within cardiac muscle, chronic ischemia promotes angiogenesis, but the relationships between the processes that stimulate development of collateral vessels in the ischemic heart and those that trigger the angiogenic response within tonically contracting skeletal muscles is unknown at this time.

Mechanical Stretch

Contractile activity obviously places sarcolemmal and cytoskeletal components of myocytes, as well as the extracellular matrix, under mechanical tension. Elegant studies of cardiomyocytes cultured on flexible supports have elucidated several of the intracellular and extracellular events provoked by mechanical stimulation, which include: activation of phospholipases to release phosphatidylinositol messengers and diacylglycerol (86, 132), stimulation of several intracellular protein kinases (132), induction of immediate early gene expression (85, 133), and increased global rates of protein synthesis (85, 133). This conversion of a mechanical signal to a hypertrophic response in cardiomyocytes is, at least in part, mediated through autocrine and paracrine effects of peptide hormones (notably angiotensin II), the secretion of which is stimulated by mechanical tension (134). Angiotensin II, via its receptor, triggers several different signal transduction pathways that converge to stimulate DNA binding of serum response factor (and associated proteins) to the serum response element of the c-*fos* promoter.

Stretch-induced events in skeletal myofibers are not as well characterized, but many sequelae of both sustained and rhythmic stretch of cultured skeletal myotubes appear to be similar to the responses evoked in cardiomyocytes (163). Stretch-induced alterations in Na^+-K^+-ATPase and phospholipase activity as well as growth factor–mediated events have been observed in skeletal myotubes (163). The specific growth factors involved in the hypertrophic response of skeletal myofibers are probably different, however, than in the heart, with insulin-like growth factors assuming a prominent role.

Mechanical signals also evoke selective effects on expression of specific genes in developing and adult skeletal muscle. Immobilization of the fast-twitch tibialis anterior muscle in the stretched position induces expression of the slow MHC gene (33, 49) and represses expression of the fast-twitch IIb MHC gene (49). Of particular interest are the gene switching events that occur when the tibialis anterior muscle is subjected to both stretch and electrical stimulation. This combination induces hypertrophy (within

4 days) that is accompanied by fast-to-slow transformation in the pattern of expression of contractile protein genes (48, 49). Similar shifts in contractile protein gene expression are induced by electrical stimulation of unloaded muscle, but are less rapid (122), and are associated with fiber atrophy rather than hypertrophy. Thus, signaling events initiated by mechanical load are likely to participate in the overall regulatory response to exercise training.

Receptor Linked Signaling Pathways

As shown in Figure 25.1, contracting myofibers are exposed to a variety of extracellular hormones and factors that recognize specific sarcolemmal receptors and trigger intracellular signaling events that ultimately may control expression of specific genes. Several factors are released directly from motor nerve terminals (e.g., CGRP); others are released from sympathetic nerve terminals or reach the myocyte via the systemic circulation (e.g., catecholamines); while others (e.g., fibroblast growth factor [FGF]) are derived from storage sites in the extracellular matrix, from different cell types within the muscle (paracrine source), or from myofibers themselves (autocrine source).

Catecholamines, acting via the β_2 adrenergic receptor, activate adenylate cyclase to generate cyclic adenosine monophosphate (cAMP), a prototypic second messenger in many signaling cascades. Skeletal myofibers express receptors for calcitonin gene-related peptide (CGRP), which are also coupled via G proteins to adenylate cyclase (92). Gene regulation by cAMP via protein kinase A is a well-studied phenomenon that involves phosphorylation of transcription factors, including but not limited to CREB and related proteins (31, 32). cAMP-dependent regulation has been demonstrated for the cytochrome *c* gene, induction of which is dependent upon binding activity of CREB to cAMP response element sequences within the cytochrome *c* promotor (52). This effect, however, is present in BALB/3T3 (52) but not in COS-1 cells (40), and has not been directly tested in skeletal muscle cell lines for any of the genes prominently regulated by muscle contractions. Nevertheless, cAMP is elevated in tonically active skeletal muscles (89), and may have some as yet undefined role in the adaptive responses to muscle contractions. In muscles stimulated via the motor nerve, cAMP falls acutely, but subsequently exhibits a sustained elevation (89), contemporaneous with many of the gene-switching events described earlier under EXPERIMENTAL SYSTEMS AND MODELS OF STUDY OF GENE REGULATION BY CONTRACTILE ACTIVITY and under WHAT GENES ARE REGULATED BY CONRACTILE ACTIVITY? This chronic, stable elevation of cAMP in continuously contracting muscles is not dependent on catecholamine drive, since it also occurs in animals receiving high doses of a β-adrenergic receptor antagonist (89). It remains to be determined, however, whether the elevated concentrations of cAMP within the muscle fibers is an epiphenomenon, or a determinant of important remodeling events. Denervation also increases cAMP levels and protein kinase A activity (22), but induces effects on gene expression that are opposite to many of those evoked by motor nerve stimulation.

A considerable body of other literature has assessed the potential role of the β-adrenergic receptor in the endurance training response. Some reports have asserted that concurrent administration of β-adrenergic receptor antagonists during a period of training significantly blunts the acquisition of the major physiological hallmarks of the trained state (80). In addition, the chronic administration of adrenergic agonists has been reported to induce muscle hypertrophy or increased respiratory capacity (149). Other studies, however, present a different picture and indicate that endurance training effects, including skeletal muscle remodeling, are modified only marginally by β-adrenergic blockade (42, 64, 151). Data from the rabbit model of chronic motor nerve stimulation show that most of the important gene regulatory events triggered by tonic contractions can occur independently of β-adrenergic receptor activation (89, 90).

Peptide growth factors contact cell surface receptors and trigger multiple intracellular signaling pathways, some of which involve protein kinase C, which was discussed already with respect to Ca^{2+} as a primary messenger in contracting muscle fibers. In addition, growth factors activate tyrosine kinases, which in turn activate other kinases within signaling cascades that converge ultimately on nuclear transcription factors to regulate specific genes and sets of genes (7). Only a few studies, however, have examined the potential role of peptide growth factors and protein kinase/phosphatase cascades in mediating adaptive responses to work activity in skeletal fibers. Expression of FGFs is induced in skeletal muscles subjected to chronic motor nerve stimulation (111), but the role of FGFs as primary messengers in this process is undefined. In view of recent data defining important functions of peptide growth factors in cardiac and skeletal muscle hypertrophy (134), this would appear to be a fruitful area for future investigations.

SPECIAL PATHWAYS FOR CONTROL OF MITOCHONDRIAL GENES

The major increases in mitochondrial mass that are evoked in skeletal muscles by endurance training or chronic motor nerve stimulation require coordinated induction of many nuclear genes encoding mitochondrial proteins, as well as increased expression of genes located within mitochondrial DNA (mtDNA). In animal cells, the 16 kB circular mitochondrial genome encodes 12 essential protein subunits of respiratory chain complexes of the mitochondrial inner membrane, as well as two ribosomal RNA subunits, and the complete set of transfer RNAs required for protein translation within the mitochondrial matrix (28). Notably, all of the remaining enzymatic components required for replication and transcription of mtDNA; for RNA processing to produce mature mRNA, rRNA, and tRNA species, and for translation, folding, and assembly of mitochondrial proteins are generated as products of nuclear genes and imported into mitochondria.

Each strand of the mitochondrial genome is transcribed from a single promoter to produce a polycistronic primary transcript. The rRNA, tRNA, and mRNA products of mitochondrial DNA are then released by endonuclease cleavage of these primary transcripts. Therefore, relative differences in abundance of specific mitochondrial gene transcripts result primarily from variations in stability, and not from differential rates of transcription. The one exception to this principle is the preferential transcription of the two rRNA genes found on the mitochondrial heavy strand, by comparison to protein coding regions. This difference results from transcriptional termination, mediated by a DNA-binding protein that blocks progression of the RNA polymerase (27). The factors that determine stability of specific mitochondrial gene products appear to be subject to physiological regulation in some cells, but are not known to be altered by contractile activity in skeletal muscle. The transcriptional pausing event that determines the ratio of mitochondrial rRNA and mRNA, however, may be sensitive to signals arising in contracting muscle (5).

A major event leading to up-regulation of expression of mitochondrial genes in response to changing work demands in skeletal muscle appears to be an augmented number of copies of mtDNA per cell (5). This amplification of mtDNA is presumed to result from an increased rate of DNA replication, and indeed, the specific activity of the mtDNA polymerase in rabbit skeletal muscle is increased by motor nerve stimulation (5). It seems likely, therefore, that signals generated within contracting myofibers that regulate mitochondrial gene expression may do so, at least in part, by altering the expression of nuclear genes, products of which are rate limiting to replication of mtDNA. At a minimum, such products may include the mitochondrial DNA polymerase itself; factors governing priming and initiation of mtDNA replication, or factors governing processivity of mtDNA replication.

Priming of mtDNA synthesis currently is thought to be dependent on the generation of short RNA primers by a sequence-specific endoribonuclease termed MRP (157). Interestingly, MRP activity requires a small RNA subunit (MRP-RNA) that is encoded by a nuclear gene. The expression of MRP-RNA in skeletal muscles is stimulated markedly by changes in tonic contractile activity, with a time course that proceeds in parallel to the up-regulation of mtDNA copy number and expression of products of the mitochondrial genome (119, 172). Further studies are required to determine whether there is a causal relationship between these events.

With respect to processivity, mtDNA replication in animal cells proceeds by way of a displacement loop (D-loop) but, curiously, most replication events terminate abortively at specific points 500–1000 nucleotides downstream from the origin. Neither the mechanism nor the biological significance of this premature replicative termination is known. The relative frequency of complete vs. incomplete replication of mtDNA, however, appears to be regulated (5), and presents a potential control point for modulating mtDNA copy number.

CONCLUSIONS

Recent studies have provided a wealth of descriptive information concerning regulation of gene expression by contractile activity in skeletal muscles, and work extending over several decades has established the physiological importance of these adaptive responses. To a more limited degree, investigators in this field have begun to define biochemical and molecular mechanisms by which muscle cells sense changes in work demand and respond by altering expression of specific genes. Empowered with the increasingly powerful tools of modern molecular biology, we can reasonably expect further progress in this task, despite its complexity.

REFERENCES

1. Abate, C., L. Patel, F.3. Rauscher, and T. Curran. Redox regulation of fos and jun DNA-binding activity in vitro. *Science* 249: 1157–1161, 1990.

2. Abu-Shakra, S. R., A. J. Cole, and D. B. Drachman. Nerve stimulation and denervation induce differential patterns of immediate early gene mRNA expression in skeletal muscle. *Brain Res. Mol. Brain Res.* 18: 216–220, 1993.
3. Agron, P. G., G. S. Ditta, and D. R. Helinski. Oxygen regulation of nifA transcription in vitro. *Proc. Natl. Acad. Sci. U. S. A.* 90: 3506–3510, 1993.
4. Annex, B. H., W. E. Kraus, G. L. Dohm, and R. S. Williams. Mitochondrial biogenesis in striated muscles: rapid induction of citrate synthase mRNA by nerve stimulation. *Am. J. Physiol.* 260 (*Cell Physiol.* 29): C266–C270, 1991.
5. Annex, B. H., and R. S. Williams. Mitochondrial DNA structure and expression in specialized subtypes of mammalian striated muscle. *Mol. Cell. Biol.* 10: 5671–5678, 1990.
6. Aoyagi, T., and S. Izumo. Mapping of the pressure response element of the c-fos gene by direct DNA injection into beating hearts. *J. Biol. Chem.* 268: 27176–27179, 1993.
7. Avruch, J., X. F. Zhang, and J. M. Kyriakis. Raf meets Ras: completing the framework of a signal transduction pathway. *Trends Biochem. Sci.* 19: 279–283, 1994.
8. Baldwin, K. M., R. H. Fitts, F. W. Booth, W. W. Winder, and J. O. Holloszy. Depletion of muscle and liver glycogen during exercise. Protective effect of training. *Pflugers Arch.* 354: 203–312, 1975.
9. Bar, A., J. A. Simoneau, and D. Pette. Altered expression of myosin light-chain isoforms in chronically stimulated fast-twitch muscle of the rat. *Eur. J. Biochem.* 178: 591–594, 1989.
10. Bassel-Duby, R., M. D. Hernandez, Q. Yang, J. M. Rochelle, M. F. Seldin, and R. S. Williams. Myocyte nuclear factor, a novel winged-helix transcription factor under both developmental and neural regulation in striated myocytes. *Mol. Cell. Biol.* 14: 4596–4605, 1994.
11. Benjamin, I. J., S. Horie, M. L. Greenberg, R. J. Alpern, and R. S. Williams. Induction of stress proteins in cultured myogenic cells. Molecular signals for the activation of heat shock transcription factor during ischemia. *J. Clin. Invest.* 89: 1685–1689, 1992.
12. Benjamin, I. J., B. Kroger, and R. S. Williams. Activation of the heat shock transcription factor by hypoxia in mammalian cells. *Proc. Natl. Acad. Sci. U. S. A.* 87: 6263–6267, 1990.
13. Bessereau, J. L., B. Fontaine, and J. P. Changeux. Denervation of mouse skeletal muscle differentially affects the expression of the jun and fos proto-oncogenes. *New Biol.* 2: 375–383, 1990.
14. Bessereau, J. L., L. D. Stratford-Perricaudet, J. Piette, C. Le Poupon, and J. P. Changeux. In vivo and in vitro analysis of electrical activity-dependent expression of muscle acetylcholine receptor genes using adenovirus. *Proc. Natl. Acad. Sci. U. S. A.* 91: 1304–1308, 1994.
15. Booth, F. W. Cytochrome c protein synthesis rate in rat skeletal muscle. *J. Appl. Physiol.* 71: 1225–1230, 1991.
16. Booth, F. W., and C. R. Kirby. Changes in skeletal muscle gene expression consequent to altered weight bearing. *Am. J. Physiol.* 262 (*Regulatory Integrative Comp. Physiol.* 31): R329–R332, 1992.
17. Booth, F. W., and D. B. Thomason. Molecular and cellular adaptation of muscle in response to exercise: perspectives of various models. *Physiol. Rev.* 71: 541–585, 1991.
18. Buckenmeyer, P. J., A. H. Goldfarb, J. S. Partilla, M. A. Pineyro, and E. M. Dax. Endurance training, not acute exercise, differentially alters beta-receptors and cyclase in skeletal fiber types. *Am. J. Physiol.* 258 (*Endocrinol. Metab.* 27): E71–E77, 1990.
19. Buller, A. J., J. C. Eccles, and R. M. Eccles. Interactions between motoneurons and muscles in respect of the characteristic speeds of their responses. *J. Physiol. (Lond.)* 150: 417–439, 1960.
20. Byrd, S. K., L. J. McCutcheon, D. R. Hodgson, and P. D. Gollnick. Altered sarcoplasmic reticulum function after high-intensity exercise. *J. Appl. Physiol.* 67: 2072–2077, 1989.
21. Carey, J. O., P. D. Neufer, R. P. Farrar, J. H. Veerkamp, and G. L. Dohm. Transcriptional regulation of muscle fatty acid-binding protein. *Biochem. J.* 3: 613–617, 1994.
22. Chahine, K. G., E. Baracchini, and D. Goldman. Coupling muscle electrical activity to gene expression via a cAMP-dependent second messenger system. *J. Biol. Chem.* 268: 2893–2898, 1993.
23. Chahine, K. G., W. Walke, and D. Goldman. A 102 base pair sequence of the nicotinic acetylcholine receptor delta-subunit gene confers regulation by muscle electrical activity. *Development* 115: 213–219, 1992.
24. Chau, C. M., M. J. Evans, and R. C. Scarpulla. Nuclear respiratory factor 1 activation sites in genes encoding the gamma-subunit of ATP synthase, eukaryotic initiation factor 2 alpha, and tyrosine aminotransferase. Specific interaction of purified NRF-1 with multiple target genes. *J. Biol. Chem.* 267: 6999–7006, 1992.
25. Chrzanowska-Lightowlers, Z. M. A., T. Preiss, and R. N. Lightowlers. Inhibition of mitochondrial protein synthesis promotes increased stability of nuclear-encoded respiratory gene transcripts. *J. Biol. Chem.* 269: 27322–27328, 1994.
26. Chung, A. B., G. Stepien, Y. Haraguchi, K. Li, and D. C. Wallace. Transcriptional control of nuclear genes for the mitochondrial muscle ADP/ATP translocator and the ATP synthase beta subunit. Multiple factors interact with the OXBOX/REBOX promoter sequences. *J. Biol. Chem.* 267: 21154–21161, 1992.
27. Clayton, D. A. Nuclear gadgets in mitochondrial DNA replication and transcription. *Trends Biochem. Sci.* 16: 107–111, 1991.
28. Clayton, D. A. Transcription and replication of animal mitochondrial DNAs. *Int. Rev. Cytol.* 141: 217–232, 1992.
29. Cohen, P. The structure and regulation of protein phosphatases. *Annu. Rev. Biochem.* 58: 453–508, 1989.
30. Dash, P. K., K. A. Karl, M. A. Colicos, R. Prywes, and E. R. Kandel. cAMP response element-binding protein is activated by Ca^{2+}/calmodulin-as well as cAMP-dependent protein kinase. *Proc. Natl. Acad. Sci. U. S. A.* 88: 5061–5065, 1991.
31. de Groot, R. P., and P. Sassone-Corsi. Hormonal control of gene expression: multiplicity and versatility of cyclic adenosine 3′,5′-monophosphate-responsive nuclear regulators [published erratum appears in *Mol. Endocrinol.* 1993 Apr; 7:603]. *Mol. Endocrinol.* 7: 145–153, 1993.
32. Delmas, V., C. A. Molina, E. Lalli, R. de Groot, N. S. Foulkes, D. Masquilier, and P. Sassone-Corsi. Complexity and versatility of the transcriptional response to cAMP. *Rev. Physiol. Biochem. Pharmacol.* 124: 1–28, 1994.
33. Dix, D. J., and B. R. Eisenberg. Redistribution of myosin heavy chain mRNA in the midregion of stretched muscle fibers. *Cell Tissue Res.* 263: 61–69, 1991.
34. Duclert, A., J. Piette, and J. P. Changeux. Induction of acetylcholine receptor alpha-subunit gene expression in chicken myotubes by blocking electrical activity requires ongoing protein synthesis. *Proc. Natl. Acad. Sci. U. S. A.* 87: 1391–1395, 1990.

35. Dusterhoft, S., and D. Pette. Effects of electrically induced contractile activity on cultured embryonic chick breast muscle cells. *Differentiation* 44: 178–184, 1990.
36. Ecob-Prince, M. S., M. Jenkison, G. S. Butler-Browne, and R. G. Whalen. Neonatal and adult myosin heavy chain isoforms in a nerve-muscle culture system. *J. Cell. Biol.* 103: 995–1005, 1986.
37. Eftimie, R., H. R. Brenner, and A. Buonanno. Myogenin and MyoD join a family of skeletal muscle genes regulated by electrical activity. *Proc. Natl. Acad. Sci. U. S. A.* 88: 1349–1353, 1991.
38. Egginton, S., and B. D. Sidell. Thermal acclimation induces adaptive changes in subcellular structure of fish skeletal muscle. *Am. J. Physiol.* 256 (*Regulatory Integrative Comp. Physiol.* 25): R1–R9, 1989.
39. Etgen, G. J., Jr., R. P. Farrar, and J. L. Ivy. Effect of chronic electrical stimulation on GLUT4 protein content in fast-twitch muscle. *Am. J. Physiol.* 264 (*Regulatory Integrative Comp. Physiol.* 33): R816–R819, 1993.
40. Evans, M. J., and R. C. Scarpulla. Interaction of nuclear factors with multiple sites in the somatic cytochrome c promoter. Characterization of upstream NRF-1, ATF, and intron Sp1 recognition sequences. *J. Biol. Chem.* 264: 14361–14368, 1989.
41. Falduto, M. T., A. P. Young, and R. C. Hickson. Exercise interrupts ongoing glucocorticoid-induced muscle atrophy and glutamine synthetase induction. *Am. J. Physiol.* 263 (*Endocrinol. Metab.* 26): E1157–E1163, 1992.
42. Fell, R. D., S. E. Terblanche, W. W. Winder, and J. O. Holloszy. Adaptive responses of rats to prolonged treatment with epinephrine. *Am. J. Physiol.* 241 (*Cell Physiol.* 10): C55–C58, 1981.
43. Fitch, C. D., M. Jellinek, and E. J. Mueller. Experimental depletion of creatine and phosphocreatine from skeletal muscle. *J. Biol. Chem.* 249: 1060–1063, 1974.
44. Fontaine, B., and J. P. Changeux. Localization of nicotinic acetylcholine receptor alpha-subunit transcripts during myogenesis and motor endplate development in the chick. *J. Cell. Biol.* 108: 1025–1037, 1989.
45. Freerksen, D. L., N. A. Schroedl, G. V. Johnson, and C. R. Hartzell. Increased aerobic glucose oxidation by cAMP in cultured regenerated skeletal myotubes. *Am. J. Physiol.* 250 (*Cell Physiol.* 19): C713–C719, 1986.
46. Gilles-Gonzalez, M. A., G. S. Ditta, and D. R. Helinski. A haemoprotein with kinase activity encoded by the oxygen sensor of Rhizobium meliloti. *Nature* 350: 170–172, 1991.
47. Goldman, D., H. R. Brenner, and S. Heinemann. Acetylcholine receptor alpha-, beta-, gamma-, and delta-subunit mRNA levels are regulated by muscle activity. *Neuron* 1: 329–333, 1988.
48. Goldspink, G., A. Scutt, P. T. Loughna, D. J. Wells, T. Jaenicke, and G. F. Gerlach. Gene expression in skeletal muscle in response to stretch and force generation. *Am. J. Physiol.* 262 (*Regulatory Integrative Comp. Physiol.* 31): R356–R363, 1992.
49. Goldspink, G., A. Scutt, J. Martindale, T. Jaenicke, L. Turay, and G. F. Gerlach. Stretch and force generation induce rapid hypertrophy and myosin isoform gene switching in adult skeletal muscle. *Biochem. Soc. Trans.* 19: 368–373, 1991.
50. Goldspink, G., L. Turay, E. Hansen, S. Ennion, and G. Gerlach. Switches in fish myosin genes induced by environment temperature in muscle of the carp. *Symp. Soc. Exp. Biol.* 46: 139–149, 1992.
51. Gollnick, P. D., P. Korge, J. Karpakka, and B. Saltin. Elongation of skeletal muscle relaxation during exercise is linked to reduced calcium uptake by the sarcoplasmic reticulum in man. *Acta. Physiol. Scand.* 142: 135–136, 1991.
52. Gopalakrishnan, L., and R. C. Scarpulla. Differential regulation of respiratory chain subunits by a CREB-dependent signal transduction pathway. Role of cyclic AMP in cytochrome c and COXIV gene expression. *J. Biol. Chem.* 269: 105–113, 1994.
53. Gordon, T., and M. C. Pattullo. Plasticity of muscle fiber and motor unit types. In: *Exercise and Sport Science Reviews*, edited by J. O. Holloszy and K. B. Pandolf. Baltimore, MD: Williams & Wilkins, 1990, p. 331–362.
54. Green, H. J., S. Dusterhoft, L. Dux, and D. Pette. Metabolite patterns related to exhaustion, recovery and transformation of chronically stimulated rabbit fast-twitch muscle. *Pflugers Arch.* 420: 359–366, 1992.
55. Gundersen, K., J. R. Sanes, and J. P. Merlie. Neural regulation of muscle acetylcholine receptor epsilon- and alpha-subunit gene promoters in transgenic mice. *J. Cell. Biol.* 123: 1535–1544, 1993.
56. Hahn, C. G., and J. Covault. Neural regulation of N-cadherin gene expression in developing and adult skeletal muscle. *J. Neurosci.* 12: 4677–4687, 1992.
57. Haraguchi, Y., A. B. Chung, S. Neill, and D. C. Wallace. OXBOX and REBOX, overlapping promoter elements of the mitochondrial F0F1-ATP synthase beta subunit gene. OXBOX/REBOX in the ATPsyn beta promoter. *J. Biol. Chem.* 269: 9330–9334, 1994.
58. Hayashi, T., Y. Ueno, and T. Okamoto. Oxidoreductive regulation of nuclear factor kappa B. Involvement of a cellular reducing catalyst thioredoxin. *J. Biol. Chem.* 268: 11380–11388, 1993.
59. Helfman, T., and V. Falanga. Gene expression in low oxygen tension. *Am. J. Med. Sci.* 306: 37–41, 1993.
60. Helgren, M. E., S. P. Squinto, H. L. Davis, D. J. Parry, T. G. Boulton, C. S. Heck, Y. Zhu, G. D. Yancopoulos, R. M. Lindsay, and P. S. DiStefano. Trophic effect of ciliary neurotrophic factor on denervated skeletal muscle. *Cell* 76: 493–504, 1994.
61. Henriksen, E. J., K. J. Rodnick, and J. O. Holloszy. Activation of glucose transport in skeletal muscle by phospholipase C and phorbol ester. Evaluation of the regulatory roles of protein kinase C and calcium [published erratum appears in *J. Biol. Chem.* 1990 Apr 5;265:5917]. *J. Biol. Chem.* 264: 21536–21543, 1989.
62. Henriksen, E. J., K. J. Rodnick, C. E. Mondon, D. E. James, and J. O. Holloszy. Effect of denervation or unweighting on GLUT-4 protein in rat soleus muscle. *J. Appl. Physiol.* 70: 2322–2327, 1991.
63. Henriksson, J., M. M. Chi, C. S. Hintz, D. A. Young, K. K. Kaiser, S. Salmons, and O. H. Lowry. Chronic stimulation of mammalian muscle: changes in enzymes of six metabolic pathways. *Am. J. Physiol.* 251 (*Cell Physiol.* 20): C614–C632, 1986.
64. Henriksson, J., J. Svedenhag, E. A. Richter, N. J. Christensen, and H. Galbo. Skeletal muscle and hormonal adaptation to physical training in the rat: role of the sympatho-adrenal system. *Acta. Physiol. Scand.* 123: 127–138, 1985.
65. Hentze, M. W., T. A. Rouault, J. B. Harford, and R. D. Klausner. Oxidation-reduction and the molecular mechanism of a regulatory RNA-protein interaction. *Science* 244: 357–359, 1989.
66. Hofmann, S., and D. Pette. Low-frequency stimulation of rat fast-twitch muscle enhances the expression of hexokinase II and both the translocation and expression of glucose transporter 4 (GLUT-4). *Eur. J. Biochem.* 219: 307–315, 1994.

67. Holloszy, J. O., and F. W. Booth. Biochemical adaptations to endurance exercise in muscle. *Annu. Rev. Physiol.* 38: 273–291, 1976.
68. Holloszy, J. O., and E. F. Coyle. Adaptations of skeletal muscle to endurance exercise and their metabolic consequences. *J. Appl. Physiol.* 56: 831–838, 1984.
69. Holloszy, J. O., and W. W. Winder. Induction of delta-aminolevulinic acid synthetase in muscle by exercise or thyroxine. *Am. J. Physiol.* 236 (*Regulatory Integrative Comp. Physiol.* 5): R180–R183, 1979.
70. Hood, D. A., and G. Parent. Metabolic and contractile responses of rat fast-twitch muscle to 10-Hz stimulation. *Am. J. Physiol.* 260 (*Cell Physiol.* 29): C832–C840, 1991.
71. Hood, D. A., and D. Pette. Chronic long-term electrostimulation creates a unique metabolic enzyme profile in rabbit fast-twitch muscle. *FEBS Lett.* 247: 471–474, 1989.
72. Hood, D. A., J. A. Simoneau, A. M. Kelly, and D. Pette. Effect of thyroid status on the expression of metabolic enzymes during chronic stimulation. *Am. J. Physiol.* 263 (*Cell Physiol.* 32): C788–C793, 1992.
73. Hood, D. A., R. Zak, and D. Pette. Chronic stimulation of rat skeletal muscle induces coordinate increases in mitochondrial and nuclear mRNAs of cytochrome-c-oxidase subunits. *Eur. J. Biochem.* 179: 275–280, 1989.
74. Horie, S., O. Moe, Y. Yamaji, A. Cano, R. T. Miller, and R. J. Alpern. Role of protein kinase C and transcription factor AP-1 in the acid-induced increase in Na/H antiporter activity. *Proc. Natl. Acad. Sci. U. S. A.* 89: 5236–5240, 1992.
75. Huang, C. F., B. E. Flucher, M. M. Schmidt, S. K. Stroud, and J. Schmidt. Depolarization-transcription signals in skeletal muscle use calcium flux through L channels, but bypass the sarcoplasmic reticulum. *Neuron* 13: 167–177, 1994.
76. Huang, C. F., Y. S. Lee, M. M. Schmidt, and J. Schmidt. Rapid inhibition of myogenin-driven acetylcholine receptor subunit gene transcription. *EMBO J.* 13: 634–640, 1994.
77. Huang, R. P., and E. D. Adamson. Characterization of the DNA-binding properties of the early growth response-1 (Egr-1) transcription factor: evidence for modulation by a redox mechanism. *DNA Cell Biol.* 12: 265–273, 1993.
78. Izumo, S., B. Nadal-Ginard, and V. Mahdavi. Protooncogene induction and reprogramming of cardiac gene expression produced by pressure overload. *Proc. Natl. Acad. Sci. U. S. A.* 85: 339–343, 1988.
79. Jackson, R. J. Cytoplasmic regulation of mRNA function: the importance of the 3′ untranslated region. *Cell* 74: 9–14, 1993.
80. Ji, L. L., D. L. Lennon, R. G. Kochan, F. J. Nagle, and H. A. Lardy. Enzymatic adaptation to physical training under beta-blockade in the rat. Evidence of a beta 2-adrenergic mechanism in skeletal muscle. *J. Clin. Invest.* 78: 771–778, 1986.
81. Kadowaki, T., and Y. Kitagawa. Hypoxic depression of mitochondrial mRNA levels in HeLa cell. *Exp. Cell Res.* 192: 243–247, 1991.
82. Kaufmann, M., J. A. Simoneau, J. H. Veerkamp, and D. Pette. Electrostimulation-induced increases in fatty acid-binding protein and myoglobin in rat fast-twitch muscle and comparison with tissue levels in heart. *FEBS Lett.* 245: 181–184, 1989.
83. Kerppola, T. K., and T. Curran. DNA bending by Fos and Jun: the flexible hinge model. *Science* 254: 1210–1214, 1991.
84. Kirschbaum, B. J., J. A. Simoneau, A. Bar, P. J. Barton, M. E. Buckingham, and D. Pette. Chronic stimulation-induced changes of myosin light chains at the mRNA and protein levels in rat fast-twitch muscle. *Eur. J. Biochem.* 179: 23–29, 1989.
85. Komuro, I., T. Kaida, Y. Shibazaki, M. Kurabayashi, Y. Katoh, E. Hoh, F. Takaku, and Y. Yazaki. Stretching cardiac myocytes stimulates protooncogene expression. *J. Biol. Chem.* 265: 3595–3598, 1990.
86. Komuro, I., Y. Katoh, T. Kaida, Y. Shibazaki, M. Kurabayashi, E. Hoh, F. Takaku, and Y. Yazaki. Mechanical loading stimulates cell hypertrophy and specific gene expression in cultured rat cardiac myocytes. Possible role of protein kinase C activation. *J. Biol. Chem.* 266: 1265–1268, 1991.
87. Kong, X., J. Manchester, S. Salmons, and J. J. C. Lawrence. Glucose transporters in single skeletal muscle fibers. Relationship to hexokinase and regulation by contractile activity. *J. Biol. Chem.* 269: 12963–12967, 1994.
88. Korge, P., S. K. Byrd, and K. B. Campbell. Functional coupling between sarcoplasmic-reticulum-bound creatine kinase and Ca(2+)-ATPase. *Eur. J. Biochem.* 213: 973–980, 1993.
89. Kraus, W. E., T. S. Bernard, and R. S. Williams. Interactions between sustained contractile activity and beta-adrenergic receptors in regulation of gene expression in skeletal muscles. *Am. J. Physiol.* 256 (*Cell Physiol.* 25): C506–C514, 1989.
90. Kraus, W. E., J. P. Longabaugh, and S. B. Liggett. Electrical pacing induces adenylyl cyclase in skeletal muscle independent of the beta-adrenergic receptor. *Am. J. Physiol.* 263 (*Endocrinol. Metab.* 26): E226–E230, 1992.
91. Lai, M. M., and F. W. Booth. Cytochrome c mRNA and alpha-actin mRNA in muscles of rats fed beta-GPA. *J. Appl. Physiol.* 69: 843–848, 1990.
92. Laufer, R., and J. P. Changeux. Calcitonin gene-related peptide elevates cyclic AMP levels in chick skeletal muscle: possible neurotrophic role for a coexisting neuronal messenger. *EMBO J.* 6: 901–906, 1987.
93. Laufer, R., and J. P. Changeux. Activity-dependent regulation of gene expression in muscle and neuronal cells. *Mol. Neurobiol.* 3: 1–53, 1989.
94. Lawrence, J., Jr., and W. J. Salsgiver. Evidence that levels of malate dehydrogenase and fumarase are increased by cAMP in rat myotubes. *Am. J. Physiol.* 247 (*Cell Physiol.* 16): C33–C38, 1984.
95. Lewis, S. F., and R. G. Haller, Skeletal muscle disorders and associated facors that limit exercise performance. In: *Exercise and Sport Science Reviews*, edited by K. B. Pandolf. Baltimore, MD: Williams & Wilkins, 1989, p. 67–114.
96. Li, K., J. A. Hodge, and D. C. Wallace. OXBOX, a positive transcriptional element of the heart-skeletal muscle ADP/ATP translocator gene. *J. Biol. Chem.* 265: 20585–20588, 1990.
97. Li, K., C. K. Warner, J. A. Hodge, S. Minoshima, J. Kudoh, R. Fukuyama, M. Maekawa, Y. Shimizu, N. Shimizu, and D. C. Wallace. A human muscle adenine nucleotide translocator gene has four exons, is located on chromosome 4, and is differentially expressed. *J. Biol. Chem.* 264: 13998–14004, 1989.
98. Li, L., and E. N. Olson. Regulation of muscle cell growth and differentiation by the MyoD family of helix-loop-helix proteins. *Adv. Cancer Res.* 58: 95–119, 1992.
99. Li, L., J. Zhou, G. James, R. Heller-Harrison, M. P. Czech, and E. N. Olson. FGF inactivates myogenic helix-loop-helix proteins through phosphorylation of a conserved protein kinase C site in their DNA-binding domains. *Cell* 71: 1181–1194, 1992.
100. Liu, F., M. A. Thompson, S. Wagner, M. E. Greenberg, and M. R. Green. Activating transcription factor-1 can mediate

Ca(2+)- and cAMP-inducible transcriptional activation. *J. Biol. Chem.* 268: 6714–6720, 1993.
101. Matsushita, S., and D. Pette. Inactivation of sarcoplasmic-reticulum Ca(2+)-ATPase in low-frequency-stimulated muscle results from a modification of the active site. *Biochem. J.* 285: 303–309, 1992.
102. McBride, A. A., R. D. Klausner, and P. M. Howley. Conserved cysteine residue in the DNA-binding domain of the bovine papillomavirus type 1 E2 protein confers redox regulation of the DNA-binding activity in vitro. *Proc. Natl. Acad. Sci. U. S. A.* 89: 7531–7535, 1992.
103. Megeney, L. A., P. D. Neufer, G. L. Dohm, M. H. Tan, C. A. Blewett, G. C. Elder, and A. Bonen. Effects of muscle activity and fiber composition on glucose transport and GLUT-4. *Am. J. Physiol.* 264 (*Endocrinol. Metab.* 27): E583–E593, 1993.
104. Mendelzon, D., J. P. Changeux, and H. O. Nghiem. Phosphorylation of myogenin in chick myotubes: regulation by electrical activity and by protein kinase C. Implications for acetylcholine receptor gene expression. *Biochemistry* 33: 2568–2575, 1994.
105. Merlie, J. P., J. Mudd, T. C. Cheng, and E. N. Olson. Myogenin and acetylcholine receptor alpha gene promoters mediate transcriptional regulation in response to motor innervation. *J. Biol. Chem.* 269: 2461–2467, 1994.
106. Michel, J. B., G. A. Ordway, J. A. Richardson, and R. S. Williams. Biphasic induction of immediate early gene expression accompanies activity-dependent angiogenesis and myofiber remodeling of rabbit skeletal muscle. *J. Clin. Invest.* 94: 277–285, 1994.
107. Moe, O. W., R. T. Miller, S. Horie, A. Cano, P. A. Preisig, and R. J. Alpern. Differential regulation of Na/H antiporter by acid in renal epithelial cells and fibroblasts. *J. Clin. Invest.* 88: 1703–1708, 1991.
108. Moerland, T. S., N. G. Wolf, and M. J. Kushmerick. Administration of a creatine analogue induces isomyosin transitions in muscle. *Am. J. Physiol.* 257 (*Cell Physiol.* 20): C810–C816, 1989.
109. Monson, E. K., M. Weinstein, G. S. Ditta, and D. R. Helinski. The FixL protein of Rhizobium meliloti can be separated into a heme-binding oxygen-sensing domain and a functional C-terminal kinase domain. *Proc. Natl. Acad. Sci. U. S. A.* 89: 4280–4284, 1992.
110. Morrison, P. R., R. B. Biggs, and F. W. Booth. Daily running for 2 wk and mRNAs for cytochrome c and alpha-actin in rat skeletal muscle. *Am. J. Physiol.* 257 (*Cell Physiol.* 26): C936–C939, 1989.
111. Morrow, N. G., W. E. Kraus, J. W. Moore, R. S. Williams, and J. L. Swain. Increased expression of fibroblast growth factors in a rabbit skeletal muscle model of exercise conditioning. *J. Clin. Invest.* 85: 1816–1820, 1990.
112. Mosser, D. D., P. T. Kotzbauer, K. D. Sarge, and R. I. Morimoto. In vitro activation of heat shock transcription factor DNA-binding by calcium and biochemical conditions that affect protein conformation. *Proc. Natl. Acad. Sci. U. S. A.* 87: 3748–3752, 1990.
113. Neufer, P. D., and G. L. Dohm. Exercise induces a transient increase in transcription of the GLUT-4 gene in skeletal muscle. *Am. J. Physiol.* 265 (*Cell Physiol.* 34): C1597–C1603, 1993.
114. Neufer, P. D., M. H. Shinebarger, and G. L. Dohm. Effect of training and detraining on skeletal muscle glucose transporter (GLUT4) content in rats. *Can. J. Physiol. Pharmacol.* 70: 1286–1290, 1992.
115. Neuhold, L. A., and B. Wold. HLH forced dimers: tethering MyoD to E47 generates a dominant positive myogenic factor insulated from negative regulation by Id. *Cell* 74: 1033–1042, 1993.
116. Nicholson, C. D., D. Angersbach, and R. Wilke. The effect of physical training on rat calf muscle, oxygen tension, blood flow, metabolism and function in an animal model of chronic occlusive peripheral vascular disease. *Int. J. Sports Med.* 13: 60–64, 1992.
117. O'Doherty, R. M., D. P. Bracy, H. Osawa, D. H. Wasserman, and D. K. Granner. Rat skeletal muscle hexokinase II mRNA and activity are increased by a single bout of acute exercise. *Am. J. Physiol.* 266 (*Endocrinol. Metab.* 29): E171–E178, 1994.
118. O'Malley, J. P., R. G. Mills, and J. J. Bray. Effects of electrical stimulation and tetrodotoxin paralysis on antigenic properties of acetylcholine receptors in rat skeletal muscle. *Neurosci. Lett.* 120: 224–226, 1990.
119. Ordway, G. A., K. Li, G. A. Hand, and R. S. Williams. RNA subunit of mitochondrial RNA-processing enzyme is induced by contractile activity in striated muscle. *Am. J. Physiol.* 265 (*Cell Physiol.* 34): C1511–C1516, 1993.
120. Peleg, S., W. T. Schrader, and B. W. O'Malley. Differential sensitivity of chicken progesterone receptor forms to sulfhydryl reactive reagents. *Biochemistry* 28: 7373–7379, 1989.
121. Pette, D., and S. Dusterhoft. Altered gene expression in fast-twitch muscle induced by chronic low-frequency stimulation. *Am. J. Physiol.* 262 (*Regulatory Integrative Comp. Physiol.* 31): R333–R338, 1992.
122. Pette, D., and G. Vrbova. Adaptation of mammalian skeletal muscle fibers to chronic electrical stimulation. *Rev. Physiol. Biochem. Pharmacol.* 120: 115–202, 1992.
123. Pognonec, P., H. Kato, and R. G. Roeder. The helix-loop-helix/leucine repeat transcription factor USF can be functionally regulated in a redox-dependent manner. *J. Biol. Chem.* 267: 24563–24567, 1992.
124. Preiss, T., and R. N. Lightowlers. Post-transcriptional regulation of tissue-specific isoforms. A bovine cytosolic RNA-binding protein, COLBP, associates with messenger RNA encoding the liver-form isopeptides of cytochrome c oxidase. *J. Biol. Chem.* 268: 10659–10667, 1993.
125. Pugh, C. W., C. C. Tan, R. W. Jones, and P. J. Ratcliffe. Functional analysis of an oxygen-regulated transcriptional enhancer lying 3′ to the mouse erythropoietin gene. *Proc. Natl. Acad. Sci. U. S. A.* 88: 10553–10557, 1991.
126. Reichmann, H., H. Hoppeler, O. Mathieu-Costello, F. von Bergen, and D. Pette. Biochemical and ultrastructural changes of skeletal muscle mitochondria after chronic electrical stimulation in rabbits. *Pflugers Arch.* 404: 1–9, 1985.
127. Reichmann, H., R. Wasl, J. A. Simoneau, and D. Pette. Enzyme activities of fatty acid oxidation and the respiratory chain in chronically stimulated fast-twitch muscle of the rabbit. *Pflugers Arch.* 418: 572–574, 1991.
128. Ren, J. M., and J. O. Holloszy. Adaptation of rat skeletal muscle to creatine depletion: AMP deaminase and AMP deamination. *J. Appl. Physiol.* 73: 2713–2716, 1992.
129. Rodnick, K. J., E. J. Henriksen, D. E. James, and J. O. Holloszy. Exercise training, glucose transporters, and glucose transport in rat skeletal muscles. *Am. J. Physiol.* 262 (*Cell Physiol.* 31): C9–C14, 1992.
130. Rodnick, K. J., and B. D. Sidell. Cold acclimation increases carnitine palmitoyltransferase I activity in oxidative muscle of striped bass. *Am. J. Physiol.* 266 (*Regulatory Integrative Comp. Physiol.* 35): R405–R412, 1994.
131. Roy, R. R., K. M. Baldwin, and V. R. Edgerton, The plasticity of skeletal muscle: effects of neuromuscular activity.

In: *Exercise and Sport Science Reviews*, edited by J. O. Holloszy. Baltimore, MD: Williams & Wilkins, 1991, p. 269–312.

132. Sadoshima, J., and S. Izumo. Mechanical stretch rapidly activates multiple signal transduction pathways in cardiac myocytes: potential involvement of an autocrine/paracrine mechanism. *EMBO J.* 12: 1681–1692, 1993.
133. Sadoshima, J., L. Jahn, T. Takahashi, T. J. Kulik, and S. Izumo. Molecular characterization of the stretch-induced adaptation of cultured cardiac cells. An in vitro model of load-induced cardiac hypertrophy. *J. Biol. Chem.* 267: 10551–10560, 1992.
134. Sadoshima, J., Y. Xu, H. S. Slayter, and S. Izumo. Autocrine release of angiotensin II mediates stretch-induced hypertrophy of cardiac myocytes in vitro. *Cell* 75: 977–984, 1993.
135. Sahlin, K., A. Katz, and J. Henriksson. Redox state and lactate accumulation in human skeletal muscle during dynamic exercise. *Biochem. J.* 245: 551–556, 1987.
136. Saito, M., J. Nguyen, and Y. Kidokoro. Inhibition of nerve- and agrin-induced acetylcholine receptor clustering on Xenopus muscle cells in culture. *Brain Res. Dev. Brain Res.* 71: 9–17, 1993.
137. Salmons, S., and G. Vrbova. The influence of activity on some contractile characteristics of mammalian fast and slow muscles. *J. Physiol. (Lond.)* 201: 535–549, 1969.
138. Saltin, B., and P. D. Gollnick, Skeletal muscle adaptability: significance for metabolism and performance. In: *Handbook of Physiology, Skeletal Muscle, Skeletal Muscle*, edited by L. D. Peachey. Bethesda, MD: Am. Physiol. Soc., 1983, p. 555–631.
139. Sapega, A. A., R. B. Heppenstall, D. P. Sokolow, T. J. Graham, J. M. Maris, A. K. Ghosh, B. Chance, and A. L. Osterman. The bioenergetics of preservation of limbs before replantation. The rationale for intermediate hypothermia. *J. Bone. Joint. Surg. Am.* 70: 1500–1513, 1988.
140. Schreck, R., P. Rieber, and P. A. Baeuerle. Reactive oxygen intermediates as apparently widely used messengers in the activation of the NF-kappa B transcription factor and HIV-1. *EMBO J.* 10: 2247–2258, 1991.
141. Schulte, L. M., J. Navarro, and S. C. Kandarian. Regulation of sarcoplasmic reticulum calcium pump gene expression by hindlimb unweighting. *Am. J. Physiol.* 264 (*Cell Physiol.* 33): C1308–C1315, 1993.
142. Semenza, G. L., P. H. Roth, H. M. Fang, and G. L. Wang. Transcriptional regulation of genes encoding glycolytic enzymes by hypoxia-inducible factor 1. *J. Biol. Chem.* 269: 23757–23763, 1994.
143. Semenza, G. L., and G. L. Wang. A nuclear factor induced by hypoxia via de novo protein synthesis binds to the human erythropoietin gene enhancer at a site required for transcriptional activation. *Mol. Cell. Biol.* 12: 5447–5454, 1992.
144. Sheng, M., M. A. Thompson, and M. E. Greenberg. CREB: a Ca(2+)-regulated transcription factor phosphorylated by calmodulin-dependent kinases. *Science* 252: 1427–1430, 1991.
145. Silva, C. M., and J. A. Cidlowski. Direct evidence for intra- and intermolecular disulfide bond formation in the human glucocorticoid receptor. Inhibition of DNA binding and identification of a new receptor-associated protein. *J. Biol. Chem.* 264: 6638–6647, 1989.
146. Slentz, C. A., E. A. Gulve, K. J. Rodnick, E. J. Henriksen, J. H. Youn, and J. O. Holloszy. Glucose transporters and maximal transport are increased in endurance-trained rat soleus. *J. Appl. Physiol.* 73: 486–492, 1992.
147. Sreter, F. A., J. R. Lopez, L. Alamo, K. Mabuchi, and J. Gergely. Changes in intracellular ionized Ca concentration associated with muscle fiber type transformation. *Am. J. Physiol.* 253 (*Cell Physiol.* 22): C296–C300, 1987.
148. Storz, G., L. A. Tartaglia, and B. N. Ames. Transcriptional regulator of oxidative stress-inducible genes: direct activation by oxidation. *Science* 248: 189–194, 1990.
149. Sullivan, M. J., P. F. Binkley, D. V. Unverferth, J. H. Ren, H. Boudoulas, T. M. Bashore, A. J. Merola, and C. V. Leier. Prevention of bedrest-induced physical deconditioning by daily dobutamine infusions. Implications for drug-induced physical conditioning. *J. Clin. Invest.* 76: 1632–1642, 1985.
150. Sundberg, C. J. Exercise and training during graded leg ischaemia in healthy man with special reference to effects on skeletal muscle. *Acta. Physiol. Scand. Suppl.* 615: 1–50, 1994.
151. Svedenhag, J., J. Henriksson, and A. Juhlin-Dannfelt. Beta-adrenergic blockade and training in human subjects: effects on muscle metabolic capacity. *Am. J. Physiol.* 247 (*Endocrinol. Metab.* 10): E305–E311, 1984.
152. Takahashi, M., and D. A. Hood. Chronic stimulation-induced changes in mitochondria and performance in rat skeletal muscle. *J. Appl. Physiol.* 74: 934–941, 1993.
153. Takahashi, M., D. T. McCurdy, D. A. Essig, and D. A. Hood. Delta-aminolaevulinate synthase expression in muscle after contractions and recovery. *Biochem. J.* 291: 219–223, 1993.
154. Taylor, D. A., V. B. Kraus, J. J. Schwarz, E. N. Olson, and W. E. Kraus. E1A-mediated inhibition of myogenesis correlates with a direct physical interaction of E1A12S and basic helix-loop-helix proteins. *Mol. Cell Biol.* 13: 4714–4727, 1993.
155. Termin, A., and D. Pette. Changes in myosin heavy-chain isoform synthesis of chronically stimulated rat fast-twitch muscle. *Eur. J. Biochem.* 204: 569–573, 1992.
156. Toledano, M. B. and W. J. Leonard. Modulation of transcription factor NF-kappa B binding activity by oxidation-reduction in vitro. *Proc. Natl. Acad. Sci. U. S. A.* 88: 4328–4332, 1991.
157. Topper, J. N., J. L. Bennett, and D. A. Clayton. A role for RNAase MRP in mitochondrial RNA processing. *Cell* 70: 16–20, 1992.
158. Town, G. P., and D. A. Essig. Cytochrome oxidase in muscle of endurance-trained rats: subunit mRNA contents and heme synthesis. *J. Appl. Physiol.* 74: 192–196, 1993.
159. Tsay, H. J., and J. Schmidt. Skeletal muscle denervation activates acetylcholine receptor genes. *J. Cell. Biol.* 108: 1523–1526, 1989.
160. Turinsky, J. Phospholipids, prostaglandin E2, and proteolysis in denervated muscle. *Am. J. Physiol.* 251 (*Regulatory Integrative Comp. Physiol.* 20): R165–R173, 1986.
161. Underwood, L. E., and R. S. Williams. Pretranslational regulation of myoglobin gene expression. *Am. J. Physiol.* 252 (*Cell Physiol.* 21): C450–C453, 1987.
162. van Deursen, J., A. Heerschap, F. Oerlemans, W. Ruitenbeek, P. Jap, H. ter Laak, and B. Wieringa. Skeletal muscles of mice deficient in muscle creatine kinase lack burst activity. *Cell* 74: 621–631, 1993.
163. Vandenburgh, H. H. Mechanical forces and their second messengers in stimulating cell growth in vitro. *Am. J. Physiol.* 262 (*Regulatory Integrative Comp. Physiol.* 31): R350–R355, 1992.
164. Virbasius, J. V., and R. C. Scarpulla. Activation of the human mitochondrial transcription factor A gene by nuclear respiratory factors: a potential regulatory link between nu-

clear and mitochondrial gene expression in organelle biogenesis. *Proc. Natl. Acad. Sci. U. S. A.* 91: 1309–1313, 1994.

165. Walke, W., J. Staple, L. Adams, M. Gnegy, K. Chahine, and D. Goldman. Calcium-dependent regulation of rat and chick muscle nicotinic acetylcholine receptor (nAChR) gene expression. *J. Biol. Chem.* 269: 19447–19456, 1994.
166. Wang, G. L., and G. L. Semenza. Characterization of hypoxia-inducible factor 1 and regulation of DNA binding activity by hypoxia. *J. Biol. Chem.* 268: 21513–21518, 1993.
167. Weber, F. E., and D. Pette. Contractile activity enhances the synthesis of hexokinase II in rat skeletal muscle. *FEBS Lett.* 238: 71–73, 1988.
168. Weber, F. E., and D. Pette. Changes in free and bound forms and total amount of hexokinase isozyme II of rat muscle in response to contractile activity. *Eur. J. Biochem.* 191: 85–90, 1990.
169. Weber, F. E., and D. Pette. Rapid up- and down-regulation of hexokinase II in rat skeletal muscle in response to altered contractile activity. *FEBS Lett.* 261: 291–293, 1990.
170. Whitelaw, P. F., and J. E. Hesketh. Expression of c-myc and c-fos in rat skeletal muscle. Evidence for increased levels of c-myc mRNA during hypertrophy. *Biochem. J.* 281: 143–147, 1992.
171. Wicks, K. L., and D. A. Hood. Mitochondrial adaptations in denervated muscle: relationship to muscle performance. *Am. J. Physiol.* 260 (*Cell Physiol.* 29): C841–C850, 1991.
172. Williams, R. S. Mitochondrial gene expression in mammalian striated muscle. Evidence that variation in gene dosage is the major regulatory event. *J. Biol. Chem.* 261: 12390–12394, 1986.
173. Williams, R. S., and I. J. Benjamin. Stress proteins and cardiovascular disease. *Mol. Biol. Med.* 8: 197–206, 1991.
174. Williams, R. S., M. G. Caron, and K. Daniel. Skeletal muscle beta-adrenergic receptors: variations due to fiber type and training. *Am. J. Physiol.* 246 (*Endocrinol. Metab.* 9): E160–E167, 1984.
175. Williams, R. S., M. Garcia-Moll, J. Mellor, S. Salmons, and W. Harlan. Adaptation of skeletal muscle to increased contractile activity. Expression nuclear genes encoding mitochondrial proteins. *J. Biol. Chem.* 262: 2764–2767, 1987.
176. Williams, R. S., S. Salmons, E. A. Newsholme, R. E. Kaufman, and J. Mellor. Regulation of nuclear and mitochondrial gene expression by contractile activity in skeletal muscle. *J. Biol. Chem.* 261: 376–380, 1986.
177. Winter, B., T. Braun, and H. H. Arnold. cAMP-dependent protein kinase represses myogenic differentiation and the activity of the muscle-specific helix-loop-helix transcription factors Myf-5 and MyoD. *J. Biol. Chem.* 268: 9869–9878, 1993.
178. Witzemann, V., and B. Sakmann. Differential regulation of MyoD and myogenin mRNA levels by nerve induced muscle activity. *FEBS Lett.* 282: 259–264, 1991.
179. Xanthoudakis, S., and T. Curran. Identification and characterization of Ref-1, a nuclear protein that facilitates AP-1 DNA-binding activity. *EMBO J.* 11: 653–665, 1992.
180. Yao, K. S., S. Xanthoudakis, T. Curran, and P. J. O'Dwyer. Activation of AP-1 and of a nuclear redox factor, Ref-1, in the response of HT29 colon cancer cells to hypoxia. *Mol. Cell. Biol.* 14: 5997–6003, 1994.
181. Zhou, J., and E. N. Olson. Dimerization through the helix-loop-helix motif enhances phosphorylation of the transcription activation domains of myogenin. *Mol. Cell. Biol.* 14: 6232–6243, 1994.

26. Cellular, molecular, and metabolic basis of muscle fatigue

ROBERT H. FITTS | *Department of Biology, Marquette University, Milwaukee, Wisconsin*

CHAPTER CONTENTS

THEORIES REGARDING THE CELLULAR MECHANISMS OF MUSCLE FATIGUE ABOUND. This topic was recently described in detail elsewhere (111), and the reader is referred to that review for an in-depth discussion of the original data. The known alterations in muscle mechanics associated with fatigue, and the possible causative agents, will be discussed here. Although in a few cases original data are reprinted, for the most part diagrams are used to illustrate the cellular disturbances associated with a particular fatigue agent. Differences in the susceptibility to fatigue depending on muscle fiber type will be emphasized.

DEFINITION AND CURRENT THEORIES OF FATIGUE

By definition, muscle fatigue is a loss of peak force and power output (10, 100, 253). Additionally, a decline in the rate of tension development (dP/dt) and a slowing of relaxation would contribute to fatigue by reducing the force and power obtained early in the contraction cycle and the frequency of activation cycles per second, respectively. Edwards (101) defined fatigue as "failure to maintain the required or expected power output." This definition recognizes that the ability to sustain a given work rate without decrement requires the maintenance of both force and velocity. Although progress has been made, the etiologies of muscle fatigue have not been clearly established. One roadblock has been the lack of basic information on the mechanisms of excitation-contraction (E-C) coupling and the cross-bridge cycle. Recently, considerable progress has been made in understanding these basic mechanisms of muscle contraction (38, 124, 232), and this in turn has led to a better understanding of how a particular fatigue agent might disrupt the contractile process. Nevertheless, the problem is complex, since multiple factors are clearly involved; the relative importance of each depends on the fiber-type composition of the contracting muscle(s); the intensity, type, and duration of the contractile activity; and the individual's degree of fitness. For example, fatigue in marathon running or other endurance activities may be related to muscle glycogen depletion, low blood glucose, or dehydration, whereas such factors are clearly not involved during short-term, high-intensity exercise (111).

Figure 26.1 is a redrawing of a scheme originally published by Bigland-Ritchie (26) in which she identified the major potential sites of fatigue: (*1*) excitatory input to higher motor centers, (*2*) excitatory drive to lower motoneurons, (*3*) motoneuron excitability, (*4*) neuromuscular (N-M) transmission, (*5*) sarcolemma (S_L) excitability, (*6*) excitation-contraction coupling, (*7*) contractile mechanism, and (*8*) metabolic energy supply and metabolite accumulation. Considerable controversy exists regarding the role of these sites, in particular, the relative importance of central and N-M transmission (sites 1–4) vs. peripheral (sites 5–8) mechanisms in the etiology of muscle fatigue (26, 100, 104, 155). Although muscle fatigue may in some cases result from deleterious alterations occurring proximal to the muscle S_L (111), the preponderance of evidence suggests that the primary sites of fatigue lie within the muscle itself (100, 101). Although failure in N-M transmission has been observed, it is generally associated with unphysiologically high stimulation frequencies (170, 172). Additionally, high-intensity exercise is frequently associated with a reduced neural drive and α motor nerve activation frequency; however, rather than precipitate fatigue this change is thought to protect against its development (28, 30).

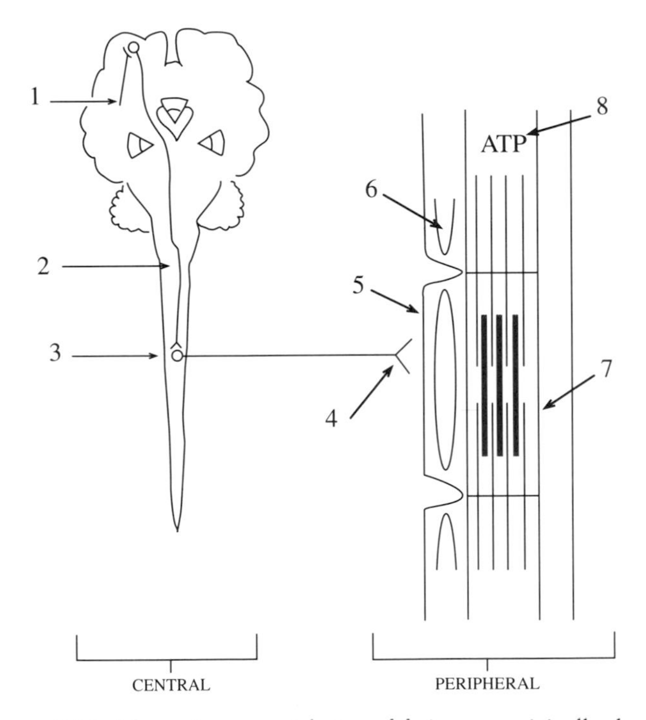

FIG. 26.1. The major potential sites of fatigue as originally described by Bigland-Ritchie (26) are shown. The neural components are: *1*, excitatory input to higher motor centers; *2*, excitatory drive to lower motoneurons; *3*, motoneuron excitability; and *4*, neuromuscular transmission. The peripheral factors within the muscle cell include: *5*, sarcolemma excitability; *6*, excitation-contraction coupling to include T-tubular and SR Ca^{2+} release and reuptake events; *7*, contractile mechanisms; and *8*, metabolic energy supply and metabolic accumulation.

The focus of this chapter is on the cellular aspects of muscle fatigue, and thus emphasis will be placed on the putative fatigue factors located distal to the neuromuscular junction. This topic has received considerable attention. In addition to the recent comprehensive review cited above (111), reviews have been published on specific topics, such as alterations in excitation-contraction coupling (27, 283), the role of ionic changes (182, 251, 255), disturbances in cell metabolism (101, 152, 164, 190, 236, 247, 266), or alterations in cell ultrastructure (8, 47, 199). Although numerous mechanisms have been suggested as causative in muscle fatigue, most are related to alterations in excitation or cell metabolism. The most prominent involve changes in: (*1*) the amplitude and propagation of the sarcolemma and T-tubular action potential; (*2*) T-tubular dihydropyridine receptor (charge sensor); (*3*) the sarcoplasmic reticulum (SR) Ca^{2+} release channel; and (*4*) metabolic factors affecting the SR, the thin filament regulatory proteins, and the cross-bridge.

MUSCLE FIBER-TYPE COMPOSITION

One factor affecting the speed and extent of muscle fatigue is the fiber-type composition of the muscle or muscles employed in the exercise task. Adult mammalian skeletal muscles contain at least three distinct fiber types classified on the basis of their functional and metabolic properties as fast glycolytic (FG), fast oxidative glycolytic (FOG), and slow oxidative (SO). The FG and FOG fiber types are fast-twitch fibers characterized by high SR and myofibrillar adenosine triphosphatase (ATPase) activities, correspondingly short isometric twitch durations, and high maximal shortening velocities (V_o) (62, 226). In contrast, the SO fiber possesses a low SR and myofibrillar ATPase activity, prolonged twitch duration, and low V_o compared to the fast-twitch fiber types (35, 40, 62, 250). Each fiber type contains a specific isozyme for the contractile protein myosin, and fibers are frequently identified on the basis of their histochemically determined myosin ATPase activity as slow type I, fast type IIa, or fast type IIb (35, 40). Recently, adult skeletal muscle has been shown to contain a third fast fiber type containing a specific myosin isozyme identified as IIx or IId (35). In addition to the different isozymes for myosin, the three main fiber types can be distinguished by specific isozymes for a number of muscle proteins, and by their mitochondrial enzyme content. In the context of muscle fatigue, this latter property is particularly important. The FOG and SO fibers contain a high mitochondrial content and thus are relatively fatigue resistant compared to the FG fiber type. Consequently, the soleus and deep region of the gastrocnemius containing primarily SO and FOG fibers, respectively, are considerably more fatigue resistant than muscle or muscle regions containing primarily the FG fiber type. The fact that the FG fiber type contains the highest adenosine triphosphate (ATP) utilization rates, and lowest efficiency likely contributes to their susceptibility to fatigue (250). The hierarchy of fatigability is perhaps best demonstrated by an analysis of single motor units. Larsson et al. (179) showed the type IIb single motor unit to fatigue first and most extensively followed by the IIx unit, while the type IIa unit showed little fatigue, and the type I unit was fatigue resistant.

Many studies evaluating the etiology of muscle fatigue have employed frog limb muscle (94, 98, 114, 115, 175–177, 184, 272). For the most part, these muscles are fast-twitch and contain a high glycolytic but poor oxidative capacity (268). Although the fast-twitch fibers of the frog show some diversity as regards their myosin isozyme content, all appear to have V_o values at leat as high as the mammalian FG fiber type (96, 98, 268).

MECHANICAL PROPERTIES

Each contractile property (e.g., maximal shortening velocity, twitch duration, peak force) is dependent on specific cellular and molecular events associated with the cross-bridge cycle. The exact mulecular events of the cross-bridge interaction responsible for tension development and sarcomere shortening are as yet unknown. Figure 26.2 presents a block diagram that reflects the current model of the actomyosin ATP hydrolysis reaction (cross-bridge cycling) in skeletal muscle, and how the products and reactants of the various steps are altered by high-intensity exercise. The diagram was modeled after the scheme published by Metzger and Moss (210), and represents their adaptation of the current models of ATP hydrolysis, which in turn were derived from modifications of the model originally proposed by Lymn and Taylor (187). Force production depends on the binding of the myosin head (M) to actin (A). Inorganic phosphate (P_i) release (Fig. 26.2, step 2) is thought to be coupled to the transition in actomyosin binding from a weakly bound, low-force state (AM-ADP-P_i) to the strongly bound, high-force state (AM′-ADP). This latter state is likely the dominant cross-bridge form during a peak isometric contraction (210). Brenner (38) and Metzger et al. (206) have suggested that this step limits the peak rate of tension development (dP/dt). Peak dP/dt can be mea-

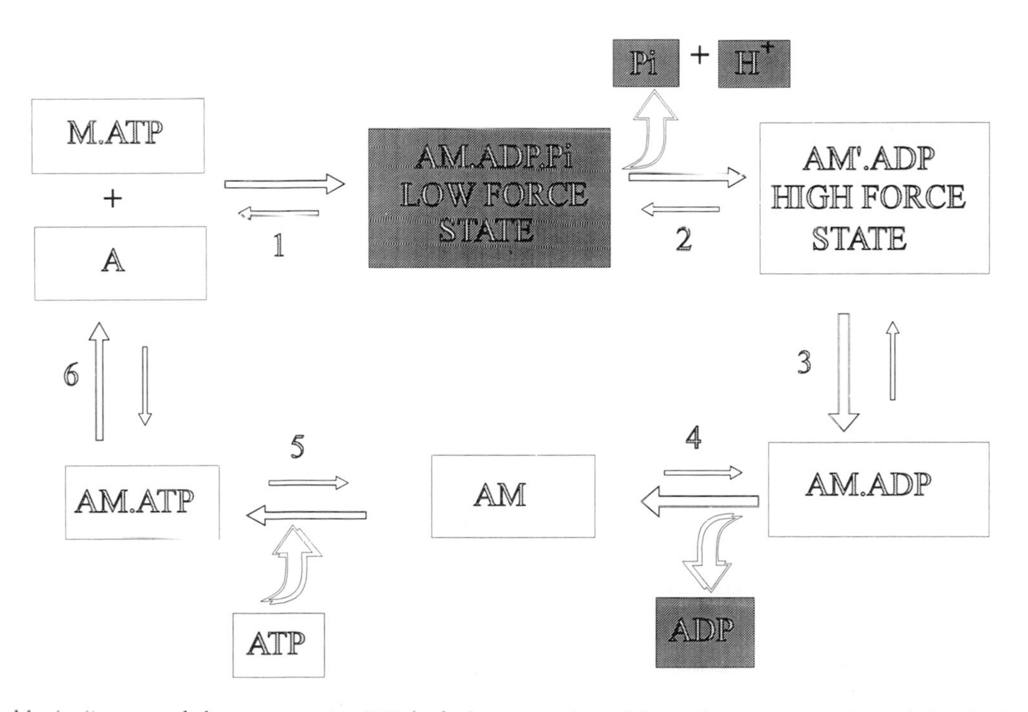

FIG. 26.2. A block diagram of the actomyosin ATP hydrolysis reaction during contraction in skeletal muscle, where *A* is actin and *M* is heavy meromyosin or myosin S1. The scheme is adapted from the current models of ATP hydrolysis (see 210). The *shaded blocks* represent the cross-bridge state and products of the reaction thought to increase with muscle fatigue.

sured experimentally by determining the rate of tension redevelopment following an imposed slack-unslack protocol (rapid release to zero force followed by re-extension to the initial optimal length) in a fully activated fiber (39). By employing this technique, Metzger and Moss (211) recently showed a seven-fold higher rate constant of tension redevelopment (k_{tr}) in fast- compared to slow-twitch fibers. The k_{tr} is also Ca^{2+} sensitive, thus the peak k_{tr} was reduced at suboptimal Ca^{2+} concentrations (39, 211). This Ca^{2+} sensitivity may result from a direct effect of Ca^{2+} on the forward apparent rate constant of step 2 of the cross-bridge reaction scheme (Fig. 26.2).

The maximal velocity of shortening in skeletal muscle (V_o) is highly correlated with, and thought to be limited by, the rate of ATP hydrolysis by myosin (14, 250). V_o is obtained during maximal unloaded contractions where the requirement for the strongly bound, high-force states of the cross-bridge (Fig. 26.2) is low and the overall cycle rate is maximal. In contrast to dP/dt, where the rate of cross-bridge transition from the weakly to the strongly bound state appears to be limiting, V_o is thought to be limited by the rate of cross-bridge dissociation (124, 208). The rate-limiting step in cross-bridge detachment is unknown, but the possibilities include steps 3–6 of the scheme shown in Figure 26.2. Fiber V_o can be determined by the slack test method (96) or from extrapolation of the force–velocity relation to zero load (145). The slack test is the preferred method, as the force–velocity technique appears to underestimate V_o (162).

The ability of humans and other vertebrates to perform work depends on the capacity to displace a load, and thus an important consideration is the power output of a muscle or muscle group. The power spectrum for a single fiber, a muscle, or a muscle group can be calculated from the force–velocity relationship. From the analysis of force-velocity curves, it is known that peak power output is obtained at intermediate velocities (86, 281).

In muscle fatigue, force, V_o, and power are all depressed. These changes can be related to alterations in specific steps of the cross-bridge cycle (Fig. 26.2). In the following section, the fatigue-induced alterations in contractile function will be reviewed, and the etiology of the observed changes will be related to specific disturbances in the cross-bridge scheme (Fig. 26.2).

The Isometric Contractile Properties

The changes in the isometric and isotonic contractile properties with fatigue are summarized in Figure 26.3. Regardless of the fiber type or stimulation conditions, the isometric twitch contraction generally shows: (*1*) a reduced peak twitch tension (P_t), (*2*) a prolonged contraction time (CT) or time to peak tension (TPT), (*3*) a prolonged relaxation time [generally measured as one-half relaxation time (1/2 RT], (*4*) a reduced rate of tension development (+dP/dt), and (*5*) a reduced rate of tension decline (−dP/dt). Each of these alterations reflects disturbances in one or more of the sites shown in Figure 26.1, steps 5–8. Although peak P_t has frequently been used to assess the degree of fatigue, the best indicator of the number of high-force cross-bridges is peak tetanic tension (P_o). P_o decreases with contractile activity (4, 115, 272), with shortening contractions at optimal length producing the largest decline (5, 75). The ex-

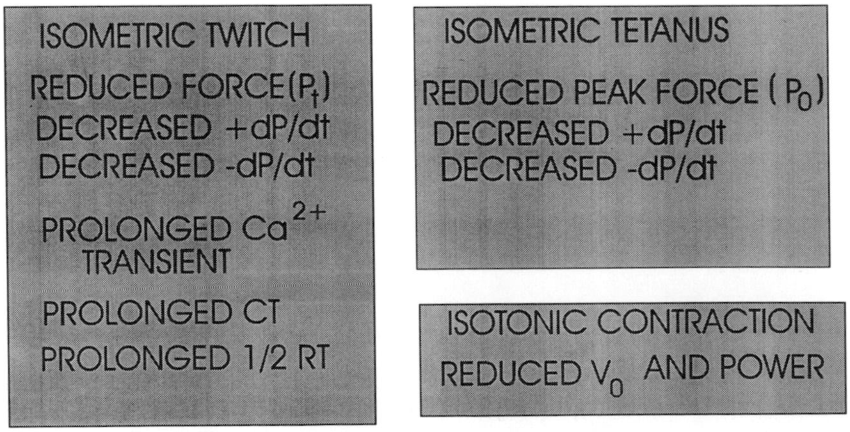

ISOMETRIC TWITCH
REDUCED FORCE (P_t)
DECREASED +dP/dt
DECREASED -dP/dt
PROLONGED Ca^{2+} TRANSIENT
PROLONGED CT
PROLONGED 1/2 RT

ISOMETRIC TETANUS
REDUCED PEAK FORCE (P_0)
DECREASED +dP/dt
DECREASED -dP/dt

ISOTONIC CONTRACTION
REDUCED V_0 AND POWER

FIG. 26.3. A summary of the known changes in the isometric twitch and tetanus, and isotonic contractions with fatigue. +dP/dt and −dP/dt represent the peak rate of tension development and decline, respectively. CT, isometric twitch contraction time; 1/2 RT, twitch one-half relaxation time; V_o, maximal velocity of unloaded shortening.

tent of the decline in P_o is generally used as an indicator of the severity of fatigue (100, 111). The fall in −dP/dt is greater than that observed for +dP/dt (204). In most cases, the reduced dP/dt (in grams per millisecond per square centimeter) is largely due to the decreased force output. Thus, when the dP/dt is corrected for the changes in tension [(dP/dt)/P_o], the observed decrease is attenuated (204). The recovery of both P_t and P_o following fatigue generally occurs in two phases (95, 115, 175,204, 216): a rapid phase complete within 1 min, followed by a slow (30–60 min) recovery to the prefatigue tension. However, under some conditions recovery from fatigue in amphibian muscle is slowed by a period of reduced tension (278, 279). Weserblad and Lännergren (278, 279) have referred to this condition as postcontraction depression (PCD), the etiology of which is entirely unknown. However, it is apparent that it is not caused by S_L inactivation, as the resting and action potentials were unaltered during PCD (176).

Recently, Lännergren et al. (174) observed a similar but somewhat different phenomenon during recovery from fatigue following in situ stimulation of single motor units in the rat. Consistent with whole-muscle experiments, single motor units showed prolonged contraction and relaxation times, reduced rates of tension development and decline, and a lowered shortening speed following fatigue (45, 46, 135, 136, 172). These stimulation-induced changes in contractile function were most apparent in the fast type IIb motor units.

Isolated single fibers appear to fatigue less rapidly than whole muscles, but consistent with whole muscles they show accelerated fatigue under anaerobic conditions (178). Recently, Lännergren and Westerblad (178) and Westerblad and Lännergren (280) showed the tetanic force of single mouse fibers to decline in three phases (Fig. 26.4). Phase 1 occurred in the initial 8 to 14 tetani (*a* to *b*, Fig. 26.4), and was followed by a comparatively long period of nearly steady tension (phase 2, *b* to *c*, Fig. 26.4), and finally by a rapid decline in tension (phase 3, *c* to *d*, Fig. 26.4). It is also apparent from Figure 26.4 that relaxation slowed with fatigue. The initial linear component of relaxation underwent the greatest prolongation, and the maximum reduction occurred at the end of phase 2 (Fig. 26.4).

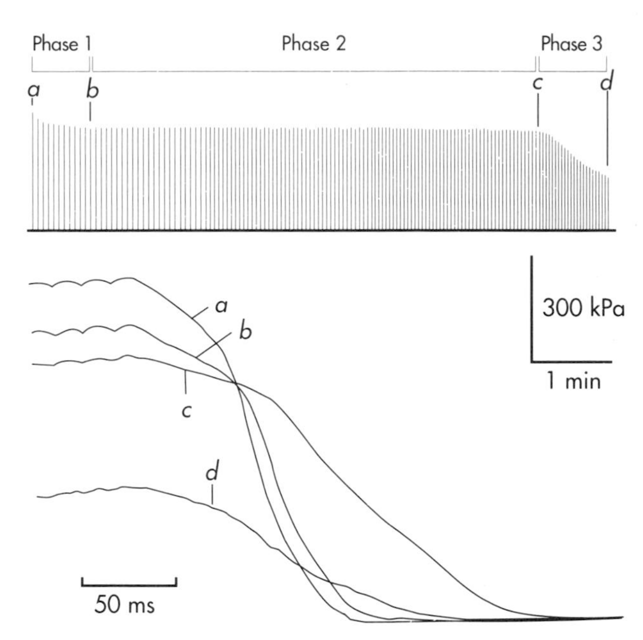

FIG. 26.4. Slowing of relaxation during fatiguing stimulation of a single fiber isolated from the mouse flexor brevis muscle. A typical fatigue curve is shown in the upper part. Each tetanus appears as a *vertical line*. The lower part displays the relaxation of the tetani indicated above the fatigue curve (*a*–*d*). The tension bar refers to the upper part only. [Reprinted with permission from Westerblad, H., and J. Lännergren. *J. Physiol.* 434: 323–336, 1991 (280).]

The Maximal Shortening Speed and Peak Power

Edman and Mattiazzi (98) observed a progressive decline in V_o with the development of fatigue. However, V_o did not significantly change until P_o had fallen by at least 10% of the prefatigued tension. In general, muscle fatigue is characerized by a greater fall in P_o than V_o (86, 98, 115, 268). Thompson et al. (268) showed the P_o and V_o of the frog semitendinosus to decline with electrical stimulation to 9% and 37% of the prefatigue value, respectively. Similar results were obtained recently in the single-fiber studies of Westerblad and Lännergren (281). They observed P_o and V_o of frog single cells to decline to 36% and 43% of the prefatigue value, respectively. Similar to peak force, Hatcher and Luff (140) observed V_o to recover from fatigue in an initial rapid phase followed by a slower phase. De Haan et al. (86) and Westerblad and Lännergren (281) demonstrated that peak power is compromised even more than P_o or V_o. Additionally, in the fatigued muscle the optimal velocity for peak power is reduced (86).

The Force–Frequency Relationship

Alterations in the force–frequency relationship during the development of fatigue could have important functional implications. It is generally accepted that the α-motoneuron firing rate declines with fatigue (28). Thus, if the force–frequency relationship shifts left (higher relative force at low frequencies), the reduced neuronal firing rate would reduce the extent of fatigue. Muscle fatigue is known to increase the duration of the Ca^{2+} transient and thus prolong the relaxation time (6, 276). The prolonged twitch relaxation would in itself cause an increased fusion of tension at low frequencies and thus explain the commonly observed left shift in the force–frequency curve (205, 268). This is consistent with the observation that the optimal stimulation frequency for peak force has been shown to decline with the development of fatigue (155, 156, 204, 268).

In some situations, a selective loss of force at low frequencies has been observed, such that the force–frequency relationship moved right with fatigue. When Cooper et al. (67) and Edwards et al. (99) studied human, and Jones et al. (157) evaluated animal as well as human muscle, they observed that fatigue in response to low frequencies of stimulation persisted after force in response to high frequencies had fully recovered. Since skeletal muscle is generally activated by low-frequency (10–30 Hz) stimulation (34, 103), the greater decline in force at low frequencies could have important functional implications. Edwards et al. (99) referred to this selective effect as low-frequency fatigue (LFF) and suggested that it was mediated by disturbances in E-C coupling, whereby Ca^{2+} release was preferentially depressed in response to a single stimulus (muscle twitch) or to low frequencies compared to high frequencies. To date, such an effect (selective inhibition of Ca^{2+} release at low frequencies) has not been demonstrated; however, it is consistent with the hypothesis that twitch tension has in some situations been shown to decline considerably more than force in response to higher frequencies (29).

Metzger and Fitts (204) reexamined the effect of high- and low-frequency stimulation on force recovery at both ends of the force–frequency relationship. They observed force to recover more rapidly at low- compared to high-frequency stimulation. Furthermore, in the fatigued state the muscle generated considerably more force during low- (5 Hz) compared to high- (75 Hz) frequency stimulation. These results were similar to those reported earlier by Jones et al. (155, 156) and Bigland-Ritchie et al. (26). It is not clear why Edwards et al. (99) found a right shift; however, their measurements were restricted to a few stimulation frequencies elicited after an hour or more of recovery. Consequently, the prolonged relaxation time associated with fatigue, which is responsible for the left shift in the force–frequency relationship, may have recovered (204, 268). Alternately, LFF may be a result of muscle damage. This possibility was first suggested by Jones et al. (155), who hypothesized that mechanical damage to the SR might result in less Ca^{2+} release in response to each action potential. Consequently, low frequencies of stimulation would produce lower than normal intracellular Ca^{2+} and thus fatigue. At high frequencies of stimulation, enough Ca^{2+} would be released from the SR (perhaps from the undamaged vesicles) to permit muscles to reach near-normal tensions. This hypothesis is supported by the frequent association of deleterious structural changes following eccentric contractions (7, 196), and also by the observation that LFF is more pronounced following eccentric compared to isometric or concentric contractions (78, 159). Davies and White (78) studied the effect of box stepping in humans and found considerably more LFF (based on 20:50 Hz force ratio) in the lead compared to the trail leg. The former conducts primarily eccentric work as it absorbs the weight of the body on return to the floor. Studies in which the force–frequency relationship in human muscle shifted to the right following fatigue all elicited contraction via percutaneous electrical stimulation (31, 101, 159, 220). Thus, in addition to muscle damage, these data could be explained by a decreased membrane excitability following fatigue, such that the applied stimulation frequencies actually elicited considerably fewer muscle action potentials. (12).

The etiology of the depressed mechanical function is complex and clearly involves multiple factors acting at various sites within the cell (Fig. 26.1). For example, the depressed P_o reflects a reduction in the numbr of cross-bridges in the strong binding state and/or a reduced force per cross-bridge (Fig. 26.2). The reduced force could result from deleterious alterations in E-C coupling producing a reduced Ca^{2+} release from the SR, changes in the extent of regulatory protein activation of the thin filament, and/or to direct effects acting at the cross-bridge. In the following sections of this chapter, the cellular sites of fatigue (Fig. 26.1, sites 5–8) will be reviewed and potential interactions between fatigue agents discussed.

EXCITATION-CONTRACTION COUPLING

Sarcolemma and T-Tubular Membranes

The first step in E-C coupling beyond the neuromuscular junction is the generation and propagation of the S_L action potential. In nonfatigued muscle cells, the resting S_L membrane potential (V_m) is approximately −80 mV, and with activation the action potential spike height approaches +20 mV (Fig. 26.5, *#1*). The action potential duration is short (1–1.5 ms), and the membrane is capable of responding to stimulation frequencies in excess of 150

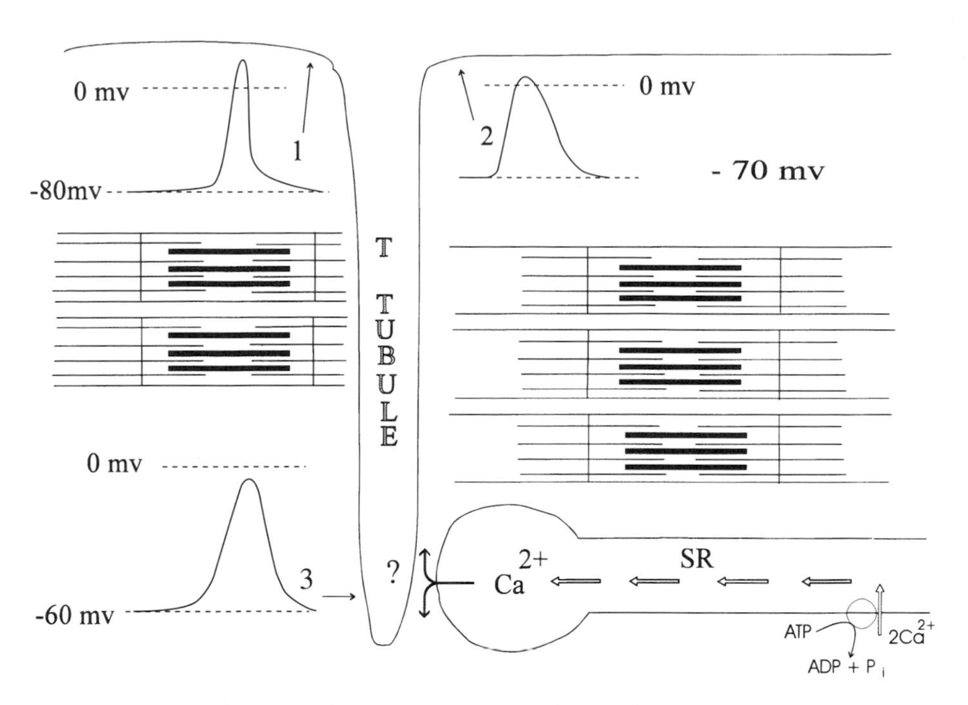

FIG. 26.5. A schematic representation of E-C coupling showing a representative sarcolemma action potential (AP) at rest (*#1*) and following fatigue (#2). It is unknown how fatigue affects the AP in the depths of the T-tubule (*#3*), hence the displayed record is theoretical and not an actual measured AP. The question mark (?) indicates that the composition of the extracellular fluid in the depths of the T-tubule in a fatigued muscle is currently unknown. The *dotted line* across each AP represents the resting and zero overshoot potentials.

Hz. With the development of fatigue, the surface membrane potential (both resting and action potential) shows characteristic changes. The resting potential becomes depolarized by 10–20 mV, and the action potential spike height declines by a similar magnitude. Additionally, the duration of the action potential becomes prolonged (Fig. 26.5, #2). Currently, it is unknown whether any of these changes in the resting and/or action potentials contribute to fatigue. A major problem in interpreting the importance of these changes is the lack of knowledge concerning the extent to which the T-tubular membrane is altered. The intracellular microelectrodes used to monitor the resting and action potentials reflect primarily the surface S_L, and thus the extent of T-tubular depolarization and the decline in the T-tubular action potential spike height is unknown. A reasonable hypothesis is that the T-tubular changes may be somewhat more extensive than those observed for the S_L. Figure 26.5 (*#3*) presents a possible scenario during fatigue in which the resting potential has depolarized to −60 mV, and the action potential spike fails to reach 0 mV. The worst-case scenario is that the action potential would fail to propagate into the depths of the T-tubule. In this case, only the superficial regions of the fiber would be activated (121).

Cell Depolarization. Some (182, 255) have suggested that alterations in sarcolemma function induce muscle fatigue by preventing cell activation. The general theory is that K^+ efflux and inhibition of the Na^+-K^+ pump (or its inability to keep pace with K^+ efflux and Na^+ influx) causes cell depolarization, a reduced action potential amplitude and, in some cells, complete inactivation. Edwards (100) suggests that cell depolarization would provide a safety mechanism to protect the cell against ATP depletion and Ca^{2+} accumulation. The uncoupling of activation at the first step in E-C coupling rather than latter steps, such as the cross-bridge cycle, would prevent activation of subsequent ATP-utilizing steps and increases in intracellular Ca^{2+}. The latter might activate Ca^{2+}-sensitive proteases and phospholipases, leading to the disruption of the sarcolemma and intracellular organelle (8). Lindinger and Sjøgaard (182) speculate that the membrane mechanism of fatigue would allow contractions at reduced rates and forces while preventing catastrophic changes in cellular homeostasis that might lead to cell damage. Although cell depolarization of 10–20 mV is commonly observed in fatigued muscle cells (139, 160, 175, 176, 267), it is not established that this change affects the propagation of the sarcolemma action potential into the T-tubules or subsequent steps in E-C coupling. Lännergren and Westerblad (175) did observe a steep decline in tension once V_m fell below −60 mV. The evidence linking K^+ efflux and cell depolarization to muscle fatigue was reviewed recently (111). Additionally, a number of detailed reviews on this topic have been published (182, 251, 255).

Muscle cells clearly lose K^+ and gain Na^+ during the development of fatigue. The amount of K^+ lost from muscle cells during contractile activity appears to exceed that explaind by the K^+ efflux attributable to the sarcolemma action potentials (255). Consequently, it has been suggested that the V_m depolarization frequently observed in fatigued muscle cells results from the combined effects of a reduced intracellular potassium ($[K^+]_i$), elevated extracellular potassium ($[K^+]_o$), and an increased K^+ conductance (182, 255). The increased K^+ conductance could result from activation of the ATP-dependent and/or the Ca^{2+}-dependent K^+ channel (55, 108, 109). Recently, Davies et al. (79) employed patch clamp methods to study the ATP-dependent K^+ channels (K_{ATP} channels) in frog skeletal muscle. At intracellular pH (pH_i) 7.2, the K_{ATP} channel showed little activity at 1 mM and was essentially inactive at 3 mM ATP; however, at pH_i 6.3, the K_{ATP} channel activity was detectable at both ATP concentrations. Thus, the possibility exists that K^+ efflux increases as the pH_i falls during high-intensity exercise. This would contribute to V_m depolarization and to a reduced action potential amplitude, and perhaps depolarization block of the sarcolemma or T-tubular action potential (54, 78, 93, 255). Although Light et al. (181) provided evidence for K_{ATP} channel activation during fatigue, they suggested it protected against the development of fatigue. Application of the K_{ATP} inhibitor glibenclamide increased fatigue and both slowed and reduced the extent of recovery in the sartorius muscle of the frog (181). It is also possible that K^+ conductance increases during contractile activity by activation of Ca^{2+}-dependent K^+ channels (255). K^+ conductance of metabolically poisoned and mechanically exhausted frog skeletal muscle fibers increased 100-fold (109). This increase was prevented by the electrophoretic injection of the Ca^{2+} chelating agent H_2EGTA^{2-}. From these observations, Fink et al. (129) concluded that internal free Ca^{2+} promoted the activation of K^+ conductance in exhausted muscle fibers. The observations that extracellular markers were not found in the myoplasm, that the membrane capacitance was unaltered, and that the conductance was inhibited by K^+ channel blockers in the exhausted fibers (55, 109) led several (55, 109) to conclude that the increased K^+ conductance occurred without any disruption in the structural integrity of either the surface or T-tubular membranes. Fink et al. (108) and Lüttgau and Wettwer (186) suggested that the lack of metabolic energy (low ATP) increased the probability of Ca^{2+}-activated K^+ conductance. This suggestion was based on their observation that membrane conductance did not increase during caffeine contracture or electrical stimulation of normal (nonpoisoned) fibers. Since cell ATP rarely falls by more than 30%, even in highly fatigued muscle fibers (110), it seems unlikely that Ca^{2+}-activated K^+ channels contribute to cell depolarization under physiological conditions. More recently, Castle and Haylett (55) proposed that the increased K^+ conductance of electrically stimulated and poisoned muscle fibers was predominantly due to activation of ATP-sensitive channels. This proposal was based on the observation that specific blockers of ATP- but not Ca^{2+}-sensitive K^+ channels inhibited the increased K^+ conductance. The apparent conflict between these results and those of Fink and colleagues (108, 109, 129) could be reconciled if depletion of cell metabolites induced a Ca^{2+} dependence of the ATP-sensitive K^+ channel.

Hicks and McComas (144) have questioned the hypothesis that cell depolarization mediates fatigue. Following in situ stimulation of the rat soleus (4 s at 20 Hz every 5 s for 5 min), they observed membrane hyperpolarization and an increased amplitude of the muscle fiber action potential. When ouabain was added to the bathing medium the fibers no longer exhibited a hyperpolarization in the recovery period. This result supports the authors' conclusion that the hyperpolarization resulted from stimulation of the Na^+-K^+ pump. Hicks and McComas (144) suggest that the depolarization observed by others (138, 160) can be attributed to unphysiologically high stimulation frequencies, and to the absence of protein in the bathing media, which they suggest may be necessary for the normal operation of the Na^+-K^+ pump. However, many have observed an increase in plasma K^+ in exercising humans (50, 61, 161, 238, 251, 254). An increase in venous K^+ draining contracting muscles suggests that the $[K^+]_o$ must increase, and the increase is likely to be greatest close to the surface membrane (256). More than half of the exercise-induced increase in plasma K^+ can be attributed to hemoconcentration (271), which results from a shift of water from the plasma into the interstitial and intracellular compartments of contracting muscle (257). Nevertheless, continuous release of K^+ has been observed during prolonged exercise (238, 256). One group found the arteriovenous plasma K^+ concentration difference to become increasingly negative near exhaustion (238). The highest level of K^+ efflux was found during maximal exercise (256). Vyskocil et al. (274) used a K^+-sensitive electrode, and observed that $[K^+]_o$ increased from 4.5 mmol/liter to 9.5 mmol/liter during maximal voluntary contractions in humans. The work of Creese et al. (73) suggests that cell depolarization with contractile activity is greater in centrally located fibers. This observation is not surprising, in that increases in $[K^+]_o$ in the interstitium and T-tubules is likely to be higher in the core of the muscle. This suggested to some (182, 255, 256) that fatigue may be related to changes in the K^+ gradient across muscle cells, and that the rapid recovery following brief rest periods reflects partial restoration of the resting membrane potential.

The Na^+-K^+ Pump and the Sarcolemma Action Potential. The increase in intracellular Na^+ and extracellular K^+ with fatigue indicates that the activity of the sarcolemma Na^+-K^+ pump is insufficient. Possibly the pump density may not be high enough to compensate fully for the ionic fluxes during the action potentials (251). This condition would be exacerbated in the T-tubules, where the Na^+-K^+ pump density is lower than that of the sarcolemma membrane (251). Insufficient pump activity might be fostered by an unfavorable microenvironment at the ATPase sites, such that locally high ADP or low ATP develops (see discussion below on functional coupling between the cell ATPases and the creatine kinase reaction). Alternately, the increase in K^+ efflux may have little effect on the Na^+-K^+ pump activity because of a relatively low K_m for $[K^+]_o$ (>1 mM) (251). The increased $[Na^+]_i$ associated with muscle fatigue would stimulate the pump, but maximal activity may require 10 mM internal sodium (251). Medbo and Sejersted (201) showed that both the rise of plasma potassium concentration during maximal exercise in man and its decline during recovery followed exponential time courses with a half-time of 25 s. After exercise, the plasma K^+ content fell below the preexercise level by 0.5 mmol/liter, which suggests that the sensitivity of the pump had been stimulated by the exercise (106). It is apparent from these results that fatigue resulting from cell depolarization (increased $[K^+]_o$) would rapidly reverse within a few minutes after exercise. Thus, the membrane theory cannot explain the slowly recovering phase of muscle fatigue (111).

With fatigue, the S_L action potential shows a reduced spike amplitude, a prolonged duration, and an increased amplitude of the early negative afterpotential (18, 136, 138, 139, 175). Additionally, the S_L action potential frequency declines. Brown and Burns (41) and Krnjevic and Miledi (170) observed a reduced sarcolemma action potential frequency with fatigue, and Lüttgau (184) found action potentials to drop out without effect on mechanical force when frog muscle fibers were stimulated at frequencies above 40 Hz. Collectively, the data demonstrate that the S_L action potential frequency definitely declines with fatigue that is induced by high-frequency stimulation. However, because the force–frequency curve generally shifts left, the reduced activation frequency does not contribute to the decline in force. In fact, Jones et al. (156) and others (26, 205) have shown an increased force when the frequency of stimulation was reduced following high-frequency fatigue. Additionally, at the maximal in vivo activation rate of ~50 Hz (87), the action potential dropout rate would be small and unlikely to fall below the optimal for force development (184).

The question remains whether any of the S_L effects reviewed here actually contribute to fatigue. If the amplitude of the action potential was reduced enough, it would fail to initiate or at least reduce the T-tubular charge movement, which in turn would inhibit both SR Ca^{2+} channel opening and Ca^{2+} release (232, 233). The results of Bezanilla et al. (18) and Grabowski et al. (136) argue against this possibility. They found that a reduction in the size of the spike amplitude, even to the point of no overshoot (0 mV), had no effect on peak tension. Furthermore, Metzger and Fitts (203) showed that the peak force (P_o) was significantly more depressed after high- compared with low-frequency stimulation, yet the action potential amplitudes were reduced the same amount. The action potential recovered from fatiguing stimulation considerably faster than force (171, 203). Sandow (249) observed no fixed relationship between the size of the action potential and force output, and concluded that a considerable "safety factor" exists relative to the extent of depolarization necessary for full activation. Nevertheless, as reviewed above, the extent of membrane depolarization and decline in the action potential spike height in the depths of the T-tubule are not established (Fig. 26.5, #3). Furthermore, neither the ionic environment in the depths of the T-tubular lumen nor how it changes with fatigue is known [indicated by question mark (?) in Fig. 26.5]. A large buildup of K^+ in this region could depolarize the cell to the extent that either the action potential is blocked or the T-tubular charge sensor inactivated. In either case, Ca^{2+} release in that portion of the cell would be inhibited.

T-Tubular–Sarcoplasmic Reticulum Junction and Calcium Release

Recent progress has been made in elucidating the cellular and molecular mechanisms by which the T-tubular action potential leads to Ca^{2+} release from the SR. It is now generally believed that the T-tubular action potential is sensed by an intramembranous T-tubular protein [dihydropyridine receptor (DHPr)], which during activation undergoes a voltage-driven conformational change (T-tubular charge movement) that in turn somehow triggers Ca^{2+} release from adjacent SR Ca^{2+} channels (231, 232, 233). The structural relationship between the T-tubular DHPr and the SR Ca^{2+} release channel (the ryanodine receptor) is shown in Figure 26.6. Although the exact mechanism of transduction of the activation signal across these structures is unknown, their morphological relationship supports the hypothesis that the main mechanism involves mechanical or allosteric coupling (231, 232, 233).

The E-C coupling process requires an optimal ionic environment, both intracellular and extracellular. As shown in Figure 26.6, the T-tubular voltage sensor of E-C coupling (DHPr) has as essential Ca^{2+} binding site on its extracellular (T-tubular lumen) side (42, 233). Consequently, metal-free conditions in the extracellular fluid suppress intramembranous T-tubular charge and the amplitude of the Ca^{2+} transient (42, 227, 233). Function of the ryanodine receptor is also dependent on Ca^{2+}. Micromolar intracellular Ca^{2+} activates the channel, whereas high Ca^{2+} inhibits channel opening (153, 188). Channel opening also depends on the presence of ATP, whereas increased amounts of H^+ and Mg^{2+} have been shown to inhibit channel activity and thus Ca^{2+} release.

The main evidence that disturbances in E-C coupling contribute to fatigue is the depressed amplitude of the Ca^{2+} transient (6, 33, 137, 276, 282). Allen et al. (6) and Westerblad and Allen (276) observed that the major decline in Ca^{2+} release occurred late in fatigue (Fig. 26.7). In both studies, the amplitude of the Ca^{2+} transient initially increased as force declined, after which both force and the Ca^{2+} signal declined. In the early phases of fatigue (phases 1 and 2, Fig. 26.4), little change occurred in the amplitude of the Ca^{2+} transient. The general conclusion was that fatigue was initially elicited by metabolic factors, while alterations in E-C coupling were important in the latter stages of fatigue (178, 276, 280). Recently, Westerblad and Lännergren (281) suggested that fatigue in phase 1 (Fig. 26.4) (characterized by a decline in P_o but not V_o) was mediated by an elevated P_i resulting from the rapid breakdown of phosphocreatine (PCr) and increased ATP turnover during the initial stages of contractile activity. They hypothesized that the decline in force during phase 2 (Fig. 26.4) was primarily caused by an increased H^+, whereas the reduced V_o associated with

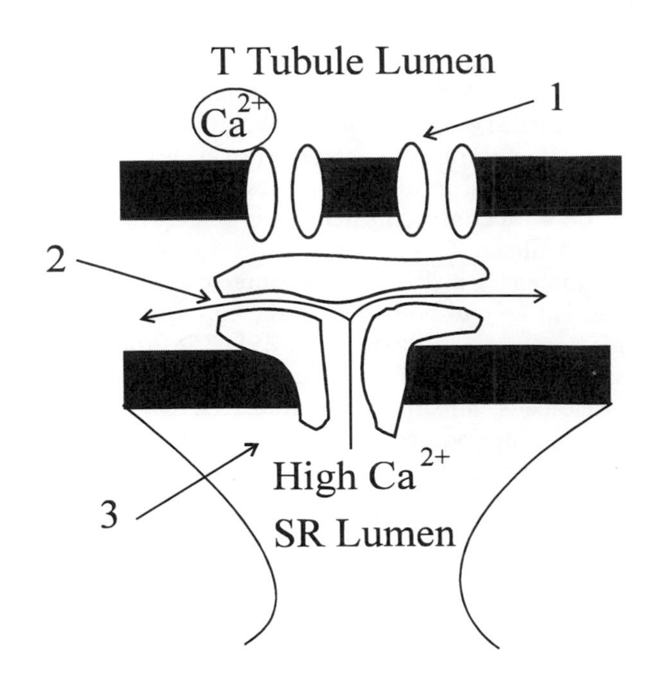

FIG. 26.6. A schematic drawing of the T-tubular SR junction showing the T-tubular dihydropyridine receptor or charge sensor (site 1), the calcium release channel (site 2), and the lumen of the SR (site 3). Disturbances in E-C coupling could result from fatigue-induced alterations in any or all of the three sites. See text for possible factors affecting each site. (The figure was modified from that presented previously [233].)

this phase of fatigue was attributed to an increase in both H^+ and ADP (281). Allen et al. (6) and Westerblad and Allen (276) attributed the early rise in tetanic $[Ca^{2+}]_i$ to a saturation of the myoplasmic Ca^{2+} buffers rather than to an increased Ca^{2+} release from the SR. As stimulation continued, a reduced Ca^{2+} release became quantitatively more important in the fatigue process (276). The observation that 10 mM caffeine had little effect early in fatigue but greatly increased both the $[Ca^{2+}]_i$ and force late in fatigue (Fig. 26.7) supports their contention that the depression of Ca^{2+} release and its contribution to fatigue develop after the initiation of fatigue by Ca^{2+}-independent factors acting directly at the cross-bridge.

The T-Tubular Charge Sensor. The reduced Ca^{2+} release is strong evidence that alterations in E-C coupling play some role in eliciting fatigue; however, the nature and site(s) of the disturbance have yet to be elucidated. Sites 1, 2, and 3 of Figure 26.6, representing: *(1)* the T-tubule lumen and DHPr, *(2)* the SR Ca^{2+} release channel, and *(3)* the SR lumen could all be involved. Regarding site 1, the DHP receptor is voltage dependent, and a maintained depolarization to levels less negative than -60 mV would be expected to inactivate the sensor such that the Ca^{2+}

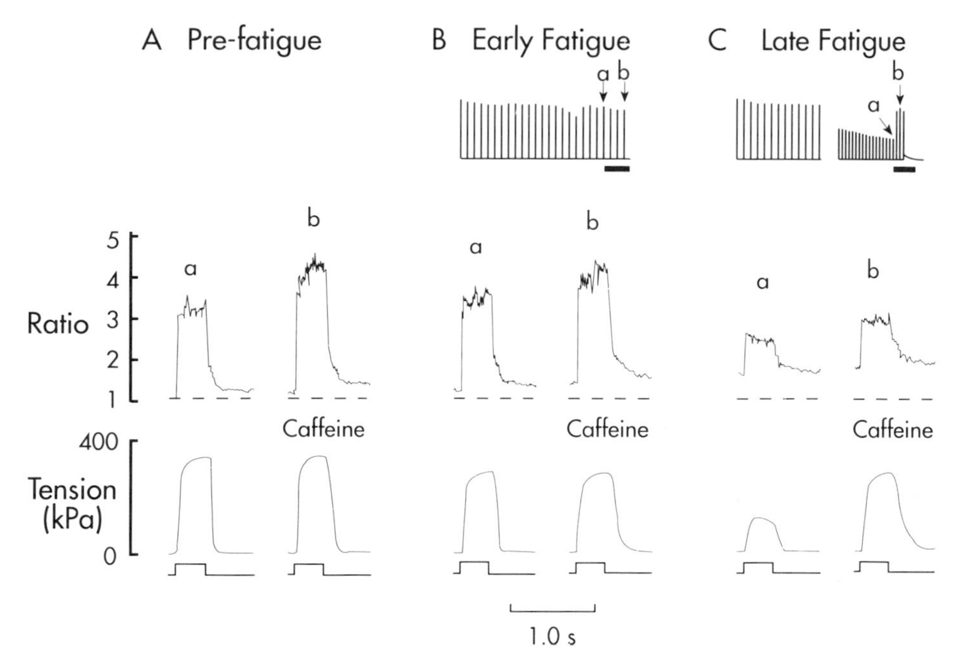

FIG. 26.7. Application of 10 mM caffeine in control (*A*) and during two successive fatigue runs (*B* and C). Bars below tension records in the top panels indicate caffeine exposure during fatiguing stimulations; caffeine was applied after 22 fatiguing tetani (*B*) and when tetanic tension was depressed to 0.36 P_o by 187 tetani (*C*). Fluorescence ratio (representative of the intracellular free Ca^{2+}) and tension records from tetani elicited before application of caffeine (*a*) and in the presence of caffeine (*b*) are shown in the two lower panels. *Dashed lines* represent resting ratio in control; stimulation periods are displayed below tension records. Note that the tetanic ratio increase induced by caffeine in late fatigue was accompanied by a substantially enhanced tension production, whereas tension was not markedly affected by the increased ratios in the other two states. [Reprinted with permission from Westerblad, H., and D. G. Allen. *J. Gen. Physiol.* 98: 615–635, 1991 (276) by copyright permission of the Rockefeller University Press.]

release channels would not be opened (227). The extracellular surface of the DHP receptor requires cation binding for proper function, and Ca^{2+} is the preferred ion (227). As Figure 26.5 indicates, we do not know what happens to the ionic environment of the T-tubular lumen with fatigue. Because the electrochemical gradient favors Ca^{2+} influx, and the T-tubular calcium channels are opened by depolarization to 0 mV (15), the possibility exists that T-tubular calcium drops with fatigue. Lüttgau et al. (185) employed the voltage-clamp technique to study the effects of zero $[Ca^{2+}]_o$ on the activation of frog single fibers. They showed that the dependence of force inactivation on the steady-state potential shifted to more negative potentials. If T-tubular depolarization develops with fatigue, it would be more likely to cause inactivation if T-tubular Ca^{2+} was reduced (42, 185). Lüttgau et al. (185) suggested that $[Ca^{2+}]_o$ might stabilize the T-tubular membrane, and that depolarization might reduce the affinity of Ca^{2+} at "a force-controlling system in the T-tubular membrane." Rios and co-workers (42, 227) have identified this site as the DHPr or the charge sensor of the T-tubular membrane. They demonstrated that charge movement and Ca^{2+} release were inhibited in zero $[Ca^{2+}]_o$. In other experiments, V_m depolarized from −80 or −90 mV to −50 mV with fatigue (175). In normal Ca^{2+}, the effect of depolarization of this magnitude on intramembranous T-tubular charge movement would be negligible; however, in low Ca^{2+} considerable inactivation of charge movement and Ca^{2+} release would exist (42, 43), and severe inhibition of force would be expected (185).

An important component in the regulation of T-tubular Ca^{2+} would be the density and activity of the T-tubular Ca-ATPase pumps. Although the T-tubular membranes of skeletal muscle are known to contain Ca-ATPase pump sites (24, 25, 251), their activity during the development of muscle fatigue is unknown. The increase in resting $[Ca^{2+}]_i$ associated with fatigue (6) would be expected to activate the pump sites, but other factors, such as an increased intracellular H^+, might inhibit the Ca-ATPase pumps.

Bianchi and Narayan (24) reported that electrical stimulation increased T-tubular Ca^{2+}, and calculated that T-tubular Ca^{2+} could reach 28 mM following as few as 120 twitches. However, they failed to consider the movement of Ca^{2+} out of the T tubules via diffusion either into the cell or intercellular space.

Nevertheless, the possibility exists that the Ca^{2+} content of the T-tubular lumen increases with fatigue. A modest increase in T-tubular Ca^{2+} (increases of 5–10 mM) would stabilize the DHPr, thus preserving charge movement and reducing the likelihood of fatigue (42, 227, 233). In a classic paper, Lüttgau (183) demonstrated that the resting V_m was depolarized and the peak K^+ contracture tension reduced in low extracellular Ca^{2+} (0.2 mM), and the latter was inhibited completely in zero $[Ca^{2+}]_o$. Perhaps more importantly, he observed the threshold potential to be altered by $[Ca^{2+}]_o$. Low $[Ca^{2+}]_o$ shifted the activation threshold to the left with weak contractions recorded at 10–20 mM $[K^+]_o$ or a V_m of −60 mV. Increasing extracellular calcium from the control value of 1.8 to 5 mM increased the threshold potential from −35 mV to −18 mV (183). Consistent with this observation, Shlevin (252) observed high external Ca^{2+} to shift the T-tubular charge–voltage relationship to the right, such that the half maximal charge (V) was obtained at more depolarized potentials. Additionally, following a 190 mM KCl contracture, fibers in 5 mM $[Ca^{2+}]_o$ were able to reprime to a greater extent at a given level of depolarization. For example, in 1.8 and 5.0 mM $[Ca^{2+}]_o$ repriming reached 50% at −37 and −25 mV, respectively. The effects of extracellular calcium on the activation threshold was confirmed by Frankenhaeuser and Lännergren (117). Recent data from Rios and co-workers (227, 233) demonstrate that high $[Ca^{2+}]_o$ would also increase the rate of repriming. Grabowski et al. (136) have shown that the activation threshold was shifted by about 20 mV more positive following fatigue. In addition, the peak contracture elicited by 190 mM KCl was reduced in the fatigued fibers (136). The rightward shift in the activation threshold in the fatigued fibers would be expected if T-tubular $[Ca^{2+}]_o$ increased (42, 183, 252). However, if T-tubular calcium does not exceed 5 mM, the threshold for activation would be reached by −20 mV and full activation obtained at 0 mV (132, 183, 252). Since the action potential spike height generally reaches 0 mV even in extreme fatigue (139, 175, 176), this shift in the voltage–tension relationship should not contribute to fatigue. The high T-tubular Ca^{2+} might help prevent fatigue both by stabilizing the resting V_m and by decreasing the likelihood of inactivation that might occur with depolarization. Although the spike height of the S_L action potential does not appear to decline enough to prevent activation, the amplitude could be considerably less in the depths of the T-tubule, such that incomplete activation occurs in the core of the fiber.

Howell and two co-workers (148, 150) suggested that an activity-induced increase in T-tubular Ca^{2+} might slow the T-tubular action potential conduction velocity to the point of conduction block, thereby producing incomplete activation of the axial core of the fiber. High Ca^{2+} altered the early afterpotential, the origin of which has been attributed to T-tubular conduction events (147, 148). Howell and co-workers (148, 149) also observed myofibril waviness in the axial core of fibers activated in 10 mM Ca^{2+}, and attributed this to a failed conduction of the T-tubular action potential. Recently, Garcia et al. (121) found a similar condition following electrical stimulation of single frog muscle fibers. The extent of wavy myofibril formation increased in parallel with the development of muscle fatigue, and caffeine contracture eliminated wavy myofibrils and restored tension. Previously, Taylor and Rüdel (264) observed wavy myofibrils in nonfatigued fibers at short sarcomere lengths; however, Garcia et al. (121) report that wavy myofibrils were never seen in prefatigued fibers. They concluded that fatigue was caused by either a failure of the tubular action potential or by the conduction signal between the T system and the terminal cisternae. Others (133, 258) found the preferential development of vacuoles in the T system of fatigued muscle fibers, and with recovery the vacuoles disappeared. In their recent work, Garcia et al. (121) suggested that the activation failure may occur at the site of tubular vacuolation. Consistent with the theory of T-tubular conduction block, Westerblad et al. (282) found high-frequency stimulation to produce a spatial gradient of $[Ca^{2+}]_i$ with higher concentrations near the edges of the fiber. The authors attributed the low Ca^{2+} in the fiber center to action potential conduction block in the T-tubule network. To contribute significantly to the decline in force, T-tubular Ca^{2+} would have to approach 15 mM during contractile activity [see Fig. 2 in Howell and Snowdowne (150)].

SR Calcium Release Channel. A second potential site for the failure of E-C coupling is the SR Ca^{2+} release channel (site 2, Fig. 26.6). The positive feedback effects of Ca^{2+} on both the ryanodine and dihydropyridine receptors might be inhibited during the development of fatigue. For example, the H^+ ion, known to increase with intense contractile activity, might inhibit the release process. Following reconstitution of the purified ryanodine receptor channel into a lipid bilayer, Ma et al. (188) studied the pH dependence of the release channel. Reducing pH on either side of the bilayer decreased the frequency and duration of channel openings. "Open-probability" of the channel was maximum at pH 7.4 and decreased to almost null at pH 6.5. Acidification (pH 7.4–6.6) of the myoplasmic side of the SR lipid bilayers decreased the open probability of the Ca^{2+} release channel, whereas acidification of the luminal side decreased channel conductance but not the open-probability (234). They suggested that the rate of protonation might change the affinity of the Ca^{2+} activating binding sites. Recently, Ma and Zhao (189) reconstituted into lipid bilayers not only the isolated release channel protein but also the other proteins associated with SR terminal cisternae. This system mimics more closely the in vivo situation; nevertheless, the results were identical to those obtained with the isolated release channel. As pH was reduced the channel open-probability declined, and at pH 6.2 it was near zero. We recently found that a decline in pH to 6.0 does not affect the extent of T-tubular charge moved in response to cell depolarization (E. M. Balog and R. H. Fitts, unpublished observation). Thus, the pH effect on E-C coupling appears to be restricted to inhibition of the SR Ca^{2+} release channel. This conclusion is consistent with the observation that there is no decline in T-tubular charge movement despite a significant reduction in the amplitude of the Ca^{2+} transient during fatiguing stimulations of single frog fibers (137). Reduced Ca^{2+} transient was attributed to a direct inhibition of the SR Ca^{2+} release channel and not to disturbance in T-tubular action potential or the DHP charge sensor (137).

During contractile activity, Ca^{2+} is redistributed from the SR release site (site 3, Fig. 26.6) to other intracellular sites, particularly the Ca^{2+}-binding protein parvalbumin and the SR pump. This redistribution would decrease the driving force for Ca^{2+} release, and thus reduce the rate and extent of Ca^{2+} release. The saturation of intracellular calcium buffers likely occurs early during contractile activity, and this would in turn place an increased load on the reuptake process. This hypothesis is supported by the observation that the rate of $[Ca^{2+}]_i$ reuptake following a tetanic contraction declined as the tetanic duration increased (53), and also by the observation that the prolonged relaxation generally occurs early before the major decline in force (280). Additionally, the SR Ca^{2+} pump rate may be slowed by elevated H^+ in fatigued muscle fibers (49, 218).

The reduced driving force associated with the redistribution of Ca^{2+} during contractile activity undoubtedly contributes to the reduced amplitude of the Ca^{2+} transient. However, the observation that caffeine, a compound stimulating direct release of Ca^{2+} from the SR reverses most of the tension loss in fatigued fibers demonstrates that depletion of $Ca^{2+}$from the SR release site cannot be of primary importance (95). This observation has since been confirmed by several groups (121, 136, 177, 219, 272, 276) (see Fig. 26.7). Furthermore, fatigued muscles exposed to high K^+ respond with high levels of Ca^{2+} release and force contracture (6, 136). If fatigue was caused by depletion of SR Ca^{2+}, caffeine and K^+ contracture would fail to produce significant tension. Additionally, electron probel analysis also supports the theory that the SR Ca^{2+} stores were not depleted with stimulation to fatigue (133). Thus, in summary, it appears that the primary site involved in the disturbance of E-C coupling with fatigue is the SR Ca^{2+} release site (site 2, Fig. 26.6).

LACTIC ACID, INTRACELLULAR pH AND FATIGUE

Muscle Lactate

The relationship between muscle lactate and the development of muscle fatigue during exercise at various intensities was recently reviewed (111). Although a high inverse correlation exists between the increase in muscle lactate and the decline in force and performance during high-intensity exercise, it is now generally believed that the increase in lactate itself plays little or no role in the fatigue process (111). With fatigue, the osmotic pressure within muscle rises, causing an increased intracellular water and cell swelling (13, 237). The increased muscle water with exercise was caused by an increase in extra- as well as intracellular water content, and the intracellular water change was highly correlated with the increase in lactate (237, 242). The lactate-induced fiber swelling would affect the lateral spacing of the contractile filament lattice, and this could reduce peak force. This effect is likely to be small, however, as skinned fibers, known to swell by approximately 20% compared to living fibers, showed only a small increase in P_o when cell width was compressed by dextran (122, 208). High muscle lactate could significantly increase ionic strength, which in turn would depress peak force (134). However, the observation of Chase and Kushmerick (56) that 50 mM lactate had no effect on the P_o of single rabbit psoas fibers provides direct evidence that the lactate ion does not directly induce fatigue in limb skeletal muscle. Sahlin et al (237, 242) found a high correlation between the fall in muscle pH and the increase in lactate and pyruvate content following dynamic exercise in man. It is now generally recognized that the high inverse correlation between lactate and force is, for the most part, dependent on the high correlation between lactate and the free hydrogen ion, and that the force-depressing agent is the hydrogen ion and not lactate (207, 237).

Hydrogen Ion and Muscle Fatigue

Table 26.1 shows representative values for muscle pH at rest and following fatigue produced by high-intensity contractile activity. In a wide variety of limb skeletal muscles, the pH of a nonfatigued muscle cell is 7.0. With exercise, the higher the intensity of work the greater the decline in intracellular pH (pH_i), with the highest fall observed in the FG fiber type. It is not uncommon for pH_i to fall to 6.1, and the mean value obtained in fast-twitch fibers is generally 6.2–6.3 (Table 26.1). Although a consensus exists that cell pH_i declines with high-intensity exercise, some question whether the pH_i change is causative in fatigue (191, 229, 240, 277, 279). The major arguments against a role for H^+ in the etiology of fatigue are the observations that (*1*) pH_i recovers at a different rate than tension following fatigue, and (*2*) reduction in pH_i to levels observed in fatigued fibers by carbon dioxide exposure yields an inhibition of force considerably less than that observed in fatigue. Westerblad and Lännergren (279) argue that intracellular acidification is unlikely to be a major cause of fatigue, as they observed a large variation in pH_i in fibers fatigued to the same standardized tension loss, and secondly, pH_i recovered considerably faster than tension. Metzger and Fitts (205) and Thompson et al. (267) also observed pH_i to recover before tension, but nonetheless the correlation between pH_i and force was high. These authors interpreted the data to imply that although pH_i was an important fatigue agent, other factors (such as P_i, alterations in the free energy of ATP hydrolysis, and disturbances in E-C coupling) must also be involved. Following a 50 s isometric contraction of the knee extensors at 66% of maximal voluntary contraction (MVC) in man, Sahlin and Ren (245) observed force to recover in 2 min, during which time-calculated pH_i (based on muscle lactate) remained low. They concluded that the high intracellular concentration of H^+ did not limit the capacity to generate force in vivo. Under their experimental conditions only a modest level of fatigue was obtained (decrease from 66% to 50% MVC); the rapid recovery of force suggests that the fatigue was elicited by alterations in E-C coupling. It is not clear why the low pH_i did not inhibit force in this experiment, but perhaps the calculated pH_i was lower than the actual pH_i.

Nuclear magnetic resonance (NMR) technology has shown a good correlation between the decline in pH_i and force during either in situ or in vivo contractile activity in slow- as well as fast-twitch skeletal muscles (1, 215, 286). However, Adams et al. (1) found no significant effect of hypercapnia (70% carbon dioxide) on P_o in either slow or fast muscles of the cat. Although pH_i was as low as that obtained with electrical stimulation, the Ca^{2+} distribution within the fibers was entirely different. Large decreases in pH_i would have less effect when Ca^{2+}release (and thus the amplitude of the Ca^{2+} transient) is high as it would be in the hypercapnic condition. Furthermore, none of the other factors thought to be involved in muscle fatigue, or any H^+ interactions with such factors, were likely present in the hypercapnic condition. As the authors point out, they have not examined the effects of hypercapnic acidosis on force during fatiguing stimulation. Under these conditions, Ca^{2+} release would be reduced and the effects of H^+ on the regulatory protein troponin and cross-bridge kinetics would become magnified. In contrast to the NMR results, Sahlin et al. (239) found high carbon dioxide to decrease pH_i (0.34 units) and force (55% of initial), approximately the same amount as electrical stimulation. Further, Hultman et al. (151) reported a 75 s contraction of the quadriceps femoris in man to produce a greater decline in cell pH (6.54 vs. 6.70) and force (44.6% vs. 55.4% of initial) after induced metabolic acidosis compared to control conditions. The work of Mainwood and Renaud (191) clearly points out the quantitative difference in the effect of pH_i on muscle force when H^+ is produced by hypercapnia as opposed to contractile activity. With equal cellular H^+ concentration, tension declined by 30% and 70% following hypercapnia and electrical stimulation, respectively. Wilson et al. (286) conducted an experiment in which 2 min of submaximal exercise preceded maximal wrist flexion exercise in man. The submaximal

TABLE 26.1. *Skeletal Muscle pH**

Method	Rest Value	Fatigue Value	Reference
Muscle homogenate	6.92 ± 0.03	6.41 ± 0.04	142
Calculated from HCO_3^- + P_{CO_2}	7.04 ± 0.05	6.37 ± 0.11	237
Microelectrode	7.06 ± 0.04	6.33	205
Microelectrode	7.00 ± 0.02	6.42 ± 0.12	267
NMR method	6.99 ± 0.04	6.17 ± 0.33	286

*Values are means ± SE except for Sahlin et al. (237), where ± SD are listed.

exercise reduced pH_i, so that during the subsequent maximal exercise a given percentage decline in force was associated with a lower pH_i than observed in a control maximal exercise bout. From this experiment and those employing hypercapnia, one cannot conclude that H^+ lacks a direct effect on muscle fatigue, but only that the magnitude of the effect is dependent on other factors. During hypercapnia, a particularly important factor is the amplitude of the Ca^{2+} transient, which is surely higher than that observed in fatigued fibers.

Perhaps the most convincing evidence that low pH_i contributes to fatigue is the observation that acidosis depresses force in isolated skinned fibers (91, 107, 202, 204, 207). Fast-twitch fibers were more sensitive to the acidotic depression of tension than were the slow muscle fibers (56, 91, 207). The mechanism by which an increased H^+ could induce fatigue is multifactorial. In addition to the inhibition of SR Ca^{2+} release (reviewed above), a reduced pH could depress force by inhibiting (*1*) Ca^{2+} activation of the thin filament, (*2*) the transition of the cross-bridge from the low- to the high-force state, (*3*) SR ATPase activity and Ca^{2+}reuptake into the SR, (*4*) the Na^+-K^+ ATPase activity, and (*5*) glycolysis. Additionally, low pH_i reduced V_o (98, 207), and this, coupled with the reduced force, will inhibit peak power. Many of these possibilities are shown diagrammatically in Figure 26.8. Insufficient Na^+-K^+ pump activity would lead to cell depolarization and a reduced action potential spike potential. As described above, these factors could induce fatigue by blocking E-C coupling at the DHP receptor site in the T-tubular membrane.

H^+, Troponin, and the Cross-Bridge Cycle. The observation that decreasing pH from 7.0 to 6.2 increased the free Ca^{2+} required for the initiation of contraction (activation threshold) and shifted the force–pCa curve to the right such that higher free Ca^{2+} was required to reach a given tension suggests that H^+ inhibits Ca^{2+} binding to troponin (91, 107). However, controversy surrounds this suggestion. Blanchard et al. (32) concluded that lowering pH from 7.0 to 6.2 reduced the affinity of Ca^{2+} binding to troponin, whereas others have found no direct effects of pH on the affinity of Ca^{2+}-binding sites on troponin (224). The tension–pCa curve is less steep in slow- compared to fast-twitch fibers, a phenomenon attributed to greater cooperativity in the Ca^{2+}

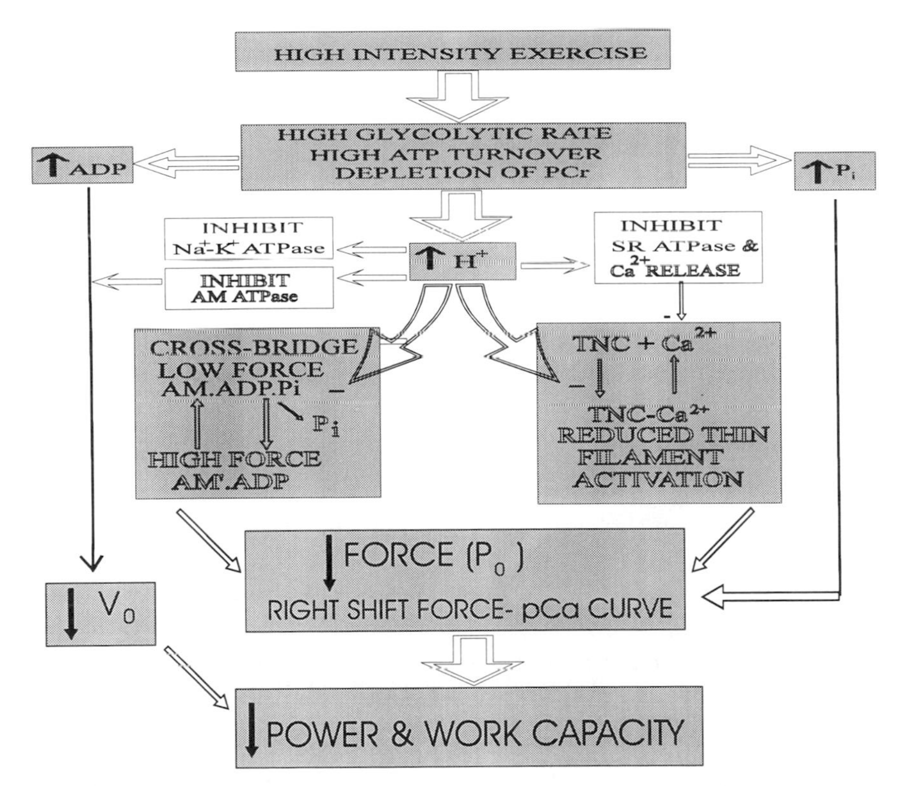

FIG. 26.8. Schematic representation of mechanisms by which increases in H^+, inorganic phosphate (P_i), and ADP could contribute to fatigue during high-intensity exercise. An *upward* or *downward arrow* indicates an increased or decreased response for the indicated variable, respectively [an exception is the arrows indicating the cross-bridge and troponin C (TNC) reactions]. A *negative sign* indicates inhibition at the site indicated. AM, actomyosin cross-bridge.

activation of tension in the fast fiber type (37, 207). Low pH_i appears to affect the positive cooperativity in fiber-type–specific ways, with slow and fast fibers showing an increased and decreased cooperativity, respectively (207). However, in both slow- and fast-twitch fibers, decreasing pH from 7.0 to 6.2 increased the free Ca^{2+} required for the initiation of tension development (threshold activation) and for half-maximal tension (pCa_{50}) (207). Alterations in the tension–pCa relationship are likely to be caused by a combination of factors induced by low pH. These include a direct inhibition of Ca^{2+} binding to troponin, reduced cooperativity between adjacent regulatory subunits, and a reduced cooperativity caused by fewer active cross-bridges (207, 210).

The observation that low pH still inhibits force at saturating levels of free Ca^{2+} suggests that the effect cannot be entirely attributable to a simple H^+ interference of Ca^{2+} binding to troponin (107, 207). Fabiato and Fabiato (107) observed a 33% reduction in maximal rigor tension of the frog semitendinosus when pH was reduced from 7.0 to 6.2. A similar effect was observed in mammalian fast and slow fibers (209). Both groups interpreted this as evidence for a direct effect of H^+ on the contractile proteins. It is currently thought that H^+ directly inhibits force by reducing the cross-bridge transition from the low- to the high-force state. This concept is diagrammed in Figure 26.8. The cross-bridge transition from the low- to the high-force state corresponds to the release of P_i and H^+, and thus a buildup in either of these compounds would be expected to reduce the transition from low to high force; this in turn would inhibit force development of the contracting muscle.

A direct effect of pH on the cross-bridge could involve: (*1*) a reduction in the number of cross-bridges, and/or (2) a reduction in the force per cross-bridge. The number of attached cross-bridges can be estimated from fiber stiffness measured during high-frequency length oscillations of a fully activated fiber (209). When pH_i was reduced with high cardon dioxide, peak force decreased 24% and 30% for the mouse soleus and extensor digitorum longus (EDL) muscles, but stiffness only decreased 9% and 14%, respectively (230). These results suggest that the primary effect of low pH is to reduce the force per cross-bridge. More recently, Edman and Lou (97) established this to be true in living single fibers. During development of moderate levels of muscle fatigue (75% of initial force), they observed only a 9% reduction in fiber stiffness. In nonfatigued fibers, stiffness reached its peak before force, and following fatigue this difference was magnified as the rate of rise of force (+dP/dt) was markedly depressed while the rate of stiffness development remained unchanged. This result implies that fatigue altered the rate of transition from the cross-bridge attached state (reflected by stiffness) to the high-force state of the cross-bridge. Intracellular acidification by high carbon dioxide altered cell function in a manner similar to that observed with fatigue. However, for a given fall in tension, stiffness fell less with acidosis compared to fatigue. Unlike fatigue, the rate of rise of stiffness showed a progressive decline as acidosis developed. This result suggests that other factors unique to fatigue (such as P_i or the amplitude of the Ca^{2+} transient) modified the pH effect on the cross-bridge kinetics. In skinned fiber studies, Metzger and Moss (209) showed low pH to decrease the number of cross-bridges in fast- but not slow-twitch fibers. Additionally, they observed a high H^+ to reduce the force per cross-bridge in both slow- and fast-twitch fibers.

In addition to the decline in tension, fatigue is associated with a reduced +dP/dt (116). Part of the decline in +dP/dt can be explained by the decrease in the number of active cross-bridges acting in parallel. The latter is caused by incomplete activation (inhibition of E-C coupling) or direct inhibition of the cross-bridge. Consequently, when data for post-fatigue +dP/dt were corrected for the fall in force [$(+dP/dt)/P_0$] the observed decrease in +dP/dt was attenuated (204). If the peak +dP/dt in an intact muscle is limited by the cross-bridge transition rate from the weakly bound low-force state to the strongly bound high-force state or step 2 in Figure 26.2 (as it appears to be in fully activated single fibers), then the rate constant for cross-bridge binding may be reduced in the fatigued cell. Alternatively, the rate-limiting step in the rate of force development in intact muscles may be limited by other factors (such as the rate of Ca^{2+} release) or the limiting step may switch with fatigue from cross-bridge binding to Ca^{2+} release. This could occur if the E-C coupling process was altered such that fewer SR Ca^{2+} release channels were opened (188, 234). Regardless of what limits +dP/dt, several lines of evidence suggest that its decline with fatigue is at least partially caused by the development of low pH_i. We have recently observed a high correlation between +dP/dt and pH_i during the recovery from fatigue (267). Furthermore, Edman and associates (97, 98) found a similar fall in peak force and +dP/dt with fatigue and acidosis induced by carbon dioxide exposure in single intact fibers. Finally, at suboptimal Ca^{2+} concentrations (pCa >5.0), Metzger and Moss (210) showed low pH to inhibit the rate constant of tension redevelopment (k_{tr}) in both slow- and fast-twitch single skinned fibers. These authors observed no effect of low pH on the k_{tr} during maximal Ca^{2+} activation (pCa = 4.5). However, since the amplitude of the intracellular Ca^{2+} transient is known to be reduced with fatigue, the pH effect on the k_{tr} could be of physiological importance.

An increased H^+ concentration has also been shown to reduce V_o in isolated skinned fibers. This effect has been observed in fast and slow rabbit and rat fibers, with the fast fiber type showing the largest depression (56, 64, 207). Consistent with the skinned fiber observations, Edman and Mattiazzi (98) demonstrated a significant decrease in V_o of fatigued frog skeletal muscle fibers; however, V_o never declined until force fell by at least 10%. They suggested that the decline in V_o was mediated by an increased myoplasmic H^+ concentration, since unstimulated fibers incubated in high Pco_2, showed a similar reduction in force and V_o. The fibers with the highest initial velocity (presumably fast-twitch) showed the greatest drop in V_o. The decline in V_o with fatigue has also been observed in whole muscles, but not until force has fallen by at least 30% (115, 268). The fact that an elevated H^+ concentration depresses P_o and V_o suggests that this ion may affect more than one step of the cross-bridge cycle (Fig. 26.2).

H^+ and SR Function. A prolonged relaxation time and Ca^{2+} transient is a consistent feature of fatigued muscle, and the slowed relaxation has frequently been attributed to an incrased H^+ (51, 76, 77, 240, 241). The observation of a significant correlation between pH_i and ½ RT time during the recovery from fatigue supports this hypothesis (267). Relaxation from a peak contraction shows an initial linear phase followed by a nonlinear, almost exponential, decline to the resting tension (77, 276). The major prolongation of relaxation occurs in the initial linear phase (77, 280). During contractile activity, Ca^{2+} is redistributed from the SR release site to the Ca^{2+}-binding proteins troponin C, parvalbumin, and the SR pump, therefore placing a greater load on the reuptake process. With contractile activity, parvalbumin becomes rapidly saturated and thus likely does not contribute to the slowing of relaxation beyond the first few seconds of contractile activity (23, 53, 280). Both fatigue and acid pH produced by high carbon dioxide slow relaxation; however, the latter is not accompanied by a slowed Ca^{2+} transient (6). Westerblad and Lännergren (280) hypothesized that the inhibition of relaxation with fatigue was due to the combined effect of an altered cross-bridge kinetics and an impaired ability of the SR to resequester Ca^{2+}. Since acidic pH did not alter the Ca^{2+} transient, they concluded that the pH effect was mediated through a direct effect on cross-bridge kinetics. Considerable evidence suggests that a reduced pH_i is in part responsible for the prolongation of relaxation associated with fatigue. Fibers showing the largest decline in pH_i consistently show the greatest prolongation of relaxation, and lactic acidosis prolongs relaxation (192, 277). Iodoacetic acid–poisoned muscles underwent a 50% fall in tension with stimulation, but no change in pH_i or relaxation time (235, 241). Although these data are consistent with a role for H^+ in the prolongation of relaxation, it is clear that additional factors are involved. One such factor may be the reduced free energy of ATP, which has been correlated with a prolonged relaxation time in fatigued muscle (see HIGH-ENERGY PHOSPHATES AND THE FREE ENERGY OF ATP HYDROLYSIS). Cady et al. (51) observed a differential effect of muscle fatigue on the relaxation rate of the first dorsal interosseous in control and myophosphorylase-deficient (MPD) subjects. For the control subjects, pH_i fell to 6.5, and the rate constant for relaxation was reduced to 24% of its initial value. In contrast, the MPD subjects showed no significant change in pH_i; however, the relaxation rate declined although less than that observed in the control subjects. Additionally, the relaxation rate recovered considerably faster in the MPD than in the control subjects. Furthermore, in the first few minutes following fatigue, the relaxation rate increased, while pH_i remained acidic, and later in the recovery period pH_i returned to the control value at a time when relaxation was only partially recovered (51, 267).

Skinned fiber experiments of Fabiato and Fabiato (107) and Lamb et al. (173) showed acidic pH to reduce the extent of Ca^{2+} reloading into the SR, while the latter group concluded that Ca^{2+} release was not inhibited. This conclusion was based on the observation that the force decreased in acidic pH the same regardless of whether contraction was induced by depolarization or direct Ca^{2+} activation. The observation that acidic pH inhibits Ca^{2+} reuptake is not consistent with the hypothesis of Westerblad and Allen (277) that the pH-dependent effect on relaxation primarily acts on the cross-bridge cycle. Considerable evidence suggests that H^+ compromises the functional capacity of the SR pump protein. Both the ATPase activity and Ca^{2+} reuptake capacity of the SR are known to be depressed following high-intensity exercise (49). The inhibition could in part be mediated by H^+, as the SR ATPase has an optimal pH of 7.0 and its activity decreases with lowered pH (154, 193). Additionally, acidic pH has been shown to depress SR Ca^{2+} reuptake, presumably by inhibiting both the formation and cleavage of the phosphorylated enzyme intermediate (154).

H^+ and Muscle Glycogenolysis. A number of observations suggest that low pH inhibits glycolysis. Hill found that lactate formation during muscle stimulation stopped when the intracellular pH dropped to 6.3 (146). Additionally, Hermansen and Osnes (142) measured the pH of muscle homogenates and observed no change during a 60 s measurement period for the most acidic homogenates of fatigued muscle; the pH values of the homogenates from resting muscle fell markedly owing to significant glycolysis during the measurement period. A decrease in cell pH could inhibit both glycogenolysis and glycolysis by inhibiting phosphorylase and phosphofructokinase (57, 228, 260). In fact, a number of studies have demonstrated the glycogenolytic rate to decline with fatigue during high-intensity exercise (195, 261). The important question is whether the reduced glycogenolytic rate contributes to fatigue by limiting ATP production or alternatively if glycogenolysis is reduced in response to a lowered ATP requirement as fatigue develops. Although H^+ inhibition of glycolysis might be a limiting factor for performance (102, 237), this suggestion seems unlikely in that cell ATP rarely falls below 70% of the prefatigued value during intense exercise (110, 269). It seems more likely that the inhibitory effects of H^+ are countered by increases in AMP, inosine monophosphate (IMP), and inorganic phosphate, all of which are known activators of phosphorylase and phosphofructokinase (57, 228, 260). The high correlation between glycogenolysis and the ATP turnover rate during the development of fatigue supports the hypothesis that the former declines in response to the reduced energy requirement of the fatigued muscle.

INORGANIC PHOSPHATE AND MUSCLE FATIGUE

Total Phosphate and the Diprotonated Form

During contractile activity, P_i increases stoichiometrically with the decrease in PCr, and both are significantly correlated with the development of fatigue (74, 80–82, 215, 275). Following fatigue, both P_i and PCr recover with similar time courses that are generally related to the recovery in P_o (215, 268). These observations plus the demonstration that P_i inhibits force in skinned fibers (64, 66, 166, 194, 214, 222, 225) provide strong evidence that this ion contributes to the development of fatigue in high-intensity exercise. However, the active species of P_i in the etiology of fatigue remains controversial (214, 225, 285). Wilkie (285) plotted the data of Dawson et al. (82) as total P_i and the $H_2PO_4^-$ form vs. fatigue and observed a simple inverse linear relation between the latter and force with zero force attained at a $H_2PO_4^-$ concentration of approximately 20 mmol/kg wet weight. From this observation, Wilkie (285) and Dawson et al. (84) hypothesized that the diprotonated form of P_i was contributory to fatigue. This hypothesis was supported by others (215, 222, 275) who observed a similar inverse linear relation between $H_2PO_4^-$ and force. For example, Nosek et al. (222) reported skinned fiber force to approach zero at 30–35 mM $H_2PO_4^-$. This agrees well with the relationship between diprotonated P_i and force in human skeletal muscle (215, 275).

In contrast, others (66, 214, 225) found the decline in force to be linearly related to the logarithm of the average P_i concentration. Millar and Homsher (214) found the slope of the relative tension vs. log $[P_i]$ to be the same at pH 7 and 6.2. This result confirmed the earlier finding of Chase and Kushmerick (56), who reported the relative force at 15 mM P_i (normalized to that at 1 mM P_i) to be the same at pH 7.1 and 6.0. This observation led Chase and Kushmerick (56) to reject the hypothesis (82, 285) that $H_2PO_4^-$ is the primary causative agent in muscle fatigue. Pate and Cooke (225) argue that if tension depends on the logarithm of P_i concentration, then the question cannot be answered by determining the relationship between P_i (total or the $H_2PO_4^-$ form) and force, as both forms will increase by the same factor as fatigue develops.

Recently, Nosek et al. (223) reevaluated the effect of P_i on force developed by skinned fibers and concluded that the diprotonated form correlated with force in the fast-twitch psoas, but not in slow-twitch or cardiac fibers. This result agreed with that of Kentish (168), who found total but not the diprotonated form of P_i to be correlated with reduced force in cardiac muscle. In addition to the species of phosphate, the range of P_i required to induce fatigue has not been clearly established. Studies employing skinned fibers show the inhibition of force to be particularly sensitive to increases in P_i between 1 and 15 mM (64–66), whereas NMR analysis of muscles contracting in vivo or in vitro reveal little effect on force until P_i exceeds 20 mM (1, 52, 82, 198). The reason for this discrepancy is not apparent. In a recent study, Thompson and Fitts (269) evaluated the relationship between P_i and force during the recovery from fatigue in the frog semitendinosus. These authors determined P_i chemically and found 49 and 103 mmol/kg dry weight P_i (~10 and 20 mM P_i wet weight) to be associated with a P_o of 50% and 37% of the prefatigued value, respectively. The latter value was obtained at 5 min of recovery when intracellular pH was 6.5. This result shows considerable agreement wiht the data of Cooke and Pate

(65), who observed a relative tension of 30% with activation of skinned fibers in 20 mM P_i and pH 6.5. When the entire recovery period was considered, Thompson and Fitts (269) observed a significant inverse correlation between both the diprotonated and total P_i and force; however, during the second slow phase of recovery only the $H_2PO_4^-$ form was significantly correlated with force. The effect of P_i on tension is greater in fast- than in slow-twitch fibers. Stienen et al. (263) found 15 mM P_i to reduce force to 58% and 78% of the control situation in single skinned fibers isolated from the fast psoas and slow soleus, respectively.

It is clear that fatigue results from a number of factors (e.g., disturbances in E-C coupling, elevated H^+, and P_i) acting at various sites within the cell. Consequently, the relationship between P_i and force is not always correlated. Miller and colleagues (215, 275) observed P_i to increase more rapidly than the decline in the peak force of a maximal voluntary contraction (MVC), and following 2 min of contraction to plateau while the peak force continued to fall. Dawson (80) observed a high correlation between the decline in force and the increase in the diprotonated ($H_2PO_4^-$) form of P_i in frog skeletal muscle. Wilson (286) and McCully et al. (197, 198) reported a similar response in human muscle when the exercise consisted of 1 s maximal voluntary contractions every 5 s. However, when a ramp of increasing work rate was employed, no correlation was observed between $H_2PO_4^-$ and muscle fatigue (197, 198).

Mechanisms of Phosphate Action

In addition to the decline in force, the increase in P_i may affect relaxation time. Bergstrom and Hultman (22) demonstrated a high correlation between the increase in $H_2PO_4^-$ and relaxation time during the development of and recovery from fatigue. However, a causative effect of an increased P_i on relaxation time has not been established. It has been hypothesized that the increased P_i reduces the free energy of ATP hydrolysis, which in turn might inhibit the rate of SR pump activity and thus Ca^{2+} reuptake (83; see also later under HIGH-ENERGY PHOSPHATES AND THE FREE ENERGY OF ATP HYDROLYSIS).

As reviewed above, the decline in fiber V_o with fatigue is at least in part caused by an elevated H^+; however, V_o does not appear to be effected by the increased P_i. In skinned fiber experiments, Cooke and co-workers (64, 65, 225) found increases in P_i up to 20 mM to have no effect on V_o. An increased P_i has been shown to depress fiber ATPase activity, but not as much as tension (64, 166). Consequently, the tension cost (ATPase/tension ratio) increased with increasing P_i. Kawai et al. (166) suggest that the decreased hydrolysis rate at high P_i concentrations was not caused by a reduced cross-bridge cycle rate, but simply reflected the mobilization of fewer cross-bridges. Pate and Cooke (225) observed P_i in excess of 10 mM to depress V_o, but only at low ATP concentrations. They proposed that P_i competitively inhibited the binding of MgATP to the myosin nucleotide site at the end of the cross-bridge power stroke, which prevented the dissociation of myosin from actin and slowed fiber velocity. However, even in cases of extreme fatigue, cell ATP concentration rarely falls by more than 30% of its concentration before fatigue. Consequently, it seems unlikely that high P_i contributes to the fatigue-induced decline in V_o. Dawson et al. (84) and Wilkie (285) hypothesized that rather than acting directly on the cross-bridges, the deleterious effects of low intracellular pH might be mediated by producing an inhibitory high concentration of $H_2PO_4^-$. Since high H^+ but not P_i depresses V_o, this hypothesis seems unlikely.

An important problem is understanding the mechanism by which high P_i inhibits force. In the cross-bridge cycle, P_i is thought to be released from the actin-myosin complex during the transition of cross-bridges from a low- to a high-force state (Fig. 26.2, step 2). This transition is associated with a large reduction in free energy, and thus this step is generally believed to be the "power stroke" that results in force generation (167, 225). Hibberd et al. (143) observed 10 mM P_i in the presence of Ca^{2+} to increase the rate of force redevelopment; at the same time the P_i reduced the steady-state tension following the release of ATP from a caged precursor compound in single skinned rabbit psoas fibers. During the steady-state phase of contraction, P_i decreased tension more than stiffness (143, 166, 194). When Ca^{2+} was absent, Hibberd et al. (143) observed high P_i to increase the rate of final relaxation from rigor upon the release of caged ATP. Accordingly, they hypothesized that P_i release was closely associated with the power stroke and that an increased P_i concentration increased the rate constant for tension redevelopment by increasing the rate of reversal of step 2, Figure 26.2. Force declined due to a redistribution of cross-bridges from the strong to the weak binding state. The observation that high P_i did not affect rigor tension suggests that P_i had no direct effect on strong cross-bridge binding (143). A second possibility is that P_i acts to accelerate cross-bridge detachment by increasing the rate of the forward reactions 3 and 4 (Fig. 26.2). Hibberd et al. (143) suggest that this is unlikely, as ATP hydrolysis would increase markedly and, in fact, high P_i has been shown to decrease fiber ATPase activity (166).

High P_i shifts the force–pCa relationship to the right and increases the Hill coefficient or slope (n) (214). Millar and Homsher (214) found P_o, pK, and n to all vary linearly with log [P_i]. P_i had its greatest effect on tension as Ca^{2+} was reduced. This has functional importance, as the amplitude of the Ca^{2+} transient is known to be depressed in the fatigued muscle cells (6). A P_i-induced decrease in strongly bound cross-bridges would reduce thin filament activation, leading to a further decline in tension, particularly at suboptimal Ca^{2+} (214). This effect would explain the rightward shift in the force–pCa curve and also the reduced pK in the absence of a direct effect of P_i on calcium binding to troponin (194).

HIGH-ENERGY PHOSPHATES AND THE FREE ENERGY OF ATP HYDROLYSIS

ATP and Muscle Fatigue

Depletion of Cell ATP. Since ATP is the direct source of energy for the cross-bridge as well as the sarcolemma, SR, and mitochondrial ATPases, its depletion to critical levels during intense exercise could be causative in muscle fatigue. However, muscle cells possess multiple mechanisms for the production of ATP (oxidative phosphorylation, glycolysis, and the creatine kinase and adenylate kinase reactions), and consequently ATP rarely falls below 60% of its concentration prior to fatigue (results reviewed in 110). Even in conditions where force declined by more than 80%, the muscle ATP concentration remained high (114, 269). Thus, it appears that other factors reduce the ATP utilization rate before ATP becomes limiting (22, 111). The possibility exists that ATP is compartmentalized, such that ATP declines considerably more than the cell average in regions of high ATP consumption (cross-bridges of the myofibrils, SR, and S_L pump sites). However, a number of observations suggest that fatigue is not caused by the direct effect of insufficient ATP. Nassar-Gentina et al. (219) demonstrated that fatigued frog semitendinosus muscles, containing 70% of their initial ATP, could still generate considerable extra tension with activation by caffeine. Also, these muscles could further deplete more than 50% of the remaining ATP. Furthermore, when glycolysis is blocked by iodoacetate, skeletal muscle hydrolyzes up to 75% of the cell ATP (44, 92). Additionally, no correlation exists between ATP and force in frog (114), rat (270), or human (21) skeletal muscle. Also, Karlsson and Saltin (165) observed the same depletion of ATP in the first few minutes of work irrespective of whether the load was exhaustive or not. If ATP became limiting at the cross-bridge, resting muscle tension would increase as rigor bridges developed. Yet resting tension does not change in skeletal muscles fatigued in vitro, and Spriet et al. (262) found no occurrences of rigor despite one of the largest decreases in muscle ATP (average 57% with a low of 33% of resting content) concentration reported in healthy men. Additionally, even in highly fatigued fibers, ATP concentration is over 100-fold higher than the micromolar amounts required for peak force (110, 269). Thus, for compartmentalization to be a factor, more than 99% of the cell ATP would have to be unavailable to the cross-bridge.

The Free Energy of ATP Hydrolysis. The data reviewed above suggest that fatigue is unlikely to originate directly from insufficient ATP. However, an alteration in the high-energy state of the cell could contribute to fatigue by reducing the free energy of ATP hydrolysis below that required for optimal cell function (83, 244). Sahlin et al. (244) found the free energy of ATP hydrolysis to decrease from 54 kJ/mol to 50 kJ/mol, and they suggested that the actual decrease must have been considerably higher inasmuch as the value was calculated from an ATP/ADP ratio in biopsy tissue obtained 4–6 s after exercise (244). Dawson et al. (83) found no correlation between the decline in force and the reduction in free energy; however, the latter was well correlated with the prolongation of muscle relaxation. Kammermeier (163) suggested that ion transport processes, such as the SR Ca^{2+} pump, might be more susceptible to a reduced free energy of ATP hydrolysis. The free energy available in the cytoplasm (G′) is calculated by

$$G' = G^{\circ} - RT \ln [ATP]/[ADP][P_i]$$

where G° is the standard Gibbs free energy change, R is the ideal gas constant, and T is absolute temperature. In a resting muscle cell, the free energy of ATP hydrolysis is approximately 55 kJ/mol, which is approximately equal to that required for the proper operation of the SR Ca^{2+} pump (163). Consequently, even a small decline in cytosolic free energy could compromise the pump and prolong muscle relaxation time. The large increase in P_i coupled with the modest rise in ADP known to occur with fatigue could reduce the available free energy even if ATP remained constant. The sole purpose of the creatine kinase reaction is to maintain cell ATP and prevent increases in ADP. However, during intense contractile activity, PCr declines rapidly (110, 114, 195), and thus ADP might increase significantly, particularly in the ATP-utilizing regions of the cell. Saks et al. (246) suggest that a significant restriction to ADP diffusion exists and this could contribute to a reduction in cytosolic free energy. In resting cells, creatine and PCr are in high concentration relative to ADP, and their diffusion between the mitochondria and the energy-utilizing sites of the cell is apparently not restricted (246). The creatine kinase reaction serves two purposes: *(1)* to facilitate diffusion of ADP and ATP, and *(2)* to provide a high-energy store in the form of PCr to ensure that adequate ATP is maintained. This is particularly important in the first few seconds of intense contractile activity before peak activation of glycolysis occurs. Possibly the depletion in PCr with intense contractile activity slows the creatine kinase reaction and thereby increases ADP in the region of the proteins of the ATPase ion pump. Such a mechanism could explain the selective inhibition of the SR Ca^{2+} reuptake process. However, Korge et al. (169) demonstrated that small increases in ADP (from 30 μm to 100 μM) stimulated SR Ca^{2+} uptake even with PCr as low as 1 mM.

Even if the free energy of ATP hydrolysis declines with intense exercise, it apparently does not fall enough to directly alter P_o (83). The results of Godt and Nosek (123) provide a possible explanation for this apparent paradox. They employed the skinned fiber to mimic the conditions observed in fatigued cells, and observed that the decline in ATP to 1 mM actually increased P_o. Furthermore, increases in ADP and AMP also increased force, and when the affinity for ATP hydrolysis was reduced to reflect that observed in fatigued cells, they found no effect on P_o. These data suggest that any reduction in force caused by a low cytosolic free energy is compensated for by the force-enhancing effects of the elevated ADP.

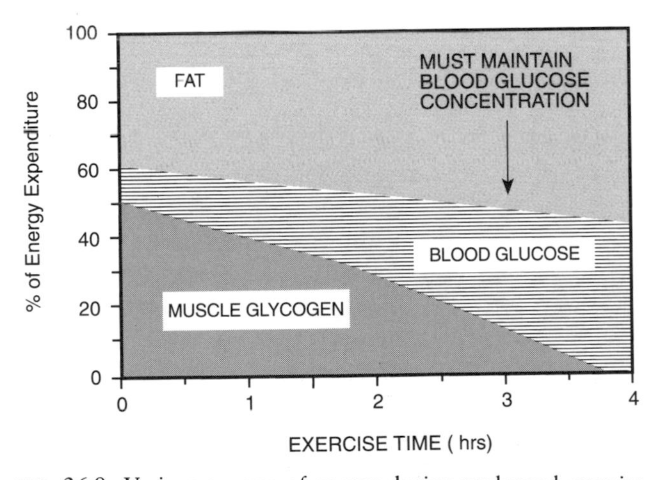

FIG. 26.9. Various sources of energy during prolonged exercise at 79% VO_{2max}. Note that blood glucose becomes the predominant source of carbohydrate energy during the latter stages of exercise and thus it is important to maintain blood glucose concentration by eating carbohydrates. [Reprinted with permission from Coyle, E. F. Carbohydrate metabolism and fatigue. In: *Muscle Fatigue: Biochemical and Physiological Aspects*, edited by G. Atlan, L. Beliveau, and P. Bouissou. Paris: Masson Pub., 1991, p. 153–164 (70).]

In addition to low pH, an increase in ADP has been shown to reduce V_o (65). Consequently, if cell ADP increased with intense exercise it could contribute to a reduced power. Additionally, De Haan and co-workers (85, 284) suggested that IMP or some compound formed in the conversion of ATP to IMP caused fatigue. Although IMP has been shown to increase with contractile activity (213, 236), to date there is no evidence that the increase induces fatigue. During the production of IMP from AMP, ammonia (NH_3) is generated and rises in both muscle and blood. The largest increase was observed in the fast-twitch muscle (212). Although NH_3 is toxic, there is no convincing evidence that it plays a role in muscle fatigue (217).

BLOOD GLUCOSE AND MUSCLE GLYCOGEN

Hypoglycemia and Performance

In the past decade, the primary attention and thus the greatest progress has been made in elucidating the causative factors of fatigue during high-intensity exercise (111). These factors (reviewed above) include alterations in E-C coupling, and disturbances in cross-bridge interaction caused by increases in H^+ and P_i. High-intensity exercise elicits fatigue within minutes, and thus depletion of stored muscle glycogen or blood glucose is not a factor. However, during prolonged exercise performed between 65% and 90% of maximal oxygen uptake (VO_{2max}), hypoglycemia and muscle glycogen depletion can occur (2, 3, 19, 20, 70). In fact, muscle fatigue during prolonged exercise is highly correlated with muscle glycogen depletion (2, 19, 20, 141, 248), and in some cases with hypoglycemia (3, 70). During the early minutes of prolonged exercise, carbohydrates contribute approximately 60% of the total energy output, with muscle glycogen providing more than 80% of this total (Fig. 26.9). Later, as muscle glycogen becomes depleted, blood glucose metabolism becomes more important in providing energy (Fig. 26.9). Without oral glucose intake during the exercise, hypoglycemia ensues and causes premature fatigue due to the deleterious effects of low blood glucose on the central nervous system (3, 70). If exercise occurs in a hot environment, the resulting dehydration can reduce blood volume to a point where blood flow to the muscles and other vital organs falls. The importance of ingesting a water/carbohydrate drink throughout the exercise period has been recognized since the early part of this century. In the 1930s, Dill et al. (88) and Christensen and Hansen (59) demonstrated the importance of carbohydrate supplementation during exercise. The latter group, who studied human subjects, found glucose feedings during exercise to prevent hypoglycemia and improve performance. However, they observed only a small increase in the respiratory quotient (RQ), which suggested to them that the main beneficial effect was the prevention of low blood glucose and the symptoms of neuroglucopenia.

The major metabolic changes associated with prolonged exercise are shown in Figure 26.10. As muscle glycogen is depleted, the uptake and utilization of blood glucose by the muscle cell become increasingly important. Without oral intake of glucose, this process is compromised by the depletion of liver glycogen and the corresponding decline in splanchnic glucose production. Coyle and colleagues (63, 71, 72) conducted a series of studies to evaluate the importance of maintaining blood glucose in endurance exercise. They compared subjects drinking a placebo (noncarbohydrate) to those ingesting a carbohydrate drink. The placebo group developed hypoglycemia and a reduced carbohydrate oxidation rate; exercise stopped after 3 h. In contrast, the carbohydrate-ingesting group maintained their blood glucose concentration and their carbohydrate oxidation rate, and they continued to exercise for an additional hour (70, 71). In agreement with earlier observations (2, 20), the glucose ingestion had no effect on the rate of muscle glycogen depletion. The additional hour of exercise occurred with little further decline in muscle glycogen—apparently the carbohydrate metabolism was maintained almost entirely by the oxidation of blood glucose. Thus, those who did not receive oral glucose developed fatigue as a consequence of hypoglycemia (blood glucose declined from 4.5 mM to 2.5–3 mM) and the decline in carbohydrate oxidation. The reason for fatigue in the carbohydrate-fed group was a mystery, as plasma glucose and the carbohydrate oxidation rate remained unchanged throughout exercise.

Carbohydrate Metabolism and Muscle Fatigue

The general consensus is that a certain level of carbohydrate metabolism is required for the mainte-

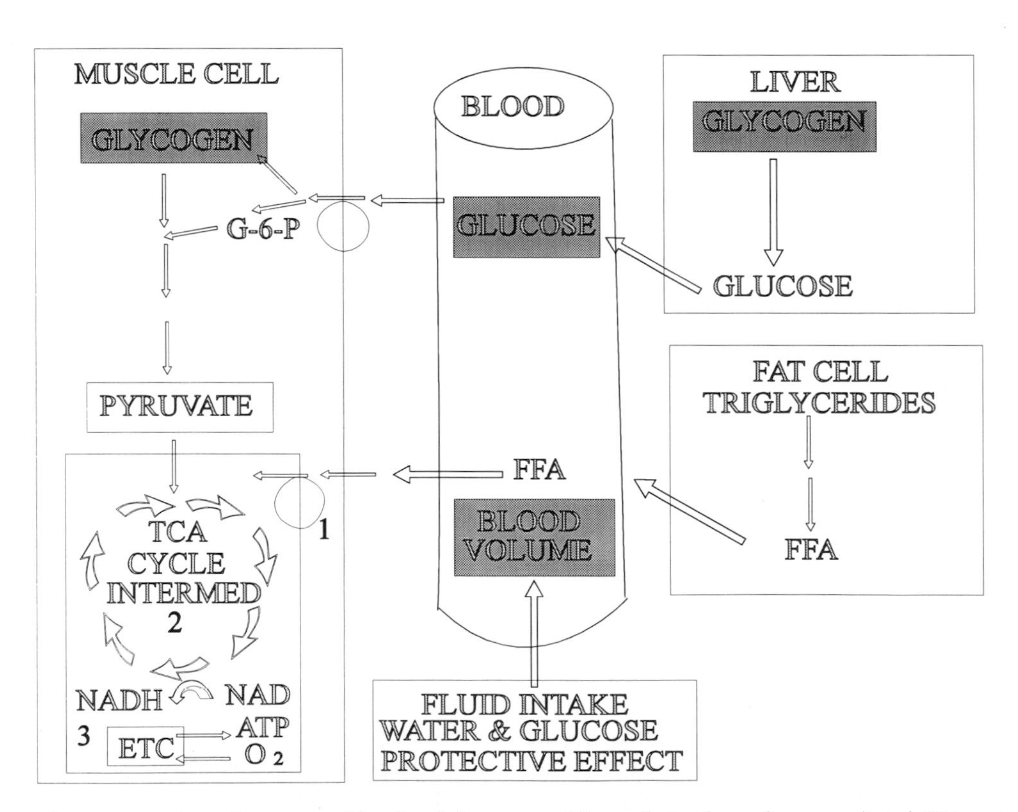

FIG. 26.10. Schematic representation of important blood and tissue changes with prolonged exercise. The *shaded boxes* indicate substances known to decline during prolonged exercise. Depletion of muscle glycogen, dehydration, and hypoglycemia have all been linked to fatigue in prolonged exercise. Sites 1–3 represent carnitine palmitoyltransferase-mediated FFA uptake into mitochondria, concentrations of tricarboxylic acid cycle intermediates, and the production rate of NADH, respectively. Disturbances in all three sites have been linked to fatigue during endurance exercise (see text).

nance of prolonged exercise at moderate to high intensities, and that glucose ingestion protects against fatigue by maintaining carbohydrate metabolism above the critical level (70). Currently, there is no cellular explanation for this apparent obligatory oxidation of carbohydrates. The possibilities include: (*1*) high muscle oxidation rates cannot be maintained without a carbohydrate fuel source; (*2*) carbohydrates supply critical metabolic intermediates such that carbohydrate depletion reduces the oxidation rate of available fats and proteins; or (*3*) carbohydrate oxidation is not obligatory, but rather carbohydrate depletion is correlated with (and perhaps causative of) changes in other cellular events that in turn elicit fatigue. At present, however, the only undisputed point is that muscle glycogen depletion (coupled with a declining blood glucose) is highly correlated with fatigue in endurance exercise (2, 19, 20,70, 141). Additionally, factors that reduce the rate of glycogen depletion delay the onset of fatigue. For example, endurance exercise training increases the oxidation of free fatty acids (FFA), reduces liver and muscle glycogen utilization, and delays the onset of fatigue (112, 248).

Figure 26.10 (*#1–3*) shows a few possibilities that may link a reduced carbohydrate oxidation with fatigue. With the decline in carbohydrates, the contracting muscle cell must depend more on FFA oxidation. This involves an increased FFA uptake and transport into the mitochondria for subsequent β oxidation. The mitochondrial transport process requires the enzyme carnitine acyltransferase I (CAT I), and this step is thought to limit the rate at which active muscle can oxidize FFA. Possibly, this process fails to keep up with the increased demand for fat oxidation in the latter stages of prolonged exercise (Fig. 26.10, *#1*). If this were to occur, one would expect tissue ATP levels, cell respiration, and whole-body $\dot{V}O_2$ to decline. At the end of prolonged exercise, work rate generally declines before exhaustion is complete. Consequently, it is difficult to assess whether a decline in whole-body $\dot{V}O_2$ results from insufficient substrate supply (inability to transport FFA across mitochondrial membrane) or fatigue caused by other factors. The observation that carnitine administration delayed fatigue in the isolated soleus muscle supports the hypothesis that fatigue results from an inhibitory process at the FFA transport step (36). However, carnitine administration did not alter the rate of glycogen depletion either in the isolated contracting soleus or in the intact exercising human (36, 273). Nevertheless, the carnitine effect may not be important until the onset of glycogen depletion and the obligatory increase in FFA oxidation. A second possibility is that a certain rate of carbohydrate oxidation is required to maintain either the optimal production of NADH and electron transport (Fig. 26.10, *#3*) or optimal concentration of tricarboxylic acid cycle (TCA) intermediates (Fig. 26.10, *#2*). Some evidence supports this latter possibility (243, 259). Sahlin et al. (243) found TCA intermediates to decline during cycle exercise to fatigue, and Spencer et al. (259) reported that carbohydrate feedings reduced the fall in TCA intermediates.

An important question is whether any particular fiber type is especially susceptible to the fatigue-inducing effects of glycogen depletion. The answer is that the rate of glycogen depletion in a muscle or fiber depends directly on the degree of recruitment. Consequently, prolonged running on a level terrain depletes muscle glycogen in calf muscles more than in the quadriceps, whereas bicycle exercise depletes mainly quadriceps muscle glycogen (69, 105). During prolonged exercise of moderate intensity, the first fibers recruited (the slow type I and fast type IIa) show selective glycogen depletion (68, 125, 128, 131). In contrast, the fast type IIb fibers show a delayed onset of glycogen depletion, which reflects the recruitment of this fiber type late in the exercise when the type I and IIa fibers fatigue (125, 128). On the other hand, during high-intensity exercise all fiber types are recruited, and the fast type IIb fibers with the highest glycolytic and lowest oxidative capacity have the fastest rate of glycogen utilization (126). However, as stated earlier, fatigue in this type of exercise occurs within minutes and long before glycogen depletion begins. Nevertheless, glycogen depletion could contribute to fatigue during repeated, short bouts of high-intensity exercise. In this case, fatigue during the final bout of exercise could involve glycogen depletion in the fast type IIb fibers, but the earlier bouts would have to be explained by other factors (11, 58).

Although hypoglycemia, muscle glycogen depletion, and a reduced carbohydrate oxidation are frequently correlated with fatigue during prolonged exercise, it seems unlikely that these factors are exclusively involved in the fatigue process. In the experiments of Coyle and colleagues (63, 70), the carbohydrate supplement delayed but did not prevent fatigue, despite a maintained blood glucose concentration and carbohydrate oxidation rate. Possibly, muscle glycogen depletion is causative in fatigue via mechanisms independent of its role in energy production. For example, a certain content of cell glycogen may be important for the integrity of various cell organelle, such as the SR or lysosomal membranes. Alternatively, the correlation between muscle glycogen and fatigue may in some instances be coincidental. In such cases, fatigue may result from independent deleterious changes in the structure of important cell organelle.

ULTRASTRUCTURAL CHANGES AND MUSCLE FATIGUE

Muscle Damage and Exercise Intensity

Exercise can clearly induce structural damage in the myofibrils, mitochondria, and SR (8, 127, 129, 133). Furthermore, the likelihood of such damage increases with exercise involving a high component of eccentric contraction (9, 199). Two important questions are whether the tissue damage occurs during the exercise or afterwards, and whether a particular fiber type is selectively affected. If the damage occurs during the exercise, it would be likely to contribute to the loss of peak force and power and to the development of muscle fatigue. Recently, numerous reviews, have focused on the relationship between muscle injury and performance (8, 60), and the relationship between fatigue and injury has been discussed in detail (111). It is clear from the published literature that injury can occur during exercise, and can result from high-intensity short-duration as well as prolonged work (7, 118, 180, 196, 199). Muscle fiber injury is restricted to the recruited fibers, and occurs more readily during eccentric contractions. The degree of injury appears to be related to the force or strain developed, so that during high-intensity exercise it occurs early in the exercise period when these factors are greatest (180, 199). It is generally thought that the damage is a direct result of mechanical disruption of the sarcomeres and in some cases the sarcolemma membrane (118, 180, 196, 199). Subsequent to the cell membrane disruption, Ca^{2+} influx would increase and activate cell proteases and phospholipases. These changes in turn would contribute further to the disruption of the cell and compromise its mechanical function (8, 158). Prolonged endurance exercise is less likely to directly disrupt the surface membrane, and damage from this type of exercise likely develops late in the exercise period. One possibility is that prolonged exercise leads to inhibition of the SR pump, and thus to an increased cytosolic Ca^{2+} (48, 113). Again, this type of exercise is associated with glycogen depletion, but it is not known whether the disruption in the function of SR or other organelle is somehow linked to the depletion of glycogen or occurs via a totally independent mechanism. During endurance exercise, slow fibers are preferentially recruited and thus show the highest degree of damage (7). However, during high-intensity exercise, despite the fact that all fibers types are recruited, the fast-twitch fibers show preferential damage (119, 180). This likely results from the fact that fast fibers are generally larger, with higher peak forces and thus susceptibility to mechanical damage.

Organelle Susceptibility to Damage

The structures most susceptible to damage appear to be membrane systems, such as mitochondria, and the SR. Although ultrastructural damage occurs to myofibrils following exercise with a high eccentric component, the damage is generally confined to fewer than 10% of the fibers (7, 16, 118). Although alterations in cross-bridge function definitely contribute to fatigue during high-intensity exercise, these changes are thought to be mediated by alterations in H^+ and P_i (reviewed above) and not primarily by structural damage.

The question of whether mitochondrial damage contributes to fatigue is controversial. Gollnick and King (129) and Dohm and co-workers (89, 90) reported structural alterations in mitochondria and a reduced oxidative capacity in rat muscle after prolonged endurance exercise. Furthermore, the mitochondrial yield obtained from the gastrocnemius and quadriceps was reduced (89, 90). These structural alterations were confirmed by others (200, 221). Gollnick et al. (129) also reported a reduced mitochondrial respiratory capacity following high-intensity exercise. In contrast, Terjung et al. (265) and Gale (120) observed no structural change in mitochondria following endurance exercise, and the former also found no change in mitochondrial respiration.

Vacuoles have been reputed to arise from swollen T-tubules in fatigued frog fibers (133), and swollen SR with altered functional properties have also been reported following exhaustive endurance exercise (16, 17, 48, 200). SR vesicles isolated from rat slow and fast twitch red muscle following a prolonged swim showed normal ATPase activity, but a reduced Ca^{2+} uptake (113). In this study, and in a more recent report by Byrd et al. (48), the SR isolated from fast white muscle was unaltered by exhaustive endurance exercise. High-intensity exercise has also been shown to inhibit SR Ca^{2+} uptake in horses and humans (49, 130). These results suggest that both high-intensity and prolonged endurance exercise can induce a reduced SR pump capacity, and it is reasonable to conclude that this direct effect on the SR membrane contributes to the prolonged relaxation observed in fatigued muscle.

SUMMARY AND CONCLUSIONS

The etiology of muscle fatigue is complex in that it involves multiple elements acting at multiple sites within the contracting muscle. The causative factors appear to act primarily within the muscle, and do not for the most part involve the central nervous system or the N-M junction. The nature, speed of onset, and extent of fatigue are all dependent on the fiber type, exercise intensity, and general fitness level of the exercising individual. The slow-twitch oxidative fibers show the highest resistance to fatigue, followed by the oxidative fast red (type IIa), fast type IIx, and the least resistant fast-twitch white (type IIb) fiber. Additionally, the causative events in high-intensity exercise are clearly different from those eliciting fatigue in prolonged work. Despite this, both high-intensity short-duration and prolonged exercise induce somewhat similar alteration in the mechanical properties of the muscle cell. These include a reduction in peak force, velocity, and power, with the force change occurring earlier and to a greater extent than the velocity change. Additionally, the peak rate of force development (dP/dt) is depressed and the relaxation time prolonged in fatigued muscle. During high-intensity exercise, these changes can primarily be attributed to disturbances in E-C coupling and/or metabolic disturbances that directly inhibit the cross-bridge. The alterations in E-C coupling may involve depolarization of the surface and T-tubular membrane, failure of the action potential to propagate into the depths of the T-tubule, inactivation of the T-tubular charge sensor, disturbances in the linking mechanism between the T-tubular membrane DHPr and the SR Ca^{2+} release channel, or direct inhibition of the release channel. In some cases, a metabolic disturbance may inhibit both E-C coupling and the cross-bridge. An example is the increase in intracellular H^+. Figure 26.8 shows the multiplicity of factors by which an increased H^+ might elicit fatigue. The most important factors likely involve the inhibitory effects of H^+ on the SR Ca^{2+} release channel, and the cross-bridge transition from the low- to the high-force state. This latter process is also inhibited by P_i, which is known to increase during high-intensity exercise.

Fatigue in single muscle fibers has been characterized by three phases (Fig. 26.4). In the initial phase, force shows a rapid drop with little change in V_o. This has been attributed to a rapid rise in P_i with the onset of contraction and the increased ATP turnover. The second phase shows a slow, rather modest decline in P_o as well as the initial decline in V_o. During this phase, H^+ has risen to a level that contributes to the depression of force and velocity, while the small increase in ADP contributes to the reduced V_o. Since ADP is known to increase force, it may in part explain the rather slow decline in tension during this phase. Finally, during the last phase SR Ca^{2+} release is inhibited; this could be caused by direct effects of H^+ on the SR Ca^{2+} release channel or by disturbances in E-C coupling preceding the activation of the release channel. In whole-muscle preparations, force shows a more rapid drop during the middle phase of fatigue. This effect could be due to an earlier inhibition of SR Ca^{2+} release. For example, in whole muscles contracting in vitro or in vivo, the buildup in extracellular K^+ would likely be larger, which would lead to a greater T-tubular membrane depolarization. Thus, in these situations, the cell would be more susceptible to depolarization block of the action potential or inactivation of the DHPr.

Fatigue during prolonged endurance exercise is less understood. A high correlation has been observed between the depletion of muscle glycogen and fatigue in this type of work, but this is unlikely to be the sole contributing factor. In certain situations, dehydration and/or hypoglycemia develop and these factors are known to exacerbate fatigue. A certain level of carbohydrate metabolism appears necessary to prevent fatigue, but the mechanism of this requirement is unknown.

Although considerable progress has been made in understanding the etiology of skeletal muscle fatigue, a number of important questions remain unanswered. For example, it will be important to determine why carbohydrate metabolism appears to be obligatory to the maintenance of prolonged exercise, and to establish the cellular mechanisms of the observed alterations in E-C coupling.

REFERENCES

1. Adams, G. R., M. J. Fisher, and R. A. Meyer. Hypercapnic acidosis and increased $H_2PO_4^-$ concentration do not decrease force in cat skeletal muscle. *Am. J. Physiol.* 260 (*Cell Physiol.* 29): C805–C812, 1991.
2. Ahlborg, B., J. Bergström, L-G. Ekelund, and E. Hultman. Muscle glycogen and muscle electrolytes during prolonged physical exercise. *Acta Physiol. Scand.* 70: 129–142, 1967.
3. Ahlborg, G., P. Felig, L. Hagenfeldt, R. Hendler, and J. Wahren. Substrate turnover during prolonged exercise in man: splanchnic and leg metabolism of glucose, free fatty acids, and amino acids. *J. Clin. Invest.* 53: 1080–1090, 1974.
4. Aljure, E. F., and L. M. Borrero. The evolution of fatigue associated with isometric contraction in toad sartorius. *J. Physiol. (Lond.)* 194: 289–303, 1968.
5. Aljure, E. F., and L. M. Borrero. The influence of muscle length on the development of fatigue in toad sartorius. *J. Physiol. (Lond.)* 199: 241–252, 1968.

6. Allen, D. G., J. A. Lee, and H. Westerblad. Intracellular calcium and tension during fatigue in isolated single muscle fibers from *Xenopus laevis*. *J. Physiol. (Lond.)* 415: 433–458, 1989.
7. Armstrong, R. B., R. W. Ogilvie, and J. A. Schwane. Eccentric exercise-induced injury to rat skeletal muscle. *J. Appl. Physiol.* 54: 80–93, 1983.
8. Armstrong, R. B., G. L. Warren, and J. A. Warren. Mechanisms of exercise-induced muscle fiber injury. *Sports Med.* 12: 184–207, 1991.
9. Asmussen, E. Observations on experimental muscular soreness. *Acta Rheum. Scand.* 2: 109–116, 1956.
10. Asmussen, E. Muscle fatigue. *Med. Sci. Sports Exerc.* 11: 313–321, 1979.
11. Åstrand, P.-O., E. Hultman, A. Juhlin-Danfelt, and G. Reynolds. Disposal of lactate during and after strenous exercise in humans. *J. Appl. Physiol.* 61: 338–343, 1986.
12. Balog, E. M., L. V. Thompson, and R. H. Fitts. Role of sarcolemma action potentials and excitability in muscle fatigue. *J. Appl. Physiol.* 76: 2157–2162, 1994.
13. Bangsbo, J., P. D. Gollnick, T. E. Graham, C. Juel, B. Kiens, M. Mizuno, and B. Saltin. Anaerobic energy production and O_2 deficit-debt relationship during exhaustive exercise in humans. *J. Physiol. (Lond.)* 422: 539–559, 1990.
14. Bárány, M. ATPase activity of myosin correlated with speed of muscle shortening. *J. Gen. Physiol.* 50: 197–218, 1967.
15. Beam, G., and C. M. Knudson. Calcium currents in embryonic and neonatal mammalian skeletal muscle. *J. Gen. Physiol.* 91: 781–798, 1991.
16. Belcastro, A. N., W. Parkhouse, G. Dobson, and J. S. Gilchrist. Influence of exercise on cardiac and skeletal muscle myofibrillar proteins. *Mol. Cell. Biochem.* 83: 27–36, 1988.
17. Belcastro, A. N., M. Rossiter, M. P. Low, and M. M. Sopper. Calcium activation of sarcoplasmic reticulum ATPase following strenuous activity. *Can. J. Physiol. Pharmacol.* 59: 1214–1218, 1981.
18. Benzanilla, F., C. Caputo, H. González-Serratos, and R. A. Venosa. Sodium dependence of the inward spread of activation in isolated twitch muscle fibers of the frog. *J. Physiol. (Lond.)* 223: 507–523, 1972.
19. Bergström, J., L. Hermansen, E. Hultman, and B. Saltin. Diet, muscle glycogen and physical performance. *Acta Physiol. Scand.* 71: 140–150, 1967.
20. Bergström, J., and E. Hultman. A study of the glycogen metabolism during exercise in man. *Scand. J. Clin. Lab. Invest.* 19: 218–228, 1967.
21. Bergström, J., and E. Hultman. Energy cost and fatigue during intermittent electrical stimulation of human skeletal muscle. *J. Appl. Physiol.* 65: 1500–1505, 1988.
22. Bergström, M., and E. Hultman. Relaxation and force during fatigue and recovery of the human quadriceps muscle: relations to metabolite changes. *Pflugers Arch.* 418: 153–160, 1991.
23. Berquin, A., and J. Lebacq. Parvalbumin, labile heat and slowing of relaxation in mouse soleus and extensor digitorum longus muscles. *J. Physiol. (Lond.)* 445: 601–616, 1992.
24. Bianchi, C. P., and S. Narayan. Muscle fatigue and the role of transverse tubules. *Science* 215: 295–296, 1982.
25. Bianchi, C. P., and S. Narayan. Possible role of the transverse tubules in accumulating calcium released from the terminal cisternae by stimulation and drugs. *Can. J. Physiol. Pharmacol.* 60: 503–507, 1982.
26. Bigland-Ritchie, B. Muscle fatigue and the influence of changing neural drive. *Clin. Chest Med.* 5: 21–34, 1984.
27. Bigland-Ritchie, B., F. Bellemare, and J. J. Woods. Excitation frequencies and sites of fatigue. In: *Human Muscle Power*, edited by N. L. Jones, N. McCarney, and A. J. McComas. Champaign, IL: Human Kinetics Publishers, Inc., 1986, p. 197–214.
28. Bigland-Ritchie, B., N. J. Dawson, R. S. Johansson, and O. C. J. Lippold. Relflex origin for the slowing of motoneuron firing rates in fatigue of human voluntary contractions. *J. Physiol. (Lond.)* 379: 451–459, 1986.
29. Bigland-Ritchie, B., F. Furbush, and J. J. Woods. Fatigue of intermittent submaximal voluntary contractions: central and peripheral factors. *J. Appl. Physiol.* 61: 421–429, 1986.
30. Bigland-Ritchie, B., D. A. Jones, and J. J. Woods. Excitation frequency and muscle fatigue: electrical responses during human voluntary and stimulated contractions. *Exp. Neurol.* 64: 414–427, 1979.
31. Binder-Macleod, S. A., and L. R. McDermond. Changes in the force frequency relationship of the human quardriceps femoris muscle following electrically and voluntarily induced fatigue. *Phys. Ther.* 72: 95–104, 1992.
32. Blanchard, E. M., B.-S. Pan, and R. J. Solaro. The effect of acidic pH on the ATPase activity and troponin Ca^{2+} binding of rabbit skeletal myofilaments. *J. Biol. Chem.* 259: 3181–3186, 1984.
33. Blinks, J. R., R. Rüdel, and S. R. Taylor. Calcium transients in isolated amphibian skeletal muscle fibers: detection with aequorin. *J. Physiol. (Lond.)* 277: 291–323, 1978.
34. Borg, J., L. Grimby, and J. Hannerz. The fatigue of voluntary contraction and the peripheral electrical propagation of single motor units in man. *J. Physiol. (Lond.)* 340: 435–444, 1983.
35. Bottinelli, R., S. Schiaffino, and C. Reggiani. Force-velocity relations and myosin heavy chain isoform compositions of skinned fibers from rat skeletal muscle. *J. Physiol. (Lond.)* 437: 655–672, 1991.
36. Brass, E. P., A. M. Scarrow, L. J. Ruff, K. A. Masterson, and E. V. Lunteren. Carnitine delays rat skeletal muscle fatigue *in vivo*. *J. Appl. Physiol.* 75: 1595–1600, 1993.
37. Bremel, R. D., and A. Weber. Cooperation within actin filament in vertebrate skeletal muscle. *Nat. New Biol.* 238: 97–101, 1972.
38. Brenner, B. Mechanical and structural approaches to correlation of cross-bridge action in muscle with actomyosin ATPase in solution. *Ann. Rev. Physiol.* 49: 655–672, 1987.
39. Brenner, B. Effect of Ca^{2+} on cross-bridge turnover kinetics in skinned single psoas fibers: implication for regulation of muscle contraction. *Proc. Natl. Acad. Sci. U. S. A.* 85: 3265–3269, 1988.
40. Brooke, M. H., and K. K. Kaiser. Muscle fiber types: how many and what kind? *Arch. Neurol.* 23: 369–379, 1970.
41. Brown, G. L., and B. D. Burns. Fatigue and meuromuscular block in mammalian skeletal muscle. *Proc. R. Soc. B.* 136: 182–195, 1949.
42. Brum, G., R. Fitts, G. Pizarro, and E. Rios. Voltage sensors of the frog skeletal muscle membrane require calcium to function in excitation-contraction coupling. *J. Physiol. (Lond.)* 398: 475–505, 1988.
43. Brum, G., E. Rios, and E. Stefani. Effects of extracellular calcium on calcium movements of excitation-contraction coupling in frog skeletal muscle fibers. *J. Physiol. (Lond.)* 398: 441–473, 1988.
44. Brumback, R. A., J. W. Gerst, and H. R. Knull. High energy phosphate depletion in a model of defective muscle glycolysis. *Muscle Nerve* 6: 52–55, 1983.

45. Burke, R. E., D. N. Levine, P. Tsairis, and F. E. Zajac, III. Physiological types and histochemical profiles in motor units of the cat gastrocnemius. *J. Physiol (Lond.)*. 234: 723–748, 1973.
46. Burke, R. E., and P. Tsairis. Anatomy and innervation ratios in motor units of cat gastrocnemius. *J. Physiol. (Lond.)* 234: 749–765, 1973.
47. Byrd, S. K. Alterations in the sarcoplasmic reticulum: a possible link to exercise-induced muscle damage. *Med. Sci. Sports Exerc.* 24: 531–536, 1992.
48. Byrd, S. K., A. K. Bode, and G. A. Klug. Effects of exercise of varying duration on sarcoplasmic reticulum function. *J. Appl. Physiol.* 66: 1383–1389, 1989.
49. Byrd, S. K., L. J. McCutcheon, D. R. Hodgson, and P. D. Gollnick. Altered sarcoplasmic reticulum function after high-intensity exercise. *J. Appl. Physiol.* 67: 2072–2077, 1989.
50. Byström, S., and G. Sjøgaard. Potassium homeostasis during and following exhaustive submaximal static handgrip contractions. *Acta Physiol. Scand.* 142: 59–66, 1991.
51. Cady, E. B., H. Elshove, D. A. Jones, and A. Moll. The metabolic causes of slow relaxation in fatigued human skeletal muscle. *J. Physiol. (Lond.)* 418: 327–337, 1989.
52. Cady, E. B., D. A. Jones, J. Lynn, and D. J. Newham. Changes in force and intracellular metabolites during fatigue of human skeletal muscle. *J. Physiol. (Lond.)* 418: 311–325, 1989.
53. Cannell, M. B. Effect of tetanus duration on the free calcium during the relaxation of frog skeletal muscle fibers. *J. Physiol. (Lond.)* 376: 203–218, 1986.
54. Caputo, C., P. Bolaños, and G. F. González. Effect of membrane polarization on contractile threshold and time course of prolonged contractile responses in skeletal muscle fibers. *J. Gen. Physiol.* 84: 927–943, 1984.
55. Castle, N. A., and D. G. Haylett. Effect of channel blockers on potassium efflux from metabolically exhausted frog skeletal muscle. *J. Physiol. (Lond.)* 383: 31–43, 1987.
56. Chase, P. B., and M. J. Kushmerick. Effects of pH on contraction of rabbit fast and slow skeletal muscle fibers. *Biophys. J.* 53: 935–946, 1988.
57. Chasiotis, D., K. Sahlin, and E. Hultman. Regulation of glycogenolysis in human muscle at rest and during exercise. *J. Appl. Physiol.* 53: 708–715, 1982.
58. Cheetham, M. E., L. H. Boobis, S. Brooks, and C. Williams. Human muscle metabolism during sprint running. *J. Appl. Physiol.* 61: 54–60, 1986.
59. Christensen, E. H., and O. Hansen. Hypoglykamie, arbeitsfahigkeit and Ermudung. *Scand. Arch. Physiol.* 81: 172–179, 1939.
60. Clarkson, P. M., K. Nosaka, and B. Braun. Muscle function after exercise-induced muscle damage and rapid adaptation. *Med. Sci. Sports Exerc.* 24: 512–520, 1992.
61. Clausen, T., and M. E. Everts. Regulation of the Na, K-pump in skeletal muscle. *Kidney Int.* 35: 1–13, 1989.
62. Close, R. I. Dynamic properties of mammalian skeletal muscles. *Physiol. Rev.* 52: 129–197, 1972.
63. Coggan, A. R., and E. F. Coyle. Reversal of fatigue during prolonged exercise by carbohydrate infusion or ingestion. *J. Appl. Physiol.* 63: 2388–2395, 1987.
64. Cooke, R., K. Franks, G. B. Luciani, and E. Pate. The inhibition of rabbit skeletal muscle contraction by hydrogen ions and phosphate. *J. Physiol. (Lond.)* 395: 77–97, 1988.
65. Cooke, R., and E. Pate. The effects of ADP and phosphate on the contraction of muscle fiber. *Biophys. J.* 48: 789–798, 1985.
66. Cooke, R., and E. Pate. Addition of phosphate to active muscle fibers probes actomyosin states within the powerstroke. *Pflugers Arch.* 414: 73–81, 1989.
67. Cooper, R. G., R. H. T. Edwards, H. Gibson, and M. J. Stokes. Human muscle fatigue: frequency dependence of excitation and force generation. *J. Physiol. (Lond.)* 397: 585–599, 1988.
68. Costill, D. L., P. D. Gollnick, E. D. Jansson, B. Saltin, and R. B. Stein. Glycogen depletion pattern in human muscle fibers during distance running. *Acta Physiol. Scand.* 89: 374–383, 1973.
69. Costill, D. L., E. Jansson, P. D. Gollnick, and B. Saltin. Glycogen utilization in the leg muscles of men during level and uphill running. *Acta Physiol. Scand.* 94: 475–481, 1974.
70. Coyle, E. F. Carbohydrate metabolism and fatigue. In: *Muscle Fatigue: Biochemical and Physiological Aspects*, edited by G. Atlan, L. Beliveau, and P. Bouissou. Paris: Masson, 1991, p. 153–164.
71. Coyle, E. F., A. R. Coggan, M. K. Hemmert, and J. L. Ivy. Muscle glycogen utilization during prolonged strenuous exercise when fed carbohydrate. *J. Appl. Physiol.* 61: 165–172, 1986.
72. Coyle, E. F., J. M. Hagberg, B. F. Hurley, W. H. Martin, A. A. Ehsani, and J. O. Holloszy. Carbohydrate feedings during prolonged strenuous exercise can delay fatigue. *J. Appl. Physiol.* 55: 230–235, 1983.
73. Creese, R., S. E. E. Hashish, and N. W. Scholes. Potassium movements in contracting diaphragm muscle. *J. Physiol. (Lond.)* 143: 307–324, 1958.
74. Crow, M. T., and M. J. Kushmerick. Chemical energetics of slow- and fast-twitch muscles of the mouse. *J. Gen. Physiol.* 79: 147–166, 1982.
75. Cummins, M. E., R. S. Soomal, and N. A. Curtin. Fatigue of isolated mouse muscle due to isometric tetani and tetani with high power output. *Q. J. Exp. Physiol.* 74: 951–953, 1989.
76. Curtin, N. A. Intracellular pH and relaxation of frog muscle. *Adv. Exp. Med. Biol.* 226: 657–669, 1988.
77. Curtin, N. A., and K. A. P. Edman. Effects of fatigue and reduced intracellular pH on segment dynamics in isometric relaxation of frog muscle fibers. *J. Physiol. (Lond.)* 413: 159–174, 1989.
78. Davies, C. T. M., and M. J. White. Muscle weakness following eccentric work in man. *Pflugers Arch.* 392: 168–171, 1981.
79. Davies, N. W., N. B. Standen, and P. R. Stanfield. The effect of intracellular pH on ATP-dependent potassium channels of frog skeletal muscle. *J. Physiol. (Lond.)* 445: 549–568, 1992.
80. Dawson, M. J. The relation between muscle contraction and metabolism: studies by ^{31}P nuclear magnetic resonance spectroscopy. *Adv. Exp. Med. Biol.* 226: 433–448, 1988.
81. Dawson, M. J., D. G. Gadian, and D. R. Wilkie. Contraction and recovery of living muscles studied by ^{31}P nuclear magnetic resonance. *J. Physiol. (Lond.)* 267: 703–735, 1977.
82. Dawson, M. J., D. G. Gadian, and D. R. Wilkie. Muscular fatigue investigated by phosphorus nuclear magnetic resonance. *Nature* 274: 861–866, 1978.
83. Dawson, M. J., D. G. Gadian, and D. R. Wilkie. Mechanical relaxation rate and metabolism studied in fatiguing muscle by phosphorus nuclear magnetic resonance. *J. Physiol. (Lond.)* 299: 465–484, 1980.
84. Dawson, M. J., S. Smith, and D. R. Wilkie. The [$H_2PO_4^{-1}$]

may determine cross-bridge cycling rate and force production in living fatiguing muscle. *Biophys. J.* 49: 268a, 1986.
85. De Haan, A. High-energy phosphates and fatigue during repeated dynamic contractions of rat muscle. *Exp. Physiol.* 75: 851–854, 1990.
86. De Haan, A., M. A. N. Lodder, and A. J. Sargeant. Age-related effects of fatigue and recovery from fatigue in rat medial gastrocnemius muscle. *Q. J. Exp. Physiol.* 74:715–726, 1989.
87. De Luca, C. J., R. S. Lefever, M. P. McCue, and P. Xenakis. Behavior of human motor units in different muscles during linearly varying contractions. *J. Physiol. (Lond.)* 329: 113–128, 1982.
88. Dill, D. B., R. G. Edwards, and J. H. Talbott. Factors limiting the capacity for work. *J. Physiol. (Lond.)* 77: 49–62, 1932.
89. Dohm, G. L., H. Barakat, T. P. Stephenson, S. N. Pennington, and E. B. Tapscott. Changes in muscle mitochondrial lipid composition resulting from training and exhaustive exercise. *Life Sci.* 17: 1075–1080, 1975.
90. Dohm, G. L., R. L. Huston, E. W. Askew, and P. C. Weiser. Effects of exercise on activity of heart and muscle mitochondria. *Am. J. Physiol.* 223: 783–787, 1972.
91. Donaldson, S. K., and L. Hermansen. Differential, direct effects of H^+ and Ca^{2+}-activated force of skinned fibers from the soleus, cardiac and adductor magnus muscle of rabbits. *Pflugers Arch.* 376: 55–65, 1978.
92. Dudley, G. A., and R. L. Terjung. Influence of aerobic metabolism on IMP accumulation in fast-twitch muscle. *Am. J. Physiol.* 248 (*Cell Physiol.* 17): C37–C42, 1985.
93. Dulhunty, A. F. Effects of membrane potentials on mechanical activation in skeletal muscle. *J. Gen. Physiol.* 79:233–251, 1983.
94. Eberstein, A., and A. Sandow. Fatigue in phasic and tonic fibers of frog muscle. *Science* 134: 383–384, 1961.
95. Eberstein, A., and A. Sandow. Fatigue mechanisms in muscle fibers. In: *The Effect of Use and Disuse of Neuromuscular Function*, edited by E. Gutmann, and P. Hnik. Prague: Czechoslovak Acad. Sci., 1963, p. 515–526.
96. Edman, K. A. P. The velocity of unloaded shortening and its relation to sarcomere length and isometric force in vertebrate muscle fibers. *J. Physiol. (Lond.)* 291: 143–159, 1979.
97. Edman, K. A. P., and F. Lou. Changes in force and stiffness induced by fatigue and intracellular acidification in frog muscle fibers. *J. Physiol. (Lond.)* 424: 133–149, 1990.
98. Edman, K. A. P., and A. R. Mattiazzi. Effects of fatigue and altered pH on isometric force and velocity of shortening at zero load in frog muscle fibers. *J. Muscle Res. Cell Motil.* 2: 321–334, 1981.
99. Edwards, R. G., D. K. Hill, and D. A. Jones. Fatigue of long duration in human skeletal muscle after exercise. *J. Physiol. (Lond.)* 272: 769–778, 1977.
100. Edwards, R. H. T. Human muscle function and fatigue. In: *Ciba Foundation Symposium 82: Human Muscle Fatigue: Physiological Mechanisms*, edited by R. Porter. and J. Whelan. London: Pitman Medical, 1981, p. 1–18.
101. Edwards, R. H. T. Biochemical bases of fatigue in exercise performance: catastrophe theory of muscular fatigue. In: *Biochemistry of Exercise*, edited by H. G. Knuttgen. Champaign, IL: Human Kinetics, 1983, p. 3–28.
102. Edwards, R. H. T., R. C. Harris, E. Hultman, L. Kaijser, D. Hoh, and L.-O. Nordesjö. Effect of temperature on muscle energy metabolism and endurance during successive isometric contractions sustained to fatigue, of the quadriceps muscle in man. *J. Physiol. (Lond.)* 220: 335–352, 1972.
103. Enoka, R. M., G. A. Robinson, and A. R. Kossev. Task and fatigue effects on low-threshold motor units in human hand muscle. *J. Neurophysiol.* 62: 1344–1359, 1989.
104. Enoka, R. M., and D. G. Stuart. Neurobiology of muscle fatigue. *J. Appl. Physiol.* 72: 1631–1648, 1992.
105. Essen, B. Intramuscular substrate utilization during prolonged exercise. *Ann. N. Y. Acad. Sci.* 301: 30–44, 1977.
106. Everts, M. E., K. Retterstol, and T. Clausen. Effects of adrenaline on excitation-induced stimulation of the sodium-potassium pump in rat skeletal muscle. *Acta Physiol. Scand.* 134: 189–198, 1988.
107. Fabiato, A., and F. Fabiato. Effects of pH on the myofilaments and the sarcoplasmic reticulum of skinned cells from cardiac and skeletal muscles. *J. Physiol. (Lond.)* 276: 233–255, 1978.
108. Fink, R., S. Hase, H. C. Lüttgau, and E. Wettwer. The effect of cellular energy reserves and internal calcium ions on the potassium conductance in skeletal muscle of the frog. *J. Physiol. (Lond.)* 336: 211–228, 1983.
109. Fink, R., and H. C. Lüttgau. An evaluation of the membrane constants and the potassium conductance in metabolically exhausted muscle fibers. *J. Physiol. (Lond.)* 263: 215–238, 1976.
110. Fitts, R. H. Substrate supply and energy metabolism during brief high intensity exercise: importance in limiting performance. In: *Perspectives in Exercise Science and Sports Medicine, Vol 5: Energy Metabolism in Exercise and Sport*, edited by D. R. Lamb and C. V. Gisolfi. Dubuque, IA: Brown & Benchmark, 1992, p. 53–99.
111. Fitts, R. H. Cellular mechanisms of muscle fatigue. *Physiol. Rev.* 74: 49–94, 1994.
112. Fitts, R. H., F. W. Booth, W. W. Winder, and J. O. Holloszy. Skeletal muscle respiratory capacity, endurance, and glycogen utilization. *Am. J. Physiol.* 228: 1029–1033, 1975.
113. Fitts, R. H., J. B. Courtright, D. H. Kim, and F. A. Witzman. Muscle fatigue with prolonged exercise: contractile and biochemical alterations. *Am. J. Physiol.* 242 (*Cell Physiol.* 11): C65–C73, 1982.
114. Fitts, R. H., and J. O. Holloszy. Lactate and contractile force in frog muscle during development of fatigue and recovery. *Am. J. Physiol.* 231: 430–433, 1976.
115. Fitts, R. H., and J. O. Holloszy. Effects of fatigue and recovery on contractile properties of frog muscle. *J. Appl. Physiol.* 45: 899–902, 1978.
116. Fletcher, W. M. The relation of oxygen to the survival metabolism of muscle. *J. Physiol. (Lond.)* 28: 474–498, 1902.
117. Frankenhaeuser, B., and J. Lännergren. The effect of calcium on the mechanical response of single twitch muscle fibers of *Xenopus laevis*. *Acta Physiol. Scand.* 69: 242–254, 1967.
118. Friden, J., and R. L. Lieber. Structural and mechanical basis of exercise-induced muscle injury. *Med. Sci. Sports Exerc.* 24: 521–530, 1992.
119. Friden, J., R. L. Lieber, and L.-E. Thornell. Subtle indications of muscle damage following eccentric contractions. *Acta Physiol. Scand.* 142: 523–524, 1991.
120. Gale, J. B. Mitochondrial swelling associated with exercise and method of fixation. *Med. Sci. Sports Exerc.* 6: 182–187, 1974.
121. Garcia, M. D. C., H. González-Serratos, J. P. Morgan, C. L. Perreault, and M. Rozycka. Differential activation of myofibrils during fatigue in phasic skeletal muscle cells. *J. Muscle Rev. Cell Motil.* 12: 412–424, 1991.
122. Godt, R. E., and D. W. Maughan. Influence of osmotic compression on calcium activation and tension in skinned

muscle fibers of the rabbit. *Pflugers Arch.* 391: 334–337, 1981.

123. Godt, R. E., and T. M. Nosek. Changes of intracellular milieu with fatigue or hypoxia depress contraction of skinned rabbit skeletal and cardiac muscle. *J. Physiol. (Lond.)* 412: 155–180, 1989.
124. Goldman, Y. E. Kinetics of the actomyosin ATPase in muscle fibers. *Annu. Rev. Physiol.* 49: 637–654, 1987.
125. Gollnick, P. D., B. Armstrong, C. W. Saubert, IV, W. L. Sembrowich, R. E. Sheppard, and B. Saltin. Glycogen depletion patterns in human skeletal muscle fibers during prolonged work. *Pflugers Arch.* 344: 1–12, 1973.
126. Gollnick, P. D., B. Armstrong, W. L. Sembrowich, R. E. Shepherd, and B. Saltin. Glycogen depletion pattern in human skeletal muscle fibers after heavy exercise. *J. Appl. Physiol.* 34: 615–618, 1973.
127. Gollnick, P. D., L. A. Bertocci, T. B. Kelso, E. H. Witt, and D. R. Hodgson. The effect of high-intensity exercise on the respiratory capacity of skeletal muscle. *Pflugers Arch.* 415: 407–413, 1990.
128. Gollnick, P. D., J. Karlsson, K. Piehl, and B. Saltin. Selective glycogen depletion in skeletal muscle fibers of man following sustained contractions. *J. Physiol. (Lond.)* 241: 59–67, 1974.
129. Gollnick, P. D., and D. W. King. Effect of exercise and training on mitochondria of rat skeletal muscle. *Am. J. Physiol.* 216: 1502–1509, 1969.
130. Gollnick, P. D., P. Korge, J. Karpakka, and B. Saltin. Elongation of skeletal muscle relaxation during exercise is linked to reduced calcium uptake by the sarcoplasmic reticulum in man. *Acta Physiol. Scand.* 142: 135–136, 1991.
131. Gollnick, P. D., K. Piehl, and B. Saltin. Selective glycogen depletion pattern in human muscle fibres after exercise of varying intensity and at varying pedaling rates. *J. Physiol. (Lond.)* 241: 45–57, 1974.
132. Gomolla, M., G. Gottschalk, and H. C. Lüttgau. Perchlorate-induced alterations in electrical and mechanical parameters of frog skeletal muscle fibers. *J. Physiol. (Lond.)* 343: 197–214, 1983.
133. González-Serratos, H., A. V. Somlyo, G. McClellan, H. Shuman, L. M. Borrero, and A. P. Somlyo. Composition of vacuoles and sarcoplasmic reticulum in fatigued muscle: electron probe analysis: *Proc. Natl. Acad. Sci. U. S. A.* 75: 1329–1333, 1978.
134. Gordon, A. M., R. E. Godt, S. K. B. Donaldson, and C. E. Harris. Tension in skinned frog muscle fibers in solution of varying ionic strength and neutral salt composition. *J. Gen. Physiol.* 62: 550–574, 1973.
135. Gordon, D. A., R. M. Enoka, G. M. Karst, and D. G. Stuart. Force development and relaxation in single motor units of adult cats during a standard fatigue test. *J. Physiol. (Lond.)* 421: 583–594, 1990.
136. Grabowski, W., E. A. Lobsiger, and H. C. Lüttgau. The effect of repetitive stimulation at low frequencies upon the electrical and mechanical activity of single muscle fibers. *Pflugers Arch.* 334: 222–239, 1972.
137. Gyorke, S. Effects of repeated tetanic stimulation on excitation-contraction coupling in cut muscle fibers of the frog. *J. Physiol. (Lond.)* 464: 699–710, 1993.
138. Hanson, J. The effects of repetitive stimulation on the action potential and the twitch of rat muscle. *Acta Physiol. Scand.* 90: 387–400, 1974.
139. Hanson, J., and A. Persson. Changes in the action potential and contraction of isolated frog muscle after repetitive stimulation. *Acta Physiol. Scand.* 81: 340–348, 1971.
140. Hatcher, D. D., and A. R. Luff. Force-velocity properties of fatigue-resistant units in cat fast-twitch muscle after fatigue. *J. Appl. Physiol.* 63: 1511–1518, 1987.
141. Hermansen, L., E. Hultman, and B. Saltin. Muscle glycogen during prolonged severe exercise. *Acta Physiol. Scand.* 71: 129–139, 1967.
142. Hermansen, L., and J. Osnes. Blood and muscle pH after maximal exercise in man. *J. Appl. Physiol.* 32: 304–308, 1972.
143. Hibberd, M. G., J. A. Dantzig, D. R. Trentham, and Y. E. Goldman. Phosphate release and force generation in skeletal muscle fibers. *Science* 228: 1317–1319, 1985.
144. Hicks, A., and A. McComas. Increased sodium pump activity following repetitive stimulation of rat soleus muscles. *J. Physiol. (Lond.)* 414: 337–349, 1989.
145. Hill, A. V. The heat of shortening and dynamic constants of muscle. *Proc. Roy. Soc. B.* 126: 136–195, 1938.
146. Hill, A. V. The influence of the external medium on the internal pH of muscle. *Proc. Roy. Soc. B.* 144: 1–22, 1955.
147. Hodgkin, A. L., and P. Horowicz. Potassium contractures in single muscle fibers. *J. Physiol. (Lond.)* 153: 386–403, 1960.
148. Howell, J. N., and H. Oetliker. Effects of repetitive activity, ruthenium red, and elevated extracellular calcium on frog skeletal muscle: implications for t-tubule conduction. *Can. J. Physiol. Pharmacol.* 65: 691–696, 1987.
149. Howell, J. N., A. Shankar, S. G. Howell, and F. Wei. Evidence for t-tubular conduction failure in frog skeletal muscle induced by elevated extracellular calcium concentration. *J. Muscle Res. Cell Motil.* 8: 229–241, 1987.
150. Howell, J. N., and K. W. Snowdowne. Inhibition of tetanus tension by elevated extracellular calcium concentration. *Am. J. Physiol.* 240 (*Cell Physiol.* 9): C193–C200, 1981.
151. Hultman, E., S. Del Canale, and H. Sjöholm. Effect of induced metabolic acidosis on intracellular pH, buffer capacity and contraction force of human skeletal muscle. *Clin. Sci.* 69: 505–510, 1985.
152. Hultman, E., and H. Sjöholm. Biochemical causes of fatigue. In: *Human Muscle Power*, edited by N. L. Jones, N. McCartney, and A. J. McComas. Champaign, IL: Human Kinetics Publishers, Inc., 1986, p. 215–238.
153. Imagawa, T., J. S. Smith, R. Coronado, and K. P. Campbell. Purified ryanodine receptor from skeletal muscle sarcoplasmic reticulum is the Ca^{2+}-permeable pore of the calcium release channel. *J. Biol. Chem.* 262: 16636–16643, 1987.
154. Inesi, G. Calcium and proton dependence of sarcoplasmic reticulum ATPase. *Biophys. J.* 44: 271–280, 1983.
155. Jones, D. A. Muscle fatigue due to changes beyond the neuromuscular junction. In: *Ciba Foundation Symposium 82. Human Muscle Fatigue: Physiological Mechanisms*, edited by R. Porter and J. Whelan. London: Pitman Medical, 1981, p. 178–196.
156. Jones, D. A., B. Bigland-Ritchie, and R. H. T. Edwards. Excitation frequency and muscle fatigue: mechanical responses during voluntary and stimulated contractions. *Exp. Neurol.* 64: 401–413, 1979.
157. Jones, D. A., S. Howell, C. Roussos, and R. H. T. Edwards. Low-frequency fatigue in isolated skeletal muscle and the effects of methylxanthines. *Clin. Sci.* 63: 161–167, 1982.
158. Jones, D. A., M. J. Jackson, G. McPhail, and R. G. Edwards. Experimental mouse muscle damage: the importance of external calcium. *Clin. Sci.* 66: 317–322, 1984.
159. Jones, D. A., D. J. Newham, and C. Torgan. Mechanical influences on long-lasting human muscle fatigue and delayed-onset pain. *J. Physiol. (Lond.)* 412: 415–427, 1989.

160. Juel, C. Potassium and sodium shifts during *in vitro* isometric muscle contraction, and the time course of the ion-gradient recovery. *Pflugers Arch.* 406: 458–463, 1986.
161. Juel, C., J. Bangsbo, T. Graham, and B. Saltin. Lactate and potassium fluxes from human skeletal muscle during and after intense, dynamic, knee extensor exercise. *Acta Physiol. Scand.* 140: 147–159, 1990.
162. Julian, F. J., and R. L. Moss. Effects of calcium and ioninc strength on shortening velocity and tension development in frog skinned muscle fibres. *J. Physiol. (Lond.)* 311: 179–199, 1981.
163. Kammermeier, H. Why do cells need phosphocreatine and a phosphocreatine shuttle. *J. Mol. Cell. Cardiol.* 19: 115–118, 1987.
164. Karlsson, J. Lactate and phosphagen concentrations in working muscle of man. *Acta Physiol. Scand.* 81: 1–72, 1971.
165. Karlsson, J., and B. Saltin. Lactate, ATP, and CP in working muscles during exhaustive exercise in man. *J. Appl. Physiol.* 29: 598–602, 1970.
166. Kawai, M., K. Güth, K. Winnikes, C. Haist, and J. C. Ruegg. The effect of inorganic phosphate on the ATP hydrolysis rate and the tension transients in chemically skinned rabbit psoas fibers. *Pflugers Arch.* 408: 1–9, 1987.
167. Kawai, M., and H. R. Halvorson. Two step mechanism of phosphate release and the mechanism of force generation in chemically skinned fibers of rabbit psoas muscle. *Biophys. J.* 59: 329–342, 1991.
168. Kentish, J. C. The effects of inorganic phosphate and creatine phosphate on force production in skinned muscles from rat ventricles. *J. Physiol. (Lond.)* 370: 585–604, 1986.
169. Korge, P., S. K. Byrd, and K. B. Campbell. Functional coupling between sarcoplasmic-reticulum-bound creatine kinase and Ca^{2+}-ATPase. *Eur. J. Biochem.* 213: 973–980, 1993.
170. Krnjevic, K., and R. Miledi. Failure of neuromuscular propagation in rats. *J. Physiol. (Lond.)* 140: 440–461, 1958.
171. Kugelberg, E., and L. Edström. Differential histochemical effects of muscle contractions on phosphorylase and glycogen in various types of fibers: relation to fatigue. *J. Neurol. Neurosurg. Psychiatry* 31: 415–423, 1968.
172. Kugelberg, E., and B. Lindegren. Transmission and contraction fatigue of rat motor units in relation to succinate dehydrogenase activity of motor unit fibres. *J. Physiol. (Lond.)* 288: 285–300, 1979.
173. Lamb, G. D., E. Recupero, and D. G. Stephenson. Effect of myoplasmic pH on excitation-contraction coupling in skeletal muscle fibres of the toad. *J. Physiol. (Lond.)* 448: 211–224, 1992.
174. Lännergren, J., L. Larsson, and H. Westerblad. A novel type of delayed tension reduction observed in rat motor units after intense activity. *J. Physiol. (Lond.)* 412: 267–276, 1989.
175. Lännergren, J., and H. Westerblad. Force and membrane potential during and after fatiguing, continuous high-frequency stimulation of single *Xenopus* muscle fibres. *Acta Physiol. Scand.* 128: 350–368, 1986.
176. Lännergren, J., and H. Westerblad. Action potential fatigue in single skeletal muscle fibres of *Xenopus*. *Acta Physiol. Scand.* 129: 311–318, 1987.
177. Lännergren, J., and H. Westerblad. Maximum tension and force-velocity properties of fatigued, single *Xenopus* muscle fibers studied by caffeine and high K^+. *J. Physiol. (Lond.)* 409: 473–490, 1989.
178. Lännergren, J., and H. Westerblad. Force decline due to fatigue and intracellular acidification in isolated fibers from mouse skeletal muscle. *J. Physiol. (Lond.)* 434: 307–322, 1991.
179. Larsson, L., L. Edström, B. Lindegren, L. Gorza, and S. Schiaffino. MHC composition and enzyme-histochemical and physiological properties of a novel fast-twitch motor unit type. *Am. J. Physiol.* 261 (*Cell Physiol.* 30): C93–C101, 1991.
180. Lieber, R. L., T. M. Woodburn, and J. Friden. Muscle damage induced by eccentric contractions of 23% strain. *J. Appl. Physiol.* 70: 2498–2507, 1991.
181. Light, P. E., A. S. Comtois, and J. M. Renaud. The effect of glibenclamide on frog skeletal muscle: evidence for K^{+}_{ATP} channel activation during fatigue. *J. Physiol. (Lond.)* 475: 495–507, 1994.
182. Lindinger, M. I., and G. Sjøgaard. Potassium regulation during exercise recovery. *Sports Med.* 11: 382–401, 1991.
183. Lüttgau, H. C. The action of calcium ions on potassium contractures of single muscle fibers. *J. Physiol. (Lond.)* 168: 679–697, 1963.
184. Lüttgau, H. C. The effect of metabolic inhibitors on the fatigue of the action potential in single muscle fibers. *J. Physiol. (Lond.)* 178: 45–67, 1965.
185. Lüttgau, H. C., G. Gottshalk, and D. Berwe. The effect of calcium and Ca antagonists upon excitation-contraction coupling. *Can. J. Physiol. Pharmacol.* 65: 717–723, 1987.
186. Lüttgau, H. C., and E. Wettwer. Ca^{2+}-activated potassium conductance in metabolically exhausted skeletal muscle fibers. *Cell Calcium* 4: 331–341, 1983.
187. Lymn, R. W., and E. W. Taylor. Mechanism of adenosine triphosphate hydrolysis by actomyosin. *Biochemistry* 10: 4617–4624, 1971.
188. Ma, J., M. Fill, C. M. Knudson, K. P. Campbell, and R. Coronado. Ryanodine receptor of skeletal muscle is a gap junction-type channel. *Science* 424: 99–102, 1988.
189. Ma, J., and J. Zhao. Highly cooperative and hysteretic response of the skeletal muscle ryanodine receptor to changes in proton concentrations. *Biophys. J.* 67: 626–633, 1994.
190. Maclaren, D. P. M., H. Gibson, M. Parry-Billings and R. H. T. Edwards. A review of metabolic and physiological factors in fatigue. In: *Exercise and Sport Sciences Reviews*, edited by K. B. Pandolf. Baltimore: Williams & Wilkins, 1989, p. 29–66.
191. Mainwood, G. W., and J. M. Renaud. The effect of acid-base balance on fatigue of skeletal muscle. *Can. J. Physiol. Pharmacol.* 63: 403–416, 1985.
192. Mainwood, G. W., J. M. Renaud, and M. J. Mason. The pH dependence of the contractile response of fatigued skeletal muscle. *Can. J. Physiol. Pharmacol.* 65: 648–658, 1987.
193. Martonosi, A. Sarcoplasmic reticulum. *J. Biol. Chem.* 244: 613–620, 1969.
194. Martyn, D. A., and A. M. Gordon. Force and stiffness in glycerinated rabbit psoas fibers. *Pflugers Arch.* 99: 795–816, 1992.
195. McCartney, N., L. L. Spriet, G. J. F. Heigenhauser, J. M. Kowalchuk, J. R. Sutton, and N. L. Jones. Muscle power and metabolism in maximal intermittent exercise. *J. Appl. Physiol.* 60: 1164–1169, 1986.
196. McCully, K. K. Exercise-induced injury to skeletal muscle. *Federation Proc.* 45: 2933–2936, 1986.
197. McCully, K. K., B. Boden, M. Tuchler, M. R. Fountain, and B. Chance. Wrist flexor muscles of elite rowers measured with magnetic resonance spectroscopy. *J. Appl. Physiol.* 67: 926–932, 1989.

198. McCully, K. K., B. J. Clark, J. A. Kent, J. Wilson, and B. Chance. Biochemical adaptations to training: implications for resisting muscle fatigue. *Can. J. Physiol. Pharmacol.* 69: 274–278, 1991.
199. McCully, K. K., and J. A. Faulkner. Characteristics of lengthening contractions associated with injury to skeletal muscle fibers. *J. Appl. Physiol.* 61: 293–299, 1986.
200. McCutcheon, L. J., S. K. Byrd, and D. R. Hodgson. Ultrastructural changes in skeletal muscle after fatiguing exercise. *J. Appl. Physiol.* 72: 1111–1117, 1992.
201. Medbo, J. I., and O. M. Sejersted. Plasma potassium changes with high intensity exercise. *J. Physiol. (Lond.)* 421: 105–122, 1990.
202. Metzger, J. M. Mechanism of chemomechanical coupling in skeletal muscle during work. In: *Perspectives in Exercise Science and Sport Medicine, Vol 5: Energy Metabolism in Exercise and Sport*, edited by D. R. Lamb and C. V. Gisolfi. Dubuque, IA: Brown & Benchmark, 1992, p. 1–44.
203. Metzger, J. M., and R. H. Fitts. Fatigue from high- and low-frequency muscle stimulation: role of sarcolemma action potentials. *Exp. Neurol.* 93: 320–333, 1986.
204. Metzger, J. M., and R. H. Fitts. Fatigue from high- and low-frequency muscle stimulation: contractile and biochemical alterations. *J. Appl. Physiol.* 62: 2075–2082, 1987.
205. Metzger, J. M., and R. H. Fitts. Role of intracellular pH in muscle fatigue. *J. Appl. Physiol.* 62: 1392–1397, 1987.
206. Metzger, J. M., M. L. Greaser, and R. L. Moss. Variations in cross-bridge attachment rate and tension with phosphorylation of myosin in mammalian skinned skeletal muscle fibers. *J. Gen. Physiol.* 93: 855–883, 1989.
207. Metzger, J. M., and R. L. Moss. Greater hydrogen ion-induced depression of tension and velocity in skinned single fibers of rat fast than slow muscles. *J. Physiol. (Lond.)* 393: 727–742, 1987.
208. Metzger, J. M., and R. L. Moss. Shortening velocity in skinned single muscle fibers. *Biophys. J.* 52: 127–131, 1987.
209. Metzger, J. M., and R. L. Moss. Effects on tension and stiffness due to reduced pH in mammalian fast- and slow-twitch skinned skeletal muscle fibers. *J. Physiol.* 428: 737–750, 1990.
210. Metzger, J. M., and R. L. Moss. pH modulation of the kinetics of a Ca^{2+}-sensitive cross-bridge state transition in mammalian single skeletal muscle fibers. *J. Physiol. (Lond.)* 428: 751–764, 1990.
211. Metzger, J. M., and R. L. Moss. Calcium-sensitive cross-bridge transitions in mammalian fast and slow skeletal muscle fibers. *Science* 247: 1088–1090, 1990.
212. Meyer, R. A., G. A. Dudley, and R. L. Terjung. Ammonia and IMP in different skeletal muscle fibers after exercise in rats. *J. Appl. Physiol.* 49: 1037–1041, 1980.
213. Meyer, R. A., and R. L. Terjung. Differences in ammonia and adenylate metabolism in contracting fast and slow muscle. *Am. J. Physiol.* 237 (*Cell Physiol.* 6): C111–C118, 1979.
214. Millar, N. C., and E. Homsher. The effect of phosphate and calcium on force generation in glycerinated rabbit skeletal muscle fibers. *J. Biol. Chem.* 265.: 20234–20240, 1990.
215. Miller, R. G., M. D. Boska, R. S. Moussavi, P. J. Carson, and M. W. Weiner. ^{31}P nuclear magnetic resonance studies of high energy phosphates and pH in human muscle fatigue. *J. Clin. Invest.* 81: 1190–1196, 1988.
216. Miller, R. G., D. Giannini, H. S. Milner-Brown, R. B. Layzer, A. P. Koretsky, D. Hooper, and M. W. Weiner. Effects of fatiguing exercise on high energy phosphates, force, and EMG: evidence for three phases of recovery. *Muscle Nerve* 10: 810–821, 1987.
217. Mutch, B. J. C., and E. W. Banister. Ammonia metabolism in exercise and fatigue: a review. *Med. Sci. Sports Exerc.* 15: 41–50, 1983.
218. Nakamaru, Y., and A. Schwartz. The influence of hydrogen ion concentration on calcium binding and release by skeletal muscle sarcoplasmic reticulum. *J. Gen. Physiol.* 59: 22–32, 1972.
219. Nassar-Gentina, V., J. V. Passonneua, and S. I. Rapoport. Fatigue and metabolism of frog muscle fibers during stimulation and in response to caffeine. *Am. J. Physiol.* 241 (*Cell Physiol.* 10): C160–C166, 1981.
220. Newham, D. J., K. R. Mills, B. M. Quigley, and R. H. T. Edwards. Pain and fatigue after concentric and eccentric muscle contractions. *Clin. Sci.* 64: 55–62, 1983.
221. Nimmo, M. A., and D. H. Snow. Time course of ultrastructural changes in skeletal muscle after two types of exercise. *J. Appl. Physiol.* 52: 910–913, 1982.
222. Nosek, T. M., K. Y. Fender, and R. E. Godt. It is diprotonated inorganic phosphate that depresses force in skinned skeletal muscle fibers. *Science* 236: 191–193, 1987.
223. Nosek, T. M., J. H. Leal-Cardoso, M. Mclaughlin, and R. E. Godt. Inhibitory influence of phosphate and arsenate on contraction of skinned skeletal and cardiac muscle. *Am. J. Physiol.* 259 (*Cell Physiol.* 28): C933–C939, 1990.
224. Ogawa, Y. Calcium binding to troponin C and troponin: effects of Mg^{2+} ionic strength and pH. *J. Biol. Chem.* 97: 1011–1023, 1985.
225. Pate, E., and R. Cooke. A model of crossbridge action: the effects of ATP, ADP and Pi. *J. Muscle Res. Cell Motil.* 10: 181–196, 1989.
226. Peter, J.B. Histochemical, biochemical, and physiological studies of skeletal muscle and its adaptation to exercise. In: *Contractility of Muscle Cells and Related Processes*, edited by R. J. Podolsky. Englewood Cliffs, NJ: Prentice-Hall, Inc., 1971, p. 151–173.
227. Pizarro, G., R. Fitts, I. Uribe, and E. Rios. The voltage sensor of excitation contraction coupling in skeletal muscle. Ion dependence and selectivity. *J. Gen. Physiol.* 94: 405–428, 1989
228. Ren, J.-M., and E. Hultman. Regulation of phosphorylase activity in human skeletal muscle. *J. Appl. Physiol.* 69: 919–923, 1990.
229. Renaud, J. M. Is the change in intracellular pH during fatigue large enough to be the main cause of fatigue? *Can. J. Physiol. Pharmacol.* 64: 764–767, 1986.
230. Renaud, J. M., R. B. Stein, and T. Gordon. The effects of pH on force and stiffness development in mouse muscles. *Can. J. Physiol. Pharmacol.* 65: 1798–1801, 1987.
231. Rios, E., and G. Brum. Involvement of dihydropyridine receptors in excitation-contraction coupling in skeletal muscle. *Nature* 325: 717–720, 1987.
232. Rios, E., J. Ma, and A. Gonzlez. The mechanical hypothesis of excitation-contraction (EC) coupling in skeletal muscle. *J. Muscle Res. Cell Motil.* 12: 127–135, 1991.
233. Rios, E., and G. Pizarro. The voltage sensor of excitation-contraction coupling in skeletal muscle. *Physiol. Rev.* 71: 849–908, 1991.
234. Rousseau, E., and J. Pinkos. pH modulates conducting and gating behavior of single calcium release channels. *Pflugers Arch.* 415: 645–647, 1990.
235. Sahlin, K. Effect of acidosis on energy metabolism and force generation in skeletal muscle. In: *International Series on Sport Sciences, Biochemistry of Exercise*, edited by

H. G. Knuttgen, J. A. Vogel, and J. Poortmans. Champaign, IL: Human Kinetics Publishers, Inc., 1983, p. 151–160.

236. Sahlin, K. Metabolic changes limiting muscle performance. In: *International Series on Sport Sciences, Biochemistry of Exercise VI*, edited by B. Saltin. Champaign, IL: Human Kinetics Publishers, Inc., 1986, p. 323–344.
237. Sahlin, K., A. Alverstrand, R. Brandt, and E. Hultman. Intracellular pH and bicarbonate concentration in human muscle during recovery from exercise. *J. Appl. Physiol.* 45: 474–480, 1978.
238. Sahlin, K., and S. Broberg. Release of K^+ from muscle during prolonged dynamic exercise. *Acta Physiol. Scand.* 136: 293–294, 1989.
239. Sahlin, K., L. Edström, and H. Sjöholm. Fatigue and phosphocreatine depletion during carbon dioxide-induced acidosis in rat muscle. *Am. J. Physiol.* 245 (*Cell Physiol.* 14): C15–C20, 1983.
240. Sahlin, K., L. Edström, and H. Sjöholm. Force, relaxation and energy metabolism of rat soleus muscle during anaerobic contraction. *Acta Physiol. Scand.* 129: 1–7, 1987.
241. Sahlin, K., L. Edström, H. Sjohölm, and E. Hultman. Effects of lactic acid accumulation and ATP decrease on muscle tension and relaxation. *Am. J. Physiol.* 240 (*Cell Physiol.* 9): C121–C126, 1981.
242. Sahlin, K., R. C. Harris, B. Nylind, and E. Hultman. Lactate content and pH in muscle samples obtained after dynamic exercise. *Pflugers Arch.* 367: 143–149, 1976.
243. Sahlin, K., A. Katz, and S. Broberg. Tricarboxylic acid cycle intermediates in human muscle during prolonged exercise. *Am. J. Physiol.* 259 (*Cell Physiol.* 28): C834–C841, 1990.
244. Sahlin, K., G. Palmskog, and E. Hultman. Adenine nucleotide and IMP contents of the quadriceps muscle in man after exercise. *Pflugers Arch.* 374: 193–198, 1978.
245. Sahlin, K., and J. M. Ren. Relationship of contraction capacity to metabolic changes during recovery from a fatiguing contraction. *J. Appl. Physiol.* 67: 648–654, 1989.
246. Saks, V. A., Y. O. Belikova, A. V. Kuznetsov, Z. A. Khuchua, T. H. Branishte, M. L. Semenovsky, and V. G. Naumov. Phosphocreatine pathway for energy transport: ADP diffusion and cardiomyopathy. *Am. J. Physiol. Suppl.* 261: 30–38, 1991.
247. Saltin, B., and B. Essen, Muscle glycogen, lactate, ATP, and CP in intermittent exercise. In: *Advances in Experimental Medicine and Biology, Muscle Metabolism During Exercise*, edited by B. Pernow and B. Saltin. New York: Plenum Press, 1971, p. 419–424.
248. Saltin, B. and J. Karlsson, Muscle glycogen utilization during work of different intensities. In: *Advances in Experimental Medicine and Biology, Muscle Metabolism During Exercise*, edited by B. Pernow and B. Saltin. New York: Plenum Press, 1971, p. 289–299.
249. Sandow, A. Excitation-contraction coupling in muscular response. *Yale J. Biol. Med.* 25: 176–201, 1952.
250. Schluter, J. M., and R. H. Fitts. Shortening velocity and ATPase activity of rat skeletal muscle fibers: effects of endurance exercise training. *Am. J. Physiol.* 266 (*Cell Physiol.* 35): C1699–C1713, 1994.
251. Sejersted, O. M. Electrolyte imbalance in body fluids as a mechanism of fatigue during exercise. In: *Perspectives in Exercise Science and Sport Medicine, Energy Metabolism in Exercise and Sport*, edited by D. R. Lamb and C. V. Gisolfi. Dubuque, IA: Brown & Benchmark, 1992, p. 149–200.
252. Shelvin, H. H. Effects of external calcium concentration and pH on charge movement in frog skeletal muscle. *J. Physiol. (Lond.)* 288: 129–158, 1979.
253. Simonson, E. *Physiology of Work Capacity and Fatigue*, Springfield, IL: Charles C Thomas, 1971.
254. Sjøgaard, G. Muscle energy metabolism and electrolyte shifts during low-level prolonged static contraction in man. *Acta Physiol. Scand.* 134: 181–187, 1988.
255. Sjøgaard, G. Exercise-induced muscle fatigue: the significance of potassium. *Acta Physiol. Scand. Suppl.* 593: 1–63, 1990.
256. Sjøgaard, G., R. P. Adams, and B. Saltin. Water and ion shifts in skeletal muscle of humans with intense dynamic knee extension. *Am. J. Physiol.* 248 (*Regulatory Integrative Comp. Physiol.* 17): R190–R196, 1985.
257. Sjogaard, G., and B. Saltin. Extra- and intracellular water spaces in muscles of man at rest and with dynamic exercise. *Am. J. Physiol.* 243 (*Regulatory Integrative Comp. Physiol.* 12): R271–R280, 1982.
258. Somlyo, A. V., H. González-Serratos, G. McClellan, H. Shuman, L. M. Borrero, and A. P. Somlyo. Electron probe analysis of the sarcoplasmic reticulum and vacuolated T-tubule system of fatigued frog muscles. *Ann. N. Y. Acad. Sci.* 307: 232–234, 1978.
259. Spencer, M. K., Z. Yan, and A. Katz. Carbohydrate supplementation attenuates IMP accumulation in human muscle during prolonged exercise. *Am. J. Physiol.* 261 (*Cell Physiol.* 30): C71–C76, 1991.
260. Spriet, L. L. Phosphofructokinase activity and acidosis during short-term tetanic contractions. *Can. J. Physiol. Pharmacol.* 69: 298–304, 1991.
261. Spriet, L. L., M. I. Lindinger, R. S. McKelvie, G. J. F. Heigenhauser, and N. L. Jones. Muscle glycogenolysis and H^+ concentration during maximal intermittent cycling. *J. Appl. Physiol.* 66: 8–13, 1989.
262. Spriet, L. L., K. Söderlund, M. Bergström, and E. Hultman. Skeletal muscle glycogenolysis, glycolysis, and pH during electrical stimulation in men. *J. Appl. Physiol.* 62: 616–621, 1987.
263. Stienen, G. J. M., P. G. A. Versteeg, Z. Papp, and G. Elizinga. Mechanical properties of skinned rabbit psoas and soleus muscle fibers during lengthening: effects of phosphate and Ca^{2+}. *J. Physiol. (Lond.)* 451: 503–523, 1992.
264. Taylor, S. R., and R. Rüdel. Striated muscle fibers: inactivation of contraction induced by shortening. *Science* 167: 882–884, 1970.
265. Terjung, R. L., K. M. Baldwin, P. A. Mole, G. H. Klinkerfuss, and J. O. Holloszy. Effect of running to exhaustion on skeletal muscle mitochondria: a biochemical study. *Am. J. Physiol.* 223: 549–554, 1972.
266. Terjung, R. L., G. A. Dudley, and R. A. Meyer. Metabolic and circulatory limitations to muscular performance at the organ level. *J. Exp. Biol.* 115: 307–318, 1985.
267. Thompson, L. V., E. M. Balog, and R. H. Fitts. Muscle fatigue in frog semitendinosus: role of intracellular pH. *Am. J. Physiol.* 262 (*Cell Physiol.* 31): C1507–C1512, 1992.
268. Thompson, L. V., E. M. Balog, D. A. Riley, and R. H. Fitts. Muscle fatigue in frog semitendinosus: alterations in contractile function. *Am. J. Physiol.* 262 (*Cell Physiol.* 31): C1500–C1506, 1992.
269. Thompson, L. V., and R. H. Fitts. Muscle fatigue in the frog semitendinosus: role of the high-energy phosphate and Pi. *Am. J. Physiol.* 263 (*Cell Physiol.* 32): C803–C809, 1992.
270. Troup, J. P., J. M. Metzger, and R. H. Fitts. Effect of high-intensity exercise training on functional capacity of limb skeletal muscle. *J. Appl. Physiol.* 60: 1743–1751, 1986.

271. Van Beaumont, W., J. C. Strand, J. S. Petrosfsky, S. G. Hipskind, and J. E. Greenleaf. Changes in total plasma content of electrolytes and proteins with maximal exercise. *J. Appl. Physiol.* 34: 102–106, 1973.
272. Vergara, J. L., S. I. Rapoport, and V. Nassar-Gentia. Fatigue and posttetanic potentiation in single muscle fibers of the frog. *Am. J. Physiol.* 232 (*Cell Physiol.* 1): C185–C190, 1977.
273. Vukovich, M. D., D. L. Costill, and W. J. Fink. Carnitine supplementation: effect on muscle carnitine and glycogen content during exercise. *Med. Sci. Sports Exerc.* 26: 1122–1129, 1994.
274. Vyskocil, F., P. Hnik, H. Rehfeldt, R. Vejsada, and E. Ujec. The measurement of K^+ concentration changes in human muscles during volitional contractions. *Pflugers Arch.* 399: 235–237, 1983.
275. Weiner, M. W., R. S. Moussavi, A. J. Baker, M. D. Boska, and R. G. Miller. Constant relationships between force, phosphate concentration, and pH in muscles with differential fatigability. *Neurology* 40: 1888–1893, 1990.
276. Westerblad, H., and D. G. Allen. Changes of myoplasmic calcium concentration during fatigue in single mouse muscle fibers. *J. Gen. Physiol.* 98: 615–635, 1991.
277. Westerblad, H., and D. G. Allen. Changes of intracellular pH due to repetitive stimulation of single fibers from mouse skeletal muscle. *J. Physiol. (Lond.)* 449: 49–71, 1992.
278. Westerblad, H., and J. Lännergren. Force and membrane potential during and after fatiguing, intermittent tetanic stimulation of single *Xenopus* muscle fibers. *Acta Physiol. Scand.* 128: 369–378, 1986.
279. Westerblad, H., and J. Lännergren. The relation between force and intracellular pH in fatigued, single *Xenopus* muscle fibers. *Acta Physiol. Scand.* 133: 83–89, 1988.
280. Westerblad, H., and J. Lännergren. Slowing of relaxation during fatigue in single mouse muscle fibers. *J. Physiol. (Lond.)* 434: 323–336, 1991.
281. Westerblad, H. and J. Lännergren. Changes of the force-velocity relation, isometric tension and relaxation rate during fatigue in intact, single fibers or *Xenopus* skeletal muscle. *J. Muscle Res. Cell Motil.* 15: 287–298, 1994.
282. Westerblad, H., J. A. Lee, J. A. Lamb, S. R. Bolsover, and D. G. Allen. Spatial gradients of intracellular calcium in skeletal muscle during fatigue. *Pflugers Arch.* 415: 734–740, 1990.
283. Westerblad, H., J. A. Lee, J. Lannergren, and D. G. Allen. Cellular mechanisms of fatigue in skeletal muscle. *Am. J. Physiol.* 261 (*Cell Physiol.* 30): C195–C209, 1991.
284. Westra, H. G., A. De Haan, E. Van Doorn, and E. J. De Haan. IMP production and energy metabolism during exercise in rats in relation to age. *Biochem. J.* 239: 751–755, 1986.
285. Wilkie, D. R. Muscular fatigue: effects of hydrogen ions and inorganic phosphate. *Federation Proc.* 45: 2921–2923, 1986.
286. Wilson, J. R., K. K. McCully, D. M. Mancini, B. Boden, and B. Chance. Relationship of muscular fatigue to pH and diprotonated P_i in humans: a ^{31}P-NMR study. *J. Appl. Physiol.* 64: 2333–2339, 1988.

Index